C0-CEE-326

DVD Video Contents

Trauma Problems: Lower Extremities
Hip Joint

Surgical hip dislocation in the treatment of degenerative hip joint	Siebenrock
Hip joint arthroscopy in the treatment of degenerative hip joint	Steimer
Pipkin fractures – anterior approach	Gänsslen
Surgical hip dislocation in the treatment of Pipkin fractures	Mella

Mal and Non Union of Proximal Femur Fractures

Arthroplasty following proximal femur fractures	Seekamp
Proximal femur replacement following proximal femur fractures	Bastian
Management of non unions of the proximal femur	Krettek
Failed osteosynthesis and infection	Raschke

Femur Fractures

Antegrade Nailing with conventional entry point	Gösling
Antegrade Nailing with lateral entry point	Stecher
Retrograde Nailing	Ostermann
C-Arm based navigated femoral nailing	Hüfner

Battle Pro & Contra: Patient positioning for femoral nailing:

Pro supine	Gösling
Pro lateral decubitus	Woltmann

New Techniques:

Locking Screw Interlocking Nails	Höntzsch
Angle stable nail-secrew fixations	Höntzsch
CT based Navigation	Regazzoni

Osteoporotic Femur Fractures: Fixation Techniques:

Locking plates / Reduction techniques	Babst
Locking plates: Where, how many and which screws?	Sommer

Periprosthetic Femur Fractures:

Periprosthetic femur fractures: Locking plate	Mittlmeier
Periprosthetic femur fractures: Retrograde nail	Ostermann

Management of Complications and Correction of Lower Limb Deformities I:

When the nail breaks	Mittelmeier
Leg lengthening with Ilizarov fixator	Blattert
Leg lengthening with monorail technique	Raschke
Leg lengthening with intramedullary device	Hankemeier

Expert | CONSULT

Online + Print

Online access activation instructions

This Expert Consult title comes with access to the complete contents online. **Activate your access today** by following these simple instructions:

1. Gently scratch off the surface of the sticker below, using the edge of a coin, to reveal your **activation code.**

2. Visit **www.expertconsultbook.com** and click on the **"Register"** button.

3. **Enter your activation code** along with the other information requested...and begin enjoying your access.

It's that easy! For technical assistance, email **online.help@elsevier.com** or **call 800-401-9962** (inside the US) or **+1-314-995-3200** (outside the US).

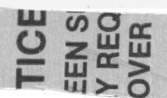

SKELETAL TRAUMA

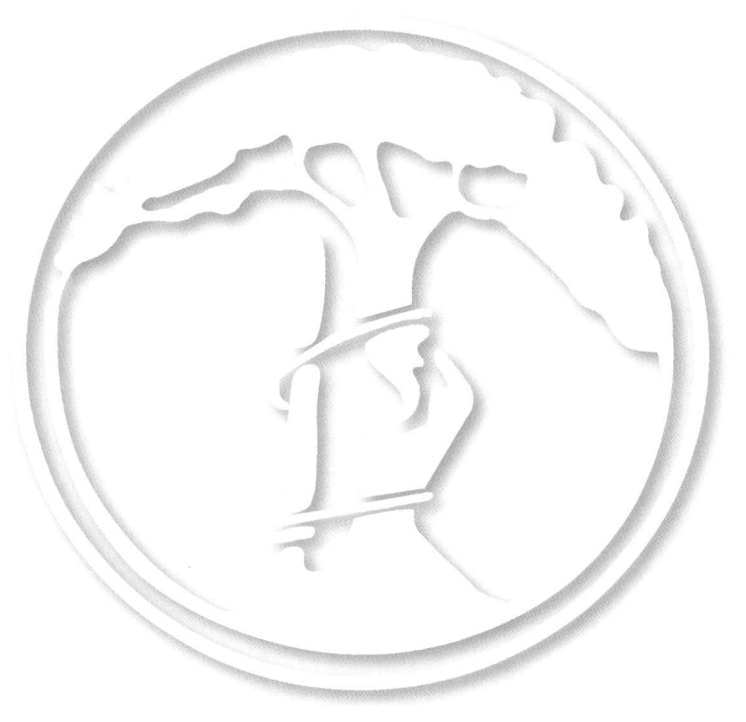

MEDICAL ILLUSTRATORS

The editors would like to thank Matrix Art Services who created all of the new artwork
for this edition and Michael Carcel at Elsevier who so efficiently processed it.

The editors would also like to recognize the work of the medical illustrators listed below who created
the beautiful art for the first edition, much of which has been retained for this new edition:

Phillip Ashley and Denis Lee in association with

Leona Allison	Theodore Huff
Marie Chartrand	Christine Jones
Megan Costello	John Klausmeyer
Charles Curro	Valerie Loomis
Glenn Edelmayer	Larry Ward

The editors espically wish to thank Theodore Huff, who created all of the new artwork for the last edition.

SKELETAL TRAUMA

Basic Science, Management, and Reconstruction

VOLUME ONE

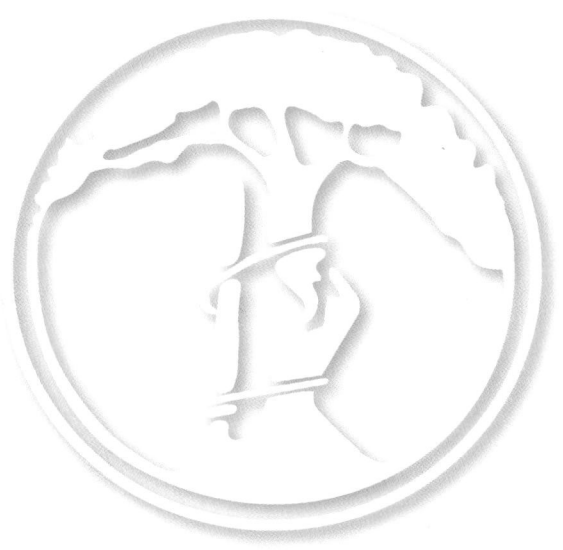

FOURTH EDITION

Bruce D. Browner, M.D., M.S., F.A.C.S.

Gray-Gossling Chair
Professor and Chairman Emeritus
Department of Orthopaedic Surgery
University of Connecticut Health Center
Director, Department of Orthopaedics
Hartford Hospital
Hartford, Connecticut

Jesse B. Jupiter, M.D.

Director, Orthopaedic Hand Service
Massachusetts General Hospital
Hansjörg Wyss/AO Professor
Harvard Medical School
Boston, Massachusetts

Alan M. Levine, M.D.

Director, Alvin and Lois Lapidus Cancer Institute
Sinai Hospital
Baltimore, Maryland

Peter G. Trafton, M.D., F.A.C.S.

Professor of Orthopaedics
The Warren Alpert Medical School of Brown University
Former Surgeon-in-Charge
Orthopaedic Trauma, Rhode Island Hospital
Providence, Rhode Island

Christian Krettek, M.D., F.R.A.C.S., F.R.C.S.Ed.

Professor and Director of the Department of
   Trauma & Orthopaedics
Hannover Medical School (MHH), Germany

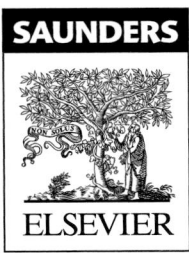

SAUNDERS

ELSEVIER

SAUNDERS
ELSEVIER

1600 John F. Kennedy Blvd.
Ste 1800
Philadelphia, PA 19103-2899

SKELETAL TRAUMA: BASIC SCIENCE, MANAGEMENT, AND
RECONSTRUCTION, 4E

Expert Consult: Online and Print: ISBN: 978-1-4160-2220-6

Volume 1: Part no. 9996004635

Volume 2: Part no. 9996004694

Expert Consult: Online and Print: Skeletal Trauma 2-Volume Set and Green: Skeletal Trauma in Children:
ISBN: 978-1-4160-4839-8

Expert Consult Premium Edition: Enhanced Online Features: Skeletal Trauma 2-Volume Set and Green:
Skeletal Trauma in Children: ISBN: 978-1-4160-4840-4

NOTICE

Knowledge and best practice in this field are constantly changing. As new research and experience broaden our knowledge, changes in practice, treatment, and drug therapy may become necessary or appropriate. Readers are advised to check the most current information provided (i) on procedures featured or (ii) by the manufacturer of each product to be administered, to verify the recommended dose or formula, the method and duration of administration, and contraindications. It is the responsibility of the practitioner, relying on their own experience and knowledge of the patient, to make diagnoses, to determine dosages and the best treatment for each individual patient, and to take all appropriate safety precautions. To the fullest extent of the law, neither the Publisher nor the Editors assume any liability for any injury and/or damage to persons or property arising out of or related to any use of the material contained in this book.

The Publisher

Previous editions copyrighted 2003, 1998, 1992

Library of Congress Cataloging-in-Publication Data
Skeletal trauma: basic science, management, and reconstruction / [edited by] Bruce D. Browner . . . [et al.]. – 4th ed.
   p. ; cm.
   Includes bibliographical references and index.
   ISBN 978-1-4160-2220-6
   1. Musculoskeletal system–Wounds and injuries. 2. Fractures. I. Browner, Bruce D.
   [DNLM: 1. Fractures, Bone. 2. Bone and Bones–injuries. 3. Dislocations. 4. Ligaments–injuries.
WE 175 S6267 2008]
   RD731.S564 2008
   617.4'7044–dc22

          2008039526

Publishing Director: Kim Murphy
Developmental Editor: Janice M. Gaillard
Project Manager: David Saltzberg
Design Direction: Steven Stave
Marketing Manager: Catalina Nolte

Printed in Canada
Last digit is the print number: 9 8 7 6 5 4 3 2 1

Contributors

Joseph A. Abate, III, M.D.
Associate Professor, University of Vermont,
Department of Orthopaedics and Rehabilitation,
Burlington, Vermont
Dislocations and Soft Tissue Injuries of the Knee

Albert J. Aboulafia, M.D.
Assistant Clinical Professor, Department of
Orthopaedic Surgery, University of Maryland School
of Medicine; Co-Director, Sarcoma Service, Alvin
and Lois Lapidus Cancer Center, Sinai Hospital,
Baltimore, Maryland
Pathologic Fractures

Annunziato Amendola, M.D., F.R.C.S.(C.)
Associate Professor, University of Western Ontario,
London, Ontario, Canada
Compartment Syndromes

Caesar A. Anderson, M.D., M.P.H.
Fellow, Yale–New Haven Hospital,
New Haven, Connecticut
Substance Abuse Syndromes: Recognition, Prevention, and Treatment

Paul A. Anderson, M.D.
Professor, Department of Orthopedic Surgery and
Rehabilitation, University Hospital,
Madison, Wisconsin
Injuries of Lower Cervical Spine

Michael T. Archdeacon, M.D.
Vice-Chairman and Associate Professor,
Department of Orthopaedic Surgery,
University of Cincinnati; Director, Division of
Musculoskeletal Traumatology,
University Hospital,
Cincinnati, Ohio
Patella Fractures and Extensor Mechanism Injuries

Terry S. Axelrod, M.D.
Associate Professor of Surgery, University of Toronto
Faculty of Medicine; Head, Division of Orthopaedic
Surgery, Sunnybrook and Women's College Health
Sciences Centre, Toronto, Ontario, Canada
Fractures and Dislocations of the Hand

Rahul Banerjee, M.D.
Assistant Professor, Texas Tech University Health
Sciences Center; Chief of Orthopaedic Trauma,
William Beaumont Army Medical Center, El Paso, Texas
Foot Injuries

Craig S. Bartlett, III, M.D.
Assistant Clinical Professor, Orthopaedic Trauma
Service, Department of Orthopaedics, University of
Vermont College of Medicine, Burlington, Vermont
Fractures of the Tibial Pilon

Rebecca M. Bauer, M.D., M.P.H.
Research Coordinator, Division of Orthopedic Trauma,
Vanderbilt Orthopedic Institute, Nashville, Tennessee
Outcomes Research in Orthopaedics

Michael R. Baumgaertner, M.D.
Professor, Department of Orthopaedics and
Rehabilitation, Yale University School of Medicine;
Chief, Orthopaedic Trauma Service, Yale–New Haven
Hospital, New Haven, Connecticut
*Medical Management of the Patient with Hip Fracture;
Intertrochanteric Hip Fractures*

Fred F. Behrens, M.D.*
Fractures with Soft Tissue Injuries

Mark R. Belsky, M.D.
Associate Clinical Professor of Orthopaedic Surgery,
Tufts University School of Medicine, Boston; Chief of
Orthopaedic Surgery, Newton-Wellesley Hospital,
Newton, Massachusetts
Fractures and Dislocations of the Hand

Daniel R. Benson, M.D.
Professor, Department of Orthopaedics, University of
California, Davis, School of Medicine; Orthopaedic
Surgeon, University of California, Davis, Medical
Center, Sacramento, California
*Initial Evaluation and Emergency Treatment of the
Spine-Injured Patient*

Daniel J. Berry, M.D.
Professor of Orthopaedic Surgery, Mayo Clinic College
of Medicine; Consultant, Department of Orthopaedics,
Mayo Clinic, Rochester, Minnesota
Periprosthetic Fractures of the Lower Extremity

*Deceased.

Mohit Bhandari, M.D., M.Sc., F.R.C.S.C
Clinical Research Fellow, St. Michael's Hospital, Toronto, Ontario, Canada
Fractures of the Humeral Shaft

Christopher T. Born, M.D., F.A.A.O.S., F.A.C.S
Professor, Department of Orthopaedic Surgery, The Alpert Medical School, Brown University; Director, Orthopaedic Trauma Service, Rhode Island Hospital, Providence, Rhode Island
Disaster Management

Michael J. Bosse, M.D.
Orthopaedic Trauma Surgeon, Department of Orthopaedic Surgery, Carolinas Medical Service, Charlotte, North Carolina
Damage Control Orthopaedic Surgery: A Strategy for the Orthopaedic Care of the Critically Injured Patient

Robert T. Brautigam, M.D., F.A.C.S.
Associate Professor of Surgery, School of Medicine, University of Connecticut, Farmington, Connecticut; Director of the Surgical Program, American College of Surgeons Comprehensive Education Institute; Associate Director, Neuroscience, Neurosurgery/Trauma Intensive Care Unit; Associate Director, Surgical Intensive Care Unit, Department of Surgery, Hartford Hospital, Hartford, Connecticut
Evaluation and Treatment of the Multiple-Trauma Patient

Mark R. Brinker, M.D.
Clinical Professor of Orthopaedic Surgery, Tulane University School of Medicine, New Orleans, Louisiana; Clinical Professor of Orthopaedic Surgery, Baylor College of Medicine; Director of Acute and Reconstructive Trauma, Fondren Orthopedic Group, Texas Orthopedic Hospital, Houston, Texas
Nonunions: Evaluation and Treatment

Bruce D. Browner, M.D., M.S., F.A.C.S.
Gray-Gossling Chair,
Professor and Chairman Emeritus,
Department of Orthopaedic Surgery,
University of Connecticut Health Center;
Director, Department of Orthopaedics,
Hartford Hospital, Hartford, Connecticut
Principles of Internal Fixation; Surgical Site Infection Prevention; Chronic Osteomyelitis

Ryan P. Calfee, M.D.
Fellow of Orthopaedic Trauma, Department of Orthopaedic Surgery, Brown University School of Medicine; Fellow of Orthopaedic Trauma, Department of Orthopaedic Surgery, Rhode Island Hospital, Providence, Rhode Island
Disaster Management

Jason H. Calhoun, M.D.
Department of Orthopaedics and Rehabilitation, University of Texas Medical Branch, Galveston, Texas
Surgical Site Infection Prevention

Andrew E. Caputo, M.D.
Clinical Assistant Professor, Department of Orthopaedic Surgery, University of Connecticut Health Sciences Center, Farmington; Co-Director, Hand Surgery Service, Hartford Hospital and Connecticut Children's Medical Center, Hartford, Connecticut
Principles of Internal Fixation

James B. Carr, M.D.
Associate Clinical Professor, Department of Orthopaedic Surgery, University of South Carolina, Columbia, South Carolina; Attending Orthopedic Surgeon, Lewis Gale Medical Center, Salem, Virginia
Malleolar Fractures and Soft-Tissue Injuries of the Ankle

Charles Cassidy, M.D.
Chairman, Department of Orthopaedics, Henry H. Banks Associate Professor of Orthopaedic Surgery, Tufts–New England Medical Center, Boston, Massachusetts
Fractures and Dislocations of the Carpus

Mark S. Cohen, M.D.
Professor, Director, Hand and Elbow Section, Director, Ortopaedic Education, Department of Orthopaedic Surgery, Rush University Medical Center, Chicago, Illinois
Fractures of the Distal Radius

Peter A. Cole, M.D.
Associate Professor, Department of Orthopaedic Surgery, University of Minnesota, Minneapolis, Minnesota; Chief, Department of Orthopaedic Surgery, Regions Hospital, Saint Paul, Minnesota
Tibial Plateau Fractures

Christopher L. Colton, M.D., F.R.C.S., F.R.C.S.Ed.
Senior Consultant in Orthopaedic Trauma, Nottingham University Hospital, Nottingham, England
The History of Fracture Treatment

Leo M. Cooney, Jr., M.D.
Humana Foundation Professor of Geriatric Medicine, Professor and Chief, Section of Geriatrics, Yale University School of Medicine, New Haven, Connecticut
Medical Management of the Patient with Hip Fracture

Brian W. Cooper, M.D., F.A.C.P.
Director, Division of Infectious Disease, Allergy, and Immunology, Hartford Hospital; Professor of Clinical Medicine, University of Connecticut School of Medicine, Farmington, Connecticut
Avoidance of Occupationally Acquired Blood-Borne Pathogens

Charles N. Cornell, M.D.
Associate Professor, Orthopaedic Surgery, Cornell University Joan and Sanford I. Weill Medical College and Graduate School of Medical Sciences, New York; Chairman, Department of Orthopaedic Surgery, New York Hospital Medical Center of Queens and Flushing Hospital Medical Center, Flushing, New York
Osteoporotic Fragility Fractures

Jerome M. Cotler, M.D.
Professor of Orthopaedic Surgery, Thomas Jefferson University Hospital, Philadelphia, Pennsylvania
Fractures in the Stiff and Osteoporotic Spine

Bradford L. Currier, M.D.
Mayo Clinic Department of Orthopaedic Surgery, Rochester, Minnesota
Complications in the Treatment of Spinal Trauma

Joseph P. DeAngelis, M.D.
Department of Orthopaedic Surgery, University of Connecticut School of Medicine, Farmington, Connecticut
Principles of Internal Fixation

Christopher W. DiGiovanni, M.D.
Assistant Professor, Department of Orthopaedic Surgery, Brown University School of Medicine; Director, Foot and Ankle Service, Rhode Island Hospital, Providence, Rhode Island
Foot Injuries

Mark E. Easley, M.D.
Assistant Professor, Division of Orthopaedic Surgery, Duke University Medical Center, Durham, North Carolina
Foot Injuries

Robert K. Eastlack, M.D.
Clinical Instructor, Department of Orthopaedic Surgery, University of California–San Diego; Orthopaedic Spine Surgeon, Orthopaedic Medical Group, Sharp Memorial Hospital, San Diego, California
Complications in the Treatment of Spinal Trauma

Thomas A. Einhorn, M.D.
Professor of Orthopaedic Surgery and Biomedical Engineering, Chairman, Department of Orthopaedic Surgery, Boston University School of Medicine, Boston, Massachusetts
Biology and Enhancement of Skeletal Repair

Frank Eismont, M.D.
Professor and Vice-Chairman, Department of Orthopaedic Surgery, University of Miami School of Medicine; Co-Director, Acute Spinal Cord Injury Unit, Jackson Memorial Hospital, Miami, Florida
Thoracic and Upper Lumbar Spine Injuries; Gunshot Wounds of the Spine

Nathan K. Endres, M.D.
Assistant Professor, Department of Orthopaedics and Rehabilitation, University of Vermont; Orthopaedic Surgeon, Fletcher Allen Health Care, Burlington, Vermont
Fractures of the Tibial Pilon

David V. Feliciano, M.D.
Professor of Surgery, Emory University School of Medicine; Chief of Surgery, Chief of Vascular Surgery, Grady Memorial Hospital, Atlanta, Georgia
Evaluation and Treatment of Vascular Injuries

Theodore Fischer, M.D., M.S.
Orthopaedic Spine Surgeon, Illinois Bone and Joint Institute, Chicago, Illinois
Spinal Orthoses

John C. France, M.D.
Professor, Orthopaedics, West Virginia University, Morgantown, West Virginia
Injuries of the Cervicocranium

Robert Frigg
Chief Technology Officer, Synthes GmBH, Bettlach Solothurn, Switzerland
Locking Plates: Development, Biomechanics, and Clinical Application

Richard H. Gannon, Pharm.D.
Adjunct Clinical Professor, School of Pharmacy, University of Connecticut, Storrs, Connecticut; Clinical Specialist, Pain Management, Department of Pharmacy Services, Hartford Hospital, Hartford, Connecticut
Pharmacologic Management of the Orthopaedic Trauma Patient

Steven R. Garfin, M.D.
Professor and Chair, Department of Orthopaedics, University of California, San Diego, San Diego, California
Thoracic and Upper Lumbar Spine Injuries

Peter V. Giannoudis, M.D.
Professor of Trauma and Orthopaedics, The University of Leeds, The General Infirmary at Leeds, Leeds, West Yorkshire, United Kingdom
Femoral Shaft Fractures

Gregory E. Gleis, M.D.
Associate Clinical Professor, Department of Orthopaedic Surgery, University of Louisville School of Medicine, Louisville, Kentucky
Diagnosis and Teatment of Complications

Ryan T. Gocke, M.D.
Department of Orthopaedics, West Virginia University, Morgantown, West Virginia
Injuries of the Cervicocranium

James A. Goulet, M.D.
Professor, Department of Orthopaedic Surgery, University of Michigan Medical School; Director, Orthopaedic Trauma Service, University of Michigan Hospital, Ann Arbor, Michigan
Hip Dislocations

Andrew Green, M.D.
Associate Professor, Department of Orthopaedic Surgery, Brown Medical School; Chief of Shoulder and Elbow Surgery, Orthopaedic Surgery, Rhode Island Hospital, Providence, Rhode Island
Proximal Humerus Fractures and Glenohumeral Dislocations

Stuart A. Green, M.D.
Clinical Professor, Orthopaedic Surgery, University of California, Irvine, School of Medicine, Irvine, California
Principles and Complications of External Fixation

Neil Grey, M.D.
Department of Endocrinology, Hartford Hospital, Hartford, Connecticut
Surgical Site Infection Prevention

Munish C. Gupta, M.D.
Associate Professor, Department of Orthopaedics, University of California, Davis, School of Medicine; Orthopaedic Surgeon, University of California, Davis, Medical Center, Sacramento, California
Initial Evaluation and Emergency Treatment of the Spine-Injured Patient

George J. Haidukewych, M.D.
Division of Adult Reconstruction and Orthopedic Trauma, Florida Orthopedic Institute and Tampa General Hospital, Temple Terrace, Florida
Post-Traumatic Reconstruction of the Hip Joint

Sigvard T. Hansen, Jr., M.D.
Professor and Chairman Emeritus, Department of Orthopaedic Surgery, University of Washington School of Medicine; Director, Foot and Ankle Institute, Harborview Medical Center, Seattle, Washington
Post-Traumatic Reconstruction of the Foot and Ankle

Wilson C. Hayes, Ph.D.
Professor, Nutrition and Exercise Science, College of Health and Human Science, Oregon State University; Adjunct Professor, Mechanical Engineering, College of Engineering, Oregon State University, Corvallis, Oregon
Biomechanics of Fractures

John A. Hipp, Ph.D.
Department of Orthopedic Surgery, Baylor College of Medicine, Houston, Texas
Biomechanics of Fractures

Lenworth M. Jacobs, M.D., M.P.H., F.A.C.S.
Professor of Surgery, University of Connecticut School of Medicine, Farmington; Director, Traumatology, Hartford Hospital, Hartford, Connecticut
Evaluation and Treatment of the Multiple-Trauma Patient

Jesse B. Jupiter, M.D.
Director, Orthopaedic Hand Service, Massachusetts General Hospital; Hansjörg Wyss/AO Professor, Harvard Medical School, Boston, Massachusetts
Fractures and Dislocations of the Hand; Fractures of the Distal Radius; Diaphyseal Fractures of the Forearm; Trauma to the Adult Elbow and Fractures of the Distal Humerus; Injuries to the Shoulder Girdle

Sanjeev Kakar, M.D., M.R.C.S.
Orthopaedic Research Associate, Department of Orthopaedic Surgery, Boston University School of Medicine; Orthopaedic Surgery Resident, Orthopaedic Surgery, Boston Medical Center, Boston, Massachusetts
Biology and Enhancement of Skeletal Repair

Steven P. Kalandiak, M.D.
Assistant Professor of Clinical Orthopaedics Surgery of the Shoulder and Elbow, Department of Orthopaedics and Rehabilitation, Miller School of Medicine, University of Miami, Miami, Florida
Gunshot Wounds to the Musculoskeletal System

Timothy L. Keenen, M.D.
Clinical Associate Professor of Orthopaedic Surgery, Oregon Health Sciences University School of Medicine, Portland, Oregon
Initial Evaluation and Emergency Treatment of the Spine-Injured Patient

James F. Kellam, M.D., F.R.C.S.(C.), F.A.C.S., F.R.C.S.(I.)
Director, Orthopaedic Trauma Program and Fellowships, Vice Chairman, Department of Orthopaedic Surgery, Carolinas Medical Center, Charlotte, North Carolina
Damage Control Orthopaedic Surgery: A Strategy for the Orthopaedic Care of the Critically Injured Patient; Pelvic Ring Disruptions; Diaphyseal Fractures of the Forearm

Gino M.M.J. Kerkhoffs, M.D., Ph.D.
Orthopedic Surgeon, University of Amsterdam; Orthopedic Surgeon, Department of Orthopaedic Surgery, Academic Medical Center, Amsterdam, The Netherlands
Malunions and Nonunions About the Knee

Choll W. Kim, M.D., Ph.D.
Assistant Professor, Orthopaedic Surgery, University of California–San Diego, San Diego, California
Complications in the Treatment of Spinal Trauma

Ioannis P. Kioumis
Center for Anti-Infective Research and Development, Aristotle University of Thessaloniki, Medical Faculty, Thessaloniki, Greece
Antibiotic Therapy: General Considerations

Christian Krettek, M.D.
Director, Trauma Department, Hannover Medical School, Hannover, Germany
Fractures of the Distal Femur

Joseph L. Kuti, Pharm. D.
Associate Director, Clinical and Economic Studies Center for Anti-Infective Research and Development, Hartford Hospital, Hartford, Connecticut
Antibiotic Therapy: General Consderations

Brian K. Kwon, M.D., Ph.D., F.R.C.S.(C.)
Combined Neurosurgical and Orthopaedic Spine Program, Department of Orthopaedics, University of British Columbia, Vancouver, British Columbia, Canada
Injuries of Lower Cervical Spine

Joseph M. Lane, M.D.
Professor of Orthopaedic Surgery, Assistant Dean, Weill College of Medicine of Cornell University; Chief, Metabolic Bone Disease Service, Attending, Orthopaedic Trauma Service, Hospital for Special Surgery, New York, New York
Osteoporotic Fragility Fractures

Yu-Po Lee, M.D.
Assistant Clinical Professor, Orthopedic Surgery, University of California–San Diego, San Diego, California
Thoracic and Upper Lumbar Spine Injuries

Alan M. Levine, M.D.
Director, Alvin and Lois Lapidus Cancer Institute, Sinai Hospital, Baltimore, Maryland
Pathologic Fractures; Spinal Orthoses; Low Lumbar Fractures; Fractures of the Sacrum

Bruce A. Levy, M.D.
Assistant Professor, Department of Orthopaedic Surgery, University of Minnesota, Minneapolis, Minnesota; Vice Chief of Orthopaedic Surgery, Regions Hospital, St. Paul, Minnesota
Tibial Plateau Fractures

Frank A. Liporace, M.D.
Assistant Professor, Department of Orthopaedics—Trauma Division, New Jersey Medical School; Assistant Professor, Department of Orthopaedics—Trauma Division, University of Medicine and Dentistry of New Jersey, Newark, New Jersey
Fractures with Soft Tissue Injuries

Susan MacArthur, R.N., C.I.C., M.P.H.
Infection Control Practitioner, Clinical Quality Management Specialist, Hartford Hospital, Hartford, Connecticut
Avoidance of Occupationally Acquired Blood-Borne Pathogens; Surgical Site Infection Prevention

Luke Madigan, M.D.
Attending Spine Surgeon, Knoxville Orthopaedic Clinic, Knoxville, Tennessee
Fractures in the Stiff and Osteoporotic Spine

René K. Marti, M.D.
Department of Orthopaedic Surgery, Academic Medical Center, Amsterdam, The Netherlands
Malunions and Nonunions About the Knee

Peter J. Mas, M.S., D.A.B.M.P.
Medical Health Physicist and Radiation Safety Officer, Hartford Hospital, Hartford, Connecticut
Optimal and Safe Use of C-Arm X-Ray Fluoroscopy Units

Jeffrey W. Mast, M.D.
Northern Nevada Medical Center, Sparks, Nevada
Principles of Internal Fractures

Keith A. Mayo, M.D.
Orthopaedic Center, Tacoma, Washington
Pelvic Ring Disruption

Augustus D. Mazzocca, M.D.
Assistant Professor, Department of Orthopaedic Surgery, University of Connecticut Health Sciences Center, Farmington, Connecticut
Principles of Internal Fixation

Michael D. McKee, M.D.
Associate Professor, Division of Orthopaedics,
Department of Surgery, University of Toronto;
Staff Surgeon, Division of Orthopaedic Surgery,
St. Michaels Hospital, Toronto, Canada
Trauma to the Adult Elbow and Fractures of the Distal Humerus

Michael W. Mendes, M.D.
Attending Physician, McLeod Regional Medical
Center, Florence, South Carolina
Principles of Internal Fixation

Stuart E. Mirvis, M.D., F.A.C.R.
Professor, Department of Radiology, University of
Maryland School of Medicine; Director, Trauma and
Emergency Radiology, Diagnostic Radiology,
University of Maryland Medical Center, Baltimore,
Maryland
Spinal Imaging

Victor A. Morris, M.D.
Assistant Professor of Medicine, General Medicine;
Director, Hospital Service; Director, Medicine Consult
Service; Director, Medicine Consult Service,
Yale University School of Medicine, New Haven,
Connecticut
Medical Management of the Patient with Hip Fracture

Amir Mostofi, M.D.
Resident, University of Connecticut, Farmington,
Connecticut
Surgical Site Infection Prevention

David P. Nicolau, Pharm.D., F.C.C.P.
Center for Anti-Infective Research and Development,
Hartford Hospital, Hartford, Connecticut
Antibiotic Therapy: General Considerations

Florian Nickisch, M.D.
Assistant Professor of Orthopaedic Surgery,
Department of Orthopaedics, University of Utah,
Salt Lake City, Utah
Foot Injuries

Sean E. Nork, M.D.
Associate Professor, Orthopaedics and Sports
Medicine, University of Washington; Associate
Professor, Orthopaedics and Sports Medicine,
Veterans' Hospital, Seattle, Washington
Subtrochanteric Fractures of the Femur

Tom R. Norris, M.D.
Orthopaedic Surgery, California Pacific Medical
Center, San Francisco, California
Proximal Humerus Fractures and Glenohumeral Dislocations

William T. Obremskey, M.D., M.P.H.
Associate Professor, Department of Orthopaedics and
Rehabilitation, Division of Orthopaedic Trauma,
Vanderbilt University Medical Center, Nashville,
Tennessee
Outcomes Research in Orthopaedics

Daniel P. O'Connor, Ph.D.
Assistant Professor, University of Houston,
Houston, Texas
Nonunions: Evaluation and Treatment

Matthew E. Oetgen, M.D.
Resident, Orthopaedic Surgery, Yale–New Haven
Hospital, New Haven, Connecticut
Intertrochanteric Hip Fractures

Patrick W. Owens, M.D.
Assistant Professor of Clinical Orthopaedics,
Department of Orthopaedics, Miller School of
Medicine, University of Miami, Miami, Florida
Gunshot Wounds to the Musculoskeletal System

Dror Paley, M.D., F.R.C.S.C.
Director, Rubin Institute for Advanced Orthopaedics,
Co-Director, International Center for Limb-
Lengthening, Sinai Hospital of Baltimore, Baltimore,
Maryland
Principles of Deformity Correction

George A. Perdrizet, M.D., Ph.D., F.A.C.S.
University of Connecticut; Staff Surgeon, Hartford
Hospital, Hartford, Connecticut
Substance Abuse Syndromes: Recognition, Prevention, and Treatment

Ed Pesanti, M.D., F.A.C.P.
Professor, Department of Medicine, University of
Connecticut School of Medicine; University
of Connecticut Health Center, Farmington,
Connecticut
Chronic Osteomyelitis

Michael S. Pinzur, M.D.
Professor, Department of Orthopaedic Surgery and
Rehabilitation, Loyala University Medical Center,
Maywood, Illinois
Amputations in Trauma

Ryan M. Putnam, M.D.
Clinical Instructor, Orthopaedic Surgery and
Rehabilitation, University of Vermont; Clinical
Instructor, Orthopaedic Surgery and Rehabilitation,
Fletcher Allen Health Care, Burlington, Vermont
Fractures of the Tibial Pilon

Mark C. Reilly, M.D.
Department of Orthopaedic Surgery, Newark, New Jersey
Subtrochanteric Fractures of the Femur

David Ring, M.D., Ph.D.
Assistant Professor, Orthopaedic Surgery, Harvard Medical School; Medical Director and Director of Research, Orthopaedic Hand and Upper Extremity Service, Massachusetts General Hospital, Boston, Massachusetts
Injuries to the Shoulder Girdle

Craig S. Roberts, M.D.
Professor, Residency Program Director, University of Louisville School of Medicine, Louisville, Kentucky
Diagnosis and Treatment of Complications

Kenneth J. Robinson, M.D., F.A.C.E.P.
Associate Professor of Emergency Medicine, University of Connecticut School of Medicine, Farmington, Connecticut; Medical Director, Program Director, LIFE STAR Helicopter Program; Chief, Prehospital Services, Department of Emergency Medical Services/Trauma, Hartford Hospital, Hartford, Connecticut
Evaluation and Treatment of the Multiple-Trauma Patient

Craig M. Rodner, M.D.
Assistant Professor, University of Connecticut Department of Orthopaedics, Farmington, Connecticut
Chronic Osteomyelitis

Jonathan G. Roper, M.D.
Department of Orthopaedic Surgery, Kaiser Permanente Medical Center, San Diego, California
Gunshot Wounds of the Spine

Milton Lee (Chip) Routt, Jr., M.D.
Professor, Orthopaedics and Sports Medicine, University of Washington; Professor, Orthopaedics and Sports Medicine, Harborview Medical Center, Seattle, Washington
Surgical Treatment of Acetabular Fractures

Leonard K. Ruby, M.D.
Professor of Orthopaedic Surgery, Tufts University School of Medicine; Senior Staff, Hand Surgery, Department of Orthopaedic Surgery, New England Medical Center, Boston, Massachusetts
Fractures and Dislocations of the Carpus

Roy W. Sanders, M.D.
Clinical Professor of Orthopaedics, University of South Florida College of Medicine, Tampa, Florida
Patella Fractures and Extensor Mechanism Injuries

Richard A. Saunders, M.D.
Orthopedic Surgeon, The Glens Falls Hospital, Glens Falls, New York
Physical Impairment Ratings for Fractures

Joseph Schatzker, M.D.
Professor, University of Toronto Faculty of Medicine; Orthopaedic Surgeon, Sunnybrook Health Science Center, Toronto, Ontario, Canada
Tibial Plateau Fractures

Emil H. Schemitsch, M.D., F.R.C.S.C.
Professor and Head, Division of Orthopaedic Surgery, St. Michael's Hospital, Toronto, Ontario, Canada
Fractures of the Humeral Shaft

David Seligson, M.D.
Department of Orthopaedic Surgery, University of Louisville, Louisville, Kentucky
Diagnosis and Treatment of Complications

Richard Sheppard, M.D.
Sub-specialty Chair, Orthopaedics and Anesthesia, Hartford Anesthesiology Associates, Hartford, Connecticut
Evaluation and Treatment of the Multiple-Trauma Patient

Randy Sherman, M.D.
Professor of Surgery, Orthopedics, and Neurologic Surgery, Chief, Division of Plastic Surgery, Keck School of Medicine, University of Southern California; Chair, Department of Surgery, Associate Medical Director, Surgical Services, Los Angeles County and U.S.C. Medical Center, Los Angeles, California
Soft Tissue Coverage

Michael S. Sirkin, M.D.
Associate Professor, University of Medicine and Dentistry of New Jersey Medical School; Chief, Orthopaedic Trauma Service, University Hospital, Newark, New Jersey
Fractures with Soft Tissue Injuries

Raymond Malcolm Smith, M.D., F.R.C.S.
Chief, Orthopaedic Trauma Service, Massachusetts General Hospital; Associate Professor in Orthopaedics, Harvard Medical School, Boston, Massachusetts
Femoral Shaft Fractures

Michael D. Stover, M.D.
Director, Division of Orthopaedic Surgery, Loyola University Medical Center, Maywood, Illinois
Pelvic Ring Disruption

Marc F. Swiontkowski, M.D.
Professor and Chair, University of Minnesota,
Department of Orthopaedic Surgery, Minneapolis,
Minnesota
*Outcomes Research in Orthopaedics; Intracapsular Hip
Fractures*

Max Talbot, M.D., F.R.C.S.
1 Canadian Field Hospital, Canadian Forces
Fractures of the Humeral Shaft

Cary Templin, M.D.
Staff Surgeon, Hinsdale Orthopaedic Associates,
Hinsdale, Illinois
Thoracic and Upper Lumbar Spine Injuries

Peter G. Trafton, M.D.
Professor of Orthopaedics, The Warren Alpert Medical
School of Brown University; Former Surgeon-in-
charge, Orthopaedic Trauma, Rhode Island Hospital,
Providence, Rhode Island
Tibial Shaft Fractures

Bruce C. Twaddle, M.D., F.R.A.C.S.
Director of Orthopaedic Trauma, Auckland Hospital,
Auckland, New Zealand
Compartment Syndromes

Elizabeth E. C. Udeh, Pharm.D., B.C.P.S.
Assistant Clinical Professor, University of Connecticut
School of Pharmacy, Storrs, Connecticut; Clinical
Pharmacy Coordinator, Department of Pharmacy,
Hartford Hospital, Hartford, Connecticut
Anticoagulation

Michael A. Wagner, M.D.
Professor and Director, Division of Trauma Surgery
and Sports Medicine, Wilhelmin Hospital, Vienna,
Austria
*Locking Plates: Development, Biomechanics, and Clinical
Application*

J. Tracy Watson, M.D.
Professor of Orthopaedic Surgery, Wayne State
University School of Medicine; Vice Chief of
Orthopaedics, Divison of Orthopaedic Traumatology,
Detroit Receiving Hospital, Detroit Medical Center,
Detroit, Michigan
Tibial Plateau Fractures

Brent B. Wiesel, M.D.
Instructor, Orthopaedic Surgery, University of
Pennsylvania, Philadelphia, Pennsylvania
Physical Impairment Ratings for Fractures

Sam W. Wiesel, M.D.
Professor and Chair, Department of Orthopaedics,
Georgetown University Medical Center,
Washington, D.C.
Physical Impairment Ratings for Fractures

Susan L. Williams, M.D.
Orthopaedic and Spine Surgery, Roseburg, Oregon
Spinal Orthoses

Luther H. Wolff, III, M.D.
Mayo Clinic, Rochester, Minnesota
Periprosthetic Fractures of the Lower Extremity

Michael J. Yaszemski, M.D., Ph.D.
Professor, Departments of Orthopedic Surgery and
Biomedical Engineering, Mayo Clinic College of
Medicine; Consultant, Orthopedic Spine Surgery,
Department of Orthopaedic Surgery, Mayo Clinic,
Rochester, Minnesota
Complications in the Treatment of Spinal Trauma

Gregory A. Zych, D.O.
Christine E. Lynn Distinguished Chair in
Orthopaedic Trauma, Associate Chairman for
Clinical Affairs, Department of Orthopaedics and
Rehabilitation, Miller School of Medicine at the
University of Miami; Chief, Orthopaedic Trauma,
Ryder Trauma Center, Jackson Memorial Hospital,
Miami, Florida
Gunshot Wounds to the Musculoskeletal System

Foreword

It is a pleasure for me to be asked to write the foreword to the latest edition of Skeletal Trauma edited by Browner et al. This textbook, since its inception and subsequent additions, has become the reference text of record for the diagnosis, treatment, and rehabilitation of musculoskeletal trauma patients.

In this edition the editors have divided the text into diagnostic and anatomical groupings starting with general principles including the principles of fracture repair, biomechanics and broad-based principles of treatment including the role of skeletal repair in the management of the multiple trauma patient and have added important chapters on the use of locking plates, the emerging concept of damage control orthopaedics and the management of mass casualties. They also include important material on outcomes which most now recognize as central to appropriate care of trauma patients.

The sections begin with spine and move on to pelvis; this is followed by upper extremity and lower extremity injury. Throughout the text each section consists of a number of focused chapters written by recognized experts in the field. Each of these chapters is clearly written and profusely illustrated demonstrating not only the principles of care but also specific surgical techniques to achieve the optimal outcome for each of these individual injuries. A number of new authors have been invited to participate in this edition and their contributions are clearly recognized and have improved the text.

Skeletal trauma continues to be a leading cause of disability in every society. Although the trauma problem in North America continues to be significant with dozens of unnecessary deaths occurring daily as a consequence of road traffic injury and industrial trauma, our problems pale in comparison to those of the emerging world. The rapid industrialization of these societies is often occurring without the concomitant or concurrent changes in industrial plant safety and worker protection. Furthermore, rapid industrialization brings with it urbanization and a proliferation of motor vehicles. It is estimated that there were one million fatalities from motor vehicle accidents in 2007 and this number will double within the next five years unless we make dramatic inroads in both trauma prevention and trauma treatment.

An international survey encompassing most of the emerging world completed over the past year has revealed five significant problems relating to trauma prevention and trauma care. Among those five are things which we as individuals can do very little such as improved road infrastructure or driver education. Among the top five, however, is the need to improve the quality of trauma care which in turn will minimize the disability of the trauma patient. It is increasingly recognized that the optimum treatment of skeletal trauma will not only shorten the period of acute disability for patients but the quality of care is directly proportional to the quality of their outcome and therefore determines the residual disability experienced by the patient following successful healing of their skeletal injury. Optimum care of skeletal trauma is the most important factor diminishing residual disability for these patients everywhere in the world and therefore continued efforts to refine our ability and to teach others so as to improve patient care results and in turn improve patient outcome.

I commend the editors and their authors for their efforts to refine old ideas and bring new ideas to us as practicing orthopaedic surgeons to enable us to improve patients' welfare.

This is a stellar effort and I hope you enjoy the fruits of their labours.

James P. Waddell, M.D., F.R.C.S.C
Professor, Division of Orthopaedic Surgery
University of Toronto

Preface

FIRST EDITION

The first edition of *Skeletal Trauma: Fractures, Dislocations, Ligamentous Injuries* was written between 1988 and 1991. This represented a unique window for the creation of this text, coinciding with the increased recognition of the special needs of trauma victims. By the mid-1980s, more than 500 regional trauma centers had been established throughout the United States and Canada. The volume and acuity of blunt trauma and associated musculoskeletal injuries reached a high-water mark. The editors and contributing authors for *Skeletal Trauma* had been on the front lines working in the major trauma centers throughout this period. They helped to develop a new operative approach to the treatment of these injuries that stressed early skeletal fixation and rapid mobilization. The incomparable first-hand experience that they gained helped shape their contributions to the text.

In the early 1990s, many states adopted the child restraint device and seat belt legislation. Successful initiatives to control driving under the influence of alcohol significantly lowered incidence of motor vehicle crashes. Improvements in automotive design, such as airbags and strengthened bodies, continued to reduce the incidence and severity of blunt trauma and complex musculoskeletal injuries. Although there was an alarming increase in injuries and deaths from gunshots in our major cities, penetrating trauma does not usually result in the multiplicity and complexity of skeletal injuries that are caused by vehicular crashes. In addition, managed care contracting practices resulted in the dispersion of trauma patients to community hospitals, often reducing the number of injuries seen in trauma centers. In retrospect, the 1980s provided a unique opportunity for the creation of this text.

The excellent manuscripts provided by our contributing authors and the beautiful illustrations created by the artists were assembled into an outstanding text by the W.B. Saunders production department. In the year of its publication, 1992, it won first prize in medical sciences from the Association of American Publishers as the best new medical book. The text was widely embraced by orthopaedic and trauma surgeons throughout the world for its clarity and its utility. They consistently expressed their appreciation of our approach, which stressed the discussion of problem-focused clinical judgment and proven surgical techniques. The textbook was regarded by surgeons in training and practicing physicians to be a practical resource that helped guide them through the management of the musculoskeletal injuries with which they are confronted.

SECOND EDITION

We retained and strengthened the basic philosophy and organization of the original text in the second edition that was published in 1998. We added new chapters to cover important subjects that were not addressed adequately in the first edition.

In the years since the publication of the second edition of *Skeletal Trauma*, major new global epidemiologic trends have been noted that influence the character of musculoskeletal injuries throughout the world. In the developed market economies, decreased birth rates and increasing longevity have resulted in the aging of the population. Osteoporosis and associated fragility fractures have grown in number and significance. Road safety improvements in these countries, such as pediatric restraint devices, seat belts, drunken driving control, airbags, vehicle design improvements, and enhanced law enforcement, have decreased the number and severity of road traffic injuries. In the developing world, however, there is a growing epidemic of road traffic injuries. Vulnerable travelers such as pedestrians, bicyclists, motorcycle riders, and passengers on overcrowded buses and trucks are the main victims. Annually, 1.2 million people die on the world's roads and an estimated 24 to 33 million are severely injured or disabled.

To raise awareness of the burden of these and other musculoskeletal disorders, empower patients, expand research and improvements for prevention and treatment of these problems, and engender multidisciplinary cooperation, the years 2000-2010 have been declared the "Bone and Joint Decade" by U.N. Secretary General Kofi Annan. The movement has also been endorsed by the World Health Organization, the World Bank, and the governments of forty nations.

THIRD EDITION

The third edition of *Skeletal Trauma*, published in 2003, was written in recognition of the challenges of the era and was dedicated to the improvement of musculoskeletal trauma care throughout the world in keeping with the spirit of the "Bone and Joint Decade." Although there have been dramatic advances in biology, pharmaceuticals, technology, and fixation to improve the care of patients with musculoskeletal disorders in wealthy countries, a large portion of the world's population lacks basic health care and has very limited orthopaedic services available. Road traffic injuries and deaths have risen to epidemic proportions in the developing countries. With the leadership of the country of Oman and its UN Mission, the UN implemented an international road safety program in 2004. The WHO serves as a coordinating agency is working with UN regional commissions and member countries to address this major global health problem. Prevention is the primary focus of this initiative, but serious injuries will continue to occur, so capacity building for treatment in developing countries is essential.

For many years, the *Skeletal Trauma* editorial group had discussed the possibility of creating a separate volume for skeletal trauma reconstruction. Our contributing authors and others had gained wide experience in post-trauma reconstruction, but there were no comprehensive texts written on this subject. In conjunction with our publisher, we made a decision to incorporate this material into the third edition. As we were limited by the established size of the two volumes, some basic science chapters were deleted and other information was condensed to make room for the new reconstructive material. New chapters were added on perioperative pain management, osteoporotic fragility fractures, chronic osteomyelitis, gunshot wounds of the spine, fractures in the stiff and osteoporotic spine, medical management of patients with hip fractures, total hip arthroplasty after failed primary treatment of fractures involving the hip joint, acute foot injuries, foot injury reconstruction, lower extremity alignment, periprosthetic fractures, and amputations for trauma. Some of the authors from previous editions continued but made major revisions to revitalize their work. In other cases, new authors were recruited to add international perspective and broaden the base of expertise. Minimally invasive plating, an important new technique, was covered by one of its major developers in the chapter on the distal femur. New biologic agents are addressed in an expanded chapter on enhancement of fracture healing.

In addition to discussing the treatment of acute injuries, the authors of the anatomic chapters were asked to expand their scholarly writing to include the management of nonunions, malunions, bone loss, osteomyelitis, and fixation in osteoporotic bone. The use of fusion and arthroplasty in post-traumatic arthritis was described in detail.

FOURTH EDITION

The publication of the fourth edition in 2008 brings a number of new features and an important addition to the editorial team. Many surgical texts have begun to include videos of surgical techniques and lectures that are provided in a companion DVD or via a website. To add this dimension to *Skeletal Trauma*, we turned to Professor Christian Krettek, Chairman of the Department of Traumatology at Hannover Medical University in Hannover Germany. An outstanding trauma surgeon, educator, investigator and innovator, he has been a leader in the use of videos in orthopaedic and trauma education. He has utilized an annual educational meeting involving guest lecturers and his faculty as a platform to develop a phenomenal library of surgical videos and lectures. Selected videos from this collection that are relevant to the subject of the text have been included in a special companion DVD and made accessible through the website developed for *Skeletal*

Trauma Ed 4. To recognize this contribution and the leadership that Professor Krettek has provided for the assembly, production and translation of these videos, we have made him a member of our editorial team. As members of his department have served as contributing authors for previous editions and his predecessor, Professor Harald Tscherne wrote the forward to the third edition, this represents an even closer affiliation. Surgeons from Europe have contributed greatly to the development of musculoskeletal trauma management. The growing connection with this important European center and inclusion of other authors from the continent reflects our move to internationalize the text.

In recognition of the contemporary movement by younger physicians to acquire increasing amounts of information electronically via the internet, the 4th editon will be offered as an 'Expert Consult' title with online and print components. The Publisher of this text, Elsevier, has published more than 70 text/web product packages across the medical and surgical specialties since release of the first such product in March 2003. This combination of text and web product has been very well received in the market and is now a mature and well organized offering. The publisher's objective in marketing and branding the concept is to provide currency and portability of information, and counter the charges that print texts are 'out of date' upon publication. Many studies acknowledge that this generation of residents and fellows have fully embraced online access to information. Premium features of the web components include full text search; link through to full text articles in Pub Med and Cross Ref; all images and figures downloadable to Power Point, video components; and, the most popular feature, content updates.

The editors have been gratified by comments from surgeons around the world indicating that *Skeletal Trauma* has been adopted by many trauma centers and orthopaedic training programs as the principal fracture text. We have welcomed their constructive criticism as well as their accolades. Many of the changes in the current edition were made in response to comments from these surgeons and our own residents.

We are grateful to our contributing authors, whose high level of scholarship and dedication to their chapter writing and video production makes this such a readable and useful reference. The pressures of modern medical practice have made these surgeons busier than they were during the writing of the second and third editions, so they should be afforded special recognition for the devotion they have shown communicating to other surgeons about their subject. Together we have refashioned our text to better address readers' needs for information concerning basic science, acute injury management, and post-traumatic reconstruction.

Bruce D. Browner, M.D.
Jesse B. Jupiter, M.D.
Alan M. Levine, M.D.
Peter G. Trafton, M.D.
Christian Krettek, M.D.

Acknowledgments

We have had the pleasure of working with another group of people who have carried on the tradition of excellence established in the first, second, and third editions. We particularly wish to acknowledge Kim Murphy, Publishing Director, Global Surgery, the driving force behind the project, and Janice Gaillard, our Senior Developmental Editor, the glue that kept the work on track. Additionally, we acknowledge the work of our Project Manager, David Saltzberg, the switchmaster that coordinated the flow of production. Without their efforts, we could not have hoped to maintain this level of excellence.

No staff was hired by the editors for the production of this text. Again, we relied on the hard work and dedication of our own personal staffs. We recognize that without their help we could not have upheld our commitment to this project.

Bruce Browner would like to recognize the assistance of Kaye Straw, his Administrative Assistant in the Hartford Hospital office, who assisted him in communicating with the authors in his section during multiple phases of the development and editing of the fourth edition. He would also like to thank Sue Ellen Pelletier, his Executive Assistant at the University of Connecticut office, for her help in contacting the authors, editors, and publisher during the creation of the fourth edition. Finally, he would like to thank his colleagues, residents, physicians' assistants, nurse practitioners, and students whose constructive feedback has helped to improve this edition of the text.

Alan Levine would like to express his appreciation to Sylvia Horasek, his research assistant, for her tireless efforts in completing this edition by proofreading manuscripts, page proofs, and checking citations. He would also like to acknowledge the tremendous effort of his office administrator, Joanne Barker, who has kept him organized, focused, and assisted him in communication with the many people necessary to complete this edition. Finally, he would like to thank all of the residents, fellows, and staff at both Sinai Hospital and at the Maryland Shock Trauma Unit without whom he would never have garnered the experience necessary to effectively contribute to the preparation of this book.

Peter Trafton gratefully acknowledges the continued support of his colleagues and the staff of University Orthopaedics, the stimulus and candor of the Brown University Orthopaedic Surgery Residents, and particularly Brown University's Orthopaedic Trauma fellows, whose quest for surgical expertise and understanding will always be a daily inspiration.

Christian Krettek would like to express his strong appreciation to Daniela Koss from the TRAUMASTIF-TUNG for her tremendous efforts in coordinating the entire video editing and translation process. He would also like to acknowledge the continued support of the entire staff of the Department of Trauma & Orthopaedics of the Hannover Medical School (MHH), especially the efforts of Dr. Stefan Hankemeier, M.D., Dr. Michael Klein, Jacob Huefner, and Kurt Singelmann. Strong appreciation is given especially to the numerous contributors of the Hannover VIDEOSYMPOSIUM, who spent enormous time and efforts to produce the videos and agreed to share their expertise and video material with the readers of *Skeletal Trauma*.

Table of Contents

---

* Dr. Behrens is deceased

*Deceased.

General Principles

Section Editor: Bruce D. Browner, M.D., M.S., F.A.C.S.

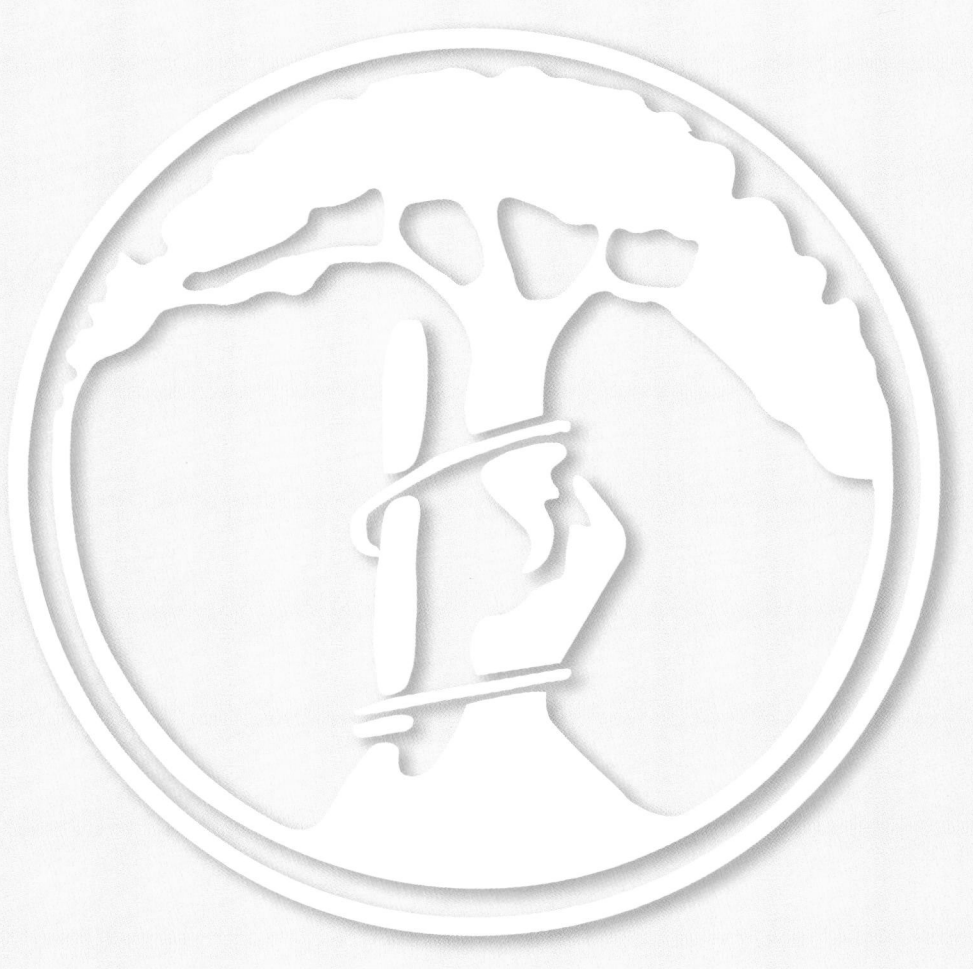

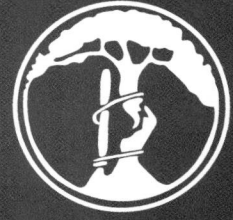

CHAPTER 1

The History of Fracture Treatment

Christopher L. Colton, M.D., F.R.C.S., F.R.C.S.Ed.

EARLY SPLINTING TECHNIQUES

Humans have never been immune from injury, and doubtless the practice of bonesetting was not unfamiliar to our most primitive forebears. Indeed, given the known skills of Neolithic humans at trepanning the skull,[49] it would be surprising if techniques of similar sophistication had not been brought to bear in the care of injuries. However, no evidence of this remains.

The earliest examples of the active management of fractures in humans were discovered at Naga-ed-Der (about 100 miles north of Luxor in Egypt) by Professor G. Elliott Smith during the Hearst Egyptian expedition of the University of California in 1903.[74] Two specimens were found of splinted extremities. One was an adolescent femur with a compound, comminuted midshaft fracture that had been splinted with four longitudinal wooden boards, each wrapped in linen bandages. A dressing pad containing blood pigment was also found at approximately the level of the fracture site. The victim is judged to have died shortly after injury, as the bones show no evidence whatsoever of any healing reaction (Fig. 1-1). The second specimen was of open fractures of a forearm, treated by similar splints, but in this case a pad of blood-stained vegetable fiber (probably obtained from the date palm) was found adherent to the upper fragment of the ulna, evidently having been pushed into the wound to stanch bleeding. Again, death appears to have occurred before any bone healing reaction had started. The Egyptians were known to be skilled at the management of fractures, and many healed specimens have been found. The majority of femoral fractures had united with shortening and deformity, but a number of well-healed forearm fractures have been discovered.

Some form of wooden splintage bandaged to the injured limb has been used from antiquity to the present day. Certainly, both Hippocrates and Celsus described in detail the splintage of fractures using wooden appliances,[54] but a fascinating account of external splintage of fractures is to be found in the work of El Zahrawi (AD 936 to 1013). This Arab surgeon, born in Al Zahra, the royal city 5 miles west of Cordova in Spain, was named Abu'l-Quasim Khalas Ibn'Abbas Al-Zahrawi, commonly shortened to Albucasis. In his 30th treatise, "The Surgery," he described in detail the application of two layers of bandages, starting at the fracture site and extending both up and down the limb, after reduction of the fracture. He continued:

> Then put between the bandages enough soft tow or soft rags to correct the curves of the fracture, if any, otherwise put nothing in. Then wind over it another bandage and at once lay over it strong splints if the part be not swollen or effused. But if there be swelling or effusion in the part, apply something to allay the swelling and disperse the effusion. Leave it on for several days and then bind on the splint. The splint should be made of broad halves of cane cut and shaped with skill, or the splints may be made of wood used for sieves, which are made of pine, or of palm branches, or of brier or giant fennel or the like, whatever wood be at hand. Then bind over the splints another bandage just as tightly as you did the first. Then over that tie it up with cords arranged in the way we have said, that is with the pressure greatest over the site of the fracture and lessened as you move away from it. Between the splints there should be a space of not less than a finger's breadth.

It is of interest that the brother of the celebrated French surgeon Bérenger Féraud, an interpreter with the French army in Algeria, wrote in 1868 that all Arab bonesetters (*tebibs* [a tebib is an Arab medicine man, whence the modern French slang word *toubib,* meaning quack or doctor]) carried with them "sticks of *kelar,* a sort of fennel, well dried and of extreme lightness, which are used as splints." Albucasis then went on to describe various forms of plaster that may be used as an alternative, particularly for women and children, recommending "mill dust, that is the fine flour that sticks to the walls of a mill as the grindstone moves. Pound it as it is, without sieving, with egg white to a medium consistency, then use." He suggested as an alternative plaster a mixture of various gums, including gum mastic, acacia, and the root of *mughath* (*Glossostemon bruguieri*), pounded fine with clay of Armenia or Asia Minor and mixed with water of tamarisk or with egg white.[76]

In 1517, Gersdorf[25] beautifully illustrated a novel method of binding wooden splints, using ligatures around the assembled splint that are tightened by twisting them with cannulated wooden toggles, with a wire then passed down the hollow centers of the toggles to prevent them from untwisting (Fig. 1-2). In this book, he also illustrated the use of an extension apparatus for

FIGURE 1-1 *A* and *B,* Specimen of a fracture of an adolescent femur from circa 300 BC, excavated at Naga-ed-Der in 1903. This injury was an open fracture, and the absence of any callus (arrow in *A*) indicates early death.

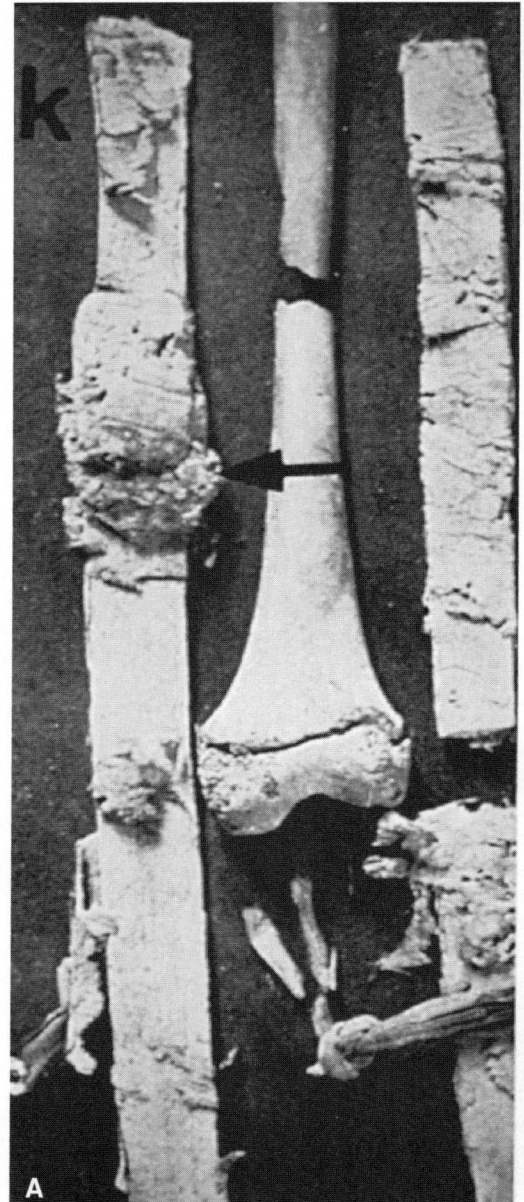
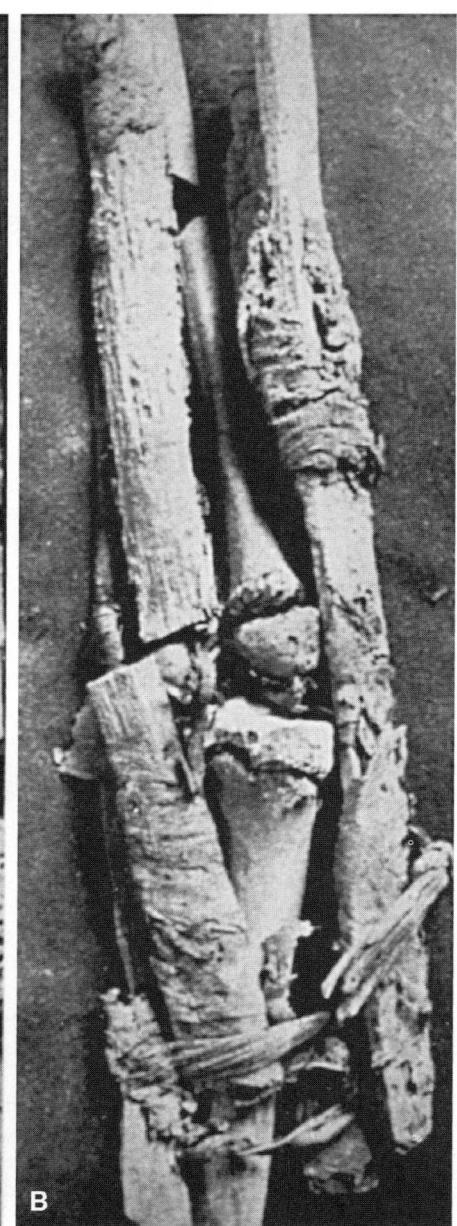

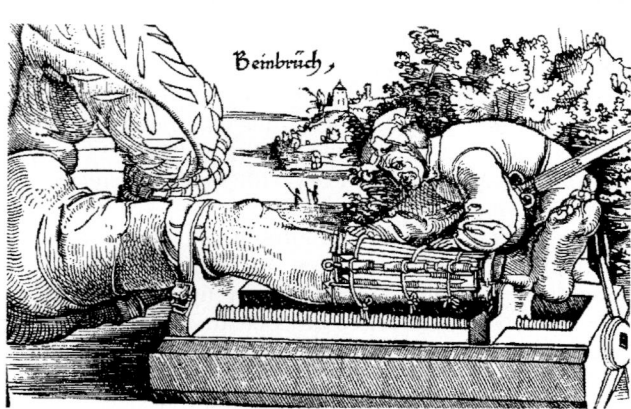

FIGURE 1-2 *Illustration of wooden splintage from Gersdorf (1517). Note the cannulated toggles used to tighten the bindings.*

overcoming overriding of the fractures of the bones, although similar machines had been in use for centuries according to the descriptions of Galen, Celsus, and Paulus Aegineta.[54]

Gersdorf's technique of tightening a circumferential splint ligature was plagiarized by Benjamin Gooch,[26] who in 1767 described what must be regarded as the first functional brace (Fig. 1-3), designed as it was to return the worker to labor before the fracture had consolidated. Gooch fashioned shape splints for various anatomic sites; these consisted of longitudinal strips of wood stuck to an underlying sheet of leather that could then be wrapped around the limb and held in place with ligatures and cannulated toggles. I recollect Gooch splintage still being used for temporary immobilization of injured limbs by ambulance crews as late as the 1960s. Gooch's are perhaps the most sophisticated wooden splints ever devised. The 19th century literature abounds with descriptions of many types of wooden fracture apparatus, none of which is as carefully constructed or apparently efficient as those of Gooch.

The use of willow board splints for the treatment of tibial shaft fractures and Colles' fractures in modern times has been described in great detail by Shang T'ien-Yu and colleagues[72] in a fascinating description of the integration of modern and traditional Chinese medicine in the treatment of fractures. Amerasinghe and Veerasingham continued to use shaped bamboo splints, held in place by circumferential rope ligatures, in the functional bracing of tibial fractures in Sri Lanka (Fig. 1-4).[1] They reported 88% of their patients to be weight bearing and freely mobile by 10 weeks, with a 95% union rate, and less than half an inch of shortening in 85% of patients. The Liston wooden board splint for fractures of the femoral shaft is currently in use in one institution in Scotland for the management of this injury in children.

PRECURSORS OF THE PLASTER BANDAGE

As indicated previously, El Zahrawi, probably drawing from the work of Paulus Aegineta, described the use of both clay gum mixtures and flour and egg white for casting materials. In AD 860, the Arab physician Rhazes Athuriscus wrote, "But if thou make thine apparatus with lime and white of egg it will be much handsomer and still more useful. In fact it will become as hard as stone and will not need to be removed until the healing is complete."[3]

William Cheselden (1688 to 1752), the famous English surgeon and anatomist, as a schoolboy sustained an elbow fracture that was treated in this manner. In his book *Anatomy of the Human Body,* he recorded, "I thought of a much better bandage which I had learned from Mr. Cowper, a bonesetter at Leicester, who set and cured a fracture of my own cubit when I was a boy at school. His way was, after putting the limb in a proper posture, to wrap it up in rags dipped in the whites of eggs and a little wheat flour mixed. This drying grew stiff and kept the limb in good posture. And I think there is no way better than this in fractures, for it preserves the position of the limb without strict [tight] bandage which is the common cause of mischief in fractures."[55] Cheselden was later reputed to have been able to perform a lithotomy procedure in 68 seconds; it would appear that his functional result was excellent. A more precise use of the technique of Rhazes was introduced into France by Le Dran in the late 18th century; he stiffened his bandage with egg white, vinegar, and powder of Armenian clay or plaster.[80]

The technique of pouring a plaster-of-Paris mixture around an injured limb would appear to have been used in Arabia for many centuries and was brought to the attention of European practitioners by Eaton, a British diplomat in Bassora, Turkey. In 1798 he wrote:

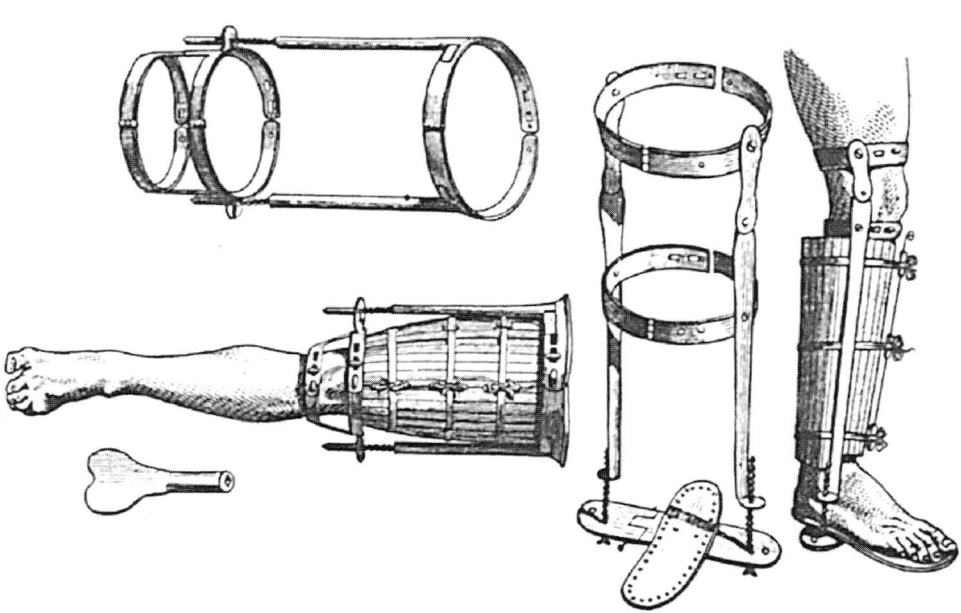

FIGURE 1-3 *Benjamin Gooch described the first functional brace in 1767. Note the similarity to Gersdorf's bindings.*

FIGURE 1-4   ***A*** *and* ***B,*** *Bamboo functional bracing currently in use in Sri Lanka. (Courtesy of Dr. D. M. Amerasinghe.)*

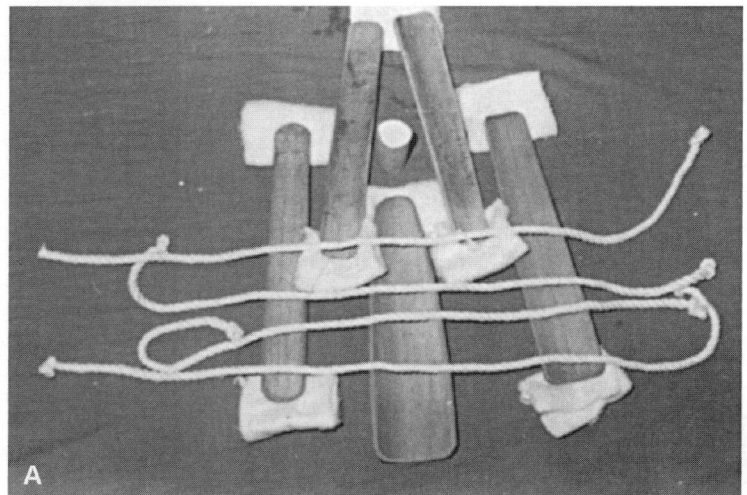

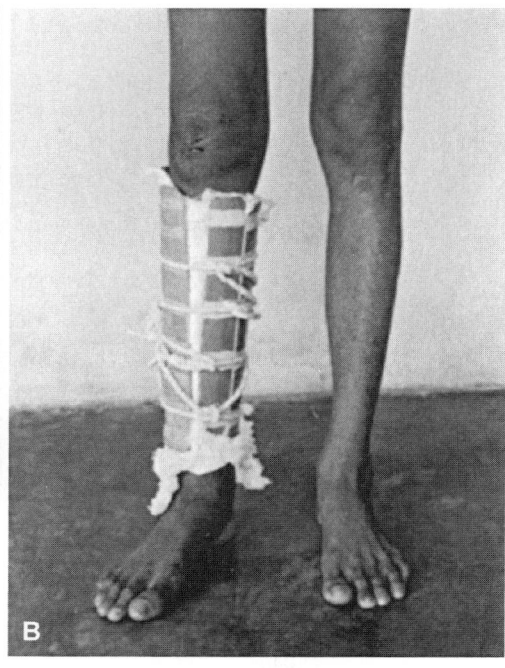

I saw in the eastern parts of the Empire a method of setting bones practised, which appears to me worthy of the attention of surgeons in Europe. It is by inclosing [*sic*] the broken limb, after the bones are put in their places, in a case of plaster of Paris (or gypsum) which takes exactly the form of the limb without any pressure and in a few minutes the mass is solid and strong [Fig. 1-5]. This substance may be easily cut with a knife and removed and replaced with another. When the swelling subsides, [and] the cavity is too large for the limb, a hole or holes being left, liquid gypsum plaster may be poured in which will perfectly fill up the void and exactly fit the limb. A hole may be made at first by placing oiled cork or a bit of wood against any part where it is required and when the plaster is set it is to be removed. There is nothing in gypsum injurious if it be free from lime. It will soon become hard and light and the limb may be bathed with spirits which will penetrate through the covering. I saw a case of a most terrible compound fracture of the leg and thigh by the fall of a cannon. The person was seated on the ground and the plaster case extended from below the heel to the upper part of his thigh, where a bandage fastened into the plaster went round his body.[22]

This technique of *plâtre coulé* was enthusiastically embraced in Europe in the early 19th century. Malgaigne[52] recorded in detail the various techniques of its use, stating that he found it first employed by Hendriksz at the Nosocomium Chirurgicum of Groningen in 1814. Shortly afterward Hubenthal,[38] believing himself to be its inventor, described *plâtre coulé* in the *Nouveau Journal de Médecine.* In 1828, Keyl, working with Dieffenbach at the Charity Hospital in Berlin, finally succeeded in calling general attention to it. Although the Berlin surgeons applied the method only to fractures of the leg,

Hubenthal had described its use in fractures of the forearm, the hand, and the clavicle, mixing the plaster powder with unsized paper (similar to blotting paper). He encased the limb in a trough made of pasteboard, closed

FIGURE 1-5   Plâtre coulé *such as Eaton recorded seeing in Turkey in the 18th century.*

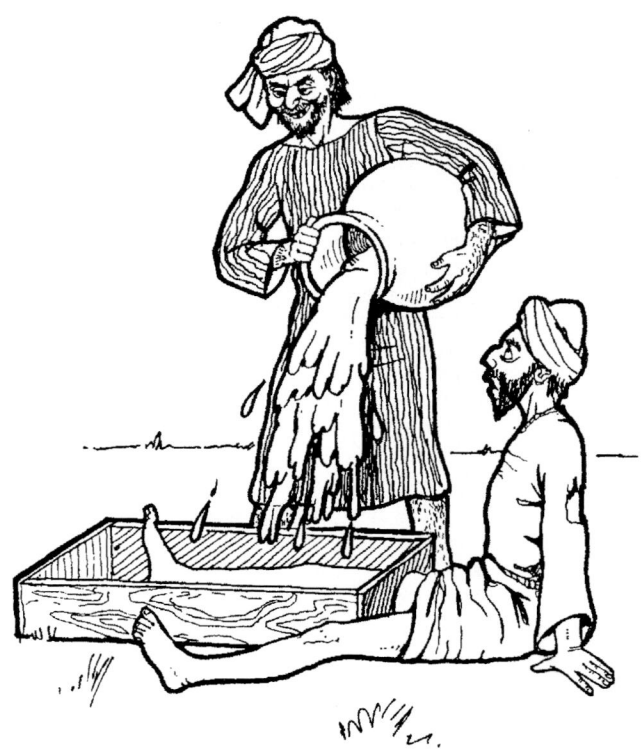

at the top and bottom with toweling, and first poured in the mixture to encase only the posterior half of the limb. After this posterior cast was allowed to set, the edges were smoothed, notched, and then oiled so that a second anterior cast could be created by applying the paste to the front of the limb, thus ending up with two halves of a cast, which could be bandaged together, yet easily separated for wound inspection or to relieve any tension.[51] Malgaigne himself was not keen on *plâtre coulé* and after having problems with swelling within a rigid cast, albeit incomplete over the crest of the tibia, he abandoned the technique in favor of albuminated and starched bandages of the type recommended by Seutin—bandage amidonné.[71]

A great variety of other apparatuses have been devised over the centuries for the management of fractures, notably the copper limb cuirasse described by Heister[32] and what Malgaigne called "the great machine of La Faye." The latter was made of tin and consisted of longitudinal pieces that were hinged together so that it could be laid flat beneath the limb and then wrapped around. It was described as confining "at once the pelvis, thigh, leg and foot, hence it ensured complete immobility." Bonnet of Lyons went one stage further by producing an apparatus for the management of fractures of the femur that enveloped both legs, the pelvis, and the trunk up to the axillae.[10] The great disadvantage of all these extensive and heavy forms of immobilization of the limb was that the patient was largely confined to bed during the whole period of fracture healing. This disadvantage was particularly emphasized by Seutin,[55] who, in recommending his bandage amidonné, or starched bandage, wrote:

> It has not yet been well understood that complete immobility of the body, whilst being recommended by authors as an adjunct to other curative methods, is truly but a last resort which one would be better to avoid than to prescribe. One has not previously dared to say that the consolidation of the bony rupture is certainly more sure and prompt than the injured person's recovery of movements and (ability) to forget thereby his affliction, in order to take up again at least part of his ordinary occupation. Early mobilization causes neither accident nor displacement of the fragments. In permitting the patient to distract himself and take himself out into the fresh air, instead of remaining nailed to his bed, it has the happiest influence on the formation and consolidation of callus.

Again we see the roots of the concept of functional bracing. Seutin showed a man with a light starched bandage on his leg, the limb suspended by a strap around his neck, and walking with crutches.

In the first half of the 19th century, battle lines were drawn between the European surgeons who prescribed total immobilization and those who followed Seutin's *déambulation* regimen, and much intellectual effort was wastefully expended in fruitless argument. Seutin's emphasis on the importance of joint motion was also appreciated by others. In 1875 Sir James Paget wrote, "With rest too long maintained the joint becomes stiff and weak, even though there be no morbid process in it; and this mischief is increased if the joint hath been too long bandaged." A little later, Lucas-Championnière[50] wrote:

> The immobilisation of the members, which was dogma not open for discussion in the treatment of fractures and as well articular lesions, has been practised with such contentment by the authors of the immovable apparatuses, that we threw ourselves with abandon into all forms of immobilisation. It was forbidden even to discuss such immobilisation and to criticise it in the name of healthy physiology. When I attacked, at the Society of Surgery, this forced immobilisation, I was called by Verneuil an "*ankylophobe*" and I remained practically alone in protesting against these practises, which are so contrary to the interests of the injured and the ill. . . . Absolute immobilisation is not a favourable condition for bony repair. . . . [A] certain quantity of movement, regulated movement, is the best condition for this process of repair.

He then described animal experiments that confirm this view and went so far as to recommend massage of the injured limb to produce some degree of movement between the fragments. He was particularly vitriolic in his condemnation of prolonged immobilization of children and became the great champion of early and graduated controlled mobilization, not only to achieve union of the fracture but also to prevent edema, muscle atrophy, and joint stiffness, later to be christened *fracture disease.*

THE PLASTER BANDAGE AND ITS DERIVATIVES

The battle of minds between the mobilizers and the immobilizers was neither won nor lost but rather forgotten with the advent of the plaster-of-Paris bandage. In Holland in 1852, Antonius Mathijsen (1805 to 1878) published a new method for the application of plaster in fractures.[53] As a military surgeon, he had been seeking an immobilizing bandage that would permit the safe transport of patients with gunshot wounds to specialized treatment centers. He sought a bandage that could be used at once, would become hard in minutes, could be applied so as to give the surgeon access to the wound, was adaptable to the form of the extremity, would not be damaged by wound discharge or humidity, and was neither too heavy nor too expensive. His exact technique was described by van Assen and Meyerding[2] as follows:

> He cut pieces of double folded unbleached cotton or linen to fit the part to be immobilized. Then the pieces were fixed and held in position by woollen thread or pins. The dry plaster which was spread between the layers remained two finger breadths within the edges of the cloth. The extremity was then placed on the bandage, which was moistened with water. Next the edges of the bandage were pulled over so that they overlapped one another and they were held by pins. When an opening in the bandage was necessary, a piece of cotton wool the size of the desired opening was placed between the compresses so that this area remained free of plaster. In cases in which it was found necessary to enlarge the cast, enlargement could be achieved by the application of cotton bandages, four inches wide, rubbed with plaster and moistened.

Mathijsen introduced his plaster bandage in 1876 at the Centennial Exhibition in Philadelphia at the invitation of his friend Dr. M. C. Gori. The use of plaster-of-Paris bandages for the formation of fracture casts became widespread after Mathijsen's death and replaced most other forms of splintage.

Although the fire of the intellectual contest between the mobilizers and the immobilizers was reduced to mere embers, it was not extinguished, and the early functional concepts of Gooch, Seutin, Paget, Lucas-Championnière, and many others continued for decades to be regarded by surgical orthodoxy as heretical. In Britain, the great advocate of rest—enforced, prolonged, and uninterrupted—in the management of skeletal disorders, both traumatic and nontraumatic, was Hugh Owen Thomas (Fig. 1-6), who came from a long line of unqualified bonesetters residing in the Isle of Anglesey. Hugh Thomas's father, Evan Thomas, left his home and agricultural background to work in a foundry in Liverpool. His native skills as a bonesetter rapidly became legendary, and he opened consulting rooms in Liverpool, developing an extensive practice. His eldest son, Hugh Owen, broke with family tradition and qualified in medicine in 1857. His attempt at a partnership with his father failed, and

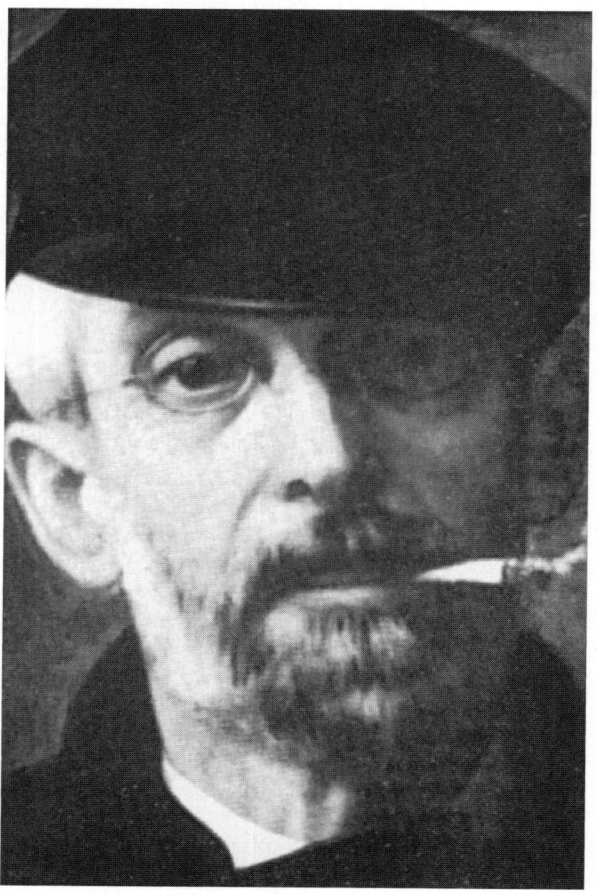

FIGURE 1-6 *Hugh Owen Thomas (1834 to 1891), the father of British orthopaedics. (Courtesy of Prof. L. Klenerman, Department of Orthopaedic Surgery, University of Liverpool.)*

he set himself up as a general practitioner in the slums of Liverpool, where he worked for 32 years, reputedly taking only 6 days of vacation. He died in 1891 at the age of 57.[77]

There cannot be an orthopaedic surgeon in the world who is not familiar with the Thomas splint, still in current use in many centers throughout the world in the management of fractures of the femur, although it was originally designed to assist in the management of tuberculous disease of the knee joint (Fig. 1-7). As discussed later, the use of this splint in World War I saved many lives. Not the least of the contributions of this industrious, single-minded, chain-smoking eccentric was to fire his nephew with enthusiasm for orthopaedic surgery. Robert Jones, later to be knighted, practiced with his uncle Hugh for many years in Liverpool before becoming one of the best known orthopaedic surgeons in the English-speaking world. Hugh Owen Thomas and Robert Jones were the two men to whom Watson Jones dedicated his classical work *Fractures and Joint Injuries*, writing of them, "They whose work cannot die, whose influence lives after them, whose disciples perpetuate and multiply their gifts to humanity, are truly immortal." Watson Jones remained greatly influenced by Hugh Owen Thomas's belief in enforced, uninterrupted, and prolonged rest, and in the preface to the fourth edition of his book,[81] he described one of its chapters as

> . . . a vigorous attack upon the almost universally accepted belief that contact compression, lag screws, slotted plates, compression clamps, and early weight bearing promote the union of fractures. I do not accept a word of it. Forcible compression of bone is pathological rather than physiological and it avails in the treatment of fractures only insofar as it promotes immobility and protects from shear. In believing this and denying the view that is held so widely, I reiterate the observations of Hugh Owen Thomas. Moreover, I believe that gaps between the fragments of a fractured bone are always filled if immobility is complete. . . . I still believe firmly that, apart from interposition of muscle and periosteum, the sole important cause of nonunion is inadequate immobilisation.

TRACTION

Although longitudinal traction of the limb to overcome the overriding of fracture fragments had been described as early as the writings of Galen (AD 130 to 200), in which he described his own extension apparatus, or *glossocomium* (Fig. 1-8), this traction was immediately discontinued once splintage had been applied. The use of continuous traction in the management of diaphyseal fractures seems to have appeared around the middle of the 19th century, although Guy de Chauliac (1300 to 1367) wrote in *Chirurgia Magna*, "After the application of splints, I attach to the foot a mass of lead as a weight, taking care to pass the cord which supports the weight over a small pulley in such a manner that it shall pull on the leg in a horizontal direction (*Ad pedum ligo pondus plumbi transeundo chordam super parvampolegeam; itaque tenebit tibiam in sua longitudinae*).[27]

FIGURE 1-7 *Early Thomas splint.*

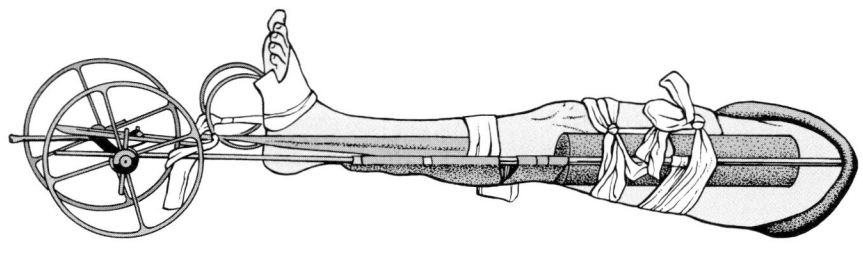

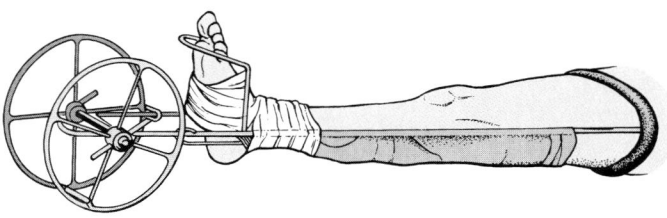

FIGURE 1-8 *The glossocomium, here illustrated from the works of Ambroise Paré (1564).*

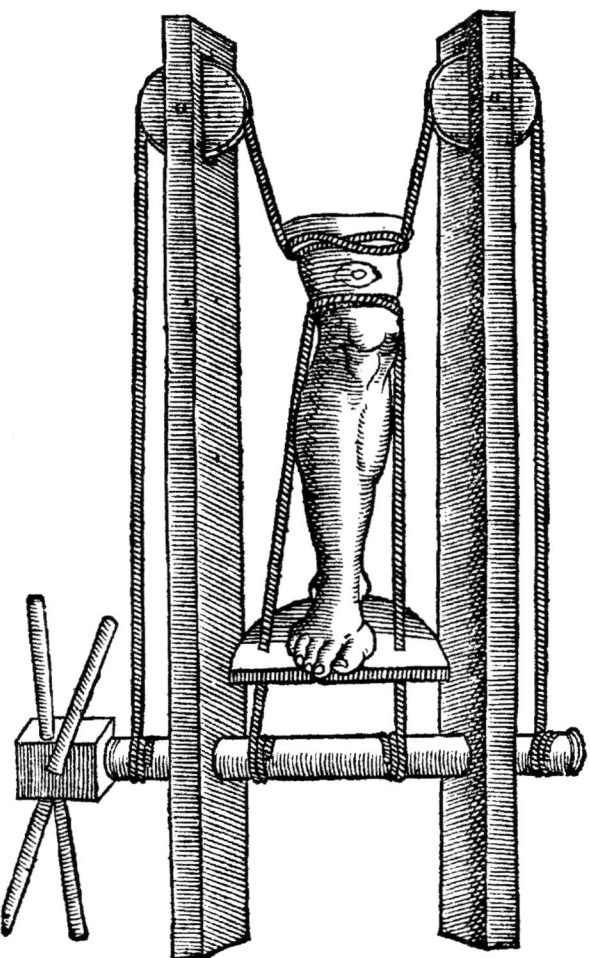

Whereas Sir Astley Cooper in his celebrated treatise on dislocations and fractures of the joints illustrated the method of treating simple fractures of the femur on a double inclined plane with a wooden splint strapped to the side of the thigh, there is no mention in his work of the use of traction.[17] On the other hand, in his book on fractures and dislocations published in 1890, Albert Hoffa of Wurzburg (where Roentgen discovered x-rays) liberally illustrated the use of traction for many types of fractures—not only of the femur in adults and children but also of the humerus.[35] Straight arm traction for supracondylar and intercondylar fractures of the distal humerus recently so in vogue was clearly described and illustrated by Helferich in 1906 (Fig. 1-9).[33]

Certainly one of the earliest accounts of the use of continuous skin traction in the management of fractures must be that of Dr. Josiah Crosby of New Hampshire. He described the application of "two strips of fresh spread English adhesive plaster, one on either side of the leg, wide enough to cover at least half of the diameter of the limb from above the knee to the malleolar processes." Over these he laid a firm spiral bandage before applying weight to the lower ends of the adhesive straps. He recorded the use of this method in a fracture of the femur, an open fracture of the tibia, and, surprisingly, two cases of fracture of the clavicle in 2-year-old children. The technique of Dr. Crosby was illustrated in detail by Hamilton in his treatise on military surgery.[29] Billroth, describing his experiences between 1869 and 1870, gave the alternatives of plaster-of-Paris bandages or extension in the management of fractures of the shaft of the femur. He stated, "On the whole, I far prefer extension by means of ordinary strapping. This I apply generally on Volkmann's plan."[7] It is interesting to note that in the early descriptions of traction for the management of fractures of the femoral shaft, when no other form of splintage was used, union was usually said to

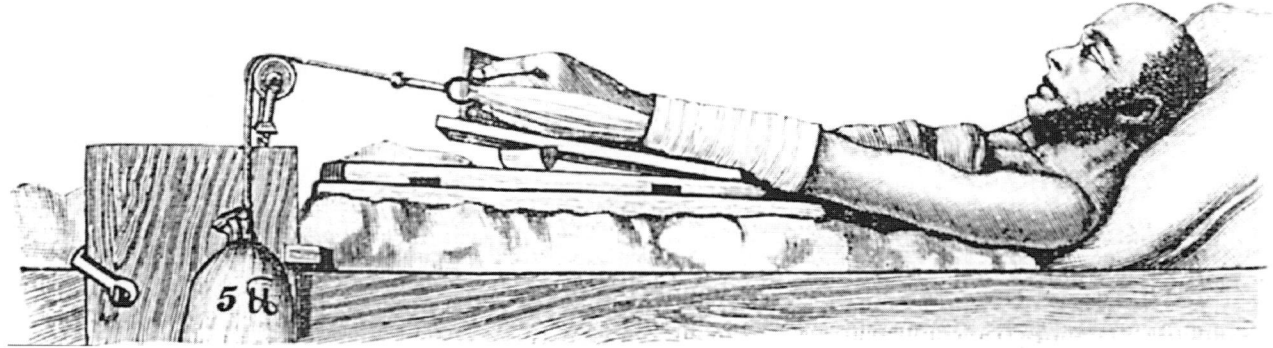

FIGURE 1-9 *Forearm skin traction for the treatment of T fractures of the distal humerus. (From Helferich, H. Frakturen und Luxationen. München, Lehmann Verlag, 1906.)*

have been consolidated by 5 or 6 weeks, in comparison with the 10 to 14 weeks that later came to be regarded as the average time to femoral shaft union using traction in association with external splintage.

The rapid consolidation of femoral shaft fractures was, of course, stressed by Professor George Perkins of London in the 1940s and 1950s, when he abandoned external splintage and advocated straight simple traction through an upper tibial pin and immediate mobilization of the knee, using a split bed (so-called Pyrford traction). This was in some ways a development and simplification of the traction principles outlined by R. H. Russell (who also remarked on rapid consolidation with early movement), describing his mobile traction in 1924.[67] In the same year, Dowden, speaking mainly of upper limb fractures, wrote, "The principle of early active movement in the treatment of practically all injuries and in most inflammations will assuredly be adopted before long."[21] Perkins, like Dowden and the many others before, was a great advocate of movement, both active and passive, of all the joints of the involved limb as being more important than precise skeletal form.

FUNCTIONAL BRACING

Given that Gooch's description in 1767 of the first tibial and femoral functional braces was to remain obscure for more than two centuries, it is surprising that after the intense discussion of the technical minutiae and principles of splintage in the 19th century, there was no real modification of the "standard" plaster-of-Paris cast until the work of Sarmiento,[69] published 200 years after that of Gooch. Following experience with patellar tendon-bearing below-knee limb prostheses, Sarmiento developed a patellar tendon-bearing cast for the treatment of fractures of the tibia, applied after initial standard cast treatment had been used to permit the acute swelling to settle. This heralded the renaissance of functional bracing, and in 1970 Mooney and colleagues[56] described hinged casts for the lower limb in the management of femoral fractures treated initially with some 6 weeks of traction.

Since the mid-1970s, the development of a variety of casting materials and the use of thermoplastics in brace construction have extended the ideas of these pioneers of the 1960s and 1970s to the point where functional bracing, certainly for shaft fractures of the tibia and certain lower femoral fractures, is accepted without question as the natural sequel to early management by plaster casting or traction. The widespread use of functional bracing has liberated countless patients from prolonged hospitalization and permitted early return to function and to gainful employment.

OPEN FRACTURES

Until about 150 years ago, an open fracture was virtually synonymous with death and generally necessitated immediate amputation. Amputation itself carried with it a very high mortality rate, usually with death resulting from hemorrhage or sepsis. Until the 16th century, the traditional method of attempting to control the hemorrhage after amputation was cauterization of the wound, either with hot irons or by the application of boiling pitch. This in itself may well have caused tissue necrosis and encouraged infection and secondary hemorrhage. The famous French surgeon Ambroise Paré (1510 to 1590), who served as surgeon to the Court of Henry II and Catherine de Medici and is rightfully regarded as the father of military surgery, was in 1564 the first to describe the ligation of the bleeding vessels after amputation. He developed an instrument that he called the "crow's beak" (*bec de corbin*) for securing the vessels and pulling them out of the cut surface of the amputation stump in order to ligate them (Fig. 1-10). Notwithstanding this advance, Le Petit, who in 1718 described the use of the tourniquet to control hemorrhage

FIGURE 1-10 Bec de corbin—*crow's beak—devised by Paré for pulling out vessel ends during amputation to facilitate their ligature.*

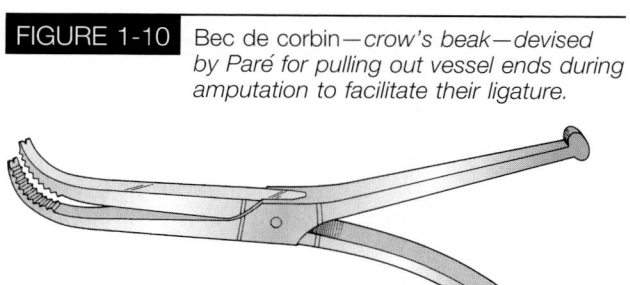

during amputation,[61] is reputed to have claimed that his invention reduced the mortality rate from amputation of the lower limb from 75 percent to 25 percent.

In the history of the open fracture, Ambroise Paré[58] features again in documenting for the first time the conservation of a limb after an open fracture. He in fact described his own injury, sustained on May 4, 1561, when, while crossing the Seine on a ferry to attend a patient in another part of Paris, his horse, startled by a sudden lurch of the vessel, gave him "such a kick that she completely broke the two bones of the leg four fingers above the junction of the foot." Fearing that the horse would kick him again and not appreciating the nature of the injury, he took an instinctive step backward "but sudden falling to the earth, the fractured bones leapt outwards and ruptured the flesh, the stocking and the boot, from which I felt such pain that it was not possible for man (at least in my judgment) to endure any greater without death. My bones thus broken and my foot pointing the other way, I greatly feared that it would be necessary to cut my leg to save my life." He then described how, with a combination of prayer, splintage, and dressing of the open wound with various astringents, coupled with the regular use of soap suppositories, he survived the initial infection and by September, "finally thanks to God, I was entirely healed without limping in any way," returning to his work that month (Fig. 1-11).

Nevertheless, in insisting on conservative management of his open fracture rather than amputation, Paré was flying in the face of orthodox surgical practice, as indeed was the English surgeon Percival Pott, who in 1756 was thrown from his horse while riding in Kent Street, Southwark, and suffered a compound fracture of the lower leg. Aware of the dangers of mishandling such an injury, he would not permit himself to be moved until he had summoned his own chairmen from Westminster to bring their poles, and it is said that while lying in the January cold awaiting them, he bargained for the purchase of a door, to which his servants subsequently nailed their poles

and thereby carried him on a litter to Watling Street near St. Paul's cathedral. There he was attended by an Edward Nourse, a prominent contemporary surgeon, who expressed the view that because of the gentle handling of the limb, no air had entered the wound and therefore there was a chance of preserving the leg, which otherwise was destined for amputation. Finally, success attended a long period of immobilization and convalescence.

As late as the 19th century, not all victims of open fracture were so fortunate. Even in circumstances considered ideal at the time, the mortality rate associated with open injuries remained high. Billroth[7] recorded four patients with compound dislocations of the ankle who came under his care in Zurich, with one dying of pyemia, one of septicemia, and a third of overwhelming infection after amputation for suppuration on the 36th day after injury. The fourth patient recovered. Of 93 patients with compound fractures of the lower leg whom he treated in Zurich, 46 died. Recovery from open fracture of the femur was, in Billroth's experience, so unusual that, describing the case of a woman of 23 who recovered from such an injury, he stated, "The following case of recovery is perhaps unique."

Gunshot wounds producing fracture were particularly notorious and generally treated with immediate amputation, certainly until the early part of the 20th century. The results of this policy, however, were in certain instances quite horrifying. Wrench recorded that in the Franco-Prussian War (1870 to 1871), the death rate from open fracture was 41 percent, and open fractures of the knee joint carried a 77 percent mortality rate.[82] On the French side, of 13,172 amputees, some 10,006 died. On the other hand, in the American Civil War, the overall mortality rate for nearly 30,000 amputations was on the order of 26 percent, although for thigh amputations it reached 54 percent (Fig. 1-12). The difference in the mortality rates for different theaters of war around that time was probably related to the postoperative management, as very often the suppurating amputation stump was sponged daily with a solution from the same "pus bucket" used for

FIGURE 1-11 *Illustration from Paré's surgical text of 1564 of his own open tibial fracture treated by splintage and open care of the wound. This is the first well-documented cure of an open limb fracture without amputation.*

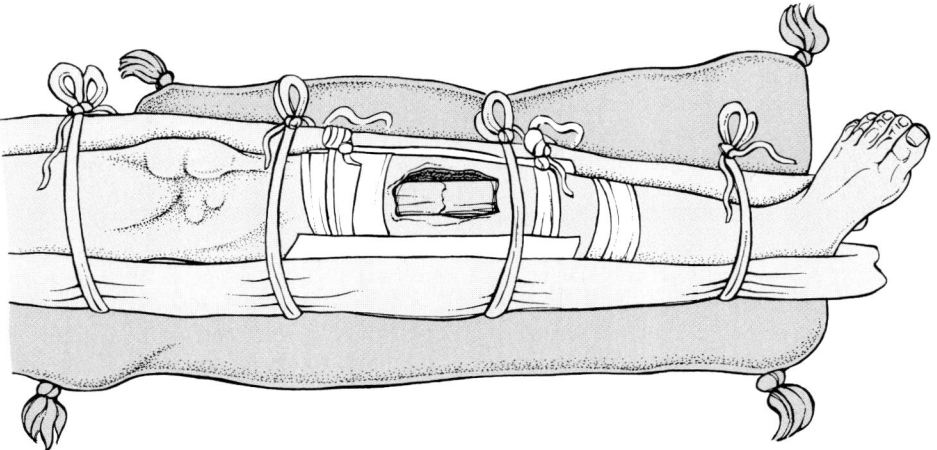

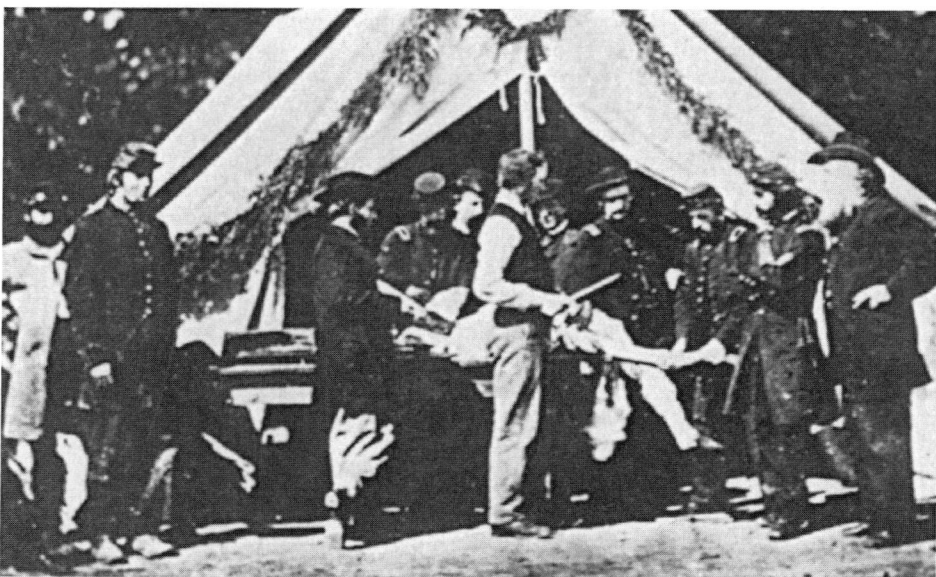

FIGURE 1-12 *Amputation scene at General Hospital during the American Civil War. Stereoscopic slide. (Courtesy of the Edward G. Miner Library, Rochester, New York.)*

all the patients. It has been said of that era that it was probably safer to have your leg blown off by a cannonball than amputated by a surgeon!

During World War I, gunshot wounds of the femur carried a very high mortality rate in the early years. In 1916 the death rate from gunshot wound of the femur was 80 percent in the British army. Thereafter it became policy to use the Thomas splint, with fixed traction applied via a clove hitch around the booted foot, before transportation to the hospital. Robert Jones reported in 1925 that this simple change of policy resulted in a reduction of the mortality rate to 20 percent by 1918. With progressive understanding of bacterial contamination and cross-infection after the pioneering work of Pasteur, Koch, Lister, and Semmelweis; the use of early splintage, as learned by the British forces in World War I; and the application of open-wound treatment following wound extension and excision as advocated first by Paré and later by Larrey (Napoleon's surgeon and inventor of the *ambulance*),[57,78] the scourge of the open fracture, even from a femoral gunshot wound, has been greatly reduced.

EARLY FRACTURE SURGERY

Wire Fixation

It is generally believed that the earliest technique of internal fixation of fractures was that of ligature or wire suture and, according to Malgaigne, the first mention of the ligature dates back to the early 1770s. A. M. Icart, surgeon of the Hôtel Dieu at Castres, claimed to have seen it used with success by Lapujode and Sicre, surgeons of Toulouse. This observation came to light when, in 1775, M. Pujol accused Icart of bringing about the death of a young man with an open fracture of the humerus in whom Icart was alleged to have performed bone ligature using brass wire. In his defense, Icart cited the experience of the Toulouse surgeons in the earlier part of the decade, although denying that he himself had personally used this technique in the case in dispute.[39,63,64] In a scholarly discussion of Pujol versus Icart, Evans has called into question whether this type of operation was any more than the subject of surgical theory at that time,[24] but Icart's contention was widely accepted by so many French observers in the 19th century that it is highly probable that bone ligature was performed at least by Lapujode (if not Sicre) around 1770.

On July 31, 1827, Dr. Kearny Rodgers of New York is recorded as having performed bone suture.[31] He resected a pseudarthrosis of the humerus and, finding the bone ends to be most unstable, drilled a hole in each and passed a silver wire through to retain coaption of the bone fragments. The ends of the wire were drawn out through a cannula that remained in the wound. Although on the 16th day the cannula fell from the wound with the entire wire loop, the bones remained in their proper position and union was said to have occurred by 69 days after the operation. The patient was not allowed to leave his bed for 2 months after the operation!

In the introduction to his *Traité de l'Immobilisation Directe des Fragments Osseux dans les Fractures* (the first book ever published on internal fixation),[6] Bérenger Féraud recounted that, at the beginning of his medical career when he was an intern at the Hôtel Dieu Saint Esprit at Toulon in 1851, he was involved in the treatment of an unfortunate workman who had sustained a closed, comminuted fracture of the lower leg in falling down a staircase. Initial splintage was followed by a period of infection and suppuration, requiring several drainage procedures; eventually, after many long weeks, amputation was decided on. At the last moment, the poor patient begged to be spared the loss of his leg, so Dr. Long, Bérenger Féraud's chief, exposed the bone ends, freshened them, and held them together with three lead wire ligatures (cerclage) "as one would reunite the ends of a broken stick, and to our great astonishment then guided the patient to perfect cure without limp or shortening of the member, which for so long had appeared to be irrevocably lost." The patient survived, and the lead wires were removed 3 weeks later; the fracture united, and the workman left the hospital 105 days after his accident and resumed work 6 months after the operation. Bérenger Féraud went on to say:

> I assisted at the operation and I bandaged with my own hands the injured for many long weeks. Can anyone understand how this extraordinary cure struck me? The strange means of producing and maintaining solid coaptation of the bony fragments by encircling them with a metallic ligature fascinated me as during my childhood I had heard tales of this technique being performed by Arab surgeons and, until then, had considered this to be a mere product of a barbaric empiricism. . . . In my childhood, in 1844 and 1845, I heard an old *tebib* renowned in the environs of Cherchell, in Algeria, for his erudition and his experience, recount to my father who, a surgeon impassioned with our art, avidly questioned native practitioners of French Africa, in order to sort out, from their experiences and their therapeutic means, the scientific principles, which had been passed down to them from their ancestors, amidst some of the ordinary practices of a more or less coarse empiricism. I tell you, I heard him say that in certain cases of gunshot wounds, or when a fracture had failed to unite, the ancient masters advised opening the fracture site with a cutting instrument, ligating the fragments one to another with lead or iron wire . . . and only to remove the wire once the fracture was consolidated.

It therefore seems that there is some anecdotal evidence to suggest that such techniques had been used in the early part of the 19th century or even before. Bérenger Féraud himself cited the example of Lapujode and Sicre mentioned earlier. Commeiras[15] reported native Tahitian practitioners to be skilled in the open fixation of fractures using lengths of reed.

Screw Fixation

The use of screws in bone probably started around the late 1840s. Certainly in 1850, the French surgeons Cucuel and Rigaud described two cases in which screws were used in the management of fractures.[19] In the first case, a man of 64 sustained a depressed fracture of the superior part of his sternum, into which a screw was then inserted to permit traction to be applied to elevate the depressed sternal fragment into an improved position. In the second case, a distracted fracture of the olecranon, Rigaud inserted a screw into the ulna and into the displaced olecranon, reduced the fragments, and wired the two screws together (*vissage de rappel*), thereafter leaving the arm entirely free of splintage and obtaining satisfactory union of the fracture. Rigaud also described a similar procedure for the patella. In his extraordinarily detailed and comprehensive treatise on direct immobilization of bony fragments, Bérenger Féraud made no mention of interfragmentary screw fixation, which was probably first practiced by Lambotte (see following section).

Plate Fixation

The first account of plate fixation of bone was probably the 1886 report by Hansmann of Hamburg entitled "A new method of fixation of the fragments of complicated fractures."[30] He illustrated a malleable plate, applied to the bone to span the fracture site, the end of the plate being bent through a right angle so as to project through the skin. The plate was then attached to each fragment by one or more special screws, which were constructed with long shanks that projected through the skin for ease of removal (Fig. 1-13). He recorded that the apparatus was removed approximately 4 to 8 weeks after insertion and described its use in 15 fresh fractures, 4 pseudarthroses, and 1 reconstruction of the humerus after removal of an enchondroma.

George Guthrie[28] discussed the current state of direct fixation of fractures in 1903 and quoted Estes as having described a nickel steel plate that he had been using to maintain coaption in compound fractures for many years. This plate, perforated with six holes, was laid across the

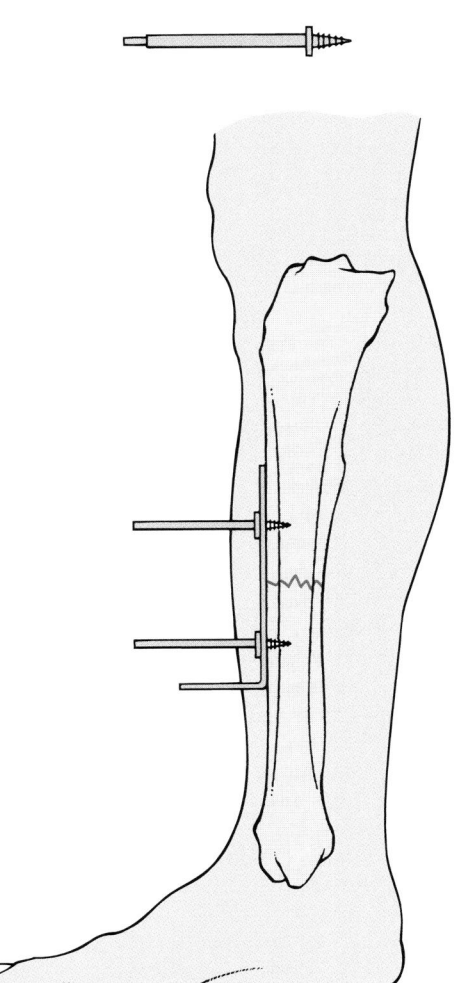

FIGURE 1-13 *Redrawn from Hansmann's article of 1886, "A new method of fixation of the fragments of complicated fractures," the first publication on plate fixation of fractures. The bent end of the plate and the long screw shanks were left protruding through the skin to facilitate removal after union.*

fracture, and holes were drilled into the bone to correspond to those of the plate. The plate was fixed to the bone by ivory pegs, which protruded from the wound. Removal was accomplished 3 or 4 weeks later by breaking off the pegs and withdrawing the plate through a small incision. Guthrie reported that in a recent letter Dr. Estes had said, "The little plate has given me great satisfaction and has been quite successful in St. Luke's Hospital." Guthrie also quoted Steinbach as reporting four cases of fractured tibia in which he had used a silver plate by this method and obtained good results. He removed the plate using local anesthesia. Silver was greatly favored at this time as an implant metal, as it was believed to possess antiseptic properties. Interestingly, in this article, Guthrie referred to the use of rubber gloves during surgery, seemingly antedating the reputed first use of gloves by Halstead.

The man who coined the term *osteosynthesis* was Albin Lambotte (1866 to 1955), although Bérenger Féraud referred to the restoration of bone continuity by ligature or bone suture as *synthèsisation*. It is believed, however, that by osteosynthesis Lambotte meant *stable* bone fixation rather than simply suture. Lambotte is generally regarded as the father of modern internal fixation, and in his foreword to a book commemorating the works of Lambotte, Dr. Elst briefly discussed the early attempts in the 19th century at surgical stabilization of bone and then continued, "Thus at the end of the last century, the idea was floating among surgeons. As always in the field of scientific progress, comes the right man in the right place, a genial mind who collects the items spread here and there, melts them into a solid block and forges the whole together. So did Albin Lambotte in Belgium, a pioneer of osteosynthesis."[23]

Lambotte (Fig. 1-14), the son of a professor of comparative anatomy, biology, and chemistry at the University of Brussels, was taught almost exclusively by his brother Elie, a brilliant young surgeon, who sadly died prematurely. Albin had worked under the direction of his brother at the Schaerbeek Hospital in the suburbs of Brussels and then in 1890 became assistant surgeon at the Stuyvenberg Hospital in Antwerp, rapidly progressing to become the head of the surgical department. From 1900, he tackled the surgical treatment of fractures with great enthusiasm and much innovation. He manufactured most of his early instruments and implants in his own workshop, developing not only plates and screws for rigid bone fixation in a variety of materials but also an external fixation device similar in principle to the ones in use today. He met with much intellectual opposition, but his excellent results were persuasive. In 1908, he reported 35 patients who had made a complete recovery after plate fixation of the femur. His classical book on the surgical treatment of fractures was published in 1913.[42] His legendary surgical skill was the product not only of a keen intellect but also of his extraordinary manual dexterity, which was also channeled into his great interest in music. He became a skilled violinist, but this was not enough for him, and he subsequently trained as a lute maker. He, in fact, made 182 violins and his name is listed in Vanne's *Dictionnaire Universel des Luthiers*. Elst related the following anecdote as an indication of Lambotte's manual skills:

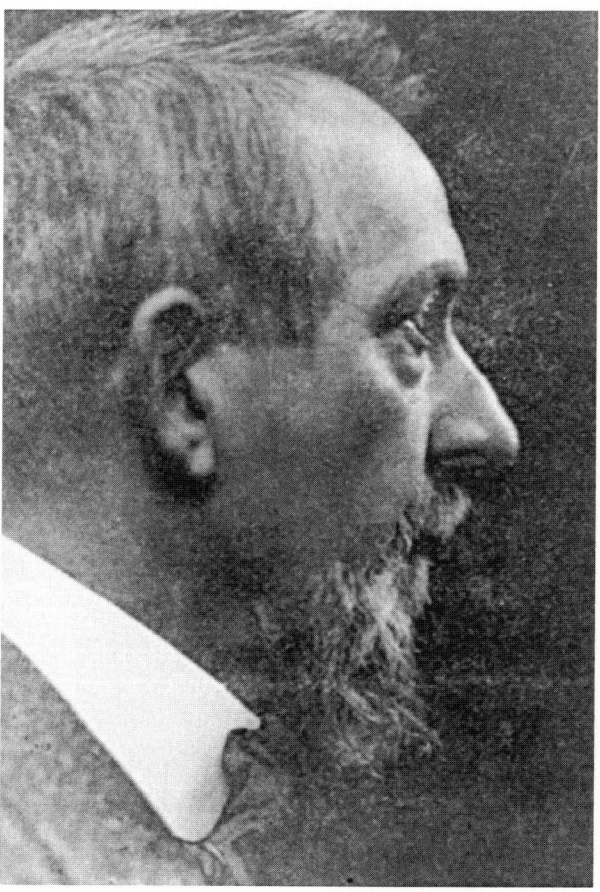

FIGURE 1-14   *Albin Lambotte (1866 to 1955), the father of osteosynthesis. (Courtesy of la Société Belge de Chirurgie Orthopédique et de Traumatologie.)*

One day Lambotte was in Paris staying at the Hôtel Louvois, at that time, and even nowadays, the Belgian headquarters in Paris. One morning he was on his way to the Avenue de l'Opéra, accompanied by a young colleague who was the one who told me the story. As he made his way through the old narrow streets, lined with windows and workshops belonging to every type of craftsman, Lambotte would enter one or two, admiring each one's dexterity and set of tools and discussing their methods like an expert. All of a sudden he stopped short, gazing with marvel at the instruments of a shoemaker. The idea of a new type of forceps had struck him. Suddenly inspired, he strode quickly towards the famous manufacturer of surgical instruments, the Collin factory, neighbouring the area that he was in. With great gestures and explanations, he tried to describe the instrument he desired. It seemed as if nobody could understand him, and not being able to endure it any longer he took off his jacket and rolled up his sleeves. Before a flabbergasted audience, he began to forge, file, hammer, strike, model and so finish off the piece of iron. They were all stunned with admiration and one of them came up to him and said "I have been here for forty two years sir, and never have I seen anybody work like you." Lambotte went away deeply moved, confiding in his companion "That is the highest prize I have ever received. It moves me as much as all the academic titles."

As if these qualities were not enough, he is also recorded as being an extremely hard-working and kind man, noted for his devotion to his patients; a patron of the arts; and a great surgical teacher. Indeed, before World War I, the brothers Charles and William Mayo would take turns coming and spending several weeks in Antwerp. It is said that as soon as they disembarked, they devoted all their time in Europe to Lambotte and left only when their work in Rochester called them back. As an indication of the esteem in which he was held, among the many international figures attending his jubilee celebration in Antwerp in 1935 were René Leriche, Fred Albee, Ernest Hey Groves, and Vittorio Putti. The Lambotte instrumentarium remained in regular use until the 1950s (Fig. 1-15).

Contemporaneous with the work of Lambotte in Belgium was that of the other great pioneer of internal fixation, William Arbuthnot Lane (Fig. 1-16) of Guy's Hospital, London. The tradition in the late 19th century at this hospital was that fracture patients be admitted under the surgeon of the day and, after discharge, then be reviewed as outpatients by his assistant. Lane, working as the assistant to Clement Lucas, was most unhappy with the results of fracture management. In his biography of Lane, Layton[46] recorded:

Before Lane's time, the criteria of a good result in a fracture were indefinite and vague. They were aesthetic rather than practical. Firm union went without saying, but when a false joint, a nonunion or a weak fibrous one resulted, it was rather the patient's fault than the surgeon's. Given a firm union, the rest was an aesthetic problem, affecting the reputation of the surgeon rather than the way in which the patient could use his limb. "Pay great attention to your fracture cases" was the tradition—"with them alone the grave does not cover your mistakes."

Lane had told Layton of a stevedore, who said:

Mr. Lucas thinks this is a good result. He says there is not much displacement and it looks all right. But I can't work with it. My job is carrying a sack of flour, weighing two hundredweight, up a plank from a barge to the wharfside and I can't do it. The foreman won't have me and I am still out of work.

Lane then went down to the docks and discovered that the stevedore had been telling the truth. Any slip from the plank from the barge to the wharf would have resulted in a fall onto the dock between the barge and the wharfside or between two barges. Lane observed that a man whose foot was in the slightest degree out of alignment could very easily fall. Lane thus became greatly impressed with the need for accuracy and maintenance of good reduction. Initially he started work with wires, and then in 1893 he is recorded as having used screws across a fracture site. Shortly afterward, he devised his first plate. Beginning in 1892, Lane made it his practice, whenever he could, to perform open reduction and fixation in all cases of simple fracture. This practice, however, met opposition from his chief, Mr. Lucas, and it was not until 1894, when Lucas was off work for 6 months after an attack of typhoid, that

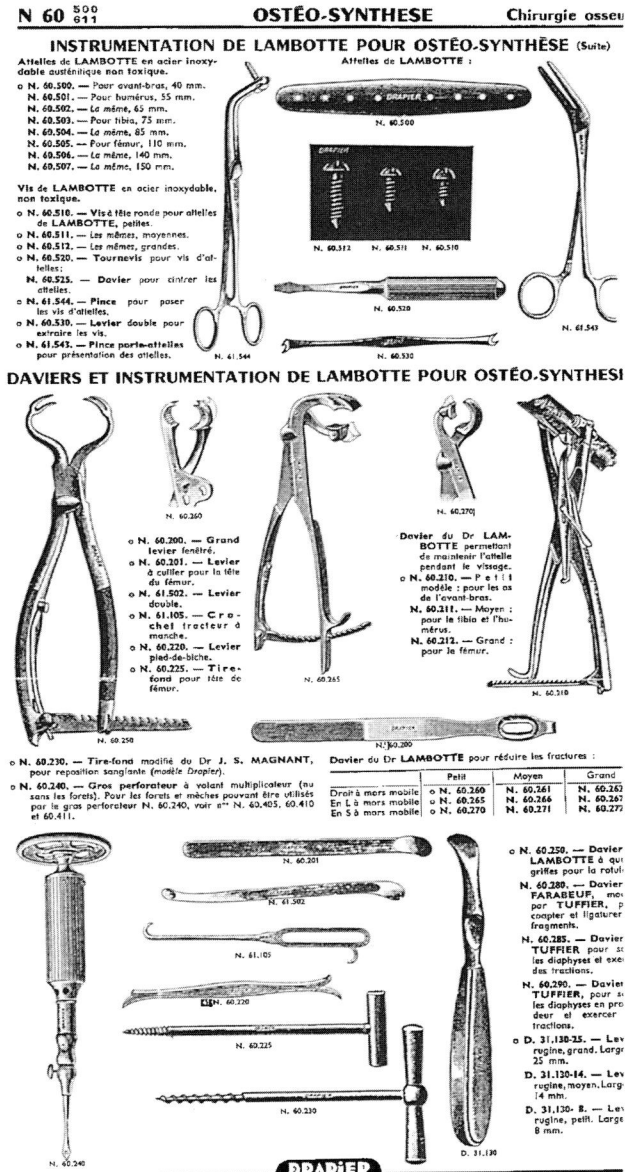

FIGURE 1-15 *Instruments and implants designed by Lambotte featured in a surgical catalogue of Drapier (Paris) in the early 1950s.*

Lane had his chance to operate on a large series of simple fractures.

Although his attempts at internal fixation of compound fractures were almost universally a failure, Layton recorded that not one case of internal fixation of a simple fracture became infected during this period. During these 6 months of intensive internal fixation, Lane was using Lister's antiseptic techniques, and his dresser, Dr. Beddard, told that Lane and his associates wallowed in carbolic almost from dawn until dusk, with half of them passing black urine from the carbolic absorbed through their skins. At this time Lane insisted on his own variant of the antiseptic technique. Everyone wore long mackintoshes up to

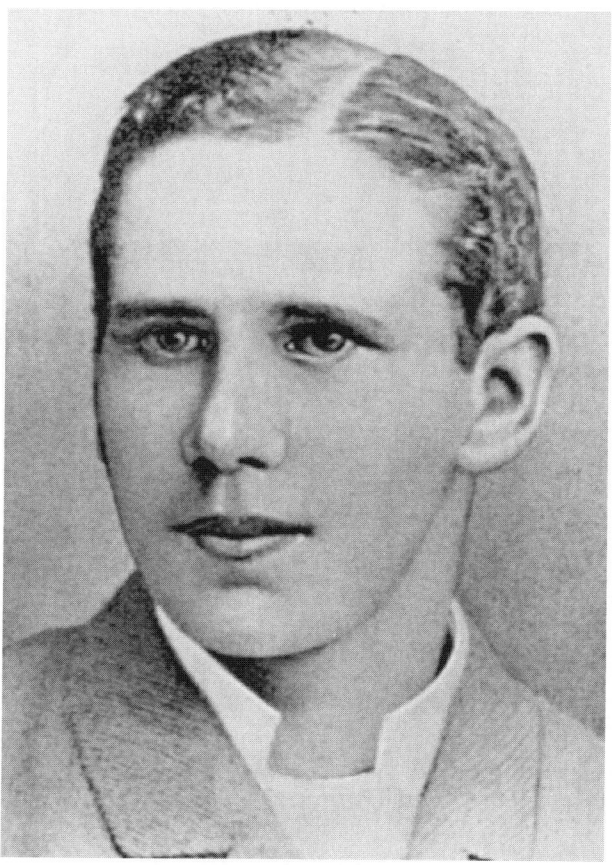

FIGURE 1-16 *William Arbuthnot Lane (1856 to 1943), seen here shortly after qualifying at Guy's Hospital, London. (From Layton, T.B. Sir William Arbuthnot Lane, Bt. Edinburgh, E. & S. Livingstone, 1956.)*

the neck, over which they applied gowns wet with carbolic or Lysol solution, and similarly the patients were draped with antiseptic towels introduced by Lane around 1889. The instruments were also soaked in Lysol, but by 1904 dry sterilization of the gowns and the instruments was Lane's routine.

Interestingly, Layton recorded the postmortem exploration of a fracture plated by Lane; the patient subsequently died of an unrelated septicemia. Layton said, "I cut down onto the bone and found this firmly joined without the throwing out of any callus around it. The plate was well in place, the screws all firmly fixed without a suspicion of any inflammation of the bone into which they had been put."[46] This surely must have been the first observation of healing without external callus formation in the presence of rigid fixation. In addition, Lane is credited with developing the nontouch technique of bone surgery and devised many instruments to enable him to hold implants without handling them directly. Of operative technique, Lane wrote:

I will now relate the several steps which are involved in an operation for simple fracture. I will do so in some detail as apart from manual dexterity and skill the whole secret of success in these operations depends on the most rigid asepsis. The very moderate degree of cleanliness that is adopted in operations generally will not suffice when a large quantity of metal is left in a wound. To guarantee success in the performance of these operations the surgeon must not touch the interior of the wound even with his gloved hand for gloves are frequently punctured, especially if it be necessary to use a moderate amount of force, and the introduction into the wound of fluid which may have been in contact with the skin for some time may render the wound septic. All swabs introduced into the wound should be held with long forceps and should not be handled in any way. The operator must not let any portion of an instrument which has been in contact with a cutaneous surface or even with his glove enter the wound. After an instrument has been used for any length of time or forcibly it should be resterilised.[45]

He then went on to describe the preparation of the skin with tincture of iodine and the use of skin toweling. By 1900 he had invented a huge variety of different-shaped plates for particular fracture problems, and in 1905 he wrote his classical work on the operative treatment of fractures, in which he illustrated both single and double plating and the use of intramedullary screw fixation for fractures of the neck of the femur.[44] In 1905 and 1906 Lambotte had also performed intramedullary screw fixation in four cases of femoral neck fracture, but this technique was not in fact new. In 1903 Guthrie quoted from Bryant's *Operative Surgery*:

Koenig operated in a case of recent fracture, making a small incision over the outer side of the trochanter major and drilled a hole through it with a metal drill in the direction of the head of the bone, applied extension to the limb to the extent necessary to overcome the deformity and then drove a long steel nail through the canal in the trochanter into the head of the bone and left it there. The limb was then immobilised and extended for 6 weeks. Good union and free motion of the joint were obtained. Cheyne, in a case of recent fracture, exposed the fragments through a longitudinal incision made over the anterior aspect of the joint, exposed the fracture, made extension and internal rotation of the limb, and with the fingers in the wound, manipulated the fragments into place. Then a small longitudinal incision was made over the outer side of the trochanter major and two canals drilled through the fragments at a distance of half an inch apart. Ivory pegs were then driven through the holes made by the drill and the limb immobilised. Good union and motion were obtained.[28]

It is understood that this procedure was in fact first suggested to Koenig by von Langenbeck, who is reputed to have treated fractures of the neck of the femur by drilling across them with a silvered drill and then leaving the drill bit in place.

Most of the screws used in plating procedures at this time were close derivatives of the traditional wood screw, with its tapered thread, although the later designs of both Lambotte and Lane were of screws with parallel threads, probably inspired by the classical publication of Sherman in 1926.[73] While stressing "the most scrupulous aseptic techniques" along the lines recommended by

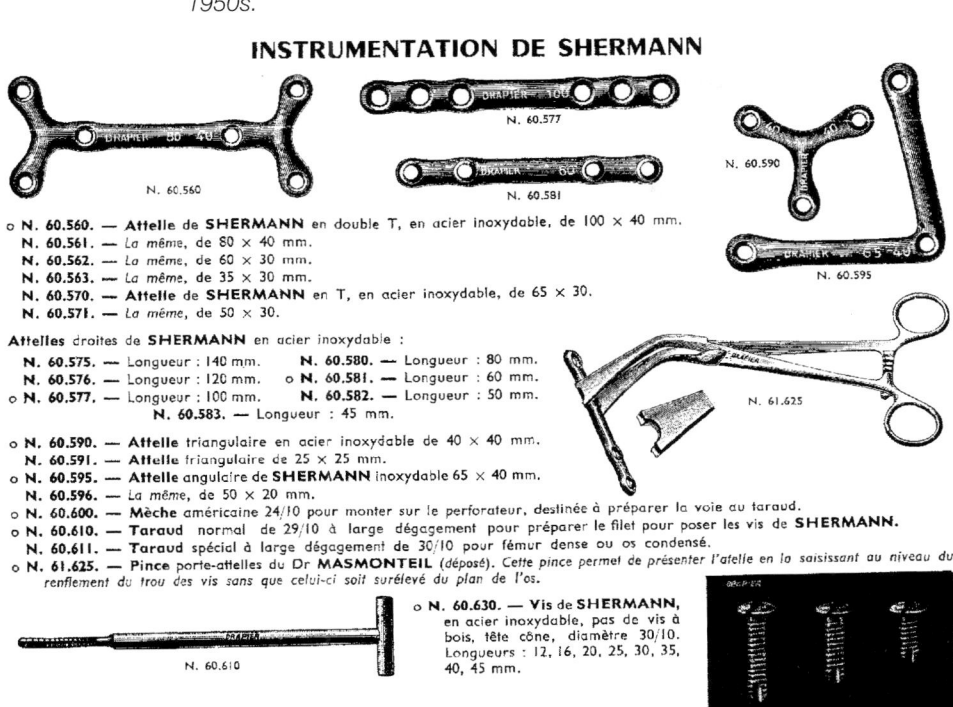

FIGURE 1-17 *Sherman instrumentation from the Drapier (Paris) catalogue of the early 1950s.*

Lane, Sherman designed his own series of plates and also drew attention to the superior holding power of parallel threaded screws of a self-tapping, fine pitch design (Fig. 1-17). He pointed out that these had something like four times the holding power of a wood or carpenter's screw. He also introduced the use of corrosion-resistant vanadium steel. In addition, he emphasized particularly that the fixation should be firm enough to permit early functional rehabilitation. In describing his postoperative regimen for femoral fracture fixation, he recommended the following:

> Immediately following the operation, the leg is placed in a Thomas' splint, flexed by the use of the Pierson attachment and then swung from a Balkan frame. Plaster is never used. The clips are removed on the fourth day and passive movements of the knee joint begun on the third or fourth day and continued daily. With immobilization of the fracture by transfixion screws, active and passive motion can be freely indulged in without any danger whatsoever of disturbing the position. ... Early mobilization is the most valuable adjunct in the postoperative treatment and should be instituted within the first few days. Great care should be taken not to permit weight bearing until the union is firm and callus hard.

Sherman reported a series of 78 cases of plating of the femoral shaft with only one death (caused by a pulmonary embolism 2 days after operation), no amputations, and no cases of nonunion; in only two patients was it necessary to remove the plates and screws because of infection, both nonetheless ending in an excellent functional result after treatment by immediate wound débridement and intermittent irrigation of the cavity with 0.5% sodium hypochlorite. He also cited the reported experience of Hitzrot, who had plated approximately 100 cases of femoral fracture, with one death and only two infections; in the remainder there were no nonunions, no stiff knees, no plates needed to be removed, and "no appreciable changes in function or anatomy. ..."[34]

Although now superseded by superior implant design, the Sherman plate is still in current use in hospitals throughout the world. In the 1930s and 1940s, a great variety of plate designs, some bizarre, were reported but with no great conceptual innovations. The so-called slotted plated splint of Egger, designed to hold the fracture fragments in alignment while allowing them to slide toward each other under the influence of weight bearing and muscle force, was neither new nor predictably successful: Lambotte had described, and later abandoned, a slotted plate as early as 1907. It was indeed the work of Danis in the 1940s that heralded the modern era of internal fixation, as will be discussed further on.

EXTERNAL FIXATION

Traditionally, the first external fixation device was the *pointe métallique* conceived by Malgaigne in 1840 and subsequently documented in 1843 in the *Journal de Chirurgie*.[5] This apparatus consisted of a hemicircular metal arc that could be strapped around the limb in such a manner that a finger screw, passing through a slot in the arc, could be positioned over any projecting fragment threatening the overlying skin, the screw then being tightened to press the fragment into a position of reduction. Although this apparatus and modifications of it, such as those of Roux, Ollier, and Valette, gained such a prominent place in contemporary surgery that the chapter on their use in the treatise of Bérenger Féraud occupies 126 pages, it is probably incorrect to regard it as an external fixation device in that it simply pressed one of the fragments into place but did not in itself result in any stability of the fracture.

Nevertheless, Malgaigne still retains the credit for the design of the first external fixator, for in 1843 he also described his *griffe métallique*, or metal claw, which consisted of two pairs of curved points, each pair attached to a metal plate, one plate sliding within grooves on the other and the two components being capable of approximation using a turnbuckle type of screw (Fig. 1-18). This device was designed for use on distracted fractures of the patella, and it was commonly perceived that Malgaigne proposed that the metal points were driven into the bony fragments of the patella in order to approximate them. This, in fact, is incorrect. Malgaigne's concept was that the metal points would engage in the aponeurotic substance of the quadriceps and patellar tendons and thereby obtain purchase in this tough tissue alongside the bone. This concept becomes evident from reading the discussion of Cucuel and Rigaud in which they say, "M. Malgaigne has recommended several years ago a pair of claws to maintain the fragments of the patella, but his claws were only supposed to press upon the fragments. I have gone further. I have driven the claws just inside the substance of the patella and have maintained the fragments, thus hooked, using two *vis de rappel*."[19] The *vis de rappel* was in fact the technique of inserting a screw into each fragment and then binding these screws together with twine as Rigaud described for the olecranon, as mentioned previously. Thus, the metal claw device of Malgaigne became a true external fixator. It is interesting to note in later publications[61] that this device was also used indirectly to approximate fragments of the patella by drawing together molded gutta percha splints (Fig. 1-19).

An ingenious modification of Malgaigne's metal claw was proposed in 1852 by Chassin[13] for use on displaced fractures of the clavicle. It consisted of two pairs of points of claws, smaller than but similar in design to the Malgaigne device, but also incorporating two finger screws that could, in addition, be advanced down on the fragments to correct anteroposterior displacements (Fig. 1-20). These additional

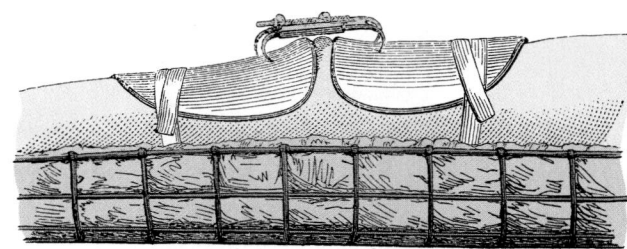

FIGURE 1-19 *The Malgaigne claw device (1870), here used to control gutta percha splints for a fractured patella.*

pointed screws were admitted by Chassin to be inspired by the other device of Malgaigne, *la pointe métallique*. In describing this device in his treatise, Bérenger Féraud gave a glimpse of his vision of the future, saying, "Could one not say by varying the form of the claws, surgeons would be able to apply them to a great quantity of bones of the skeleton and I am persuaded that before long we will have observations of fractures of the metacarpus, the metatarsus, the radius or the ulna, the ribs, the apophyses of the scapula treated in this manner. Who knows even if one would not be able to make claws sufficiently powerful, whilst remaining narrow enough, to maintain fragments of the tibia, the femur, or the humerus." Was he not indeed foreseeing the development in the 20th century of the widespread use of external fixation?

Hitherto, these devices had simply punctured the surface of the bone, and it was a British surgeon at the West London Hospital, Mr. Keetley,[40] who first described an external fixation device deliberately implanted into the full diameter of the bone. In 1801, Benjamin Bell wrote that "an effectual method of securing oblique fractures in the bones of the extremities and especially of the thigh bone, is perhaps one of the greatest desiderata of modern surgery. In all ages the difficulty of this has been confessedly great and frequent lameness produced by shortened limbs arising from this cause evidently shows that we are still deficient in our branch of practice."[4]

FIGURE 1-18 *The* griffe métallique, *or claw, of* Malgaigne (1843).

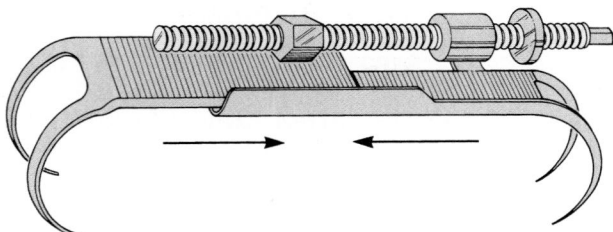

FIGURE 1-20 *Chassin's clavicular fixator (1852).*

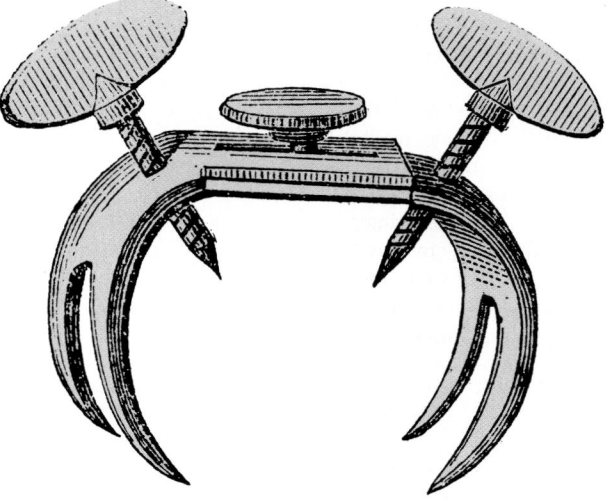

FIGURE 1-21   *The external fixation device invented by Keetley of the West London Hospital, England—probably the first to be drilled into the substance of the bone. (Redrawn from Lancet, 1893.)*

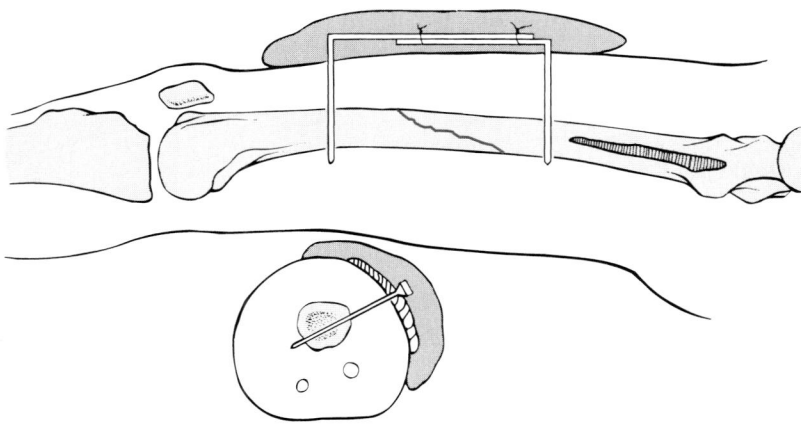

Inspired by these words, Keetley produced a device to hold the femur out to length in cases of oblique fracture. "A carefully purified pin of thickly plated steel, made to enter through a puncture in the skin, cleansed with equal care" was passed through drill holes, one in each main fragment, and then the two horizontal arms of each device, suitably notched along the edges, were united by twists of wire, the whole then being dressed with a wrapping of iodoform gauze (Fig. 1-21). This device obviously inspired Chalier, who described his *crampon extensible*, an apparatus very similar in principle but perhaps a little more sophisticated in design.[12] Something approaching the type of external fixation device with which we are today familiar was documented in 1897 by Dr. Clayton Parkhill of Denver, Colorado (Fig. 1-22). He recounted that, in 1894, he devised a new method of immobilization of bones, initially for the treatment of a young man with a pseudarthrosis of the humerus following a gunshot wound 11 months previously. He described the device (Fig. 1-23) as

> . . . a steel clamp made up of separable pieces in order to secure easy and accurate adjustment. It is heavily plated with silver in order to secure the antiseptic action of that metal. Clamps of different sizes are made to correspond with the bone upon which they are used; the largest sizes for the femur, the intermediate sizes for the humerus and tibia, the smallest sizes for radius, ulna, fibula and clavicle. The instrument consists essentially of four screws, or shafts. On these are cut threads at the lower end and also near the upper end. The extreme upper end, however, is made square so that the screw may be governed by a clock key. Two sets of wing plates are attached to these screws, a shorter pair corresponding to the inner screws and a longer pair to the outer. Each is attached to its screws by two nuts, one above the plate and the other below for accuracy of adjustment. When in position, one wing plate overlies the other in each half of the instrument. When ready to be clamped these plates lie side by side. They are fastened together by a steel clamp with a screw at either end.

In 1898, he recorded the use of his device in 14 cases, mainly of pseudarthrosis or malunion of the femur,

humerus, forearm, and tibia, although there was one case of a refracture of a previously united patella treated by immediate application of the Parkhill clamp.[60] He claimed that union had been secured in every case in which the clamp had been employed, the clamp was easy to use and

FIGURE 1-22   *Dr. Clayton Parkhill of Denver, Colorado. (Courtesy of Dr. Walter W. Jones and the Denver County Medical Society.)*

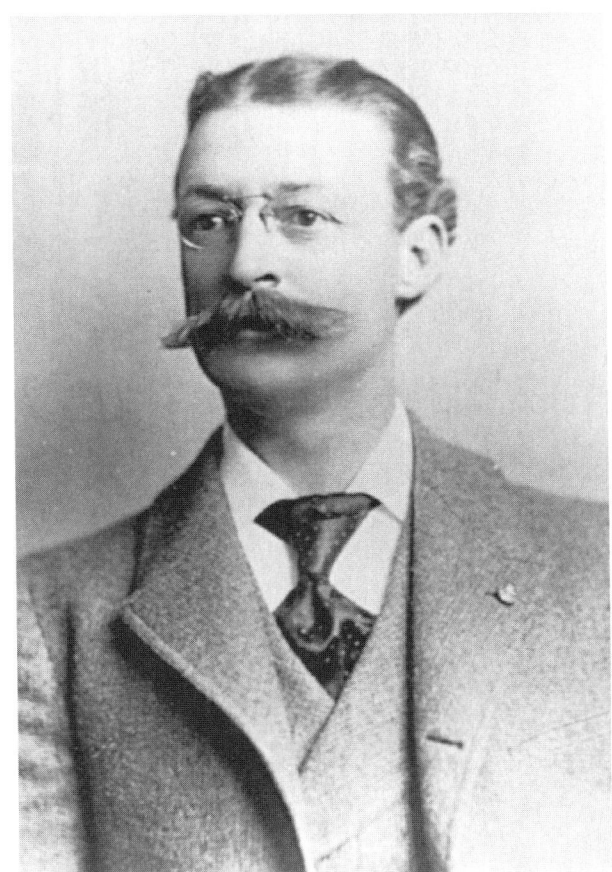

FIGURE 1-23   *The external fixation device of Parkhill (1894). (Redrawn from Annals of Surgery, 1898.)*

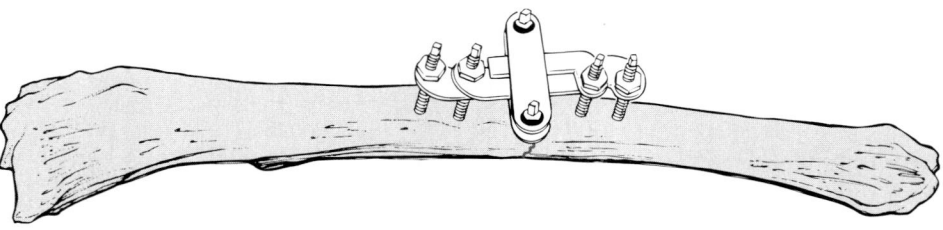

prevented motion between the fragments, the screws inserted into the bone stimulated the production of callus, no secondary operation was necessary, and after removal nothing was left in the tissues "that might reduce their vitality or lead to pain and infection."

It was only a few years later, across the Atlantic, on April 24, 1902, that Albin Lambotte first used his own external fixation device. This device was fairly primitive, consisting of pins screwed into the main fragments of a comminuted fracture of the femur, two above and two below, with the pins then clamped together by sandwiching them between two heavy metal plates bolted together. Subsequently, he devised a more sophisticated type of external fixator

in which the protruding ends of the screws were bolted to adjustable clamps linked with a heavy external bar (Fig. 1-24). Lambotte recorded the use of his external fixator in many sites, including the clavicle and the first metacarpal.

Over the next few decades a number of devices were described, two of which were particularly notable for their ingenuity. In 1919, Crile[18] described a method of maintaining the reduction of femoral fragments that consisted of (1) a peg driven into the neck of the femur via the outer face of the greater trochanter, this peg bearing externally a metal sphere; (2) a metallic caliper bearing double points that were driven into the condyles of the distal femur that also bore a metal sphere to form part of a ball joint; and (3) an external

FIGURE 1-24   *Some of the instruments of Lambotte in the collection of the University Hospital of Ghent, Belgium, including a Lambotte fixateur externé.*

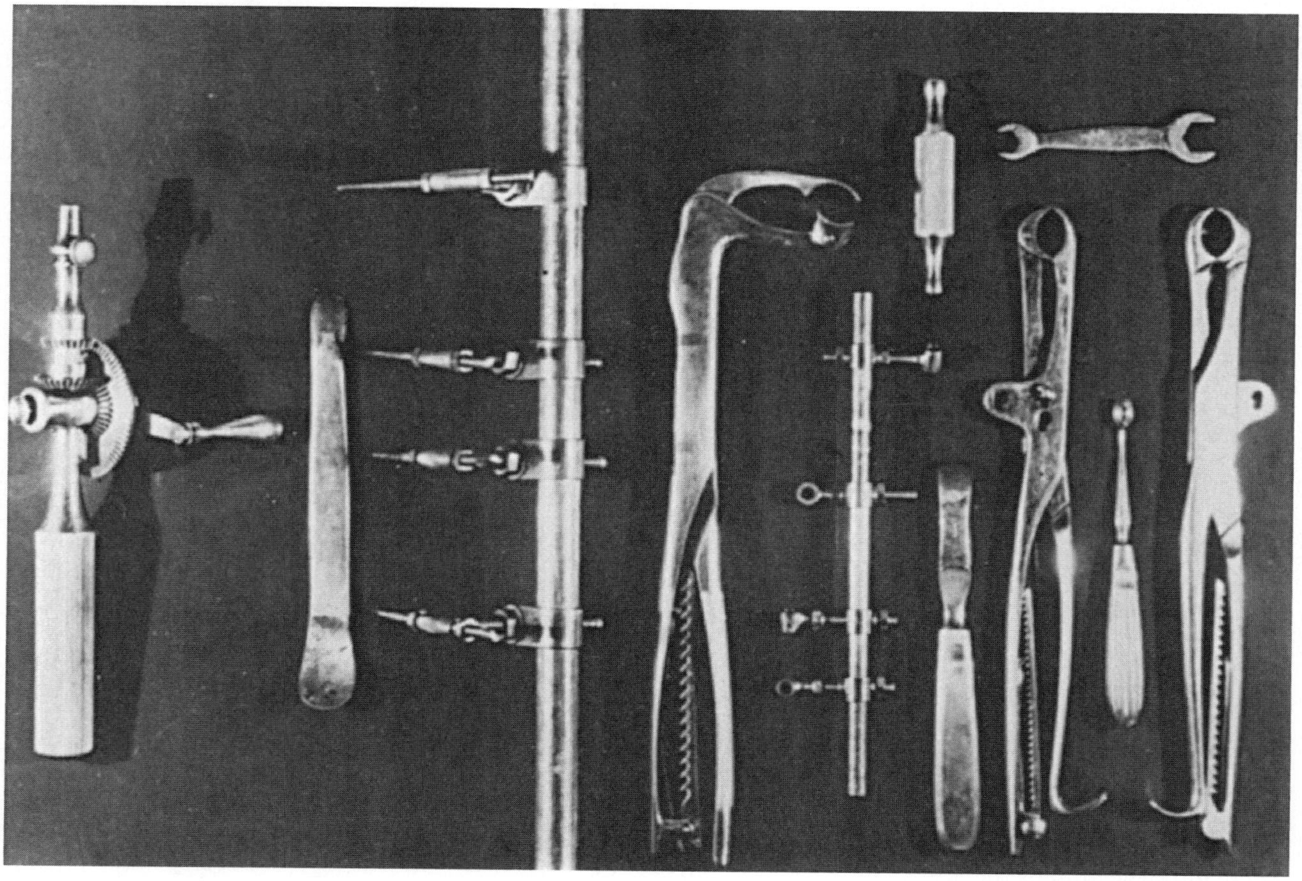

linking device with a universal joint at each end capable of being clamped onto the metal spheres and also capable itself of extension via a lengthening screw (Fig. 1-25). He described its use in only one case, that of a gunshot wound of the femur sustained by a young soldier in 1918. This wound had been particularly contaminated and, using his device after a period of initial traction with a Thomas splint, Crile succeeded in gaining control of the soft tissue infection and securing early union of the fracture. The soldier was discharged to England 9 weeks after injury following removal of the apparatus. In 1931, Conn[16] described an articulated external linkage device that consisted of two Duralumin slotted plates linked in the center by a lockable ball-and-socket joint. Half pins were then driven into the bone fragments, two above the fracture and two below, with the pins then bolted to the slotted plates and the fracture adjusted at the universal joint before locking it with a steel bolt. He reported 20 cases with no delay in union and emphasized that the early motion of the joints of the limb, permitted by his device, had allowed prompt return to function. Conn also emphasized scrupulous pin tract care, recommending daily removal of dried serum and application of alcohol.

Hitherto, all external fixation devices had relied on half pins and a single external linkage device. The first fracture apparatus using transfixion pins with a bilateral frame was that of Pitkin and Blackfield.[62] In the 1930s and 1940s, Anderson of Seattle experimented with a great variety of external fixation configurations, enclosing the whole of the apparatus in plaster casts. He emphasized the benefits of early weight bearing and joint mobilization, but contrary to the advice of Conn, he recommended that wounds should not be dressed or disturbed "even though there is present some discharge and odour." His ideas were by no

FIGURE 1-25 *The external fixation apparatus of Crile.*

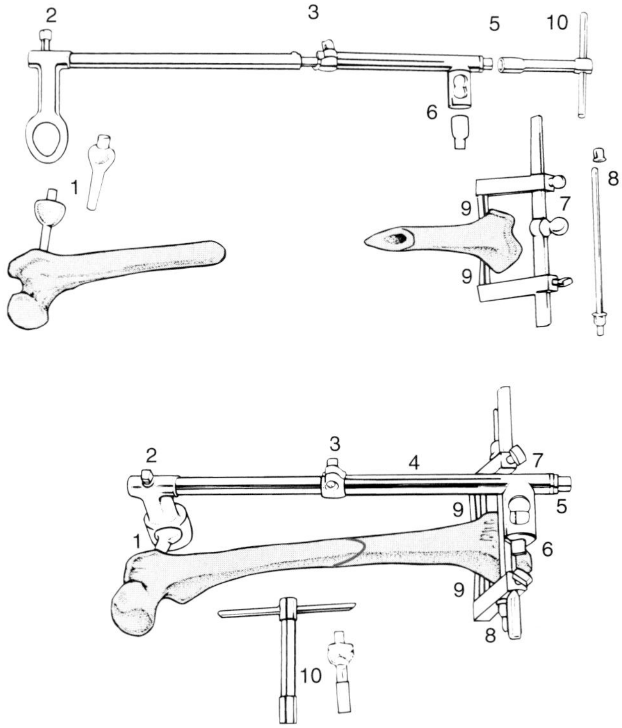

means universally accepted, and indeed in World War II, the advice given to American army surgeons working in the European theater was that "the use of Steinmann pins incorporated in plaster of Paris or the use of metallic external fixation splints leads to gross infection or ulceration in a high percentage of cases. This method of treatment is not to be employed in the Third Army."[14]

In Switzerland, Raoul Hoffmann of Geneva was developing his own system of external fixation, the early results of which he published in 1938.[36] Although many devices had been invented for external fixation and the literature abounded with reports of series of cases treated in this manner, it was not until the 1960s that, building on the groundwork of Hoffman, both Burny and Bourgois[11] and Vidal and co-workers[79] started to outline the biomechanical principles on which external fixation was based. This led the way to the universal acceptance of this method of fracture management. An interesting by-product of improved external fixation has been the opportunity for surgical lengthening of bones, although it has to be pointed out that this was first described in 1921 by Vittorio Putti, who used a transfixion device.[65]

INTRAMEDULLARY FIXATION

As previously discussed, pioneers such as von Langenbeck, Koenig, Cheyne, Lambotte, and Lane had all used intramedullary screw fixation in the management of fractures of the neck of the femur. In addition, there are a number of reported instances of intramedullary devices in the neck of the femur being used for the management of nonunion, including the extensive operation of Gillette, who used the transtrochanteric approach to perform an intracapsular fixation of ununited femoral neck fractures using intramedullary bone pegs.[27] Curtis used a drill bit—as, reputedly, had Langenbeck—in the neck of the femur, and Charles Thompson used silver nails in 1899.[7] Lambotte also recorded the use of a long intramedullary screw in the management of a displaced fracture of the neck of the humerus in 1906.

In the late 19th century, attempts were made to secure fixation of fractures using intramedullary ivory pegs, and Bircher is credited with their first use in 1886.[8] Short intramedullary devices of beef bone and of human bone were also used by Hoglund.[37] Toward the end of the first decade of the century, Ernest Hey Groves, of Bristol, England, was using massive three- and four-flanged intramedullary nails for the fixation of diaphyseal fractures of the femur, the humerus, and the ulna.[66] Hey Groves's early attempts at intramedullary fixations of this type were complicated by infection, earning him the epithet "septic Ernie" among his West Country colleagues. Metallic intramedullary fixation of bone was not at that time generally accepted. In the late 1920s the work of Smith-Peterson,[75] who used a trifin nail for the intramedullary fixation of subcapital fractures of the femur, represented a great step forward in the management of what has since been referred to as the *unsolved fracture*, and that remained the standard management for this type of injury for some 40 years.

The use of stout wires and thin solid rods in the intramedullary cavities of long bones was recommended by Lambrinudi in 1940.[43] This technique was further developed in the

United States by the brothers Rush,[68] who subsequently developed a system of flexible nails, still in occasional use.

The concept of a long metallic intramedullary device that gripped the endosteal surface of the bone—so-called elastic nailing—was the brainchild of Gerhardt Küntscher working in collaboration with Professor Fischer and the engineer Ernst Pohl at Kiel University in Germany in the 1930s. Küntscher originally used a V-shaped nail but then changed to a nail with a cloverleaf cross section for greater strength and designed to follow any guide pin more faithfully. Küntscher published his first book on intramedullary nailing at the end of World War II. Although it was written in 1942, the illustrations for it were destroyed in the air raids on Leipzig, so the book was not published until 1945.[41] For reasons that are not entirely clear, this outstanding German surgeon was virtually banished to Lapland from 1943 until the end of the European war. He was dispatched as head of the medical office at the German Military Surgical Hospital in Kemi, northern Finland. It is interesting to note that he departed Kemi in something of a hurry in September 1944 by air and left behind him a huge stock of intramedullary nails that became available for the Finnish surgeons to use.[48]

Küntscher was a brilliant technical surgeon, and his results, being so impressive, caused a somewhat overenthusiastic adoption of intramedullary nailing in Europe in the early years after World War II. According to Lindholm, this was reflected in the comments of the leading European trauma surgeon, Professor Lorenz Böhler of Vienna (Fig. 1-26). In 1944, Böhler[9] said:

Küntscher in his publication has briefly, thoroughly and with clarity described the techniques and indications for closed marrow nailing of fresh uncomplicated fractures of the thigh, lower leg and upper arm. He has also pointed out how to perform nailing of fresh, complicated, inverate and nonhealed fractures. It has been an enormous surprise compared with our experiences to see a man with such a serious femoral fracture walk without a plaster cast or any bandage with reasonably moving joints only fourteen days after the accident.

A year later, he wrote in the preface to the next edition of his book,

Later experience has revealed that the risks with marrow nailing are much greater than first predicted. We therefore use it as a rule only in femoral fractures. . . . Marrow nailing of other long bones which I have also recommended is shown by long term follow ups often to be more deleterious than profitable.

Britain appeared somewhat slow to adopt the teachings of Küntscher, possibly as a result of the influence of Hey Groves's early experiments with metallic intramedullary fixation. The January 3, 1948, issue of *Lancet* contained a somewhat flippant and puerile commentary by a "peripatetic correspondent" on the techniques of Küntscher, in which Lorenz Böhler, by that time advocating caution in relation to intramedullary nailing, was described as the "Moses of the Orthopaedic Sinai"! It is not surprising that the author chose to remain anonymous. In 1950, Le Vay,

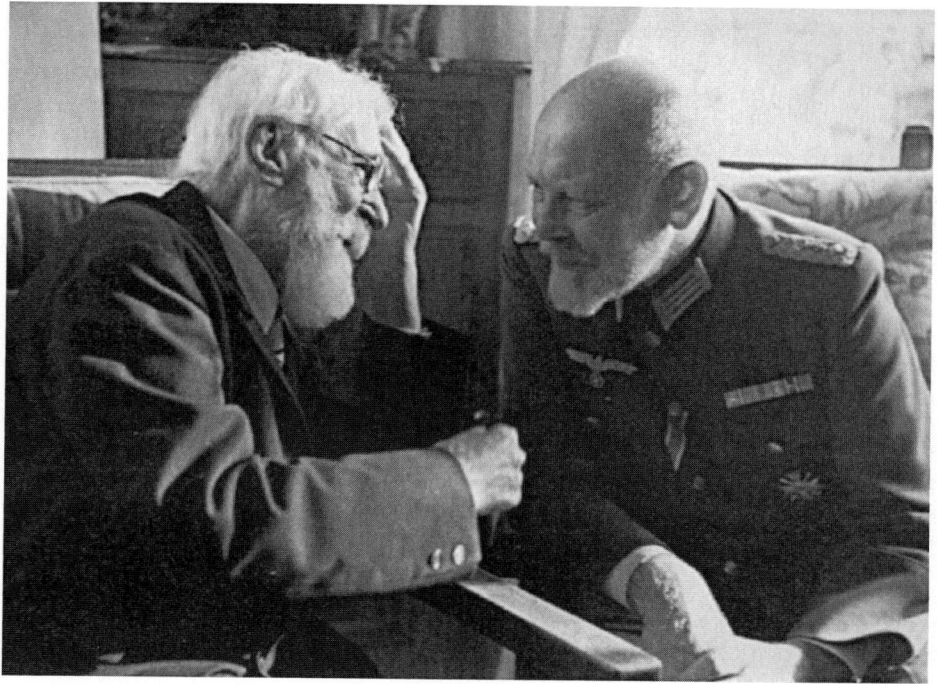

FIGURE 1-26 *Professor Lorenz Böhler (in uniform) photographed during World War II, talking to Adolph Lorenz.*

of London, published an interesting account of a visit to Küntscher's clinic, but in summing up his general impressions of Küntscher's technique, he wrote:

> It was clear that Küntscher disliked extensive open bone operations or any disturbance of the periosteum and he stated that every such intervention delayed healing. He believed that the advantage of closed nailing lay in the avoidance of such disturbance and the fact that surgical intervention could be limited. All his procedures reflected this attitude: refusal to expose a simple fracture for nailing, avoidance of bone grafting operations, dislike of plates and screws and his very limited approach for arthrodesis of the knee joint. One was bound to conclude that such methods were evolved under the pressure of circumstances—the shortage of skilled nurses, the lack of penicillin, the need for immediate fixation without transfer, and above all the total lack of certainty as to the duration of postoperative stay in hospital determined by the doubtful number of hospital beds that would be available. A virtue was made of necessity.[47]

Sadly, such smug complacency and self-satisfaction were not totally uncharacteristic of the British approach to innovation in fracture surgery at that time. In contrast, Milton Silverman in the *Saturday Evening Post* in 1955 said that Küntscher's invention was the most significant medical advance to come out of Germany since the discovery of sulfonamide. Küntscher developed interlocking femoral and tibial nails, an intramedullary bone saw for endosteal osteotomy, an expanding nail for the distal tibia, the "signal arm" nail for trochanteric fractures, cannulated flexible powered intramedullary reamers, and an intramedullary nail to apply compression across fracture sites. All this was done in collaboration with his engineer, Ernst Pohl, and his lifetime technical assistant, Gerhardt Breske, whom I had the great fortune to visit in his home in 1985. Herr Breske told me that Küntscher was a great lover of life: he swam every day, he enjoyed humor and parties and was a great practical joker, but never married, according to Herr Breske, because "he was far too busy." Gerhardt Küntscher (Fig. 1-27) died in 1972 at his desk, working on yet a further edition of his book on intramedullary nailing. He was found slumped over his final manuscript by Dr. Wolfgang Wolfers, chief of surgery at the St. Franziskus Hospital of Flensberg, where from 1965 onward Küntscher had worked as a guest surgeon.

The pioneering work of Küntscher was taken further by modifications of design and technique made by the AO group (see following section), and the distillation of this great experience resulted in the work in the 1960s and 1970s of Klemm, Schellmann, Grosse, and Kempf in the development of the current generation of interlocking nailing systems. Aside from this mainstream of development of intramedullary nailing following on the work of Küntscher, there have been a multitude of different designs of intramedullary fixation devices, such as those of Soeur, Westborne, Hansen and Street, Schneider, and Huckstep. The only other device to have achieved anything like widespread acceptance, however, has been that of Zickel, which incorporates at its upper end a trifin nail to secure purchase in the proximal femur in the management of fractures in the high subtrochanteric region.

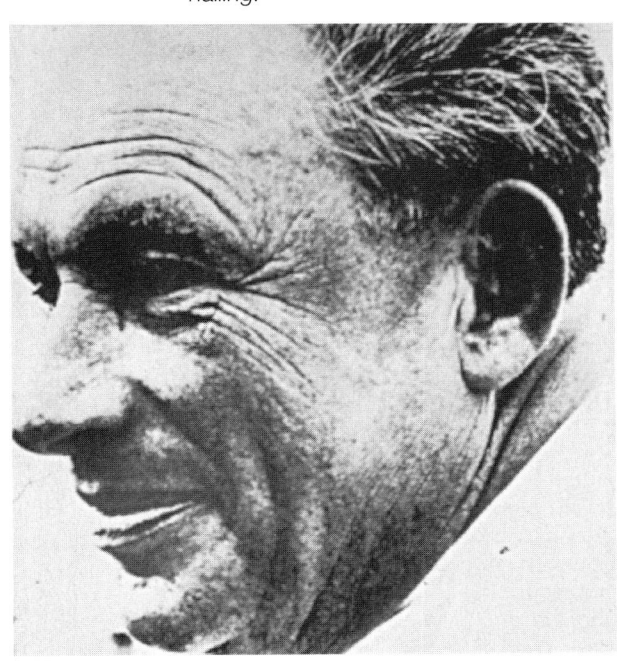

Gerhardt Küntscher (1900 to 1972), the great German pioneer of intramedullary nailing.

ROBERT DANIS AND THE DEVELOPMENT OF THE AO GROUP

Robert Danis (1880 to 1962) (Fig. 1-28) must be regarded as the father of modern osteosynthesis. Graduating from the University of Brussels in 1904, he practiced as a general surgeon, his early interests being in thoracic and vascular surgery. He became professor of theoretical and practical surgery at the University of Brussels in 1921 and while there developed a great interest in internal fixation of fractures. Although there is no direct evidence, one cannot help but feel that he must have been profoundly influenced by the mobilizers—Seutin, Paget, Lucas-Championnière, Lambotte, Lane, and Sherman, to mention but a few—in developing his concepts of immediate stable internal fixation to permit functional rehabilitation. His vast experience in this field was brought together in his monumental publication *Théorie et Pratique de l'Ostéosynthèse.*[20] In the first section of this book on the aims of osteosynthesis, he wrote that an osteosynthesis is not entirely satisfactory unless it attains the three following objectives:

1. The possibility of immediate and active mobilization of the muscles of the region and of the neighbouring joints
2. Complete restoration of the bone to its original form
3. The *soudure per primam* (primary bone healing) of the bony fragments without the formation of apparent callus

Danis devised numerous techniques of osteosynthesis based principally on interfragmentary compression, using screws and a device that he called his *coapteur*, which was basically a plate designed to produce axial compression

FIGURE 1-28 *Robert Danis (1880 to 1962), the only known photograph. (Courtesy of his son, Dr. A. Danis.)*

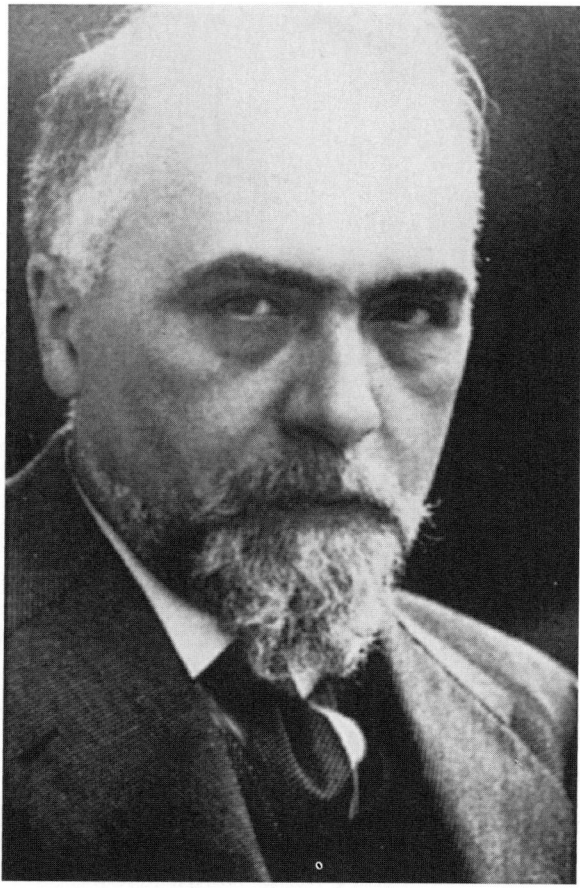

FIGURE 1-29 *The compression plate, or* coapteur, *of Danis (1949).*

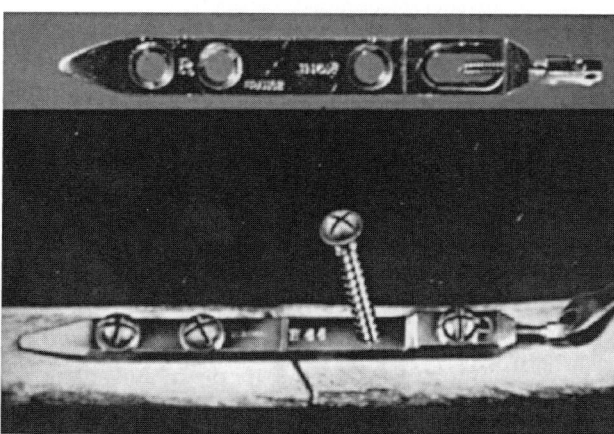

In the first section of his book, in discussing direct bone healing, Danis made the prophetic statement, "This *soudure autogène* which occurs as discretely as in the case of an incomplete fissure fracture certainly merits experimental study to establish in detail what are the modifications brought about by an ideal osteosynthesis of the phenomena of consolidation."

Robert Danis could not have realized how comprehensively this suggestion would be taken up or the profound influence that it would have on the evolution of the surgical management of fractures over the ensuing 40 years.

On March 1, 1950, a young Swiss surgeon, Dr. Maurice Müller, who had read Danis's work, paid the great surgeon a visit in Brussels. This visit left such an impression on young Dr. Müller, to whom Robert Danis presented an autographed copy of his book, that the young Swiss returned to his homeland determined to embrace and develop the principles of the ideal osteosynthesis, as outlined by Danis, and to investigate the scientific basis for his observations. Over the next few years, Müller inspired a number of close colleagues to share his passion for the improvement of techniques for the internal fixation of fractures (Fig. 1-30), gathering around himself particularly Hans Willenegger of Liestal, Robert Schneider of Grosshöchstetten, and subsequently Martin Allgöwer of Chur, who together laid the intellectual and indeed practical groundwork for a momentous gathering in the Kantonsspital of Chur on March 15 to 17, 1958. The other guests at this meeting were Bandi, Baumann, Eckmann, Guggenbühl, Hunzicker, Molo, Nicole, Ott, Patry, Schär, and Stähli. Over the 3 days, a number of scientific papers on osteosynthesis were presented, and the assembled surgeons formed a study group to look into all aspects of internal fixation—*Arbeitsgemeinschaft für Osteosynthesefragen,* or AO. This was indeed a very active group that built on Danis's work in an industrious and productive way.

There were basically three channels of activity. First, a laboratory for experimental surgery was set up in Davos, Switzerland, initially under the direction of Martin Allgöwer and subsequently Herbert Fleisch, who was succeeded by the current director, Stefan Perren, in

between two main bone fragments (Fig. 1-29). It would appear from his writings that Danis's primary aim was to produce fracture stabilization that was so rigid that he could ignore the broken bone and preserve the function of the other parts of the injured limb. In achieving such sound stabilization of the fracture by anatomic reduction and interfragmentary compression, he also produced, possibly by serendipity, the biomechanical and anatomic environment that permitted the bone to heal by direct remodeling of the cortical bone, without external callus. Having observed this type of healing, which he called *soudure autogène* (self-welding), he took this as an indication that his osteosynthesis had achieved its primary objective. The other side of this coin, however, was that if callus did appear, it was an indication that he had failed to produce the environment of stability that he had wished. He cannot initially have set out to produce direct bone healing before he had personally observed it, so he seems finally to have turned an observation of a secondary effect into the third aim of osteosynthesis as outlined previously, later causing some confusion of attitudes to callus. It is interesting to note, however, that Danis was not the first to observe healing of a diaphyseal fracture without external callus, as this was recorded by Layton in one of Arbuthnot Lane's cases.

| FIGURE 1-30 | *Hans Willenegger, Maurice Müller, and Martin Allgöwer, three of the founders of Arbeitsgemeinschaft für Osteosynthesefragen (AO), pictured in the late 1950s. (Courtesy of Professor Müller.)* |

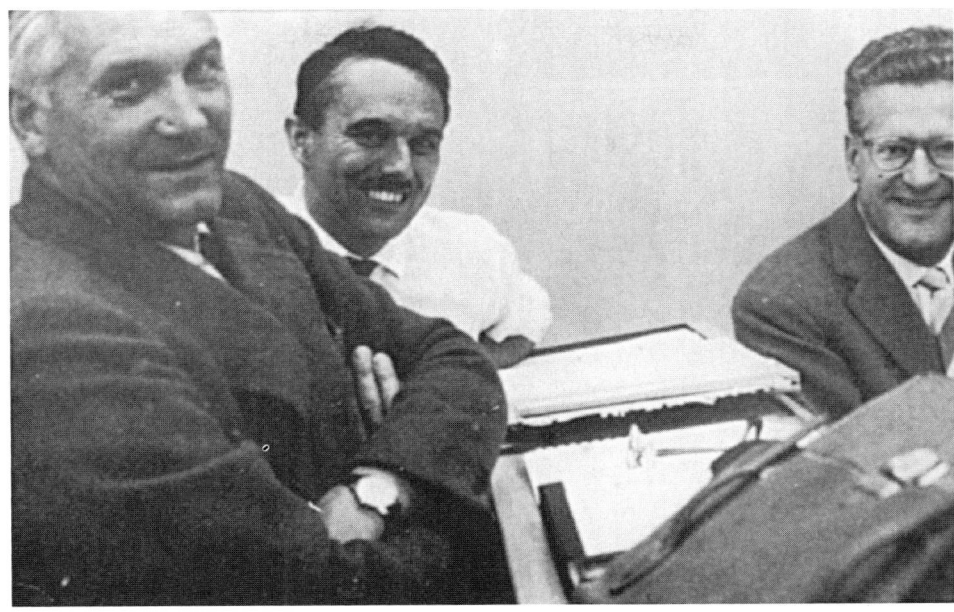

1967. These workers, in collaboration with Robert Schenk, professor of anatomy at the University of Bern, instituted, and have since continued, an ever-expanding experimental program that early on clearly defined the exact process of direct bone healing and the influence of skeletal stability on the pattern of bone union, laying the foundation for our modern understanding of bone healing in various mechanical environments. Second, the group also set out, in collaboration with metallurgists and engineers in Switzerland, to devise a system of implants and instruments to apply the biomechanical principles emerging from their investigations and so enable them to produce the skeletal stability necessary to achieve the objectives enunciated by Danis. Third, they decided to document their clinical experience, and a center was set up in Bern, which continues to the present day with the documentation of osteosyntheses from all over the world.

It was not long before the work of this group, and of the other surgeons who over the years became associated with them, bore fruit and laid the foundation for our current practice of osteosynthesis. It became necessary to educate surgeons in both the scientific and the technical aspects of this new system of osteosynthesis, and combined theoretical and practical courses in AO techniques were held from 1960 onward in Davos, Switzerland, continuing annually to the present day (Fig. 1-31). Since 1965, courses have been held in many other institutions, and scholarships have allowed surgeons to visit centers of excellence throughout the world.[70] No other single group of surgeons, coming together to pursue a common scientific and clinical aim, has had such an influence on the management of fractures. It is therefore entirely fitting that this account of the history of the care of fractures should include consideration of this group, which as the AO Foundation, the umbrella under which the clinical, scientific, and educational activities of AO continue, remains at the forefront of the development of scientific thought and technical progress in this field.

Just before Christmas 1999, Hans R. Willenegger passed away. As the head of the Kantonsspital Liestal in 1958, he played a pivotal role in the creation of the AO. Thanks to his initiative, links were forged with Straumann, a metallurgical research institute, which helped solve problems with the implant material. Out of this collaboration arose the industrial production of Synthes implants and instruments with a scientific background. Parallel with this, Willenegger made contact with R. Schenk, at that time professor at the Institute of Anatomy at Basel, who contributed histologic knowledge to their experimental work in bone healing. Soon Willenegger realized that performing an osteosynthesis in a suboptimal way could create a catastrophic complication. Being willing to help such patients, Liestal became a center for the treatment of post-traumatic osteomyelitis, pseudarthrosis, and malunion.

This experience led Willenegger to initiate the worldwide teaching of the AO principles. He became the first president of AO International in 1972. This event marked the starting point of many years of global traveling, teaching AO in all five continents. Countless are the slides he gave to future AO teachers, carefully explaining the basic principles underlying each one. Worldwide, many of us recall a personal souvenir of a direct contact with him and are conscious that we have lost a friend.

FIGURE 1-31   *Martin Allgöwer instructing the late Professor John Charnley at one of the earliest Arbeitsgemeinschaft für Osteosynthesefragen (AO) instructional courses in Davos, Switzerland, circa 1961.*

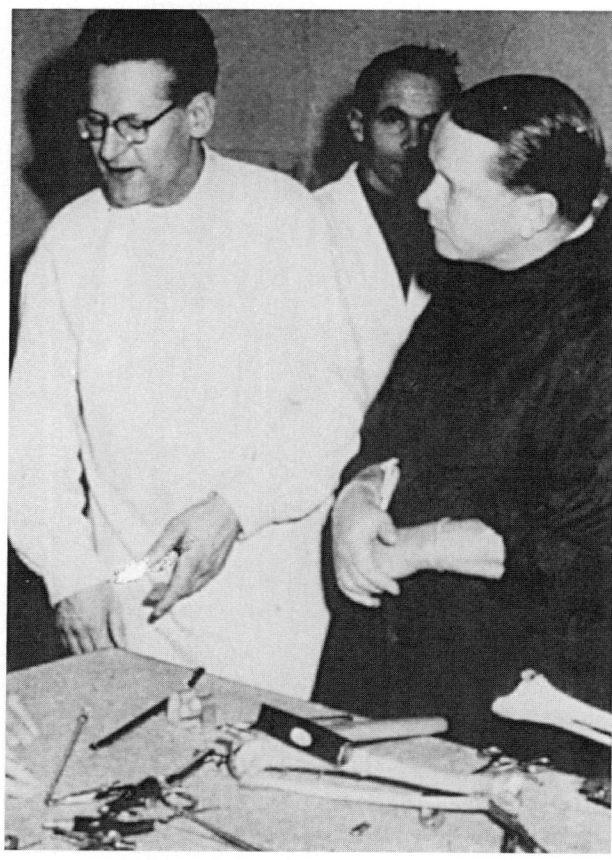

GAVRIIL A. ILIZAROV AND THE DISCOVERY OF DISTRACTION OSTEOGENESIS

Stuart A. Green, M.D.

In the 1950s, Gavriil A. Ilizarov, a Soviet surgeon working in the Siberian city of Kurgan, made a serendipitous discovery: slow, steady distraction of a recently cut bone (securely stabilized in an external fixator) leads to the formation of new bone within the widening gap. At the time, Ilizarov was using a circular external skeletal fixator that he had designed in 1951 to distract knee joints that had developed flexion contractures after prolonged plaster cast immobilization (during World War II). The device consisted of two Kirschner wire traction bows connected to each other by threaded rods.

Ilizarov originally developed his fixator to stretch out the soft tissues gradually on the posterior side of a contracted knee joint. One patient, however, had bony, rather than fibrous, ankylosis of his knee in the flexed position. After performing a bone-cutting osteotomy on this patient through the knee, Ilizarov had the patient gradually straighten out the limb by turning nuts on the fixator surrounding his limb. Ilizarov intended to insert a bone graft into the resulting triangular bone defect when the knee was straight. To his surprise, Ilizarov found a wedge-shaped mass of newly regenerated bone at the site of osteotomy when distraction was finished.

Extending his observations, Ilizarov after that time developed an entire system of orthopaedics and traumatology based on his axially stable tensioned wire circular external fixator and the bone's ability to form a "regenerate" of newly formed osseous tissue within a widening distraction gap.

Employing his discovery of distraction osteogenesis, Ilizarov used various modifications of his apparatus to elongate, rotate, angulate, or shift segments of bones gradually with respect to each other. The fixation system's adaptability also permits the reduction and fixation of many unstable fracture patterns.

Until his death in 1992, Professor Ilizarov headed a 1000-bed clinical and research institute staffed by 350 orthopaedic surgeons and 60 scientists with Ph.D. degrees, where patients from Russia and the rest of the world come for the treatment of birth defects, dwarfism, complications of traumatic injuries, and other disorders of the musculoskeletal system.

For many years, Professor Ilizarov and his co-workers have trained surgeons from socialist countries in his techniques. Around 1980, Italian orthopaedists learned of Ilizarov's methods when others from their country returned from Yugoslavia and nearby Eastern European countries with circular fixators on their limbs. Soon thereafter, Italian, other European, and, more recently, North American orthopaedic surgeons have ventured to Siberia for training in the Ilizarov method.

The techniques and applications of the Ilizarov method have continued to improve with time, both in Russia and around the world. One important advance in the technique of fixator application consists of the substitution of titanium half pins for stainless steel wires in many locations, thereby adding to patients' comfort and acceptance of the apparatus.

Nevertheless, much clinical and scientific work investigating the Ilizarov method remains to be done. Biomechanical and histochemical studies are needed. The health care insurance industry has been slow to recognize the magnitude of Ilizarov's discoveries. They must be educated. A generation of orthopaedic surgeons requires training in the method. With time, however, Ilizarov's discoveries will become fully integrated into modern clinical practice.

EMILE LETOURNEL AND THE SURGERY OF PELVIC AND ACETABULAR FRACTURES

Joel M. Matta, M.D.

Emile Letournel (Fig. 1-32) was born on the French island territory of St. Pierre et Miquelon, situated between Newfoundland and Nova Scotia. Thus, he was born in France and also in North America. This small fishing territory is completely under French control, including the economy and language.

As he developed an interest in orthopaedic surgery, it became necessary for him to apply for a postgraduate

FIGURE 1-32 *Professeur Emile Letournel.*

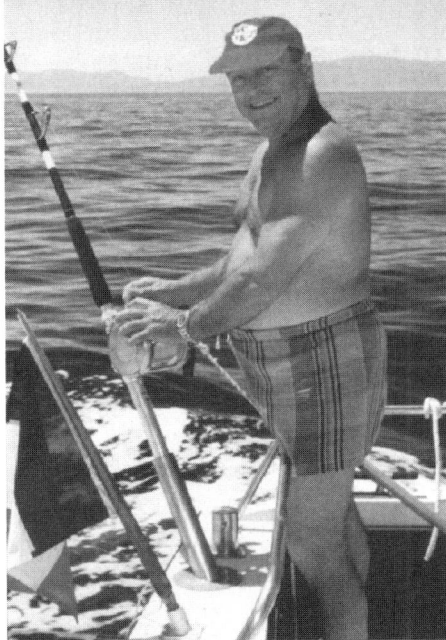

position to continue his education. The application process required the applicant to visit all the professors who were offering training positions. Being from St. Pierre, Letournel had no letters of support to contend adequately for the available orthopaedic positions. He was very concerned about not being able to acquire an orthopaedic position, when a friend suggested he meet with Professor Robert Judet. He did this out of desperation, without any hope of obtaining a position. The meeting with Judet was very brief. Professor Judet asked Letournel for his letters of recommendation, of which he had none, but Letournel indicated to him his sincere desire to obtain Judet's training position. Judet told him that he had a 6-month opening the following year. The 6-month position lasted 12 months, and Letournel then became Judet's assistant in his private clinic and advanced to associate professor and professor in 1970. He did not leave Judet until Judet's retirement in 1978. Letournel then became head of the Department of Orthopaedic Surgery at the Centre Medico-Chirurgie de la Port de Choisy in southeastern Paris. He remained there until his retirement from academic medicine in October 1993. He subsequently went into private practice at the Villa Medicis, Courbevoie, France, a suburb of Paris.

It was during his time at Choisy that physicians from North America had their greatest contact with Professeur Letournel. The importance of his work, inspired and begun by Robert Judet, was not widely recognized until the 1980s. Despite this long delay in acceptance and recognition, North America was actually one of the first areas to understand and adopt his techniques, which was a fact he certainly recognized and appreciated through his continued contact with us.

An intelligent and creative surgeon is typically able to contribute only a few components of new discoveries

during the course of his or her career, but Emile Letournel accomplished much more. He completely revolutionized the way we conceptualize and treat acetabular fractures. Judet recognized problems with nonoperative treatment of acetabular fractures and inspired Letournel to begin the work that would define the surgical anatomy of the acetabulum, the pathologic anatomy of fresh fractures, and the radiographic interpretation to define these injuries. Following this, he developed surgical approaches. First, Judet combined the Kocher and Langenbeck approaches to make the Kocher-Langenbeck. Later, Letournel developed the ilioinguinal and finally the iliofemoral approach. Techniques of reduction as well as internal fixation were developed. Finally, the radiographic, clinical, and statistical documentation of immediate and long-term results of the surgical treatment became a lifelong passion of Letournel.

Letournel was committed to the idea of creating a comprehensive instructional course that taught the surgical treatment of fractures of the acetabulum and pelvis. Although he had been received so positively in North America, he felt he remained incompletely recognized in France. Therefore, the first course in 1984 was held in Paris but with faculty from North America and England, and he conducted the course in English. Letournel's Paris course set the standard and educational model for acetabulum and pelvis courses to follow. In all, there were nine courses consisting of lectures with intense study of radiographs. Surgical technique was taught with lectures, plastic bones, and live surgery, and there was always a day at the historic Paris anatomy institute, the Fer à Moulin. Every course included a black-tie banquet, always with the same fine musicians and Letournel singing "La Prune" and, if the spirit was right, the "Marseillaise." His Paris meetings culminated in the May 1993 first international symposium on the results of the surgical treatment of fractures of the acetabulum. His radiographic description and classification system, which was originally established in 1960 and by this time was well established worldwide, was used throughout the symposium for clear understanding of the statistical results.

Professeur Emile Letournel died relatively suddenly after an illness of only 2 months. Up to this time, he maintained his busy surgical schedule, traveled, and taught. We, his pupils and patients throughout the world, are fortunate to have enjoyed his great persona and contributions.

KLAUS KLEMM AND INTERLOCKING NAILING AND LOCAL ANTIBIOTIC BEAD CHAIN THERAPY

David Seligson, M.D.

Dr. Klaus Klemm (1932 to 2001): Who was he, and why remember him in a book about skeletal trauma?

Dr. Klaus Klemm (Figs. 1-33 and 1-34) developed two important techniques for fracture care—interlocking nailing and local antibiotic bead chain therapy. These advances are appreciated by thousands of injured patients who benefit from his ideas. Klemm always said that his third great passion after interlocking nails and bead chains was chocolate, but it was really his wife, Dr. Brigitte

FIGURE 1-33   *Klaus Klemm at Reingau.*

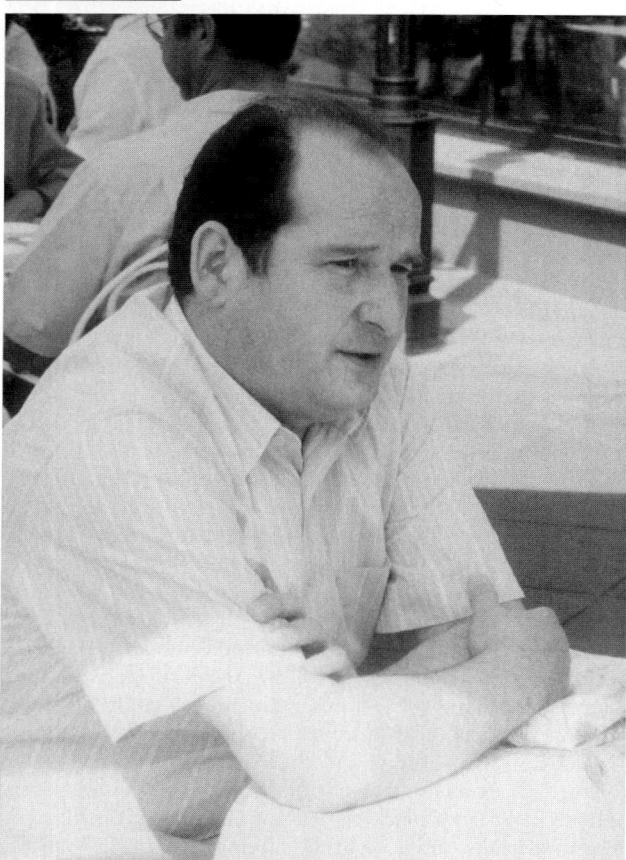

FIGURE 1-34   *Klaus Klemm at Grant's Pass.*

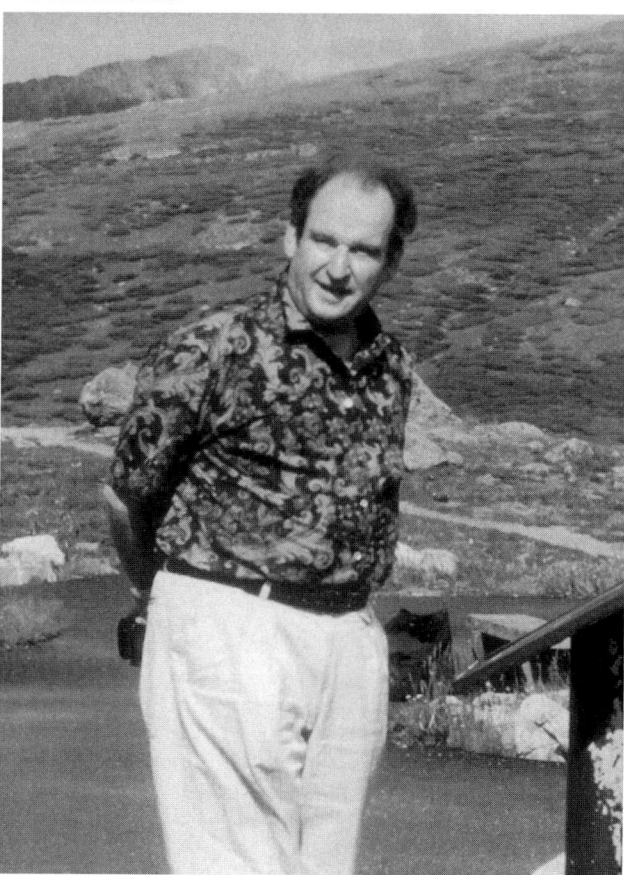

Winter-Klemm. Let me share with you some of my memories of Dr. Klemm and look more into his story so you will understand his importance to those in traumatology whom he influenced.

Klaus Klemm was born into a comfortable Frankfurt am Main family on May 19, 1932. He spent some of World War II as part of a youth group at a rail station in the Black Forest. He entered medical school in Frankfurt/Main in 1952, took a semester in Freiburg, and finished his medical degree in 1958. He then went to the Northern Westchester Hospital in Mount Kisco, New York, from 1958 to 1960 and returned to Germany, where he was licensed as a physician in 1962. Next, he took a position as an assistant to Professor Junghans in the new Workman's Hospital (BG) Frankfurt. At the BG, he was part of the new Septic Unit. From 1966 to 1969, he took his training in Surgery at St. Markus Hospital, Frankfurt/Main, and became Oberarzt and Chief of the Septic Unit at BG/Frankfurt first under Prof. Junghans and later with Prof. Contzen and finally until his retirement in 1999 under the direction of his student, Professor Börner.

Therefore, Dr. Klemm trained during the confusion of postwar Germany, spoke good English because of his 2 years in Westchester County, and accepted the task of treating bone infection with limited resources in a rebuilding country. Conventional treatment for osteomyelitis was

implant removal, bed rest, suction drainage, and long courses of intravenous antibiotics. Klemm pioneered interlocking nailing as a method for fracture stabilization, and antibiotic implants as a way to provide ambulatory antibacterial therapy. Indeed, he corresponded with Küntscher about the "Detensor" and was advised not to use the term interlocking nailing but went ahead anyway, working with W. D. Schellmann to make a practical system for intramedullary locked nailing.

Antibiotic bead chains evolved from antibiotic bone cement implants. The bead chains have been commercially available in Europe since 1978 but were never, to Klaus's frustration, approved by the U.S. Food and Drug Administration (FDA). It was ironic in those days in the 1980s to visit with Klemm in the U.S. military hospital down the Friedberger Landstraße from the BG. The Americans were trying to educate Germans in basic hygiene such as handwashing and were treating femur fractures in cast braces.

Klemm was not a great speaker, nor did he write a great deal. One learned from Klaus by being around him. He operated frequently, and saw his patients personally. If you spent time with him, you always picked up tips such as the "free hand" method for placing locking screws or how to take a bone graft from the proximal tibia. Klemm always included his guests either at dinner at Claudio's, a restaurant near his home on the Marbachweg, or at home or perhaps for an evening with his team at his retreat in

Eichelsachsen. At one such evening, I asked Guy Jenny how long one could leave antibiotic bead chains in a patient. Dr. Jenny replied, "I don't really know, my first chains are still in place after twenty years."

Klemm was a great supporter of the Gerhard Küntscher Society and its Secretary for more than a decade. Though quintessentially German at a time when it was not fashionable to be nationalistic, he nurtured connections throughout Europe and the United States. However, his relationship with the BG became more problematic as his career grew toward retirement. After all, the visitors to the clinic came to see Klaus, not the Chief. Furthermore, the development of competing nail systems did not help matters. At his retirement, we all gathered again in Frankfurt/Main at the Römer. It was a magical evening. Many of the younger colleagues present had served in menial roles during the years of American occupation. Here in the refurbished Ratskeller in the basement, the beer flowed, his friends and family were there, everyone toasted Klaus, and the old German songs rang out.

Retirement was not kind to Klemm. Klaus developed symptomatic lumbar spondylosis. He had back surgery. The site became infected. Ironically, the most innovative surgeon for the treatment of bone infection died of sepsis in the intensive care unit at the BG, where he had worked for three decades.

SUMMARY
Christopher L. Colton, M.D.

As technology advances, so do the severity and frequency of traumatic insult, and the demand for ever-increasing skill on the part of the fracture surgeon grows likewise. It is only by the study of the history of our surgical forebears and by keeping in mind how they have striven, often in the face of fierce criticism, to achieve the apparently unattainable that young surgeons will continue to be inspired to emulate them and so carry forward the progress they have achieved.

Any consideration of the history of 5000 years of endeavor, confined of necessity within the strictures of a publication such as this, is perforce eclectic. Nevertheless, in deciding to highlight the achievements of some, I have not in any way set out to minimize the pioneering work of those whose activities have not been specifically detailed in this overview, and with respect to these necessary omissions I ask the reader's indulgence.

REFERENCES

1. Amerasinghe, D.M.; Veerasingham, P.B. Early weight bearing in tibial shaft fractures protected by wooden splints. Proc Kandy Med Soc 4:(pp. unnum.), 1981.
2. Assen, J. van; Meyerding, H.W. Antonius Mathijsen, the discoverer of the plaster bandage. J Bone Joint Surg Am 30:1018, 1948.
3. Bacon, L.W. On the history of the introduction of plaster of Paris bandages. Bull Soc Med Hist 3:122, 1923.
4. Bell, B. System of Surgery, 7th ed., Vol. 2. Edinburgh, Bell and Bradfute, 1801, p. 21.
5. Bérenger Féraud, L.J.B. De l'emploi de la pointe de Malgaigne dans les fractures. Rev Ther Medicochir 15:228, 256, 1867.
6. Bérenger Féraud, L.J.B. Traité de l'Immobilisation Directe des Fragments Osseux dans les Fractures. Paris, Delahaye, 1870, p. 371.
7. Billroth, W. Clinical Surgery. London, The New Sydenham Society, 1881.
8. Bircher, H. Eine neue Methode unmittelbarer Retention bei Frakturen der Roehrenknochen. Arch Klin Chir 34:91, 1886.
9. Böhler, L. Vorwort zur 1 bis 4 Auflage, Wien, im Januar 1944. Technik der Knochenruchbehandlung im Frieden und im den Kriege, 1944, pp. IV-V.
10. Bonnet Mémoire sur les fractures du fémur. Gaz Med Paris, 1839.
11. Burny, F.; Bourgois, R. Étude bioméchanique de l'ostéotaxis. In: La Fixation Externe en Chirurgie. Brussels, Imprimerie Médicale et Scientifique, 1965.
12. Chalier, A. Nouvel appareil prothétique pour ostéosynthèse (crampon extensible). Presse Med 25:585, 1907.
13. Chassin Thèse de Paris, 1852, p. 63.
14. Cleveland, M. Surgery in World War II: Orthopedic Surgery in the European Theater of Operations. Washington, DC, Office of the Surgeon General, Dept. of the Army, 1956, p. 77.
15. Commeiras. J Soc Med Montpellier, 1847.
16. Conn, H.R. The internal fixation of fractures. J Bone Joint Surg 13:261, 1931.
17. Cooper, A. Treatise on Dislocations and on Fractures of the Joints. London, Longman, Hurst, Rees, Orme, Brown and Green, 1822.
18. Crile, D.W. Fracture of the femur: A method of holding the fragments in difficult cases. Br J Surg 4:458, 1919.
19. Cucuel; Rigaud. Des vis métalliques enfoncées dans le tissue des os pour le traitement de certaines fractures. Rev Medicochir Paris 8:113, 1850.
20. Danis, R. Théorie et Pratique de l'Ostéosynthèse. Paris, Masson, 1949.
21. Dowden, J.W. The Principle of Early Active Movement in Treating Fractures of the Upper Extremity. London, Oliver & Boyd, 1924.
22. Eaton, W. Survey of the Turkish Empire. London, 1798.
23. Elst, V.E. Les débuts de l'ostéosynthése en Belgique. Private publication for Société Belge de Chirurgie Orthopédique et de Traumatologie. Brussels, Imp des Sciences, 1971.
24. Evans, P.E.L. Cerclage fixation of a fractured humerus in 1775: Fact or fiction? Clin Orthop 174:138, 1983.
25. Gersdorf, H. von. Feldtbuch der Wundartzney. Strasbourg, 1517.

26. Gooch, B. Cases and Practical Remarks in Surgery. Norwich, W. Chase, 1767.

27. Guthrie, D. A History of Medicine. London, T. Nelson, 1945, p. 124.

28. Guthrie, G. Direct fixation of fractures. Am Med March:376, 1903.

29. Hamilton, F.H. Treatise on Military Surgery and Hygiene. New York, Baillière, 1865.

30. Hansmann. Eine neue Methode der Fixirung der Fragmente bei complicirten Fracturen. Verh Dtsch Ges Chir 15:134, 1886.

31. Hartshorne, E. On the causes and treatment of pseudarthrosis and especially that form of it sometimes called supernumerary joint. Am J Med Sci 1:121, 1841.

32. Heister, L. Chirurgie Complète. Paris, 1739.

33. Helferich, H. Atlas and Grundriss der traumatischen Frakturen und Luxationen. München, Lehmann Verlag, 1906, p. 170.

34. Hitzrot. Transactions of New York Surgical Society. Ann Surg 83:301, 1926.

35. Hoffa, A. Lehrbuch der Fracturen und Luxationen für Arzte und Studierende. Wurzburg, 1896.

36. Hoffmann, R. Rotules à os pour la réduction dirigée, non sanglante, des fractures (ostéotaxis). Helv Med Acta 6:844, 1938.

37. Hoglund, E.J. New intramedullary bone transplant. Surg Gynecol Obstet 24:243, 1917.

38. Hubenthal. Nouveau manière de traiter les fractures. Nouv J Med 5:210, 1817.

39. Icart, J.F. Lettre à réponse au mémoire de M. Pujol. Médicin de Castres et de l'Hôtel-Dieu, sur une amputation naturelle de la jambe avec des réflexions sur quelques autres cas rélatifs a cette operation, 1775.

40. Keetley, C.B. On the prevention of shortening and other forms of malunion after fracture, by the use of metal pins passed into the fragments subcutaneously. Lancet June 10:137, 1893.

41. Küntscher, G. Die Technik der Marknagelung gemeinsam mit B. Maatz. Leipzig, Thieme, 1945.

42. Lambotte, A. Chirurgie Opératoire des Fractures. Paris, Masson, 1913.

43. Lambrinudi, C. Intramedullary Kirschner wires in the treatment of fractures. Proc R Soc Med 33:153, 1940.

44. Lane, W.A. Clinical remarks on the operative treatment of simple fractures. BMJ 2:1325, 1905.

45. Lane, W.A. Operative Treatment of Fractures, 2nd ed. London, 1914, p. 126.

46. Layton, T.B. Sir William Arbuthnot Lane, Bt. C.B., M.S. An Enquiry into the Mind and Influence of a Surgeon. Edinburgh, Livingstone, 1956.

47. Le Vay, A.D. Intramedullary nailing in the Küntscher clinic. J Bone Joint Surg Br 32:698, 1950.

48. Lindholm, R.V. The bone nailing surgeon: G.B.G. Küntscher and the Finns. Acta Universitatis Ouluensis B10 Historica 5.

49. Lucas-Championnière, J. Trépanation Néolithique, Trépanation Pré-Colombienne des Kabyles, Trépanation Traditionelle. Paris, Steinheil, 1912.

50. Lucas-Championnière, J. Les dangers l'immobilisation des membres—Fragilité des os—Altération de la nutrition du membre—Conclusions pratiques. J Med Chir Prat 78:8187, 1907.

51. Malgaigne, J.F. Traitement des fractures de la jambe par le platre coulé, suivant la méthode de M. Dieffenbach de Berlin. Gaz Med Paris, 1832.

52. Malgaigne, J.F. A Treatise of Fractures. Philadelphia, J.B. Lippincott, 1859.

53. Mathijsen, A. Nieuwe Wijze van Aanwending van het Gipsverband. Eene Bijdrage Tot de Militaire Chirurgie. Haarlem, van Loghen, 1852.

54. Milne, J.S. The apparatus used by the Greeks and the Romans in the setting of fractures and the reduction of dislocations. Interstate Med J 16:3, 1909.

55. Monro, J.K. The history of plaster of Paris in the treatment of fractures. J Bone Joint Surg 23:257, 1935.

56. Mooney, V., Nickel, V.L., Harvey, J.P., Snelson, R. Cast brace treatment for fractures of the distal part of the femur. J Bone Joint Surg Am 52:1563, 1970.

57. Orr, H.W. Wounds and Fractures. A Clinical Guide to Civil and Military Practice. London, Baillière, Tindall & Cox, 1941.

58. Paré, A. Dix Livres de la Chirurgie avec le Magasin des Instruments Necessaires à Icelle, Vol. 7. Paris, Jean le Royer, 1564, Chap. 13.

59. Parkhill, C. A new apparatus for the fixation of bones after resection and in fractures with a tendency to displacement. Trans Am Surg Assoc 15:251, 1897.

60. Parkhill, C. Further observations regarding the use of the boneclamp in ununited fractures, fractures with malunion, and recent fractures with a tendency to displacement. Ann Surg 27:553, 1898.

61. Petit, J Le. D'un nouveau instrument de chirurgie. Mem Acad R Sci 1718, p. 254.

62. Pitkin, H.C.; Blackfield, H.M. Skeletal immobilization in difficult fractures of shafts of long bones: New method of treatment as applied to compound, comminuted and oblique fractures of both bones of the leg. J Bone Joint Surg 3:589, 1931.

63. Pujol, A. Mémoire sur une amputation naturelle de la jambe avec des réflexions sur quelques autre cas rélatifs à l'amputation. J Med Chir Pharm (Paris) 43:160, 1775.

64. Pujol, A. Eclaircissements en réponse à la lettre de M. Icart, chirurgien. J Med Chir Pharm (Paris) 45:167, 1776.

65. Putti, V. The operative lengthening of the femur. JAMA 77:934, 1921.

66. Ratliff, A.H.C. Ernest William Hey Groves and his contributions to orthopaedic surgery. Ann R Coll Surg Engl 65:203, 1983.

67. Russell, R.H. Fracture of the femur. A clinical study. Br J Surg 11:491, 1924.

68. Rush, L.V.; Rush, H.L. Technique for longitudinal pin fixation of certain fractures of the ulna and of the femur. J Bone Joint Surg 21:619, 1939.

69. Sarmiento, A. A functional below the knee cast for tibial fractures. J Bone Joint Surg Am 49:855, 1967.

70. Schneider, R. 25 Jahre AO Schweiz. Arbeitsgemeinschaft für Osteosynthesefragen 1958–1983. Biel, Gassmann AG, 1983.

71. Seutin. Traité de la Méthode Amovo-Inamovible. Brussels, 1849.

72. Shang T'ien-Yu; Fang Hsien-Chih; Ku Yun-Wu; Chow Ying Ch'ing. The integration of modern and traditional Chinese medicine in the treatment of fractures. Chin Med J 83:419, 1964.

73. Sherman, W.O'N. Operative treatment of fractures of the shaft of the femur with maximum fixation. J Bone Joint Surg 8:494, 1926.

74. Smith, G. The most ancient splints. BMJ 28:732, 1903.

75. Smith-Peterson, M.N.; Cave, E.F.; Vangarder, G.H. Intracapsular fractures of the neck of the femur; treatment by internal fixation. Arch Surg 23:715, 1931.

76. Spink, M.S.; Lewis, G.L. Albucasis on Surgery and Instruments. London, Wellcome Institute of the History of Medicine, 1973.

77. Thomas, G. From bonesetter to orthopaedic surgeon. Ann R Coll Surg Engl 55:134, 1974.

78. Trueta, J. An Atlas of Traumatic Surgery: Illustrated Histories of Wounds of the Extremities. Oxford, Blackwell, 1949.

79. Vidal, J.; Rabischong, P.; Bonnel, F. Étude biomécanique du fixateur externe dans les fractures de jambe. Montpelier Chir 16:43, 1970.

80. Walker, C.A. Treatment of fractures by the immoveable apparatus. Lancet 1:553, 1839.

81. Watson Jones, R. Preface. In: Wilson, J.N., ed. Fractures and Joint Injuries. Edinburgh, Livingstone, 1952, pp. v-vi.

82. Wrench, G.T. Lord Lister: His Life and Work. London, Fisher Unwin, 1914.

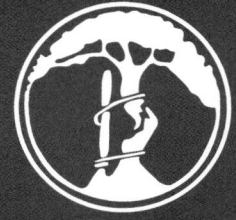

CHAPTER 2

Biology and Enhancement of Skeletal Repair

Sanjeev Kakar, M.D., M.R.C.S. and Thomas A. Einhorn, M.D.

INTRODUCTION

For nearly a half-century, the field of skeletal trauma surgery has benefited from a refined understanding of the biological and biomechanical principles that underlie the healing of bone and its associated soft tissues. For the most part, these principles have focused on rigid internal fixation leading to so-called *primary* cortical healing as described Schenk and Willenegger.[123] However, with advances in intramedullary skeletal fixation, external skeletal fixation, small pin fixation (distraction osteogenesis), and "less invasive" locking-plate technology, the healing of many of the fractures treated by trauma surgeons involves pathways that are predominantly driven by endochondral ossification.

Despite most fractures healing uneventfully, approximately 5 to 10 percent of the fractures occurring annually in the United States exhibit some degree of impaired healing.[35] In many instances, the cause is unknown and may be related to inadequate reduction, instability,[20] the systemic state of the patient,[36,93] or the nature of the traumatic insult itself.[108,136] In these circumstances, enhancement of fracture repair would be beneficial to ensure rapid restoration of skeletal function. This chapter reviews the current understanding of the biology of fracture healing and methods that can be used to stimulate this process when indicated.

BIOLOGY OF FRACTURE REPAIR

Fracture healing is a highly orchestrated process comprising a series of biological repair stages intimately linked with one another. The result is near complete biochemical and biomechanical restoration of the original bony substance. Fracture of a long bone involves not only rupture of calcified and soft tissue structures but also the transfer and dissipation of energy at the fracture site. This leads to a healing response among four major tissue types: cortical bone, periosteum, bone marrow, and external soft tissues. *Primary cortical* healing involves anatomic reduction of the fracture fragments, optimization of the strain environment, and a biological response in which the cortex directly attempts to reestablish its own continuity with the aid of so-called

"cutting cones."[56] These are remodeling units consisting of osteoclasts that resorb cortical bone, thereby permitting angiogenesis and stem cell deposition into the fracture site, and progenitor cells differentiate into osteoblasts that secrete matrix and bridge the fracture gap.[123] This process enlists minimal participation from the periosteum, external soft tissues, and the bone marrow.[96]

If rigid internal fixation is not provided and micromotion exists at the fracture site, *secondary* bone healing occurs. The response of the periosteum and neighboring soft tissues to bony injury forms the basis of secondary fracture healing through which the majority of fractures heal. It involves both intramembranous and endochondral ossification that proceed concurrently. Intramembranous bone formation occurs on either side of the fracture, and the cells that drive this process are derived from periosteum.[56] The endochondral response is also dependent on the periosteum,[105] but the cells in the neighboring soft tissues additionally contribute to this process.[71,73]

To study endochondral fracture healing, a model was developed in which a standard closed transverse femoral fracture was produced in the rat femur. This fracture was then stabilized with an intramedullary pin.[36] Characterization of this model shows that within the first 7 days after fracture, an inflammatory response takes place at the fracture site as demonstrated by the invasion of macrophages, polymorphonuclear leukocytes, and lymphocytic cells. These cells secrete proinflammatory cytokines including interleukin-1, interleukin-6, and tumor necrosis factor-α (TNF-α).[38,84] At the same time, peptide signaling molecules such as members of the transforming growth factor-beta (TGF-β) super gene family, including all of the bone morphogenetic proteins (BMPs), as well as platelet-derived growth factor, are triggered. The relationship between the proinflammatory cytokines and the triggering of these peptide signaling, growth-promoting molecules is unknown at this time.

Once the fracture healing events are initiated, the first 7 to 10 days of healing involve a process of chondrogenesis in which two major biochemical constituents are secreted: type II collagen and a variety of proteoglycans. Type II collagen provides the initial structure of the fracture callus while the proteoglycans mediate hydration of the newly formed tissue and control the rate and physical chemistry of the mineralization process. By 14 days, protein synthesis is complete and hypertrophic chondrocytes release calcium into the extracellular matrix in order to precipitate with phosphate ions.[34] High-energy phosphate bonds contained in phosphate esters in the extracellular matrix (e.g., ATP) are hydrolyzed by protein-degrading enzymes released from chondrocyte membranes. As proteoglycans inhibit mineralization, their degradation by these enzymes is a way by which chondrocytes control the rate and physical chemistry of this mineralization process. In simple terms, preliminary fracture callus is composed largely of cartilage; that cartilage must develop a critical mass before it is ready to calcify; that goal is achieved by the presence of proteoglycans, which prevent mineralization; and once enough cartilaginous callus is formed, mineralization takes place by the removal of the proteoglycan inhibitors.[37]

By 3 to 4 weeks after fracture, the callus is composed mostly of calcified cartilage, also known as *primary spongiosa* (Fig. 2-1). This tissue becomes a target for chondroclasts, multinucleated cells specialized in the resorption of calcified tissues. The removal of calcified cartilage includes not only resorption of the mineralized matrix but also removal of the chondrocytes themselves. Lee et al.[88] have shown that chondrocytes undergo programmed cell death (apoptosis) during endochondral fracture healing and this process is identical to that which occurs in the lower hypertrophic zone of the growth plate. Thus, the transition from cartilage to bone involves a highly programmed series of events involving cellular removal and matrix modification.

As chondroclasts remove the calcified cartilage, blood vessels penetrate the tissue and bring perivascular mesenchymal stem cells that differentiate into osteoprogenitor cells and then bone-forming osteoblasts. This remodeling of the primary spongiosa to secondary spongiosa, or woven bone, results in fracture union by approximately 28 to 35 days (Fig. 2-2). At this time, osteoclasts populate the tissue and remodel the callus, converting it to lamellar bone.

FIGURE 2-1 | *Low-power histologic image of fracture callus at 3 weeks after injury. Note the abundant calcified cartilage (primary spongiosa) (4 ×; all sections stained with Safranin O/fast green, which stains chondrogenic cells orange).*

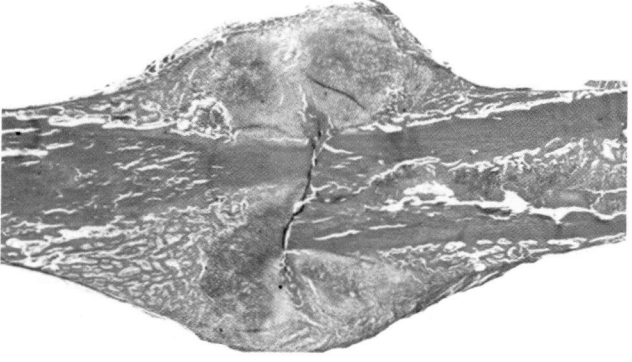

FIGURE 2-2 | *Low-power histologic image of fracture callus at 4 weeks after injury demonstrating remodeling of primary spongiosa to secondary spongiosa or woven bone (4 ×, Safranin O/fast green stain).*

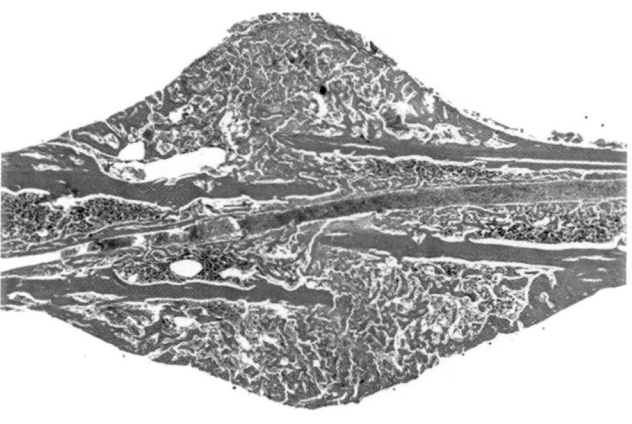

MOLECULAR MECHANISMS OF SKELETAL REPAIR: CURRENT KNOWLEDGE

Several growth factors and cytokines are involved in the process of skeletal tissue repair and remodeling. The function of these growth factors is to interact in a coordinated fashion and to influence each other's expression. A recent investigation by Cho et al.[19] studied the expression of members of the TGF-β superfamily during fracture healing. This family of growth factors, which includes all of the TGF-βs, BMPs, and growth and differentiation factors (GDFs), controls a number of processes during skeletal development and repair. In fracture healing, expression of BMP-2 and GDF-8 on the first day after fracture suggests their role as early response genes. BMP-2 most likely induces both chondrogenesis and periosteal osteogenesis, leading to the initiation of the endochondral healing response and intramembranous ossification. GDF-8, a known negative regulator of myogenic differentiation, may function to direct undifferentiated mesenchymal cells toward a chondro-osteogenic lineage as opposed to a myogenic pathway. GDF-5 and TGF-βs 2 and 3 show maximal expression on day 7 after fracture, suggesting their role during chondrogenesis. BMPs 3, 4, 7, and 8 show restricted expression between days 14 and 21, when calcification of callus cartilage is most active. Although these findings do not prove any specific function, the reproducible identification of expression at specific times after fracture suggests further experimentation to elucidate their roles.

The remodeling of fracture callus to form a mechanically competent structure is essential to the successful treatment of a skeletal injury. While the major cell type responsible for fracture callus remodeling is the osteoclast, it is the interaction between osteoblastic and osteoclastic function that leads to successful remodeling. Recent evidence suggests that cells in the osteoblastic lineage, including mesenchymal stromal cells, secrete factors that induce fully differentiated osteoblasts to express ligands that regulate the activity of osteoclasts. One of these, receptor activator of NFκB ligand (RANKL), has been shown to be essential in the development of osteoclast precursors. When the hemopoietic mononuclear osteoclast precursor binds the osteoblast through the interaction of RANKL and RANK, these mononuclear cells are induced to fuse and form multinucleated osteoclasts with bone-resorbing capacity. Recent data show that RANKL is expressed at very low levels in unfractured intact bone but is strongly induced by a fracture to increase its activity.[55] The co-regulation of this process takes place through the action of macrophage colony stimulating factor (M-CSF), which shows a peak in expression at day 14 after fracture, just before calcified cartilage removal begins. Research by Gerstenfeld et al.[55] using transgenic mice that are unable to express these molecules shows prolonged fracture healing with enlarged calluses and an inability to transition from a stage of calcified cartilage formation to the formation of bone.[55] Because many nonunions demonstrate the presence of a gritty, calcified cartilaginous tissue at the nonunion site, it is possible that deficiencies associated with fracture healing in humans are related to the failure of or mis-expression of some of these factors.

The events of fracture healing involve a well-coordinated series of events leading to chondrogenesis, the removal of calcified cartilage, its replacement with bone, and the remodeling of that bone to a lamellar bone structure with the capacity to support mechanical loads. While the molecular basis for fracture healing is far from understood, key regulators such as angiogenic factors (VEGF and Hif1-α), the chondrogenic and osteogenic factors (BMPs and GDFs), and the regulators of bone remodeling (members of the TNF-α family) are involved in a coordinated manner. The ability to further elucidate these mechanisms and to develop technologies to control their function could play an important role in the future of fracture management.

ENHANCEMENT OF FRACTURE HEALING

The enhancement of fracture repair can be broadly classified into *biological* and *physical* modalities. Biological stimulation involves the introduction of *osteoinductive, osteoconductive,* or *osteogenic* factors into the local environment, whereas physical perturbation includes electrical and ultrasound stimulation of the fracture site.

BIOLOGICAL METHODS
Bone Grafting

Each year, more than 2.2 million bone grafts are performed worldwide for treatment of delayed unions, failed joint replacements, spinal and long bone arthrodeses, limb salvage reconstructions for malignant bone tumors, and complex spine reconstructions for instability and deformity.[89] Autogenous bone graft is still considered the gold standard, as it naturally provides the basic components required to stimulate skeletal repair. These include osteoinductive growth factors, an osteoconductive extracellular matrix, and osteogenic stem cells present in bone marrow elements. *Osteoinduction* is the process by which

pluripotent mesenchymal stem cells are recruited from the surrounding host tissues and differentiate into bone-forming osteoprogenitor cells. This is mediated by graft-derived growth factors such as bone morphogenetic proteins and other signaling molecules such as platelet-derived growth factors, interleukins, fibroblast growth factors, and insulin-like growth factors.[129,139] An *osteoconductive* material is one that acts as a scaffold, supporting ingrowth of capillaries, perivascular tissue, and osteoprogenitor cells from the recipient bed. This occurs in an ordered sequence determined by the three-dimensional structure of the graft, the local blood supply, and the biomechanical forces exerted on the graft and surrounding tissues.[129] *Osteogenesis* refers to the process of bone formation. In terms of bone grafting, an osteogenic material is one that contains living cells capable of differentiating into bone.

Despite the effectiveness of autogenous bone graft, several shortcomings exist including donor site morbidity, nerve or arterial injury, and infection rates of 8 to 10 percent associated with graft harvesting.[5,46,60,144] These limitations have prompted the use of an alternative graft material such as allogeneic bone. However, despite its ready availability, the risk of disease transmission, diminished biologic and mechanical properties in comparison with autogenous bone, and increased cost have limited its use.[111] For these reasons, development of effective bone graft substitutes and strategies for tissue engineering of bone have led to a new field of study for the future of fracture management.

AUTOLOGOUS BONE

Autologous bone graft (also known as autograft, autogenous graft) is bone harvested from and implanted into the same individual and includes cancellous bone, cortical bone (nonvascularized and vascularized grafts), and bone marrow. Although much has been written about its use in skeletal reconstruction, relatively little attention has been paid to its application in the healing of fresh fractures.

The main contribution of the graft is as an osteoinductive and osteoconductive substrate. It provides the necessary physical and chemical properties to support the attachment, spreading, division, and differentiation of normal osteoblastic or osteoblast-like cells to form bone. The quality of the tissues at the host site, including their vascularity, is particularly important in influencing the rate and extent of graft union. An avascular bed or one that is deficient in endothelial or connective tissue cell precursors will be less able to respond to the osteoinductive and osteoconductive signals emanating from the graft. This may occur in patients who have undergone previous radiation therapy or who are exposed to a therapeutic or nontherapeutic agent such as glucocorticoid or nicotine, which impairs cell function. Moreover, if mechanical instability exists at the implantation site, granulation and fibrous tissue will develop at the graft-host interface, thereby preventing bony union.[7]

AUTOLOGOUS CANCELLOUS BONE GRAFT The host response to cancellous bone grafts differs from that to cortical bone in terms of its rate and completeness of repair. Cancellous bone, with its large surface area covered by quiescent lining cells or active osteoblasts, has the potential to induce more new bone than cortical bone.[49]

Bone formation and resorption occur concomitantly. Osteoblasts secrete osteoid onto the surface of necrotic bone, while osteoclasts gradually resorb the dead trabeculae. This process of *creeping substitution*[59] is characteristic of the late phase of autogenous cancellous bone grafting. Therefore, although a cancellous graft does not provide much, if any, immediate structural support, it incorporates quickly and is completely replaced by host bone and marrow after 1 year (Table 2-1).

Cancellous bone graft is usually harvested in fragments from sites such as the iliac crest, distal radius, greater trochanter, and proximal tibial and distal femoral metaphyses.[85,109] It is an excellent choice for the treatment of conditions that do not require structural integrity from the graft.[43,44,99] This was demonstrated by Ring and colleagues[116] in the treatment of 35 patients with atrophic diaphyseal nonunions of the forearm (16 radius, 11 with ulna, 8 both bones) with 3.5 mm plate and screw fixation with autogenous cancellous bone grafts. Segmental bone defects averaging 2.2 cm (range, 1–6 cm) were present in each patient. All fractures healed within 6 months, and after 43 months had achieved range of motion of 121° in the forearm, 131° at the elbow, and 137° at the wrist, with an average grip strength of 83 percent compared with the contralateral limb. The ability of autogenous bone to stimulate repair was further highlighted by Kesemenli et al.[79] in the treatment of 20 grade III open tibia fractures (8 grade IIIa, 11 grade IIIb, 1 grade IIIc) in patients who underwent primary autogenous bone grafting at the time of débridement and external fixator application. Two patients required myocutaneous flap coverage, 4 underwent delayed primary closure, and 14 were split skin grafted. After an average of 43 months follow-up, 1 patient experienced a delayed union and 1 developed an infection. Union occurred at an average of 28 weeks in the remaining fractures (range, 19–45 weeks), demonstrating that primary bone grafting performed at the time of skeletal stabilization enhances the speed to union without having an adverse affect on the infection rate.

AUTOLOGOUS CORTICAL BONE GRAFT Cortical bone grafts are usually harvested from the ribs, fibula, or shell of the ilium and can be transplanted with or without their vascular pedicle. They are mostly osteoconductive with few or no osteoinductive properties (Table 2-1). The thickness of the matrix of cortical bone limits the diffusion of nutrients to support the survival of any useful fraction of osteocytes after transplantation, thereby limiting its osteogenic properties.[29]

Cortical autografts proceed through a similar sequence of incorporation as seen with cancellous grafts. However, because of the density of cortical bone, the rate of revascularization is substantially slower.[15,58,115] This is more commonly seen with nonvascularized grafts, where vascular penetration is primarily the result of peripheral osteoclastic resorption and vascular invasion of Volkmann's and haversian canals.[42]

Vascularized cortical grafts function relatively independently of the host bed,[29] as they are implanted with their own functional blood supply. The three main sources for free vascularized bone grafts are the fibula, iliac crest, and rib. The fibula may be isolated on its peroneal vessels, the iliac crest graft uses the deep circumflex iliac artery and vein, and the rib uses the posterior intercostal artery and vein. Once the vessels are successfully anastomosed, greater than 90 percent of the osteocytes survive the transplantation procedure. Consequently, graft-host union occurs much more rapidly without substantial bone resorption and remodeling as is seen with nonvascularized grafts.[58] This lack of resorption and revascularization results in the vascularized grafts providing superior strength during the first 6 weeks after implantation.[29] As with cancellous bone, these grafts still require internal or external fixation to provide mechanical stability while they incorporate into the host bed.

Nonvascularized autologous cortical bone grafts can be used to treat segmental bone defects of up to 6 cm in length that require immediate structural support.[44] There are no definitive reports regarding the use of nonvascularized grafts for defects of between 6 and 12 cm in length. For defects greater than 12 cm, vascularized grafts are recommended.[54] The harvesting of these large grafts, however, is not without problems. Tang et al.[132] examined donor site morbidity in 39 patients with avascular necrosis of the femoral head treated by curettage and transplantation of free ipsilateral fibular grafts. Subjective complaints were common and included weakness of great toe flexion in 29 percent of patients while 43 percent experienced difficulty with toe extension.

AUTOLOGOUS BONE MARROW

Bone marrow contains osteogenic precursor cells[8,23] and may become a prime material in the future for use in tissue

Table 2-1			
Properties of Autologous Bone Grafts			
Property	**Cancellous Bone**	**Nonvascularized Cortical Bone**	**Vascularized Cortical Bone**
Osteoconduction	+++	+	+
Osteoinduction	++*	+/−	+/−
Osteoprogenitor cells	+++	−	+
Immediate strength	−	+++	+++
Strength at 6 mo	++	++, +++	+++
Strength at 1 yr	+++	+++	+++

*Although cancellous bone is widely believed to be osteoinductive, there is no evidence to critically demonstrate that inductive proteins and cytokines are active in autologous cancellous bone graft.
Reprinted with permission from Finkemeier, C.G. Bone grafting and bone graft substitutes. J Bone J Surg Am 2002,84:454–464.

engineering of bone.[104] In the treatment of bony defects, Connolly and Shindell[22] first reported its clinical use in the management of tibial nonunions. Injecting freshly harvested bone marrow into the defects resulted in clinical and radiographic union by 6 months. Others have described similar successes.[53,62] Khanal and colleagues[81] conducted a prospective study in which 40 patients with closed tibia shaft fractures were randomized to two injections of 15 mL of autologous bone marrow at the fracture site and casting or conventional casting. Bony union was determined by the lack of clinical tenderness and mobility at the fracture site as well as by plain radiographs at 3, 4, and 5 months of treatment. Results demonstrated a significant increase in the speed to union ($P=0.0004$) in the patients receiving bone marrow injections with similar complication rates and costs incurred compared with the control group.

One of the major setbacks associated with bone marrow use is its limited number of osteoprogenitor stem cells. Muschler et al.[103] noted that the mean prevalence of colony-forming units expressing alkaline phosphatase (CFU-APs), a marker of osteoblast progenitors, is 55 per million nucleated cells. These values undergo a significant age-related decline for both men and women ($P=0.002$). Muschler and co-workers[102] noted that the volume of aspirate used for grafting procedures also can affect the number of CFU-APs. As the aspirate volume increases, so does the number of CFU-APs. Contamination of the sample by peripheral blood, however, also grows as the aspiration volume increases. The investigators noted that an increase in the aspiration volume from 1 to 4 mL causes approximately a 50 percent decrease in the final concentration of CFU-APs. On the basis of these data, the authors recommended that the volume of aspiration from any one site should not be greater than 2 mL. In addition, four 1-mL aspirates will provide almost twice the number of CFU-APs as would one 4-mL aspirate.

Since the success of bone marrow grafting depends on the transfer of sufficient numbers of osteoprogenitor cells, investigators have tried to increase the concentrations of these cells. Takigami et al.[131] described a technique involving the use of a cell retention system that selectively retains osteoblastic stem cells and progenitors within an implantable graft material. Bone marrow aspirates from the posterior superior iliac spine are taken in 2-mL aliquots and made to flow through a customized allograft matrix using the selective cell retention processing system. The resulting graft–bone marrow composite can then be used as an adjunct to stimulate bone formation. In a series of four patients, the authors used this technique to treat tibial, clavicular, and femoral neck nonunions. Results demonstrated stimulation of bony repair, thereby providing surgeons with an alternative to iliac crest autograft, which eliminates pain, blood loss, and other surgical complications associated with autogenous bone graft harvesting. In a larger clinical series, Hernigou and co-workers[64] treated 60 atrophic tibial nonunions with 20 cm³ of autogenous concentrated bone marrow aspirates. The number of progenitor cells transplanted was estimated from the numbers of fibroblast colony-forming units. In the 53 successful unions, the bone marrow that had been injected contained greater than 1500 progenitor cells per cm³ at an average of $54,962\pm17,431$

progenitors. Of the 7 patients who did not heal, the concentration (634 ± 187 progenitors per cm³) and the total number of progenitor cells injected ($19,324 \pm 6843$) were significantly lower, suggesting that stem cell concentration is of vital importance for percutaneous autologous marrow injections to be effective.

ALLOGENEIC BONE

The use of allograft bone accounts for approximately one third of bone grafts performed in the United States.[11] It is an attractive alternative to autogenous bone because it avoids donor site morbidity and its relative abundance permits it to be tailored to fit the defect size. Despite its use in other areas of orthopaedics, such as in spinal surgery[32] and joint arthroplasty,[101] considerably less is known about its use in the repair of fresh fractures or nonunions. This may be in part related to the risk of blood-borne disease transmission[45] and suboptimal clinical results compared with autograft.[9] These findings may be attributed to storage and sterilization procedures such as freeze-drying or freezing that are used to lower disease transmission. Freeze-drying or lyophilization involves removal of water and vacuum packing of the tissue. Although this reduces the immunogenicity,[50] Pelker et al.[112] demonstrated that it also reduces the mechanical integrity of the graft, thereby reducing its load-bearing properties. In addition, freeze-drying reduces the allograft osteoinductive potential by inducing the death of its osteogenic cells. Freezing allografts to temperatures of $-60°C$ or below lowers their immunogenicity by diminishing the degradation of enzymes without altering the biomechanical properties.

DEMINERALIZED BONE MATRIX Allogeneic bone is available in many preparations including morselized and cancellous chips, corticocancellous and cortical grafts, osteochondral segments, and demineralized bone matrix (DBM).[44] DBM is produced by acid extraction of allograft bone.[138] It contains type I collagen, noncollagenous proteins, and osteoinductive growth factors but provides little structural support.[92] The bioavailability of the growth factors contained in DBM results in its greater osteoinductive potential than that of conventional allografts.[45] These properties can be affected by different storage, processing, and sterilization procedures.

Tiedeman et al.[134] reported a case series on the use of DBM in conjunction with bone marrow in the treatment of 48 patients with bony disorders such as comminuted fractures with associated bone loss. Of these 48 patients, 39 were available to follow up and review. Thirty of thirty-nine patients demonstrated bony union. Patients with fracture nonunion represented the most recalcitrant group clinically, with union being achieved in only 61 percent of these cases. Because no control patients were included in the study, the efficacy of the DBM–bone marrow composite could not be determined.

Numerous DBM formulations exist based on refinements of the manufacturing techniques. They are available as a freeze-dried powder, granules, gel, putty, and strips. All have osteoinductive effects in animal studies, but no randomized controlled trials have been performed in patients. However, since these materials were originally developed as reprocessed human tissues, clearance for marketing was achieved without the need for randomized controlled trials comparing their efficacy to autologous bone. For this reason, it is unclear how well any of these products perform as bone graft substitutes. Because currently marketed formulations of these products include carrier substances such as glycerol, the U.S. Food and Drug Administration (FDA) now plans to regulate DBM products as Class II medical devices. Currently marketed DBM products will most likely be reclassified using the 510K pathway requiring demonstration of substantial equivalence to a predicate device but still not requiring demonstration of efficacy comparable to that achieved with autologous bone graft.

Ziran and colleagues[147] compared the efficacy of two of the commercially available DBM formulations, Grafton and Orthoblast, in the treatment of long bone nonunions in patients who were reported to be heavy smokers (greater than a half-pack of cigarettes a day). Grafton was used in 25 patients and Orthoblast in 13 patients. Results demonstrated successful healing rates without the need for any other secondary procedures at 52 percent in the Grafton group compared with 85 percent in the Orthoblast treated patients. The authors propose that the unique thermal properties of the latter compound may enhance DBM osteoinduction, leading to the greater success rates.

BONE GRAFT SUBSTITUTES

The ideal bone graft substitute would provide scaffolding for osteoconduction, growth factors for osteoinduction, and progenitor cells for osteogenesis.[140] The currently available materials, including calcium phosphate ceramics, calcium sulfate, bioactive glass, biodegradable polymers,[89] recombinant human BMPs (OP-1 and BMP-2), and autologous bone marrow cells, each fulfil only one of these criteria. However, there is great interest in improving these materials, since the availability of an effective bone graft substitute would avoid some of the current limitations associated with the use of autologous bone.

CALCIUM PHOSPHATE CERAMICS Calcium phosphate ceramics are osteoconductive materials produced by a sintering process in which mineral salts are heated to over 1000°C. Sintering reduces the amount of carbonated apatite, an unstable and weakly soluble form of hydroxyapatite. A good osteoconductive scaffold should have the appropriate three-dimensional structure to allow for osteointegration and invasion by cells and blood vessels. It should also be biocompatible and biodegradable, with biomechanical properties similar to those of the surrounding bone. Many of the ceramics used as bone grafts enable osteoconduction to occur.[39,141] Despite this, their brittleness and poor tensile strength limit their use as bone graft materials.

The first clinical use of calcium phosphate ceramics for the repair of bony defects was reported by Albee in 1920.[2] Since then, several animal studies have reported favorable results. Despite these early experiments, it was not until the 1970s that calcium phosphates, and in particular hydroxyapatite, were synthesized, characterized, and used clinically.[72,95,118]

HYDROXYAPATITE From a functional perspective, calcium phosphate ceramics can be classified as slow- or rapid-resorbing ceramics.[45] Hydroxyapatite (HA) is a slow-resorbing compound derived from marine coral.[18] A simple hydrothermal treatment process converts it to the more mechanically stable hydroxyapatite form with pore diameters of between 200 and 500 μm, a structure similar to human trabecular bone.

Interpore (Interpore International, Irvine, CA) is a coralline hydroxyapatite and was the first calcium-phosphate-based bone graft substitute approved by the FDA. Bucholz et al.[14] investigated its use to treat tibial plateau fractures. Forty patients with metaphyseal defects needing operative reduction were randomized into a control group treated with autogenous bone graft or a group treated with Interpore hydroxyapatite. Indications for surgery included valgus instability of the knee secondary to a lateral tibial plateau fracture, varus instability due to a medial plateau injury, articular incongruence of 10 mm or greater, and translation of the major condylar fragment of more than 5 mm. After insertion of the graft, cortical fracture fragments were reduced and a standard AO interfragmentary screw and plate fixation device was used to stabilize the reduction. With an average of 15.4 months for the autograft and 34.5 months for the Interpore-treated groups, radiological and functional knee joint assessments revealed no differences between the two groups. No evidence of ceramic resorption was found in the radiographic follow-up 3 years following implantation, highlighting the potential use of HA as a bone filler.

In light of its ability to promote osseointegration, HA has been used as a coating of external fixator pins to enhance fixation.[100] In a highly loaded animal study, three tapered pins (uncoated, HA-coated, titanium-coated) were tested in terms of insertion and exertion torque. Results demonstrated a 13-fold increase in extraction torque of the HA-coated pins compared with uncoated pins and a 2-fold increase compared with titanium-coated pins. Extraction torque was significantly lower compared with the corresponding insertion torque in both the uncoated and titanium-coated pins, whereas with the HA pins, there was no difference between the extraction and insertion torque. The authors further conducted a prospective, randomized clinical study of osteoporotic wrist fractures and further demonstrated higher extraction torques of the HA-coated pins compared with standard pins ($P<0.0001$).

TRICALCIUM PHOSPHATE Tricalcium phosphate (TCP) is a fast-resorbing ceramic that undergoes partial conversion to HA once implanted into the body. The HA is resorbed more slowly and will remain in place for years.

Reports have demonstrated the efficacy of TCP as a bone graft substitute. McAndrew et al.[95] investigated the suitability of TCP to treat bony defects in a case series of 43 patients with 33 fractures and 13 nonunions. Patients were followed for an average of 1 year. Healing was demonstrated in 90 percent of the fracture patients and 85 percent of those with nonunions. Radiographic analysis showed complete resorption of TCP between 6 and 24 months after implantation.

CALCIUM PHOSPHATE–COLLAGEN COMPO-SITES Collagen is the most abundant protein in the extracellular matrix of bone and promotes mineral deposition by providing binding sites for matrix proteins. Types I and III collagen have been combined with HA, TCP, and autologous bone marrow to form a graft material devoid of structural support but able to function as an effective bone graft substitute or bone graft expander to augment fracture healing. This was demonstrated by Chapman et al.,[17] who conducted a multicenter prospective, randomized, controlled study comparing autogenous bone graft and a composite of bovine collagen, calcium phosphate, and autogenous bone marrow (Collagraft, Zimmer, Warsaw, IN) in the treatment of acute long bone fractures. Two hundred forty-nine fractures were grafted and followed for a minimum of 2 years. The authors observed no significant differences between the two treatment groups in terms of union rates, functional outcomes, and impairments of activities of daily living. The prevalence of complications was similar in the two groups except for higher infection rates in patients receiving autogenous bone grafts. Antibodies to the bovine collagen developed in 12 percent of patients in the Collagraft-treated group, but no specific allergic problems were identified. Similar results using this material have been reported by others.[26]

CALCIUM SULPHATE Calcium sulphate, or plaster of Paris, was first used as a bone filler in the early 1900s.[33] It acts as an osteoconductive material that completely resorbs as newly formed bone remodels and restores anatomic features and structural properties.

Moed et al.[98] investigated its ability as a bone graft substitute in a prospective nonrandomized clinical study for the treatment of acetabular fractures with intra-articular comminution, marginal impaction, or both. Thirty-one patients (32 fractures) were treated with calcium sulphate pellets. Radiographic analysis demonstrated that the majority of fractures healed successfully, with most of the pellets being replaced by bone. Two groups of investigators reported the use of calcium sulphate as a material that augments or extends the use of autologous bone graft. In a prospective nonrandomized multicenter study, Kelly et al.[77] treated 109 patients with bone defects with calcium sulphate pellets alone or mixed with bone marrow aspirate, demineralized bone, or autograft. After 6 months, radiographic results for all patients showed that 99 percent of the pellets were resorbed and 88 percent of the defects were filled with trabeculated bone. Borrelli et al.[10] treated 26 patients with persistent long bone nonunions or osseous defects after an open fracture with a mixture of autogenous iliac crest bone graft and medical-grade calcium sulphate. Twenty-two patients achieved healing after primary surgery, while a further two demonstrated union after a second procedure. Persistent nonunions were seen in two patients. Despite these encouraging reports, there have been no randomized, controlled trials to study the efficacy of calcium sulphate in the treatment of skeletal injuries.

CALCIUM PHOSPHATE CEMENTS Calcium phosphate cements (CPCs) can be used to fill bony defects in conjunction with the treatment of acute fractures. This involves the combination of inorganic calcium and phosphate to form an injectable paste that can be delivered into the fracture site. Under physiologic conditions, the material begins to harden within minutes, forming a mineral known as dahllite. By 12 hours, dahllite formation is nearly complete, providing the cement with an ultimate compressive strength of 55 MPa. Studies in animals have shown that it is remodeled in vivo and, in some cases, completely resorbed and replaced by host bone.[24] However, while CPCs are osteoconductive and therefore may seem to function as bone graft substitutes, their major contribution in the treatment of skeletal injuries is to function as adjuncts of fixation and thereby shorten the time to functional recovery and full weight-bearing.

Sanchez-Sotelo et al.[119] conducted a prospective, randomized controlled study examining the use of a commercially available calcium phosphate paste, Norian SRS (Norian, Cupertino, CA), in the treatment of distal radius fractures. One hundred ten patients, who were between 50 and 85 years of age and had sustained either an AO type A3 or C2 distal radius fracture, were enrolled. Patients were prospectively randomized to receive either closed reduction with a short arm cast for 6 weeks or closed reduction and stabilization with Norian SRS for 2 weeks. They were followed for a 12-month period and assessed by radiography, range of motion, and grip strength. The results showed improved functional and radiographic outcomes in the patients treated with Norian SRS. In a subsequent randomized, controlled study, Cassidy et al.[16] compared the use of Norian SRS and closed reduction versus closed reduction and application of a cast or external fixator in 323 patients with intra- or extra-articular fractures of the distal radius. Significant clinical differences were seen at 6 to 8 weeks postoperatively, with better grip strength, wrist and digit range of motion, and hand function and less swelling in the patients treated with Norian SRS. By 1 year, these differences had normalized.

In light of the promising results seen with distal radius fractures, Norian SRS has been used to treat other bony injuries. Schildhauer et al.[124] reported its use in the treatment of complex calcaneal fractures. Thirty-six joint depression fractures were treated with Norian SRS after standard open reduction and internal fixation. Patients were allowed to bear weight fully as early as 3 weeks postoperatively. Results demonstrated no statistical difference in clinical outcome scores in patients who bore full weight before or after 6 weeks postoperatively, suggesting that this cement may permit early full weight-bearing after treatment of this fracture.

Lobenhoffer and co-workers[91] used Norian SRS in the treatment of 26 tibial plateau fractures (OTA types B2, B3, and C3) followed for a mean period of 19.7 months. Successive radiographs were taken and clinical parameters measured using Lysholm's and Tegner's knee scores. Twenty-two fractures healed without any displacement or complications (two cases required early wound revision secondary to sterile drainage, and two cases developed partial loss of fracture reduction between 4 and 8 weeks postoperatively requiring revision surgery). The high mechanical strength of the cement allowed earlier weight-bearing after a mean postoperative period of 4.5 weeks. Similar results supporting the use of Norian SRS for filling metaphyseal defects in the treatment of displaced tibial plateau fractures have been reported by others[67] (Fig. 2-3).

Simpson and Keating[128] compared the use of Norian SRS and minimal internal fixation to buttress plating and bone grafting in 13 patients with lateral tibial plateau fractures. All patients were followed for a minimum of 1 year and compared in terms of operative time, quality of reduction, and maintenance of reduction. Compared with the buttress-plated patients, those treated with Norian SRS demonstrated quicker operative times (55 minutes Norian SRS vs. 101 minutes buttress plate), better anatomic reductions on postoperative radiographs (13 excellent reductions in Norian SRS vs. 9 in buttress plate), and less plateau depression at 1 year (0.7 mm with Norian SRS vs. 4 mm in buttress group).

More recently, Mattsson and colleagues[94] conducted a prospective randomized multicenter study of 112 unstable trochanteric fractures investigating whether the fixation using a sliding hip screw combined with Norian SRS could improve clinical, functional, and radiographic results compared with fractures treated with the sliding hip screw alone. Six weeks after surgery, patients in the Norian SRS group had significantly lower functional pain scores ($P<0.003$), improved activities of daily living (ADLs) ($P<0.05$), and improved SF-36 scores compared with the control patients. This trend continued for up to 6 months after surgery.

Growth Factors and Related Molecules

Growth factors are proteins secreted by cells that function as signaling molecules. They comprise a family of molecules having autocrine, paracrine, or endocrine effects on appropriate target cells. In addition to promoting cell differentiation, they have direct effects on cell adhesion, proliferation, and migration by modulating the synthesis of proteins, other growth factors, and receptors.[74]

BONE MORPHOGENETIC PROTEINS

Since the discovery of the osteoinductive properties of bone morphogenetic protein (BMP),[137] attention has focused on the role of these proteins in embryologic development and bone repair in the postnatal skeleton.[19,74,117] BMPs are a group of noncollagenous glycoproteins that belong to the TGF-β superfamily. They are synthesized locally and predominantly exert their effects by autocrine and paracrine mechanisms. Fifteen different human BMPs have been identified and their genes cloned.[28] For clinical applications, the most extensively studied among these are BMP-2 and BMP-7 (Osteogenic Protein 1).

The importance of BMPs in bone repair has been the subject of much investigation. Cho et al.[19] characterized the temporal expression of BMPs during murine fracture healing, defining specific periods when individual BMPs may exert important roles in normal skeletal repair. BMP-2 showed maximal expression on day 1 after fracture, suggesting its role as an early response gene in the cascade of healing events. BMP-3, -4, -7, and -8 exhibited a restricted period of expression from days 14 through 21, when the resorption of calcified cartilage and osteoblastic recruitment was most active. BMP-5 and -6 were constitutively expressed from days 3 to 21.

To determine whether BMPs are likely to play a key role during fracture healing in patients, Kloen et al.[82] demonstrated the presence of BMPs and their various receptors in human fracture callus. Tissue was obtained from the fracture site of malunions in five patients who were undergoing revision fracture treatment. Immunohistochemical analysis demonstrated consistent positive staining for all BMPs and receptors, with immunoreactivity most intense for BMP-3 and -7. These findings indicate that components of the BMP signaling cascade are expressed in human fracture callus and that modulation of the repair process may be mediated by BMP signaling.

Over the past 20 years, investigators have tested the use of purified or recombinant BMPs in the treatment of several musculoskeletal conditions.[87] While these studies have reported encouraging results, only two randomized, controlled studies and one subgroup analysis have been reported in the treatment of fractures.

In a large prospective, randomized, controlled, partially blinded, multicenter study, Friedlaender et al.[51] assessed the efficacy of rhBMP-7 (OP-1) versus iliac crest bone graft in the treatment of 122 patients with 124 tibial nonunions. All nonunions were at least 9 months old and had shown no progress toward healing for the 3 months prior to patient enrollment. Patients were randomized to receive either standard treatment with reduction and fixation with an intramedullary nail and autologous bone graft, or reduction and fixation with an intramedullary nail and implantation of rhBMP-7 (OP-1) on a type I collagen carrier. Nine months after surgery, 81 percent of the 63 patients treated with BMP-7 and 85 percent of 61 patients treated with autologous bone grafting had achieved clinical union. Radiographic assessments suggested healing in 75 and 84 percent of these patients, respectively. As these results

---

FIGURE 2-3 *Radiograph demonstrating the filling of a metaphyseal defect with Norian SRS in a tibial plateau fracture.*

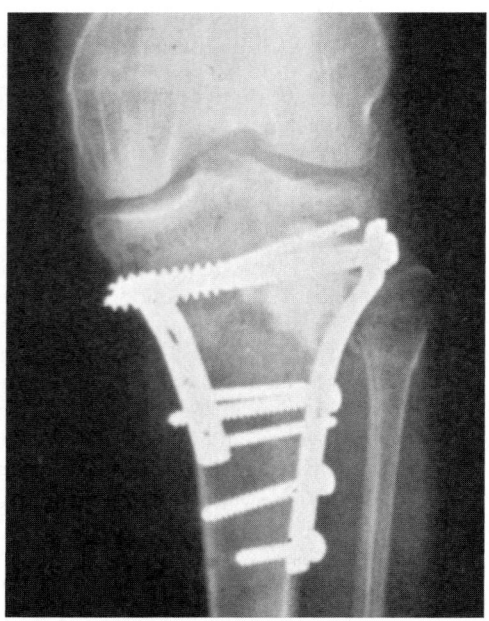

showed equivalent efficacy between OP-1 and autogenous bone graft, the authors concluded that OP-1 was a safe and effective alternative to bone graft in the treatment of tibial nonunions (Fig. 2-4).

Dimitriou et al.[31] reported on the use of recombinant BMP-7 on the treatment of persistent fracture nonunions in 25 patients with 10 tibial, 8 femoral, 3 humeral, 3 ulnar, 1 patellar, and 1 clavicular nonunion. The average number of procedures performed prior to using BMP-7 was 3.2, with autologous bone graft and bone marrow injections being used in 10 cases. Results demonstrated that BMP-7 application was associated with clinical and radiographic union in 24 (92.3%) of the cases, thereby providing further support for this compound as an adjunct to facilitate repair in challenging clinical conditions.

Recently, the BMP-2 Evaluation in Surgery for Tibial Trauma (BESTT) Study Group reported on a large prospective, randomized, controlled multicenter trial evaluating the effects of rhBMP-2 in the treatment of open tibial fractures.[61] Four hundred fifty patients with these injuries were randomized to receive either initial irrigation and débridement followed by treatment with intramedullary (IM) nail fixation alone or IM fixation plus an implant containing either 0.75 mg/kg or 1.5 mg/kg of rhBMP-2 at the time of definitive treatment. The implant was placed over the fracture site at the time of wound closure. After 1 year, there were fewer secondary interventions (returns to the operating room for additional treatment) in the group treated with 1.5 mg/kg rhBMP-2. In addition, those patients treated with 1.5 mg/kg rhBMP-2 had accelerated times to union, improved wound healing, and reduced infection rates (Fig. 2-5).

FIGURE 2-5 *Radiographs of a Gustilo-Anderson type IIIB tibia fracture treated with an unreamed intramedullary nail and a 1.50 mg/mL rhBMP-2 implant. The fracture was considered to be clinically healed by 20 weeks and radiographically healed by 26 weeks. (Reprinted with permission from Govender, S.; Csimma, C.; Genant H.K.; et al. Recombinant human bone morphogenetic protein 2 for treatment of open tibial fractures. A prospective, controlled, randomized study of four hundred and fifty patients. J Bone Joint Surg Am 2002, 84:2123–2134).*

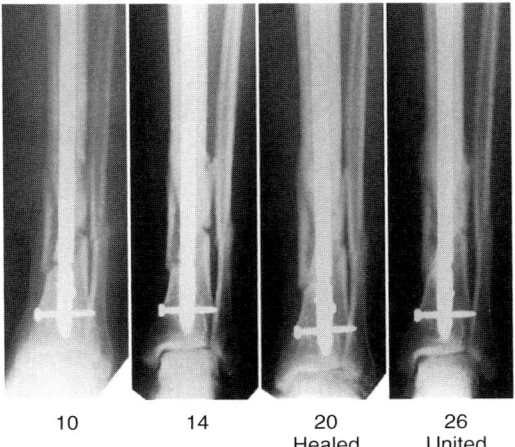

| 10 | 14 | 20 Healed | 26 United |

Swiontkowski et al.[130] conducted a subgroup analysis combining the data from two prospective, randomized studies of 510 patients with open tibia fractures who were treated with intramedullary nail fixation and routine soft tissue management with or without placement of an absorbable collagen sponge impregnated with rhBMP-2 over the fracture site at the time of definitive wound closure. The authors noted that in the 131 patients with Gustilo-Anderson type IIIA or IIIB open tibia fractures, patients who received rhBMP-2 had significantly better results with fewer bone grafting procedures ($P=0.0005$), fewer invasive secondary surgeries ($P=0.0065$), a lower infection rate ($P=0.0234$), and an earlier time to weight-bearing by an average of 32 days compared with the control group. In contrast, in the 113 patients treated with reamed intramedullary nailing, no significant difference was noted between the control and rhBMP-2 patients. These results appear to support the use of rhBMP-2 in the treatment of the more severe grade III injuries rather than in all open tibia fractures. Not only do these patients appear to demonstrate maximal clinical benefit but in a recent economic model based on the BESTT study, their treatment costs were reduced when rhBMP-2 was reserved for only type IIIA and IIIB tibia fractures.[75]

Despite these promising results, the outcomes in human studies are not so impressive as those seen in animals, where greater bone formation and healing has been noted. Diefenderfer et al.[30] noted that one reason may be

FIGURE 2-4 *Radiographs taken postoperatively at 9 months and 24 months later of a tibial nonunion treated with OP-1 (BMP-7). Note the abundant bridging callus resulting in tibial union. (Reprinted with permission from Friedlaender, G.E.; Perry, C.R.; Cole, J.D.; et al. Osteogenic protein 1 [bone morphogenetic protein 7] in the treatment of tibial nonunions. J Bone Joint Surg Am 2001; 83 Suppl 1[pt 2]:151–158.)*

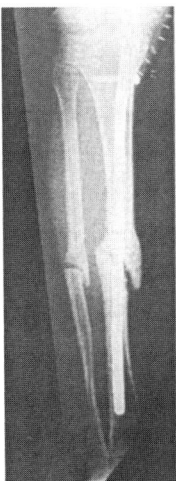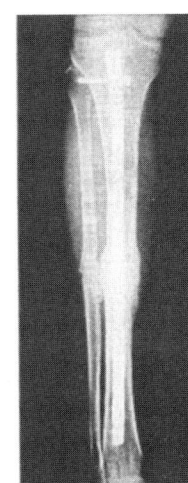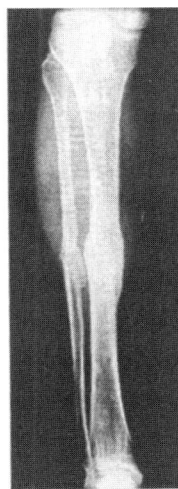

a differential response of human bone marrow stromal cells to BMPs. Bone marrow cells isolated from patients undergoing hip replacement were cultured, grown to confluence with or without dexamethasone, and treated with BMPs. The results demonstrated no significant osteogenic response to BMP-2, -4, or -7 as determined by alkaline phosphatase induction, unless cells were pretreated with dexamethasone. Moreover, even when cells were pretreated, the alkaline phosphatase response to BMPs was only about 50 percent of that measured in murine bone marrow cell cultures. The authors concluded that the ability of human bone marrow cells to respond to BMPs may differ substantially from that which exists in lower mammalian species.

TRANSFORMING GROWTH FACTOR BETA

Transforming growth factor-beta (TGF-β) influences a number of cell processes including the stimulation of mesenchymal stem cell (MSC) growth and differentiation and the enhancement of collagen and other extracellular matrix (ECM) protein synthesis, and it also functions as a chemotactic factor for fibroblast and macrophage recruitment.[80]

Lind et al.[90] tested two doses of TGF-β in rabbits in which tibial defects had undergone unilateral plate fixation. After 6 weeks of healing, mechanical testing showed improved bending stiffness only in the group treated with the low dose, and no improvement in the group treated with the high dose. Critchlow et al.[27] performed a study of tibial defect healing in rabbits to test the hypothesis that the anabolic effects of TGF-β on bony repair are dependent on the mechanical stability at the fracture site. Under stable mechanical conditions, a low dose of TGF-$β_2$ had an insignificant effect on callus development, whereas the higher dose led to a larger callus.

To elucidate a relationship between mitogens of the TGF-β superfamily and fracture repair, Zimmermann et al.[145] analyzed the serum concentrations of BMP-2, BMP-7, and TGF-$β_1$ in patients with delayed and normal fracture healing. One hundred three patients with diaphyseal long bone fractures were prospectively recruited and had blood samples taken at standardized time points over a 6-month period. Delayed union was diagnosed if there was impaired healing after 4 months. Results demonstrated an increase in TGF-$β_1$ serum levels up to 2 weeks after fracture in both groups with a return to normal values after 6 weeks of injury. In the patients with delayed union, however, the decline in serum concentration occurred much earlier, and by 4 weeks after trauma, serum TGF-$β_1$ levels were significantly lower in patients exhibiting impaired fracture healing. Serum levels of BMP-2 and -4 were below detection levels in all patients. These findings suggest that TGF-$β_1$ has an important role during fracture healing, with events during the consolidation phase being somewhat dependent on its concentration.

From these studies, TGF-β appears to have some efficacy in augmenting fracture healing; however, the effects are highly dose-dependent and not especially robust. To our knowledge, no studies are under way or planned to test the use of TGF-β in human fracture healing.

Systemic Enhancement
PARATHYROID HORMONE

Parathyroid hormone (PTH) is an 84-amino-acid polypeptide involved in the regulation of calcium and phosphate metabolism. Its role in mineral homeostasis is to increase serum calcium levels by enhancing gastrointestinal calcium absorption, increase renal calcium and phosphate reabsorption, liberate calcium from the skeleton in response to systemic needs, and participate in the regulation of vitamin D metabolism.[76] Although the effects of this hormone are usually associated with bone resorption, the responses of osteoclasts to PTH are most likely mediated via osteoblastic activity as receptors for PTH are found on osteoblast membranes.[76] Indeed, while continual exposure to PTH leads to an increase in osteoclast activity and density, intermittent exposure stimulates osteoblasts and results in an increase in bone formation.[65,114]

Clinically, PTH has been approved by the FDA for its use in the treatment of osteoporosis in postmenopausal women and men. Several recent clinical trials have demonstrated that daily systemic treatment with PTH increases bone mineral density (BMD) and reduces fracture risk in osteoporotic patients. In 2001, Neer et al.[107] published the results of a study of 1637 postmenopausal women with prior vertebral fractures who received either parathyroid hormone or placebo. Patients were evaluated based on the occurrence of new fractures and BMD measurements over a median observation period of 21 months. PTH treatment was associated with a significant reduction in the risk of both vertebral and nonvertebral fractures. Treatment with PTH also resulted in a significant dose-dependent increase in bone mineral density of the spine, total hip, femoral neck, and total body.

In light of the observed skeletogenic effects of intermittent PTH (1–34) administration, several investigators have begun to examine its impact upon fracture repair. Andreassen et al.[4] reported the results of the first study on the influence of intermittent PTH (1–34) administration on callus formation and mechanical strength in tibia fractures in healthy sexually mature adult rats after 40 days of healing. Compared with controls, fracture callus volume and mechanical properties were significantly enhanced within the PTH (1–34) treated animals. Similar outcomes have been reported by others.[3,4,66,106] Recently, Alkhiary et al.[3] investigated the effect of recombinant PTH on fracture healing in 270 rats that underwent standard, closed femoral fractures and received doses of PTH similar to those shown to be effective in the treatment of osteoporosis in postmenopausal women. Using biomechanical tests, histomorphometry, and quantitative microcomputed tomography, results demonstrated that daily systemic administration of both a 5 µg/kg/day and a 30 µg/kg/day dose enhanced fracture healing by increasing bone mineral density, bone mineral content, and total osseous tissue volume. These findings have supported the initiation of clinical trials to study the role of systemic administration of PTH (1–34) in fracture patients.

PHYSICAL ENHANCEMENT OF SKELETAL REPAIR

The mechanical environment has a direct impact on fracture healing. Direct mechanical perturbation as well as biophysical modalities such as electrical and ultrasound stimulation have been shown to affect fracture healing. To enhance fracture repair by these mechanical measures it is necessary to develop a fundamental understanding of the ways in which the mechanical environment impacts cellular and molecular signaling.

Mechanical Stimulation

The fracture repair process can be modulated by mechanical forces. By controlling the weight-bearing status of a limb, the resultant load at the fracture site will influence the stress environment. Sarmiento and associates[121] found that early weight-bearing accelerates the fracture healing process. Standardized femoral fractures were produced in rats and stabilized by nonrigid intramedullary fixation. The animals either were allowed to bear weight at an early stage or were kept non-weight-bearing by cast immobilization. Histologic, radiologic, and mechanical differences were present by the second week after fracture. These differences became progressively greater during the next 3 weeks. The authors attributed these findings to early mobilization facilitating the maturation of callus tissue produced by endochondral ossification.

Several investigators have attempted to modulate fracture healing by altering the mechanical strain environment. In a prospective, randomized clinical trial, Kenwright et al.[78] compared the effects of controlled axial micromotion on tibial diaphyseal fracture healing in patients who were treated with external fixation and stratified according to fracture severity and extent of soft tissue injury. A specially designed pneumatic pump was attached to the unilateral frame of one group of patients and delivered a cyclical axial displacement of 1.0 mm at 0.5 Hz for 20 to 30 minutes a day. Fracture healing was assessed clinically, radiologically, and by measurement of the mechanical stiffness of the fracture. Both clinical and mechanical healing were enhanced in the group subjected to micromovement, compared with those treated with frames without micromotion. The differences in healing times were statistically significant and independently related to the treatment method. There was no difference in complication rates between treatment groups.

DISTRACTION OSTEOGENESIS

Distraction osteogenesis generates new tissue through the application of tensile forces to developing callus via a controlled osteotomy.[21,68,69,97] It is characterized by three separate stages: (1) the latency phase that immediately follows osteotomy; (2) the active or distraction phase, which permits active separation of bony segments; and (3) the consolidation phase, in which active distraction has ended and healing of the callus begins.[70,122,133] The period of time for each stage varies depending on anatomic site and size of the osseous defect needing repair.

To delineate the molecular mechanisms by which distraction osteogenesis promotes new bone formation, Pacicca et al.[110] studied the expression of angiogenic factors during this process. They demonstrated the expression of several of these molecules localizing to the leading edge of the distraction gap, where nascent osteogenesis

was occurring. Expression of these factors was greatest during the active phase of distraction. Weiss et al.[142] further tried to delineate which angiogenic factors were involved during distraction by collecting the serum from patients undergoing callus distraction for limb lengthening and comparing it to the serum of osteotomy patients undergoing elective axis correction, prior to and up to 6 months after the procedures. During distraction, significantly elevated serum concentrations were recorded for proMMP1, MMP9, TIMP1, angiogenin, and VEGF, indicating that these may be the key regulatory factors during this process.

Several investigators have utilized the technique of distraction osteogenesis to stimulate new bone formation in the clinical setting. Kocaoglu et al.[83] treated 16 patients with hypertrophic nonunions with the Ilizarov distraction method (Fig. 2-6). All patients had at least 1 cm shortening, three patients had a deformity in one plane, and the remainder had a deformity in two planes. All nonunions healed at an average follow-up of 38.1 months, with correction of all preoperative length inequalities and limb angulation to normal anatomic alignment (Fig. 2-6). Sen et al.[126] reported on the efficacy of distraction in the management of patients with grade III open tibia fractures. Twenty-four patients who had open tibia fractures with bone (mean bone defect of 5 cm) and

FIGURE 2-6 *Radiographs of a 23-year-old woman with a hypertrophic nonunion of the distal femur with a history of a previous open reduction and internal fixation and a 13-month period of nonunion. **A,** Preoperative anteroposterior radiograph. **B,** Callus formation during distraction osteogenesis using an Ilizarov fixator. **C,** Three months after frame removal, the radiograph demonstrates correction of preoperative length inequalities and limb angulation to normal anatomic alignment. (Reprinted with permission from Kocaoglu, M.; Eralp, L.; Sen C.; et al. Management of stiff hypertrophic nonunions by distraction osteogenesis: a report of 16 cases. J Orthop Trauma 2003;17:543–548).*

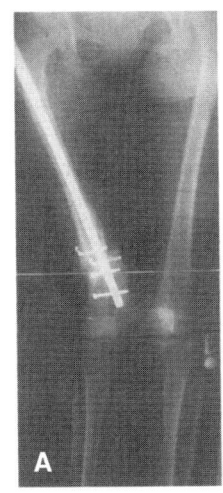
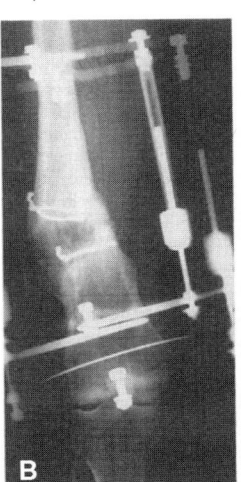
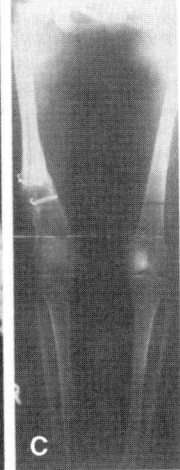

soft-tissue (mean, 2.5 × 3.5 cm) loss and a Mangled Extremity Severe Score of 6 and below were selected and treated with compression-distraction osteogenesis using the Ilizarov type circular external fixator. After an average of 30 months follow-up, bone assessment results were excellent in 21 and good in 3 patients. Functional assessment scores were excellent in 19, good in 4, and fair in 1 patient. These findings demonstrate that distraction osteogenesis is a safe, reliable, and successful method for the treatment of acute open tibia fractures with bone and soft-tissue loss.

Sangkaew[120] used the principles of distraction osteogenesis to treat 21 patients (9 infected open fractures, 12 infected nonunions) with tibial bone loss using a conventional external fixator. After corticotomy, the bone was distracted at 1 mm every 48 hours and patients were followed for a mean of 18.7 months (range, 6–108 months) after the frame was removed. Results showed that average new bone gained was 7.4 cm (range, 2–17 cm) with union being achieved with acceptable alignment (<7° angulation) and limb length difference (<2.5 cm) in 86 percent of patients. Total wound infection was resolved in 90.5 percent of patients with 11 of the 12 nonunions uniting. Eighteen patients had an excellent and three a good functional outcome.

Electrical Stimulation

Fukada and Yasuda[52] first reported the occurrence of piezoelectric potentials in mechanically loaded dry bone in 1957. Since then, many investigators have studied the influence of electrical stimulation on bone formation and growth.[12,48] Currently available devices for electrical stimulation can be categorized as one of three types: constant direct-current stimulation with the use of percutaneous or implanted electrodes (invasive), capacitive coupling (noninvasive), and time varying inductive coupling produced by a magnetic field (noninvasive). In direct-current stimulation, stainless steel cathodes are placed in the tissues and electrically induced osteogenesis exhibits a dose-response curve in relation to the amount of current that is delivered. Currents below a certain threshold result in no bone formation while those above a certain level lead to cellular necrosis.[47] With electromagnetic stimulation, an alternating current produced by externally applied coils leads to a time varying magnetic field that, in turn, induces a time varying electrical field in bone. In capacitative coupling, an electrical field is induced in bone by an external capacitor (i.e., two charged metal plates are placed on either side of a limb and are attached to a voltage source).[13]

In terms of its applicability to orthopaedics, electrical stimulation has primarily been used in the treatment of nonunions. Brighton and co-workers[13] reported on the treatment of 178 nonunions in 175 patients with direct current. Solid bone union was seen in 84 percent of patients. Patients with a history of osteomyelitis had a healing rate of nearly 75 percent. The presence of previously inserted metallic fixation devices did not affect the healing rate. When this study was expanded to include other centers, an additional 58 of 89 nonunions achieved similar results. Review of the nonunions treated unsuccessfully with constant direct current suggested that inadequate electricity, the presence of a synovial pseudarthrosis

or infection, and dislodgement of the electrodes were the causes of failure with this procedure. Complications of direct current were minor, and no deep infections resulting from this procedure in patients without previous osteomyelitis were noted. The authors concluded that given proper electrical parameters and proper cast immobilization, a rate of bone union comparable to that seen with bone-graft surgery was achieved.

Similar results were reported by Scott and King[126] in a prospective, double-blind trial using capacitive coupling in patients with established nonunions. In a population of 21 patients, 10 were actively managed and 11 were treated with a placebo unit. Results showed healing in 60 percent of the patients who had received electrical stimulation. None of the patients managed with the placebo unit demonstrated any bone formation.

Bassett et al.[6] reported on the use of pulsed electromagnetic fields (PEMF) in the treatment of un-united tibial diaphyseal fractures. One hundred twenty-five patients with 127 nonunions underwent long-leg plaster cast immobilization. Patients were treated with nonweight-bearing ambulation and a total of 10 hours of PEMF stimulation daily. The authors reported an overall fracture healing rate of 87 percent, with success being independent of the age or sex, number of previous surgeries, presence of infection, or metal fixation.

Despite the promising results seen in patients with nonunions, the application of this technology to the treatment of fresh fractures has not been clearly defined. Although some studies have shown that pulsed electromagnetic fields favorably influence fracture healing in experimental animals,[47] other studies have failed to demonstrate this effect.[1] At this time, there is a paucity of published clinical studies showing that electrical stimulation enhances the healing of fresh fractures.

An important question concerning the use of electrical stimulation for fractures is whether it is possible to accelerate repair when healing has been slow or when there is early evidence that a nonunion may be developing. Sharrard[127] conducted a double-blind, multicenter trial of the use of pulsed electromagnetic fields in patients who had developed delayed union of tibial fractures. Forty-five tibial fractures that had not united for more than 16 weeks but less than 32 weeks were treated with immobilization in a plaster cast that incorporated the coils of an electromagnetic stimulation unit. The unit was activated for 20 of these fractures and was not turned on for 25. Radiographs showed evidence of union in nine of the fractures that had had active electromagnetic stimulation and in only three of the fractures in the control group (P=0.02).

Ultrasound Stimulation

Low-intensity pulsed ultrasound (LIPUS) has been shown to promote fracture repair and increase the mechanical strength of fracture callus in both animal[113,143] and clinical studies.[63,86] In a prospective, randomized double-blind trial, Heckman et al.[63] examined the use of US as an adjunct to conventional treatment with a cast in 67 patients with closed or open grade I tibial shaft fractures. Thirty-three fractures were treated with the active device and thirty-four with placebo. Using clinical and radiographic criteria, the authors noted a statistically significant decrease in the time to union (86 ± 5.8 days in the US treatment group compared with 114 ± 10.4 days in the control group) and in the time to overall healing (96 ± 4.9 days in the US treatment group versus 154 ± 13.7 days in the controls). There were no issues with patient compliance in the treatment group and no serious complications reported with its use.

In a subsequent multicenter, prospective, randomized, double-blind study, Kristiansen and co-workers[86] evaluated the efficacy of LIPUS in the treatment of dorsally angulated distal radius fractures that had been treated with manipulation and a cast. Time to union was significantly shorter for the fractures that were treated with US compared with the controls (61 ± 3 days compared with 98 ± 5 days). The authors further noted that treatment with US was associated with a significantly smaller loss of reduction (20 ± 6% vs. 43 ± 8%) as determined by the degree of volar angulation as well as with a significant decrease in the mean time until the loss of reduction ceased (12 ± 4 days compared with 25 ± 4 days).

In a study by Cook et al.,[25] the ability of low-intensity US to accelerate the healing of tibial and distal radius fractures in smokers was evaluated. In this patient group, the usual healing time for tibial fractures was 175 ± 27 days and for distal radius fractures 98 ± 30 days. The investigators were able to show a statistically significant reduction in healing time with the use of US, with 103 ± 8.3 days reported in the tibial fracture group and 48 ± 5.1 days in the patients with distal radius fractures. Treatment with US also substantially reduced the incidence of delayed unions in tibias in smokers and nonsmokers. These results are important because they suggest that US can override some of the detrimental effects that smoking has on fracture healing.

In addition to enhancing the rate of fracture repair, ultrasound has been used as an adjunct to speed up the rate of distraction osteogenesis. El-Mowafi and Mohsen[40] treated 20 patients with tibial defects ranging from 5 to 8 cm with Ilizarov external fixators. After completing the distraction phase, 10 patients received daily 20-minute treatments of LIPUS onto the bone lengthening site, whereas rigid fixation was maintained in the remaining patients. The LIPUS group healed at 30 days (range, 27–36 days) while the control group united at 48 days (range, 42–75 days). Similar results have been reported by others,[135] suggesting that LIPUS is highly effective in accelerating the maturation of bone during the consolidation phase, thereby reducing the time of distraction osteogenesis.

In contrast to the above findings, Emami et al.[41] noted that ultrasound did not appear to have a stimulatory role on tibial fracture repair. In a prospective, randomized, double-blind controlled study, patients with fresh tibial fractures who were treated with a reamed and statically locked intramedullary rod were divided into an ultrasound group and a placebo group. They all used a US device 20 minutes daily for 75 days without knowing whether it was active or inactive. Standardized radiographs were taken every third week until healing and at 6 and 12 months. Results showed that low-intensity US treatment did not shorten the healing time.

CONCLUSION AND EXPECTATIONS

The process of fracture healing involves a well-coordinated series of events leading to a return of skeletal integrity and load-carrying capacity. With improved understanding of the key components involved in this delicate repair process, the field of tissue engineering is developing rapidly and expanding in its applications to stimulate healing when difficulties arise.

To date, strategies have met with limited success within the clinical setting. With ongoing research to enhance the osteogenic potential of cell concentrates and to develop better delivery systems and gene therapy applications for growth factors and osteoinductive substances, this technology will add to current treatment modalities and greatly enhance the management of musculoskeletal injuries and diseases in the future.

REFERENCES

1. Akai, M.; Yabuki, T.; Tateishi, T.; et al. Mechanical properties of the electrically stimulated callus: An experiment with constant direct current in rabbit fibulae. Clin Orthop 18(8):293–302, 1984.
2. Albee, F.H. Studies in bone growth: Triple CaP as a stimulus to osteogenesis. Ann Surg 71:32–36, 1920.
3. Alkhiary, Y.M.; Gerstenfeld, L.C.; Krall, E.; et al. Enhancement of experimental fracture healing by systemic administration of recombinant human parathyroid hormone (PTH 1–34). J Bone Joint Surg Am 87:731–741, 2005.
4. Andreassen, T.T.; Ejersted, C.; Oxlund, H. Intermittent parathyroid hormone (1-34) treatment increases callus formation and mechanical strength of healing rat fractures. J Bone Miner Res 14:960–968, 1999.
5. Banwart, J.C.; Asher, M.A.; Hassanein, R.S. Iliac crest bone graft harvest donor site morbidity: A statistical evaluation. Spine 20:1055–1060, 1995.
6. Bassett, C.A.L.; Mitchell, S.N.; Gaston, S.R. Treatment of ununited tibial diaphyseal fractures with pulsing electromagnetic fields. J Bone Joint Surg Am 63:511–523, 1981.
7. Bauer, T.W.; Muschler, G.F. Bone graft materials: An overview of the basic science. Clin Orthop 37(1):10–27, 2000.
8. Beresford, J.N. Osteogenic stem cells and the stromal system of bone and marrow. Clin Orthop 240:270–280, 1989.
9. Betz, R.R. Limitations of autograft and allograft: New synthetic solutions. Orthopaedics 25(5 suppl):561–570, 2002.
10. Borrelli, J., Jr.; Prickett, W.D.; Ricci, W.M. Treatment of nonunions and osseous defects with bone graft and calcium sulfate. Clin Orthop 41(1):245–254, 2003.
11. Boyce, T.; Edwards, J.; Scarborough, N. Allograft bone: The influence of processing on safety and performance. Orthop Clin North Am 30:571–581, 1999.

12. Brighton, C.T. Current concepts review: The treatment of nonunions with electricity. J Bone Joint Surg Am 63:847–851, 1981.

13. Brighton, C.T.; Black, J.; Friedenberg, Z.B.; et al. A multicenter study of the treatment of non-union with constant direct current. J Bone Joint Surg Am 63:2–131981.

14. Bucholz, R.W.; Carlton, A.; Holmes, R. Interporous hydroxyapatite as a bone graft substitute in tibial plateau fractures. Clin Orth Rel Res 240:53–62, 1989.

15. Burchardt, H. The biology of bone graft repair. Clin Orthop 42:28–42, 1983.

16. Cassidy, C.; Jupiter, J.B.; Cohen, M.; et al. Norian SRS cement compared with conventional fixation in distal radius fractures. J Bone Joint Surg Am 85:2127–2137, 2003.

17. Chapman, M.W.; Bucholz, R.; Cornell, C. Treatment of acute fractures with a collagen calcium phosphate graft material. J Bone Joint Surg Am 79:495–502, 1997.

18. Chiroff, R.T.; White, E.W.; Weber, K.N.; et al. Tissue ingrowth of replamineform implants. J Biomed Mater Res 9:29–45, 1975.

19. Cho, T.-J.; Gerstenfeld, L.C.; Einhorn, T.A. Differential temporal expression of members of the TGF-B superfamily during murine fracture healing. J Bone Miner Res 17:513–520, 2002.

20. Claes, L.; Augat, P.; Suger, G.; et al. Influence of size and stability of the osteotomy gap on success of fracture healing. J Orthop Res 15:577–584, 1997.

21. Codivilla, A. On the means of lengthening in the lower limbs, the muscles and tissues which are shortened through deformity. Am J Orthop Surg 2:353, 1905.

22. Connolly, J.F.; Shindell, R. Percutaneous marrow injection for an ununited tibia. Nebr Med J 71:105–107, 1986.

23. Connolly, J.F.; Guse, R.; Tiedeman, J.; et al. Autologous marrow injection as a substitute for operative grafting of tibial nonunions. Clin Orthop 266:259–270, 1991.

24. Constantz, B.R.; Ison, I.C.; Fulmer, M.T.; et al. Skeletal repair by in situ formation of the mineral phase of bone. Science 267:1796–1799, 1995.

25. Cook, S.D.; Ryaby, J.P.; McCabe, J.; et al. Acceleration of tibia and distal radius fracture healing in patients who smoke. Clin Orthop 337:198–207, 1997.

26. Cornell, C.N. Initial clinical experience with the use of Collagraft as a bone graft substitute. Tech Orthop 7:55, 1992.

27. Critchlow, M.A.; Bland, Y.S.; Ashhurst, D.E. The effect of exogenous transforming growth factor β2 on healing fractures in the rabbit. Bone 16:521–527, 1995.

28. Croteau, S.; Rauch, F.; Silvestri, A.; et al. Bone morphogenetic proteins in orthopaedics: From basic science to clinical practice. Orthopaedics 22:686–695, 1999.

29. Dell, P.C.; Burchardt, H.; Glowczewskie, F.P., Jr. A roentgenographic, biomechanical and histological evaluation of vascularized and non-vascularized segmental fibula canine autografts. J Bone Joint Surg Am 67:105–112, 1985.

30. Diefenderfer, D.L.; Osyczka, A.M.; Garino, J.P.; et al. Regulation of BMP induced transcription in cultured human bone marrow stromal cells. J Bone Joint Surg Am 85(Suppl 3):19–28, 2003.

31. Dimitriou, R.; Dahabreh, Z.; Katsoulis, E.; et al. Application of recombinant BMP-7 on persistent upper and lower limb nonunions. Injury 36(Suppl 4): S51–S59, 2005.

32. Dodd, C.A.F.; Fergusson, C.M.; Freedman, L.; et al. Allograft versus autograft bone in scoliosis surgery. J Bone Joint Surg Br 70:431–434, 1988.

33. Dreesman, H. Ueber Knochenplombierung. Bietr Klin Chir 9:804–810, 1892.

34. Einhorn, T.A. The cell and molecular biology of fracture healing. Clin Orthop 355:S7–S21, 1998.

35. Einhorn, T.A. Current concepts review: Enhancement of fracture healing. J Bone Joint Surg Am 77:940–956, 1995.

36. Einhorn, T.A.; Bonnarens, F.; Burnstein, A.H. The contributions of dietary protein and mineral to the healing of experimental fractures: A biomechanical study. J Bone Joint Surg Am 68:1389–1395, 1986.

37. Einhorn, T.A.; Hirschman, A.; Kaplan, C.; et al. Neutral protein-degrading enzymes in experimental fracture callus: A preliminary report. J Orthop Res 7:792–805, 1989.

38. Einhorn, T.A.; Majeska, R.J.; Rush, E.B.; et al. The expression of cytokine activity by fracture callus. J Bone Miner Res 10:1272–1281, 1995.

39. Ellies, L.G.; Nelson, D.G.; Featherstone, J.D. Crystallographic structure and surface morphology of sintered carbonated apatites. J Biomed Mater Res 22:541–553, 1988.

40. El-Mowafi, H.; Mohsen, M. The effect of low intensity pulsed ultrasound on callus maturation in tibial distraction osteogenesis. Int Orthop 29:121–124, 2005.

41. Emami, A.; Petren-Mallmin, M.; Larsson, S. No effect of low-intensity ultrasound on healing time of intramedullary fixed tibial fractures. J Orthop Trauma 13:252–257, 1999.

42. Enneking, W.F.; Burchardt, H.; Puhl, J.J.; et al. Physical and biological repair in dog cortical bone transplants. J Bone Joint Surg Am 57:237–252, 1975.

43. Enneking, W.F.; Eady, J.L.; Burchardt, H. Autogenous cortical bone grafts in the reconstruction of segmental skeletal defects. J Bone Joint Surg Am 62:1039–1058, 1980.

44. Finkemeier, C.G. Bone grafting and bone graft substitutes. J Bone Joint Surg Am 84:454–464, 2002.

45. Fleming, J.E., Jr.; Cornell, C.N.; Muschler, G.F. Bone cells and matrices in orthopaedic tissue engineering. Orthop Clin North Am 31:357–374, 2000.

46. Fowler, B.L.; Dall, B.E.; Rowe, D.E. Complications associated with harvesting autogenous iliac bone graft. Am J Orthop 24:895–903, 1995.

47. Friedenberg, Z.B.; Andrews, E.T.; Smolenski, B.I.; et al. Bone reaction to varying amounts of direct current. Surg Gynecol Obstet 131:890–891, 1970.

48. Friedenberg, Z.B.; Harlow, M.C.; Brighton, C.T. Healing of nonunion of the medial malleolus by means of direct current: A case report. J Trauma 11:883–885, 1971.

49. Friedlaender, G.E. Current concepts review: Bone grafts. J Bone Joint Surg Am 69:786–790, 1987.

50. Friedlaender, G.E. Immune responses to osteochondral allografts: Current knowledge and future directions. Clin Orthop 174:58–68, 1983.

51. Friedlaender, G.E.; Perry, C.R.; Cole, J.D.; et al. Osteogenic protein 1 (bone morphogenetic protein 7) in the treatment of tibial nonunions. J Bone Joint Surg Am 83:S151–S158, 2001.

52. Fukada, E.; Yasuda, I. On the piezoelectric effect of bone. J Phys Soc Japan 12:1158, 1957.

53. Garg, N.J.; Gaur, S.; Sharma, S. Percutaneous autogenous bone marrow grafting in 20 cases of ununited fracture. Acta Orthop Scand 64:671–672, 1993.

54. Gazdag, A.R.; Lane, J.M.; Glaser, D.; et al. Alternatives to autogenous bone graft: Efficacy and indications. J Am Acad Orthop Surg 3:1–8, 1995.

55. Gerstenfeld, L.C.; Cho, T.-J.; Kon, T.; et al. Impaired fracture healing in the absence of tumor necrosis factor-α signaling: The role of TNF-α in endochondral cartilage resorption. J Bone Miner Res 18:1584–1592, 2003.

56. Gerstenfeld, L.C.; Cullinane, D.M.; Barnes, G.L.; et al. Fracture healing as a post-natal development process: Molecular, spatial and temporal aspects of its regulation. J Cell Biochem 88:873–884, 2003.

57. Goldberg, V.M.; Shaffer, J.W.; Field, G.; et al. Biology of vascularized bone grafts. Orthop Clin North Am 18:179–185, 1987.

58. Goldberg, V.M.; Stevenson, S. The biology of bone grafts. Semin Arthroplasty 7:12, 1996.

59. Goldberg, V.M.; Stevenson, S.; Shaffer, J.W. Biology of autografts and allografts. In: Friedlaender, G.E.; Goldberg, V.M., eds. Bone and Clinical Applications. Park Ridge, IL, American Academy of Orthopaedic Surgeons, 1991, pp. 3–12.

60. Goulet, J.A.; Senunas, L.E.; DeSilva, G.L.; et al. Autogenous iliac crest bone graft: Complications and functional assessment. Clin Orthop 339:76–81, 1997.

61. Govender, S.; Csimma, C.; Genant, H.K.; et al. Recombinant human bone morphogenetic protein 2 for treatment of open tibial fractures: A prospective, controlled, randomized study of four hundred and fifty patients. J Bone Joint Surg Am 84:2123–2134, 2002.

62. Healey, J.H.; Zimmerman, P.A.; McDonnell, J.M.; et al. Percutaneous bone marrow grafting of delayed union and nonunion in cancer patients. Clin Orthop 256: 280–285, 1990.

63. Heckman, J.D.; Ryaby, J.P.; McCabe, J.; et al. Acceleration of tibial fracture-healing by non-invasive, low-intensity pulsed ultrasound. J Bone Joint Surg Am 76:26–34, 1994.

64. Hernigou, P.H.; Poignard, A.; Beaujean, F.; et al. Percutaneous autologous bone marrow grafting for nonunions. J Bone Joint Surg Am 87:1430–1437, 2005.

65. Hock, J.M.; Gera, I.J. Effects of continuous and intermittent administration and inhibition of resorption on the anabolic response of bone to parathyroid hormone. J Bone Miner Res 7:65–72, 1992.

66. Holzer, G.; Majeska, R.J.; Lundy, M.W.; et al. Parathyroid hormone enhances fracture healing: A preliminary report. Clin Orthop 366:258–263, 1999.

67. Horstmann, W.G.; Verheyen, C.C.; Leemans, R. An injectable calcium phosphate cement as a bone graft substitute in the treatment of displaced lateral tibial plateau fractures. Injury 34:141–144, 2003.

68. Ilizarov, G.A.; Khelimskii, A.M.; Saks, R.G. Characteristics of systemic growth regulation of the limbs under the effects of various factors influencing their growth and length [in Russian]. Ortop Travmatol Protez 8:37–41, 1978.

69. Ilizarov, G.A.; Pereslitskikh, P.F.; Barabash, A.P. Closed directed longitudino-oblique or spinal osteoclasia of the long tubular bones (experimental study) [in Russian]. Ortop Travmatol Protez 11:20–23, 1978.

70. Isefuko, S.; Joyner, C.J.; Simpson, H.R.W. A murine model of distraction osteogenesis. Bone 27:661–665, 2000.

71. Iwata, H.; Sakano, S.; Itoh, T.; et al. Demineralized bone matrix and native bone morphogenetic protein in orthopaedic surgery. Clin Orthop 395:99–109, 2002.

72. Jarcho, M.; Kay, J.; Gumaer, K.; et al. Tissue: Cellular and subcellular events at a bone-ceramic hydroxyapatite interface. J Bioengineering 1:79–92, 1977.

73. Jingushi, S.; Urabe, K.; Okazaki, K.; et al. Intramuscular bone induction by human recombinant bone morphogenetic protein 2 with beta tricalcium phosphate as a carrier: In vivo bone banking for muscle pedicle autograft. J Orthop Sci 7:490–494, 2002.

74. Johnson, E.E.; Urist, M.R.; Finerman, G.A. Repair of segmental defects of the tibia with cancellous bone grafts augmented with human bone morphogenetic protein: A preliminary report. Clin Orthop 236:249–257, 1988.

75. Jones, A.L.; Swiontkowski, M.F.; Polly, D.W.; et al. Use of rhBMP-2 in the treatment of open tibial shaft fractures: Do improved clinical outcomes outweigh the additional expense of rhBMP-2? Presented as a poster exhibit at the Annual Meeting of the Orthopaedic Trauma Association, October 8–10, 2004, Hollywood, FL.

76. Juppner, H.; Kronenberg, H.M. Parathyroid hormone. In: Favus, M.J., ed. Primer on the Metabolic Bone Diseases and Disorders of Mineral Metabolism, 5th ed. Washington, D.C., American Society for Bone and Mineral Research, 2003, pp. 117–124.

77. Kelly, C.M.; Wilkins, R.M.; Gitelis, S.; et al. The use of a surgical grade calcium sulfate as a bone graft substitute: Results of a multicenter trial. Clin Orth Rel Res 382:42–50, 2001.

78. Kenwright, J.; Richardson, J.B.; Cunningham, J. L.; et al. Axial movement and tibial fractures: A controlled randomised trial of treatment. J Bone Joint Surg Br 73:654–659, 1991.

79. Kesemenli, C.C.; Kapukaya, A.; Subasi, M.; et al. Early prophylactic autogenous bone grafting in type III open tibial fractures. Acta Orthop Belg 70:327–331, 2004.

80. Khan, S.N.; Bostrom, M.P.; Lane, J.M. Bone growth factors. Orthop Clinic 31:375–388, 2000.

81. Khanal, G.P.; Garg, M.; Singh, G.K. A prospective randomized trial of percutaneous marrow injection in a series of closed fresh tibial fractures. Int Orthop 28:167–170, 2004.

82. Kloen, P.; Di Paola, M.; Borens, O.; et al. BMP signaling components are expressed in human fracture callus. Bone 33:362–371, 2003.

83. Kocaoglu, M.; Eralp, L.; Sen, C.; et al. Management of stiff hypertrophic nonunions by distraction osteogenesis: A report of 16 cases. J Orthop Trauma 17:543–548, 2003.

84. Kon, T.; Cho, T.-J.; Aizawa, T.; et al. Expression of osteoprotegrin, receptor activator of NF-KB ligand (osteoprotegrin ligand) and related pro-inflammatory cytokines during fracture healing. J Bone Miner Res 16:1004–1014, 2001.

85. Krause, J.O.; Perry, C.R. Distal femur as a donor site of autogenous cancellous bone graft. J Orthop Trauma 9:145–151, 1995.

86. Kristiansen, T.K.; Ryaby, J.P.; McCabe, J.; et al. Accelerated healing of distal radial fractures with the use of specific, low-intensity ultrasound: A multicenter, prospective, randomized, double-blind, placebo-controlled study. J Bone Joint Surg Am 79:961–973, 1997.

87. Lee, F.Y.; Sinicropi, S.M.; Lee, F.S.; et al. Treatment of congenital pseudoarthrosis of the tibia with recombinant human bone morphogenetic protein-7 (rhBMP-7): A report of five cases. J Bone Joint Surg Am 88:627–633, 2006.

88. Lee, F.Y.H.; Choi, Y.W.; Behrens, F.F.; et al. Programmed removal of chondrocytes during endochondral fracture healing. J Orthop Res 16:144–150, 1998.

89. Lewandrowski, K.; Gresser, J.D.; Wise, D.L.; et al. Bioresorbable bone graft substitutes of different osteoconductivities: A histologic evaluation of osteointegration of poly(propylene glycol-co-fumaric acid)-based cement implants in rats. Biomaterials 21:757–764, 2000.

90. Lind, M.; Schumacker, B.; Soballe, K.; et al. Transforming growth factor β enhances fracture healing in rabbit tibiae. Acta Orthop Scand 64:553–556, 1993.

91. Lobenhoffer, P.; Gerich, T.; Witte, F.; et al. Use of an injectable calcium phosphate bone cement in the treatment of tibial plateau fractures: A prospective study of twenty six cases with twenty month mean follow-up. J Orthop Trauma 16:143–149, 2002.

92. Ludwig, S.C.; Boden, S.D. Osteoinductive bone graft substitutes for spinal fusion: A basic science summary. Orthop Clin North Am 30:635–645, 1999.

93. Macey, L.R.; Kana, S.M.; Jingushi, S.; et al. Defects of early fracture healing in experimental diabetes. J Bone Joint Surg Am 71:722–733, 1989.

94. Mattsson, P.; Alberts, A.; Dahlberg, G.; et al. Resorbable cement for the augmentation of internally fixed unstable trochanteric fractures. J Bone Joint Surg Br 87:1203–1209, 2005.

95. McAndrew, M.P.; Gorman, P.W.; Lange, T.A. Tricalcium phosphate as a bone graft substitute in trauma: Preliminary report. J Orthop Trauma 2:333–339, 1988.

96. McKibbin, B. The biology of fracture healing in long bones. J Bone Joint Surg Br 60:150–162, 1978.

97. Meyer, U.; Meyer, T.; Wiesmann, H.P.; et al. Mechanical tension in distraction osteogenesis regulates chondrocyte differentiation. Int J Oral Maxillofac Surg 30:522–530, 2001.

98. Moed, B.R.; Willson Carr, S.E.; Craig, J.G.; et al. Calcium sulfate used as bone graft substitute in acetabular fracture fixation. Clin Orthop 410:303–309, 2003.

99. Moore, J.R.; Weiland, A.J.; Daniel, R.K. Use of free vascularized bone grafts in the treatment of bone tumors. Clin Orthop 175:37–44, 1983.

100. Moroni, A.; Pegreffi, F.; Cadossi, M.; et al. Hydroxyapatite coated external fixation pins. Expert Rev Med Devices 2:465–471, 2005.

101. Moucha, C.S.; Einhorn, T.A. Enhancement of skeletal repair. In: Browner, B.D.; Jupiter, J.B.; Levine, A.M.; et al., eds. Skeletal Trauma: Basic Science, Management and Reconstruction, 3rd ed. Philadelphia, W.B. Saunders, 2003, p. 639.

102. Muschler, G.F.; Boehm, C.; Easley, K. Aspiration to obtain osteoblast progenitor cells from human bone marrow: The influence of aspiration volume. J Bone Joint Surg Am 79:1699–1709, 1997.

103. Muschler, G.F.; Nakamoto, C.; Griffith, L.G. Engineering principles of clinical cell-based tissue engineering. J Bone Joint Surg Am 86:1541–1558, 2004.

104. Muschler, G.F.; Nitto, H.; Boehm, C.A.; et al. Age- and gender-related changes in the cellularity of human bone marrow and the prevalence of osteoblastic progenitors. J Orthop Res 19:117–125, 2001.

105. Nakahara, H.; Bruder, S.P.; Haynesworth, S.E.; et al. Bone and cartilage formation in diffusion chambers by subcultured cells derived from the periosteum. Bone 11:181–188, 1990.

106. Nakajima, A.; Shimoji, N.; Shiomi, K.; et al. Mechanisms for the enhancement of fracture healing in rats treated with intermittent low-dose human parathyroid hormone (1-34). J Bone Miner Res 17:2038-2047, 2002.

107. Neer, R.M.; Arnaud, C.D.; Zanchetta, J.R.; et al. Effect of parathyroid hormone (1-34) on fractures and bone mineral density in postmenopausal women with osteoporosis. N Engl J Med 344:1434–1441, 2001.

108. Nicoll, E.A. Fractures of the tibial shaft: A survey of 705 cases. J Bone Joint Surg Br 46:373–387, 1964.

109. O'Keefe, R.M., Jr.; Riemer, B.L.; Butterfield, S.L. Harvesting of autogenous cancellous bone graft from the proximal tibial metaphysis: A review of 230 cases. J Orthop Trauma 5:469–474, 1991.

110. Pacicca, D.M.; Patel, N.; Lee, C.; et al. Expression of angiogenic factors during distraction osteogenesis. Bone 33:889–898, 2003.

111. Parikh, S.N. Bone graft substitutes: Past, present and future. J Postgrad Med 48:142–148, 2002.

112. Pelker, R.R.; Friedlaender, G.E.; Markham, T.C.; et al. Effects of freezing and freeze drying on the biomechanical properties of rat bone. J Orthop Res 1:405–411, 1984.

113. Pilla, A.A.; Mont, M.A.; Nasser, P.R.; et al. Noninvasive low-intensity pulsed ultrasound accelerates bone healing in the rabbit. J Orthop Trauma 4:246–253, 1990.

114. Podbesek, R.; Edouard, C.; Meunier, P.J.; et al. Effects of two treatment regimes with synthetic human parathyroid hormone fragment on bone formation and the tissue balance of trabecular bone in greyhounds. Endocrinology 112:1000–1006, 1983.

115. Ray, R.D. Vascularization of bone graft and implants. Clin Orthop 87:43–48, 1972.

116. Ring, D.; Allende, C.; Jafarnia, K.; et al. Ununited diaphyseal forearm fractures with segmental defects: Plate fixation and autogenous cancellous bone grafting. J Bone Joint Surg Am 86:2440–2445, 2004.

117. Ripamonti, U.; Duneas, N. Tissue morphogenesis and regeneration by bone morphogenetic proteins. Plast Reconstr Surg 101:227–239, 1998.

118. Roy, D.; Linnehan, S. Hydroxyapatite formed from coral skeletal carbonate by hydrothermal exchange. Nature 247:220–222, 1974.

119. Sanchez-Sotelo, J.; Munuera, L.; Madero, R. Treatment of fractures of the distal radius with a remodellable bone cement: A prospective, randomized study using Norian SRS. J Bone Joint Surg Br 82:856–863, 2000.

120. Sangkaew, C. Distraction osteogenesis with conventional external fixator for tibial bone loss. Int Orthop 28:171–175, 2004.

121. Sarmiento, A.; Schaeffer, J.F.; Beckerman, L.; et al. Fracture healing in rat femora as affected by functional weight-bearing. J Bone Joint Surg Am 59:369–375, 1977.

122. Sato, M.; et al. Mechanical tension stress induces expression of bone morphogenetic protein (BMP) 2 and BMP 4, but not BMP6, BMP7 and GDF5 mRNA during distraction osteogenesis. J Bone Miner Res 14:1084, 1999.

123. Schenck, R.; Willenegger, H. On the histological picture of so-called primary healing of pressure osteosynthesis in experimental osteotomies in the dog. Experientia 19:593–595, 1963.

124. Schildhauer, T.A.; Bauer, T.W.; Josten, C.; et al. Open reduction and augmentation of internal fixation with an injectable skeletal cement for the treatment of complex calcaneal fractures. J Orthop Trauma 14:309–317, 2000.

125. Scott, G.; King, J.B. A prospective, double-blind trial of electrical capacitive coupling in the treatment of non-union of long bones. J Bone Joint Surg Am 76:820–826, 1994.

126. Sen, C.; Kocaoglu, M.; Eralp, L.; et al. Bifocal compression-distraction in the acute treatment of grade III open tibia fractures with bone and soft-tissue loss: A report of 24 cases. J Orthop Trauma 18:150–157, 2004.

127. Sharrard, W.J.W. A double blind trial of pulsed electromagnetic fields for delayed union of tibial fractures. J Bone Joint Surg Br 72:347–355, 1990.

128. Simpson, D.; Keating, J.F. Outcome of tibial plateau fractures managed with calcium phosphate cement. Injury 35:913–918, 2004.

129. Stevenson, S. Biology of bone grafts. Orthop Clin North Am 39:543–552, 1999.

130. Swiontkowski, M.F.; Aro, H.T.; Donell, S.; et al. Recombinant human bone morphogenetic protein 2 in open tibial fractures: A subgroup analysis of data combined from two prospective randomized studies. J Bone Joint Surg Am 88:1258–1265, 2006.

131. Takigami, H.; Matsukura, Y.; Muschler, G.F. Osteoprogenitor cell enriched bone grafts prepared using selective cell retention technology: Clinical application in four patients. DePuy AcroMed, 2003.

132. Tang, C.L.; Mahoney, J.L.; McKee, M.D.; et al. Donor site morbidity following vascularized fibular grafting. Microsurgery 18:383–386, 1998.

133. Tay, B.K.; Le, A.X.; Gould, S.E.; et al. Histochemical and molecular analysis of distraction osteogenesis in a mouse model. J Orthop Res 16:636–642, 1998.

134. Tiedeman, J.J.; Garvin, K.L.; Kile, T.A.; et al. The role of a composite, demineralized bone matrix and bone marrow in the treatment of osseous defects. Orthopaedics 18:1153–1158, 1995.

135. Tsumaki, N.; Kakiuchi, M.; Sasaki, J.; et al. Low intensity pulsed ultrasound accelerates maturation of callus in patients treated with opening wedge high tibial osteotomy by hemicallotasis. J Bone Joint Surg Am 86:2399–2405, 2004.

136. Uhthoff, H.K.; Rahn, B.A. Healing patterns of metaphyseal fractures. Clin Orthop 160:295–303, 1981.

137. Urist, M.R. Bone: Formation by autoinduction. Science 150:893–899, 1965.

138. Urist, M.R.; Silverman, B.F.; Buring, K.; et al. The bone induction principle. Clin Orthop 53:243–283, 1967.

139. Urist, M.R. Bone transplants and implants. In: Urist, M.R., ed. Fundamental and Clinical Bone Physiology. Philadelphia, J.B. Lippincott, 1980, pp. 331–368.

140. Vaccaro, A.R. The role of the osteoconductive scaffold in synthetic bone graft. Orthopedics 25 (5 Suppl):s571–s578, 2002.

141. Vaes, G. Cellular biology and biochemical mechanism of bone resorption: A review of recent developments on the formation, activation and mode of action of osteoclasts. Clin Orthop 231:239–271, 1988.

142. Weiss, S.; Zimmermann, G.; Baumgart, R.; et al. Systemic regulation of angiogenesis and matrix degradation in bone regeneration: Distraction osteogenesis compared to rigid fracture healing. Bone 37:781–790, 2005.

143. Yang, K.H.; Parvizi, J.; Wang, S.J.; et al. Exposure to low-intensity ultrasound increases aggrecan gene expression in a rat femur fracture model. J Orthop Res 14:802–809, 1996.

144. Younger, E.M.; Chapman, M.W. Morbidity at bone graft donor sites. J Orthop Trauma 3:192–195, 1989.

145. Zimmermann, G.; Henle, P.; Kusswetter, M.; et al. TGF-beta1 as a marker of delayed fracture healing. Bone 36:779–785, 2005.

146. Ziran, B.; Cheung, S.; Smith, W.; et al. Comparative efficacy of 2 different demineralized bone matrix allografts in treating long bone nonunions in heavy tobacco smokers. Am J Orthop 34:329–332, 2005.

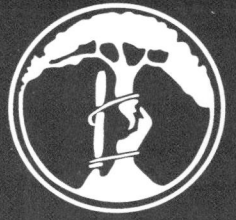

CHAPTER 3

Biomechanics of Fractures

John A. Hipp, Ph.D. and Wilson C. Hayes, Ph.D.

Bone is a remarkable material with complex mechanical properties and a unique ability for self-repair, making it a fascinating structural material from both clinical and engineering perspectives. Bone fails when overloaded, initiating a complex series of biological and biomechanical events directed toward repair and restoration of function. There are now tools that can help predict if a bone is likely to fail, with particular relevance to the problem of osteoporotic or pathologic fractures. Once a fracture has occurred, both the biological and mechanical environments must be controlled to optimize the healing process. Tremendous progress is being made toward understanding, controlling, and enhancing the biological aspects of fracture healing. The mechanical environment will always be a crucial element of fracture healing, with strong interactions between biological and mechanical factors. Clinical management of fractures must influence both the biological and mechanical conditions so that the original load-bearing capacity of the bone is restored as quickly as possible. There are thus three principal aspects to the biomechanics of fractures and their treatment: (1) the biomechanical factors that determine when and how a bone will fracture, (2) the biomechanical factors that influence fracture healing, and (3) control of the biomechanical environment by fracture treatments.

The biomechanical factors that determine whether a bone will fracture include the loads applied and the mechanical properties of bone and bone tissue. Humans engage in many activities resulting in a broad range of loads. For normal bone, the loads that result in fracture are typically extremes, whereas severely osteoporotic or pathologic bone may fracture during normal activities of daily living. In addition, the mechanical properties of bone vary over a wide range, and several pathological processes can alter bone properties. Therefore, our first objective is to review the mechanical properties of bone, the changes in mechanical properties that accompany aging and certain disease processes, and the fracture risk for normal and diseased bone.

Bone tissue possesses a unique ability for repair, frequently restoring the original load-bearing capacity in weeks to months. However, this repair process is influenced by the mechanical environment to which the healing bone is subjected and bone healing will fail under adverse conditions. The rate at which the load-bearing capacity is restored is affected by the stability of the fracture site. The second objective of this chapter is to review the biomechanics of fracture healing and the influence of the mechanical environment on the biology of fracture healing.

Successful fracture treatment requires control of both the biological and mechanical aspects of fracture healing. Different approaches to fracture treatment will control the mechanical environment in different ways and can influence the rate at which load-bearing capacity is restored. The third objective of this chapter is therefore to review the biomechanics of fracture treatment, particularly in relation to the stability these approaches provide to healing fractures. Fracture biomechanics; repair technology; and supporting scientific evidence that is specific to a unique region, such as the femur, tibia, distal radius, and so on, are covered in other chapters. This chapter deals with fracture repair concepts and supporting literature common to most all fractures. Methods that can help determine the optimal fracture treatment would be of great clinical benefit, and recent progress in computer simulation of fracture healing may help reach this goal. These measurements may help promote a fracture-healing process that provides the most rapid restoration of the load-bearing capacity. Quantitative measurements are being developed that may help determine the stability of a fracture and may also help determine the optimal timing for removal of fixation. The optimal treatment plan could be objectively selected by combining these measurements with known mechanical properties of a variety of fracture treatment approaches. The final objective is to review progress toward developing objective clinical tools for selecting and monitoring fracture treatment.

BONE PROPERTIES AND FRACTURE RISK

From a mechanical viewpoint, bone can be examined at two levels. At the first level, bone can be viewed as a material with mechanical properties that can be measured in the laboratory. These properties include the amount of deformation that occurs under load, the mechanism and rate at which damage accumulates in the bone, and the maximum loads that the material can tolerate before catastrophic failure. At a higher level, a bone can be viewed as a structure composed of a tissue organized into a geometry that has evolved for specific mechanical functions. Relevant structural properties include the amount of deformation that occurs during physiologic loading and the loads that cause failure either during a single load event or during cyclic loading. Both the material properties of bone as a tissue and the structural properties of bone as an organ determine the fracture resistance of bone and influence fracture healing. Thus, this section begins with a discussion of the relevant mechanical properties of bone as a material. This is followed by a review of the structural properties of whole bones. The section closes with a review of several important clinical applications in which the biomechanics of fracture and the risk of fracture have been studied.

Material Properties of Bone

CORTICAL BONE

The mechanical properties of bone tissue are typically determined by measuring the deformation of small, uniform specimens during application of simple, well-defined loads. Figure 3-1 illustrates a typical test that involves subjecting a machined cortical bone specimen to tensile loads. Dumbbell-shaped tensile specimens are typically used so that failure occurs in a reproducible location. Two parameters are monitored during the tensile test: (1) the applied force, and (2) the displacement between two points along the long axis of the specimen. The resulting force displacement curve provides an indication of the stiffness and failure load of the bone specimen, but the data are useful only for specimens with the same geometry as the one tested. To provide material property data that can be applied to any specimen geometry, the force and displacement data are converted to stress and strain. This is a normalization process that eliminates the influence of specimen geometry. The *stress* in the bone specimen is calculated as the applied force divided by the cross-sectional area, and the *strain* is measured as

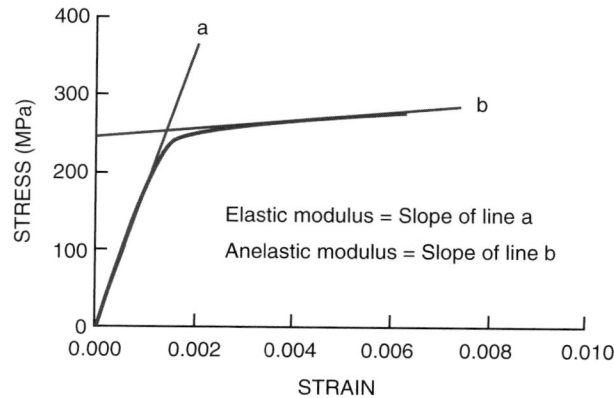

FIGURE 3-2 *Typical stress-strain curve for human cortical bone showing the curve regions where the elastic and anelastic moduli are calculated.*

Elastic modulus = Slope of line a

Anelastic modulus = Slope of line b

the percent change in length of a defined length of the specimen. A typical stress-strain curve for a tensile test of cortical bone is shown in Figure 3-2. The *elastic modulus* of bone tissue or structural materials such as stainless steel, titanium, or polymethylmethacrylate is determined from the slope of the initial, linear part of the curve. The point at which the slope of the stress-strain curve decreases and deviates from the initial linear behavior is the yield point of the bone, and the maximum recorded stress is the ultimate strength of the tissue. After the bone has yielded, the slope of the stress-strain curve drops to a new value termed the anelastic modulus.[70] The area under the stress-strain curve reflects the capacity of bone to absorb energy. The capacity to absorb energy increases with yield strength, but the greatest energy absorption is typically seen for bones with high ultimate strains, where substantial energy is absorbed during postyield deformation. Numerous published studies of bone tested under controlled loading conditions provide data to document the properties of cortical bone in tension, compression, torsion, and bending.

Bone is loaded cyclically during many activities of daily living, and the load that causes bone to fail can be dramatically lower if the load is applied repeatedly. The number of cycles of stress that bone can tolerate decreases as the stress level increases. This property of bone is measured using stress versus number of cycles to failure (SN) curves. These curves depend on the type of loading (axial, bending, or torsion), the loading rate, and the physical composition of the bone. The internal mechanisms in bone that determine its behavior under various loads are becoming understood.[32,95]

Several factors influence the material properties of cortical bone. For instance, the properties are dependent on the rate at which the bone tissue is loaded. Materials such as bone whose stress-strain characteristics are dependent on the applied strain rate are termed viscoelastic or time-dependent materials. However, the strain rate dependency of bone is relatively modest, with the elastic modulus and ultimate strength of bone approximately proportional to the strain rate raised to the 0.06 power[12] (Figs. 3-3 and 3-4). Over a

FIGURE 3-1 *Simple uniaxial tensile test with a dumbbell-shaped specimen. P is the applied load, and (L2 − L1)/L1 is the strain between two points along the specimen's axis.*

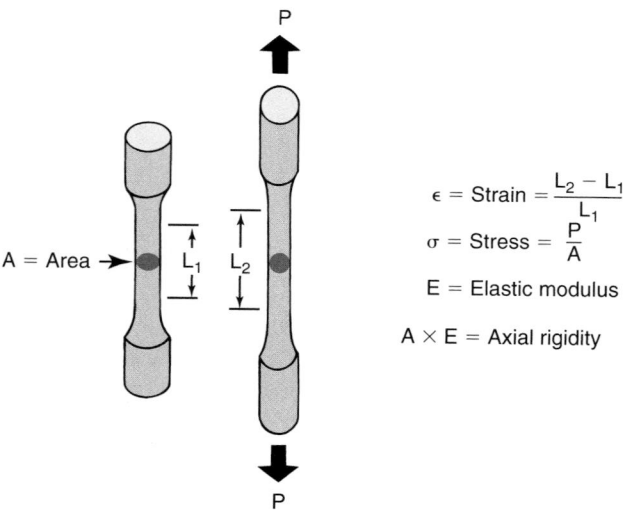

$\epsilon = \text{Strain} = \dfrac{L_2 - L_1}{L_1}$

$\sigma = \text{Stress} = \dfrac{P}{A}$

E = Elastic modulus

A × E = Axial rigidity

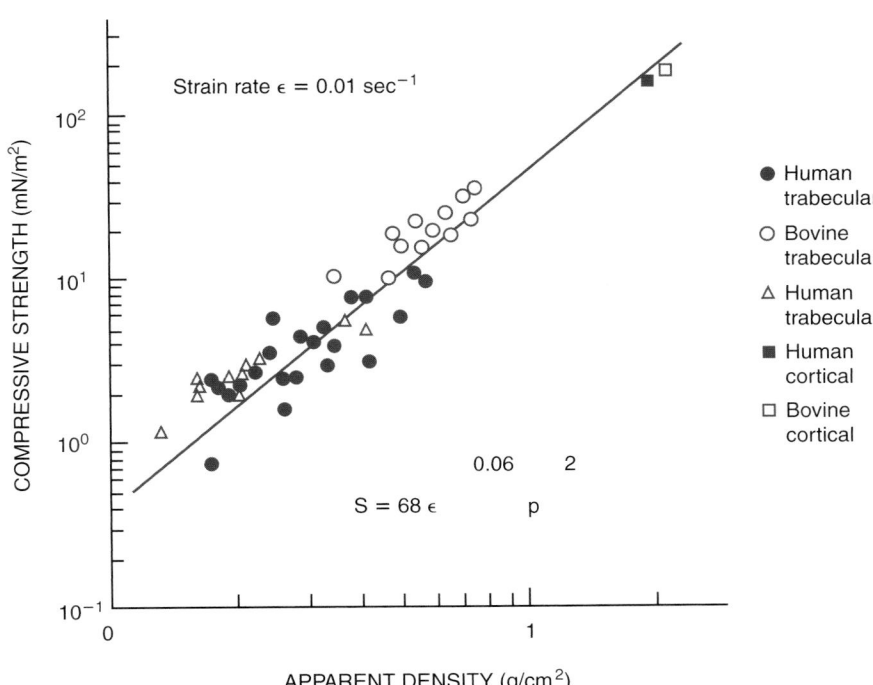

FIGURE 3-3 *Compressive strength as a function of apparent density for human and bovine trabecular and cortical bone. (Data from Carter, D.R.; Hayes, W.C. Bone compressive strength: the influence of density and strain rate. Science 194 (4270):1174–1176, 1976.)*

wide range of strain rates, the yield strength changes by 20 to 30 percent and can be predicted by computer models that represent the internal structure of bone.[98]

The stress-strain behavior of cortical bone is also strongly dependent on the orientation of bone microstructure with respect to the loading direction.[27] Several investigators have shown that cortical bone is both stronger and stiffer in the longitudinal direction (the predominate orientation of osteons) than in the transverse direction. Materials such as bone whose mechanical properties depend on

FIGURE 3-4 *Compressive modulus as a function of apparent density for human and bovine trabecular and cortical bone. (Data from Carter, D.R.; Hayes, W.C. The compressive behavior of bone as a two-phase porous structure. J Bone Joint Surg Am 59(7):954–962, 1977.)*

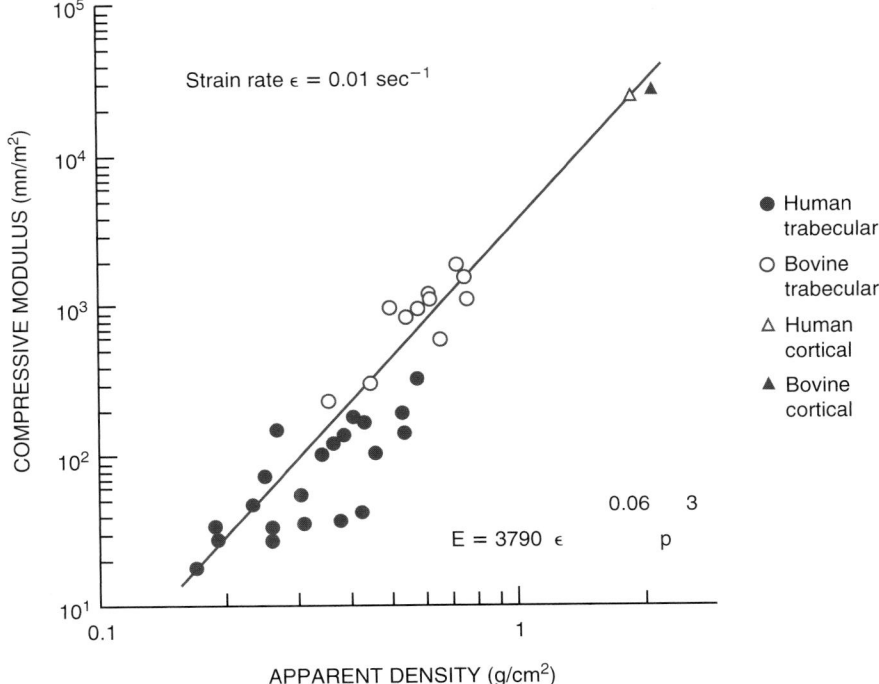

Table 3-1	
Anisotropic Material Properties for Human Cortical Bone*	
Loading Direction	**Modulus (GPa)**
Longitudinal	17.0
Transverse	11.5
Shear	3.3

*In comparison, moduli for common isotropic materials used in orthopedic implants are stainless steel, 207 GPa; titanium alloys, 127 GPa; bone cement, 2.8 GPa; ultra-high molecular weight polyethylene, 1.4 GPa.
Mean values from Reilly, D.T.; Burstein, A.H. The elastic and ultimate properties of compact bone tissue. J Biomech 8(6):393–405, 1975.

the loading direction are said to be anisotropic. The anisotropy and viscoelasticity of bone distinguish it as a complex material, and both the strain rate and loading direction must be specified when describing the material properties of bone tissue. Table 3–1 provides representative anisotropic material properties for human cortical bone, and ultimate strengths of cortical bone from adult femora for longitudinal and transverse loads are summarized in Table 3–2.

TRABECULAR BONE

The major physical difference between trabecular bone and cortical bone is the increased porosity exhibited by trabecular bone. The bone tissue that makes up the individual trabeculae is just slightly less stiff and strong than the bone tissue within cortical bone.[6] This increased porosity is quantified by measurements of the apparent density (i.e., the mass of bone tissue divided by the bulk volume of the test specimen, including mineralized bone and marrow spaces). In the human skeleton, the apparent density of trabecular bone ranges from approximately 0.1 g/cm^3 to 1.0 g/cm^3, while the apparent density of cortical bone is about 1.8 g/cm^3. A trabecular bone specimen with an apparent density of 0.2 g/cm^3 has a porosity of about 90 percent.

The compressive stress-strain properties of trabecular bone are markedly different from those of cortical bone and are similar to the compressive behavior of many porous engineering materials that absorb energy on impact.[89] Stress-strain curves (Fig. 3-5) for trabecular

Table 3-2	
Ultimate Strength Values for Human Femoral Cortical Bone	
Ultimate Loading Mode	**Strength (MPa)***
Longitudinal	
Tension	135 (15.6)
Compression	205 (17.3)
Shear	71 (2.6)
Transverse	
Tension	53 (10.7)
Compression	131 (20.7)

*Standard deviations in parentheses.
Mean values from Reilly, D.T.; Burstein, A.H. The elastic and ultimate properties of compact bone tissue. J Biomech 8(6):393–405, 1975.

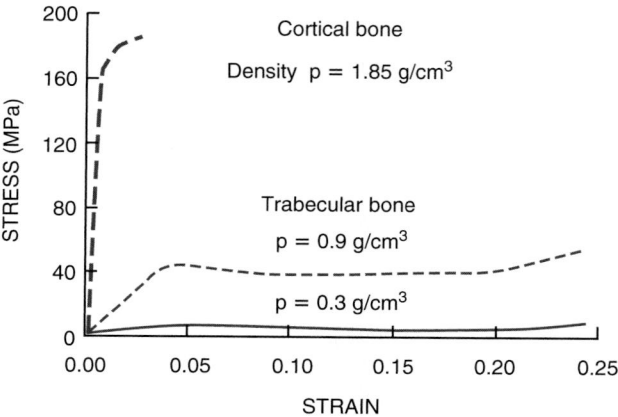

FIGURE 3-5 | *Compressive stress-strain curves for cortical and trabecular bone of different densities.*

bone in compression exhibit an initial elastic region followed by yield. The slope of the initial elastic region ranges from one to two orders of magnitude less than cortical bone. Yield is followed by a long plateau region created as more trabeculae fracture. The fractured trabeculae begin to fill the marrow spaces at approximately 50 percent strain. Further loading of the specimen after the pores are filled is associated with a marked increase in specimen modulus.

Both the compressive strength and compressive modulus of trabecular bone are markedly influenced by the apparent density of the tissue (see Figs. 3-3 and 3-4). The regressions presented in Figures 3-3 and 3-4 include cortical bone, with an apparent density of approximately 1.8 g/cm^3, as well as trabecular bone specimens from several species representing a wide range of apparent densities.[13] Since the early work in this area, many studies have shown a highly significant relationship between bone density and mechanical properties. However, it has also been shown by many investigators that density alone cannot predict all of the variation in the mechanical properties and that the way the bone is organized and the variations in the internal structure of tissue within the bone are also important determinants of the strength and stiffness of bone.[41]

These relationships between mechanical properties and the apparent density of bone tissue are important. First, they suggest that bone tissue can generate large changes in modulus and strength through small changes in bone density. Conversely, subtle changes in bone density result in large differences in strength and modulus. This is an important consideration when we note that bone density changes are usually not radiographically evident until the bone density has been reduced by 30 to 50 percent. The power law relationships of Figures 3-3 and 3-4 indicate that such reductions in bone density result in nearly an order of magnitude reduction in bone stiffness and strength.

Structural Properties of Whole Bones

When the skeleton is exposed to trauma, some regions are subjected to extreme loads. Fracture occurs when the local stresses or strains exceed the ultimate strength or strain of bone in that region. Bone fracture can therefore be viewed as an event that is initiated at the material level and then affects the load-bearing capacity of bone at the structural level. The major difference between behavior at the material level and at the structural level relates to inclusion of geometric features at the structural level and their exclusion at the material level. Thus, the structural behavior includes the effects of both bone geometry and material properties, whereas material behavior occurs without the effects of complex bone geometries. Any attempt to predict the structural behavior of a skeletal region must therefore reflect both the material properties of different types of bone in that region and the geometric arrangement of the bone.

There are several aspects of bone cross-sectional geometry, such as cross-sectional area and moment of inertia, that can be used to predict the structural properties. The cross-sectional area is straightforward. Subjected to axial loads and assuming similar bone material properties, a large, thick-walled bone is more resistant to fracture simply because it distributes the internal forces over a larger surface area, resulting in lower stresses. The moment of inertia expresses the shape of the cross-section and the particular distribution of tissue or material with respect to applied bending loads. The moment of inertia must be expressed in relation to a particular axis, since bending can occur in many different planes. Equations for calculating the moment of inertia of several regular geometric cross-sections are shown in Figure 3-6. From these equations, it is apparent that the moment of inertia is highly sensitive to the distribution of area with respect to an axis. Material that is at a greater distance from the axis is more efficient at resisting bending with respect to that axis. A simple example of this principal is that a yardstick turned on an edge is more resistant to bending than when turned horizontally.

FIGURE 3-6 *Some simple geometric cross-sections and the corresponding formulas for calculating the moments of inertia with respect to the x-axis.*

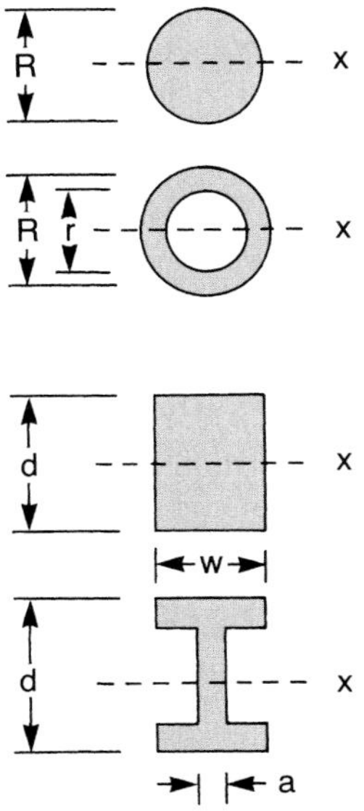

$$I_{xx} = \pi r^4/4$$

$$I_{xx} = \pi(R^4 - r^4)/4$$

$$I_{xx} = wd^3/12$$

$$I_{xx} = \frac{wd^3 - (w - a)(d - 2a)^3}{12}$$

An I-beam is a particularly efficient cross-sectional shape for resisting bending in one direction, since it distributes most of its area at a great distance from the bending axis.

If bones were subjected to bending in only one direction, their cross-sectional area probably would have evolved to something like an I-beam. Instead, long bones are loaded by axial loads, bending in several planes, and torsion. Under these conditions, a semitubular structure is most efficient. Diaphyseal bone cross-sectional geometries are roughly tubular in some regions but highly irregular elsewhere. The moment of inertia for an irregular bone cross-section can be determined from traces of the periosteal and endosteal surfaces by means of simple numerical techniques.[64] The moment of inertia partially determines the risk of fracture. For example, small cross-sectional areas and moments of inertia of the femoral and tibial diaphysis predispose military trainees to stress fractures.[9]

Although bones are typically subjected to a variety of complex loads, it is instructive to evaluate the strength of a bone or fracture treatment method for simple, well-defined loads. Three types of loading are typically considered in laboratory experiments: axial, bending, and torsion. For each load case, the behavior of the structure is described by a rigidity term that is a combination of both material stiffness (represented by a modulus) and a geometric factor (area or moment of inertia). Structures with high rigidity deform little under a load. For axial loads, the important parameters that govern the mechanical behavior of a structure are the cross-sectional area and the modulus of elasticity (see Fig. 3-1). The product of area and modulus is the axial rigidity. For bending, the applied loads are expressed as a moment with dimensions of force times distance. The important structural parameters in a bending test are the moment of inertia and the elastic modulus (Fig. 3-7), and their product is the bending (or flexural) rigidity. Torsional loads are also expressed as a force times a distance. The cross-sectional distribution of bone and the shear modulus of bone determine the torsional properties (Fig. 3-8). Just as the moment of inertia describes the distribution of material about the bending axis, for a cylindrical bone, the polar moment of inertia describes the distribution of material about the long axis of the structure being tested. The product of shear modulus and polar moment of inertia gives the torsional rigidity. For noncircular cross-sections, and structures with cross-sections that vary along the length, a simple polar moment of inertia can be inaccurate. For these structures, various formulae and simple analytical models can be used to calculate the structural properties under torsional loads.[58]

The various loading modes that occur in whole bones can result in characteristic fracture patterns (Fig. 3-9). When loaded in tension, diaphyseal bone normally fractures owing to tensile stresses along a plane that is approximately perpendicular to the direction of loading. When loaded in compression, a bone will typically fail along planes that are oblique to the bone's long axis. With compressive loads, high shear stresses develop along oblique planes that are oriented at about 45 degrees from the long axis. These maximum shear stresses are approximately one half the applied compressive stress. However,

FIGURE 3-7   *Representation of a four-point bending test of a beam. The original shape is shown by the dashed line while the deformed shape is indicated by the solid lines (deformations are exaggerated).*

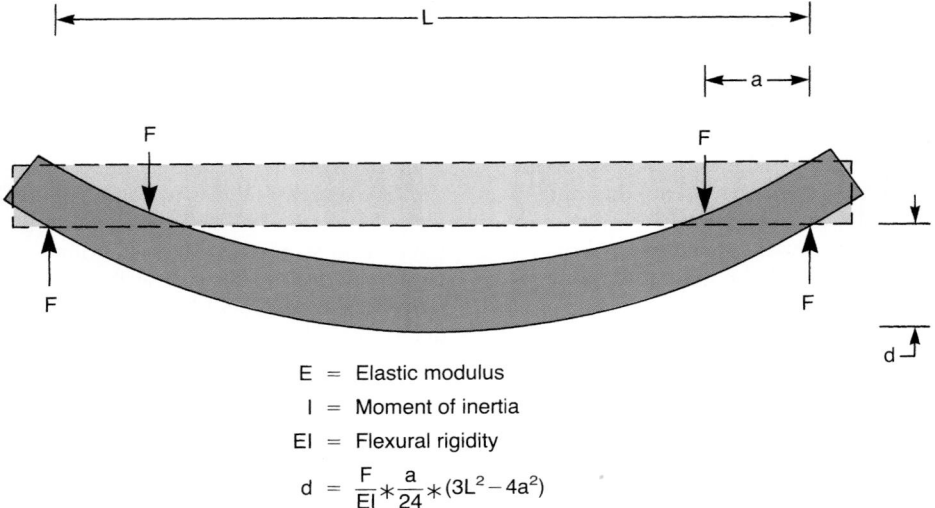

$$E = \text{Elastic modulus}$$
$$I = \text{Moment of inertia}$$
$$EI = \text{Flexural rigidity}$$
$$d = \frac{F}{EI} * \frac{a}{24} * (3L^2 - 4a^2)$$

since the shear strength of cortical bone is much less than the compressive strength (Table 3–2), fracture occurs along the oblique plane of maximum shear. Thus, compressive failures of bone occur along planes of maximum shear stress while tensile fractures occur along planes of maximum tensile stress.

When a bone is subjected to bending, high tensile stresses develop on the convex side, while high compressive stresses develop on the concave side. The resulting fracture pattern is consistent with that observed during axial compressive and tensile loading of whole bones. A transverse fracture surface occurs on the tensile side, while an oblique fracture surface is found on the compressive side. Two fracture surfaces commonly occur on the compressive side, creating a loose wedge of bone that is sometimes referred to as a "butterfly" fragment. The fracture pattern is more complex when a bone is subject to torsion. Fractures usually begin at a small defect at the bone surface and then the crack follows a spiral pattern through the bone along planes of high tensile stress. The final fracture surface appears as an oblique spiral that characterizes it as a torsion fracture.

The fracture patterns discussed for idealized loading conditions are consistent with some fractures seen clinically. However, with many traumatic loading conditions, bone is subject to a combination of axial, bending, and torsional loading, and the resulting fracture patterns can be complex combinations of the above patterns. Additionally, high loading rates often result in additional comminution of the fracture caused by the branching and propagation of numerous fracture planes. Bone may tolerate higher loads if the loads are applied rapidly,[23] although the ability of bone to absorb energy may not change with loading rate. In addition, fractures can occur owing to a single load that is greater than the load-bearing capacity of the bone, and these loads are commonly called the ultimate failure load. Repeated application of loads smaller than the ultimate failure load can fatigue the bone, resulting in the accumulation of microcracks in the bone, and can eventually lead to failure.[3] Fatigue failures of bone are common in military training and in athletes. If the loading is stopped or sufficiently reduced before gross failure of the bone, then each microcrack will be repaired through direct cortical remodeling.

Engineering tools that were originally developed to design bridges, cars, and so on, provide powerful tools to study the structural mechanics of bone, skeletal fractures, and fracture treatments. Valuable insight into the biomechanics of fractures can be obtained with simple analytical models that can be solved on paper with the help of a calculator.[87] However, the most commonly applied engineering tool is the finite element method. The finite element

FIGURE 3-8   *Simple torsion test of a cylinder. The angular deformation is indicated along with relevant formulae.*

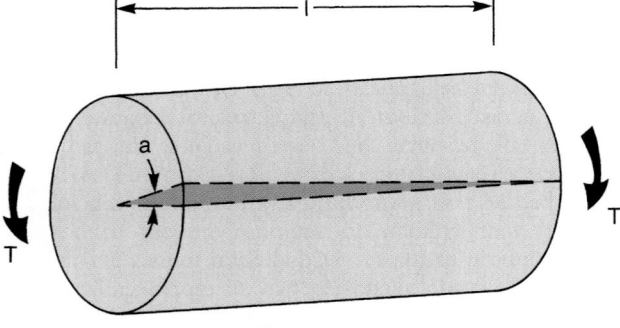

$$T = \text{Torque}$$
$$G = \text{Shear modulus}$$
$$J = \text{Polar moment of inertia}$$
$$GJ = \text{Torsional rigidity}$$
$$a/l = T/GJ$$

FIGURE 3-9 | *Characteristic fractures typically found for bones loaded to failure with "pure" loading modes.*

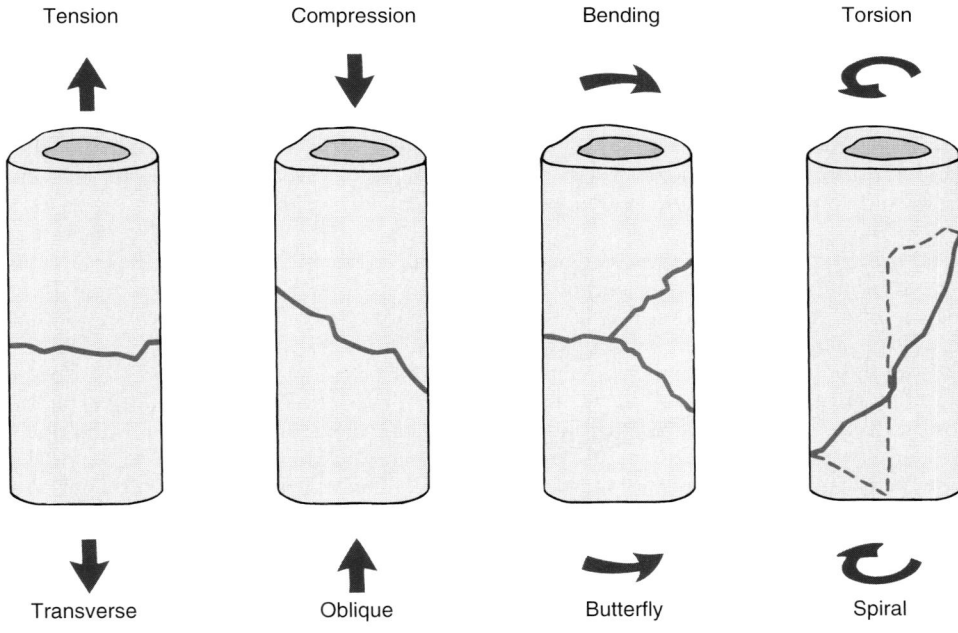

method is a powerful engineering modeling tool that is routinely used to investigate complex structures subject to varied loads and supports. The method involves forming a mathematical model of the bone from small elements of simple geometry (such as bricks or tetrahedrons). Figure 3-10 shows representative views of a finite element mesh used to model the proximal femur. The material properties of each element are specified along with the applied loads and support conditions. The model is then analyzed by a computer to predict the deformations and stresses within the structure. Thus, the behavior of bone at both the material and structural levels can be investigated using the finite element method. The finite element method allows parametric investigation of material properties, geometry, and loading conditions and has been applied in many orthopaedic biomechanical analyses.[63] Several applications of the finite element method in orthopaedic biomechanics will be discussed in this chapter. In particular, the finite element method is being developed as a useful method for understanding and predicting fracture risk and for simulating bone remodeling under a range of conditions.

Age-related and Pathological Bone Property Changes

With increasing age, the mechanical properties of bone tissue slowly degrade while geometric changes provide additional alterations to the structural characteristics of bones. Age-related changes occur in both cortical and trabecular bone, and changes in both regions can result in increased fracture risk. Changes in bone mineral mass, density, mechanical properties, and histology associated with aging have been the subject of intensive investigation. The picture to emerge from this research is a progressive net loss of bone mass with aging, becoming of clinical importance in the fifth decade and proceeding at a faster rate among women. Concurrent with this general loss of bone mass, bone tissue becomes more brittle and less able to absorb energy. The major clinical consequence of these skeletal changes is an age-related increase in fracture incidence.

At the tissue level, several age-related changes in the material properties of femoral cortical bone have been demonstrated.[99] A small decrease in elastic modulus

FIGURE 3-10 | *Different views of a finite element mesh of a proximal femur. (Adapted from J. C. Lotz, Ph.D. dissertation, Massachusetts Institute of Technology, 1988.)*

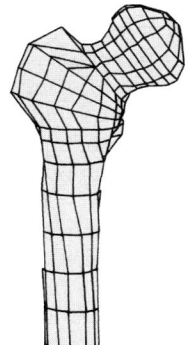 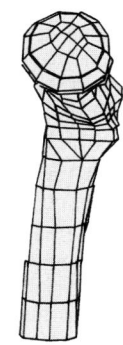 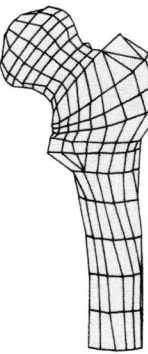

occurs with age (2.3% per decade), but the most significant change occurs in the ease with which a fracture progresses through bone. With aging, the ultimate strength decreases at approximately 4 percent per decade. The energy required to fracture a bone is reflected in the area under the stress-strain curve. Since the elastic modulus does not decrease as much, the energy to failure is predominantly reduced by age-related decreases in ultimate strain. Thus, with aging, the bone behaves more like a brittle material, and the capacity of bone to absorb the energy and resist fracture propagation from a traumatic event decreases.

Studies of skeletal aging typically focus on bone density and often do not consider the overall geometry and distribution of bone tissue. In a study of femoral density and geometry of thousands of men and women, a loss of bone density was clearly seen in both sexes, in both the femoral neck and in the diaphysis. In addition, the femurs expanded in periosteal diameter, but the cortical thickness decreased. When density and geometry were factored together into a parameter called the section modulus, it was shown that males tend to maintain overall structural properties past the fifth decade of life, but losses were recorded in women after the fifth decade.[8] Compared with bone changes that have been measured from the bones of past civilizations, bone properties have declined relative to body size, suggesting that relatively low activity levels of modern civilization may not stimulate optimal bone remodeling throughout life and thus may contribute to higher fracture risk in the contemporary aged.[25]

The preceding discussion examined age-related changes in cortical bone. Trabecular bone plays an important structural role in many bones, and the age-related changes in trabecular bone clearly contribute to the increased fracture risk in the elderly. Trabecular structure and the changes that can occur with aging have been extensively studied. Even in young people, there are wide variations in trabecular bone between individuals and between anatomic sites within an individual. The important variables include the thickness of trabeculae, the orientation of trabeculae with respect to the primary loading direction(s), the spacing between vertebrae, the morphology of the trabeculae (rods vs. plates), and how the vertebrae are connected together. All these variables have been studied by multiple investigators.[48] Although the primary focus of most of this research has been to understand osteoporosis, the knowledge gained is also being used to help design implants and in tissue engineering. Quantitative studies of trabecular bone morphology document that the thickness of trabeculae decreases while the spacing between trabeculae increases. There are surprisingly few fundamental differences in trabecular bone between the sexes other than that bone is lost faster in females between the ages of 50 and 85. These age-related morphological changes significantly reduce the strength of vertebrae, the proximal femur, and other bones, contributing to the observed increased fracture incidence in the elderly.

Fracture Risk

A bone will fail when the applied loads exceed the load-bearing capacity, so both the applied loads and the load-bearing capacity must be known to calculate fracture risk. Most structures, such as a bridge or a building, are designed to withstand loads several times greater than expected. Similarly, the normal human skeleton can support loads much higher than expected during activities of daily living. The ratio of load-bearing capacity over load-bearing requirement is frequently termed the safety factor. The inverse of this ratio has been termed the factor of risk for fracture. For loads approximating the midstance phase of gait, the average load-bearing capacity of mature and osteoporotic human femurs averages around 9000 N (2000 lb) with a standard deviation of around 3000 N.[19] Peak loads at the hip joint have been recorded to be as high as 3 to 5 times body weight during high-demand activities such as stair-climbing. Therefore, a 600 N (140 lb) individual who applies 5 times body weight to his or her femur has a femoral load-bearing capacity from less than 1 to 5 times as strong as needed, depending on the properties of the femur. For the tibia, axial loads while walking are estimated to be 3 to 6 times body weight,[83] and the greatest bending moment applied during restricted weight-bearing is estimated to be about 79 newton-meters in men.[57] Intact human tibiae loaded in three-point bending failed at from 57.9 to 294 newton-meters, so the bending strength of the tibia is also 1 to 4 times the maximum applied bending loads. The maximum torque that the tibia can tolerate was estimated to be about 29 newton-meters. Under torsional loads, tibiae failed at from 27.5 to 89.2 newton-meters, and this is 1 to 3 times the maximum applied torques. These calculations are only valid for particular types of loading. Nevertheless, these estimated factors of risk may help determine when a healing femoral fracture can tolerate moderate weight-bearing, or when a femur with a bone defect requires prophylactic stabilization.

There are several groups in whom fractures are prevalent and for whom prevention may be possible if fracture mechanisms and the patients at greatest risk can be identified. One group is the growing aged population in which age-related fractures are prevalent. Another group is cancer patients with metastatic bone disease in which prophylactic stabilization of impending fractures may increase the patients' quality of life. The next few sections will discuss the fracture risk and methods for predicting fracture risk due to aging and metastatic bone lesions.

FRACTURE RISK WITH OSTEOPOROSIS

The epidemiology of age-related fractures suggests a relation between osteoporosis and increased fracture risk, and the risk factors associated with hip fractures have been the subject of much research. The effects of age and gender have been documented, but these factors are confounded by comorbid conditions and an increased propensity for falls in the elderly.[77] Fractures related to osteoporosis are commonly associated with falls, and the frequency of falls increases with age, and this increase is partially associated with comorbid conditions and associated medications. Additionally, falls are more common in elderly women than men, and fracture rates are also greater in women than men.[72] Common sites for fall-related fractures are the proximal femur and distal forearm. Vertebral fractures are also frequently associated with traumatic loading such as backward falls, although relatively nontraumatic vertebral fractures may be much more common than nontraumatic femoral fractures.

When age- and sex-specific incidence rates are compared for all major fractures of different skeletal regions, considerable variability is observed. This may in part be due to varying proportions of cortical and trabecular bone at different sites and to the difference in pattern of bone loss of these two types.[73] The type and direction of loads during a fall (Fig. 3-11) are quite different from the loads during activities of daily living. Since the femur is adapted to support activities of daily living, it may be particularly sensitive to the abnormal loads during a fall. These factors emphasize both the complex interactions that occur between age-related bone loss and skeletal trauma and the need for improved understanding of the biomechanics of fracture risk in specific skeletal sites. Reduced skeletal resistance to trauma and the increased propensity for falling are co-factors in determining hip fracture risk. This leads to the conclusion that both bone loss and trauma are necessary, but not independently sufficient, causes of age-related hip fractures.

Fractures of the proximal femur are a significant public health problem and a major cause of mortality and morbidity among the elderly,[49] and attempts to reduce the incidence of age-related hip fractures have primarily focused on preventing or inhibiting excessive bone loss associated with osteoporosis. As a result, many noninvasive measures of bone density have been developed in the hope of identifying individuals with the greatest fracture risk. Ex vivo studies have shown that the load-bearing capacity of the proximal femur can be predicted from measurements of bone density and femoral geometry.[19,62] Excellent correlation was found between the ultimate failure load and quantitative computed tomography (CT) measurements made at intertrochanteric sites[62] (Fig. 3-12). The best correlation was found for the product of average trabecular CT number and the total bone cross-sectional area. The use of this parameter could result in improved assessment of the degree of osteoporosis and the associated risk of hip fracture.

Lotz et al.[61] analytically studied the proximal femur subject to various load configurations including one-legged stance and fall. The finite element models (Fig. 3-10) suggest that the joint load is transferred from the femoral head to the cortex of the calcar region through the primary compressive group of trabeculae during gait. These results contradict the current belief that the loads are distributed in proportion to the bone volume fractions. Instead, there is a shift in the distribution of load from mainly trabecular bone near the femoral head to cortical bone at the base of the femoral neck. This result, along with the observation that fractures of the proximal femur usually occur in the subcapital region, supports the hypothesis that fractures in osteoporotic bone result from reduced strength of trabecular bone. Finite element models created from CT data provide a relatively accurate and precise tool for predicting femoral failure loads.[55]

FIGURE 3-11   *Contact loads at the femoral head and greater trochanter representing a fall to the side. (Adapted from J. C. Lotz, Ph.D. dissertation, Massachusetts Institute of Technology, 1988.)*

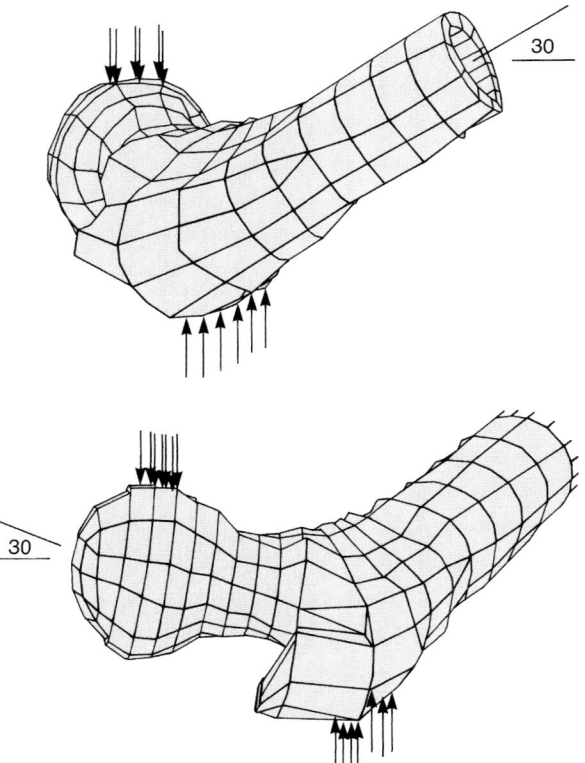

FIGURE 3-12   *Quantitative computed tomography (QCT) scan locations used to compare QCT data with in vitro failure strengths of proximal femurs. (Adapted from J. C. Lotz, Ph.D. dissertation, Massachusetts Institute of Technology, 1988.)*

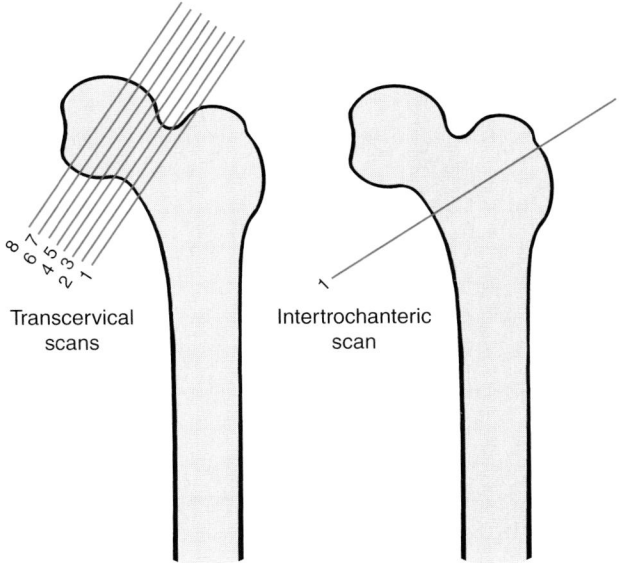

Transcervical scans   Intertrochanteric scan

FRACTURE RISK WITH METASTATIC AND BENIGN DEFECTS IN BONE

Metastatic lesions frequently occur in the axial and appendicular skeleton of breast, prostate, and other cancer patients. Benign bone tumors occur in as many as 33 percent of asymptomatic children evaluated by random radiographs of long bones.[33] These lesions can represent a significant fracture risk. Approximately 5 percent of patients receiving radiation therapy for painful bone metastases suffer a pathological fracture.[37] Prophylactic fixation of an impending fracture has several advantages over treating a pathological fracture, including relief of pain, decreased hospital stay, reduced operative difficulty, reduced risk of nonunion, and reduced morbidity. On the other hand, operations that do not reduce the overall morbidity must be avoided. Clinicians are thus faced with the task of determining whether or not a defect requires prophylactic stabilization. Commonly used clinical guidelines can provide contradictory indications for prophylactic stabilization, and the specificity of these guidelines is poor.[80] These guidelines likely overestimate the risk of pathological fracture.[90] There are many aspects of metastatic and benign defect geometry and material properties that determine the structural consequences of the lesion. In common sites of osseous metastases such as the proximal femur, even experienced orthopaedic oncologists cannot predict the strength reduction due to the defect from radiographs or from qualitative observation of CT examinations.[43]

Numerous laboratory research studies have been reported that specifically address the structural consequences of

metastatic defects in axial and appendicular skeleton.[43,80,81] In general, these studies demonstrate that finite element models and other analytical methods can be used to account for bone density and geometry and predict the structural consequences of metastatic lesions in bone. In all experiments, good agreement was found between the computer model predictions and actual measurements of strength reductions due to the defects. Existing guidelines for determining when to prophylactically stabilize long bones with metastatic lesions can overestimate the actual risk of fracture in some cases[90] but can place a bone at significant risk of fracture in others. Based on our data, the strength of bones with simulated endosteal metastatic defects is proportional to defect size (Fig. 3-13) but is highly dependent on the type of loading. For example, a 65 percent reduction in bending strength was determined for transcortical lesions destroying 50 percent of the cortex, whereas the same lesion reduces torsional load-bearing capacity by 85 percent. The finite element models show that the material properties of bone along the border of a defect can significantly increase the structural consequences of a metastatic defect. Many metastatic lesions are associated with bone resorption along the border of the lesion that extends beyond the radiographically evident lysis. Thus, for osteolytic metastatic lesions, the structural consequences may be significantly greater than predicted from plain radiographs. The finite element models also demonstrated that for endosteal defects, a critical geometric parameter is the minimum cortical wall thickness. For example, an asymmetric defect that compromises

---

FIGURE 3-13 *Percentage of intact bone bending strength as a function of endosteal defect size. Endosteal defect size is expressed as the ratio of reduced wall thickness to intact cortical wall thickness. Both experimental and analytical results are shown. (Adapted from Hipp, J.A.; McBroom, R.J.; Cheal E.J.; et al. Structural consequences of endosteal metastatic lesions in long bones. J Orthop Res 76:828–837, 1989.)*

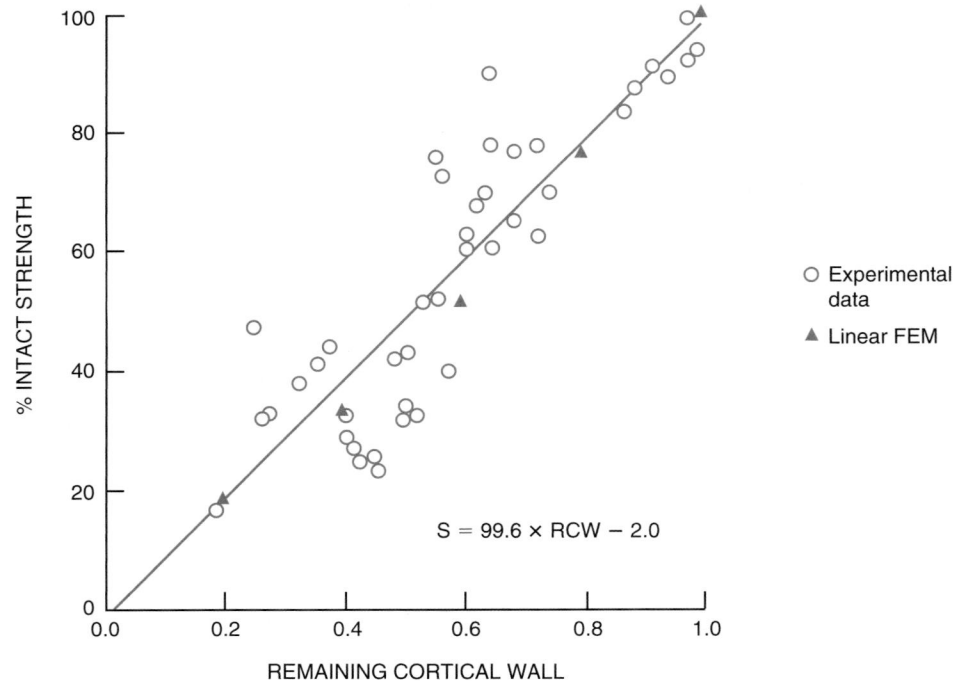

S = 99.6 × RCW − 2.0

80 percent of the cortical wall at one point but only 20 percent of the wall on the opposite side will be only 2 percent stronger in torsion than a bone with a defect that compromises 80 percent of the cortical wall around the entire circumference. Even biplanar radiographs will fail to detect critical geometric parameters if the critical defect geometry is not aligned with respect to the radiographic planes. In a retrospective study of 516 metastatic breast lesions using anteroposterior radiographs, Keene et al.[50] could not establish a geometric criterion for lesions at risk of fracture, perhaps because critical geometric parameters were missed using plain radiographs. Results of ex vivo experiments with simulated defects suggest that CT scans at small consecutive scan intervals could facilitate evaluation of the fracture risk due to metastatic or benign lesions.

Strength reductions due to long bone or vertebral defects can be determined from CT data using relatively simple engineering models.[80,81,91] These CT-based measurements require placing a phantom under the patient during the examination so that CT attenuation data can be converted to bone density. Known relations between bone density and bone modulus are then used to convert the bone density data to modulus. For each cross-section through the bone, the product of area and modulus is summed over the entire cross-section, excluding posterior elements. The lowest axial rigidity of all cross-sections was linearly related to the measured failure load, and predicted almost 90 percent of the variability in the measured failure loads in a laboratory study.[94] In a similar study using the same CT-based technique, a one-to-one correspondence between measured and predicted failure load was found, although this study looked at a wider range of defect locations and was able to predict only 74 percent of the variation in measured failure loads.[91]

In a clinical study, the CT-based rigidity of a bone with a benign defect has been shown to be significantly more sensitive and specific to pathological fracture than criteria based on defect size.[80] In this study, the rigidity of a bone with a benign lesion was normalized to corresponding sections through the contralateral bone. A combination of the minimum bending and torsional rigidities calculated from the CT data provided was 100 percent sensitive and 94 percent specific in distinguishing between the 18 patients who sustained a pathological fracture and the 18 nonfracture patients. In contrast, x-ray based criteria were 28 to 83 percent sensitive and 6 to 78 percent specific.

The power of computers has improved to the point at which individualized finite element models can now be relatively easily created from CT data and used to predict the load-bearing capacity of a bone. In one study, approximately 90 percent of the variability in fracture load could be predicted from individualized finite element models of femoral diaphyses with simulated defects.[54]

The technology to predict pathological fracture risk is now well proven in many laboratory studies and a few clinical trials. However, additional large-scale clinical trials are needed to fully understand the strengths and limitations of this technology in clinical practice. In addition, U.S. Food and Drug Administration approval and a mechanism to make the technology widely accessible would be required before this technology can be effective in routine clinical practice.

BIOMECHANICS OF FRACTURE HEALING

Fracture healing can be viewed as a staged process that gradually restores the load-bearing capacity of bone, eventually returning it to approximately the original stiffness and strength. Remodeling of a fracture site continues long after a fracture treatment is discontinued. In fact, bone that has fused with abnormal angulation can remodel to correct the abnormality. However, during the early phases of fracture healing, the mechanical environment to which a healing fracture is exposed profoundly affects the biology and radiographic appearance of the fracture-healing process. Conversely, the biology of fracture healing profoundly affects the biomechanical progression of healing, and many interacting factors play a role in this interface between biology and mechanics.[5] This section addresses in vivo studies in which fracture healing was examined under controlled biomechanical environments. These in vivo animal studies document how the biomechanical environment provided by various fracture treatment devices can alter fracture-healing biology and the rate of fracture healing.

Two general biological mechanisms have been identified by which bone can repair itself. Close approximation and rigid immobilization of the fracture fragments result in localized remodeling at the fracture site, a process termed *direct cortical reconstruction*. If a small gap exists between fracture fragments, direct cortical reconstruction is preceded by radial filling of the gap with woven bone, a process called *gap healing*. This intermediate process is followed by direct cortical reconstruction. It is likely that in most clinical situations using rigid fixation, both gap healing and direct cortical reconstruction are at work.

The conventional, more common mechanism of fracture repair is by secondary osseous repair or "natural healing." With less rigid immobilization, such as in casts or cast-braces, fracture repair is characterized by callus formation. The periosteal callus forms from the fracture site hematoma with formation of a collar of fibrous tissue, fibrocartilage, and hyaline cartilage around the fracture fragments. Subperiosteal new bone is formed some distance from the fracture site and, through a process similar to endochondral ossification, advances toward the central and peripheral region of the callus. A similar, less prolific response occurs at the endosteal surface. Over time, the callus is remodeled from randomly oriented woven bone to mature cortical bone. Direct cortical reconstruction and repair by callus formation alter the temporal changes in mechanical properties of the fracture in unique patterns.

Healing by Direct Cortical Reconstruction

Fundamental differences in direct cortical reconstruction versus fracture healing by callus formation can be clearly seen in histologic preparations, as reviewed in a previous chapter. With direct cortical reconstruction, there is little evidence of resorption of fracture surfaces. If a small gap exists between bone fragments, a layer of bone forms within the gap. Once any gap has been filled, haversian remodeling directly crosses the fracture. The vascular supply for the osteonal remodeling units is generally endosteal although some periosteal contribution is also common.[67]

Healing by Callus Formation

In contrast to direct cortical healing, fracture healing by callus formation typically involves resorption of fracture surfaces along with prolific woven bone formation originating primarily from the periosteal surface although some callus also originates from the endosteal surface. After the fracture has united through the callus, osteonal remodeling occurs across the fracture and the periosteal callus is remodeled and resorbed to some extent.

Callus formation, especially periosteal callus, offers basic mechanical advantages for a healing fracture. With reference to Figures 3-6 and 3-7, the moment of inertia (and thus the bending rigidity) for a tubular structure depends on the fourth power of the radii. If we represent the femoral shaft as a tubular structure with a normal medullary diameter of 1.5 cm and a normal periosteal diameter of 3 cm, Figure 3-14A shows that the moment of inertia increases by almost 10 times if the periosteal diameter is increased to 5 cm. Figure 3-14B shows that reduction in endosteal diameter offers substantially less improvement. Although bone formed in a callus may not be as strong or stiff as normal bone, the large increase in moment of inertia provides a biomechanical advantage for periosteal callus formation.

Biomechanical Stages of Fracture Healing

That fracture healing occurs in biomechanically unique stages was first described by White et al.[92] For fracture healing involving periosteal callus, the biomechanical stages of fracture healing have been studied in animals.

White and co-workers[66,92] used an externally fixed rabbit osteotomy model to correlate radiographic and histologic information with the torsional stiffness and failure strength at several postfracture time periods. They identified four biomechanical stages of fracture healing (Fig. 3-15). The first indication of increasing stiffness occurred after 21 to 24 days. At this stage the fracture exhibited a rubbery type of behavior characterized by large angular deflections for low torques. The bone fails through the fracture site at low loads. This stage corresponds to bridging of the fracture gap by soft tissues. At approximately 27 days, a sharp increase in stiffness identified the second stage, where failures occurred through the fracture site at low loads. Stiffness approached that of intact cortical bone. The third biomechanical stage is characterized by failure occurring only partially through the fracture site, with a stiffness similar to cortical bone but below normal strength. The final stage is achieved when the site of failure is not related to the original experimental fracture, and the stiffness and strength are similar to those of intact bone.

In a related study, Panjabi et al.[65] compared radiographic evaluation of fracture healing with the failure strength of healing osteotomies. They applied nine different radiographic measures of fracture healing (Fig. 3-16). The best radiographic measure was cortical continuity (No. 4 in Fig. 3-16), where the correlation coefficient between the radiographic measure and bone strength was 0.8 (r = 0.8). The lowest correlation between radiographic and physical measurements was found for callus area (r = 0.17). The general conclusion of this study was that even under laboratory conditions, radiographic information is not sufficient to accurately decide the biomechanical condition of a healing fracture. This is an important result, since radiographic diagnosis is commonly applied to assessing fracture healing, though few studies have objectively tested the predictive capability of this practice. Thus, the methods for in vivo biomechanical assessment of fracture healing previously discussed have particular clinical significance.

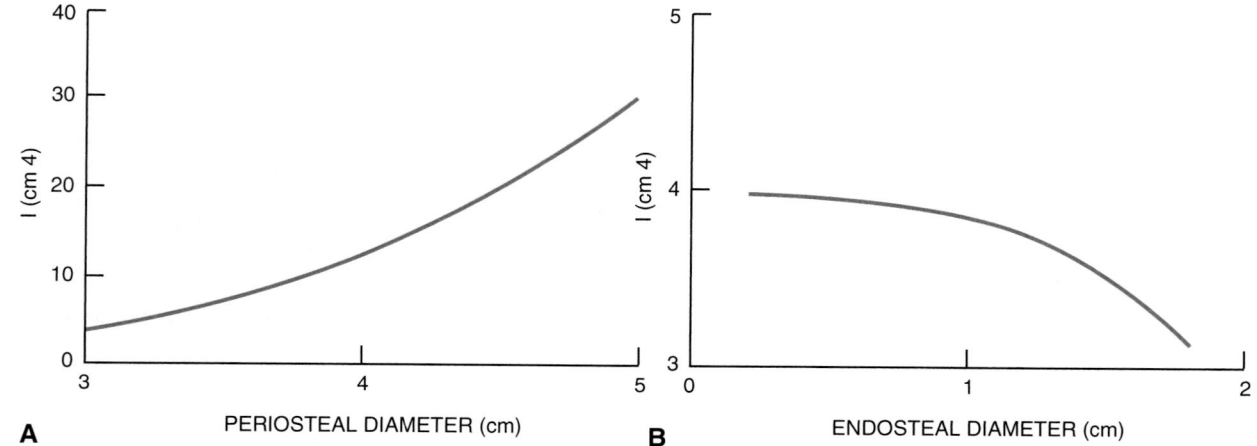

FIGURE 3-14 ***A* and *B,*** *Increase in moment of inertia afforded by changes in periosteal and endosteal diameters resulting from fracture callus. Both figures assume a tubular cross-section. Figure **A** assumes a constant 1.5 cm endosteal diameter, and Figure **B** assumes a constant 3 cm periosteal diameter.*

FIGURE 3-15 | *Angular displacement of healing osteotomies in rabbit femora as a function of applied torque. Data are shown for animals tested after several postfracture time periods. (Data from White, A.A. III; Panjabi, M.M.; Southwick, W.O. The four biomechanical stages of fracture repair. J Bone Joint Surg Am 59(2):188–192, 1977.)*

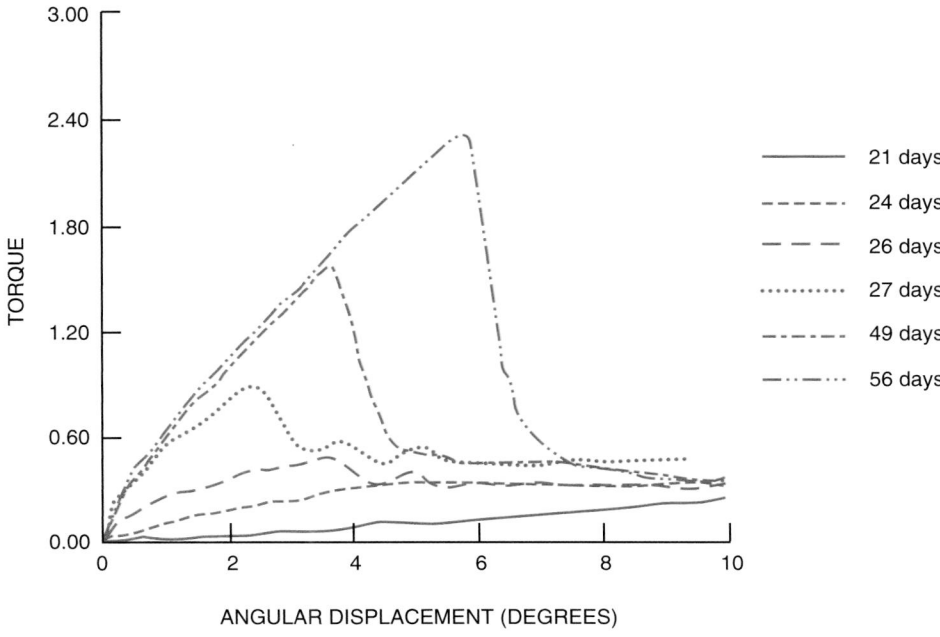

FIGURE 3-16 | *Radiographic measures that were compared to mechanical tests of partially healed fractures to evaluate the efficacy of radiographic evaluation of fracture healing. (Data from Panjabi, M.M.; Walter, S.D.; Karuda, M.; et al. Correlations of radiographic analysis of healing fractures with strength: a statistical analysis of experimental osteotomies. J Orthop Res 3(2):212–218, 1985.)*

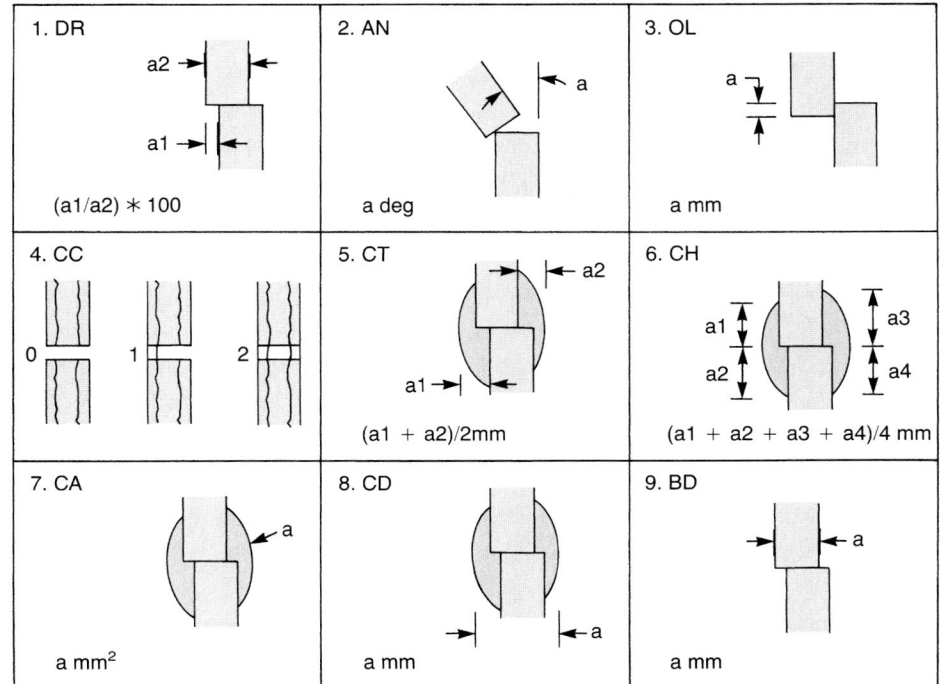

Several other animal experiments have shown similar biomechanical stages of fracture healing,[10,24] and the time at which each stage of fracture healing is achieved is dependent on several factors. Using a canine model, Davy and Connolly[24] experimentally produced fractures in weight-bearing (radii) and presumed non-weight-bearing bones (ribs). Healing bones were tested using four-point bend tests at 2 to 12 weeks. Both weight-bearing and non-weight-bearing bones healed with formation of periosteal callus. For non-weight-bearing bones, bending strength increased more rapidly than stiffness, whereas stiffness increased more rapidly than strength with the weight-bearing bones. This result also shows that the stiffness of a healing fracture does not necessarily correlate with the bone strength. They further demonstrated that bone and periosteal callus geometry can theoretically account for observed changes in fracture properties. However, radiographic criteria have not been shown to predict the strength or stiffness of a healing fracture. Under bending loads, the failure mechanism appears to be delamination of repair tissue from the bone fragments, suggesting that the adhesive bond between repair tissue and bone fragments determines the structural properties.[10]

Optimal Mechanical Environment for Fracture Healing

One primary goal of fracture treatment is to continually control the mechanical environment so that it is optimal for each stage of fracture healing. While it is known that the mechanical environment can alter the bone healing process, the conflicting results for studies that investigate the effect of fixation rigidity on fracture healing leave the question of optimum fixation rigidity unsolved. Perren and co-workers describe a hypothesis and supporting evidence that help explain how fracture healing is controlled by the local mechanical environment.[67] They postulated that a tissue can be formed only in the interfragmentary region of a healing fracture if the involved tissues can tolerate the local mechanical strain. The tissues that formed will, in turn, contribute to the fracture rigidity, making possible the next step in tissue differentiation. For example, formation of granulation tissue may reduce the strain to a level where fibrocartilage formation is possible. They further hypothesized that the fracture gap is widened by resorption of the bone ends until the local tissue strain falls below a certain limiting value. Resorption of fragment ends may reduce the strain sufficiently to permit completion of a bridging callus. Interfragmentary strain may influence fracture healing in several ways. Local deformations may disrupt vascularization and interrupt blood supply to developing osteons. Deformation of cells may alter their permeability to macromolecules and increase biological activity. Strains may also induce changes in the electrical signals within the healing fracture site or elicit a direct cellular response. In all likelihood, there exists a multifactorial relationship at various stages of the healing process.

The interfragmentary strain hypothesis has been tested by several authors using animal and computer models, and the basic premise is now fairly well established.[17] However, this hypothesis is complicated by the complexity of stresses and strains at a fracture site. Cheal et al. used computer models to show that complex three-dimensional strain fields exist, even within a relatively simple fracture gap, and that the simple longitudinal strains considered by Perren et al. underestimate the true strains experienced by the interfragmentary tissues.[26] The analytical models show that the strain in tissue is greatest at the endosteal and periosteal surfaces of the bone fragments (Fig. 3-17). These are also the areas of early bone resorption observed in the experimental animals. The models also demonstrate the asymmetric distribution of strains that occur within the tissues at the gap between plated fracture fragments.

Although the strains within a healing fracture may be complex, these strains currently must be considered in more simple terms during the clinical management of fracture healing in patients. One strategy is to consider the apparent axial and shear components of the strain across a fracture gap. Fracture fixation methods that result in shear motion within a fracture gap can significantly degrade fracture healing, at least in an animal model.[4] Shear can result in less bone bridging across a fracture gap and a lower percentage of gaps with any bone bridging across the gap. Shear can additionally reduce the amount of callus and therefore the rigidity of the healing fracture. However, it is important to note that even in the presence of shear strains and shear forces, some fractures will heal, although slower than they would under ideal conditions. Unfortunately, a validated method that can be used to calculate loads and strains across fracture in routine clinical practice does not exist, so clinicians must now estimate conditions to the best of their ability and adjust fixation if deemed necessary. Once the ideal conditions for a healing fracture have been validated in a clinical study, technology can be developed to help clinicians achieve these conditions in clinical practice. The optimal mechanical environment that a fracture fixation system should facilitate has not been determined. Some motion has been shown by multiple authors to facilitate fracture healing,

FIGURE 3-17 *Factors important in intramedullary fracture fixation.*

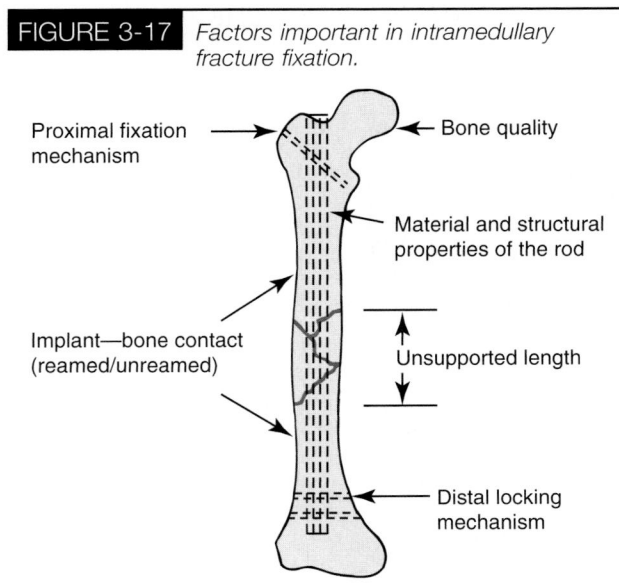

Proximal fixation mechanism

Bone quality

Material and structural properties of the rod

Implant—bone contact (reamed/unreamed)

Unsupported length

Distal locking mechanism

but others authors have demonstrated ranges of motions and loads that degrade fracture healing when applied across a fracture gap.[5]

It is also important to note that along with the evidence of central nervous system control of bone formation and resorption[30] there is also evidence that innervation of the fracture site is a requirement for timely and competent fracture repair.[60] In general, it is assumed (or hoped for) that reinnervation of a healing fracture will follow a parallel course with revascularization, but this hypothesis is not yet well supported by scientific evidence.

BIOMECHANICS OF FRACTURE TREATMENT

Many techniques are currently available for treatment of skeletal fractures, and many factors are important in choosing the best fixation. Many of these clinical factors are discussed in other chapters, but one factor that is crucial to all fractures is the need for sufficient stability to achieve fracture healing. Each method of fixation imparts specific levels of stability to a fracture, thus directly influencing fracture-healing biology. When a fracture treatment method is evaluated, the healing bone and fracture treatment device should be considered as a mechanical system, with both tissue and device contributing to the biomechanical behavior. The biomechanical behavior of the system can thus be altered by changes in tissue properties (such as resorption at fracture surfaces, osteopenia under plates), changes to the fracture treatment device (such as dynamization of external fixation), or changes to the mechanical connection between device and tissue (such as pin or bone screw loosening). Additionally, bones are subject to diverse loads that can be a combination of axial, bending, and torsional loads. Thus, the axial, bending, and torsional stability of a fracture treatment method should be considered. Technology now exists to create and apply a computer model of each individual fracture and then to use this model to test different fixation strategies and to select a system that will create a specific mechanical environment for assumed load-bearing requirements. However, there is no evidence that this would be cost-effective, and clinicians must therefore assimilate existing scientific evidence and their own experience and intuition in selecting a fracture fixation strategy. This section addresses the basic mechanical characteristics of fracture treatment techniques and the effect of each device on fracture healing.

Internal Fixation

INTRAMEDULLARY RODS

Intramedullary rods have several advantages in fracture treatment, including restoration of bony alignment and early recovery of weight-bearing. The good clinical results and low rates of nonunion suggest that many current clinical applications of these devices provide a mechanical environment that facilitates fracture repair for selected fractures. It is therefore useful to consider the stability of this treatment method as an example of a successful mechanical construct.

Intramedullary rods are intended to stabilize a fracture by acting as an internal splint, forming a composite structure in which both the bone and the rod contribute to fracture stability. This load-sharing property of rods is fundamental to their design and should be recognized when used for fracture treatment. Consequently, intramedullary rod design must be evaluated both on the structural properties of the rod and the mechanics of rod-bone interaction. Figure 3-18 illustrates factors that determine the mechanical stability of a femoral fracture stabilized by intramedullary fixation.

Biomechanical complications with intramedullary rods include permanent deformation of the rod and fatigue fractures, both of which are now rare, largely because currently available rods have been properly designed following FDA guidelines and ASTM standards. Delayed union and nonunion after intramedullary nailing are also complications resulting from mechanical factors.

There are several material and structural properties of intramedullary rods that alter their axial, bending, and torsional rigidities. These parameters include cross-sectional geometry, rod length, the presence of a longitudinal slot, and the elastic modulus of the material. The cross-sectional geometry can greatly affect all rigidities. Rods with the same nominal outside diameter and similar shape from different manufacturers vary in bending rigidity by more than a factor of two (Figs. 3-19 A and B) and vary in torsional rigidity by more than a factor of three (Fig. 3-19C).[84] This variation was attributed differences in cross-sectional geometry. The data also show that there is not always a simple relationship between rod size and rigidities. The rigidity increases significantly with rod diameter because the moment of inertia is approximately proportional to the fourth power of the rod radius (refer to Fig. 3-6). However, the magnitude of change varies with different manufacturers, in part because the wall thickness (with hollow rods) may be different for different rod diameters. Reaming will increase the rod diameter that can be used, but it may reduce the strength of the bone and further compromise blood supply.

The unsupported length of intramedullary fixation describes the distance between implant-bone contact at the proximal and distal–most extent of the fracture. This distance will effectively change as the fracture heals. During the initial stages of fracture healing, two different

---

FIGURE 3-18 *Representation of the strains experienced by tissues within a uniform osteotomy when the fractured bone is subjected to bending loads. (Data from DiGioia, A.M. III; Cheal, E.?J,; Hayes, W.C. Three-dimensional strain fields in a uniform osteotomy gap. J Biomech Eng 108(3): 273–280, 1986.)*

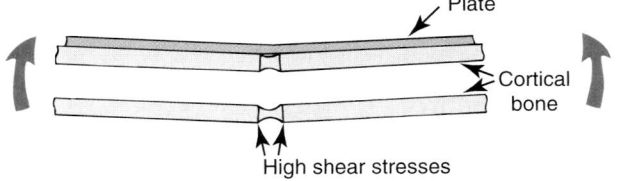

FIGURE 3-19   ***A–C***, *Anteroposterior and medial-lateral bending rigidities and torsional rigidities of slotted intramedullary rods as a function of nominal rod diameter for five commercially available rods from different manufacturers. Rods were oriented with the slot in the anteroposterior plane. (Data from Tencer, A.F.; Sherman, M.C.; Johnson, K.D. Biomechanical factors affecting fracture stability and femoral bursting in closed intramedullary rod fixation of femur fractures. J Biomech Eng 107(2):104–111, 1985.)*

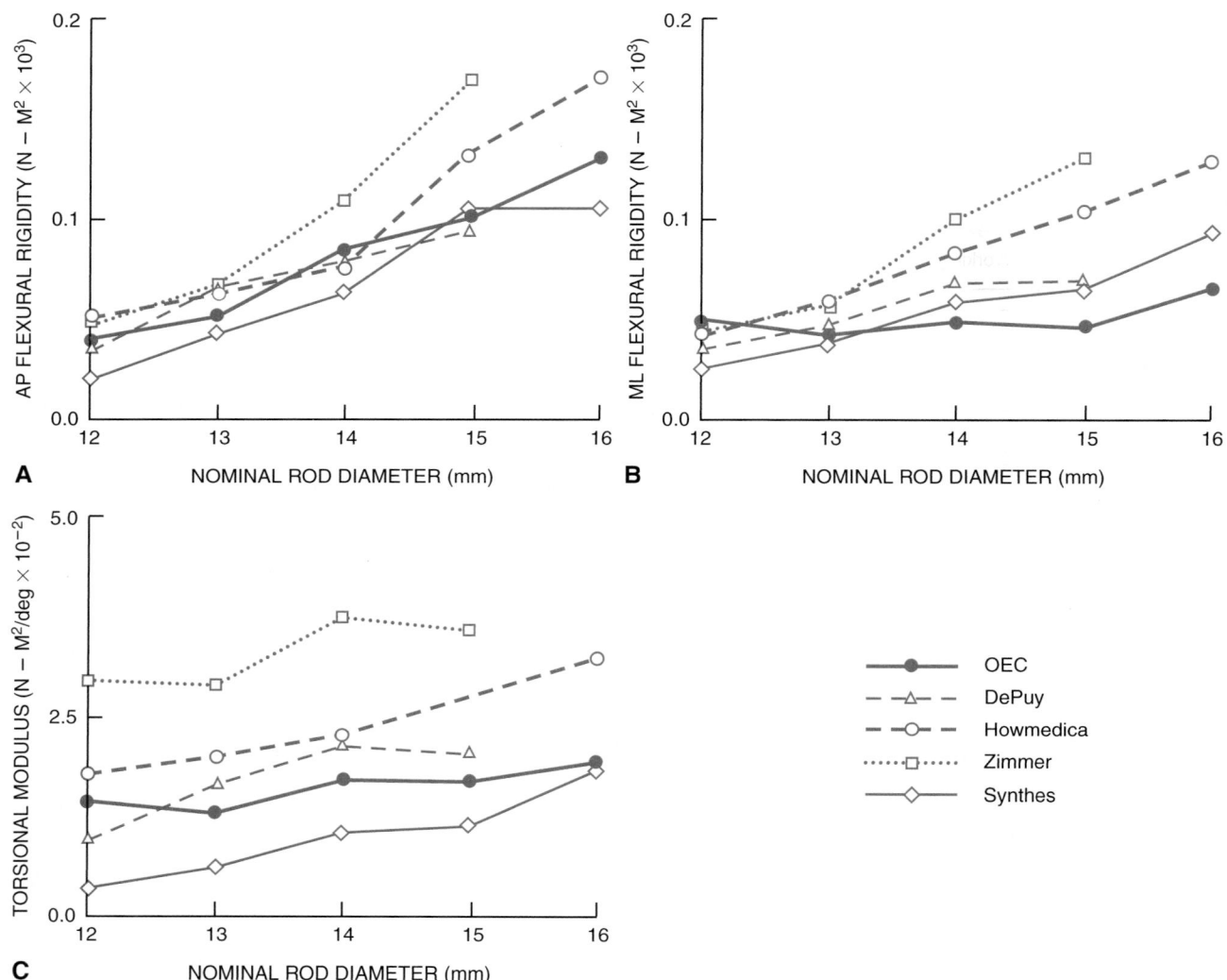

unsupported lengths are important with intramedullary rods: the unsupported length in bending and the unsupported length in torsion. Figure 3-20 illustrates the significance of unsupported length in bending. This length is determined by the points of bone-implant contact on the proximal and distal sides of the fracture and could be different depending on the direction of bending. For a simple, well-reamed transverse fracture, this distance will be small, whereas for a severely comminuted fracture, the unsupported length can be great. The unsupported length is a site where rods have failed clinically.[46] When bending loads are applied, the rod is typically loaded in approximately four-point bending (analogous to Fig. 3-7), so the nominal interfragmentary motion is proportional to the square of the unsupported length. Therefore, a small increase in unsupported length can lead to a larger increase in interfragmentary motion.

With torsional loading, the unsupported length will be determined by the points at which sufficient mechanical interlocking occurs between bone and implant to support torsional loads. Simple rod designs that do not include proximal or distal locking mechanisms have lower resistance to torsion. For rod designs that employ proximal and distal locking mechanisms, the unsupported length is typically determined by the distance between the proximal and distal locking points. Mechanical interlocking may also occur between rod and bone at other places within the medullary canal. Relative motion between fracture fragments during torsional loading is roughly proportional to the unsupported length (calculated according to Fig. 3-8).

Many rod designs have a longitudinal slot, either partially or fully along their length. The slot allows the cross-section to be compressed like a stiff spring when inserted into a medullary canal. This elastic compression

FIGURE 3-20 *The unsupported (or working) length of an intramedullary device can be much greater for a comminuted versus a simple transverse fracture.*

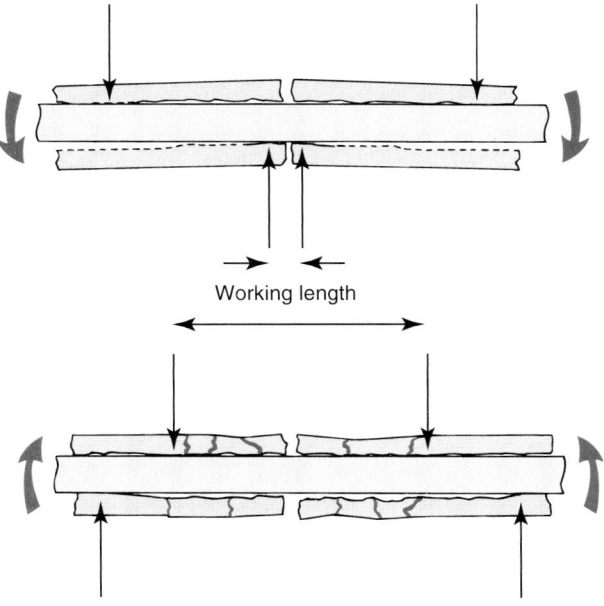

Working length

can help promote a tight fit between rod and bone. However, with torsional loads the slot creates an "open section" geometry that is theoretically 400 times less stiff than a closed section.[74] Reduced torsional rigidity can have both positive and negative value. Reduction in rod stiffness allows the rod to conform to minor discrepancies between rod and medullary geometry. Reduced rigidity may also allow twisting of the rod during insertion, easing insertion but compromising the use of external aiming devices used to locate the distal locking points. With a partially slotted rod design, stress concentrations at the end of the slot where the cross-section becomes continuous can theoretically result in failures at this location.

Intramedullary rod designs that provide mechanisms for locking the rod proximally and/or distally have increased the indications for intramedullary rod use. Proximal and distal locking mechanisms will affect the torsional, axial, and bending properties of a fracture fixed with an intramedullary rod. The use of a locking mechanism on one side of the fracture only (proximal or distal) can increase the forces transmitted between fracture fragments during limb loading. The use of both proximal and distal locking can prevent axial displacement of bone along the rod and can provide additional torsional rigidity. Several different types of distal locking mechanisms are currently available, including transverse screws and wings designed to engage cortical or cancellous bone. The strength of these locking mechanisms depends in part on the quality of supporting bone. In osteoporotic bone, a 95-degree blade plate has been shown to provide more rigid and stronger fixation than antegrade or retrograde nails for supracondylar fractures.[56]

In combination, the presence of both proximal and distal locking mechanisms helps control the axial stability of a fracture. Without both locking mechanisms, the bone can

glide axially along the implant. Thus, the combination of proximal and distal locking can maintain axial separation and bone length or can facilitate application of compression between bone fragments. The compression will be lost if the resorption occurs at the points of contact between fracture fragments.

The mechanical interaction between bone and the implant shaft can also influence the stability of an intramedullary fixed fracture. The mechanical interlock between implant and bone depends on the cross-sectional geometry of the bone and on the geometry of the medullary canal. The geometry of the medullary canal is frequently changed by reaming, in which case surgical technique and nail size together will establish the initial fit of implant in bone. In a stable fracture, a small-diameter rod can provide adequate stabilization, but with an unstable fracture, close contact between bone and rod provides improved stability.[31]

Several tests have demonstrated that torsional resistance is a primary shortcoming of some intramedullary rods, with intramedullary rod fixed femurs achieving only 13 to 16 percent of intact femoral torsional strength. To improve torsional properties, designs incorporating flutes and ribs to increase contact between rod and bone in torsion, and designs that use screws or wings to engage cortical or cancellous bone, have been developed. The use of proximal and distal locking mechanisms will also increase the torsional rigidity, but this has not been exhaustively tested.

FRACTURE HEALING WITH INTRAMEDULLARY RODS The issue of ideal intramedullary rod flexibility has been studied with animal and computer models by many investigators, but scientific evidence from human clinical trials is sparse. Utvag et al.[88] assessed femoral fracture healing in 100 rats. Twenty rats served as controls, and groups of 20 rats were fixed with steel nails, cannulated steel nails, titanium nails, or polyethylene nails. The investigators found that the bending rigidity, failure load, energy to failure, and bone mineral density (BMD) in the callus region were all highest with the titanium nails, which most closely match the stiffness of normal bone.

The optimal fixation technique must allow transfer of forces between bone and implant without causing gross failure of either the bone or the implant. For example, failure of bone has been observed with many rigid nail-plate devices used for fractures of the proximal femur. Sliding screws that allow load transmission between bone fragments as well as load transmission between bone and implant reduce, but do not eliminate, penetration of the implant into the femoral head. This penetration is associated with improper placement of the sliding screw in the proximal femur, and with osteoporotic bone. Quantitative measurements of bone density in the femoral head can help determine the load-bearing capacity of fractured proximal femurs following fixation with a sliding hip screw or with standard pins and screws and may also help identify when augmentation is required for distal interlocking in osteoporotic bone.[78,79] The load required to cause penetration of the sliding hip screw superiorly into the femoral head may be insufficient to support activities of daily living in osteoporotic patients. For example, hip screw penetration loads as low as 750 N have been recorded[79] in osteoporotic femurs. Allowing for contact forces of 3.3 times body weight during gait, load-bearing capacities greater than 1300 N would be required in a very light weight person. Quantitative measurements of bone density may therefore be beneficial to ensure that fixation will not fail because of failure of bone around the fixation system, although sensitive and specific guidelines have yet to be developed.

In combination with bone density measurements, new implant designs and implantation techniques can potentially reduce complications from overloading bone around the implant. For example, augmenting screw fixation by first injecting bone cement into surrounding osteoporotic bone can dramatically improve fixation strength.[22]

BONE PLATES

As with intramedullary devices, several basic biomechanical principals are important to fracture fixation using bone plates. Figure 3-21 illustrates some important parameters. It is crucial to realize that the plate and the bone together form a mechanical construct with some load supported by the plate and some load passing between bone fragments. Therefore, changes in the plate, the bone, or the interface between plate and bone can dramatically influence the mechanical environment of a fracture. The interaction between plate and bone is also load dependent; the plate may improve stability for one type of loading much more than for other types of loads.

The bending stiffness of a bone plate with a rectangular cross-section is related to the third power of the plate thickness, whereas the bending rigidity is directly proportional to the width or elastic modulus of the plate. Therefore, plate rigidity can be changed more by plate thickness than plate width or modulus, with the limitation that thick plates may not be possible in regions with limited overlying soft-tissue thickness.

The mechanical properties of bone will also affect the behavior of the plate-bone system. For example, less stiff bone will increase the load sharing contribution of the plate. In addition, osteoporosis, osteopetrosis, or other bone diseases may affect bone remodeling at the plate-bone or screw-bone interfaces and thus affect the

mechanical performance of the plated bone. However, the role of bone properties in fracture fixation with bone plates has yet to be investigated. Most in vivo animal studies and ex vivo studies of plate fixation examined the biomechanics of plates applied to osteotomized bones in which reduction and compression of bone fragments could be achieved. In cases of highly comminuted fractures or when bone defects need to be stabilized, adequate reduction and stability are more difficult to achieve. In these cases, the mechanical demands on the plate will be increased, since load transmission between bone fragments may not be possible and all loads must pass through the plate.

Loads can be transmitted between plate and bone through the bone screws and through mechanical interlocking or frictional forces between the plate surface and bone. The coupling between plates and bone depends on how much force is applied by the bone screws, it changes as tissues remodel following surgery, and the micromotion that can occur between plate and bone is reduced by stiffer plates.[20]

The concept of working length introduced with intramedullary devices is also applicable to bone plates. The working length of the plate, especially in the bending open configuration, is greater when the inner screws are not placed (Fig. 3-22). Maximum plate deflection is approximately proportional to the square of the working length (refer to Fig. 3-7), so large decreases in bending rigidity occur when the inner screws are not used.

Cheal et al. investigated the biomechanics of plate fixation using a combined experimental and theoretical approach.[15] The experimental model consisted of an intact plexiglass tube with an attached six-hole stainless steel compression plate. Several parameters, including friction between plate and bone, and screw pretension induced by tightening the bone screws, were investigated using finite element models (Fig. 3-23). Several load cases were considered including axial loads, off-axis loads, and bending. Excellent agreement was obtained between the theoretical and experimental models. The analytical models showed that stress shielding of bone should be limited to the central region between the inner screws. This agrees with radiographic findings from animal studies of bone changes beneath plates. Static preloads, applied by compression plate techniques, can negate any reduction in axial stress levels beneath the plate, but these preloads decay rapidly and have not been shown to affect the long-term fracture-healing process. For fractures fixed with compression plates, the experimental studies showed the importance of placing the plate on the tensile aspect of the bone, since the plated bone is particularly weak under loads that bend open the fracture. Finally, experiments have shown that the outer screws received the highest stresses.[20]

The location of the plate (tension vs. compressive side of the bone) is an important factor in the biomechanics of bone plates. This is because application of a bone plate will change the moment of inertia of the plate-bone system compared with an intact bone. With uniform axial loads, the stress throughout a cross-section of intact bone will be relatively constant. With application of a bone plate, a combination of bending and axial stresses will be

---

FIGURE 3-21   *Factors affecting the stability of a plated fracture.*

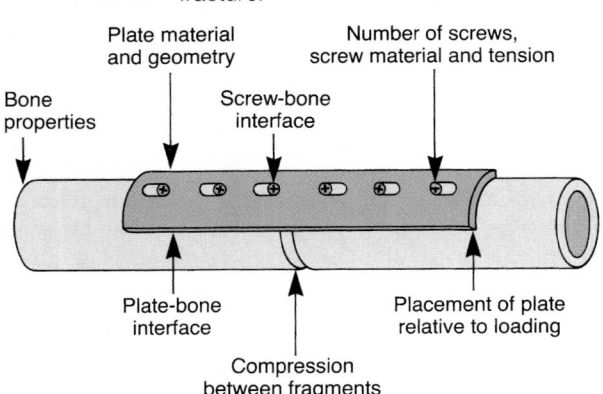

Plate material and geometry

Number of screws, screw material and tension

Bone properties

Screw-bone interface

Plate-bone interface

Placement of plate relative to loading

Compression between fragments

FIGURE 3-22 *Different bending configurations for a plated fracture. This figure also illustrates the concept of working length with bone plates and the value of using all screws.*

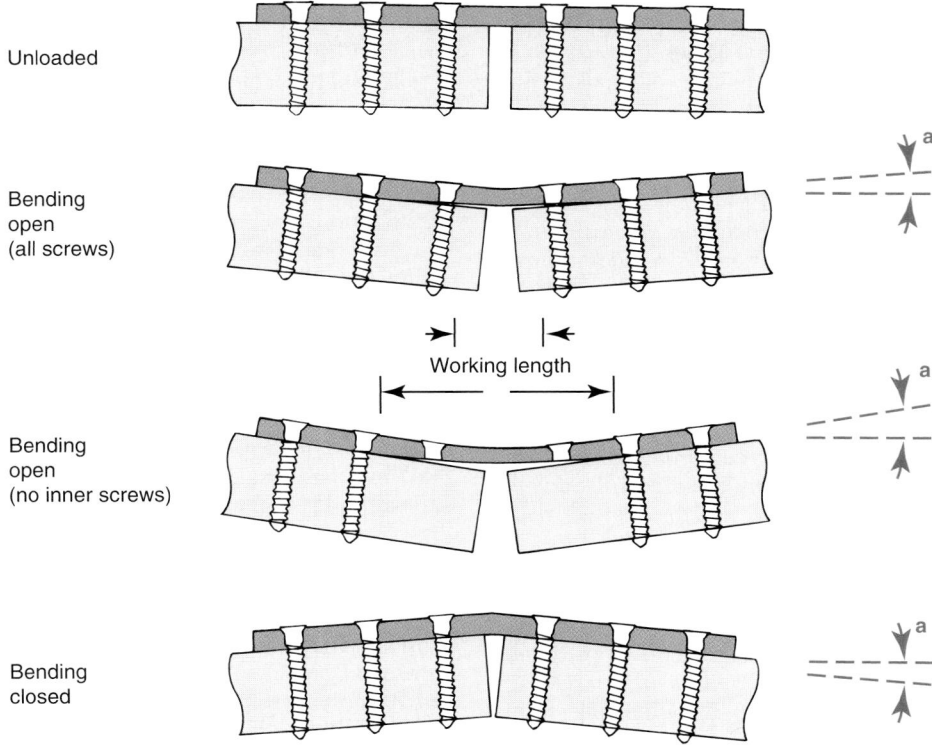

Unloaded

Bending
open
(all screws)

Working length

Bending
open
(no inner screws)

Bending
closed

realized in the same cross-section of bone. Subjected to bending loads, a plated bone can be in a bending open or bending closed configuration (see Fig. 3-22). The placement of the plate relative to the loading direction will determine the proportion of the loads supported by the plate.[82] Hayes and Perren[39] tested osteotomized, plated sheep tibia in four-point bending. They tested the

FIGURE 3-23 *Three-dimensional finite element mesh of a compression-plated tube used to analytically study the mechanical performance of plate-bone systems. Only one quarter of the plated tube needs to be modeled owing to the symmetry of the problem. (Data from Cheal, E.J.; Hayes, W.C.; White, A.A. III; et al. Stress analysis of compression plate fixation and its effects on long bone remodeling. J Biomech 18(2):141–150, 1985.)*

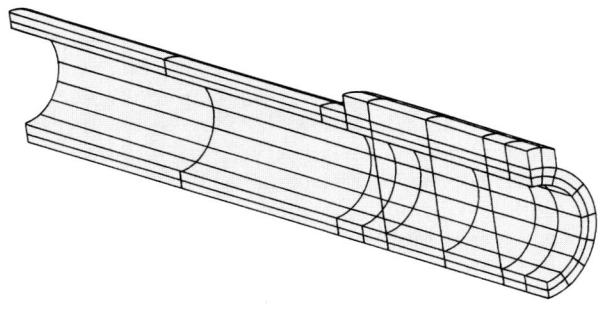

composite plate-bone system in bending open and bending closed directions, both with and without application of compression between bone fragments. Figure 3-24 shows typical results from these tests. The results clearly show that the composite plate-bone system is stiffer in the bending closed direction and that application of compression also increases the stiffness. Other investigators have also shown that application of a compression plate on the side of the bone normally loaded in tension produces the stiffest fixation.[82] Although experimental efforts have shown that preloading a fracture gap through compression plating can increase fracture stability, a static preload does not necessarily affect the pattern of bone remodeling, with the main difference being prevention of motion-induced resorption at the fracture gap that can occur if the fracture gap opens and closes with loading.[82] The size of the callus formed has been shown to be related to the proportion of the loads that are supported by the plate.[82]

The local mechanics within an oblique or comminuted fracture are significantly more complicated than with a transverse osteotomy. Insufficient bone to support ideal compression plate fixation can compromise bone healing.[82] If contact between bone fragments cannot be achieved, there are situations in which the risk of plate failure will be reduced if the plate is applied to the compression side of the bone.

FRACTURE HEALING WITH BONE PLATES The biomechanical factors that can affect fracture healing of a plated bone have been previously discussed. Several of these factors have been investigated with animal and

FIGURE 3-24 | *Maximal deflection versus bending moment for plated sheep tibiae. Tibiae were plated with or without compression and were tested in both bending open and bending closed configurations. (Data from Hayes, W.C. Biomechanics of fracture healing. In: Heppenstall, R.B., editor. Fracture Treatment and Healing. Philadelphia: W.B. Saunders, 1980, pp. 124–172.)*

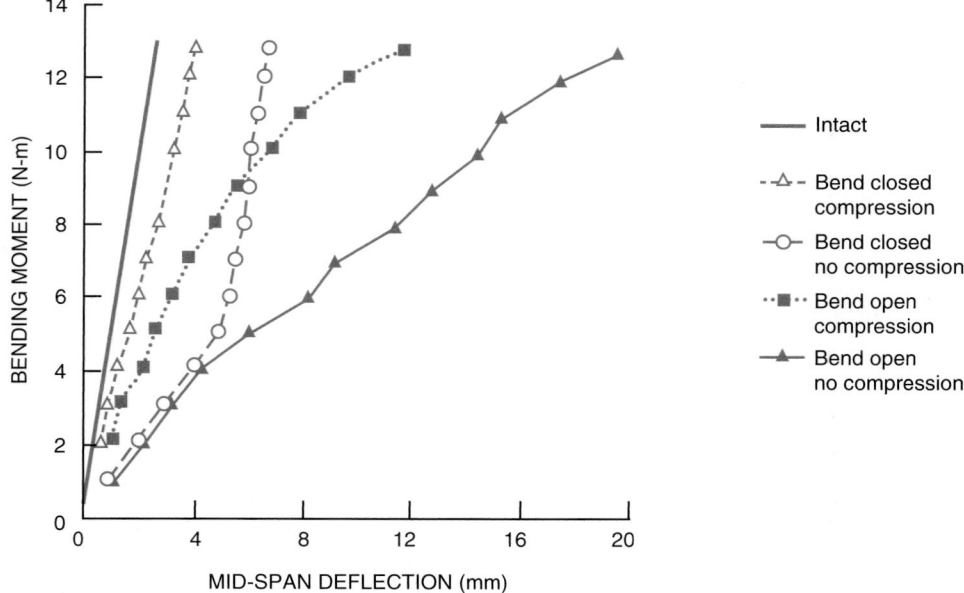

computer models. The effect of plate stiffness on fracture healing has been studied by many investigators with variable conclusions, and a consensus has yet to be reached on how this information should be used in clinical practice. Akeson et al. compared the failure strength of osteotomies at 4 months treated with stainless steel and less rigid composite internal fixation plates and found no significant difference.[1] In contrast, Bradley et al. found increased structural strength and material strength after treatment of an osteotomy with a less rigid fixation plate in comparison to a more rigid fixation plate.[11] The observation that interfragmentary relative motion influences the fracture-healing pattern of cortical bone has led to several studies that examine the healing of fractures treated with plates of varying stiffness. Woo et al. noted that there are several aspects to the structural properties of bone plates. They examined the axial, bending, and torsional stiffness of plates and designed two plates that allowed comparison of plates with high axial stiffness to plates with high bending and torsional stiffness.[96] Terjesen and Apalset investigated bone healing of rabbit tibial osteotomies fixed with plates that were 13, 17, 61, or 74 percent as stiff in bending as the intact bone. After 6 weeks of plate fixation, the amount of periosteal callus was inversely related to plate stiffness. Bones treated with the stiffest plate tended to have lower rigidity and strength than bones treated with less stiff plates. The authors also noted that no relationship was found between the amount of periosteal callus and bone strength at the 6-week time period.[85]

Rigid internal fixation depends on force transmission between implant and bone and between fractured bone ends. Bone necrosis between implant and bone or between bone fragments will compromise fixation stability. To better understand the reaction of living bone to compression

plate fixation, Perren and Rahn designed a strain-gauged, four-hole compression plate that enabled them to monitor the compression applied to the bone fragments by the plate.[68] The plates were applied to both intact and osteotomized bones in sheep. The tensile stress in the plate was measured at weekly intervals for 12 weeks following plate application. Plate tension for the intact bone group is shown in Figure 3-25. There was a gradual decrease in plate tension over 12 weeks after a steeper decrease in

FIGURE 3-25 | *Force applied by a bone plate to the bone as a function of time postcompression plating for plates applied to intact canine tibiae in vivo. (Adapted from Perren, S.M.; Rahn, B.A. Biomechanics of fracture healing. Can J Surg 23(3): 228–232, 1980 with permission.)*

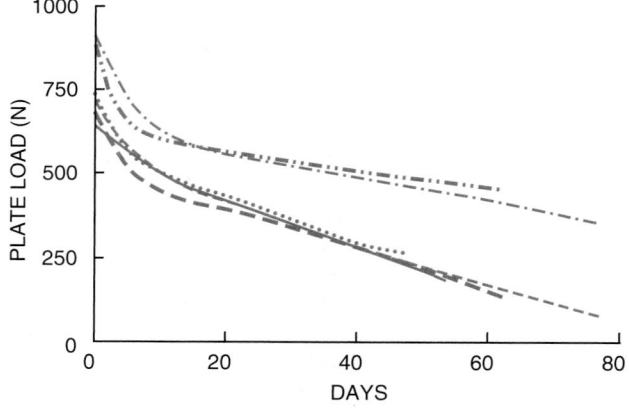

the first few days following surgery. The same general trends were found for the osteotomized group as were found for the intact bones. These results show that rigid internal fixation can maintain compression between bone fragments for several weeks. This suggests that there is no pressure necrosis between bone fragments or at the interface between implant and bone, since if a layer of bone 10 to 20 μm thick were resorbed, tensile forces in the plate would drop to zero.

Histologic analysis confirmed the radiographic indication of direct cortical reconstruction. In spite of full weight-bearing immediately after plate application, the osteotomies were bridged by direct haversian remodeling. The histologic pattern of bone remodeling suggests a mechanism for the slow decrease in plate tension. It is postulated that bone remodeling at the osteotomy site results in local reductions in bone stiffness, reducing the compressive loads maintained by the plate.

Several studies have concluded that early porosis noted beneath bone plates during the first 6 months is due to the plate shielding bone from functional stresses, although it is also attributed to the effect of the plate on the blood supply.[82] Early in fracture healing, the porosis noted beneath bone plates is likely due to disruption of the blood supply to the bone caused by the contact between bone and plate.[82] Plate-bone contact has been shown to result in porosis by 1 month after surgery. There are four arguments in support of vascular disruption as the cause of porosis beneath bone plates. First, the porosis beneath plates appears to be a temporary, intermediate stage in bone remodeling in response to surgery. Second, the bone-remodeling pattern is better explained by the pattern of vascular disruption than by the stress distribution beneath the plate. Third, in a comparative study of plastic plates and steel plates, more porosis was noted beneath the plastic plate, even though the steel plate should provide substantially more stress shielding. The fourth supporting argument is that porosis beneath bone plates can be substantially reduced by use of plates that provide for improved circulation.

EXTERNAL FIXATION

Current external fixation devices provide a wide range of frame configuration and fracture stability options, making external fixation adaptable to many clinical situations. External fixation devices also provide a convenient way to alter fixation rigidity during the course of healing and offer potential for monitoring the biomechanical progression of fracture healing. The stability provided by an external fixation device depends on both the frame configuration and the interaction between frame and bone fragments. Callus formation may be essential to the stability of a healing fracture with many frame configurations.[47] Huiskes and Chao have shown that external fixator rigidities can be altered by several orders of magnitude through changes in frame configuration.[44]

As shown in Figures 3-26 and 3-27, several geometric, material, and technical factors as well as loading directions can play a role in the biomechanics of externally fixed fractures. The relative contributions of several of these factors have been quantified using computer models.[44,47] Most biomechanical studies of external fixators examine the effect of various parameters on the rigidity under several types of loading. It must be strongly emphasized that if the clamps or other connectors used in an external fixation system become loose, the stability of the fixation will be severely compromised.[28] These connections may also actually fail under relatively low loads.

The percutaneous pins are typically the weakest component of an external fixation system. High stresses can occur in the pins, possibly resulting in permanent deformation of the pin, especially when the fracture site is unstable.[45] The bending rigidity of each pin is theoretically proportional to the fourth power of the pin diameter, so increasing the pin diameter from 4 to 6 mm increases the bending stiffness of each pin by 5 times. Pin diameter has been shown to be one of the most important parameters that determines fixator stiffness.[45] The bending stiffness of each pin is also proportional to the cube of the sidebar-to-bone distance, so small changes in the sidebar-to-bone distance cause large changes in pin rigidity.

FIGURE 3-26 *Factors affecting the stability of an externally fixed fracture.*

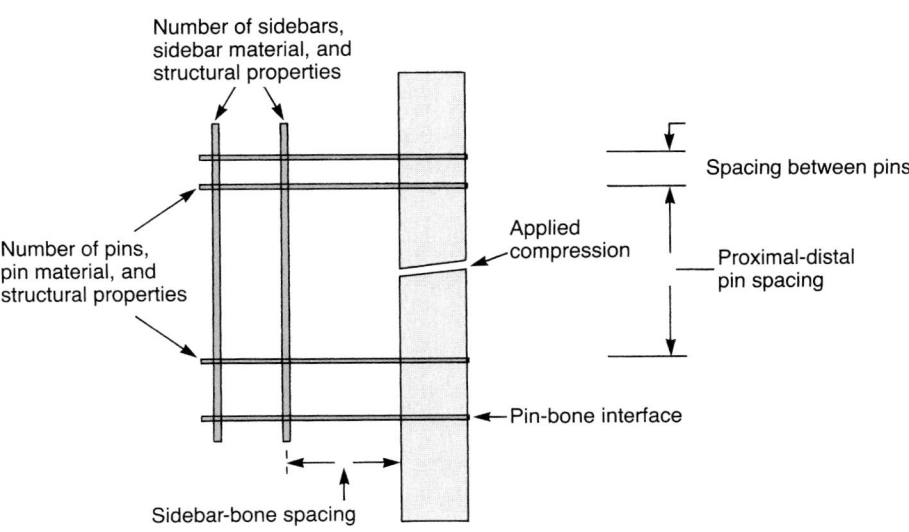

FIGURE 3-27 *Various loading modes that must be considered when evaluating the mechanical behavior of an externally fixed fracture.*

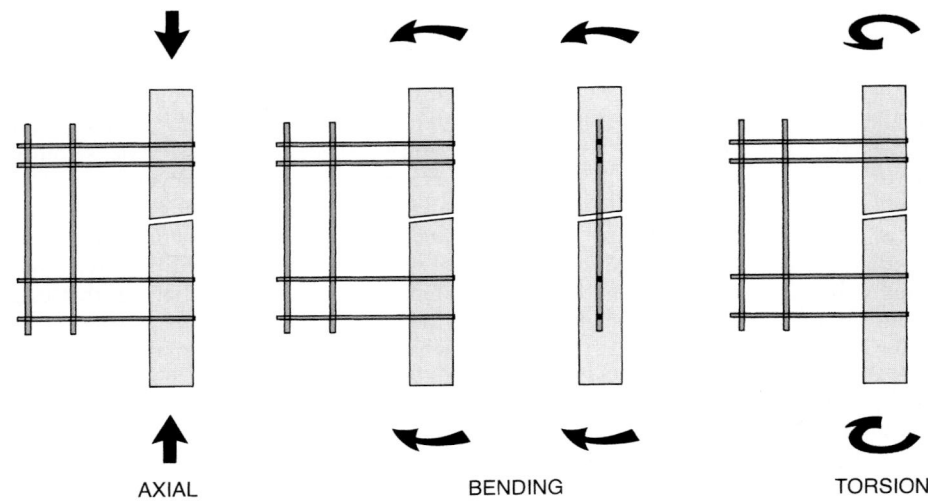

AXIAL   BENDING   TORSION

The relationship between pin diameter or sidebar-to-bone distance and fixator rigidity is more complicated in most fixators where several fixation pins are used and the fractures are subject to a variety of loads. Figures 3-28A–D illustrate this point using data from Chao and Hein[14] for a standard Orthofix external fixator tested ex vivo using an artificial fracture model. In this model, a single-plane external fixator is mounted in a plane identified as medial-lateral (ML). The axial stiffness data of Figure 3-28A show that, for example, a four-pin Orthofix fixator with a 4 mm sidebar-to-bone span will have an axial stiffness of about 3000 N/cm. Thus, a 600 N individual bearing half his weight on the fixed limb will cause approximately 1 mm displacement at the fracture site if a gap exists between the bone fragments. Experimental studies have found gap displacements up to 2 mm for a 600 N load, and these displacements are strongly dependent on the fixation system and the presence of callus.[47] Direct measurement of axial motion in externally fixed tibial diaphyseal fractures have found that displacements reached a maximum of 0.6 mm after 7 to 12 weeks of healing.[53]

Comparing Figures 3-28B and C demonstrates that the ML bending stiffness is more than 4 times the anteroposterior (AP) bending stiffness for the unilateral single-plane Orthofix fixator. The figures also show that the stiffness increases with the number of pins and decreases with sidebar-to-bone spacing under all loading configurations. However, the effect of sidebar-to-bone spacing is most pronounced with axial loads. A six-pin fixator is significantly stiffer than a four-pin fixator with axial and torsional loads, whereas the six-pin fixator is less rigid with bending loads applied in the plane of the fixator. Chao and Hein attribute this to uneven clamping pressure on the pins, causing some pins to carry more load than others.[14] If each pin carried the same load, the fixator stiffness should increase by a factor of 6/4 when comparing a six-pin to a four-pin frame.[44] The data for Figure 3-28 show that this is not the case for the Orthofix fixator, reinforcing the hypothesis that some pins must be supporting more load than others and thus may be more susceptible to pin loosening or pin failure.

External fixation is used both in situations where contact between bone fragments can be achieved (fracture reduction) and in situations where a gap remains initially between bone fragments (e.g., limb lengthening, severely comminuted fractures). These two situations provide substantially different biomechanical requirements for external fixation. Bone contact allows load sharing between bone and fixator for compressive, torsional, and certain bending loads. Without bone contact, the external fixator must support the full load, and this can have a significant effect on fracture healing. It is also possible to apply compression across a fracture gap using an external fixator. The amount of compression that can be applied depends in part on the rigidity of the external fixator. With transverse fractures, application of compression across the fracture site can greatly increase the stiffness of the frame-bone system.

Fixation pin loosening is a common problem with external fixators. Clinical and analytical studies have demonstrated that the pin-bone interface is potentially a weak link in the stability of an external fixation system.[45] Loose pins can substantially decrease the stability of an externally fixed fracture and lead to soft tissue problems. Commonly cited reasons for pin loosening include pin design and pin placement, pin tract infection, necrosis due to surgical trauma during pin placement, and necrosis due to unfavorable bone stress and contact pressure at the pin-bone interface. Suggested solutions to the pin loosening problem include changes in surgical technique, use of a hydroxyapatite coating, changes in pin properties and thread design, and changes in frame rigidity. However, rigorous human clinical studies of suggested solutions have yet to be reported.

FRACTURE HEALING WITH EXTERNAL FIXATION Experimental evidence suggesting that fracture fixation rigidity significantly affects the biology of bone healing has prompted several studies that compare bone healing with various external fixation rigidities. Wu et al. used a canine tibial osteotomy model to examine bone healing with a rigid six-pin versus a less rigid four-pin

FIGURE 3-28 ***A–D,*** *Fixator stiffness as a function of the distance between bone and sidebar for four different loading configurations. Data for both four- and six-pin fixator configurations are shown. The bending stiffness data of Chao et al. were converted to bending rigidities using the formulas from Figure 3-7. (Data from Chao, E.Y.; Hein, T.J. Mechanical performance of the standard Orthofix external fixator. Orthopedics 11(7):1057–1069, 1988.)*

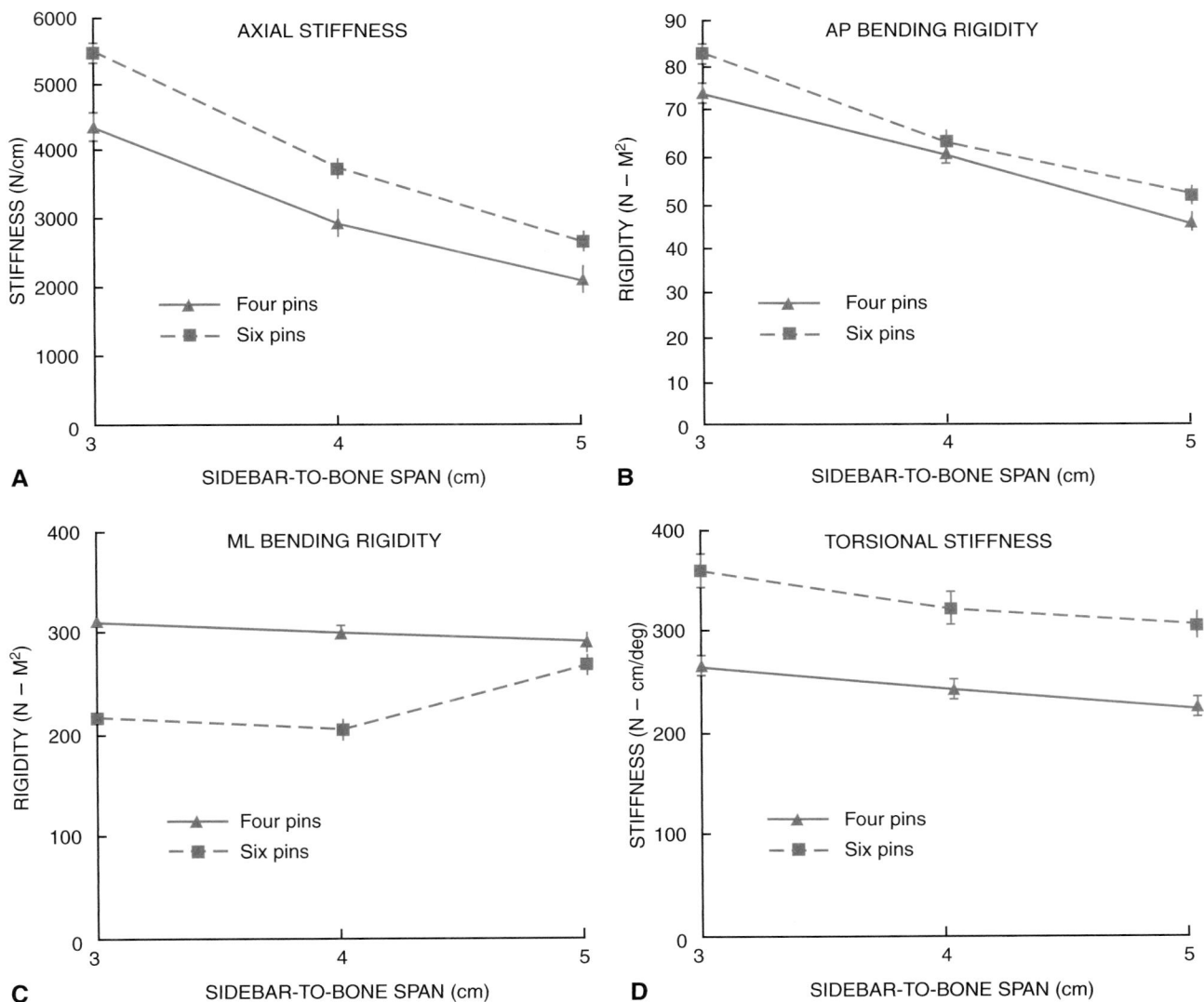

unilateral frame.[97] Union was achieved with all osteotomies; however, the clinical characteristics of bone healing depended on fixator rigidity. Bone union was clinically and biomechanically evident earlier with the more rigid frame. There was greater periosteal callus formation at 90 and 120 days and a higher incidence of pin loosening with less rigid frames. However, at 120 days after osteotomy, the torsional strength and torsional stiffness were not statistically different for the different frame rigidities. The fracture pattern noted during torsion testing suggested that the more rigidly fixed osteotomies had reached a more mature stage of fracture healing. The increased periosteal callus formation would provide torsional strength and stiffness for the less rigidly fixed tibiae. Thus, although the repair tissue formed with less rigidly fixed fractures

may be weaker as a material, the geometric distribution of the tissue provides structural stability. Histologic examination suggested that fracture healing occurred by direct cortical reconstruction with the rigid frames, whereas periosteal callus formation characteristic of secondary bone healing was evident with less rigid fixation.

The same general conclusions were realized in a study by Williams et al. that compared canine tibial osteotomies treated by one or two planes of external fixation.[93] The two-plane fixators were significantly more rigid in bending and torsion than the single-plane fixator while the axial stiffness of the fixators was similar. Bone union was achieved with both fixators. Higher fracture site stiffness early in the fracture-healing process and less callus formation were noted with the more rigid two-plane fixators.

However, after 13 weeks, the stiffness and radiographic characteristics of healing fractures were the same for the two external fixation frames. This study supports that of Wu et al.[97] in demonstrating that osteotomy union can be achieved with a range of external fixator rigidities, that more stiff external fixation frames result in more rapid return of fracture site stiffness, and that externally fixed osteotomies converge to similar biomechanical levels during later stages of fracture healing with various fixator rigidities.

External fixators that apply compression across the fracture provide more rigid fixation than those without compression. Hart et al. created tibial osteotomies bilaterally in dogs.[36] Both sides were treated with external fixators, but compression was applied on only one side. After 90 days, fracture healing was evaluated biochemically, histologically, and biomechanically. All of the osteotomies had healed after 90 days. The investigators found no significant differences in the blood flow, histology, or strength between the groups. They concluded that although compression increases the rigidity of externally fixed transverse osteotomies, it has little effect on the biological or biomechanical state of fracture healing at the time period studied.

Goodship and Kenwright investigated the influence of induced interfragmentary motion on the healing of tibial osteotomies in sheep.[34] They compared rigid fixation of an osteotomy with a 3 mm gap to a similar situation with the addition of a 1 mm axial deformation applied over 17-minute periods daily. They found a significant improvement in healing with the applied micromotion, as measured radiographically and by fracture stiffness. This improvement was evidently due to greater callus formation with the controlled motion. Kenwright et al. extended this study to examine alternate levels of applied micromotion and found that 2 mm deformations were detrimental to the healing, while 0.5 mm deformations enhanced the healing in later stages (8–12 weeks).[52] Kenwright used similar regimens of micromotion in a clinical study and found that fracture healing occurred earlier than in patients who received rigid external fixation with no applied micromotion.[51] In support of the value of limited micromotion, Goodship et al. have also shown that increasing the external fixation frame stiffness by moving the sidebars closer to the bone slowed down fracture healing in an ovine model of tibial fractures.[35]

Although numerous studies have shown that the rigidity of fracture fixation influences bone healing, most of these studies used experimental designs in which fixation rigidity was held constant throughout the study. Considering the interfragmentary strain hypothesis of Perren and co-workers leads immediately to the hypothesis that rigid fixation may be desirable early during healing to reduce the strain levels to a point where bone cells can survive. After osseous union has begun, it might be desirable to increase load transfer across the fracture site to stimulate bone remodeling. This concept is in common clinical practice where increased weight-bearing is prescribed following a period of reduced weight-bearing. External fixators provide a convenient method for altering fixation rigidity during the course of healing. This has prompted several recent studies in which fixation rigidity was altered during the course of fracture healing.

Dynamization is a term used to describe mechanisms that decrease the stiffness of a fixation device or mechanisms that allow increased motion between fracture fragments. A few devices specifically allow motion along one axis (axial dynamization). Dynamization is intended to accelerate fracture healing by allowing more load transfer across the fracture site following the initial stages of fracture healing.

To examine the effect of destabilization on unstable osteotomies, Egger et al. externally fixed bilateral oblique osteotomies in adult canine tibias.[29] In this case, a 2 mm gap was left between fracture fragments. After 6 weeks, the rigidity of fixation was reduced on one side. After 12 weeks, the "destabilized" tibia had significantly greater torsional strength (but not stiffness) than the tibia with constant rigid fixation. The difference was attributed to more advanced bone remodeling of the initial bone healing response. It is also noteworthy that the differences were not radiographically evident.

The benefits of dynamization were also demonstrated by Claes et al. in 12 sheep.[18] They created osteotomies with a 0.6 mm gap and stabilized them with a specially designed high bending and torsional stiffness external ring fixator. Axial movement across the osteotomy of less than 0.06 mm was allowed in six sheep while dynamic axial movement of between 0.15 and 0.34 mm was allowed in the other six sheep. With healing, callus formation around the osteotomy reduced motion across the gap. After 9 weeks, compared with the rigidly fixed osteotomies, the dynamized osteotomies had approximately 41 percent more callus formation and 45 percent greater tensile strength.

Dynamization increases the load that is transferred across the fracture and may allow increased micromotion between fragments. The effect of micromotion on fracture healing is not clear. Kershaw et al. have shown in a prospective clinical study that imposing micromotion reduced healing time for tibial diaphyseal fractures.[53] In contrast, Aro et al. applied Orthofix unilateral fixators to transverse osteotomies bilaterally in dogs.[3] After 15 days, axial motion was allowed on one side while rigid fixation was maintained contralaterally. After 90 days, the periosteal callus was more uniformly distributed on the side where axial freedom was allowed; however, the torsional stiffness and strength were the same for both bones.

In a sheep model of fracture healing, micromotion at an osteotomy site was controlled by applying external fixators that allowed controlled amounts of micromotion.[16] Micromotions of approximately 0.2 mm were allowed in one group, and 1 mm micromotion was allowed in the other. There was significantly more bone and a greater number of blood vessels in the group with small micromotions at 9 weeks after surgery. The osteotomy gap used in that study was 2 mm wide, so 1 mm of micromotion would cause 50 percent nominal strain across the gap, and this may not have been compatible with the later stages of fracture healing, as described in Perren's interfragmentary strain hypothesis.

Further studies are needed to determine which types of fractures benefit from delayed reduction in fixation rigidity, what magnitude of rigidity reduction is optimal, what the optimal time to change rigidity is, and how rigidity or other parameters can be noninvasively monitored.

Comparative Studies of Healing with Different Types of Fixation

The preceding discussions have examined the wide range of fracture fixation stability that can be obtained with various treatments and the different types of healing that occur with rigid versus less rigid fixation. However, the relative merits of the different healing patterns are widely debated, and little quantitative evidence is available for comparison on other than clinical grounds. Micromovement between bone fragments facilitates fracture healing, but the acceptable range of micromotion and the optimal range of micromotion have not been determined.

Although nonmechanical clinical aspects of a fracture may dictate the best fracture treatment approach, there are cases for which several options exist, and mechanical considerations are important in selecting a fixation method. Several animal studies have been reported that compare fracture healing with different types of fixation (plates vs. rods, internal vs. external fixation, etc.). Rand et al. compared compression plates and reamed, fluted intramedullary rods using the canine transverse tibial osteotomy model.[69] They evaluated blood flow, fracture site morphology, and bone strength at various times up to 120 days postfracture. Clinical union was evident in all dogs after 42 days. Blood flow to the fracture site reached higher levels and it remained high longer in osteotomies treated with reaming and intramedullary rods. There was significantly more new bone formation with intramedullary fixation, with most of the new bone formed in periosteal callus. With compression plating, most of the new bone formed was endosteal. Plated bones were significantly stronger and stiffer than rod fixed bones at 42 and 90 days but not at 120 days. The study demonstrated different healing mechanisms with the two treatments studied, but the time required to establish normal strength and stiffness was not different.

Sarmiento et al. compared rigid compression plating to functional braces for closed, nondisplaced fractures and found that the fractures treated with functional braces produced abundant callus and had greater torsional strength than the rigidly fixed fractures.[76] However, Lewallen et al. radiographically, histologically, and biomechanically compared osteotomies fixed by compression plating to those stabilized by external fixators using the canine tibia model.[59] Initially, the less rigid externally fixed osteotomies were significantly less stiff than those fixed by the more rigid compression plating. Dogs applied more load sooner to the compression-plated leg than to the contralateral externally fixed limb. After 120 days, bone union occurred in most animals independently of fixation method. However, compression-plated bones were significantly stronger and stiffer in torsion than those that were externally fixed. Histologically, the total amount of new bone was similar for the two fixation methods, but there was significantly more resorbed bone and intracortical porosity with externally fixed bones and more intracortical new bone on the compression-plated side. In addition, there was greater blood flow to externally fixed osteotomy sites, consistent with other results suggesting increased bone remodeling with the less stable fixation.

Terjesen and Svenningsen utilized transverse tibial osteotomies in rabbits to compare fracture healing with metal plates to that with plaster casts and to examine the role of limb loading in fracture healing with the different treatments.[86] Four experimental groups were studied: (1) plate fixation, (2) plate fixation with a long plaster cast, (3) long plaster cast, and (4) short plaster cast. The long plaster casts were intended to restrict loads on the healing bone. Callus area, bending strength, and bending stiffness were evaluated after 6 weeks. Fractures that were treated with the long plaster cast, both with and without plating, were significantly weaker and less stiff. More periosteal callus developed with both long and short cast treatments than with plated fractures. The authors made the very important and clinically relevant observation that weight-bearing and muscular activity are more effective at promoting bony union than fixation stiffness.

MONITORING FRACTURE HEALING

Because bones are structural members whose functions are to support the body and permit skeletal motions necessary for survival, it seems natural that fracture healing should be evaluated by the return of prefracture stiffness and strength. Instead, however, clinical assessments of fracture healing are typically made by radiographic criteria that are known to be imprecise, by subjective assessments of pain, and by reference to previous clinical experience. As a result, little is known about the return of stiffness and strength to healing bones. Noninvasive imaging techniques may also allow objective assessment of fracture healing,[25] but the sensitivity and specificity of these techniques are largely unknown in clinical practice.

Several research groups have proposed or implemented noninvasive physical tests for monitoring the biomechanical progression of fracture healing. The general approach is to apply loads across the fracture gap and measure the resultant deflections. Many of these methods are directed toward externally fixed fractures, since the external fixation pins provide a direct mechanical connection to the fractured bone (assuming that the pins have not loosened). As the fracture heals, the slope of the load versus displacement curve increases, representing a return to the original stiffness of the bone. The goal is to monitor the load versus displacement curve to determine whether the union is proceeding normally. There are two advantages to this information. First, in the case of delayed union, corrective action can be taken earlier than would be allowed using radiographic information alone. Second, the biomechanics of the fracture treatment can be "fine tuned" to provide the optimal mechanical environment for fracture healing.

One clinical objective of fracture treatment is to restore the load-bearing capacity of the bone. In the laboratory, bone from animal models of fracture healing can be removed and both the stiffness and the load-bearing capacity can be measured. In contrast, only the stiffness of healing bones can be measured in patients. It is therefore important to understand the relationships between stiffness and load-bearing capacity of healing fractures. Henry et al. demonstrated that caution is needed when bone stiffness is used to determine the strength of a healing fracture.[40] They utilized a rabbit osteotomy model. Fractures were fixed by intramedullary rodding, plating, or no surgical intervention. Bones were tested using four-point bending 5 to 10 weeks post-osteotomy. All fracture treatments resulted in similar biomechanical results, so the data were pooled. Figure 3-29 shows the relationship between bone strength and bone stiffness 5 weeks after osteotomy. Both strength and stiffness values are expressed as the ratio of fractured bone to intact bone. The regression line for the data indicates a slope of about 0.5, suggesting that bone strength returns more slowly than bone stiffness.

Proposed methods for monitoring externally fixed fracture healing can be divided into two groups: (1) methods that involve application of quasi-static loads across the fracture, and (2) methods that utilize dynamic or vibration type loads. Beaupre et al. demonstrated the application of fracture site monitoring using static loads.[7] A Hoffman-Vidal external fixation system was applied to an idealized fracture model ex vivo. The model consisted of Plexiglass cylinders representing a long bone with neoprene disks of various stiffness placed between the ends of the cylinders representing the healing fracture gap. Loads were applied to the fixation pins, and the deflection across the fracture gap was monitored. They also utilized an analytical (finite element) model of the external fixator in which changes in the fracture site stiffness could be altered. Both the experimental and analytical results demonstrated that the stiffness of a fracture gap could be evaluated by this method.

The relationships between external fixator pin displacement and the mechanical properties of the fracture site are nonlinear[7] and dependent on the applied load characteristics. Thus, it is important to document the relationship between pin displacement and fracture site

stiffness for each external fixator frame configuration before interpreting the data. For most loading configurations, there is a relatively steep decrease in pin displacement for initial increases in fracture site stiffness (0–10% of intact bone stiffness). During later stages of fracture healing, the decrease in pin displacement is small for large increases in fracture site stiffness (Figure 3-30B). If the connectors in the external fixation frame become loose, it will be difficult to separate this effect from the effects of fracture healing.

Richardson et al. measured the bending stiffness of externally fixed tibial fractures in 212 patients.[71] They demonstrated that the refracture rate in patients was less when the fixators were removed and weight-bearing allowed based on measured fracture stiffness. They used a threshold of 15 newton-meters per degree (measured by a load cell under the heal and strain gauges on the sidebar or by an electronic goniometer) as their threshold to classify a fracture as sufficiently healed.

Fracture site monitoring using dynamic tests typically involves application of an oscillating or impulse load across the fracture gap and monitoring the acceleration or displacement of the bone at one or more locations. An example of a dynamic system for monitoring fractures is the bone resonance analysis (BRA) method, developed and tested by Cornelissen et al. for monitoring tibial fractures.[21] This technique is designed to measure the lowest resonant frequency of a fractured tibia. The basis for the BRA method is that the resonant frequency of a tibia will decrease significantly owing to fracture and will then increase as the fracture heals. Small, 30 to 300 Hz cyclic, axial loads are applied to the medial malleolus and below the tibial tuberosity. The acceleration of a point along the anterior surface of the tibia is monitored. The resonant frequency of the limb is determined as the vibration frequency that results in the greatest tibial mobility. In clinical practice, the resonant frequency of the fracture limb is monitored during the course of fracture healing. This technique requires that loads be transmitted across soft tissues. Along with the presence of joints and variable muscle tension, interpretation of BRA test results is complicated. For this reason, the absolute values of measured resonant frequencies are not reliable and the data must be analyzed for temporal changes in resonant frequencies. Comparative measurements using a normal contralateral limb serve as a reference. No significant difference between resonant frequencies of normal left and right limbs was observed in tests of over 50 normal individuals.

Tibial refractures following external fixation occur in a significant number of patients, as described in Chapter 58. Quantitative measurement of structural properties can help determine the optimal time to remove the fixator and may thereby reduce the refracture rate.[71] The sensitivity of the stiffness measurement was 100 percent, but the specificity was 78 percent. Several potential difficulties must be considered. For example, fixation pin loosening significantly alters the stability of an externally fixed fracture. Pin loosening could also lead to misleading results if pin displacements are used to monitor fracture biomechanics. Thus, it is important to monitor pin loosening in studies in which pin displacements are employed to monitor fracture healing. Similarly, all connections in

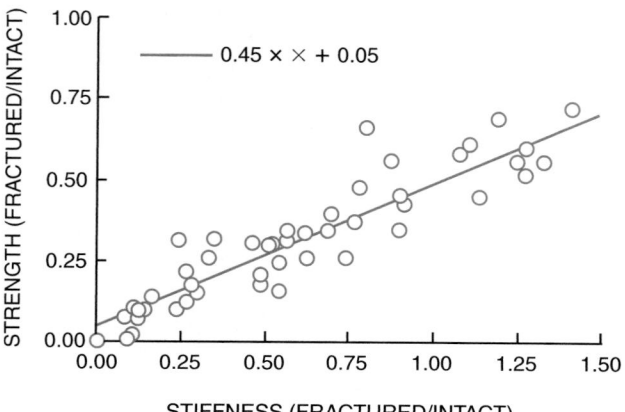

FIGURE 3-29   *Bone strength versus fracture stiffness for rabbit tibial osteotomies after 5 weeks of healing with several different fracture treatment methods. (Data from Henry, A. N.; Freeman, M.A.; Swanson, S.A. Studies on the mechanical properties of healing experimental fractures. Proc R Soc Med 61(9):902–906, 1968.)*

FIGURE 3-30 ***A*** and ***B***, Analytical results for an idealized model of an externally fixed fracture. The pin displacement during application of distraction and bending loads to the bone is shown as a function of fracture site stiffness. (Data from An, K.N.; Kasman, R.A.; Chao, E.Y. Theoretical analysis of fracture healing monitoring with external fixators. Eng Med 17(1):11–15, 1988.)

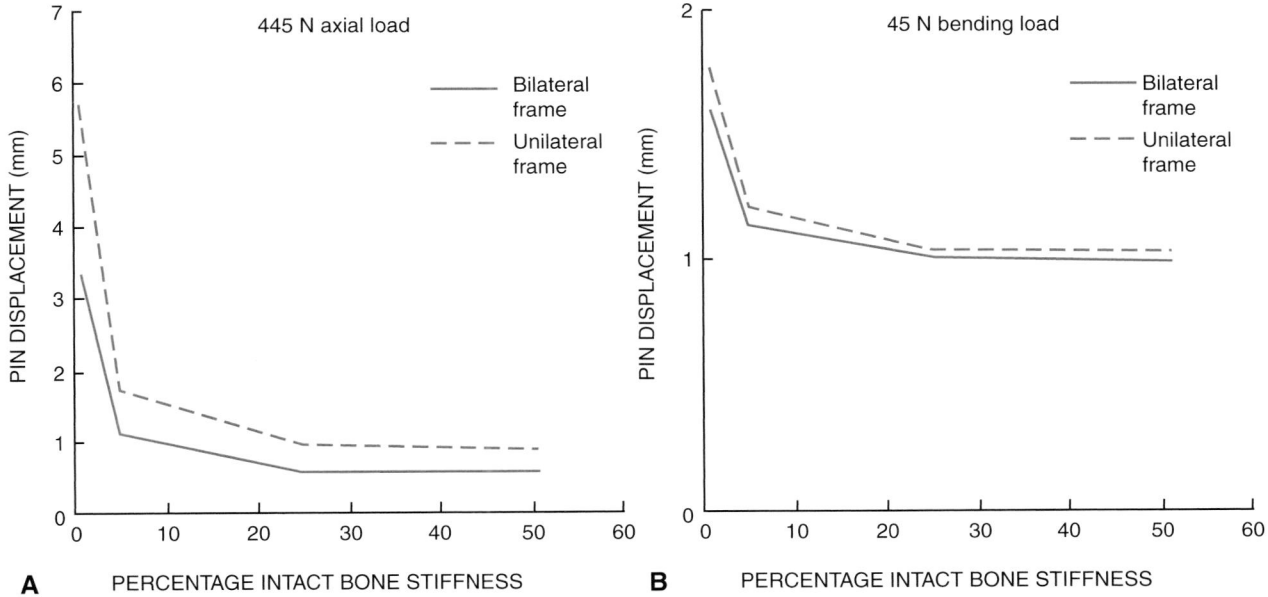

the external fixation system must not be allowed to loosen, since this will lead to misleading results. Additionally, few studies have adequately characterized the sensitivity of the monitoring techniques to determine the resolution of the in vivo biomechanical measurements and how clinical alterations in frame configurations affect data over the treatment period. Finally, additional clinical data are required to biomechanically characterize "normal" fracture-healing patterns in humans, since standard curves are needed to identify abnormal temporal sequences in fracture healing.

SUMMARY

Biomechanical studies of the material and structural properties of bones have provided a basic understanding of bone properties and the alterations in bone properties that can accompany aging and some bone pathologies. This information has been applied in several experimental and analytical studies that are enhancing our ability to predict fracture risk associated with aging and metastatic bone disease. This basic understanding of bone biomechanics also facilitates understanding of the fracture treatment biomechanics, since the mechanical properties of bone and the mechanical properties of the fracture treatment together determine the biomechanics of a fixation system.

Two basic types of fracture-healing biologies have been identified, and it has been well established that biomechanical factors influence fracture healing but also that they interact strongly with biologic factors such as the vascularity. Numerous animal studies have demonstrated that the return of bone stiffness and strength

can be altered by fixation rigidity. However, consensus has not been established on the optimal fixation rigidity for different types of fractures, nor has consensus been reached on whether or how fixation rigidity should be altered as the fracture heals. It is clear that the optimal type and rigidity of fixation depend on the type of fracture. The literature does provide information that can facilitate clinical management of orthopaedic fractures, and computer models are showing great promise for accurate and reliable simulation of the fracture-healing process. Selection of the optimal fracture management involves balancing sometimes conflicting requirements. Several studies have demonstrated that a wide range of fixation stabilities are available through numerous internal and external fixation device designs and applications. Frequently, several basic mechanical principles can be used to understand the degree of fixation rigidity provided by each treatment method. When specific biomechanical fixation requirements can be identified, sufficient engineering tools are available to choose a treatment method. One application of biomechanical analyses of fracture treatment is the monitoring of the biomechanical progression of fracture healing. Methods are being developed that will allow noninvasive biomechanical monitoring. Further research may provide noninvasive and objective measures to select treatment methods, alter treatment during the course of healing, and time the removal of the fixation for optimal return of normal weight-bearing.

However, the medical and scientific community would have to undertake a very large scale, coordinated effort to establish rigorous, evidence-based clinical guidelines for selecting optimal fixation for a specific fracture.

REFERENCES

1. Akeson, W.H.; Woo, S.L.; Rutherford, L.; et al. The effects of rigidity of internal fixation plates on long bone remodeling: A biomechanical and quantitative histological study. Acta Orthop Scand 47(3):241–249, 1976.
2. An, K.N.; Kasman, R.A.; Chao, E.Y. Theoretical analysis of fracture healing monitoring with external fixators. Eng Med 17:11–15, 1988.
3. Aro, H.T.; Kelly, P.J.; Lewallen, D.G.; et al. The effects of physiologic dynamic compression on bone healing under external fixation. Clin Orthop Rel Res 25(6):260–273, 1990.
4. Augat, P.; Burger, J.; Schorlemmer, S.; et al. Shear movement at the fracture site delays healing in a diaphyseal fracture model. J Orthop Res 21(6):1011–1017, 2003.
5. Augat, P.; Simon, U.; Liedert, A.; et al. Mechanics and mechano-biology of fracture healing in normal and osteoporotic bone. Osteoporos Int 16(Suppl 2):S36–S43, 2005.
6. Bayraktar, H.H.; Morgan, E.F.; Niebur, G.L.; et al. Comparison of the elastic and yield properties of human femoral trabecular and cortical bone tissue. J Biomech 37(1):27–35, 2004.
7. Beaupre, G.S.; Hayes, W.C.; Jofe, M.H. Monitoring fracture site properties with external fixation. J Biomech Eng 105(2):120–126, 1983.
8. Beck, T.J.; Looker, A.C.; Ruff, C.B.; et al. Structural trends in the aging femoral neck and proximal shaft: Analysis of the Third National Health and Nutrition Examination Survey dual-energy X-ray absorptiometry data. J Bone Miner Res 151(2):2297–2304, 2000.
9. Beck, T.J.; Ruff, C.B.; Shaffer, R.A.; et al. Stress fracture in military recruits: Gender differences in muscle and bone susceptibility factors. Bone 27(3):437–444, 2000.
10. Black, J.; Perdigon, P.; Brown, N.; et al. Stiffness and strength of fracture callus: Relative rates of mechanical maturation as evaluated by a uniaxial tensile test. Clin Orthop Rel Res 18(2):278–288, 1984.
11. Bradley, G.W.; McKenna, G.B.; Dunn, H.K.; et al. Effects of flexural rigidity of plates on bone healing. J Bone Joint Surg Am 61(6):866–872, 1979.
12. Carter, D.R.; Hayes, W.C. Bone compressive strength: The influence of density and strain rate. Science 194(4270):1174–1176, 1976.
13. Carter, D.R.; Hayes, W.C. The compressive behavior of bone as a two-phase porous structure. J Bone Joint Surg Am 59(7):954–962, 1977.
14. Chao, E.Y.; Hein, T.J. Mechanical performance of the standard Orthofix external fixator. Orthopedics 11(7):1057–1069, 1988.
15. Cheal, E.J.; Hayes, W.C.; White, A.A. III; et al. Stress analysis of compression plate fixation and its effects on long bone remodeling. J Biomech 18(2):141–150, 1985.
16. Claes, L. The effect of mechanical stability on local vascularization and tissue differentiation in callus healing. J Orthop Res 20(5):1099–1105, 2002.
17. Claes, L.E.; Heigele, C.A.; Neidlinger-Wilke, C.; et al. Effects of mechanical factors on the fracture healing process. Clin Orthop Rel Res 355(suppl):S132–S147, 1984.
18. Claes, L.E.; Wilke, H.J.; Augat, P.; et al. Effect of dynamization on gap healing of diaphyseal fractures under external fixation. Clin Biomech (Bristol, Avon) 10:227–234, 1995.
19. Cody, D.D.; Gross, G.J.; Hou, F.J.; et al. Femoral strength is better predicted by finite element models than QCT and DXA. J Biomech 321(0):1013–1020, 1999.
20. Cordey, J.; Borgeaud, M.; Perren, S.M. Force transfer between the plate and the bone: Relative importance of the bending stiffness of the screws and the friction between plate and bone. Injury 31:21–28, 2000.
21. Cornelissen, P.; Cornelissen, M.; Van der Perre, G.; et al. Assessment of tibial stiffness by vibration testing in situ: II. Influence of soft tissues, joints and fibula. J Biomech 19(7):551–561, 1986.
22. Cornell, C.N. Internal fracture fixation in patients with osteoporosis. J Am Acad Orthop Surg 11(2):109–119, 2003.
23. Courtney, A.C.; Wachtel, E.F.; Myers, E.R.; et al. Effects of loading rate on strength of the proximal femur. Calcif Tissue Int 55(1):53–58, 1994.
24. Davy, D.T.; Connolly, J.F. The biomechanical behavior of healing canine radii and ribs. J Biomech 15(4):235–247, 1982.
25. den Boer, F.C.; Bramer, J.A.M.; Patka, P.; et al. Quantification of fracture healing with three-dimensional computed tomography. Arch Orthop Trauma Surg 117(6):345–350, 1998.
26. DiGioia, A.M. III; Cheal, E.J.; Hayes, W.C. Three-dimensional strain fields in a uniform osteotomy gap. J Biomech Eng 108(3):273–280, 1986.
27. Dong, X.N.; Guo, X.E. The dependence of transversely isotropic elasticity of human femoral cortical bone on porosity. J Biomech 37(8):1281–1287, 2004.
28. Drijber, F.L.; Finlay, J.B. Universal joint slippage as a cause of Hoffmann half-frame external fixator failure [corrected]. J Biomed Eng 14(6):509–515, 1992.
29. Egger, E.L.; Gottsauner-Wolf, F.; Palmer, J.; et al. Effects of axial dynamization on bone healing. J Trauma 34(2):185–192, 1993.
30. Elefteriou, F.; Ahn, J.D.; Takeda, S.; et al. Leptin regulation of bone resorption by the sympathetic nervous system and CART. Nature 434(7032):514–520, 2005.
31. Frankle, M.; Cordey, J.; Sanders, R.W.; et al. A biomechanical comparison of the antegrade inserted universal femoral nail with the retrograde inserted universal tibial nail for use in femoral shaft fractures. Injury 30(suppl 1):A40–A43, 1999.

32. George, W.T.; Vashishth, D. Damage mechanisms and failure modes of cortical bone under components of physiological loading. J Orthop Res 23(5):1047–1053, 2005.

33. Gitelis, S.; Wilkins, R.; Conrad, E.U. Benign bone tumors. Instr Course Lect 45:425–446, 1996.

34. Goodship, A.E.; Kenwright, J. The influence of induced micromovement upon the healing of experimental tibial fractures. J Bone Joint Surg Br 67(4):650–655, 1985.

35. Goodship, A.E.; Watkins, P.E.; Rigby, H.S.; et al. The role of fixator frame stiffness in the control of fracture healing: An experimental study. J Biomech 269:1027–1035, 1993.

36. Hart, M.B.; Woo, J.J.; Chao, E.Y.; et al. External skeletal fixation of canine tibial osteotomies: Compression compared with no compression. J Bone Joint Surg Am 67:598–605, 1985.

37. Hartsell, W.F.; Scott, C.B.; Bruner, D.W.; et al. Randomized trial of short- versus long-course radiotherapy for palliation of painful bone metastases. J Natl Cancer Inst 97(11):798–804, 2005.

38. Hayes, W.C. Biomechanics of fracture healing. In: Heppenstall, R.B., ed. Fracture Treatment and Healing. Philadelphia, W.B. Saunders, 1980, pp. 124–172.

39. Hayes, W.C.; Perren, S.M. Flexural rigidity of compression plate fixation of fractures. (Abstract.) Proceedings of the Second Nordic Meeting on Medical and Biological Engineering, Oslo, Norway, 1971.

40. Henry, A.N.; Freeman, M.A.; Swanson, S.A. Studies on the mechanical properties of healing experimental fractures. Proc R Soc Med 61(9):902–906, 1968.

41. Hernandez, C.J.; Keaveny, T.M. A biomechanical perspective on bone quality. Bone 39:1173–1187, 2006.

42. Hipp, J.A.; McBroom, R.J.; Cheal, E.J.; et al. Structural consequences of endosteal metastatic lesions in long bones. J Orthop Res 76:828–837, 1989.

43. Hipp, J.A.; Springfield, D.S.; Hayes, W.C. Predicting pathologic fracture risk in the management of metastatic bone defects. Clin Orthop Rel Res 31(2):120–135, 1995.

44. Huiskes, R.; Chao, E.Y.S. Guidelines for external fixation frame rigidity and stresses. J Orthop Res 41:68–75, 1986.

45. Huiskes, R.; Chao, E.Y.; Crippen, T.E. Parametric analyses of pin-bone stresses in external fracture fixation devices. J Orthop Res 33:341–349, 1985.

46. Hutson, J.J.; Zych, G.A.; Cole, J.D.; et al. Mechanical failures of intramedullary tibial nails applied without reaming. Clin Orthop Rel Res 31(5):129–137, 1995.

47. Juan, J.A.; Prat, J.; Vera, P.; et al. Biomechanical consequences of callus development in Hoffmann, Wagner, Orthofix, and Ilizarov external fixators. J Biomech 25(9):995–1006, 1992.

48. Keaveny, T.M.; Yeh, O.C. Architecture and trabecular bone: Toward an improved understanding of the biomechanical effects of age, sex and osteoporosis. J Musculoskelet Neuronal Interact 23:205–208, 2002.

49. Keene, G.S.; Parker, M.J.; Pryor, G.A. Mortality and morbidity after hip fractures. BMJ 307(6914):1248-1250, 1993.

50. Keene, J.S.; Sellinger, D.S.; McBeath, A.A.; et al. Metastatic breast cancer in the femur: A search for the lesion at risk of fracture. Clin Orthop Rel Res 20(3):282–288, 1986.

51. Kenwright, J.; Richardson, J.B.; Cunningham, J.L.; et al. Axial movement and tibial fractures: A controlled randomised trial of treatment. J Bone Joint Surg Br 73(4):654–659, 1991.

52. Kenwright, J.; Richardson, J.B.; Goodship, A.E.; et al. Effect of controlled axial micromovement on healing of tibial fractures. Lancet 2(8517):1185–1187, 1986.

53. Kershaw, C.J.; Cunningham, J.L.; Kenwright, J. Tibial external fixation, weight bearing, and fracture movement. Clin Orthop 29(3):28–36, 1993.

54. Keyak, J.H.; Kaneko, T.S.; Rossi, S.A.; et al. Predicting the strength of femoral shafts with and without metastatic lesions. Clin Orthop Rel Res 43(9):161–170, 2005.

55. Keyak, J.H.; Kaneko, T.S.; Tehranzadeh, J.; et al. Predicting proximal femoral strength using structural engineering models. Clin Orthop Rel Res 43(7):219–228, 2005.

56. Koval, K.J.; Kummer, F.J.; Bharam, S.; et al. Distal femoral fixation: A laboratory comparison of the 95 degrees plate, antegrade and retrograde inserted reamed intramedullary nails. J Orthop Trauma 10(6):378–382, 1996.

57. Laurence, M.; Freeman, M.A.; Swanson, S.A. Engineering considerations in the internal fixation of fractures of the tibial shaft. J Bone Joint Surg Br 51(4):754–768, 1969.

58. Levenston, M.E.; Beaupre, G.S.; van der Meulen, M.C. Improved method for analysis of whole bone torsion tests. J Bone Miner Res 99:1459–1465, 1994.

59. Lewallen, D.G.; Chao, E.Y.; Kasman, R.A.; et al. Comparison of the effects of compression plates and external fixators on early bone-healing. J Bone Joint Surg Am 66:1084–1091, 1984.

60. Li, J.; Ahmad, T.; Spetea, M.; et al. Bone reinnervation after fracture: A study in the rat. J Bone Miner Res 16(8):1505–1510, 2001.

61. Lotz, J.C.; Cheal, E.J.; Hayes, W.C. Stress distributions within the proximal femur during gait and falls: Implications for osteoporotic fracture. Osteoporos Int 54:252–261, 1995.

62. Lotz, J.C.; Hayes, W.C. The use of quantitative computed tomography to estimate risk of fracture of the hip from falls. J Bone Joint Surg Am 72(5):689–700, 1990.

63. Mackerle, J. Finite element modeling and simulations in orthopedics: A bibliography, 1998–2005. Comput Methods Biomech Biomed Engin 93:149–199, 2006.

64. Nagurka, M.L.; Hayes, W.C. An interactive graphics package for calculating cross-sectional properties of complex shapes. J Biomech 13(1):59–64, 1980.

65. Panjabi, M.M.; Walter, S.D.; Karuda, M.; et al. Correlations of radiographic analysis of healing fractures with strength: A statistical analysis of experimental osteotomies. J Orthop Res 3(2):212–218, 1985.

66. Panjabi, M.M.; White, A.A. III; Southwick, W.O. Temporal changes in the physical properties of healing fractures in rabbits. J Biomech 10(11):689–699, 1977.

67. Perren, S.M. Evolution of the internal fixation of long bone fractures: The scientific basis of biological internal fixation: Choosing a new balance between stability and biology. J Bone Joint Surg Br 84(8):1093–1110, 2002.

68. Perren, S.M.; Rahn, B.A. Biomechanics of fracture healing. Can J Surg 23(3):228–232, 1980.

69. Rand, J.A.; An, K.N.; Chao, E.Y.; et al. A comparison of the effect of open intramedullary nailing and compression-plate fixation on fracture-site blood flow and fracture union. J Bone Joint Surg Am 63:427–442, 1981.

70. Reilly, D.T.; Burstein, A.H. The elastic and ultimate properties of compact bone tissue. J Biomech 86:393–405, 1975.

71. Richardson, J.B.; Cunningham, J.L.; Goodship, A.E.; et al. Measuring stiffness can define healing of tibial fractures. J Bone Joint Surg Br 76(3):389–394, 1994.

72. Riggs, B.L.; Melton, L.J. III; Robb, R.A.; et al. Population-based analysis of the relationship of whole bone strength indices and fall-related loads to age- and sex-specific patterns of hip and wrist fractures. J Bone Miner Res 21(2):315–323, 2006.

73. Riggs, B.L.; Melton, I.L. III; Robb, R.A.; et al. Population-based study of age and sex differences in bone volumetric density, size, geometry, and structure at different skeletal sites. J Bone Miner Res 19(12):1945–1954, 2004.

74. Roark, R.J.; Young, W.C. Formulas for Stress and Strain, 5th ed. New York, McGraw-Hill, 1975.

75. Ruff, C.B. Mechanical determinants of bone form: Insights from skeletal remains. J Musculoskelet Neuronal Interact 53:202–212, 2005.

76. Sarmiento, A.; Mullis, D.L.; Latta, L.L.; et al. A quantitative comparative analysis of fracture healing under the influence of compression plating vs. closed weight-bearing treatment. Clin Orthop 14(9):232–239, 1980.

77. Sartoretti, C.; Sartoretti-Schefer, S.; Ruckert, R.; et al. Comorbid conditions in old patients with femur fractures. J Trauma 43(4):570–577, 1997.

78. Sjostedt, A.; Zetterberg, C.; Hansson, T.; et al. Bone mineral content and fixation strength of femoral neck fractures: A cadaver study. Acta Orthop Scand 652:161–165, 1994.

79. Smith, M.D.; Cody, D.D.; Goldstein, S.A.; et al. Proximal femoral bone density and its correlation to fracture load and hip-screw penetration load. Clin Orthop Rel Res 28(3):244–251, 1992.

80. Snyder, B.D.; Hauser-Kara, D.A.; Hipp, J.A.; et al. Predicting fracture through benign skeletal lesions with quantitative computed tomography. J Bone Joint Surg Am 88(1):55–70, 2006.

81. Spruijt, S.; van der Linden, J.C.; Dijkstra, P.D.; et al. Prediction of torsional failure in 22 cadaver femora with and without simulated subtrochanteric metastatic defects: A CT scan–based finite element analysis. Acta Orthop 77(3):474–481, 2006.

82. Stoffel, K.; Klaue, K.; Perren, S.M. Functional load of plates in fracture fixation in vivo and its correlate in bone healing. Injury 31(suppl 2):S50, 2000.

83. Taylor, W.R.; Heller, M.O.; Bergmann, G.; et al. Tibio-femoral loading during human gait and stair climbing. J Orthop Res 22(3):625–632, 2004.

84. Tencer, A.F.; Sherman, M.C.; Johnson, K.D. Biomechanical factors affecting fracture stability and femoral bursting in closed intramedullary rod fixation of femur fractures. J Biomech Eng 107(2):104–111, 1985.

85. Terjesen, T.; Apalset, K. The influence of different degrees of stiffness of fixation plates on experimental bone healing. J Orthop Res 62:293–299, 1988.

86. Terjesen, T.; Svenningsen, S. The effects of function and fixation stiffness on experimental bone healing. Acta Orthop Scand 59(6):712–715, 1988.

87. Turner, C.H.; Burr, D.B. Basic biomechanical measurements of bone: A tutorial. Bone 14(4):595–608, 1993.

88. Utvag, S.E.; Reikeras, O. Effects of nail rigidity on fracture healing: Strength and mineralisation in rat femoral bone. Arch Orthop Trauma Surg 11(8):7–13, 1998.

89. Vajjhala, S.; Kraynik, A.M.; Gibson, L.J. A cellular solid model for modulus reduction due to resorption of trabeculae in bone. J Biomech Eng 12(25):511–515, 2000.

90. van der Linden, Y.M.; Dijkstra, P.D.; Kroon, H.M.; et al. Comparative analysis of risk factors for pathological fracture with femoral metastases. J Bone Joint Surg Br 86(4):566–573, 2004.

91. Whealan, K.M.; Kwak, S.D.; Tedrow, J.R.; et al. Noninvasive imaging predicts failure load of the spine with simulated osteolytic defects. J Bone Joint Surg Am 82(9):1240–1251, 2000.

92. White, A.A. III; Panjabi, M.M.; Southwick, W.O. The four biomechanical stages of fracture repair. J Bone Joint Surg Am 59(2):188–192, 1977.

93. Williams, E.A. The early healing of tibial osteotomies stabilized by one-plane or two-plane external fixation. J Bone Joint Surg Am 69:355–365, 1987.

94. Windhagen, H.J.; Hipp, J.A.; Silva, M.J.; et al. Predicting failure of thoracic vertebrae with simulated and actual metastatic defects. Clin Orthop Rel Res 34(4):313–319, 1997.

95. Winwood, K.; Zioupos, P.; Currey, J.D.; et al. Strain patterns during tensile, compressive, and shear fatigue of human cortical bone and implications for bone biomechanics. J Biomed Mater Res A 79:289–297, 2006.

96. Woo, S.L.Y.; Lothringer, K.S.; Akeson, W.H.; et al. Less rigid internal fixation plates: Historical perspectives and new concepts. J Orthop Res 14:431–449, 1983.

97. Wu, J.J. Comparison of osteotomy healing under external fixation devices with different stiffness characteristics. J Bone Joint Surg Am 66:1258–1264, 1984.

98. Yeni, Y.N.; Fyhrie, D.P. A rate-dependent micro-crack-bridging model that can explain the strain rate dependency of cortical bone apparent yield strength. J Biomech 36(9):1343–1353, 2003.

99. Zioupos, P.; Currey, J.D. Changes in the stiffness, strength, and toughness of human cortical bone with age. Bone 22(1):57–66, 1998.

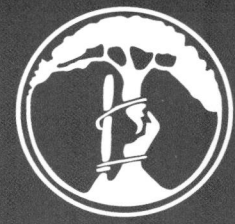

CHAPTER 4

Principles of Internal Fixation

**Augustus D. Mazzocca, M.D., Joseph P. DeAngelis, M.D.,
Andrew E. Caputo, M.D., Bruce D. Browner, M.D., M.S., F.A.C.S.,
Jeffrey W. Mast, M.D., and Michael W. Mendes, M.D.**

A mind that can comprehend the principles will devise its own methods.

N. Andry

In orthopaedic trauma, the energy that causes fractures generates a zone of injury owing to the injury to both the bone and the surrounding soft tissue.[5,19,39,92] In the resultant inflammatory reaction, vasoactive substances are released that mediate a beneficial increase in the local circulation as well as the detrimental effects of edema and pain. Additionally, these inflammatory substances and neural reflexes cause involuntary contraction of skeletal muscle groups around the fracture to splint the injured extremity, reduce painful motion, and facilitate fracture healing. As a result, early observations of the pain relief associated with external splinting led to the belief that fractures were best treated by immobilization and prolonged rest of the injured part. In this way, optimal cast immobilization included the joints both above and below the affected bone.[22] Fractures of the spine, pelvis, and femur were often treated with bed rest and traction for many weeks, followed by months of spica or body cast immobilization. Unfortunately, this approach focused on the achievement of bony union.

Although fractures usually healed with these nonoperative treatments, the inability to directly control the position of fracture fragments within the soft tissue envelope led to problems with malunion and nonunion. Additionally, long periods of immobilization required profound restriction of muscle activity, joint mobilization, and weight-bearing. In turn, the patients experienced considerable muscle atrophy, joint stiffness, disuse osteoporosis, and persistent edema—a complex of problems termed *fracture disease*.[68] At the same time, prolonged periods of immobilization sometimes led to psychologic changes, including depression, dependency, and perceived disability.[36] In light of these phenomena, it became clear that fracture treatment must focus on both fracture healing and restoration of preinjury function. Therefore, the ideal method should achieve the desired bony alignment and stabilization while permitting early function, mobilization, weight-bearing, and independence. Treatment methods that impart sufficient skeletal stability to facilitate return to functional activity include functional bracing (nonoperative), the Ilizarov method (a limited operative technique),

external fixation devices (used principally in treatment of severe open fractures), and internal fixation.

This chapter is divided into three major sections: metallurgy, hardware, and techniques of internal fixation. Because most of the implants currently used for internal fixation are made of metal, it is important to have a basic understanding of metallurgy.

METALLURGY

Metal implants are successful in fracture stabilization because they reproduce the supportive and protective functions of bone without impairing bone healing, remodeling, or growth. In an internal fixation construct, the metal implant is able to withstand tension, unlike the fractured bone, which is strongest in compression; the most efficient biomechanical internal fixation takes advantage of this difference by loading the bone in compression and the metal in tension. However, because there is no perfect material for use in internal fixation, a variety of issues must be examined when specific metals are considered as surgical implants: (1) biocompatibility—the material must be systemically nontoxic, nonimmunogenic, and noncarcinogenic; (2) strength parameters—tensile, compressive, and torsional strength; stiffness; fatigue resistance; and malleability are all important aspects; (3) resistance to degradation and erosion; (4) ease of integration when appropriate; and (5) minimal adverse effects on imaging.

Basic Metallurgy

Metal atoms form unit cell configurations based on their inherent atomic properties. These unit cells associate as a latticework or crystalline formation. As molten metal cools and solidifies, the crystals line up next to each other and interdigitate to determine the mechanical and chemical properties of the metal. Microscopic defects or impurities alter the crystalline structure and can change the mechanical properties. The differences in the mechanical behavior of metals are explained by their different atomic structures; for example, crystals of stainless steel are face-centered cubic, and titanium crystals are hexagonal close-packed (Fig. 4-1). Processing metals with chemical, thermal, or physical means changes the structure of the metal and affects its physical and mechanical properties.

FIGURE 4-1 *Unit cell configuration for three basic crystalline structures.* **A,** *Body-centered cubic.* **B,** *Face-centered cubic.* **C,** *Hexagonal close packed. (Redrawn from Ralls, K.M.; Courtney, T.H.; Wulff, J. Introduction to Materials Science and Engineering. New York, John Wiley & Sons, 1976. Reprinted by permission of John Wiley & Sons, Inc.; redrawn from Simon, S. R., ed. Orthopaedic Basic Science. Rosemont, IL, American Academy of Orthopaedic Surgeons, 1994.)*

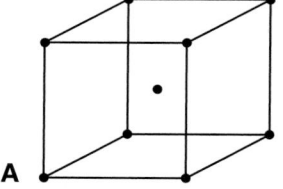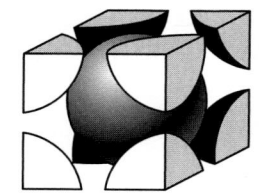

A

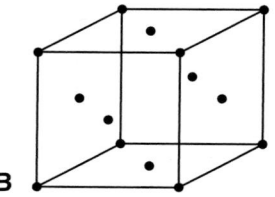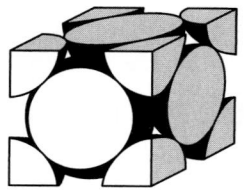

B

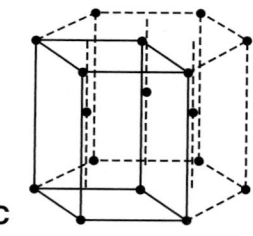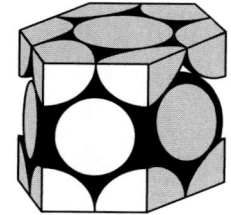

C

Metal Processing

Iron-based alloys are either cast or wrought. *Casting* is the process of pouring liquid metal into a mold of a specific shape. With this technique, problems arise when impurities migrate into the grain boundaries, resulting in areas of mechanical weakness. *Wrought iron* is made by mechanical processing of cast metal via rolling, extruding, or heat force. *Forging* is a process by which a piece of metal is heated and has a force applied through an open or closed die that represents the inverse geometry of the product being manufactured. This process refines the grain structures, increases strength and hardness, and decreases ductility. Vacuum re-melting and electroslag re-melting are processes that remove impurities and produce a purer grade of metal, which is desirable for surgical implants.

Further processing may be accomplished by cold-working. This technique requires repetitive application of a stress greater than the elastic limit of the metal. These load cycles increase the hardness and elastic limit of the material through elongation of the grains in the direction of the stress. The increased grain boundary area results in a stronger material (Fig. 4-2).

Two practical examples of cold-working are shot-peening of the surface of intramedullary nails (Zimmer, Warsaw, IN) and cold-forging of dynamic hip screw plates (Smith and Nephew Orthopaedics, Memphis, TN). The shot-peening process involves bombardment of the outer surfaces of the metal with a high-velocity stainless steel cut wire. The impact causes residual compressive stress, which reduces surface tensile stress. Shot-peening thus minimizes fatigue cracks, which usually begin on the surface and can cause fracture of the metal. The cold-forging process uses substantially more cold-working to achieve a higher degree of deformation. This step is coupled with a stress-relieving process to make a cold-forged steel of exceptionally high strength.

Passivation

Passivation is a process that allows spontaneous oxidation on the surface of the metal or treats the metal with acid or electrolysis to increase the thickness or energy level of the oxidation layer. Commonly, the process involves immersion of the implant in a strong nitric acid solution, which dissolves embedded iron particles and generates a dense oxide film on the surface. This step generally improves the biocompatibility of the implant. Passivation also enhances the corrosion resistance of the finished implant device (see Fig. 4-8).

Corrosion

Corrosion is the degradation of material by electrochemical attack. All metals used for surgical implantation undergo corrosion. The driving force for corrosion is also

FIGURE 4-2 *Cold-working. A load cycle that involves stress above the elastic limit of the metal increases the magnitude of stress necessary to achieve the subsequent elastic limit, producing a material that is harder and stronger. (Redrawn from Olsen, G.A. Elements of Mechanics of Materials, 2nd ed. Upper Saddle River, NJ, Prentice-Hall, 1966, p. 62. Reprinted by permission.)*

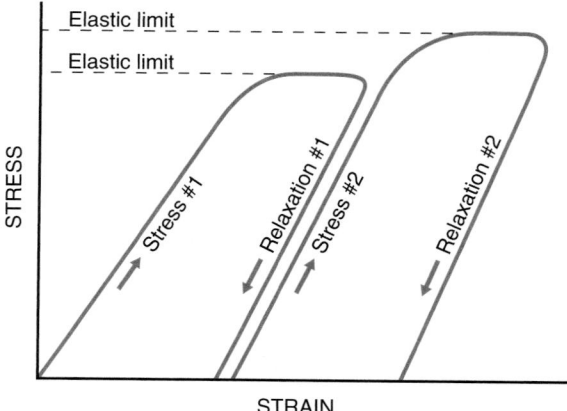

the basis of the electrical storage battery, which employs materials with two different levels of reactivity. Electrical energy is produced when ions of a more reactive material are released and partial consumption of the material occurs. This electrochemical consumption is termed *corrosion.* Corrosion or galvanic attack can occur if metals of different electrochemical potentials are placed in contact with each other (e.g., the inappropriate use of a titanium plate with stainless steel screws).

Corrosion can occur within a single type of metal or between implants made of the same metal when the reactivity differs from one area to another within the same implant. Differences in local reactivity are seen in areas of higher stress, lower oxygen tension, and crevices. The natural tendency of the base metal to corrode is decreased by the surface oxide coating from the passivation process. Scratches on the surface of the plate can disrupt the protective surface oxide coating and substantially increase corrosion. Crevices can develop from a scratch on the surface or develop macroscopically between a screw and a plate. The metal in this area is subjected to compressive forces, leading to high stress concentration. Oxygenated extracellular fluid cannot circulate in this area, resulting in a local decrease in oxygen tension. All these factors can cause differences in local reactivity and subsequent corrosion.

Mechanics

STRESS-STRAIN RELATIONSHIPS

A basic knowledge of mechanical terms is fundamental to understanding comparisons between different materials. Mechanical characteristics are based on the ability of a material to resist external forces, as expressed by stress-strain curves (Fig. 4-3A).

The *ultimate stress* of a material is the force required to make it fail or break. The *yield point* of a material is the force required to induce the earliest permanent change in shape or deformation.

Elasticity is the material's ability to restore its original shape after a deforming force lower than the yield point is removed. This is quantified by the *modulus of elasticity,* which is the slope of the elastic region of the stress-strain curve. *Stiffness* is defined as the resistance to deformation; it is proportional to the modulus of elasticity.

Plastic deformation is a permanent change in structure of a material after the stress is relieved. Ductility and brittleness are relative characteristics and not numerically quantified. *Ductility* is the ability of a material to further deform beyond the yield point before fracture. A *brittle material* has minimal deformation before failure. These characteristics are explained by the shape of the plastic (permanent deformation) curve past the yield point; a longer curve implies a more ductile substance.

Toughness is the total energy required to stress a material to the point of fracture (see Fig. 4-3B). It is defined as the area under both the elastic and the plastic parts of the stress-strain curve or as the energy to failure. *Hardness* is the ability to resist plastic deformation at the material surface only. For many materials, the mechanical properties at the surface differ from those found in the bulk of the material.

Metal has a variety of mechanical properties. Some are a function of its chemical composition and do not change with further processing; others are strongly affected by the relative orientation of the crystals and therefore are altered by processing. The elastic moduli in tension and compression do not change with processing, but yield strength, ultimate strength, and fatigue strength can be altered significantly by small changes in chemical composition and processing.[6]

FATIGUE

Fatigue is caused by cyclical (repetitive) stressing of a material. In cyclical loading, the maximal force required to produce failure decreases as the cycle number increases until the endurance limit is reached. The resulting fatigue curve shows the force necessary to cause failure of a material at each specific cycle number (Fig. 4-4). The higher the overall stress, the fewer the cycles required to produce failure (loading to the ultimate stress produces failure in one cycle). The *endurance limit* is the lowest point on the fatigue curve and represents a cyclical applied force below which the material will not have failed after 10 million (1×10^7) cycles. If the material has not failed at this point, in theory, it never will. By choosing different materials and altering implant geometry, manufacturers attempt to design implants that will tolerate cyclical loads without failure.

The *fatigue strength* (point of fatigue failure) of a material is defined as a single stress value on the fatigue curve for a specific number of cycles. In practice, certain points on a metal implant reach the fatigue failure level before others because of localized concentrations of stress (stress risers). Fatigue failure at these points results in the initiation of a crack that can propagate, causing the entire implant to fracture. On the basis of anatomic location, implants are subject to varying loads and varying frequency of stress cycles. The usual design estimate of cyclical load for orthopaedic implants is 2×10^6 stress cycles per year.[6]

Fatigue fractures of implants result from a high number of cycles of relatively low stress. Single-cycle and low-cycle failures are caused by high stress. Implants that have failed as a result of fatigue can be distinguished from single-cycle failures because they display a series of concentric fatigue striations over the fracture surface (Fig. 4-5). These striations appear to radiate from certain initiation points, which represent areas in which the overall peak tensile stress combined with the presence of stress risers (e.g., cracks, scratches, holes) exceeds the material's local resistance to failure. If the average peak stresses are large, then the striations have more distance between them. When these striations have propagated a sufficient distance to decrease the cross-sectional area of the implant, ultimate strength is reduced, leading to complete failure. This area of final failure is called the *tear zone,* and it can provide clues to the type of failure. High-stress, low-cycle failure produces a larger tear zone than low-stress, high-cycle failure. Implants must be designed to withstand these anticipated loads and cycles. If failure of an implant occurs, it should be examined to determine the failure pattern.

FIGURE 4-3 | **A,** *Stress-strain curve. The red line is an example of a ductile material; it can be stressed beyond the yield point. If a stress lower than the yield point is applied and released, the object will return to its original shape. The plastic or permanent deformation area is the portion of the curve between the amount of stress needed to reach the yield point and the amount of stress needed to reach the ultimate failure point.* **B,** *Toughness is defined as the area underneath the stress-strain curve. The two materials illustrated in this diagram have vastly different characteristics; however, they both have the same toughness because of equivalent areas under their respective curves. (Redrawn from Simon, S.R., ed. Orthopaedic Basic Science. Rosemont, IL, American Academy of Orthopaedic Surgeons, 1994.)*

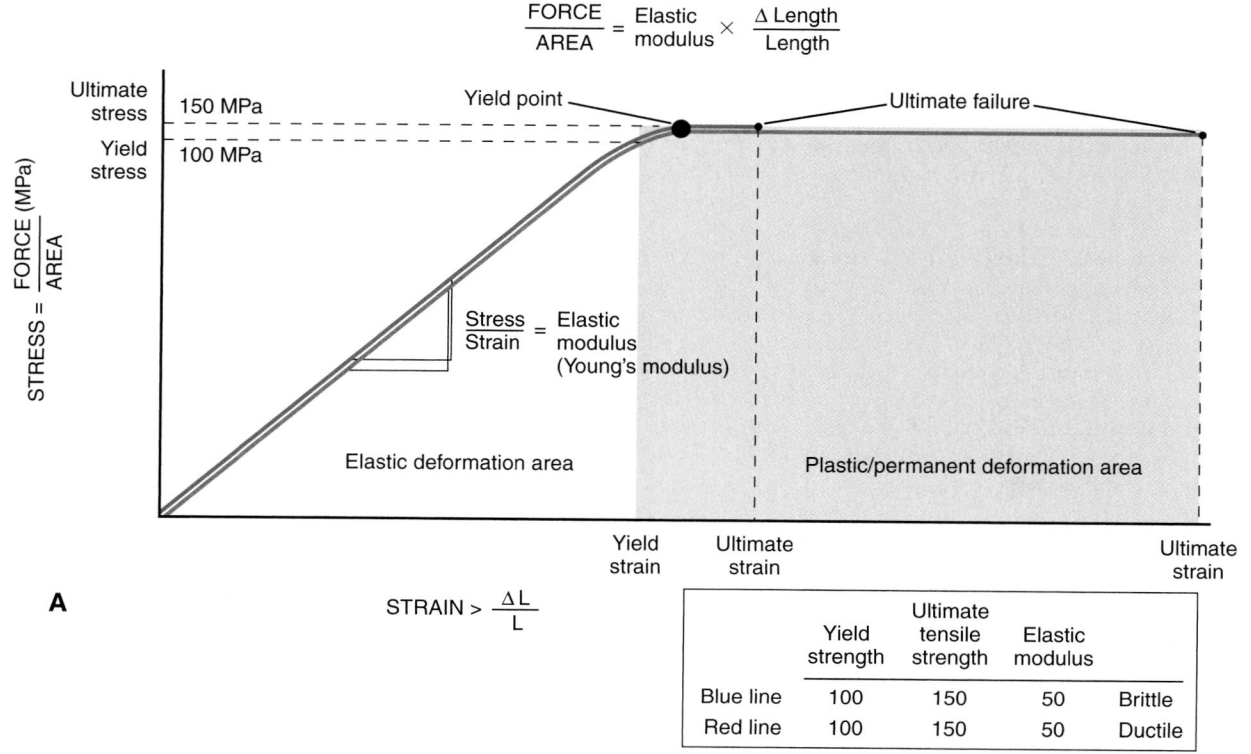

	Yield strength	Ultimate tensile strength	Elastic modulus	
Blue line	100	150	50	Brittle
Red line	100	150	50	Ductile

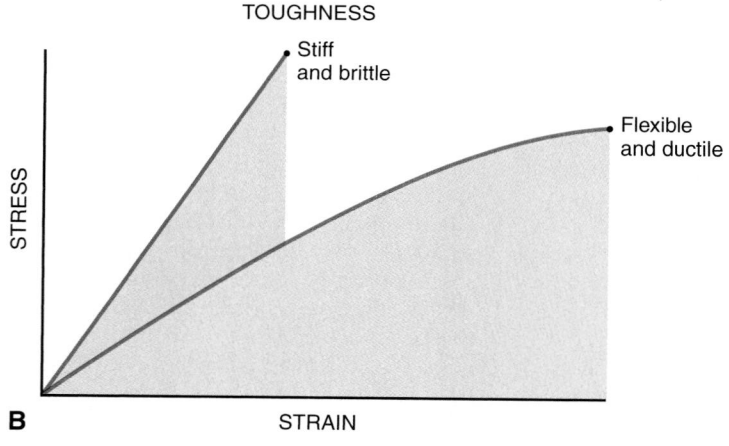

The American Society for Testing and Materials (ASTM) and the American Iron and Steel Institute (AISI) are two groups that test and monitor materials. Among other functions, these groups serve as independent sanctioning boards. Materials purchased by implant manufacturers are certified under their specifications. If a company wants to use a material that has not been sanctioned, it must go through rigorous biocompatibility and material testing procedures and submit the results to the U.S. Food and Drug Administration (FDA) for approval.

Types of Metals

The characteristics of various implant materials are shown in Figure 4-6 and Table 4-1.[8]

FIGURE 4-4 *Fatigue curve. Fatigue curve illustrating the ultimate tensile stress, the failure zone, and the endurance limit. (Redrawn from Perren, S.M. The concept of biological plating using the limited contact-dynamic compression plate [LCDCP]: Scientific background, design, and application. Injury 22[suppl 1]:1–41, 1991; with permission from Elsevier Science Ltd., The Boulevard, Langford Lane, Kidlington OX5 1GB, U.K.)*

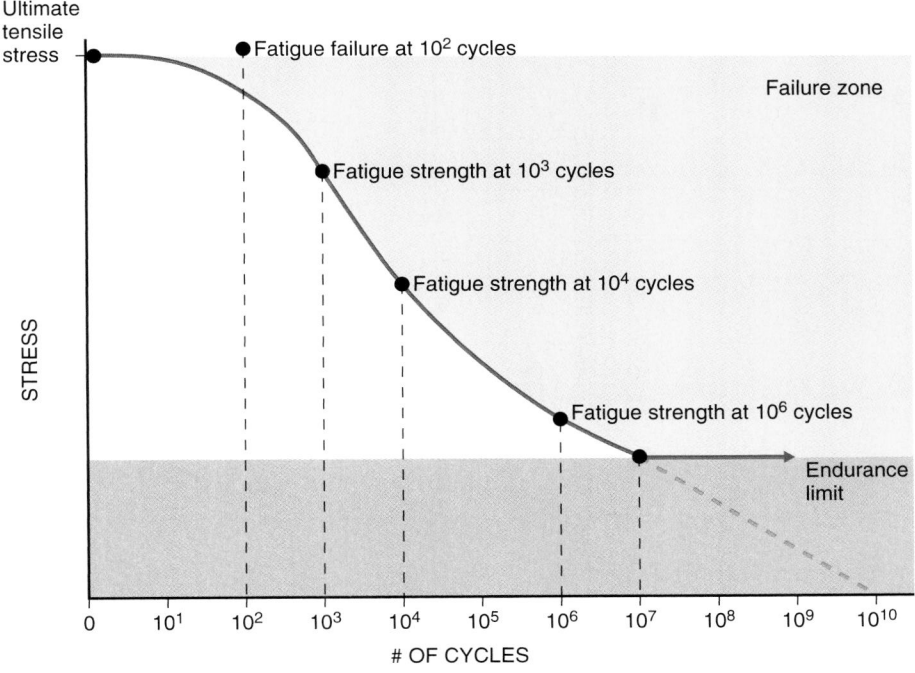

FIGURE 4-5 *Types of fatigue failure in fixation plates.* ***A,*** *High-stress, low-cycle failure.* ***B,*** *Low-stress, high-cycle failure. (Redrawn from Black, J. Orthopaedic Biomaterials in Research and Practice. New York, Churchill Livingstone, 1988.)*

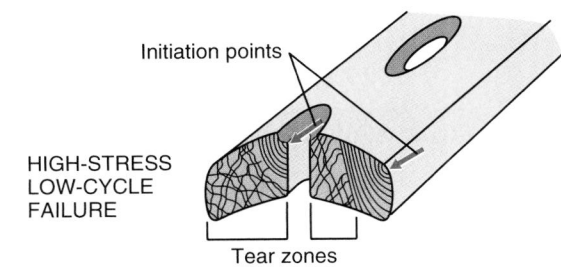

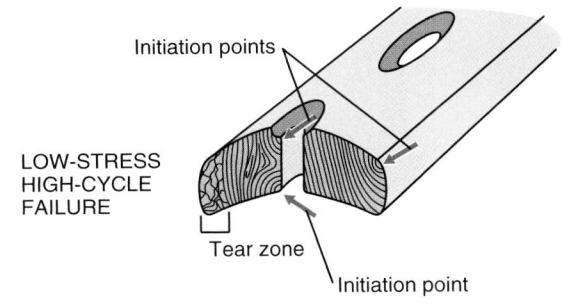

STAINLESS STEEL

Stainless steel is a combination of iron and chromium. The 316L stainless steel as specified by ASTM F-138 and F-139 is a standard for surgical implants. The number 316 is part of a modern classification system by AISI for metals and represents certain standards that allow the metal to be used for clinical application. The three-digit system separates the iron into four main groups based on composition: series 200 (chromium, nickel, and manganese), series 300 (chromium and nickel), series 400 (chromium), and series 500 (low chromium). The last two digits designate the particular type, and a letter represents a modification of the type (L stands for low carbon).

Stainless steel is further modified for use in surgical implantation by the addition of a variety of other elements to improve the alloy. The 316L stainless steel contains nickel (13% to 15.5%), which is added to increase corrosion resistance, stabilize crystalline structures, and stabilize the austenitic phase of the iron crystals at room temperature. The terms *austenitic* and *martensitic* describe specific crystallographic arrangements of iron atoms. The austenitic phase is associated with superior corrosion resistance and is favored in biologic implants. The martensitic stainless steels are hard and tough and are favored in the manufacture of osteotomes and scalpel blades. The 316L stainless steel also contains chromium (17% to 19%), which is added to form a passive surface oxide, thus contributing to corrosion resistance. Molybdenum (2% to 3%) prevents pitting and crevice corrosion in salt water. Manganese (about 2%) improves crystalline stability. Silicon controls

FIGURE 4-6 *Compilation of general material characteristics for various implant materials. **A–D,** Graphic representations of various characteristics. Abbreviations: AN, annealed; ASTM, American Society for Testing and Materials; C, cast; CF, cold-forged; CP, cold-processed; CW, cold-worked; F, forged; HF, hot-forged; SS, stainless steel. (Data from Bronzino, J. The Biomedical Engineering Handbook. Boca Raton, FL, CRC Press, 1995, with permission.)*

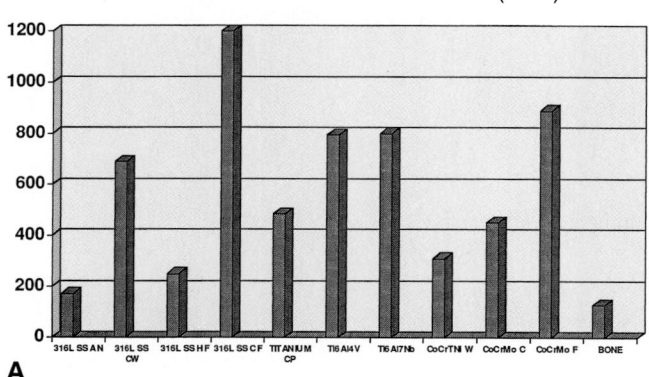

METAL VS YIELD STRENGTH (MPa)

A

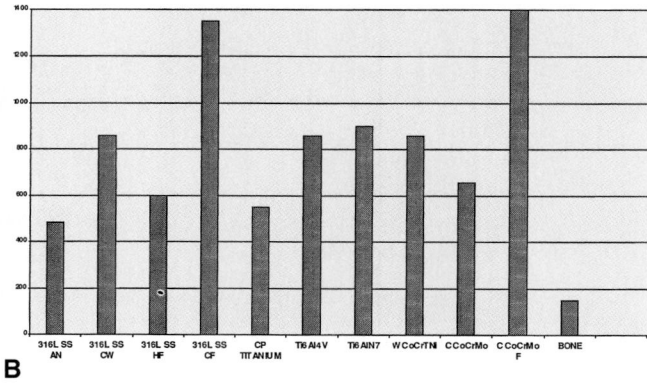

METAL VS ULTIMATE TENSILE STRESS (MPa)

B

METAL VS FATIGUE STRENGTH (MPa) X 10⁷ CYCLES

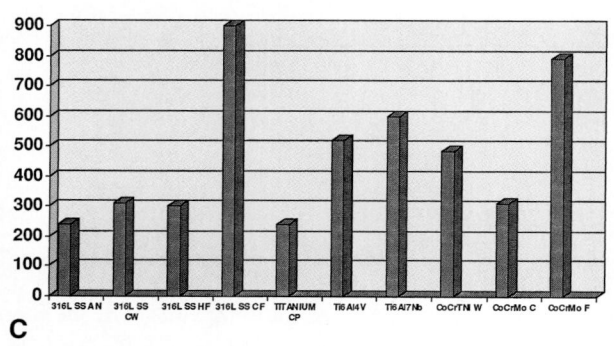

C

METAL VS ELASTIC MODULUS (GPa)

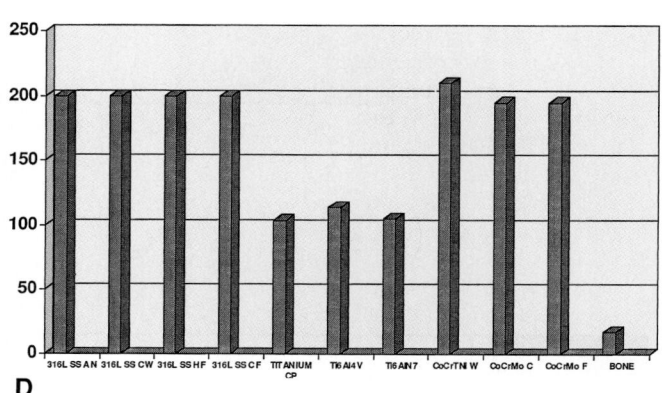

D

Table 4-1
Choice of Metals for Internal Fixation

Metal	Yield Strength (MPa)	Ultimate Tensile Stress (MPa)	Fatigue Strength (MPa) (10^7 cycles)	Elastic Modulus (GPa)
316L SS (AN)	172	485	240	200
316L SS 30% CW	690	860	310	200
316L SS HF	250	600	300	200
316L SS CF	1200	1350	900	200
CP titanium (ASTM F-67)	485	550	240	104
Ti6Al4V (ASTM F-136)	795	860	520	114
Ti6Al7Nb (ASTM F-1295)	800	900	600	105
Wrought CoCrNiMo (F-562)	310	860	485	210
Cast CoCrMo (F-76)	450	655	310	195
Cast CoCrMo (F-75) F	890	1400	793	195
Cortical bone	130	150	–	17

crystalline formation in manufacturing. The 316L stainless steel has a carbon content of 0.03%, whereas 316 stainless steel contains 0.08% carbon. Carbon is added during the smelting process and must be taken out in refining, because the carbon segregates from the major elements of the alloy, taking with it a substantial amount of chromium in the form of chromium carbide precipitate. The corrosion resistance of the final alloy is lessened by the depletion of chromium. Therefore, steel with a lower carbon content has greater corrosion resistance. Stainless steel has good mechanical strength with excellent ductility, and it can be worked by rolling, bending, or pounding to increase its strength. Steel is available in different degrees of strength corresponding to the proposed function of the implant.

TITANIUM AND TITANIUM ALLOYS

Titanium is an allotropic material that exists in both alpha and beta phases, which have a hexagonal close-packed crystal structure and a body-centered cubic structure, respectively. It is the least dense of all metals used for surgical implantation. The density of titanium is 4.5 g/cm^3, whereas that of 316 stainless steel is 7.9 g/cm^3 and that of cobalt-chromium alloy is 8.3 g/cm^3.

The four grades of commercially pure titanium that are available for surgical implantation are differentiated by the amount of impurities in each grade. The microstructure of commercially pure titanium is all-alpha titanium with relatively low strength and high ductility. Oxygen has a great influence on the ductility and strength: increasing the oxygen content of a particular grade of titanium makes it stronger and more brittle. Grade 4 titanium contains the most oxygen and is therefore the strongest of the commercially pure titaniums. The material may be cold-worked for additional strength, but it cannot be strengthened by heat treatment because it has only a single phase.

One titanium alloy (Ti6Al4V) is widely used for surgical implantation. The additional elements of the alloy are aluminum (5.5% to 6.5%), which stabilizes the alpha phase, and vanadium (3.5% to 4.5%), which stabilizes the beta phase. The beta phase is stronger because of its crystallographic arrangement, whereas the alpha phase is good for welding. For applications in which high strength and fatigue resistance are required, the material is annealed, corresponding to a universal distribution of alpha and beta phases. The Ti6Al4V alloy can be heat-treated because it is a two-phased alloy and not a single-phase commercially pure titanium. Titanium alloy has greater specific strength per unit density than any other implant material. The most recently developed titanium alloy is Ti6Al7Nb; the niobium produces mechanical characteristics similar to those of the titanium-vanadium alloy but with less toxicity.

COBALT-CHROMIUM ALLOYS

Two cobalt-chromium alloys are currently used for manufacture of surgical implants. The first is CoCrMo (ASTM F-75), which is cast, and the second is CoCrNiMo (ASTM F-562), which is wrought. Cobalt is the main component in both alloys. The cast CoCrMo was originally called Vitallium (Howmedica, Inc., Rutherford, NJ), and this name is sometimes used incorrectly to describe all the cobalt-based alloys. Chromium (7% to 30%) provides good corrosion resistance by forming chromic oxide at the surface. Molybdenum (5% to 7%) increases strength by controlling crystalline size and also increases corrosion resistance. Nickel (1%), manganese (1%), and silicon (1%) are added to improve ductility and hardness. The most attractive feature of these alloys is their excellent corrosion resistance and biocompatibility. The mechanical properties (tensile strength and fatigue resistance) of the wrought CoCrNiMo alloy make it desirable for implants that must withstand a long period of loading without fatigue failure. For this reason, this material has been chosen for the manufacture of stems for hip prostheses.

Comparison of Metals

MECHANICAL PROPERTIES

The mechanical properties of a metal vary depending on whether it is used as a pure base metal or as an alloy with other metals. They also can be altered significantly by processing (e.g., cold-working, hot-forging, annealing). The mechanical demands of the implant help determine the appropriate materials and processing methods. Fracture fixation implants require high yield strength and high fatigue resistance. The metals that can best meet these requirements are 316L stainless steel and titanium alloys. The yield stress of Ti6Al4V alloy is greater than that of unprocessed 316L stainless steel, both CoCr alloys, and commercially pure titanium. However, cold-working of stainless steel results in a material with a higher yield stress and fatigue resistance than Ti6Al4V alloy. Stainless steel is an attractive implant material because it has moderate yield and ultimate strengths, is relatively low in cost, is easy to machine, and maintains high ductility, even with large amounts of cold-forging. Ti6Al4V is more difficult to machine, more expensive, and sensitive to external stress risers (scratches), which can dramatically shorten its fatigue life. Its lower ductility results in less forewarning of failure when a screw is over-tightened (Fig. 4-7A). Stainless steel has favorable fatigue characteristics in the relatively low cycles, but in the higher cycles titanium alloy is more resistant to fatigue (see Fig. 4-7B).

Clinical studies have shown that there is no significant advantage in healing time with steel- or titanium-based dynamic compression (DC) plates used for internal fixation of 256 tibial fractures.[62] Both Ti6Al4V and cold-worked 316L stainless steel are used for implants that must withstand unusually high stresses (e.g., intramedullary nails designed for fixation of subtrochanteric fractures). The Russell-Taylor reconstruction nail (Smith and Nephew) and the ZMS reconstruction nail (Zimmer) are made from cold-worked stainless steel; the Uniflex reconstruction nail (Biomet, Warsaw, IN), the CFX nail (Howmedica), and the TriGen nail system (Smith and Nephew) are made from titanium alloy.

The process of casting the CoCrMo (F-75) alloy is expensive and leaves minute defects, which significantly reduce its strength, ductility, and fatigue life. It has superior corrosion resistance. The yield strength of wrought CoCrNiMo (F-562) can range from 600 MPa for fully annealed alloy to 1400 MPa for severely cold-drawn wire. The molybdenum is added to produce finer

FIGURE 4-7   *Titanium (Ti) versus stainless steel (SS).* **A,** *Torque versus torsion angle of screws, showing earlier failure of titanium screws.* **B,** *Fatigue curve showing that SS is stronger in low-cycle stress and Ti is more fatigue resistant in high-cycle stress.* **C,** *The Ti plate deforms nearly twice as much as the SS plate under similar loading conditions. This is explained by the lower elastic modulus of Ti. (Redrawn from Perren, S.M. The concept of biological plating using the limited contact-dynamic compression plate [LCDCP]: Scientific background, design, and application. Injury 22[Suppl 1]:1–41, 1991; with permission from Elsevier Science Ltd, The Boulevard, Langford Lane, Kidlington OX5 1GB, U.K.)*

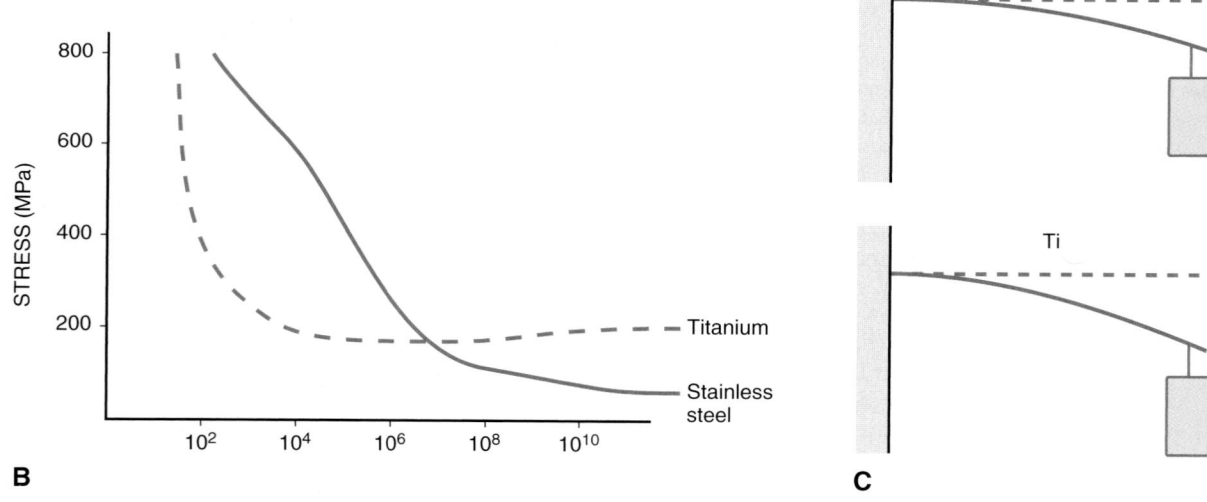

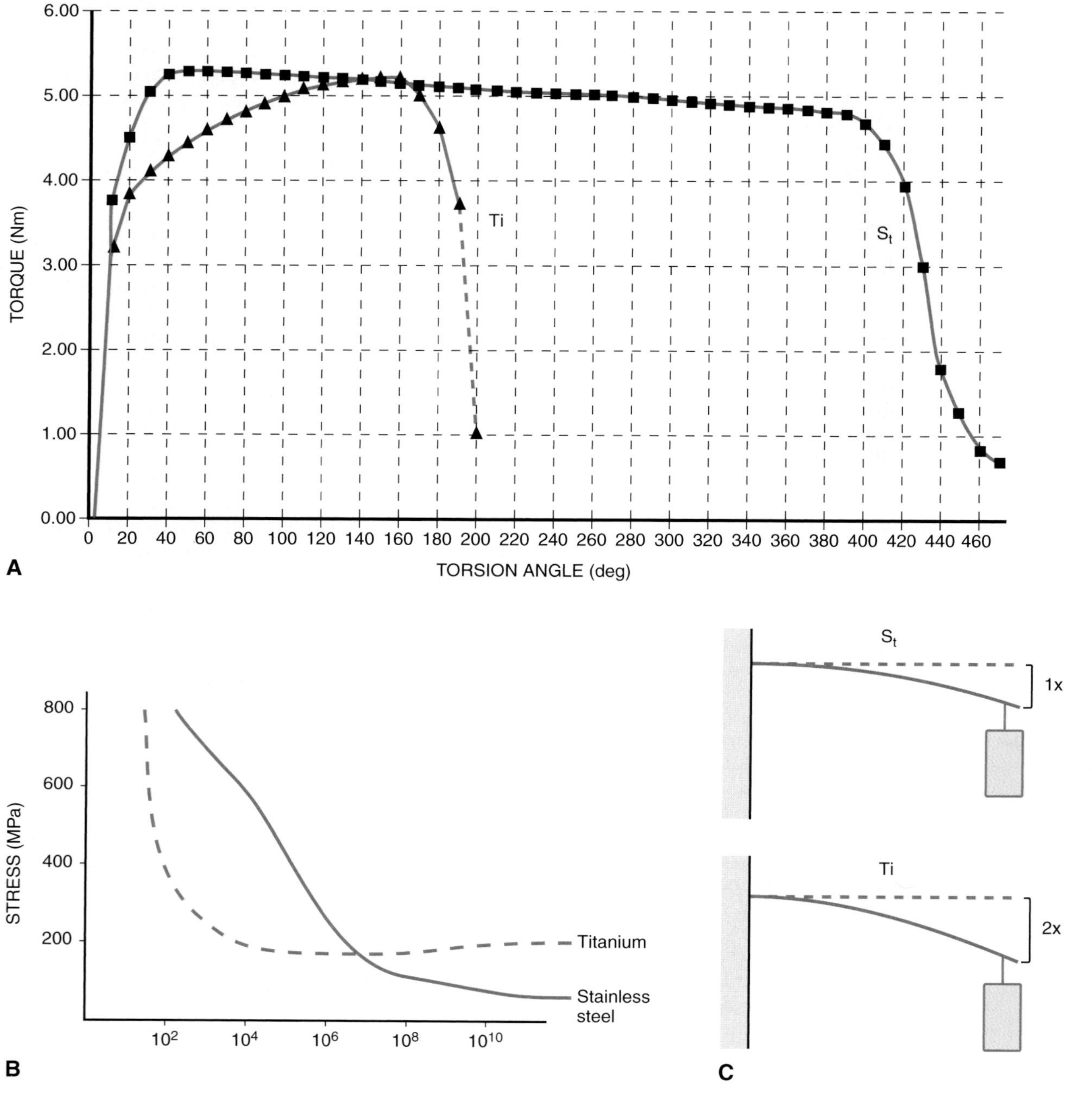

grains, which results in higher strength after casting and forging. Cobalt-chromium alloys are difficult and expensive to machine because they have high intrinsic hardness. They also have lower ductility (i.e., they are very brittle), and their base alloy costs are significantly higher. For these reasons, cobalt-chromium alloys are not generally used to make fracture fixation implants, but because of their superior fatigue resistance, long-term corrosion resistance, and biocompatibility, they are used for stems of hip prostheses.

Although the discussion thus far has emphasized the importance of implant strength and fatigue resistance, it is not possible simply to maximize size and stiffness of implants to meet the mechanical demands of fracture fixation. Bone is a living tissue that responds to mechanical loads. Both maintenance of bone mineral content and fracture healing require that the bone experience load transmission; if bone is deprived of load by the implant, stress shielding occurs. It is therefore essential that the internal fixation implant be designed to distribute stress to both the implant and the bone, often referred to as *load sharing*. Furthermore, to prevent stress concentrations and stress shielding, the elastic modulus of the implant should be similar to that of bone.[28] The elastic modulus of titanium alloys is 6 times greater than that of cortical bone, but the elastic modulus of stainless steel is 12 times greater, so titanium is the better implant material for prevention of stress shielding (see Fig. 4-7C).

BIOCOMPATIBILITY

Biocompatibility is the ability of a metal and the body to co-exist. Ideally, an implanted metal will experience minimal corrosion and minimal host reactivity. In 1972, ASTM adopted a biocompatibility standard (F-361) to assess the effect of all implant metals on the body. Every metal eventually corrodes in every environment; those metals that are deemed acceptable for implantation should demonstrate only a small amount of corrosion over a long period. For optimal biocompatibility, the products of this corrosion should cause minimal inflammatory reaction. Titanium has the greatest corrosion resistance because it rapidly forms titanium oxide on its surface. The oxide layer is tightly adherent and resistant to breakdown; if it is damaged, it re-forms in milliseconds. While implants made of other metals are typically surrounded by a thin fibrous capsule, implants made of titanium and its alloys demonstrate a remarkable ability to form an intimate interface directly with bone. From evaluation of tissue reactivity of implanted materials, Perren[75] found no avascular zone with titanium and a 0.02-mm avascular zone with stainless steel. Additionally, titanium promotes bone ingrowth, which can be a problem if late extraction of the implant is necessary.[95]

A small percentage of the population is sensitive to nickel and chromium. These persons cannot tolerate implants made of metals such as stainless steel or chromium cobalt alloy, which contain these elements. Commercially pure titanium, however, can be used in patients who are sensitive to nickel and chromium.

Stainless steel implants have localized areas of corrosion, mostly at microfracture sites, crevices, and abrasion sites (screw-plate interfaces). A capsule forms around stainless steel implants, indicating poor integration at the surface-tissue interface. Stainless steel is compatible but does not promote bone ingrowth at the surface of the implant.[64] This fact confers some advantage in the design of devices that eventually will be removed from the body. Cast CoCrMo (F-75) has excellent corrosion resistance compared with stainless steel, and its fatigue strength can be increased by various forging and pressing techniques, making it an excellent material for high-cycle, high-stress environments such as the femoral stem of a hip prosthesis.

Infection is a major concern with internal fixation. Although overt infection is a multifactorial problem, the adherence of bacteria to biomaterials may be an initial step in the process of implant loosening and ultimate implant failure. Minimal clinical research exists comparing bacterial adherence with various biomaterials in humans. The AO (*Arbeitsgemeinschaft für Osteosynthesefragen*)/ASIF (Association for Study of Internal Fixation) group retrospectively evaluated 1251 titanium DC plates and 25,000 stainless steel plates implanted into humans and did not find significant differences in infection rates. Bacteria have a natural tendency to adhere to inert surfaces (Fig. 4-8). Bacteria that produce significant amounts of glycocalyx have a greater adherence to biomaterials.[91] Fibronectin is a serum and matrix protein that binds to various biomaterials. The presence of fibronectin on the surface of these metals is an important determinant of colonization by staphylococci.[26] Chang and Merritt[20] found that the in vitro and in vivo adherence of *Staphylococcus epidermidis* was greatest for stainless steel, followed by commercially pure titanium. Stainless steel was also found to inhibit polymorphonuclear cell production of superoxide, thereby decreasing the bactericidal activity of these leukocytes. No effect on superoxide production was found with commercially pure titanium, Ti6Al4V, or cobalt-chromium alloy.[71]

IMAGING

Concerning plain radiographs, titanium alloy produces much less attenuation (scatter of x-rays) than stainless steel or cobalt-chromium and only slightly more than calcium. For computed tomography (CT), titanium alloys have the least amount of scatter and do not lead to image disruption.[29] Cast CoCrMo (F-75) exhibits the greatest artifact on CT, and stainless steel causes moderate artifact. Concerning magnetic resonance imaging (MRI) compatibility, commercially pure titanium, titanium alloy, and cobalt-chromium alloy do not have magnetic characteristics and can be imaged with minimal attenuation problems. Surgical manipulations with stainless steel can induce areas of ferromagnetic potential that could either move the implant or cause an electrical current.[28]

A common question is whether orthopaedic implants are perceived by metal detectors. These machines work by detecting eddy currents that depend on a material's conductivity and permeability (ability to temporarily magnetize). Modern orthopaedic implants have both low permeability and poor conductivity and therefore are detected infrequently.[4]

RADIATION THERAPY

Although penetration characteristics are much stronger for external beam irradiation than for diagnostic radiography, implants still cause a significant amount of bulk reflection. Reflected radiation in front of the plate increased the radiation dose by 25% for stainless steel and 15% for titanium; absorption behind the plate reduced the dose by 15% and 10%, respectively.[78] If plates and screws are being placed in an area that will be irradiated, use of the lowest density material (e.g., titanium) and a small, susceptible configuration will best reduce the effects of reflection and attenuation.

Summary

The design and manufacture of internal fracture fixation devices are changing constantly. The choice of material

FIGURE 4-8 *Biofilm containing bacteria on a metal implant. The biofilm or (slime) is made up of the implant passivation layer, host extracellular macromolecules (fibrinogen, fibronectin, collagen), and bacterial extracellular glycocalyx (polysaccharide). Staphylococci are bonded on the implant, which inhibits phagocytosis. Failure of the glycopeptide antibiotics to cure prosthesis-related infection is not caused by poor penetration of drugs into the biofilm but probably by the diminished antimicrobial effect on bacteria in the biofilm environment.*

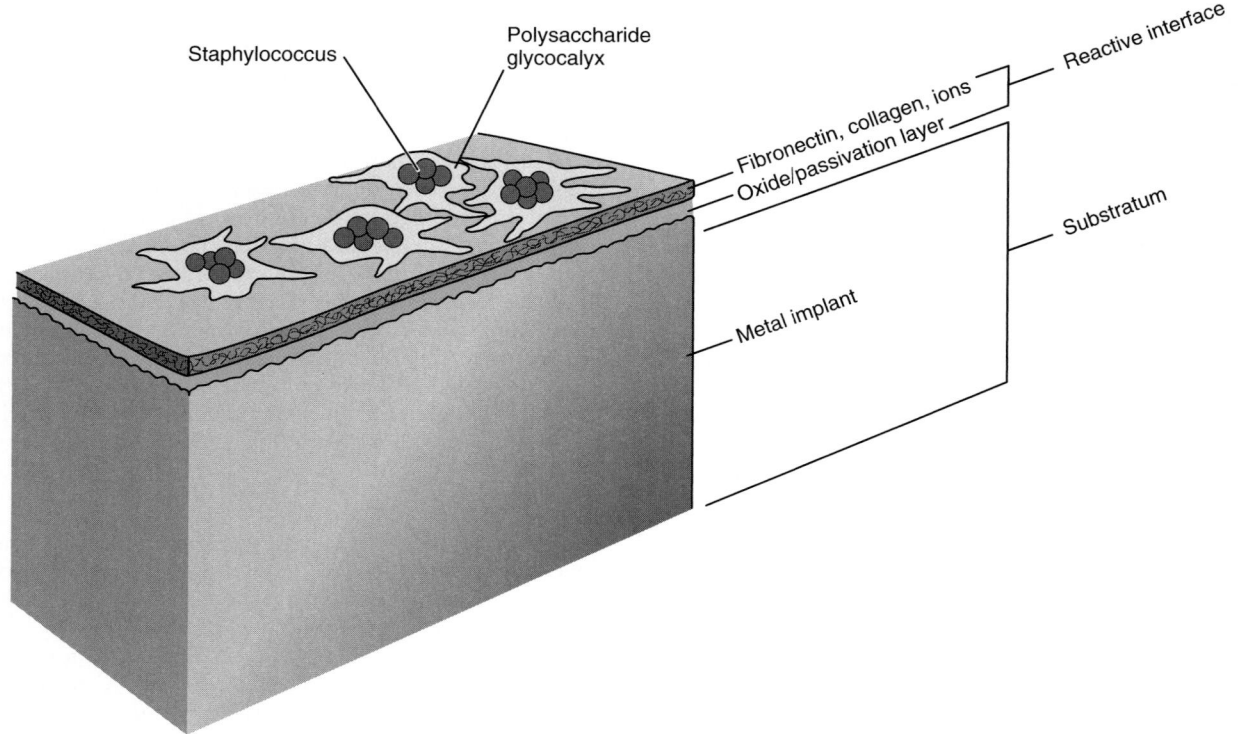

depends on its mechanical and biocompatibility properties as well as the cost of processing and machining. There is no single ideal metal for internal fixation. Although metals are an imperfect implant material, they predominate in current orthopaedic practice. The rigorous requirements imposed by the FDA for premarket demonstration of safety and efficacy of new implant materials and devices may delay or forestall the introduction of metal substitutes, such as resin-fiber composites, indefinitely.

HARDWARE

Internal fixation is based on the implantation of various appliances to assist with the body's natural healing process. The following sections describe the basic anatomy, biomechanics, and types of hardware, including screws, drills, taps, plates, intramedullary nails, and reamers.

Screws

Any discussion about different types of screws and their applications should be based on an understanding of basic screw design (Fig. 4-9). The *outer diameter* is defined as the outermost diameter of the threads. *Pitch* is defined as the longitudinal distance between the threads. The bending strength and shear strength of a screw depend on its *root*, or *core, diameter*. This dimension is the solid section of the screw from which the threads protrude. The core diameter also determines the size of the drill bit used for the pilot hole. Many screws have a common core diameter. For example, the 4.5-mm cortical, 6.5-mm cancellous, and 4.5-mm malleolar screws all have the same core diameter (3.0 mm). The core diameter of a screw determines its strength in bending because strength is a function of the cross-sectional moment of inertia, which is proportional to the third power of the radius. If the thickness of the core is increased, a significant increase in bending strength is obtained. The core or root diameter is often confused with the *shaft diameter*, which is the unthreaded portion of the screw between the head and the screw threads.

A screw can break in two ways (Fig. 4-10).[88] The first is through the application of a torque that exceeds the shear strength of the screw. Von Arx determined the range of torque applied by surgeons during insertion to be 2.94 to 5.98 N-m.[94] This force can break a screw with a root diameter of 2.92 mm or less if it becomes incarcerated. The second way is through application of bending forces when a load is applied perpendicularly to the long axis of the screw. If the screws fixing the plate to the bone are not secure enough, the plate will slide between the bone and the screw head. This sliding permits application of an excessive bending force perpendicular to the axis of the screw, which ultimately can result in fatigue failure of the screw.[93] In the clinical setting, the screw must be tight enough to avoid plate sliding but not so tight as to exceed the maximal shear strength of the screw itself. Several factors affect how tight the screw-plate-bone interface can be made, including the

FIGURE 4-9 *Configuration of screws.*

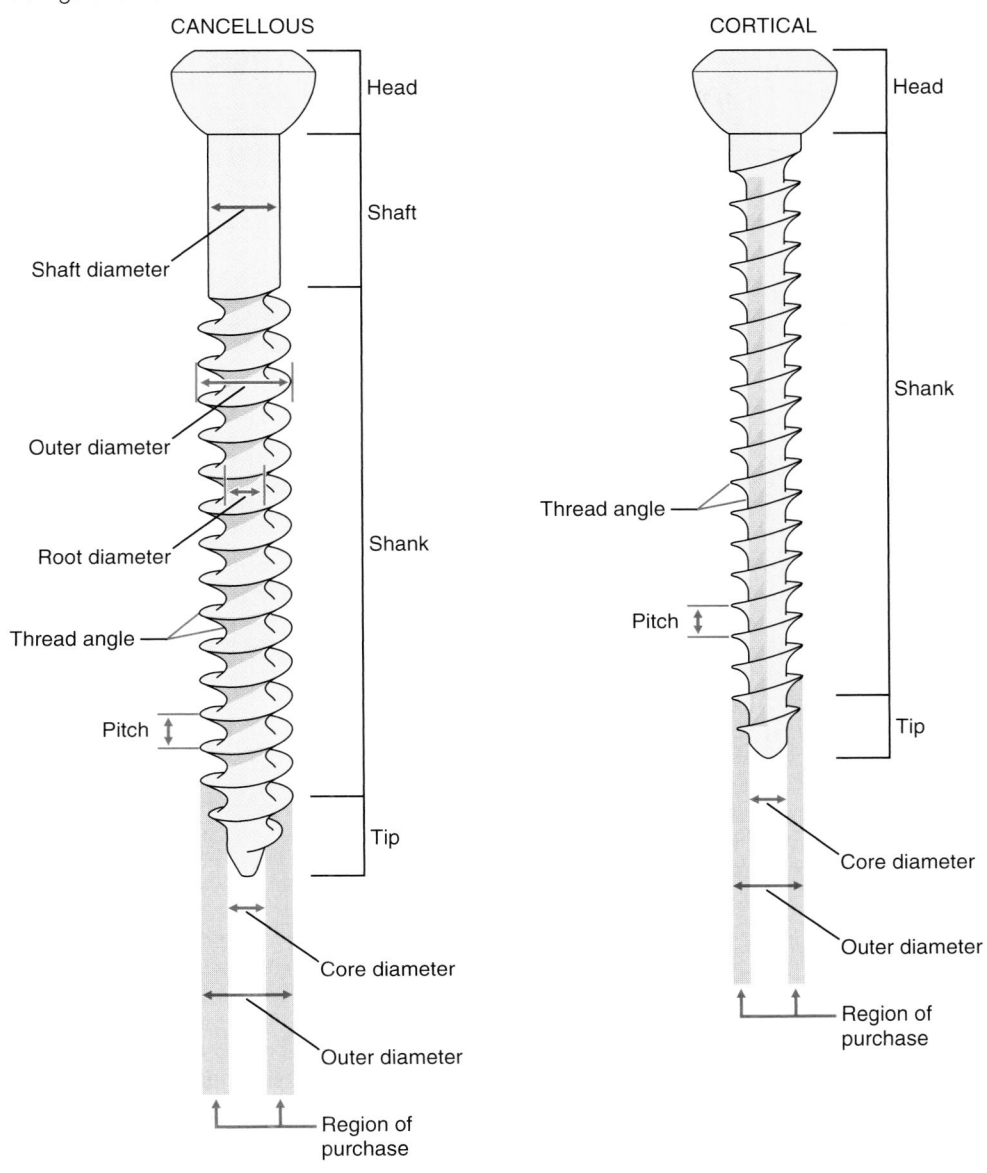

maximal torque applied during insertion, thread design, and bone quality. Because of the variation in bone quality among individuals and among anatomic locations, it is not possible to determine the insertional torque necessary to optimally tighten all screws. For this reason, a torque screwdriver cannot be used, and screw purchase is best assessed empirically. *Purchase* is defined as the perception that the screw is meeting resistance and becoming tight rather than slipping and spinning.

The design of the threads can also influence the strength of the screw and its resistance to breakage. Stress on the core can be increased if the surfaces of adjoining threads intersect with the core at a sharp angle. This sharp notch acts as a stress concentrator, increasing the possibility of screw failure. To minimize this problem, bone screws are designed so that the intersection of the thread

surfaces with the core contains curves without a sharp angle (Fig. 4-11A).

Although bending strength and shear strength are important mechanical features, the pullout strength of a screw is of even greater significance in internal fixation. The ability of a screw to achieve interfragmentary fixation or stable attachment of a plate relates to its ability to hold firmly in bone and resist pullout. The *pullout strength* of a screw is proportional to the surface area of thread that is in contact with bone. There are two methods to increase this surface contact. The first is to increase the difference between the core and the external diameters; this maximizes the amount of screw thread surface that is in contact with bone, resulting in stronger fixation. The second method is to increase the number of threads per unit length—that is, to decrease the point-to-point distance

FIGURE 4-10 *Screw failure. **A,** Bending failure secondary to a loose junction between the plate and the screw. **B,** Shear failure secondary to excessive torque.*

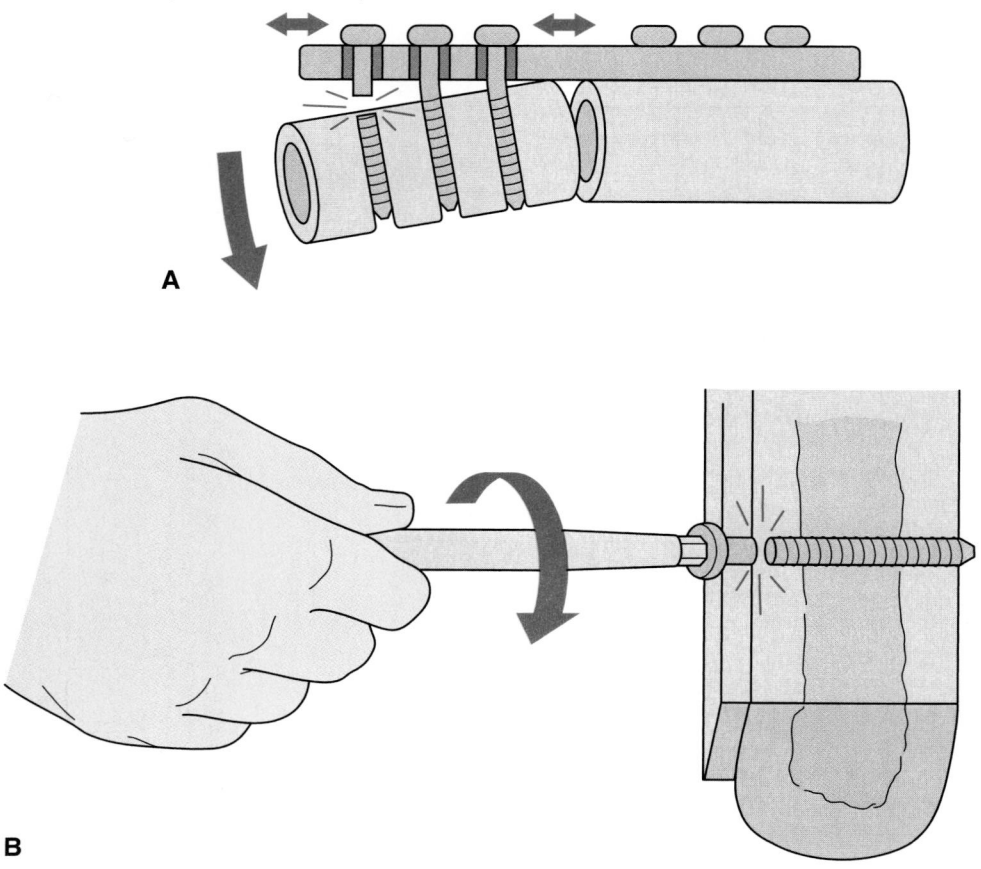

between successive threads (pitch). The smaller the pitch, the greater the number of threads that can engage in the bone, and the more secure the fixation (see Fig. 4-11B).

The size, shape, and quality of bone and the physiologic stress on the fracture site determine the number of screws required for adequate fixation. The AO/ASIF group has performed retrospective clinical reviews of large numbers of fracture fixations.[67] These studies have empirically determined the number of screws that should be used to attach a plate to each long bone. Because the diaphysis of long bones is tubular, it is possible to achieve thread purchase in the cortex on one or both sides of the intramedullary canal. The screw purchase required for stable plate fixation in each long bone is described in the *Manual of Internal Fixation* as a specific number of cortices.[68] The recommended number of cortices on each side of the fracture is seven in the femur, six in the tibia or humerus, and five in the radius or ulna.

Circumstances may dictate the use of a longer plate that has more holes than required. The question arises whether all of the holes should be filled. Placement of a screw limits micromotion and reduces stress by increasing the area of surface contact between the plate and the bone. On the other hand, every drill hole in bone represents a site

of stress concentration and a point of potential fracture (Fig. 4-12). Brooks and colleagues[9] found that a single hole can reduce overall bone strength by 30%. However, leaving screw holes empty may cause concern about plate failure. Plates can fail because of stress concentration caused by the fracture type or by the screw hole itself. A short defect has an increased stress concentration because the forces are distributed over a smaller area than with a longer, more oblique defect. In addition, the screw hole is the plate's weakest portion because it has the highest stress concentration. Stress equals force divided by area; the presence of a screw hole reduces the area of the plate, so the stress on the plate is greater at the screw hole. Although each hole in the plate acts as a stress concentrator, the load experienced at each hole relates to its location in terms of the fracture site and the shape and stability of the fracture. Empty holes at the ends of the plate experience less stress than those closer to the fracture. Pawluk and associates[74] reported bending strains for screws proximal to the fracture at 240 $\mu\epsilon$ and for those distal to the fracture at 87 $\mu\epsilon$ under bone-to-bone contact conditions. Filling of these holes is of limited value because the screw does not reinforce the plate and may needlessly increase the risk of fracture at the screw site. When a long plate

FIGURE 4-11 | *Effects of thread design. **A,** A sharp intersection between the screw core and the threads acts as an area of stress concentration, increasing the possibility of screw failure. **B,** The effect of thread pitch on the linear advance of a screw for a single turn. (Redrawn from Tencer, A.F.; et al. In: Asnis, S.E.; Kyle, R.F., eds. Cannulated Screw Fixation: Principles and Operative Techniques. New York, Springer Verlag, 1996. Used with permission.)*

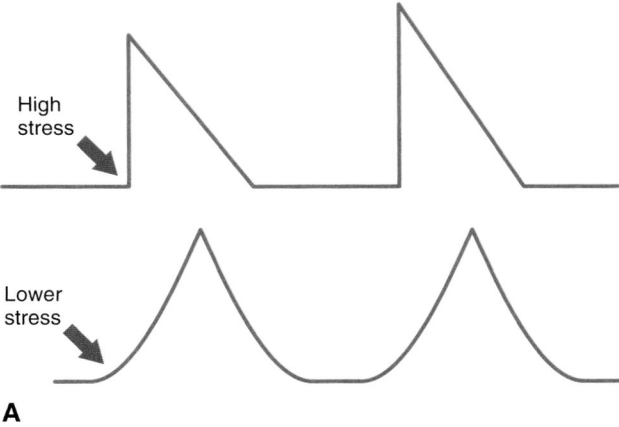

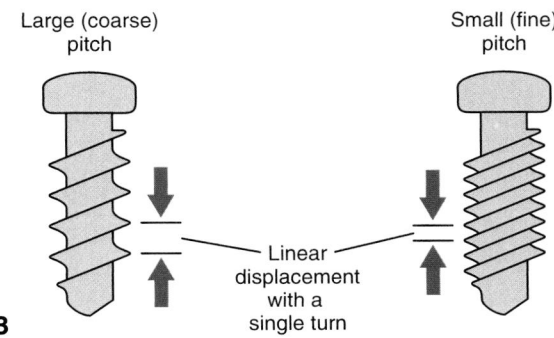

is used, it is desirable to intersperse screws and open holes at the ends of the plate while concentrating screw placement close to the fracture site.

Empty screw holes in bone, both those drilled but not filled and those left after screw removal, weaken the bone. Burstein and co-workers[18] reported 1.6 times greater stresses around empty holes than in the surrounding bone when in torsion. Within approximately 4 weeks, these holes are filled with woven bone, which eliminates the stress-concentrating effect. This point is important for postoperative management after implant removal.

Drills

Fundamental to screw placement is proper preparation of the bone with drilling. The most important aspect of this process is the design of the drill bit. The configuration of a drill bit is shown in Figure 4-13 and is relatively simple. The central tip is the first area to bite into the bone. The sharper the tip, the better the bite and the less skive or shift in the proposed drill site. The *cutting edge*, located at the tip of the drill bit, performs the actual cutting and is crucial to efficient penetration. *Flutes* are helical grooves along the sides of the bit that direct the bone chips away from the hole. Failure to remove bone debris could cause the drill bit to deviate from its intended path, decreasing drilling accuracy. The *land* is the surface of the bit between adjacent flutes. The *reaming edge* is the sharp edge of the helical flutes that runs along the entire surface, clearing the drill hole of bone debris while performing no cutting

function. Disruption of these edges diminishes reaming performance. The *rake* or *helical angle* is the angle made by the leading edge of the land and the center axis of the drill bit. A larger rake angle reduces the cutting forces regardless of the direction in which the bone is cut. This angle can be positive, negative, or neutral. Positive rake angles cut only when rotated clockwise.

Most drill bits are constructed with two flutes; they are used with rotary-powered drills and are provided in standard fracture fixation sets. To limit drilling damage to the soft tissues adjacent to bone, an attachment has been developed that converts a drill's action from rotary to oscillating drive. With the oscillating drive, there is less tendency for the drill bit to damage neighboring soft tissue. An oscillating drill bit can be placed on skin and will not cut it because of the skin's elasticity. A three-fluted drill bit has been developed for use with oscillating drill attachments. To work effectively, a two-fluted drill bit must rotate beyond 180°. Because the excursion of the oscillating device is less than 180°, a three-fluted drill bit must be used to achieve cutting. This drill bit also provides an added advantage when drilling on an oblique angle. Although the oscillating three-fluted drill bit may be safer for soft tissue, the two-fluted rotary drill bit cuts through bone more efficiently and is used more commonly.

Drilling into bone is different from drilling into wood because bone is a living tissue. The process of drilling in bone must minimize physiologic damage. Jacob and Berry[41] determined the optimal drill bit design and

FIGURE 4-12 | *Stress is concentrated at the equator of the hole and at the bottom of the notch. A sharp notch will concentrate the stress further. (Redrawn from Radin, E.L.; et al. Practical Biomechanics for the Orthopaedic Surgeon. New York, John Wiley & Sons, 1979.)*

FIGURE 4-13 | *Configuration of the drill bit.*

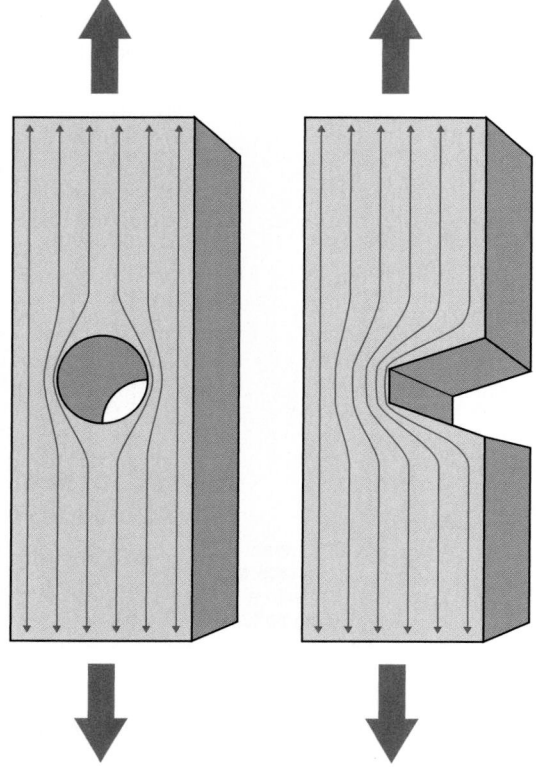

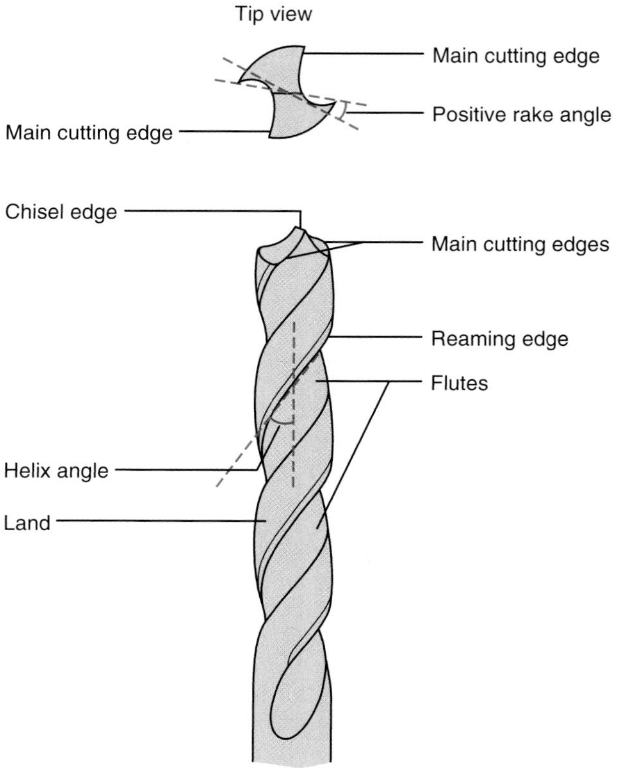

method for bone drilling. They found that the cutting forces are higher at lower rotational speeds and suggested a physiologic bone drilling method that includes the following: (1) bone drill bits with positive rake angles between 20° and 35°; (2) a point on the drill to avoid walking (skiving); (3) high torque and relatively low drill speeds (750 to 1250 rpm) to take advantage of a decrease in flow stress of the material; (4) continuous, copious irrigation to reduce friction-induced thermal bone necrosis; (5) reflection of the periosteum to prevent bone chips from being forced under the tissue, clogging the drill flutes; (6) drill flutes that are steep enough to remove chips at any rake angle; (7) sharp and axially true drill bits to decrease the amount of retained bone dust; and (8) drilling of the thread hole exactly in the direction in which the screw is to be inserted for accuracy and strength. These techniques reduce local bone damage significantly.

Most drill bits are constructed with high-carbon stainless steel and are heat-processed for increased hardness. Damaged or dull bits decrease drilling efficiency significantly and may cause local trauma to bone. A damaged drill bit can increase drilling time by a factor of 35.[77] Damage is frequently caused by contact with other metal (plate or drill sleeve). AO/ASIF recommends certain procedures to decrease drill bit damage. The first is to drill

only bone. Pohler[77] found that drilling of 110 bone cortices had a negligible effect on the bit itself. The second is to always use the drill guide. This minimizes bending, which is the leading cause of drill failure. The drill guide or sleeve should be of correct size; an excessively large guide results in a larger hole because of wobbling of the drill. The third recommendation is to start the drill only after the drill bit has been inserted into the drill guide. This technique limits contact with the drill guide and consequent damage to the cutting and reaming edges. These recommendations combined with the defined physiologic bone drilling method limit local damage to bone and result in optimal holes for screw fixation.

Most standard fracture fixation sets provide specific drill bits that are used to drill tap and glide holes appropriate for all screws contained in the set. Drill bits are named by their diameter and, because they should always be used with soft tissue protective sleeves, they have both a total and an effective length, the latter being the portion of the bit that extends past the drill sleeve and is responsible for cutting. The diameters of drill bits correspond to specific screws in the fracture fixation set. Generally, the size of the drill bit used to make the pilot hole for the screw threads is 0.1 to 0.2 mm larger than the core diameter of the corresponding screw. The size of the drill bit used to make glide holes is the same size as the diameter of the shaft of a shaft screw or the outer diameter of a fully threaded cortical screw. The cutting edge of the bit is at its tip; it should always be protected and should frequently be examined for flaws.

Taps

Taps are designed to cut threads in bone that resemble exactly the profile of the corresponding screw thread. The process of tapping facilitates insertion and enables the screw to bite deeper into the bone. This allows the torque applied to the screw to be used for generating compressive force instead of being dissipated by friction and cutting of threads (Fig. 4-14). Tapping also removes additional material from the hole, thereby enlarging it. The screw pullout strength depends on the material density. The larger hole created by the tap does not decrease pullout strength in cortical bone because of its density; in less dense trabecular or osteopenic bone, the larger hole has a progressively larger effect and can decrease pullout strength by as much as 30%.[88]

Taps are threaded throughout their length and increase gradually in height up to the desired thread depth. A flute extends from the tip through the first 10 threads to facilitate clearing of bone debris, which can collect and jam the tap. Proper technique calls for two clockwise and one counterclockwise turn to facilitate bone chip removal. The entire far cortex should always be tapped, because screw pullout strength increases substantially with full cortical purchase. The tap size, which corresponds to its outer

diameter, should be the same as the outer diameter of the screw. For example, a 4.5-mm cortical screw has an outside diameter of 4.5 mm and uses a 4.5-mm tap; a 6.5-mm cancellous screw with an outside diameter of 6.5 mm uses a 6.5-mm tap (Fig. 4-15).

Screw Types

In practice, screws are most commonly referred to by the outer diameter of the threads (3.5, 4.5, 6.5, and 7.3 mm). Screws are also described as self-tapping or non-self-tapping, solid or cannulated, cortical or cancellous, and fully or partially threaded. The final variables are the overall length of the screw and the thread length of a partially threaded screw. The following sections describe self-tapping, non-self-tapping, cortical, shaft, cancellous, cannulated, and malleolar screws.

SELF-TAPPING SCREWS

Self-tapping screws are designed to cut their own thread path during insertion without prior use of a tap (see Fig. 4-14). The feature that differentiates these screws from others is the tip shape and design. Most commonly, the tip has cutting flutes that allow the leading threads to cut a path. Because the flutes are only at the tip and do not

FIGURE 4-14 *Self-tapping versus non-self-tapping screws. **A,** In a non-self-tapping screw, the majority of the torque applied to the screw is used in generating compression. **B,** In a self-tapping screw, the pilot hole is larger and the majority of the torque applied to the screw is used in cutting threads and generating friction, not in generating compression. In addition, the threads do not penetrate as deeply into the bone. **C,** To maximize screw thread purchase into the cortical bone, self-tapping screws should be inserted so that the cutting threads extend beyond the far cortex. (Redrawn from Perren, S.M.; et al. Int J Orthop Trauma 2:31–48, 1992; redrawn from Tencer, A.F.; et al. In: Asnis, S.E.; Kyle, R.F., eds. Cannulated Screw Fixation: Principles and Operative Techniques. New York, Springer Verlag, 1996. Used with permission.)*

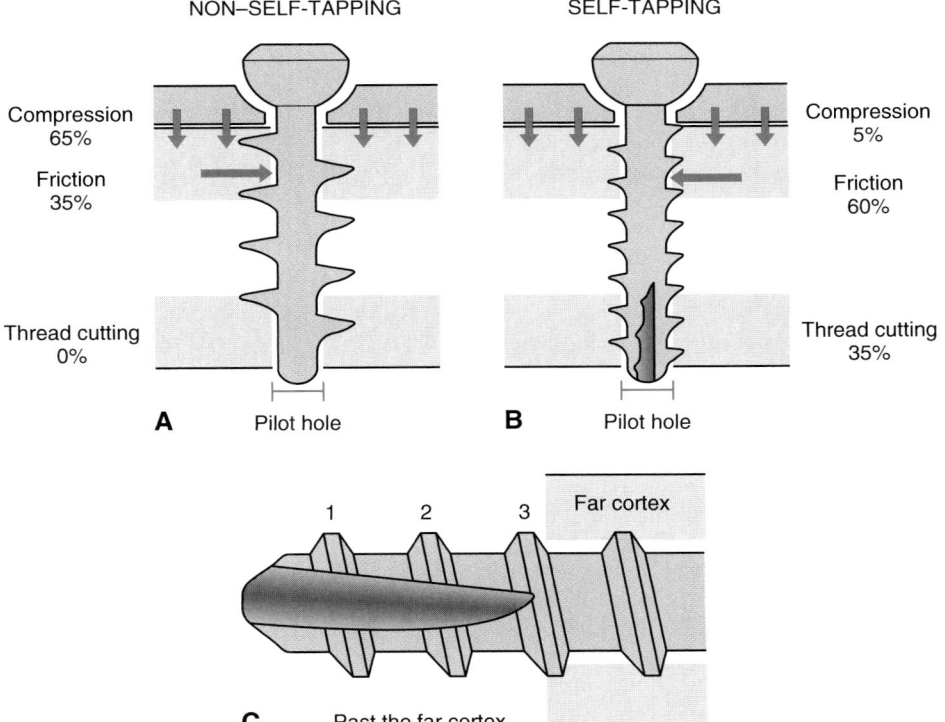

Taps and their corresponding screws. ***A,*** *A 4.5-mm cortical screw has an outside diameter of 4.5 mm and uses a 4.5-mm tap.* ***B,*** *A 6.5-mm cancellous screw has an outside diameter of 6.5 mm and uses a 6.5-mm tap. (Redrawn from Texhammar, R.; Colton, C. AO/ASIF Instruments and Implants: A Technical Manual. New York, Springer Verlag, 1995.)*

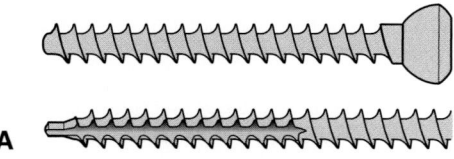

A

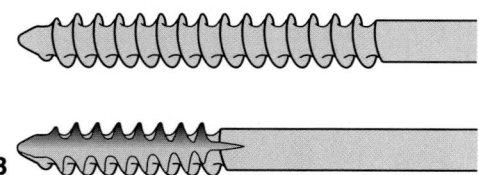

B

extend the full length of the screw, debris cannot be removed completely and is instead impacted into the thread path. These fluted-tipped, self-tapping screws are designed primarily for use in cortical bone. Some screws are designed to drill the pilot hole and tap the threads. These screws usually have a trochar, diamond-shaped tip as well as flutes. This design is most commonly used in cannulated screw systems.

Although not designated as self-tapping screws, cancellous screws are commonly inserted without tapping of the cancellous bone. The thread tip of these screws has a corkscrew pattern with a gradually increasing thread diameter. The corkscrew shape impacts the bone around the sides of the pilot hole rather than cutting and removing debris. The purchase of the cancellous screw is enhanced by this impaction. Tapping of the entire length of the cancellous threads removes essential bone, reducing the pullout strength.

An advantage of self-tapping screws is that the number of steps necessary for the operation is reduced, decreasing the operative time. An intimate fit of the screw thread in the bone occurs because the screw cuts its own thread and bone is impacted in the thread path. A disadvantage of self-tapping screws is the increased torque required for screw insertion. Ansell and Scales[1] found that three flutes extended over three threads required the least torque for insertion (see Fig. 4-14). However, these flutes weaken the pullout strength of this portion of the screw because the fluted threads have 17% to 30% less thread surface than threads farther up the screw. Therefore, the screw should be advanced so that the cutting flutes protrude beyond the far cortex.[2] Because additional axial load and torque are necessary for insertion of self-tapping screws,

fracture displacement may occur. This is one reason why self-tapping screws are not recommended for interfragmentary lag screw fixation.[67]

NON-SELF-TAPPING SCREWS

Non-self-tapping screws do not have flutes and are designed with a blunt tip. These screws require a predrilled pilot hole and threads cut with a tap. The most important advantage of non-self-tapping screws is that less axial load and torque are applied during tapping and screw insertion than with self-tapping screws (see Fig. 4-14). This difference allows the screws to be used more effectively for interfragmentary compression, lessening the chance of fracture displacement. In addition, unlike self-tapping screws, these screws can be replaced accurately because they cannot cut their own channel.

COMPARISON OF SELF-TAPPING AND NON-SELF-TAPPING SCREWS

Baumgart and colleagues[3] evaluated the insertion torque, pullout force, and temperature on insertion of a self-tapping screw and compared the results with those of non-self-tapping screws with or without the process of proper tapping. They found that 1 to 1.5 N-m of insertion torque was required to insert a 4.5-mm self-tapping screw into human cortical bone. This value is slightly more than the torque required to insert a non-self-tapping screw into a pretapped hole. Placement of a non-self-tapping screw into an untapped pilot hole required twice the torque. The pullout force of a self-tapping screw is 450 to 500 N per millimeter of cortex, which is less than but not significantly different from the pullout force of a tapped screw in cortical bone. The heat generated during introduction of the self-tapping screw causes an increase in temperature at the screw tip, but little heat is transferred to the surrounding bone. The increase in temperature does not depend on the rate of insertion as long as the insertion is not hindered.

The discussion so far has focused on differentiating screws according to their specific biomechanical function. In the following sections, screws are differentiated based on the type of bone in which they are used.

CORTICAL SCREWS

Cortical screws are made with a shallow thread, small pitch, and relatively large core diameter (Fig. 4-16). The large core diameter increases the strength of the screw, which is important for attachment of plates to bone and for resistance to the deforming loads experienced by interfragmentary compression. These screws are fully threaded throughout their length and are commonly non-self-tapping. The thread and the polished surface allow easy removal and replacement if incorrect insertion has been performed.

SHAFT SCREWS

The shaft screw is a partially threaded cortical screw in which the shaft diameter equals the external diameter of the thread (see Fig. 4-16). This screw is used for interfragmentary compression, either in bone alone or positioned through a plate. The nonthreaded shaft presents a smooth

FIGURE 4-16 *Comparison of the inner and outer diameters of cannulated, cortical, cancellous, shaft, and malleolar screws. (Redrawn from Synthes Equipment Ordering Manual. Paoli, PA, Synthes USA, 1992.)*

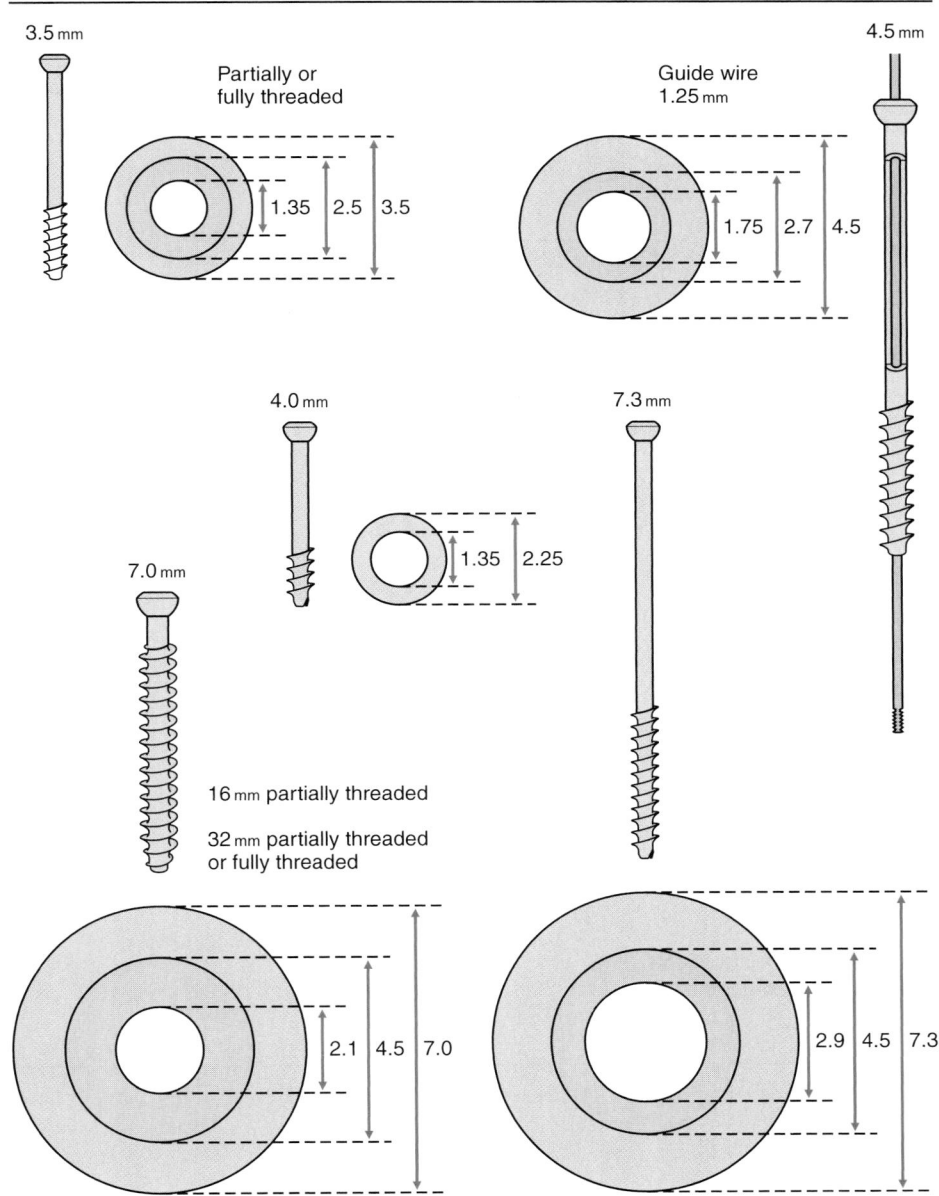

CANNULATED SCREWS

(Continued)

surface to sit in the glide hole, eliminating binding. Klaue and associates reported that almost 40% of the compressive effect of a fully threaded cortical lag screw through a plate may be lost because of binding of the screw on the side of the glide hole in the proximal cortex.[52] They termed this binding phenomenon *parasitic force.* The absence of binding removes the parasitic force, resulting in a 60% improvement in lag screw compression (Fig. 4-17).

CANCELLOUS SCREWS

Cancellous screws are characterized by a thin core diameter and wide, deep threads (see Fig. 4-16). The higher ratio of outer to core diameter increases the holding power, which is especially important for cancellous trabeculae commonly found at the epiphysis and metaphysis. Cancellous screws are available in either fully or partially threaded forms with variable thread lengths. The choice of the specific thread length depends on fracture configuration and bone anatomy. When a cancellous screw is used as a lag screw, the entire length of thread must be contained within the fracture fragment. Allowing the thread to cross the fracture site inhibits compression and may cause distraction. Choosing the correct thread length is critical to ensure maximal purchase while avoiding displacement. Compression of cancellous bone by screw threads does not cause resorption but actually causes hypertrophy and

FIGURE 4-16   *(Continued)*

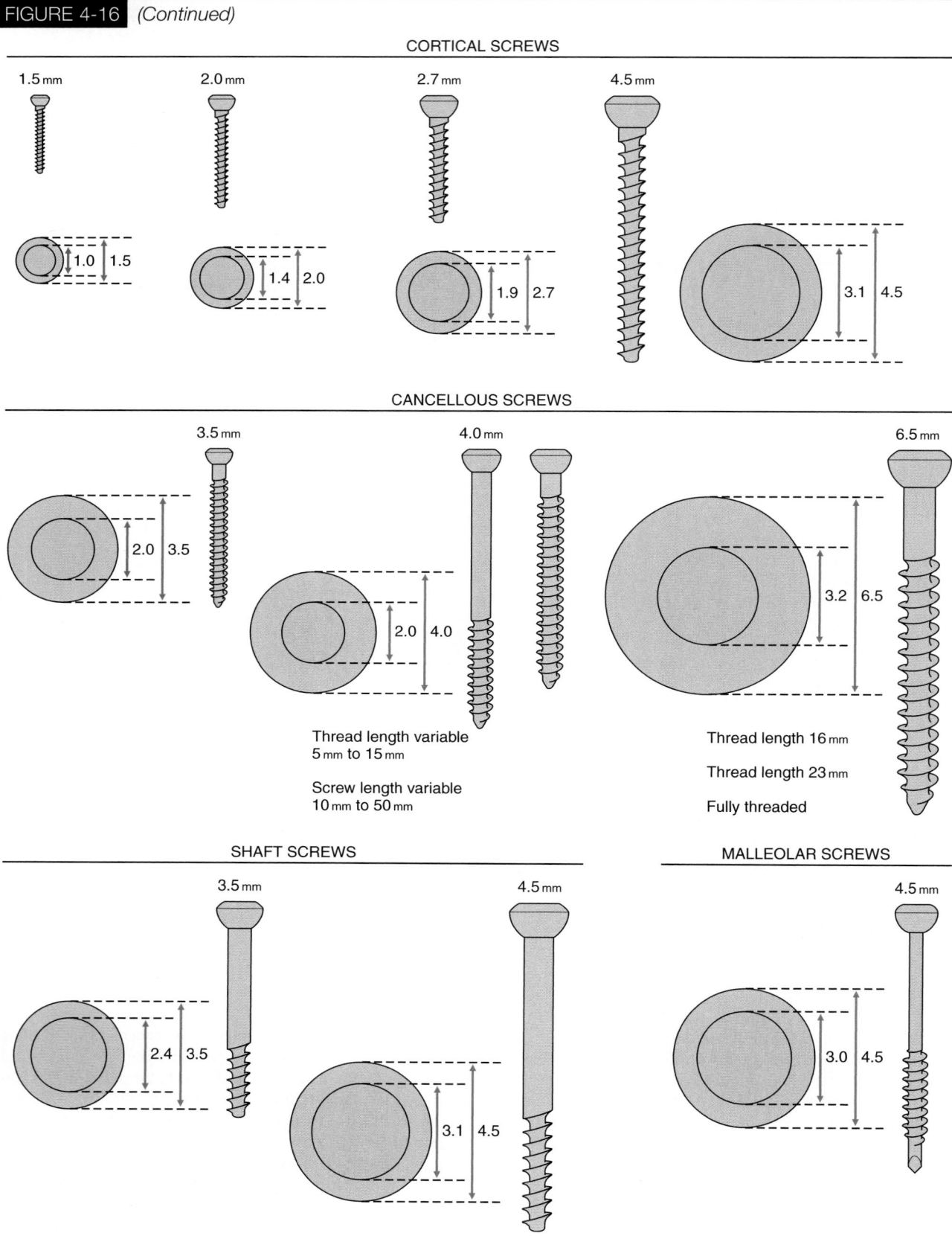

CORTICAL SCREWS

1.5 mm   2.0 mm   2.7 mm   4.5 mm

1.0 | 1.5   1.4 | 2.0   1.9 | 2.7   3.1 | 4.5

CANCELLOUS SCREWS

3.5 mm   4.0 mm   6.5 mm

2.0 | 3.5   2.0 | 4.0   3.2 | 6.5

Thread length variable
5 mm to 15 mm

Screw length variable
10 mm to 50 mm

Thread length 16 mm

Thread length 23 mm

Fully threaded

SHAFT SCREWS

3.5 mm   4.5 mm

2.4 | 3.5   3.1 | 4.5

MALLEOLAR SCREWS

4.5 mm

3.0 | 4.5

FIGURE 4-17 *Loss and recovery of lag screw compression.* **A,** *With a fully threaded lag screw applied in an inclined position, wedging of the threads within the gliding hole can occur, causing a 40% loss of the compression effect.* **B,** *The use of a partially threaded shaft screw avoids this wedging problem.* **C,** *The differences between the measured values of compression for the standard fully threaded lag screw* (blue bars) *and the shaft screw* (red bars). *The newer shaft screw is 60% more efficient than the fully threaded inclined lag screw. (Redrawn from Perren, S.M. The concept of biological plating using the limited contact-dynamic compression plate [LCDCP]: Scientific background, design, and application. Injury 22[Suppl 1]:1–41, 1991; with permission from Elsevier Science Ltd., The Boulevard, Langford Lane, Kidlington OX5 1GB, U.K.)*

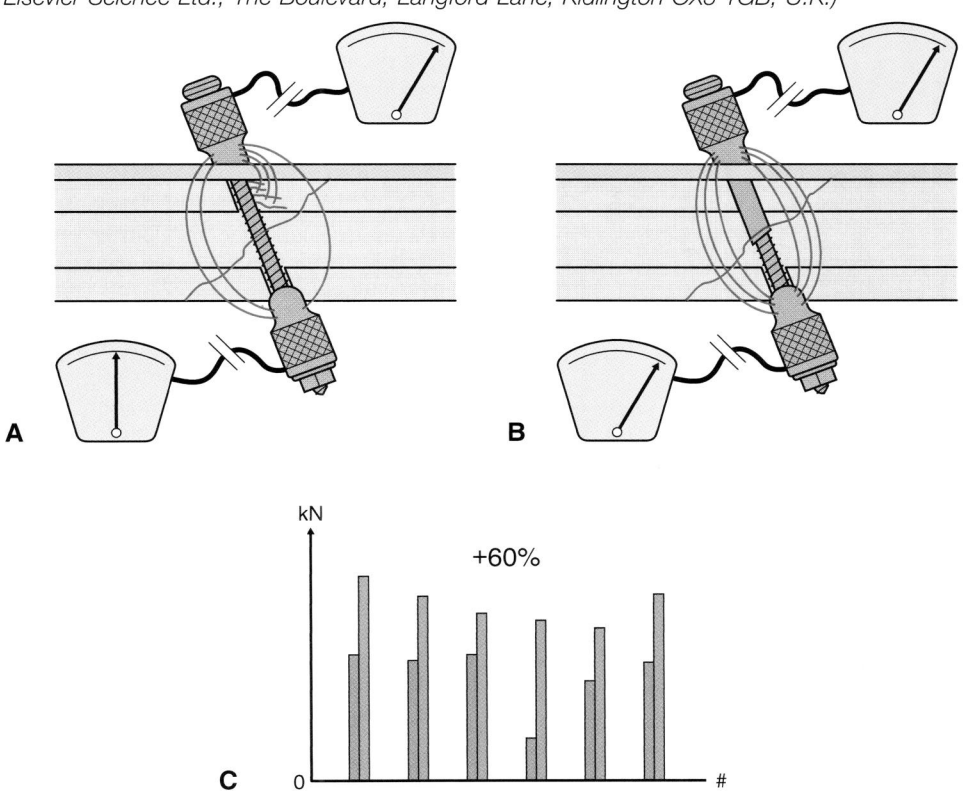

realigns the trabeculae with the force on the side exposed to pressure.[96] The design of a cancellous screw takes into account the fact that cancellous bone is softer than the denser cortical bone. The root diameter is decreased, allowing for increased thread depth. This configuration results in greater holding capacity at the expense of loss of bending and shear strength.

CANNULATED SCREWS

A cannulated screw has a hollow center that allows it to be passed over a guide wire (see Fig. 4-16). The root diameter is increased to account for placement of the screw over the wire. The increased size of the screw is necessary to account for the cannulation wire, which must be of adequate strength to hold steady in bone without bending. The screw cannot be too large or it would remove too much bone and decrease the strength of the construct. Guide pins are used to determine the optimal screw position and aid in the fracture reduction. The guide pin makes a relatively small defect in the bone, allowing modification with little effect on the ability of the screw to compress and hold bone. It is threaded to aid in its fixation and to prevent migration when the screw is inserted. The guide pin also makes the pilot hole for the cannulated screw. When combined with fluoroscopic imaging,

cannulation improves the precision of cancellous screw placement significantly. This method is important in areas where errant placement could result in catastrophic complications. Once the guide pin is in position, the screw is advanced through the soft tissues in a counterclockwise fashion to avoid tissue damage. At the proximal cortex, the screw is turned clockwise and self-tapped to the desired level of insertion. Cannulated screw systems are commonly used in areas with abundant cancellous bone; tapping of this type of bone decreases the pullout strength.[2]

The mechanics of a cannulated screw are different from those of solid screws. The most important factor in maximizing the overall pullout strength of a cannulated screw is the host material density (Fig. 4-18), followed by outer diameter, pitch, and root diameter. Pullout strength depends on two basic parameters: screw fixation and screw design. The patient's variable bone density is the primary factor affecting screw fixation. There are many variables to screw design. The larger the outer diameter, the greater the pullout strength. A 6.4-mm screw has significantly greater holding power than a 4.5-mm screw in bone of comparable density. A smaller pitch also increases holding power. This variable is limited because as the number of threads per inch increases, they become tight and remove too much bone.

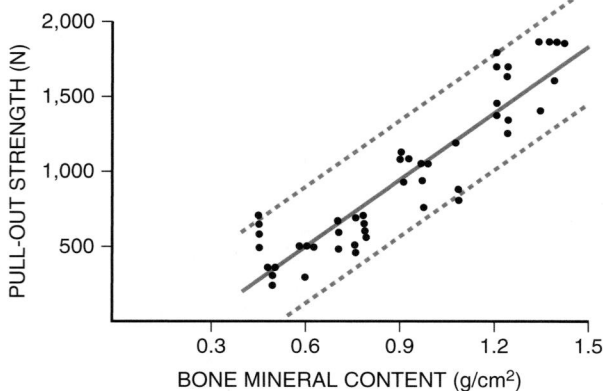

COMPARISON OF CORTICAL, CANCELLOUS, AND CANNULATED SCREWS

A cortical screw can handle four times the stress of a cancellous screw of similar size and 1.7 times the stress of a cannulated screw. The thread design and larger root diameter enable it to handle 6.2 and 1.7 times the maximal bending stress of a solid cancellous or cannulated screw, respectively. The increase in strength caused by increased root diameter comes with the disadvantage of decreased thread depth (see Fig. 4-16). However, this decrease in thread depth does not decrease holding power in cortical bone.[2] The resistance of a screw to bending stresses does increase with the root diameter.

For screws to have cannulation, the root diameter must be increased. In relation to solid screws of the same external diameter, the thread depth of a cannulated screw is decreased and the root diameter is increased, resulting in the decreased pullout strength of cannulated screws. Leggon and coworkers[57] found a 20% decrease in holding power between cannulated and solid screws of similar diameter. To compensate for this difference, larger diameter cannulated screws are recommended. Hearn and colleagues[40] found no significant difference in pullout strength between solid 6.5-mm cancellous screws and 7.0-mm cannulated cancellous screws.

MALLEOLAR SCREWS

Malleolar screws were originally designed for the fixation of the medial malleolus. They are partially threaded cortical screws with a trephine tip that allows them to cut their own path in cancellous bone. To achieve stable fixation of the malleolar fragment, two points of fixation are necessary. Medial malleolar fractures often have distal fragments that are too small to permit fixation with two of these screws; the large size of the screw often shatters these small fragments. The prominence of the large screw head at the tip of the medial malleolus also causes excessive patient discomfort.

Summary

Proper drilling, tapping, and insertion of screws are critical in internal fixation. Surgeons use different screws based on the design, application, and anatomy of the fracture. This section has addressed the basic geometry, design, and function of screws, drills, and taps to offer a general understanding that can be further applied to specific fractures.

Plates

Plates are a fundamental element of internal fixation. They are principally differentiated by the biomechanical function they perform. Examples of these functions are neutralization, buttressing, compression, bridging, formation of a tension band, and anti-glide. Additionally, plates can be categorized by their specific designs: dynamic compression (DC), limited contact-dynamic compression (LCDC), tubular, reconstruction, angled, and sliding screw plates. Certain specially designed plates can be modified to perform different biomechanical functions according to anatomic need. In addition, some plates have evolved with specific names based on their location (e.g., lateral tibial head plate). Various plates can be used or adapted on the basis of function, design, or anatomic location. This section discusses the basic biomechanical functions of plates and some specific plate designs. The application of particular plates to certain injuries is discussed in other parts of this book.

BIOMECHANICAL FUNCTIONS OF PLATES

NEUTRALIZATION A neutralization plate is used to protect lag screw fixations from various external forces. Torsional and bending forces on long bone fractures are too great to be overcome by lag screw stabilization alone. A plate can protect the interfragmentary compression achieved with the lag screw from torsional, bending, and shear forces exerted on the fracture. This technique achieves fracture fixation that is sufficiently stable to allow early motion. When comparing two plates of the same design, a longer plate provides greater neutralization capability (Fig. 4-19).

BUTTRESSING The buttress plate is used to counteract bending, compressive, and shearing forces at the fracture site when an axial load is applied. Buttress plates are used commonly to stabilize intra-articular and periarticular fractures at the ends of long bones. Without fixation or with lag screw fixation alone, epiphyseal and metaphyseal fragments can displace when they are subjected to axial compression or bending forces. The buttress plate supports the underlying cortex and effectively resists displacement and the resulting angular deformity of the joint. In this manner, the plate acts as a buttress or retaining wall (Fig. 4-20A).

To minimize the potential for angular deformity, the screws attaching the plate to the bone must be inserted in such a manner that when a load is applied there will

FIGURE 4-19 *Neutralization plate.* **A,** *Interfragmentary screw fixation without a neutralization plate.* **B,** *Interfragmentary screw fixation without a neutralization plate in a loaded position, resulting in construct failure.* **C,** *Interfragmentary screw fixation with a neutralization plate effectively resisting an external load.*

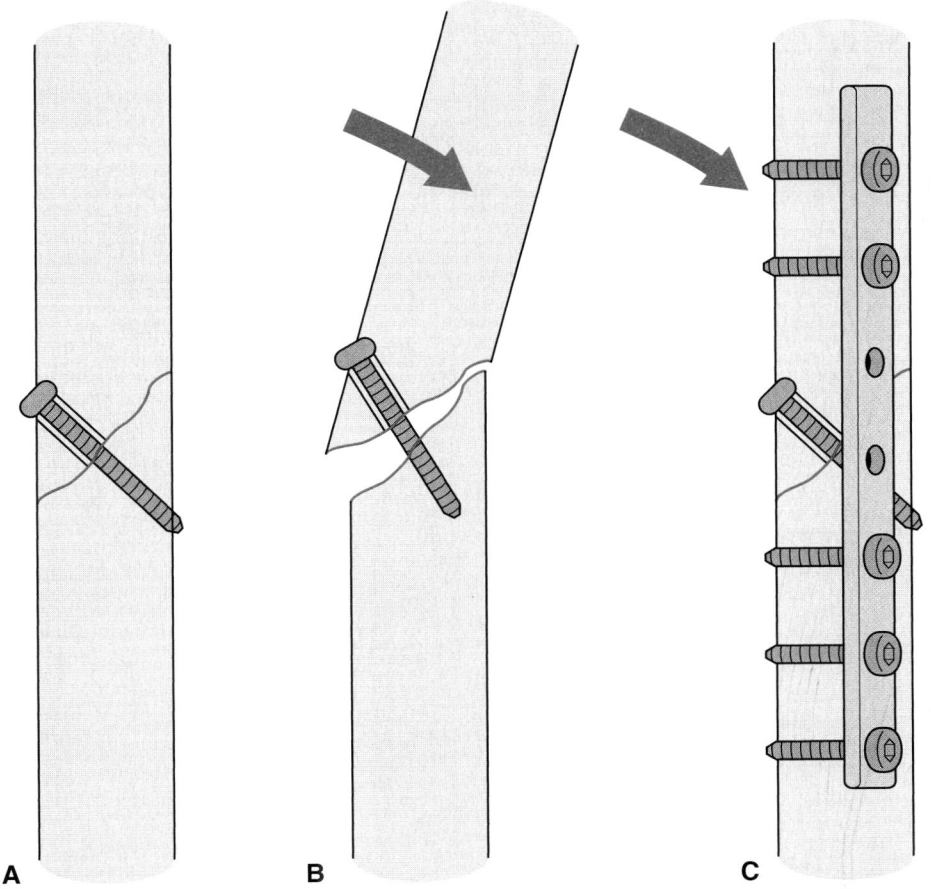

be no shift in the position of the plate in relation to the bone. A screw inserted through an oval hole closest to the fracture is said to be in *buttress mode*. This mode minimizes axial movement at the fracture site. To avoid the possibility of displacing the fracture fragment during application of the plate, the plate should be accurately contoured to match the anatomy of the underlying cortex. Screw placement in a buttress mode does not always imply that the plate is functioning as a buttress plate. A buttress plate applies force to the bone in a direction normal (perpendicular) to the flat surface of the plate, in contrast to a compression plate application, in which the direction of stress is parallel to the plate. Buttress plates are designed to fit specific anatomic locations (see Fig. 4-20B). If the fracture extends from the metaphysis into the diaphysis, a long plate with a condylar end can be used to combine buttressing with other plate functions. A spring plate is a specialized form of buttress in which the plate is affixed with screws to only one of the two fracture fragments (see Fig. 4-20C).

Plates designed to provide compression (DC or LCDC plates) can be used as buttress plates with proper contouring. Other plates are designed specifically to function as buttress plates in particular locations. Some examples of buttress plates by design are the T-buttress plate for lateral tibial plateau fractures, the spoon plate for treatment of anterior metaphyseal fractures of the distal tibia, the cloverleaf plate for the medial distal tibia, and the distal femoral condylar buttress plate (see Fig. 4-20B).

COMPRESSION Compression plates can be used to reduce and stabilize transverse or short oblique fractures when lag screw fixation alone is inadequate. The plate can produce static compression in the direction of the long axis of bone in three ways: by over-bending of the plate, by application of a tension device, and by a special plate design that generates axial compression by combining screw hole geometry with screw insertion (Fig. 4-21).

BRIDGING A bridge plate is intended to maintain length and alignment of severely comminuted and segmental fractures. It is called a *bridge plate* because its fixation is out of the main zone of injury at the ends of the plate to avoid additional injury in the comminuted zone. During fracture fixation, the bridge plate can be used as a reduction device to limit the dissection in the zone of injury. This fixation method limits devitalization of bone fragments and thereby allows for a better healing environment (Fig. 4-22A).

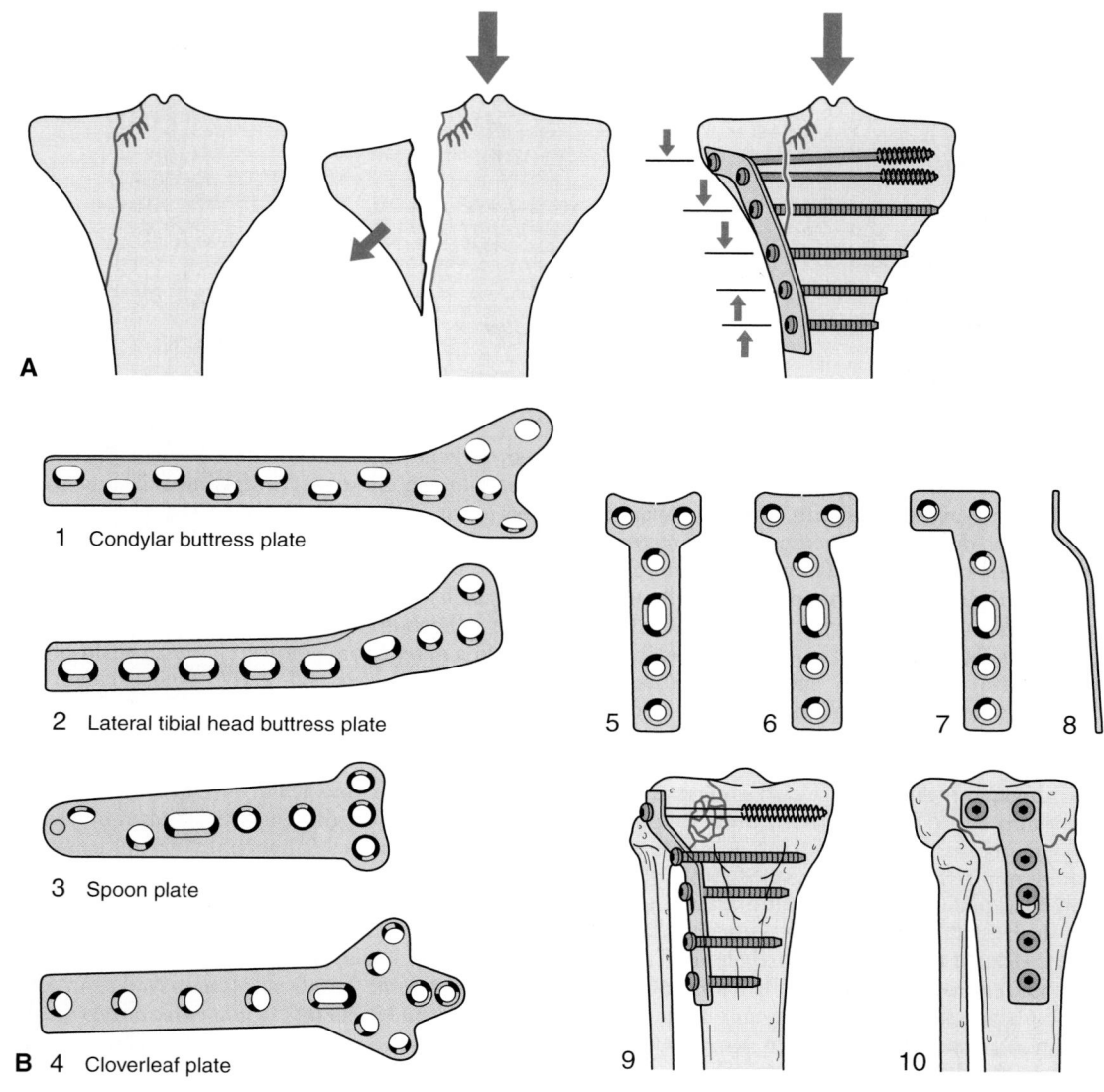

Buttress plates. **A,** *Buttress plate supporting the underlying cortex and effectively resisting displacement, which otherwise would result in angular deformity of the joint. The plate acts as a buttress or retaining wall.* **B,** *Examples of various buttress plates designed for specific anatomic locations. (1) Condylar buttress plate; (2) lateral tibial head buttress plate; (3) spoon plate; (4) cloverleaf plate; (5) medial T plate; (6) lateral T plate; (7) lateral L plate; (8) profile of lateral L plate; anteroposterior (9) and lateral (10) views of lateral L plate used in conjunction with cancellous bone graft to buttress a lateral tibial plateau fracture.*

(Continued)

The *wave plate* is similar to a bridge plate; it is primarily used in areas of delayed healing (see Fig. 4-22B). The wave plate is contoured away from the comminuted area or pseudarthrosis to be bridged.[15] This contour leaves some distance between the cortex of bone and the plate, where autologous bone graft can be placed. In the treatment of nonunions, this space allows for better ingrowth of vessels into the graft beneath the plate. The bending of the plate distributes force over a greater area, decreasing local stress at the fracture site. The plate also can act as a tension band, creating compression on the opposite cortex. These factors make the wave plate an efficient tool in the treatment of nonunions.

TENSION BAND Pauwels adopted the tension band principle from classical mechanics.[72,73] It is best understood by examining the forces that occur at discontinuity in an I-beam (Fig. 4-23). The stretching and compressing of springs can be used to demonstrate the different forces. As shown in this analogy, forces applied in line with the central axis of the I-beam produce uniform compression in both springs on either side of the neutral axis and uniform closure of the discontinuity in the beam. In contrast, when the force is applied eccentrically at a distance from the central axis to the beam, a bending moment is created. This bending moment produces tension on the opposite side of the beam. This change is demonstrated

FIGURE 4-20 *(Continued)* **C,** *The use of spring plates to buttress small, thin fragments of the acetabular rim. Fork-ended plates are fashioned by cutting into the last hole of a one-third tubular or semi-tubular plate. The forked prongs, which are bent at 90°, are impaled into the small fragments to improve fixation. By creating a mismatch between the contour of the plate and the bone (1), the plate is pulled down and springs against the bone as the screws are tightened (2, 3). (***B*** *[1–4], Redrawn from Synthes Equipment Ordering Manual. Paoli, PA, Synthes USA, 1992.* ***C,*** *Redrawn from Mast, J.; et al. Planning and Reduction Technique in Fracture Surgery. New York, Springer Verlag, 1989, p. 244.)*

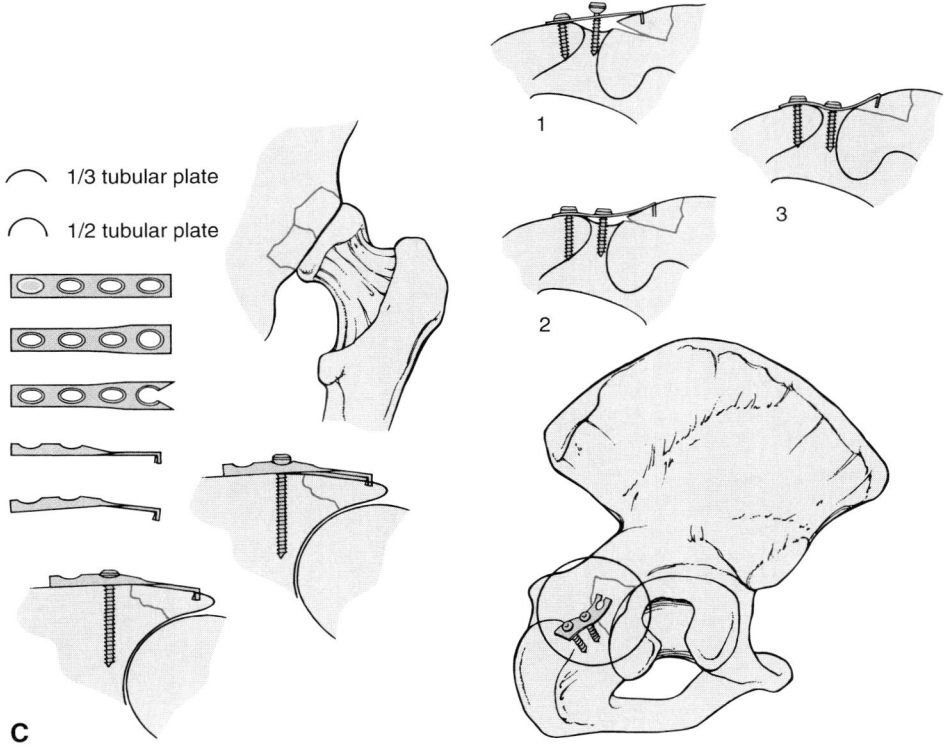

by opening of the discontinuity and spring distraction. On the same side of the beam on which the weight is applied, the moment creates compression, as evidenced by closing of the discontinuity with spring compression. In anticipation of this eccentrically applied weight, an unyielding band can be applied to the side on which tension will be created by the bending moment. This band is used to create a small amount of compression, which results in partial closure of the discontinuity and compression of the spring on the same side as the band. Under these conditions, the application of an asymmetric force to the opposite side of the beam leads to uniform compression on both sides of the discontinuity, further closing of the space and compression of the springs. This technique, which is placed before the functional application of the eccentric load, is called the *tension band*.

Wires, cables, nonabsorbable sutures, and plates can be used to perform the function of the tension band. Practically speaking, tension band implants can be used to fix fractures in only certain limited locations in the body. Some examples are the greater trochanter of the femur, the olecranon, and the patella. In these situations, the eccentric pull of the muscles forces the joint surface of the fractured bone against the corresponding joint surface of another bone, which acts as a fulcrum. The extensor muscle usually provides the major deforming force causing

the bending moment at the discontinuity. A wire or cable is frequently used as a tension band in these situations. It is applied to the surface of the bone, which is subjected to tensile loads during active motion. The wire is tensioned to apply slight compression to the site of the fractures. This creates a small gap on the opposite side. When dynamic forces are applied during subsequent contractions of these antagonistic deforming muscles, the tension band resists the tendency for distraction of the opposite side of the bone, producing uniform compression at the fracture site. Parallel longitudinal Kirschner wires, Steinmann pins, or cancellous lag screws are used as adjunctive fixation to prevent displacement of the fracture site through shearing, translation, or rotation. Because they are placed in parallel orientation, the smooth pins or screw shafts act as rails along which the bone fragment can slide during dynamic compression.

In fractures of the patella and olecranon, dynamic compression is achieved through antagonistic muscle function during active flexion of the knee and elbow. The intercondylar grooves of the distal femur and humeral trochlea act as a fulcrum over which the antagonistic muscle groups apply bending forces to the patella and olecranon. Fractures or osteotomies of the greater trochanter of the femur and greater tuberosity of the humerus can also be fixed in a similar fashion using the tension band principle. The

FIGURE 4-21 | *Application of a compression plate to the lateral aspect of the femur demonstrates the combination of static and dynamic compression. **A,** Immediately after the plate is applied, static compression is achieved at the fracture site. **B,** After functional loading of the curved bone, additional dynamic compression is obtained at the fracture site because of the effect of the laterally placed plate, which acts as a tension band.*

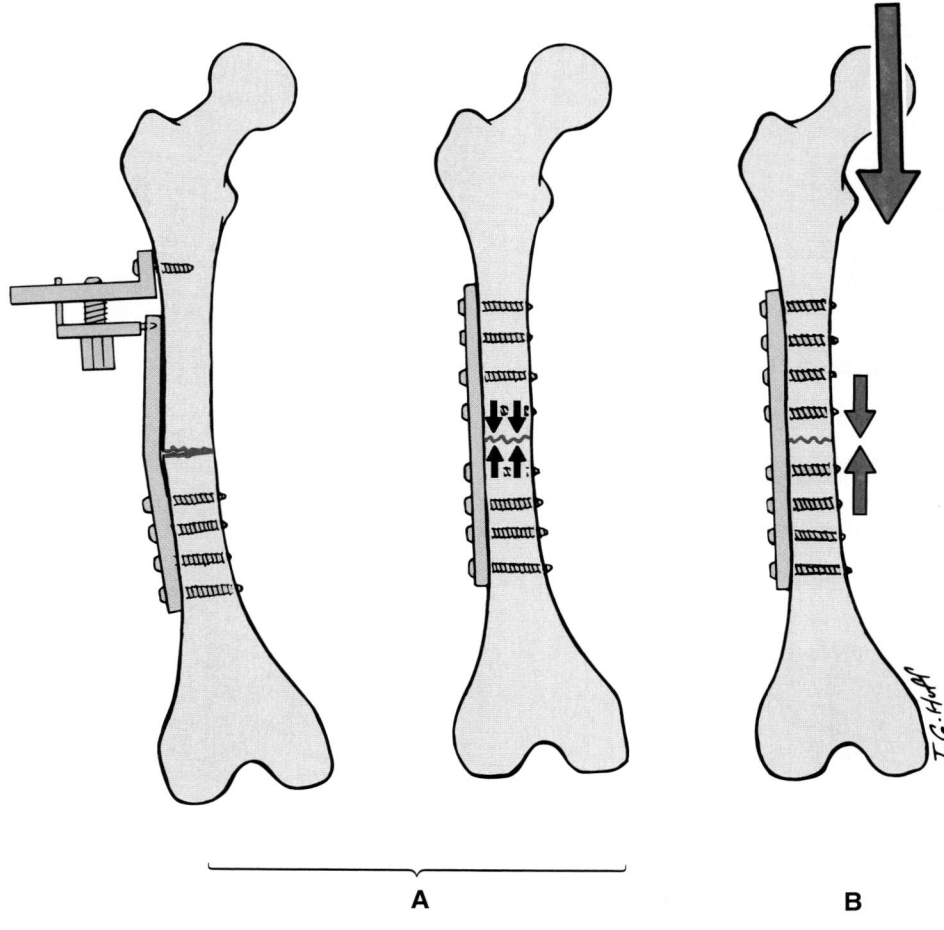

A

B

FIGURE 4-22 | *Bridging. **A,** The bridge plate maintains length and alignment by fixing to bone away from the comminution and preserving critical blood supply to that area by limiting surgical dissection. **B,** The wave plate is used primarily in areas of delayed healing. The added space created by the bend allows for better ingrowth of vessels into the graft. (Redrawn from Texhammar, R.; Colton, C. AO/ASIF Instruments and Implants: A Technical Manual. New York, Springer Verlag, 1995.)*

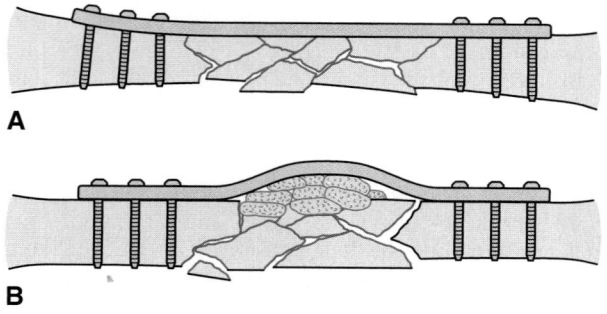

A

B

antagonistic pull of the gluteal and abductor musculature, using the hip joint as a fulcrum, causes a bending moment at the site of discontinuity between the greater trochanter and the remaining femur. In a similar fashion, the antagonistic pull of the supraspinatus and pectoralis major, using the glenohumeral joint as a fulcrum, causes a bending moment at the site of discontinuity between the greater tuberosity and the remaining humerus. Optimal compression is achieved with this method only during functional activity that results in eccentric loading and the production of bending moments.

PREVENTION OF GLIDE The anti-glide plate is another example of the dynamic compression principle.[16,82] Although there are many potential applications, the construct is most commonly used for oblique, Weber type B fractures of the distal fibula (Fig. 4-24). A plate applied to the posterior surface of the proximal fragment forms an axilla into which the spike of the distal fragment fits. The axial loads of walking are converted into compression of the surfaces of the two fracture fragments. The plate acts as a buttress to prevent external rotation of the distal fragment.

FIGURE 4-23 *Tension band principles. **A,** (1) An interrupted I-beam connected by two springs. (2) The I-beam is loaded with a weight (Wt) placed over the central axis of the beam; there is uniform compression of both springs at the interruption. (3) When the I-beam is loaded eccentrically by placing the weight at a distance from the central axis of the beam, the spring on the same side compresses, whereas the spring on the opposite side is placed in tension and stretches. (4) If a tension band is applied prior to the eccentric loading, it resists the tension that would otherwise stretch the opposite spring and thus causes uniform compression of both springs. **B,** The tension band principle applied to fixation of a transverse patellar fracture. (1) The anteroposterior view shows placement of the parallel Kirschner wires and anterior tension band. (2) The lateral view demonstrates antagonistic pull of the hamstrings and quadriceps, causing a bending moment of the patella over the femoral trochlea. An anterior tension band transforms this eccentric loading into compression at the fracture site. **C,** The tension band principle applied to fixation of a fracture of the ulna. The antagonistic pull of the triceps and brachialis causes a bending moment of the ulna over the humeral trochlea. The dorsal tension band transforms this eccentric load into compression at the fracture site. **D,** The tension band principle applied to fixation of a fracture of the greater trochanter. With the hip as a fulcrum, the antagonistic pull of the adductors and abductors causes a bending moment in the femur. The lateral tension band transforms this eccentric load into compression at the greater trochanteric fracture site. **E,** The tension band principle applied to fixation of a fracture of the greater tuberosity of the humerus. Using the glenoid as a fulcrum, the antagonistic pull of the pectoralis major and supraspinatus causes a bending moment of the humerus. The lateral tension band transforms this eccentric load into compression at the greater tuberosity fracture site.*

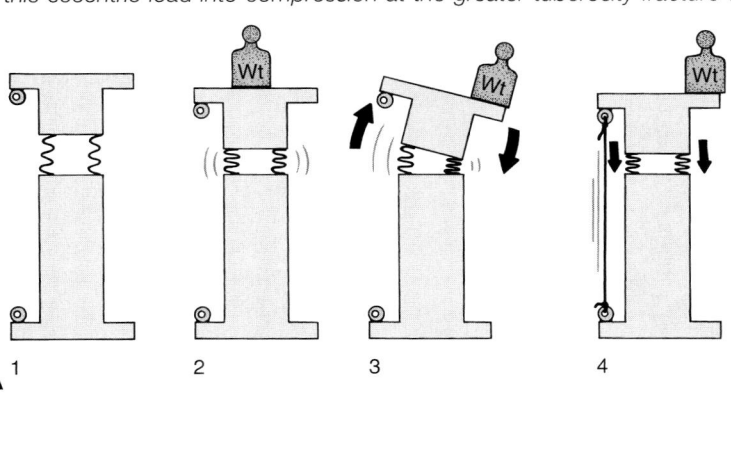

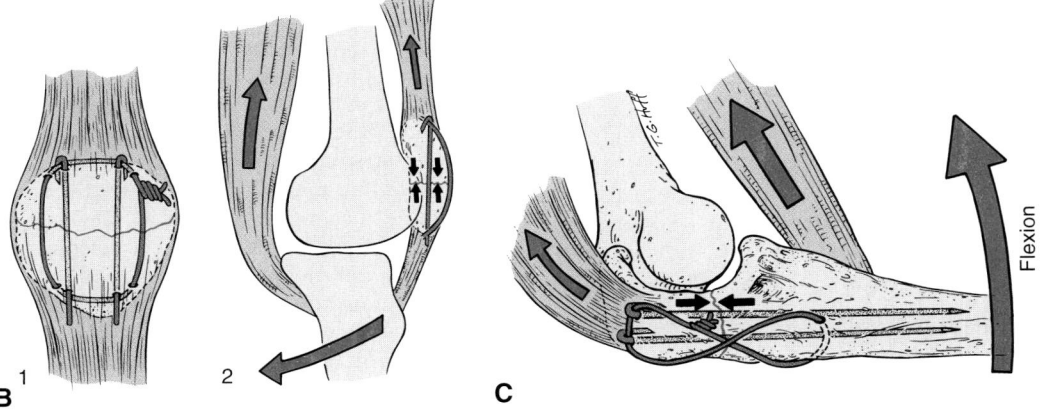

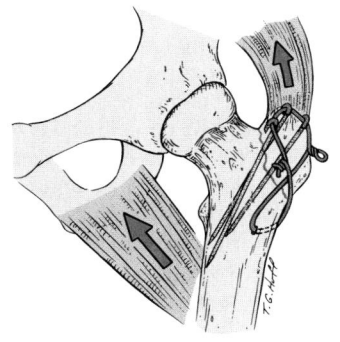

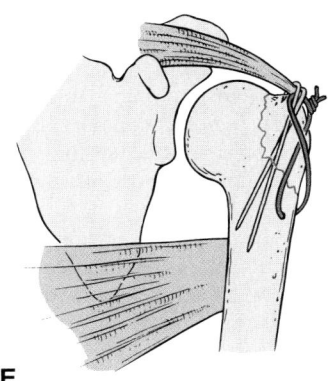

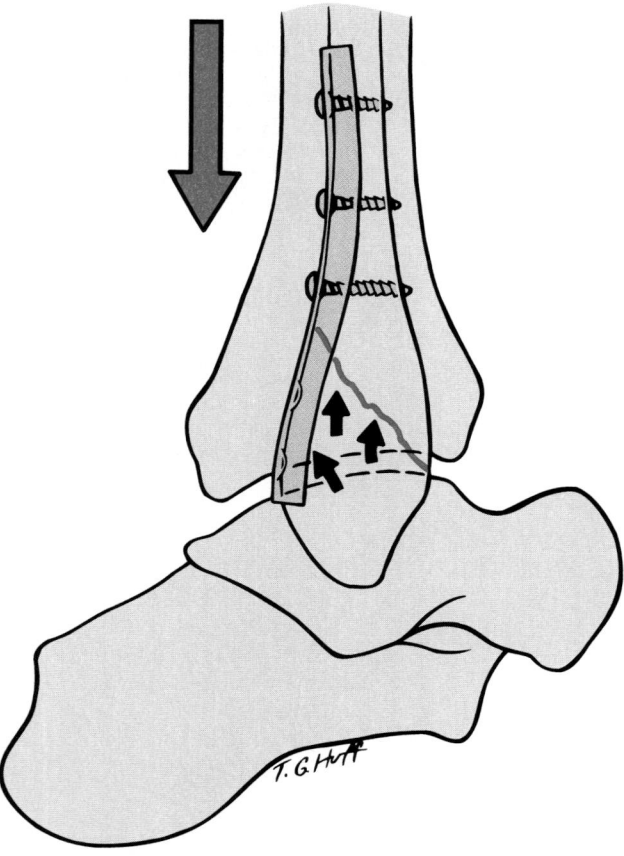

FIGURE 4-24 *Dynamic compression—an antiglide plate. Because of the obliquity of the typical Weber type B fracture, a one-third tubular plate, fixed proximally only to the posterior surface of the fibula, acts as an antiglide plate. Dynamic compression is achieved on weight-bearing because the distal fragment is trapped between the fracture site and the plate.*

SPECIFIC PLATE DESIGNS

The discussion thus far has dealt with the biomechanical application of plates. An important concept is that different plates can be used for various biomechanical problems. Some plates are specifically designed for function; others can be functionally modified for the same application. The idea of design versus function versus anatomic location is important for the general understanding of plates. For example, the LCDC plate is designed primarily as a self-compression plate, but it can also be used as a bridging plate or tension band plate or further modified as a medial femoral condylar buttress plate. Therefore, depending on anatomic location and bending modification, it can function in most other biomechanical applications.

To understand the decisions orthopaedic surgeons make in using different plates for different applications, it is important to have a general understanding of the different types of plates manufactured and the mechanics of their designs. This section includes the basic designs such

as DC plates, LCDC plates, point contact (Schuhli) plates, semi-tubular and one-third tubular plates, reconstruction plates, angled plates, and sliding screw plates. Locking plates are addressed separately.

DC PLATE The special geometry of the DC plate hole allows for two basic functions: independent axial compression and the ability to place screws at different angles of inclination. Perren and colleagues[76] designed a screw housing in which an inclined and a horizontal cylinder meet at an obtuse angle, permitting a downward and horizontal movement of the screw head for axial compression in one direction (Fig. 4-25A). Sideways movement of the screw head is impossible. A screw placed at the inclined plane (i.e., eccentrically in the load position) moves the plate horizontally in relation to the bone until the screw head reaches the intersection of the two circles. *Eccentric position* refers to circles with different centers, whereas *concentric position* refers to circles with the same center. The act of compression is accomplished through the merging of two eccentric circles to become concentric. At this point, the screw has optimal contact with the hole, ensuring maximal stability and producing axial compression of the bone and tension on the plate. There are three areas in which to place a screw in an oval hole: one at each end (eccentrically) and one in the middle (concentrically).

The plate can be placed for neutralization, compression, or buttressing, depending on the insertion of the screw (see Fig. 4-25B). In the neutral mode, the screw is placed in a relatively central position. In actuality, this neutral position is 0.1 mm eccentric, causing horizontal displacement of the plate that results in minimal axial compression.

In the compressive mode, the screw is inserted 1.0 mm eccentrically to its final position in the hole on the side away from the fracture site. When the screw is tightened, its head slides down along the inclined plane, merging the eccentric circles and causing horizontal movement of the plate (1.0 mm). This results in fracture compression, assuming that a plate screw has previously been inserted to affix the plate into the other fracture fragment. This procedure can produce a maximum of 600 N of axial compression if anatomic reduction of the fragments is accomplished.[75] One screw in compression produces 1 mm of displacement, and the horizontal track in the hole still permits a further 1.8 mm of gliding. A second load screw can therefore be inserted into the next hole without being blocked by the first screw, producing another 1.0 mm of horizontal movement.[64] This is sometimes referred to as *double loading* (see Fig. 4-25C).

In buttress mode, the screw is placed eccentrically in the horizontal tract closest to the fracture. This position results in no horizontal movement of the plate when an axial load is placed. Under certain circumstances, the screw position may not be perpendicular to the plate. The design of the DC plate allows for inclined insertion of the screw head up to angles of 25° longitudinally and 7° laterally. The DC plate can be modified for use in most biomechanical applications of fracture fixation, and its use is based on fracture pattern and location.

Certain shortcomings of the DC plate have been discovered through the years. These include a large area of

FIGURE 4-25 *The dynamic compression (DC) plate. **A,** Perren designed the screw housing in which an inclined and a horizontal cylinder meet at an obtuse angle, permitting a downward and horizontal movement of the screw head for axle compression in one direction. **B,** The plate can be placed in neutral, compression, or buttress modes depending on the placement of the screw in the gliding hole. In a neutral mode, the screw is placed in a relatively central position. In actuality, this neutral position is 0.1 mm eccentric. In the compression mode, the screw is inserted 1.0 mm eccentric to its final position in the hole on the side away from the fracture site. When the screw is tightened, its head slides down along the inclined plane, merging the eccentric circles and causing horizontal movement of the plate (1.0 mm). This results in fracture compression. In buttress mode, the screw is placed eccentrically in the horizontal track close to the fracture. Note that the DC plate allows for incline insertion of the screw head up to angles of 25° longitudinally and 7° laterally. **C,** One screw in compression produces 1 mm of displacement while the horizontal track in the hole still permits a further 1.8 mm of gliding. A second load screw can, therefore, be inserted into the next hole without being blocked by the first screw, producing another 1.0 mm of horizontal movement. This is sometimes referred to as double loading. (**A,** left, Redrawn from Synthes Equipment Ordering Manual. Paoli, PA, Synthes USA, 1992, Figs. 2–45, 2–46, 2–65, 2–67, p. 84; right, Redrawn from Texhammar, R; Colton, C. AO/ASIF Instruments and Implants: A Technical Manual. New York, Springer Verlag, 1995. **B,** Redrawn from Muller, M.E.; Allgöwer, M.; Schneider, R.; Willenegger, H., eds. Manual of Internal Fixation, 3rd ed. New York, Springer Verlag, 1995. **C,** Redrawn from Texhammar, R; Colton, C. AO/ASIF Instruments and Implants: A Technical Manual. New York, Springer Verlag, 1995.)*

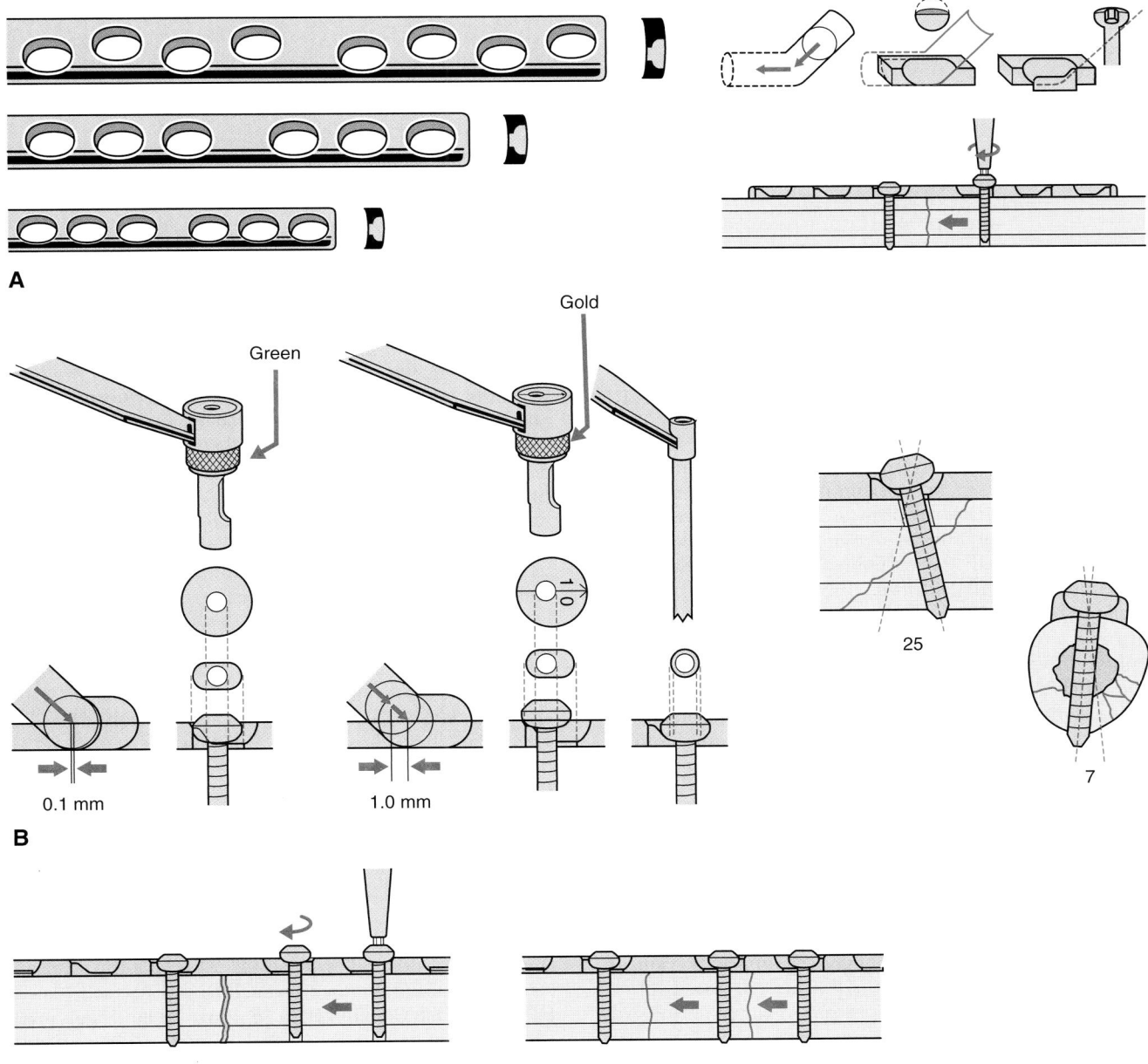

undersurface contact, which can lead to an interference with the periosteal blood supply (Fig. 4-26A). This effect is thought to be the main reason for plate-induced osteoporosis[33] and the possible danger that a sequestrum could form underneath the plate. Also, a soft spot in fracture healing can occur where the periosteal surface of the bone is in contact with the plate. This defect may act as a stress riser because it increases the mechanical stress locally; therefore, the possibility of refracture after plate removal is increased.[75]

Another shortcoming is that the design of the plate limits static compression to one site. This occurs because the orientation of the inclined planes within the screw holes points in one direction on either side of the plate center. The *plate center* is defined as a small area of the plate with no screw hole. These inclines oppose each other, so compression can occur only at a single site.

Because the plate is of uniform width, the holes produce areas of increased stress and decreased stiffness, causing uneven stiffness in the entire plate. With contouring, the plate bends preferentially through the holes rather than

with even distribution, further increasing stress at the screw holes and the risk of implant failure (see Fig. 4-26B).

LCDC PLATE The LCDC plate is a modification that attempts to correct some of the design shortcomings of the DC plate. Based on work by Klaue and Perren, there are three main differences in design.[51] First, the sides of the plate are inclined to form a trapezoidal cross section interrupted by undercuts that form arcs (Fig. 4-27A). This design reduces the area of contact between the plate and the periosteal surface of the bone, decreasing the disturbance of the blood supply and allowing for periosteal callus formation under the plate- decreasing stress concentration at an unhealed fracture gap.[75] Second, the screw hole is made up of two inclined and one horizontal cylinder; they meet at the same angle, permitting compression in both directions (see Fig. 4-27B). As a result, compression can be achieved at multiple sites between screw holes, which is of value in treating certain segmental and comminuted fractures. Third, because of the undercut design, the stiffness between screw holes is relatively similar to that across the screw holes. As a result, stress is more equally distributed, less deformation occurs at the screw holes when contouring, and fewer stress risers exist within the plate. The more uniform cross-sectional area along the plate decreases the amount of stress concentrated at the screw holes. The undercuts also allow for an increase to 40° of screw horizontal tilt. The biomechanical uses and applications of the LCDC plate are the same as those for the DC plate.

POINT CONTACT (SCHUHLI) DEVICES A Schuhli device consists of a three-pronged nut and a washer (Fig. 4-28). It functions to lock a cortical screw to a plate if pullout failure due to osteopenic bone is a concern, and to elevate the plate from the bone, decreasing periosteal blood flow compromise. It elevates the plate from the periosteal surface farther than the LCDC plate does. The nut engages the screw and locks it to the plate at a 90° angle, producing a fixed angle construct. This device has been shown to be effective in withstanding both axial and torsional loads to failure.[55] Matelic and associates[61] reported its use in treatment of femoral nonunions in which the lateral cortex of the femur was deficient.

SEMI-TUBULAR, ONE-THIRD TUBULAR, AND QUARTER-TUBULAR PLATES The semi-tubular plate was the first AO self-compression plate designed in the shape of a half-tube (Fig. 4-29). It provides compression through eccentrically placed oval plate holes. It maintains its rotational stability with edges that dig into the side of the periosteum under tension. The semi-tubular plate is 1 mm thick and very malleable, so it is prone to fatigue and fracture, especially in areas of high stress. Its main indication is for tension resistance, as in the treatment of open-book injury of the pelvis.[67] The one-third tubular plate is commonly used as a neutralization plate in the treatment of lateral malleolar fractures. The quarter-tubular plates have been used in small bone fixation (e.g., in hand surgery).

RECONSTRUCTION PLATE This plate is designed with notches in its side so that it can be contoured in any plane (Fig. 4-30). It is mainly used in fractures of

FIGURE 4-26 *Dynamic compression plate.* **A,** *Plate-induced osteoporosis is a temporary stage of intense remodeling and is related to vascular damage produced by both the injury and the presence of the implant.* **B,** *Since the plate is of uniform width, the holes produce areas of increased stress and decreased stiffness, causing uneven stiffness in the entire plate. With contouring, the plate bends preferentially through the holes rather than with an even distribution. This further increases stress at the screw hole and the risk of implant failure.* (**A,** *Redrawn from Texhammar, R.; Colton, C. AO/ASIF Instruments and Implants: A Technical Manual. New York, Springer Verlag, 1995.* **B,** *Reprinted from Perren, S.M. The concept of biological plating using the limited contact-dynamic compression plate [LCDCP]: Scientific background, design, and application. Injury 22[suppl 1]:1–41, 1991; with permission from Elsevier Science Ltd., The Boulevard, Langford Lane, Kidlington OX5 1GB, U.K.)*

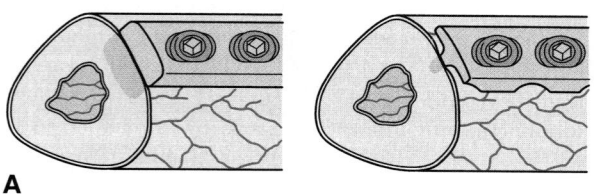

A

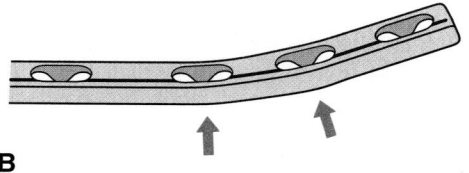

B

FIGURE 4-27 | *The limited contact-dynamic compression (LCDC) plate. **A,** The sides of the plate are inclined to form a trapezoidal cross section interrupted by undercuts that form arcs. **B,** In contrast to the DC plate, the LCDC plate's screw holes are designed with two horizontal cylinders that allow for compression in different directions along a single plate. (Redrawn from Muller, M.E.; Allgöwer, M.; Schneider, R.; Willenegger, H.; eds. Manual of Internal Fixation, 3rd ed. New York, Springer Verlag, 1995.)*

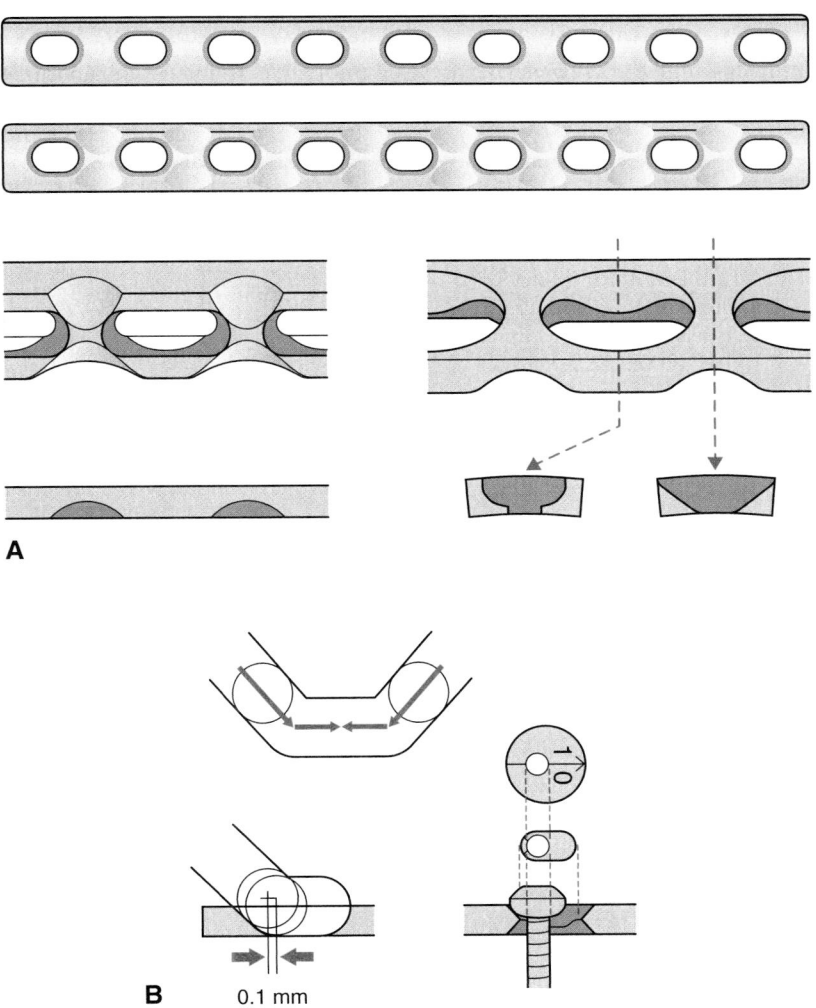

the pelvis, where precise contouring is important in reduction. It can also be used for fixation of distal humerus and calcaneal fractures. The plate has relatively low strength, which is further diminished with contouring. It offers some compression because of its oval screw holes.

ANGLED PLATES Angled plates were developed in the 1950s for the fixation of proximal and distal femur fractures. They are a one-piece design with a U-shaped profile for the blade portion and a 95° or 130° fixed angle between the blade and the plate. The shaft is thicker than

the blade and can withstand higher stress. This detail is important because the subtrochanteric region is the most highly stressed region of the skeleton, a fact that predisposes the region to fixation failure. The forces applied in this area exceed 1200 lb/in.[2], with the medial cortex exposed to compression combined with greater stress and the lateral cortex exposed to tension.[31]

The 130° Blade Plate
The 130° blade plate was originally designed for fixation of proximal femur fractures and has different lengths to

FIGURE 4-28 *The Schuhli device is a three-pronged nut and washer that locks in a cortical screw and elevates the plate from the bone. This not only facilitates periosteal blood flow but also creates a fixed angle construct. (Redrawn from Synthes, AO/ASIF Newsletter. Paoli, PA, Synthes USA, November 1996.)*

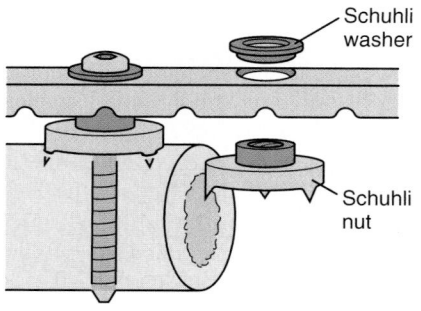

accommodate different fracture patterns. The 4- and 6-hole plates are used for fixation of intertrochanteric fractures, while the 9- to 12-hole plates are used for treatment of subtrochanteric fractures. The placement of the blade is critical; improper placement can lead to various healing deformities. In the femoral head, there is a zone where the tension and compression trabeculae intersect. The plate is inserted so it is below this trabecular intersection (6 to 8 mm above the calcar) and in the center of the neck, with no anterior or posterior angulation. The use of this device depends on the specific biomechanics and angulation of the fracture site. It has been replaced for the most part by the dynamic hip screw, which allows for compression of the fragments.

The 95° Condylar Blade Plate

The 95° condylar blade plate was designed for use with supracondylar and bicondylar distal femur fractures, and the length employed is also fracture specific (Fig. 4-31). It can be used for subtrochanteric fractures where more purchase on the fracture fragment can be gained with a sharper angled plate. With the 130° blade plate, the blade enters the proximal femoral fragment close to the subtrochanteric fracture site, precluding insertion of plate screws into the proximal fragment. In contrast, the blade of the 95° blade plate can be introduced into the proximal fragment just below the tip of the greater trochanter, allowing placement of screws proximal to the fracture site into the calcar for added stability. Although the device is strong and provides stable fixation, its insertion is technically demanding. The need for precise alignment in all three planes demands careful preoperative planning and intraoperative radiographic control.

SLIDING SCREW AND COMPRESSION PLATES

Compression/Telescoping Hip Screw

The compression/telescoping or sliding hip screw system is designed for internal fixation of basicervical, intertrochanteric, and selected subtrochanteric fractures.[24,30,42,44,85] It uses the principle of dynamic compression, which modifies functional physiologic forces into compression at the fracture site. The implant consists of two major parts: a wide-diameter cannulated lag screw that is inserted into the femoral head and a

FIGURE 4-29 *Examples of semi-tubular (A), one-third tubular (B, C), and one-quarter tubular (D) plates. (Redrawn from Muller, M.E.; Allgöwer, M.; Schneider, R.; Willenegger, H.; eds. Manual of Internal Fixation, 3rd ed. New York, Springer Verlag, 1995.)*

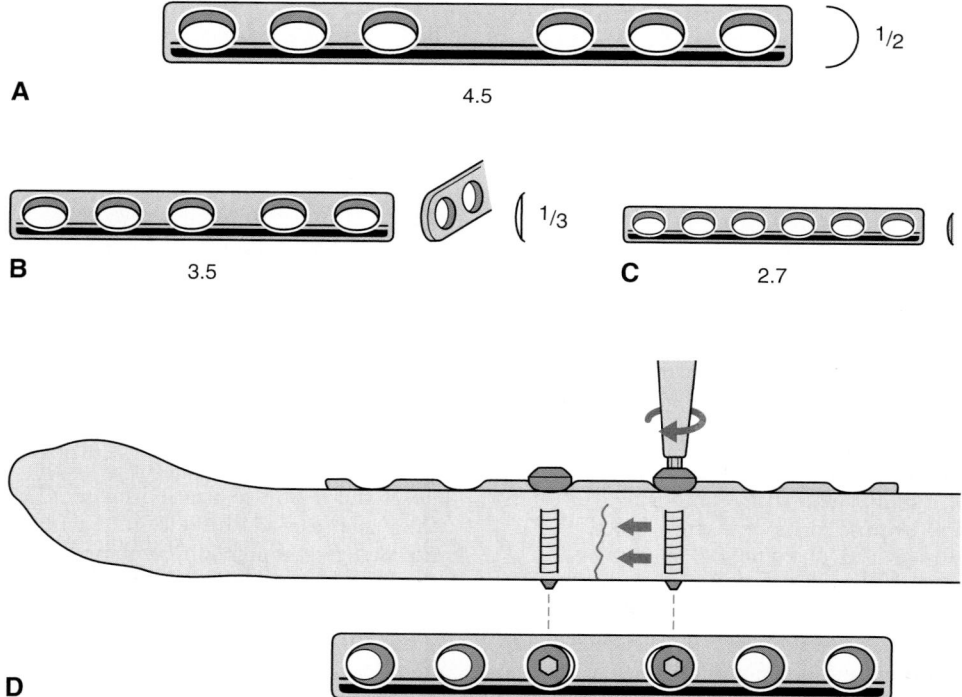

FIGURE 4-30   ***A,*** *Examples of reconstruction plates. Note that the notches in the sides are placed there so the plates can be contoured in all dimensions.* ***B,*** *Reconstruction plate for fixation of a posterior wall acetabular fracture. (Redrawn from Muller, M.E.; Allgöwer, M.; Schneider, R.; Willenegger, H., eds. Manual of Internal Fixation, 3rd ed. New York, Springer Verlag, 1995.)*

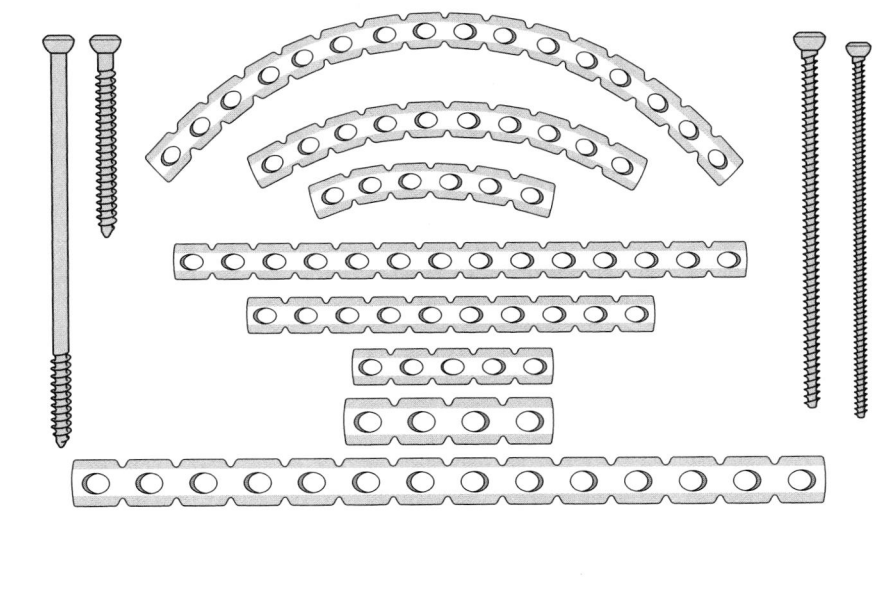

A

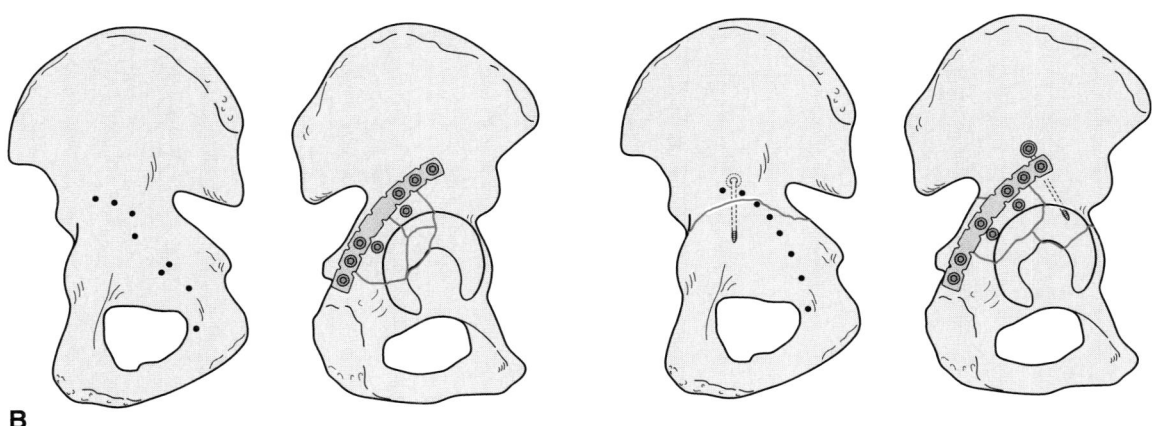

B

side plate with a barrel at a set angle that is attached to the femoral shaft (Fig. 4-32). Weight-bearing and abductor muscle activity cause the screw shaft to slide through the barrel, resulting in impaction of the fracture surfaces and, optimally, a stable load-sharing construct.

Two basic principles must be recognized when using a sliding hip screw. The first is that fracture compression can occur only if the lag screw and barrel are inserted across the fracture site. This occurs when a sliding hip screw is used to fix a fracture at the base of the femoral neck or in the intertrochanteric area. In contrast, when a sliding hip screw is used to fix a high subtrochanteric fracture, the lag screw and barrel are located exclusively in the proximal fragment and do not cross the fracture site. In these circumstances, the lag screw acts only as a fixation device and does not contribute to fracture compression by sliding.

The second principle is that the lag screw must slide far enough through the barrel to allow the fracture gap to

close sufficiently for the proximal and distal fragments to impact completely. Sliding does not occur as desired if the bending forces (from weight-bearing and muscle contraction) on the lag screw cause it to impinge and bind. The lag screw slides more predictably through a longer barrel because it provides more support. Some sliding hip screw systems include two side plates, with one long and one short barrel. Usually, the long barrel is chosen to ensure adequate support and unimpeded lag screw sliding. Lag screws are available in varying lengths (60 to 120 mm) to accommodate patient anatomy and fracture configuration. If a lag screw of 80 mm or smaller is used, there may not be enough space between the base of the threads on the screw and the tip of the long barrel to allow full impaction of the fracture. In this small proportion of cases, the short-barrel side plate should be used. Some of these systems are slotted and provide rotational control as a result. However, the fragment still may rotate around the screw itself despite implant geometry. Various

FIGURE 4-31   *The 95° blade plate. **A,** T profile. **B,** U profile. **C,** Use of a blade plate in proximal femoral fixation, as for subtrochanteric fractures. Note placement of the tip of the blade at the intersection of the primary compressive and the primary tensile trabeculae. (**A** and **B,** Redrawn from Synthes Equipment Ordering Manual. Paoli, PA, Synthes USA, 1992.)*

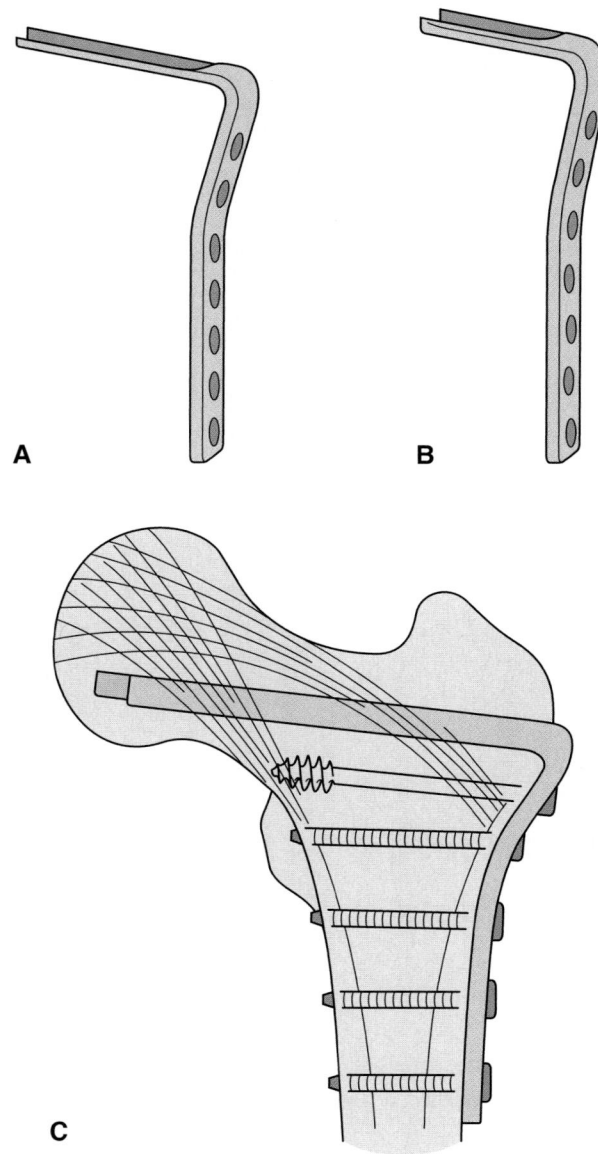

manufacturers produce systems containing a range of side plate-lag screw angles; the angle used depends on the fracture configuration and the patient's anatomy. The basic principle of these devices is that they collapse and shorten to accommodate comminution, osteopenia, and bone lysis at the fracture site.

Dynamic Condylar Screw

The condylar compression screw system has basically the same design as the 95° condylar blade plate except that the blade is replaced by a cannulated screw (Fig. 4-33). The angle between screw and plate is fixed at 95°, in contrast to the sliding hip screw, which allows different angles to be selected. The compression generated by the large

cannulated screw placed across the femoral condyles permits greater compression of the fracture fragments than can be achieved with a blade plate. The plate is contoured to fit the distal end of the femur. It is a two-piece device that can allow for some correction in the lateral and coronal planes after the lag screw is inserted, unlike a blade plate. This system is used for fixation of low, supracondylar, and intercondylar T- and Y-fractures.

Precise positioning of the implants is critical for fixation and proper alignment. If the screw is inserted in a valgus position (angled away from the midline), a varus deformity will develop on healing. Conversely, if the plate is angled in varus (toward the midline), a valgus deformity will develop. The screw systems allow for some correction

FIGURE 4-32 *Dynamic compression-sliding hip screw. Functional loading of a sliding hip screw causes dynamic compression at the fracture site. With functional loading, the screw slides through the barrel of the side plate, allowing the fracture to impact or compress. Note placement of the cannulated screw in the inferior third of the femoral neck.*

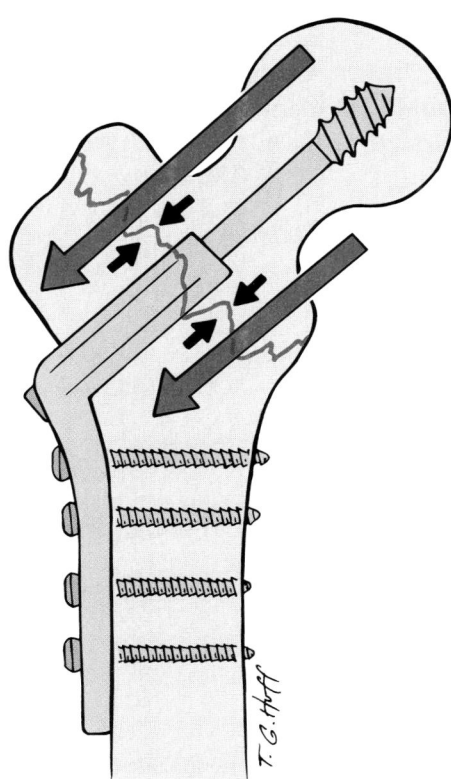

of alignment, whereas blade plates do not, and, correspondingly, are technically more forgiving.

PLATE FAILURE

Internal fixation is frequently viewed as a race between fracture healing and implant failure. This paradigm is especially true when a fracture is fixed with a plate and there is a cortical gap opposite the plate. When the bone-implant complex is loaded by physiologic muscle forces and weight-bearing, repetitive opening and closing of the gap can occur, subjecting the plate to cyclical bending stresses. The longer this process continues, the greater the chance that the plate will fail. This cyclical bending of the plate continues until the gap on the opposite cortex is bridged with callus. If the cyclical bending continues long enough, the fatigue limit will be exceeded and the plate will break. Healing of the fracture on the side opposite the plate can be impaired if the bone fragments are devascularized by the injury or during surgery. Fracture healing in the gap can be optimized by protection of remaining periosteal blood supply and addition of bone graft or other inductive substances. Bone grafts speed healing in the gap, compared with unassisted callus formation. Biologically,

bone graft is osteoconductive and osteoinductive; it both provides support for bone formation and brings potential osteogenic cells and growth factors to the site. Cancellous bone has more osteoblastic cells and loose-knit trabeculae, giving it the potential for a remodeling rate three times faster than that of cortical grafts, and is generally revascularized within 7 days.[32,84] Persistent micromotion and cyclical implant loading in the absence of fracture union ultimately lead to failure of any implant regardless of its size and strength.

Summary

The basic biomechanical functions of plates in fracture fixation have been discussed, as well as some of the major plate designs and examples of plates modified for use in specific anatomic areas. It is important to realize that specific design features of plates can be used to fulfill biomechanical needs based on the particularities of the fracture. Research in this area continues to improve fracture fixation techniques and instrumentation.

Intramedullary Nails

Intramedullary nails are internal fixation devices designed for use in bridging or splinting of fractures of long bones (e.g., femur, tibia, humerus). In contrast to plates and screws, which are placed on the cortical surface, these devices are placed within the medullary canal.

CONFIGURATION

The basic configuration of an intramedullary nail is depicted in Figure 4-34. Nails are constructed of various metal alloys, and are described by their outer diameter and their overall length. By definition, cannulated nails are hollow to allow them to be placed using a guide wire.

BIOMECHANICS OF INTRAMEDULLARY NAILS

Rigidity and strength are the most important characteristics of an intramedullary nailing system. The nail's geometry is responsible for its strength, rigidity, and interaction with the bone. Four main shape characteristics are commonly evaluated, each of which has two main categories. An understanding of these basic features is necessary when evaluating any intramedullary nailing system.

LONGITUDINAL CURVATURE Long bones have variable amounts of anatomic curvature. Early intramedullary nails were straight, and as a result, there was a significant mismatch between these straight implants and the normal curve of the femur. Insertion of straight nails was possible only with the use of rigid shaft reamers and small-diameter implants. Also, the anatomic bow of the intact femur was reduced by breaking it into two or more fragments, thus creating a straighter path for the nail. The introduction of the curved anterior bow on the femoral nails and the associated use of flexible shaft reamers permitted a better fit with the normal anatomy of the femur. These reamers reduced the amount of bone that had to be removed and simplified implant insertion. However, most modern femoral intramedullary nails are designed with a curvature that is less than the curvature of the average femur. This results in a slight mismatch, which actually improves frictional fixation.

FIGURE 4-33 *Dynamic condylar screw (DCS).* **A,** *Basic components of the DCS system.* **B,** *Here the DCS is used to generate compression of a T-type supracondylar fracture of the distal femur. Note the anatomic fit to the lateral femoral cortex. (Redrawn from DHS/DCS Dynamic Hip and Condylar Screw System: Technique Guide. Paoli, PA, Synthes USA, 1990.)*

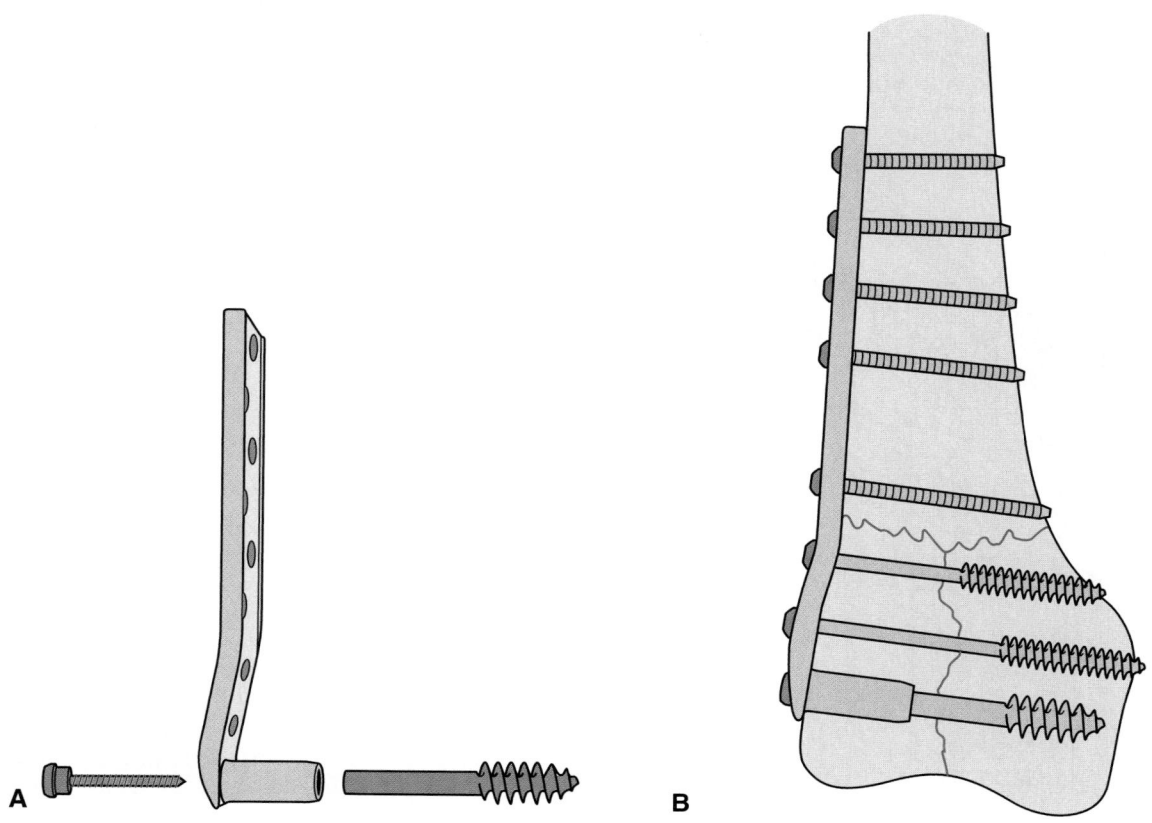

Translation, rotation, and angulation of fracture fragments are partially controlled by frictional contact between bone and nail at a number of locations, including the entry portal, the endosteal surface of the diaphysis, and the cancellous

FIGURE 4-34 *Basic configuration of an intramedullary nail. The proximal end has an internally threaded opening for adaptation of driver/extractor instrumentation. It has a longitudinal bow that approximates that of the femur. Proximal and distal screw holes are placed in the nail for interlocking fixation.*

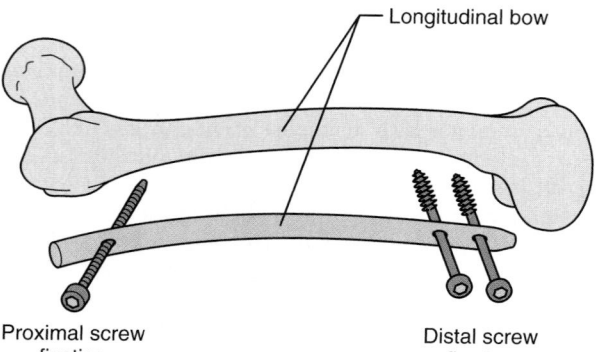

Longitudinal bow

Proximal screw fixation

Distal screw fixation

bone at the tip of the nail. Frictional stability is of greater importance in a nonlocked nail than in a locked nail.

CROSS-SECTIONAL SHAPE The early intramedullary nails developed by Küntscher had a V-shaped cross-section, which allowed the sides of the nail to compress and fit tightly in the canal. The design was modified to a cloverleaf shape with a longitudinal slot running the length of the implant to increase the strength of the nail and permit insertion over a guide wire (Fig. 4-35A). As with the V-design, the two halves of the cloverleaf are compressed into the slot as the nail is driven into the medullary canal. Because the amount of compression is within the elastic zone of the nail, the nail springs open and presses on the endosteal surface, increasing the frictional contact in the medullary canal (see Fig. 4-35B). Conversely, having a slot running down the nail decreases the nail's torsional rigidity.[81] When the nail-bone complex is loaded, the decreased torsional rigidity permits a small amount of motion, which promotes callus formation. The decreased torsional rigidity also allows the nail to accommodate to the bone and is therefore said to be more forgiving. If the nail does not match the shape of the medullary canal exactly, an accommodative will decrease the likelihood of iatrogenic fracture. If the nail is too stiff and does not deform on insertion, the bone can shatter. The cloverleaf shape has been used extensively for decades with great

FIGURE 4-35 | *Geometric features of an intramedullary nail that influence its performance.* **A,** *Note the cloverleaf, fluted, solid, and open designs. All these examples have the same diameter but different wall thicknesses.* **B,** *Similar to the way a nail achieves fixation in wood through elastic compression of the wood, the cloverleaf Küntscher nail achieves fixation in the isthmus through the elastic expansion of the compressed nail. (**A,** Redrawn from Bechtold, J.E.; Kaayle, R.F.; Perren, S.M. In: Browner, B.D.; Edwards, C.C.; eds. The Science and Practice of Intramedullary Nailing, 2nd ed. Baltimore, Williams & Wilkins, 1996.* **B,** *Redrawn from Street, D.M. In: Browner, B.D.; Edwards, C.C., eds. The Science and Practice of Intramedullary Nailing, 2nd ed. Baltimore, Williams & Wilkins, 1996.)*

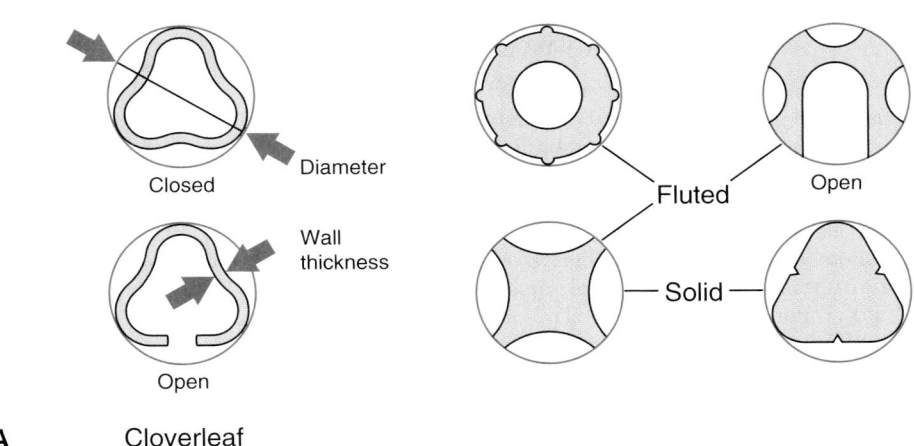

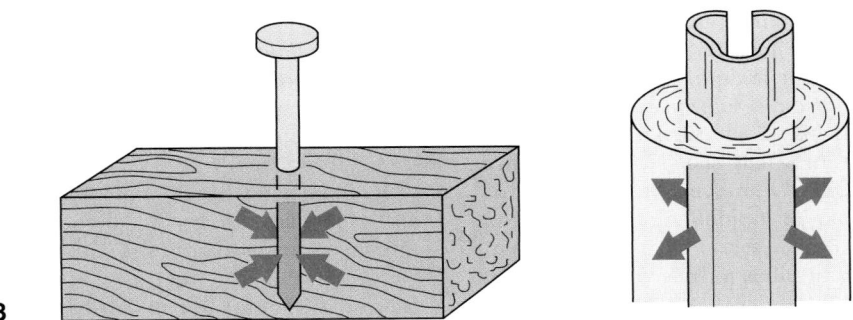

success. The design has been successful because it has adequate torsional rigidity to permit fracture union but sufficient elasticity to adapt to bone anatomy on insertion.

In contrast to the slotted cloverleaf shape, nails have been designed with no slots and a variety of other cross-sectional shapes. Removal of the slot significantly increases the torsional rigidity of the nail. This design is desirable when a small-diameter nail is used. Small nails are used when the medullary canal is small or its enlargement is contraindicated. Closed-section locking nails were designed for the femur to avoid excessive torsional deformation of the nail on insertion, which complicated distal screw fixation. The torsional stiffness of any implant can be increased substantially by the addition of spines that run the entire length of the nail. The curved indentation in the surface of the nail between the spines is called a *flute*. The edges of the spines can be designed to cut into the bone, increasing frictional resistance at the nail-bone interface. However, this contact can increase the difficulty of implant removal.

The medullary blood supply of a long bone is destroyed by reaming and the insertion of a canal-filling implant. However, the medullary blood supply reconstitutes rapidly if some space is allotted between the implant and the endosteal surface. The cloverleaf and fluted designs both provide the space critical for revascularization.

DIAMETER The medullary canals of long bones have a narrow central region called the *isthmus*. Before reaming was developed, the diameter of intramedullary nails was limited to the narrowest diameter of the medullary cavity at the isthmus (Fig. 4-36). With reaming, larger implants can be introduced and, when compared to nails with a smaller diameter, large-diameter nails with the same cross-sectional shape are stiffer and stronger. In practice, the relationship between diameter and strength is not linear. The nail stiffness can be kept constant by changing the wall thickness. For example, a 12-mm diameter nail

FIGURE 4-36   *The effect of reaming on cortical contact area.* **A,** *The isthmus is the narrowest portion of the intramedullary canal of the femur. Without reaming, the isthmus limits the size of the nail to be placed and the area of cortical contact with the nail.* **B,** *Reaming widens and lengthens the isthmic portion of the intramedullary canal.* **C,** *After reaming, a larger diameter nail may be placed and greater cortical contact area achieved.*

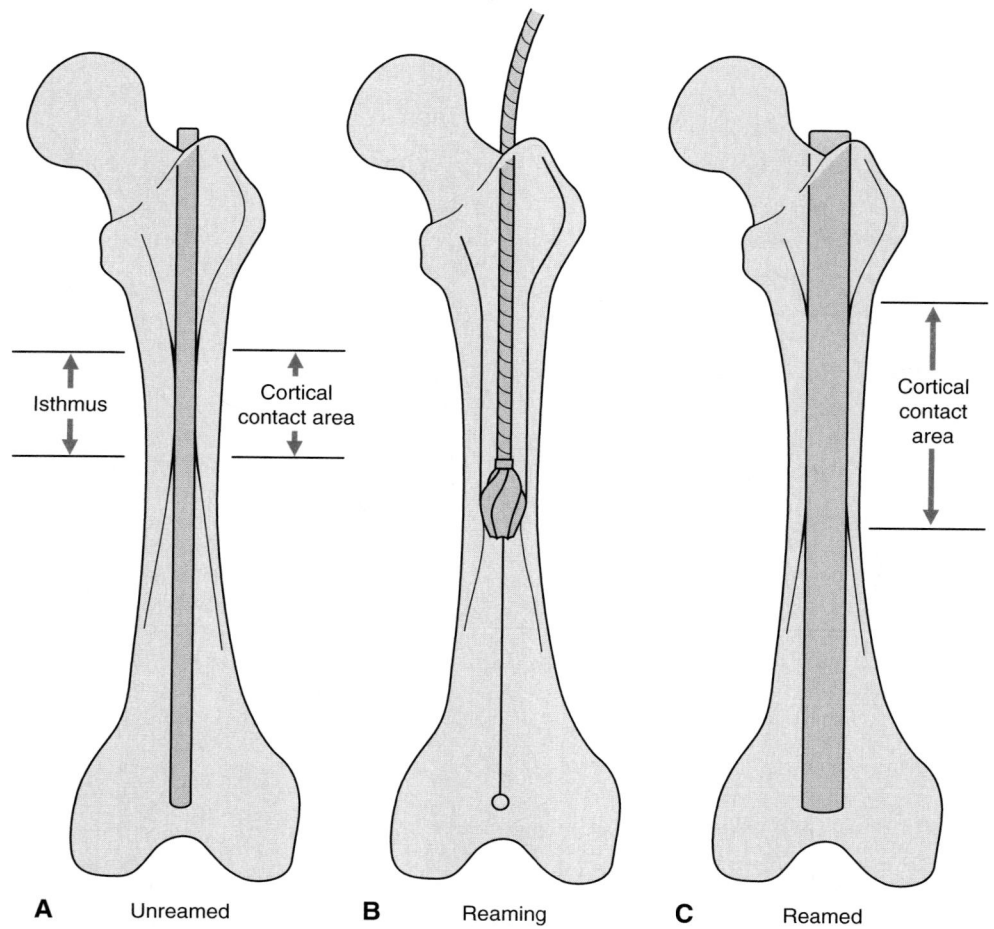

Isthmus	Cortical contact area		Cortical contact area
A Unreamed	**B** Reaming		**C** Reamed

has a wall thickness of 1.2 mm while for 14- and 16-mm nails it is decreased to 1.0 mm.

CANNULATION   The final nail construction characteristic is the core geometry. A hollow-core, or cannulated, nail allows insertion of the nail over a guide wire. In general, a curved-tip guide wire can be maneuvered across a displaced fracture site more easily than a solid intramedullary nail. Another advantage of the cannulated nail may be a reduction in intramedullary pressure. Haas and co-workers found a 42 percent increase in compartment pressures when introducing a solid nail, compared with 1.6 percent for a cannulated nail.[35] The clinical significance of this difference has yet to be determined.

Flexural Rigidity

The cross-sectional shape, diameter, and material of the nail all influence its flexural rigidity. Flexural rigidity is defined as the cross-sectional moment of inertia (CSMI) multiplied by the elastic modulus. The CSMI describes the distribution of the cross-sectional area with respect to the central axis. The elastic modulus is a reflection of the inherent material properties. The moment-of-inertia

geometry differentiates nails with the same outside diameter and shape. Tencer and colleagues reported that nails can differ in bending rigidity by a factor of two and in torsional rigidity by a factor of three based on their different moments of inertia.[89] A basic understanding of the characteristics of intramedullary nails is essential for effective evaluation of different implant systems.

Working Length

Bone healing after intramedullary nailing will occur if the motion at the fracture site falls within an acceptable range. The exact specifications of this motion are not known, but it has been observed that small amounts of motion promote callus formation while excessive motion delays union. Fracture motion results from loading in bending and torsion. The amount of motion that occurs at the fracture site is described in part by the concept of working length. The working length is the portion of the nail that is unsupported by bone under forces of bending or torsion (Fig. 4-37).

The unsupported length of nail differs in bending and in torsion.[21,87] In bending, the major bone fragments come

FIGURE 4-37 *Working length (WL). WL describes the length of the nail that is unsupported by bone when loaded. This unsupported length differs based on the mode of testing.* **A,** *In compression, WL is the distance between the intact proximal and the intact distal fragments, spanning the comminuted section of the fracture.* **B,** *In bending, the proximal and distal portions of the main bone fragments come into contact with the nail. Therefore, WL is the maximal distance between the sites at which the nail is in contact with the bone proximally and distally, which can be equal to the length of the fracture gap.* **C,** *When comminution exists, the main bone fragments do not resist torsion. In this situation, WL is the distance between the proximal and the distal locking points. Torsional rigidity is inversely proportional to WL, whereas rigidity in bending is inversely proportional to the square of WL. (Redrawn from Browner, B.; Cole, J.D. Current status of locked intramedullary nailing: a review. J Orthop Trauma 1[2]:186, 1987.)*

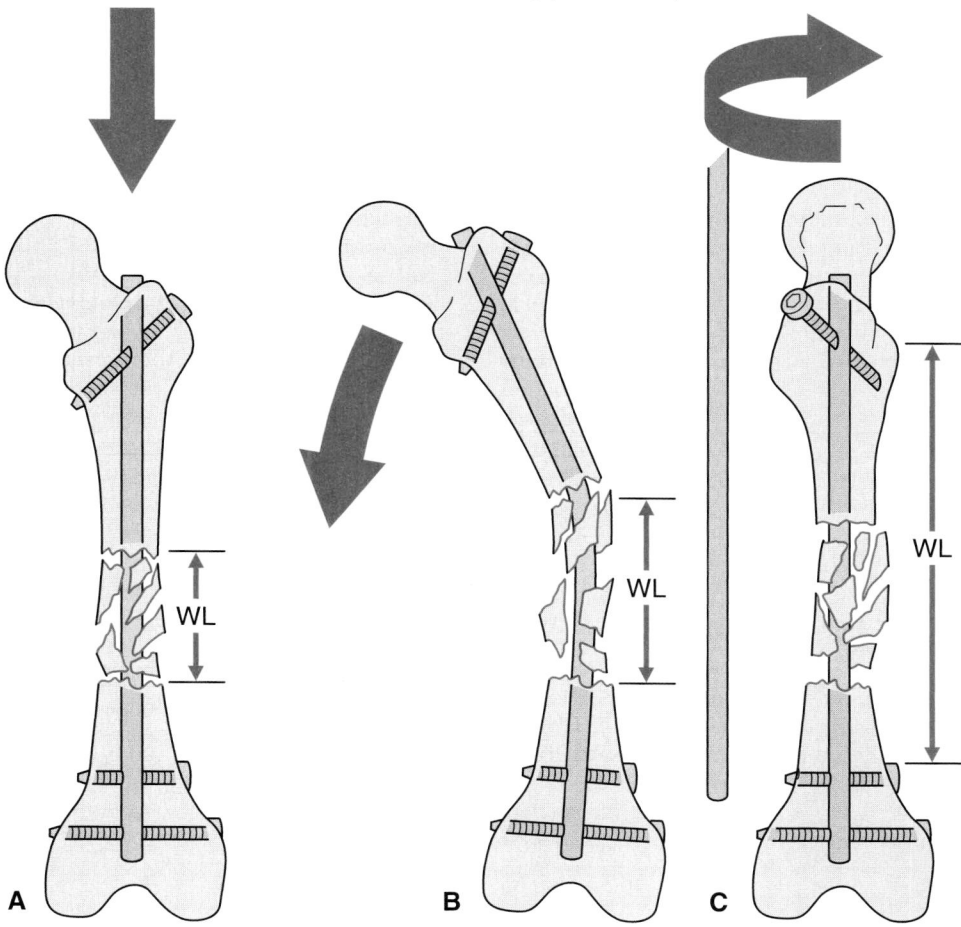

into contact with the nail, and therefore the unsupported length is the distance between the proximal and the distal fracture fragments, the fracture gap or comminution. In other words, it is the portion of the fixation that is not supported by bone, where the nail can bend independently. As the bone heals, this distance decreases. In torsion, the major bone fragments do not stabilize the nail. Because reamed nails are inserted with space between the implant and the endosteal surface, there is limited frictional contact between the nail and the bone. As a result, the locking screws are the primary restraint to torsion, and the unsupported length in torsion extends the full distance between the two locking screws. Because the working length in torsion is the distance between the proximal and the distal points of fixation, it is always greater than the working length in bending.

From the four-point bending equation, interfragmentary motion in bending is proportional to the square of the working length (see Fig. 3-7), and increases in bending working length significantly increase the likelihood of delayed healing. For locked nails, interfragmentary motion in torsion is directly proportional to working length as defined by the torsional load equation (see Fig. 3-8). In an unlocked nail, torsional motion is dependent on friction at the nail-bone interface. Unlocked nails do not significantly resist torsion and are generally not used for comminuted or rotationally unstable fractures.

There are many different designs and types of intramedullary nails. The following sections describe the basic applications of intramedullary nailing.

INTRAMEDULLARY REAMING

Küntscher initially attempted intramedullary fixation of fractures with implants that were designed to fit within the normal medullary canal. Dissatisfied with the high rates of malunion, nonunion, and implant failure obtained with these small-diameter nails, he developed the technique of reaming to enlarge the intramedullary canal.[45] This method produced a more uniform canal diameter and increased the potential surface area for contact between the implant and the endosteum. Increased contact facilitated better alignment of the fracture fragments and enhanced the rotational stability of fracture fixation. Additionally, larger canal diameters permitted insertion of larger nails with greater stiffness and fatigue strength. The successful use of larger diameter intramedullary nails paved the way for the production of nails containing holes through which transfixion screws could be inserted.

To enlarge the medullary canal, reamers are passed within the bone. They were developed for industry to precisely size and finish an already existing hole without removing large amounts of material. They have a larger caliber than drill bits because their main purpose is to enlarge an already existing hole. Reamers are designed to be end cutting, side cutting, or both (Fig. 4-38). The tip design of most reamers is a truncated cone called a *chamfer*. The *chamfer angle* is the angle between the central axis of the reamer and the cutting edge at its end. With end-cutting reamers, the majority of the cutting is accomplished by the chamfer. Additional flutes are added along the sides of the reamer to increase the cutting surface and distribute the force more evenly. If additional relief or angle is added to the land (the area between the flutes), it provides for a longitudinal cutting edge. This change permits an increase in accuracy but weakens the cutting edge. If cutting is performed primarily by the longitudinal edges, the reamer is said to be side cutting. Generally, end-cutting reamers are used only for the initial passes. An end-cutting reamer has the potential to cut eccentrically when reaming across displaced fractures because it cuts its own path (Fig. 4-39). Most reamers used for orthopaedic applications are side cutting.

The process of reaming is relatively straightforward. A small-diameter reamer head is selected, and then heads of gradually increasing size are used until the desired medullary canal diameter is reached. The reamer's speed of rotation is usually two thirds of the speed used for drilling. *Chatter* is uneven cutting that causes vibration of the reamer head, which can lead to reamer dullness or damage. Chatter is reduced with slower rotational speeds. Reamers

FIGURE 4-38 *Reamers. **A,** Note the starting taper of the front-cutting reamer used to initiate a path in bone. **B,** The side-cutting reamers have a sharper chamfer angle and a shorter chamfer length and therefore are used for increasing the size of the path, not for creating a new path. **C,** A combination front- and side-cutting reamer. **D,** A front-cutting reamer tip attached to a flexible shaft. (**A–C,** Redrawn from Donaldson, C.; Le Cain, G.H., eds. Tool Design, 3rd ed. New York, McGraw-Hill, 1973. With permission. **D,** Reproduced with permission from Zimmer, Inc., Warsaw, IN.)*

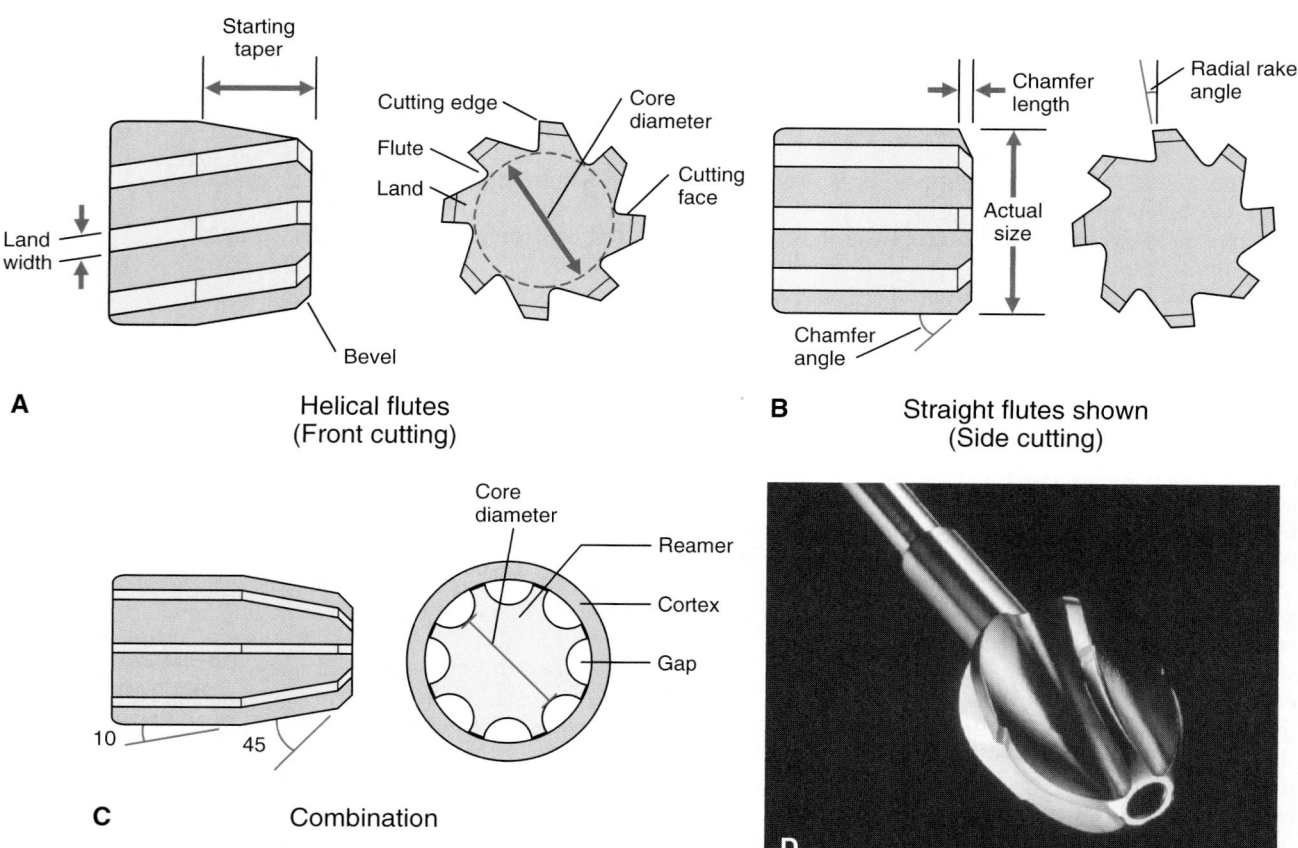

FIGURE 4-39 *Example of a front-cutting reamer.* **A,** *Eccentric reaming of distal fragment resulting from poor guide pin placement.* **B,** *Splitting of the cortex may follow nail impaction.* **C,** *Central placement of the guide pin using a small (90 mm) Küntscher nail avoids this problem. (Redrawn from Crenshaw, A.H., ed. Campbell's Operative Orthopaedics, 8th ed. St. Louis, Mosby-Year Book, 1992; redrawn from Rascher, J.J.; Nahigian, S. H.; Macys, J.R.; Brown, J.E. J Bone Joint Surg Am 54:534, 1972.)*

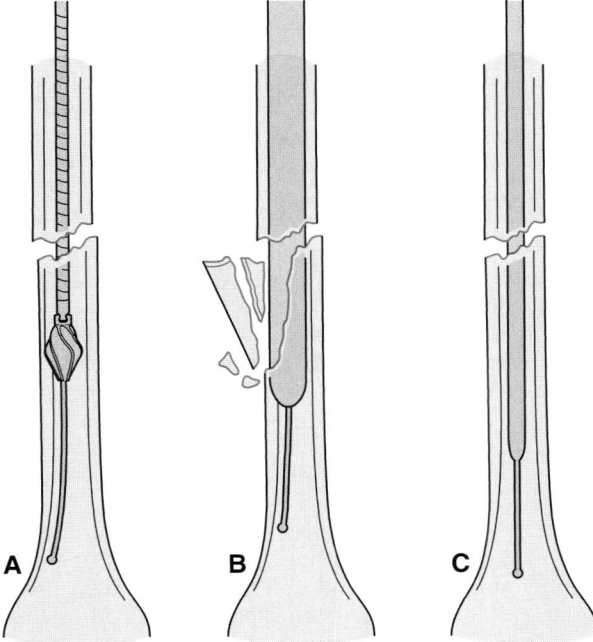

used for orthopaedic applications are of variable design; manufacturers attempt to maximize size and strength of reamers while minimizing physiologic damage.

The process of reaming causes an increase in medullary pressure and an elevation in cortical temperature. The former has been linked to an increase in extruded marrow products and the latter to cortical and medullary vascular damage. Design modifications can decrease the amount of physiologic stress sustained. Three main parts of a reamer apparatus influence the amounts of pressure and temperature generated: the reamer head, which is responsible for the actual cutting; the reamer shaft, which is usually flexible and drives the reamer head; and the bulb tip, which is the diameter inside the reamer head connection to the shaft. These components require space in the medullary canal and form a gap with the endosteal cortex. The reamer system acts like a piston and increases pressure in the relatively closed environment of a long bone. The amount of gap or space through which exhaust passes influences the build-up of medullary pressure. This concept has been quantified by a formula modified by Brown and Winquist[10]:

$$\Delta P = 3\mu \times Dm \times Vo/h^3$$

where ΔP is the change in medullary pressure; μ is the viscosity of the fluid or substance that is being reamed (it usually is highest on the initial reaming pass and thereafter reduced by bleeding in the canal); Dm is the midflute-to-midflute distance, which is influenced by the design of the reamer and the flute depth; Vo is the velocity of advancement, which is influenced by the speed of rotation (faster rotation allows for quicker cutting and faster advancement but causes increased intramedullary pressure; proper reaming procedure is slow advancement of the reamer with frequent pullback to clear debris); and h^3 is the flute depth, which is critical in determining the increase in intramedullary pressure. The flute allows for passage, or exhaust, of pressure behind the reamer head as it collects and clears the bone. The deeper the flute, the lower the pressure generated. This formula can be applied to both the shaft and the bulb tip. If the reamer head has shallow flutes, then the shaft takes on greater importance in increasing intramedullary pressure. Conversely, a large-diameter bulb decreases the intramedullary pressure.

Temperature increases during reaming have been reported to occur in stepwise increments with the successive use of larger diameter reamers. It was also reported that blunt reamers produce significantly greater temperature increases than sharp reamers do.[67] Several factors contribute to the elevation in bone temperature, including the presence or absence of flutes in the reamer head. Deep flutes that clear large amounts of bone attenuate the rise in bone temperature, whereas reamers with shallow or no flutes lead to greater increases in temperature. Sharp cutting edges and slow advancement of the reamer head decrease the rise in temperature. Blood flow to the area reduces the overall temperature increase through conductive heat transfer.

Reamer heads are constructed of 455 stainless steel, which is harder than 316L stainless steel, in an attempt to keep the cutting edge sharp longer. This class of stainless steel has increased corrosive properties, so most reamer heads are coated. However, the coating dulls the edge slightly but prolongs reamer head life. Coatings are made of titanium nitride (gold color), diamond black, and ME-92. The overall clinical significance of reamer design is still being investigated, but a basic understanding of the principles is important in evaluating these tools.

Destruction of the medullary contents by reaming has both local and systemic consequences. Reaming obliterates the remaining medullary blood supply after injury. This vascular system reconstitutes in 2 to 3 weeks.[79] Disruption of the medullary blood supply and intracortical intravasation of medullary fat during reaming result in necrosis of a variable amount of endosteal bone. If the medullary canal becomes infected before the bone is revascularized, the entire area of dead bone can become involved and act as a sequestrum in continuity. The long bones of adults contain primarily fatty marrow, with a large reserve of hematopoietic tissue in the marrow cavities of flat bones. Therefore, destruction of marrow during reaming does not produce anemia. During medullary reaming, a communication is temporarily created between the marrow cavity and the intravascular space. Use of reamers in the medullary space is somewhat like the insertion of a piston into a rigid cylinder. Exceedingly high canal pressures during medullary broaching before insertion of a femoral total hip component have been found in animals and humans.[69] Unlike the total joint broach, the medullary reamers used to prepare the canal before nail insertion are cannulated. This difference may offer some decompression of the pressure in the distal canal, but the communication is partially occluded by the guide wire and the pressurized marrow contents. Sampling of femoral vein blood during intramedullary reaming of the femur reveals embolization of fat and tissue thromboplastin. In the early days of reamed intramedullary nailing, there was great concern regarding the danger of death from fat embolization syndrome and shock. Although reamed nailing does result in embolization of marrow contents into the pulmonary circulation, this process is well tolerated if the patient has had adequate fluid resuscitation and receives appropriate hemodynamic and ventilatory support during surgery.[69]

In addition to obliterating the soft tissue in the marrow space, reaming shaves cancellous and cortical bone from the inner aspect of the cortex. This mixture of finely morcellized bone and marrow elements has excellent osteoinductive and osteoconductive potential. The rich osseous autograft is delivered by the increased interosseous pressure and by mechanical action of the reamer directly into the fracture site. In the open nailing technique, this material is exuded during reaming, but it can be collected and applied to the surface of the bone at the fracture site after the wound is irrigated, but before wound closure.

TYPES OF INTRAMEDULLARY NAILS

UNLOCKED INTRAMEDULLARY NAILS Unlocked or first-generation nails consist of intramedullary implants that are not rigidly stabilized with screw or pin fixation. This type of fixation is termed *splintage* and is defined as a construct that allows sliding of the implant-bone interface. The implant assists fracture healing by supporting bending while allowing axial loads to be transmitted to the surrounding bone. In this mode, the nail cannot control axial or rotational loading and is sometimes referred to as a *flexible gliding implant*. This type of fixation is indicated if the reduced fracture has inherent stability and will not twist or shorten when loaded.

LOCKING INTRAMEDULLARY NAILS The first locking intramedullary nail was developed by Modny in 1952.[66] This nail had an X-beam design and contained a regularly spaced series of holes that passed through the axilla of the beam on all four sides, allowing screws to be introduced from any direction. Because the holes were placed close together and had a larger diameter than the screws, they could be located with the drill without the use of a target device. The nail was straight and noncannulated and, therefore, was not suited to the closed nailing technique; it was better inserted after open reduction. Although this design was copied by other developers, locking nails did not gain widespread acceptance until Klemm and Schellman perfected a locking nail based on the cloverleaf Küntscher nail.[54] This implant was cannulated, was curved, and had a tapered tip, allowing for insertion with the closed nailing technique. Holes for transfixion screws were placed in the extreme ends of the

nail, minimizing the invasion of the fracture zone and increasing the range of fractures that could be stabilized with this device. Subsequent versions of this type of cannulated locking nail contained a cylindrical proximal end with an internally threaded core to allow firmer attachment of the driver, extractor, and proximal target device. Other minor changes were made in the location and orientation of the screw holes. These nailing systems have now been used successfully to stabilize comminuted and rotationally unstable fractures of the femur and tibia.[12,25,43,46,47,53,90,97,99,101]

SECOND-GENERATION LOCKING NAILS Standard first-generation locking nails have been very effective for the stabilization of comminuted fractures of the femoral shaft extending from 1 cm below the lesser trochanter to 10 cm above the articular surface of the knee. Because of the high stresses seen in trochanteric fractures and the proximal location of many pertrochanteric fracture lines, these nails have not provided ideal stabilization for fractures above the lesser trochanter. Most of these nails contain a proximal diagonal screw that is normally inserted in a downward and medial direction. Use of the nail intended for the opposite side allows the screw to be inserted up into the femoral head and neck. The strength of these implants is still not adequate to provide secure, lasting fixation for subtrochanteric fractures, and because the proximal screw is threaded into the nail, no gliding of the screw can occur. This design prevents impaction of bone fragments of intertrochanteric and femoral neck fractures. To overcome these problems, a second generation of locking nail was developed (Fig. 4-40). These nails have an expanded proximal end that contains two tunnels for large-diameter, smooth-shank lag screws. The increase in proximal nail diameter and wall thickness combined with the screw design provides greater fixation and strength for subtrochanteric fractures. The combination of sliding proximal lag screws and distal transfixion screws allows excellent fixation of ipsilateral femoral neck or intertrochanteric fractures and comminuted fractures of the shaft.

TECHNIQUES

To this point, the chapter has dealt with fundamental principles of metallurgy and hardware. The following sections describe the application of metallurgy and hardware to the basic techniques of internal fixation.

Basic Modes of Internal Fixation

Internal fixation has three basic modes: interfragmentary compression, splintage, and bridging. Mechanical characteristics of the bone implant fixation construct vary depending on the consistency of bone, the fracture pattern and location, the specific implant, and the mode of application. The advantages of mechanical stability of the final construct must be balanced against the detrimental surgical trauma associated with fracture reduction and implant insertion. Maintenance of sufficient blood flow to injured soft tissue and bone is essential to avoid infection and facilitate the healing process. Internal fixation also must be applied in a way that provides the desired anatomic reconstruction with adequate mobilization to reduce pain and permit full activity while facilitating fracture union

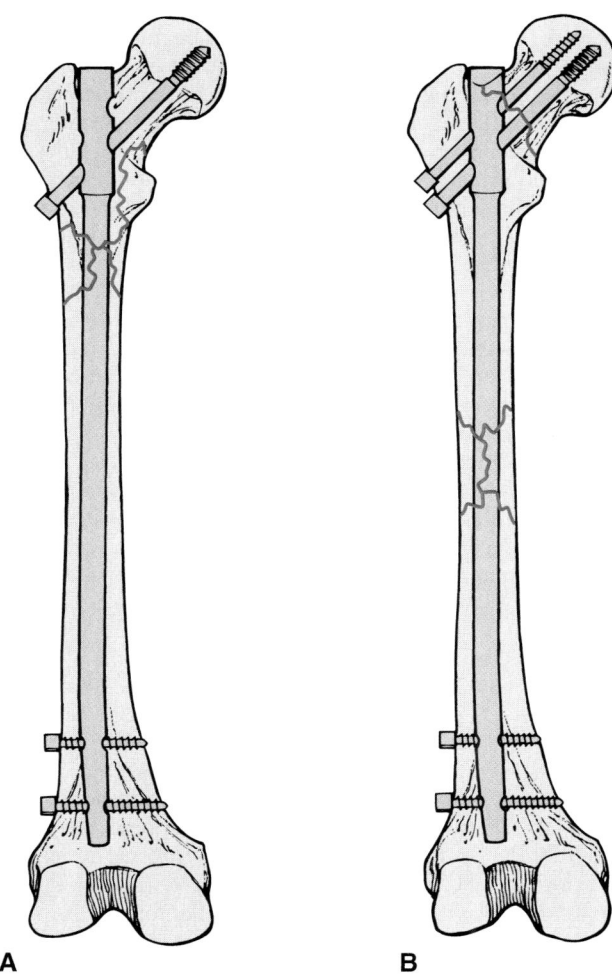

FIGURE 4-40 *Schematic representation of second-generation femoral locking nails and their primary indications.* **A,** *Fixation of a comminuted subtrochanteric fracture.* **B,** *Fixation of an ipsilateral neck and comminuted shaft fracture.*

A   **B**

and soft tissue healing. The relationship between these two major considerations can be expressed in the statement of Tscherne and Gotzen[92]: "Stability is the mechanical basis and vascularity the biologic basis of uncomplicated fracture healing."

The amount of motion at the fracture site in any fixation construct varies according to the mechanical characteristics of the construct and the direction and magnitude of the forces applied. The term *stability* has many definitions and is therefore a source of confusion. ASIF/AO considers stable fixation as that achieved in a fixation construct and subjected to loads of functional muscle activity and joint motion without any movement at the fracture site. This method is often termed *rigid fixation*. An alternative definition would hold that a fracture construct is stable when it allows pain-free functional activity even though a small amount of motion is present at the fracture site.

Additional clarity is given to the consideration of stability when the level of functional activity (e.g., active motion exercises versus weight-bearing) is specified. Under conditions of loading, there is a range of micromotion at the fracture site within which bony union will progress but above which nonunion will occur. Within this safe zone, the histologic pathway to fracture healing varies depending on the relative motion between fracture fragments.[34,49,63] If there is motion, the body supplements the immobilization provided by the implant through the development of callus. This small amount of skeletal material laid down at a distance from the central axis of the bone provides an effective method of bridging and immobilizing the main fracture fragments. The amount of callus is roughly proportional to the amount of motion. If there is complete elimination of motion between fracture fragments, callus formation is not necessary, and healing occurs more directly through intracortical osteogenesis.[83] Small gaps between fragments are filled by woven bone. Where fracture fragments are in direct contact, new intracortical haversian systems drill across the fracture site, producing direct union. This has been termed *primary union*, which suggests that it is inherently superior to the fracture union that occurs with the production of callus. Although intracortical union does progress more directly to an advanced stage of fracture remodeling, the mechanical strength and therefore the functional capability of this type of bone union are not superior to that of fracture healing through callus formation.

Both types of fracture union are functional, and the selection of an internal fixation method should pursue the fixation construct most appropriate for the specific fracture pattern. This decision must include consideration of the patient's general state of health, associated injuries, grade of the soft tissue injury, consistency of the bone, location and pattern of the displacement of the fracture, the technical expertise of the surgeon, and the physical and human resources available. We now consider the major fixation techniques that fit within each of the three modes of fixation and discuss their properties, primary indications, basic hardware, and correct technical application.

INTERFRAGMENTARY COMPRESSION

In interfragmentary compression, the fracture fragments are restored to their anatomic position and held together under compression by a metal implant. This compression improves the interference fit and increases friction at the fracture interface, enabling the final bone-implant construct to resist the deforming forces produced by functional activity. The compression of the bone fragments achieved by application of tension to the implant results in a completed construct that is said to have been *prestressed*. This term means that the stress that has been applied to the construct during application precedes the stress to which it is exposed when the fixation construct is loaded during functional activity. One result of prestressing is that the bone component of the construct is better able to share a functional load with the implant and thereby partially protect the metal from cyclical deformation and fatigue failure. Also, load sharing exposes the bone to a mechanical stimulus for fracture healing and maintenance of mineralization. The compression force or prestress on implants must be sufficient to resist the deforming forces to which the fixation construct is exposed during functional activity. If compression is applied incorrectly, excessive micromotion of the fracture fragments occurs, resulting in resorption of the bone ends and formation of small amounts of callus. Even though this occurrence is a protective physiologic response, in this circumstance, it is a warning sign of loosening and fatigue of the implant system. If steps are not taken to reverse this condition, the continued loading will lead to implant failure and nonunion.

The compression applied across the fracture surfaces can be static, dynamic, or both. *Static compression* results from pretensioning of the implants. *Dynamic compression* is achieved by harnessing forces that act on the skeleton during normal physiologic loading. In addition, implants can be applied in such a way as to combine static and dynamic compression. These concepts are discussed individually in the following sections.

STATIC COMPRESSION The lag screw is a classic example of applied static compression. The screw is tensioned across the fracture line, and the fracture is compressed. The screw has a small length of thread at its tip and a smooth shank between the head and the tip. Tension results when the screw threads bite into the cortex on one side of the fracture and the screw head blocks its progression into the bone on the other. This method is called a lag screw *by design*. These screws are usually employed to achieve interfragmentary compression between two fragments of cancellous bone (as in a metaphysis or epiphysis) (Fig. 4-41). It is critical that threads not cross the fracture site. After the hole is drilled across the fracture, threads in the near cortex must be cut with a tap. The threads of the screw spiral through the cancellous bone, which should be tapped only in the very dense cancellous bone of large, young patients. This type of screw fixation can be used only when the two cancellous surfaces make contact or become impacted. Gaps that remain in the cancellous bone after reduction of fragments will be filled by connective tissue, precluding reliable union. Therefore, a cancellous bone graft should be used to fill these gaps when they occur.

Interfragmentary compression can also be applied with simple, fully threaded screws. This technique is usually used in cortical bone. The cortex near the screw head is over-drilled so that the screw thread gains purchase only in the far cortex (Fig. 4-42A). This is called a lag screw *by application*. The over-drilled hole in the cortex near the screw head is called the *glide hole*, and the hole in the far cortex is called the *thread hole*. Cancellous type lag screws are not used to achieve interfragmentary compression in the cortex, because new cortical bone will fill the space between the drill hole and the smooth screw shank, making screw extraction difficult. Extraction is facilitated in the presence of the continuous thread of the cortical screw. Interfragmentary compression can be accomplished in the cortex with lag screws placed independently or through a plate.

Any cortical lag screw used to affix a plate that crosses a fracture site should be applied with the cortex near the screw head over-drilled as a glide hole. A screw that crosses the fracture line and threads into both cortices

prevents compression of the fracture fragments (see Fig. 4-42B). Optimal fixation with a cortical lag screw is achieved by correctly following the steps for screw insertion (Fig. 4-43). The best compression is obtained by aiming the screw into the center of the opposite fragment (Fig. 4-44A–C).

In addition to applying compression across the fracture surface, a screw fixing a simple fracture in a long bone must prevent the shear that would occur in oblique fractures under axial loading. Insertion of the screw perpendicular to the long axis of the bone best prevents shearing and fracture displacement. Therefore, this method provides the preferred orientation for screw fixation for most fractures, despite the fact that maximal compression of the fracture surfaces is achieved by lag screws oriented perpendicular to the fracture plane. When butterfly fragments are present, however, equal attention must be given to the need for interfragmentary compression at the fracture surfaces. For this reason, screw orientation halfway between perpendicular to the fracture surface and perpendicular to the long axis of the bone is used (Fig. 4-45; see also Fig. 4-44D and E).

Static compression can also be applied using plates. After fracture reduction, the plate is fixed to one fracture fragment. Tension is then applied to the opposite end of the plate, leading to compression at the fracture site. Compression may be accomplished using an external tension device or plates with specially designed screw holes that cause tensioning of the implant (Fig. 4-46). With this technique, it is helpful to initially affix the plate to the fragment that creates an axilla between the plate and the screw (Fig. 4-47A). This orientation facilitates fracture reduction and compression. Plates with specially designed screw holes that permit pretensioning include the Dynamic Compression Plate (DCP; Synthes, Paoli, PA), the Limited Contact Dynamic Compression Plate (LCDCP; Synthes), and the European Compression Technique (ECT; Zimmer, Warsaw, IN). *Dynamic compression plate* is an unfortunate name for an implant designed to provide static compression as defined here and in the AO manual. When a single plate is used, the application of tension to the plate tends to cause eccentric compression, with close apposition of the bone under the plate and slight gapping at the side of the bone away from the plate. This complication can be prevented by over-bending the plate before application (see Fig. 4-47B).

The optimal construct utilizes an interfragmentary lag screw placed through the plate to achieve greater fracture compression (see Fig. 4-46). Interfragmentary compression created by the screw fixation of the cortex opposite the plate reduces the shearing of this fracture surface that could otherwise occur with torsional forces. This combination of lag screw and plate should be used for most simple, oblique diaphyseal fractures. A pretensioned plate can be applied as the primary mode of compression in a transverse fracture in which lag screws are impractical. If the fracture includes at least one major butterfly fragment, the fracture planes between the butterfly fragment and the major diaphyseal fragments are best fixed with individual interfragmentary screws placed outside of the plate. The strength of this fixation is not great enough to

FIGURE 4-41 *Typical indications for cancellous lag screws. **A,** Two 6.5-mm cancellous screws with a 32-mm thread, used with washers to fix a lateral femoral condyle fracture. **B,** A 4.0-mm cancellous screw inserted from front to back to fix the posterior lip fragment of the distal tibia. **C,** Two 4.0-mm cancellous screws used to fix a medial malleolus fracture. **D,** A 4.0-mm cancellous screw used to fix a fragment from the anterior aspect of the distal tibia carrying the syndesmotic ligament. **E,** A 4.0-mm cancellous screw used to fix an epiphyseal fracture of the distal tibia. **F,** Two 4.0-mm cancellous screws used to fix an oblique fracture of the medial malleolus. **G,** A malleolar screw inserted obliquely to fix a short, oblique fracture of the distal fibula. This direction of insertion allows cortical purchase with an increased compression force. **H,** A 4.0-mm cancellous screw used to fix the vertical component of a supracondylar Y fracture of the distal humerus.*

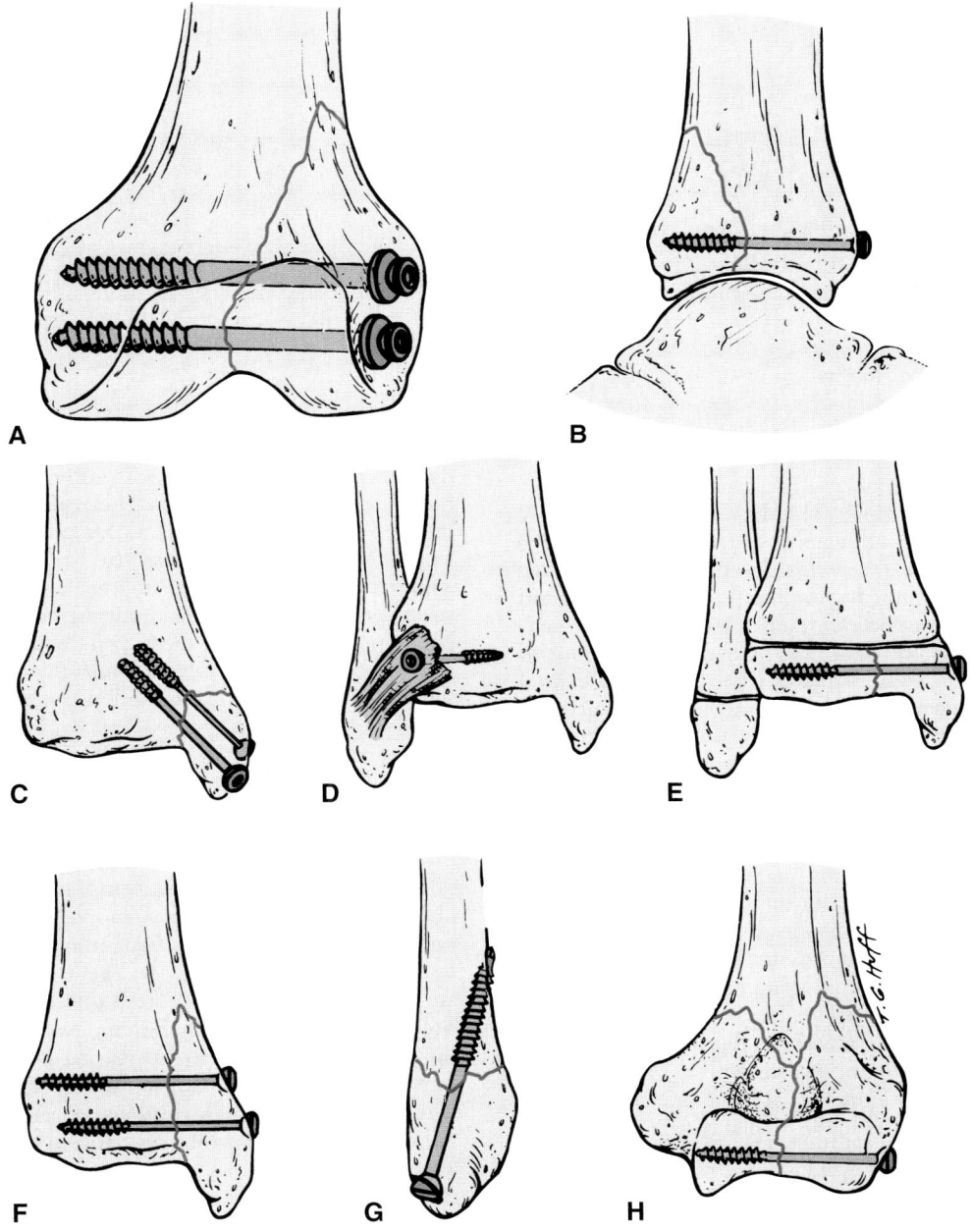

resist all torsional bending and axial loading forces, and it must be supplemented with a plate that spans the fracture site to neutralize the other forces that would disrupt the unprotected compression lag screw fixation. This use of plates is described later.

DYNAMIC COMPRESSION Stated simply, *dynamic compression* (DC) is a phenomenon by which an implant can transform or modify functional physiologic forces into compression of a fracture site. There is little or no prestress on the bone when the limb is at rest. Four typical examples

FIGURE 4-42 | *Lag screws by application. **A,** Over-drilling the near-cortex to produce a glide hole allows a cortical screw to act as a lag screw. **B,** In the absence of a glide hole, a cortical screw inserted across the fracture site will maintain fracture gapping.*

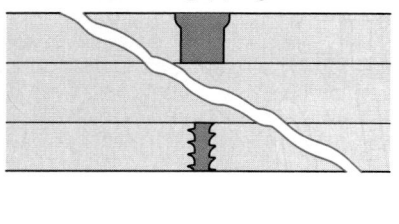

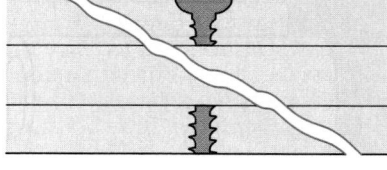

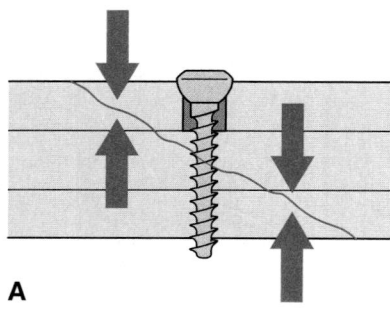

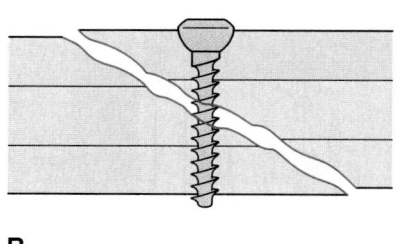

A

B

of DC constructs are the tension band, the antiglide plate, splintage by noninterlocked intramedullary nails, and the telescoping hip screw.

COMBINED STATIC-DYNAMIC COMPRESSION

Plates can be applied as tension bands if applied to the tension side of a fracture or nonunion. In addition to the anatomic situations noted previously, definite tension and compression sides can be identified at locations where anatomic or pathologic curvature or angulation of the bone or fracture results in loading that is eccentric to the central axis of the bone with weight-bearing and muscle activity. Because of its normal curvature, the femur is under tension anterolaterally and compression posteromedially. When a plate is placed on the lateral surface of the bone, it functions as a tension band. Subsequent weight-bearing and muscle activity result in dynamic compression at the fracture site. In a varus nonunion of the tibia, the abnormal angulation results in a significant bending moment. By placement of a tensioned plate in the lateral aspect of this bone, it is possible to capitalize on the abnormal eccentric loading to produce dynamic compression with weight-bearing and muscle activity (see Fig. 4-21).

In some situations, fractures and nonunions present conditions that allow their fixation with a combination of static and dynamic compression. This approach is usually accomplished through the use of plates that are pretensioned to provide static compression. In these situations, conditions permit the identification of a clear tension and compression side of the fracture. When placed on the tension surface, the plate also acts as a tension band. When functional activity is commenced, weight-bearing and muscle forces cause dynamic compression that supplements the static compression produced by pretensioning the implants.

SPLINTAGE

INTRAMEDULLARY NAILING In contrast to the relatively rigid fixation achieved with interfragmentary compression, standard nonlocking intramedullary nails provide fixation through splintage. *Splintage* may be defined as a construct in which sliding can occur between the bone and the implant. Nails extend from entry portals in the bone through the medullary canal over most of its length and allow axial loads to be transmitted to the apposed ends of the fracture fragments. Intramedullary fixation is much less rigid than interfragmentary compression but is no less effective when properly applied. Because a greater amount of motion occurs at the fracture site with functional activity, callus formation is regularly observed.

CLOSED NAILING The technique of closed nailing involves the reduction of long bone fractures by closed manipulation with the aid of a specialized traction table and fluoroscopy. The technique avoids the direct surgical exposure of the fracture site that occurs during open reduction. Because the overlying skin and muscle envelope is left intact, the periosteal vascular supply to the bone at the fracture site is preserved, and the additional surgical trauma to the surrounding soft tissue is minimized. Nails are inserted through entry portals distant from the fracture site at the end of the bone. Reaming is accomplished with the use of flexible reamers, increasing in diameter by 0.5-mm increments. The reamers are inserted over a guide wire that extends across the fracture site. These reamers follow the normal curvature of the bone. Nails inserted after reaming have a similar curvature and are cannulated to allow insertion over a guide wire. To aid their safe passage into the distal fragment, nails are designed with tapered tips, and a larger guide wire that more completely fills the internal diameter of the nail is used for nail introduction. These two factors help to keep the nail centered in the canal, preventing comminution of the cortex at the fracture site.

In the absence of direct visualization of the fracture, correct rotational alignment of the bone fragments must be inferred from proper positioning of the distal limb

FIGURE 4-43 *Steps for insertion of a cortical lag screw after reduction of a fracture. **A,** A 4.5-mm tap sleeve and a 4.5-mm drill bit are used to create a glide hole in the near-cortex. **B,** The top hat drill sleeve (58-mm long, 4.5-mm outer diameter, and 3.2-mm inner diameter) is inserted into the 4.5-mm glide hole until the serrated teeth abut the cortex. This ensures centering of the drill bit used to make the thread hole, even when the screw hole is drilled at an oblique angle. **C,** A 3.2-mm drill bit is inserted through the top hat guide to make the thread hole in the far cortex. **D,** A countersink with a 4.5-mm tip is inserted and used to produce a recess to accept the screw head. **E,** A depth gauge is used to accurately measure the length of screw needed. **F,** A 4.5-mm tap with a short threaded area is used to tap the thread hole in the far cortex. **G,** The 4.5-mm cortical screw is inserted and tightened lightly to create compression.*

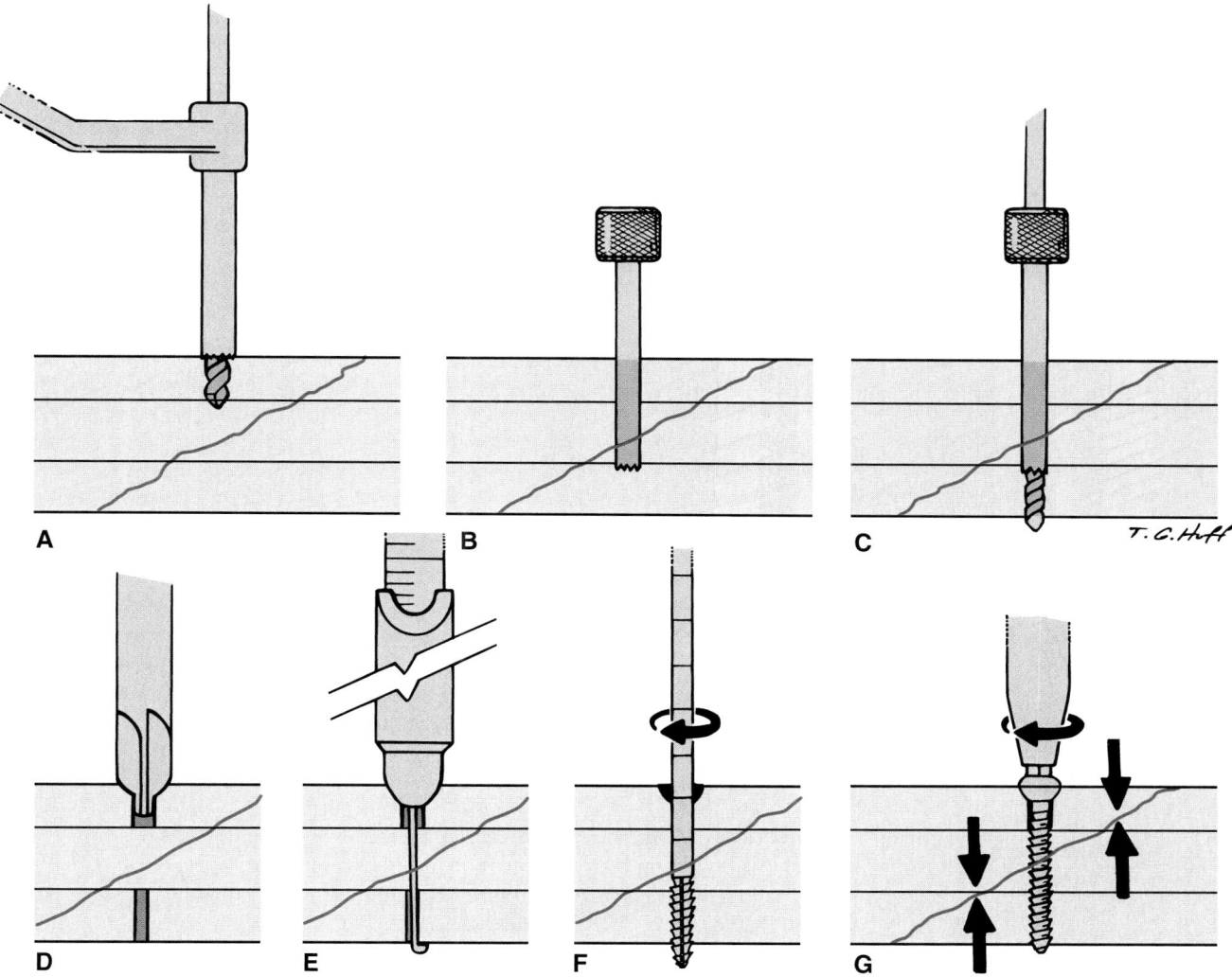

segment on the fracture table. With the pelvis flat in the supine position, the lower leg is positioned so that the patella is pointing directly at the ceiling. In fractures of the mid-diaphysis in which adequate endosteal contact is obtained with the nail on both sides of the fracture site, alignment occurs automatically on nail insertion. Conversely, very proximal or distal fractures that contain the entire diaphysis in one fragment have the potential for angulation during nailing. In these cases, lack of endosteal contact in one fragment allows the possibility of angular deformity and malunion. In noncomminuted fractures, correct length of the bone is reestablished and maintained through the abutment of the major proximal and distal fragments. If comminution results in reduction

of less than 50% of the normal surface contact between the two fragments, loss of abutment and resultant shortening can occur. Standard nonlocked nails serve only as intramedullary splints; they do not provide fixation that can prevent shortening caused by the axial pull of muscles and the forces of weight-bearing. When unrestricted by adequate cortical abutment, these forces tend to produce shortening and implant protrusion.

Standard nonlocking, closed intramedullary nailing has been employed with excellent results in the treatment of simple and minimally comminuted midshaft fractures of the femur and tibia.[7,23,37,93] Healing occurs through the callus pathway. Sharing of the load between bone and implant results in a strong union, after which repeat

---

FIGURE 4-44   *Orientation of screws for fixation of a simple spiral fracture. **A,** Screws are oriented so that the tip passes through the middle of the opposite fragment. **B,** Correct orientation of the screws with their tips passing through the center of the opposite fragment is best seen on cross-sectional views. **C,** On tightening of a screw that is not centered in the middle of the opposite fragment, the fracture fragments displace. **D,** Insertion of the screw at a right angle to the fracture plane results in the best interfragmental compression but offers inadequate resistance to axial loading. **E,** Insertion of a cortical lag screw at right angles to the long axis of the bone provides the best resistance to fracture displacement under axial loading.*

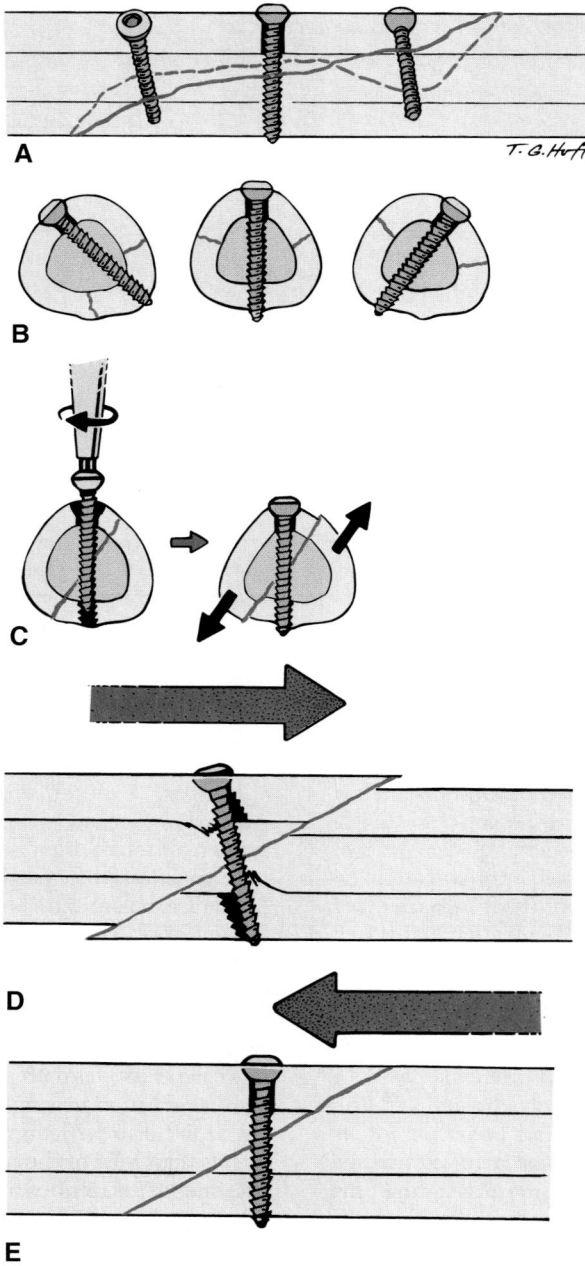

fractures are rarely encountered. Periosteal cortical osteoporosis is not observed after intramedullary nailing, although it can be seen during plating. After plate removal, the screw holes represent areas of stress concentration until new bone fills in the outer portion of the hole. After nonlocking intramedullary nailing, there are no screw holes through which fractures can propagate.

For appropriately selected fractures, nonlocking intramedullary nailing results in sufficient stability to permit early mobility of adjacent joints and early weight-bearing. Avoidance of surgical trauma to the overlying soft tissue through the use of the closed nailing technique promotes early muscle rehabilitation and results in an infection rate of less than 1%, compared with 3.2% for open nailing.[56] Provision of

FIGURE 4-45 *Screw fixation of a diaphyseal fracture with a single butterfly fragment. The center screw (a) connects the two main fragments. The outer two screws (b) fix the butterfly fragment to the two main fragments. These screws are inserted at an angle that bisects the angle formed between the perpendiculars to the fracture surface and to the long axis of the bone. Final tightening of all three screws should be completed after all are inserted.*

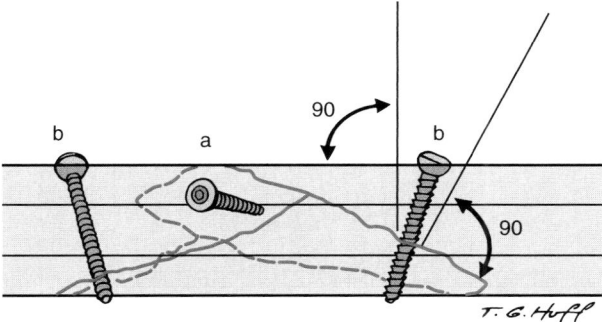

stable fixation through intramedullary nailing precludes the use of skeletal traction and lengthy periods of bed rest, resulting in a substantially shortened hospital stay.

BRIDGING

Both interfragmentary compression and splinting through intramedullary nailing require contact between the fracture fragments to achieve stability. They are best applied to simple fractures and with minimal comminution. Achieving apposition of all fragments in a markedly comminuted fracture is impractical and potentially harmful. These fractures most often result from the rapid dissipation of large amounts of energy into the trauma patient. The fracture occurs like an explosion, with great fragmentation of the bone and wide radial displacement of the individual fragments into the surrounding soft tissue. Elastic recoil of the remaining soft tissue envelope causes a reduction in the displacement that occurred at the moment of impact. The injury is considered more severe if it results in an open wound that breaches the soft tissue envelope and communicates directly with the fracture site. If this pattern has not occurred, the presence of a great degree of comminution and marked fragment displacement indicates that there has been significant injury to the soft tissue surrounding the bone.

Because the bone fragments are of variable size and are often rotated and impaled in the surrounding muscle, reduction requires direct surgical exposure and manipulation. Dissection and retraction of the injured soft tissue further compromise its damaged circulation. The use of clamps and reduction forceps to reposition and hold the bone fragments disrupts the tenuous muscle attachments that carry the remaining blood supply to these individual islands of bone. Further devascularization of soft tissue and bone increases the risk of infection and impairs fracture healing. When fracture healing is prevented or delayed, extended cyclical loading of the implants may exceed their fatigue limit and lead to failure.

To avoid these consequences, it is necessary to choose a fixation method that achieves the goals of internal fixation without causing severe damage to the vascularity of bone and surrounding soft tissue. This fixation can be provided by the technique of bridging. Bridging is accomplished by the insertion of implants that extend across the zone of soft tissue injury and fracture but are fixed to the major bone fragments proximal and distal to the fracture site. Bridging fixation can be accomplished with locked intramedullary nails inserted with a closed technique or with plates using indirect reduction.

Although fractures often appear to be held in distraction by bridging fixation with a locking intramedullary rod or plate, healing through periosteal callus is the usual outcome. These methods protect the viability of bone fragments by sparing their vascular supply and provide a favorable mechanical environment for bone formation. The metals from which most rods and plates are manufactured are somewhat elastic. This material property, combined with the structural geometry of the implants, results in a range of fracture motion consistent with callus formation. The implants allow restoration and preservation of alignment and permit functional activity. Because these tissues remain viable and a limited amount of motion is permitted at the fracture site during functional activity, a favorable environment for callus formation is present.

CLOSED LOCKING INTRAMEDULLARY NAILING

Fracture reduction and implant insertion follow the same steps outlined previously for standard nonlocking, closed intramedullary nailing. Additional attention must be given to the choice of implant length and final position on insertion, because the transfixion screws must be placed precisely. In comminuted fractures in which this bridging technique is used, additional attention must be paid to reduction to establish the correct length, rotation, and alignment.

Reducing butterfly fragments is an unreliable method for establishing the correct length of the bone. Because the patients are usually placed in skeletal traction on the fracture table, this method often results in over-lengthening of the bone. Fractures usually heal in spite of this over-distraction, and the added limb length is a noticeable annoyance to the patient. In these situations, it is necessary to make a reference length measurement from the opposite intact bone, using obvious landmarks such as the adductor tubercle and the tip of the greater trochanter on the femur. A bead-tip guide wire of known length can then be used as an intraoperative measuring device to reestablish the correct length of the fractured bone (Fig. 4-48). In nailing diaphyseal fractures proximal to the isthmus, correct alignment of the short conical proximal fragment is achieved by accurate placement of the entry portal. Insertion of the nail eccentric to the central axis of the medullary canal will result in angulation of this fragment (Fig. 4-49).

During nailing of fractures distal to the isthmus, a short, conical fragment with a wide medullary canal can easily become angulated because there is insufficient endosteal surface contact to produce or maintain alignment. The diameter of the medullary canal at the proximal end of this distal fragment is often larger than the diameter of the medullary nail. Careful reduction of this fragment is necessary to avoid comminution of the fracture

FIGURE 4-46 *The combination of axial compression with a plate and interfragmentary compression with a screw through the plate. **A,** Three methods of drilling the interfragmentary screw hole. (1) The glide hole is drilled first from the outside with a 4.5-mm drill. (2) The glide hole is drilled first from the inside with a 4.5-mm drill. (3) The thread hole is drilled first from the inside with a 3.2-mm drill. **B,** After initial drilling of the glide hole, the plate is applied. Fracture reduction and plate position are held with a clamp. To avoid slipping of the plate while drilling the first plate screw, the 3.2-mm drill guide is inserted through the plate into the hole for the interfragmentary screw. The first plate screw is drilled using the green drill guide. Note that the insertion of the first screw on this side of the fracture creates an axilla between the fracture surface and the plate that will trap the other fragment when it is compressed by placing the plate under tension. **C,** After removal of the drill sleeve, a second screw hole in the plate is drilled, using the yellow load guide. This guide locates the screw hole eccentrically with respect to the hole in the plate. **D,** Tightening of this screw results in tension in the plate and compression at the fracture site. The 3.2-mm drill sleeve is now reinserted in the glide hole and the opposite cortex is drilled. **E,** Insertion of an interfragmentary lag screw through this hole will dramatically increase compression at the fracture site. **F,** The remaining screws are now inserted through the plate, using the neutral green drill guide.*

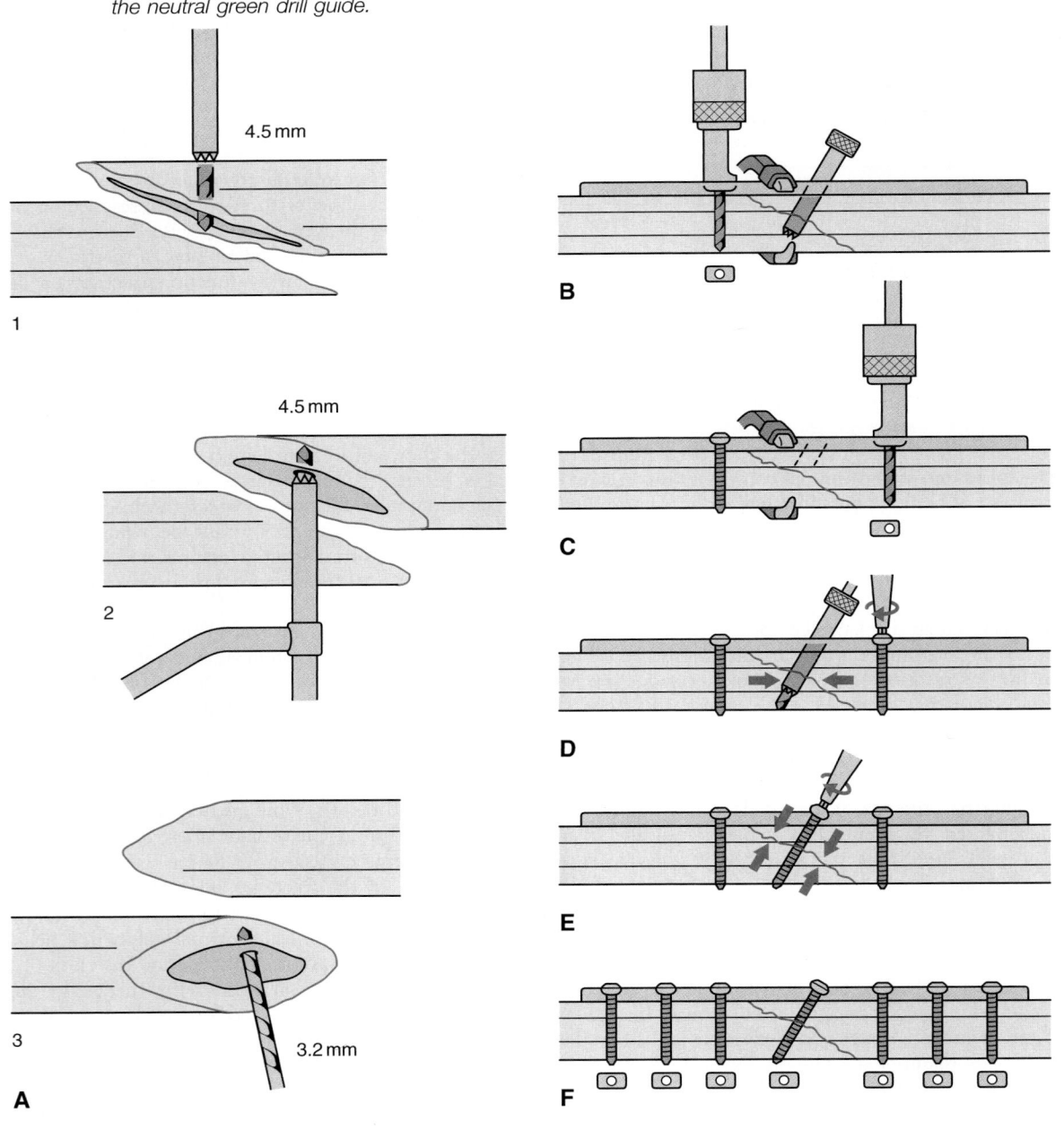

FIGURE 4-47 **A,** *The plate as a reduction tool. (1) Axilla formation. During compression, horizontal shifting of the plate on the bone may occur with displacement of the fracture as the nonstationary fragment slides down the oblique fracture plane. (2) The neutral screw should create an axilla between the bone and the plate. This will force the opposite fragment into the side to help ensure adequate compression. Fracture reduction and compression are facilitated when a stable axilla is created between the plate and one of the fracture fragments.* **B,** *Prebending of the plate. (1) Compression generated across the near-cortices and slight gapping of the far cortices result if the plate is not prebent. (2) Even fracture compression is facilitated with prebending of the plate before fixation.*

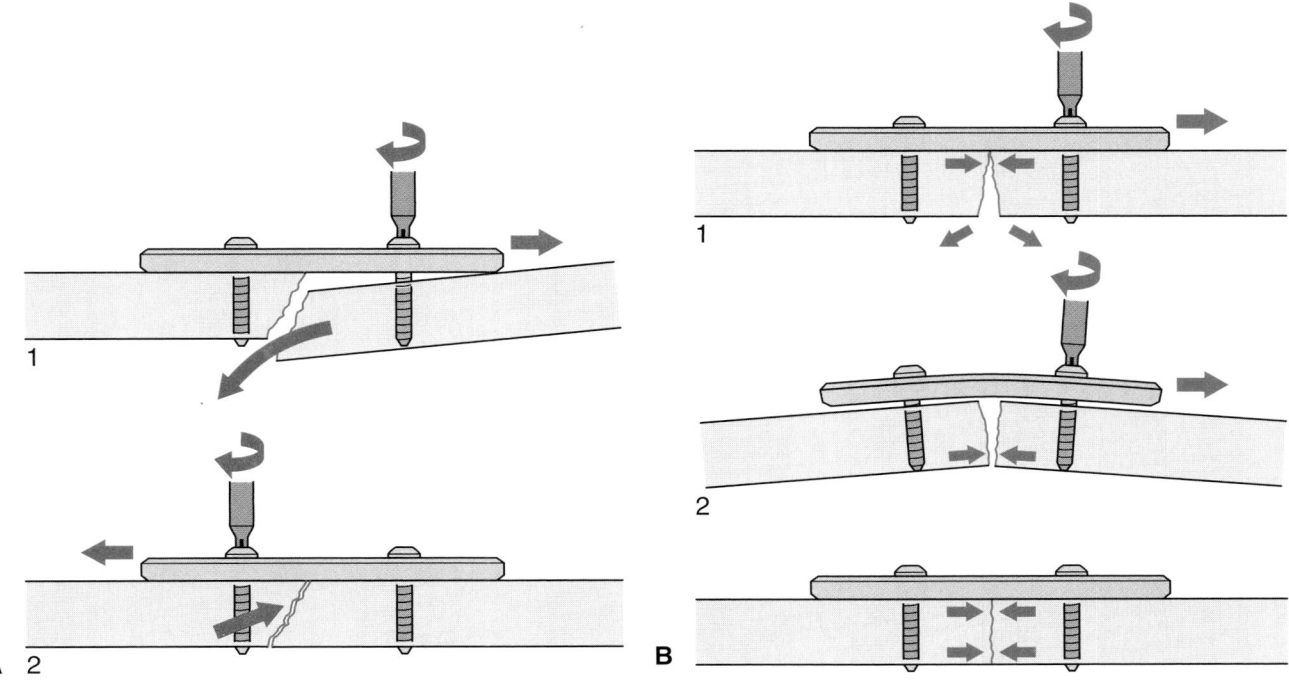

on nail insertion or abnormal angulation (Fig. 4-50). Under these circumstances, it is necessary to use two screws to transfix this distal fragment. Failure to do so will allow the fragment to toggle or rotate around a single locking screw, often causing unacceptable motion at the fracture site that can lead to nonunion and implant failure (Fig. 4-51).

Biomechanical studies indicate that placement of the proximal distal hole within 5 cm of a femoral fracture produces excessive stress on the nail, resulting in fatigue failure at this hole. The screw hole acts as a stress riser, producing stress in the nail that is greater than its fatigue endurance limit.[17] When proper closed nailing technique is used and the necessary precautions for correct reduction and implant placement are observed, excellent results can be obtained using this bridging technique for treatment of complex diaphyseal fractures of the femur and tibia.

PROXIMAL SCREW INSERTION Developers have attempted to produce locking nail systems that allow predictable percutaneous insertion of transfixion screws through the holes in both ends of the implants that is quick and easy. They have come closer to achieving this goal with the devices for providing proximal screw insertion. Many current nail designs allow drill and screw targeting devices to be firmly bolted onto the top of the nail in a desired position of rotational alignment.

DISTAL SCREW INSERTION Greater difficulty has been encountered in developing satisfactory methods for insertion of distal screws. A number of different methods have been employed with varying success. A target device mounted on the image intensifier has been used by Kempf and colleagues.[46] This device consists of a guide similar to a gun sight that is inserted into a holder attached to the image intensifier. After the x-ray beam is aligned coaxially with the tunnel through the nail, as evidenced by a perfectly round hole seen on the monitor of the image intensifier, the guide is folded down in line with the beam and maneuvered against the bone. After the position of the guide is fine-tuned to ensure alignment with the hole, it can be used to guide drilling and screw insertion. This device is used most effectively when it is attached to a rigid C-arm assembly. Many surgeons have found it easy to displace this guide if it is attached to the end of the more flexible C-arm fluoroscope.

There have been many attempts to design guides for the distal screw holes that attach to the threaded proximal end of the nail. This type of guide requires precise alignment with the distal transfixion holes before insertion of the implant. After implant insertion and proximal locking, the distal target device is reattached to the top of the nail in the hope that the guide will then align with the distal screw holes and facilitate drilling and insertion. However, nails that contain an open section over most of their length frequently undergo some deformation on insertion. This

FIGURE 4-48   *Diagrammatic representation of the recommended method of establishing the correct length (L) of a femur with a comminuted fracture. After making a reference measurement from the contralateral intact femur, traction is adjusted intraoperatively, and length is measured using a guide wire (GW) of known length. (Redrawn from Browner, B.; Cole, J.D. Current status of locked intramedullary nailing: a review. J Orthop Trauma 1[2]:192, 1987.)*

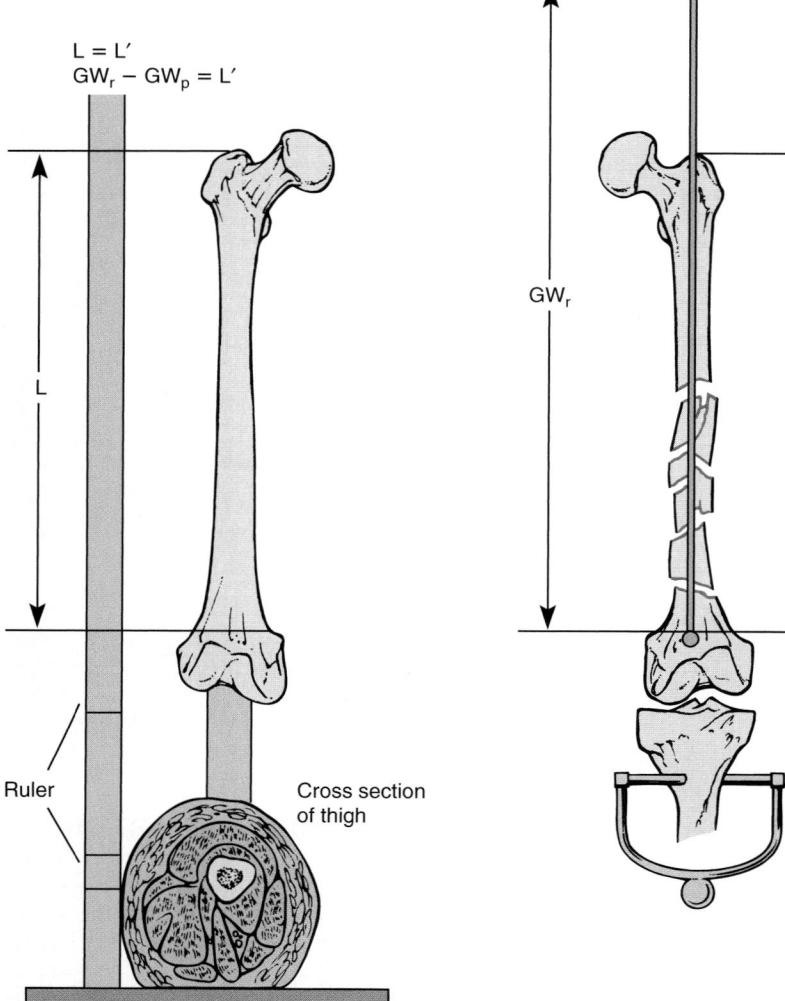

$$L = L'$$
$$GW_r - GW_p = L'$$

L

Ruler

Cross section of thigh

GW_p

GW_r

L'

changes the relation between the plane of the distal transfixion screw tunnels and the top of the nail and prohibits correct alignment of the proximally mounted target device. Because these guides often extend for a distance of more than 40 cm between their point of proximal attachment and the distal holes, the problem of malalignment is further aggravated by the tendency of the guide to sag toward the floor when used on the femur or tibia with the patient in the supine position.

The most reliable and most frequently used method for distal screw insertion is the freehand method.[13,59,65] The tip of an awl, Steinmann pin, or drill is held at an angle and aligned with the center of the hole using the monitor of the image intensifier. With the radiation off, this device is then brought in line with the x-ray beam and driven through the cortex of the femur or tibia (Fig. 4-52). An alternative method uses some form of hand-held guide to aid direct insertion of the drill. After detachment of the

Steinmann pin or drill bit from the power drill, passage through the hole in the nail is confirmed radiographically. The opposite cortex is then drilled, the screw length measured with a depth gauge, and the appropriate screw inserted. There has been great concern regarding possible excessive radiation exposure to the surgeon's hands during this portion of the procedure. Measurement of radiation by radiosensitive dosimeter rings worn during locking intramedullary nailing indicates that the surgeon's hands receive very small amounts of radiation, provided that they do not enter the beam.[58,86] This method is now the most widely used technique for distal screw insertion.

STATIC VERSUS DYNAMIC LOCKING The presence of screw holes at both ends of the nail offers the option to insert screws at only one or at both ends. Insertion of screws at both ends interlocks the nail and the major proximal and distal fragments. This fixation controls

FIGURE 4-49 *In proximal femoral fractures, insertion of straight nails, eccentric to the central axis of the medullary canal, through a lateral trochanteric entry portal, causes varus angulation of the proximal fragment.*
A, *Correct entry portal over the medullary axis.* ***B,*** *Incorrect entry portal, eccentric to the medullary axis.*

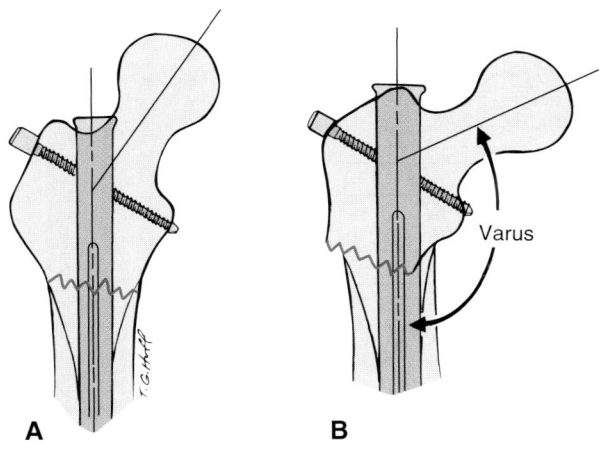

A　　　　　**B**

both the length of the bone and the rotation of the fragments. Because the screws prevent the sliding together of the two main fragments, this method of fixation is called the *static mode* (Fig. 4-53). It is a true example of the bridging mode of fixation and is used in fractures with marked comminution and bone loss. Although callus formation is regularly observed with this type of fixation, it

FIGURE 4-50 *Problems caused by malreduction of a short distal femoral fragment.*
A, *Translation resulting in comminution of the distal cortex during nail passage.*
B, *Failure to correctly position the distal fragment with a large medullary canal results in fixation in an angulated position.*

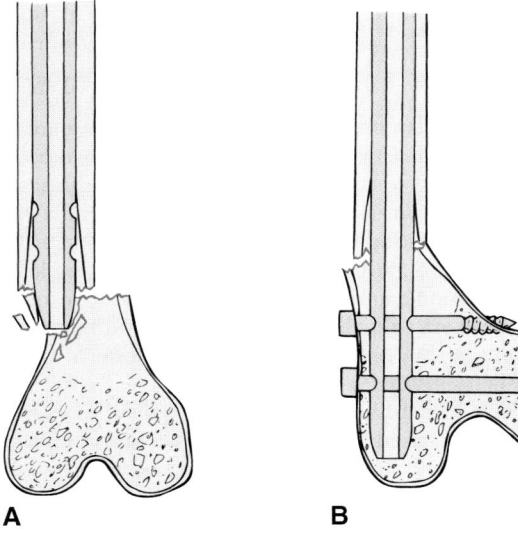

A　　　　　**B**

was originally feared that the presence of screws at both ends of the nail would prevent axial impaction and impair the ultimate remodeling of the fracture zone. Therefore, it was suggested that the screw or screws at one end of the nail be removed within 8 to 12 weeks after callus was radiographically observed.[11,45,48,90,100] However, the callus seen on radiographs of some healing fractures is not strong enough to withstand the axial loading that occurs after the transfixion is removed from one end of the nail. Therefore, screw removal can lead to shortening and implant protrusion.[11,14,46,90,100] Subsequent studies have shown that dynamization by removal of transfixion at one end of the nail is not necessary for satisfactory fracture healing and remodeling.[14]

When screws are inserted at only one end of the nail, the fixation is termed *dynamic.* This type of fixation is used to maintain rotational control of the short, conical, epiphyseal-metaphyseal fragment that occurs in fractures or nonunions that are proximal or distal to the diaphysis of the femur or tibia. This type of fixation is appropriate only when the area of contact between the two main fragments is at least 50% of the cortical circumference.[98] The unlocked end of the nail fits into the reamed medullary canal with the long fragment containing the diaphysis and achieves fixation in the splinting mode (Fig. 4-54). Displacement and subsequent instability can occur if dynamic fixation is chosen for fractures with insufficient contact between the two main fragments. Axial forces resulting from muscle activity and weight-bearing can lead to rotation or displacement of fracture fragments, with resultant loss of abutment and fracture shortening. Because the static or bridging mode of fixation results in predictable fracture healing, it is best to limit the use of dynamic fixation.

INDIRECT REDUCTION AND BRIDGE PLATING

Comminuted fractures involving the articular surface or metaphysis are often inappropriate for locking nail fixation. In these cases, fixation of articular fragments can often be accomplished with the use of interfragmentary lag screws and a plate that is attached to that fragment and that extends across the fracture zone to the diaphysis. After the plate has been fixed to the articular component, it can be used as a handle. An articulating tension device or a lamina spreader and clamp can be used between the plate and an isolated screw in the diaphysis to maneuver the articular fragment to the desired position (Fig. 4-55). This technique, which avoids direct exposure and further muscle stripping of the many small bone fragments in the comminuted fracture zone, is called *indirect reduction.*[50,60] Because of distraction across the fracture zone, the bone fragments are reduced through generation of tension in their soft tissue attachments. Alternatively, tension can be applied with the AO distractor.

The high-energy forces that produce comminuted fractures result in a major bony discontinuity. Deformities then occur as a result of the original deforming forces in combination with the unopposed pull of muscles attached to the major bone fragments. A highly variable combination of translational, angular, and rotational malalignment is often present, and shortening is almost always a feature.

FIGURE 4-51   *Failure to insert both distal transfixion screws in a short, distal femoral fragment in which the medullary canal is larger than the diameter of the nail produces continued toggling of the fragment on the single screw, resulting in nonunion and implant failure.* **A,** *Diagrammatic representation of fragment motion around the single screw.* **B,** *Distal femoral fracture fixed with a nail not sunk deeply enough into the femur and with the use of only one screw.* **C,** *Continued motion of the distal femoral fragment results in nonunion and implant failure.*

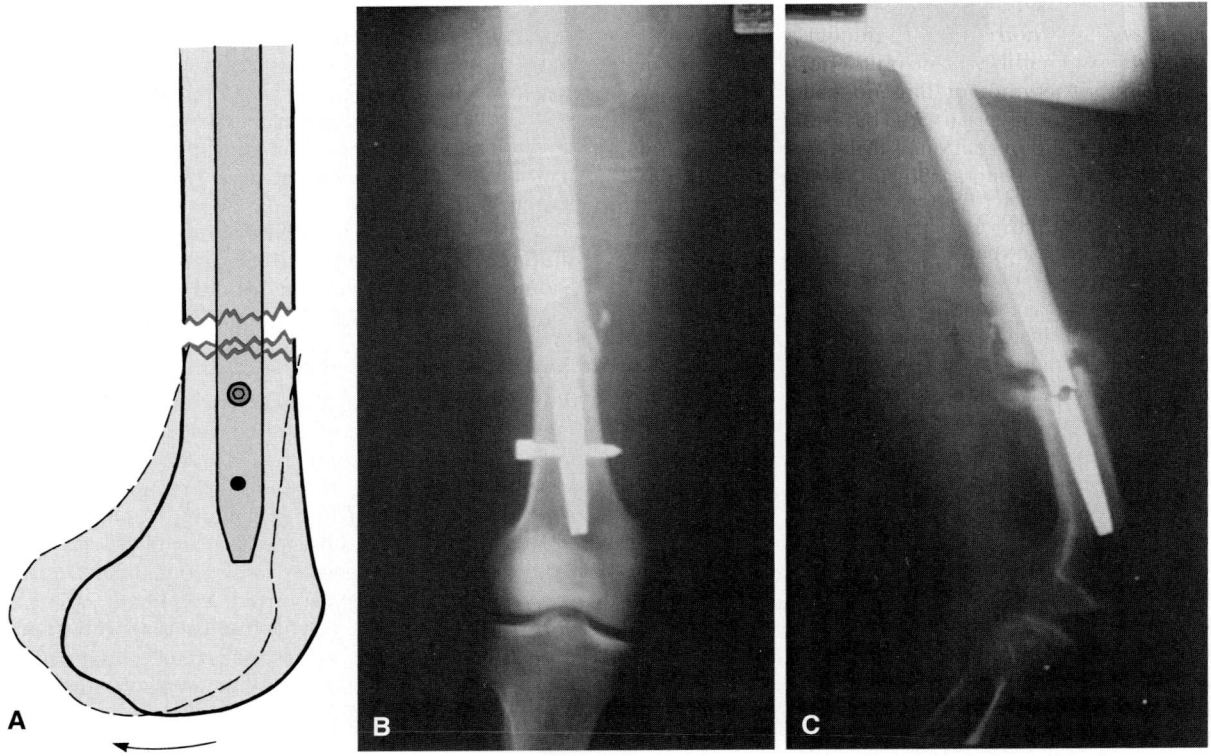

FIGURE 4-52   *Freehand technique for insertion of distal transfixion screws with femoral locking nails.* **A,** *Correct positioning of the image intensifier and use of the awl. Using the image intensifier, the tip of the awl is positioned opposite the hole, as seen on the screen. Fluoroscopy is then stopped, and the awl is brought in line with the beam and perpendicular to the nail.* **B,** *As an alternative, a drill guide can be aligned with the hole to correctly locate the awl or a drill bit.* **(A,** *Redrawn from Browner, B.; Edwards, C. The Science and Practice of Intramedullary Nailing. Philadelphia, Lea & Febiger, 1987, p. 248.)*

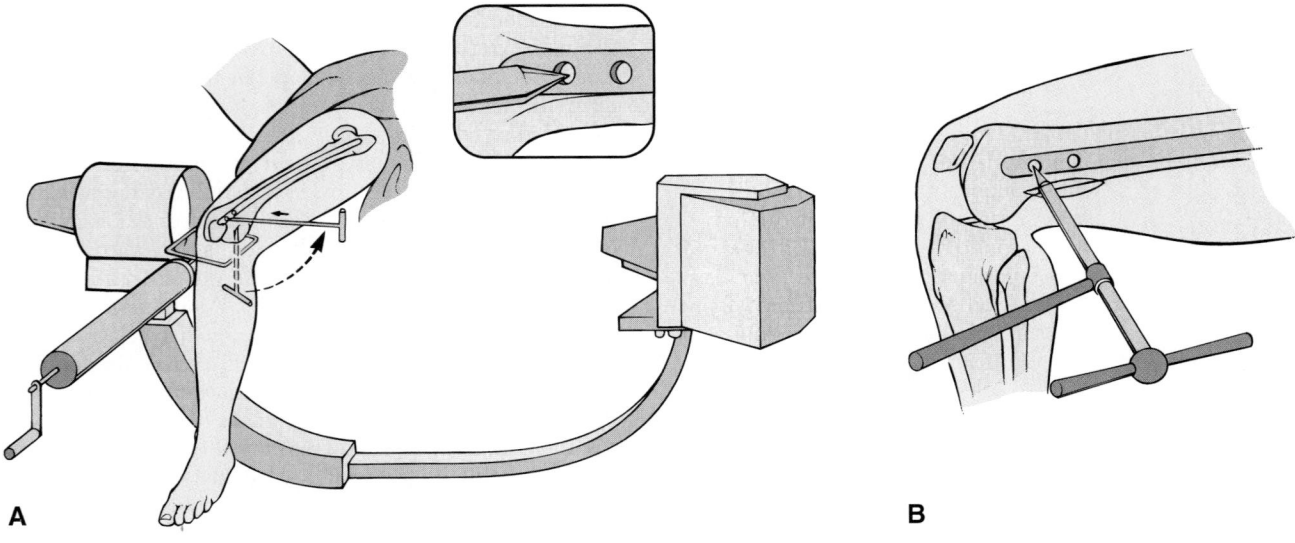

FIGURE 4-53 | *The static mode of fixation. Screws on both sides of the fracture fix the two main fragments to the nail, preventing them from rotating or sliding together. A small amount of elastic bending and torsion of the nail produces limited motion at the fracture site. This fixation is "static" only with respect to its resistance to shortening and rotation. (Redrawn from Browner, B.; Edwards, C. The Science and Practice of Intramedullary Nailing. Philadelphia, Lea & Febiger, 1987, p. 235.)*

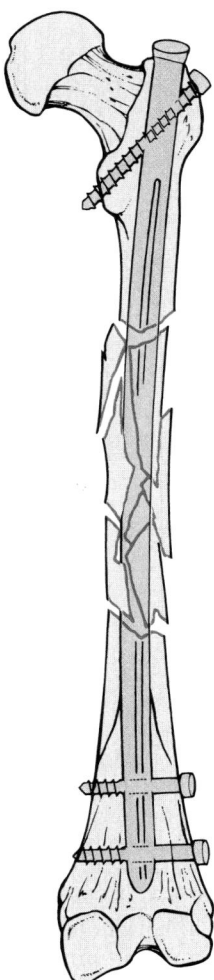

with a dental pick. If extensive intercalary comminution is present, axial compression cannot be applied, and the resulting bridge plate maintains anatomic length via distraction of the proximal and distal fragments.

Fixation of Osteopenic Bone

The treatment of fractures involving osteopenic bone will become more prevalent as the aging population increases. Routine internal fixation techniques may not be adequate to obtain stability. There are three basic concepts that should be considered when dealing with osteopenic bone.

FIGURE 4-54 | *The dynamic mode of fixation. Screws are inserted in only one end of the nail. Abutment of the main fragments prevents shortening. Contact between the endosteum and the nail in the long fragment prevents rotation of that fragment. It allows axial sliding of this fragment with impaction at the fracture site and with loading from muscle forces and weight-bearing. **A,** Use of a proximal screw controls only rotation of the short proximal fragment in a closed subtrochanteric fracture. **B,** Two screws are inserted to control the motion of the short distal femoral fragment with the large medullary canal. (Redrawn from Browner, B.; Edwards, C. The Science and Practice of Intramedullary Nailing. Philadelphia, Lea & Febiger, 1987, p. 237.)*

Restoration of bone length with proper consideration for rotational alignment will approximate the reduction in most fracture patterns. As with the indirect reduction technique, the application of longitudinal traction to the soft tissues facilitates their realignment.

In the attempt to align diaphyseal fractures, tension is transmitted through the muscular and fascial attachments to the bone. In a similar fashion, periarticular fractures can be partially realigned by generating tension in the ligaments and capsule attached to the articular fragment. Once the correct alignment, rotation, and length of the bone are restored by one of these indirect reduction maneuvers, the smaller bone fragments can be teased into place

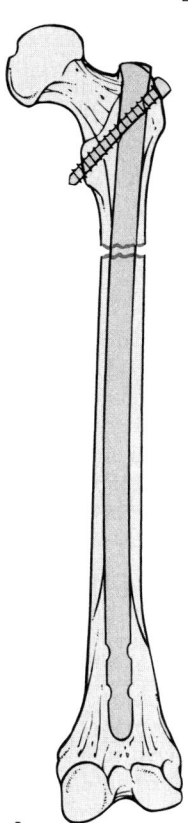

A

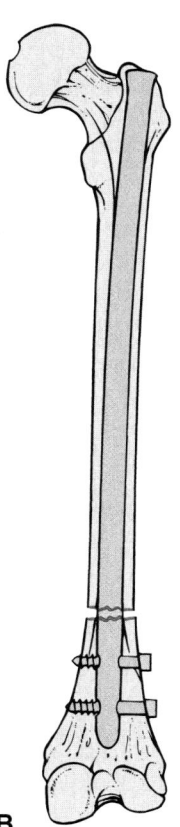

B

Avoid iatrogenic comminution of the fracture. Fracture reduction and fixation should proceed with caution to avoid increased comminution of the fragile, fragmented osteopenic bone.

Bone-to-implant stability and strength should be enhanced in three ways.

1. Use longer implants (plate or rod) to avoid failure at the junction of implant and osteopenic bone.[80]

2. Use additional screws when plating, increase the number of locking screws when using intramedullary rods, and use increased pins when applying external fixators to distribute the force over a greater area, thus unloading the osteopenic bone slightly.

3. Use fixed angled devices, which prevent pull-out. Bone implant stability can be increased by using fixed angled devices such as locking plates, blade plates, and Schuhli washers.[70] Prevention of implant

FIGURE 4-55 *Indirect reduction technique demonstrated during plating of a pillion fracture of the distal tibia. **A,** The plate is contoured to fit the bone. **B,** The plate is affixed first to the distal articular fragment. **C,** The plate is held against the shaft with the Verbrugge clamp. **D,** An articulating tension device is fixed to the diaphysis above the plate with a single screw. The device is turned so that its jaws open, causing the partially fixed plate to distract the fracture. Bone graft is applied to the impaction defects. **E,** Articular fragments that have been realigned by the pull of the attached soft tissues are now provisionally fixed with Kirschner wires. **F,** Slight compression is applied. **G,** The plate is fixed to the diaphysis above the fracture. (Redrawn from Mast, J.; Jakob, R.; Ganz, R. Planning and Reduction Technique in Fracture Surgery. New York, Springer Verlag, 1989, pp. 73, 74.)*

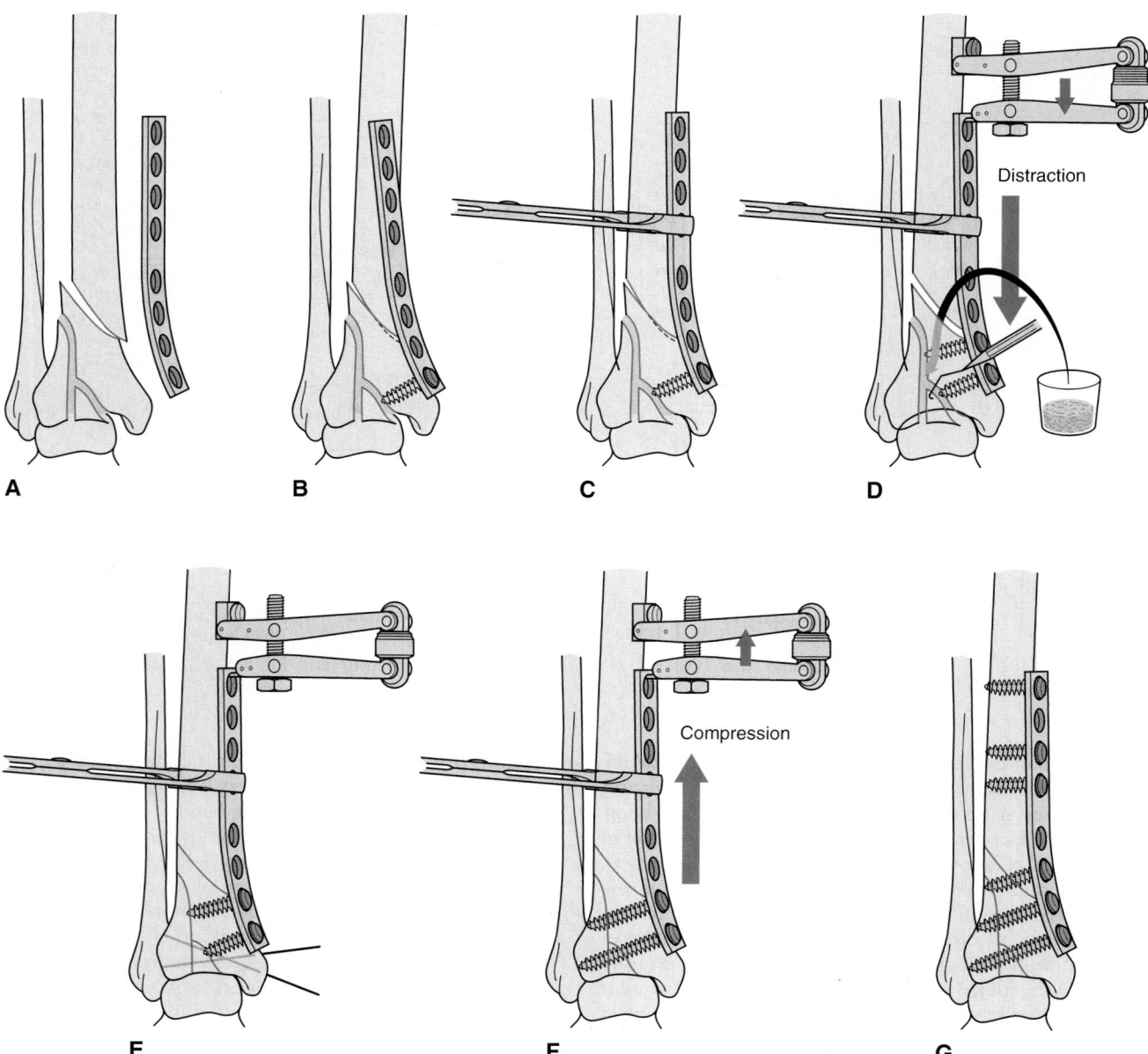

A   B   C   D

E   F   G

to bone failure can be accomplished by attaching a screw to the plate with a threaded hole or by attaching the screw to the plate with a specialized nut.

Augment weakened bone with various substances. The osteopenic bone itself can be augmented at certain areas with the use of polymethylmethacrylate (PMMA) or biodegradable calcium phosphate bone substitutes.[27,38]

Screw stability or holding strength is directly related to the cross-sectional area of the screw thread in the material and the density of material. PMMA and calcium phosphate bone substitutes both increase the density for greater screw holding strength and can also improve fracture stability by acting as an intramedullary strut.

Preoperative Planning

The development of a preoperative plan requires decision-making on a number of essential issues.

FIXATION

The choice of interfragmentary compression, splinting, or bridging fixation is based on analysis of the fracture pattern and location and the nature and extent of associated injury to the soft tissues and to other bones and organ systems. This decision leads to a specific selection of implants.

When screw and plate fixation is selected for interfragmentary compression or bridging fixation in fractures with multiple fragments, optimal placement of the implants can be facilitated by the creation of a preoperative blueprint. This plan is a diagram that shows the exact location of the plate and all screws and their relations to the various bone fragments when fixed in their final position of reduction. The shape of each bone fragment is drawn on tracing paper or clear x-ray film from the original injury film. The individual pieces are then assembled like a jigsaw puzzle into a whole bone. This method is accomplished by placing the pieces within the outline of the intact whole bone taken from a radiograph of the opposite side. Alternatively, cutouts of these individual fragments can be assembled over line drawings of the anatomic axis of the appropriate bone. A composite tracing is then made of the whole bone, showing all reduced fracture lines. Radiographs used in planning should be taken with the x-ray tube at 1 m from the subject. Under these conditions, images on the radiograph represent a 10 percent magnification of the real dimensions of the bone. Templates are available carrying an outline of certain plates with the same magnification. These templates can be used with the composite bone drawings to create a blueprint showing the optimal position of the implants. Once completed, this blueprint serves as an important reference during the surgery to guide proper placement of the plate and screws.

REDUCTION

The choice of reduction method also depends on the quality of bone, fracture pattern and location, and extent of associated soft tissue injury. A constant goal in fracture surgery is the preservation of bone viability by minimization of surgical trauma to muscle and fascial attachments that provide vascular supply to bone. Because these tissues are connected to the bone fragments, the application of longitudinal tension results in alignment of the fragments. The surgeon must decide whether traction will be applied manually, using a fracture table or a distractor, or through an indirect reduction technique. If a fracture table or distractor is used, the exact placement of traction or fixation pins must be chosen. If open reduction is planned, the surgeon should consider which special forceps and clamps will be necessary to achieve, and provisionally hold, the reduction. The surgeon must also decide whether an image intensifier or serial radiographs will be necessary to guide the reduction and implant insertion.

SURGICAL APPROACH

The fixation and reduction methods, the anatomy of the fractured part, and the condition of the overlying skin and muscle envelope must be considered when selecting the surgical approach. Review of descriptions of standard surgical approaches and practice of these in cadaver dissection improve the surgeon's ability to perform the surgery. The need for special retractors and other instruments must be considered based on the patient's size and the specific surgical approach.

POSITIONING, DRAPING, AND SPECIAL EQUIPMENT

Decisions regarding fixation, reduction, and surgical approach dictate patient positioning and draping. The surgeon should consider whether a pneumatic tourniquet will be used. In contrast, the expectation of large blood loss may indicate the need for a cell saver device or packed red blood cells and other blood components. The surgeon should also consider the need for special intraoperative monitoring such as somatosensory evoked potentials.

PERIOPERATIVE MANAGEMENT

Medical conditions that require intervention before surgery may be disclosed through the patient's history and physical examination. Drugs such as corticosteroids and anticoagulants should be discontinued or adjusted accordingly. A decision must be made regarding use of parenteral antibiotics, including their schedule and duration. The use of an epidural catheter for postoperative pain management should be determined preoperatively to allow patient and family education and consultation with the anesthesiology department.

PRIORITIZATION IN POLYTRAUMA

The presence of multiple injuries to several organ systems and different areas of the skeleton requiring a variety of procedures demands an organized approach to examination, decision-making, and implementation. Surgical teams should work simultaneously on different areas of the body to shorten the total anesthesia time. The general surgeon and anesthesiologist should oversee and coordinate the total patient care during resuscitation and initial surgical intervention. The orthopaedic surgeon plays an important role in this early treatment period, and the preoperative plan should be communicated to other specialists with primary responsibility for the patient.

Summary

Collectively, these considerations constitute preoperative planning. By proceeding through these categories sequentially, the necessary decisions can be made in a logical manner. This method allows the surgeon to present a more organized explanation to the patient and family, operating room staff, and colleagues. Exact requirements for the operating table, instruments, implants, associated devices, table positioning, draping, and medications can then be transmitted to the operating room staff and anesthesiologists. The blueprints created during the planning phase can be hung on the x-ray view box during the actual procedure to orient the entire surgical team. Effective planning and successful surgery are best accomplished through a clear understanding of the principles of internal fixation.

ACKNOWLEDGMENT

Preparation of this chapter would not have been possible without the support provided by the residents in the Department of Orthopaedic Surgery at the University of Connecticut Health Center. Their experience and encouragement are extremely appreciated.

REFERENCES

1. Ansell, R.; Scales, J. A study of some fractures which affect the strength of screws and their insertion and holding power in bone. J Biomech 1:279–302, 1968.
2. Asnis, S.; Kyle, R., eds. Cannulated Screw Fixation: Principles and Operative Techniques. New York, Springer-Verlag, 1996.
3. Baumgart, F.W.; Morikawa, C.K.; Morikawa, S.M.; et al. AO/ASIF Self-Tapping Screws (STS). Davos, Switzerland, AO/ASIF Research Institute, 1993.
4. Beaupre, G.S. Airport detectors of modern orthopaedic implant metal (Comment). Clin Orthop 303:291–292, 1994.
5. Bennett, A.; Harvey, W. Prostaglandins in orthopaedics (Editorial). J Bone Joint Surg Br 63:152, 1981.
6. Black, J. Orthopaedic Biomaterials in Research and Practice. New York, Churchill Livingstone, 1988.
7. Bone, L.B.; Johnson, K.D. Treatment of tibial shaft fractures by reaming and intramedullary nailing. J Bone Joint Surg Am 68:877–887, 1986.
8. Bronzino, J. The Biomedical Engineering Handbook. Hartford, CT, CRC Press, 1995.
9. Brooks, D.B.; Burstein, A.H.; Frankel, V.H. The biomechanics of torsional fractures: The stress concentration effect of a drill hole. J Bone Joint Surg Am 52:507–514, 1970.
10. Brown, G.; Winquist, R.A. Personal communication, 1996.
11. Browner, B.D. The Grosse-Kempf locking nail. Contemp Orthop 8:17–25, 1984.
12. Browner, B.D.; Boyle, M.; Morvant, R.; et al. Grosse-Kempf nailing of unstable femoral fractures: The initial North American experience—Orthopaedic transactions of American Orthopaedic Association. J Bone Joint Surg Am 8:405, 1984.
13. Browner, B.D.; Wiss, D.A. The Grosse-Kempf locking nail for the femur. In Browner, B.D.; Edwards, C.C., eds. The Science and Practice of Intramedullary Nailing. Philadelphia, Lea & Febiger, 1987, pp. 233–252.
14. Brumback, R.J.; Uwagie-Ero, S.; Lakatos, R.P.; et al. Intramedullary nailing of femoral shaft fractures. Part II: Fracture healing with static interlocking fixation. J Bone Joint Surg Am 70:1453, 1988.
15. Brunner, C.F.; Weber, B.G. Internal fixation plates with a specialized form and function. In Brunner, C.F.; Weber, B.G.; eds. Special Techniques in Internal Fixation. New York, Springer-Verlag, 1982, pp. 151–152.
16. Brunner, C.F.; Weber, B.G. Special Techniques in Internal Fixation. New York, Springer-Verlag, 1982.
17. Bucholz, R.W.; Ross, S.E.; Lawrence, K.L. Fatigue fracture of the interlocking nail in the treatment of fractures of the distal part of the femoral shaft. J Bone Joint Surg Am 69:1391, 1987.
18. Burstein, A.H.; Currey, J.; Frankel, V.; et al. Bone strength. J Bone Joint Surg Am 54:1143, 1972.
19. Canalis, E. Effect of growth factors on bone cell replication and differentiation. Clin Orthop 193:246, 1985.
20. Chang, C.C.; Merritt, K. Infection at the site of implanted materials with and without preadhered bacteria. J Orthop Res 12:526–531, 1994.
21. Chapman, M.W. The role of intramedullary nailing in fracture management. In Browner, B.D.; Edwards, C.C., eds. The Science and Practice of Intramedullary Nailing. Philadelphia, Lea & Febiger, 1987, pp. 17–24.
22. Charnley, J. The Closed Treatment of Common Fractures, 3rd ed. New York, Churchill Livingstone, 1961.
23. Clawson, D.K.; Smith, R.F.; Hansen, S.T. Closed intramedullary nailing of the femur. J Bone Joint Surg Am 53:681, 1971.
24. Cobelli, N.J.; Sadler, A.H. Ender rod versus compression screw fixation of hip fractures. Clin Orthop 201:123–129, 1985.
25. Cross, A.; Montgomery, R.J. The treatment of tibial shaft fractures by the locking medullary nail system. J Bone Joint Surg Br 69:489, 1987.
26. Delmi, M.; Vaudaux, P.; Lew, D.P.; et al. Role of fibronectin in staphylococcal adhesion to metallic surfaces used as models of orthopaedic devices. J Orthop Res 12:432–438, 1994.
27. Elder, S.; Frankenburg, E.; Goulet, J.; et al. Biomechanical evaluation of calcium phosphate cement–augmentation fixation of unstable intertrochanteric fractures. J Orthop Trauma 14:386–393, 2000.
28. Ellerbe, D.M.K.; Frodel, J.L. Comparison of implant materials used in maxillofacial rigid internal fixation. Otolaryngol Clin North Am 28:2, 1995.
29. Eppley, B.C.; Spartis, C.; Herman, I. Effects of skeletal fixation on craniofacial imaging. J Craniofac Surg 4:67–73, 1993.

30. Esser, M.P.; Kassab, J.V.; Jones, D.H. Trochanteric fractures of the femur: A randomised prospective trial comparing the Jewett nailplate with the dynamic hip screw. J Bone Joint Surg Br 68:557–560, 1986.

31. Frankel, V.H.; Burstein, A.H. Orthopaedic Biomechanics. Philadelphia, Lea & Febiger, 1970.

32. Frost, H.M. Bone Remodeling Dynamics. Springfield, IL, Charles C. Thomas, 1963.

33. Gautier, F. Belastungsveran derung des knochens durch platterosteosynthese (Dissertation). Bern, Switzerland, 1988.

34. Goodship, A.E.; Kelly, D.J.; Rigby, H.S.; et al. The effect of different regimes of axial micromovement on the healing of experimental tibial fractures. Trans Orthop 11:285, 1987.

35. Haas, N.; Krettek, C.; Schandelmaier, P.; et al. A new solid unreamed tibial nail for shaft fractures with severe soft tissue injury. Injury 24:49–54, 1993.

36. Hansen, S.T. The type IIIC tibial fracture. J Bone Joint Surg Am 69:799–800, 1987.

37. Hansen, S.T.; Veith, R.G. Closed Küntscher nailing of the tibia. In Browner, B.D.; Edwards, C.C., eds. The Science and Practice of Intramedullary Nailing. Philadelphia, Lea & Febiger, 1987, pp. 267–280.

38. Harrington, K.D. The use of methylmethacrylate as an adjunct in the internal fixation of unstable comminuted intertrochanteric fractures in osteoporotic patients. J Bone Joint Surg Am 57:744–750, 1975.

39. Hauschka, P.V.; Chen, T.L.; Mavrakos, A.E. Polypeptide growth factors in bone matrix. CIBA Found Symp 136:207–225, 1988.

40. Hearn, T.C.; Schatzker, J.; Wolfson, N. Extraction strength of cannulated cancellous bone screws. J Orthop Trauma 7:138–141, 1993.

41. Jacob, C.H.; Berry, J.T. A study of the bone machining process: Drilling. J Biomech 9:343, 1976.

42. Jacobs, R.R.; Armstrong, J.H.; Whittaker, J.H.; et al. Treatment of intertrochanteric hip fractures with a compression hip screw and a nail plate. J Trauma 16:599, 1976.

43. Johnson, K.D.; Johnston, D.W.C.; Parker, B. Comminuted femoral shaft fractures: Treatment by roller traction, cerclage wires and an intramedullary nail, or an interlocking intramedullary nail. J Bone Joint Surg Am 66:1222–1235, 1984.

44. Kaufer, H. Mechanics of the injured hip. Clin Orthop 146:53–61, 1980.

45. Kellam, J.F. Early results of the Sunnybrook experience with locked intramedullary nailing. Orthopedics 8:1387–1388, 1985.

46. Kempf, I.; Grosse, A.; Beck, G. Closed locked intramedullary nailing: Its application to comminuted fractures of the femur. J Bone Joint Surg Am 67:709, 1985.

47. Kempf, I.; Grosse, A.; Lafforgue, D. L'enclouage avec blocage de la rotation on "clou bloque": Principes, technique, indications et premiers resultats: Communication a la journée d'hiver. SOFCOT, 1976.

48. Kempf, I.; Grosse, A.; Lafforgue, D. L'apport due verrouillage dans l'enclouage centromidullaire, des os longs. Rev Clin Orthop 64:635–651, 1978.

49. Kenwright, J.; Goodship, A.E. Controlled mechanical stimulation in the treatment of tibial fractures. Clin Orthop 241:36, 1989.

50. Kinast, C.; Bolhofner, B.R.; Mast, J.W.; et al. Subtrochanteric fractures of the femur. Clin Orthop 238:122–130, 1989.

51. Klaue, H.; Perren, S.M. Fixation interne des fractures pas lensemble plaque: Vis a compression conjuguée (DVC). Helv Chir Acta 49:77–80, 1982.

52. Klaue, K.; Perren, S.M.; Kowalski, M. Internal fixation with a self-compressing plate and lag screw: Improvements of the plate hole and screw design. 1. Mechanical investigations. J Orthop Trauma 5:280, 1991. Original work: Klaue, K., Frigg, R., Perren, S.M. Die entlastung der osteosyntheseplatte durch interfragmentare plattenzugschraube. Helv Chir Acta 52:19–23, 1985.

53. Klemm, K.W.; Borner, M. Interlocking nailing of complex fractures of the femur and tibia. Clin Orthop 212:89–100, 1986.

54. Klemm, K.W.; Schellman, W. Dynamische und statische Verriegelung des Marknagels. Unfallheilkunde 75:568, 1972.

55. Kolodziej, P.; Lee, F.S.; Ashish, P.; et al. The Biomechanical Evaluation of the Schuhli Nut. Detroit, MI, Wayne State University, 1992.

56. Küntscher, G. Praxis der Marknagelung. Stuttgart, Germany, Schattauer, 1962.

57. Leggon, R.; Lindsey, R.W.; Doherty, B.J.; et al. The holding strength of cannulated screws compared with solid core screws in cortical and cancellous bone. J Orthop Trauma 7:450, 1993.

58. Levin, P.E.; Schoen, R.W.; Browner, B.D. Radiation exposure to the surgeon during closed interlocking intramedullary nailing. J Bone Joint Surg Am 69:761, 1987.

59. MacMillan, M.; Gross, R.H. A simplified technique of distal femoral screw insertion for the Grosse-Kempf interlocking nail. Clin Orthop 226:253–259, 1988.

60. Mast, J.; Jakob, R.; Ganz, R. Planning and Reduction Technique in Fracture Surgery. New York, Springer-Verlag, 1989.

61. Matelic, T.M.; Monroe, M.T.; Mast, J.W. The use of endosteal substitution in the treatment of recalcitrant nonunions of the femur: Report of seven cases. J Orthop Trauma 10:1–6, 1996.

62. Matter, P.; Holzach, P. Behandlungsergebnisse von 221 Unterschenkel-Osteosynthesen mit schmalen dynamischen Kompressionsplatten (DCP) aus Stahl oder Titan. Unfallheilkunde 80:195–196, 1977.

63. McKibbin, B. The biology of fracture healing in long bones. J Bone Joint Surg Br 60:150, 1978.

64. Mears, J. Materials and Orthopaedic Surgery. Baltimore, Williams & Wilkins, 1979.

65. Medoff, R.J. Insertion of distal screws in interlocking nail fixation of femoral shaft fractures. J Bone Joint Surg Am 68:1275–1277, 1986.

66. Modny, M.T. The perforated cruciate intramedullary nail: Preliminary report of its use in geriatric patients. J Am Geriatr Soc 1:579, 1953.

67. Muller, M.E.; Allgöwer, M.; Schneider, R.; et al. Manual of Internal Fixation: Techniques Recommended by the AO/ASIF Group. New York, Springer-Verlag, 1995. Corrected 3rd printing.

68. Muller, M.E.; Allgöwer, M.; Schneider, R.; et al. Manual of Internal Fixation, 2nd ed. New York, Springer-Verlag, 1979.

69. Olerud, S. The effect of intramedullary reaming. In Browner, B.D.; Edwards, C.C., eds. The Science and Practice of Intramedullary Nailing. Philadelphia, Lea & Febiger, 1987, pp. 71–74.

70. Palmer, S.H.; Hanley, R.; Willett, K. The use of interlocked "customized" blade plates in the treatment of metaphyseal fractures in patients with poor bone stock. Injury 31:187–191, 2000.

71. Pascal, A.; Tsukayama, D.T.; Wicklund, B.H.; et al. The effect of stainless steel, cobalt-chromium, titanium alloy, and titanium on the respiratory burst activity of human polymorphonuclear leukocytes. Clin Orthop 280:281–287, 1992.

72. Pauwels, F. Der Schenkelhalsbruch: Ein Mechanisches Problem. Stuttgart, Germany, Enke, 1935.

73. Pauwels, F. Gessammelte Abhandlungen zur Funktionellen Anatomie des Bewegungsapparates. Berlin, Springer-Verlag, 1965.

74. Pawluk, R.J.; Musso, E.; Tzitzikalakis, G.I. The effects of internal fixation techniques on alternating plate screw strain distributions. Orthop Trans 9:294, 1985.

75. Perren, S.M. The concept of biological plating using the limited contact-dynamic compression plate (LCDCP): Scientific background, design and application. Injury 22(1):1–41, 1991.

76. Perren, S.M.; Russenberger, M.; Steinemann, S.; et al. A dynamic compression plate. Acta Orthop Scand Suppl 125:31–41, 1969.

77. Pohler, O. Unpublished study conducted at Strauman Metallurgical Research Institute, Switzerland. In AO/ASIF Drill Bits: Synthes Update Bulletin No. 87-2. Paoli, PA, Synthes USA, 1987.

78. Postlethwaite, K.R.; Philips, J.G.; Booths, M.D. The effects of small plate osteosynthesis on postoperative radiotherapy. Br J Oral Maxillofac Surg 27:375–378, 1989.

79. Rhinelander, F.W.; Wilson, J.W. Blood supply to developing, mature and healing bone. In Sumner-Smith, G., ed. Bone in Clinical Orthopedics: A Study in Comparative Osteology. Philadelphia, W.B. Saunders, 1982, pp. 81–158.

80. Ring, D.; Perey, B.H.; Jupiter, J.B. The functional outcome of preoperative treatment of ununited fractures of the humeral diaphysis in older patients. J Bone Joint Surg Am 81:177–190, 1999.

81. Russel, T.A.; Taylor, J.C.; Lavelle, D.G.; et al. Mechanical characterization of femoral interlocking intramedullary nailing systems. J Orthop Trauma 5:332–340, 1991.

82. Schaffer, J.J.; Manoli, A. The antiglide plate for distal fibular fixation. J Bone Joint Surg Am 69:596, 1987.

83. Schenk, R.; Willenegger, H. Zur histologie der primaren knockenheilung. Langenbecks Arch Klin Chir 308:440, 1964.

84. Schweber, L. Experimentelle untersuchungen von knochertransplantation vit unvermdeter und mit denaturierter mochengrandsubstat. Hefte Unfallheilhd 103:1–70, 1976.

85. Sherk, H.H.; Foster, M.D. Hip fractures: Condylocephalic rod versus compression screw. Clin Orthop 192:255–259, 1985.

86. Skjeldal, S.; Backe, S. Interlocking medullary nails: Radiation doses in distal targeting. Arch Orthop Trauma Surg 106:179, 1987.

87. Tarr, R.R.; Wiss, D.A. The mechanics and biology of intramedullary fracture fixation. Clin Orthop 212:10–17, 1986.

88. Tencer, A.F.; Asnis, S.E.; Harrington, R.M.; et al. Biomechanics of cannulated and noncannulated screws. In Asnis, S.E.; Kyle, R.F., eds. Cannulated Screw Fixation: Principles and Operative Techniques. New York, Springer-Verlag, 1997.

89. Tencer, A.F.; Sherman, M.C.; Johnson, K.D. Biomechanical factors affecting fracture stability and femoral bursting in closed intramedullary rod fixation of femur fractures. J Biomech Eng 107:104–111, 1985.

90. Thoresen, B.O.; Alho, A.; Ekeland, A.; et al. Interlocking intramedullary nailing in femoral shaft fractures: A report of forty-eight cases. J Bone Joint Surg Am 67:1313, 1985.

91. Tsai, C.L.; Liu, T.H.; Hung, M.H. Glycocalyx products and adherence of *Staphylococcus* to biomaterials. Acta Med Okayama 46:11–16, 1992.

92. Tscherne, H.; Gotzen, L. Fractures with Soft Tissue Injuries. New York, Springer-Verlag, 1984.

93. Velazco, A.; Whitesides, T.E.; Fleming, L.L. Open fractures of the tibia treated with the Lottes nail. J Bone Joint Surg Am 65:879–885, 1983.

94. Von Arx, C. Schubebertragung durch reiburg bei der plattenosteosynthese: Dissertation. Basel, Switzerland, 1973.

95. Vresilovic, E.J.; Spindler, K.P.; Robertson, W.W.; et al. Failures of pin removal after in situ pinning of slipped capital femoral epiphyses: A comparison of different pin types. J Pediatr Orthop 10:764–768, 1990.

96. Wagner, H. Die Einbettung der metallschrauben in Knocher und die Heilungsvorgänge des Knochergewebes unter dem Einfluss der Stabilen Osteosynthese. Langenbecks Arch Klin Chir 305:28–40, 1963.

97. Werry, D.G.; Boyle, M.R.; Meck, R.N.; et al. Intramedullary fixation of tibial shaft fractures with AO and Grosse-Kempf locking nails: A review of 70 consecutive patients. J Bone Joint Surg Br 67:325, 1985.

98. Winquist, R.A.; Hansen, S.T. Segmental fractures of the femur treated by closed intramedullary nailing. J Bone Joint Surg Am 60:934, 1978.

99. Wiss, D.A.; Fleming, C.H.; Matta, J.M.; et al. Comminuted and rotationally unstable fractures of the femur treated with an interlocking nail. Clin Orthop 212:35, 1986.

100. Wolf, J.W.; White, A.A. III ; Panjabi, M.M.; et al. Comparison of cyclic loading versus constant compression in the treatment of long bone fracture in rabbits. J Bone Joint Surg Am 63:805–810, 1981.

101. Zinghi, G.F.; Specchia, L.; Montanari, G.; et al. The Grosse-Kempf locked nail in the treatment of diaphyseal and meta diaphyseal fractures of the tibia. Ital J Orthop Traumatol 12:365, 1986.

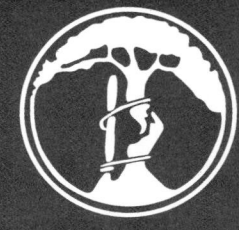

CHAPTER 5

Locking Plates: Development, Biomechanics, and Clinical Application

Michael A. Wagner, M.D. and Robert Frigg

DEVELOPMENT AND BACKGROUND

Evolution of the Concepts of Fracture Fixation

Historically, the most notable development in the treatment of diaphyseal fractures has been a shift away from the mechanical aspects of internal fixation toward the biological aspects. The emphasis in the fixation of diaphyseal fractures today is on the biology of the bone and on preserving the blood supply to the bone fragments.[6,32,37]

It has been recognized that open direct anatomic reduction, that is, direct manipulation of bone fragments, as was generally carried out during internal fixation procedures (compression method with conventional plates) to achieve interfragmentary compression, was a major cause of devitalization of the bone fragments.[28]

Imaginative thinking led to the development of the wave plate[4] and bridge plate. The basic idea is to leave the fracture zone and its fragments undisturbed by fixing the plate to the intact part of the bone on the proximal and distal sides of the fracture zone.

The technique of bridge plating (splinting method with plates) was developed to help prevent the devitalization of fragments in multifragmentary fractures.[19,38] The fracture is first reduced by indirect technique. The fragmentation zone is then bridged with a plate that is fixed to the main proximal and distal fragments. This maintains length, rotation, and axial alignment. This type of internal fixation is a form of splinting. It is not absolutely stable, and union occurs through callus formation. This plating technique is indicated for the fixation of multifragmentary fractures.

To minimize damage to the vascularization of osseous tissue and the surrounding soft tissues, indirect reduction techniques have become as popular as open reduction and internal fixation.[28] The alternative approach was advocated by Mast and colleagues,[30] who introduced indirect reduction methods and biological solutions such as bridge plating for diaphyseal fracture fixation.

While investigating the biological effects of conventional compression plates[1] on the underlying cortex, Perren and colleagues[34] made the important discovery that plates interfere significantly with the blood supply to the underlying cortex. Porotic bone formation appeared to be directly related to the amount of necrosis occurring beneath the plate. This observation led to the development of plates that ensure limited contact between the bone and the implant, for example, the limited-contact dynamic compression plate (LC-DCP) and the later development of noncontact plates.

In the 1990s, Krettek et al.[26,27] popularized minimally invasive percutaneous plate osteosynthesis techniques using conventional implants inserted through small incisions and submuscular tunnels. Cadaveric studies demonstrated better preservation of the periosteal vasculature with these minimally invasive methods than with standard open exposures for internal fixation.[10,11]

The principle of biological internal fixation consists of minimizing the biological damage caused by indirect reduction, by the surgical approach, and by contact between the implant and the bone.[3,32,37] Minimizing such damage can be achieved, but it implies less precise reduction and less stable, more flexible fixation.

Background and Development of the Technology of Locked Plates

The Zespol system, the first plate that functioned as a fixator for stabilizing long bones, was developed in the 1970s in Poland.[16] It functions mechanically as an external fixator, and the locked plate is above the skin.

SCHUHLI NUT

Several 95° fixed-angle devices, such as the blade plate or dynamic condylar screw, have been used successfully to manage such injuries; however, these devices cannot be used in all situations. This shortcoming necessitated the development of other methods to achieve fixed-angle or "locked" internal fixation constructs. Early attempts to gain angular stability of conventional screws placed through commercially available plates led to the development of the Schuhli nut (Synthes, Paoli, PA).[22] This device, essentially a threaded washer, served two purposes: it allowed screws to lock into the plate, thereby preventing screw toggle, and it limited the contact of the plate with the underlying bone in an attempt to preserve periosteal perfusion. The results of biomechanical studies and clinical series have documented the improved stability and clinical utility of these devices in managing difficult nonunions and malunions.[21]

RATIONALE BEHIND LOCKED INTERNAL FIXATORS (LIFs)

Toward the end of the 1980s, the AO (*Arbeitsgemeinschaft für Osteosynthesefragen*)/ASIF (Association for Study of Internal Fixation) started to examine internal fixator systems to further develop their plates. The key to these internal fixators is the locking mechanism of the screw in the implant, which provides angular stability. This technical detail means that there is no need to induce compression forces at the bone surface to stabilize the bone–implant construct. The lack of compression improves fracture healing, and the locking head screws obtain excellent anchorage even in osteoporotic bone. This turns a plate into an internal fixator. It functions mechanically as an external fixator but is implanted beneath the skin. This method of internal extramedullary locked splinting, which reduces mobility at the fracture site but does not eliminate it, is designed to keep the bone fragments vital and to induce indirect bone healing by callus formation.

POINT CONTACT FIXATOR

The point contact fixator (PC-FIX; Synthes, Paoli, PA) was developed in a joint venture by the AO Research Institute and the AO Development Institute. This implant has minimal contact with the bone and is secured by monocortically inserted screws. The screw's tapered head ensures that it jams in the plate hole and provides the required angular stability. Minimal contact between the plate and the bone is still necessary to ensure axial stability. Like the limited-contact dynamic compression plate (LC-DCP), the PC-Fix has shown to disrupt the underlying blood supply significantly less than the dynamic compression plate[7] (Fig. 5-1); the monocortical screws appear to damage the endosteal blood supply less than conventional bicortical screws.

The point contact fixator device (PC-Fix; Synthes, Paoli, PA) incorporates monocortical screws that lock into a plate using a Morse cone mismatch that prevents screw toggle as the screws are tightened to the plate.[33] The undersurface of the plate is undercut to allow minimal points of contact with the bone, further reducing bony devascularization. The clinical success of this type of treatment was astonishing: indirect healing resulted in early and reliable solid union. At the same time, the severity of complications declined, as there was a shift away from biological complications due to necrosis with sequestration of bone and soft tissues toward rare complications resulting from inadequate mechanical stability.

Multiple European clinical series have documented high union rates and low complication rates using the PC-Fix for fractures of the forearm.[17,31]

Locking plate technology has also been used successfully in both oral maxillofacial surgery and spinal surgery, where stability is required without bicortical screw purchase.[20,36]

DEVELOPMENT OF LOCKING HEAD SCREWS

PC-Fix was the first type of plate fixator in which angular stability was achieved by establishing a conical connection between the screw heads and screw holes. However, the tapered screw–plate connection does not provide axial anchorage of the screw in the plate, so that point contact between the plate and the bone is still required to achieve stability. A new type of thread connection between the screw head and screw hole, resulting in angular and axial stability, was therefore developed so that no contact at all is required for stability. The screw simply functions as a Schanz screw. Angular stable implants and especially angular stable noncontact plates are called locked internal fixators (LIFs). Their distinguishing mechanical feature lies mainly in the fact that stability is not achieved by friction between the undersurface of the plate and the bone, with all the associated disadvantages, but rather by connecting elements between the extramedullary load carrier and the main fragments of the bone. The rigid connection of the pins, blades, or bolts/screws to the load

---

| FIGURE 5-1 | *Comparing the Limited Contact Dynamic Compression Plate (LC-DCP)* **(B)** *with the Dynamic Compression Plate (DCP)* **(A)** *the contact area of the plate underside (shown in red), with the bone surface has been reduced and later minimized to only points with the Point Contact Fixator (PC-FIX)* **(C)**. |

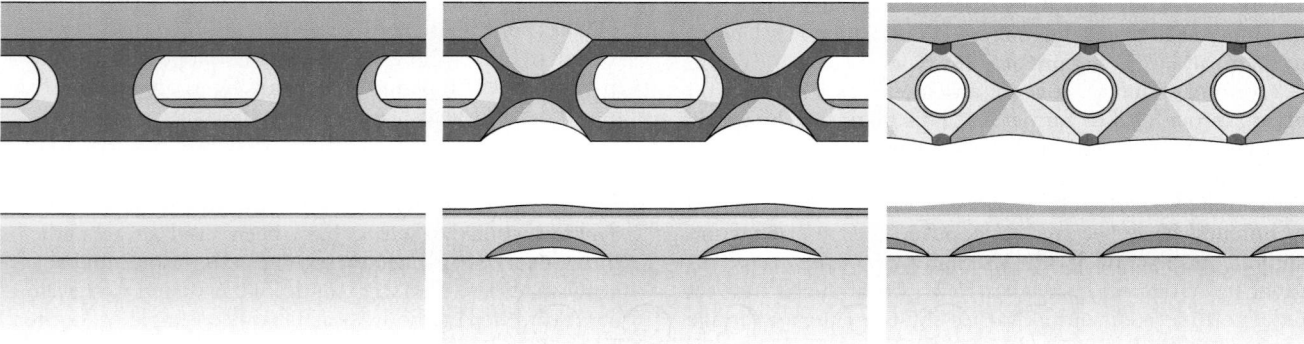

A　　　　　　　　　　**B**　　　　　　　　　　**C**

FIGURE 5-2 | *A* and *B*, *Force distribution of a plate osteosynthesis without angular stability: The screw tightening moment leads to surface pressure between the plate and bone. The friction thus created in the plate-bone contact zone stabilizes the bone fragment in relation to the load carrier. This system only becomes statically secure after bicortical screw fixation. Typical distribution of forces for a LIF osteosynthesis with angular stability: This configuration is statically secure with only monocortical fixation since the locking head screw (LHS) is anchored in a mechanically stable manner in the load carrier.*

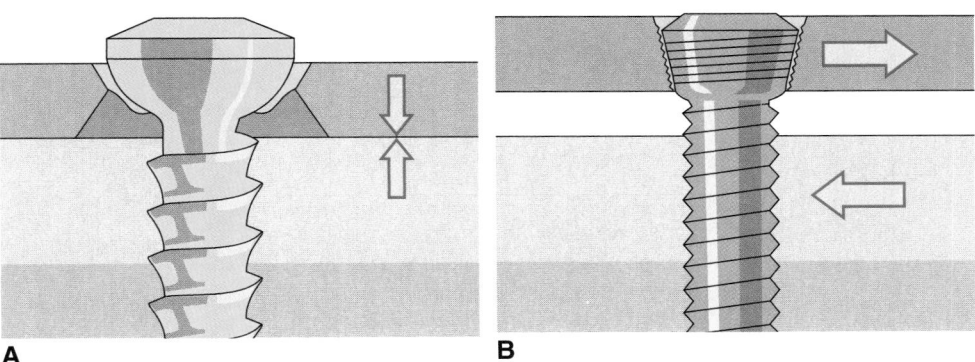

A   **B**

carrier facilitates the mechanical bridging of the fracture zone without creating friction between the load carrier and the bone. This mechanical concept is similar to external fixators (Fig. 5-2).

This type of thread connection has been incorporated into the new AO internal fixation systems—the less invasive stabilization system (LISS) and the locking compression plate (LCP). The aim of the basic locked internal fixation technique is to achieve flexible elastic fixation to trigger spontaneous healing, including the induction of callus formation, supporting the principle of minimally invasive plate osteosynthesis (MIPO).

Development of LISS

The less invasive stabilization system (LISS) for the management of distal femoral fractures and proximal lateral tibial fractures makes it possible to use a minimally invasive surgical technique, applying the principle of fracture fixation with relative stability. LISS is an anatomically preshaped internal fixator that can be inserted percutaneously by means of an adaptable insertion guide. Combined with a trocar assembly, the handle also serves as an aiming instrument for exact percutaneous placement of the self-drilling, self-tapping locking head screws. Based on extensive anatomic studies, the orientation of the individual screws is predetermined and cannot be changed. The reason for this is the angular stable screw–plate connection that is achieved with the outer thread of the screw head and the inner thread of the plate hole, which does not allow variable orientation of the screw (Fig. 5-3).

LISS for the distal femur (LISS DF) and the proximal lateral tibia (LISS-PLT) are implants that act as splints. LISS acts mechanically as an internal fixator. This device is a 100 percent locked internal fixator because only locking head screws (LHSs) are used. LISS is designed for percutaneous insertion. A less invasive approach also is possible. Closed indirect reduction and pure splinting of the fracture zone are important. Internal fracture fixation with locked fixators is a new technology in which the aim is to preserve biological conditions.*

————————————
*See references 9,10,11,14,15,18,29,35,38,41,42 and 44.

Development of the Locking Compression Plate (LCP)

LISS was originally designed as a device that would provide angular stability and accommodate only locking head screws; all of the plate holes are threaded. However, clinicians found that this technology was too restrictive in some cases and that an all-purpose implant system would offer greater flexibility. Research and development work

FIGURE 5-3 | *A* and *B*, *The less invasive stabilization system. LISS DF LISS PLT.*

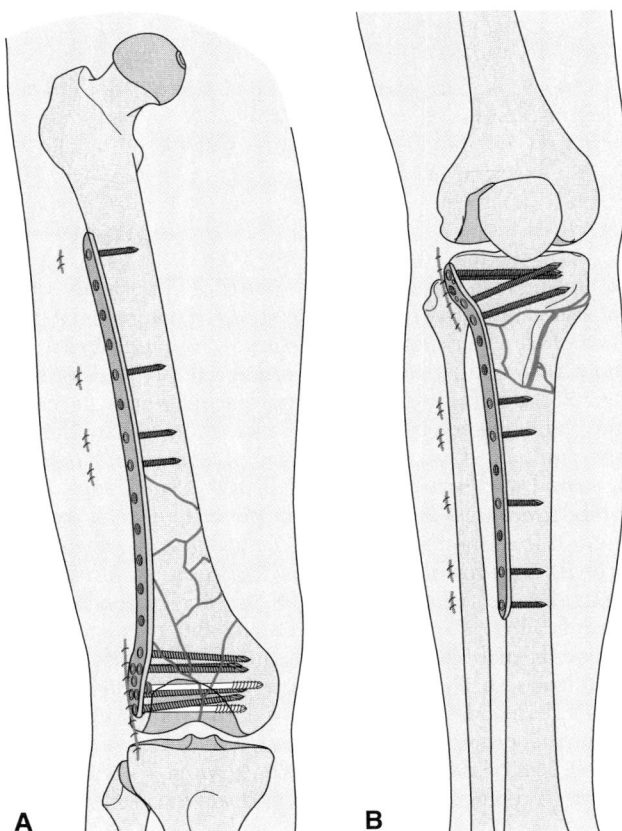

A   **B**

FIGURE 5-4   ***A–C,*** *Locking compression plate with combination hole. LCP combination hole combining two proven elements. One half of the hole has the design of the DC/LC-DCP dynamic compression unit (DCU) for conventional screws. The other half is conical and threaded to accept the matching thread of the locking head screw providing angular stability.*

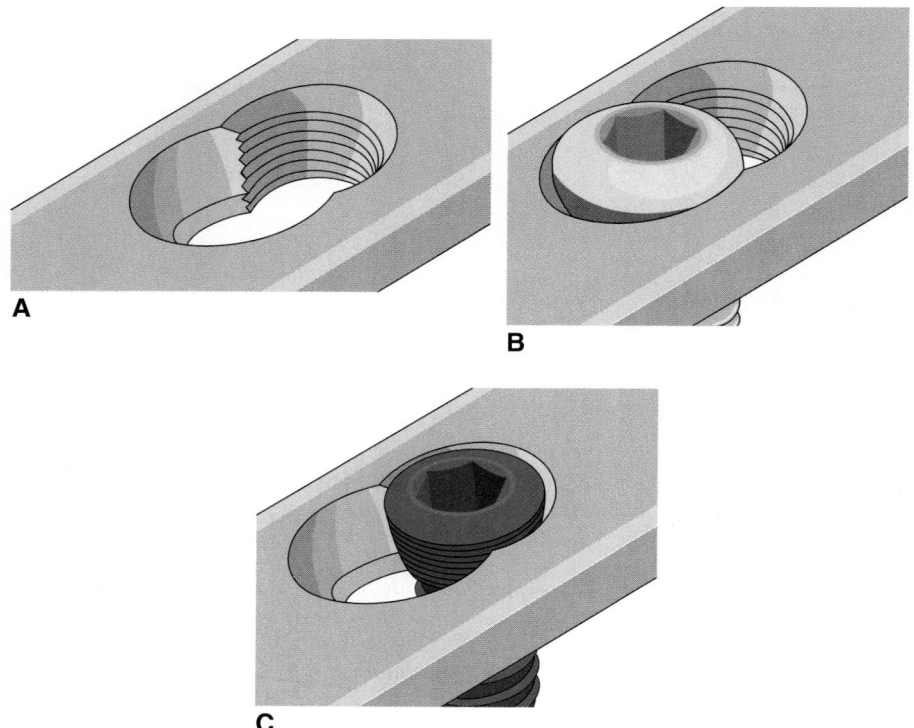

in this area—with multidisciplinary collaboration among clinicians, researchers, developers, and manufacturers—ultimately led to the concept of a combination hole, which has been incorporated into the most recent type of plate—the locking compression plate, or LCP—a single-plate system that allows the surgeon more choices.[12,13,46,47] The LCP combination hole (Fig. 5-4) allows internal fixation to be achieved by the insertion of either conventional screws (into the unthreaded part of the hole) or locking head screws with angular stability (into the threaded part of the figure-eight hole). The LHS can be inserted only at right angles into the plate. The LCP hole also makes it possible to insert different screw types into the same plate so that the surgeon can choose the type depending on intraoperative requirements. In retrospect, combining two completely different anchorage techniques into a single implant was a logical approach and a straightforward, practical solution. With the LCP, the surgeon has two plating methods to choose from and is able to select the more appropriate. With its newly designed combination hole, the LCP makes it possible to implement the methods of both compression and splinting for fracture stabilization in the same implant. The option of using the LCP either as a compression plate or as an internal fixator provides ideal plate anchorage that can be adapted to individual requirements. This significantly extends the range of indications in minimally invasive plate osteosynthesis.

Two versions of the LCP with combination holes are available: a 4.5/5.0 large-fragment version and a 3.5 small-fragment version. Special plates also are available for many anatomic regions. These LCPs are anatomically preshaped to fit the average shape of specific bones and can be inserted using open or minimally invasive techniques.

Other Technical Solutions for Locking a Screw in a Plate Hole

There are many technical possibilities for locking a screw into a plate hole. A threaded interface between plate hole and screw head creates a geometrical strong angular and axial stable interlocking of the screw with the plate. The disadvantage of a threaded interface is the predefined insertion axis of the screw in generic plates.

So-called polyaxial locking head screws have the advantage that the insertion axis of the screw can be adapted to the anatomy. This is an advantage for the use of generic plates, which are shaped intraoperatively to compensate for the changed screw direction after the plate has been adapted to the bone surface.

Solutions used to mechanically lock polyaxial locking head screws in plates are based on friction or plastic deformation of the screw–plate interface. If friction is used to lock a screw into a plate, the angular and axial stability of the locking head screw in the plate relies on the friction generated during screw insertion or on tightening an additional locking element. There are two current methods of achieving this:

1. The locking element can be part of the plate hole (e.g., Polyax, DePuy, Raynham, MA; Numelock II, Stryker, Allendale, NJ). The Polyax system is shown as an example (Fig. 5-5A). When it is not locked

FIGURE 5-5 *A–C,* Polyax system.

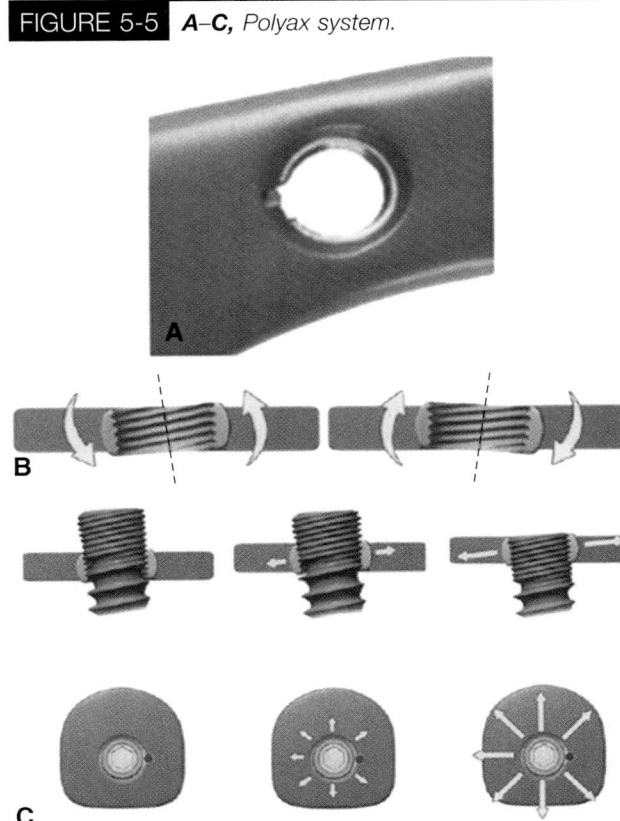

FIGURE 5-6 *A* and *B,* NCB system.

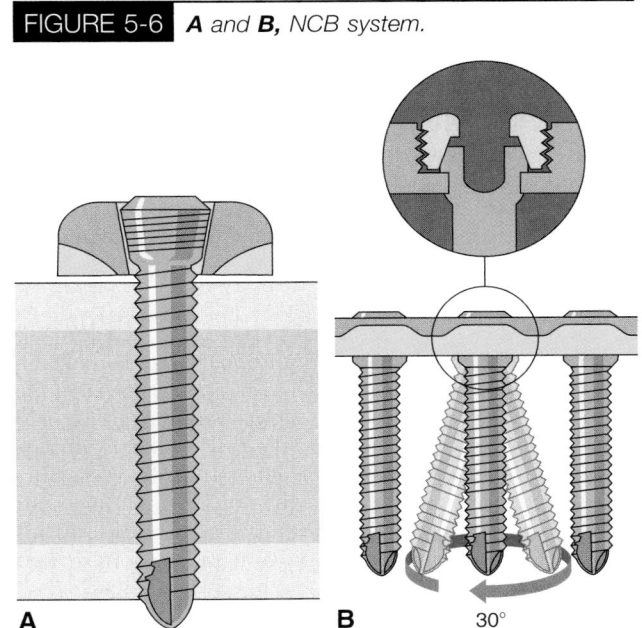

(see Fig. 5-5B), the bushing can toggle to a certain extent. The system is locked by the screw exerting a radial force (see Fig. 5-5C) on the bushing. In such systems the angular stability is related to the frictional surface area (the thickness of the plate and the screw angulation) and the force exerted.

2. Another possibility is to use a specially designed cap that is inserted on top of the bone screw head and screwed into the plate hole (e.g., NCB, Zimmer, Warsaw, IN) (Fig. 5-6A). The screw itself can toggle (Fig. 5-6B) to a certain extent and will be locked at the desired angle. Here the angular stability is related to the tightening force of the locking cap and the screw angulation.

Plastic deformation of the screw–plate interface is another well-known technique. It permits the locking head screw to be fixed off-axis to the plate hole to some degree. The plate material used to allow this deformation must be "softer" than the screw material (e.g., Litos). The plate hole has a lip (Fig. 5-7A), which, during screw insertion, is deformed, creating geometric fit (see Fig. 5-7B).

The advantages of polyaxial locking head screws must be compensated by plate size, implant material, or reduced angular stability. Depending on the clinical indication, these compromises can be acceptable. Until now, only systems with a threaded screw–plate interface could be used for basically any plate thickness, size, and implant material. In combination with the possibility to apply dynamic fracture compression through the same screw hole, basically any plate indication can be covered with one system.

In alignment with clinical preferences, more and more plates are anatomically preshaped, internal fixators having the advantage of not having to be perfectly adapted to the bone surface. Screw placement and screw directions in those anatomically preshaped plates are predefined on the basis of anatomic studies. The goal of these studies is to obtain the best screw placement, safest screw direction,

FIGURE 5-7 *A* and *B,* Litos system.

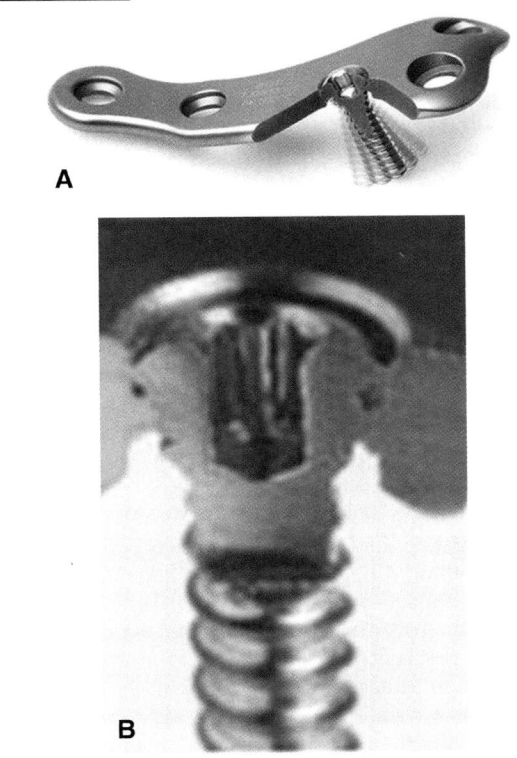

and strongest anchorage in the bone. In combination with external aiming arms, predefined screws can be placed in minimally invasive fashion through these aiming arms, through the anatomic preshaped plates, and into the bone.

Where polyaxial systems will show real clinical benefits is still in discussion, especially with the tendency toward anatomically preshaped plates. However, in pelvic fractures and periprosthetic factures, these technologies could be beneficial.

BIOMECHANICS

The more recent locked internal fixators, such as LISS and LCP with LHS, consist of plate and screw systems in which the screws are locked into the plate. The locking process minimizes the compressive forces exerted on the bone by the plate. This method of angle stable screw–plate fixation means that the plate does not have to touch the bone at all (noncontact plates), which is particularly advantageous for minimally invasive plate osteosynthesis. With these new screws, precise anatomic contouring of a plate is no longer necessary and the plate does not have to be pressed onto the bone to achieve stability. This prevents intraoperative primary displacement of the fracture caused by inexact contouring of a plate and plate fixation with conventional screws. LISS and special anatomic LCPs are preshaped to match the average anatomic form of the relevant site and require no further intraoperative alteration. The basic locked internal fixator technique aims to achieve flexible elastic fixation to stimulate spontaneous healing, including the induction of callus formation. In addition, for the compression method of conventional plating technique, the use of locking head screws are a great advantage.

Different Screws and Different Fixation of Plates onto the Bone

CONVENTIONAL SCREWS

When conventional bicortical screws are applied through a plate, the tightening of the screws compresses the plate onto the bone. The stability of this construct results from friction between the undersurface of the plate and the bone[12–14,48,49] (see Fig. 5-4A–C).

If a conventional cortex or cancellous bone screw is inserted into the bone and tightened, axial preload of the threads in the bone will be achieved. This procedure prevents the micromovements that can lead to bone resorption and, consequently, to screw loosening.

Conventional plating techniques for fracture fixation require adequate plate-bone contact and screw tightening to achieve stability between the plate and one surface. Loss

of reduction, delayed union, and nonunion are complications encountered with conventional plating techniques.

With compression plating, stress risers caused by remaining screw holes and avascular bone under the plate may lead to refracture after implant removal. The LC-DCP with partial preservation of osseous blood supply may limit this complication.

LOCKING HEAD SCREWS

All locking head screws (LHSs) provide angular and axial stability inside the plate hole. They act more like bolts than screws, and there is a complete absence of axial preloading within the screw during its insertion. The advantages of LHSs include improved anchorage in bone resulting from the slight increase in the outer screw diameter and the altered loading conditions. Under functional loading they are loaded in bending and in axial load depending on the external loading condition. LHSs cannot be used as lag screws. From a biological point of view, they have the additional advantage of no contact between the plate and bone, thereby protecting the blood supply to the bone (see Fig. 5-4A–C).

Two different types of LHS are available: self-drilling and self-tapping only for monocortical use and self-tapping for bicortical use (Fig. 5-8A and B). Each design has distinct indications, contraindications, and pitfalls.

SELF-DRILLING, SELF-TAPPING LHS

Self-drilling, self-tapping LHSs are used only as monocortical screws in the diaphyseal segment of bone when excellent bone quality is present. The cutting tip of the screw prevents destruction of the bone thread in the near cortex when there is a narrow medullary cavity because the screw tip is able to penetrate the opposite cortex. When a self-drilling, self-tapping LHS is anchored in both cortices, the drilling unit protrudes well into the soft tissues, with a potential risk of damage to the neurovascular structures in that area. Furthermore, inserting a self-drilling, self-tapping LHS by percutaneous freehand technique (i.e., without an aiming device) sometimes results in imperfect centering of the screw tip in the hole and angulation of the LHS. Accordingly, bicortical purchase is less important than with nonlocking plates. Avoiding bicortical drilling also theoretically minimizes further damage to the endosteal circulation and may decrease the risk of refracture after plate removal.[14,48,49] Current locking plate designs have used self-drilling, self-tapping monocortical screws (less invasive stabilization system, or LISS; Synthes); this has eliminated the need to measure the length for percutaneous screw insertion, decreased inventory, and minimized surgical time.

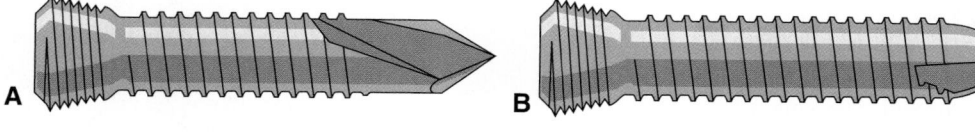

FIGURE 5-8 *A and B, Different types of locking head screws. Self-drilling, self-tapping locking head screw. Self-tapping locking head screw.*

A   B

SELF-TAPPING LHS

Self-tapping LHSs are used in the epiphyseal, metaphyseal, and diaphyseal segments of the bone when the insertion of a bicortical LHS or the longest possible LHS is planned. The self-tapping LHS has a blunt rather than a sharp cutting tip. To provide good anchorage of the screw threads in both cortices, the self-tapping LHS should protrude slightly beyond the far cortex.

Self-tapping LHSs need predrilling through the threaded drill sleeve. If this technique is performed correctly, the mono- or bicortical self-tapping LHS is always perpendicular and in the center of the threaded conical part of the combination hole.

In the presence of osteoporosis, the bone cortex is usually thin. In these conditions, the working length of a monocortical LHS is short, so that poor anchorage is obtained even with locking head screws (Fig. 5-9A–D) This difficulty can lead to complete loss of screw anchorage, resulting in instability of the fixation—a common situation in bones that are subjected to mainly torsional loading (e.g., the humerus). The use of bicortical self-tapping LHSs is recommended in all segments for all osteoporosis-associated fractures. This approach improves the working length and avoids potential problems at the interface between the screw thread and bone (Fig. 5-10). Even the shortest monocortical self-tapping LHS will destroy the bone thread if the screw tip touches the opposite cortex before the screw head has locked into the plate hole. If this occurs, the LHS should be replaced with a bicortical self-tapping LHS, which will ensure anchorage in the opposite cortex (Fig. 5-11A–C). The problem can be avoided at an early stage of the procedure by drilling both cortices (e.g., in bones of small diameter such as forearm or fibula).

MONOCORTICAL OR BICORTICAL LHS

Monocortical LHSs can be used only in the diaphyseal segment of long bones when the bone quality is normal, when the cortex is thick enough to allow anchorage of the screw with a sufficient working length of the thread, and when the specific bone has a low loading level in torque.

Bicortical LHSs are recommended in the following situations: weak osteoporotic bone, thin bone cortex that does not provide a sufficient working length for the screw, high torsional loading in the plated bone segment, a short main fragment that only allows a limited number of screws, in bones of small diameter, when a previous cortical reduction screw is replaced by an LHS, and after destruction of the bone thread in the near cortex due to incorrect insertion of the LHS.

SELECTING THE TYPE OF SCREW[47,49]

Four different types of screws can be used with the LCP. Careful analysis of the intended function is required to ensure optimal use of the different types (Table 5-1).

- Cortex screw, self-tapping cortex screw, cortex shaft screw
- Cancellous bone screw
- Self-drilling, self-tapping locking head screw (for monocortical use only)
- Self-tapping locking head screw (for mono- or bicortical use)

The following factors are critical for the appropriate choice of screw:

- The mechanical principle of fixation required:
  - Locked splinting versus interfragmentary compression method
  - Locked internal fixator versus standard plating technique
  - Plate fixation to the bone with LHS (noncontact plate) or standard screw compression
- Technique of reduction and plate insertion:
  - Minimally invasive plate osteosynthesis (MIPO) technique versus open reduction and internal fixation (ORIF)
  - Epiphyseal area versus diaphyseal/metaphyseal area

Cancellous bone screws and cortex screws are designed to create compression. They can be used as position

---

FIGURE 5-9 *A–D, The working length of monocortical screws depends on the thickness of the bone cortex. In normal bone, this working length is sufficient. In osteoporotic bone, by contrast, the cortex is usually very thin so that the working length of a monocortical screw is insufficient. This difference in working length is important when osteoporotic bones such as the humerus have to be stabilized. In normal bone, the length of anchorage of the screw thread is sufficient enough to withstand rotational displacement. When there is osteoporosis, the working length is very short due to the thin cortex, and under torque the bone thread will quickly wear out, leading to secondary displacement and instability.*

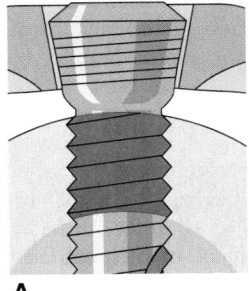

A

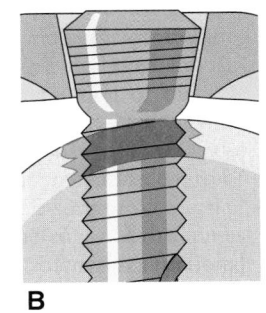

B

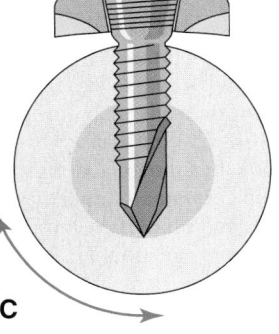

C

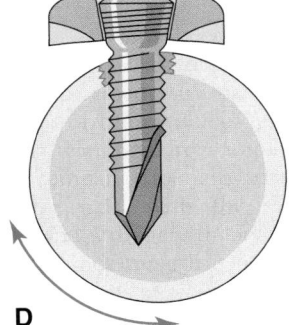

D

FIGURE 5-10 *Improvement of the working length. In osteoporotic bone with a very thin cortex, the standard use of bicortical screws is recommended, as the longer working length leads to a much better torque resistance.*

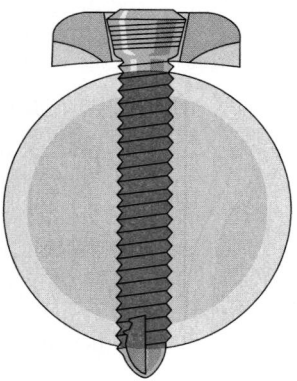

screws, to compress the plate to the bone surface, or as lag screws—plate-dependent, inserted through a plate hole, or plate-independent—to create interfragmentary compression. In combination with a plate, these screws are also used as eccentric compression screws or as fixation screws. Their use is recommended when the screw has to be inserted at an angle in cases of axial malalignment between the bone and plate axis, to avoid screw penetration into a joint, whenever interfragmentary compression with eccentric screw insertion or a lag screw is required, or with a bridge plating technique with good bone quality. Cancellous bone screws or cortex screws are also used for reduction of a fragment onto the plate. These screws are usually anchored in both cortices; monocortical screw insertion is only carried out exceptionally.

Cancellous bone screws and cortex screws have the advantage that they can be angulated within the plate hole, making it possible to reduce fragments onto the plate. Their disadvantage is that they compromise the blood supply to the bone cortex owing to the need for direct contact between the plate and the bone to allow load transmission by a friction force (Table 5-2).

Earlier AO guidelines recommending specific numbers of screws or cortices in each fragment should no longer be the only deciding factor for anchoring a plate in the main fragments. For adequate stabilization, it is more important to insert a few screws with high plate leverage (e.g., a long plate with enough distance between the LHSs in each main fragment) to reduce the load on the screws.

From a purely mechanical point of view, two monocortical LHS screws in each main fragment in the shaft area are the minimum requirement to keep the construct stable. However, this type of construct will fail if one screw breaks owing to overloading or if bone resorption occurs at the interface between the bone cortex and the screw thread, leading to loosening (screw pull-out). The use of two bicortical screws in each fragment does not improve the situation in relation to screw fatigue failure, but it does enhance the working length of the screw and thus improve

FIGURE 5-11 ***A–C,*** *Danger of insertion of monocortical self-tapping LHS. In bones with a small diameter, the tip of the screw can contact the opposite bone cortex before the screw head has engaged in the thread of the plate hole. This leads to the destruction of the bone thread in the near cortex and complete loss of anchorage of the screw. The situation can be resolved by using a threaded drill sleeve; the opposite cortex is drilled in the correct axis, inserting a self-tapping bicortical LHS to obtain anchorage in the opposite cortex.*

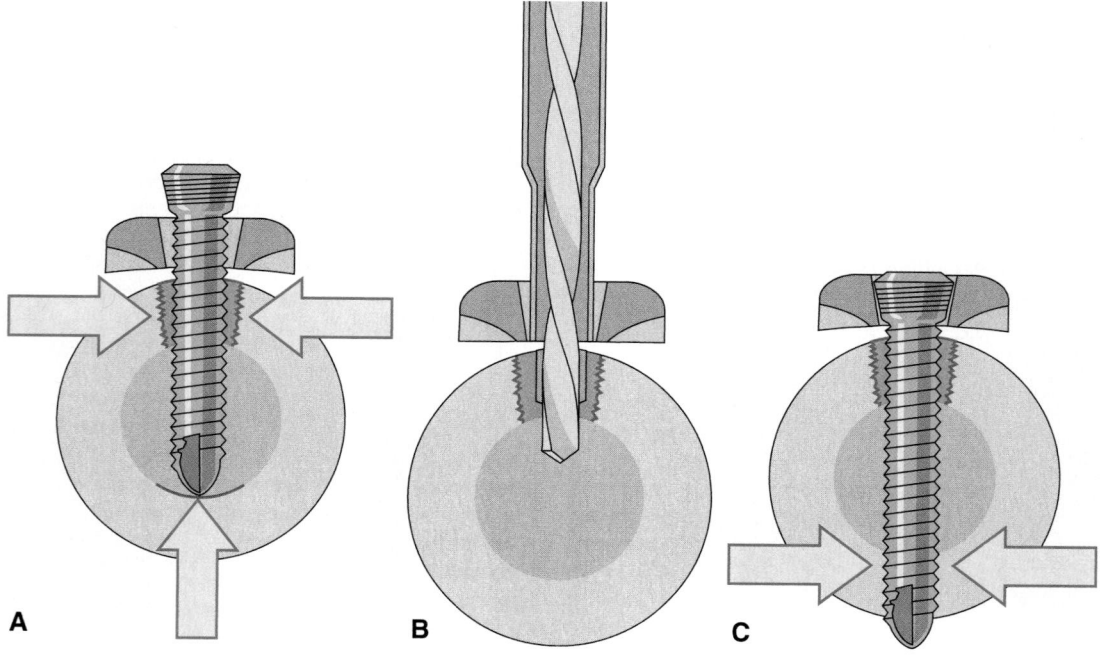

A   **B**   **C**

Table 5-1
Select the Correct Screw Type

Type of Screw	Bone Segment	Function of Screw	Anchorage
Cancellous bone screw: partially (i.e., cancellous shaft screw) or fully threaded	Epiphysis Metaphysis	Free, plate-independent lag screws* Plate lagging screws* Plate fixation screw	As long as possible
Cortex screw, self-tapping cortex screw	Diaphysis Epiphysis Metaphysis	Free, plate-independent lag screw Plate lagging screw Plate fixation screw Position screw Reduction screw	Monocortical or bicortical
Cortex shaft screw partially threaded	Diaphysis	Free, plate-independent lag screw Plate lagging screw	Monocortical
Self-tapping locking head screw	Epiphysis Metaphysis Diaphysis	Plate fixation screw Plate-dependent position screw	Monocortical or bicortical (in metaphysis and epiphysis as long as possible)
Self-drilling, self-tapping locking head screw	Diaphysis	Plate fixation screw	Monocortical

*Only partially threaded cancellous screws can be used as lag screws.

the anchorage at the interface between the screw thread and the bone. Even when the surgeon ensures that all of the screws are inserted correctly, this type of construct can only be used in bone of good quality. For safety reasons, a minimum of three screws per main fragment is recommended in all other cases.

When fractures are being fixed in the epiphyseal and metaphyseal areas, neither the length of the plate nor the number of screws should be chosen on the basis of mechanical considerations alone. The longest possible LHSs are recommended, but penetration of the articular surface must be avoided. The local anatomy and the length of the epiphyseal and/or metaphyseal fragment are also relevant to the decision. In these cases, the use of metaphyseal plates or anatomically preshaped plates is recommended to achieve balanced fixation, with load bearing being distributed equally between the proximal and distal plate segments anchored in the two main fragments.

Table 5-2
Different Functions and Rules of Screws

Function	Type of Screw	Effect	Prerequisites
Lag screw – free, plate-independent – plate lagging screw	Cortex screw* Cortex shaft screw† Cancellous shaft screw#	Interfragmentary compression	Gliding hole, threaded hole for a fully threaded screw or partially threaded
Eccentric screw = compression screw	Cortex and self-tapping cortex screw Cancellous bone screw	Interfragmentary compression	Dynamic compression unit (DCU) and hemispheric screw head of conventional screw
Plate fixation screw	Cortex and self-tapping cortex screw Cancellous bone screw Self-tapping LHS	Friction between bone and plate Locking	For conventional screws, good bone quality and prebending of the plate
Position screw – free, plate-independent – through a plate hole	Cortex and self-tapping cortex screw Cancellous full threaded bone screws Self-tapping LHS	Holds the relative position between two fragments	Threaded hole in each fragment Only plate dependent
Reduction screw	Cortex screw and self-tapping cortex screw LHS/Fine tunning	Reduction onto the plate Reduction of a butterfly fragment	No interfragmentary compression LHS + screwdriver, screw hold sleeve

*Self-tapping screws are not recommended for use as lag screws.
† and # partially threaded.

FIGURE 5-12   *A and **B**, Load transfer from bone to splint. Plate and cortex screws (compression). Plate and locking head screws.*

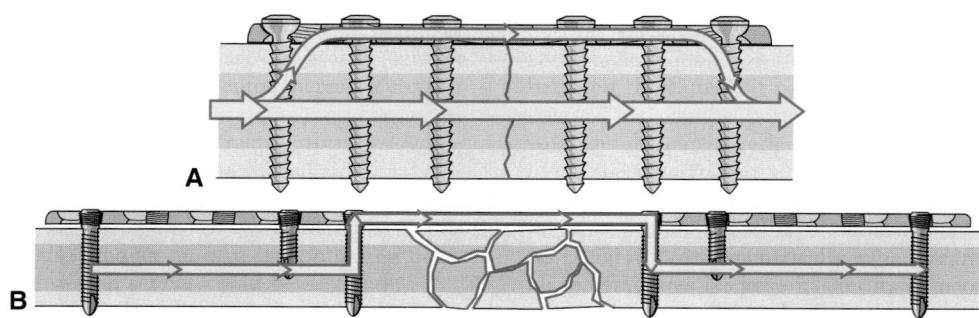

Because the standard screws are free to toggle in the plate, stability requires bicortical purchase of these screws. However, with a locking plate construct, threads on the screw head lock into corresponding threads in the screw hole of the plate (see Fig. 5-2A and B), thus eliminating toggle. The forces are transferred from the bone to the plate across the screw–plate threaded connection[13,14,48,49] (Fig. 5-12A and B). Compression of the plate to the underlying bone therefore is not required to achieve construct stability, and the blood supply to the bone directly under the plate is preserved.

Full understanding of the mechanics of locking plates and monocortical screws requires an appreciation of the prevailing forces these fixation constructs must withstand in different anatomic regions of a bone. Bone quality is less dense in the metaphysis than in the diaphysis. Therefore, locked screws are usually placed in long rows perpendicular to the applied load and the limb axis. When, in a medial bony defect, a cantilever bending force is applied, multiple locking head screws function like small blade plates, resisting the bending moment. Under the same circumstances, conventional screw–plate fixation allows toggle and thus progressive varus deformity. In the diaphysis, locked screws can also be inserted perpendicular to the axial load, but they are then more commonly loaded in shear, similar to the prevailing conditions when half pins are inserted for external fixation.[14]

The pull-out strength of a monocortical locked screw is about 60 percent of the strength of a standard bicortical screw.[14] In fact, a locked screw–plate construct can be thought of as being similar to an implanted external fixator. Studies of the biomechanics of monolateral external fixation have shown improved stability of constructs that incorporate wide spacing of half pins and placement of the connecting bar as close to the bone as possible. A locking plate construct might be considered the ultimate external fixator, with minimal soft tissue dissection, wide screw spacing, locked screws, and the plate functioning as the connecting bar, placed extremely close to the mechanical axis of the bone. Although a direct comparison has not been made, the ability to move the plate closer to the mechanical axis should markedly increase stability compared with a monolateral external fixator, in which the

bar is far from the limb axis, creating a large bending moment.

Since locking head screws are not tightened in the bone but in the plate instead, no axial preload will occur within the bone. The locking head screws cannot be over-tightened even in poor bone structures. Nevertheless, a so-called press-fit technique through radial preload, as used for pin-type connections, is applied to prevent harmful micromovements.

The advantages of angular stability become far clearer for a system comprising several screws in a plate. In a plate–screw configuration with nonlocking screws, conventional screws are stand-alone screws, and sequential loosening of the screws occurs when force is applied. The lack of angular stability permits each screw to align along the axis of force. This leads to gradual loosening with pull-out of the individual screws. In the case of fixed-angle application, en bloc fixation is achieved. The LHS can no longer be regarded as a stand-alone screw, and the fixed-angle connection between the plate and the screw head prevents screw orientation along the axis of force. Pull-out can occur only en bloc (Fig. 5-13A–E).

The effect of en bloc fixation can be reinforced by convergent or divergent positioning of the screws, an approach applied chiefly in metaphyseal areas. Several screws inserted in convergent or divergent positions and in fixed-angle technique achieve such a high level of stability that failure can only be due to pull-out of the entire system or to plate failure.

The aspects of load transmission across a fracture stabilized with a locking screw plate device in comparison to existing devices demonstrates the theoretical, practical, and comparative advantages of the locking plate. To understand this comparison requires an appreciation of the concepts of working length, mechanics of standard plate stability, and the effect of cantilever bending.

The working length of a plate-bone construct is the length of plate unsupported by bone because of comminution, segmental bone loss, or other reasons.[4] Bridge plates span large areas of comminution and thus typically have long working lengths.[4] Although biologically advantageous because they help preserve soft tissue, such constructs are often at a mechanical disadvantage, especially when they

FIGURE 5-13 *A–E, Pull-out of standard screws and locking head screws (LHS). Fixation with cortex screws. Pull-out of cortex screws by a bending load. Sequential screw loosening. Fixation with LHS, en bloc fixation. LHS provides greater resistance against bending loads. Pull-out of LHS with axial loading.*

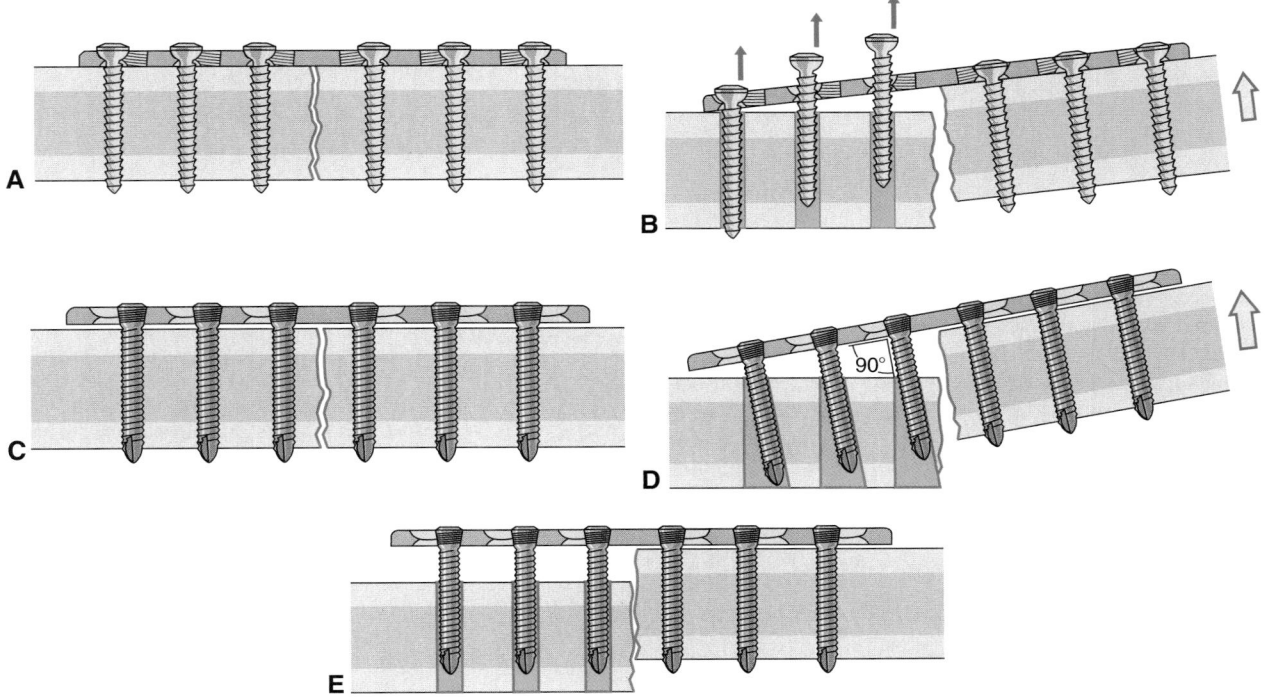

are used for periarticular injuries, a common application. These fractures frequently have short periarticular fragments and long working lengths; the result is coronal plane instability and consequent collapse when standard non-locking plates are used. To avoid this, a fixed angle must be provided between the plate and the fixation into the periarticular segment. This can be achieved with 95° fixed-angle devices. The locking screw–plate design facilitates a similar mechanical advantage with multiple points of screw fixation. This is most important in fractures with long working lengths, short periarticular segments, and the absence of bony support on the side of the fracture opposite the plate.

LENGTH OF THE IMPLANT

The development of locking plates has resulted in relatively unusual fixation constructs of long plates that use few, often monocortical, screws. Understanding the design rationale and potential clinical applications of such unconventional plates requires a basic understanding of the biomechanics of plate fixation.

The choice of the appropriate length of the LCP (and of all plates) is one of the most important steps in internal fixation. It depends on the fracture pattern and the method and mechanical principle being used for fixation. In intramedullary nailing, there is no question regarding the length of the nail, which is more or less equal to the complete length of the fractured bone from one epiphysis to the other (Fig. 5-14).

The external fixator also bridges almost the entire length of the bone. In contrast, the length of the plate was a matter of controversy for some time. In the past, a short (or too short) plate was often chosen to avoid a long skin incision and extensive soft tissue dissection. With the newer techniques of indirect reduction, with subcutaneous or submuscular insertion of the implant and the new locked splinting method to bridge the fracture zone, the plate length can be increased without additional soft tissue dissection. Little or no additional biological damage is caused, and the plate length can be adapted to the mechanical requirements of the specific fracture. From the mechanical point of view, plate loading and screw loading should be kept as low as possible to avoid fatigue failure of the plate due to cyclic loading or pull-out of the screws due to excessive single overloading. A long plate should be used.

Three segments of the plate can be distinguished: the middle segment at the fracture site between the two innermost screws, and the proximal and distal plate segments anchoring the implant onto the proximal and distal main fragments. The length of the plate and the positioning of the screws influence the loading conditions in the plate and screws. The length of the middle plate segment and the method of spanning the fracture are responsible for the biological response of fracture healing (indirect healing, direct healing, or failure to heal) (Fig. 5-15).

FIGURE 5-14   *Prerequisites for using the LCP as a locked internal fixator: long plate/fixator; adequate space between the LHS in each main fragment. Avoid stress concentration while leaving out three or four plate holes without screws in the fracture zone.*

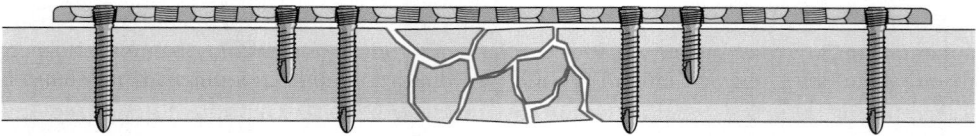

The ideal length for the internal fixator can be determined using two values: the plate-span ratio and the plate–screw density.[49] The plate-span ratio is the ratio of plate length to overall fracture length. It was found empirically that the plate-span ratio should be greater than 2:1 or 3:1 in multifragmentary fractures and greater than 8:1, 9:1, or 10:1 in simple fractures. The plate–screw density is the proportion of the number of screws inserted to the number of plate holes. Values below 0.5 to 0.4 are recommended, indicating that fewer than half of the plate holes are occupied by screws.

Locking Plates and the Splinting Method

Bridge plating can be carried out with both standard screws and locking head screws. The method of splinting the fracture zone with standard plates and conventional screws, using a "no-touch" technique combined with indirect reduction, was a great step forward when it was introduced. Only the main fragments were fixed to the plate. With conventional screws, it was necessary to preshape the plate to fit the main fragment.

However, LHSs are preferable for bridge plating procedures, since it is easier to carry out the MIPO technique because there is no need to preshape the plate and the fragments do not pull on the plate, resulting in primary loss of reduction. In addition, there is no disturbance—or only minimal disturbance—to the periosteal blood supply. It is possible to use both conventional screws and LHSs in normal-quality bone. In soft osteoporotic bone, LHSs should be used for additional stability. Technically, the locked splinting method (pure splinting) can be carried out either with an open approach or with the MIPO technique and indirect closed approximate reduction. LISS and LCP with LHS look like plates but, biomechanically, they are locked splints or fixators (locked internal fixators) (Fig. 5-16A and B).

Locking Plates and the Compression Method

CONVENTIONAL PLATING TECHNIQUE WITH LOCKING PLATES

Despite the advantages of locked internal fixators, there is still a need for the anatomic reconstruction and absolute stability that are provided by conventional plates and

FIGURE 5-15   *Importance of the plate-span ratio and plate–screw density in bridge plating technique. The schematic drawing shows a mechanically sound fixation of a multifragmentary diaphyseal fracture in the lower leg. The ratio between the length of the plate and the length of the fracture is known as the plate-span ratio. In this case, the ratio is high enough—that is, approximately 3, indicating that the plate is three times longer than the overall fracture area. The plate–screw density is shown for all the three bone segments. The proximal main fragment has a plate–screw density of 0.5 (three out of six holes occupied); the segment over the fracture has a density of 0 (none of four holes occupied); and the distal main fragment has a density of 0.75 (three out of four holes occupied). The higher plate–screw density in the distal main fragment has to be accepted, since for anatomic reasons there is no way of reducing it. The overall plate–screw density for the construct in this example is 0.43 (six screws in a 14-hole plate).*

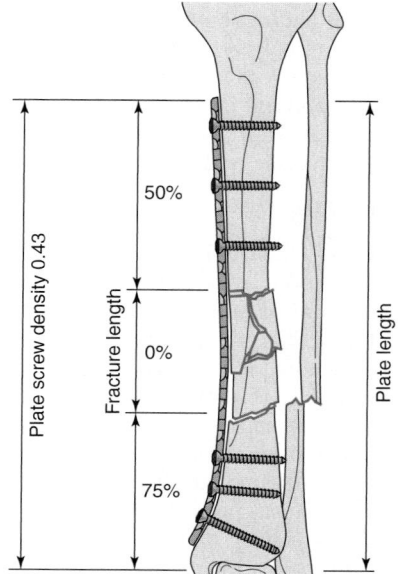

FIGURE 5-16 *A* and *B,* Bridging the fracture zone with a long plate. The bridging plate is only fixed to the main fragments proximally and distally. Fixation with conventional screws presses the plate against the bone, and the shape of the plate has to be adapted to the bone. Locked internal fixator: LHSs are angular and axial stable. No compression of the plate onto the bone is required to achieve stability.

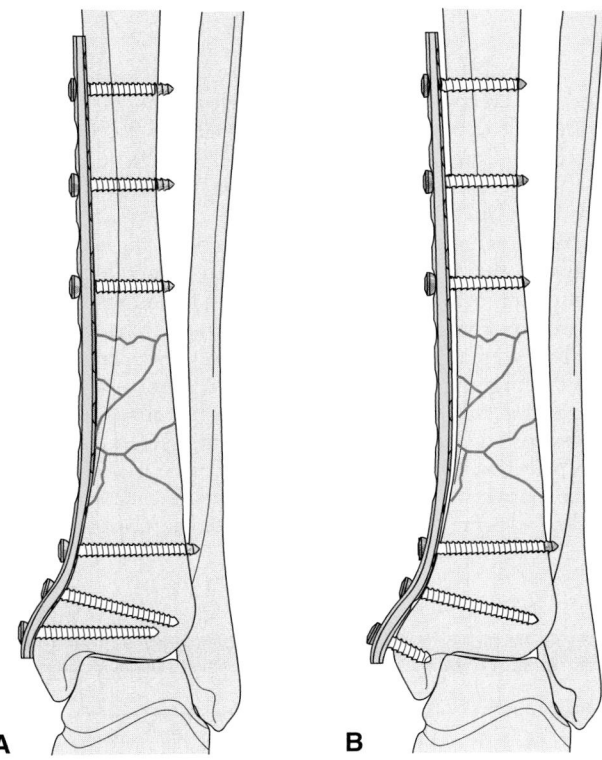

A   B

screws. Appropriate indications for the latter include intra-articular fractures, osteotomies, complex bone reconstruction procedures, pseudarthroses, and fractures with traumatic damage to the blood supply. A lag screw can also be placed independently from the plate, with a protection plate being fixed with locking head screws (Fig. 5-17A and B). This technique is much easier to perform than trying to insert a lag screw through a plate hole. There is no risk of primary loss of reduction. In soft osteoporotic bone, LHSs find a better hold and there is less or no risk of screw loosening.

The method of interfragmentary compression can be also achieved using the LCP as a compression plate for axial compression (Fig. 5-18).

CLINICAL APPLICATION, INDICATIONS, AND TECHNIQUES
Concepts of Fracture Fixation

The theoretical principles underlying fracture fixation are the establishment of stability—either absolute or relative stability, meaning maximal or less mechanical stability after osteosynthesis. The two methods applied to achieve these goals are compression (static or dynamic) and splinting (locked or unlocked). A variety of techniques and implant technologies are applied in the steps required to carry out these two methods (Fig. 5-19 and Table 5-3).

Plate osteosynthesis has changed in the last decades. The last milestone is the locking of screws in the plate hole. In some situations the locked non-contact plates have biological and biomechanical advantages over the compression method with conventional compression plating technique. These advantages of the locking compression plate can be used best in combination with the methodological principle of locked extramedullary splinting.

Less Invasive Stabilization System

The LISS approach is based on the use of anatomically shaped buttress plates that are anchored by the insertion of self-drilling and self-tapping monocortical locking head screws.

The system consists of instruments required to join the fixator and insertion guide together. These include the stabilization bolt, fixation bolt, and drill sleeve. The other instruments have been designed to facilitate the temporary positioning of the fixator, the adjustment of its position, and reduction before the first screws are inserted to attach the fixator to the bone. These include K-wires that can be inserted through the insertion guide and the aiming device for K-wires.

The LISS plate is designed for the distal lateral femur aspect (LISS-DF) and the proximal lateral tibia (LISS-PLT) and acts as an anatomically shaped buttress plate anchored with self-drilling, self-tapping monocortical locking head screws. The screws are connected to the plate by a thread on the outer edge of the screw head and on the inner edge of the plate hole. LISS is an anatomically pre-shaped internal fixator that can be inserted percutaneously by means of an adaptable insertion guide. As a true internal fixator, the applied LISS fixation construct must be longer than conventional plates. The LISS-DF and the LISS-PLT are available in three lengths (5, 9, and 13 holes), right

FIGURE 5-17 *A* and *B,* Protection plate with independent lag screw.

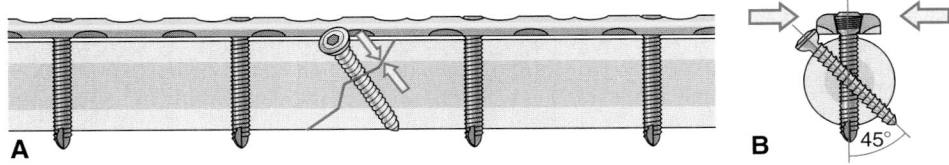

A   B   45°

FIGURE 5-18 *A* and *B,* Compression plate. After reduction of this fracture, the plate is fixed with LHS to one fragment. Then an eccentric cortex screw is inserted in the dynamic compression part of the combination hole at the other end of the plate. Finally, stabilization with an additional LHS. No compression to the periosteum in the fracture zone. Interfragmentary compression plating using dynamic compression unit.

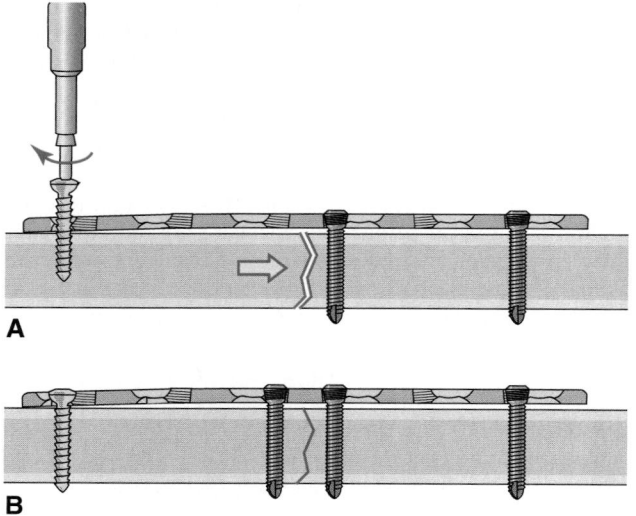

A

B

FIGURE 5-19 *Spectrum of stability.*

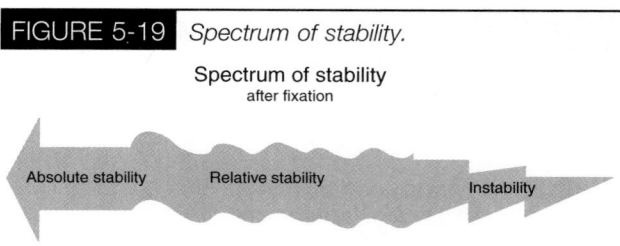

Spectrum of stability
after fixation

Absolute stability   Relative stability   Instability

Stability is a spectrum from
total to none
In other words
absolute to relative

and left versions. With the development of the LCP combination hole, anatomically preshaped LCP-DF and LCP-PLT are also available (Fig. 5-20A–D).

The screws are connected to the plate by a thread on the outer surface of the screw head and a mating thread on the inner surface of the plate hole. The angular stability between the screws and the plate no longer requires any compression between the plate and the bone to ensure secure anchorage. LISS is a noncontact plate. Each self-drilling, self-tapping screw requires a new sharp drill bit for drilling and a sharp tap to cut the thread, after which the screw follows into the precisely prepared hole. The monocortical self-drilling, self-tapping screws lock into the plate and fasten the proximal and distal main fragments after indirect reduction has been carried out. Owing to the locking design, the LHS does not need to obtain purchase

Table 5-3				
Different Concepts of Fracture Fixation				
Principle of Fracture Fixation = Grade of Stabilization	**Method**		**Technique and Implant Function**	**Bone Healing**
Absolute stability = high	**Compression**		Lag screw (conventional screw)	**Direct**
	Static*		Lag screw and protection plate	
			Compression plate	
			Tension band	
	Dynamic†		Tension band plate	
			Buttress plate‡	
	Splinting	External splinting	External fixator**	
		Intramedullary splinting	Intramedullary nail**	
	Locked#			
		Internal extramedullary splinting	Bridging with standard plate	
			Bridging with locked internal fixator	
		External splinting	Conservative fracture treatment (cast, traction)	
	Unlocked§	Intramedullary splinting	Elastic nail	
Relative stability = low		K-wire		**Indirect**

*Fracture under compression—implant under tension.
†Compression under function.
#Locked splinting with control of length, alignment, and rotation.
§Splinting with limited control of length, alignment, and rotation.
**Can be changed to dynamic compression in case of a dynamically locked nail or dynamic external fixator.
‡Using an angular stable plate–screw construct (i.e., LISS or LCP with LHS) as buttress plate, the plate acts as a blade plate. Occasionally a buttress plate may be considered as a splint.

FIGURE 5-20 | *A–D, Different types of internal fixators for the distal femur and the proximal lateral tibia. LISS-DF plate LCP-DF plate LISS-PLT plate LCP-PLT plate.*

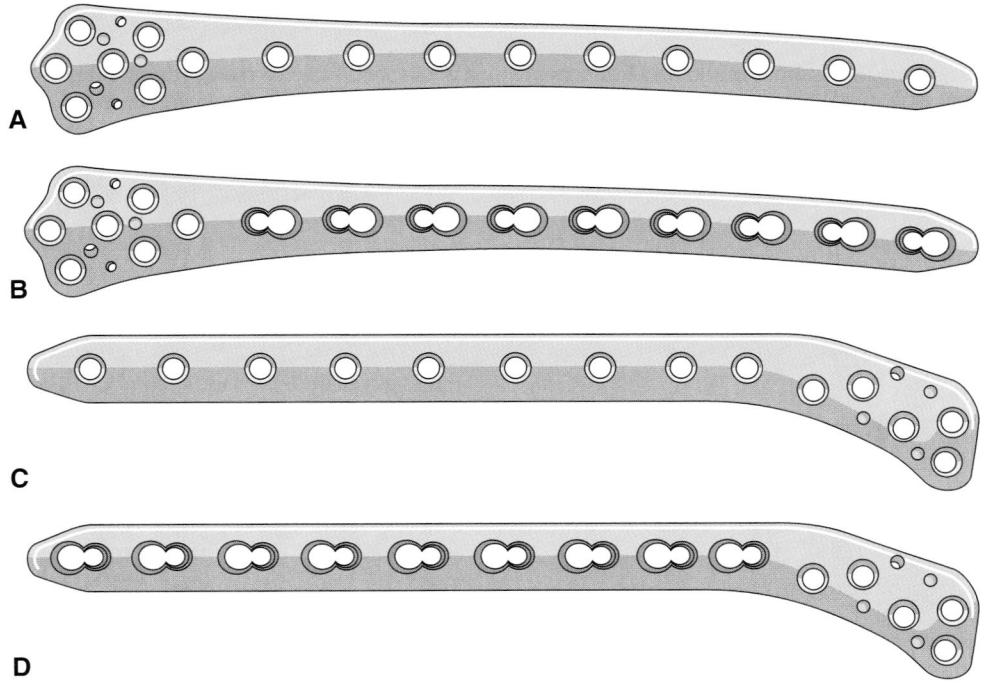

in the second cortex and can easily be inserted percutaneously and by self-drilling. This produces a better bone-plate construct compared with the use of conventional screws. The stability of the bone-implant construct results from the angular stability of the plate–screw interface rather than from the friction generated between the plate and bone, as with conventional implants. This has mechanical advantages and avoids problems related to the bone-implant interface, such as the "windshield wiper" effect.

LISS resembles a plate but functions as a fully implanted fixator offering "biological" internal fixation. The primary objectives are to minimize biological damage due to surgical intervention, to provide an improved implant anchoring especially in osteoporotic bones and immediate postoperative active or passive motion of the adjacent joints, resulting in an uneventful fracture healing.

LESS INVASIVE STABILIZATION SYSTEM FOR THE DISTAL FEMUR

INDICATIONS The indications for LISS DF include all extra-articular (supracondylar, distal shaft) and intra-articular fractures that cannot be treated with screws alone, for example, Müller AO classification 33-A1–A3 and 33-C1–C3 fractures of the distal femur (Table 5-4).[2,18,25,35,42,49] The LISS technique is advantageous in severe intra-articular fractures,[32] since it allows free placement of lag screws and does not additionally disrupt the condylar complex after reconstruction. It preserves the soft tissues in the metaphyseal and diaphyseal regions as a result of minimally invasive insertion and closed reduction.[3,10,11,26,30,45] LISS also makes it possible to stabilize fractures where

Table 5-4
Indications for LISS DF in Femoral Fractures
• Supracondylar fractures (33-A1–A3)
• Articular fractures (33-C1–C3)
• Distal shaft fractures (32-B1–B3 and 32-C1–C3 if nailing is not possible)
• Periprosthetic fractures (distal to hip prosthesis or proximal to knee prosthesis)
• Repeated fracture with implants in place
• Fractures in osteoporotic bone
• Pathological fracture

implants are already in situ (e.g., total knee replacements[6]) whether or not they have a medullary stem. Since screws can be inserted into all seven distal screw holes, LISS offers a high degree of stability and reliability in osteoporotic bone. No other implant currently available has such a wide range of applications. There are certain cases for which LISS provides a unique answer, especially when the distal femoral block is short. These include multiplane, complex distal articular injuries, especially with a short distal segment, osteoporotic fractures, and fractures above a total knee arthoplasty.

APPROACHES The surgical procedure essentially depends on whether or not an intra-articular fracture requires open reduction. In nonarticular fractures (Müller AO classification A1–A3) and fractures with simple articular involvement (Müller AO classification C1 and C2), a lateral approach to the distal femur is used. A lateral para-patellar approach is preferable for multiplane articular involvement, medial-based intercondylar splits, additional Hoffa fractures, and separate intercondylar notch fragments. The surgeon utilizes the approach needed to view the articular surface, and traditional lag screw fixation of the articular surface is carried out.

For all displaced intra-articular fractures of the distal femur (not only complex ones), a lateral parapatellar approach should be selected that ensures an optimal overview of the articulation. The joint capsule can then be divided in line with the split in the iliotibial ligament. The technique of LISS fixation in displaced intra-articular fractures starts with direct visualization and stable internal fixation of the articular surface. Priority is always given to precise anatomic reconstruction of the articular surface (Figs. 5-21A and B and 5-22).

LESS INVASIVE STABILIZATION SYSTEM FOR THE PROXIMAL LATERAL TIBIA

INDICATIONS The indications for LISS PLT include fractures of the proximal shaft, the metaphysis, and intra-articular fractures in which treatment with screws alone is not possible (Table 5-5). The principle of angular stable screw fixation gives the LISS PLT system distinct biomechanical advantages over comparable devices for similar indications. Once the system has been applied to the lateral aspect of the tibia, it prevents varus collapse in metaphyseal/diaphyseal fractures and in fractures of the tibial plateau with medial condyle involvement. This means that the LISS PLT can also be used in the treatment of proximal tibial fractures that involve both the lateral and medial condyles, that is, condylar fractures (Müller AO classification type 41-A2, A3, C1–C3 and all proximal 42-type

fractures). In the Schatzker classification for tibial plateau fractures, the indications include Schatzker type V and VI fractures.

The LISS fixator is not specifically indicated for isolated fractures of the tibial diaphysis in the mid-third but is quite useful for segmental shaft fractures involving the proximal half of the tibia and for ipsilateral diaphyseal and bicondylar tibial plateau fractures. Other less common conditions in which the LISS PLT has been used include pathologic lesions with impending fracture of the proximal tibia and periprosthetic fractures.

A lateral approach to the tibial head is recommended for the treatment of extra-articular fractures of the proximal tibia. Access along the proximal contour of the tibia should be extended in a medial direction to detach the anterior tibial muscle close to the bone with part of the muscle fascia on the bone being left intact to ensure easier refixation of the muscle. The LISS PLT device is inserted by sliding it onto the proximal tibia from the proximal side in a distal direction under the anterior tibial muscle. Attention should be given to correct positioning in the condylar area and, particularly, on the tibial shaft. K-wires are used to fix this position and are advanced through the insertion guide, and the self-drilling, self-tapping LHSs are mounted in the trocar assemblies (Fig. 5-23).

IMPLANT-SPECIFIC PROBLEMS AND COMPLICATIONS

One of the complications specific to LISS DF is proximal screw pull-out. Possible predisposing factors include failure to place the LISS DF on the shaft laterally and possibly incorrect rotation, which causes tangential placement of the screws in the shaft cortex so that the screws gain purchase only in a small section close to the tip of the

---

FIGURE 5-21 | *A* and *B, In the case presented here, a lateral parapatellar approach with inclusion of the soft tissue injury was chosen.*

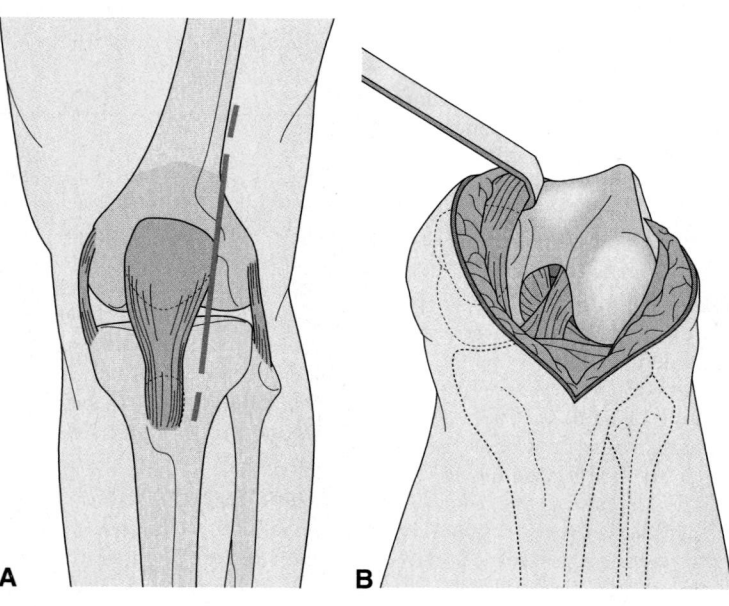

A   B

FIGURE 5-22 *Clinical case LISS-DF.*

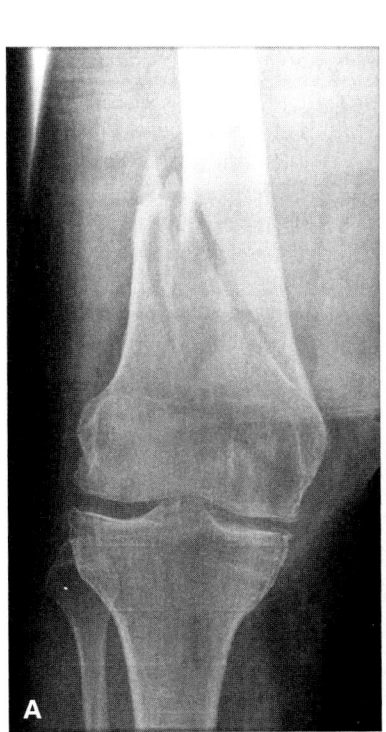

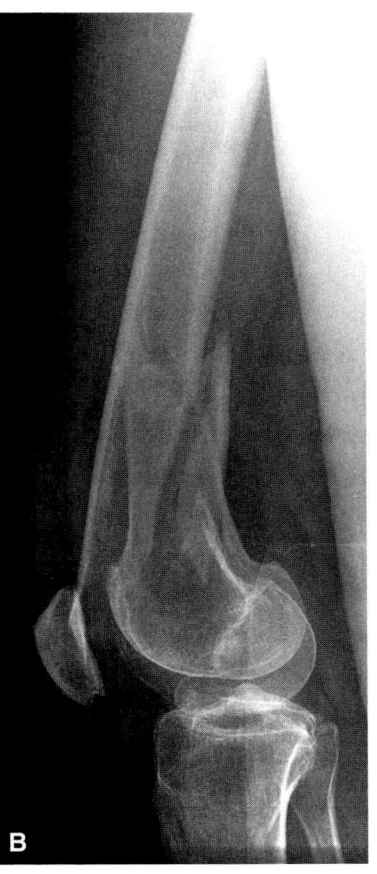

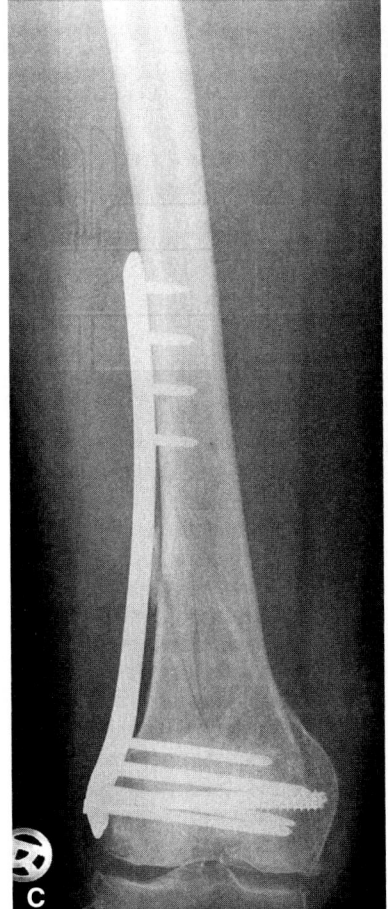

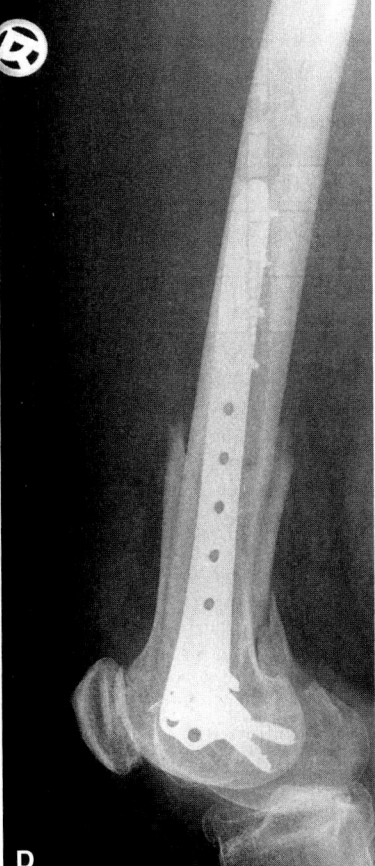

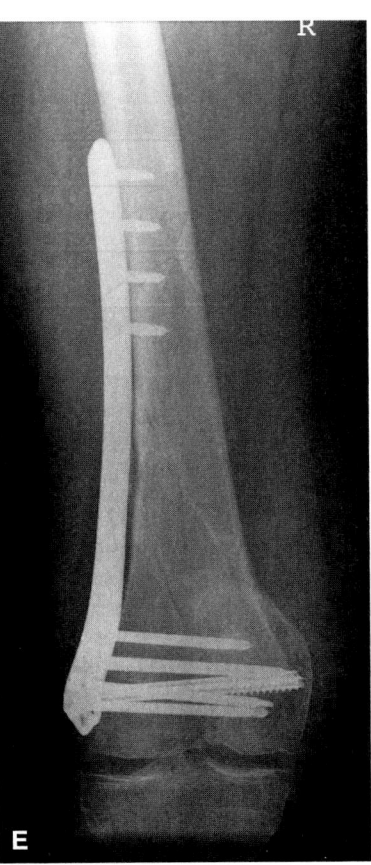

Table 5-5

Indications for LISS PLT in Proximal Tibial Fractures

- Metaphyseal fractures (multifragmentary)
- Proximal shaft fractures (multifragmentary, not nailable)
- Segmental shaft fractures (not nailable)
- Articular fractures (41-A2, A3, C1, C2, C3)
- Fractures in osteoporotic bone
- Pathological fractures
- Periprosthetic fractures

screw. Pull-out occurs typically after approximately 6 to 8 weeks, that is, as soon as the patient increases weight-bearing (Fig. 5-24).

If the plate lies too far toward the anterior or posterior aspects, the screws will not be centered in the medullary canal and will not have adequate purchase. Incorrect positioning of the LISS DF on the lateral condyle of the femur may result in soft tissue irritation.

Bending and twisting of the LISS plate is not recommended, since this results in malalignment of the holes on the insertion guide with the corresponding plate holes.

FIGURE 5-23 *Clinical case LISS-PLT.*

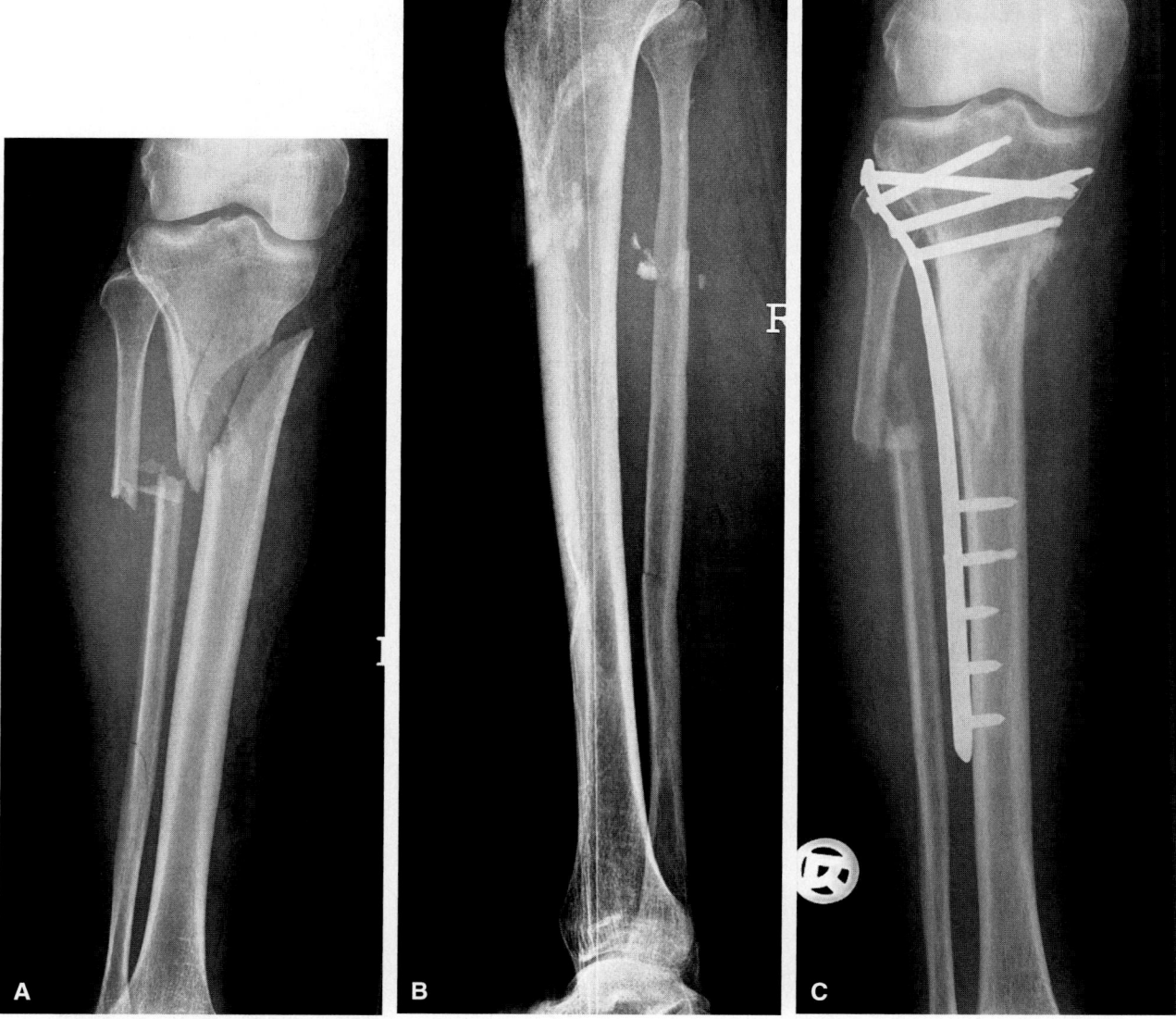

FIGURE 5-23 *(Continued)*

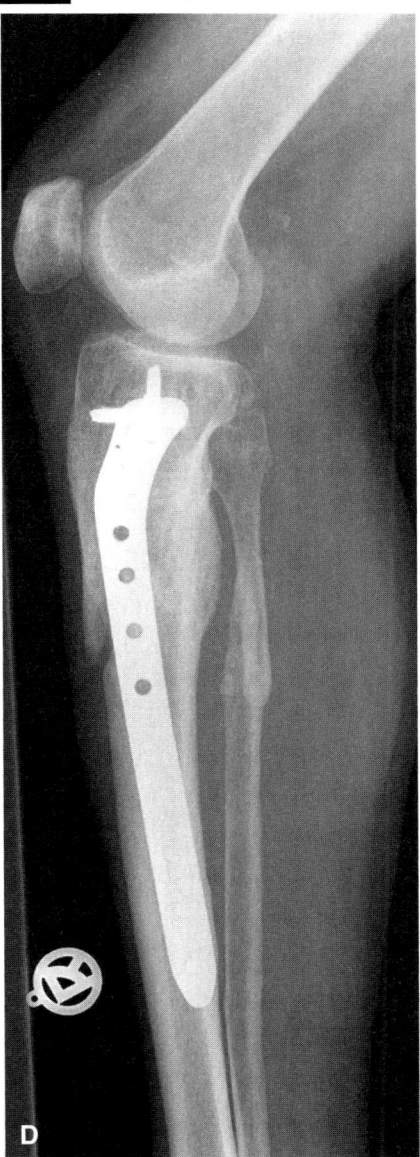

D

CLINICAL EXPERIENCE

The current indications for locking plate fixation are complex periarticular fractures, especially those with comminution of the metaphyseal region. Comminuted distal femoral fractures with multiplanar articular involvement are excellent indications[24] (see Fig. 5-22). Locking plates allow the surgeon more options for fixed-angle fixation while avoiding previously placed lag screws or fracture lines, such as the coronal (Hoffa) fracture of the distal femur. In the past, these obstacles sometimes precluded the use of traditional fixed-angle devices, such as the blade plate or the dynamic condylar screw. Bicondylar tibial plateau fractures, in which coronal plane stability is required, may benefit from this type of fixation[22,25] (see Fig. 5-23).

In some patients, use of a lateral locking plate is an alternative to double-plating techniques. Locked plating may also provide an alternative to external fixation, thus minimizing associated complications such as pin-site infection and patient tolerance. The importance of anatomic reduction of the articular surface with lag screw fixation remains paramount. The metaphyseal comminution is then "bridged" by the plate with locked screw fixation of the articular segment and with either locked or conventional bicortical screw fixation of the diaphyseal segment. Great care is taken to preserve soft tissue integrity and, therefore, bone viability in the metaphyseal region, regardless of whether an open or a percutaneous submuscular plate application technique is chosen.

Other potential indications for locking plate technology include periprosthetic fractures when total knee arthroplasty is involved.[2,23] Retrograde intramedullary fracture fixation is difficult to use with posterior cruciate ligament–substituting total knee arthroplasty designs because of the closed femoral housing. Lugs, stems, or other portions of the femoral component may also preclude the use of fixed-angle devices, such as the blade plate or dynamic condylar screw. Locking plates afford fixed-angle stability and permit the use of multiple distally locked screws, which often can be inserted around such obstacles and provide stable distal fixation even for very short distal fragments.

In some series, extra-articular or simple intra-articular fractures of the distal femur and proximal tibia with short periarticular fragments have demonstrated unacceptable rates of malalignment with intramedullary nailing.[35] The use of locked plating constructs may provide improved fixation in these patients and result in less malalignment. If intramedullary nailing cannot be used for selected long bone fractures with long working lengths, a bridge plate technique with locked screw fixation may be a viable alternative. Other evolving applications for locking plate technology include fixation of corrective osteotomies, malunions, and nonunions as well as applications for orthopaedic oncology; however, published clinical data for these applications are lacking.

LISS DF and LISS PLT procedures have been in clinical use since 1995. Several studies and a large number of articles have been published on these procedures, reporting both biomechanical and clinical advantages. The published data show that LISS is a valuable treatment option for fractures of the distal femur[23–25,29,35,38,40–42,45,51] and the proximal tibia.[5,15,35,40]

Most published clinical studies of locking plate fixation have focused on the results of the LISS plate in fractures of the distal femur and proximal tibia. This device is an externally targeted plate designed for submuscular, extraperiosteal application, with all screws locking to the plate. In one prospective trial that included nine European trauma centers, 112 patients with 116 fractures of the distal femur were treated.[42] Ninety-six patients with 99 fractures completed the study (mean follow-up, 14 months). Twenty-nine percent of fractures were open; 91 percent of fractures healed. Six patients required bone grafting to achieve union, and four infections were reported. Average knee flexion at union was 107°. Deviations greater than 5°

FIGURE 5-24 **A–D,** *Malalignment between the bone axis and plate leads to an eccentric plate position* **(A).** *At the far end of the plate, a monocortical locking head screw will not anchor in the bone in these conditions* **(B).** *To overcome the problem of insufficient anchorage of a monocortical self-drilling, self-tapping screw when the plate is positioned eccentrically, it is recommended either to insert* **(C)** *a long bicortical self-tapping screw or* **(D)** *a cortex screw that allows angulation in the plate hole.*

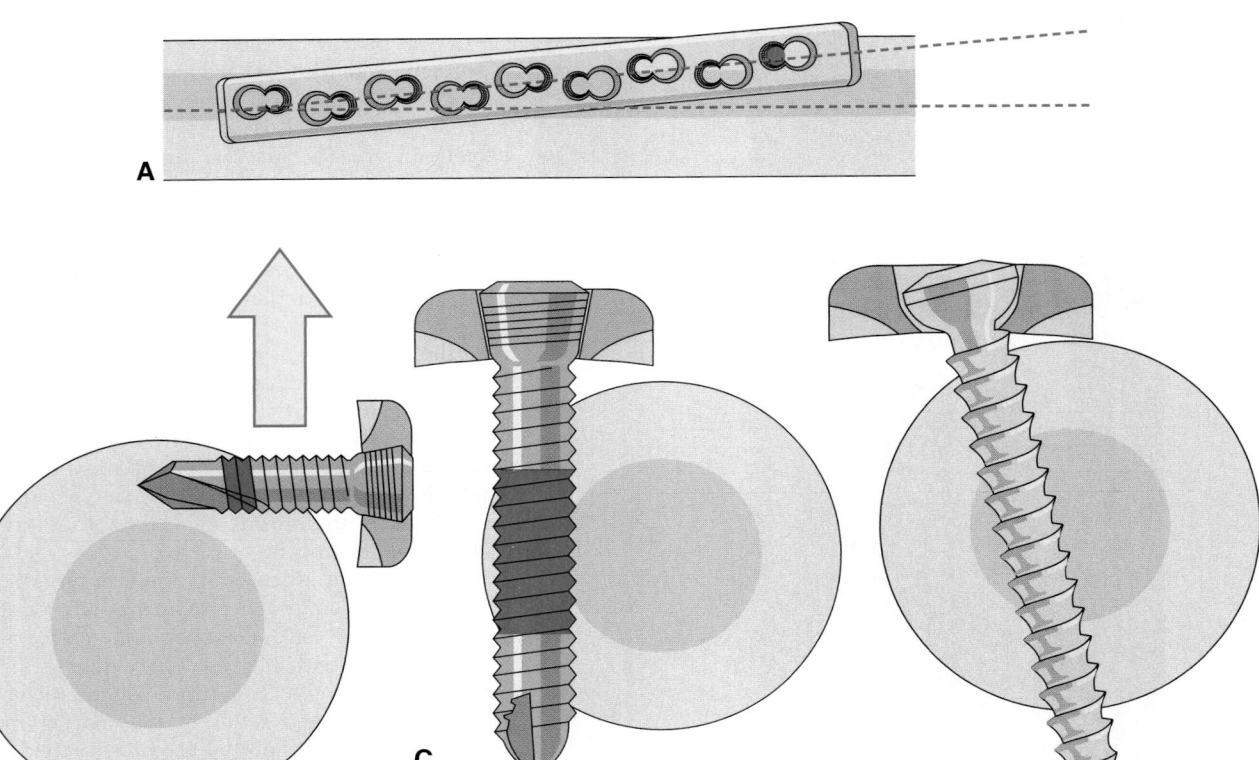

from normal coronal or sagittal alignments were noted on approximately 40 percent of postoperative radiographs.

In a series of 66 patients with fractures of the distal femur treated with the LISS plate, all fractures healed without loss of distal femoral fixation.[24] Only three fractures (5%) required bone grafting to achieve union. Three patients (5%) had malalignments greater than 5° in any plane. In another study, 54 fractures of the distal femur were treated with the LISS DF plate.[38] Four had loss of proximal fixation, attributed to errors in surgical technique resulting in incorrect implant placement on the femoral diaphysis. Two infections and three delayed unions were reported. Of the 27 patients who completed a minimum 1-year follow-up, 20 (74%) had good or excellent results; 7 (26%) had alignment deviations greater than 5° in any plane.

When the femoral LISS was used for 13 periprosthetic fractures above total knee arthroplasties, only one patient required bone grafting to achieve union.[23] No cases of varus collapse or distal fixation failure were noted. In another study, 46 complex intra-articular and extra-articular fractures of the proximal tibia (45 patients) were treated with the tibial LISS plate. Of the 16 open fractures, there was one infection. One patient required bone grafting to achieve union; no varus collapse or loss of proximal fixation was reported. Six of the 46 fractures (13%)

had malalignment greater than 5°. Gosling et al.[15] and Ertl and Smith[8] reported encouraging results using lateral locked plating as an alternative to double plating in bicondylar tibial plateau fractures.

An obvious interdependence has developed between locked internal fixation technology and minimally invasive techniques of plate application. Although impressive union rates have been reported, this may be the result of improved soft tissue handling techniques, a favorable biological environment, and the improved mechanical stability provided by locking plate technology. Additionally, it appears that monocortical fixation is adequate to achieve union; in the absence of errors in surgical technique, reported rates of fixation failure are low. When percutaneous techniques are used, malalignments are more common, but the operations are technically demanding. With increased experience and the development of new techniques to improve the accuracy of closed reduction, the frequency of such malunions should decrease. The long-term clinical significance of the malalignments remains unknown.

LOCKING COMPRESSION PLATE

Using the LCP, the surgeon is free to select the best treatment method—either the compression method or the

Table 5-6

Biomechanical Aspects of Plate and Screw Fixation

Fixation Method	Fracture Configuration After Reduction	Fixation Technique	Screw Type*
Compression (static or dynamic)	Simple fracture type > full contact between the main fragments	Lag screw and protection plate	Cortex screw as lag screw; cortex screws (1) neutral position or LHS (2) as plate screws
		Compression plate (and lag screw)	Cortex screws in eccentric position or axial compression with a tension device and cortex screws (1) in neutral position or LHS (2) as plate screws
		Tension band plate	Plate position important support vis-à-vis support is important, cortex screws in neutral position or LHS (2) as plate screws
		Buttress plate	Cortex screws (1) in neutral position or LHS (2) as plate screws
Splinting	Multifragmentary fracture > partial or no contact between the main fragments	Bridge plating or locked internal fixator	Cortex screws (1) in neutral position or LHS (2) as plate screws
	Simple fracture type (in exceptional cases) > full or partial contact between the main fragments	Bridge plating or locked internal fixator	Cortex screws (1) in neutral position as plate screws or LHS (2) as plate screws

LHS, locking head screw(s).
*Bone quality: (1) Normal, (2) Poor, (2) Also for technical reason: no primary loss of reduction, accurate shaping of the plate is not needed, MIPO easier.

locked splinting method—to bridge the fracture zone in the individual patient. The type, number, and position of screws used dictate the method and technique and must be appropriate to the fracture situation (Table 5-6). LCP functions in accordance with the latest plating techniques, the aim of which is to achieve an optimal anchoring of the implant to the bone, to maintain fracture reduction throughout the fracture healing process, while reducing the amount of surgery-related soft-tissue trauma and maintaining the bone vascularity.

The LCP combination hole allows internal fixation to be achieved by the insertion of either standard screws (into the unthreaded part of the hole) or locking head screws with angular stability (into the threaded part of the figure-eight hole). LHSs can only be inserted at right angles to the plate. The LCP hole also makes it possible to insert different screw types into the same plate so that the surgeon is able to choose the type depending on intraoperative requirements. In retrospect, combining two completely different anchorage techniques into a single implant was a logical approach and a straightforward, practical solution.

The option of using the LCP either as a compression plate or as an internal fixator provides ideal plate anchorage that can be adapted to individual requirements. This significantly extends the range of indications in minimally invasive plate osteosynthesis. With the LCP, the surgeon has two plating methods to choose from and is able to select the more appropriate.

LCP IN CONVENTIONAL COMPRESSION PLATING

Compression Method Conventional Plating Technique

Despite the advantages of locked internal fixators, there is still a need for the anatomic reconstruction and absolute stability that are provided by conventional plates and screws. Appropriate indications for the latter include intra-articular fractures, osteotomies, complex bone reconstruction procedures, pseudarthroses, and fractures with traumatic damage to the blood supply.

The compression method of fracture fixation, aiming for absolute stability, involves open reduction and internal fixation (ORIF) using plates and cortex and/or cancellous bone screws. This approach, the principles of which are outlined above, became established as a standard and successful technique for treating bone fractures. The success of the technique depends on the precision of the reduction and the degree of stabilization. Wide surgical exposure is necessary to achieve reduction, and soft tissues were often stripped from fracture fragments.

With experience, it became increasingly evident that there was a biological price for precise reduction and absolutely stable fixation. Handling, and even cleaning, of the bone fragments before and during reduction was likely to result in dead bone that might only revascularize slowly and require long-term protection.

In some fracture situations, the LCP with combination holes can be used with a conventional plating technique, that is, fracture fixation using the compression method based on the principle of achieving absolute stability and direct bone healing. The surgical technique and instruments are similar to those used in conventional plating with DCP or LC-DCP.

Indications
- Simple fractures of the diaphysis and metaphysis: cases in which precise anatomic reduction is necessary for the functional outcome; simple transverse or oblique fractures with little soft-tissue compromise and good bone quality (compression plating or protection plating in combination with a lag screw or tension-band plate)
- Intra-articular fractures (buttress plate)
- Delayed union or nonunion
- Closed-wedge osteotomies
- Complete avascularity of the bone fragments

The following conditions have to be met for the use of the compression method:

- Precise reduction of the fragments—in most cases requiring open, direct reduction
- Precise anatomic preshaping of the plate (when the protection plate is fixed with cortical screws)
- Good bone quality, to ensure adequate anchorage of cortex or cancellous bone screws
- Minor soft-tissue damage

Technique

The method of interfragmentary compression can be achieved using the following approaches:

- Compression plate for axial compression (in transverse fractures)
- Lag screw and protection plate (in oblique fractures)
- Tension band principle using a plate
- Buttress plate and lag screw

The guidelines for the compression method–conventional plating technique are shown in Table 5-7.

Axial Compression After open and direct precise anatomic reduction of the fracture and preshaping of the plate, interfragmentary compression is applied using the eccentric cortex screw option in the dynamic compression unit (DCU) of the LCP's combination hole. Fracture compression can also be applied using a tensioning device. Osteosynthesis is then completed with cortex screws inserted in the neutral position.

If different screws are combined in compression plating, the cortex screws should be inserted in the middle of the plate in their eccentric positions first, to achieve fracture compression. As a modification, the LCP can initially be fixed to one of the main fragments with one or two LHSs. Subsequently, compression can be applied by inserting one eccentric screw into the other fragment or by applying the tensioning device. Osteosynthesis is then completed with locking head screws.

Table 5-7

Guidelines for Plate Fixation in Simple and Multifragmentary Fractures

	Simple Fracture		Multifragmentary Fracture
Biomechanical principle	Interfragmentary compression	Splinting in exceptional cases without lag screw	Splinting
Reduction technique	Mainly direct	Indirect or percutaneous direct*	Preferably indirect
Insertion	At least partly open	Open, less invasive, MIPO	Closed, minimally invasive
Shaping of the plate	Has to be fitted to bone surface	Accurate shaping not needed with LHSs	Accurate shaping not needed with LHSs
Plate-span ratio (see text) = Plate length/fracture length	>8:10/1	>2:3/1	>2:3/1
Screw type/function	• Cortex or cancellous screw as plate-dependent lag screw • Cortex screws in eccentric position for compression • Cortex screw in neutral position or LHS for plate fixation	• Cortex screws or LHS in good bone • LHS in poor bone and with MIPO technique	• Cortex screws or LHS in good bone • LHS in poor bone and with MIPO technique
Monocortical/bicortical screw anchorage:			
Conventional screw	• Bicortical; lag screw monocortical	• Bicortical	• Bicortical
LHS in the diaphysis	• Self-drilling, self-tapping monocortical *or* self-tapping bicortical	• Self-drilling/self-tapping monocortical *or* self-tapping bicortical	• Self-drilling/self-tapping monocortical *or* self-tapping bicortical
LHS in the epiphysis/metaphysis	• Self-tapping bicortical, as long as possible	• Self-tapping bicortical, as long as possible	• Self-tapping bicortical, as long as possible
Plate screw density (see text)	≤0.4–0.3	≤0.5–0.4	≤0.5–0.4
Screws per main fragment (*n*)	≥3;2 exceptionally	≥3;2 exceptionally	≥3;2 exceptionally
Cortices per main fragment (*n*)	3–5	≥4	≥4
Screw position in the plate	Short middle segment without screws	Middle segment without screws, without lag screws; splinting method required or unprecise reduction*	Long middle segment without screws
Empty plate holes over the fracture	0–3	>2–3	≥3

LHS, locking head screw; MIPO, minimally invasive plate osteosynthesis.
*Splinting of simple fractures should respect the biomechanical rules according to the strain theory.

Lag Screw and Protection Plate Interfragmentary compression of a simple fracture in the metaphyseal or diaphyseal segment, or of an intra-articular fracture, can also be accomplished using a lag screw inserted through the plate.

The additional cortex screws are again used to increase the friction between plate and bone. If there is good bone quality and an open approach is possible so that accurate plate contouring can be carried out, then cortex or cancellous bone screws can be inserted. This protection plate construct helps protect the fractured bone from bending and torsional forces.

Conventional compression plating requires precise adaptation of the implant to the bone to maintain precise reduction; the screws apply a compressive preload at the interface between the plate and the bone, and the fragments are pulled toward the implant (see Fig. 5-4B). Using the LCP with cortex or cancellous bone screws therefore requires accurate shaping of the plate in the same way as with a conventional LC-DCP. Imperfect shaping of the plate leads to a mismatch between plate and bone surface resulting in primary loss of reduction when cortex or cancellous bone screws are tightened. If LHSs are inserted to support the reduction and compression being maintained by the lag screws, no uncontrollable forces due to pressure of the plate on the bone surface will be created. This way the risk of primary reduction loss is eliminated. In osteoporotic bone the use of locking head screws improves the anchoring of the implant by its angular and axial stability provided by the threaded screw head – plate hole interface. This improved anchoring can be very beneficial to protect the lag screw placed through a plate hole or for the anchoring of a so-called neutralization or protection plate after the placement of a plate independent lag screw.

The lag screw can also be placed independently from the plate, with a protection plate being fixed with locking head screws (see Fig. 5-17). There is no risk of a primary loss of reduction. This technique is much easier than placing a lag screw through a plate hole (Fig. 5-25).

LOCKED SPLINTING WITH LOCKED INTERNAL FIXATORS

LOCKING COMPRESSION PLATE WITH SPLINTING

Internal Extramedullary Locked Splinting Method—Principle of Relative Stability

New methods involving minimal risk were developed to accelerate bone regeneration and bone healing in difficult fractures. Whereas anatomic reduction of the fracture was the goal in the conventional plating technique, the aim in bridging plate osteosynthesis for multifragmentary shaft fractures has been to reduce vascular damage to the bone. The use of indirect reduction, as advocated by Mast and colleagues,[30] was intended to take advantage of the soft-tissue attachments on the bone fragments, which align spontaneously when traction is applied to the main fragments.

Bridge plating can be carried out with both standard screws and locking head screws. The method of bridging the fracture zone with standard plates and standard screws, using a "no-touch" technique combined with indirect reduction, was a great step forward when it was introduced. Only the main fragments were fixed to the plate. For the plate fixation with standard screws, it was necessary to pre-shape the plate to fit the main fragment. It is possible to use both standard screws and LHSs in normal-quality bone. In areas with reduced bone mass the anchoring of the locking compression plate will be enhanced with the use of locking head screws. Bridge plating procedures in combination with the MIPO technique, locking head screws are very helpful to compensate for the lack of the plate shape to the anatomical bone shape. In contrast with compression

---

FIGURE 5-25 *A–E, Clinical case LCP compression method.*

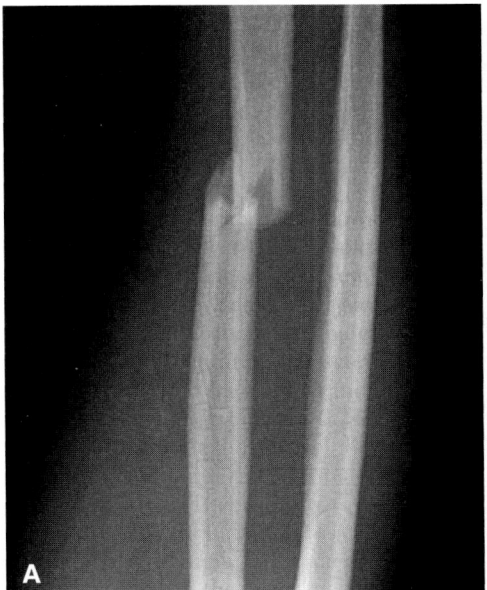
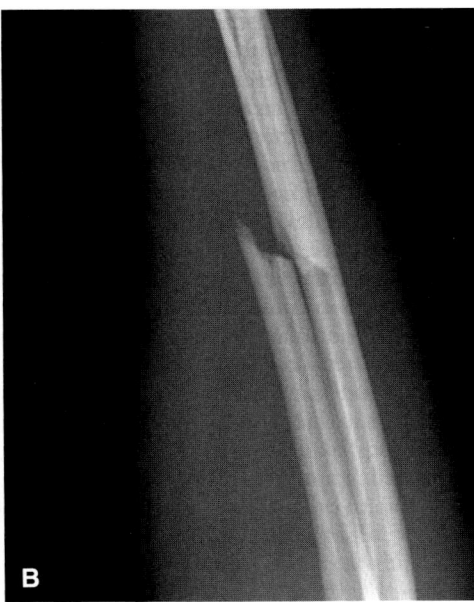

(Continued)

FIGURE 5-25 *(Continued)*

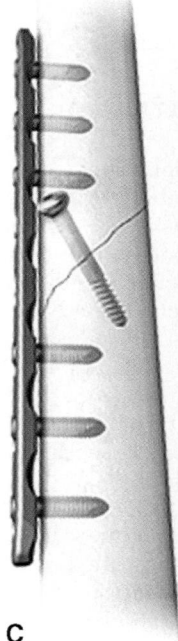 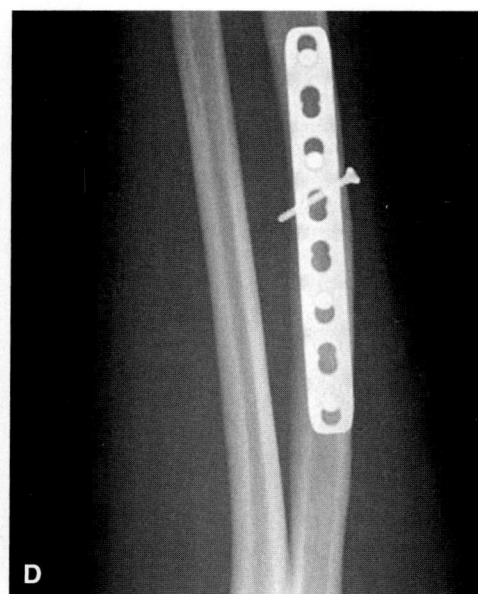 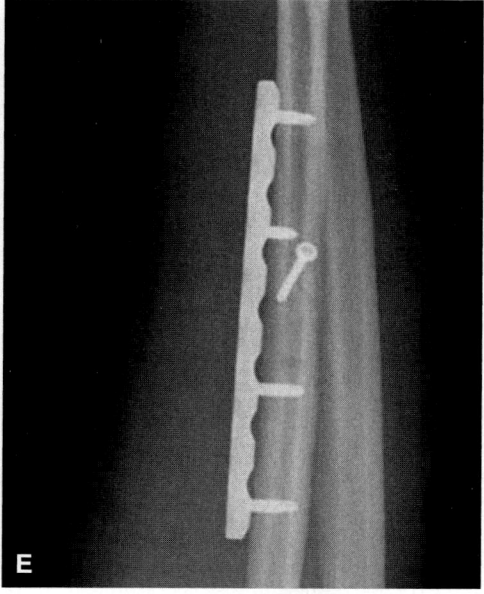

C D E

screws, the use of locking head screws will maintain the pre-reduced fracture alignment.

In addition, there is no disturbance—or only minimal disturbance—to the periosteal blood supply. Technically, the locked splinting method (pure splinting) can be carried out either using an open approach or with the MIPO technique and indirect, closed, approximate reduction.

The LCP is used as a locked internal fixator to bridge the fracture zone in a less invasive or MIPO technique, that is, the locked splinting method with an internal fixator, based on the principle of relative stability, is applied in the following cases:

- Multifragmentary fractures of the diaphysis and metaphysis (Fig. 5-26)
- Simple fractures of the diaphysis and metaphysis (in cases in which approximate reduction is adequate for the functional outcome, although it is important to strictly observe the biomechanical principles of strain tolerance)
- Fractures in problem zones when there are relative contraindications to intramedullary nailing, for example, shaft fractures with anomalies of the medullary morphology, fractures in children and adolescents with open epiphyses, shaft fractures in children, shaft fractures in patients with multiple injuries (polytrauma, chest and traumatic brain injury)
- Open-wedge osteotomies (e.g., in the proximal tibia)
- Periprosthetic fractures (Fig. 5-27)
- Other implants in situ
- Secondary fractures or redislocation, instability after intramedullary nailing
- Delayed conversion from an external fixator to the definitive internal fixation

- LCP as an external fixator in emergency situations
- Tumor surgery

Technique (see Table 5-7)
There are two prerequisites for using the LCP as a locked internal fixator:

- The bridging plate has to be long—the longer the plate, the better.
- The space between the locking head screws has to be adequate.

Locking the screw into the fixator increases stability, and avoids the risk of primary dislocation of the fragment toward the plate induced by tightening the screws, and decreases the risk of secondary fracture displacement due to toggling of the screw within the plate hole. The advantages of locking head screws are that the screw length can be reduced to a monocortical size and that self-drilling screws can be used, thus eliminating the need for length measurement. In good-quality bone, monocortical LHSs are adequate, but at least three screws should be inserted into each main fragment on either side of the fracture. In osteoporotic bone, it is strongly recommended that at least three LHSs should be inserted into each main fragment on either side of the fracture, and that at least one or two of these LHSs should be inserted bicortically.

Bicortical insertion of LHS is recommended in the following circumstances:

- Osteoporosis
- Thin cortex
- High torsional forces during rehabilitation and physical therapy
- Short main fragment
- Small medullary diameter

FIGURE 5-26 | **A–F,** *Clinical case LCP splinting method.*

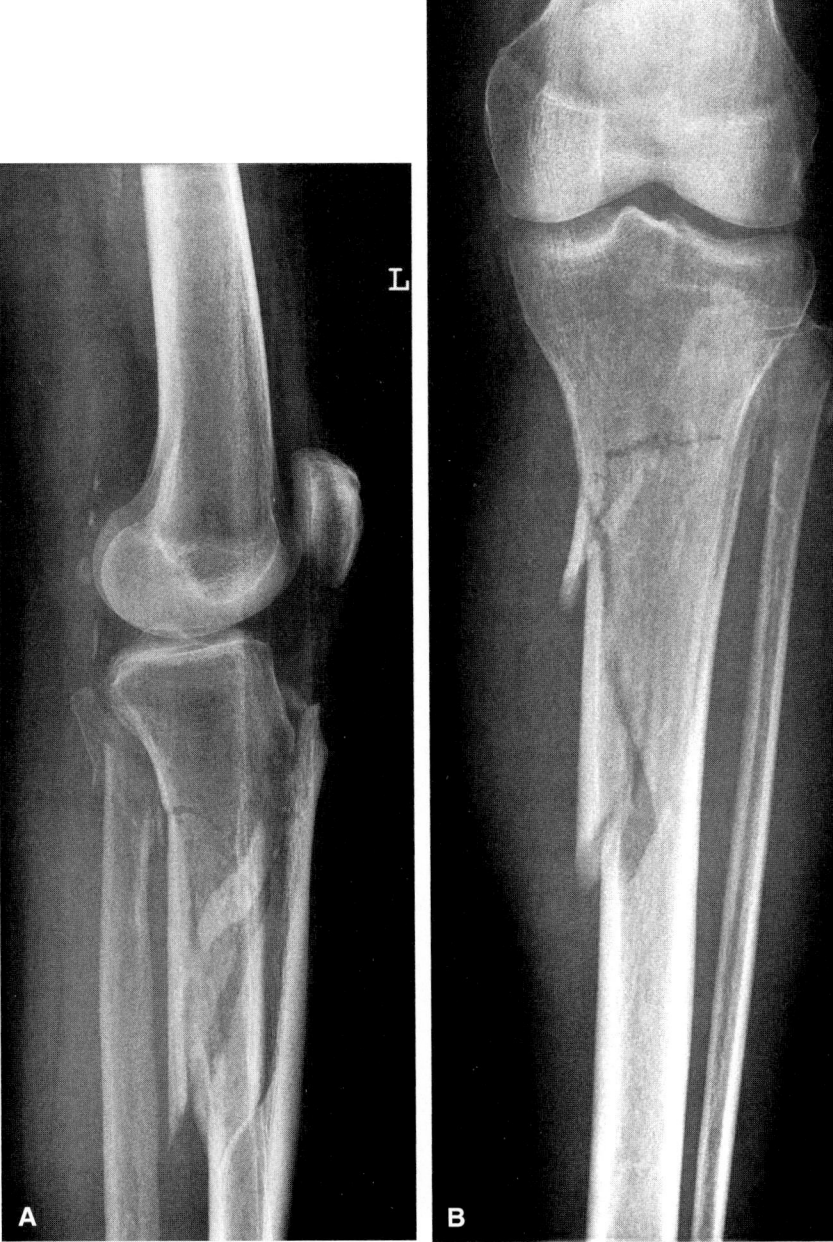

(Continued)

It is important to avoid stress concentrations at the fracture site, and this can be achieved by leaving two or three plate holes without screws in the fracture zone. Stress distribution is an important feature of the internal fixator technique as stress concentration and implant failures are avoided.

LCP WITH A COMBINATION OF THE TWO METHODS The compression method and splinting method should be used in combination only in situations in which the bone has been fractured in two different places. In these cases, the two biomechanical principles—absolute

stability through interfragmentary compression and relative stability by splinting with an internal fixator—can be combined.

INDICATIONS

- Segmental fractures with two different fracture patterns (one simple and one multifragmentary). In these cases, conventional interfragmentary compression is used to stabilize the simple fracture while splinting with an internal fixator stabilizes the multifragmentary fracture area.

FIGURE 5-26 *(Continued)*

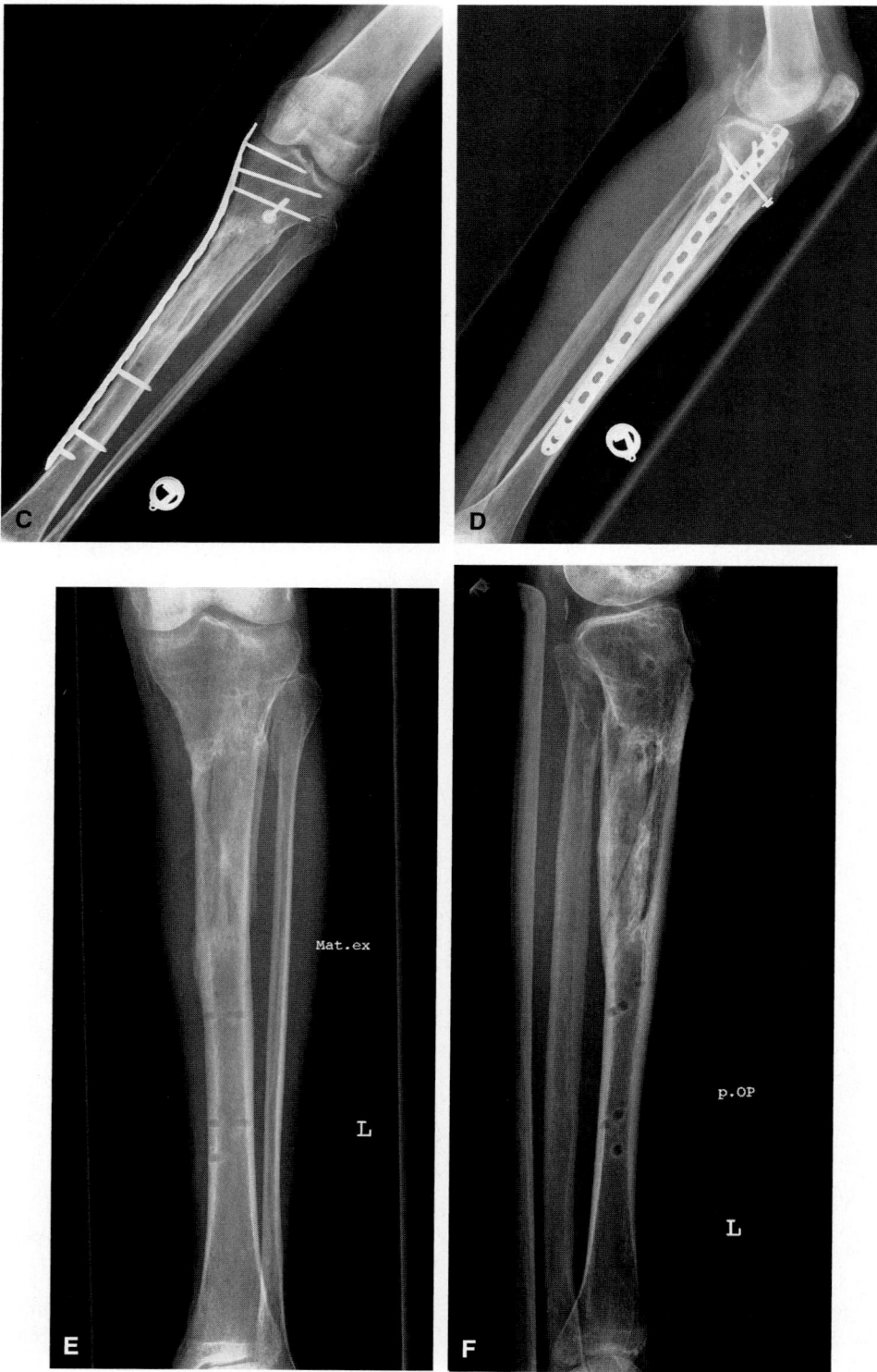

FIGURE 5-27 **A–F,** Clinical case LCP periprosthetic fracture.

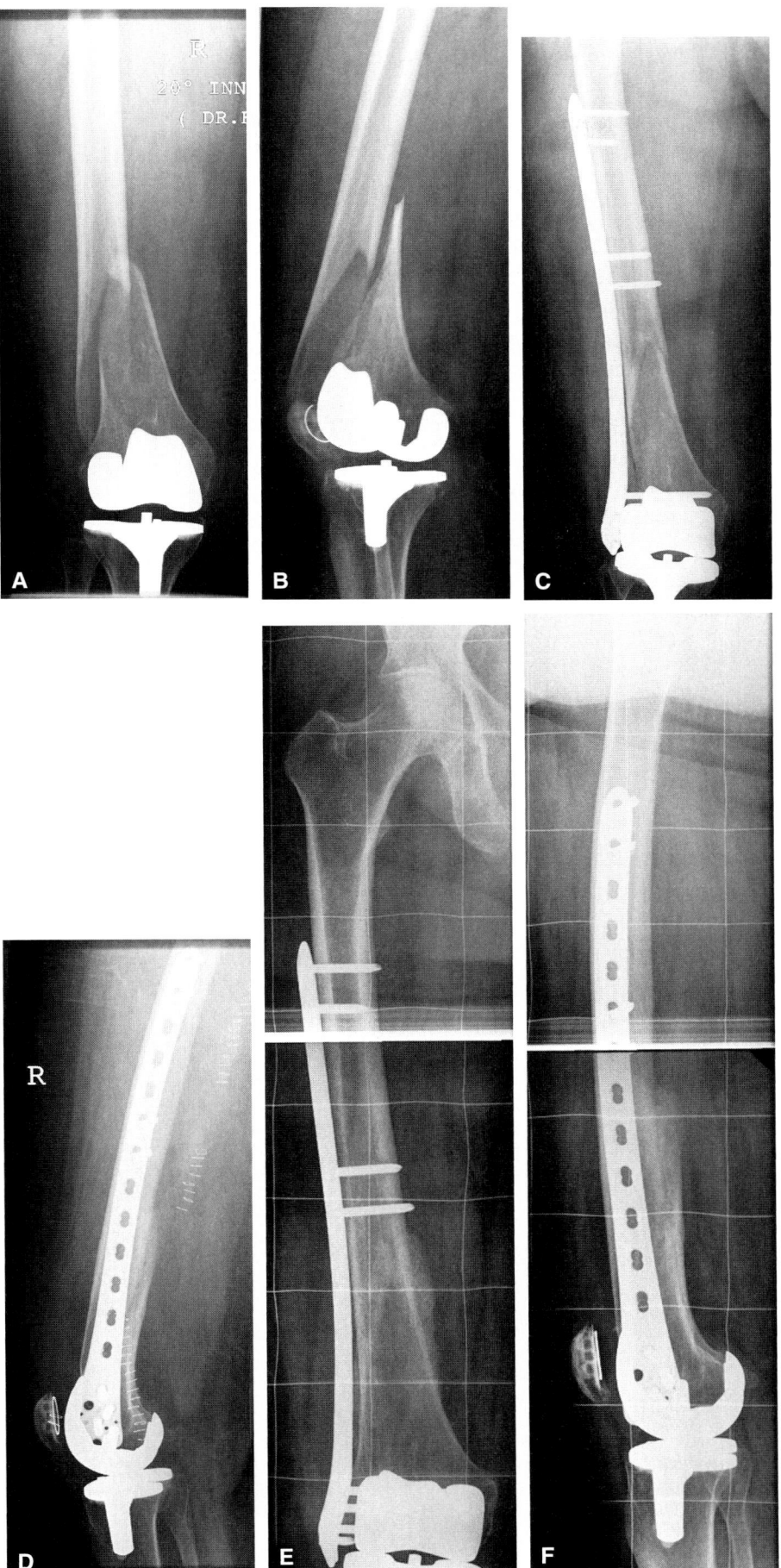

● Intra-articular fractures with a multifragmented extension into the diaphysis. In these cases, the anatomic reduction and interfragmentary lag screw compression of the articular component are combined with a bridging fixation from the reconstructed joint block to the diaphysis (Fig. 5-28).

COMBINATIONS OF DIFFERENT SCREWS It is possible to combine the two plating techniques—simultaneously applying compression with standard screws and locking head fixation using a single plate—and this can be valuable, depending on the indication. It is important to be familiar with the different features of both techniques. Probably the most frequent use of a combination technique will be in the treatment of fractures adjacent to the joint, with locking head screws being used to fix the fragment close to the joint and standard screws being used to apply axial compression between the metaphysis and the diaphysis in a simple fracture type (individual blade plate) (Fig. 5-29).

The splinting method can be carried out with an internal fixator and an additional reduction screw (reducing the plate onto the bone or reducing a displaced fragment) or positioning screw. In addition, the conventional screw-plating technique (the compression method) can be used, but with fixation of the protection plate using locking head screws (see Fig. 5-18).

MINIMALLY INVASIVE PLATE OSTEOSYNTHESIS

The newly developed locked internal fixators used in the LISS and LCP are based on the principles of biological internal fixation and minimally invasive plate osteosynthesis (MIPO) (Table 5-8). The MIPO approach is possible with conventional plates, but there are additional advantages if the MIPO technique is combined with the use of a locked internal fixator—there is no need for precise contouring of the plate, drilling, measuring, or tapping, because self-drilling, self-tapping monocortical LHSs are used. These screws lend themselves optimally to monocortical fixation, in which it is not necessary to select the length of the screw precisely and a protruding screw tip is not able to damage or irritate the soft tissues, tendons, or muscles.

Only small incisions are necessary to insert the plate in MIPO technique—with benefits including not only improved cosmetic results but, above all, protection of the fracture zone. "The skin protects the fracture zone from the surgeon."

The technology developed for the blind insertion and application of internal fixators can also be used with open approaches. The open approach, using an aiming device, can help the surgeon become accustomed to the more demanding technique of aligning the internal splint. The locked monocortical screws require alignment of the implant and the bone axis within comparatively narrow limits. Open procedures can be used for initial training in the techniques.

FIGURE 5-28   **A–F,** *Clinical case LCP combining two methods.*

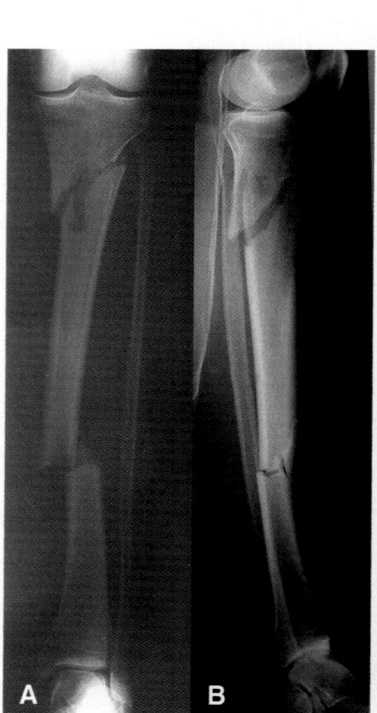
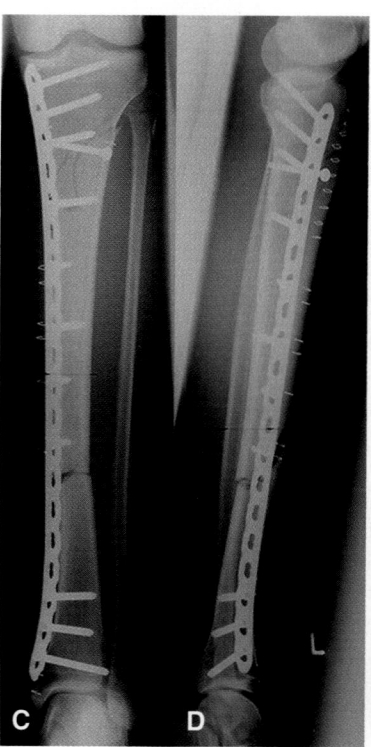
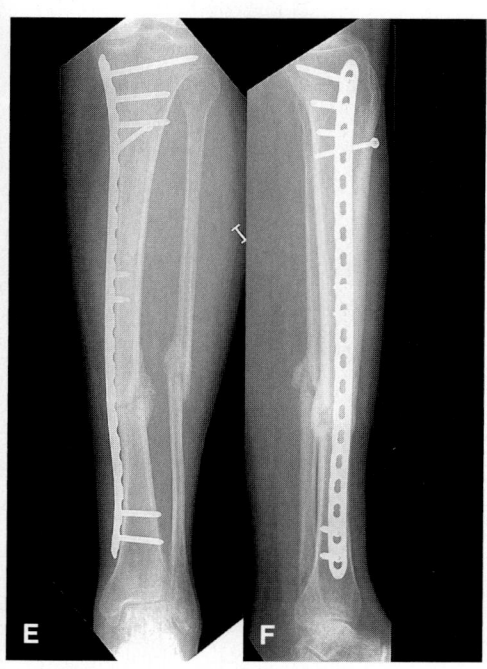

FIGURE 5-29 **A–F,** *Clinical case LCP individual blade plate.*

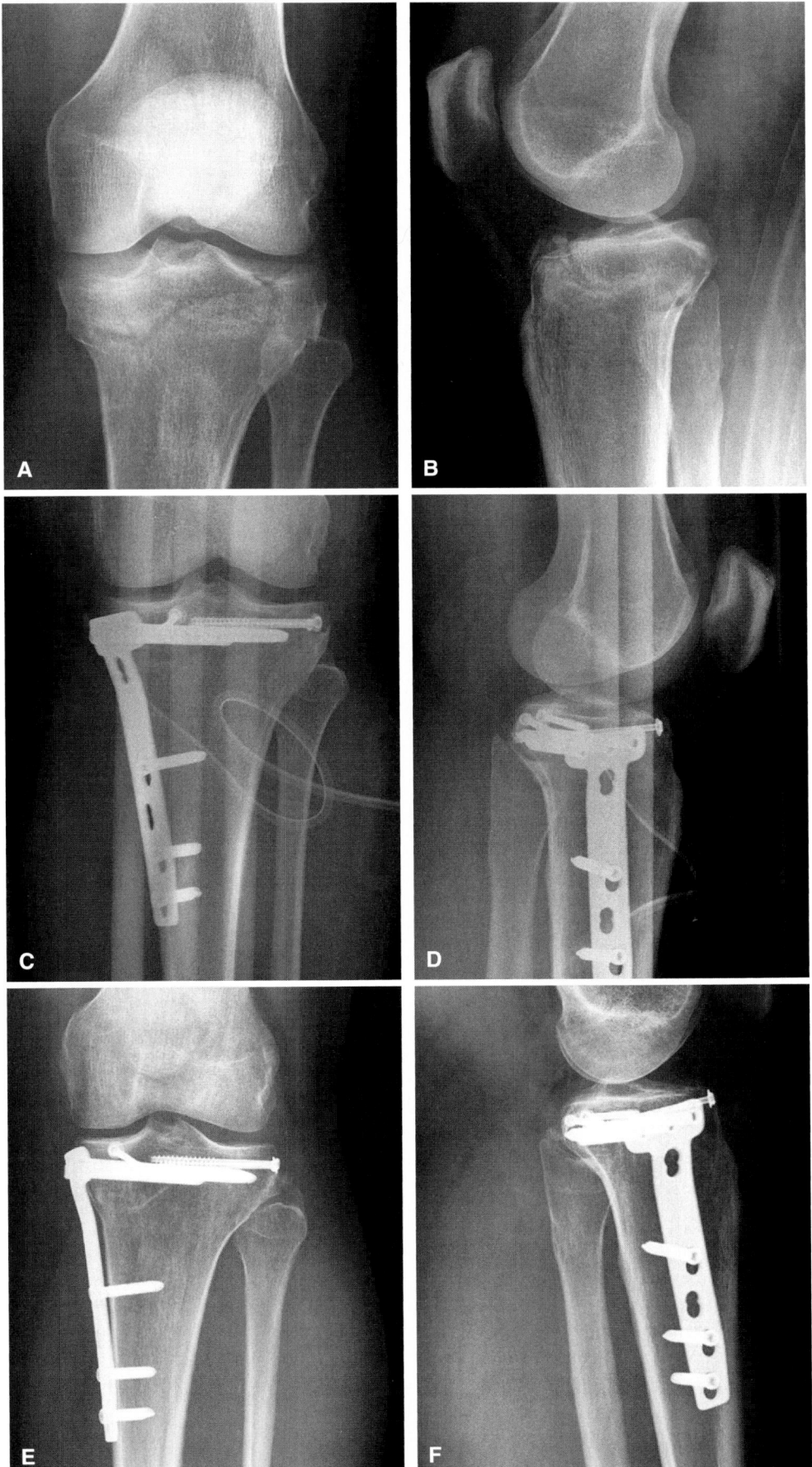

Table 5-8
Definition of MIPO
Access to the bone through soft tissue windows (not only small skin incisions but also careful gentle handling of deep layers of the soft tissue).
Minimal trauma to the soft tissue and the bone by indirect reduction.
Minimal additional trauma at the fracture site when direct reduction is necessary.
Reduction tools which cause "small footprints."
Implants with adequate bone-implant interface:
• Noncontact plates, angular stable screws • Monocortical screw fixation
Optimized screw placement according to the anatomical region.

In addition, using LCP with LHS as a locked internal fixator (locked splinting method) in the MIPO technique has many technical and biological advantages.

ADVANTAGES

- Biological internal fixation avoids the need for precise reduction, especially of the intermediate fragments, and takes advantage of indirect reduction.
- The aim of indirect reduction is to align the proximal and distal main fragments. This avoids exposure of the individual bone fragments.
- Submuscular/subcutaneous slide insertion techniques are possible.
- Minimization of biological damage caused by the surgical approach, the reduction, and at the implant-bone interface (MIPO). This is achieved at the expense of precise reduction and rigid fixation.
- Flexible elastic fixation to stimulate spontaneous healing, including the induction of callus formation.
- Locked internal fixators are noncontact plates; no compression of the plate onto the bone is required.
- There is no need for shaping when applying LISS or anatomically preshaped LCPs.
- There is no need for exact preshaping of the LCP to match the bone anatomy.
- There is no need for drilling, measuring, or tapping, since self-drilling monocortical LHSs are used.
- Preservation of all blood supply to the bone including periosteal blood supply.
- There is a reduced risk of secondary loss of reduction.
- Locking the screw into the plate ensures angular as well as axial stability and eliminates any unwanted movement of the screw (secondary loss of reduction).
- The technique works well in osteoporotic bone.
- For treatment of multifragmentary, complex fractures.
- MIPO is easier using locked noncontact plates.
- There is improved local resistance to infection.
- Less risk of refracture.

PREREQUISITES

- Indirect closed reduction without exposure of the fracture.
- Small incisions for insertion of the implants.
- Implants that have minimal bone contact (e.g., LISS and LCP). The internal fixators are slightly raised above the bone surface to eliminate any mismatch between the preshaped implant and the anatomy of the bone.
- Elastic bridging of the fracture zone (principle of relative stability stimulates callus formation).
- Plates/fixators are used as pure splints, that is, without the additional lag screw effect.
- Self-drilling, self-tapping locking head screws can be used for monocortical insertion; self-tapping locking head screws can be used for monocortical or bicortical insertion.

In LISS alone, a geometric correlation has to be achieved between the aiming device and the plate for closed application.

SHORTCOMINGS AND DISADVANTAGES

- The stability of the fracture fixation depends on the stiffness of the construct.
- Closed reduction and intraoperative control of alignment are not easy.
- Minimally invasive plate application and fixation are not easy.
- With the predetermined screw orientation, possible difficulties can arise when a locking head screw is inserted (penetration of articular surface).
- Reduction toward the plate can be achieved only with special instruments or bumps or standard screws.
- Excessive demands on the system: the bone is not carrying any load because it has not been precisely reduced.
- Delayed healing in the diaphyseal region when bone fragments are stripped of the periosteum after the injury or due to iatrogenic disturbance of the blood supply (wrong reduction and fixation).

BENEFITS OF MINIMALLY INVASIVE TECHNIQUES (MIPO) WITH LOCKED PLATES (TABLE 5-9)

It was originally argued that the tunneling required to achieve blind insertion of the plate would result in the same amount of damage as the open surgical approach. However, studies conducted by Krettek's group on the effect of ligating the perforating arteries, for example, during open surgical procedures for femoral fractures, disproved this argument.[10,11,27] Although MIPO techniques can be used with plates and compression screws, the advantages of the technique using locked splints and monocortical self-drilling screws are greater.

In surgical approaches involving access through contused areas of skin in which stability is required, the minimally invasive approach offers considerable advantages.

Table 5-9
Anatomically Preshaped Plates
Strong demands for anatomically preshaped plates
Advantages for anatomically preshaped plates:
• No intraoperative shaping of the plate required • Plate helps achieve the anatomical reduction • Aiming blocks to insert the locking head screws • Clear indications for a given implant • Defined placement for a given implant • Clear rules of how to use the given implant • Optimized screw placement according to the anatomical region

The mechanical benefits of these systems (i.e., locked noncontact plates) are as follows. There is no need for precise anatomic preshaping of the plate—a procedure which is in any case hardly possible with blind, minimally invasive techniques. LCP used as an internal fixator with LHSs are noncontact plates. This feature considerably facilitates the MIPO procedure. The preshaped plates supplied by the manufacturer are based on measurements of the average shape required, using computed tomography data and cadaver bones. Since the plate does not need to be pressed onto the bone when it is being used as an internal fixator, minor variations in the bone will result in areas of plate stand-off from the bone. Anatomically preshaped LCPs are available for certain metaphyseal areas (the proximal/distal humerus, olecranon, distal radius, distal femur, and proximal and distal tibia), and LISS devices are available for the treatment of fractures of the distal femur and the proximal lateral tibia. An additional advantage of the anatomically preshaped plates is that they make it possible to insert the screw in an appropriate direction to suit the anatomic conditions, allowing optimal anchorage. The guiding blocks help ensure the correct axial insertion of the drill sleeves and locking head screws. If required, standard screws can be inserted before the guiding block is positioned.

Less experienced surgeons can also use this technique with an open, but less invasive, approach. The fracture zone remains untouched. The MIPO technique is a great step forward in minimally invasive surgery (MIS) to treat fractures. To avoid complications and to shorten the learning curve, a reasonably invasive surgery (RIS) is recommended.

DISADVANTAGES AND COMPLICATIONS OF LOCKED SCREWS/PLATES

Several potential disadvantages of locking plate fixation exist. One is that the surgeon may completely lose the feel for the quality of the bone during screw insertion and tightening, when the screw head engages in the conically threaded plate hole. When tightening the screws, the surgeon has no tactile feedback as to the quality of screw purchase in the bone. Because the screws lock into the plate holes, they all abruptly stop advancing when the threads are completely seated in the plate, regardless of bone quality. Transcutaneous insertion of short monocortical LHSs in the diaphyseal area is critical at the end of the plate,

when there is some malalignment between the long bone axis and the plate. In these situations, anchorage is not obtained with a short screw, despite the surgical sensation that there is good tightening. Technically, the problem can be solved either by inserting a long self-tapping LHS or by using an angulated cortex or cancellous bone screw. The problem can be avoided at an early stage of the procedure by using the drill bit to center the screw and feel the bone cortex before the monocortical self-drilling screw is inserted. Alternatively, a small incision can be made at the plate end and the position of the plate can be assessed on the lateral side of the bone by manual palpation.

In addition, current locking plate designs can be used to maintain fracture reduction but only with anatomically preshaped locked plates and a specific technique. For example, for the complex distal femoral fracture, the distal fragment can be prepared to accept a LISS-DF or LCP DF by placing the second from most distal LHS exactly parallel to the knee joint. When the side plate is applied, limb alignment will be correct. With a nonanatomically preshaped locking plate design, the fracture must be reduced and limb alignment, length, and rotation set properly before placement of any locked screws. Once a locked screw has been placed above and below a fracture line, no further reduction adjustment is possible unless the screws are completely removed. Locked screws will not "pull" the plate down to the bone. This reduction maneuver is possible with special instruments or a temporary reduction screw. This lack of construct reduction capability, combined with percutaneous plating techniques, can result in higher rates of fracture malalignment than occur with formal open reduction and internal fracture fixation. New techniques are evolving to facilitate the accuracy of closed reduction of such difficult fractures. Surgeons contemplating a percutaneous approach should be experienced in conventional open techniques and be cognizant of their differences.

Another concern is the rigidity of a locked screw plate construct. For example, in diaphyseal or metadiaphyseal areas, any fracture distraction at the time of reduction or fracture resorption during healing will be held rigidly by such constructs and potentially result in delayed union or nonunion. In this situation, no load-sharing can occur with locked screws on either side of a fracture. If the fracture is repetitively loaded, the plate may eventually fracture or fixation may be lost. This is true in cases of simple fracture patterns and fracture fixation in a diastasis. The internal fixator will keep the diastasis and as a consequence may delay the fracture healing. This can lead to the risk of a cyclic overload of the plate and of the fracture bridging segment of the plate, between the two closest to the fracture placed screws, spans over less than 2–3 empty screw holes. Because of these concerns and the additional cost of a locking plate compared with an equivalent but nonlocking plate, locking plates probably should be used selectively for fractures that have demonstrated high failure rates with conventional plating techniques.

The lack of angulation within a nonanatomically preshaped plate can be a disadvantage in the epiphyseal bone segment. The disadvantage of current locking plate design is the inability of the surgeon to alter the angle of the screw within the hole and still achieve a locked screw.

The use of certain screw holes in the plate potentially could be blocked by lag screws placed for articular reduction, unique fracture geometry, anatomic variations, or implanted components of a joint arthroplasty. Exact preoperative planning is needed.

Any attempt to contour locked plates could potentially distort the screw holes and adversely affect screw purchase.

When locking plates are used, hardware removal may be more difficult, especially if locked screws become osteointegrated or were overtightened to the plate. Current systems offer torque-limiting screwdrivers that may minimize this concern.

SUMMARY

"Bridging plate osteosynthesis" using a locked plate is the technique of spanning the fracture site with an internal fixator without exposing the fracture site, and it was developed to preserve fragment vascular supply. This technique requires stabilization of the bone proximal and distal to the fracture site to achieve bone healing without direct manipulation of fracture fragments, and it is ideal for comminuted diaphyseal fractures and metadiaphyseal fracture patterns, particularly in osteoporotic bone.

Locked plating systems provide both angular and axial construct stability through a threaded interface between the screw heads and the plate body, which obviously avoids pressing the plate directly to a bony surface, thereby preserving blood supply and reducing the need for plate contouring. Furthermore, the angular and axial stability of locked plates minimizes the risk of secondary loss of reduction. Primary loss of reduction is minimized, since exact plate contouring is not required.

Bicortical locked screws are superior to unicortical locked screws in all modes of loading owing to the increased working length, or amount of bone purchase, present.

Locked plating allows for stable fracture fixation without the need for plate contouring or direct contact with bone. To maintain osseous blood supply, the plate is placed in an extraperiosteal position and will likely have no direct contact with bone.

Initial clinical data demonstrate excellent union rates, low rates of fixation failure, and few associated complications with the use of locking plates for internal fixation of fractures, particularly periarticular fractures. Locking plate technology will undoubtedly proliferate for fractures in other anatomic locations. Hybrid plates offering the versatility of either a locked or unlocked screw will probably enjoy widespread use. The clinical success of these implants is probably the result of the improved biological environment provided by minimally invasive plate insertion as well as the stable mechanical environment. As with all new technology, caution is warranted. Because these implants are used for difficult fractures, complications both old (e.g., malalignment, infection) and new (e.g., difficult hardware removal, incorrectly placed screws, pull-out) will occur. When such plates are inserted percutaneously, malalignment is common. Further clinical and biomechanical research on locking plate technology are needed to define fully its place alongside existing technology in orthopaedic trauma.

REFERENCES

1. Allgöwer, M.; Ehrsam, R.; Ganz, R.; et al. Clinical experience with a new compression plate "DCP." Acta Orthop Scand 125(Suppl):45–61, 1969.
2. Althausen, P.L.; Lee, M.A.; Finkemeier, C.G.; et al. Operative Stabilization of supracondylar femur fractures above total knee arthroplasty: A comparison of four treatment methods. Arthroplasie 18:834–839, 2003.
3. Bolhofner, B.R.; Carmen, B.; Clifford, P. The results of open reduction and internal fixation of distal femur fractures using a biologic (indirect) reduction technique. Orthop Trauma 10:372–377, 1996.
4. Brunner, C.; Weber, B.G. Special Techniques in Internal Fixation. Berlin, Springer-Verlag, 1982.
5. Cole, P.A.; Zlowodzki, M.; Kregor, P.J. Treatment of proximal tibia fractures using the less invasive stabilization system: surgical experience and early clinical results in 77 fractures. J Orthop Trauma 18(8):528–535, 2004.
6. Collinge, C.A.; Sanders, R.W. Percutaneous plating in the lower extremity. J Am Acad Orthop Surg 8(4):211–216, 2000.
7. Eijer, H.; Hauke, C.; Arens, S.; et al. PC-Fix and local infection resistance—influence of implant design on postoperative infection development, clinical and experimental results. Injury 32(Suppl 2):B38–43, 2001.
8. Ertl, W.; Smith, D.G. Bicondylar tibial plateau fractures: Comparison of early results with a locking plate compared with medial and lateral plating. In: Orthopaedic Trauma Association 18th Annual Meeting Final Program. Rosemont, IL: Orthopaedic Trauma Association, 2002, pp 170–171.
9. Fankhauser, F.; Gruber, G.; Schippinger, G.; et al. Minimal-invasive treatment of distal femoral fractures with the LISS (Less Invasive Stabilization System): a prospective study of 30 fractures with a follow up of 20 months. Acta Orthop Scand 75(1):56–60, 2004.
10. Farouk, O.; Krettek, C.; Miclau, T.; et al. Minimally invasive plate osteosynthesis and vascularity: preliminary results of a cadaver injection study. Injury 28(Suppl 1):A7–12, 1997.
11. Farouk, O.; Krettek, C.; Miclau, T.; et al. Minimally invasive plate osteosynthesis: Does percutaneous plating disrupt femoral blood supply less than the traditional technique? J Orthop Trauma 13(6):401–406, 1999.
12. Frigg, R. Locking Compression Plate (LCP): An osteosynthesis plate based on the Dynamic Compression Plate and the Point Contakt Fixator (PC-Fix). Injury 31 (Suppl 2):B63–B66, 2001.
13. Frigg, R. Development of the Locking Compression Plate. Injury 34(Suppl 1):B6–10, 2003.
14. Frigg, R.; Appenzeller, A.; Christensen, R.; et al. The development of the distal femur less invasive stabilization system (LISS). Injury 32:SC24–31, 2001.

15. Gosling, T.; Schandelmaier, P.; Müller, M.; et al. Single lateral locked screw plating of bicondylar tibial plateau fractures. Clin Orthop Relat Res 439:207–214, 2005.

16. Granowski, R.; Ramotowski, W.; Kaminski, E.; et al. "Zespol"—a new type of osteosynthesis, I: An internal self-compressing stabilizer of bone fragments. Chir Narzadow Ruchu Orthop Pol 49(4):301–305, 1984.

17. Haas, N.; Hauke, C.; Schütz, M.; et al. Treatment of diaphyseal fractures of the forearm using the Point Contact Fixator (PC-Fix): Results of 387 fractures of a prospective multicentric study (PC-Fix II). Injury 32(Suppl 2):B51–B62, 2001.

18. Hahn, U.; Prokop, A.; Jubel, A.; et al. LISS versus condylar plate. Kongressbd Dtsch Ges Chir Kongr 119:498–504, 2002.

19. Heitemeyer, U.; Hierholzer, G. Bridging osteosynthesis in closed compound fractures of the femur shaft. Aktuelle Traumatol 15:205–209, 1985.

20. Herford, A.S.; Ellis, E. III. Use of a locking reconstruction bone plate/screw system for mandibular surgery. Oral Maxillofac Surg 56:1261–1265, 1998.

21. Kassab, S.S.; Mast, J.J.; Kummer, F.J.; et al. Distal femoral fixation: A biomechanical comparison of the standard condylar buttress plate, a locked buttress plate, and the 95-degree blade plate. Orthop Trauma II:521–524, 1997.

22. Kolodziej, P.; Lee, F.S.; Patel, A.; et al. Bio-mechanical evulation of the Schuhli nut. Clin Orthop Relat Res 347:79–85, 1998.

23. Kregor, P.J.; Hughes, J.L.; Cole, P.A. Fixation of distal femoral fractures above total knee arthroplasty utilizing the Less Invasive Stabilization System (LISS). Injury 32(Suppl 2):SC64–SC75, 2001.

24. Kregor, P.J.; Stannard, J.; Zlowodzki, M.; et al. Distal femoral fracture fixation utilizing the Less Invasive Stabilization System (LISS): The technique and early results. Injury 32(Suppl 3):SC32–SC47, 2001.

25. Kregor, P.J.; Stannard, J.A.; Zlowodzki, M.; et al. Treatment of distal femur fractures using the less invasive stabilization system: Surgical experience and early clinical results in 103 fractures. J Orthop Trauma 18(8):509–520, 2004.

26. Krettek, C.; Müller, M.; Miclau, T. Evolution of minimally invasive plate osteosynthesis (MIPO) in the femur. Injury 32(Suppl 3):SC14–SC23, 2001.

27. Krettek, C.; Schandelmaier, P.; Miclau, T.; et al. Minimally invasive percutaneous plate osteosynthesis (MIPPO) using the DCS in proximal and distal femoral fractures. Injury 28(Suppl 1):A20–A30, 1997.

28. Leunig, M.; Hertel, R.; Siebenrock, K.A.; et al. The evolution of indirect reduction techniques for the treatment of fractures. Clin Orthop Relat Res 375:7–14, 2000.

29. Markmiller, M.; Konrad, G.; Südkamp, N. Femur-LISS and distal femoral nail for fixation of distal femoral fractures: Are there differences in outcome and complications? Clin Orthop Relat Res 426:252–257, 2004.

30. Mast, J.; Jakob, R.; Ganz, R. Planning and Reduction Technique in Fracture Surgery. Heidelberg, Springer, 1989.

31. Miclau, T.; Remiger, A.; Tepic, S.; et al. A mechanical comparison of the dynamic compression plate, limited contact-dynamic compression plate, and point contact fixator. Orthop Trauma 9:17–22, 1995.

32. Perren, S.M. Evolution of the internal fixation of long bone fractures: The scientific basis of biological internal fixation: Choosing a new balance between stability and biology. J Bone Joint Surg [Br] 84(8):1093–1110, 2002.

33. Perren, S.M.; Buchanan, J.S. Basic concepts relevant to the design and development of the Point Contact Fixator (PC-Fix). Injury 26(Suppl 2):B1–B4, 1995.

34. Perren, S.M.; Cordey, J.; Rahn, B.A.; et al. Early temporary porosis of bone induced by internal fixation implants: A reaction to necrosis, not to stress protection? Clin Orthop Relat Res 232:139–151, 1988.

35. Ricci, A.R.; Yue, J.J.; Taffet, R.; et al. Less Invasive Stabilization System for treatment of distal femur fractures. Am J Orthop 33(5):250–255, 2004.

36. Richter, M.; Wilken, H.J.; Kluger, P.; et al. Biomechanical evaluation of a newly developed monocortical expansion screw for use in anterior internal fixation of the cervical spine: In vitro comparison with two established internal fixation systems. Spine 24:207–212, 1999.

37. Rüedi, T.P.; Sommer, C.; Leutenegger, A. New techniques in indirect reduction of long bone fractures. Clin Orthop Relat Res 347:27–34, 1998.

38. Schandelmaier, P.; Partenheimer, A.; Koenemann, B.; et al. Distal femoral fractures and LISS stabilization. Injury 32(Suppl 3):SC55–SC63, 2001.

39. Schatzker, J. Fractures of the distal femur revisited. Clin Orthop Relat Res 347:43–56, 1998.

40. Schütz, M.; Haas, N.P. LISS—internal plate fixator. Kongressbd Dtsch Ges Chir Kongr 118:375–379, 2001. German.

41. Schütz, M.; Müller, M.; Kääb, M.; et al. Less invasive stabilization system (LISS) in the treatment of distal femoral fractures. Acta Chir Orthop Traumatol Cech 70(2):74–78, 2003.

42. Schütz, M.; Müller, M.; Krettek, C.; et al. Minimally invasive fracture stabilization of distal femoral fractures with the LISS: a prospective multicenter study: Results of a clinical study with special emphasis on difficult cases. Injury 32(Suppl 3):SC48–SC54, 2001.

43. Sommer, C.; Gautier, E.; Müller, M.; et al. First clinical results of the Locking Compression Plate (LCP). Injury 34(Suppl 2):B43–B54, 2003.

44. Stannard, J.P.; Wilson, T.C.; Volgas, D.A.; et al. Fracture stabilization of proximal tibial fractures with the proximal tibial LISS: early experience in Birmingham, Alabama (USA). Injury 34(Suppl 1):A36–A42, 2003.

45. Stover, M. Distal femoral fractures: Current treatment, results and problems. Injury 32(Suppl 3):SC3–SC13, 2001.

46. Syed, A.A.; Agarwal, M.; Giannoudis, P.V.; et al. Distal femoral fractures: long-term outcome following stabilisation with the LISS. Injury 35(6):599–607, 2004.

47. Wagner, M. General principles for the clinical use of the LCP. Injury 34(Suppl 2):B31–B42, 2003.

48. Wagner, M.; Frenk, A.; Frigg, R. New concepts for bone fracture treatment and the locking compression plate. Surg Technol Int 12:271–277, 2004.

49. Wagner, M.; Frigg, R. (ed) Internal Fixators. Thieme, 2006.

50. Weight, M.; Collinge, C. Early results of the less invasive stabilization system for mechanically unstable fractures of the distal femur (AO/OTA types A2, A3, C2, and C3). J Orthop Trauma 18(8):503–508, 2004.

51. Wong, M.K.; Leung, F.; Chow, S.P. Treatment of distal femoral fractures in the elderly using a less-invasive plating technique. Int Orthop 29(2):117–120, 2005.

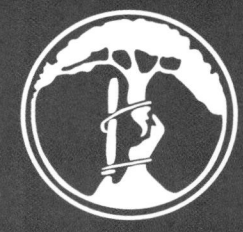

CHAPTER 6

Evaluation and Treatment of the Multiple-Trauma Patient

Robert T. Brautigam, M.D., F.A.C.S., Richard Sheppard, M.D., C.A.B.A., Kenneth J. Robinson, M.D., F.A.C.E.P., and Lenworth M. Jacobs, M.D., M.P.H., F.A.C.S.

INTRODUCTION

According to the Centers for Disease Control and Prevention's (CDC) National Center for Health Statistics (NCHS), injury remains a serious public health problem taking a toll on the health of the population while imposing enormous social and economic costs on society.[47] The NCHS data are used specifically to identify and track injury-related health problems while documenting injury's impact on the health of Americans including premature deaths and hospitalizations, and emergency department and other ambulatory visits associated with injuries. In addition, with the use of this data policymakers are able to direct health resources and interventions at the local and national levels.

In 2002, the NCHS noted there were 161,269 injury-related deaths. Hospital discharges constituted 1.8 million with 33 million emergency department visits. Outpatient visits were estimated to be approximately 82.3 million. Unintentional injuries ranked as the fifth most common cause of death. The leading causes of death by mechanism of injury in 2002 were classified as follows:

Motor-vehicle traffic: 44,065

Firearm: 30,242

Poisoning: 26,435

Fall: 17,116

These accounted for 73.1 percent of all injury deaths.

In 2005, the American College of Surgeons' (ACS) National Trauma Data Bank (NTDB) indicated the highest rate of injury between the ages of 12 to 24.[49] Deaths by age have two distinct peaks: first, around 20 years of age; and second, around 80 years. Injuries related to motor-vehicle traffic and firearms account for the first peak, and deaths from falls and motor-vehicle traffic account for the second peak.[49]

The trimodal distribution of mortality associated with trauma is categorized as immediate, early, and late.[77] Immediate deaths occur as a result of brain laceration, high spinal cord or brainstem injury, or major vessel or cardiac injury.[77] Given the poor survival from this type of injury, prevention is the best approach in reducing this distribution of fatalities. At the other end of the spectrum, late deaths occur several days to weeks following admission.[77] Eighty percent of these are secondary to head injury, and 20 percent are attributed to multiple organ failure and sepsis.[10] Early fatalities in the trimodal distribution of trauma deaths occur during the interval between injury and definitive care; this interval is crucial.[77] The American College of Surgeons Committee on Trauma Research reported that 62 percent of all in-hospital deaths occurred in the first 4 hours of admission, which emphasizes the need for expedient and definitive intervention.[6] A trauma systems approach to care of this cohort of the injured population reduced morbidity and mortality.

The Committee on Trauma Research in 1985 presented its report entitled *Injury in America*, which documented the significant impact injury has on the general population. This resulted in the federal government establishing the Center for Injury Control.[48] Funds were allocated to the Department of Transportation's National Highway Traffic Safety Administration and later assigned to the Division of Injury Epidemiology, a division of the CDC.[34] Injury Prevention Research Centers were established and charged with the responsibility to collect data and report to the CDC the results of their research investigation.[34] With government commitment to the investigation of injury, this public health problem could be specifically addressed.

Epidemiologic principles and practice were applied to the investigation of injury. This provides information that is generalized to the population, provides quantitative assessment of events, and is based on comparative analysis of observations. The study of injury in epidemiologic terms is divided into two arms: first, identification of a phenomenon to be investigated, and second, quantification based on the number of incidents in reference to severity, time, space, and concentration.[59] This process is described as descriptive epidemiology.[59] An assessment of these descriptive data is termed analytical epidemiology, which strives to identify risk factors and makes inferences as to the cause of the injury.

William Haddon was at the forefront of epidemiologic investigation for injury.[59] Following the principles of

Table 6-1

Haddon's Technical Strategies for Injury Control

1. Prevent creation of hazards in the first place.
2. Reduce the amount of hazards brought into being.
3. Prevent the release of hazards that already exist.
4. Modify the rate or spatial distribution of release of the hazard from its source.
5. Separate, in time or space, the hazard and that which is to be protected.
6. Separate the hazard and that which is to be protected by interposition of a material barrier.
7. Modify basis relevant qualities of the hazard.
8. Make what is to be protected more resistant to damage from the hazard.
9. Begin to counter the damage already done by the environmental hazard.
10. Stabilize, repair, and rehabilitate the object of the damage.

Adapted from L. Robertson. Injury Epidemiology. Copyright © 1992 by L. Robertson. Used by permission of Oxford University Press, Inc.

epidemiologic investigation, he devised a strategic plan for the control of injury and identified 10 objectives in the implementation of injury control (Table 6-1).[59] In general terms, these 10 objectives have laid the groundwork from which most epidemiologic investigations of injury originate.[59] This analysis of injuries has assisted with the development of a trauma care system aimed at prevention, resuscitation, treatment, and rehabilitation of the injured patient.

THE TRAUMA SYSTEM

Historical Perspective

Documentation of the effectiveness of a trauma systems approach to the care of the injured has been one of the goals of the Injury Prevention Research Centers of the CDC and Level I trauma centers accredited by the American College of Surgeons. Jacobs and Jacobs reported on the increased survival of trauma patients who were taken to a trauma center by rapid air transport when compared with a cohort of trauma patients taken by ground.[35] This finding was consistent with the improved outcomes of military evacuation in Korea and Vietnam when injured soldiers were immediately transported to mobile army surgical hospitals (MASH). This concept of providing definitive care as quickly as possible resulted in reduced morbidity and mortality.[25] Guidelines established by the American College of Surgeons Resources for Optimal Care of the Injured Patient[7] and by Shackford and associates[70] and Rauzz[55] demonstrated improved outcome of injured patients.

The issue of sophisticated trauma care has been challenged by the trends of managed care. In response to this challenge, Demetriades and colleagues demonstrated that the care provided by Level I trauma centers made a difference in improved survival and decreased permanent disability.[22] Miller and Levy demonstrated that states with dedicated trauma systems provide care for patients with major injuries at a reduced cost.[44] The challenge for the future will be to continue outcomes research to demonstrate that trauma systems are cost effective for the injured patient.

Structure

The Trauma Care Systems and Development Act created guidelines for the development of an inclusive trauma system integrated with the emergency medical services (EMS) system to meet the needs of acutely injured patients.[7] The objective of the system is to match the needs of patients to the most appropriate level of care.[7] This process of designation of level I, II, III, or IV is dependent on the commitment and resources of the medical staff and administration to trauma care at facilities seeking designation. The criteria for each level of designation appear in Table 6-2.

The configuration of the trauma team receiving patients is variable but includes emergency medicine physicians, nurses, allied health personnel, and the trauma surgeon as the team leader.[35] Various subspecialists in surgery, orthopaedics, neurosurgery, cardiothoracic surgery, anesthesia, and pediatrics are readily available at a Level I center.[7] The receiving facility should have a dedicated area for the resuscitation of trauma patients as well as a dedicated operating room available 24 hours a day. A resuscitation room should be well equipped with devices for the warming of fluid, rapid infusers, and appropriate surgical supplies for the performance of lifesaving procedures. Permanently fixed radiographic equipment expedites the evaluation of the injured patient in the resuscitation room. Staffing in the trauma room should be limited to those with experience in trauma resuscitation, and their duties should follow the guidelines outlined in the American College of Surgeons Committee on Trauma Resources for Optimal Care of the Trauma Patient 1999.[7]

Following the acute phase of resuscitation and operative intervention, a Level I trauma facility maintains a highly trained staff of surgical intensivists. The staff provides 24-hour coverage of the intensive care unit (ICU). These patients are susceptible to complications such as sepsis, adult respiratory distress syndrome (ARDS), and multisystem organ failure, which require the technical support provided by a Level I center. This includes, but is not limited to, jet ventilation, hemodialysis, and cardiac assist devices. Intermediate care units provide intensive supervision of the patient prior to placement on the trauma floor, which is critical for the recovery of the patient. During this time, patients receive rehabilitation to prepare for dealing with disabilities and limitations that may have changed their lives owing to their injury. The patient's physical and emotional health are evaluated, and treatment is initiated. Patients who have suffered significant injury will have special nutritional needs, given their increased caloric demands. The patient's nutritional status is assessed by nutritional services and a recommendation made to the trauma service. As the patient nears discharge, arrangements for home needs and potential placement are made by Social Services and Case Care Coordinators. The availability of and relationships with rehabilitation centers and chronic nursing facilities are essential for injured patients.

ASSESSING SEVERITY OF INJURY

Several scoring systems have been developed in an attempt to triage and classify patients both in the field and at the receiving hospital. Champion and coworkers have

Table 6-2	
Criteria for Trauma Designation	
Level	**Criteria**
Level I	
Regional resource trauma center	
	Provide leadership and total care of the trauma patient
	Participate in trauma prevention and rehabilitation
	Clinical capabilities:
	Cardiac, hand, microvascular, and pediatric surgery
	In-house general surgeon or in-house officer at postgraduate year IV level or greater in surgery
	Facility resources:
	Cardiopulmonary bypass
	Operating microscope
	Acute hemodialysis
	Nuclear scanning
	Neuroradiology
	Provide leadership in education, research, and systems development
Level II	
	Provide initial definitive trauma care
	Clinical capabilities similar to Level I, with exception of the subspecialty areas of surgery
	In absence of house staff, general surgeon may be out of house but readily available
	Education outreach, research, and prevention programs similar to Level I, but research not essential
	System flexibility to transfer complex patients to Level I facilities
Level III	
	Provide immediate assessment, resuscitation, emergency operations, and stabilization of trauma patients
	Have prearranged transfer agreements with Level I facilities
	Prompt availability of general surgeon required
Level IV	
	Provide advanced trauma life support in remote areas prior to transfer to higher level of care

Adapted from American College of Surgeons Committee on Trauma. Resources for Optimal Care of the Injured Patient: 1993. Chicago, American College of Surgeons, 1993.

classified the scoring systems into physiologic and anatomic types.[14] The Glasgow Coma Scale (GCS) for brain injury is perhaps the most widely accepted physiologic score currently utilized. This scale ranges from 3 to 15, with 15 being normal. Each section, with its weighted score, is as follows: eye movement (4 points maximum), verbal response (5 points maximum), and motor response (6 points maximum) (Table 6-3). The GCS is a part of the Revised Trauma Score (RTS), which allows inferences to patient outcome as a result of these scores. This score comprises the GCS score, systolic blood pressure, and respiratory rate (Table 6-4).[14]

PREHOSPITAL RESUSCITATION

The on-scene evaluation and treatment of trauma patients can be widely variable and are dependent on the level of training of the provider, local standards and protocols, and available resources. Each EMS system has a unique structure, but in general, there are four levels of providers: first responder, emergency medical technician (EMT),

paramedic, and prehospital critical care provider. Prehospital critical care providers include critical care trained paramedics, nurses, respiratory therapists, and physicians. These providers operate in ground and air transport systems. Although local protocols often follow nationally accepted standards there may be small variations for each specific protocol based on regional need or the local medical director's preference. In general, more densely populated areas have a greater number of EMS providers and resources. Unfortunately, as the population density decreases, EMS resources often decrease. In rural areas there may be only one ambulance and a basic EMT team for a large geographic area.

Each level of prehospital provider has specific required training that increases in conjunction with the number and complexity of the available protocols and interventions to be performed. In addition, the education and training in the EMS system are cumulative, with each of the preceding levels often being a building block of the knowledge for the next level. For example, the knowledge base and skills of the first responder level are the foundation for EMT training.

Table 6-3	
Glasgow Coma Scale	
Response	**Score**
A. Eye opening	
Spontaneous	4
To voice	3
To pain	2
None	1
B. Verbal response	
Oriented	5
Confused	4
Inappropriate words	3
Incomprehensible sounds	2
None	1
C. Motor response	
Obeys commands	6
Localized pain	5
Withdraw to pain	4
Flexion to pain	3
Extension to pain	2
None	1

Total GCS points (A + B + C) 3–15

Adapted from Teasdale, G.; Jennett, B. Assessment of coma and impaired consciousness. A practical scale. Lancet 2:81–84, © by The Lancet Ltd, 1974.

The U.S. Department of Transportation (DOT) establishes the National Standard Curricula (NSC) as the minimum standards for each level and recommends the range of required training hours. In this section, each level of provider will be defined, the required training will be described, and the evaluation and care of a multiple trauma patient for each level will be discussed.[53]

Table 6-4		
Revised Trauma Score (RTS)		
Response	**Variables**	**Score**
A. Respiratory rate (breaths/min)	10–29	4
	>29	3
	6–9	2
	1–5	1
	0	0
B. Systolic blood pressure (mm Hg)	>89	4
	76–89	3
	50–75	2
	1–49	1
	0	0
C. Glasgow Coma Scale score conversion	13–15	4
	9–12	3
	6–8	2
	4–5	1
	3	0
Revised Trauma Score = Total of A + B + C		

Adapted from Champion, H.R.; Sacco, W.J.; Copes, W.S.; et al. A revision of the Trauma Score. J Trauma 29:623–629, 1989.

First Responders

First responders are often the first people to arrive at the scene of an emergency. These providers are often public safety personnel such as police officers or fire fighters. The DOT curriculum for a first responder includes a total of 40 hours of education and training.[53]

The first responder evaluation of a trauma patient begins with an evaluation of the scene. This is followed by an initial assessment, including the ABCs (airway, breathing, and circulation), then a rapid trauma assessment. Cervical spine protection is maintained at all times. The airway is assessed for patency. If the airway is not open, then a basic airway maneuver, like the jaw thrust, is used. If respirations are abnormal, inadequate, or absent, rescue breathing is initiated. The assessment of circulation includes a search for obvious bleeding, a check of central and peripheral pulses, and determination of skin color, temperature, and capillary refill. If bleeding is discovered, it is controlled with direct pressure and then a dressing is applied.[1,74]

The rapid trauma assessment involves a head-to-toe physical examination searching for injuries. Vital signs are determined, and the head, neck, chest, abdomen, pelvis, back, neurologic status, and extremities are examined. If a back injury is suspected, full spinal immobilization is employed. All obvious or suspected extremity injuries are splinted, and pelvic fractures are stabilized with a pneumatic antishock garment or a sheet tied tightly around the patient's pelvis.

Splinting is initially taught at the first responder level. Some commonly accepted guidelines for splinting include the following: expose the injured area, remove clothing and jewelry from the injured area, assess neurovascular status of the injured limb before and after applying the splint, dress open wounds, splint the extremity as it is found with a padded splint that immobilizes the joint above and below the injured area, and splint the extremity before transport unless the patient has other life-threatening injuries that necessitate immediate transportation.[2,64]

The splints utilized can be made from a variety of materials and may be custom made or commercially available. Air casts are available in sizes that fit most extremities. A suspected femur fracture is most commonly immobilized with a bipolar traction splint (Hare), which provides stabilization of the entire leg and traction of the foot to obtain realignment of the femur fracture. When traction splints are employed for lower extremity injuries, the pulses in the foot are to be continuously assessed.[2] Once the patient has been assessed and properly immobilized, transport is initiated.

Besides medical care, first responders are also trained in scene safety. They are often invaluable in establishing and maintaining control of chaotic scenes, directing rescue resources, and calming family and bystanders.[53]

Emergency Medical Technicians

The EMT level includes EMT-Basic (EMT-B) and EMT-Intermediate (EMT-I). The total hours of training for an EMT-B are approximately 115 hours and the required training for an EMT-I ranges from 300 to 400 total hours. This training includes didactic and clinical components and an optional internship.[53]

The skills and interventions an EMT-B is able to provide include the scope of first responder practice; advanced history, noting mechanism of injury; vital sign assessment; oxygen administration; application of an automatic external defibrillator (AED); on-scene triage; splinting and immobilization; extrication and transport; administration of activated charcoal, epinephrine auto-injectors, and oral glucose; and assisting patients in taking their own nitroglycerin and inhalation medications. The EMT-I is able to initiate intravenous access, endotracheally intubate or place a Combitube, place a nasogastric tube, manually defibrillate, initiate cardiac pacing, and administer the following medications: aspirin, atropine, adenosine, bronchodilators, diazepam, epinephrine, Lasix, lidocaine, morphine, Narcan, nitroglycerin, and dextrose (D_{50}).[53]

The EMT assessment of a trauma victim also begins with the assessment of the adequacy of the airway, breathing, and circulation (ABC). The airway is assessed. If indicated, an attempt is made to open the airway employing various methods such as suctioning foreign material or manual positioning of the airway. Because of the potential for cervical spine injuries in trauma patients, the jaw-thrust maneuver is preferred to the chin-lift. If the patient is having difficulty breathing and the airway is open, oxygen is applied and ventilation is assisted with a bag-valve mask (BVM). In the event that the BVM is not successful, an advanced airway adjunct (ETT, LMA, or Combitube) may be employed. Blood pressure and heart rate are determined, and intravenous fluids are initiated if indicated. Any major external bleeding is identified and controlled. A cervical collar is placed, and cervical spine immobilization is maintained. Cardiopulmonary resuscitation (CPR) is initiated as needed, and an AED can be applied as well.[50]

Once the evaluation of the ABCs and any necessary interventions are completed, a more thorough physical examination is performed. The mechanism of injury is considered and helps direct this assessment. Full spinal immobilization is maintained, and the head and neck are inspected for injuries. The chest is assessed for presence and quality of breath sounds, and the abdomen is palpated. The back, pelvis, and extremities are inspected, and any injuries (obvious or suspected) are immobilized as described above. Long bone injuries that have resulted in cyanosis or loss of pulses may have gentle, constant traction applied. If there is resistance to the traction, the limb is immobilized as it was found. Once the assessment is complete, appropriate treatments have been initiated, and proper immobilization has been performed, the patient is transported to the appropriate hospital.[50]

Paramedic

Paramedic (EMT-P) training is more extensive and includes didactic and clinical components, an internship, and a practical lab, totaling approximately 3000 hours.[53] The paramedic scope of practice includes that of an EMT-I and includes a more sophisticated evaluation, endotracheal intubation, cricothyrotomy, needle thoracostomy, 12-lead electrocardiogram (ECG), selective cervical spine immobilization, termination of resuscitation, and a significantly wider array of medications.[53] As always, the scope of practice can vary from region to region and depends on local medical direction.

The paramedic evaluation of a trauma victim on scene is similar to but more comprehensive than that of an EMT-I.[62] The care of musculoskeletal trauma is similar except that the paramedic can provide intravenous analgesia and sedation. The paramedic may also be permitted to more fully properly align the injured extremity in order to enhance circulation, reduce further injury, and improve patient comfort.[63]

Prehospital Critical Care Provider

This category of provider covers a wide range of disciplines including critical care trained paramedics, respiratory therapists, nurses, and physicians. These providers are often required to have a certain amount of in-hospital critical care experience before joining a transport team. Commonly they receive further training, both didactic and practical, as part of an orientation to the transport program. Each critical care transport program (air or ground) has a unique training regimen, and the most advanced teams receive 2 to 6 months of training after joining the transport team.

The scope of practice of these providers is often dictated by their license. Most can perform rapid sequence intubation and other high-risk interventions. These practitioners have more clinical experience and a higher level of understanding of pathophysiology and pharmacology. They operate with greater autonomy and are able to administer many of the same medications that are administered in a hospital critical care unit or emergency department.

This group of practitioners provides the highest level of care outside of the hospital setting. The assessment of a trauma patient is generally the same as described above but may involve more attention to detail. The interventions follow the same general principles but are often more aggressive, including intravenous fluid resuscitation and administration of analgesia. The same principles for immobilization are utilized, and the patient is transported to the hospital.[60]

The training, assessment skills, and level of care provided by EMS personnel are variable and depend on the EMS system. In every system, the goal of evaluation and treatment of the trauma patient in the field is to evaluate airway, breathing, and circulation; provide spinal immobilization; initiate appropriate resuscitation; perform a secondary survey; properly prepare the patient for transport; and minimize time on scene. The specific standards or protocols are determined by the regulatory agency governing that region and local medical control.

HOSPITAL RESUSCITATION

Once the trauma patient has reached the trauma center, resuscitation is continued according to the principles of a primary, secondary, and tertiary survey as established by the American College of Surgeons Committee on Trauma. The primary survey encompasses the ABCs, disability, and exposure. The secondary survey involves a head-to-toe evaluation of the patient's injuries and implementation of appropriate interventions. The tertiary survey involves serial reevaluation of the patient's status during his or her hospital course. This section reviews the process of trauma resuscitation and diagnostic modalities and treatment options for specific injuries.

PRIMARY SURVEY

Airway

The first objective is to evaluate, manage, and secure the airway. Inspection of the airway for foreign bodies such as broken teeth, foodstuff, emesis, and clotted blood is essential prior to placing an artificial airway. In all Basic Life Support courses, the emphasis on chin lift and jaw thrust cannot be overemphasized as the initial treatment.[46] This simple maneuver moves the tongue away from the back of the throat and in many instances reestablishes a patent airway. At this point an oral airway may need to be placed. This is a semicircular plastic device that is placed into the oropharynx in such a fashion as to prevent the tongue from occluding the oropharynx. Appropriate size selection is essential to prevent the complication of airway obstruction. The nasopharyngeal airway is a device that is placed through the nasal passage into the back of the oropharynx to prevent the tongue from occluding the airway. Prior to its placement it is lubricated to facilitate its passage.

Once this maneuver has been performed, the airway may need to be definitively controlled in patients who are unresponsive or have an altered mental status (GCS ≤8), are hemodynamically unstable, or have multiple injuries including to the head and neck. Of utmost importance remains cervical spine protection while the optimal airway is maintained, with in-line cervical spine stabilization. This maneuver minimizes iatrogenic injuries to the spine and/or spinal cord during the process of definitive airway control.

Whenever the decision is made to emergently secure an airway, it must be accomplished in as quick and safe a method as possible. Pharmacologic agents must be chosen that will allow the safe placement of an airway while minimizing the risk to the patient. The most rapidly acting agents with the shortest duration along with an acceptable side effect profile should be chosen. In all circumstances, the practitioner must avoid the situation in which a long-acting agent has been given and the airway cannot be intubated or ventilated with a bag mask device.

In the case of the standard rapid sequence induction, the patient should be preoxygenated, then a hypnotic agent is immediately followed by the paralytic agent. Mask ventilation is not attempted, and it is hoped that the immediate successful placement of the endotracheal tube will proceed. Proper placement is verified by auscultation of the lungs bilaterally, lack of gastric sounds with ventilation, and the presence of end-tidal carbon dioxide at the proximal end of the endotracheal tube.

Thermal injuries to the airway initially may not be symptomatic or present as hypoxia for some time after the insult. During the initial survey, documentation of singed hair, soot, or burns around the air passages should be noted. The decision may be made to secure an airway with an endotracheal tube prophylactically, before significant edema and swelling may make securing the airway much more difficult.

As the anesthetic induction is begun, an assistant should apply enough pressure onto the cricoid cartilage so as to occlude the esophagus, which lies directly posterior. This technique should be employed in any patient in whom there is the risk of aspiration of gastric contents.[31,69] It should be remembered that trauma, pain, and the use of narcotics may all delay gastric emptying. Release of cricoid pressure occurs only after proper positioning of the endotracheal tube has been verified.

Pharmacologic Agents

HYPNOTIC AGENTS

Etomidate has been available for clinical use since 1972. Its popularity is due to its cardiovascular and cerebrovascular profile. Etomidate lowers intracranial pressure (ICP)[20] and intraocular pressure (IOP)[23] and has minimal effects on respiratory response to carbon dioxide.[56] At a dose of 0.3 mg/kg it produces minimal changes in mean arterial pressure or heart rate. Duration is for 5 to 15 minutes. It does not produce histamine release. For these reasons, it is often the drug of choice for induction of a patient with known or suspected cardiovascular disease, hypovolemia, or elevated ICP.

When given via a small peripheral vein, etomidate is associated with significant pain on injection and the potential for phlebitis. It is also associated with significant myoclonic activity, which may be confused with seizure activity (especially if given in conjunction with succinylcholine associated fasciculations) and postoperative nausea or vomiting.[57]

Finally, even one dose has been associated with the inhibition of steroid synthesis within the adrenal gland.[79] This may present as an Addisonian crisis some time later when the patient may be in an ICU setting and develops hypotension and/or shock from no obvious cause.

KETAMINE

Ketamine produces dissociative anesthesia when given at a dose of 0.5 to 2 mg/kg intravenously or 4 to 6 mg/kg intramuscularly. It is chemically related to phencyclidine ("angel dust").[45] A single dose lasts about 10 to 15 minutes with complete arousal after about 30 minutes. Profound analgesia with moderate amnesia is provided while respiration is maintained along with eyelid and cough reflexes. Activity begins within 1 minute of injection and is associated with the onset of nystagmus.

Ketamine increases ICP and the metabolism of cerebral tissues.[26] It should be avoided in patients with an elevated ICP or a history of seizures. Because of the associated tachycardia and hypertension, it is best avoided in patients with suspected ischemic heart disease. Prior hyperventilation may attenuate the rise in ICP caused by ketamine.[71] It reduces the activity of bronchial smooth muscle and may improve pulmonary compliance.[32] Increased upper airway secretions may be reduced by pretreatment with an agent such as glycopyrrolate. Ketamine elevates heart rate and blood pressure and is, therefore, often used for induction in patients who may be suspected of having hypovolemia.[58] These effects are mediated through a central nervous system pathway. The direct effect of ketamine in the periphery is actually as a depressant.[17] Therefore, in a patient who may have had a long extrication in the field and may have had endogenous catecholamines depleted, ketamine may actually act as a cardiovascular depressant and exacerbate any hypotension. It is an excellent choice for patients with cardiac tamponade or restrictive pericarditis, since it maintains spontaneous ventilation and supports cardiac contractility. The management of cardiac tamponade is described later in this chapter. The drug is associated with some undesirable psychological side effects, among them delusions, vivid dreams, and paranoia. These are more common in adults and can be minimized by the prior use of benzodiazepines.

PROPOFOL

Propofol initially contained soybean oil and egg phosphatide. One formulation contains sulfite as a preservative. Known allergy to any of these components may necessitate the use of another drug. Unlike barbiturates, it does not have anti-analgesia properties.[12] At an induction dose of 2 to 3 mg/kg, the effects last about 5 to 10 minutes, and it is metabolized by the liver.[73] It reduces ICP[75] while maintaining the response to serum carbon dioxide. Propofol produces apnea for a longer period than most other induction agents[76] and is also associated with a significant drop in cardiac index as well as systolic and diastolic pressures. It decreases both preload and afterload and is also associated with mild myocardial depression.[27] It is therefore a poor choice for cardiac tamponade. It may not be the drug of choice for a patient with borderline cardiovascular reserve. Like etomidate, it is associated with myoclonic activity and pain if injected through a small peripheral vein. Its popularity as an induction agent is due to its pharmacokinetic profile. It is rapidly cleared, with minimal complaints of nausea and vomiting. It is easily given as a continuous infusion for sedation (25–100 µg/kg/min), together with a narcotic and/or benzodiazepine. It is often combined with ketamine as an infusion for procedures that require the patient to maintain spontaneous ventilation, respond to inquiries, and tolerate pain (e.g., facial cosmetic surgery).

PARALYTIC AGENTS

Paralytic agents, as a general rule, should not be injected unless the ability to ventilate the patient by mask has been established. In a trauma scenario, where rapid placement of a secure endotracheal tube is paramount to protect the airway, this may not be practical. Therefore, a careful examination of the airway should be done and Mallampati classification[78] should be identified. If the patient is obese, proper positioning is critical while in-line cervical spine stabilization is maintained. If this is uncertain, a short-acting paralytic agent should be utilized. Once the airway is secure, a longer acting agent may be utilized.

SUCCINYLCHOLINE Depolarizing paralytic agents, such as succinylcholine, are rapidly acting paralytic agents of short duration (usually 3–5 minutes). The drug is metabolized by serum cholinesterases (pseudocholinesterase). Pseudocholinesterase is not present at the neuromuscular junction; therefore, the duration of activity of the drug that does reach the motor endplate is dependent on its diffusion away from the neuromuscular junction.

Because pseudocholinesterase is synthesized by the liver, patients with significant hepatic disease may have lower levels of the enzyme, which may result in a prolonged duration of activity of the drug. High estrogen levels are also associated with reduced levels of pseudocholinesterase, as may occur in the third trimester of pregnancy.

Certain drugs also affect the activity of the enzyme. Anticholinesterase drugs used in the treatment of myasthenia gravis, glaucoma, and insecticides are some of the more common agents.

There is also a genetic predisposition for altered activity of pseudocholinesterase. About one in 3200 people is homozygous for an atypical form of pseudocholinesterase. These people may have duration of activity for succinylcholine that may last several hours. About one in 480 people are heterozygous for the atypical form of the enzyme and may have only a slightly prolonged duration of the drug.

Several known side effects of succinylcholine may actually contraindicate its use. Because it is a depolarizing agent, the drug can cause significant fine muscle fasciculations, which may result in significant myalgias in the immediate postoperative period. They may also produce a rise in intraocular and intragastric pressure, making aspiration more likely. Succinylcholine has been shown to produce myoglobinuria in pediatric patients. The increased muscle activity may produce significant elevations in serum carbon dioxide, which in turn may affect cerebral blood flow. Studies have shown an increase of ICP of about 5 mm Hg when succinylcholine is used in patients with space-occupying lesions of the brain.

The drug may also be associated with approximately a 1 mEq/L elevation in serum potassium levels. This effect is exaggerated in certain disease states. These include any trauma patient with crushing muscle injuries; third-degree burns, especially 10 to 60 days after the initial burn;[66] and any neurological injury resulting in chronic muscle denervation, such as an upper or lower motor neuron lesion.[21] It is thought that the denervated muscle tissue produces excessive acetylcholine receptors. These receptors react in an exaggerated way to succinylcholine to produce excessive muscle fasciculations with resultant large releases of potassium. Therefore, succinylcholine may be contraindicated in any patient with suspected high levels of serum potassium, such as with renal failure or rhabdomyolysis. The result could be sudden cardiac arrest due to hyperkalemia.

Because of the rise in carbon dioxide and fasciculations of fine muscles, succinylcholine is also associated with the potential rise in intraocular pressure. This may be of concern with any open eye injury, since the fasciculations may have the potential to cause the extrusion of intraocular contents. This theoretical risk has been minimized by the prior use of "de-fasciculating" doses of nondepolarizing agents.[38]

Repeated doses of succinylcholine within a short time period are associated with bradycardic episodes. The most life-threatening complication of succinylcholine use is the production of malignant hyperthermia (MH) in susceptible people. This has a genetic pattern and, if possible, a careful family history should be taken. If after injection, trismus-masseter spasm occurs with peripheral flaccidity, MH should be suspected. The clinical signs of tachycardia, hypercarbia, and pyrexia may not present for several hours. If MH is undiagnosed, the outcome is poor. If it is diagnosed early and treated appropriately with dantrolene sodium, there is usually a good outcome. The Malignant Hyperthermia Association of the United States (MHAUS) can be reached at 1-209-634-4917, 24 hours a day.

VECURONIUM Nondepolarizing paralyzing agents, such as vecuronium (0.1 mg/kg) and rocuronium (0.6 mg/kg), have gained popularity because of their relatively quick onset (2–3 minutes) and intermediate duration (30 minutes), together with their minimal effects on the cardiovascular system. They show minimal or no release of histamine and can be used as "de-fasciculating agents" prior to the use of succinylcholine.

Atracurium (0.5 mg/kg) and cisatracurium (0.2 mg/kg) last about 30 minutes and 45 minutes, respectively. Their onset of action takes several minutes, and they are probably not the drugs of choice for rapid sequence inductions. However, they both have a unique pharmacokinetic characteristic: they undergo spontaneous Hoffman degradation in the plasma. As a result they are independent of both renal and liver function for their elimination. They are excellent choices for long-term use in end-stage renal or hepatic disease.

ADJUVANTS The prior use of a nondepolarizing paralytic agent 3 to 4 minutes prior to the use of succinylcholine has been shown in certain studies to reduce the incidence of significant fasciculations and their accompanying complications. Vecuronium (0.01 mg/kg) or d-tubocurarine (0.06 mg/kg) has been used in this regard. Some patients may become symptomatic by these small doses and may complain of dyspnea prior to the initiation of the intubation process. Curare may cause the release of histamine.

Lidocaine (1.5 mg/kg) given 3 to 4 minutes prior to induction has been shown to reduce the response to laryngoscopy,[30] thereby minimizing the risk of elevations in blood pressure and ICP. Small doses (40–60 mg) given just prior to propofol or etomidate have been shown to reduce the pain on injection if given through small peripheral veins. Laryngoscopy alone is associated with an increased ICP of up to 10 to 20 mm Hg. The use of beta-blockers (e.g., esmolol, labetalol) prior to induction to ablate the cardiovascular response to laryngoscopy is also helpful.

In any induction process, the judicious use of narcotics (e.g., fentanyl) and/or benzodiazepines (e.g., midazolam) is often beneficial.

If time allows and there is no risk of aspiration, hyperventilation after injection of the hypnotic agent may reduce the risk of hypercarbia associated with succinylcholine.

Airway Supplements

The use of the laryngeal mask airway (LMA) has gained popularity because of the relative ease of placement and relatively low cardiovascular stress that the patient undergoes compared with standard endotracheal intubation. It must be remembered that the LMA does not technically protect the airway from aspiration and was designed to be used in spontaneously breathing patients.

The LMA may be used emergently for the patient to whom a paralytic agent has been given but successful intubation has not been achieved, or prior to the injection of the paralytic agent if mask ventilation is not adequate. In this manner, it acts as a bridge to allow for adequate ventilation in a patient who is no longer spontaneously breathing and cannot be intubated or mask-ventilated.

A recent design has modified the classic LMA—the ProSeal LMA. This device has a second tube placed directly posterior to the airway tube, which ventilates the trachea. In this manner, the posterior placed tube sits at the origin of the esophagus. An orogastric tube can be placed into the stomach to aspirate gastric contents. This should minimize the risk of passive or active aspiration.

Another device is the Combitube. This device is placed "blindly" like the LMA but is designed quite differently. The Combitube has two balloons, which are inflated once it is placed. The distal balloon is smaller and is situated just proximal to the end of the Combitube. Just proximal to the distal balloon are fenestrations that allow for ventilation to occur. Proximal to the fenestrations is a second larger balloon. The fenestrations and the distal end of the Combitube can be ventilated by separate proximal tube connections. Because the Combitube is placed blindly, if the distal end of the tube is situated within the esophagus and the small distal balloon is expanded, the esophagus is occluded and the trachea can be ventilated via the fenestrations in the proximal part of the Combitube between the two balloons. If the distal end of the tube is placed within the trachea, the distal balloon can be expanded and traditional ventilation can occur. The position of the distal end of the Combitube is verified by serial auscultation.

It is not uncommon to place a nasotracheal tube once continuity of the airway has been established. It is often helpful to coat a nasal trumpet with topical anesthetic lubricant and nasal decongestant prior to placement into one or both nares. After a few minutes, a warmed, flexible endotracheal tube can be slowly passed via one of the nares into the posterior pharynx. Under direct laryngoscopy, the tube can be placed into the trachea, or assisted with a McGill forceps. A "blind nasal" intubation can be achieved if the patient is adequately sedated by slowly passing the nasotracheal tube into the posterior pharynx and listening for air sounds at the proximal end of the tube. As the tube approaches the glottic opening, the sounds become more intense and the tube is passed "blindly" into the trachea.

Surgical Airway

In the rare instance when an airway cannot be obtained by the above methods, a surgical airway may need to be created.[33] The standard emergency adult surgical airway procedure is cricothyroidotomy (Fig. 6-1). This surgical airway procedure requires a vertical incision to be made in the skin over the cricothyroid membrane, followed by a transverse incision into the trachea through this

FIGURE 6-1 *Technique for cricothyroidotomy. (Adapted from Bone, L.B. In: Browner, B.D.; Jupiter, J.B.; Levine, A.M.; et al. (eds.). Skeletal Trauma, 1st ed. Philadelphia, W.B. Saunders, 1992.)*

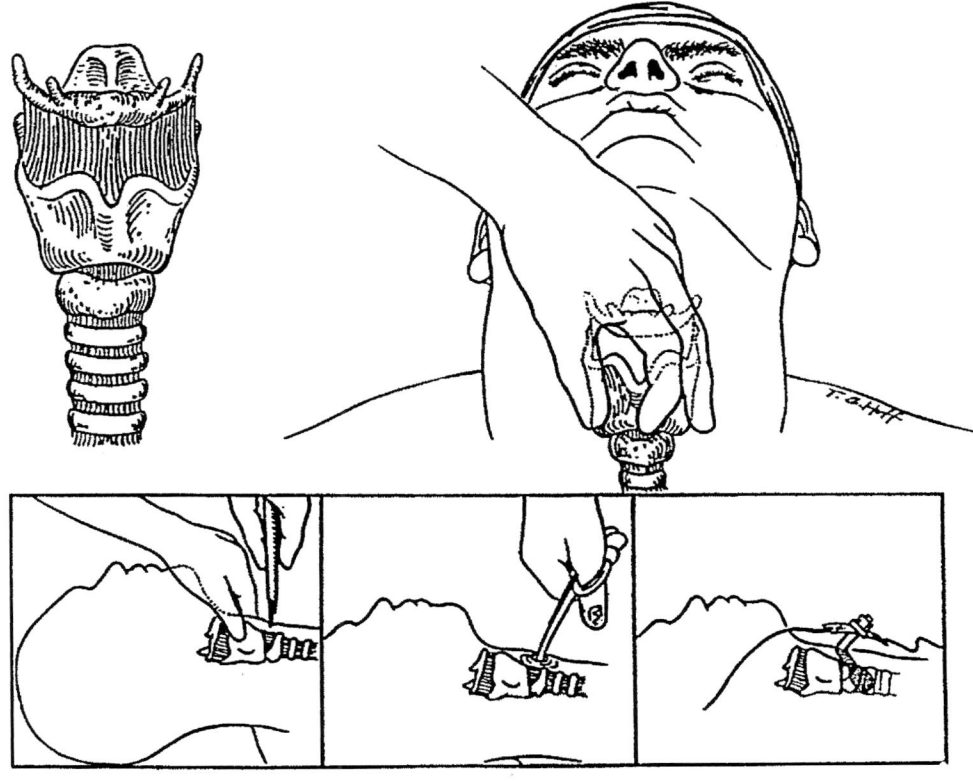

membrane. An endotracheal or tracheostomy tube is then placed into the trachea and secured to provide ventilation and oxygenation.

A needle cricothyroidotomy may be performed in some instances with positive pressure ventilation as a bridge to the definitive surgical airway. This involves placing a large angiocatheter (14-gauge) through the cricothyroid membrane and ventilating with 30 to 60 pounds per square inch (psi) of pressurized oxygen. This allows for oxygenation but is inadequate for the treatment of hypercarbia if used for more than 45 minutes.

Once the airway is secured, supplemental oxygen must be given to begin the process of providing adequate tissue oxygenation.[29]

Breathing

A wide range of breathing devices is currently available. The use of SteriShields or more sophisticated mouth-to-mask breathing devices have introduced an element of safety for the resuscitator. These devices are small and are found in first responder mobile units as a standard approach to resuscitation. Some of these devices allow for supplemental oxygen to be used in the resuscitation. This can be accomplished utilizing various ranges of oxygen concentration. Hyperoxygenation is essential for cardiopulmonary stabilization and resuscitation.

At the more advanced level, the use of bag valve ventilation via an endotracheal tube provides the most effective method of oxygen delivery. Another method of ventilation is the use of portable and stationary ventilators, which have the added benefit of allowing more sophisticated control of ventilatory mechanics.

After the airway has been secured, the patient's chest, neck, and breathing pattern must be assessed. Respiratory rate, depth of respiration, use of accessory muscles, presence of abdominal breathing, chest wall symmetry, and the presence of cyanosis must all be evaluated. Life-threatening injuries causing tension pneumothorax, open pneumothorax, flail chest, and massive hemothorax are identified and treated immediately.

It is imperative to remember that positive pressure ventilation will worsen a pneumothorax unless a thoracostomy tube is placed to prevent a tension pneumothorax. Tension pneumothorax is diagnosed by the identification of jugular vein distention (not always present in the hypovolemic patient), tracheal deviation (toward the contralateral side), decreased breath sounds (on the ipsilateral side), hyperresonance to percussion (on the ipsilateral side), respiratory distress, hypotension, tachycardia, hypoxia, and cyanosis. In addition, a high level of suspicion must be present to identify this injury. Emergent treatment is life saving and consists of a needle thoracostomy (14-gauge needle, 2¼-in. length) at the second intercostal space at the midclavicular line on the affected side. This procedure is always followed by placement of a chest tube (40 F) at the fifth intercostal space, anterior to the midaxillary line (Fig. 6-2).

FIGURE 6-2 *Technique for chest tube thoracotomy. (Adapted from Bone, L.B. In: Browner, B.D.; Jupiter, J.B.; Levine, A.M.; et al. (eds.). Skeletal Trauma, 1st ed. Philadelphia, W.B. Saunders, 1992.)*

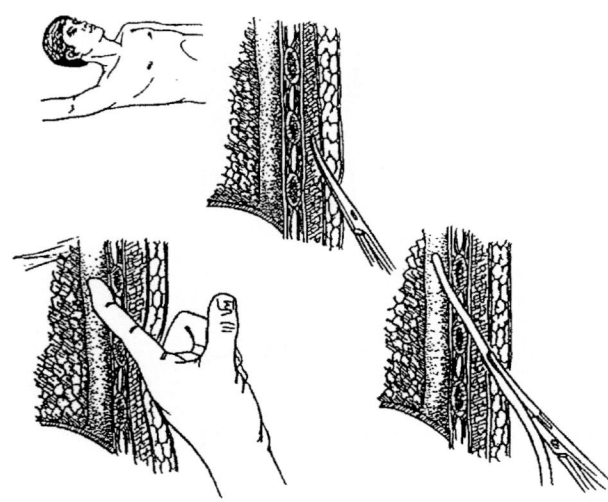

Open pneumothorax (sucking chest wound) is initially treated with a three-sided occlusive dressing, thereby preventing a tension pneumothorax, followed by chest tube placement (40 F) as described above. It should be noted that the chest tube should not be placed through the injury but through a separate incision. The need for intubation and surgical closure of the defect is based on the severity of the defect, associated injuries, the ability to provide adequate oxygenation, and the patient's overall condition.

Flail chest, described as more than two consecutive rib fractures with multiple fractures in each rib resulting in a loss of chest wall integrity, will result in the development of paradoxical chest wall movement and respiratory embarrassment. This condition usually is associated with underlying pulmonary contusion, which will worsen for the first 24 hours. The paradoxical chest wall movement with its resulting ventilation-perfusion mismatch and pulmonary contusion leads to hypoxia. Intubation with mechanical ventilation will "splint" the flail segment and recruit alveoli, allowing for more effective alveolar ventilation and more efficient oxygenation. It is essential to provide adequate analgesia to provide comfort and facilitate aggressive pulmonary toilet whether or not the patient is intubated. In some cases, placement of chest tubes may be required to prevent the development of a pneumothorax if high levels of ventilator support are needed or a hemopneumothorax already exists.

Massive hemothorax, described as $\geq$1500 mL of blood from the injured hemithorax or >200 mL of blood per hour for 4 consecutive hours, requires surgical intervention.

Circulation

Maintaining adequate circulation and controlling hemorrhage for the prevention or reversal of shock are of utmost importance in the resuscitation of the trauma patient. Shock is defined as a compromise in circulation resulting in inadequate oxygen delivery to meet a given tissue's oxygen demand. The most common cause of shock in the trauma patient is hypovolemia secondary to hemorrhage. The initial management of the patient should include establishing two intravenous (IV) lines (16 gauge or greater), one in each antecubital fossa vein. Central access in the form of an introducer (8.5 Fr, intravenous line) may be necessary for more rapid infusion of crystalloids and blood products in the unstable patient. These lines should be placed in the femoral or subclavian vein depending on the patient's injuries. Resuscitation with 2 L of lactated Ringer's or normal saline solution is recommended, followed by blood if indicated.[5]

If possible, rapid infusion devices, which warm all fluids, should be utilized. Hypothermia may be exacerbated by the infusion of room temperature or colder fluids, which in turn may hinder the normal activity of platelets and worsen the coagulopathy.

If the patient remains unstable after the infusion of 2 L of a balanced salt solution, then blood should be given.[72] The type of blood product in part depends on the urgency with which the transfusion must be given. Typed and crossmatched packed red blood cells are the product of choice, but the cross-matching process may take up to an hour. Type-specific packed red blood cells are the second choice; however, it takes approximately 20 minutes to perform a rapid cross-match. Universal donor O-positive or O-negative blood (for female patients of childbearing years) is usually well tolerated when given to trauma victims in severe shock. Approximately 200,000 units of O-negative is used each year in emergency situations.[67] Autotransfusion has also been utilized in the trauma setting but requires special equipment. This equipment should be assembled prior to the initiation of resuscitation.

There is continuing research in the area of blood substitutes. Early investigations with perfluorocarbon derivatives failed to show superiority to balanced salt solutions. Preclinical investigations utilizing stroma-free hemoglobin derived from outdated red blood cells (RBCs) either in cross-linked or liposome bound forms have shown these materials to produce oxygen dissociation curves similar to those produced by RBCs.[13]

In the trauma patient, hemorrhage or hypovolemia is the most common cause of shock.[29] Hemorrhagic shock has been classified as follows[4]:

Class I hemorrhage: loss of 15% of blood volume, or up to 750 mL; clinical symptoms are minimal, and blood volume is restored by various intrinsic mechanisms within 24 hours

Class II hemorrhage: loss of 15–30% of blood volume, or 750 to 1500 mL; tachycardia; tachypnea; decrease in pulse pressure; mild mental status changes

Class III hemorrhage: 30–40% blood loss, or 1500 to 2000 mL; significant tachycardia; tachypnea; mental status changes; and decrease in systolic blood pressure

Class IV hemorrhage: >40% blood loss, or greater than 2000 mL; severe tachycardia; decreased pulse pressure; obtundation; or coma

Patients who have sustained minimal blood loss (<20%) will require a minimal volume of fluid to stabilize their blood pressure. A 20 to 30 percent blood loss will require at least 2 L of a balanced salt solution, but blood may not be required. Blood loss greater than 30 percent usually requires blood for stabilization.[80] Patients who stabilize initially but then become hemodynamically unstable usually have ongoing bleeding and require further investigation and/or operative intervention.

Patients who are identified as having ongoing hemorrhage are treated with direct pressure and elevation if applicable. Hemorrhage can be obvious and external or contained in body cavities (chest, abdomen, retroperitoneum, or pelvis) or surrounding a fractured bone. Radiographs of the chest and pelvis can quickly rule out these areas as a source of hemorrhage. Hemothorax is managed as previously described. Blood contained in the pelvis secondary to a fracture is best controlled by stabilization of the pelvis, as described in detail in this textbook. This is perhaps the only remaining role for the use of the pneumatic antishock garment (PASG). Pelvic binders, bed sheets, or operative stabilization in the resuscitation suite utilizing external fixators immediately returns the pelvis to its original size. This decreases the volume of the pelvis and compresses the pelvic hematoma. The resultant rise in intrapelvic pressure compresses the pelvic vasculature and stops the hemorrhage. This is an excellent way to control pelvic venous hemorrhage but is not as effective for pelvic arterial bleeding. The use of pelvic angiography and embolization provides a method for identifying and treating arterial pelvic bleeding.[3] Other contained areas of significant bleeding occur with long bone fractures. These injuries should be managed by a splint to decrease the potential space into which hemorrhage can occur. Realignment is advantageous to extremity viability and restoration of arterial circulation, as evidenced by a return of distal pulses and perfusion. Blood loss associated with intra-abdominal injuries is discussed later in the chapter.

Perhaps the most insidious and lethal of circulatory insults secondary to trauma is cardiac tamponade. Cardiac tamponade occurs more commonly with penetrating injuries and is rare with blunt injuries.[4] The degree of tamponade depends on the size of the defect, the rate of bleeding, and the chamber involved. Tamponade may be caused by as little as 60 to 100 mL of blood in the pericardial space. Progression from compensated to uncompensated tamponade can be sudden and severe. Cardiac tamponade should be suspected in hypotensive patients when there is evidence of a penetrating injury in the "danger zone," which includes the precordium, epigastrium, and superior mediastinum. Beck's triad, which includes distended neck veins, quiet heart tones, and hypotension, may be present only 10 to 40 percent of the time. Diagnostic options in a stable patient include a two-dimensional echocardiogram or transesophageal echocardiogram. The type of injury, presence of distended neck veins, distant heart sounds, and hypotension should raise the possibility of the diagnosis of cardiac tamponade. If the patient is in shock, subxiphoid needle decompression of the pericardial space is indicated (Fig. 6-3). The removal of 10 to 50 mL of blood from the pericardial space can significantly improve survival. Pericardiocentesis may provide a stabilizing

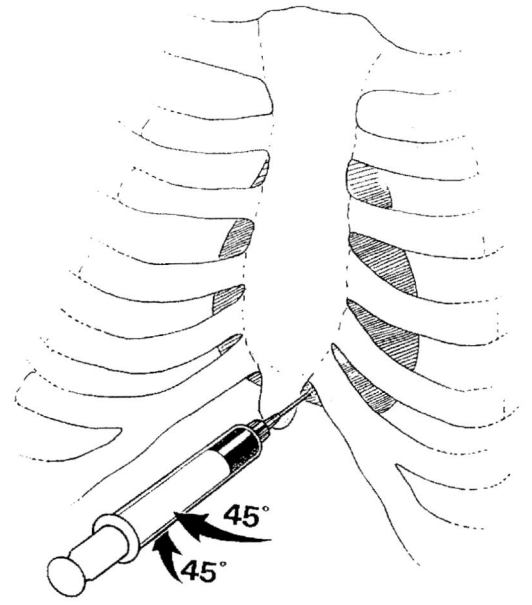

FIGURE 6-3   *Pericardiocentesis. (Adapted from Ivatury, R.R. In: Feliciano, D.V.; Moore, E.E.; Mattox, K.L. (eds.). Trauma, 3rd ed. Stamford, CT, Appleton & Lange, 1996.)*

option in the unstable patient but is by no means a definitive treatment. This procedure should be followed by emergent operative decompression and repair of underlying cardiac or great vessel injury.

Disability

An initial brief neurologic evaluation should be performed to ascertain the level of consciousness, pupillary response, and whether there is any gross neurologic deficit either centrally or in any of the four extremities. Any progression of a neurologic deficit may require an immediate therapeutic maneuver or operative procedure.[4,72] A quick way to describe the level of consciousness is using the acronym AVPU (*a*lert, responds to *v*oice commands, responds to *p*ain, *u*nresponsive).[4] The GCS is a more detailed assessment of the level of consciousness. Patients with a GCS score of 3 to 8 are considered to have a severe head injury and will require airway control. A score of 9 to 13 signifies a moderate head injury, and a score of 14 to 15 is consistent with a minor head injury.[5]

The cervical, thoracic, and lumbar spines are protected from injury by being placed on a long board with cervical spine immobilization. Detailed management of the spine-injured patient may be found in subsequent chapters in this textbook.

Exposure/Environmental Control

A head-to-toe examination of the patient must be performed. All clothing should be removed from the patient to facilitate a complete examination. Once this examination has been completed, the patient should be covered with a warm blanket for protection from hypothermia.[4,39]

Patients with hypo- or hyperthermia require immediate intervention to return to normothermia. The patient should be removed from the exposure as quickly as possible. In cold exposure, gradual rewarming is preferred to avoid the potential problem of dysrhythmias. Patients with thermal burns should have any burned clothing rapidly removed to prevent further injury from continued heat transmission. It is essential to determine the type, concentration, and pH of any contaminating agent that has had contact with the patient. The agent should be removed and the area either irrigated with water or saline, or neutralized. The skin should be constantly reexamined to be sure that contamination or burning is not continuing. The area is then covered with sterile dry dressings.

Hazardous materials create a special problem, not only for the victims but also for caregivers, especially in cases of radiation or chemical exposure. The most important step is developing a plan prior to the event. Prehospital protocols established in conjunction with receiving facilities capable of handling such emergencies are necessary to protect the staff and other noninvolved patients at that facility. These protocols should be available in the "disaster manual," which should be immediately available in the emergency department. Decontamination protocols are important in the initial phase of any treatment in patients who have been exposed to toxic materials.[35]

As the trauma surgeon completes the primary survey and life-threatening injuries are identified and treated, a secondary survey is then initiated. In addition, the placement of a pulse oximeter, an electrocardiogram, and initiation of blood pressure monitoring provide continuous monitoring of vital signs. The placement of a naso- or orogastric tube, placement of a Foley catheter, chest and pelvic radiographs, and FAST (focused assessment by sonography in trauma) are then performed.

SECONDARY SURVEY

The secondary survey begins once the primary care survey is completed. This involves a complete head-to-toe evaluation, combined with definitive diagnosis and treatment of injuries. If indicated, more extensive tests such as ultrasound, diagnostic peritoneal lavage, computed tomography (CT) scan, angiography, and imaging of suspected bone injuries should be performed. The basic evaluation and management of commonly incurred injuries are discussed here.

Trauma to the Cranium

Closed head injury is a significant contributor to the morbidity and mortality associated with the multi-traumatized patient. It is estimated that approximately 50 percent of traffic fatalities involve associated head injuries.[52] The most common mechanism of injury for head trauma in adults is motor vehicle crashes, followed by falls. The CT scan is the diagnostic modality of choice.

Brain injury may be classified in terms of primary and secondary injury. Primary injury is due to the mechanical damage that occurs at the time of insult as a result of the contact between the brain parenchyma and vascular structures and the interior of the cranium or a foreign body entering the cranium. The brain undergoes distortion from shearing forces, leading to contusions and lacerations of the parenchyma, and disruption of the arterial and venous arcades. This may result in subarachnoid hemorrhages and epi- and subdural hematomas.

Four categories of primary brain injury have been described.[40] First, a contusion involves injury to the brain parenchyma in the form of a coup injury, in which there is direct brain injury at the point of impact, and/or a countercoup injury, in which the injury occurs at a site opposite the point of impact.[40] Clinically, the patient may be asymptomatic or may present with neurologic deficits. Second, diffuse axon injury is caused by damage to the white matter, resulting in clinical sequelae ranging from confusion to complete coma.[40] Third, a foreign object, such as a gunshot injury, lacerates and destroys brain parenchyma. Finally, skull fractures occur when a force has been applied to the cranium that results in disruption of the continuity of the cranial bones. This may or may not be associated with underlying brain injury and/or neurologic deficits. Associated periorbital hematoma, or "raccoon eyes," indicates an anterior cranial fossa injury. The presence of cerebrospinal fluid (CSF) in the external auditory canal (otorrhea) or nasal canal (rhinorrhea) is usually indicative of a basilar skull fracture or middle cranial fossa injury. A mastoid hematoma, or Battle's sign, indicates an injury to the posterior cranial fossa.

Secondary brain injury with continuing neural damage is caused by cerebral hypoxia, hypo- and hypercapnia, increased intracerebral pressure, decreased cerebral blood flow, hyperthermia, and electrolyte and acid/base abnormalities.[16] Interventions are geared toward preventing or lessening the neurologic destruction by optimizing cerebral perfusion and oxygenation. Ventriculostomy catheters may be placed to monitor intracranial pressures and maintain pressures less than 20 mm Hg. Monitors to assess the oxygen partial pressure may be placed to assess cerebral oxygenation.[41] Hemodynamic monitors should also be placed to assess and assist with the maintenance of adequate intravascular volume and mean arterial pressure (MAP). The ultimate goal is to maintain cerebral perfusion pressure (CPP) greater than 60 mm Hg. CPP is the difference between MAP and ICP.[19] Acid-base balance, electrolytes, and coagulopathy should be evaluated and corrected. Failure to do so may result in significant morbidity or even death.

Qureshi et al. have shown that administration of intravenous hypertonic saline (3% saline) has demonstrated beneficial effects by decreasing ICP in patients with cerebral edema secondary to trauma.[54]

Intracranial hematomas also cause secondary brain damage and are classified as epidural, subdural, or intracerebral. Epidural hematomas (EDHs) occur usually secondary to a skull fracture with subsequent laceration of the middle meningeal artery. They appear on CT scan in a characteristic lentiform or lens shape. Patients may have a classic lucid period, followed by an alteration in mental status. Subdural hematomas (SDHs) occur as a result of injury to bridging veins. This type of hematoma is more common and may cause greater morbidity than epidural hematomas because of the associated cerebral contusions.[41] They appear on CT scan as concave shapes that do not cross the midline. Causes of intracerebral hematomas include penetrating injuries, depressed skull fractures, or shearing forces sufficient enough to tear the brain parenchyma. The hematoma and accompanying cerebral edema can cause a mass that results in a shift of the cerebrum and herniation.

Early evacuation of an intracranial hematoma has been associated with an improved outcome.[40] The extent of the procedure depends on the type and severity of the injury. Subdural hematomas require a large craniotomy to permit adequate evacuation. Epidural hematomas may be evacuated through a more limited craniotomy. Guidelines for the management of severe head injury are more specifically outlined by Chestnut.[15]

Neck Trauma

Penetrating neck injuries account for up to 11 percent of deaths. To better aid in the diagnosis and treatment of neck injuries, the neck can be divided into three zones, referred to as Monson's divisions (Fig. 6-4). Zone I is inferior to the cricoid cartilage. Zone II extends from the cricoid cartilage to the angle of the jaw. Zone III is located between the angle of the mandible and the base of the skull. These anatomic regions become important in the evaluation and treatment of neck injuries. Vascular injuries in zones I and III pose difficult technical surgical challenges to obtaining proximal and distal control; therefore, it is essential to delineate the vascular structures by angiography. Treatment of injuries in these areas may require interventional radiologic techniques or open operative procedures. Zone II vascular structures are more easily accessible and can be evaluated by angiography or by direct surgical exploration.[8]

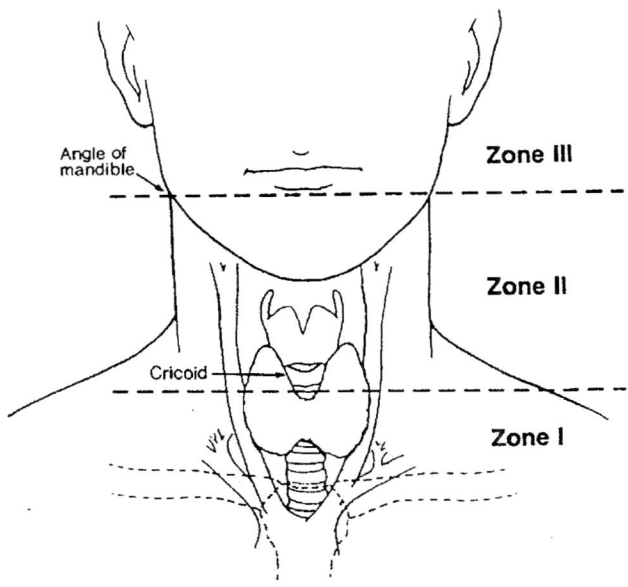

FIGURE 6-4 *Monson's anatomic zones for penetrating injury to the neck. (Adapted from Thal, E.R. In: Feliciano, D.V.; Moore, E.E.; Mattox, K. L. (eds.). Trauma, 3rd ed. Stamford, CT, Appleton & Lange, 1996.)*

For patients with suspected esophageal injuries, the combination of esophagography and rigid esophagoscopy in the operating room has proven to be effective in confirming the presence or absence of an injury.[8,81] If a tracheal injury is suspected, the use of fiberoptic or rigid bronchoscopy will assist with diagnosis. Injuries to the cervical spine in zones I, II, or III of the neck are addressed in detail in this textbook.

There are several indications for performing a formal neck exploration in patients with injuries penetrating the platysma. Vascular indications include substantial blood loss; persistent bleeding; and pulsatile, expanding hematoma. Respiratory indications include hemoptysis, crepitus, and dysphonia. Digestive indications include hematemesis, dysphagia, and crepitus, and nervous system indications include neurologic defects.[40]

Repair of vascular, tracheal, and esophageal injuries is addressed later in this chapter.

Thoracic Trauma

Serious injuries to the thorax result in significant morbidity and mortality.[42] Injuries to the respiratory, vascular, and digestive systems must be ruled out in patients with blunt and penetrating injuries to the thorax. Injuries that require immediate lifesaving therapeutic intervention include tension pneumothorax, open pneumothorax, flail chest, massive hemothorax, and pericardial tamponade, as previously described.[4] The use of CT scan, bronchoscopy, angiography, and esophagoscopy/esophagram further delineates injured structures.

Definitive treatment is performed in the operating room. Known tracheal, cardiac, and great vessel injuries may be managed through a median sternotomy, but this approach does not allow access to the descending aorta and the esophagus. Another incision that can be rapidly performed in an emergency situation is a left anterolateral thoracotomy through the fifth intercostal space (Fig. 6-5). This provides access to the heart, left lung, esophagus, and aorta. To gain additional access, the incision may be extended across the sternum. Exposure to the distal esophagus and right lung may be performed through a right lateral thoracotomy.

Injuries to the trachea may be primarily repaired or, if needed, resected and a primary anastomosis performed. Care must be taken not to compromise the vascular supply. Bronchial injuries may be primarily repaired or, if needed, resected and a primary anastomosis performed.

Pulmonary parenchyma injuries are usually treated effectively with a tube thoracostomy but may require primary repair, wedge resection, or in extreme cases, pneumonectomy.

Vascular injuries are usually repaired primarily or, if significant vessel wall destruction is present, may require placement of an interposition graft. In the management of these injuries, as with all vascular injuries, it is essential to obtain proximal and distal control of the vessel prior to starting the repair.

Cardiac injuries may temporarily be controlled with direct pressure, skin staples, or a Foley catheter, using the balloon to stop the bleeding. The wound is then repaired primarily with pledgeted sutures.[36]

Trauma to the esophagus should be primarily repaired and covered with pleura, stomach, or an intercostal muscle

FIGURE 6-5 *Anterolateral thoracotomy/emergency room thoracotomy. (Adapted from Ivatury, R.R. In: Feliciano, D.V.; Moore, E.E.; Mattox, K.L. (eds.). Trauma, 3rd ed. Stamford, CT, Appleton & Lange, 1996.)*

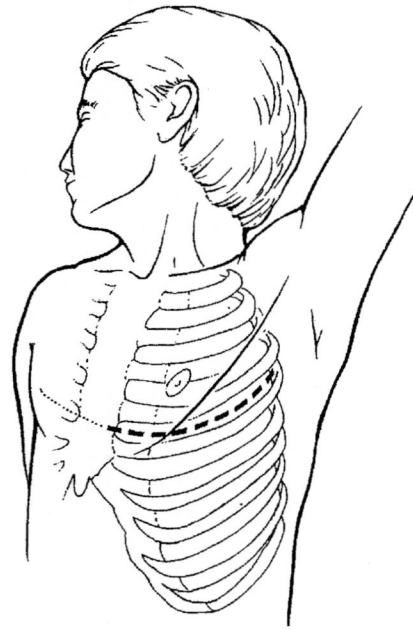

flap. A drain is placed adjacent to the repair to prevent the development of an abscess in the event of an esophageal leak. The repair should be performed as soon as possible. If there is a delay in making the diagnosis, then surgical débridement, drainage of the injured area with diversion, and esophageal exclusion may be indicated. In either case, broad-spectrum antibiotics should be provided.

Abdominal Trauma

Intra-abdominal injury should be suspected in any victim of a high-speed motor vehicle crash, fall from a significant height, or penetrating injury to the trunk. Up to 20 percent of patients with hemoperitoneum may not manifest peritoneal signs.[4] The major goal during trauma resuscitation is not to diagnose a specific intra-abdominal injury but to confirm the presence of an injury. The diagnosis of abdominal injury should begin with the physical examination during the secondary survey. This should include inspection, auscultation, percussion, and palpation. A rectal examination and examination of the genitalia should also be performed. A nasogastric tube and Foley catheter must be placed to aid in diagnosing an esophagogastric or urinary tract injury.

Patients with penetrating injuries to the abdomen, especially from gunshot wounds, and trauma patients with obvious peritoneal signs (rebound tenderness, involuntary guarding), presence of a foreign body, hemodynamic instability, and evisceration of omentum or bowel should undergo exploratory laparotomy because of the high likelihood of intra-abdominal injury. Victims of blunt trauma, stable stab-wound victims, patients with an equivocal abdominal examination due to CNS impairment, and multiply injured patients require further diagnostic

evaluation. Diagnostic options include abdominal ultrasound, abdominal/pelvis CT scan, diagnostic peritoneal lavage (DPL), angiography, and diagnostic laparoscopy. An extensive diagnostic evaluation should be omitted when there are clear indications for celiotomy.

FAST has gained popularity in the United States although it has been in use in Europe for many years. It has been demonstrated to have sensitivity of 93.4 percent, specificity of 98.7 percent, and accuracy of 97.5 percent when used by trauma surgeons to detect hemoperitoneum and visceral injury.[61] The FAST ultrasound machine should be kept in the trauma suite to assist with obtaining results rapidly in the unstable patient. Four basic areas are evaluated for fluid. The subcostal view evaluates the heart motion and pericardium. The morison's pouch view visualizes the right upper quadrant at the interface between the liver and right kidney. The splenorenal view evaluates the left upper quadrant between the spleen and kidney. The pouch of Douglas view allows evaluation for fluid around the bladder.

The abdomen/pelvis CT scan provides the ability to evaluate for intraperitoneal and retroperitoneal injuries. CT has sensitivity of 93 to 98 percent, specificity of 75 to 100 percent, and accuracy of 95 to 97 percent. Its major drawback is the low sensitivity for identifying intraperitoneal bowel injuries.[43] A CT scan is indicated in stable patients with no indications for immediate abdominal exploration. The major disadvantage of a CT scan is the need to transport the patient from the trauma suite to the CT scan room; thus, it should be performed only in the hemodynamically stable patient.

DPL has sensitivity of 98 to 100 percent, specificity of 90 to 96 percent, and accuracy of 98 to 100 percent.[43] It is also useful in the evaluation of intraperitoneal solid and hollow viscous injury.[24] The procedure may be performed in one of three ways: open, semi-open, or closed. Details of this procedure may be found in the ACS ATLS manual. Positive DPL results for blunt injury include more than 10 mL of gross blood on initial aspiration, or cell count of >100,000 red blood cells or >500 white blood cells, or evidence of enteric contents after removal of warmed crystalloid previously instilled for the procedure.

Angiography can be both diagnostic and therapeutic. Diagnostic angiography is useful in detecting injury, defining the precise site of injury, evaluating patency of the vessel, and assessing collateral flow.[68] There are four categories of vascular insults from trauma that can be treated angiographically. These include therapeutic embolization, stent-graft placement for arterial disruptions, pseudoaneurysms, and arteriovenous fistulae, as well as retrieval of embolized foreign objects.[68] Transcatheter embolization has been reported to be successful in 85 to 87 percent of cases.[37,51,65]

Indications for angiography in patients with pelvic fractures include transfusion of >4 units of packed red blood cells (PRBCs) in a 24-hour period, a negative DPL in an unstable patient, and/or a large retroperitoneal hematoma.[68] Controversy still exists in regard to the indications and optimal timing of angiography and intervention in unstable severe pelvic trauma patients. When a trauma patient undergoes celiotomy, opening the abdominal cavity through a standard midline incision can increase pelvic volume. This maneuver may release the tamponade and exacerbate pelvic bleeding. Some authors recommend that embolization be considered a secondary treatment after external fixation.

The multidisciplinary approach to the management of grades IV and V liver injuries has shown a significant improvement in survival. The use of surgery, endoscopic retrograde cholangiopancreatography (ERCP), biliary stenting, CT scan-guided procedures, and angiography has decreased mortality.[9]

Scalifani and associates introduced the concept of splenic embolization with a high success rate of approximately 98.5 percent with proximal embolization. Overall, the success rate still seems to be significant at 80 percent for grades IV and V splenic injuries.[28]

Diagnostic laparoscopy is useful in evaluating the presence of penetration of the peritoneum from penetrating injury, and it has utility in evaluating the diaphragm for injury.[82] It offers no advantage over DPL or CT scan for the diagnosis of other intra-abdominal injuries.

Liver injuries are more challenging to manage intraoperatively, and the use of angiography and embolization shows significant benefit in management of high-grade liver injuries, as noted above. Intraoperative management of injuries to the spleen may be treated with a wide range of therapeutic interventions ranging from direct pressure to splenorrhaphy and splenectomy. Simple injuries to the bowel may be closed primarily. If there are multiple wounds or if they involve more than 50 percent of the circumference of the bowel, these areas should be resected.

Retroperitoneal Injuries

The duodenum, pancreas, parts of the colon, great vessels, and urinary system are retroperitoneal structures. Injuries to these organs can be missed by physical examination, FAST, and DPL but may be diagnosed with CT scan of the abdomen and pelvis or intraoperatively.

Three fourths of duodenal injuries are penetrating injuries, whereas the majority of pancreatic injuries are due to blunt trauma. Injuries to both organs may be diagnosed with a CT scan of the abdomen or intraoperatively. DPL with elevated amylase levels is nonspecific but can contribute to an increased level of suspicion of an injury to one of these organs. ERCP is useful for evaluating injuries to the duodenum, biliary system, and pancreatic duct.[18] Treatment of duodenal injuries varies depending on the extent and location of the injury. The procedures range from simple primary repair to bypass, and pyloric exclusion of the severely injured duodenum. Drains should be placed adjacent to the repair to prevent the development of an abscess and/or control a fistula in the event of a duodenal leak. Injuries to the proximal pancreas require wide closed suction drainage if the duodenum and pancreatic ampulla are intact. Injuries to distal pancreatic duct (distal to the superior mesenteric artery and vein) are best treated with distal pancreatectomy and drainage. More complex injuries involving the duodenum, ampulla, and pancreatic head may require pancreaticoduodenectomy with placement of adjacent drainage catheters.

When considering management options, one must separate the nature of injury according to blunt and penetrating causes of retroperitoneal hematoma. For retroperitoneal hematomas from blunt causes in hemodynamically stable patients with no other reason for exploratory celiotomy, treatment is conservative. A massive or rapidly expanding hematoma on CT scan may require an arteriogram of the abdomen and pelvis with injured vessel embolization. When exploratory celiotomy is warranted, decision-making is centered on anatomic considerations based on zones, of which there are three (Fig. 6-6).

Zone I extends from the diaphragm to the sacral promontory. The aorta, vena cava, proximal renal vessels, portal vein, pancreas, and duodenum are located in this area. In general, a retroperitoneal hematoma in this area should be explored for both blunt and penetrating injuries. Proximal and distal control of the vessels to be explored must always be accomplished before entering the hematoma or attempting to repair an injured vessel.

Zone II includes the right and left flanks and contains the kidneys, adrenal glands, suprapelvic ureters bilaterally, and hilum of the vascular pedicle to the kidney. Retroperitoneal hematomas in zone II usually do not require exploration when resulting from blunt trauma unless there is a colon injury, expanding hematoma involving Gerota's fascia, or a urinoma. Penetrating injuries should be explored.

FIGURE 6-6 *Anatomical zones for retroperitoneal hematomas. (Adapted from Meyer, A.A.; Kudsk, K.A.; Sheldon, G.F. In: Blaisdell, F.W., Trunkey, D.D. (eds.). Abdominal Trauma, 2nd ed. New York, Thieme Medical Publishers, 1993.)*

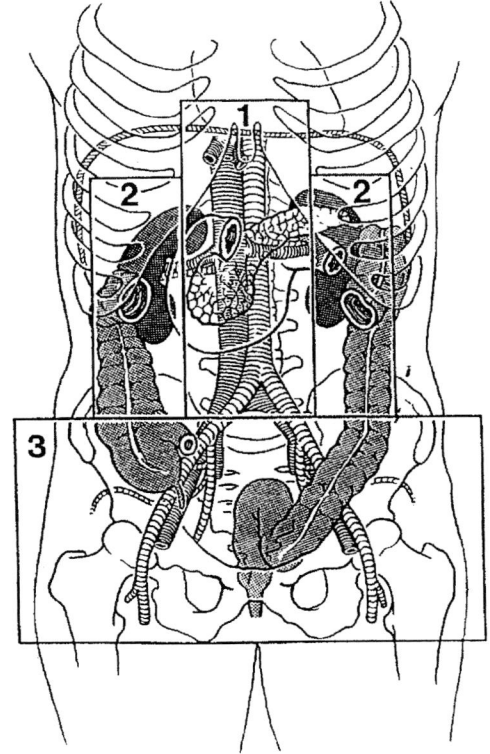

Zone III is the pelvis and contains the iliac vessels, distal sigmoid colon, rectum, bladder, and distal pelvic segment of the ureters. Zone III hematomas associated with pelvic fractures and hemodynamic instability may require reduction and fixation of the pelvis to control bleeding and may require angiography, as described earlier. Nonexpanding hematomas are observed. Hematomas resulting from penetrating injuries are explored once proximal and distal vascular control is obtained.

Genitourinary Injuries

Hematuria in the setting of significant blunt abdominal trauma, penetrating trauma, or pelvic fractures should signal that there might be significant injury to the genitourinary tract. Placement of a Foley catheter is important during the initial resuscitation of the trauma patient. Prior to placement of the Foley catheter, a digital rectal examination and visual inspection of the urethral meatus, scrotum, or labia should be performed. Blood at the urethral meatus or scrotal or labial hematomas may be indicative of a pelvic fracture or urethral injury. In this case, a retrograde urethrogram must be performed in male trauma patients prior to Foley catheter placement to rule out a urethral injury.

Further evaluation of significant hematuria may include a cystogram with filling, voiding, and postvoiding radiographs to diagnose bladder injuries. Additionally, CT scan of the abdomen and pelvis with intravenous contrast may assist with the diagnosis of a renal or ureteral injury. A penetrating injury to the abdomen may warrant a "one-shot" intravenous pyelogram (IVP) in the setting of hematuria to help evaluate renal excretory function of the ipsilateral and contralateral kidney, but this is being less frequently done.

The majority of blunt injuries to the genitourinary tract do not require surgical intervention. In the event that significant disruption of the renal parenchyma, ureter, bladder, or urethra is identified, definitive treatment is warranted. Depending on the extent of the injury, treatment may range from primary repair to resection of the injured area and adequate closed suction drainage.

Musculoskeletal Injuries

Detailed management of specific bony injuries is addressed in this textbook. Fractures with significant displacement may be associated with significant soft tissue injury. For example, patients with rib, scapular, clavicular, or sternal fractures may have great vessel or cardiac injuries that may require angiography or duplex ultrasound and possibly operative intervention. Fractures of the axial skeleton may have associated neurologic, vascular, or visceral injury that may take priority in the management scenario of a patient. Pelvic and long bone fractures may be associated with vascular injuries that result in hemorrhagic shock. Early reduction and fixation will contribute significantly to hemodynamic stabilization of the patient. The stabilization results in significant improvement in the patient's overall pulmonary status, rehabilitation, hospital course, and length of stay. With any fracture of an extremity in a trauma patient, there must be an awareness of the possibility of a compartment syndrome or vascular injury that may result in limb ischemia. Expeditious diagnosis and treatment of concomitant injuries may avert a potentially catastrophic result.

TERTIARY SURVEY

The tertiary survey consists of a repeat head-to-toe evaluation of the trauma patient along with reevaluation of available laboratory data and review of radiographic studies. Any change in the patient's condition must be promptly evaluated and treated. The most expeditious method to accomplish this task is to begin with the ABCs of the primary survey followed by the secondary survey. Any newly discovered physical findings are further investigated. Injuries often missed during earlier assessments include minor fractures, lacerations, and traumatic brain injury. Emphasis on repeated physical examinations and evaluation of newly obtained laboratory and radiology studies will continue to impact positively on patient outcome. Implementation of a standardized tertiary survey has been shown to decrease missed injuries by 36 percent.[11]

SUMMARY

Successful identification, resuscitation, and treatment of the multiple-injured patient require a carefully systematic, thorough approach. Special priority and attention have to be given to addressing injuries that are life threatening. Once the primary survey has been completed and lifesaving interventions are initiated, a secondary survey that is designed to identify other injuries has to be rapidly performed. An appropriate management plan can be rapidly developed and implemented so that no injuries are missed. Finally, a tertiary survey should be performed to detect any latent problems that present hours after the patient has been admitted to the hospital. A comprehensive, careful approach to management will afford the severely injured patient the best possible outcome.

ACKNOWLEDGMENT

We thank Randy Edwards, M.D., for his help in collecting data and reviewing the chapter.

REFERENCES

1. Aehlert, B. Injuries to muscles and bones. In Aehlert, B. (ed.). Emergency Medical Responder. New York, McGraw-Hill, 2007, pp. 394–413.
2. Aehlert, B. Patient assessment. In Aehlert, B. (ed.). Emergency Medical Responder. New York, McGraw-Hill, 2007, pp. 252–265.
3. Agolini, S.F.; Shah, K.; Jaffe, J.; et al. Arterial embolization is a rapid and effective technique for controlling pelvic fracture hemorrhage. J Trauma 43:395–399, 1997.
4. American College of Surgeons Committee on Trauma. Advanced Trauma Life Support. Chicago, American College of Surgeons, 1997.
5. American College of Surgeons Committee on Trauma. Advanced Trauma Life Support. Chicago, American College of Surgeons, 2004.

6. American College of Surgeons Committee on Trauma. Major Outcome Study. Chicago, American College of Surgeons, 1993.

7. American College of Surgeons Committee on Trauma. Resources for Optimal Care of the Injured Patient. Chicago, American College of Surgeons, 1999.

8. Asensio, J.A. Management of penetrating neck injuries: The controversy surrounding Zone II injuries. Surg Clin North Am 71:267–295, 1991.

9. Asensio, J.A.; Roldan, G.; Petrone, P.; et al. Operative management and outcomes in 103 AAST-OIS Grade IV and V complex hepatic injuries: Trauma surgeons still need to operate, but angioembolism helps. J Trauma 54:647–654, 2003.

10. Baker, C.C.; Oppenheimer, L.; Stephens, B.; et al. Epidemiology of trauma deaths. Am J Surg 140:144, 1980.

11. Biffl, W.; Harrington, D.; Cioffi, W. Implementation of a tertiary survey decreases missed injury. J Trauma 54:38–44, 2003.

12. Briggs, L.P.; Dundee, J.W.; Bahar, M.; et al. Comparison of propofol and thiopentone in response to somatic pain. Br J Anaesth 54:307, 1982.

13. Carrico, C.J.; Mileski, W.J.; Kaplan, H.S. Transfusion, autotransfusion, and blood substitutes. In Feliciano, D.V.; Moore, E.E.; Mattox, K.L. (eds.). Trauma, 3rd ed. Stamford, CT, Appleton & Lange, 1996, pp. 181–191.

14. Champion, H.R.; Sacco, W.J.; Copes, W.S. Trauma scoring. In Feliciano, D.V.; Moore, E.E.; Mattox, K.L. (eds.). Trauma, 3rd ed. Stamford, CT, Appleton & Lange, 1996, pp. 53–67.

15. Chesnut, R.M. Guidelines for the management of severe head injury: What we know and what we think we know. J Trauma 42(5 Suppl):S19–S22, 1997.

16. Chesnut, R.M. Secondary brain insults after head injury: Clinical perspectives. New Horiz 3(3):366–375, 1995.

17. Chodoff, P. Evidence for central adrenergic action of ketamine. Anesth Analg 51:247, 1972.

18. Clements, R.H.; Reisser, J.F. Urgent endoscopic retrograde pancreatography in the stable trauma patient. Am Surg 62:446–448, 1996.

19. Cohen, S.M.; Marion, D.W. Traumatic brain injury. In Fink, M.P.; Abraham, E.; Vincent, J.L.; et al. (eds.). Textbook of Critical Care, 5th ed. Philadelphia, Elsevier/Saunders, 2005, pp. 377–389.

20. Cold, G.E.; Eskesen, V.; Ericksen, H.; et al. CBF and CMRO2 during continuous etomidate infusion supplemented with N2O and fentanyl in patients with supratentorial cerebral tumor: A dose-response study. Acta Anesthesiol Scand 29:490, 1985.

21. Cooperman, L.H. Succinylcholine-induced hyperkalemia in neuromuscular disease. JAMA 213:1867, 1970.

22. Demetriades, D.; Berne, T.V.; Belzberg, H.; et al. The impact of a dedicated trauma program on outcome in severely injured patients. Arch Surg 130:216–220, 1995.

23. Donlon, J.V., Jr. Anesthesia and eye, ear, nose and throat surgery. In Miller, R.D. (ed.). Anesthesia, 3rd ed. Philadelphia, Churchill-Livingstone, 1990, p. 2005.

24. Fabian, T.C.; Croce, M.A. Abdominal trauma, including indications for celiotomy. In Feliciano, D.V.; Moore, E.E.; Mattox, K.L. (eds.). Trauma, 3rd ed. Stamford, CT, Appleton & Lange, 1996, pp. 441–459.

25. Franklin, J.; Doelp, A. Shock Trauma. New York, St. Martin's Press, 1980.

26. Fukuda, S.; Murakawa, T.; Takeshita, H.; et al. Direct effects of ketamine on isolated canine cerebral and mesenteric arteries. Anesth Analg 62:553, 1983.

27. Grounds, R.M.; Twigley, A.J.; Carli, F.; et al. The hemodynamic effects of thiopentone and propofol. Anaesthesia 40:735, 1985.

28. Haan, J.; Bochicchio, G.; Kramer, N.; et al. Nonoperative management of blunt splenic injury: A 5-year experience. J Trauma 58:492–498, 2005.

29. Halvorsen, L.; Holcroft, J.W. Resuscitation. In Blaisdell, F.W.; Trunkey, D.D. (eds.). Abdominal Trauma, 2nd ed. New York, Thieme, 1993, pp. 13–31.

30. Hamill, J.F.; Bedford, R.F.; Weaver, D.C.; et al. Lidocaine before endotracheal intubation: Intravenous or laryngotracheal? Anesthesiology 55:578–581, 1981.

31. Herman, N.L.; Carter, B.; Van Decar, T.K. Cricoid pressure: Teaching the recommended level. Anesth Analg 83:859–863, 1996.

32. Huber, F.C.; Reves, J.G.; Gutierrez, J.; et al. Ketamine: Its effect on airway resistance in man. South Med J 65:1176, 1972.

33. Isaacs, J.H., Jr.; Pedersen, A.D. Emergency cricothyroidotomy. Am Surg 63:346–349, 1997.

34. Jacobs, B.B.; Jacobs, L.M. Injury epidemiology. In Moore, E.E.; Mattox, K.L.; Feliciano, D.V.; et al. (eds.). Trauma, 2nd ed. Stamford, CT, Appleton & Lange, 1991, p. 15.

35. Jacobs, B.B.; Jacobs, L.M. Emergency medicine: A comprehensive review. In Kravis, T.C.; Warner, C.G.; Jacobs, L.M. (eds.). Prehospital Emergency Medical Services. New York, Raven Press, 1993, p. 1.

36. Jacobs, L.; Gross, R.; Luk, S. The cardiac and vascular system. In Jacobs, L.; Gross, R.; Luk, S. (eds.). Advanced Trauma Operative Management: Surgical Strategies for Penetrating Trauma. Woodbury, CT, Cine-Med, 2004.

37. Jander, H.P.; Russinovich, N.A.E. Transcatheter gel foam embolization in abdominal, retroperitoneal, and pelvic hemorrhage. Radiology 136:337, 1980.

38. Konchigeri, H.N.; Lee, Y.E.; Venugopal, K. Effects of pancuronium on intra-ocular pressure induced by succinylcholine. Can Anaesth Soc J 26:479, 1979.

39. Krantz, B.E. Initial assessment. In Feliciano, D.V.; Moore, E.E.; Mattox, K.L. (eds.). Trauma, 3rd ed. Stamford, CT, Appleton & Lange, 1996, pp. 123–140.

40. Kreiger, A.J. Emergency management of head injuries. Surg Rounds Feb: 57–78, 2004.

41. Lang, E.W.; Czosnyka, M.; Mehdorn, H.M. Tissue oxygen reactivity and cerebral autoregulation after severe traumatic brain injury. Crit Care Med 31:267–271, 2003.

42. Mattox, K.L.; Wall, M.J.; Pickard, L.R.; et al. Thoracic trauma: General considerations and indications for thoracotomy. In Feliciano, D.V.; Moore, E.E.; Mattox, K.L. (eds.). Trauma, 3rd ed. Stamford, CT, Appleton & Lange, 1996, pp. 345–354.

43. Mendez, C.; Jurkovich, G.J. Blunt abdominal trauma. In Cameron, J.L. (ed.). Current Surgical Therapy, 6th ed. St. Louis, Mosby, 1998, pp. 928–933.

44. Miller, T.R.; Levy, D.T. The effect of regional trauma care systems on costs. Arch Surg 130:188–193, 1995.

45. Morrow, J.S. Laryngeal (superior and recurrent) nerves. In Hahn, M.B.; McQuillan, P.M.; Sheplock, G.J.; et al. (eds.). Regional Anesthesia. St. Louis, Mosby, 1995, p. 83.

46. Mulder, D.S. Airway management. In Feliciano, D.V.; Moore, E.E.; Mattox, K.L. (eds.). Trauma, 3rd ed. Stamford, CT, Appleton & Lange, 1996, pp. 141–157.

47. National Center for Health Statistics: Injury Data and Resources Fact Sheet 2002. Centers for Disease Control and Prevention. Available at: www.cdc.gov/nchs/injury.htm.

48. National Committee for Injury Prevention and Control: Injury Prevention: Meeting the Challenge. New York, Oxford University Press, 1989.

49. National Trauma Data Bank Report 2005: American College of Surgeons Trauma Registry. Available at: www.facs.org/trauma/ntdb.html.

50. North Central Connecticut EMS Council Regional EMT: Intermediate Protocols. 2001, pp. 32–38. Available at: www.northcentralctems.org/nccems_policies.htm.

51. Panetta, T.; Scalifani, S.J.A.; Goldstein, A.S.; et al. Percutaneous transcatheter embolization for arterial trauma. J Vasc Surg 2:54, 1985.

52. Pitts, L.H.; Martin, N. Head injuries. Surg Clin North Am 62:47–60, 1982.

53. Pointer, J.E.; McGuire, T.J. Levels of providers. In Kuehl, A.E. (ed.). Prehospital Systems and Medical Oversight, 3rd ed. Dubuque, IA, Kendall/Hunt, 2002, pp. 106–113.

54. Qureshi, A.I.; Suarez, J.I.; Bhardwaj, A.; et al. Use of hypertonic (3%) saline/acetate infusion in the treatment of cerebral edema: Effect on intracranial pressure and lateral displacement of the brain. Crit Care Med 26:440–446, 1998.

55. Rauzz, A.I. The Maryland emergency medical services system: An update. Md Med J 37:517–520, 1988.

56. Renou, A.M.; Vernhiet, J.; Macrez, P.; et al. Cerebral blood flow and metabolism during etomidate anaesthesia in man. Br J Anaesth 50:1047, 1978.

57. Reves, P.S.; Glass, A. Non-barbiturate intravenous anesthetics. In Miller, R.D. (ed.). Anesthesia, 3rd ed. Philadelphia, Churchill-Livingstone, 1990, p. 262.

58. Reves, P.S.; Glass, A. Non-barbiturate intravenous anesthetics. In Miller, R.D. (ed.). Anesthesia, 3rd ed. Philadelphia, Churchill-Livingstone, 1990, p. 257.

59. Robertson, L. Injury Epidemiology. London, Oxford University Press, 1992.

60. Robinson, K.J. Orthopedic trauma: Amputations and deformities. In Association of Air Medical Services: Guidelines for Air Medical Crew Education. Alexandria, VA, AAMS, 2004, pp. 1–7.

61. Rozycki, G.S.; Shackford, S.R. Ultrasound: What every trauma surgeon should know. J Trauma 40:1–4, 1996.

62. Sanders, M.J.; McKenna, K.; Lewis, L.M. Musculoskeletal trauma. In Sanders, M.J.; McKenna, K.; Lewis, L.M.; et al. (eds.). Mosby's Paramedic Textbook, 3rd ed. St. Louis, Mosby, 2005, pp. 652–671.

63. Sanders, M.J.; McKenna, K.; Lewis, L.M. Patient assessment. In Sanders, M.J.; McKenna, K.; Lewis, L.M.; et al. (eds.). Mosby's Paramedic Textbook, 3rd ed. St. Louis, Mosby, 2005, pp. 281–289.

64. Santoro, V.M. Musculoskeletal care. In Browner, B.D.; Pollack, A.N.; Gupton, C.L. (eds.). Emergency Care and Transportation of the Sick and Injured, 8th ed. Boston, Jones and Bartlett, 2002, pp. 641–679.

65. Scalifani, S.J.A.; Cooper, R.; Shaftan, G.W.; et al. Arterial trauma: Diagnostic and therapeutic angiography. Radiology 161:165, 1986.

66. Schaner, P.J.; Brown, R.L.; Kirskey, T.D.; et al. Succinylcholine-induced hyperkalemia in burned patients. Anesth Analg 48:764, 1969.

67. Schulman, C.I.; Cohn, S.M. Transfusion in surgery and trauma. Crit Care Clin 20:281–297, 2004.

68. Schwarcz, T.H. Therapeutic angiography in the management of vascular trauma. In Flanigan, D.P. (ed.). Civilian Vascular Trauma. Philadelphia, Lea & Febiger, 1992, pp. 336–345.

69. Sellick, B.A. Cricoid pressure to control regurgitation of stomach contents during induction of anaesthesia. Lancet 2:404–406, 1961.

70. Shackford, S.R.; MacKensie, R.C.; Hoyt, D.B.; et al. Impact of a trauma system on outcome of a severely injured patient. Arch Surg 1221:523, 1987.

71. Shapiro, H.M.; Wyte, S.R.; Harris, A.B. Ketamine anesthesia in patients with intracranial pathology. Br J Anaesth 44:1200, 1972.

72. Shires, G.T. III. Trauma. In Schwartz, S.I.; Shires, G.T.; Spencer, F.C. (eds.). Principles of Surgery, 6th ed. New York, McGraw-Hill, 1994, pp. 175–224.

73. Simons, P.J.; Crockshott, I.D.; Douglas, E.J.; et al. Blood concentrations, metabolism and elimination after a subanesthetic dose of propofol to male volunteers (abstract). Postgrad Med J 61:64, 1985.

74. Smith, M.; Bourn, S. Patient assessment. In Browner, B.D.; Pollack, A.N.; Gupton, C.L. (eds.). Emergency

Care and Transportation of the Sick and Injured, 8th ed. Boston, Jones and Bartlett, 2002, pp. 238–279.

75. Stephen, H.; Sonntag, H.; Schenk, H.D.; et al. Effects of disoprivan on cerebral blood flow, cerebral oxygen consumption, and cerebral vascular reactivity. Anaesthetist 36:60, 1987.

76. Taylor, M.B.; Grounds, R.M.; DuRooney, P.D.; et al. Ventilatory effects of propofol during induction of anesthesia: Comparison with thiopentone. Anaesthesia 41:816, 1986.

77. Trunkey, D.D.; Blaisdell, F.W. Epidemiology of Trauma. Sci Am 4:1–7, 1988.

78. Tse, J.C.; Rimm, E.B.; Hussain, A. Predicting difficult endotracheal intubation in surgical patients scheduled for general anesthesia: A prospective blind study. Anesth Analg 81:254–258, 1995.

79. Wagner, R.I.; White, P.F. Etomidate inhibits adrenocortical function in surgical patients. Anesthesiology 60:647, 1984.

80. Weigelt, J.A. Resuscitation and initial management. Crit Care Clin 9:657–671, 1993.

81. Weigelt, J.A.; Thal, E.R.; Snyder, W.H.; et al. Diagnosis of penetrating cervical esophageal injuries. Am J Surg 154:619–622, 1987.

82. Zantut, L.F.; Ivatury, R.R.; Smith, R.S.; et al. Diagnostic and therapeutic laparoscopy for penetrating abdominal trauma: A multi-center experience. J Trauma 42:825–831, 1997.

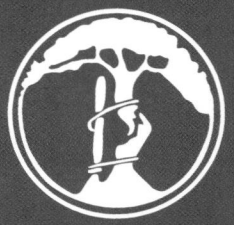

CHAPTER 7

Damage Control Orthopaedic Surgery: A Strategy for the Orthopaedic Care of the Critically Injured Patient

Michael J. Bosse, M.D. and James F. Kellam, M.D.

We must guard against dogmatism in our teaching. We allow things that are not solidly supported by known, published facts to creep into our "standard of care." It is detrimental to be dogmatic when teaching about fracture care. Young colleagues believe us. Older colleagues believe us. Examination boards believe us, to the detriment of our trainees who do not automatically accept the dogma. Sometimes, the courts believe us to the detriment of our colleagues and their malpractice premiums. And, unfortunately, we begin to believe ourselves. We are not practicing a religion, we are practicing medicine!

Robert Meek, M.D.[42]

Debate surrounding the appropriate timing of non-lifesaving orthopaedic surgical procedures in the care of the multiply injured patient continues. Early total care (ETC) of extremity trauma, particularly femoral fractures, was advanced in the early 1980s.* Early in the evolution of this trend, however, some surgeons recognized a distinct subset of critically injured patients that often required orthopaedic care other than prescribed by the aggressive ETC protocols. In the mid-1980s, Burgess suggested that this cohort of the most severely injured trauma patients might be "too sick" for definitive fracture fixation techniques. He advocated the concept of provisional skeletal fixation of the femur fracture via external fixation devices—"traveling traction."

The second edition (1998) of this textbook included a chapter entitled "Orthopaedic Management Decisions in the Multiple Trauma Patient."[9] The authors (us) critically reviewed the literature advocating ETC and concluded that the level of evidence supporting immediate definitive orthopaedic care of the severely injured patient was not robust. Furthermore, assessment of the early trauma patient's physiologic

stresses, consideration of the care needed for the optimal recovery of a traumatic brain injury, and the impact of anesthesia and surgery on the early stability of the patient suggested that an immediate aggressive definitive surgical approach was likely to be counterproductive to the goals of the resuscitation and recovery of a brain injury. Delay in surgery until the patient's physiologic condition was optimized, followed by the use of temporary external fixation in selected cases, was recommended. This concept was controversial at that time. Publication of the chapter was permitted, but only after the authors agreed to attach a disclaimer at the front of the chapter. When the chapter was revised for the third edition (2003), the disclaimer was no longer required—recognition of the need to titrate the amount of orthopaedic care to the specific patient's physiology was now commonly accepted.

This chapter is a refinement of our previous philosophy regarding the appropriate timing and techniques of orthopaedic care in the critically injured patient. This approach is now referred to as "damage control orthopaedic surgery" (damage control orthopaedics, DCO). Note that this chapter is without a disclaimer. The opinions expressed in this chapter, however, may be as controversial as the "disclaimer chapter" in the second edition. Orthopaedic trauma care trends seem to snowball in use and importance. We need to remember, as we start to consider this topic, prior popular treatment strategies—ETC, the unreamed nail, and emergent pelvic external fixation—as examples. The application of these techniques has been modified or abandoned based on critical research and clinical experience. Likely, the "damage control" concept will similarly evolve. DCO surgery appears to be the hot orthopaedic treatment philosophy of this decade. The initial concept of advocating early provisional external fixation of femur fractures for a very select group of critically ill patients has evolved to include even the application of simple spanning external fixators to

*See references 3, 5, 7, 16, 27, 35, 37, 43, 64, 65, 75

FIGURE 7-1 *Trauma patient survival—claiming the credit.*

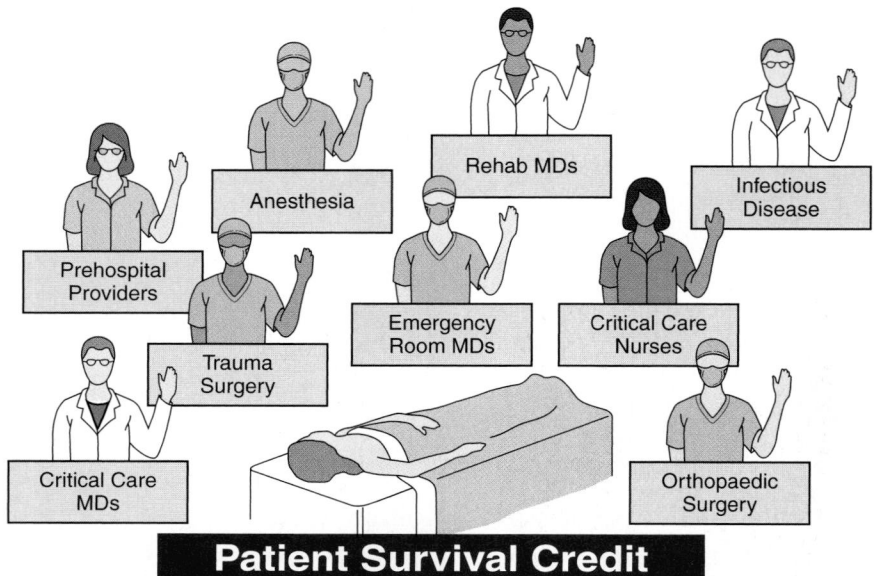

provisionally stabilize isolated complex articular injuries in both critically ill and isolated injury patients.[13]

As orthopaedic surgeons consider the place of damage control in their own practices, these points should be considered. Most importantly, DCO refers to the care of femur fracture, major pelvic fractures, and significant soft tissue injuries that are present in patients in critical condition. The reader needs to consider that the application of the damage control care concept to all critical trauma patients might be counterproductive to the goals of initial trauma critical care resuscitation in some of those patients. Additionally, damage control concepts applied to the care of the isolated extremity injury may have no positive clinical or functional effect. The total cost of care, however, with additional operating room (OR) exposures and the use of temporary external fixation, might be significantly increased. This chapter will not serve as a grand endorsement of the damage control concept or argue for its expansion to all facets of fracture care. Rather, it will attempt to critically examine the available literature and suggest considerations for the timing and titration of care offered to the critically injured patient.

In the context of the current enthusiasm of the orthopaedic surgeon for a "damage control" approach, we need to critically consider these issues:

> If the trauma patient isn't already in the operating room for the care of life-threatening injuries, should the orthopaedic team take the patient to the OR simply to apply an external fixator?
>
> Is bedside application of external fixation of clinical value? Is provisional skeletal traction for 36 to 72 hours detrimental to the outcome of the severely injured patient?
>
> Can a traction pin be considered as a damage control technique that provides provisional stability during the initial resuscitation period?

> Are there sufficient data to support early non-lifesaving surgery, of any kind, in a patient with a significant traumatic brain injury?

As was recognized in the critical assessment of the literature that advocated early total care, the retrospective assessment of patient outcomes and the assignment of benefit to any one therapy cannot be valid unless all other therapies provided by other caring services are held constant during the same period. In the case of the trauma patient, outcomes of early or late surgery for orthopaedic injuries coincide with advances occurring in prehospital care, acute resuscitation, critical intensive care, infection control, ventilation philosophies and technology, nursing care, nutritional support, head injury care, and so on (Fig. 7-1). During any 5- to 10-year assessment period, all trauma care specialties are advancing the care of the patient in their specific field of interest. The combined efforts, likely, are the reasons for observed decreases in morbidity and mortality. No one technique, technology, or philosophy can be implicated as the generator of the improved outcome without an evaluation of the impact of all other changes in patient care that occurred during the same period.

THE DAMAGE CONTROL CONCEPT

"Damage control" is a U.S. Navy shipboard doctrine developed to control fire and flooding in order to save the ship. Predetermined and practiced maneuvers are initiated in the event of a ship casualty (Fig. 7-2). Flooding control (internal hemorrhage), fire suppression (inflammation), and shoring of bulkheads, decks, and frames to prevent structural collapse (fracture fixation) are simultaneously engaged to prevent sinking (death) of the vessel. The adoption of this term to describe the initial events in the care of the trauma patient first appeared in the general

FIGURE 7-2   *Flooding around the propeller shaft of the USS Cole was controlled by aggressive "packing."*

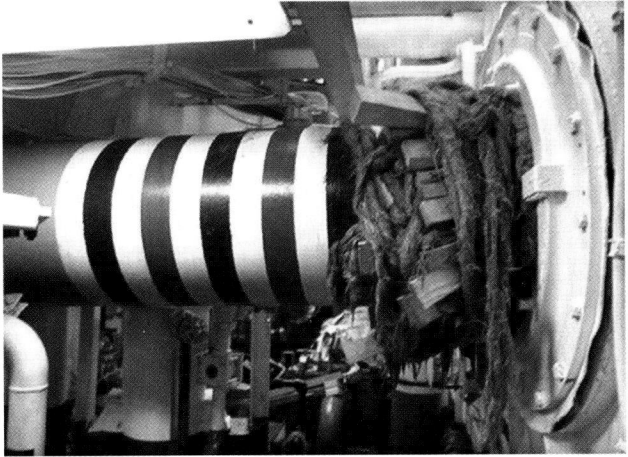

surgery literature. Rotondo et al. described the early termination of trauma laparotomy after emergent control of bleeding and contamination. Definitive reconstruction was later performed after the patient was physiologically stabilized.[69] This approach recognized and respected the critical triad of hypothermia, coagulopathy, and acidosis. Recognizing the importance of short, focused early surgeries specifically aimed at preserving life; the damage control philosophy evolved to the current standard in general surgery and was adopted by other surgical specialties.

Damage control surgery is not a new topic in orthopaedic surgery. Components of this practice have been advocated since the early 1980s. Scalea and colleagues from the R Adams Cowley Shock Trauma Center, Baltimore, are credited with first recognizing the importance of this concept and coining the provisional treatment of a femur fracture in the most injured patients with an external fixator as damage control orthopaedics.[72] In general, patients considered as candidates for DCO have high injury severity scores, severe and on-going hemorrhage, coagulopathic profiles, significant base deficits, hypothermia, chest trauma, and traumatic brain injury. These patients represent only a *small portion* of the typical orthopaedic trauma practice profile. Damage control practices, therefore, are not germane to most of our patients. In general surgery, only 10 percent of patients who required emergent celiotomy need a damage control approach.[44,69] Similar low percentages should be expected in orthopaedic surgery. Scalea confirmed this and noted the DCO practice was employed in only 13 percent of the Baltimore patients in the late 1990s. O'Toole recently reassessed the Baltimore experience (2000–2005) and again found that only 13 percent of patients with femur fracture required a DCO approach.[49,72]

Defining the patient and the patient parameters that trigger the surgeon to consider damage control care is important to understanding and applying this concept. The orthopaedic surgeon is tasked to provide care to patients who fall into three broad categories: stable patients with isolated extremity trauma, stable patients with visceral and major orthopaedic injuries, and physiologically unstable or marginally stable trauma patients and/or traumatic brain injury patients with orthopaedic injuries. The orthopaedic injuries in these patients can be subclassified as life- or limb-threatening (emergent), urgent (open fractures, femur fractures, major joint dislocations, and significant soft tissue wounds), or semi-elective (most other fractures). On the basis of the presence and severity of other injuries, the systemic physiology, and the urgency of the orthopaedic intervention, decisions are made regarding type and timing of treatment. In the context of orthopaedic care, *damage control surgery can be best defined as treatment techniques that enhance the immediate survival of the patient with the least stress to the patient's physiologic condition.*

THE ORTHOPAEDIC DEBATE: TIMING OF CARE FOR LONG BONE FRACTURES

Evolution of the Care of the Multiply Injured Patient

Early definitive fixation of major unstable fractures in the multiply injured patient (MIP) has been credited with resultant reductions in mortality rates, intensive care unit (ICU) and ventilator days, incidence of adult respiratory distress syndrome (ARDS), sepsis, multiple organ dysfunction, fracture complications, length of hospital stay, and overall cost of care. Proponents of early definitive care claim that the stabilization of major fractures decreases the output of inflammatory mediators, reduces catecholamine release, lowers analgesic requirements, facilitates ICU care through earlier mobilization, and is cost effective.[5]

Beginning in 1977, a series of clinical papers concluded that the aggressive management of long bone fractures had a significant positive effect on patients, decreasing overall morbidity and mortality.[3,6–9,11,14,15,18,87] Early fixation evolved from "within 2 weeks"[65] to 48 hours[3,7] to within 24 hours of injury.[10,16,26,35] Riska and co-workers[65] were among the first authors to note a correlation of systemic outcome with the timing of surgical care. They considered early operative care to be within 2 weeks of injury and attributed the 15 percent to 0 percent reduction in the incidence of fat embolism syndrome to the increase in operative intervention on the fractures in their population of patients from 23 to 66 percent. In a small retrospective series, Goris and associates[27] argued that fixation within 24 hours reduced the mortality, ARDS, and sepsis rates.

Building on the "early fracture fixation–reduced mortality" concept, other authors attempted to solidify the relationship between the timing of fracture care and the outcome of the trauma patient. In a small injury- and age-matched retrospective trauma series, Meek and colleagues demonstrated superior outcomes for patients in the early fracture fixation group.[43] Johnson and co-workers[35] retrospectively reviewed 132 patients with an injury severity score (ISS) of 18 or greater and with two major fractures, attempting to define a relationship between ARDS and the timing of fracture surgery. A fivefold increase in ARDS was noted in patients with fracture fixation delayed beyond 24 hours, and the severely injured patients had an ARDS rate of 75 percent when treatment was delayed compared with 17 percent when it was within 24 hours. This study, however, was likely biased by the fact that the unstable patients probably experienced surgical delays as they were being optimized for surgical fracture fixation. ARDS was defined as a Pao_2 of less than 70 with an Fio_2 of 40 percent and ICU admission for 4 days with ventilator support. The definition of ARDS is currently more stringent.

The only randomized prospective research on the effect of the timing of fracture fixation on subsequent outcomes was performed by Bone and associates; 178 patients with femoral fractures were entered into an early fixation (<24 hours) or a delayed fixation (>48 hours) group.[6] The incidence of pulmonary complications (ARDS, fat embolism, or pneumonia) was higher, the hospital stay was longer, and ICU requirements increased when femoral fixation was delayed in the MIP although the differences were not statistically significant. The only significant difference between the groups was the total cost of care. This paper, revolutionary for its time, still persists as an orthopaedic "silver bullet" used by those needing to argue for early fracture fixation. The project, however, had major flaws and likely would not be accepted for publication in current journals. The randomization process was not clearly defined, and 10 of 37 MIPs (10 of the 11 total patients in the whole series) in the delayed treatment group had pulmonary parenchymal injuries, compared with only 1 of 46 in the early treatment group. Patients who were taken to the OR emergently within the first 24 hours for the care of lifesaving or open fractures were randomized to the delayed treatment cohort. Their return time to the OR for fixation of the femur fracture was greater than 48 hours, but the criteria for return were not well defined. Other authors have found that the pulmonary injury predisposes the patient to the development of both pneumonia and ARDS.[10,29,63]

Bone and colleagues later studied the effect of the timing of orthopaedic injuries on patient outcomes with a retrospective multicenter study design. The outcomes of 676 patients with an ISS greater than 18 and major pelvic or long bone injury, or both, treated under an early fixation (<48 hours) protocol at six major U.S. trauma centers were compared with historical records of 906 patients obtained from the American College of Surgeons' Multiple Trauma Outcome Study (MTOS) database. The patients in the MTOS database were assumed to have been treated by a nonaggressive orthopaedic fracture protocol. The mortality rate was significantly reduced in patients who had early fracture stabilization.[7]

Although the findings are perhaps true, the study design significantly biases the MTOS group of patients. Since the MTOS patients were historical control subjects treated in a different time frame at potentially dissimilar institutions, their increased mortality rate could be related to the overall clinical expertise of the MTOS hospital and not to the timing of the fracture fixation. In addition, the authors assumed that early fixation of fractures was not a practice in the MTOS pool of patients, essentially stating that long bone fractures in the control group were managed nonoperatively for prolonged periods of time. If this assumption is not true, the authors' conclusion could be reversed: early fracture care at less experienced clinical

centers might result in worse outcomes, possibly secondary to critical care and neurosurgical issues. Parallel advances in associated trauma subspecialty care were not investigated as possible confounders in the study design. Perhaps the effects of the evolution of trauma care—improved prehospital, resuscitative, orthopaedic, and critical care—may have combined to lower the mortality rate at the major trauma centers; the timing of the orthopaedic care might have been a less important variable in the overall care of the patients.

Rogers and co-workers[68] challenged the practice of immediate (within 24 hours) femoral fracture fixation in patients with isolated injury. In a retrospective review of 67 patients with ipsilateral femoral shaft fractures, three groups were identified: immediate fixation (within 24 hours), early fixation (24 to 72 hours), and late fixation (>72 hours). Pulmonary and infectious complications were significantly increased in the late fixation group. Operative time was longer in the immediate fixation group, when all the cases were performed as "emergencies." When compared with the immediate fixation group, the early fixation group had significantly shorter operating times and a significant reduction in resource utilization (50% of the expense of immediate fixation), with no difference in pulmonary or infectious outcomes.

Trauma Patients, Femur Fractures, and ARDS

The practice of early definitive reamed intramedullary (IM) nailing for the MIP with a femur fracture and associated chest injuries was challenged by Pape and associates, who found a higher ARDS rate in patients treated acutely as opposed to those whose treatment was delayed.[51] Small numbers in the subgroups of patients ($n = 25$) and exclusion of deaths resulting from hemorrhage and closed head injury in the delayed fixation cohort weaken the conclusions that surgery should be delayed until the patient is more stable or that alternatives to reamed IM nails should be considered for patients with femoral fractures and pulmonary injuries if the treatment is to be acute. Pape and associates theorized that embolized marrow products from the reaming initiated an inflammatory cascade in the lung that tipped the injured lung into ARDS. Subsequent animal studies have both supported and refuted this theory.[14,45,47,52,53,74,88–90] Despite the very weak clinical evidence to support the concept that medullary contents embolize to the lungs with reamed nail techniques and that these products cause subsequent pulmonary dysfunction, industry and clinician enthusiasm for the theory fueled the development and explosive clinical use of unreamed nails.

Pape's study was repeated, with alterations in design, at other centers. Charash and colleagues noted that the overall pulmonary complication rate was 56 percent in a group of patients with thoracic and femoral fractures treated more than 24 hours after injury, contrasted with 16 percent if patients with similar injuries were treated acutely.[16] They concluded that delayed surgical fixation was associated with a higher pulmonary complication rate independent of the presence of blunt thoracic trauma.

Ziran and colleagues[91] attempted to clarify the relationship between skeletal injuries, the timing of fracture fixation, and mortality or pulmonary morbidity in patients with and without chest injury. Their analysis of 226 patients concluded that the combination of skeletal and chest injuries does not amplify the pulmonary morbidity or mortality compared with that of patients with isolated chest injuries. The quantity of skeletal injury and the timing of fixation of structures that affected the patient's mobilization (spine, pelvic, and femur fractures), however, were found to have a significant effect on pulmonary morbidity. The authors acknowledged a major weakness in their study, in common with all prior studies on the same topic—the uncontrolled reason for surgical delays of long bone fixation in the MIP. These delays were most commonly associated with unfavorable patient physiologic parameters. They were likely delayed as a result of prolonged resuscitation.

A review of patients in Vancouver with chest injuries with and without femur fractures treated by early IM nail fixation did not find a difference in the death rate from serious pulmonary complications.[42] Bone et al.[4] also looked at the MIP with thoracic injuries, with and without femur fractures. Femur fracture fixation was stratified by nail or plate fixation technique. No increase in ARDS was identified in the reamed nail cohort (0/24 patients vs. 15/55 [27%] without femoral fractures). Carlson[15] found that the rate of ARDS, the rate of pneumonia, and the duration of mechanical ventilation were similar in patients with isolated chest injuries and chest injuries with an associated femur fracture treated with reamed IM nailing.

Bosse and co-workers could not find a difference in ARDS, pneumonia, multiple organ dysfunction syndrome (MODS), or death rates in MIPs with femur fractures and pulmonary injury treated acutely with either reamed nails or plates.[10] The choice of operative procedure did not appear to potentiate or lessen the risks of ARDS (<3% overall). Turchin and associates[82] examined trauma patients with pulmonary contusion with or without fracture. Outcome appeared to be related more to the presence of the pulmonary contusion than to the fracture. Handolin et al. found no difference in pulmonary outcome for patients treated with immediate IM and pulmonary injury compared with pulmonary injury alone.[29]

Different Treatment Approach for Selected Patients

Not all centers subscribe to the urgent long bone fixation protocols for MIPs. The timing of the surgical fixation is weighed against ongoing systemic instabilities and the severity of the patient's associated injuries. Non-lifesaving surgical procedures are delayed until the patient's condition is stabilized to a point at which operative exposure involves less risk. The patient is admitted to the surgical ICU, where abnormalities in coagulation, core temperature, hypoxia, and base deficit are corrected.

Reynolds and colleagues[63] believe that fixation of all long bone fractures within the first 24 hours is not the primary determinant of outcome for the severely traumatized patient. In a study to assess the effect of the timing of IM femoral fixation, records of 424 consecutive trauma patients were reviewed. One hundred five of the patients had an ISS of 18 or higher. A definitive early long bone fixation protocol was not followed at the trauma center. Femur fractures were generally stabilized on the day of admission if the patient was systemically stable. Femoral fixation was typically delayed if the patient required a long resuscitative effort or had a lingering base deficit or an excess serum lactate level indicating under-resuscitation (the "borderline patient"). Surgery was also delayed for patients with hypothermia; coagulopathic conditions; significant intrapulmonary shunting; and severe head, pulmonary, or pelvic injuries. Fracture fixation was often delayed in MIPs with long bone fractures who had already experienced a significant "lifesaving" operative exposure. Surgery was usually delayed beyond 36 hours to avoid surgical procedures during the period of the patient's anticipated maximal inflammatory response to the initial trauma.

A significant rise in pulmonary complications was noted by Reynolds and colleagues in patients with an ISS lower than 18 with progressive surgical delays. No relationship, however, was found between pulmonary complications and timing of femoral fixation in patients with an ISS of 18 or higher. The data suggest that the severity of the injuries, not the timing of the fracture fixation, determined the MIP's pulmonary outcome. Reynolds and colleagues found no significant difference in pulmonary morbidity related to early versus delayed femoral fixation in the MIP. The incidence of pulmonary complications was found to parallel the frequency of initial thoracic injury.

Reynolds and colleagues argued that the theoretical concerns raised by supporters of immediate long bone fixation involve interpretation of data from an era when fractures were routinely treated with prolonged immobilization. There are no data to support fracture fixation immediately or at 12, 24, or 36 hours after injury. Patients with severe closed head injuries or major pulmonary flail segments routinely require prolonged immobilization and ventilatory support. Because of advances in surgical ICUs and the development of critical care subspecialties, these patients, who previously succumbed with multiple comorbidities, including deep vein thrombosis, pulmonary embolism, decubitus ulcer formation, atelectasis, pneumonia, sepsis, and thrombophlebitis, are currently efficiently managed and preemptively monitored and treated to prevent these conditions. Attention to positioning of the patient, pulmonary toilet, skin care, nutritional support, and sepsis surveillance has significantly reduced the morbidity and mortality of trauma patients since the mid-1980s.

Reynolds et al. believe that clinical judgment regarding the timing of long bone fixation was the most important determinant of the patient's outcome. Delays in femoral fixation that were made to stabilize the patient or to treat associated injuries did not appear to affect the patient's outcome adversely. Pulmonary complications were found to be related to the severity of the injury, not to the timing of fracture fixation.

Boulanger and co-workers[11] were unable to detect a difference in outcomes when comparing patients with femur fractures, with and without pulmonary injury, treated with either early or late IM fixation. Although the authors concluded the study did not demonstrate an increased morbidity or mortality associated with early IM nail fixation in the presence of thoracic trauma, the opposite can also be stated—neither did a delay in fracture fixation.

A critical review of the timing of long bone fractures was undertaken by the EAST Practice Management Guidelines Work Group in 2000.[22] An evidence-based medicine analysis concluded that trauma patients undergoing long-bone stabilization within 48 hours of injury have no improvements in outcomes compared with those receiving later stabilization, but these patients may have a reduction in days of mechanical ventilation, ICU days, and hospital stay as well as a reduction in the incidence of ARDS, pulmonary complications, pneumonia, and systemic infections. When the analysis was directed to the patients with chest injuries, the group found no compelling evidence that early long-bone stabilization in patients with chest injury either enhanced or worsened outcomes.

The Harborview Group also examined the association between the timing of femur fracture fixation and outcomes in patients with concomitant chest and head injuries.[12] They conducted a retrospective trauma registry review of 1362 patients admitted to their Level I trauma center over a 12-year period. Patients were grouped by the timing of the femur fracture fixation: 867 patients' femurs were fixed within 24 hours (group 1); 155 patients were treated between 24 and 48 hours (group 2), 37 patients from 48 to 120 hours (group 3), 22 patients greater than 120 hours (group 4), and 281 patients were not surgically fixed (group 5). Patients treated beyond 120 hours and those not surgically treated had significantly higher injury severity scores and chest injury scores. The mortality in the operative patient was 1.9 percent and was not different between the groups. The mortality in the nonoperative group was 29 percent ($P < 0.0001$); however, 82 percent of the deaths occurred within 1 day of admission. ARDS, pneumonia, length of stay, and ICU days were lowest in the patients fixed within 24 hours—even in patients with associated head and chest injuries. There was a significantly increased incidence of ARDS, pneumonia, and fat embolism syndrome in the patients with concurrent chest trauma in the cohort fixed between 2 and 5 days. Glasgow Coma Scale (GCS) scores were highest in the cohort fixed within 24 hours. The time of operative fixation had no impact on mortality. On the basis of these findings, the authors concluded that chest and head trauma is not a contraindication to early femur fixation with a reamed IM nail.

To critically assess these conclusions, we need to consider the quality and history of the institution. This study occurred in the era when Harborview subscribed to an early total orthopaedic care protocol. The authors analyzed their series and found that the timing of fracture fixation was consistent through the period. They emphasize that their patients were adequately resuscitated and hemodynamically and physiologically normal before anesthesia and fracture fixation. Only 65 percent met parameters to allow surgery within 24 hours. Given this fact, the cohorts *are not* similar. The correct interpretation of these data should be that despite prolonged resuscitation and

hemodynamic instability, patients who required delay in fracture fixation beyond 24 hours had no difference in mortality. *The observed increased incidence in pulmonary complications is more likely related to the condition that necessitated the surgical delay rather than the delayed surgical fixation.*

Importantly, analysis of chest and head injuries included patients with abbreviated injury score (AIS) equal to or greater than 2. The effect of more severe head or chest injuries (AIS=3) is not reported. The authors also conclude that early fracture fixation was tolerated by head-injured patients without negatively impacting neurologic outcome. Since the early group likely had higher initial GCS scores and were later discharged with high scores, no data conclusively support that interpretation. As in other studies assessing the impact of the timing of non-lifesaving surgery on recovery of a head injury, the authors are using the GCS score as a surrogate for functional recovery. The GCS score is an assessment of gross brain function and has no correlation to final cognitive recovery.

The Polytrauma Study Group of the German Trauma Society also analyzed the body of evidence-based medicine related to the initial care of the femur fracture. They identified 37 studies that supported early definitive fracture fixation and 18 studies that advocated late definitive fixation. Another 8 papers were "indifferent." A detailed analysis of outcomes and all patients' injury factors *did not* identify superiority of either early or late femur fracture fixation strategy nor did it find worse outcomes in patients with chest or brain injuries treated by early fixation. Analysis of the prospective German trauma registry identified the major "risk factors" for the use of initial external fixation. The primary factors were the GCS score, AIS_{thorax}, and prothrombin time. They were able to conclude that the initial operative stabilization of a femur fracture in the multiple trauma patients appeared to be advantageous. Insufficient and contradictory results from the literature showed no definitive advantage or disadvantage to "early definitive" fracture stabilization, even if patient subgroups that included brain and thoracic injuries were included.[66]

On the basis of this review, Rixen et al. suggested that rather than attempt to clearly define "early" or "late" surgery or the methods for those surgeries, clinical studies should assess the concept of "risk-adapted damage control orthopaedic surgery," since no study has demonstrated the efficacy of the concept or identified the variables that should be considered in the patient care decision process.

A Critical Element: Defining "Early" Fracture Care

The problem with the definition of early fracture fixation and the analysis of outcomes based on an arbitrary time assignment suggests that 24 hours from injury is better than 25, 28, or 36 hours. In most retrospective studies reported over the last 15 years, all the reporting centers typically subscribed to the early long bone fracture fixation dogma. Given that, patients delayed beyond the 24-hour care ceiling likely were different from patients treated prior to 24 hours—for some reason not identified by review of the medical records, the surgical team determined that the patient was incapable of safely undergoing femur fracture fixation before that point. *The physiologic problems that caused the delayed fixation, more than likely, also drove related adverse outcomes—not the timing of the fixation of the fracture!*

MULTIPLY INJURED PATIENTS: BASIC PHYSIOLOGY AND THE INFLAMMATORY PROCESS

Systemic Effects

To understand the systemic effects of trauma, the injury or injuries sustained by the patient can be considered as a wound. This wound stimulates a variety of responses that must be coped with by the MIP if he or she is to survive. The wound (injury) consists of necrotic or devitalized tissue in an ischemic hypoxic region that will start an inflammatory process.[87] The patient's ability to resolve this inflammatory insult is dependent on the magnitude of the injury, the patient's systemic metabolic response, the treatment, and the resolution of the inflammatory process.

The systemic metabolic response to this wounding mechanism is temporal and represented early by the *ebb phase,* which is dominated by cardiovascular instability, alterations in circulating blood volume, impairment in oxygen transport, and heightened autonomic activity. Hypovolemic shock is a typical example of this phase and requires emergent resuscitation. After effective resuscitation and restoration of oxygen transport, a secondary group of responses, the *flow phase,* occurs. Hyperdynamic circulatory changes, fever, glucose intolerance, and muscle wasting are responses of this period.

In response to the ebb phase, the initial need for oxygen delivery is rapidly met by management of the airway and breathing problems through appropriate use of endotracheal intubation and ventilation with appropriate oxygenation. Hypovolemic or traumatic shock is recognized by the clinical manifestations of adrenergic nerve stimulation and increased levels of angiotensin and vasopressin, causing constricture of the vasculature to the skin, fat, skeletal muscle, gastrointestinal tract, and kidneys. This condition is characterized by a usually orderly progression of cutaneous pallor and clamminess with cool extremities, oliguria, tachycardia, hypotension, and finally cerebral and cardiac signs. These clinical manifestations of the compensatory mechanisms occur as the neuroendocrine adrenergic nervous system's vasoactive volume conserving and metabolic hormones cause the peripheral capacitance vessels to constrict and displace residual peripheral blood to the organ systems that require it for the maintenance of life.[32]

Increased heart rate and myocontractility are a second response to the epinephrine released by the neuroendocrine axis. There is also a fluid shift from the interstitial space to the intravascular space, which adds hypo-osmotic fluids. Release of epinephrine, cortisol, and glucagon increases glucose concentration and extracellular osmolarity, thus pulling water out of the cells and into the extracellular space and subsequently forcing it back through the lymphatics and into the vascular space. Without adequate resuscitation, however, these compensatory mechanisms may also

have adverse effects. Ongoing ischemia to arterial or smooth muscle may cause dilatation of the arterioles while the postcapillary sphincters are in spasm, resulting in engorgement of the capillaries and extravasation of fluid into the interstitium.[32] Release of endorphins may cause dilatation of the venules and arterioles, counteracting any positive effect they have by increasing deep spontaneous breathing, which in effect increases cardiac return. In addition, the coagulation and inflammatory responses, both at the site of injury and remotely, are stimulated. In the flow phase, the wound creates an intense metabolic load on the patient. Large arteriovenous shunts, which increase cardiac work, are required to support the profound metabolic changes necessary for this repair process. Glucose, the main fuel for wound healing, is metabolized to lactate, which can then be used by the liver to form more glucose. Gluconeogenesis using alanine obtained from muscle produces more glucose at the expense of muscle. Significant muscle wasting, nitrogen loss, and accelerated protein breakdown occur. This phenomenon was first described by Cuthbertson,[21] who observed it in patients with long bone fractures. The gut also begins to use glutamine as a principal fuel, converting it to alanine, which is transported through the portal circulation to the liver for gluconeogenesis. The increased portal circulation, along with gastrointestinal mucosal damage, permits entry of bacteria and toxins, which worsen the response (gut hypothesis).[85] A state of hypermetabolism increases the core body temperature, changing thermal regulation in these patients so that they cannot tolerate cold environments and require a higher ambient temperature.

The central nervous system also plays a significant role in the regulation of the hypermetabolic flow phase responses. It appears that an intact central nervous system is required for full expression of the metabolic responses after injury, and it is thought that this occurs through a neuroendocrine reflex arc. The central nervous system is particularly important in the ebb phase for early response to injury, as pain, hypovolemia, acidosis, and hypoxia stimulate the neural afferent signals to the central nervous system. During the flow phase this relationship is not totally understood.[85]

INFLAMMATORY RESPONSE

As well as the physiologic response, inflammation plays a major role in determining the outcome. This response is primarily responsible for the development of the major complications of trauma: adult respiratory distress syndrome and the multiple organ dysfunction syndrome and subsequently death.[24] Table 7-1 lists the principal mediators of the inflammatory response.

The inflammatory response consists of two components: a proinflammatory process known as the systemic inflammatory response (SIR) and an anti-inflammatory response known as the counter-regulatory anti-inflammatory response (CAR).[77] These two processes work in conjunction to assure that the inflammatory process is controlled and focused on improving the patient's condition. Should the balance be lost, significant complications will occur (Fig. 7-3).

Table 7-1	
Inflammatory Mediators	
Acute-phase Reactants	
Lipopolysaccharide-binding protein (LBP)	A protein of hepatic origin with the ability to bind bacteria lipopolysaccharide (LPS). The binding of bacterial LPS by LBP stimulates macrophage proinflammatory cytokine production (IL-6, IL-1, TNF-α). In the acute phase of trauma, the levels of LBP rise to a maximum on the second and third day. It is a nonspecific marker for infection although it may be prognostic in severe sepsis.
C-reactive protein (CRP)	Produced by hepatocytes and increased in production by cytokine stimulation. It is nonspecific with no correlation to severity of trauma. A decrease in CRP usually means the resolution of the underlying inflammatory process.
Procalcitonin (PCT)	Produced by C cells of the thyroid. Increases in the first 24 to 48 hours predict severe SIRS, sepsis, and MODS. May be useful to monitor the inflammatory process.
Markers of Mediator Activity	
Tumor necrosis factor (TNF)	An autocoid of two types: TNF-α and TNF-β. TNF-α is mainly seen in the inflammatory process. It is the central regulator of the immunoinflammatory response after trauma and is produced by monocytes, lymphocytes, Kupffer cells, macrophages, endothelial cells, and glial cells. IL-1, IL-2, and IL-12, interferon-γ, platelet-aggregating factor (PAF), and complement protein C5a stimulate the cellular release of TNF. Because its half-life is very short, it is not useful as an assayable marker of the inflammatory response.
Interleukin-1 (IL-1)	This group of peptides consists of three related polypeptides—IL-1-α, IL-1-β, and IL-1 receptor antagonist (IL-1ra)—produced primarily by monocytes. Biologically IL-1 acts with TNF-α to induce fever, hypotension, endothelial cell adhesion, and chemotaxis of polymorphonuclear leukocytes and macrophages. It has a very short half-life and hence is difficult to detect and levels do not correlate with death or MODS.
Interleukin-6 (IL-6)	This mediator, produced by T and B cells and endothelial cells, is the best prognostic marker concerning the outcome of patients with SIRS, sepsis, and MODS. It induces a proliferation of B lymphocytes with increased production of immunoglobulins and T lymphocyte proliferation. An increased level of IL-6 (>500 pg/dL) has the potential to identify patients who will develop MODS and die.
Interleukin-10 (IL-10)	This anti-inflammatory cytokine synthesized mainly by T lymphocytes is a macrophage deactivation factor. The plasma concentration of IL-10 is elevated in patients with trauma and correlates with severity of injury.
Interleukin-18 (IL-18)	Formerly called interferon-γ. It is commonly elevated in septic patients and not elevated in trauma patients with nonseptic inflammation.
Markers of Cellular Activity	
Cytokine receptors	Cytokines exert their influence by interaction with a cellular membrane receptor system. The membrane-bound receptor concentration directly correlates with the rate of MODS. TNF-α and many interleukins have their activity controlled by the amount of receptors available for interaction or by antagonist-type receptor sites.
Adhesion molecules	These molecules are necessary for polymorphonuclear leukocytes (PMNs) to adhere to the capillary endothelium and start the migration to the inflammatory site. There are three types: selectins, immunoglobulins, and integrins. Each of these adhesion molecules provides a different type of adhesion, thereby facilitating the transfer of PMNs to the inflammatory site. Concentrations of these adhesion molecules appear to increase along with the amount of injury suffered but are not predictive.
Elastase	Has the capacity to degrade most extracellular proteins and important plasma proteins. Also causes the release of proinflammatory cytokines (IL-6, IL-8). Levels of elastase correlate well with severity of trauma and occurrence of MODS and ARDS.
Human leukocyte antigens, HLSA-DR class II molecules	Changes in some leukocyte cell-surface antigens correlate well with development of subsequent complications and death. Class II major histocompatibility antigen (MHC class II) expression on mononuclear cells has been associated with septic morbidity and mortality after trauma. MHC class II antigens are indispensable in the presentation of processed antigen to T cells for specific immune response. Without this activity, there is no response, and patients are immunocompromised. This is the only marker of immune reactivity that correlates with mortality and morbidity after trauma. Since it is very difficult to assay for these markers, this is not very useful in clinical practice.
DNA	Free DNA in the circulation is increased after major trauma and may be a potential marker of cellular injury. The higher its concentration is, the greater the chance for a complication.

FIGURE 7-3 *After trauma, there is a balance between the systemic inflammatory response and the counter-regulatory anti-inflammatory response. Severe inflammation can lead to acute organ failure and death. A lesser inflammatory response coupled with an excessive counter-regulatory anti-inflammatory response may also induce a prolonged immunosuppressed state that can be deleterious to the host. Abbreviations: CARS, counter-regulatory anti-inflammatory response syndrome; SIRS, systemic inflammatory response syndrome. (Redrawn from Roberts C, Pape HC, Jones AL, et al. Damage control orthopaedics: Evolving concepts in the treatment of patients who have sustained orthopaedic trauma. J Bone Joint Surg (Am) 87:434–449, 2005, with permission.)*

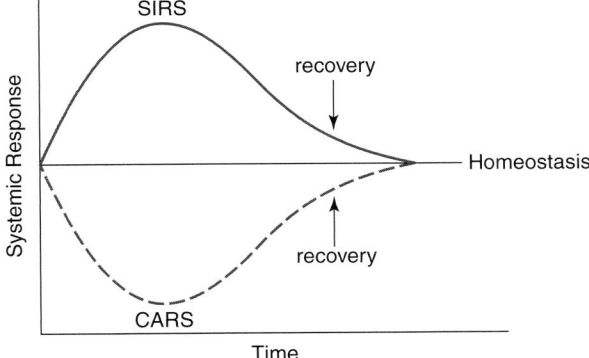

Patients with traumatic injuries may be in one of four categories[8]:

1. No or little evidence of any systemic reaction. The recovery is determined by the severity of the injury, and no organ dysfunction results.
2. A mild form of the systemic inflammatory response syndrome (SIRS) develops involving one or two organs but quickly resolves in several days.
3. Massive SIRS develops rapidly after the initial trauma, and the patients may die rapidly.
4. The initial course of SIRS is less severe but deteriorates markedly several days or more from the initial injury. This may occur after a secondary insult. The patients have organ failure and may die.

The body is designed to compensate for injury. The inflammatory defenses include macrophages and their products (tumor necrosis factor [TNF], interleukins [IL-1, -6, -8]; neutrophils and their degranulation products, platelets and the coagulation factors formed on their surfaces, derivatives of arachidonic acid, and T and B lymphocytes and their products). They interact in a complex, little understood network. Bone has proposed the following five-stage mechanism of how SIRS, MODS, and ARDS develop.[8] This can be applied to the injured patient to better understand the second-hit phenomenon and why damage control may have a role to play in certain patients.

Stage one is the local response to an insult such as an injury. Prompt release of proinflammatory mediators

occurs that limits any new damage and ameliorates whatever damage has happened by destroying damaged tissue, promoting new tissue growth, and preventing infection. To avoid the proinflammatory mediators becoming too destructive, a counter anti-inflammatory response occurs. Mediators are interleukins 4, 10, and 11; soluble TNF receptors; interleukin-1 receptor antagonists; transforming growth factors; and others. These alter monocyte function, impair antigen-presenting activity, and reduce the cells' ability to produce proinflammatory cytokines.

Stage two is the initial systemic response. If the injury is severe enough, there is an overflow of the pro- and counter-inflammatory mediators into the systemic system. They can be measured through various assays that are too imprecise and expensive to be clinically useful. This overflow signals that the local environment has been overwhelmed and cannot control the injury and help is needed. More proinflammatory cells and mediators are recruited from elsewhere, and the counterinflammatory response also heightens to contain the inflammatory response.[17,76] Little happens at this time to the patient.

Stage three is massive systemic inflammation. This occurs when the regulation of the proinflammatory state is lost. Initially the proinflammatory response results in SIRS—hypotension, abnormal body temperature, and tachycardia. Endothelial damage occurs, leading to transudation of fluids into the organs; platelet sludge blocking the microcirculation, causing maldistribution of blood flow; and activation of the coagulation system. Severe complications will occur as a result of the massive proinflammatory response overwhelming the counterinflammatory system or an insufficient counter–anti-inflammatory response, or the initial pro- and anti-inflammatory mediator balance is correct but is lost by a secondary insult (the second hit).

Stage four is excessive immunosuppression as the compensatory anti-inflammatory response becomes excessive. This stage increases the patient's susceptibility to infection as the immune system is shut down. Finally, stage five is what Bone calls immune dissonance. The patient's organs fail owing to overwhelming inflammation or immunosuppression, and death ensues. This upset of the normal balance between pro- and anti-inflammatory processes can occur as a result of a massive injury so severe that the proinflammatory response overwhelms the counterinflammatory system and SIRS and MODS occur. An alternative is when the patient is "pre-primed" to develop SIRS and/or MODS through prior illness, genetic predisposition, moderate injury, and second injury or is under-resuscitated.[17,70,76]

Giannoudis has proposed four potential mechanisms for the development of post-traumatic complications: the macrophage theory, the gut hypothesis, the two-hit theory, and the microenvironment theory.[25]

The microenvironment theory is presently felt to provide the logical cause for these complications. Essentially it results from the adherence of activated neutrophils to the endothelium creating a protected local environment for the toxic metabolites secreted by these neutrophils. These toxic products cannot be neutralized by the appropriate antioxidants and antiproteinase and so destroy the endothelial lining. The destroyed lining permits the exudation of fluid and migration of cells and toxic mediators, causing lung and other organ failure (Bone stage two).

The macrophage theory is also known as the one-hit model. In this situation, the injury is massive enough to cause an intense systemic inflammatory reaction that activates the immune system including the macrophages, neutrophils, natural killer cells, interleukin-8, and complement components C5a and C3a, which promote inflammatory cell migration into the site. This response overwhelms any counter–anti-inflammatory response, and the inflammatory process runs amok, ultimately causing MODS and death (Bone stage three).

The two-hit model occurs when the injury is less intense and the body can react with the appropriate counter–anti-inflammatory response. However, this finely balanced system can be thrown out of control by a second insult, causing SIRS to flourish or perhaps the counter–anti-inflammatory process to suppress the inflammatory process, making the patient susceptible to sepsis and ultimately MODS and death (Bone stage four). *This is the situation that the concept of damage control orthopaedics was devised to minimize.* The problem becomes determining which patients are susceptible to the second-hit phenomenon and require a DCO approach to care.[50,54,55]

Attempts to predict which of these responses will be either inadequate or overwhelming have not been successful using the plasma concentration of these markers. Our ability to determine which patient is on the verge of inflammatory collapse, therefore, has not reached the level of precise predictability. The traditional assessment of body functions by the standard tests of urinary output, oxygen saturation, blood gases, C-reactive protein, base excess, and lactate is not predictive of impending collapse, since abnormal results in these tests are predicated on the fact that the organs have already started to fail. This leaves the surgeon with the need to rely on clinical scenarios in which it is known from experience that the patient will probably be able to cope with the first hit but a further insult (the second hit) will likely precipitate a downward spiral to MODS and death.

Several other components of this secondary treatment may potentiate the second hit of surgical treatment: coagulopathy, hypothermia, and anesthesia.

COAGULOPATHY

Transfusions are often required in the acute resuscitation of the MIP, and the use of additional blood products continues through the emergent surgical procedures. Coagulation defects develop after transfusions and are usually secondary to depletion of host clotting factors and platelets and the development of hypothermia. Transfused blood is deficient in factors V and VIII and platelets. Fresh-frozen plasma and platelet replacement therapy must be anticipated if blood requirements are high, and replacement should be initiated as early as possible. Clotting abnormalities can result from intracranial injuries. The etiology of the coagulopathy is thought to be related to the release of tissue thromboplastin from the injured brain tissue. The coagulation profile should be monitored after major resuscitation or torso surgery, prior to or during the subsequent orthopaedic care. A platelet count less than 100,000/mL³, a fibrinogen level less than 1 g/L, and an abnormal prothrombin time or partial thromboplastin time are associated with a decrease in hemostasis capability and a worsening prognosis.[61]

HYPOTHERMIA

Hypothermia (<32 °C) causes platelet segregation and impairs the release of platelet factor required in the intrinsic clotting pathway. The patient's core temperature begins to drop at the accident scene with the initial administration of intravenous fluids at ambient temperature, and this temperature drop continues in the emergency department and the operating suite as ambient fluid administration continues and as larger body surfaces are exposed to ambient temperature.

ANESTHESIA

Although necessary for the conduct of lifesaving surgical procedures, the anesthetic process and the agents used have systemic effects that are counter to the desired physiologic state of the acute trauma patient and should be avoided, if possible, in certain patients. Most anesthetic agents are myocardial depressants, and cardiac output diminishes with their use. In elective procedures, crystalloid infusions are used to maintain normal cardiac output. The trauma patient often arrives in the operating room hypovolemic and marginally coagulopathic. Resuscitation with crystalloid solutions and blood products continues throughout the operative procedure. Filling pressure and cardiac output monitoring can help titrate the amount of fluid provided to the patient, but significant amounts are absorbed in the extravascular volume—the "third space" phenomenon. This tissue edema can have negative effects on patients with severe head or pulmonary injuries, or both. Despite the aggressive use of room heaters, warming blankets, and warm infusion fluids, the patient's core temperature often begins to drop. Non-lifesaving surgical procedures increase the blood loss and the demands for additional fluids and blood products and increase the time during which the patient remains anesthetized in the operating room environment.

Transportation of a critically injured or ill patient from the ICU to the operating room poses some risk. Ten percent of such transports have resulted in significant disturbance of cardiovascular or respiratory function.[33,84] Commonly recognized transport related problems include hypoxemia, hypotension, and arrhythmia.

The Decision: Damage Control Orthopaedic Surgery

The need for stabilization of the injured or fractured extremity is still an imperative in the management of the multiply injured patient for many reasons. Pain plays a significant role in the response of the patient. Because neurostimuli are an important part of the stress response, pain relief is important in the modification and modulation of this effect. Relief of pain also improves mobilization and perhaps decreases morbidity through this period. Alignment and stabilizing of the fracture decrease the ongoing muscle damage and continued stimulation of the inflammatory process. They are also important for prevention of vascular and neurologic injury. Finally, a patient with stabilized extremity injuries is easier to nurse and to provide with resuscitative and lifesaving intensive care treatment. Following an understanding of the physiologic responses to trauma, the inflammatory process induced by trauma, and other factors that may affect the injured patient, the decision of when to perform non-lifesaving orthopaedic surgery is extremely important. If surgery is undertaken, a damage control approach appears to be a reasonable clinical pathway at this time.

Damage control orthopaedic surgery is not for every patient with multiple fractures or every patient with multiple injuries and several fractures. It is for the injured patient whose inflammatory response will potentially be overwhelmed by further stimuli. These are patients with a major constellation of injuries that have been recognized as having significant impact on the inflammatory and physiologic response. These injuries are usually associated with deranged physiology that has been difficult to correct or is undercorrected, such as hypovolemic shock. Delayed manifestations of certain conditions such as lung injury are also a clue to deciding which patients may be better served by a damage control mode of care. The aim of the assessment during the initial resuscitative phase of care is to determine whether the injured patient with orthopaedic injuries can withstand early definitive surgical care for these injuries without overwhelming the inflammatory process.[67] Using the patient's history from the injury scene, ambulance transport, and resuscitative course, as well as the injury patterns, the patient may be classified into one of four groups.

THE STABLE PATIENT

This patient has never been in shock and has only minor associated injuries although there may be multiple fractures. These patients are treated with the preferred method of care for their orthopaedic injuries. Long bone fractures can be fixed with IM nails. The timing of surgery is usually in the first 24 to 36 hours, depending on local OR and surgeon availability.

THE UNSTABLE PATIENT

These patients require ongoing resuscitation to maintain their normal physiologic state. Major non-lifesaving procedures that would cause blood loss or major fluid shift must be avoided. These patients should undergo continued resuscitation. The initial treatment of the long bone fracture can be with skeletal traction. As the patient's clinical course becomes defined, early IM nailing can be performed. When the patient remains unstable, external fixation of the fractures should be considered.

THE IN EXTREMIS PATIENT

This patient has had a major insult and is never adequately resuscitated in the initial 24 hours. This patient is not a candidate for any major non-lifesaving surgical procedure in the short-term. External fixation of the long bone fractures should be considered as a bridge to definitive internal fixation. Temporary skeletal traction can be employed in the acute resuscitation period. If the patient is in the OR for lifesaving surgery, external fixation of the long bone fractures should be performed in concert with the lifesaving surgery.

THE BORDERLINE PATIENT

This patient is the most difficult to define. In general all these patients will have lower extremity long bone fractures, especially of the femur and/or a pelvic ring injury, associated with severe nonorthopaedic injuries. The initial response to injury and treatment may compromise the patient's ability to withstand the second surgical hit necessary for the management of the orthopaedic injuries. Therefore, the borderline patient has the propensity to deteriorate and develop major complications and die. Pape et al. believed that patients with the physiologic parameters listed in Table 7-2 are the ones best suited for damage control.[55,58,59]

Patients with the "at-risk" physiologic parameters demonstrate that a second hit is too much for their inflammatory response to cope with and deteriorate, developing SIRS, ARDS, MODS, and death. To assist the surgeon with the identification of the at-risk patient, the Louisville group has specified physiologic parameters to these clinical situations. They believe that damage control orthopaedic surgery is indicated if the patient has a pH of <7.24, a temperature of 32 °C to 35 °C, is undergoing an operative procedure of more than 90 minutes' duration, is coagulopathic (platelet count $<90,000$), and has received more than 10 units of packed red cells.[67] In addition to these criteria, the following orthopaedic injury complexes have also shown a trend to the development of traumatic complications. These are femoral fractures in MIPs, pelvic ring injuries with exsanguinating hemorrhage, and multiple trauma in the geriatric patient. Other clinical parameters associated with these patient types have been proposed as clues to the borderline patient. These are an unstable condition or a difficult resuscitation, especially if 25 units of packed cells are needed; the association of multiple long bone injuries and a truncal injury (AIS ≥ 2); over 6 hours of surgery; an arterial injury and hemodynamic instability (blood pressure <90 mm Hg), and finally evidence of an exaggerated inflammatory response (e.g., IL-6 >800 pg/mL).

Serum lactate levels (>2–2.5 mmol/L) may serve as a "poor man's" gauge of the relative state of a patient's resuscitation and of end-organ perfusion. Prolonged hypoperfusion has been associated with worse outcomes. Crowl et al.[20] retrospectively reviewed femur fracture patients. Fixation was performed within 24 hours. Serum lactate levels were followed, and levels greater than 2.5 mmol/L were considered to represent a hypoperfused patient. Patients exposed to femur fracture surgery while

Table 7-2
The Borderline Patient
Injury severity score (ISS) >40 without thoracic injury
ISS >20 with thoracic injury (abbreviated injury score <2)
Multiple trauma with abdominal trauma (Moore score >3 points)
Bilateral lung contusions evident on a chest radiograph
Initial mean pulmonary artery pressure >24 mm Hg
Increase in pulmonary artery pressure >6 mm Hg during intramedullary nailing

hypoperfused had a twofold higher incidence of postoperative complications. Claridge et al.[19] assessed the outcomes and complications of 381 consecutive trauma patients, of whom 118 were never hypoperfused and 263 exhibited hypoperfusion as indicated by elevated lactate levels. Patients whose lactate levels were corrected by 12 hours had an infection rate no different from that of the patient group with normal lactate levels (13.6% vs. 12.7%). The infection rate rose to 40.5 percent ($P < 0.01$) when the lactate level was corrected between 12 and 24 hours and to 65 percent ($P < 0.01$) when it was corrected after 24 hours. The mortality increased from 1.3 percent to 7.1 percent for patients with hypoperfusion for less than and more than 12 hours. Patients with prolonged hypoperfusion appear to be at risk for increased infection and mortality. The authors believe that subspecialty operations, long radiology evaluations, and the boarding of patients in units unfamiliar with trauma patient resuscitation protocols are factors that may prolong the state of hypoperfusion.

With these clinical and physiologic guidelines, the orthopaedic surgeon involved in the acute management of the injured patient with major pelvic or lower extremity fractures or open wounds now has the opportunity to individualize a treatment plan based on the potential for the patient to develop severe post-traumatic complications. Prior to undertaking non-lifesaving surgery, the patient needs to be aggressively resuscitated to a stable hemodynamic and oxygenation state, should have a decreasing to normal lactate level (<2 mmol/L), a normalized coagulation profile, a normalized temperature, and a urine output of a least 1 mL/kg/hr. Lastly, the patient should be off inotropic support. On the basis of the patient's response to the resuscitation and the magnitude of the patient's injuries, the orthopaedic surgeon needs to consider a "risk-adapted" damage control orthopaedic surgery approach.[66] Our current approach is depicted in Figure 7-4. The options for care of a patient with a femur fracture fall into three broad treatment schemes:

Early Femoral Intramedullary Nail Fracture Fixation
The use of IM nailing has the advantage of being definitive, but the operation time, reaming, and nail insertion may act as a second-hit phenomenon in these patients.

Splinting or Traction
Splinting and/or traction is performed until the patient's condition is optimized for surgery—typically IM nail fixation of the long bones. The target time for this surgery is usually within the first 36 hours. The patient's hemodynamic and pulmonary parameters are optimized during this period, and hypoperfusion is reversed.

Application of Temporary External Fixation and Later Conversion to an IM Nail
Temporary external fixation is simple and has minimal blood loss. It is postulated to reduce the systemic inflammatory response and subsequent organ dysfunction and mortality. It does require a second operation and a possible increase in the rate of infection. This approach may increase the final cost of care. The surgeon must decide, however, based on the risk factors of surgery, whether or not the patient will benefit from a surgical exposure just for the application of an external fixator. Oftentimes, these patients are not in the OR for lifesaving surgery. In many cases, bedside external fixation application could be utilized.

Damage Control Orthopaedics: The Clinical Evidence

Scalea retrospectively reported the use of external fixation as a bridge to IM nailing of femur fracture in patients with multiple injuries.[72] The practice was termed damage control orthopaedics. Forty-three of 324 patients with femur fracture (13%) initially treated with external fixation of the femur were compared with 284 patients treated with primary IM nailing of the femur. Patients provisionally treated with external fixation

---

FIGURE 7-4 *Orthopaedic damage control algorithm.*

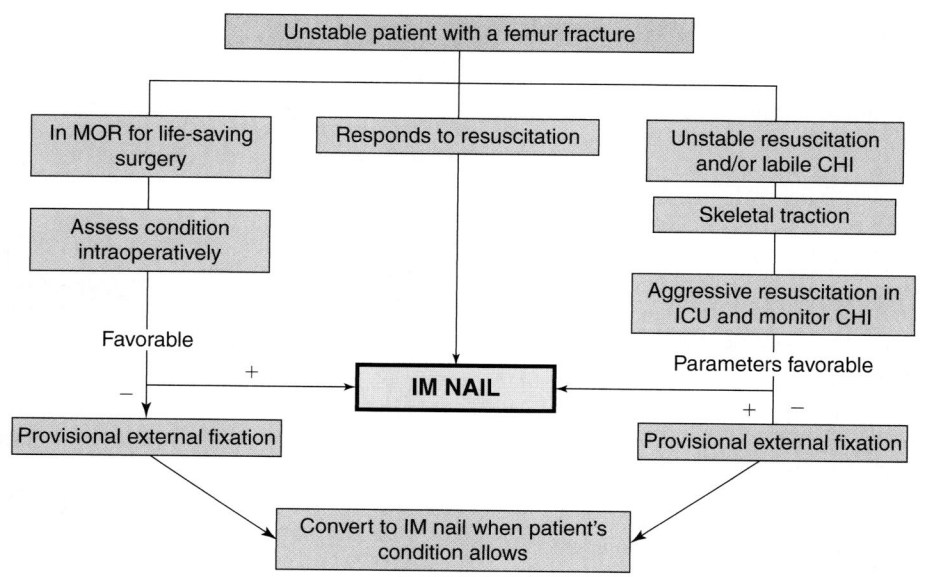

had higher ISS (26.8 vs. 16.8), lower GCS (11 vs. 14.2), and required significantly more fluid resuscitation (11.9 L vs. 6.2 L) and more blood (1.5 L vs. 1.0 L) in the first 24 hours. Noted reasons for delay in IM nailing included closed head injury (46%), hemodynamic instability (65%), thoracoabdominal injuries (51%), and other (mostly orthopaedic) serious injuries (46%). Many of the patients had more than one of the risk factors. Initial external fixation was performed in 35 minutes. Conversion to an IM nail was performed, on the average, 4.8 days later. Serum lactate levels were obtained for all patients treated with external fixation. The average admission lactate level was 4.3. Ninety-one percent of the lactate levels normalized, typically within 28 hours.

Pape et al. reviewed the outcomes of MIP with femur fractures treated at a German Level 1 trauma center.[57] In a retrospective cohort study, patients were divided according to the treatment philosophy of the trauma center: early total care (ETC) with primary nail fixation of the femur; intermediate (INT), as the treatment evolved to less nailing and more provisional external fixation; and damage control (DCO), when patients at high risk for organ failure were initially treated with external fixation, then converted to nail fixation as their conditions stabilized. External fixation was employed as the initial treatment more commonly in the DCO group (16.6% ETC, 23.9% INT, and 35.6% DCO). The incidence of multiple organ failure decreased significantly from the ETC period (1981–1989) to the DCO period (1993–2000) *regardless of the type of treatment of the femur fracture.* Patients treated with primary EF had similar post-traumatic local and systemic complications as patients treated with primary IM nailing, despite a higher ISS in the EF cohort. There was a significantly higher incidence of adult respiratory distress syndrome when primary femoral nailing (15.1%) or primary external fixation (9.1%) was employed in the DCO cohort, although the mortality rate for the groups was the same. The authors concluded that DCO was a reasonable alternative treatment strategy for the care of severely injured patients.

While these conclusions may be correct, critical assessment of the methodology and conclusions is required. This paper suffers from the same weaknesses as the papers that argued for the value of ETC. The study is retrospective, comparing dissimilar eras of trauma care: 1981–1989 versus 1993–2000. While the authors acknowledge possible confounders that include increased frequency of air rescue, transition to unreamed nails, and heightened awareness of the impact of thoracic and abdominal injuries, they fail to acknowledge or control for other variables that likely drove the observed outcomes, such as advances in the critical care of the patient, decreased use of exploratory laparotomy and more noninvasive therapy to control hemorrhage, improved care of the head injury, and significant advances in ventilator technology, infection surveillance and control. Assigning the "no difference" result between the cohorts related to the development of post-traumatic local and systemic complications as a positive result supporting DCO because of a higher ISS in the DCO/EF cohort is not acceptable, particularly given the small number of patients. ISS is recognized to underscore the

injury load, especially when more than one injury is present in a body region. The observation of a decrease in the incidence of ARDS in the DCO cohort in patients primarily treated with external fixation may be related to corresponding pulmonary or head injuries in the cohort of nailed patients. A subanalysis to explore the observed difference was not performed. Stratifying patients with and without chest or head injuries and comparing outcomes with IM nailing or EF would be a more reasonable test, since pulmonary injury and head injury are recognized as major risk factors for ARDS.[10] Pape et al. also studied the impact of IM nailing versus initial external fixation of femur fractures on immunoinflammatory parameters.[56] A sustained inflammatory response was measured after primary femoral nailing and not after initial external fixation or the conversion procedure to an IM nail. The authors believe that these observations confirm prior studies demonstrating that damage control orthopaedic surgery appears to minimize the additional systemic stress of femoral nailing.

O'Toole and colleagues[49] retrospectively analyzed the outcomes of polytrauma patients with femur fractures treated in a major North American Level 1 trauma center that did not subscribe to a dogmatic damage control protocol. Patients with femur fractures were treated with reamed IM nails after adequate resuscitation as demonstrated by normalizing lactate levels and optimized pulmonary and hemodynamic parameters. Patients who did not respond to the resuscitation efforts were treated with provisional external fixation. Only 37 patients (7%) were treated by DCO external fixation methods; 484 (97%) were treated with early reamed IM nailing. The patients were divided and evaluated in three groups: polytrauma patients with ISS >17 (*n*=249); polytrauma patients with lung injury (ISS >17 and thoracic AIS >2 [*n*=197]), and severe polytrauma patients with lung injury (ISS >28 and thoracic AIS >2 [*n*=86]). Of the 249 patients in the cohort with ISS >17, only 33 (13%) were treated with damage control external fixation. These patients had a significantly higher ISS and a higher mortality rate (18% vs. 2.3%) than the primary IM nail patients. The average time from admission to the operating room was just under 14 hours in both treatment groups. Over 52 percent of the patients were in the operating room at 8 hours from the time of admission. Patients with chest injuries (AIS >2) treated with IM nails had a 1.8 percent rate of ARDS and a 2.4 percent mortality rate. The subgroup of severely injured patients (ISS >28, AIS_{chest} >2) had a 3.1 percent rate of ARDS and a 3.1 percent mortality rate. Serum lactate levels were used to assess the degree of the patient's resuscitation at the time of surgery. In each of the subgroups, the lactate levels decreased significantly between the time of admission and the time of surgery. The patients treated with damage control external fixation had higher lactate levels at all time points.

O'Toole and colleagues concluded that the ARDS rates from their center were significantly lower than from centers that reported damage control external fixation in up to 36 percent of their cases. The primary indications for the use of damage control external fixation of femur fractures at the Baltimore Shock Trauma Center were elevated lactate levels that failed to normalize and closed head injuries with labile intracranial pressures.

Taeger et al.[80] reported on 409 patients with multiple injuries (ISS >30) where the DCO concept was applied to 75 patients with major orthopaedic injuries—75 patients with 135 fractures (49 femurs, 39 tibias, 25 pelvic, and 22 upper extremity). Of the fractures 72.6 percent were closed. They report that 84.5 percent of the cases were in the OR for other DCO procedures but report only 14 laparotomies, 3 thoracotomies, 4 hemorrhagic facial fractures, 13 craniotomies, and 2 compartment syndrome fasciotomies. If these injuries were isolated to single patients, likely only 48 percent needed DCO surgical procedures. Surgical time averaged 33 minutes per orthopaedic injury. Later conversion to internal fixation was uncomplicated. The authors concluded that DCO provides a major reduction in operating time and blood loss in the primary treatment period as compared to the later exchange procedure.

The conclusion of this study was obvious to the authors prior to the research, thus questioning the purpose of the research. External fixation takes less time and has a lower recorded blood loss than does a definitive fixation procedure. What this paper pinpoints is a major conceptual difference between European and North American trauma centers. We may not be seeing the same types of patients and may define "immediate and emergent" in different ways when considering the treatment of orthopaedic injuries. *In North America, few if any of the fractures treated in this paper by DCO would be considered as emergency procedures.* If the patient were in the OR for lifesaving surgical procedures, the femur would be externally fixed. Upper extremity, tibia, and most pelvic fractures are initially treated with splints (or binders).

Perhaps the statement made by the authors sheds some light on North American and European emergent orthopaedic care differences. Taeger et al. state, "although the necessity of early fracture fixation for reduction of pulmonary failure and other complications in the severely injured is undoubtedly accepted . . ." This statement represents a dogmatic approach that is poorly supported by the literature and is not universally accepted by senior surgeons. Surgeons must come to a clear consensus on the terms early and fracture. In this series, only 49 femur fractures were in the cohort of 135 fractures treated with DCO external fixation. DCO external fixation of tibia, pelvic, and upper extremity fractures likely provides no benefit to the resolution of the patient's immediate physiologic stress. If these patients were exposed to the OR for the sole purpose of externally fixing these fractures (i.e., not in conjunction with a lifesaving surgical procedure), it is possible that the patient was further harmed by the event.

We continue to investigate the timing of femur fracture surgery in the multiple trauma population. It appears that experiences and results from the German centers may not be generalized to North American or other trauma centers and future evaluations should be directed at determining the reason for this difference. North American centers report a low rate of ARDS (3–5%).[7,10,49,63,72,86] White et al.[86] studied the incidence of ARDS in a single center in Scotland. The addition of a thoracic injury increased the ARDS rate from 1.7 to 7.7 percent in trauma patients with femur fractures. These rates need to be compared to the higher rates experienced in the

German centers (20–35%).[51,54,57,66] This difference could be related to the mechanisms of injury (speed limits), prehospital care, initial resuscitation protocols, the timing and techniques of surgical interventions, postinjury critical care, patient population health habits (smoking), or genetic predisposition—alone or in combinations. The aggressive prehospital care described by the German trauma system might expose patients to over-resuscitation and the development of *Da Nang* (wet lung) syndrome (ARDS).[23,31,60] Pape et al.[19,57] reported that only 2 percent of 525 patients with femur fractures had surgery intervention after 8 hours from the time of admission. The cause of the different rates of ARDS between the two continents needs to be determined.

Long bone stabilization is beneficial to the patient and facilitates early mobilization and hospital discharge. The debate over early versus late fixation is misguided. Early definitive orthopaedic fixation is preferred and is determined by the patient's response to the injury, resuscitation, and the capabilities of the health care environment. When the patient has met the criteria of physiologic and inflammatory stability as defined by local trauma protocols, then definitive stabilization can be performed (early or late). Up until that point, damage control is performed in a manner best suited to the patient's expected clinical course—provisional skeletal traction or external fixation. Adjustments to definitive femoral fixation techniques and other fracture fixation protocols must be considered, however, when these injuries are present in patients with associated systemic instability or severe traumatic brain or pulmonary injury. Adherence to rigid implant and time orthopaedic protocols (for both definitive and DCO care) can be detrimental to the overall recovery of the severely injured patient. The surgical team (trauma surgeon, neurosurgeon, orthopaedic surgeon, and anesthesiologist) must agree on the general concepts of care for the patient and apply these concepts in a planned reconstructive approach tailored to the patient's specific injury constellation and immediate needs. Definitive early long bone stabilization is, of course, the optimal goal for each patient. Pursuit of the goal, however, is counter to the physiologic needs of many trauma patients. In every case, the care team should attempt to improve the patient's physical condition before performing non-lifesaving surgery and develop surgical plans that are intentionally simple, quick, and well executed.

Special Considerations in Damage Control Orthopaedics: Traumatic Brain Injury Patients

CLINICAL EXPERIENCE: FRACTURE AND THE HEAD-INJURED PATIENT

Head injury is present in up to 20 percent of all trauma patients and is the leading cause of death following injury in the developed world.[28,38,39] The mortality rate following head injury in the multiply injured patient is twice that of the isolated head-injured patient.[28,38,39] Optimal trauma care will provide treatment that protects the central nervous system as a priority due to the brain's vulnerability for primary (as a consequence of the injury) and secondary (subsequent damage not related to the injury) damage.[2,18,28] Clinical outcome information concerning the optimal care of the patient with a significant closed head injury and major fractures is inconclusive. Most of the trauma literature regarding fracture care and the head-injured patient reports on a limited number of variables to assess effectiveness—typically, mortality, ARDS, pneumonia, infection, and fracture union rates. What is lacking in most studies is a validated functional outcome or, better, a quality of life determination. Until these are developed and applied, the debate over the ideal care will continue. Therefore, the trauma surgeon, the orthopaedic surgeon, and the neurosurgeon must communicate and cooperate in planning the care of a patient with brain and orthopaedic injuries.[28]

In negotiating the care sequence of the MIP with a severe head injury, orthopaedic and trauma surgeons cite the ICU care and mobilization benefits of early surgery to support more aggressive fracture care. Every orthopaedic surgeon, however, has experienced the frustration of observing the emergently stabilized patient who is supine and pharmacologically sedated to treat the intracranial injury. Early mobilization is usually not realized in patients with severe brain or chest injuries. Employment of the mobility benefit argument to justify emergent surgery in this group of patients is difficult to support. Despite attempts by a number of authors employing retrospective techniques, a major question remains unanswered in care of trauma patients concerning the risk-to-benefit ratio of non-lifesaving emergency extremity surgery in the presence of a severe head injury.[28,34,36,79] Stein and colleagues[79] identified 123 of 253 (48.6%) new or progressive lesions (secondary brain injury) in serial computed tomography (CT) scans of head-injured patients. Fifty-five percent of these patients had coagulation abnormalities on admission, compared with 9 percent with stable or improved follow-up scans. An 85 percent risk of developing a delayed injury was calculated if the patient had at least one abnormal clotting parameter at the time of admission. Extension of this information suggests to the clinician that therapeutic interventions that affect the coagulation parameters secondary to loss of clotting factors, dilution, or development of hypothermia should be avoided in susceptible patients.

In an animal model, Schmoker and colleagues[75] showed that hemorrhage after focal brain injury caused a reduction in cerebral oxygen delivery leading to cerebral ischemia. In a retrospective study of 17 patients with a traumatic brain injury in whom an intracranial monitor was placed, reamed femoral nailing was performed. Anglen et al. was able to show that intraoperative cerebral perfusion pressure decreased as the intracranial pressure rose and mean arterial pressure dropped intraoperatively. Intraoperative systemic hypotension accounted for two thirds of the total decrease in cranial perfusion pressure. They were unable to show that this decrease had a long-term effect on neurologic recovery owing to lack of detailed follow-up data.[1] This effect in cranial perfusion pressure and intracranial pressure has been supported by an animal model in sheep exposed to hemorrhagic shock, resuscitation, and IM nailing.[1,38,39,46] McMahon and co-workers[41] compared patients with brain injury and peripheral injury (*n*=378) with patients with peripheral injury alone (*n*=2339). When combined with peripheral

injury, the risk of death from brain injury was double that attributable to peripheral injury. The authors suggested a possible bidirectional interaction between brain injury and peripheral injury—hemorrhagic shock associated with neurotrauma induces a secondary brain injury. The brain injury may affect cardiovascular control mechanisms, further reducing cerebral oxygen delivery and consumption. As well, the brain injury disrupts the blood-brain barrier mechanism, making the cerebral tissue more susceptible to fluid shifts caused by transient hypoperfusion secondary to ongoing blood loss from surgery and under-resuscitation. This situation will compound the other factors, leading to secondary brain injury.

Addressing the clinical implications of non-lifesaving trauma care in patients with closed head injuries, Hofman and Goris[30] retrospectively reviewed a consecutive series of 58 patients with major extremity fractures and GCS scores of 7 or less. Fifteen patients underwent fracture fixation on the day of injury. A lower mortality rate was noted in the early fixation group. The neurologic results were better in the early fixation group but did not reach statistical significance. On the basis of these data, it was concluded that there was no reason for concern about a negative influence of early fracture surgery in patients with severe brain injury.

Poole and co-workers[62] did not find a relationship between pulmonary complications and timing of fracture surgery in a review of records of 114 patients with head injuries and femur or tibia fractures, but they did find a significant correlation with injuries to the head and chest. They also noted that a delay in fracture fixation did not protect the brain, since the outcome appeared to be related to the severity of the initial injury. Because early fracture fixation appeared to simplify the patient's care without a negative neurologic cost, early fracture fixation was advocated.[62] In reviewing the effect of treatment of unstable pelvic fractures in patients with severe head injuries, Riemer and associates[64] demonstrated a decrease in mortality in patients with pelvic fractures associated with closed head injuries from 43 to 7 percent after initiation of a protocol involving pelvic external fixation and mobilization. Scalea and colleagues[73] reviewed trauma registry data to determine the timing of fracture care in patients with closed head injuries. No differences were found between the early and late fixation groups as measured by the discharge GCS score or mortality. The authors concluded that they found no evidence to suggest that early fracture fixation negatively influences central nervous system outcomes. Velmahos and colleagues[83] found no difference in the rate of intraoperative or postoperative hypoxic or hypotensive episodes in groups of patients with femur fractures and closed head injury treated either early or late. Final GCS scores were similar. Starr and associates[78] found that a delay in stabilization of the femur fracture increased the risk of pulmonary complication but that early fixation did not increase central nervous system complications.

Retrospective clinical studies that conclude in favor of continued early fracture fixation often do so on the basis of reliance on crude outcomes—mortality and final GCS. Unfortunately, the GCS is not a good predictor of long-term cognitive function. McKee and co-workers[40] included cognitive function, matched control groups, and long-term follow-up in their clinical study of the possible effects of timing of femur fracture fixation in patients with severe closed head injuries. They found no difference in outcomes and believed the data supported the continued practice of early IM fixation of femur fractures in patients with closed head injuries. Although it appears that early fracture stabilization in the head-injured patient is safe, two factors must be accounted for in this early care. Perioperative hypotension and hypoxemia must be guarded against. Chestnut,[18,28] using data from the Traumatic Coma Data Bank, showed that hypotension either during resuscitation or in the operating room or ICU at least doubled the mortality of those who remained normotensive. Jaicks and associates[34] confirmed this finding by reviewing 33 patients with blunt trauma with significant closed head injuries requiring operative fracture fixation. The early fixation group ($n=19$) required significantly more fluids and trended to higher rates of intraoperative hypotension and hypoxia. They concluded that these conditions may contribute to poor neurologic outcomes. Townsend and co-workers[81] studied 61 patients with femur fractures and severe brain injury. They identified an inversely proportional trend when comparing time until surgery with the percentage of patients who became hypotensive during surgery. Patients in the early femur fixation group were eight times more likely to become hypotensive during the surgery than the patients delayed at least 24 hours (43% overall). The research team concluded that operative delay beyond 24 hours may be necessary to prevent hypoxia, hypotension, and low cerebral perfusion pressure.

Kalb and colleagues[36] had similar findings, noting that patients with severe head injury undergoing early fracture fixation had a significant increase in crystalloid and blood infusion and in operative blood loss. Sarrafzadeh, in the only prospective study comparing severely brain injured patients with patients with only extracranial injuries, showed that secondary brain injury was not increased in the head-injured patients with extracranial injuries if the non-lifesaving surgery was delayed and they were under continuous monitoring of cerebral perfusion pressure and cerebral oxygenation. Long-term outcomes were not related to the multiple injuries but were dependent on the head injury when patients were managed by a targeted protocol including intracranial pressure– and cerebral perfusion pressure–guided therapy and *delayed surgery* for extracranial non-life-threatening lesions.[71]

The most recent research on the timing of noncranial surgery in a trauma patient took advantage of patient cohorts from two randomized, prospective, double-blind studies on the treatment of traumatic brain injury. These studies collected both functional and neuropsychological outcomes. Wang et al.[85] performed a cohort study to evaluate the effect of the timing of noncranial surgery on neurologic and functional outcomes and morbidity and mortality rates of the patients undergoing surgery in less than or longer than 24 hours from injury. After adjusting for potential confounders, they found that the early timing of orthopaedic and facial fracture surgery under general anesthesia was not associated with worse neuropsychological or functional outcomes when compared with delayed surgery. Above all, the authors believed that these findings contribute to equipoise regarding the timing of surgery and emphasize the need for a randomized clinical trial.

TREATMENT OF TRAUMATIC BRAIN INJURY

The general principles employed in the treatment of the brain-injured patient are simple: maintain optimal cerebral perfusion, oxygenation, and glucose delivery. MIPs with suspected brain injury are evaluated by CT scanning, and the nature and severity of the injury are defined. Brain injuries are classified as focal or diffuse and can be associated with open, closed, or depressed skull fractures. Focal injuries consist of brain contusion, hemorrhage, or hematomas. Neurosurgical care is directed toward operative or nonoperative modes on the basis of the presence or absence of open or depressed skull fractures and mass lesions.

Survival of the head-injured patient is dependent on the maintenance of adequate cerebral blood flow. Autoregulated in the normal patient, the blood flow is altered in the trauma patient by a number of factors including mean arterial pressure (MAP), intracranial pressure (ICP), pH, and the partial pressure of carbon dioxide in arterial blood ($Paco_2$). Cerebral blood flow is indirectly monitored by calculation of the cerebral perfusion pressure (CPP):

$$CPP = MAP - ICP$$

Normal ICP is 10 mm Hg or less. ICP is defined in the Monro-Kellie hypothesis in relation to the volume of the cerebrospinal fluid (CSF), the blood, and the brain matter:

$$K_{ICP} = V_{CSF} + V_{Blood} + V_{Brain}$$

CSF production is constant. CSF absorption is regulated by the ICP. Brain volume is a constant unless increased by edema or hemorrhage. Intracranial blood volume is affected by passive venous drainage and arterial blood volume autoregulation. Increased intrathoracic pressure and ICP diminish intracranial venous drainage.

Injury to the brain causes swelling, hemorrhage, or both. CSF and venous blood are removed from the intracranial compartment in an effort to accommodate the increased volume. When this adjustment mechanism is exhausted, additional volume increases the ICP. ICP greater than 20 mm Hg requires monitoring and treatment. Venous drainage is impaired with ICP in the range of 30 to 35 mm Hg, and as with an extremity compartment syndrome, brain edema is exacerbated at this level. Pressures that exceed 40 mm Hg represent severe intracranial hypertension. Cerebral perfusion pressures fall, and ischemia results. Brain death ensues when perfusion is compromised to the point at which oxygen and glucose delivery ceases.

In practical terms, after depressed injuries or mass lesions are ruled out or appropriately cared for, the patient's MAP, Pao_2, $Paco_2$, hemoglobin, and ICP and glucose levels are the variables available for manipulation to optimize recovery of the central nervous system. Cerebral oxygen content is dependent on the arterial hemoglobin level and the O_2 saturation. A Pao_2 greater than 80 mm Hg is desired in most brain-injured patients.

ICP is monitored and regulated as necessary. The patient is initially placed in a 30-degree head-up position. The neck is maintained in neutral rotation in an effort to not compress the veins necessary for intracranial drainage. Hyperventilation, fluid restriction, and hyperosmolar agents are used as required to maintain optimal ICP.

If these measures fail to control the ICP, ventriculostomy with CSF withdrawal, sedation, or barbiturate coma—and, in some institutions, selective lobectomy procedures to decrease the intracranial volume—are used to control elevations in ICP.

At present no firm recommendations can be made with regard to the timing of non-life-threatening extremity surgery in the severely head injured (GCS 3–9) patient. However, prior to any orthopaedic intervention the patient needs to be adequately resuscitated and the severity of the head injury determined. If orthopaedic procedures are required acutely for the management of multiple lower extremity fractures or for excessive blood loss, the patient must be closely monitored (ICP <20 mm Hg and CPP >60–70 mm Hg) and procedures that minimize blood loss used (damage control). It is imperative that during these procedures, hypotension and hypoxemia be avoided at all cost to minimize secondary brain injury.[28] Otherwise it is probably wise to delay extremity surgery until ICP and CPP normalize in about 7 to 10 days.[71] Patients with mild (GCS 13–15) to moderate (GCS 9–12) head injury and normal CT scans may undergo definitive extremity surgery early as long as they are fully monitored and blood pressure and oxygenation are maintained.

The Damage Control Strategy

The timing and technique of fracture fixation most likely play some role in the recovery of the critically injured patient. The magnitude and significance of the contribution are yet to be determined. The very concept of "early fixation" is poorly defined in the orthopaedic trauma literature. Initially defined as within the first 2 weeks, the current definition ranges from 12 to 36 hours (or beyond). On the basis of available knowledge of trauma physiology, animal research, and clinical experience, surgeons need to consider altering their care for a small cohort of the trauma population. A reasonable strategy is presented in Figure 7-4.

Seriously injured and unstable trauma patients quickly fall into two groups: those who need immediate lifesaving surgery in the operating room and those who do not. Those in the operating room for lifesaving surgery need coordination to ensure that the major orthopaedic injuries (femur fractures) are stabilized at the same sitting. If, after the emergent surgery, the patient's condition is stabilized, the femur can be treated with an IM nail. If the patient remains unstable, resuscitation needs to continue. An external fixator is applied to the femur as open wounds are cleaned and other fractures splinted—prior to returning the patient to the trauma ICU. As the patient's condition improves and the physiologic parameters optimize, the patient is returned to the OR for conversion of the external fixator to an IM nail and for treatment of other orthopaedic injuries.

Patients who do not need to be in the operating room for visceral lifesaving surgery present a more difficult treatment decision challenge. Resuscitation is initiated in the trauma admitting area and, if needed, continued in the ICU. If the patient responds to the resuscitation and is not acidotic, coagulopathic, or hypothermic or a borderline patient, early IM nail fixation of the femur fracture is warranted. If the patient fails to quickly respond or if the patient has a labile or evolving closed head injury,

a more prolonged stay in the ICU might be required to optimize the patient for femur fixation and other orthopaedic surgery. Skeletal traction can serve as a bridge to more definitive fracture care during this time. As the head injury stabilizes and/or if the patient's physiologic condition improves, the femur can be addressed with either an IM nail or an external fixator in the OR. If at any time in the initial course it becomes obvious that the patient's condition will not improve for formal surgery, an external fixator can be applied in the ICU and the traction pin discontinued.

The application of the external fixator must be rapid. The construct should provide enough stability at the fracture site to allow for pain relief and mobilization of the patient, usually in the ICU. This is usually appropriate turning for skin care and upright position for the chest to enhance respiratory function. The frame is constructed using two pins above the fracture and two pins below the fracture and these pin clusters are joined by a single or double bar construct depending on the fracture stability required. The frame may be applied anteriorly or laterally. If the fracture being stabilized is in the supracondylar region or proximal tibia, the pins must be placed to keep them out of the operative incision site.

Damage Control Strategy: For Other Than Femur Fractures

The femur fracture is used in this chapter as the sample injury forcing treatment decisions. We recognize that other injuries, including high-energy open fractures, contaminated wounds, and elevated compartment pressures, occur in critically injured patients and the timing of care for these patients must also be considered. As with the femur fracture, optimal care is delivered in the OR. If the patient is in the OR for lifesaving surgical procedures, clear communication with the trauma team outlining the immediate orthopaedic goals is critical. Fractures and wounds can be quickly débrided and fasciotomies performed as needed. As in the case of the femur fracture, the surgeon must decide if a trip to the OR in the early course of resuscitation is in the best interest of the patient. Often it isn't. Bedside surgery (DCO) can provide sufficient débridement of the wound to bridge the gap to a more definitive exposure in the operating room. Fasciotomies can be performed at the bedside.

Conversion to Definitive Fixation

Definitive treatment of long bone fractures with external fixation is associated with high rates of complications including malunion, shortening, nonunion, local and regional pin-related infection, and inhibited range of motion of joints in proximity. The conversion of external fixation to IM nail appears to be relatively safe in the femur. The timing of this event should be as soon as possible but not at the risk of compromising the patient's recovery. The best time is when the inflammatory response has settled and the risk that a second hit will stimulate deterioration is not likely. Since monitoring the inflammatory process through assay of the mediators has not proved useful clinically, most surgeons wait until the inflammatory process has abated, usually 6 to 8 days following the injury.

The patient must have no evidence of SIRS. A recent prospective study showed that MIPs operated on for secondary definitive surgery between days 2 and 4 have a significantly ($P<0.0001$) increased inflammatory response compared with those operated on between days 6 and 8.[58]

Nowotarski et al.[48] reported on 59 patients treated with external fixation and a planned, staged conversion to an IM nail over an 8-year period. The time in the external fixator averaged 7 days. All but four of the femurs were converted in a one-stage procedure. The four patients treated by a staged conversion had evidence of a pin tract infection. The external fixator was removed, and the patient was placed in traction to allow resolution of the pin tract infection. Ninety-seven percent of the fractures healed in 6 months. There was one deep infection. In a small German series, Harwood et al. reported a comparable infection rate in patients treated with conversion of provisional external fixation to an IM nail to those primarily treated with an IM nail.

Damage Control Strategy: Missed Opportunities

Agreement about basic concepts of care needs to be developed among the major players: trauma, neurosurgery, and orthopaedic surgery. Clear communication needs to occur throughout the course of care for a patient. Too often, DCO opportunities are missed as the trauma team crashes the patient to the OR for a lifesaving procedure, then, as an afterthought, notifies the orthopaedic team of multiple suspected fractures as the patient is in transit to the trauma ICU. Débridement and external fixation equipment need to be readily available to the trauma room. Use of a radiolucent table for the emergent care of the trauma patient allows a smooth transition from the trauma team to the orthopaedic team.

Arguments that patients cannot remain in the OR for an additional 20 minutes to allow for the application of an external fixator and débridement of contaminated wounds are difficult to understand. The OR and the trauma ICU should be equal environments, except that more help, including the anesthesia team, is present in the OR.

SUMMARY

Survival with normal cognitive function is the primary objective of the initial care of the MIP. Undoubtedly, early stabilization of long bone fractures and early mobilization of the patient have been associated with a reduction in mortality, ARDS, and pneumonia rates. This does not mean that early fracture fixation techniques must be employed in all patients or that surgery must be accomplished within the first 24 hours. Rigid treatment protocols dictating definitive fracture fixation within 24 hours are not appropriate in the orthopaedic management plans for the severely injured patient. Understanding the concepts of the care for the severely injured patient and attempting to restore physiologic homeostasis as early as possible should be the primary focus of the orthopaedic trauma team.

In place of rigid "time and implant" protocols, general treatment philosophies should be observed and outcome goals for the patient developed. On the basis of the

presence and severity of associated injuries, the resuscitative status of the patient, and the severity of the coagulopathy and pulmonary and head injuries, individualized care plans are tailored for each patient. Investigations have begun to show that the acute monitoring of the byproducts of the inflammatory response and shock, such as lactate, base, and pro-inflammatory cytokines, may help determine the timing of initial and delayed reconstruction fracture care.

In the initial care of the MIP, orthopaedic procedures and eventual musculoskeletal function are of little concern except within the context of the orthopaedic intervention required to enhance the patient's immediate survival potential. The recognition that malunions, nonunions, limb length discrepancies, joint contractures, and chronic infection can be addressed by delayed reconstruction procedures allows the orthopaedic trauma surgeon to focus on the overall immediate needs of the patient and not be distracted by concern over optimal fixation techniques for individual orthopaedic injuries.

REFERENCES

1. Anglen, J.O.; Luber, R.R.E.; Park, T. The effect of femoral nailing on cerebral perfusion pressure in head patients. J Trauma 54:1166–1170, 2003.
2. Auerbach, S.H. The pathophysiology of traumatic brain injury. In Horn, L.J.; Cope, D.N., eds. Physical Medicine and Rehabilitation: State of the Art Reviews. Philadelphia, Hanley and Belfus, 1989, pp. 1–11.
3. Behrman, S.W.; Fabian, T.C.; Kudsk, K.A.; et al. Improved outcome with femur fractures: Early vs. delayed fixation. J Trauma 30:792–798, 1990.
4. Bone, L.B.; Anders, M.J.; Rohrbacher, B.J. Treatment of femoral fractures in the multiply injured patient with thoracic injury. Clin Orthop Relat Res 347:57–61, 1998.
5. Bone, L.B.; Chapman, M.W. Initial management of the patient with multiple injuries. Inst Course Lect 39:557–563, 1990.
6. Bone, L.B.; Johnson, K.D.; Weigelt, J.; et al. Early vs. delayed stabilization of femoral fractures. J Bone Joint Surg Am 71:336–340, 1989.
7. Bone, L.B.; McNamara, K.; Shine, B.; et al. Mortality in multiple trauma patients with fractures. J Trauma 37:262–265, 1994.
8. Bone, R.C.M. Immunologic dissonance: A continuing evolution in our understanding of the systemic inflammatory response syndrome (SIRS) and the multiple organ dysfunction syndrome (MODS). Ann Intern Med 125:680–687, 1996.
9. Bosse, M.J.; Kellam, J.F. Orthopaedic management decisions in the multiple-trauma patient. In Browner, B.D.; Jupiter, J.B.; Levine, A.M.; et al., eds. Skeletal Trauma. Philadelphia, W.B. Saunders, 1998.
10. Bosse, M.J.; MacKenzie, E.J.; Riemer, B.L.; et al. Adult respiratory distress syndrome, pneumonia, and mortality following thoracic injury and a femoral fracture treated either with intramedullary nailing with

reaming or with a plate: A comparative study. J Bone Joint Surg Am 79:799–809, 1997.

11. Boulanger, B.R.; Stephen, D.; Brenneman, F.D. Thoracic trauma and early intramedullary nailing of femur fractures: Are we doing harm? J Trauma 43:24–28, 1997.

12. Brundage, S.I.; McGhan, R.; Jurkovich, G.J.; et al. Timing of femur fracture fixation: Effect on outcome in patients with thoracic and head injuries. J Trauma 52:299–307, 2002.

13. Burgess, A.R. Damage control orthopaedics. J Orthop Trauma 18:S1, 2004.

14. Buttaro, M.; Mocetti, E.; Alfie, V.; et al. Fat embolism and related effects during reamed and unreamed intramedullary nailing in a pig model. J Orthop Trauma 16:239–244, 2002.

15. Carlson, D.W.; Rodman, G.H.; Kaehr, D.; et al. Femur fractures in chest-injured patients: Is reaming contraindicated? J Orthop Trauma 12:164–168, 1998.

16. Charash, W.E.; Fabian, T.C.; Croce, M.A. Delayed surgical fixation of femur fractures is a risk factor for pulmonary failure independent of thoracic trauma. J Trauma 37:667, 1994.

17. Cheadle, W.G.; Hershman, M.J.; Wellhausen, S.R.; et al. Immune Consequences of Trauma, Shock, and Sepsis. Berlin, Springer-Verlag, 1989.

18. Chestnut, R. Secondary brain insults after head injury: Clinical perspectives. New Horizons 3:366–369, 1995.

19. Claridge, J.A.; Crabtree, T.D.; Pelletier, S.J.; et al. Persistent occult hypoperfusion is associated with a significant increase in infection rate and mortality in major trauma patients. J Trauma 48:8–14, 2000.

20. Crowl, A.C.; Young, J.; Kahler, D.; et al. Occult hypoperfusion is associated with increased morbidity in patients undergoing early femur fracture fixation. J Trauma 48:260–267, 2000.

21. Cuthbertson, D.P. The disturbance of metabolism produced by bony and nonbony injury, with notes on certain abnormal conditions of bone. Biochem J 24:1244–1263, 1930.

22. Dunham, C.M.; Bosse, M.J.; Clancy, T.V.; et al. Practice management guidelines for the optimal timing of long-bone fracture stabilization in polytrauma patients: The EAST Practice Management Guidelines Work Group. J Trauma 50:958–967, 2001.

23. Fishman, A.P. Shock lung: A distinctive nonentity. Circulation 47:921–923, 1973.

24. Giannoudis, P.V.; Hildebrand, F.; Page, H.C. Inflammatory serum markers in patients with multiple trauma: Can they predict outcome? J Bone Joint Surg Br 86:313–323, 2004.

25. Giannoudis, P.V.; Smith, R.M.; Banks, R.E.; et al. Stimulation of inflammatory markers after blunt trauma. Br J Surg 85:986–990, 1998.

26. Glenn, J.N.; Miner, M.E.; Peltier, L.F. The treatment of fractures of the femur in patients with head injuries. J Trauma 13:958–961, 1973.

27. Goris, R.J.A.; Gimbrere, J.S.F.; van Niekerk, J.L.M.; et al. Early osteosynthesis and prophylactic mechanical ventilation in the multitrauma patient. J Trauma 22:895–903, 1982.

28. Grotz, M.R.; Giannoudis, P.V.; Pape, H.C.; et al. Traumatic brain injury and stabilisation of long bone fractures: An update. Injury 35:1077–1086, 2004.

29. Handolin, L.; Pajarinen, J.; Lassus, J.; et al. Early intramedullary nailing of lower extremity fracture and respiratory function in polytraumatized patients with a chest injury. Acta Orthop Scand 75:477–480, 2004.

30. Hofman, P.A.M.; Goris, R.J.A. Timing of osteosynthesis of major fractures in patients with severe brain injury. J Trauma 31:261–263, 1991.

31. Holcomb, J.B.; Jenkins, D.; Rhee, P.; et al. Damage control resuscitation: Directly addressing the early coagulopathy of trauma. J Trauma 62:307–310, 2007.

32. Holcroft, J.W.; Robinson, M.K. Shock. In Wilmore, D.W.; Brennan, M.F.; Harken, A.H.; et al. (eds.) Care of the Surgical Patient. New York, Scientific American, Inc., 1995.

33. Insel, J.; Weissman, C.; Kemper, M.; et al. Cardiovascular changes during transport of critically ill and postoperative patients. Crit Care Med 14:539–542, 1986.

34. Jaicks, R.R.; Cohn, S.M.; Moller, B.A. Early fracture fixation may be deleterious after head injury. J Trauma 42:1–6, 1997.

35. Johnson, K.D.; Cadambi, A.; Seibert, G.B. Incidence of adult respiratory distress syndrome in patients with multiple musculoskeletal injuries: Effect of early operative stabilization of fractures. J Trauma 25:375–384, 1985.

36. Kalb, D.C.; Ney, A.L.; Rodriguez, J.L.; et al. Assessment of the relationship between timing of fixation of the fracture and secondary brain injury in patients with multiple trauma. Surgery 124:739–744, 1998.

37. LaDuca, J.; Bone, L.; Seibel, R.; et al. Primary open reduction and internal fixation of open fractures. J Trauma 20:580, 1980.

38. Lehmann, U.; Rucjets, E.; Krettek, C. Multiple trauma with craniocerebral trauma: Early definitive surgical management or long bone fractures. Unfallchirurg 104:196–209, 2001.

39. Lehmann, V.; Reif, W.; Hobbensiefken, G.; et al. Effect of primary fracture management on craniocerebral trauma in polytrauma: An animal experimental study. Unfallchirurg 93:437–441, 1995.

40. McKee, M.D.; Schemitsch, E.H.; Vincent, L.O.; et al. The effect of a femoral fracture on concomitant closed head injury in patients with multiple injuries. J Trauma 42:1041, 1997.

41. McMahon, C.G.; Yates, D.W.; Campbell, F.M.; et al. Unexpected contribution of moderate traumatic brain injury to death after major trauma. J Trauma 47:891–895, 1999.

42. Meek, R.N. The John Border Memorial Lecture: Delaying emergency fracture surgery: Fact or fad. J Orthop Trauma 20:337–340, 2006.

43. Meek, R.N.; Vivoda, E.; Crichton, A. Comparison of mortality in patients with multiple injuries secondary to method of fracture treatment. Injury 17:2–4, 1986.

44. Morris, J.A.; Eddy, V.A.; Blinman, T.A. The staged celiotomy for trauma: Issues in unpacking and reconstruction. Ann Surg 217:576–586, 1993.

45. Mousavi, M.; David, R.; Ehteshami, J.; et al. Pressure changes during reaming with different parameters and reamer designs. Clin Orthop Relat Res 373:295–303, 2000.

46. Mousavi, M.; Kolonja, A.; Schaden, E.; et al. Intracranial pressure-alterations during controlled intramedullary reaming of femoral fractures: An animal study. Injury 32:679–682, 2001.

47. Muller, C.; Baumgart, F.; Wahl, D.; et al. Technical innovations in medullary reaming: Reamer design and intramedullary pressure increase. J Trauma 49:440–445, 2000.

48. Nowotarski, P.J.; Turen, C.H.; Brumback, R.J.; et al. Conversion of external fixation to intramedullary nailing for fractures of the shaft of the femur in multiply injured patients. J Bone Joint Surg Am 82:781–788, 2000.

49. O'Toole, R.V.; O'Brien, M.; Habashi, N.; et al. Resuscitation prior to stabilization of femoral fractures limits ARDS in polytrauma patients despite low utilization of damage control orthopaedics. Paper presented at Annual Meeting of the Orthopaedic Trauma Association, Phoenix, AZ, October 5–7, 2006. Available at: http://www.hwbf.org/ota/am/ota06/ota06cov.htm.

50. Pape, H.C. Immediate fracture fixation: Which method? Comments on the John Border Memorial Lecture, Ottawa, 2005. J Orthop Trauma 20:341–350, 2006.

51. Pape, H.C.; Auf'm'Kolk, M.; Paffrath, T.; et al. Primary intramedullary femur fixation in multiple trauma patients with associated lung contusion: A cause of posttraumatic ARDS? J Trauma 34:540–547, 1993.

52. Pape, H.C.; Dwenger, A.; Grotz, M.; et al. Does the reamer type influence the degree of lung dysfunction after femoral nailing following severe trauma? J Orthop Trauma 8:300–309, 1994.

53. Pape, H.C.; Dwenger, A.; Regel, G.; et al. Pulmonary damage after intramedullary femoral nailing in traumatized sheep: Is there an effect from different nailing methods? J Trauma 33:574–581, 1992.

54. Pape, H.C.; Giannoudis, P.V.; Krettek, C. The timing of fracture treatment in polytrauma patients: Relevance of damage control orthopedic surgery. Am J Surg 183:622–629, 2002.

55. Pape, H.C.; Giannoudis, P.V.; Krettek, C.; et al. Timing of fixation of major fractures in blunt polytrauma: Role of conventional indicators in clinical decision making. J Orthop Trauma 19:551–562, 2005.

56. Pape, H.C.; Grimme, K.; van Griensven, M.; et al. Impact of intramedullary instrumentation versus damage control for femoral fractures on immunoinflammatory parameters: Prospective randomized analysis by the EPOFF Study Group. J Trauma 55:7–19, 2003.

57. Pape, H.C.; Hildebrand, F.; Pertschy, S.; et al. Changes in the management of femoral shaft fractures in polytrauma patients: From early total care to damage control orthopedic surgery. J Trauma 53:452–462, 2002.

58. Pape, H.; Stalp, M.; van Griensven, M.; et al. [Optimal timing for secondary surgery in polytrauma patients: An evaluation of 4,314 serious injury cases.] Chirurg 70:1287–1293, 1999.

59. Pape, H.C.; van Griensven, M.; Rice, J.; et al. Major secondary surgery in blunt trauma patients and perioperative cytokine liberation: Determination of the clinical relevance of biochemical markers. J Trauma 50:989–1000, 2001.

60. Pearce, F.J.; Lyons, W.S. Logistics of parenteral fluids in battlefield resuscitation. Mil Med 164:653–655, 1999.

61. Phillips, T.F.; Soulier, G.; Wilson, R.F. Outcome of massive transfusion exceeding two blood volumes in trauma and emergency surgery. J Trauma 27:903–910, 1987.

62. Poole, G.V.; Miller, J.D.; Agnew, S.G.; et al. Lower extremity fracture fixation in head-injured patients. J Trauma 32:654–659, 1992.

63. Reynolds, M.A.; Richardson, J.D.; Spain, D.A.; et al. Is the timing of fracture fixation important for the patient with multiple trauma? Ann Surg 222:470–481, 1995.

64. Riemer, B.L.; Butterfield, S.L.; Diamond, D.L.; et al. Acute mortality associated with injuries to the pelvic ring: The role of early patient mobilization and external fixation. J Trauma 35:671–677, 1993.

65. Riska, E.R.; von Bonsdorff, H.; Hakkinen, S.; et al. Primary operative fixation of long bone fractures in patients with multiple injuries. J Trauma 17:111–121, 1977.

66. Rixen, D.; Grass, G.; Sauerland, S.; et al. Evaluation of criteria for temporary external fixation in risk-adapted damage control orthopaedic surgery of femur fractures in multiple trauma patients: "Evidence-based medicine" versus "reality" in the Trauma Registry of the German Trauma Society. J Trauma 59:1375–1395, 2005.

67. Roberts, C.; Pape, H.C.; Jones, A.L.; et al. Damage control orthopaedics: Evolving concepts in the treatment of patients who have sustained orthopaedic trauma. J Bone Joint Surg Am 87:434–449, 2005.

68. Rogers, F.B.; Shackford, S.R.; Vane, D.W.; et al. Prompt fixation of isolated femur fractures in a rural trauma center: A study examining the timing of fixation and resource allocation. J Trauma 36:774–777, 1994.

69. Rotondo, M.F.; Schwab, C.W.; McGonigal, M.D. "Damage control": An approach for improved survival in exsanguinating penetrating abdominal injury. J Trauma 35:375–382, 1993.

70. Salmon, J.E.; Edberg, J.C.; Brogle, N.L.; et al. Allelic polymorphisms of human Fc gamma receptor IIA and Fc gamma receptor IIIB: Independent mechanisms for differences in human phagocyte function. J Clin Invest 89:1274–1281, 1992.

71. Sarrafzadeh, A.S.; Peltonen, E.E.; Kaisers, U.; et al. Secondary insults in severe head injury: Do multiply injured patients do worse? Crit Care Clin 29:1116–1123, 2001.

72. Scalea, T.M.; Boswell, S.A.; Scott, J.D.; et al. External fixation as a bridge to intramedullary nailing for patients with multiple injuries and with femur fractures: Damage control orthopaedics. J Trauma 48:613, 2000.

73. Scalea, T.M.; Scott, J.D.; Brumback, R.J.; et al. Early fracture fixation may be "just fine" after head injury: No difference in central nervous system outcomes. J Trauma 45:839–846, 1999.

74. Schemitsch, E.H.; Jain, R.; Turchin, D.C.; et al. Pulmonary effects of fixation of a fracture with a plate compared with intramedullary nailing: A canine model of fat embolism and fracture fixation. J Bone Joint Surg Am 79:984–996, 1997.

75. Schmoker, J.D.; Zhuang, J.; Shackford, S.R. Hemorrhagic hypotension after brain injury causes an early and sustained reduction in cerebral oxygen delivery despite normalization of systemic oxygen delivery. J Trauma 32:714–722, 1992.

76. Schulman, A.M.; Claridge, J.A.; Carr, G.; et al. Predictors of patients who will develop prolonged occult hypoperfusion following blunt trauma. J Trauma 57:795–800, 2004.

77. Smith, R.M.; Giannoudis, P.V. Trauma and the immune response. J R Soc Med 91:417–420, 1998.

78. Starr, A.J.; Hunt, J.L.; Chason, D.P.; et al. Treatment of femur fractures with associated head injury. J Orthop Trauma 12:38–45, 1998.

79. Stein, S.C.; Young, G.S.; Talucci, R.C.; et al. Delayed brain injury after head trauma: Significance of coagulopathy. Neurosurgery 30:160–165, 1992.

80. Taeger, G.; Ruchholtz, S.; Waydhas, C.; et al. Damage control orthopedics in patients with multiple injuries is effective, time saving and safe. J Trauma 59:408–415, 2005.

81. Townsend, R.N.; Lheureau, T.; Protetch, J.; et al. Timing of fracture repair in patients with severe brain injury. J Trauma 44:977–983, 1998.

82. Turchin, D.C.; Schemitsch, E.H.; McKee, M.D.; et al. A comparison of the outcome of patients with pulmonary contusion versus pulmonary contusion and musculoskeletal injuries. Paper presented at AAOS meeting, 2006.

83. Velmahos, G.C.; Arroyo, H.; Ramicone, E.; et al. Timing of fracture fixation in blunt trauma patients with severe head injuries. Am J Surg 176:324–330, 1998.

84. Venkataraman, S.T.; Orr, R.A. Intrahospital transport of critically ill patients. Crit Care Clin 8:525–531, 1992.

85. Wang, M.C.; Temkin, N.R.; Deyo, R.A.; et al. Timing of surgery after multisystem injury with traumatic brain injury: Effect on neuropsychological and functional outcome. J Trauma 62:1250–1258, 2007.

86. White, T.O.; Jenkins, P.J.; Smith, R.D.; et al. The epidemiology of posttraumatic adult respiratory distress syndrome. J Bone Joint Surg Am 86:2366–2376, 2004.

87. Wilmore, D.W.; Brennan, M.F.; Harken, A.H.; et al. Care of the Surgical Patient. New York, Scientific American, Inc., 1995.

88. Wolinsky, P.R.; Banit, D.; Parker, R.E.; et al. Reamed intramedullary femoral nailing after induction of an "ARDS-like" state in sheep: Effect on clinically applicable markers of pulmonary function. J Orthop Trauma 12:169–175, 1998.

89. Wozasek, G.E.; Simon, P.; Redl, H.; et al. Intramedullary pressure changes and fat intravasation during intramedullary nailing: An experimental study in sheep. J Trauma 36:202–207, 1994.

90. Wozasek, G.E.; Thurnher, M.; Redl, H.; et al. Pulmonary reaction during intramedullary fracture management in traumatic shock: An experimental study. J Trauma 37:249–254, 1994.

91. Ziran, B.H.; Le, T.; Zhou, H.; et al. The impact of the quantity of skeletal injury on mortality and pulmonary morbidity. J Trauma 43:916–921, 1997.

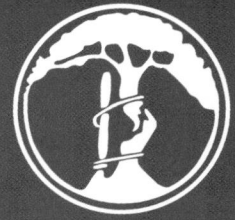

CHAPTER 8

Disaster Management

Christopher T. Born, M.D., F.A.A.O.S., F.A.C.S. and Ryan P. Calfee, M.D.

INTRODUCTION

Disasters are large-scale destructive events that disrupt the infrastructure and normal functioning of a community. Disasters are both natural (e.g., earthquakes, tornadoes, hurricanes) and man-made (e.g., industrial spills, explosions, structural collapse, a terrorist attack). Such an event presents the medical community with a large number of casualties that require rapid triage and treatment that is disproportionate to the available personnel and resources necessary for optimal care.

The increase in geopolitical acts of terrorism has changed civilian health care. Providers are now charged with having familiarity with mass casualty situations and must now understand both the pathophysiology and injury patterns produced by chemical, biologic, radiologic, nuclear, and explosive (CBRNE) devices. Civilian caregivers must learn to deliver care in a mass casualty setting with limited or compromised resources, fulfilling the basic mission of minimizing the population's morbidity and mortality.

True *mass casualty incidents* (MCIs) are rare, providing little opportunity for real-time training. No formal components of medical school or residency prepare physicians for the unique demands and approaches required for the medical care of mass casualties. Thus, most medical care providers have limited training and experience in disaster management. Furthermore, disaster preparations in both community hospitals and even trauma centers are often rudimentary at best.[28,37] However, proper disaster training and planning are nearly universal in their application to actual scenarios. Regardless of the specific event, the elements of an effective disaster response are similar. This allows for an "all-hazards approach" to the development of disaster management principles, which are then easily applied. Well-defined goals of the disaster response and a clearly delineated command structure serve as the basis for efficient and effective recovery from such an event.

DISASTER PLANNING

Effective planning is paramount to a community's ability to cope with any disaster. All hospitals and communities need well-rehearsed strategies for disaster management. It is accepted that nearly half of injured survivors from disasters reach hospitals within the first hour and that health care facilities can expect approximately 75 percent of victims within a 2-hour window. This rapid surge of patients can easily overwhelm hospital staff and resources without prearranged triage algorithms and organizational systems designed for such occurrences.

Disaster plans must have several elements. First, all levels of acute care providers and administrators should be actively involved in their design to ensure that practical aspects from all phases of the medical response to disaster victims are considered. Prehospital providers, emergency room nurses, physicians, surgeons, and anesthesiologists who routinely encounter lesser scale casualty situations add invaluable experience to the process. Once drafted, the plan requires the acceptance and endorsement of all involved to create a well-coordinated approach to an expectedly chaotic situation. Since no disaster can be perfectly predicted because of a large number of variables, disaster plans are designed to be generic and somewhat flexible. Incorporating common requirements, treatment principles, and expected barriers into disaster plans has been termed an "all-hazards" approach. This eliminates the need for numerous individual plan variations that quickly become cumbersome and risk adding confusion and inefficiency into the disaster response. It is appropriate for disaster plans to vary by region and even by community. Hazard vulnerability analysis refers to the formal evaluation of potential disasters with ranking or weighting of scenarios based on their relative probability of occurrence and the severity of impact. Such analysis, while based on both objective historical data and subjective educated projections, provides a basis upon which communities can begin focused disaster planning. Thus, hospitals in California may focus preparations on earthquakes while those in Florida concentrate on the sequelae of hurricanes, since these represent probable and highly significant foreseeable disasters. Plans should be based on injuries and lessons learned from previous disasters. Universal organizational schemes are based on predetermined leadership positions with realistic expectations for each individual. Within communities, trauma centers should provide the template for disaster planning, as they possess both the staff and resources primed to respond to casualties. Finally, disaster plans are only as effective as the ability of those involved to carry out the objectives. To avoid having a false sense of security in a written plan, hospitals must continually educate staff about disaster care and practice regular disaster drills. The plan's execution can then become routine and deficiencies remedied while still in a controlled environment. Ideally, each drill is accompanied by debriefing sessions to give feedback from drill organizers to participants and includes a critical revisiting of the plan by all involved.

DISASTER CLASSIFICATION

Disasters are classified in many ways with each adding to the detailed understanding of the event and its probable impact. This is primarily done by mechanism, with the broad categories of "natural" versus "man-made" events. This division is useful in that each type of disaster will pose unique challenges and produce varied injuries. Natural disasters can be further separated into geophysical events, such as volcanic eruptions, and weather-related events, such as floods. Man-made disasters are subdivided into intentional and accidental catastrophes.

Disasters are also described by the extent and duration of the event. Open and closed are accepted terminology for defining disaster extent. Open disasters are devastating for a large geographic area, such as the widespread flooding of the gulf coast following Hurricane Katrina in 2005. Closed disasters generally occur in easily defined and contained locations, such as the bombing of a federal building in Oklahoma City in 1995. Disaster duration is characterized as being finite or ongoing. Ongoing events do not end abruptly and produce severe prolonged effects and strains from significant disasters. Protracted military conflicts and natural disasters with extensive flooding can be considered ongoing disasters. The loss of infrastructure and increased incidence of postdisaster complications such as disease, starvation, and population displacement characterize ongoing events.

Disaster response, resource consumption, and casualty load are also used to describe mass casualty events. Understanding a disaster's response and resource requirements may help accurately depict the disaster's impact. Classification in this sense has three levels. Level I events require only the use of local resources albeit with some strain on that health care system. These are episodes of multiple casualty events that extend beyond the normal volume of daily trauma. Level II disasters require the mobilization of resources such as regional assets in addition to community efforts. Finally, level III disasters necessitate the allocation of large-scale resources from state to international organizations.

DISASTER MANAGEMENT

Disaster management is broken down into four acknowledged categories: preparedness, response, recovery, and mitigation.[65] Each stage is important in coping with a disaster and in limiting the attendant devastation produced by the event.

Preparedness refers to making a community aware of the circumstances that have the potential for disaster formation (e.g., presence of an aging dam or a nuclear power plant) and empowering it to effectively cope should such an event occur. This includes tasks such as training personnel, purchasing equipment, engaging in interagency planning, and conducting timely mass casualty exercises.[7]

Disaster response encompasses the basic elements of search and rescue, triage and initial stabilization, definitive medical care, and medical evacuation. These essential steps of the medical response must occur simultaneously as the global needs for water, food, shelter, sanitation, security, communication, and disease surveillance are also addressed. The actual disaster response is expected to progress through well-defined phases. Initially chaos predominates, while care providers are disorganized and victims are struck with early panic and fear. The more distant and less responsive the health care resources, the longer this phase continues. Minimizing this phase is critical; anecdotally, experts estimate that every 5 minutes of chaos requires an additional 30 minutes for order to be returned by the Incident Command System (ICS). Chaos is followed by the initial response and organization phase, heralded by the arrival of first responders. To effectively progress, this response requires strong leadership and implementation of an organizational framework. At this time, the scene is assessed, victims are triaged in the field, and security is established. While important for all disasters, the principle of ensuring first responders' safety before rescue efforts commence is especially relevant when facing terrorist attacks. Specifically, it is now acknowledged that terrorist tactics include initial events that precede the main attack and that first responders may be a focus for ambush. In October 2002, a suicide bomber in Bali, Indonesia, detonated a bomb in a busy business district, attracting people to the location from surrounding buildings. This event was then followed by a large, vehicle-based explosion in the street that became more lethal given the assembled crowd. First responders have themselves been targeted, for example, in bombings in Atlanta, Georgia, in 1997 when the bombing of a building was followed by an explosive device detonated 1 hour later in the parking lot as emergency personnel worked. This risk of a "second hit" must be remembered when approaching all terrorist targets. Disaster scenes with unstable buildings represent another source of a "second hit," such as in the New York World Trade Center attacks in 2001 when hundreds of potential rescuers were lost when the towers collapsed. Additionally, in any explosive event, a high index of suspicion for a "dirty bomb" should be maintained.[15] In these blast situations, an assessment of the safety and the exposure risk of rescue personnel along with the risk of contamination of health care workers and hospital facilities must be considered before rescue efforts are initiated.

First responders must be educated about nuclear, biologic, and chemical (NBC) exposure hazards and understand that sequelae of such exposure may not be immediately apparent. Proceeding cautiously and suspecting potential NBC contamination following a blast are critical. Blasts with known biologic or chemical contaminants will require appropriate protective gear for the rescuers to begin the triage efforts.[15] The administration of antidotes may be necessary in some scenarios, but the most appropriate time or place for this to commence (i.e., before or after decontamination/transfer of victims) may be difficult to assess for a given event.[15] Once the scene is deemed safe for responders, site-clearing commences with both the decontamination and physical clearing of the disaster scene as well as the transport of casualties to hospitals. Recovery is the last phase and implies a return of normalcy to the area and reconstitution of the damaged infrastructure. This may be relatively rapid in a confined, finite event or may require significant time following a large natural disaster. This phase marks a transition in the focus of disaster response from crisis management toward one of consequence management. While frequently underemphasized in disaster plans, this phase is essential for the reestablishment of the affected community. During this time, large-scale efforts to permanently replace damaged buildings, revitalize economies, or restore agricultural systems to their full predisaster production capacity are undertaken.[7]

Disaster mitigation refers to the ability to reduce the devastating effects of disasters before the actual event. Tornado warning systems or evacuations prior to hurricanes are two such examples. Mitigation can occur at any point in the disaster cycle.

Barriers to Effective Disaster Response

In any mass casualty incident, a small group of critically injured patients (typically, 5–25% of the live casualties) will be contained within the larger crowd of less severe casualties. This was well demonstrated in the 1995 Oklahoma City bombing, where of 388 victims who went to local hospitals only 72 (18.6%) required admission and 7 (2%) required intubation.[35] The core mission of a hospital disaster response system is to identify these critical casualties and to provide the requisite level of trauma care that may be acceptable under the circumstances. Failure in this task may result in the misappropriation of valuable resources away from those casualties most in need. While this task is quite manageable in daily traumas such as following motor vehicle accidents, mass casualty events add considerable complexity to attaining this goal. A key barrier is any obstacle that threatens this core mission. This includes a lack of warning, inaccessible resources, triage errors, or even a lack of disaster training. Disaster response plans must anticipate these obstacles to achieve success.

The rapid evolution of true mass casualty events poses the first key barrier. Disasters, especially the increasingly prevalent intentional attacks, may provide no warning and little lead time for hospital preparedness. Two corporate bombings in Turkey in 2003 produced 184 casualties for evaluation by a single medical center within the first hour after the incident.[55] This initial surge of patients may also place hospital facilities and personnel at risk for exposure to nuclear, biologic, or chemical toxins. Following the sarin attacks on the Tokyo subway system in March 1995, hospital workers became victims before the toxin was even suspected. This resulted in contaminated hospitals and fewer caregivers available to provide treatment. Even with a well-rehearsed disaster plan, it takes time to organize a facility into an appropriate disaster response mode and to clear physical space for victim management. Once the patient load outpaces the allotment of resources, an exponentially longer amount of time is necessary to restore the balance.

The timing of disasters can also present significant yet variable barriers. For instance, a daytime mass casualty situation may flood hospitals with victims while resources such as operating rooms are in use and therefore are not available for immediate reallocation. Meanwhile, a nighttime MCI may be met by an understaffed response capability until additional assets are made available.

Communications are another consistent source of difficulty during disasters. Whether this equates to cellular phones ceasing to function or emergency lines being inundated with calls, backup plans for communication are critical. This may include dedicated land telephone lines, computer-based systems, or satellite connections. If communication both within and between the response teams (prehospital responders, hospital providers, incident command leaders) fails, then the entire response effort suffers severely. Effective communication also encompasses the relaying of accurate information and proper instruction to the general population through the media. This can reduce panic and the gridlocking of communication and resources of hospitals. Given the requirements of coordination and efficiency in a disaster response, the failure of communications must be prevented.

Another barrier in providing disaster care is human error. Beginning at the scene, first responders will tend to overtriage, and hospital systems will be overburdened with the less severely injured. Once at the hospital, the initial wave of casualties will be treated while there is limited knowledge about the nature of the event. This will cause early errors in resource allocation. Disaster training exercises may help minimize these mistakes.

The overall lack of disaster preparedness by health care professionals poses a most formidable barrier. In any community, the majority of physicians are not involved in disaster training and planning, which will hinder an effective disaster response. This is evidenced by several recent physician surveys. Seventy-two percent (118/166) of nonurban physicians in Texas reported no CBRNE training. This mirrored a national survey in which only 21 percent of physician respondents felt prepared to treat bioterrorism victims.[37] Among trauma surgeons, only 60 percent understood the Incident Command System for disasters, and less than 50 percent of respondents were prepared to manage an exposure to nerve or biologic agents.[14] Even the manual of Advanced Trauma Life Support (ATLS) mentions the basics of blast injury on only a single page.[4] In addition to being unable to provide exposure specific treatments, untrained physicians can impede disaster responses by adding to the number of unnecessary people around intake areas without assigned duties or knowledge of mass casualty triage. Now more than ever, it seems appropriate for all members of the health care community to become versed in the language and principles of disaster management.

Disaster Response Organization— Incident Command System

The effective response to any disaster is predicated on the coordination of many individuals, teams, and organizations. This may require concerted efforts by local agencies and medical specialists or involve added dimensions of resources dedicated from geographically distanced areas. To optimize outcomes and maximize communication and efficiency during disasters, the ICS and the Hospital

Emergency Incident Command System (HEICS) were developed (Fig. 8-1). These systems provide a simple, reproducible, and adaptable organizational hierarchy to manage mass casualty situations.

Since its inception in the 1970s, the ICS concept has become standard practice as an organizational approach to managing temporary situations by safety professions.[25] In 1981, the ICS provided the basis for the National Interagency ICS Management System (NIIMS), which is the structural backbone for emergency responses by U.S. federal agencies.[9,66] This design was declared to be the "best practice" standard in 2004 by the Department of Homeland Security, and currently compliance with the ICS structure is required to receive federal disaster relief.[24]

The ICS structure is built on five major managerial tasks: command, operations, planning, logistics, and finance/administration. These are considered central to managing all disasters, with the size and scope of the situation dictating the number of individuals assigned to complete these tasks. Heading the ICS effort is the Incident Commander (IC). This individual is ultimately responsible for the entirety of the disaster response. As the ranking official, this person defines objectives, oversees all operations, and delegates responsibility. Up to seven officials will report to the Incident Commander.

The safety, public information, and liaison officers are the three officials who constitute the "command staff" and report directly to the Incident Commander. The safety officer is charged with assuring that appropriate protection is provided to first responders. With intentional terrorist activity on the rise, this officer must weigh response efforts with the risk of NBC contamination and

the chances of a "second hit." The public information officer is the reference for updated knowledge to the media and public. The liaison officer is tasked with coordinating responses of the potentially numerous agencies and organizations involved.

"General staff" perform the remaining core aspects of the ICS including operations, planning, logistics, and finance. These areas are referred to as Sections, and the head of each is titled a section chief. The assignment of individuals to these positions and the number of persons within each section depend on the nature and extent of the disaster encountered. In a small-scale event, the Incident Commander may personally oversee these additional activities. However, the modularity built into the ICS becomes important in larger disasters when individual section chiefs can be assigned to each of the above aspects with direct responsibility over teams at their disposal. These chiefs may also report directly to the Incident Commander (see Fig. 8-1).

The planning section chief works in coordination with the IC to develop the designated response. It is this individual's job to conceptualize an effective strategy to approach the given disaster. Most importantly this includes maintaining foresight to anticipate evolving needs and resource depletion. Meanwhile, the logistics section chief must obtain those resources and assets sufficient to perform the planned response. This would include gaining human resources equipment as well as the supplies to ensure a sustainable effort. Operation activities encompass the physical deployment of resources into the field. This includes rescue efforts, securing treatment areas, as well as the delivery of aid. This section chief is therefore responsible for the actual delivery of care directly to the

FIGURE 8-1 *The organizational structure of the Incident Command System (ICS) demonstrates the relationship between the command staff, general staff, and section chiefs. The modular structure allows for the ICS to be expanded or contracted according to the changing needs of a disaster situation. Additional units are added as needed under the direction of each of the section chiefs.*

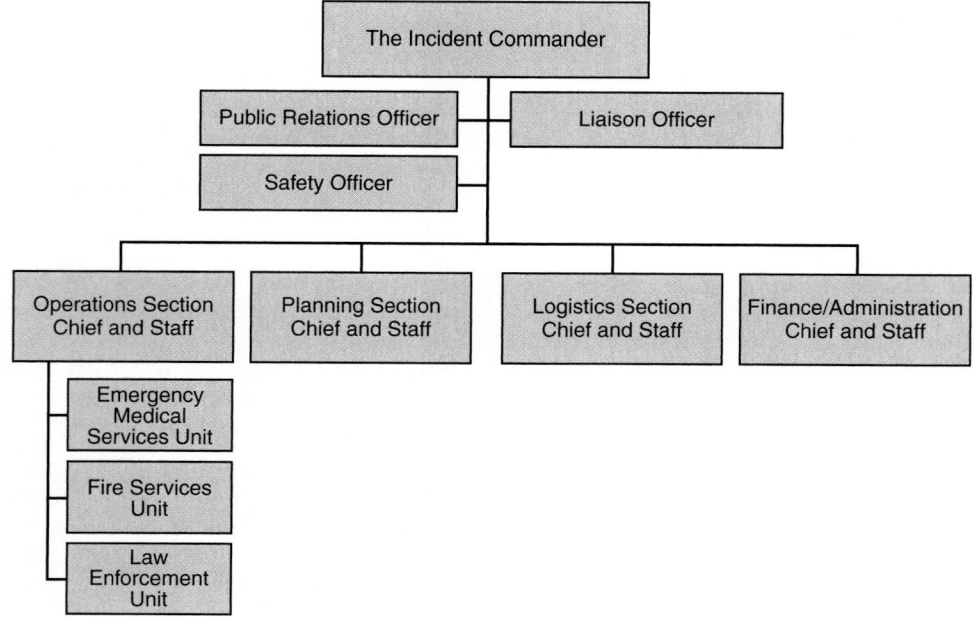

casualties involved. The finance/administrative section chief should record and analyze the monetary cost of the disaster and the ongoing response.

While the ICS is built on well-defined leadership roles as above, the overall function of the ICS depends on several general principles. As predicted, the more rapidly the ICS is established, the quicker an effective response is mounted. To this end, the terminology, titles, and working procedures are standardized to function in any mass casualty situation. Furthermore, while the specifics of each disaster may dictate the size of the ICS and the expertise of those in charge, the overlying structure of the ICS is constant. The flexibility of the ICS is in its modularity, which permits expansion and contraction of the incident command structure as needed. The key concept dictating this fluctuating size of the ICS is one of a "manageable span of control." This equates to no one person supervising more than 3 to 7 individuals to maintain the ability to effectively manage responsibility. An additional mechanism for the ICS to expand when confronted with a devastating event that will involve significant interagency efforts is to add a Unified Command (UC). The Unified Command would be composed of Incident Commanders from the primary organizations involved and allow them to coordinate efforts from a central location termed the Emergency Operations Center (EOC). This UC attempts to restore efficiency to situations where jurisdictional or functional roles of agencies overlap. Finally, all individuals involved in the response must perform within this structure. Efforts outside the ICS detract from the overall coordination of efforts and the efficient utilization of resources.

The ICS structure has also been adapted to provide a mode of operations for hospitals facing disasters. The Hospital Incident Command System (HICS) was originally presented in 1991.[56] This system follows the ICS hierarchy, principles, and structure. Ideally, this same type of organization and distributed responsibility provides the hospital with an effective paradigm to provide organized care to casualties. The only alteration to the ICS structure in the hospital is to modify operation sections into appropriate divisions such as surgical, medical, intensive, and ambulatory care services. Again, the adaptable nature of this system allows for expansion of those areas most needed while preserving the universal titles and terminology to allow for easy communication with other facilities and with those involved with other phases of the disaster response such as those transporting casualties to the care facilities.

ACCIDENTAL AND MAN-MADE DISASTERS

Although both natural and man-made disasters produce significant morbidity and mortality, most of the detailed literature on specific injury mechanisms in mass casualty situations focuses on man-made disasters. In this age of geopolitical instability, much emphasis has been placed on the potential effects of NBC agents. The fact is that blast injury accounts for the preponderance of mass casualty incidents (Fig. 8-2). Despite this, there is significantly less awareness among physicians of how to manage blast-related injuries. In a 2004 survey of the members of the Eastern Association for the Surgery of Trauma (EAST), only 73 percent of the trauma surgeons queried understood the classification and pathophysiology of blast injuries.[14] With explosive munitions becoming an increasingly common form of civilian attack, it is critical that physicians possess basic knowledge of blast injuries and NBC agents.

Nuclear and Radiologic Events

Nuclear or radiologic material may be dispersed by a detonation of a nuclear device, sabotage or meltdown of a nuclear reactor, explosion of a "dirty bomb," or a nonexplosive release of radioactive material in a public place. In approaching ionizing radiation exposure, the critical variables are time, distance, and shielding. In these situations,

---

FIGURE 8-2 *Injuries and fatalities from terrorist incidents, 1998–2005. Data from the RAND-MIPT Terrorism Incident Database show that bomb blast injuries account for 82% of all injuries caused by terrorists. (Available at: http://www.tkb.org/incidenttacticmodule.jsp.)*

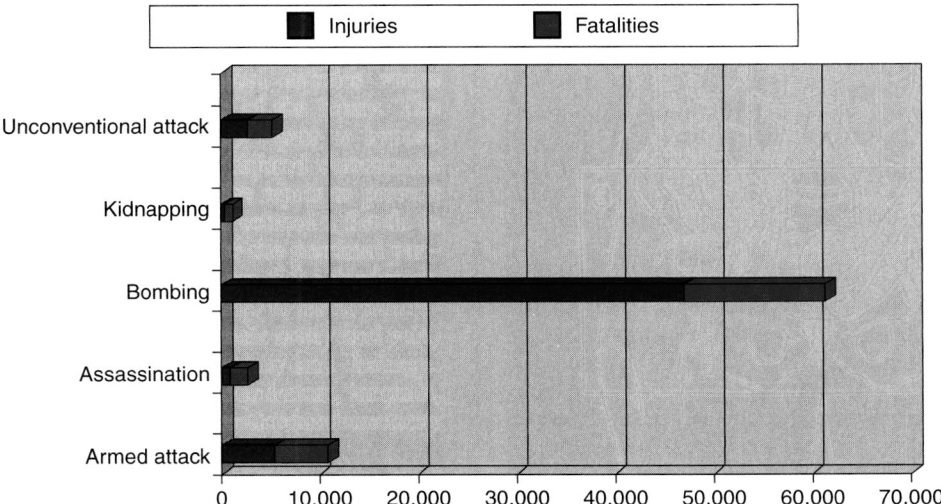

irradiated casualties are not radioactive themselves. Therefore, emergency trauma care may commence with life- and limb-threatening injuries being addressed without delay for radiologic decontamination. Eighty-five to ninety percent of external radiologic contamination is easily removed simply by removal of clothing.[22] Skin forms a useful protective barrier and any decontamination technique that could traumatize the skin should be avoided. However, if open wounds are contaminated, routine débridement and delayed closure is the rule. Radioactive debris should always be removed with instruments, and the surgery may be facilitated by the use of personal dosimeters.[60] Once radiation exposure has been verified, the radionuclides involved, amounts, and physical forms must be determined.

Time to onset of systemic symptoms is the most important factor in determining whether significant radiation exposure has taken place. Initial symptoms include nausea, vomiting, diarrhea, skin tingling, and central nervous system (CNS) signs. If there are injuries requiring surgery, the procedures are best performed in the initial 48 hours, before exposure-induced bone marrow suppression occurs. If victims remain asymptomatic for 24 hours and show no aberration in complete blood count (CBC), particularly the lymphocyte count, the patient can be safely discharged.[21]

Biological Events

One of the greatest challenges of biological terrorism is the timely identification of its use. As opposed to the overt nature of explosives, biologic weaponry can be deployed covertly without immediate effects to those exposed. Instead, identification may require syndromic surveillance using local/regional health data to identify an outbreak. With the help of the Centers for Disease Control (CDC), state and local organizations must collaborate to minimize the time needed for the detection and identification of the pathogen. Rapid biological event recognition is critical to prevent the secondary exposure of the population at large. Monitored system-level activities include school absenteeism, 911 calls, trends in sales of over-the-counter pharmaceuticals, and voluntary reporting by medical groups of apparent trends of illnesses.

The CDC has divided biological threats into groups A, B, and C. The categories are based on the ease of disease transmission, potential mortality and societal health impact, potential for inducing panic and social disruption, and the need for a specialized health response.[19] Category A sample of pathogens with the highest potential for being weaponized are listed in Table 8-1.[2,19,24,26,31,36,39,48]

Chemical Events

The use of sarin in the Tokyo subway in 1995 demonstrates the potential impact of a chemical attack. The attack, which resulted in the exposure of a number of health care providers to the neurotoxin, reinforces the importance of hospitals taking aggressive measures to preserve and protect their health care facility and resources. The most commonly used chemical agents have traditionally been pulmonary toxins with popularity among terrorists owing to their ready availability, ease of dispersal, significant clinical effects, and proven ability to disrupt and contaminate initial caregivers.

Chemical agents are categorized by their physiologic effects. The five general classes of chemical agents are nerve, blood, pulmonary, blistering (vesicants), and riot control agents. Table 8-2 summarizes the toxicity, mechanisms, clinical signs, and exposure management of common agents.[33,42,51,54,57,64]

Blast Events

Bomb detonation is the rapid chemical transformation of a solid or liquid into a gas. The gas expands radially outward as a high-pressure blast wave that exceeds the speed of sound. Air is highly compressed on the leading edge of the blast wave, creating a shock front. The body of the wave and the associated mass outward movement of ambient air (the "blast wind") follow this front (Fig. 8-3).

Under ideal conditions in an open area, the "overpressure" that results from an explosion generally follows a well-defined pressure-time curve ("Friedlander wave"). There is an initial, near-instantaneous spike in the ambient air pressure followed by a longer period of subatmospheric pressure (Fig. 8-4). The pressure-time curves are variable depending on the local topography, presence of walls/solid objects, and whether the blast is detonated indoors or outside. The blast wave can reflect off of and flow around solid surfaces. These reflected waves can be magnified by eight to nine times, causing significantly greater injury.[38,50] Blasts that occur within buildings, vehicles, or other confined spaces are more devastating and lethal because of this increased energy and slower dissipation of the complex and reflected waves.[44] The distance from the explosion's epicenter also is important, as the pressure wave decays roughly proportionally to the inverse cube of the distance.[38,67]

The velocity, duration, and magnitude of the blast wave's overpressure are dependent on several factors. These include the physical size as well as the component explosive of the charge being detonated. High-energy (HE) explosives such as TNT and nitroglycerin are much more powerful than lower order explosives such as gunpowder. However, lower energy explosives can produce conflagrations with a higher thermal output that cause severe burns. HE explosives tend to cause only superficial flash burns on exposed skin[38] (Table 8-3).

Blast wave propagation varies with the medium through which it moves. The increased density of water allows for faster propagation and a longer duration of positive pressure. Therefore, immersion blast injuries are typically more severe. Following in-water detonation, shock waves are also reflected backward off the water-air interface at the surface and admix with the incident blast wave. The resultant overpressures are greater at the 2-foot depth and cause greater injury to the lower areas of the lung and to the abdomen in the partially submerged victim who is treading water in the vertical position. A high index of suspicion should be maintained for delayed presentations of bowel injury in those injured by underwater blasts.[30]

BLAST INJURY PATHOPHYSIOLOGY

Classically, the mechanisms of injury from blast have been classified as primary, secondary, and tertiary. Quaternary, or miscellaneous, forms of injury indirectly related to the blast are now also recognized.

Table 8-1
Potential Agents of Biological Terrorism

Agent	Route of Infection	Clinical Signs and Symptoms	Management of Exposure and Treatment
Anthrax *Bacillus anthracis*	1. Inhalation of spores, most likely in a bioterrorism incident 2. Cutaneous 3. Gastrointestinal	1. Fever, flu-like symptoms, chest discomfort in 2–42 days, severe respiratory distress 2–3 days later, death 24–36 hours later; >50% mortality. 2. Black scab, dermal and lymph node involvement. 3. Nausea, vomiting; abdominal pain progresses to bloody diarrhea and sepsis.	Airborne precautions, decontamination of surfaces. Wash exposed skin. Penicillin. Centers for Disease Control and Prevention (CDC) recommends initial therapy with doxycycline or ciprofloxacin.
Botulism *Clostridium botulinum*	Food-borne illness and wound infection 1 g botulinum toxin will kill 1 million people	Symptoms begin to show in 6–7 days from impaired acetylcholine release resulting in cranial nerve deficits, descending skeletal musculature weakness, and paralysis.	Standard precautions. Ventilator support for weeks or months until patient clinically improves. Trivalent equine antitoxin is available from CDC.
Viral hemorrhagic fevers RNA viruses	Highly infectious by aerosol route from animal bites, excrement, insect vectors, and from human to human	Fever, myalgias, prostration within 4–21 days, progressing to systemic inflammatory response, petechiae, bleeding, subsequent shock, and death; >50% mortality.	Airborne and body fluids precautions. Negative pressure rooms. Treatment is supportive. No specific therapy.
Plague *Yersinia pestis*	Bubonic plague spread from fleas on rodents to humans Pneumonic plague spread by aerosol route from human to human	Bubonic plague, local inflammatory response at flea bite, swollen lymph nodes (buboes) in 1–3 days; if untreated can progress to pneumonic plague. Pneumonic plague, cough, fever, watery sputum, bronchopneumonia. If untreated, 100% mortality.	Airborne and body fluids precautions. Treatment is supportive. Antibiotics: streptomycin, combinations of gentamicin and chloramphenicol or doxycycline and fluoroquinolone. Vaccine for bubonic plague.
Smallpox Variola virus	Highly infectious by aerosol route from human to human	Fever, rigors, headache, back pain, malaise in 7–17 days. Vesicular and pustular rash leads to scabs and pitted scars. Death occurs as a result of toxemia from viral infection.	Smallpox vaccination in first week following exposure. Immediate vaccination for caregivers. Treatment is supportive.
Tularemia *Francisella tularensis*	Human infection from ticks, deerfly bites, contaminated animal products Inhalation from infectious aerosols	Ulceroglandular tularemia, fever, chills, headache, malaise, skin ulceration, painful adenopathy. Typhoidal tularemia and pneumonic tularemia result from inhalation. Symptoms include nonproductive cough and pneumonia.	Standard precautions. Antibiotic: gentamicin.

PRIMARY BLAST INJURY Primary blast injury (PBI) results from the high-pressure shock front and associated blast wave. Blast waves propagate through the body as stress, shock, and shear waves.[16] Stress waves are similar in speed to sound waves but have higher amplitude. Shock waves have a higher pressure and amplitude than sound waves. Shear waves are lower in velocity and longer in duration and travel in a transverse direction, producing gross distortions of tissue and organs. PBI occurs as the shock front and blast wave move through the body. The severity of injury depends on the overpressure to the bodily organs (Table 8-4). Density differences in the body's anatomic components (particularly at gas-fluid interfaces) render those components susceptible to spalling, implosion, inertial mismatches and pressure differentials. Spalling describes the forcible, explosive movement of fluid from more dense to less dense tissues such as in the lungs. Implosion relates to areas of gas that are rapidly compressed at the time of shock front impact and then rapidly reexpand after it passes, causing rebound expansion with attendant shearing and injury. Acceleration/deceleration can cause tearing of organ pedicles and mesentery when there is an inertial difference between organ structures.

The most susceptible organs to PBI are the ears, lungs, and gastrointestinal tract. The ears are the most sensitive organs to blast injury, and tympanic membrane rupture can be used as a marker of exposure to significant overpressure.[12,52] Tympanic injury may occur preferentially based on the orientation of the ear relative to the blast.

	Table 8-2		
Potential Agents of Chemical Terrorism			
Agent	**Toxicity and Mechanism**	**Clinical Signs and Symptoms**	**Management of Exposure and Treatment**

Nerve agents
  GA (sarin)
  GV (soman)
  GD (cyclosarin)
  GS
  VX
	Organophosphates
	Fatal at 1–10 mL (GA, GV, GD) or 1 drop of VX on skin
	Blocks acetylcholine esterase
		Cholinergic crisis: salivation, lacrimation, urination, diaphoresis, GI distress, emesis
		Bronchorrhea: excessive airway secretions
		Brochoconstriction causing respiratory distress
		Death from paralysis of diaphragm and respiratory muscles, essential apnea
			Decontamination
			Respiratory support
			Antidotes:
			Atropine—anticholinergic
			Oxime—2-PAM-Cl reactivates acetylcholine esterase
			Diazepam—anticonvulsant

Blood agents
  Hydrogen cyanide
  Cyanogen chloride
	Absorption
	  Inhalation (most toxic)
	  Ingestion
	  Percutaneous
	Concentration dependent
	Combines with iron to inhibit cytochrome oxidase pathway
		Dyspnea, tachypnea, hypertension, tachycardia, flushing (cherry red skin), vomiting, confusion, agitation, cardiac palpitation, bitter almond odor on victim
		Progress to arrhythmias, respiratory failure
		Death from inhalation within 6–8 minutes from respiratory arrest
			Remove from exposure
			Antidotes:
			Inhalation of crushed pearl of amyl nitrite (in the field)
			Sodium nitrate (intravenous)

Pulmonary agents Chlorine Phosgene	Chlorine: irritating, pungent yellow-green gas, caustic, reacts with water to form hypochlorite and hydrochloric acid Phosgene: odor of fresh-cut hay. Less soluble in water, reacts over time in distal respiratory tree.	Chlorine: cutaneous burning, ocular injury, respiratory irritation Pulmonary edema, hypoxemia, respiratory failure may result Phosgene: minor upper respiratory irritation, over time severe pulmonary edema and respiratory failure	Chlorine: remove from exposure, respiratory support, no antidote Phosgene: monitor at least 12–24 hours, management is expectant

Blistering agents / vesicants
  Mustard agents
  Lewisite
	Mustard agents: oily, garlic-onion odor
	Both: exposure dependent
	Both cutaneous, ocular, respiratory damage
	Lewisite: vapor/liquid, geranium odor
	Lewisite: increased tissue permeability, hypovolemic shock, organ damage
		Both: skin erythema, vesicles, ocular burning, respiratory eruption, potential bronchial damage, necrosis, hemorrhage
		If prolonged, pancytopenia, inability to fight infection, death from respiratory failure
		Lewisite: immediate pain, prone to tissue necrosis, sloughing, airway obstruction
			Remove from exposure
			Decontamination
			Respiratory management
			Débride cutaneous lesions
			Lewisite: British anti-lewisite skin, ophthalmic ointments

Riot control agents	Lacrimators ("tear gas"), irritants, vomiting agents	Lacrimation, sneezing, rapid heart rate, respiratory insufficiency	Supportive, self-limiting, resolving within 15 minutes

With enough energy exposure, severe pulmonary barotrauma can occur with disruption of the capillary-alveolar interface. Low-velocity stress waves may be the primary source of lung injury as they are reinforced by reflection off of the mediastinum. The ensuing complex pressure environment within the lung parenchyma promotes disruption of the alveolar/capillary membrane with the leakage of blood and interstitial fluid.[16,20] Emphysematous spaces can be created in addition to pneumothorax. The interstitial changes of blast lung can lead to adult respiratory distress syndrome (ARDS). Blast lung remains a common cause of fatality among initial survivors of the detonation.[20] In rare cases, air embolism of the vascular tree is thought to be the cause of sudden death.[18,49] Primary blast lung injury does not appear to stem from direct compression of the thorax but rather from coupling of the shock front into the lung tissue.[17]

As a gas-filled organ, the gastrointestinal tract is highly susceptible to primary blast effect. Injury to the mucosa may range from bruising and petechiae to frank hemorrhage and mesenteric shear injury caused by acceleration/deceleration. Solid organ laceration or rupture of the liver, spleen, and kidney in addition to late bowel perforation can also occur.[20] In the large bowel, shearing rather than stress wave propagation may be the primary mechanism of injury, since the large bowel is not able to dislocate to the same degree as the small intestine.

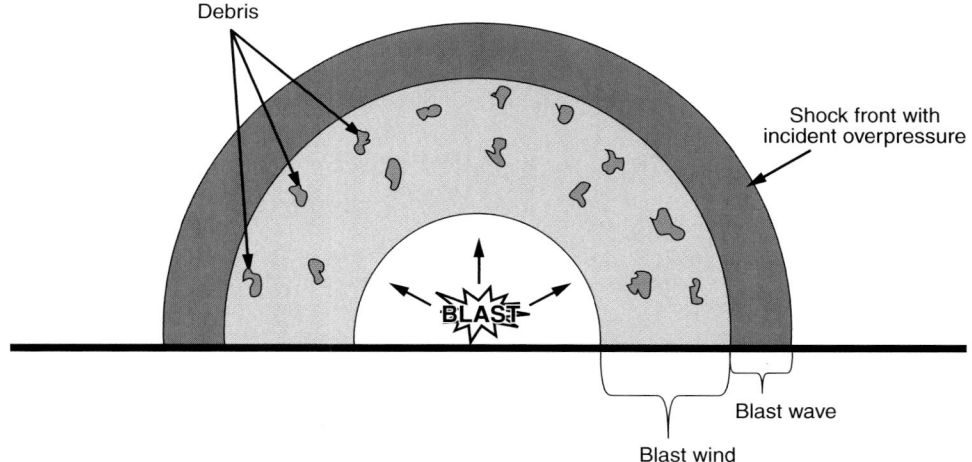

FIGURE 8-3 *Diagram of a blast wave and associated components. (Adapted from Hull, J.B. Blast: Injury patterns and their recording. J Audiov Media Med 1992;15:121–127.)*

Other organ systems (musculoskeletal, ocular, and cardio-circulatory) have varying degrees of response to injury from primary blast.[38,40] There also is evidence that blast can lead to primary CNS injury. A variety of irregular brain wave activities may be noted by electroencephalography, including hypersynchronous, discontinuous, or irregular brain activity with increased theta activity consistent with cortical dysfunction within the first 3 days. With the variety of effects on the CNS, there may be long-term changes that manifest as post-traumatic stress disorder (PTSD) and so the term shell-shocked may have a physiologic basis.[62]

Traumatic amputations from PBI are uncommon and are often considered a marker for a lethal injury. Blast-induced amputations primarily occur through the shaft rather than as disarticulations. There is evidence to suggest that these are the result of direct coupling of the blast wave into the tissues. Fracture results from axial stress to the long bone. Flailing of the extremity from the blast wind gas flow completes the amputation.[30,38]

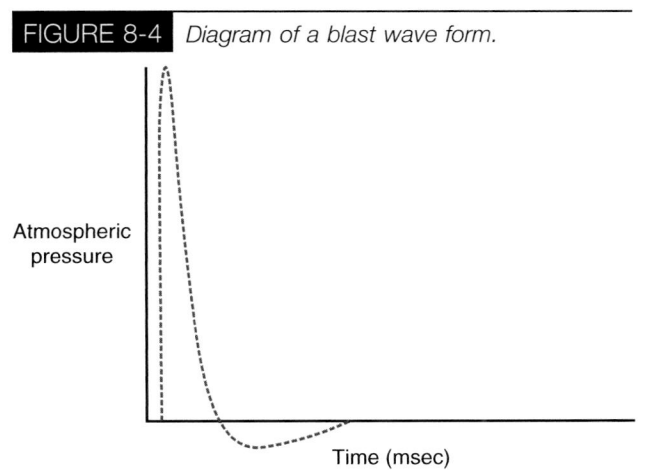

FIGURE 8-4 *Diagram of a blast wave form.*

SECONDARY BLAST INJURY Secondary blast injury results from missiles propagated by the explosion. *Primary fragmentation* can be part of the bomb casing itself or objects intentionally imbedded into the explosive such as nails, screws, or bolts designed to inflict further wounding. Nearby objects made airborne by proximity to the explosion can become projectiles (*secondary fragmentation*). Injury from glass is the most common.

TERTIARY AND QUATERNARY BLAST INJURY

Tertiary blast injury stems from the victim's body being thrown as a projectile by the blast. This can result in fractures, head trauma, and other blunt injury typically seen in the survivor population. Secondary and tertiary blast injuries are the most common wounding mechanisms seen in survivors of explosive events.[30]

Quaternary blast injury represents miscellaneous blast-related injuries. These include those from structural collapse or burn secondary to the detonation. Crush, traumatic amputation, compartment syndromes, and other blunt and penetrating injuries are common sequelae of structural collapse related to the blast. Secondary fires can cause additional burns as well as smoke and dust inhalation. Victims may also be exposed to irradiation as well as toxic gas and other chemical and biologic pathogens by a "dirty bomb."

MEDICAL MANAGEMENT OF DISASTER CASUALTIES

Triage—Concept and Principles

Triage is the prioritization of patients according to injury severity and the need for immediate care. This is a familiar concept but is not often practiced given the abundance of health care resources. Triage becomes vitally important in the face of a true mass casualty event. Triage is effective only to the extent that the triage officer has a firm understanding of the nature of the injuries likely to be seen (i.e., bodily injury; biological, chemical,

Table 8-3
Explosive Types

High-energy Explosive	Low-energy Explosive
TNT	Pipe bomb
C-4	Gun powder
Semtex	Pure petroleum-based bomb
Nitroglycerine	"Molotov cocktail"
Dynamite	
Ammonium nitrate fuel oil (ANFO)	

radiation injury), as well as comprehensive training in the unique principles of mass casualty management with limited resources. It is this knowledge base and background that determine the proper triage officer rather than a particular title. Surgeons, emergency medicine physicians, nurses, prehospital personnel, and other acute care providers all can potentially learn the skills to function in such a role. Each may possess a skill set ideal for evaluating victims of a particular disaster.

There are four widely accepted triage categories for casualties: (1) *immediate*, or the most severely injured who require urgent, lifesaving treatment; (2) *delayed*, or those who are not in immediate need of treatment, including the walking wounded; (3) *expectant*, those whose extensive injuries would require time and significant resource utilization and where elevated care requirements would jeopardize the lives of many more salvageable casualties; and (4) *dead*. It is the approach to the expectant category that differs most markedly from that of routine medical care in developed countries. These victims, while potentially salvageable, may not receive care in the interest of applying the limited resources to an entire group of more salvageable casualties, thereby ensuring maximum preservation of lives. This runs counter to the usual civilian

Table 8-4
Victim Groups According to Blast Loading

Group	Overpressure (kPa)	Blast Loading
1	<150	Minor: maximum overpressure sustained sufficient to cause ruptured tympanic membrane
2	150–350	Moderate: higher overpressure than group 1, but probably insufficient to cause primary lung damage in a significant number of casualties
3	350–550	Severe: sufficient overpressure to cause primary lung damage in a significant proportion of casualties
4	>550	Very severe: sufficient overpressure to cause severe primary lung damage with a significant incidence of death

Source: Mellor, S.G.; Cooper, G.J. Analysis of 828 servicemen killed or injured by explosion in Northern Ireland 1970–1984: The hostile action casualty system, Br J Surg 1989;76:1006–1010.

emergency care paradigm in which the most severely injured survivors would be selected early for immediate and exhaustive care. The definition of an expectant injury will differ with each event and should be determined early in the course of casualty management according to the victim load and anticipated resources available. Once casualty influx has ceased, these expectant casualties can be reassessed in the light of remaining resources and possibly cared for at that time.[59,61]

THE CHALLENGE OF INDIVIDUAL TRIAGE

In a mass casualty incident, triage decisions must be made rapidly and aim to deliver the greatest good for the greatest number. The patterns and severity of injury produced by previous disasters serve as reference for future mass casualty events. Terrorist bombings are by far the most commonly documented mass casualty events and serve as a useful model for the practice of triage. The immediate death rate tends to be quite high, ranging from 50 to 99 percent. Critical injuries occur in only 5 to 25 percent of survivors, but late deaths among survivors generally occur in this severely injured group. The most commonly injured body systems in survivors of bombings are soft tissue and musculoskeletal, most of which are not critical and not life threatening. Most deaths among initial survivors are secondary to head, abdomen, and chest trauma. Nineteen percent of all survivors with abdominal trauma, 14 percent of all survivors with chest trauma, and 10 percent of all survivors with traumatic amputation or blast lung injury ultimately die, representing the body system injuries with the highest specific mortality rates among survivors. However, these body system injuries are found in only a small (2–5%) percentage of all survivors because most victims with these injuries die immediately.[29] The minority of survivors with these injuries must be recognized early as having a high risk of death and be urgently attended. They often require prolonged intensive care unit (ICU) stays and significant resource utilization.

Efforts are ongoing to develop methods to improve the accuracy of field triage and optimize health care resource utilization following mass casualty disasters caused by explosions. Studies of soldiers in Iraq have demonstrated that the presence of two or more variables (sustained hypotension, three or more long bone fractures, penetrating head injury, and other fatalities sustained in the blast) is associated with increased mortality (86% vs. 20% for a single marker alone, $P=0.015$).[53] Similarly, in 798 victims of bombings in Israel, significant associations ($P<0.001$) with the development of blast lung were found between penetrating wounds to the head or torso, burns greater than 10 percent of the body surface area, and skull fractures.[3] Victims in fully confined spaces such as buses were also more likely to suffer blast lung effects. These findings are important because they provide rapid ways to identify patients who will likely require more intensive monitoring and resuscitative efforts even before the clinical manifestations of pulmonary compromise are apparent.

GLOBAL TRIAGE ACCURACY

The accuracy of triage has a major impact on casualty outcome. *Undertriage* is the assignment of critically injured casualties needing immediate care to a delayed category.

This leads to unnecessary deaths. It can be avoided by the proper training of triage officers to recognize life-threatening problems requiring urgent treatment. *Overtriage* is the assignment to immediate care, hospitalization, or evacuation of those casualties that are not critically injured, thus potentially displacing critically injured victims from necessary immediate care. In the routine practice of medicine, only errors in undertriage risks patients' well-being, so that overtriage (or erring on transporting seemingly less injured patients to hospitals to prevent missing a critical injury) is fully accepted.[13] However, in a true mass casualty disaster, overtriage is as life threatening as undertriage. The inundation by large numbers of noncritically injured patients into a system of scarce medical resources may prevent the timely detection of that small minority who need immediate care. To quantify this notion, computer modeling of a 700-bed Level 1 trauma center (Ben Taub General Hospital) was challenged with the profiles of 223 urban bombing victims.[34] The analysis suggests that the global level of care suffers as the critical casualty load increases. There is a point at which the facility becomes less efficient and less able to provide care as patients continue to pile up. *Surge capacity* refers to the ability of a facility to rapidly expand its patient load capacity in response to a major public health crisis and overwhelming number of patients. For this model, a surge capacity of 4.6 critical care patients per hour using present resources was decreased to 3.8 and 2.7 patients per hour when overtriage rates of 50 percent and 75 percent were trialed. Avoidance of this situation requires extensive training of triage officers. Triage accuracy—the minimizing of both undertriage and overtriage—is thus a major prognostic factor in the medical management of all disasters.[28,29]

The *critical mortality rate* is the death rate among initial survivors expressed as a percentage of the total number of *critically injured* survivors, rather than being based on the total number of survivors, most of whom are not at risk of death.[28] The medical management of a disaster and the success of triage are best assessed by looking at critical, rather than overall, mortality, and this also allows the most accurate comparison of medical outcomes between different disasters. An analysis of 1880 survivors of 10 terrorist bombing incidents treated at one institution, from which critical injuries, overtriage, and critical mortality rates could be derived, reveals the direct correlation of overtriage with the critical mortality rate in major bombing disasters (Fig. 8-5). This confirms that overtriage as much as undertriage must be minimized in this setting to maximize the salvage of surviving casualties.[28]

Decontamination

During any mass casualty event that releases dangerous chemicals, biologic agents, or radioactivity, planning for decontamination becomes critically important. Decontamination refers to physically removing particulate, liquid, or vapor contamination from victims. This halts ongoing injury to the casualty and prevents exposure to other victims, responders, or the surrounding environment.

The concept of zones within such a casualty situation defines gradations in safety for victims and rescuers.[7] The most dangerous is the "hot zone," that area within the range of immediate danger. This area may contain unstable buildings or be in immediate proximity to the release site of hazardous materials. Efforts are focused in the hot zone on the rapid evacuation of victims before medical interventions are initiated. Responders need to have the highest level of appropriate personal protective equipment and to spend only the necessary amount of time within the hot zone. Traditionally, HAZMAT (hazardous materials) personnel have been the responders trained to operate within the hot zone. However, EMS personnel are increasingly being trained and equipped to perform medically complicated extractions within this dangerous environment. The "warm zone," while posing some risk, is sufficiently removed from the scene to allow for lifesaving procedures. Generally, a reduced amount of personal protective equipment is required. To date, medical professionals such as orthopaedic surgeons have not delivered care within hot or warm zones. The "cold zone" does not pose a direct threat and is considered appropriate for providing basic medical care.

Four levels of personal protective equipment are defined by the Occupational Safety and Health Administration (OSHA).[1] Level A, while being the most protective, is bulky and permits only gross motor function when in use. It includes a disposable, full-body suit, completely impervious, with a self-contained positive-pressure breathing system. This type of equipment is employed for facing unidentified or highly concentrated hazardous substances. Level B gear provides respiratory protection but less surface protection with a liquid-resistant body suit. Dexterity is still limited. Level A and B gear is generally restricted to HAZMAT personnel. Level C equipment provides a respirator with the appropriate filters but not a self-contained or externally supplied oxygen source. This gear is much more functional and is appropriate for most warm zone

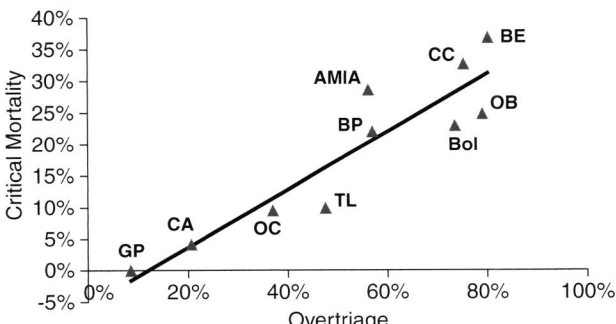

FIGURE 8-5 *Graphic relationship between overtriage rate and critical mortality rate in 10 major terrorist bombing incidents. Linear correlation coefficient (r) = 0.92. Abbreviations: GP, Guildford pubs; CA, Craigavon; OC, Oklahoma City; TL, Tower of London; BP, Birmingham pubs; Bol, Bologna; AMIA, Buenos Aires; OB, Old Bailey; CC, Cu Chi; BE, Beirut. (Reprinted with permission from Frykberg, E.R. Medical management of disasters and mass casualties from terrorist bombings: How can we cope? J Trauma 2002;53:201–212.)*

decontamination sites. Level D protective equipment is acceptable when there is little to no potential for inhalation or skin contact with hazardous concentrations of chemicals. Compliance with universal precautions during patient care is not compromised by Level D equipment.

Decontamination is usually performed in the warm zone after disasters. Ideally, this should be situated uphill and upwind from the hot zone and distanced by at least 300 yards. Contaminated clothing is removed, and victims are moved in one direction to the cold zone, where further medical treatment and evacuation decisions are made. Although removing clothing will eliminate a large percentage of contaminants, any additional visible material is also atraumatically removed from the skin.[64] Copious showering with water further dilutes any toxic residue. Since rapid and efficient decontamination is key, use of simple water, free of additives, is preferred at this stage. Showering should be performed at a minimum of 60 psi, which is within the standard range for household shower pressure. Concerns about hypothermia, the specific contaminants present, the number of victims, the amount of water available, and the number of decontamination stations affect the duration of showering.

Evacuation

The objectives of evacuation are to decompress the disaster area, to improve care for the most critical casualties, and to provide specialized care to specific casualties, such as those with burns and crush injuries. "Decompressing" the disaster scene means that critically ill casualties who are consuming the most resources (supplies, casualty care space, caregiver attention) are moved to relatively resource-rich areas. Evacuation of seriously injured casualties to off-site medical facilities not only improves their care but also allows increased attention to the remaining casualties.[7,32,45]

In planning the transportation of victims, consideration should be given to the surrounding medical facilities and their respective assets. The most common tendency is to deliver a preponderance of casualties to the geographically nearest hospital. This overburdens that single facility and may force providers to ration medical care at a time when other local hospitals' resources are being underutilized. To minimize this mismanagement and its associated potential morbidity and mortality, some recommend utilizing the nearest hospital as a triage center. This would still allow for rapid evacuation of casualties from the scene but charges the nearest hospital with distributing survivors needing significant care to surrounding facilities. Conversely, extremely well organized prehospital efforts can be made to transport equitable numbers of casualties to accepting institutions.

The primary modes of evacuation are ground, rotary-wing aircraft, and small and large fixed-wing aircraft. Ground evacuation, although available, is inefficient; only a small number of casualties can be evacuated at once. Rotary-wing aircraft and small fixed-wing aircraft are costly and similarly inefficient in the small number of casualties evacuated. They may be better utilized in the disaster area for other purposes.[47] Large fixed-wing aircraft are very costly but are more efficient in allowing medical crew to manage complex multiple casualties over long distance. Large fixed-wing aircraft provide the possibility of retrograde airlift; that is, they may be used to bring in supplies to the disaster area and to evacuate casualties as they return for more supplies.[7,32]

Evacuated patients on a long-range flight are subject to stresses from the hypobaric environment—decreased partial pressure of oxygen, turbulence, vibration, temperature control, and humidity. Clinical preparation should include a systematic review of the stresses of flight and how they will apply to each casualty.[7,32,45,47] Consideration needs to be given to how to best address oxygen therapy, mechanical ventilation, trapped gas, decompression sickness/arterial gas embolism, casts, abdominal damage control surgery, burns, and infection control.

Oxygen supply is critical. Supplemental oxygen can be given to patients with known hypoxemia, dyspnea, and anemia. For mechanical ventilation, steps must be taken to reduce the risk of tracheal injury and/or endotracheal tube cuff rupture from expansion of the cuff at altitude. The air can be removed from the cuff and replaced by normal saline solution with sufficient pressure to eliminate leakage around the cuff. If the medical crew is equipped with a cuff manometer, this could be used with an air-filled cuff to monitor and adjust cuff pressure during ascent and descent.

In general, all trapped gas within the body should be evacuated before long-range evacuation by air to eliminate the risk of tissue damage from gas expansion. For pneumothorax, a functioning chest tube should be in place with a Heimlich valve in line, in case the pleural drainage unit must be disconnected for emergency exit. Recent abdominal surgery is not a contraindication to air transport, but if the casualty has an ileus, a functioning nasogastric tube must be secured and attached to suction. Obstructed middle ear and paranasal sinuses can be assessed by the casualty's response to the Valsalva maneuver. If obstruction is present, it can generally be managed by application of a topical vasoconstrictor such as oxymetazoline. Patients with decompression sickness or arterial gas embolism should not be exposed to altitudes greater than that of the origination airfield.

Patients with casts are prone to edema formation on exposure to altitude, and this risk increases with damaged tissue and reduced plasma oncotic pressure. This edema can lead to compartment syndrome inside the cast. Casts that have been in place for less than 48 to 72 hours should be bivalved before evacuation and held closed with elastic dressings if this can be done without compromising fracture stability. If this cannot be done safely, it is imperative to follow the neurovascular status of the limb closely and to be prepared to open the cast in-flight if compartment syndrome develops.[7,45]

Abdominal damage control surgery places casualties at risk for abdominal compartment syndrome with continued volume resuscitation and as edema worsens on altitude exposure. The medical crew must be prepared to monitor abdominal compartment pressures and open the abdomen if this syndrome develops. If this is not practical, patients should be transported with their abdomen open.[7,32]

Burns place patients at risk for several flight stresses including impaired thermoregulation, increased insensible fluid loss, and difficult infection control. Blankets, sleeping bags, heat conserving dressings, and/or active warming devices should be used to prevent hypothermia. Wounds should be dressed immediately preflight and not undressed in-flight if at all possible, to reduce the risk of environmental contamination. Strong consideration should be given to performing endotracheal intubation preflight in patients with significant inhalation injury. It is difficult to monitor the airway and to perform intubation in-flight.[7,45]

Infection control is a special challenge during air evacuation. Patients with known or suspected infections requiring respiratory isolation should not be transported by air unless essential.

In all cases of medical evacuation, attention should be paid to accurate record keeping. The use of clear, concise notations and standard forms is important to prevent duplication of initial assessment efforts. Records should remain with victims at all times and provide a key tool for enhancing casualty flow in receiving institutions.

Hospital Care

Once transported to hospitals, disaster victims must be again triaged and treated according to injury severity and available resources. During the initial arrival of casualties, efforts should be made to ensure that appropriate decontamination has taken place. This may include initial evaluation bays being set up outside the facility to prevent hospital contamination. Trauma room evaluation continues to follow ATLS standards with primary surveys, first looking for life-threatening airway, breathing, or circulatory compromise. If no life- or limb-threatening injuries are identified, individual treatment then depends on the specifics of each case. Early on, when the size of the casualty load is unknown, further interventions are performed on a minimal acceptable care basis. Secondary tests and time-consuming treatments are delayed when possible until an accurate assessment of available resources is possible.

Common injury patterns include crush, environmental exposure, and dehydration. The most significant of these for the orthopaedic surgeon are crush injuries. The details of crush management are outlined in Chapter 13. While most of the injury patterns overlap with those seen in more isolated trauma and are readily recognized and treated by surgeons, blast injuries remain an entity that are largely foreign to civilian physicians and deserve a more detailed review.

BLAST INJURY

Once victims suffering from primary blast injury are identified, treatment begins with the life-sustaining measures needed for airway protection, ventilation, and circulation. Initial radiographs should include a chest radiograph. The classic "white butterfly" pattern is highly suggestive of bilateral blast lung, and free air under the diaphragm may be indicative of hollow viscus rupture.[5] In many centers, computed tomography (CT) scanning is readily available and is the test of choice to quickly evaluate the head, chest, and abdomen.

Blast lung is a well-described entity that requires substantial respiratory support. The effects of blast lung may appear within 2 hours of injury, but signs of blast lung may appear as late as 48 hours after exposure.[10] The pulmonary compromise can be severe and potentially fatal. The chest radiographic findings and physiologic consequences are similar to those of more typical pulmonary contusion. Primary blast lung should be suspected in the presence of apnea, bradycardia, and hypotension or if patients develop dyspnea, cough, or chest pain following exposure. Avidan reviewed the cases of 29 patients admitted to a Jerusalem trauma center following blast injury with blast lung manifestations.[6] Each had the typical hypoxia and radiographic chest infiltrates. Seven patients who were able to support their own ventilation had a Pao_2/Fio_2 above 200. Twenty-two (76%) of the victims required mechanical ventilation, and all were intubated within 2 hours of presentation. They remained intubated for a mean of 4 days. The highest required PEEP support reached a maximum of 15 cm H_2O with caregivers using the minimal necessary positive pressure ventilation for adequate oxygenation. Alternative modes of ventilation (high-frequency or nitric oxide) were also employed in an attempt to minimize airway pressures. During treatment, two patients were thought to suffer air embolus, and one patient died of multiple organ failure. The risk of air embolism is lessened by minimizing positive pressure ventilation, treating with supplemental oxygen, and resting in a decubitus position.[5] The supplemental oxygen is beneficial for gas exchange and allows for more efficient absorption of arterial air, which occurs when the emboli are more predominantly oxygen rather than nitrogen. Body positioning is an important consideration for these patients, since remaining upright increases CNS injury while Trendelenburg positioning has increased coronary emboli effects. If one lung has been preferentially injured in a blast, the patient should be positioned with the injured lung down in a dependent position. That will result in lower alveolar pressures with greater vascular pressures, which can lower the chances for air being forced into the bloodstream.[5] The definitive treatment for air embolism remains hyperbaric chamber therapy. Although mortality from blast lung was low in this series, other authors have reported much higher rates, with Frykberg estimating an 11 percent mortality associated with blast lung.[28]

Primary blast injury to the abdomen may cause organ edema, hemorrhage, or frank rupture and result in bleeding significant enough to cause shock. Blood pressure should be maintained with fluids without administering excess volumes, which can worsen pulmonary injury. The abdomen can be evaluated by CT scan, ultrasound, or diagnostic peroneal lavage (DPL). DPL is more sensitive but less specific than CT in detecting abdominal organ injury from blast.[5] As for the injured lung, treatment for abdominal blast injury is supportive until the severity or extent of the injury requires bowel resection.

Hearing loss is produced by several mechanisms with the most common being rupture of the tympanic membrane.[5] CDC therefore recommends that all persons exposed to blast detonations be evaluated for tympanic membrane rupture, have an otologic examination, and be followed with serial audiometry.[5] Patients should have any debris removed for the external canal and have antiseptic solution irrigation. Tympanic membranes usually heal without repair if the rupture involves less than

33 percent of its area. Finally, victims should avoid repetitive auditory stresses, since remaining in loud environments decreases the chance of regaining hearing.

Blasts also can have an impact on the ophthalmologic system. Diligent repeat examinations are required to look for globe lacerations, hypopyon, corneal ulcers, and traumatic optic nerve atrophy.[41] Ocular perforating injuries are particularly serious. In soldiers from Iraq, this type of injury was frequently grossly contaminated by a large number of small particles. Thirty-one percent of these injuries required globe excision even when eyes with minimal potential functional recovery were preserved.[46] These penetrating injuries accounted for 80 percent of globe excisions among 251 severe ocular injuries. The use of protective goggles in combat cannot be overemphasized.

Several aspects of open extremity wounds produced by blasts deserve special attention. First, most penetrating injuries caused by blast driven projectiles should be considered as contaminated and survivors given appropriate antibiotics and tetanus toxoid. Open wounds from various types of shrapnel and blast debris require detailed physical and radiologic examination. Even for small entrance wounds, surgeons should maintain a low threshold for thorough débridement, since deep contamination and devitalized tissue can produce highly morbid infectious complications. Second, these extremities should be thoroughly evaluated from a vascular standpoint.[27] In examinations of soldiers at Walter Reed Army Medical Center from 2001 to 2004, 107 vascular injuries were recorded with 64 percent resulting from explosive injuries. Remarkably, when arteriograms were ordered based solely on the injury mechanism in the absence of vascular changes on physical examination, 25 percent (7/28) were positive. Overall, two thirds of vascular injuries missed on physical examination but evident on angiography were attributable to blast. While most occult injuries remained asymptomatic, 18 percent required treatment and included arteriovenous fistulas and pseudoaneurysms. The experience at Walter Reed has led to several recommendations. It seems that the physical examination is less reliable for detecting vascular injuries due to blast than in routine civilian trauma. In the treatment of these injuries, it is important to avoid prosthetic grafts or repairs/reconstruction within contaminated zones of injury because these factors significantly increase complication rates. Most operative procedures aim to ligate expendable vessels or use autologous vein grafts for critical reconstructions. Endovascular techniques and wound vacuum-assisted closure devices have also begun to play important roles. Finally, even with ideal management, complications are expected. Forty-four percent of battlefield vascular repairs involved complications with 25 percent of these repairs subsequently requiring additional procedures.

Beyond emergent débridement and bony stabilization, the approach to reconstruction for high-velocity, high-energy extremity wounds has changed over time. Traditionally, these wounds underwent long-term dressing changes and immobilization. However, some surgeons now advocate for earlier definitive reconstruction and coverage. Celikov published a large experience covering 215 patients suffering from combat gunshot, missile, and land mine injuries of the lower extremity.[11] These patients were treated definitively from 1 to 3 weeks (mean, 9.3 days) after injury. Following a mean of 1.9 débridement procedures, final procedures were performed. Twenty-three (10.2%) were treated with primary below-knee amputation. However, a greater number of amputations were carried out at primary hospitals on limbs not transferred to the referral center in this study. The remaining 209 defects were scheduled for simultaneous bony and soft tissue reconstruction. Soft tissue coverage consisted of 18 local muscle and 208 free muscle flaps. Associated Gustilo type III open tibia fractures or bony foot defects numbered 104 and 64, respectively. These were addressed with 106 bone grafts, 25 free fibula flaps, and 14 cases of distraction osteogenesis. Overall, the results were encouraging given the severity of injuries. All patients survived their injuries, and the success of the free flaps was 91.3 percent. Bony complications included early infection in 15.4 percent, chronic infection in 3.8 percent, and union difficulty in 22 percent. Only two late amputations were performed, and at a mean follow-up of 25 months, no patients had requested amputation secondary to functional problems or pain. While this extensive series provides insight into aggressive treatment protocols, it is important to remember, as the authors point out, that their success is based on early, aggressive bony and soft tissue débridement and that these results are from a highly experienced referral trauma center.

Unique infectious risks are also associated with blast wounds. Reports of burn patients from blast attacks document the appearance of infected wounds and sepsis from multidrug resistant bacteria that are novel to treating burn centers.[41] Even in the setting of private rooms, pneumonia caused by resistant bacterial strains developed in several patients in one center. While an explosive's shrapnel and debris carry some bacteria, blast attacks are also noteworthy for increasing subsequent contamination of wounds due to conditions at the scene or during transport to the hospital in civilian vehicles (including a garbage truck in one bombing).[41] For example, blast victims from meat and vegetable marketplaces have suffered from increased incidence of candidemia.[68] Furthermore, suicide bombings have been associated with the traumatic implantation of allogenic biologic material into victims as secondary fragmentation from either the bomber or from others in proximity to the blast.[8, 23, 43] This introduces risk of significant infectious transmission, since some impaled bony fragments have tested positive for hepatitis B.[23] In response, Israel now mandates hepatitis B vaccination as part of the first-line response to suicide bombings.[58] To date, one reported transmission of the virus has occurred while bony fragments from two suicide bombers have tested positive for the virus.[23] Risk of hepatitis C and HIV inoculation may warrant screening but have not yet been reported.[41]

Summary

Physicians practicing today face an increasingly unstable political world with ongoing acts of terrorism. Both civilian attacks and natural disasters have brought increased attention to disaster care. These disasters introduce risk to first responders as well as to hospital personnel that is unseen in the delivery of routine health care. As little real-time training is available, preparation and education provide the cornerstone of any effective disaster response. The "all-hazards approach" defines the current model of generic disaster preparations, which provide uniform responses yet allow sufficient flexibility to enable adaptation to unique circumstances. It is essential that health care providers become fluent in the universal terminology of disasters as well as the Incident Command System. Physicians should appreciate the changes that disasters impose on the conventional civilian approach to triage. While MCIs are rare, their potential impact on communities or society as a whole mandate that the health care profession stand ready to deliver in the face of disasters.

REFERENCES

1. Agency for Healthcare Research and Quality, U.S. Department of Health and Human Services. Development of Models for Emergency Preparedness: Personal Protective Equipment, Decontamination, Isolation/Quarantine, and Laboratory Capacity. Rockville, MD, 2005, pp. 27–61.

2. Ales, N.C.; Katial, R.K. Vaccines against biologic agents: Uses and developments. Respir Care Clin 10:123–146, 2004.

3. Almogy, G.; Luria, T.; Richter, E.; et al. Can external signs of trauma guide management? Lessons learned from suicide bombing attacks in Israel. Arch Surg 140:390–393, 2005.

4. American College of Surgeons: Advanced Trauma Life Support for Doctors, 7th ed. Chicago, 2004, p. 330.

5. Argyros, G.J. Management of primary blast injury. Toxicology 121:105–115, 1997.

6. Avidan, V.; Hersch, M.; Armon, Y.; et al. Blast lung injury: Clinical manifestations, treatment, and outcome. Am J Surg 190:927–931, 2005.

7. Bailin, M.T.; Beninati, W.; Bohanan, A.M.; et al. Incident Command System. In Briggs, S.M.; Brinsfield, K.H., eds. Advanced Disaster Medical Response Manual for Providers. Boston, MA, Harvard Medical International Trauma and Disaster Institute, 2003, pp. 1–5, 17–26, 35–36.

8. Braverman, I.; Wexler, D.; Oren, M. A novel mode of infection with hepatitis B: Penetrating bone fragments due to explosion of a suicide bomber. Isr Med Assoc J 4:528–529, 2002.

9. Brewster, P. Clear understanding of ICS proves value for emergency management. Hazard Monthly May:7–9, 1990.

10. Caseby, N.G.; Porter, M.F. Blast injuries to the lungs: Clinical presentation, management and course. Injury 8:1–12, 1976.

11. Celikoz, B.; Sengezer, M.; Isik, S.; et al. Subacute reconstruction of lower leg and foot defects due to high velocity–high energy injuries caused by gunshots, missiles, and land mines. Microsurgery 25:3–15, 2005.

12. Cernak, I.; Savic, J.; Ignjatovic, D.; et al. Blast injury from explosive munitions. J Trauma 47:96–102, 1999.

13. Champion, H.R.; Sacco, W.J. Trauma severity scales. In Maull, K.I., ed. Advances in Trauma, Vol. 1. Chicago, Yearbook Medical, 1986, pp. 1–20.

14. Ciraulo, D.L.; Frykberg, E.R.; Feliciano, D.V.; et al. A survey assessment of the level of preparedness for domestic terrorism and mass casualty incidents among Eastern Association for the Surgery of Trauma members. J Trauma 56:1033–1041, 2004.

15. Cone, D.C.; Koenig, K.L. Mass casualty triage in the chemical, biological, radiological, or nuclear environment. Eur J Emerg Med 12:287–302, 2005.

16. Cooper, C.J.; Taylor, D.E.M. Biophysics of impact injury to the chest and abdomen. J R Army Med Corps 135:58–67, 1989.

17. Cooper, G.J.; Townsend, D.J.; Cater, S.R.; et al. The role of stress waves in thoracic and visceral injury from blast loading: Modification of stress transmission by foams and high density materials. J Biomechanics 24:273–285, 1991.

18. Coppel, D.L. Blast injury of the lungs. Br J Surg 63:735–737, 1976.

19. Darling, R.G.; Catlett, C.L.; Huebner, K.D.; et al. Threats in bioterrorism. I. CDC category A agents. Emerg Med Clin North Am 20:273–309, 2002.

20. Department of Health and Human Services, Centers for Disease Control and Prevention (CDC). Mass casualties/explosions and blast injuries: A primer for clinicians. Available at: http://www.bt.cdc.gov/mass-casualties/explosions.asp.

21. Department of Health and Human Services, Centers for Disease Control and Prevention (CDC). Response to Radiation Emergencies: Centers for Disease Control and Prevention. Available at: http://www.bt.cdc.gov/radiation.

22. Edsall, K.; Keyes, D. Personal protection and decontamination for radiation emergencies. In Keyes, D.; Burstein, J.; Schwartz, R.; et al., eds. Medical Response to Terrorism: Preparedness and Clinical Practice. Baltimore, MD, Lippincott Williams & Wilkins, 2005.

23. EshKol, Z.; Katz, K. Injuries from biologic material of suicide bombers. Injury 36:271–274, 2005.

24. Federal Emergency Management Agency (FEMA). Incident Command System. Available at: http://www.fema.gov.

25. Federal Emergency Management Agency (FEMA). National Emergency Training Center, Emergency Management Institute: Exemplary practices in emergency management: The California Firescope Program. Monograph series No. 1. Emmitsberg, MD, 1987.

26. Fly, D.E.; Schecter, W.P.; Parker, J.S. The surgeon and acts of civilian terrorism: Biologic agents. J Am Coll Surg 200:291–302, 2005.

27. Fox, C.J.; Gillespie, D.L.; O'Donnell, S.D.; et al. Contemporary management of wartime vascular trauma. J Vasc Surg 41:638–644, 2005.

28. Frykberg, E.R. Medical management of disasters and mass casualties from terrorist bombings: How can we cope? J Trauma 53:201–212, 2002.

29. Frykberg, E.R.; Tepas, J.J. Terrorist bombings: Lessons learned from Belfast to Beirut. Ann Surg 208:569–576, 1988.

30. Gans, L.; Kennedy, T. Management of unique clinical entities in disaster medicine. Emerg Med Clin North Am 14:301–325, 1996.

31. Greenfield, R.A.; Drevets, D.A.; Machado, L.V.; et al. Bacterial pathogens as biological weapons and agents of bioterrorism. Am J Med Sci 323:299–315, 2002.

32. Grissom, T.E.; Farmer, J.C. The provision of sophisticated critical care beyond the hospital: Lessons from physiology and military experiences that apply to civil disaster medical response. Crit Care Med 33 (1 Suppl):S13–S21, 2005.

33. Harrison, R. Occupational Toxicologic Emergencies. In Kravis, T.C.; Warner, C.G.; Jacobs, L.M., eds. Emergency Medicine: A Comprehensive Review, 3rd ed. New York, Raven Press, 1993, pp. 761–779.

34. Hirshberg, A.; Scott, B.G.; Granchi, T.; et al. How does casualty load affect trauma care in urban bombing incidents? A quantitative analysis. J Trauma Injury Infect Crit Care 58:686–693; discussion 58:694–695, 2005.

35. Hogan, D.E.; Waeckerle, J.F.; Dire, D.J.; et al. Emergency department impact of the Oklahoma city terrorist bombing. Ann Emerg Med 34:160–167, 1999.

36. Horn, J.K. Bacterial agents used for bioterrorism. Surg Infect [Larchmt] 4:281–287, 2003.

37. Hsu, C.E.; Mas, F.S.; Jacobson, H.; et al. Assessing the readiness and training needs of non-urban physicians in public health emergency and response. Disaster Manag Response 3:106–111, 2005.

38. Hull, J.B. Blast injury patterns and their recording. J Audiov Media Med 15:121–127, 1992.

39. Inglesby, T.B.; Henderson, D.A.; Bartlett, J.G.; et al. Anthrax as a biological weapon. JAMA 281:1735–1745, 1999.

40. Irwin, R.J.; Lerner, M.R.; Bealer, J.F.; et al. Cardiopulmonary physiology of primary blast injury. J Trauma 43:650–655, 1997.

41. Kennedy, P.J.; Haertsch, P.A.; Maitz, P.K. The Bali burn disaster: Implications and lessons learned. J Burn Care Rehabil 26:125–131, 2005.

42. Lee, E.C. Clinical manifestations of sarin nerve gas exposure. JAMA 290:659–662, 2003.

43. Leibner, E.D.; Weil, Y.; Gross, E.; et al. A broken bone without a fracture: Traumatic foreign bone implantation resulting from a mass casualty bombing. J Trauma 58:388–390, 2005.

44. Leibovici, D.; Gofrit, O.N.; Stein, M.; et al. Blast injuries: Bus versus open-air bombings—A comparative study of injuries in survivors of open-air versus confined-space explosions. J Trauma 41:1030–1035, 1996.

45. Lhowe, D.W.; Briggs, S.M. Planning for mass civilian casualties overseas: IMSuRT: International Medical/Surgical Response Teams. Clin Orthop Relat Res 422:109–113, 2004.

46. Mader, T.H.; Carroll, R.D.; Slade, C.S.; et al. Ocular war injuries of the Iraqi insurgency, January–September 2004. Ophthalmology 113:97–104, 2006.

47. Mahoney, E.F.; Harrington, D.T.; Biffl, W.L.; et al. Lessons learned from a nightclub fire institutional disaster preparedness. J Trauma 58:487–491, 2005.

48. Martin, C.O.; Adams, H.P. Neurological aspects of biological and chemical terrorism: A review for neurologists. Arch Neurol 60:21–25, 2003.

49. Maynard, R.L.; Cooper, G.J.; Scott, R. Mechanism of injury in bomb blasts and explosions. In Westby, S., ed. Trauma: Pathogenesis and Treatment. Oxford, Butterworth Heinemann, 1988, pp. 30–41.

50. Mayorga, M.A. The pathology of primary blast overpressure injury. Toxicology 121:17–28, 1997.

51. McDonough, J., Jr., McMonagle, J.; Copeland, T.; et al. Comparative evaluation of benzodiazepines for control of soman-induced seizures. Arch Toxicol 73:73–78, 1999.

52. Mellor, S.G. The relationship of blast loading to death and injury from explosion. World J Surg 16:893–898, 1992.

53. Nelson, T.J.; Wall, D.B.; Stedje-Larsen, E.T. Predictors of mortality in close proximity blast injuries during operation Iraqi freedom. J Am Coll Surg 202:418–422, 2006.

54. Newmark, J. Nerve agents: Pathophysiology and treatment of poisoning. Semin Neurol 24:185–196, 2004.

55. Rodoplu, U.; Arnold, J.L.; Tokyay, R.; et al. Impact of the terrorist bombings of the Neve Shalom and Beth Israel synagogues on a hospital in Istanbul, Turkey. Acad Emerg Med 12:135–141, 2005.

56. San Mateo County Health Services Agency, Emergency Medical Services: The Hospital Emergency Incident Command System, 3rd ed. San Mateo, CA, 1998.

57. Schecter, W.P.; Fry, D.E. The governor's committee on blood-borne infection and environmental risk of American College of Surgeons: The surgeons and act of civilian terrorism: Chemical agents. J Am Coll Surg 200:128–134, 2005.

58. Siegel-Itzkovich, J. Israeli minister orders hepatitis B vaccine for survivors of suicide bomber attacks. Br Med J 323:417, 2001.

59. Sklar, D.P. Casualty patterns in disasters. J World Assoc Emerg Disaster Med 3:49–51, 1987.

60. Smith, J.; Ansari, A.; Harper, F.T. Hospital management of mass radiological casualties: Reassessing exposures from contaminated victims of an exploded radiological dispersal device. Health Phys 89:513–520, 2005.

61. Stein, M.; Hirshberg, A. Medical consequences of terrorism: The conventional weapon threat. Surg Clin North Am 79:1537–1552, 1999.

62. Stuhmiller, J.H. Biological response to blast overpressure: A summary of modeling. Toxicology 121:91–103, 1997.

63. U.S. Army Medical Research Institute of Chemical Defense (USAM RICD): Medical Management of Chemical Casualties Handbook, 3rd ed., 2000. Available at: http://ccc.apgea.army.mil.

64. U.S. Army Soldier and Biological Chemical Command (SBCCOM): Guidelines for Mass Casualty Decontamination During a Terrorist Chemical Agent Incident. 2000, pp. 4–23. Available at: http://www.chembio.com/resource/2000/cwirp_guidelines_mass.pdf.

65. U.S. Government: National Response Plan, 2005. Available at: www.dhs.gov/xnews/releases/press_release_0581.shtm.

66. Wenger, D.; Quatrantelli, E.L.; Dynes, R.R. Is the Incident Command System a plan for all seasons and emergency situations? Hazard Monthly March:8–12, 1990.

67. Wightman, J.M.; Gladish, S.L. Explosions and blast injuries. Ann Emerg Med 37:664–678, 2001.

68. Wolf, D.G.; Polacheck, I.; Block, C.; et al. High rate of candidemia in patients sustaining injuries in a bomb blast at a marketplace: A possible environmental source. Clin Infect Dis 31:712–716, 2000.

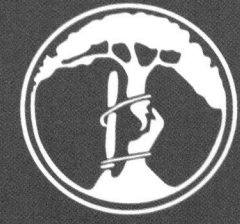

CHAPTER 9

Occupational Hazards in the Treatment of Orthopaedic Trauma

PART I
Optimal and Safe Use of C-Arm X-Ray Fluoroscopy Units

Peter J. Mas, M.S., D.A.B.M.P.

INTRODUCTION

The use of fluoroscopic imaging procedures allows the health care professional to view the examination/procedure of the patient in real-time. Modern fluoroscopic devices are greatly improved from the darkened room imaging conducted in the mid-20th century. The imaging system, or image intensifier assembly, is the central ingredient for the production of the patient image. It has grown from an approximately 6-in. diameter image intensifier to a 12-in. diameter device on mobile C-arm units. Stationary C-arm fluoroscopic units, such as those found in a busy radiology department, can come equipped with an 18-in. image intensifier, although it is more common to see an 15-in. intensifier, (Fig. 9-1).

The term C-arm refers to the letter C-shaped yoke of the x-ray tube-to-image intensifier geometry (Fig. 9-2).

In addition to the x-ray production electronics, display electronics, x-ray tube, and collimation device, the C-arm unit has an anti-scatter grid, a charge-coupled device (CCD), and a video system camera to feed the image onto the display monitors. Mobile C-arm units are equipped with wheels and a steering mechanism for transport to the procedure room or operatory where it will be used.

FEATURES

The image intensifier assembly is composed of

1. An anti-scatter grid (which reduces scattered x-rays entering the unit)
2. A vacuum tube with photo-absorptive and electro-emissive surfaces, electrostatic focusing electrodes, and an output phosphor (CCD)
3. Light focusing lenses, diaphragm, and video signal pickup
4. Electronic shielding
5. Lead-lined enclosure

The function of each component of the image intensifier system is summarized below:

1. Anti-scatter grid: The anti-scatter grid reduces the loss of image resolution due to scattered x-rays reaching the image intensifier (Fig. 9-3). Scattered x-rays are those deflected from the original "straight-on" path to the image intensifier.
2. Vacuum tube: The vacuum tube is made of glass or a nonferromagnetic material (Fig. 9-4). It provides for the accelerated travel of electrons emitted from the entrance (input phosphor-to-photocathode) surfaces and directed to the output phosphor.
3. Electrostatic focusing lenses: Changing the electrical bias on these lenses spreads out (or compresses) the beam of electrons coming from the photocathode surface, thereby causing magnification (or minification) of the resultant image being captured.
4. Output phosphor: The output phosphor produces light photons representative of the x-rays absorbed/transmitted within the patient (Fig. 9-5).
5. Video signal pickup: The image generated at the output phosphor is then viewed with the attached video system (TV camera or CCD). An automatic brightness control (ABC) feedback circuit is used to drive the x-ray generator to produce more (or less) x-rays by increasing (or decreasing) the x-ray tube energy (kVp) operating potential and/or the x-ray tube current (mA).
6. Electronic shielding: Electronic shielding reduces any possible distortion of the image production system from external sources of electric and magnetic fields.
7. Lead-lined enclosure: The image intensifier system is a primary radiation barrier. X-rays do not escape from the image intensifier back into the suite (Figs. 9-6 and 9-7).

I have not paid much attention to the x-ray tube itself, primarily because its purpose is limited: it either produces

FIGURE 9-1 *A stationary C-arm fluoroscopic x-ray unit with a 15-in. image intensifier assembly.*

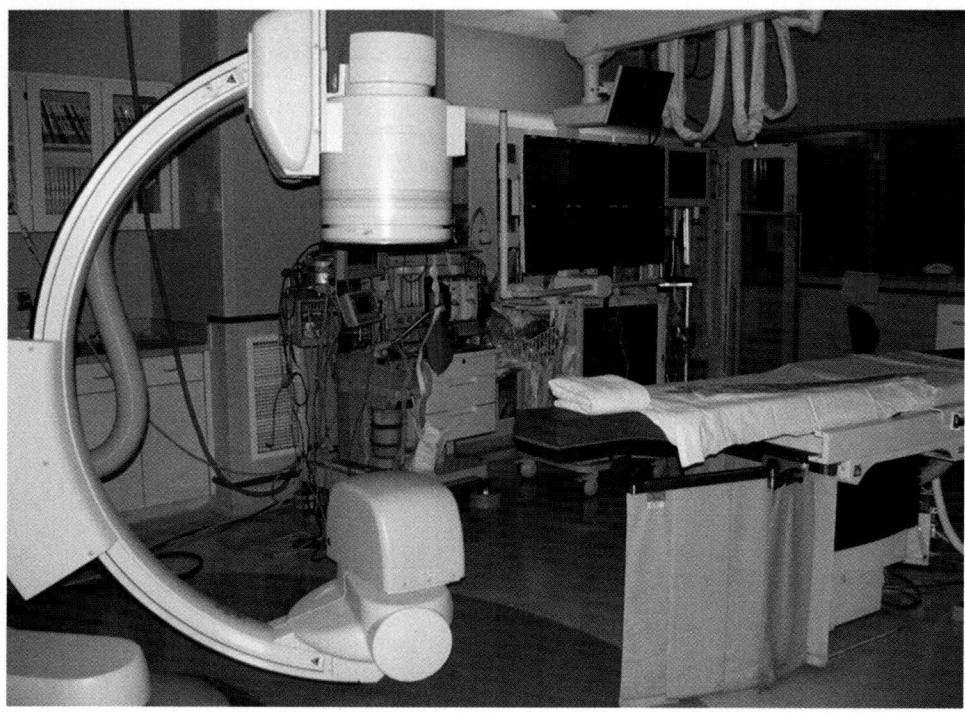

x-rays or not. The x-ray tube does not independently manage, manipulate, or modify the x-rays produced, but the x-ray tube housing is another matter. The tube housing (Fig. 9-8) is a lead-lined enclosure with three important components of the x-ray generation chain in addition to the x-ray tube itself: the x-ray beam filter(s), the beam collimation (a beam-size limiting device), and a thermal switch to sense overheating of the x-ray tube.

X-rays are produced when a stream of electrons is accelerated toward a high atomic number (Z-number) target material, such as tungsten, functioning as the anode in an electrical circuit. The collisions of the electrons with

FIGURE 9-2 *A mobile "C-arm" unit.*

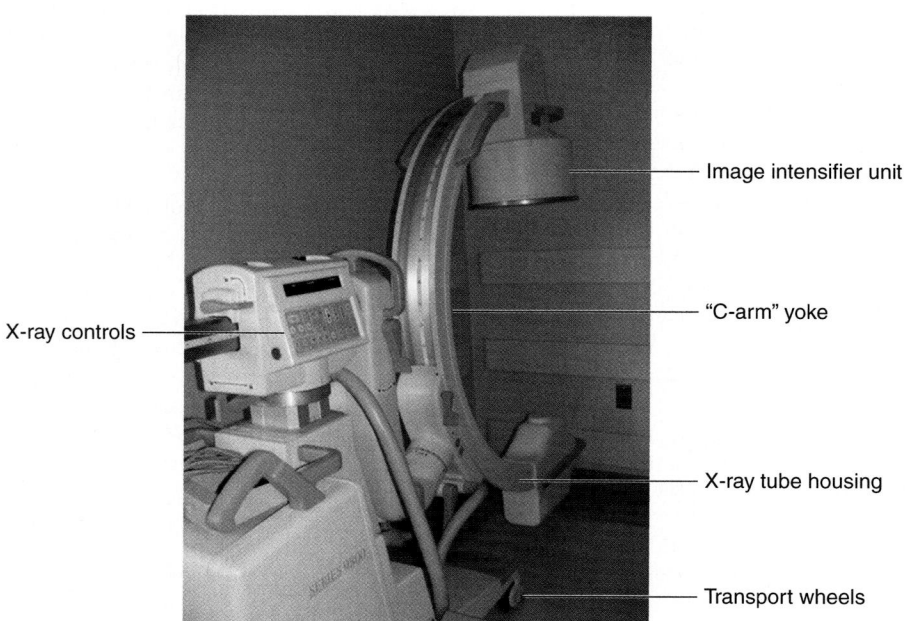

Image intensifier unit

"C-arm" yoke

X-ray controls

X-ray tube housing

Transport wheels

FIGURE 9-3 | *The complete image intensifier assembly is composed of (1) an anti-scatter grid, which reduces scattered x-rays entering the unit. (See Fig. 9-4.)*

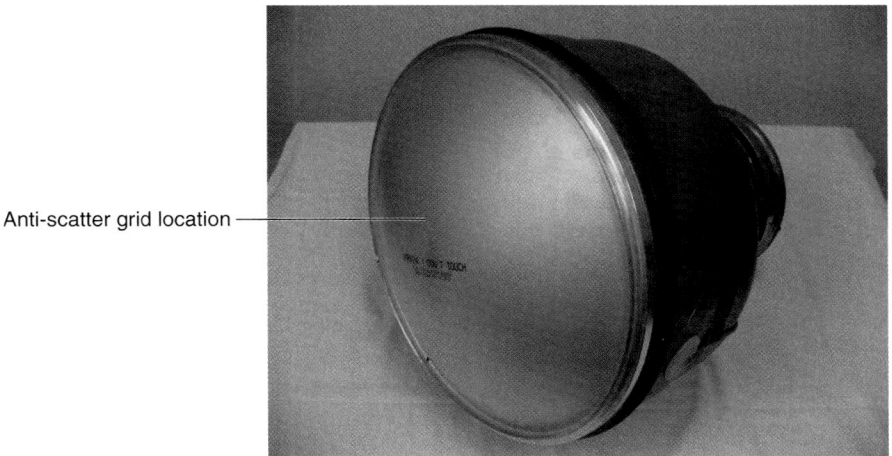

Anti-scatter grid location

the target results in x-rays, but approximately 99 percent of the collisions simply result in the heating of the target, so a thermal overload interrupt switch is a necessity. The tube housing also serves as a barrier against x-rays. By regulation of the U.S. Food and Drug Administration (FDA), x-rays escaping the tube housing ("leakage x-rays") cannot result in greater than 0.1 roentgen per hour exposure rate, measured 1 meter from the x-ray source, when operated at its maximum kVp energy and maximum continuous mA tube current.

X-rays produced in this manner are termed "polychromatic" because they cover a wide spectrum of energies; they are not monoenergetic like gamma-ray (nuclear) sources of radiation. The addition of x-ray beam filters achieves a cleaner and higher effective energy x-ray beam profile. The insertion of aluminum metal filters will remove (filter out) the lower energy x-rays that cause much greater radiation exposure to the patient and do not contribute to the creation of the diagnostic image. The higher energy x-rays continue to pass through the added aluminum filtration and reach the patient for the selective attenuation by tissues, and the imaging process begins. Higher energy x-ray imaging devices, such as computerized tomographic (CT) scanners, employ copper metal beam filtration to essentially eliminate all low-energy x-rays.

The x-ray beam collimation component is also governed by FDA regulation. The x-ray beam can never be larger (wider) than the image intensifier diameter, and

FIGURE 9-4 | *The complete image intensifier assembly is composed of (2) a vacuum tube. (See Fig. 9-3.)*

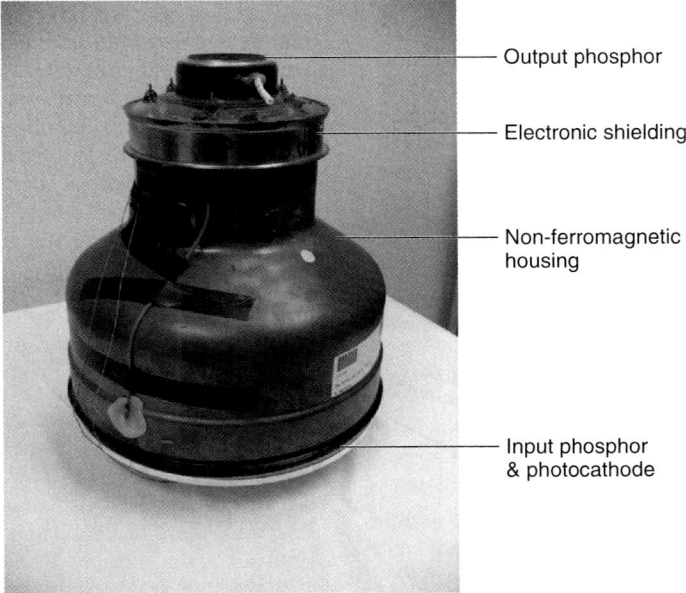

Output phosphor

Electronic shielding

Non-ferromagnetic housing

Input phosphor & photocathode

FIGURE 9-5 | *The output phosphor of the image intensifier.*

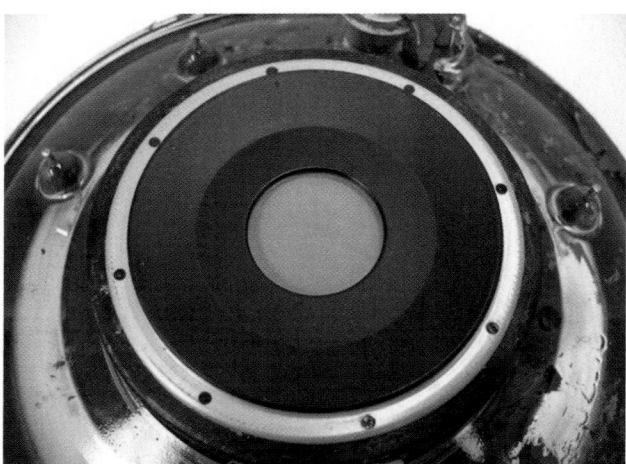

the image intensifier must be affixed to the x-ray device in such a way that it always intercepts the x-ray beam. An unattenuated, primary beam x-ray field must never extend beyond the physical size of the x-ray primary barrier that is built into the image intensifier device. In the clinical setting, such a misalignment would be comparable to standing next to a bulls-eye while the projectiles are hitting outside the intended target. Manufacturers can place a lead diaphragm (or cone) at the x-ray tube to satisfy the beam-size limiting criteria, but physical abuse or mishandling of the unit may jeopardize the x-ray beam-to-image intensifier alignment.

The final components of the imaging system are the x-ray control panel (Figs. 9-9 and 9-10), the exposure

FIGURE 9-6 | *Lead-lined housing of the image intensifier.*

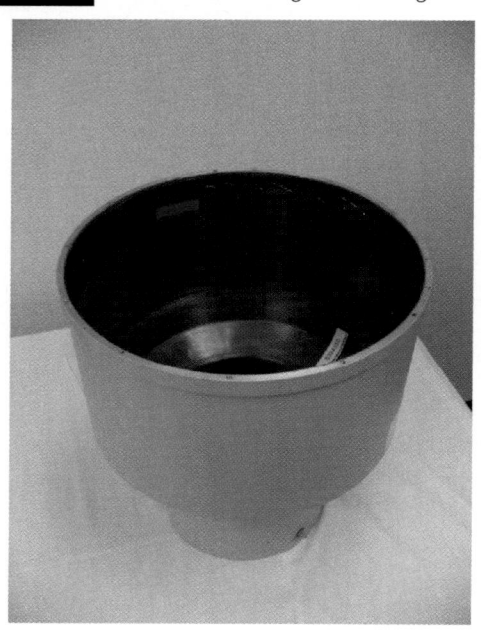

FIGURE 9-7 | *View of the interior of the intensifier housing.*

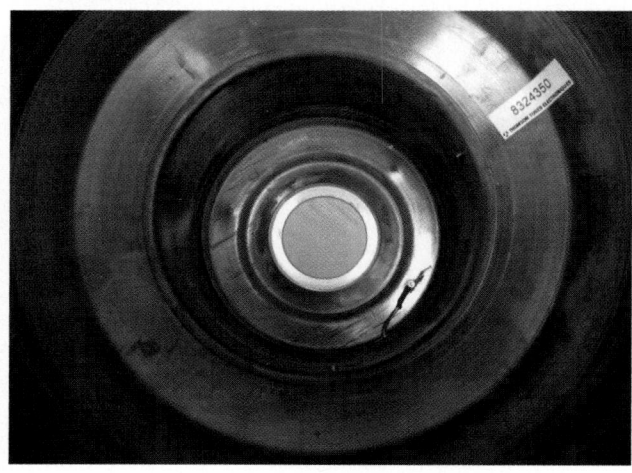

FIGURE 9-8 | *The X-ray tube housing.*

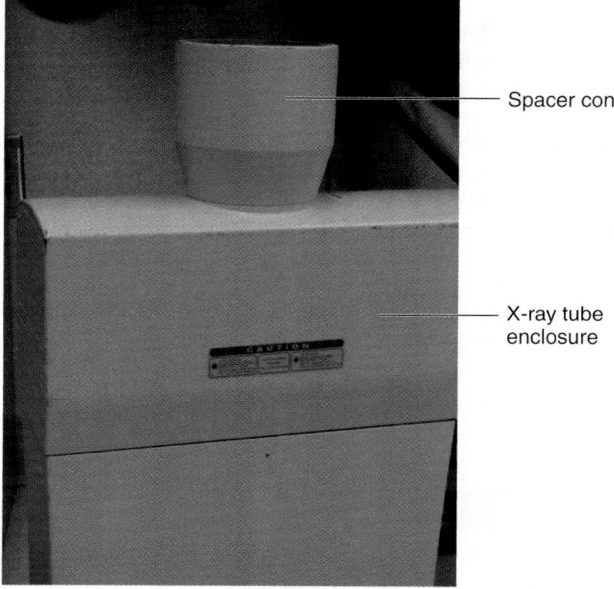

Spacer cone

X-ray tube enclosure

FIGURE 9-9 | *OEC unit x-ray control panel.*

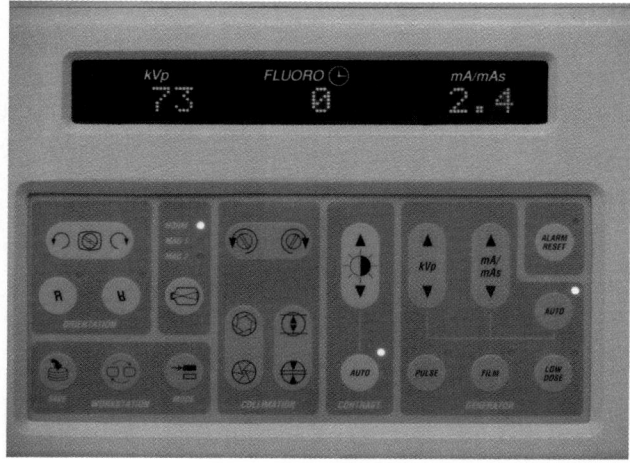

FIGURE 9-10 *Philips unit x-ray control panel.*

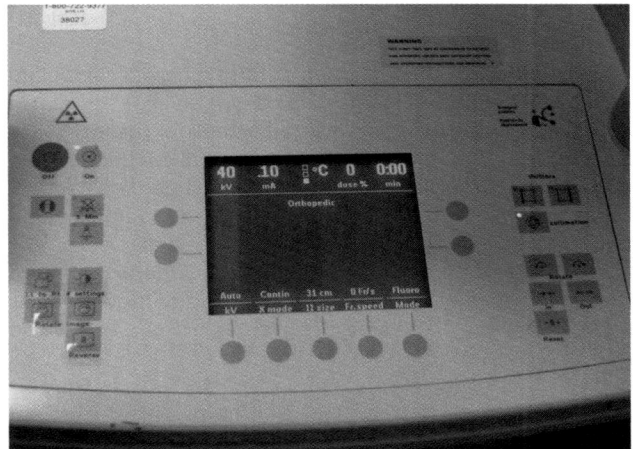

activation switches, customarily performed via a "dead man" type foot switch (Fig. 9-11), and the image display and recording device (Fig. 9-12). The x-ray control panel indicates the mode of operation of the C-arm unit. Details such as the kVp beam energy, mA tube current, elapsed time for the procedure, timer alarm reset, imaging frame rate, intensifier Mag (magnification) mode, and image display parameters are viewed and controlled at the console. Nearly each one of these has a direct bearing on the patient's (and staff's) radiation exposure (described later).

The "dead man" foot switch is so called because the operator must actively depress the switch to get the x-ray beam "on." If the operator were to drop dead during the procedure, the spring loaded foot switch would return to the "off" position and the C-arm unit would drop to zero x-ray emissions and again would be "radiation safe." The foot switch is on a long cord for placement where most convenient to the operator of the C-arm.

The image display and recording/archival device is the final leg of the diagnostic imaging process. The monitors must be of sufficient resolution and brightness to clearly display the progress of the procedure. Most C-arm units sold presently include an integrated hard drive with picture (frame) grabber hardware and software. The stored images can be called up for review and printing onto film media, but there is a finite number of images that can be stored. Depending on the hard drive capacity, that number ranges from a low of 100 to as high as 10,000, and once the storage media are filled, the unit will write over the first image in storage and continue therefrom. The advantage of a "last image hold" frame grabber is for the operator to be able to see the last recorded position of the device he or she is manipulating or inserting into the patient on the monitors. Thus, the x-ray beam does not need to be kept "on" at all times to review progress during the procedure.

REDUCTION OF RADIATION DOSE DURING C-ARM OPERATION

No two patients are exactly alike. There will be differences in size, height, weight, general shape, and anatomy, but a properly operated mobile C-arm unit does quite well for the vast majority.

Patients are routinely imaged on an operating room table, procedure table, stretcher, and even hospital bed. When the operator can choose the surface they will be imaged on, it is better to select an "x-ray compatible" table surface, plus its mattress and/or foam padding. The

FIGURE 9-11 *"Dead man" foot switch.*

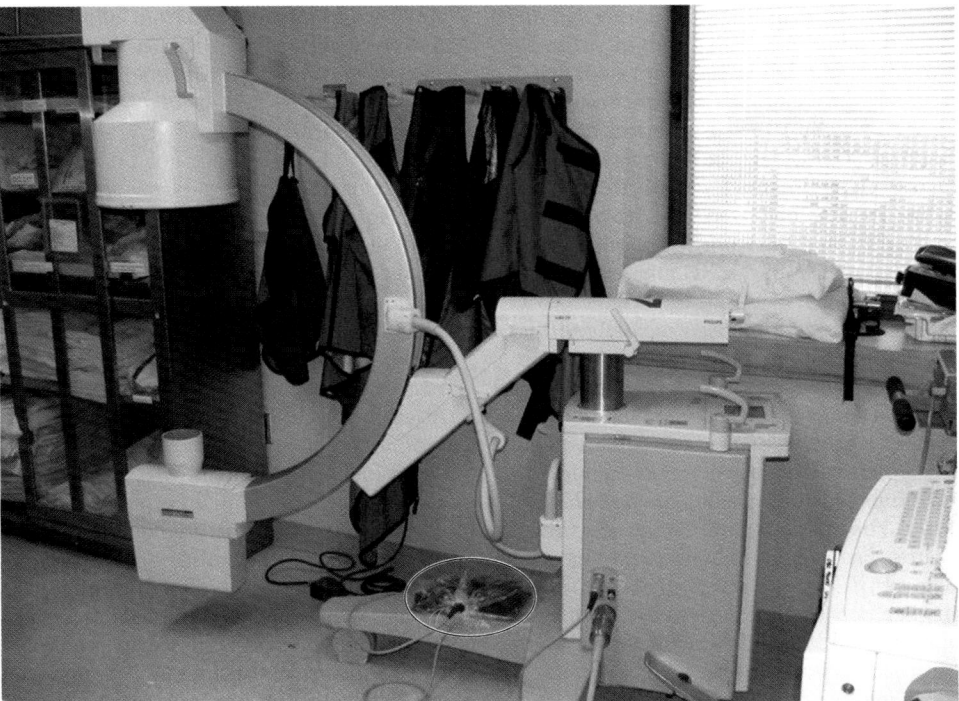

FIGURE 9-12 *C-arm unit display station.*

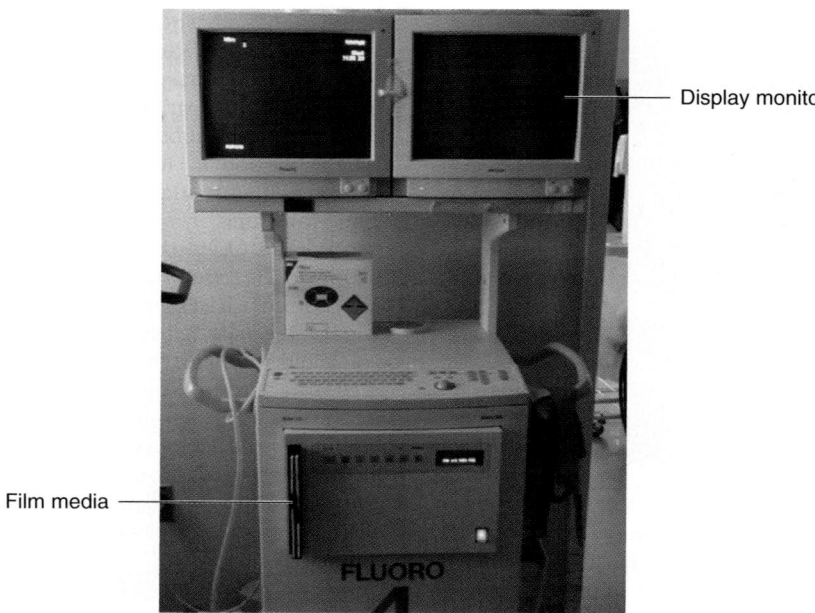

Display monitors

Film media

designation of x-ray compatible means that the table material itself is not highly attenuating of the x-ray beam. Attenuation of the x-rays results in the following:

1. Loss of object contrast. The C-arm unit will be forced to operate at a higher kVp beam energy or higher mA tube current as a result of the automatic brightness control feedback circuit. The ABC compensates for the reduced output phosphor light level due to the attenuation of the x-ray beam by the table materials. Object contrast decreases with increasing x-ray energy.
2. Greater entrance skin exposure to the patient from the increased imaging technique.
3. Greater amount of scattered radiation during the procedure.

The most desirable, but also expensive, surface is the carbon-fiber tabletop. It is the least attenuating because of its low atomic (Z-number) material composition.

A few words about "scattered radiation"—how and where it occurs with a C-arm unit. I like to use the following analogy to spatially describe the concept of scattering. Consider driving a car on a clear night. The headlights shine and easily illuminate the road ahead. Now consider driving that same car on a foggy night. There is a "halo" or "corona" of light starting at the headlight surface and radiating outward in the general direction of the road surface. This is "scattered" radiation, but radiation in the form of visible light that is being diffracted by the water molecules suspended in the air. X-rays can be scattered by striking air molecules, but the denser the material it interacts with, the greater the probability for scattering (and absorption) of the x-rays (Figs. 9-13 and 9-14).

Diagnostic imaging x-rays are a low-energy form of radiation. The scattering of the kilovoltage x-rays is predominantly directed back toward the x-ray tube. In comparison, high-energy megavoltage x-rays, like those used in cancer treatment, will scatter forward past the patient in the general direction of the treatment x-ray beam. From a radiation protection perspective, when the C-arm is positioned more parallel to the floor (shooting across the procedure table) personnel should not stand close to the x-ray tube, and it is better to stand at the image intensifier side.

We now move ahead to when the C-arm is brought to the patient's side during the orthopaedic procedure. The next exposure reduction step starts with the positioning of the C-arm at the patient. The single most important positioning criterion is to *place the image intensifier as close as possible to the patient's body* (Figs. 9-15 and 9-16). Use a sterile cover on the intensifier to maintain the sterility of the operatory field. In this orientation, three favorable things are achieved:

1. Increased sensitivity to the exiting x-rays that generate the patient's image, plus decreased scattered radiation because the image intensifier is a leaded barrier that has been placed nearer to the body that causes the scattering. When the intensifier is positioned closer to the patient, there is less scattering of x-rays beyond it into the room environment.
2. Increased image resolution. The improved imaging geometry will increase image sharpness, much like a hand will cast a sharper shadow the closer it gets to a wall or the floor (assuming the light is coming from overhead). In this analogy, the hand is the object you need to "see" clearly and the wall (or floor) is the "imaging" device.
3. Decreased entrance skin exposure at the patient because the x-ray tube is kept at the farthest distance possible from the patient's skin.

Radiation intensity follows the inverse-square law: the change in intensity is proportional to the square of the distance from the source. For example, if you double (2) the distance away from the radiation source, the intensity drops by the inverse, squared product $(\frac{1}{2}) \times (\frac{1}{2})$, which

FIGURE 9-13 *Morning fog.*

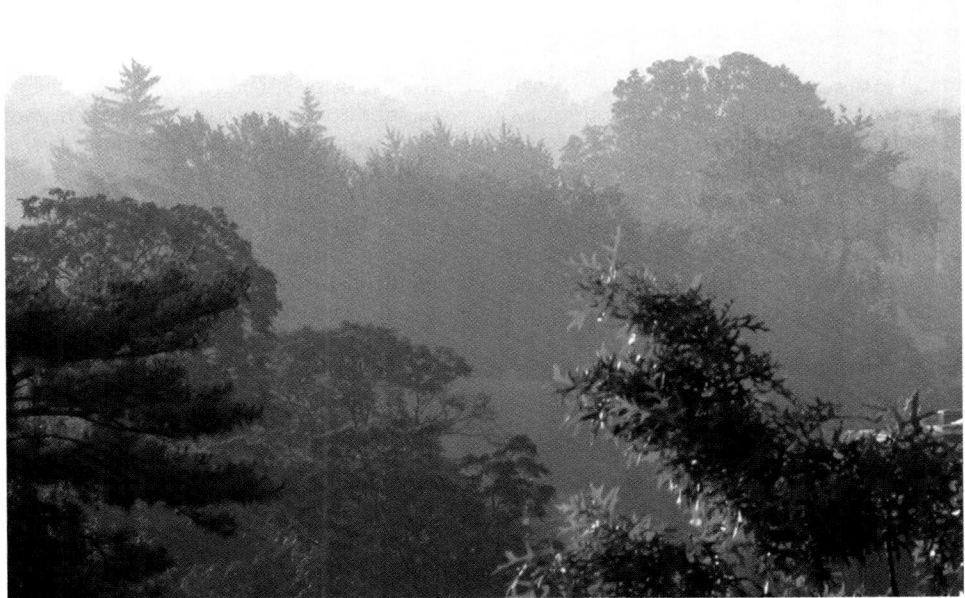

equals ¼ (25%) of the original radiation intensity. Conversely, if you halve (½) the distance from the radiation source, the intensity of the exposure is quadrupled (4). This situation is the most worrisome when you image in a truly lateral orientation. It is best to maintain the x-ray tube as far as possible from the patient's body surfaces and the image intensifier as close as possible. One FDA required component of fluoroscopic imaging systems, albeit frequently removed from the C-arm, is the spacer cone (see Fig. 9-8). The spacer cone is used to maintain 12-in. distance from the patient's body; otherwise very large radiation exposure rates and skin doses can be given to the patient. The FDA has publicized warnings to this effect and has identified the procedures most likely to cause conspicuous radiation damage to the skin of patients.

Orthopaedic surgical procedures are not on that list, but they can contribute to the deterministic effects of skin epilation and skin erythema. For more information, see the FDA Web site at http://www.fda.gov/cdrh/rsnaii.html.

FIGURE 9-15 *Proper positioning of an image intensifier; posteroanterior view.*

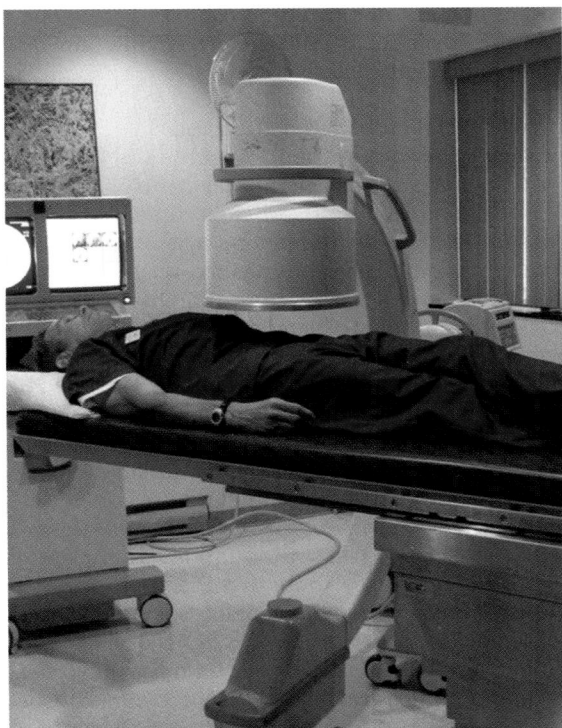

FIGURE 9-14 *Nighttime fog.*

FIGURE 9-16   *Lateral-oblique placement of the image intensifier.*

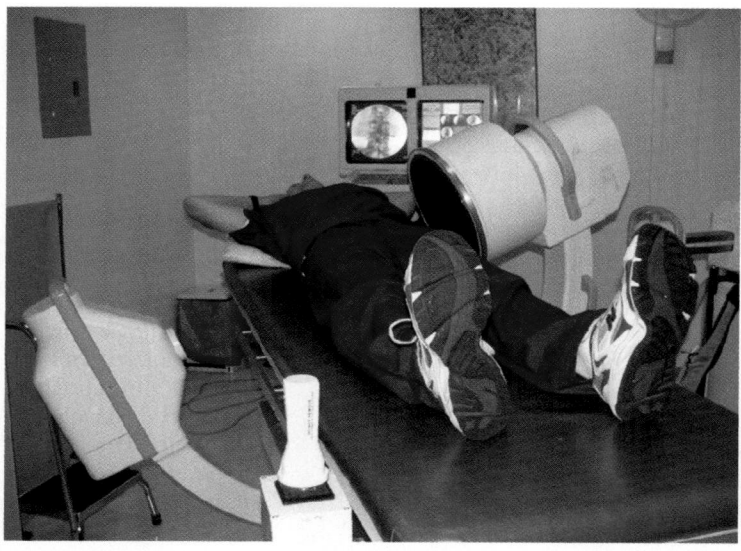

Today's C-arm units have the ability to magnify the area being imaged and are usually designed with two "mag modes" (magnification modalities) of operation. Image magnification is achieved within the intensifier by changing the bias voltage on the electrostatic focusing lenses. The electron beam traveling toward the output phosphor is forced to spread out, thereby eliminating some of the signal from the periphery of the electron stream that would have struck the output phosphor. Simultaneously, the collimator assembly narrows down the field of view because a smaller area of the patient is being imaged. The resultant effect is that less of the image intensifier input phosphor is being irradiated, and consequently fewer electrons are released into the intensifier assembly. The process is reversed when the control panel button for "normal" viewing is pressed.

Let us look at the net effect on the production of the electron stream at the input phosphor with the following images and a bit of algebra (Figs. 9-17 through 9-20) for an intensifier of 12/9/6-in. viewing modes. In "normal"

viewing mode, a 12-in. circular image intensifier is almost fully irradiated by the x-ray beam exiting the patient; the area (πr^2) of that surface equals 36π sq. in. At mag mode 1, the intensifier decreases to 9-in. diameter and surface area drops to 20.25π sq in. At mag mode 2, the intensifier decreases to 6-in. diameter and surface area drops to 9π sq in. Changing the intensifier size from 12 in. to 9 in. has a net effect of losing approximately 45 percent of the input phosphor's imaging area. Changing the intensifier size from 12 in. to 6 in. has a net effect of losing approximately 75 percent of the input phosphor's imaging area.

The decreased input phosphor area translates directly to a decreased production of electrons inside the image intensifier. The decreased number of electrons results in decreased light production by the output phosphor. The

FIGURE 9-18   *Partially open collimation for 9-in. "mag mode 1" viewing.*

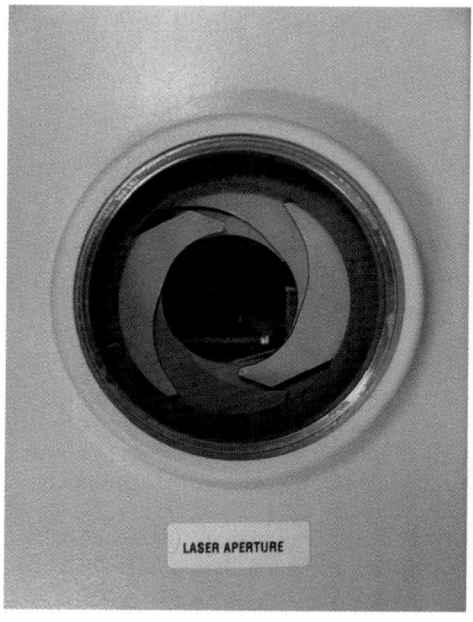

FIGURE 9-17   *Fully open collimation for 12-in. "normal" mode viewing.*

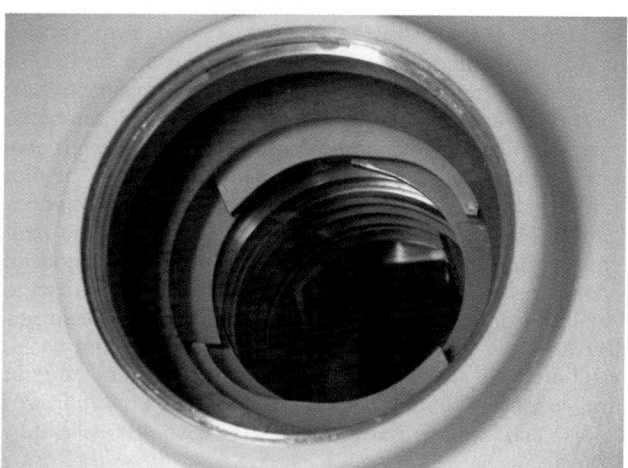

FIGURE 9-19 *Minimally open collimation for 6-in. "mag mode 2" viewing.*

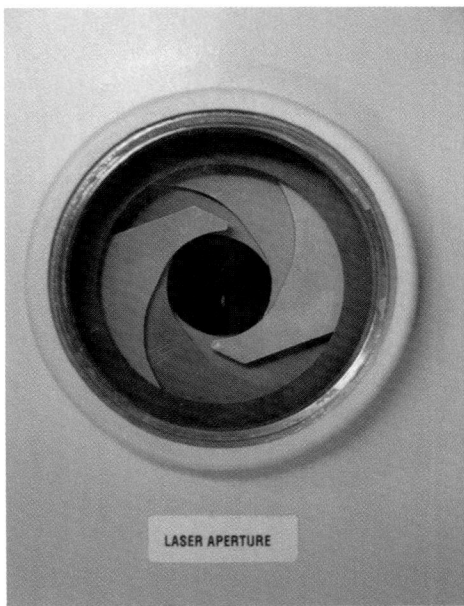

ABC feedback circuit seeks to correct the situation by calling on the x-ray generator to increase the tube energy potential (kVp) and/or the tube current (mA). A higher energy (kVp) x-ray will cause more electrons to be released by its interactions at the input phosphor. A higher tube current (mA) will cause the production of more x-rays at the x-ray tube. Ultimately, a combination of these two x-ray generator adjustments will satisfy the ABC circuitry. C-arm operation in a magnification modality is one source of significant increases in the imaging techniques (kVp, mA) and will result in the following:

1. Increased image resolution (at high mag mode); the patient object will appear larger, allowing the viewer to see the smaller details.
2. Increased patient entrance skin exposure because the x-ray tube is operating at a higher technique. If the

magnification is doubled (2 ×) the patient's exposure rate is quadrupled (4 ×).
3. Increased heat loading of the x-ray tube. The C-arm may shut down because of overheating, particularly when a lengthy procedure on a large-sized patient body is being performed.

To reduce the exposure of patient and the personnel, as well as to reduce the heating of the x-ray tube and increase its usable operating time, the magnification mode imaging features should be called upon only when necessary for the task at hand. Mag mode imaging is another tool of the C-arm but one to be used sparingly. Two other tools of the C-arm that impact image acquisition, patient exposure, and image storage are the "high-dose rate" mode fluoroscopy and the "frame rate" pulsed fluoroscopy settings found at the control panel.

The FDA limit for the patient's skin entrance exposure rate (at tabletop) is 100 mGy per minute (10 roentgens per minute in the old terminology). Fluoroscopic examinations typically yield skin entrance exposures ranging from 10 to 100 mGy/min, with 50 mGy/min being a fair estimate for routine, uncomplicated patient studies. An exception to the limit is the "high-dose rate" feature on fluoroscopic units, including C-arms. This feature may be called into use when the normal exposure rate does not produce enough x-rays for imaging an extremely large patient. The high-dose rate feature can go up to 200 mGy/min (20 R/min) skin entrance exposure rate, and a visible and audible alert must be produced by the imaging equipment when it is operated in this mode. Human skin will suffer epilation from x-rays when it has received radiation exposure as low as 1000 mGy (100 R), and skin erythema occurs with 2000 mGy (200 R) of exposure. Thus the value of a visible and audible alert with an imaging system that can cause 200 mGy/min exposure at skin entrance is clear; this patient may have to cope with radiation damage to skin at little more than 5 minutes of fluoroscopy time into the procedure.

There is another alert located on C-arm devices—the elapsed fluoroscopy time warning bell. The timer routinely alarms at 4 to 5 minutes of elapsed fluoroscopy beam "on" time and has to be reset at the control panel. This time can

FIGURE 9-20 *Active viewing area for 12/9/6-in. modes.*

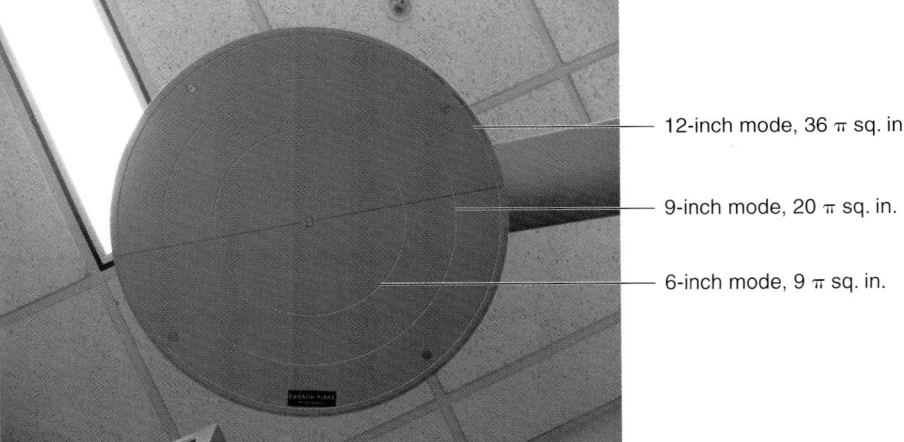

12-inch mode, 36 π sq. in.

9-inch mode, 20 π sq. in.

6-inch mode, 9 π sq. in.

be used as a marker of progress during the procedure and as a marker of the accrued total skin dose. If we assume 50 mGy/min (5 R/min) skin entrance exposure for the "normal-sized" patient, then 20 minutes of fluoroscopy approaches 1000 mGy.

The acquisition and recording of the fluoroscopic image can be changed at the control panel with the pulsed fluoroscopy feature. In contrast to real-time fluoroscopic images that are captured at a rate of 30 frames per second (33 msec imaging frame time), pulsed fluoroscopy operates with very short exposure times, usually 10 msec per pulse. Advantages of this feature are

1. Reduced patient motion blurring in the acquired image. (Picture in your mind the "frozen" and discontinuous images of dancers when a strobe light is in operation.)
2. Reduced total patient and personnel exposures.

The exposure reduction is proportional to the decrease in the image frame rate. If you drop from 30 to 15 frames per second, you have halved (½) the exposure. If you further reduce to 7.5 frames per second, you quarter (¼) the original exposure rate.

The drawback lies with the operator, who may not like seeing discontinuous images acquired at 15 frames per second and even less so at 7.5 frames per second. We are accustomed to a television video display of 30 frames per second, and real-time fluoroscopy is performed at that imaging rate. The "watching a movie" format and sense of fluid motion are lost at lower image capture rates, but bear in mind, *you are not watching television.* You are observing the gross deposition, absorption, and transmission of radiation energy within a patient. If enough energy is imparted to parts of that living body, it will cause the appearance of deterministic radiation effects, in the near future, on the patient.

A lower frame rate feature is desired when the purpose is to observe the general placement of readily observed medical devices, for example, orthopaedic screws, electric leads, and some catheters. If you need to assess the progress of your work in a millimeter-by-millimeter fashion, or you are imaging a structure with high degree of motion, you will likely prefer 15 frames per second images.

PROTECTION FROM RADIATION OF C-ARM EQUIPMENT WHEN IN OPERATION

The three tenets of radiation protection are time, distance, and shielding:

1. Time: Reduce the amount of time you are exposed to radiation and you reduce your total exposure.
2. Distance: Maintain a safe distance away from the radiation source. Remember how the inverse-square law greatly influences the intensity of radiation with changing distance.
3. Shielding: Whenever you will be working with an x-ray source, you must wear an appropriate lead-equivalent gown. Thyroid shields and leaded glasses are optional pieces of protective equipment, but in very busy or higher exposure environments, these may be required

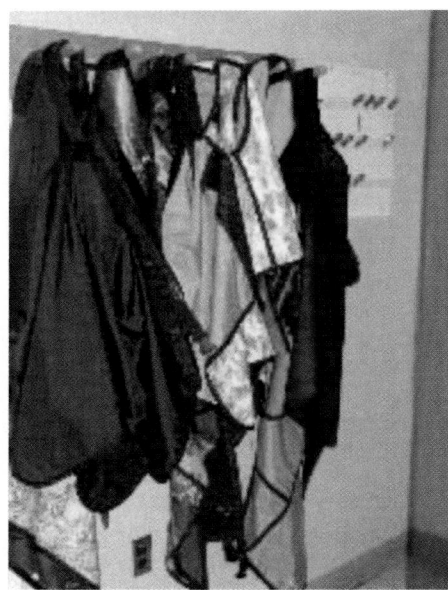

FIGURE 9-21 *Apron rack next to a procedure room alongside radiation dosimeters.*

by your medical physicist. To avoid cracking the shielding inside the protective garment, store these on suitable racks or laid out flat on a table until the next use (Fig. 9-21).

The use of radiation dosimeters may or may not be required depending on the frequency of use of C-arm units and the duration of the procedures routinely performed. An assessment of the need for dosimeters should be conducted by the medical physics/radiation safety staff. If used, dosimeters must be worn outside the lead-equivalent garment (shielded apron) in order to be exposed to whatever levels of scattered radiation are present. Placing the dosimeter underneath the shield will keep it from being exposed, while your head, hands, and feet will not be covered by the shield.

MEDICAL PHYSICS INSPECTION OF C-ARM EQUIPMENT

Joint Commission on Accreditation of Healthcare Organizations (JCAHO)–accredited institutions are required to perform safety inspections of the radiological equipment at least yearly. State and local governments may have the same or more stringent requirements, as well as the right to conduct public health inspections and examine the x-ray producing equipment. Hospital settings with large radiology, nuclear medicine, and radiation oncology departments are likely to have medical physicists on board to perform the equipment inspection tasks and to ensure that patient images are of the highest quality. A preventive maintenance program will also bring to their attention any equipment that is failing to perform as intended. These professionals are essential elements for the safe and accurate diagnostic imaging services of the institution and are a valuable resource for the clinicians and technologists who image the patients.

PART II

Prevention of Occupationally Acquired Blood-borne Pathogens

Brian W. Cooper, M.D., F.A.C.P. and Susan MacArthur, R.N., C.I.C., M.P.H.

The emergence of human immunodeficiency virus (HIV) during the 1980s had a profound effect on efforts to prevent occupational transmission of blood-borne infections. As of December 2001, the Centers for Disease Control (CDC) had received reports of 57 documented cases and 138 possible cases of occupationally acquired HIV infection among health care personnel in the United States since reporting began in 1985.[8] In 1987, the CDC published recommendations to protect health care workers from exposure to blood-borne pathogens. These recommendations introduced a concept known as "universal blood and body fluid precautions," or "universal precautions." Since medical history and examination could not reliably identify all patients infected with HIV or other blood-borne pathogens, the CDC recommended that "universal precautions" be consistently used for all patients.[5] While the CDC's recommendations were voluntarily adopted by hospitals, it was not until 1991 that the Occupational Safety and Health Administration (OSHA), urged by health care unions, promulgated the Bloodborne Pathogens Standard (BPS), which mandated health care facility compliance.[18] The OSHA Bloodborne Pathogens Standard required employers to formally establish an exposure control plan, provide education and training, institute engineering controls, provide personal protective equipment, and establish standard safety practices to assure a safe work environment. In addition, health care facilities were required to provide free hepatitis B vaccine or obtain a declination from employees whose work duties included contact with blood and other body fluids, and to provide exposure evaluation and follow-up treatment for occupationally exposed health care workers. OSHA provided compliance oversight and had the administrative authority to levy substantial fines should a health care facility fail to adhere to the Bloodborne Pathogens Standard. Although in 1991 the OSHA Bloodborne Pathogens Standard represented a significant change, health care facilities have since incorporated these requirements into standard operating procedures and today most health care workers could not imagine working without these basic protections.

Blood-borne infections in health care workers may theoretically be caused by any pathogens transmissible by blood including syphilis, trypanosomiasis, and other bacterial or protozoan parasites. But as a practical matter, the vast majority of the infectious risks after exposure to blood and body fluids are due to blood-borne viruses, chiefly, hepatitis B virus, hepatitis C virus, and human immunodeficiency virus.

HEPATITIS B VIRUS

Hepatitis B virus was once the most common blood-borne disease acquired by health care workers with blood exposure. Prior to the advent of hepatitis B vaccine, the CDC estimated that more than 12,000 health care workers per year were being infected with the hepatitis B virus (HBV). Blumberg's discovery of Australia antigen in 1967 was the first step in solving the riddle of viral "serum" hepatitis.[3] The ability to detect hepatitis B surface antigen and its antibody gave epidemiologic investigators the tools necessary to discover that health care workers, in particular surgeons, had a high rate of infection with HBV from unprotected blood exposure.

HBV is an enveloped DNA virus that consists of an outer layer of glycoprotein, the hepatitis B surface antigen (HBsAg), as well as envelope lipids. The viral nucleocapsid contains the viral genome and DNA polymerase plus a protein known as core antigen. In infected liver cells, a third core-associated antigen is known as the hepatitis B e antigen (HBeAg). HBV is transmitted by exposure to blood or body fluids primarily by the percutaneous or mucous membrane route. Among the blood-borne viruses, it is the most highly communicable. Because of its route of transmission, persons are at risk from sexual exposure and vertical transmission from a pregnant woman to her fetus in addition to percutaneous exposure.

The frequency of HBV infection differs dramatically in different regions of the world. Areas of hyperendemicity, the so-called hepatitis belt, stretch from North Asia across Africa to South America. In these areas, the primary route of exposure is vertical transmission or early childhood exposure. In contrast, in the United States and Europe, sexual transmission among adults as well as intravenous drug use has been the chief mode of spread. Health care workers were found to be highly infected with HBV in the 1970s. In fact, HBV infection is likely the leading occupationally acquired illness in health care workers.[7]

Acute Infection

After infection the incubation period until symptomatic illness varies from 6 weeks to 6 months, with an average of 12 weeks. It has been recognized that as many as half of the cases of HBV infection are clinically silent. In those that become symptomatic, common signs and symptoms include anorexia, low-grade fever, nausea, vomiting, and jaundice. Extrahepatic manifestations of illness include urticaria, arthritis, and arthralgias. HBsAg may be detected in serum 2 to 3 weeks prior to the onset of clinical illness. In uncomplicated cases, the illness resolves with clearance of the virus, clearance of HBsAg, and development of hepatitis B surface antibody, which is recognized as protective.

Chronic Disease

Chronic HBV infection is defined as persistence of HBsAg for greater than 6 months. Progression to chronic infection is higher in the pediatric age group, where 50 to 90 percent of children develop chronic infection.[14] In otherwise healthy adults, approximately 10 percent will develop chronic hepatitis B after an acute infection.

Chronic HBV infection is characterized by persistent viral replication in hepatocytes leading to increased risk for development of cirrhosis and hepatocellular carcinoma. An estimated 15 percent of adult patients who develop chronic HBV infection will develop one of these complications.

Treatment

There is no treatment other than supportive therapy for acute HBV infection. Clinicians should be alert to signs of overwhelming HBV infection, which occurs in up to 1 percent of infected individuals. Massive hepatic necrosis may lead to hepatic coma and death. In these cases, urgent liver transplantation may be lifesaving. The therapy of chronic HBV infection is continuing to evolve. Medications such as interferon alpha, the nucleoside lamivudine, and other nucleoside antiviral agents have been utilized with varying degrees of success. The goal of completely eliminating hepatitis B virus is not achieved in a substantial number of patients who are treated for chronic HBV.

Prevention

Current U.S. hepatitis B vaccines are genetically engineered preparations that utilize recombinant DNA technology. The vaccine consists of recombinant hepatitis B surface antigen. The vaccine is highly recommended for all health care workers with potential blood exposure. Hepatitis B vaccine is dosed on a 0-, 1-, and 6-month schedule; however, modified schedules such as 0, 1, 2, and 12 months may also be used. The vaccine is administered by deep intramuscular injection in the deltoid region. Administration of the vaccine in fat-bearing areas such as the gluteus has been found to decrease the immunogenicity of the vaccine response. It is important to check the antibody response 1 or 2 months after receipt of the last dose of the vaccine to assure a protective level of antibody has developed. In general, 85 to 90 percent of healthy individuals will develop a protective response to the vaccine. The response rates are lower for older individuals, the obese, and persons with chronic illness. Nonresponders to the standard three-dose series may respond to further immunization, and a number of optional follow-on immunizations schedules have been recommended.[21]

Passive Immunity

After blood exposure such as a sharps injury in a previously unimmunized individual, the combination of vaccination and passive immunotherapy with hepatitis B immune globulin has been recommended. This combination approach is highly effective at preventing hepatitis B viral infection when the source of the response is known to be infected with HBV. Hepatitis B immune globulin is administered in a dose of 0.06 mL/kg given as a deep intramuscular injection in a large muscle group, such as the gluteal region or thigh. The initial hepatitis B vaccine dose can be given simultaneously at a separate site. It is important to follow up with the subsequent hepatitis B vaccine doses on the proper schedule.

HEPATITIS C VIRUS

By the 1950s it was clear to investigators that the two major forms of viral hepatitis were "infectious" hepatitis, spread by fecal-oral contamination, and "serum" hepatitis, spread by blood and sexual exposure. With the discovery of hepatitis A, the main cause of "infectious" hepatitis and hepatitis B, it became clear that other agents were causing "serum" viral hepatitis. Hepatitis C was discovered in the early 1990s and found to be the major cause of so-called non-A, non-B hepatitis. Hepatitis C virus infection is now the most common cause of blood-borne infection in the United States. It is estimated that 1.8 percent of the U.S. population has been infected with HCV.[15] Indeed, hepatitis C–related chronic liver disease has become the most common indication for liver transplantation in the United States.

Hepatitis C is transmitted most efficiently by blood exposure. Sexual transmission has been reported but is less frequent. Transmission through blood transfusion, once common, has been dramatically reduced by blood donor serologic screening. It is estimated that injection drug use is the most common mode for infection with HCV in the United States.

Acute hepatitis C infection, as with other types of viral hepatitis, is often asymptomatic. Only 20 to 30 percent of patients develop symptoms of anorexia, malaise, and abdominal pain. Jaundice occurs in approximately 20 percent of those infected. The average incubation period is 6 weeks. Antibodies to HCV typically develop 8 to 12 weeks after exposure; however, some individuals remain seronegative for many months. Biochemical alterations in serum ALT levels, often in a fluctuating pattern, are the most frequent abnormality found. After acute infection, 10 to 15 percent of individuals clear the virus without further sequelae, leaving 85 to 90 percent with chronic hepatitis C viral infection. Among those with chronic hepatitis C viral infection, it is estimated that 10 to 15 percent will develop cirrhosis over a period of many years. As with hepatitis B, hepatocellular carcinoma is associated with some cases of chronic HCV.

Health care workers with blood exposure are at risk for infection with HCV although, relative to HBV, the risk is much lower. Numerous surveys of health care workers estimate that the seroprevalence of HCV antibodies could be similar to that in volunteer blood donors.

Screening

Antibody to hepatitis C virus is commonly detected by enzyme immunoassay (EIA). This test is highly sensitive; however, false positives have occurred, and all positive test results should be confirmed with a more specific assay, such as a recombinant immunoblot assay (RIBA). Antibody tests do not distinguish between chronic hepatitis C infection and cleared hepatitis C virus due to a prior infection. HCV RNA assays can detect HCV viral presence as early as 2 weeks after acute infection. HCV RNA assays are useful in the detection of chronic infections as well as early acute disease.

Prevention of health care–associated HCV infection centers on prevention of sharps injuries, since no vaccine or immunoglobulin has proven useful. Screening for HCV infection after a parenteral exposure is important to identify those who develop acute infection. HCV RNA assays are most useful in this setting. Serodiagnosis of HCV antibodies is less useful because of the delay in development of these antibodies. Available data indicate that early treatment of acute hepatitis C infection with interferon alpha for 24 weeks is highly effective at eradicating the virus and preventing chronic hepatitis C.[13]

HUMAN IMMUNODEFICIENCY VIRUS

Among the major transmissible blood-borne viruses that pose a potential risk to health care workers, it is clear that hepatitis B virus and hepatitis C virus make up the bulk of the risk. Although HIV accounts for substantially fewer cases of occupationally acquired infection, it elicits the most anxiety and attention from health care workers.

HIV, an RNA retrovirus, causes the acquired immunodeficiency syndrome. It is called a retrovirus because of the enzyme reverse transcriptase, which reverses the usual flow of genetic information. Instead of DNA forming messenger RNA in order to synthesize protein, reverse transcriptase catalyzes the creation of a complementary DNA copy of the virus's RNA genes.

Upon percutaneous infection, the virus bonds to specific receptors that are chiefly found on cells engaged in host defense, such as lymphocytes and macrophages. In the skin, animal models have shown that the virus binds to dendritic cells within about 24 hours after percutaneous inoculation. The dendritic cells then migrate to regional lymphatics, where lymphocytes are subsequently infected. The virus has a particular affinity for CD4-positive lymphocytes, and its subsequent life cycle leads to the slowly progressive destruction of most CD4 lymphocytes with progressive and ever worsening immunosuppression the result. As the disease progresses, infected patients are subject to a wide variety of infections by opportunistic pathogens, chronic wasting, and a host of malignancies.

The risk for occupational infection by HIV is generally low, but given the severity of illness produced by infection with HIV much attention has been focused on prevention of occupational HIV exposure and prevention of HIV infection once exposed. Studies of exposed health care workers indicate that the risk of HIV infection after percutaneous exposure to HIV-infected blood is approximately 0.3 percent.[12]

The risk after mucous membrane exposure (nonpercutaneous injury) is estimated at approximately 0.09 percent. Although cases of occupational HIV acquisition after blood exposure on intact skin have been anecdotally recorded, the magnitude of the risk is too low to establish an estimate. The magnitude of risk for transmission of HIV after exposure depends on several factors including the depth of injury, the presence of visible blood on the sharp instrument, the viral load in the source patient, and whether a hollow bore or solid needle transmitted the injury. During percutaneous needle-stick injury, the amount of blood transferred is reduced by glove use, leading to the recommendation for use of double gloving in high-risk settings.[2]

As of 2001, 57 health care workers have been reported to the CDC as being infected by HIV most likely by occupational risk. It is thought that little occult undiscovered transmission is occurring among health care workers. One way of

indirectly assessing the risk of occupational transmission of HIV in health care workers is to conduct HIV seroprevalence surveys. A 1992 survey of general surgeons, obstetricians, and orthopaedic surgeons was conducted among practices in moderate to high HIV risk areas. Among 770 physicians surveyed, only 1 was seropositive and he reported nonoccupational behavioral risks.[20] Similarly a 1991 survey of 3420 orthopaedic surgeons attending the annual meeting of the American Academy of Orthopedic Surgery found only two seropositives, both individuals who reported nonoccupational risks.[22] These studies suggest that ongoing occult transmission to surgeons is rare.

Management of Occupational Exposure to HIV

After transmission of HIV an acute retroviral syndrome resembling a mononucleosis-like illness has been a common finding in health care workers who have been occupationally infected. Symptoms such as fever, myalgias, rash, pharyngitis, and adenopathy may occur a median of 25 days after exposure, with a range of 1 to 6 weeks. HIV-specific antibodies appear from 6 weeks to 4 months after exposure in infected individuals. The average interval to development of HIV-specific antibodies has been 2 months. Serodiagnosis is accomplished by routine screening EIA followed by a Western blot for confirmation if the EIA was positive. These routine antibody measurements are usually recommended to be carried out at baseline (after exposure), 6 weeks, 3 months, and 6 months. Direct detection of viral RNA by PCR or antigenic assays such as P24 antigen may be useful as ancillary tests to serodiagnosis, but they should not be used to routinely detect infection in exposed health care workers owing to the relatively high rate of false-positive results. Serologic follow-up of exposed health care workers should also be accompanied by follow-up counseling and expert medical evaluation.

Postexposure prophylaxis with antiviral agents has become a cornerstone of management of occupational exposure to HIV since 1996. Recommendations for the choice of antiviral agents, dose, and duration have recently been updated.[6] Use of postexposure prophylaxis may be appropriate in percutaneous injury or contact of mucous membrane or nonintact skin with blood, tissue, or potentially infectious body fluids. The following fluids are considered potentially infectious: cerebrospinal, synovial, pleural, peritoneal, pericardial, and amniotic fluids. Feces, nasal secretions, saliva, sputum, sweat, tears, urine, and vomitus are not considered infectious for HIV unless they are visibly bloody. The risk of HIV transmission from these latter fluids is too low to justify postexposure antiviral prophylaxis.

Antiretroviral agents used in prophylaxis should never be used as single agents. Several classes of antiviral agents are available for use as postexposure prophylaxis, including nucleoside reverse transcriptase inhibitors, non-nucleoside reverse transcriptase inhibitors, protease inhibitors, and others. Regimens containing two drugs are usually recommended for basic postexposure prophylaxis. Most of these two drug regimens are based on azidothymidine (Zidovudine) plus lamivudine (Epivir) or Zidovudine plus emtricitabine (Emtriva), but many others are potentially useful. An enhanced regimen of three-drug prophylaxis is used for higher risk exposures and usually involves the addition of a protease inhibitor. The risk stratification of exposures is based on the nature of the injury and the status of the source HIV case.[13] Most authorities recommend starting the postexposure prophylaxis as soon as possible, preferably within hours of exposure, and continuing for 4 weeks.

These antiviral agents are potent drugs with a range of potential toxicities, including headache, nausea, bone marrow depression, diarrhea, peripheral neuropathy, rash (including Stevens-Johnson syndrome), and severe liver toxicity. Expert physicians should carefully monitor persons receiving postexposure antiviral prophylaxis.

STRATEGIES TO PREVENT OCCUPATIONAL TRANSMISSION OF BLOOD-BORNE PATHOGENS

The Hospital Infection Control Practices Advisory Committee (HICPAC), convened by the CDC, published the "Guideline for Isolation Precautions in Hospitals," which details basic infection control strategies that can significantly reduce the risk of blood-borne pathogen transmission among patients and health care workers.[9] Professional surgical organizations such as the American Association of Orthopedic Surgeons (AAOS) and the Association of Perioperative Registered Nurses (AORN) have also published specific guidelines for preventing the transmission of blood-borne pathogens. We focus here on a discussion of personal protective equipment and safe work practices because they are pivotal in preventing accidental exposures to blood and other body fluids.

Personal Protective Equipment (PPE)

In a surgical setting, gowns, gloves, masks, and hair coverings are worn to preserve the sterile field but they also serve as an effective barrier against accidental blood and body fluid exposure. Health care facilities are required by law to provide appropriate and effective personal protective equipment to employees who can reasonably anticipate exposure to blood and other body fluids during the performance of their work duties. OSHA defines personal protective equipment as "specialized clothing or equipment worn by an employee for protection against a hazard. General work clothes (e.g., uniforms, scrubs, pants, shirts, or blouses) are not considered to be personal protective equipment."

GLOVES

Gloves provide an excellent barrier to blood/body fluid exposure and represent the most common type of personal protective equipment used in health care. Gloves are available in a variety of sizes, styles, and textures and can be made of latex or synthetic materials. Gloves should be worn whenever exposure to blood/body fluids, excretions, secretions, nonintact skin, and mucous membranes is anticipated. Gerberding demonstrated that the volume of blood transmitted by a needlestick is reduced by 50 percent when the needle passes through a glove.[10] Double gloving for orthopaedic procedures is recommended by the American Academy of Orthopaedic Surgeons.[1] In addition they recommend that "during procedures where sharp instruments and devices are used, or when bone

fragments are likely to be encountered, the surgeon should consider the use of reinforced or cloth gloves that offer a greater amount of protection." Although gloves are an effective barrier, small holes may go undetected; therefore, it is important to always perform a thorough handwashing when the gloves are removed.

GOWNS

Surgical gowns protect health care workers by providing a barrier to blood and body fluids that are commonly generated during orthopaedic procedures. Gowns and aprons come in a variety of styles and are produced from a number of materials. When selecting a gown, one should consider the activity and amount of fluid likely to be encountered. Soiled gowns should be removed as promptly as possible, and hands should be washed to avoid transfer of microorganisms to other patients or environments.[9]

MASKS, EYE PROTECTION, AND FACE SHIELDS

Orthopaedic surgery frequently generates spatters and splashes of blood and other body fluids owing to the use of powered tools and the types of procedures performed. To protect the mucous membranes of the eyes, nose, and mouth against potential exposures, health care workers must wear masks and eye protection. A variety of products are available for mucous membrane protection. Surgical masks, surgical masks with attached plastic shields, face shields, goggles, and eyeglasses with side shields can provide adequate protection against exposure. Soiled masks, eye protection, and face shields should be removed as soon as possible after the procedure, and hands should be washed to avoid transfer of microorganisms to other patients or environments. Reusable protective equipment should be cleaned with an appropriate disinfectant.

OTHER PERSONAL PROTECTIVE EQUIPMENT

Traditional surgical accessories such as head and shoe covering provide additional barriers against exposure to blood and body fluids during orthopaedic procedures. Hair covering is an effective barrier against spatters and splashes, and footwear such as shoe covers or tall boots protects against the wet environment that can be experienced during orthopaedic procedures. Soiled accessories should be removed as soon as possible after the procedure, and hands should be washed to avoid transfer of microorganisms to other patients or environments.

WORK PRACTICES AND ENGINEERING CONTROLS

Assuring compliance with established guidelines can pose a difficult challenge in the surgical setting. Introducing safer work practices and changing deeply engrained behaviors is a slow but necessary process. OSHA requires that all health care workers whose job requirements expose them to blood and other body fluids receive training on the prevention of blood-borne pathogens before they begin those responsibilities. In addition, staff should be oriented to organizational policies and procedures as well as protocols specific to the perioperative setting.

Setting Expectations

Orthopaedic surgeons must set the standard for safe behavior in the operating room and insist on vigilance and compliance by the surgical team. Since surgical team members in close proximity to each other with sharp instruments are frequently required to work with blood and body fluids, inadvertent exposures may occur. For this reason, communication among team members is especially important. If an exposure does occur, the surgeon must strongly encourage reporting of the incident as soon as feasible.

Needles and Sharps

Of the 57 health care workers with documented occupationally acquired HIV infection, 51 (88%) had percutaneous injuries. The circumstances varied among the 51 percutaneous injuries, with the largest proportion (41%) occurring after a procedure, 35 percent occurring during a procedure, and 20 percent occurring during disposal of sharp objects.[8] In 2001, OSHA revised the Bloodborne Pathogens Standard, in response to the Needlestick Safety and Prevention Act.[19] The revised standard clarified the need for employers to select safer needle devices and to involve employees in identifying and choosing these devices. The number of safety needles and needle devices available on the market today is dizzying. New products should be periodically evaluated to determine whether they might reduce parenteral injury. Disposal of needles and other sharps into appropriately sized, puncture-resistant containers can reduce accidental exposures.

Needles are not the only sharp implements in orthopaedic surgery. For instance, the exposed end of all orthopaedic pins should be securely covered with a plastic cap or other appropriate device. The points of pins that have passed through soft tissue should be cut off. Specialized tools can cause cuts or abrasions if not handled properly.[20]

Hands-Free Technique (HFT)

The traditional method of passing instruments between team members is from hand to hand. To reduce potential exposures, some propose the use of a "neutral zone" to which instruments are returned during a procedure. The neutral zone can be a tray or magnetic pad that aids in the passing of surgical instruments and suture material.

Blunted Surgical Needles

"No-touch suturing techniques should be used whenever possible. Sutures should not be tied with the suture needle in the surgeon's hand. Blunt suture needles are recommended when their use is technically feasible. Two surgeons should not suture the same wound simultaneously."[1]

REGULATED MEDICAL WASTE

During the summer of 1987, New York and New Jersey beaches were closed because syringes, blood vials, and other medical waste products repeatedly washed ashore. The public's concern about HIV/AIDS transmission prompted legislators to enact the Medical Waste Tracking Act (MWTA) of 1988.[16] The MWTA amended the Solid Waste Disposal Act and promulgated regulations on the management of infectious waste. Each state was instructed to implement a medical waste tracking program that was at least as stringent as the federal demonstration program. To protect waste handlers and the general public from inadvertent exposure, medical waste was required to be segregated from other wastes and tracked in labeled containers. The specific solid wastes that require tracking are listed in Box 9-1,

---

Box 9-1 | Listing of Medical Wastes

1. Cultures and stocks of infectious agents and associated biologicals, including cultures from medical and pathological laboratories, wastes from the production of biologicals, discarded live and attenuated vaccines, and culture dishes and devices used to transfer, inoculate, and mix cultures.

2. Pathological wastes, including tissues, organs, and body parts that are removed during surgery or autopsy.

3. Waste human blood and products of blood, including serum, plasma, and other blood components.

4. Sharps that have been used in patient care or in medical, research, or industrial laboratories, including hypodermic needles, syringes, Pasteur pipettes, broken glass, and scalpel blades.

5. Contaminated animal carcasses, body parts, and bedding of animals that were exposed to infectious agents during research, production of biologicals, or testing of pharmaceuticals.

6. Wastes from surgery or autopsy that were in contact with infectious agents, including soiled dressings, sponges, drapes, lavage tubes, drainage sets, underpads, and surgical gloves.

7. Laboratory wastes from medical, pathologic, pharmaceutical, or other research, commercial, or industrial laboratories that were in contact with infectious agents, including slides and coverslips, disposable gowns, laboratory coats, and aprons.

8. Dialysis wastes that were in contact with the blood of patients undergoing hemodialysis, including contaminated disposable equipment and supplies such as tubing, filters, disposable sheets, towels, gloves, aprons, and laboratory coats.

9. Discarded medical equipment and parts that were in contact with infectious agents.

10. Biological waste and discarded materials contaminated with blood, excretion, exudates, or secretions from human beings or animals that are isolated to protect others from communicable diseases.

11. Such other waste material that results from the administration of medical care to a patient by a health care provider and is found by the administrator to pose a threat to human health or the environment.

although other types may be included in specific state plans. Health care settings have incorporated the segregation of medical waste; however, it is unclear whether this disposal has resulted in transmission prevention.

SUMMARY

Blood-borne pathogens present an uncommon but real risk to health care workers. Although risk cannot be completely eliminated, implementation of basic infection control strategies is an effective way to prevent occupational transmission. Measures such as vaccination, conscientious use of personal protective equipment, strict adherence to "universal precautions," and compliance with safe work practices can further reduce the low risk of occupational blood-borne pathogen transmission.

REFERENCES

1. American Academy of Orthopedic Surgeons. Advisory Statement: Preventing the Transmission of Bloodborne Pathogens. Available at: http://www.aaos.org/about/papers/advistmt/1018.asp.
2. Bennett, N.; Howard, R. Quantity of blood inoculated in a needle stick injury from suture needles. J Am Coll Surg 178:107–110, 1994.
3. Blumberg, B.S.; Alter, H.J.; Visnick, S. A new antigen in leukemia sera. JAMA 191:541–546, 1967.
4. Bushberg, J.T. The Essential Physics of Medical Imaging, 2nd ed. Philadelphia, Lippincott Williams & Wilkins, 2002.
5. Centers for Disease Control (CDC). Recommendations for prevention of HIV transmission in healthcare settings. MMWR 36(suppl. 2S), 1987.
6. Centers for Disease Control (CDC). Updated U.S. Public Health Service guidelines for the management of occupational exposures to HBV, HCV and HIV and recommendations for post-exposure prophylaxis. MMWR 50(RR-11), 2001.
7. Dienstag, J.L.; Ryan, D.M. Occupational exposure to hepatitis B virus in hospital personnel: Infection or immunization. Am J Epidemiol 115:115–129, 1982.
8. Do, A.N.; Ciesielski, C.A.; Metler, R.P.; et al. Occupationally acquired human immunodeficiency virus (HIV) infection: National case surveillance data during 20 years of the HIV epidemic in the United States. Infect Control Hosp Epidemiol 24(2):82–85, 2003.
9. Garner, S. Guideline for isolation precautions in hospitals. Infect Control Hosp Epidemiol 17:53–80, 1996; Am J Infect Control 24:24–52, 1996.
10. Gerberding, J.L. Current epidemiologic evidence and case report of occupationally acquired HIV and other bloodborne diseases. Infect Control Hosp Epidemiol 1(10):558–560, 1990.
11. Huda, W. Review of Radiological Physics, 2nd ed. Philadelphia, Lippincott Williams & Wilkins, 2003.
12. Ipploito, G.; Puro, B.; Decarli, G.; et al. The risk of occupational human immunodeficiency virus infections in health care workers. Arch Intern Med 153:1451–1458, 1993.
13. Jacekele, E.; Cornberg, M.; Wedemeyer, H.; et al. Treatment of acute hepatitis C with interferon alpha–2B. N Engl J Med 245:1452–1457, 2001.
14. McMahon, B.J.; Alward, W.L.; Hall, B.B. Acute hepatitis B viral infection: Relation of age to the clinical expression of disease and subsequent development of the carrier state. J Infect Dis 151:599–603, 1985.
15. McQuillan, G.M.; Alter, M.J.; Moyer, L.A.; et al. A population based serologic study of hepatitis C virus infection in the United States. In Rizzetto, M.; Purcell, R.H.; Gerin, J.L.; et al., eds. Viral Hepatitis and Liver Disease. Turin, Italy, Edizioni Minerva Medica, 1997, pp. 267–270.
16. Medical Waste Tracking Act of 1988 (H.R. 3515). 40 Code of Federal Regulations 22, 259. Mar. 24, 1989.
17. National Cancer Institute. Interventional Fluoroscopy: Reducing Radiation Risks for Patients and Staff, NIH Publication No. 05-5286, March 2005.
18. Occupational Safety and Health Administration (OSHA). Occupational exposure to bloodborne pathogens: Final rule. 29 Code of Federal Regulations 1910. Dec. 6, 1991.
19. Occupational Safety and Health Administration (OSHA). Occupational exposure to bloodborne pathogens—Needlestick and other sharps injuries: Final rule. 29 Code of Federal Regulations 1910.1030. Jan. 18, 2001.
20. Panililo, A.; Shapiro, C.; Schable, C., et al. Serosurvey of immunodeficiency virus, hepatitis B virus and hepatitis C virus infection among hospital based surgeons. J Am Coll Surg 180:16–24, 1995.
21. Poland, G.A. Hepatitis B immunization in health care workers: Dealing with vaccine nonresponse. Am J Prev Med 15:73–77, 1998.
22. Tokars, J.; Chamberland, M.; Schable, C. A survey of occupational blood contact and HIV infection among orthopedic surgeons. JAMA 268:489–494, 1992.
23. Wang, J.; Blackburn, T.J. The AAPM/RSNA Physics Tutorial for Residents: X-Ray Image Intensifiers for Fluoroscopy. Radiographics 2000;20:1471–1477.

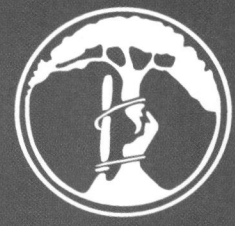

CHAPTER 10

Pharmacologic Management of the Orthopaedic Trauma Patient

PART I

Pain Management

Richard H. Gannon, Pharm.D.

Orthopaedic procedures are some of the most painful surgeries that are performed. The surgeries themselves or the trauma that preceded the surgery produce three of the most common pain syndromes: somatic, visceral, and neuropathic pain.

ASSESSMENT

Involving the patient in the pain assessment is crucial as it is the description of the patient's pain that will enable you to most effectively treat the patient's pain appropriately. The use of pain scales has helped objectify a subjective phenomenon.[19,60] An assessment/rating of the patient's mental status in conjunction with the pain scale may help avoid excessive sedation.[166] Institutions use a pain scale that best suits their patient population. Examples of pain scales include numerical (0–10), descriptive (excellent–poor), faces (smiling–sad), and behavioral for the cognitively impaired (grimacing, vocalizations, resistance to care, etc.). One of the most important questions for the patient is, "How would you describe your pain?" The importance of this question rests on the fact that if a patient has predominantly neuropathic pain (burning, muscle spasms, shooting, stabbing) then adjuvants such as anticonvulsants should be started.[29]

Whether the patient describes mostly somatic pain (aching, throbbing)/musculoskeletal pain or visceral (deep, crampy, diffuse) abdominal pain, then acetaminophen, nonsteroidal anti-inflammatory drugs (NSAIDs), and/or opioids are the medications of choice.

Patients sometimes have unrealistic expectations regarding the amount of pain they will have postoperatively, "I want to be pain free." Patient education concerning pain management during the pre- and postoperative period is very important. The goal should be to decrease a patient's pain from excruciating to mild. It is

unrealistic for a patient to expect to have no pain or that the pain will be eliminated immediately after surgery. It is important to review with a patient during preoperative teaching all the options available for pain management during the pre-, intra-, and postoperative periods.

PHARMACOTHERAPY

Nonsteroidal Anti-inflammatory Drugs

Prior to surgery a thorough medication history needs to be done. Medications that the patient is taking preoperatively may need to be held prior to surgery. Both aspirin and herbal medications need to be held for 1 week prior to surgery. Nonselective NSAIDs should be held for 3 to 4 days prior to surgery because NSAIDs cause platelet dysfunction. If an analgesic is needed, then acetaminophen or celecoxib can be used, since they do not have an effect on platelet function.[90] Recently, rofecoxib (Vioxx) was withdrawn from the market owing to an excessive risk of cardiovascular death occurring in patients taking the medication long term.[13] Valdecoxib (Bextra) also seems to cause an excess of cardiovascular deaths in patients taking the medication after open-heart surgery.[117] Higher doses of celecoxib (Celebrex), 400–800 mg/day, seem to have the side effect of increased cardiovascular death.[15]

Using NSAIDs postoperatively may decrease the use of postoperative opioids by 20 to 40 percent while maintaining the same degree of analgesia.[17,128,132] The NSAIDs appear to be equally effective when equivalent doses are used. Efficacy of NSAIDs may be patient specific so that if a patient fails to respond to one NSAID a different one can be tried. It is best to give the NSAIDs around the clock (ATC) rather than as needed (prn) because the NSAIDs are inhibiting a cascade of cytokine activation. If a patient has constant pain, ATC use of NSAIDs provides more consistent and constant analgesia. If patients develop dyspepsia from their NSAID, switching to a different NSAID may eliminate this side effect. The use of an enteric-coated product such as diclofenac (Voltaren) or a pro-drug such as sulindac (Clinoril) or nabumetone (Relafen) may also avoid dyspepsia.

There may be a pharmacodynamic interaction between aspirin and some of the nonselective NSAIDs in terms of affecting platelet function.[20] The inhibition of platelet function is a COX-1 mediated effect. If the nonselective NSAID is given on a consistent basis or before the daily dose of aspirin, the NSAID will occupy the COX-1 site on the platelet inhibiting the ability of the aspirin to cause an irreversible inhibition of platelet function. Nonselective NSAIDs will only temporarily impair platelet function. The COX-2-selective NSAIDs do not interfere with aspirin's effect on platelets.

Certain patients should not receive NSAIDs because of the high risk of precipitating congestive heart failure or acute renal failure.[42] Patients at risk have as preexisting conditions congestive heart failure, renal dysfunction, or liver disease with ascites.[173]

There is a growing amount of literature suggesting that NSAIDs have an effect on bone healing.[30] For patients with spinal fusions, nonselective NSAIDs should not be used, as they may affect the ability of the spine to fuse.[56] In one study, a short postoperative course of celecoxib, 200 mg every 12 hours for 5 days, did not seem to affect healing of the fusion and there was a decreased incidence of prolonged pain at the iliac crest bone harvesting site.[130] For patients with pain due to acute fractures, the short-term use of NSAIDs is not detrimental, but long-term use can prevent fractures from fusing. NSAIDs can be given to hip replacement and trauma patients to prevent heterotopic ossification. Naproxen, 500 mg bid for 2 weeks, has been successful.[30]

Acetaminophen

Sometimes acetaminophen, 1 g, is given as part of a preemptive analgesic regimen and then continued postoperatively as 1 g four times a day.[79] Since is the suggested maximum daily dose of acetaminophen, other acetaminophen-containing products should be avoided. Patients may have a prolongation of the international normalized ratio (INR) when high-dose acetaminophen is given while they are taking warfarin.[98] Certain patients are at risk for acetaminophen hepatotoxicity if more than 4 g/day is given. Patients who are alcoholic, have liver dysfunction, or are taking enzyme-inducing medications such as rifampin or carbamazepine have a higher potential for hepatotoxicity from acetaminophen.

Opioids

Patients may be using opioids before surgery. The amount of opioid used before surgery needs to be considered when deciding what medication and what dose should be used for postoperative analgesia. If a patient is using opioids prior to surgery, then giving just prn opioids for postoperative pain control may result in poor analgesia, adverse effects, over- or under-dosing, dosing intervals that are too long, or conflicts

between patients and provider-willingness to give pain medication. In an effort to resolve some of these issues, patient-controlled analgesia (PCA) has become popular. With this method of administering opioids, a continuous amount of opioid may be given as well as providing the patient with access to a "demand" dose of analgesic available at a specific interval, usually every 6 to 15 minutes.[64] Currently only morphine and meperidine are FDA approved and available in prefilled PCA syringes. We rarely use meperidine PCA because of its potential for metabolite (normeperidine) accumulation. Empty PCA syringes are available that can be filled with morphine at high concentrations, or other opioids may be used (fentanyl, hydromorphone, buprenorphine). Table 10-1 lists the usual PCA medications and dosing for patients who are opioid naïve or who have used low doses of opioids preoperatively. The literature suggests that demand-only dosing is just as effective and safer than continuous plus demand dosing in patients who are opioid naïve.[64]

Some patients take significant doses of opioids before surgery. If these patients are started on the "usual" doses of PCA analgesics, they will have poor pain control or opioid withdrawal. Patients using PCA can have their long-acting ATC analgesics continued, but the PCA should be used in demand mode only. These patients will require higher than usual demand dosing. Use of both the patient's own opioid and the continuous opioid from the PCA could result in side effects. What we usually do is discontinue the patient's long-acting opioid and increase the continuous dose of PCA to compensate for the long-acting opioid that has been discontinued.

Part of the education regarding PCA should include the fact that only the patient should push the demand button and not the nurse or family. Allowing family members or friends to push the demand button may cause excessive sedation.

The option exists to convert all of a patient's preoperative opioids into the PCA opioid. Table 10-2 is the opioid equivalence table that is used at Hartford Hospital. All the doses listed are equivalent to one another, both orally and parenterally. A patient's 24-hour opioid use should be totaled and converted to the equivalent opioid that will be used in the PCA. This dose should then be divided by 24 to determine the hourly continuous rate on the PCA. The demand dose is usually set at 50 to 100 percent of the hourly rate. Sometimes for slower onset analgesics (hydromorphone, morphine), the demand interval is set at 10 to 15 minutes to allow those analgesics to reach their peak effect before another demand dose is potentially available. Table 10-3 lists the suggested starting doses for PCA when patients have been on long-acting opioids.

Table 10-1					
Usual PCA Medications and Doses					
Drug	**Concentration**	**Continuous**	**Demand Dose**	**Demand Interval**	**4-hour Lockout**
Fentanyl	10 μg/mL	10 μg/hr	10 μg	5–10 min	300 μg
Hydromorphone	0.2 mg/mL	0.2 mg/hr	0.2 mg	6–15 min	6 mg
Morphine	1 mg/mL	1 mg/hr	1 mg	6–15 min	30 mg
Meperidine *(not recommended)*	10 mg/mL	10 mg/hr	10 mg	6–15 min	150 mg

Table 10-2
Opioid Equivalent Doses

Drug	Parenteral Dose	Oral Dose
Codeine	120 mg	180 mg
Fentanyl	100 µg	—
Hydrocodone	—	20 mg
Hydromorphone	2 mg	8 mg
Levorphanol	2 mg	4 mg
Meperidine	100 mg	300 mg
Methadone	2.5 mg	5 mg
Morphine	10 mg	20 mg
Oxycodone	—	15 mg
Tramadol	—	150 mg

When patients are able to take oral medication they can be switched to prn short-acting opioids or a combination of long-acting ATC opioids plus prn short-acting opioids. If sustained-release oxycodone or sustained-release morphine is used, the initial doses can be given and then the PCA discontinued 2 hours later. If a fentanyl patch is used, the patch should be applied and the PCA

discontinued 8 to 12 hours later. For some patients the transition from intravenous (IV) opioids to oral or topical opioids is difficult. To ease the transition, the ATC oral or topical opioid is started, then the PCA is changed to demand only for the next 24 hours. Appropriate adjustments in the ATC opioid can be made after reviewing the next 24-hour use of the PCA demand doses. The information in Table 10-4 can be used to switch patients from PCA to oral or topical products. The dose conversions in Tables 10-3 and 10-4 are estimates, and factors such as age, trajectory for recovery, and incomplete opioid cross-tolerance need to be considered when these calculations are done.

Patients in a methadone maintenance program should always have their methadone doses confirmed by the methadone treatment facility and have their dose continued while hospitalized. This is to make certain that the issues of opioid withdrawal, opioid addiction, and pain management are kept separate.[87] Some patients may be treated with oral buprenorphine-naloxone (Suboxone) instead of methadone as part of an opioid addiction program. Suboxone partially blocks the mu opioid receptor, making it difficult to control a patient's pain. It is probably best to discontinue the Suboxone while aggressively treating the patient's pain and then restart the Suboxone as the patient's pain subsides.[2] Opioid

Table 10-3
Preoperative Opioid Conversion

Preoperative Opioid Dose/24 hr	Hydromorphone	Morphine
Oxycodone SR 30–40 mg Fentanyl 25 µg/hr Morphine SR 60–90 mg	0.2 mg/mL; 30 mL Continuous: 0.3 mg/hr Demand: 0.3 mg q 15 min 4-hr lockout: 6 mg	1 mg/mL; 30 mL Continuous: 1.5 mg/hr Demand: 1.5 mg q 15 min 4-hr lockout: 30 mg
Oxycodone SR 60–80 mg Fentanyl 50–75 µg/hr Morphine SR 120–180 mg	0.5 mg/mL; 30 mL Continuous: 0.5 mg/hr Demand: 0.5 mg q 15 min 4-hr lockout: 10 mg	2 mg/mL; 30 mL Continuous: 2.5 mg/hr Demand: 2.5 mg q 15 min 4-hr lockout: 50 mg
Oxycodone SR 100–160 mg Fentanyl 100–125 µg/hr Morphine SR 240–320 mg	1 mg/mL; 30 mL Continuous: 1 mg/hr Demand: 1 mg q 15 min 4-hr lockout: 20 mg	5 mg/mL; 30 mL Continuous: 5 mg/hr Demand: 5 mg q 15 min 4-hr lockout: 100 mg
Oxycodone SR 180–240 mg Fentanyl 150–200 µg/hr Morphine SR 360–480 mg	1 mg/mL: 30 mL Continuous: 1.5 mg/hr Demand: 1 mg q 15 min 4-hr lockout: 30 mg	5 mg/mL; 30 mL Continuous: 7.5 mg/hr Demand: 5 mg q 15 min 4-hr lockout: 150 mg

Table 10-4
PCA Opioid Converter

Hydromorphone IV (mg/24hr)	Morphine IV (mg/24hr)	Fentanyl Patch	Oxycodone SR	Morphine SR
0–7	0–35	—	—	—
8–11	36–55	25 µg/hr	20 mg q12hr	30 mg q12hr
12–16	56–80	50 µg/hr	30 mg q12hr	45 mg q12hr
17–21	81–105	75 µg/hr	40 mg q12hr	60 mg q12hr
22–26	106–130	100 µg/hr	60 mg q12hr	90 mg q12hr

agonists/antagonists (nalbuphine, butorphanol, pentazocine) should not be given to patients taking methadone maintenance or Suboxone, since an immediate opioid withdrawal syndrome will be precipitated.

Methadone provides little to no analgesia for patients taking this medication once daily. In fact, these patients usually have a very low pain tolerance.[105] If the patient cannot be given food by mouth (NPO), the methadone should be converted to IV. The IV dose of methadone is approximately 50 percent of the oral dose. The total IV dose is divided so that equal amounts are given at 8- or 12-hour intervals. This is so the patient does not receive a large IV bolus of methadone as a single daily dose. Patients in a methadone maintenance program should have both a continuous and demand opioid during PCA treatment. Their initial doses should be at least 50 percent higher than the doses listed in Table 10-1. Patients taking high doses of methadone will require high doses of their analgesic opioid.

SELECTION OF OPIOIDS

Morphine is still the gold standard for analgesia. It is available in multiple dose forms for ease of administration: liquids (multiple concentrations), suppositories, injectable (IV, IM, SC, epidural), immediate-release tablets, and long-acting tablets/capsules (daily [qd] or every 8 to 12 hours [q8–12hr]). A new lipid-based morphine epidural formulation is available (DepoDur) for postoperative pain that provides analgesia for 48 hours.

One drawback with morphine is the production of a metabolite, morphine 6-glucuronide. This metabolite is a more potent analgesic than morphine itself; however, it does accumulate in patients who are elderly or who have renal insufficiency. Accumulation of the metabolite can cause sedation, confusion, and respiratory depression. These adverse effects are immediately reversible with naloxone. It may take 24 to 48 hours for these adverse effects to reverse once the morphine is stopped.

Hydromorphone has become our drug of choice because of its versatility and decreased incidence of side effects when used in the elderly or in patients with impaired renal function. It can be given PO, IM, IV, SC, rectally, and epidurally. An oral liquid is available as well as a concentrated injection. One of the issues with hydromorphone is that it has poor oral bioavailability. There is a difference in the equipotent doses between the oral and parenteral products. Oral hydromorphone 4 mg is equipotent to approximately 1 mg of parenteral hydromorphone.

The use of meperidine has dropped dramatically owing to the availability of safer alternatives. Meperidine has a metabolite, normeperidine, that has no analgesic activity but is a potent central nervous system stimulant. Normeperidine accumulates especially in patients with renal insufficiency. Patients may or may not show the signs of early toxicity (agitation, delirium, myoclonus) before they have the severe toxicity, which is a tonic-clonic seizure. Administration of naloxone should be avoided, since it may only precipitate more seizures. A benzodiazepine will stop the seizure, and if the meperidine is stopped the patient may not have another seizure. The half-life of normeperidine is 12 hours in patients with normal renal function. The half-life is longer in patients with renal insufficiency. If the meperidine is stopped, the adverse effects will decrease over the next 24 hours. If parenteral meperidine is used, the dose should be limited to at most 10 mg/kg/day (600–900 mg/day) for 48 hours in patients with normal renal function.[146] Intravenous meperidine is still excellent for treating postoperative and amphotericin B–induced shivering. Oral meperidine is not very potent; 50 mg provides no better analgesia than 1 g of acetaminophen or an NSAID. In fact, oral meperidine generates more normeperidine owing to the first-pass effect in the gastrointestinal tract.

Fentanyl can be used in a PCA when patients develop nausea, confusion, or pruritus from other opioids. Fentanyl does not accumulate in patients with renal insufficiency. When patients are ready to stop the parenteral fentanyl, a fentanyl patch can be applied that is equal in strength to the hourly use of fentanyl that can be determined from the PCA. The patch is applied to a nonhairy area of skin and held in place for 30 seconds. This facilitates good adherence between the patch and the patient's skin. The PCA and patch are overlapped for 8 to 12 hours, then the PCA can be stopped. Patients will usually need an oral prn short-acting opioid such as oxycodone, hydromorphone, or hydrocodone for breakthrough pain. Actiq is the fentanyl "lozenge on a stick." This is used prn but should be reserved for patients who cannot tolerate the usual oral opioids. It is expensive and somewhat difficult to use. A PCA fentanyl patch will be available soon. This device is about the size of a credit card and adheres to the skin. It delivers a dose of fentanyl via iontophoresis. Initial studies show that it is safe and effective.[86,167]

Oxycodone is safe in patients with renal insufficiency. Multiple oral dose forms of oxycodone are available: liquids, liquid concentrate, immediate-release tablets, and sustained-release tablets. With OxyContin, approximately 30 to 40 percent of the oxycodone in the tablet is immediately released with the rest being released over the ensuing 8 to 12 hours. Various oxycodone-acetaminophen combinations are available. Using the medication with the least amount of acetaminophen, usually 325 mg per tablet, should avoid acetaminophen toxicity. Patients should not ingest more than 4 g/d of acetaminophen on a chronic basis in order to avoid hepatotoxicity. Also available is an oxycodone-ibuprofen combination product (5 mg/400 mg per tablet).

Hydrocodone is not available as a stand-alone analgesic. It is combined with either acetaminophen or ibuprofen. The ibuprofen dose is 200 mg per tablet; however, the amount of acetaminophen per tablet varies widely from 325 mg up to 750 mg. A liquid formulation is available. Hydrocodone products are classified as CIII narcotics, so the prescription may be called into a pharmacy and refills may be written on the prescription.

Tramadol as an analgesic has a dual mechanism of action. Tramadol itself inhibits the reuptake of norepinephrine and serotonin while the major metabolite, desmethyltramadol, binds to the mu opioid receptor. Tramadol is not a controlled drug. There are two tablets; one is a 50 mg tablet and the other is 37.5 mg combined with acetaminophen 325 mg. A sustained-release product, which is given once daily, is available in 100, 200, and 300 mg strengths. Slow upward titration prevents the side effects of sedation, nausea, and dizziness from being problematic. The combination of tramadol and antidepressants may cause seizures or the serotonin syndrome; however, the incidence is low.

Methadone is a unique analgesic in that it has a long half-life (at least 24 hours), is inexpensive, and the (d) stereoisomer is an N-methyl D-aspartate (NMDA) receptor antagonist, which means it may have an effect on neuropathic pain. It is available as an injection (IV, IM), tablets, and a liquid. Despite the long pharmacokinetic half-life, the analgesic action persists for only 6 to 8 hours, so methadone for analgesia needs to be dosed every 6 to 8 hours. When methadone is initiated, a fixed initial dose should be started and not changed for 3 to 4 days, allowing the methadone to accumulate. Patients should have short-acting opioids for breakthrough pain. What should happen over the ensuing 3 to 4 days is that the use of the prn opioids should decrease. The conversion from other opioids to methadone can be difficult. The long half-life and the equivalency change depending on the amount of daily prior opioid use. Usually the equivalency is in the range of 10 to 25 percent of the morphine equivalent dose.

Hydroxyzine has been used as a "potentiator" of opioid analgesia for a number of years. In reality, the studies that demonstrated this effect were poorly designed as analgesic trials.[139] These studies used high doses of hydroxyzine (100 mg IM), while today the typical dose is 25 to 50 mg. It is true that hydroxyzine is an antihistamine, mild antiemetic, and potent sedative. It is very painful as an IM injection and has a long half-life (approximately 24 hours). For the most part now we avoid using hydroxyzine so that there is less of a problem with sedation.

Opioids commonly cause side effects; however, if these are promptly recognized and treated the side effects are manageable. Nausea and vomiting should be treated with antiemetics (haloperidol, metoclopramide, promethazine), and if these side effects occur frequently during the treatment, the antiemetics should be scheduled ATC. Patients will develop a tolerance to nausea and vomiting, but it may take 1 to 2 weeks. Reducing the dose of the opioid, changing the route of administration, increasing the time of infusion, or changing the opioid may all have a significant effect. Constipation is a side effect to which tolerance does not develop. Patients need to be started on a laxative that is both a softener and a stimulant. The laxatives need to be given daily so that if the patient is eating well there should be a bowel movement daily or every other day. Senokot-S, MiraLax, and lactulose can all be effective. An ileus can occur from opioids or surgery. For a postoperative ileus, if the patient is not taking opioids chronically, using buprenorphine may provide effective analgesia without aggravating the ileus. Buprenorphine is a partial mu receptor agonist. It has very little effect on smooth muscle and does not cause spasm of the sphincter of Oddi. It may precipitate opioid withdrawal in patients on methadone maintenance or in patients taking opioids chronically. For analgesic use, it is available only as an injection and can be given IM, IV, or via PCA.

Pruritus does not necessarily indicate a true allergy unless hives and a rash accompany it. Most opioids cause histamine release, which causes pruritus. Both oral and parenteral opioids will cause pruritus. It is thought that the least potent opioids (meperidine) cause more pruritus than the most potent (fentanyl). One of the treatments is to switch to a more potent opioid to relieve the pruritus. Antihistamines are somewhat effective for the pruritus.

If a patient becomes sedated, it is time to reassess the opioid therapy. Opioids will cause a decrease in respiratory rate, hypoventilation, and hypoxia. They do not cause dyspnea or tachypnea. Other causes of sedation need to be ruled out such as other medications (benzodiazepines), metabolic abnormalities, etc. Was the opioid dose titrated up too quickly? Is the patient on morphine and now has developed renal insufficiency? Unless the patient is apneic, naloxone (Narcan) should be given slowly and in a low dose to avoid a rebound in pain or opioid withdrawal. Naloxone 0.4 mg (1 mL) should be mixed with 9 mL of saline with 1 to 2 mL given by IV push every 1 to 2 minutes until the patient is awake or a satisfactory respiratory rate has been achieved. Naloxone's duration of action is short (30–60 minutes), so the patient will need to be monitored carefully for a few hours.

Myoclonus is seen most often with meperidine>morphine>hydromorphone. These involuntary, symmetrical muscle spasms occur while the patient is awake or asleep. Myoclonus occurs when the patient is being treated with high doses of opioids or the dose has been titrated up rapidly. Some adjuvants (gabapentin) also cause myoclonus. Sometimes the muscle spasms are painful, and other times it is the family that is bothered by the myoclonus. Decreasing the opioid dose or switching to a different opioid (methadone) will eliminate the myoclonus. A benzodiazepine or valproic acid will effectively decrease the number and/or intensity of the spasms.

Neuropathic pain is sometimes difficult to identify. It is important to ask patients how they would describe their pain. Words such as burning, stabbing, shooting, aching, throbbing, and electricity-like may indicate the presence of neuropathic pain. Procedures done to bone may affect the nerves that supply the bone marrow and bone matrix; therefore, neuropathic pain should be considered a component of bone pain.[114] Typically, this pain is described as being opioid resistant or insensitive. What usually happens when a patient is given an opioid for this pain is that the patient obtains some analgesia but it is of short duration. Patients also frequently have severe side effects at low doses of opioids. These are the patients who are sedated, awaken and ask for analgesics, then fall back asleep before the analgesic is administered. Typically, opioids alone are only fairly effective for neuropathic pain.[23,55] When opioids alone are used for neuropathic pain, patients tend to complain about poor pain control despite what we would consider adequate doses of opioid analgesics. The patient may then be labeled as an "addict" or as "drug seeking" when in reality if an adjuvant such as gabapentin is introduced early in therapy, the patient's pain control may be better with the combination of an opioid and gabapentin. When treating difficult neuropathic pain, multiple adjuvants may be needed, and it is best to use agents from different pharmacologic classes, for example, anticonvulsant + muscle relaxant rather than anticonvulsant + anticonvulsant.[4] The anticonvulsants are usually added first (gabapentin, oxcarbazepine, pregablin) because of their fast onset of action and their lack of significant drug interactions. A patient may have effective pain relief within 24 to 48 hours of initiation of therapy. If a patient has muscle spasms, opioids are not effective at relieving the spasm. Medications such as baclofen, lorazepam, and tizanidine are effective at relieving spasms. Diazepam and its metabolites have long half-lives so its use is minimal. Antidepressants are effective; however, they require a titration process, so their efficacy may be delayed. Usually patients respond in a shorter time and at a lower dose compared to that which is needed for an antidepressant effect. Lidocaine patch 5% (Lidoderm) is effective for topical pain syndromes. The lidocaine penetrates a few millimeters into the epidermis/dermis. The systemic blood levels are approximately one tenth of those needed to treat an arrhythmia. Table 10-5 lists the most commonly used adjuvants for neuropathic pain.

PART II

Antibiotic Therapy: General Considerations

Ioannis P. Kioumis,
Joseph L. Kuti, Pharm.D.,
David P. Nicolau, Pharm.D., F.C.C.P.

Antibiotics represent an inextricable part of infection therapy. A well-designed systematic review and meta-analysis[154] concluded that adjuvant antibiotic therapy for bone and joint infections resulted in an overall control of infection after 1 year in 78.6% of the patients while bacterial eradication was observed in 77.0% of the cases. More importantly, outcome seemed not to be influenced by the presence of acute or exacerbated chronic inflammation. Nevertheless, the use of antimicrobial agents can provide favorable results when it is appropriate, as defined by three principal elements:

Prompt initiation of the therapy

Selection of the proper agents for the pathogens of interest

Adequate dosage, including the administration scheme (quantity of the antibiotic, route and method of administration), and duration of the therapy

Table 10-5				
Neuropathic Pain Adjuvants				
Drug	**Class**	**Starting Dose**	**Dose Range**	**Side Effects/Comments**
Amitriptyline (Elavil)	Tricyclic antidepressant	10–25 mg PO at bedtime; titrate dose up every 3 days	25–150 mg daily	Sedation, anticholinergic effects, prolongation of corrected QT interval (QTc)
Baclofen	Muscle relaxant	5–10 mg PO tid; titrate dose up every 2–3 days	30–40 mg tid	Sedation, delirium, muscle weakness; avoid in renal insufficiency; withdrawal seizures
Carbamazepine (Tegretol)	Anticonvulsant	100 mg PO bid; titrate dose up every 3 days	400–1200 mg daily divided bid–tid	Sedation, SIADH, enzyme induction, bone marrow suppression; monitor serum levels for effect
Desipramine (Norpramin)	Tricyclic antidepressant	10–25 mg PO at bedtime; titrate dose up every 3 days	25–150 mg daily	Less sedation and anticholinergic effects than amitriptyline, prolongation of QTc
Duloxetine (Cymbalta)	Antidepressant (SSNRI)	20–30 mg PO daily; titrate up every 3 days	60–120 mg divided bid	Nausea, insomnia, headache, diarrhea, constipation; taper off to avoid withdrawal
Gabapentin (Neurontin)	Anticonvulsant	100–300 mg PO tid; titrate up every 24 hr	900–3600 mg divided tid	Sedation, confusion, myoclonus; decrease dose with renal impairment
Lidocaine patch 5% (Lidoderm)	Topical anesthetic	1 patch daily; on for 12 hr, off for 12 hr	1–3 patches per day depending on area needing analgesia; cut to fit	Skin irritation; apply to site of pain; effective for postherpetic neuralgia
Mexiletine	Antiarrhythmic	150 mg PO bid–tid; titrate up every 3 days	200–250 mg PO tid	Nausea, insomnia, delirium; no effect on ECG; not proarrhythmic
Oxcarbazepine (Trileptal)	Anticonvulsant	150 mg PO bid; titrate up every 2 days	300–600 mg PO bid	Sedation, SIADH
Pregabalin (Lyrica)	Anticonvulsant	75 mg PO bid; titrate up q 24 hr	75–300 mg PO bid	Somnolence, dizziness, peripheral edema
Tizanidine (Zanaflex)	Muscle relaxant	2 mg PO bid–tid; titrate up every 3 days	4–8mg PO tid	Sedation, hypotension, dry mouth
Valproic acid (Depakote)	Anticonvulsant	250–500 mg PO bid; titrate up every 3 days	500 mg–1 g PO bid; use same dose IV	Mild sedation, tremor, increased LFTs; monitor serum level
Venlafaxine (Effexor)	Antidepressant (SSNRI)	75 mg PO daily; titrate up every 3 days	150–225 mg PO daily	Nausea, headache, sedation, insomnia; taper off to avoid withdrawal

Abbreviations: SIADH, syndrome of inappropriate secretion of antidiuretic hormone; SSNRI, selective serotonin-norepinephrine reuptake inhibitor.

The significance of the appropriate initial antibiotic therapy is well recognized.[70,96,97,156] Recent data indicate that staphylococcal invasion and persistence within osteoblasts, if not prevented by early antibiotic administration, can reduce the efficacy of the subsequent antimicrobial regimen.[39] It might also emphasize that the empiric initial treatment should be de-escalated to a more targeted therapeutic regimen once susceptibility data become available. As the initial antimicrobial coverage is usually broad-spectrum, it can exert a selective pressure for the growth of multiresistant bacteria, resulting in so-called collateral damage. A further reason for de-escalating the initial empiric therapy to simpler agents is that it may also reduce the toxic potential of the initially chosen drugs, given that the duration of antimicrobial therapy for orthopaedic infections is often extremely long.

Although it is recognized that a number of host factors have to be considered in the choice of an antimicrobial agent, the most important is the site of infection. Therapy is expected to be effective only if an adequate concentration of the proper drug is delivered to the site of infection. The term "adequate" in most of the cases reflects the ability of the antibiotic concentrations to exceed multiples of the minimal inhibitory concentration (MIC) of the responsible pathogens at the site of infection and to maintain these levels for a certain period of time during which the antibiotic has to occupy a critical number of binding sites on the surface or in the microbial cell. In skeletal trauma–related infections, the therapeutic concentration of an antimicrobial agent is largely influenced by its ability to penetrate bone, the adequacy of the blood supply, the presence of pus, the local pH, and above all, the presence of foreign material. The last factor is of paramount importance, since certain bacteria are capable of creating surface-adherent microcolonies that produce a fibrous exopolysaccharide material known as glycocalyx and to organize a complex biofilm surface sufficient to protect them from the action of antibiotics. In addition, these microbes are deprived of nutrients, and therefore they remain in a static or slowly multiplying condition while being nonvulnerable to the circulating immunologic defenses as well as to the vast majority of the available antibiotics.[63,159] Effective therapy is more likely when the microbial inoculum is of limited size, so prompt initiation of the anti-infective therapy is a critical fact, especially when the infection is related to the presence of prosthetic devices. Finally, the adequacy of antibiotic therapy is also determined by the spectrum of the suspected pathogens, by the prevalence of local microbial resistance, and importantly, by the ability of the antibiotic to prevent the emergence of such resistance.

Once there is a need for therapeutic use of either a single agent or a combination of antibiotics, the antimicrobial spectrum, dose, adverse effects, and required dosage modifications in the presence of metabolic insufficiencies of each drug of interest have to be considered carefully. Table 10-6 presents the spectrum of activity for the commonly utilized parenteral therapies in orthopaedic infections. Table 10-7 describes the potential clinically significant adverse events related to these agents, and Table 10-8 provides information about the commonly utilized antibiotic dosages and dosage modifications in patients with renal or hepatic impairment.

Duration of antimicrobial therapy is usually linked to tolerability. In most cases, orthopaedic infections do not require chemotherapies exceeding 6 to 8 weeks. Agents possessing a very broad spectrum of activity are more prone to modify the patient's normal microbial flora, and this fact is more prominent with drugs having substantial antianaerobic activity. Since some antibiotics (e.g., β-lactams, linezolid) are evidently able to cause hematologic abnormalities, such as bone marrow suppression or bleeding time prolongation, and others are nephrotoxic (e.g., aminoglycosides) or hepatotoxic (e.g., certain quinolones, rifampin), patients should undergo periodic testing to allow early detection of these serious adverse effects (see Table 10-7). Plasma concentrations of aminoglycosides should be closely monitored in patients with renal impairment because of the apparent danger of toxic drug accumulation. Nevertheless, for a number of agents considerable experience regarding prolonged (or sometimes lifelong) administration, as in cases of long-term suppressive therapy, has been accumulated.

Although a variety of pathogens have been involved in orthopaedic infection, *Staphylococcus aureus* is the single most common organism causing osteomyelitis, and coagulase-negative staphylococci are more prevalent in prosthetic joint infection. It is apparent that in these cases the ideal agents should be able to combine potent in vitro activity, low toxicity potential, affordable cost, feasible administration scheme, and/or good oral bioavailability. While the choice of agents will depend in part on the local prevalence of methicillin resistance, antibiotics possessing these desirable characteristics include the following:

Fluoroquinolones
Trimethoprim-sulfamethoxazole
Rifampin
Minocycline, doxycycline
Teicoplanin, vancomycin
Linezolid
Daptomycin
Tigecycline

Oral antibiotic therapy can be as effective as parenteral treatment. Certain *fluoroquinolones* as well as *clindamycin*, agents known for their excellent bioavailability and bone penetration, can usually successfully substitute for parenteral regimens.[66,82,99] A meta-analysis of clinical studies comparing quinolones to control drugs performed by Stengel and coworkers in 2001 did not reveal any statistically significant differences in regard to efficacy,[154] but newer agents such as levofloxacin, moxifloxacin, and gatifloxacin have better in vitro activity against quinolone-susceptible staphylococci when compared with older compounds. Despite the fact that quinolones are highly appreciated for the above-mentioned advantages, it should be noted that in addition to their poor activity against enterococci, staphylococcal resistance to ciprofloxacin, levofloxacin, and moxifloxacin is increasing.[9] At the time of this writing, no controlled clinical trials of newer

Table 10-6

Antibiotic Spectrum of Activity for Commonly Utilized Parenteral Therapies in Orthopaedic Infections

Antibiotic	Gram-positive (+)*	VS Enterococci	MRSA	VR Enterococci	Gram-negative (−)†	Pseudomonas aeruginosa	Acinetobacter Species	Anaerobes
Natural penicillins: penicillin G	+	±	0	0	0	0	0	++‡
β-Lactamase-resistant penicillins: nafcillin, oxacillin	++	±	0	0	0	0	0	0
Aminopenicillins: ampicillin, amoxicillin	++	++	0	0	+§	0	0	++‡
Aminopenicillins + β-lactamase inhibitors: ampicillin/sulbactam	++	++	0	0	++	0	++	+++
Antipseudomonal β-lactams + β-lactamase inhibitors: Ticarcillin/clavulanate,	++	±	0	0	+++	+	+	+++
piperacillin/tazobactam	++	+	0	0	+++	+++	+	+++
First-generation cephalosporins: cefazolin	++	0	0	0	±	0	0	0
Second-generation cephalosporins: cefuroxime, cefamandole	+	0	0	0	+	0	0	±§
Third-generation cephalosporins: cefotaxime, ceftriaxone, ceftizoxime,	+	0	0	0	++	0	0	±§
ceftazidime	±	0	0	0	++	++	+	±§
Fourth-generation cephalosporins: cefepime	++	0	0	0	+++	++	+	0
Cephamycins: cefoxitin, cefotetan	++	0	0	0	+	0	0	+
Carbapenems: imipenem, meropenem	+++	+	0	0	+++	+++	+++	+++
ertapenem	+++	±‖	0	0	+++	0	0	+++
Monobactams: aztreonam	0	0	0	0	+++	++	0	0
Aminoglycosides: gentamicin, tobramycin, amikacin	0¶	+#	0	0	+++	++	±	0
Quinolones: ciprofloxacin, levofloxacin	+	0	0	0	++	++	±	±§
moxifloxacin	+++	+	±	0	++	0	0	++
Tetracyclines: doxycycline	+	+	+	±	±**	0	0	+
minocycline	++	+	++	±	±**	0	0	+
Glycylcyclines: tigecycline	+++	+++	++	+++	+++	0	++	++
Rifamycins: rifampin	++	0	+++	0	+**	0	0	0
Glycopeptides: vancomycin, teicoplanin	+++	+++	+++	0	0	0	0	+††
Oxazolidinones: linezolid	+++	+++	+++	+++	0	0	0	+††
Streptogramins: Quinupristin/dalfopristin	+++	++‡‡	+++	++‡‡	0	0	0	±§
Lipopeptides: daptomycin	+++	+++	+++	+++	0	0	0	+††

Table 10-6

Antibiotic Spectrum of Activity for Commonly Utilized Parenteral Therapies in Orthopaedic Infections—Cont'd

Antibiotic	Gram-positive (+)*	VS Enterococci	MRSA	VR Enterococci	Gram-negative (−)†	*Pseudomonas aeruginosa*	*Acinetobacter* Species	Anaerobes
Sulfonamide derivatives: Trimethoprim/sulfamethoxazole	+	0	+	0	+	0	0	0
Nitroimidazoles: metronidazole	0	0	0	0	0	0	0	+++
Lincosamides: clindamycin	++	0	0	+	0	0	0	++
Polymixins: colistin	0	0	0	0	+	++§§	++§§	0

Abbreviations: VS, vancomycin sensitive; VR, vancomycin resistant; MRSA, methicillin-resistant *Staphylococcus aureus*; 0, not active; ±, limited activity against few strains; +, clinically active against selected strains; ++, good activity; +++, excellent activity.

*Gram (+): streptococci group A, B, C, G, *Streptococcus pneumoniae*, methicillin-sensitive *Staphylococcus aureus*.
†Gram (−): enterobacteriaceae and other gram-negative bacteria, excluding nonfermentors (e.g., *Pseudomonas* and *Acinetobacter*).
‡Not active against *Bacteroides fragilis*.
§Limited action only against a number of species.
‖Limited action against *Enterococcus faecalis*.
¶Active against methicillin-sensitive *Staphylococcus aureus*.
#Active only in synergy.
**Action against only some species, enterobacteriaceae not included.
††Active only against gram-positive anaerobes.
‡‡Not active against *Enterococcus faecalis*.
§§Usually active against multiresistant strains.

quinolones in implant-associated infection with a sufficient follow-up period have been conducted, and moreover, the possibility of interactions of these agents with rifampin has not been systematically assessed. Clindamycin remains a valuable antistaphylococcal agent insofar as it retains activity against the most community-acquired methicillin-resistant *S. aureus* (CA-MRSA).[59]

The glycopeptide *vancomycin* has been traditionally used for the treatment of bone infections due to methicillin-resistant *S. aureus* (MRSA). Vancomycin use should be restricted to infections due to MRSA and to those patients who cannot tolerate alternative drugs. The bone penetration of this agent is marginal, especially in the cortical zone,[65] its killing rate is slow, it can be administered only intravascularly, dose adjustment is indispensable in patients with renal impairment, anaerobiosis at the site of deep infection may adversely affect its activity,[165] and its use has been correlated with an increased risk of infection recurrence.[159] Nonetheless, vast experience is present in the literature with this agent. *Teicoplanin*, another glycopeptide available in many countries outside the United States, possesses similar antistaphylococcal activity to vancomycin but has been reported to have better bone penetration.[35] An additional advantage is its potential for intramuscular administration. High-dose and prolonged therapy with teicoplanin has been associated with thrombocytopenia and neutropenia.[178]

Rifampin is of particular interest in orthopaedic infections because of its excellent action against staphylococci, independent of their susceptibility to methicillin.

This antibiotic also offers the advantage to remain active against static or slowly multiplying adherent staphylococcal populations, but it should never be used as monotherapy because in such cases resistance develops very rapidly.[115] As a component of combination therapy, rifampin appears to improve effectiveness when combined with ofloxacin, fusidic acid, trimethoprim-sulfamethoxazole, minocycline, linezolid, quinupristin/dalfopristin, and daptomycin but not with nafcillin.[36,80,116,126,136,162,182] The widely accepted fact that rifampin represents the cornerstone of antistaphylococcal combination regimens has raised interest for further investigation of novel rifamycin compounds for the treatment of implant-associated infections. **Minocycline** and **doxycycline,** both long-acting enterally available members of the tetracycline group of antibiotics, reveal good activity against many strains of MRSA and have been successfully used either alone or in combination with rifampin in a limited number of cases of relevant infections, including infections following osteosynthesis.[120,134]

For organisms resistant to oral drugs, outpatient parenteral antibiotic therapy (OPAT) has been successfully employed.[158] In these circumstances, once daily administered drugs, such as *ceftriaxone*, are preferred,[159] and teicoplanin has been administered three times weekly to treat osteomyelitis with favorable results.[63]

As a result of the difficulties related to the treatment of bone infections, the search for novel antimicrobials appears warranted. *Linezolid* is a promising antimicrobial

Table 10-7
Potential Clinically Significant Antibiotic-related Adverse Events*

Antibiotic Class	Adverse Events
Penicillins (natural penicillins, β-lacatamase–resistant penicillins, aminopenicillins, carboxypenicillins, ureidopenicillins, carbapenems, monobactams)	Hypersensitivity reactions, hematologic abnormalities (eosinophilia, neutropenia, thrombocytopenia)
	CNS reactions (seizures) possible with high doses
Cephalosporins (all generations, cefamycins)	Fewer hypersensitivity and hematologic reactions than with penicillins
Aminoglycosides	Ototoxicity, renal and vestibular toxicity
Quinolones (all generations)	CNS reactions (dizziness, headache, confusion)
	Liver function test abnormalities with some agents
	Cardiac dysrhythmias
	Drug-to-drug interactions
Tetracyclines	Phototoxicity
	Deposition in teeth
	Vestibular symptoms with minocycline
	Hepatotoxicity, pseudotumor cerebri
Glycylcyclines	Potentially severe nausea and vomiting
	Phototoxicity and deposition in teeth similar to tetracyclines
Rifamycins	Hepatic abnormalities, hepatic failure (rare)
	Headache, urine discoloration
	Drug-to-drug interactions
Glycopeptides	Ototoxicity and nephrotoxicity (rare)
	Hematologic abnormalities
	Hypersensitivity reactions
	Rapid infusion may cause histamine release (red neck syndrome)
Linezolid	Reversible myelosuppression after prolonged use
	Lactic acidosis, neuropathy, retinopathy
	Drug-to-drug interactions (inhibitor of monoamine oxidase)
Quinopristin + dalfopristin	Venous irritation, arthralgias, myalgias
	Drug-to-drug interactions
Daptomycin	Potential muscle toxicity (increased creatine phosphokinase and myalgias), hypersensitivity reactions
Trimethoprim/sulfamethoxazole	Skin reactions, photosensitivity (rare)
Metronidazole	Disulfiram-like reaction when ingested with alcohol
	Neurologic disturbances
	Urine discoloration, urticaria
Clindamycin	Hypersensitivity reactions
Colistin	Nephrotoxicity, neurotoxicity

*This listing excludes gastrointestinal (e.g., vomiting, nausea, and diarrhea) and *Clostridium difficile* enterocolitis, as these adverse effects have been observed with all antimicrobials.

agent possessing 100% bioavailability, high bone penetration, and potent activity against virtually all gram-positive cocci,[94] but data from large clinical trials, although favorable, are still scarce.[14,74] Interestingly, a few studies comparing linezolid versus vancomycin in severe infections concluded that linezolid was superior.[170,180] However, it is not clear whether this effect can be attributed to the better pharmacologic properties of linezolid or is related to *S. aureus* heteroresistance to vancomycin.[75] *Tigecycline*, a new glycylcycline antibiotic approved in the United States for complicated skin and skin structure infections, exhibits broad-spectrum activity and has also been evaluated in experimental osteomyelitis with encouraging results.[47,181] It is worthwhile to mention

that tigecycline is not active against *Pseudomonas aeruginosa*. *Daptomycin*, a cyclic lipopeptide, is rapidly bactericidal in vitro against MRSA and vancomycin-resistant staphylococci and enterococci. This agent shows efficacy in a limited number of studies involving drug-resistant gram-positive bone and joint infections[43] as well as in experimental models of staphylococcal chronic osteomyelitis[132] and foreign body infections.[137] Nonetheless, it should be pointed out that this agent is reported to display a six-fold increase in the stationary-phase MBC of *Staphylococcus epidermidis* and a low activity on adherent *S. aureus* and *S. epidermidis* in vitro as well as in tissue-cage models.[8] The orally available mixture of streptogramins A and B, *pristinamycin*, has also been tested against methicillin-resistant *S.*

Table 10-8

Generally Utilized Antibiotic Dosages and Dosage Modifications in Patients with Renal and Hepatic Impairment

Antibiotic	Dose for Normal Renal Function	Adjustment for Renal Impairment for Estimated Creatinine Clearance (CrCl) (mL/min)			Hepatic Disease Dosage Adjustment
		>50–90	10–50	<10	
Penicillin G	Low: 600,000–1.2 million U IM qd High: >20 million U IV qd	None	75%	20–50%	
Nafcillin/oxacillin	1–2 g IM/IV q4hr	None	None	50–75%	Dose reduction; specific recommendations do not exist
Ampicillin	150–200 mg/kg IV qd	None	q8–12hr	q12–24hr	
Amoxicillin/ clavulanate	500/125 mg tid PO 875/125 mg bid PO	None	250/500 mg amoxicillin q12hr	250/500 mg amoxicillin q24hr	
Ampicillin/ sulbactam	1.5–3 g IV q6hr*	None	q8–12hr	q24hr	
Ticarcillin/ clavulanate	3.1–5.2 g IV q4–6hr†	None	2.0 g q4–8hr	2.0 g q12hr	
Piperacillin/ tazobactam	3.375–4.5 g IV q6hr†	None	2.25 g q6hr	2.25 g q8hr	
Aztreonam	1–2 g q6–8hr†	None	50–75%	25%	
Imipenem	0.5–1 g IV q6–8hr†	250–500 mg q6–8hr	250 mg q6–12hr	125–250 mg q12hr	
Meropenem	0.5–2 g IV q6–8hr‡	1 g q8hr	1 g q12hr	0.5 g q24hr	
Ertapenem	1 g IM/IV q24hr	None	0.5 g q24hr	0.5 g q24hr	
Cefazolin	1 g IM/IV q6–8hr	None	q12hr	q24–48hr	
Cefuroxime	0.75–1.5 g IM/IV q8hr	None	q8–12hr	q24hr	
Cefotaxime	1–2 g IV q4–12hr	q8–12hr	q12–24hr	q12–24hr	
Cefoxitin	1–2 g IM/IV q6hr	q8hr	q8–12hr	q24–48hr	
Cefotetan	1–3 g IM/IV q12hr	None	50%	25%	
Ceftriaxone	1–2 g IV q12–24hr‡	None	None	None	Dose reduction only with concomitant severe renal failure
Ceftizoxime	1 g IV q8–12hr	None	q12–24hr	q12–24hr	
Ceftazidime	1–2 g IM/IV q8–12hr	None	q24–48hr	q48hr	
Cefepime	1–2 g IV q8–12hr†	None	2 g q12–24hr	1 g q24hr	
Amikacin	15 mg/kg q24hr	60–90% q12hr	30–70% q12–18hr	20–30% q24–48hr	
Tobramycin	5–7 mg/kg q24hr	60–90% q8–12hr	30–70% q12hr	20–30% q24–48hr	
Gentamicin	5–7 mg/kg q24hr	60–90% q8–12hr	30–70% q12hr	20–30% q24–48hr	
Ciprofloxacin	200–400 mg IV q8–12hr†	None	50–75%	50%	
Levofloxacin	250–750 mg PO/IV q24hr	None	750 mg initially, then 500 mg q48h	750 mg initially, then 500 mg q48hr	
Moxifloxacin	400 mg PO/IV q24hr	None	None	None	No dosage adjustment required in mild and moderate hepatic insufficiency
Doxycycline	100 mg PO/IV q12hr	None	None	None	
Minocycline	100 mg PO q12hr	None	None	None	No dosage adjustment in hepatic insufficiency
Tigecycline	100 mg IV initially, then 50 mg IV q12hr	None	None	None	
Rifampin	600–900 mg PO/IV q24hr	None	None	None	Administration in patients with hepatic impairment only under careful monitoring

(Continued)

Table 10-8
Generally Utilized Antibiotic Dosages and Dosage Modifications in Patients with Renal and Hepatic Impairment—Cont'd

Antibiotic	Dose for Normal Renal Function	Adjustment for Renal Impairment for Estimated Creatinine Clearance (CrCl) (mL/min)			Hepatic Disease Dosage Adjustment
		>50–90	10–50	<10	
Vancomycin	15 mg/kg q12hr§	1 g q12hr	1 g q24–96hr	1 g q4–7days	
Teicoplanin	12 mg/kg IM/IV q12–24hr	q24hr	q48hr	q72hr	
Linezolid	600 mg PO/IV q12hr	None	None	None	
Quinupristin/ dalfopristin	7.5 mg/kg q8hr¶	None	None	None	Dose reduction in patients with severe hepatic insufficiency
Daptomycin	4–6 mg/kg IV q24hr	4 mg/kg/d	CrCl <30, 4 mg/kg q48hr	CrCl <30, 4 mg/kg q48hr	
Trimethoprim/ sulfamethoxazole	8–10 mg/kg/d divided to q6, 8, or 12hr#	None	50%	Not recommended for use	
Metronidazole	7.5 mg/kg IV q6hr or 15 mg/kg IV q12hr	None	None	None	Dosage in hepatic failure: 50% q12hr
Clindamycin	600–900 mg IM/IV q8hr	None	None	None	Dose reduction only with concomitant severe renal failure
Colistin (colistimethate)	2.5 mg/kg q12hr	None	2.5 mg/kg q24hr	2.5 mg/kg q36hr	

*Dosage for *Acinetobacter* species infection is usually higher (16–24 g qd).
†High dose is used for *Pseudomonas aeruginosa* infections.
‡High dose is used for meningitis.
§Critically ill patients probably require loading dose (25 mg/kg).
¶Central line required.
#Calculations based on trimethoprim component.

aureus osteoarticular infections with fairly good results.[110] Patients having difficult-to-treat infections, including osteomyelitis, have been successfully treated in the outpatient setting by the intravenous administration of *quinupristin/dalfopristin*, another streptogramin A and B combination.[129]

Despite the existence of a wide armamentarium of antimicrobial agents against orthopaedic surgery–related infections, the outcome in many cases is still suboptimal. The development of advanced techniques for delivering antibiotics to the infection locus and the possible utilization of compounds, such as RNAIII-inhibiting peptide,[6] that act on the bacterial quorum-sensing mechanism (thereby disrupting bacterial cell-to-cell communication and subsequent biofilm formation) may present future options for the therapy of these difficult-to-treat infections.

PART III

Anticoagulation

Elizabeth E.C. Udeh, Pharm.D., B.C.P.S.

Venous thromboembolism (VTE) is a common preventable complication following orthopaedic surgery and a primary indication for use of anticoagulants in this patient population. VTE, which can manifest as deep vein thrombosis (DVT) and pulmonary embolism (PE), is a major health concern and is cited as one of the leading causes of mortality that is responsible for over 2 million deaths annually.[147] The reported annual incidence varies from 1 to 2 per 1000 worldwide.[12,57] In North America and Europe, the incidence of VTE in the general population is estimated to be 160 per 100,000 for DVT and 70 per 100,000 for PE.[12] In major orthopaedic surgery, varying rates of DVT and PE have been reported in numerous studies and range from 50 to 80 percent without prophylaxis and 10 to 25 percent with effective prophylactic protocols of venographically documented DVTs.[38,49,53,77] Death from fatal PE is estimated to be 13 percent after hip fracture surgery and up to 20 percent following hip replacement.[49] Post-thrombotic syndrome (venous insufficiency, ulcers, and pain) is a long-term complication of VTE with a reported incidence of 60 to 70 percent within 5 years after a DVT.[67] Twenty-five percent of the 300 annual cases of venous ulcers per 100,000 patients reported in the literature are associated with DVTs.[111]

Pathophysiology of Venous Thromboembolism

The clinical course of VTE is controlled by the balance between factors that promote clot formation (vascular damage, venous stasis, hypercoagulability) and the intrinsic fibrinolytic system (normal blood flow, natural thrombolytics).[69] A disruption in this balance causes thrombogenic stimuli to overwhelm the endogenous antithrombotic system, resulting in clot formation.[69] Orthopaedic surgery with its associated instrumentation predisposes patients to vascular damage, venous stasis, and hypercoagulability, making it a powerful risk factor for VTE.[10] The importance of these three factors in the pathogenesis of thromboembolism was recognized by Rudolf Virchow in the eighteenth century—Virchow's triad.[69] Vascular damage initiates platelet aggregation and the release of tissue thromboplastin. Tissue thromboplastin activates the extrinsic pathway of the coagulation cascade, while at the same time substances in the blood from the damaged vessel activate the intrinsic pathway via factors XIa and XIIa. The net effect is the activation of factor X in the common pathway with subsequent conversion of factor II (prothrombin) to factor IIa (thrombin), and then the conversion of fibrinogen to fibrin clot.[69] Most DVTs develop within the distal deep veins of the calf muscles (84%) and less frequently in the proximal veins (40%).[10] If untreated, 20 to 25 percent of calf vein thrombi will extend to the proximal vein, the origin of most pulmonary emboli.[53,57] In addition to the inherent thrombogenic potential of orthopaedic surgery, many patients undergoing major orthopaedic procedures have co-morbid conditions and risk factors that facilitate VTE. These risk factors are discussed in the following section.

Risk Factors for Venous Thromboembolism

Many clinical conditions predispose patients to VTE and also decrease survival after a VTE event (Table 10-9). These risk factors include inheritable conditions such as deficiencies in antithrombin III, protein C, and protein S; acquired hypercoagulable disorders such as hyperhomocysteinemia; elevated levels of factor VIII; hormonal therapy; and co-morbid conditions such as obesity, metabolic syndrome, malignancy, and previous VTE.[10,53,57,68] Recently long-haul air travel (>8 hours) was added to the growing list of risk factors for VTE and is associated with a 10 percent prevalence of DVT.[48] These risk factors are cumulative, and it is not uncommon for multiple risk factors to be present in a patient prior to orthopaedic surgery.[53] Several risk assessment models have been published in an effort to help clinicians stratify patients for VTE risk (low, moderate, high, and highest).[49,53] The American College of Chest Physicians (ACCP) in their 2004 guideline strongly recommended that every health institution have a program in place for assessing a patient's risk for developing VTE.[53]

Clinical Manifestations of Venous Thromboembolism

The clinical signs and symptoms that are associated with but not specific to DVT may include the following: unilateral leg pain or tenderness, swelling, discoloration, vein distention, and a palpable cord in the calf of the affected leg.[68] Pain behind the knee or calf upon dorsiflexion of the foot (Homan's sign) may be present in less than 50 percent of patients with DVT.[68] Many patients with DVT are asymptomatic while still at very high risk for PE.[68] PE can manifest with dyspnea, tachypnea, tachycardia, chest pain, cough, hemoptysis, sudden death, or no symptoms at all.[57] It is reported that 70 percent of patients with a diagnosis of PE have asymptomatic DVT while clinically silent (asymptomatic) PE is present in approximately 50 percent of patients with venographically documented DVT.[53,57]

Diagnosis of Venous Thromboembolism

The diagnosis of VTE is difficult, as many patients remain asymptomatic and the reported clinical symptoms are not specific for VTE. Noninvasive tests include imaging and nonimaging techniques. The imaging tests include radiographic duplex ultrasonography (DUS) of leg veins (Doppler, B-mode), impedance plethysmography, magnetic resonance imaging, and fibrinogen uptake scan of the leg and have all been validated for the diagnosis of DVT.[68] However, their specificity and sensitivity for detecting DVT vary depending on the experience of the examiner.[68] The only nonimaging, noninvasive diagnostic test is the whole blood D-dimer assay, which is limited by false-positive results and a negative predictive value that varies with assay sensitivity and methodology.[57,68] The gold standard test is venography (bilateral or unilateral) using radiocontrast material.[68,164] This is an invasive test that exposes the patient to contrast-induced hypersensitivity reaction.[57]

Diagnostic tests for PE include ventilation perfusion (V/Q) scanning, spiral computed tomography (CT) scanning, and selective pulmonary angiography.[57] V/Q scanning is the most widely used test but is diagnostic in only 30 to 40 percent of confirmed PE cases.[57,68] Spiral CT scanning is mostly sensitive for large clots, while pulmonary angiography, the gold standard (>90% sensitivity and specificity), is an invasive procedure associated with significant complications.[57] Overall diagnosis and initiation of treatment were made in only 25 percent of the annual estimated PE cases.[57] Abnormalities in chest radiographs, electrocardiograms, and arterial blood gases are common in patients with PE but are nonspecific.[57] Routine screening of high-risk patients with DUS to diagnose and preemptively treat asymptomatic patients was not validated in large trials and not recommended.[53] Cumulative risk assessment and stratification of the patients is a useful diagnostic aid for VTE.

Rationale for Thromboprophylaxis of Venous Thromboembolism

The rationale for VTE prophylaxis relates to the relative nonspecificity of the clinical presentation, the low

Table 10-9
Clinical Risk Factor Profile for Prevention of Venous Thromboembolism (VTE)

VTE Risk Factors

Co-morbid Conditions	Inherited or Acquired Thrombophilia
Acute infections, pneumonia, sepsis	Activated protein C resistance
Cancer/malignancies	Antiphospholipid antibodies
Cardiac disorders (heart failure, MI)	Antithrombin III deficiency
Central venous catheterization	Hyperhomocysteinemia
Cigarette smoking	Lupus anticoagulant
Immobility/paralysis/spinal cord injury	Prothrombin G20210A mutation
Inflammatory bowel disorders	Medications
Ischemic stroke	Estrogens and hormonal therapy
Major surgery in past few months	Oral contraceptive use
Metabolic syndrome	Natural
Myeloproliferative disorder	Increasing age
Nephrotic syndrome	Pregnancy or postpartum
Obesity (>20% of ideal body weight)	Others
Orthopaedic surgery in past few months	Casts and cement use in orthopaedic surgery
Previous or strong family history of VTE	Long distance air travel
Respiratory failure, severe COPD	
Thrombotic disorders, varicose veins	
Trauma, especially with fractures	

Bleeding Risks and Contraindications to Anticoagulants

Active bleeding
Coagulopathy or low platelet count of <20,000 m^3
Hypersensitivity
Intracranial bleeding
Neuraxial anesthesia/analgesia <24 hours ago
Recent brain or eye surgery
Recent trauma to brain or spinal cord
Spinal tap or lumbar puncture <24 hours ago

Data from references 12, 18, 48, 53, 57, 68, and 69.

sensitivity and specificity of the diagnostic tests, and the rather sudden and catastrophic complications of PE. VTEs are clinically silent in a large percentage of patients, and the resultant PE is often sudden with a fatal outcome.[18,53,58] The increasing number of the elderly population eligible for surgery, recurrence of VTE in about one third of patients within 10 years of the first episode, and high incidence (40–80%) and risk of VTE following orthopaedic surgery underscore the need for routine thromboprophylaxis.[38,53,57,77,142] In one report, as many as 70 to 80 percent of hospitalized patients who died of PE did not receive the diagnosis prior to their death.[53,69] Nonfatal VTE highly predisposes patients to future VTE and chronic post-thrombotic syndrome (venous insufficiency, pain, ulcers).[18,53,67] Prediction of at-risk patients who will progress to symptomatic VTE complications is virtually impossible.[53] In the absence of prophylaxis, enormous financial cost could be incurred by investigating and treating symptomatic patients.[18,53] VTE treatment also predisposes patients to risk of bleeding.[18] Finally, currently available preventive measures are highly efficacious in preventing VTE, associated complications, and cost.[18,33,53,67]

Prevention of Venous Thromboembolism

Proactive identification and prophylaxis of patients at high risk for VTE to decrease overall incidence of VTE and its associated complications are an ideal goal in orthopaedic surgery. A desirable strategy would be highly efficacious, safe, and cost effective. None of the currently available prophylactic measures are ideal for all patients, thus selection of the regimen should be based on the patient's risk stratification. The effectiveness of numerous pharmacologic and mechanical modalities has been proven in clinical studies.[18,38,46,53,77,85,89,93,104,164]

NONPHARMACOLOGIC STRATEGIES

Mechanical modalities (compression stockings, pneumatic compressors, foot pumps) and early ambulation prevent VTE by increasing the velocity of venous blood flow, thereby preventing venous stasis without the bleeding risk associated with anticoagulants. The use of mechanical prophylaxis is associated with a relative risk reduction against DVT of 20 to 70 percent; however, its effectiveness is lower than that of anticoagulant-based methods.[46,53]

An evidence-based review showed that graduated compression stockings (GCSs) reduced the relative risk of DVT by 64 percent in general surgery patients and by 57 percent following total hip replacement (THR).[1] The effect of GCSs was enhanced when combined with other anticoagulants.[1,10,73,77,145] Intermittent pneumatic compression (IPC) devices (boot and plantar foot pump) also enhance fibrinolysis and have reduced the incidence of VTE following orthopaedic surgery.[18,46,53,142] GCSs and IPC are recommended in combination with anticoagulants to enhance efficacy and for patients at high risk of bleeding.[53] Retrievable vena cava (VC) filters can be used for short-term therapy in very high risk patients and those patients with transient contraindication to anticoagulants.[53,57]

PHARMACOLOGIC STRATEGIES

In orthopaedic surgery, low-dose unfractionated heparin (LDUFH), low-molecular-weight heparins (LMWHs), pentasaccharides, vitamin K antagonists, warfarin, and aspirin have been mostly studied and compared for thromboprophylaxis despite controversies on the best markers for

efficacy and outcome.* Several newer agents are being evaluated in clinical trials for the prevention of VTE[27,40,71] (Table 10-10).

Unfractionated heparin (UFH) is a heterogeneous mixture of polysaccharide polymers that binds to antithrombin III (ATIII) to inhibit factors IXa and Xa and formation of thrombin. In a meta-analysis, heparin 5000 units every 8 to 12 hours was superior to no prophylaxis but less effective than LMWH and fondaparinux in high-risk orthopaedic patients.[46] Adjusted-dose UFH to maintain a partial thromboplastin time (PTT) in the upper normal range seems to be more effective but has been used only in small clinical trials and requires frequent monitoring.[53] In addition to bleeding risk common to all anticoagulants, heparin is associated with heparin-induced thrombocytopenia (HIT types 1 and 2).[12] LDUFH is not recommended as a single agent for thromboprophylaxis in elective hip and knee arthroplasty but can be used in hip fracture surgery.[53]

LMWHs (enoxaparin, dalteparin) are more specific for the inhibition of factor Xa and have been proven to be efficacious and safe for thromboprophylaxis in orthopaedic surgery.[58] LMWHs have a more predictable

Table 10-10			
Thromboprophylaxis in Orthopaedic Surgery			
Indication	**Recommended Medication (Grade)**	**Timing (hr)**	**Duration (days)**
Total hip arthroplasty	Dalteparin 5000 IU SC daily (1A)	12 hr presurgery or 12–14 hr postsurgery	10; extend to 28–35
	Enoxaparin 30 mg SC q12 h (1A)		
	Enoxaparin 40 mg SC daily (1A)		
	Dalteparin 2500 IU SC pre- and postsurgery; 5000 IU SC daily	<2 hr presurgery, 4–6 hr postsurgery, or daily starting next day	10; extend to 28–35
	Fondaparinux 2.5 mg SC daily (1A)	6–8 hr after surgery	10, extend to 28–35
	Adjusted-dose VKA: INR 2–3 (1A)	Presurgery or evening postsurgery	10, extend to 28–35
	LDUFH: not recommended alone (1A)		
Total knee arthroplasty	Dalteparin 5000 IU SC daily (1A)	Same as above	10, may extend if cumulative is risk high
	Enoxaparin 30 mg SC q12hr (1A)		
	Enoxaparin 40 mg daily (1A)		
	Adjusted-dose VKA: INR 2–3 (1A)		
	Fondaparinux 2.5 mg SC daily		
Hip fracture surgery	Fondaparinux 2.5 mg SC daily (1A)	Preoperatively when surgery is delayed; postoperatively when bleeding stabilizes	10, extend to 28–35
	Dalteparin 5000 IU SC daily (1C)		
	Enoxaparin 30 mg SC q12hr (1C)		
	Adjusted-dose VKA: INR 2–3 (2B)	Preoperatively when surgery is delayed; postoperatively when bleeding stabilizes	
	LDUFH 5000 IU q8hr (1B)		
Trauma with fractures	Enoxaparin 30 mg SC (NA)	Bleeding is stabilized	Base on risk stratification
	Dalteparin 500 IU SC daily (NA)		
	Fondaparinux 2.5 mg SC daily (NA)		
Elective spine ↑ risk	Heparin 5000 IU SC q8hr (1C)	Postsurgery	Base on risk stratification
	Enoxaparin 30 mg SC daily (1B)		

Abbreviations: IU, international units; SC, subcutaneously; LDUFH, low-dose unfractionated heparin; INR, international normalized ratio; VKA, vitamin K antagonist.
Data from references 12, 53, 57, and 147.

*See references 10, 12, 18, 25, 46, 53, 89, 93, 104, 111, 113, 119, 122–124.

dose-response relationship and were more effective than LDUFH.[46,53,85] They also have a lower incidence of HIT.[10,12,53] When compared with warfarin, the results are conflicting; however, a meta-analysis of two randomized trials found LMWHs more efficacious than adjusted-dose warfarin for prevention of total and proximal DVT in total knee arthroplasty (TKA) with increased bleeding risk when initiated preoperatively.[85,124] Comparative efficacy of LMWHs for thromboprophylaxis in orthopaedic surgery concluded clinical equivalence among three different LMWHs.[89,122] Enoxaparin needs dosage adjustment for patients with renal impairment.

Pentasaccharides are synthetic analogues of antithrombin-binding pentasaccharide sequences found in UFH and LMWH. Fondaparinux, the first agent in this class, selectively inhibits factor Xa activity and thus inhibits thrombin generation. A systematic review and a meta-analysis found fondaparinux, 2.5 mg subcutaneously (SC) commencing about 6 hours after surgery for up to 11 days, to be more effective than enoxaparin (relative risk reduction of 55%) in reducing VTE following total hip replacement (THR), total knee replacement (TKR), and hip fracture surgery (HFS), with a significant increase in bleeding rate.[164] Fondaparinux is approved for VTE prophylaxis following orthopaedic surgery and for extended prophylaxis following HFS but is not recommended over LMWHs or vitamin K antagonists (VKAs) by the ACCP.[53] Empiric dosage adjustment is also required for patients with renal impairment.

Warfarin and vitamin K antagonists interfere with hepatic synthesis of vitamin K–dependent clotting factors (II, VII, IX, X) and anticoagulant proteins C and S, and also prevent extension of clot.[10,69] The effectiveness of VKAs for preventing VTE in orthopaedic surgery was evaluated in a meta-analysis[104] that showed VKA to be more effective than placebo and IPC with higher rates of wound hematoma, equally effective to UFH and antiplatelet agents, and less effective than LMWHs without any significant difference in bleeding risk.[104] Adjusted-dose warfarin/VKA to a target INR of 2.5 (range, 2–3) is recommended following THR and TKR.[53] Lower target INR ranges (1.8 to 2.5) have been used to minimize postoperative hematoma.[104] Variability in response; interactions with other drugs, food, and disease states; and need for frequent monitoring are major concerns with VKA therapy.

Aspirin and antiplatelet agents prevent thrombogenesis by inhibiting cyclooxygenase activity in platelets and have been used in limited studies for VTE prophylaxis in orthopaedic surgery.[53] In data from the pulmonary embolism prevention (PEP) trial, aspirin, 160 mg administered daily for 5 weeks, reduced symptomatic DVT by 36 percent and fatal PE by 53 percent in 13,356 hip fracture and 4088 elective arthroplasty patients, with better outcome in HFS.[124] These results were confounded by concurrent use of nonpharmacologic prophylactic measures in many of the patients. Aspirin is not recommended as a single agent for VTE prophylaxis in orthopaedic surgery.[38,53]

Other agents in various stages of clinical trials for VTE prophylaxis in major orthopaedic surgery are direct thrombin inhibitors desirudin, melagatran/ximelagatran, and oral factor Xa inhibitors BAY 59–7939 and LY517717.

Natural hirudin and its recombinant form desirudin directly inhibit both free and clot-bound thrombin.[177]

The effectiveness of desirudin for VTE prevention in elective hip replacement was evaluated in three standardized multicenter studies.[177] Desirudin 15 mg twice daily was more effective than UFH 5000 U administered three times daily in preventing both total DVTs (23% vs. 7%, *P*<0.0001) and proximal DVTs (16% vs. 3%, *P*<0.0001) in THR.[177] Desirudin 15 mg twice daily significantly reduced total (18.4% vs. 26%) and proximal DVTs (4.5% vs. 7.5%) compared with enoxaparin 40 mg daily in elective hip replacement, without an increase in bleeding complication.[40]

Melagatran/ximelagatran (pro-drug) are direct thrombin inhibitors used in prospective clinical trials for prevention of VTE following orthopaedic surgery. A review article supports clinical study findings that a fixed oral dose of ximelagatran 24 mg twice daily or 2–3 mg SC, then 24 mg twice daily following THR and TKR, compares favorably with enoxaparin 40 mg daily and adjusted-dose warfarin in efficacy and safety, without need for coagulation monitoring but a higher bleeding tendency.[27] However, melagatran/ximelagatran are not currently approved for use in the United States.

Two new oral factor Xa inhibitors (BAY 59–7939 and LY517717) in early phases of clinical trials look promising for thromboprophylaxis in orthopaedic surgery.[71]

PROPHYLAXIS FOR VENOUS THROMBOEMBOLISM IN ORTHOPAEDIC SURGERY

Bleeding complications associated with anticoagulant therapy have been cited as a major reason for underutilization of thromboprophylaxis.[53] Numerous data from randomized, placebo-controlled studies documented that the risk of major bleeding is minimal with current low chemoprophylaxis doses.[53,58] However, it is equally important to evaluate a patient's risk of bleeding from anticoagulant prophylaxis and to manage patients having contraindications with a mechanical device[58] (Table 10-9).

The optimal time (pre- vs. postoperative) to initiate or continue thromboprophylaxis in major orthopaedic surgery is a subject of debate. The two opposing factors driving this controversy are the concern that venous thrombosis may begin during the surgery itself versus the need to control the bleeding risk associated with the surgical procedure and regional anesthesia. This concern has been addressed in clinical studies.[76,119,127,155] In a meta-analysis, prehospital discharge venograms revealed that preoperative initiation of LMWH-dalteparin was associated with a 10 percent DVT rate compared with 15.3 percent with postoperative initiation (*P*=0.02) and less major bleeding (0.9% vs. 3.5%) in patients receiving preoperative (*P*=0.01) than postoperative LMWH but higher than with postoperative warfarin.[76] In a systematic review, preoperative administration of LMWH was no better than postoperative therapy in reducing the incidence of VTE in elective hip surgery, with a trend toward increased bleeding.[155] Starting thromboprophylaxis between 6 and 9 hours postoperatively was effective without increasing the rate of major bleeding.[127] Delayed administration of fondaparinux in elective arthroplasty concluded that fondaparinux, 2.5 mg commencing at 18 to 24 hours postoperatively, appears to be equivalent to regimens using warfarin and enoxaparin in efficacy and safety.[119] In light of the conflicting results, it is recommended that timing of thromboprophylaxis in orthopaedic surgery be based on the efficacy-to-bleeding tradeoffs of the particular agent.[53]

The duration of thromboprophylaxis to maximize VTE prevention following major orthopaedic surgery is also controversial. There is strong evidence that ongoing activation of the coagulation cascade persists for 4 weeks or longer following THR and the risk of thrombosis continues for up to 3 months.[33,53,83,174] An epidemiologic examination of 19,586 THR and 24,059 TKA patients reported a posthospital stay, venogram-documented VTE incidence of 76 percent in THR and 47 percent in TKA cases.[174] The median time following surgery for VTE diagnosis was 7 days for TKA and 17 days for THR.[42] A meta-analysis of symptomatic outcomes showed a total DVT prevalence of 38.8 percent after knee replacement compared with 16.4 percent after hip replacement; $P < 0.001$ within 3 months of surgery.[34] Posthospital-stay continuation of thromboprophylaxis with LMWH, VKA, and fondaparinux for 4 to 5 weeks was effective in significantly reducing VTE incidence further without increased risk of bleeding.[25,123] The mounting evidence and continuous decrease in length of hospital stay support the need for extended prophylaxis following major orthopaedic surgery, and the ACCP recommendation is for 28 to 35 days following THR and HFS.[53]

Concurrent use of neuraxial anesthesia/analgesia in the presence of thromboprophylaxis is of major concern in orthopaedic surgery. Regional anesthesia was commended with the benefit of reducing the risk of VTE in major orthopaedic surgery and is commonly used.[49,53,73] The incidence of spinal hematoma with neuraxial anesthesia/analgesia is low but increases with chemoprophylaxis for VTE, as documented for LMWH.[53,73,134] Evidence supports that careful identification and exclusion of patients with a significant underlying risk for bleeding, along with meticulous caution during neuraxial procedures, permit safe, concurrent use.[53,134] The American Society of Regional Anesthesia (ASRA) consensus conference on neuraxial anesthesia and anticoagulation provides guidelines to clinicians to improve the safe use of regional anesthesia with anticoagulants.[73,134] ACCP also recommends that continuous epidural analgesia not be used concurrently with warfarin for more than 1 or 2 days and the INR should be less than 1.5 at the time of catheter removal. For LMWH and other anticoagulants, they recommend that therapy not commence for at least 2 hours after catheter removal. In patients administered LMWH or UFH, an epidural catheter should be inserted or removed at the end of the dosing interval for the specific agent.[53]

We can identify patients at high risk for VTE, but we are still not able to predict which patients will have symptomatic VTE; thus, routine thromboprophylaxis with one or more of the proven modalities is highly recommended for all patients undergoing orthopaedic surgery.[58] Other orthopaedic procedures such as elective spine surgery and below-the-knee tissue injuries and fractures show lower rates of symptomatic DTV, but patients may need chemoprophylaxis when additional risk factors are present.

PART IV

Substance Abuse Syndromes: Recognition, Prevention, and Treatment

Caesar A. Anderson, M.D.,
George A. Perdrizet, M.D., Ph.D., F.A.C.S.

The initial spiritual force in any new settlement is never the newspaper, never the Sabbath-school, never the missionary, but always the whiskey.
    Mark Twain

INTRODUCTION

Substance-dependent patients are frequently hospitalized for acute care and require surgical interventions.[45,125] This section of the chapter will assist the surgeon in answering three questions:

1. Which of my patients are at risk for the development of an acute withdrawal syndrome while hospitalized?

2. How can I recognize these individuals early?
3. What can I do to prevent this medical complication from occurring?

Alcohol syndromes will be emphasized, as they are the most common and problematic substance abuse syndromes encountered in orthopaedic, trauma, and surgical patients.[3,7,22,62,112,118] Individuals often come to acute care hospitals with injuries and illnesses that are a direct result of substance abuse. Alcohol is involved in 25 to 35 percent of nonfatal motor vehicle injuries and in 40 to 50 percent of traffic fatalities.[121] It is estimated that between 10 and 40 percent of such patients are alcohol dependent and therefore at risk of developing alcohol withdrawal syndrome (AWS) during their hospital stay.[54] Acutely intoxicated and injured patients have a 75 percent chance of having a diagnosis of chronic alcoholism.[132] The prevalent association of substance abuse and injury prompted the EAST Committee on Injury Control and Violence Prevention to publish a position paper reviewing the role that alcohol and other drugs play in the care of the injured patient.[148] Approximately 8.2 million persons in the United States are dependent on alcohol and 3.5 million are dependent on illicit drugs, including stimulants (1 million) and opiates (750,000). Each year in the United States, there are approximately 85,000 deaths and 185 billion dollars in costs related to alcohol abuse.[136] Owing to the high prevalence of substance abuse disorders, it is likely that the surgeon practicing in the acute care setting will encounter this challenging and frustrating medical condition.

A preexisting substance abuse disorder adds greatly to the risk for the development of complications following hospital admission for injury or illness.[44,78,152] The postoperative patient who develops an acute withdrawal syndrome will have a protracted and complicated hospital stay.[95,109,161] Alcohol withdrawal syndrome causes increased length of stay, morbidity, and mortality in hospitalized patients and can lead to life-threatening complications.[175] The development of delirium tremens (DTs) or acute psychoses can become life threatening.[87,107] Finally, substance abuse patients often harbor significant medical and psychiatric illnesses that must be recognized and addressed.[141,171] Chronic diseases in the form of end-organ dysfunctions secondary to the protracted nature of substance abuse are common. Cardiac, central nervous system, pulmonary, immunologic, and gastrointestinal organ dysfunction are common and further dispose these patients to a complicated postoperative and hospital course.[91,160] Many alcoholics have significant bone disease, which puts them at further risk for poor bone and wound healing.[21] Osteopenia and fractures, especially of the spine and ribs, are associated with osteoporosis. Ethanol is directly toxic to osteoblasts. Other factors contributing to bone pathology include hypogonadism, decreased calcium intake and malabsorption, increased urinary calcium excretion, decreased exercise, and altered parathyroid hormone response to hypocalcemia. Alcoholics are also at increased risk for osseous avascular necrosis.[81]

The most common substance abuse syndromes encountered in the surgical patient hospitalized for trauma are (1) alcohol intoxication, dependence, and withdrawal (40–50%); (2) opiate addiction and withdrawal (10%); (3) acute cocaine intoxication (5–10%); and (4) iatrogenic benzodiazepine withdrawal.[16,103,148]

DEFINITIONS

The term substance abuse refers to the use of alcohol or other drugs that places the individual at risk of injury, addiction, and dependence. Associated with these conditions are the related social and legal problems that often develop. To minimize confusion around disease definitions, the American Society of Addiction Medicine (ASAM) in 1990 selected and defined standard addiction terminology. A few key abuse syndrome definitions are summarized in Table 10-11. As with most medical conditions, prevention of acute withdrawal syndromes is the primary goal of managing the hospitalized, substance-dependent patient. Prevention can happen only if the physician is attuned to the potential for the problem to occur. Risk stratification and a working knowledge of the early signs and symptoms of withdrawal are critical elements in effectively managing these cases.[102]

RECOGNITION—ESTIMATING RISK

Who is at risk for the development of an acute withdrawal syndrome while hospitalized?

In general, any patient who has a measurable ethanol level (blood alcohol level, or BAL) and has suffered a traumatic injury is at moderate-to-high risk (40%) for harboring an alcohol abuse syndrome. A combination of a carefully elicited past medical history and a liberal policy of drug screening is recommended in all nonelective surgical patients. For nonalcohol substances, any patient with a known history of abuse or addiction or any patient with a positive urine toxicology screen is considered to be at significant risk for withdrawal or abstinence syndromes. Once recognition of a patient's substance abuse problem is made, this diagnosis should be clearly documented in the patient's medical record and appropriate substance abuse counseling obtained.

Table 10-11	
Alcohol Abuse Syndromes	
Syndrome	**Definition**
"At-risk use": drinks (No. female: No. male)*	For females, >3 drinks daily, >7 drinks weekly; for males, >4 drinks daily, >14 drinks weekly*
Abuse	Harmful use of a specific psychoactive substance.
Addiction	Disease process characterized by the continued use of a specific psychoactive substance despite physical, psychological, or social harm.
Tolerance	State in which an increased dose of a psychoactive substance is needed to produce a desired effect.
Withdrawal	Onset of a predictable constellation of signs and symptoms following the abrupt discontinuation of, or rapid decrease in, dosage of a psychoactive substance.
Delirium tremens	An acute organic brain syndrome due to alcohol withdrawal resulting in life-threatening delirium and autonomic hyperactivity.
Wernicke's encephalopathy	Abrupt onset of a confusional state, associated with thiamine deficiency, accompanied by unsteadiness of gait and visual disturbance.
Korsakoff's syndrome	Chronic memory impairment often associated with amnestic confabulation, with relative preservation of cognitive capacity.

Adapted from American Society of Addiction Medicine.
*1 Drink = 14 g ethanol = 12 oz beer = 5 oz wine = 1.5 oz spirits. Behavioral risk of developing alcohol abuse: >14 drinks/week (male), >7 drinks/week (female).

Box 10-1	CAGE Scoring System

C Have you ever felt you ought to cut down on your drinking?
A Have people annoyed you by criticizing your drinking?
G Have you ever felt guilty about your drinking?
E Have you ever had a drink in the morning (eye opener) to steady your nerves or get rid of a hangover?
    Scoring: One point assigned for each "yes" response; a score of 2 is considered clinically significant for alcohol abuse risk.

Alcohol

The prevalence of alcohol abuse in the general population is estimated to be 5 percent and of alcohol dependence to be 4 percent.[136] Questionnaires, surveys, and scoring systems are available for grading a person's risk for AWS. The most commonly used screening tools are the AUDIT (*A*lcohol *U*se *D*isorder *I*dentification *T*est) and CAGE (*c*ut down, *a*nnoyed, *g*uilt, *e*ye-opener) questionnaires. These clinical tools are widely utilized in the setting of alcohol detoxification programs. The CAGE questionnaire has practical utility in the setting of acute injury and illness, as it can be administered in minutes (Box 10-1). The literature is replete with examples of inadequate screening and recognition of alcohol abuse in acute care settings and has not changed over time.[143, 172] A recent report found that alcohol-related problems were addressed by physicians in only 25 percent of patients admitted to a Level I trauma center.[41] Table 10-12 lists the aspects of a medical database required to accurately identify the "at risk" patient along with common screening tools, questionnaires, and their relevant scores. Surgeons typically fail to screen their patients for alcohol abuse.[31,37] Therefore, we have created the "Surgeon's Short Form," which can be used preoperatively to identify patients likely to be alcohol abusers (Table 10-13). It has been reported that 90 percent of the patients at risk for alcohol abuse can be identified by establishing the presence of just two factors: (1) a positive past medical history for alcohol abuse syndromes and (2) the ingestion of alcohol within 24 hours of presentation. The presence of both these factors places the patient at moderate-to-high risk (40–60%) for AWS during the period of abstinence imposed by hospitalization.[11]

Opiates

Opiates are naturally occurring or synthetic agents with morphine-like properties. They elicit their effect via central nervous system (CNS) receptors, causing analgesia, respiratory depression, hallucinations, sedation, miosis, bradycardia, dysphoria, and ultimately drug dependence. Patients abusing opiates have withdrawal symptoms and a high tolerance to opiate analgesics, making their postoperative management difficult. Opiates were the primary substance of abuse for 324,000 (18%) of the 1.8 million substance abuse treatment admissions reported to SAMH-SA's Treatment Episode Data Set (TEDS) in 2003. Of these, 51,000 (3% of all admissions) were for a non-heroin opiate. Non-heroin opiates include methadone, codeine, Dilaudid, morphine, Demerol, opium, oxycodone, and any other drug with morphine–like effects.[107]

Tolerance, physiologic dependence, and psychological dependence on opioids usually occur after 3 weeks of daily usage.[52] The most commonly abused opiate is heroin. The relative risk for abuse of opiates and other drugs is variable and poorly understood. The variables are attributable to genetic, environmental, or combined factors. It is important to note that outside of stereotypical notions, many patients, especially the injured, are at risk of drug and opiate abuse, adding to the difficulty in screening and subsequent management. Regardless of an individual patient's results of a urine toxicology screen, the clinician must remain alert for the possibility of opiate abuse. Multiple factors exist that prevent drug screening from being completely reliable in the preoperative patient, including dose ingested, time interval from last dosing, innate host metabolism, associated medical co-morbidities, and the presence of polysubstance abuse. Several drug screening scales exist; however, most are complex and too cumbersome for applicability on a busy orthopaedic service. The most reliable indicator for assessing opiate abuse risk, aside from a thorough history and physical examination, is the presence of certain key signs and symptoms. Aside from signs and symptoms, the presence of infectious diseases (HIV, hepatitis B and C, sexually transmitted diseases, and tuberculosis) should also raise the suspicion of possible opiate abuse.[102]

Table 10-12	
Who Is at Risk for Alcohol Withdrawal Syndrome?	
Factor	**Sign/Symptom**
Past medical history	Abuse, withdrawal, seizures, delirium tremens, hospitalization, traumatic event with positive BAL
Social history	Previous or current family, work, or scholastic performance problems
Clinical scoring systems	CAGE ≥3
	CIWA-Ar >10
	Alcohol use score ≥20
	Addiction severity index score ≥6
Blood alcohol level (BAL)	> 150 mg/dL with clear sensorium or >300 mg/dL in any person

Table 10-13	
Preoperative Interview—Surgeon's Short Form	
Questions to Ask	**Risk of Alcohol Dependence***
1. Have you ever had[†] a drinking problem?	Yes = 70%, no = unclear implications
2. Have you had any alcohol in the past 24 hours or a positive blood alcohol level[‡]	Yes plus No.1 above = 90%

*Male gender and age >30 years further increases risk.
[†]Past tense is used, as patient is more likely to be truthful.
[‡]Any level of ethanol indicates the patient has recently consumed ethanol.

Cocaine

Cocaine, a derivative of the *Erythroxylum coca* plant, is often used in combination with heroin. It is well absorbed from snorting, smoking, or injection. Fatalities from seizures, respiratory paralysis, and cardiac arrhythmias can occur.[108] The lipid solubility of cocaine is quite high. Brain concentrations can be elevated up to 10 times that of plasma, making it extremely addictive. The National Survey on Drug Use and Health (2003) found 35 million Americans older than 12 years have reported using cocaine at least once, with 8 million of these reported to have used cocaine in crack form. Cocaine-related emergency department visits increased by 78 percent from 1990 to 1994 and by 33 percent as of 2002. Cocaine abuse was reported to be second only to alcohol abuse. It was the most frequently reported substance associated with drug abuse death by 2003 Medical Examiners/Coroners.

Recognizing patients at risk for the development of cocaine withdrawal is an important consideration in the management of the hospitalized patient. Like opiate screening, there are no clear indicators for accurately assessing risk of withdrawal. Cocaine stimulates dopaminergic release, increased sympathetic tone, blockade of serotonin reuptake, and local anesthesia as a result of neuronal sodium current inhibition.[72] Intense vasospasms leading to myocardial ischemia in patients with well-perfused coronary arteries have been reported.[28] Profound CNS effects also can occur, leading to ischemic or hemorrhagic stroke, confusion, violent behavior, and seizures. The seizures associated with cocaine abuse are typically self-limited and may occur on the very first exposure, since cocaine lowers the seizure threshold. Cocaine can also induce hyperpyrexia, hyperkinesis, and rhabdomyolysis. Cocaine abuse typically induces a psychological rather than physical dependence. Abusers typically have depleted dopamine stores in the pleasure centers of the brain. Hence, continued cocaine ingestion is required in order to enjoy basic functions (sexual drive, hunger, thirst).

Benzodiazepines

The use of benzodiazepines is as commonplace as the use of a scalpel in most orthopaedic practices. SAMSHA data suggest that from 1992 to 2002 drug-related emergency department visits involving benzodiazepine-like agents increased by 41 percent. Withdrawal from these agents is a serious complication that often goes unrecognized. Benzodiazepine withdrawal has no associated signs and symptoms that can be considered pathognomonic. As with other substance abuse syndromes, great variability exists in

its presentation. Patients at risk of developing clinically relevant withdrawal symptoms from benzodiazepines typically have been administered daily therapeutic dosages for more than 4 months or doses of more than twice the recommended level for more than 2 months. Patients who require a period of intensive care during their hospitalization, especially those who have required prolonged mechanical ventilation and continuous intravenous sedation, are at particular risk for postoperative withdrawal.

RECOGNITION—EARLY IDENTIFICATION OF SIGNS AND SYMPTOMS

How do I recognize the onset and development of withdrawal syndromes in my pre/postoperative patient?

The physician must remain alert for the development of early signs of withdrawal. Early intervention has the greatest chance for success. Because of the nonspecific nature of the signs and symptoms associated with withdrawal syndromes (i.e., agitation, tachycardia, tremor, and delirium), the development of withdrawal can easily go unrecognized.

Alcohol

Symptoms of AWS range from mild anxiety and tremors to seizures, delirium, and death. Early signs of AWS most often involve tremulousness and seizures, the former starting approximately 6 to 8 hours after a significant drop in serum ethanol level. The clinical picture is colored by excessive sympathetic or adrenergic stimulation resulting in tachycardia, diaphoresis, and severe hypertension (Fig. 10-1). Associated signs include tremors, irritability, and hyperreflexia. Tremulous patients usually have a clear sensorium. Nausea, anxiety, or insomnia may be dominant complaints but are relatively nonspecific findings in the hospitalized, injured, or postoperative patient. Once a patient begins to demonstrate signs and symptoms of withdrawal, the clinical course should be documented using the CIWA-Ar scale (Clinical Institute Withdrawal Assessment for Alcohol [revised] scale; Fig. 10-2).[157] This tool is widely available in most general hospitals and should be performed every 8 hours until signs and symptoms of AWS have resolved. This tool is also used to measure response to therapy (see below). AWS is generally (80%) mild, typically peaking at 24 to 36 hours and resolving by 72 hours, but it can last from days to longer than a week.[163] Without treatment, symptoms may last as long as 10 to 14 days.[84] However, 25 percent of patients may have an escalation in symptoms and severe manifestations

FIGURE 10-1 *Time course for alcohol withdrawal syndrome (AWS). Initial signs include tachycardia and tremor secondary to the autonomic hyperactivity. Seizure activity can occur very early in the time course of development of AWS, even while the CIWA-Ar score is relatively low, e.g., 5–10. A CIWA-Ar score of ≥15–20 signifies major AWS and requires ICU monitoring. Most AWS will be mild and peak at 2–4 days. Detoxification occurs by 5–10 days with a 10% acute relapse rate. (Redrawn from Lohr, R.H. Treatment of alcohol withdrawal in hospitalized patients. Mayo Clin Proc 1995;70:777–782, 1995.)*

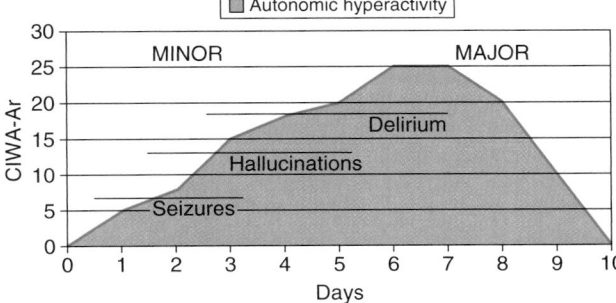

including hallucinations, acute confusion, and DTs. Currently, there is no method to predict which patients with mild AWS will progress to severe disease and DTs.

Neuropsychological symptoms include anxiety, agitation, hyperalertness, insomnia, craving for rest, self-preoccupation, inattention, and mild disorientation to time, without gross confusion. The absence of significant disorientation, confusion, and autonomic instability differentiates mild AWS from the more serious DTs. Seizures occur in 10 percent of alcoholics and are often the precipitating event that leads to injury. Alcohol-related seizures can be the *initial* sign of AWS (see Fig. 10-1).[125] Seizing-alcoholic patients are prone to falls and to hip, spinal, and rib fractures. Alcoholic seizures are precipitated mainly by hypoglycemia, hypomagnesemia, and respiratory alkalosis. They are usually generalized, tonic-clonic seizures. One third of patients who have convulsions develop DTs if not treated. Nonalcohol-related causes of seizure disorder must be investigated (metabolic, post-traumatic, and idiopathic) and ruled out before the cause is attributed to AWS. Most alcohol-associated seizures occur 6 to 48 hours following drinking cessation and are typically limited to a single event (40%). These patients can demonstrate a confusing picture, since often there is no longer any measurable alcohol in their bloodstream. Once again, a high index of suspicion is required on the part of the treating clinicians.

Delirium is a common and nonspecific acute state of confusion that complicates postoperative recovery. Delirium often goes unrecognized or misdiagnosed in the surgical patient.[179] The incidence of delirium in postoperative patients is 37 percent. Common precipitating factors include infection, hypoxia, myocardial ischemia, metabolic derangement, and anticholinergic medications. Delirium is

associated with increased rates of postoperative complications, delayed functional recovery, and increased length of hospital stay. Patients developing delirium during their hospital stay experience a two-fold increase in mortality rate. The development of DTs is the most feared complication of AWS and is seen in less than 5 percent of patients experiencing AWS. DTs are marked by autonomic hyperactivity (hypertension, tachycardia, fever, tremors, diaphoresis, and dilated pupils) and disorientation. This clinical picture can be easily confused with the presentation of a postoperative infectious complication (wound, urinary tract infection, or pneumonia). Patients can become severely agitated, uncooperative, and aggressive, thus representing a potential for harm to self and others. At this extreme stage of the disease, it is often necessary to heavily sedate and control patients with neuromuscular blockade in order to establish a safe therapeutic environment. Onset of DTs occurs 3 to 5 days following abstinence but can range from 1 to 14 days. The majority of patients (83%) recover within 3 days. Relapses occur in 10 percent of patients and can prolong the duration of the syndrome for up to 1 month. Mortality rates range from 5 to 15 percent in treated patients; however, fever and seizures are associated with the poorest outcomes. The most common causes of death are cardiac arrhythmia, pneumonia, and alcohol-related end-organ dysfunction (cardiomyopathy, pancreatitis, gastrointestinal hemorrhage, infection, and liver disease). The goal of clinical management is early recognition of AWS, prompt intervention, and prevention of DTs.

The surgeon should be alert to the need for AWS prophylaxis in any patient who is considered at risk for alcohol withdrawal and develops a mild tremor.

Opiates

Although opiate withdrawal is generally considered unlikely to cause significant morbidity or mortality, the increased level of autonomic activity often associated with this withdrawal can be life threatening in the postoperative setting. The increased demand on cardiac output and myocardial contractility can exhaust a patient's cardiac reserve and thus the ability to adequately compensate during surgery. Abrupt cessation or reduction in dosage can lead to withdrawal symptoms. These symptoms typically occur after several months of daily use. Acute opiate withdrawal typically occurs in stages. Stage one usually begins at 3 to 4 hours following abstinence and is characterized by drug craving, anxiety, and fear of withdrawal. Stage two is seen approximately 8 to 14 hours following abstinence with increased restlessness, insomnia, yawning, rhinorrhea, lacrimation, diaphoresis, mydriasis, and stomach cramps. The two final stages can occur 1 to 3 days following abstinence and are characterized by tremor, muscle spasms, vomiting, diarrhea, hypertension, tachycardia, fever, chills, piloerection, and very rarely, seizures. The early signs and symptoms of opioid withdrawal syndrome (yawning, sweating, lacrimation, rhinorrhea, anxiety, hypertension, piloerection, insomnia, and tachycardia) are generally classified as elements of autonomic hyperactivity.[102] As opiate withdrawal severity worsens, patients may then exhibit increasing restlessness, seizures, myalgias,

FIGURE 10-2 *The Clinical Institute Withdrawal Assessment for Alcohol is a clinical tool that has been recently revised— CIWA-Ar—and validated in the setting of alcohol detoxification units. This tool is widely available in general medical hospitals and is administered and recorded as part of the patient's "vital signs" by the nursing staff. The scale ranges from 0 to 50, with 15–20 representing the transition from mild to severe withdrawal symptomatology. The therapeutic goal is set at a score of ≤10. Any patient with a score >10 or with a score that is increasing with time should have AWS prophylaxis started.*

	TACTILE DISTURBANCES: Ask: "Have you any itching, pins and needles sensations, any burning, any numbness or do you feel bugs crawling on or under your skin?" Observation. 0 None 1 Very mild itching, pins and needles, burning or numbness 2 Mild itching, pins and needles, burning or numbness 3 Moderate pins and needles, burning or numbness 4 Moderately severe hallucinations 5 Severe hallucinations 6 Extremely severe hallucinations 7 Continuous hallucinations
TREMOR: Arms extended and fingers spread apart. Observation. 0 No tremor 1 Not visible, but can be felt fingertip to fingertip 2 3 4 Moderate, with patient's arms extended 5 6 7 Severe, even with arms not extended	**AUDITORY DISTURBANCES:** Ask: "Are you more aware of sounds around you? Are they harsh? Do they frighten you? Are you hearing anything that is disturbing you? Are you hearing things you know are not there?" Observation. 0 Not present 1 Very mild harshness or ability to frighten 2 Mild harshness or ability to frighten 3 Moderate harshness or ability to frighten 4 Moderately severe hallucinations 5 Severe hallucinations 6 Extremely severe hallucinations 7 Continuous hallucinations
PAROXYSMAL SWEATS 0 No sweat visible 1 Barely perceptible sweating, palms moist 2 3 4 Beads of sweat obvious on forehead 5 6 7 Drenching sweats	**VISUAL DISTURBANCES:** Ask: "Does the light appear to be too bright? Is its color different? Does it hurt your eyes? Are you seeing anything that is disturbing to you? Are you seeing things you know are not there?" Observation. 0 Not present 1 Very mild sensitivity 2 Mild sensitivity 3 Moderate sensitivity 4 Moderately severe hallucinations 5 Severe hallucinations 6 Extremely severe hallucinations 7 Continuous hallucinations
ANXIETY: Ask: "Do you feel nervous?" Observation. 0 No anxiety, at ease 1 Mildly anxious 2 3 4 Moderately anxious, or guarded, so anxiety is inferred 5 6 7 Equivalent to acute panic as seen in severe delirium or acute schizophrenic reactions	**HEADACHE, FULLNESS IN HEAD:** Ask: "Does your head feel different? Does it feel like there is a band around your head?" Do not rate for dizziness or lightheadedness. Otherwise, rate severity. 0 Not present 1 Very mild 2 Mild 3 Moderate 4 Moderately severe 5 Severe 6 Very severe 7 Extremely severe
AGITATION: Observation. 0 Normal activity 1 Somewhat more than normal activity 2 3 4 Moderately fidgety and restless 5 6 7 Paces back and forth during most of interview, or constantly thrashes about	**ORIENTATION & CLOUDING OF SENSORIUM:** Ask: "What day is this? Where are you? Who am I?" 0 Oriented and can do serial additions 1 Cannot do serial additions or is uncertain about date 2 Disoriented for date by no more than 2 calendar days 3 Disoriented for date by more than 2 calendar days 4 Disoriented for place and/or person

vomiting, diarrhea, dehydration, and abdominal pain. Intense drug craving also accompanies withdrawal. Though withdrawal is not considered life threatening, it certainly will complicate the clinical course of the postoperative patient.

The pharmacologic mechanism behind opiate withdrawal relates to decreased CNS concentrations in the opiate-tolerant individual. Receptors identified in the locus ceruleus of the limbic system are influenced by exogenous opiates, decreasing noradrenergic firing. Withdrawal results from increased sympathetic discharge and noradrenergic hyperactivity. Heroin withdrawal occurs 4 to 8 hours after the last dose with symptoms peaking 36 to 72 hours later. It may take up to 10 days for symptoms to finally subside. It is important to recognize the pharmacologic specificity of the opiate-receptors (mu, kappa) to fully appreciate the rationale and efficacy of methadone treatment and its relationship to the non-mu receptor opiate agonists in the management of acute pain. This point is addressed under the treatment of opioid withdrawal.

Cocaine

Early clinical signs and symptoms preceding cocaine withdrawal can begin as abruptly as 9 hours following last ingestion. Patients are often described as being in "crash" mode. Their symptoms include agitation, anorexia, sadness, and intense drug craving. They can then progress to early withdrawal, exhibiting drug craving and a normal mood devoid of anxiety. Once again, a thorough past medical and social history is vital to the successful management of this condition. Cocaine withdrawal symptoms are a result of depleted dopaminergic neurotransmitters, causing fatigue, hypersomnolence, hunger, anxiety, paranoid behavior, resting tachycardia, and depression.[144] There are early and late components to cocaine withdrawal. Early symptoms are typically characterized by a normal mood, low anxiety, and no evidence of drug craving. Late withdrawal, which can occur from 1 to 10 weeks following last ingestion, will present with fatigue, marked anxiety, and high drug craving. Heightened clinical suspicion remains central to early identification and treatment.

Benzodiazepines

Abrupt cessation of benzodiazepines should be avoided during hospitalization. Weaning protocols are widely employed and limit the rate at which the daily dose can be decreased. The weaning protocol employed in our institution is as follows: benzodiazepine infusion is decreased by increments of 0.1 mg/hr to a minimum of 0.1 mg/hr while the patient's sedation score is assessed. Tapering does not exceed more than 0.1 mg/hr in 8 to 12 hours.

MANAGEMENT—PROPHYLAXIS/ TREATMENT

The aim of therapeutic intervention in the moderate-to-high risk patient is to manage the severity of the AWS and permit detoxification to occur (7–10 days). Early interventions are designed to prevent the escalation of symptoms from mild and manageable to the more severe, life-threatening manifestations. Timing is

critical. The time at which abstinence is initiated should be noted and patients monitored for the appearance of early signs and symptoms of AWS. Generally speaking, several hours of abstinence are required before signs and symptoms of withdrawal appear (see Fig. 10-1). A unique caveat related to the surgical patient is the observation that general anesthetics can delay the onset of withdrawal syndromes. Thus, a patient who undergoes exploratory laparotomy on admission, followed 2 days later by operative reduction and fixation of a long bone fracture and then 2 days after that by a plastic surgical procedure, may develop AWS 7 to 10 days following initiation of abstinence.

The usual approach to AWS prevention is to provide the relevant pharmacologic agent in low-dose form *prior* to the onset of signs or symptoms of withdrawal. Titration of pharmacologic therapy is based on the patient's clinical signs and symptoms.

To standardize the objective documentation of the patient's clinical course during treatment two standardized scoring systems are widely used. The CIWA-Ar score is a measure of the patient's withdrawal symptomatology. A CIWA-Ar score ≤10, on a scale of 0–50, is the therapeutic goal.[157] The OAA/S score is a measure of the patient's alertness and is used to prevent overly sedating patients in an effort to control symptoms. An OAA/S score of ≥15, on a scale of 0–20, is the therapeutic goal.[24]

General Medical Considerations

Prior to the administration of any pharmacologic agent for the prevention or treatment of AWS, the general medical condition of the patient should be thoroughly reviewed. Type and degree of end-organ damage should be determined (Childs-Pugh classification; Box 10-2). Metabolic and electrolyte imbalances should be identified and corrected. All patients should also receive a standardized medical protocol for the metabolic management of the alcohol-dependent diagnosis that includes vitamin supplementation (folate, thiamine, B$_{12}$), magnesium sulfate for magnesium deficiency (Mg <1.5 mg/dL), sodium or potassium phosphate for phosphate deficiency (phosphate <2.7 mg/dL), haloperidol for anxiety/agitation, and nicotine replacement therapy for active tobacco users. Associated psychiatric diagnoses and treatments must also be addressed. Determination and documentation of the CIWA-Ar score should be performed every 2 to 4 hours during the initial period of hospital admission. Pharmacotherapy should include the following:

1. Folate 1 mg IV qd × 3, then 1 mg IV or PO qd thereafter
2. Thiamine 100 mg IV qd × 3, then 100 mg IV or PO qd thereafter
3. Multivitamin infusion, 1 amp IV qd × 3, then 1 amp IV or tablet PO qd thereafter
4. Nicotine replacement therapy (Nicoderm, 21 mg/ patch qd)
5. Haloperidol for management of hallucinations, 2 mg IV q4d
6. Psychiatric consultation for evaluation and treatment as well as alcohol addiction treatment and rehabilitation

Variable	A	B	C
Encephalopathy	None	Slight to moderate	Moderate to severe
Ascites	None	Slight	Moderate to large
Bilirubin (mg/dL)	<2	2–3	>3
Albumin (g/dL)	>3.5	3.0–3.5	<3.0
Prothrombin index	>70%	40–70%	<40%
Operative mortality (%)	2	10	50

Alcohol

BENZODIAZEPINE ADMINISTRATION

The benzodiazepine class of sedatives is considered the drug of choice for the treatment and prevention of AWS. Initial therapy can be administered orally or by continuous intravenous drip. A recent study in the head and neck surgical patient population found benzodiazepine prophylaxis resulted in a 13.5 percent and 9.4 percent incidence of withdrawal and DTs, respectively.[109]

BENZODIAZEPINE PROTOCOL Briefly, lorazepam (Ativan, 10 mg/100 mL D_5W) can be administered intravenously according to the following guidelines based on the CIWA-Ar scoring system. Trained nurses can carry out an evaluation in less than 2 minutes, and the interrater reliability is high (r >0.8). The titration of the lorazepam drip is based on clinical symptomatology as graded by both the CIWA-Ar score and the OAA/S score (see Fig. 10-2 and Box 10-3).

1. Loading dose: lorazepam 2 mg IV and repeat in 30 minutes if no change or an increase in CIWA-Ar scale and begin a continuous intravenous infusion, ≈0.3 mg/hr. Breakthrough coverage is provided with 2 mg IV and repeat in 30 min and q3–4hr thereafter until patient's condition stabilizes or improves.

2. **Increase** infusion by 0.1 mg/hr increments to a maximum of 0.6 mg/hr, if CIW-Ar scale increases by 5 or more points. Note: Tegretol (400 mg PO or IV q8hr) should be administered to all patients having infusion rates of ≥0.4 mg/hr (see below).

3. **Decrease** infusion by 0.1 mg/hr increments to a minimum of 0.1 mg/hr, if the patient has passed beyond 72 hours since last drink without signs of withdrawal, or the CIW-Ar scale drops 5 or more points: **do not stop the infusion completely**. Note: tapering must not exceed more than 0.1 mg/hr in 8–12 hours.

4. Once the patient has been completely weaned from the intravenous infusion, a PRN order of lorazepam should be made available.

5. Consider transferring patient to an intensive care unit environment when (a) the patient is not responding to treatment (inability to control patient's symptoms within 12–24 hours of initiation of treatment), or (b) if CIWA-Ar score is ≥25 at any time, or (c) OAA/S score is <15.

ALCOHOL REPLACEMENT

The medical administration of ethanol to prevent AWS has been used for many years. Despite the relatively wide use by surgical disciplines, very few studies or publications describe its use and therefore it is not condoned by medical practitioners.[101] This situation is, in part, due to the fact that ethanol is not considered a drug but rather a nutritional supplement (increased calories) and an appetite stimulant. Furthermore, the medical literature is deficient with respect to a description of the clinical context, safety, and efficacy of ethanol replacement therapy in the management of the alcohol-dependent hospitalized patient.

The pharmacologic gold standard for the medical management of AWS is the benzodiazepine class of sedatives. The major complication of this therapy is a generalized state of sedation. Sedation of the acutely injured or postoperative patient complicates recovery by delaying the initiation of mobilization and putting patients at risk for the development of respiratory compromise, hypoxemia, pneumonia, or deep venous thrombosis.

Box 10-3	Observer Alertness Awakeness/Sedation (OAS/S) Score			
Responsiveness	**Speech**	**Facial Expression**	**Eyes**	**Score**
Responds to name	Normal	Normal	Clear	5
Lethargic response to name	Mild slowing	Mild relaxation	Glazed with <50% ptosis	4
Responds to shouting only	Slurring	Marked relaxation/slack jaw	Glazed with >50% ptosis	3
Responds to mild prodding	Incoherent speech	None	None	2
No response to prodding	None	None	None	1

The Observer Alertness and Sedation Score was designed to monitor patients in the post-anesthesia recovery room.

Patients should be monitored in an ICU environment for scores of 3 or less.

The OAA/S Scale comprises the following categories: (a) responsiveness, (b) speech, (c) facial expression, and (d) eyes. The score is reported as a composite score, with a range of 1 (deep sleep) to 5 (alert), and reflects the lowest score obtained by the rater for any of the four assessment categories. Published literature demonstrates that composite scores of healthy volunteers equal 4.81 ± 0.31, light sedation scores equal 3.56 ± 0.78, and heavy sedation scores equal 2.44 ± 0.76. Light sedation is defined as patient being lethargic with mild slowing of speech, and heavy sedation as patient responding only to prodding or shaking plus impaired speech.

The therapeutic goals are three-fold: first, to prevent complicated AWS (efficacy); second, to permit alcohol detoxification (efficacy); and third, to avoid a state of generalized sedation (safety). This will allow the patient time to recover from injuries while avoiding the potential complications associated with AWS or generalized sedation (e.g., delirium, respiratory depression, need for physical restraint, need for transfer to higher level of care, and mechanical ventilation). Once the patient has recovered from the acute injuries, a mandatory consultation with the Substance Abuse Service, Department of Psychiatry, should be obtained, and when indicated, voluntary enrollment into a comprehensive program for alcohol addiction treatment and rehabilitation will be arranged for consenting patients.

The condition of alcohol addiction and dependence is a complicated medical disease that requires a multidisciplinary approach to provide state-of-the-art care. Although many trauma centers use ethyl alcohol to prevent the development of AWS in injured patients, this remains a poorly reported practice and as such leads to controversial issues (both medical and ethical) and misunderstanding. Numerous publications address the multiple medication protocols available for the management of AWS.[51,92,100,140] The majority of these reviews address a patient population whose primary medical problem is alcohol dependence, while the concerns of the acutely ill surgical patient go largely unaddressed. These reviews rarely mention the subject of ethanol administration in this context, and rightly so. When the issue is addressed, the administration of ethanol in the acute hospital setting is not condoned primarily because of a lack of published literature to support its use. The literature cited consists of several anecdotal reports or small observational or retrospective studies that describe the administration of ethanol but from which no valid conclusions can be made.[61,72] To our knowledge the most relevant literature addressing the problem of AWS in the acutely ill surgical patient population comes from a single author, Claudia D. Spies, M.D., from the Department of Anesthesiology and Operative Intensive Care, Benjamin Franklin Medical Center, Berlin, Germany.[150–153] These reports clearly document a difference in clinical behavior and response to therapy of AWS in the setting of acute illness and surgical care, compared with the chronic alcoholic treated in a specialized alcohol detoxification unit. One of these studies is a prospective, randomized, blinded study comparing one ethanol-based and three benzodiazepine-based protocols. This study found no significant difference among the four protocols with respect to efficacy or complications when used in the surgical intensive care unit setting. The sample sizes reported were approximately 50 patients per group, putting their conclusion of "no difference between groups" at potential risk for a type II error. Besides the Spies et al. reports, the remainder of the medical literature that addresses the use of ethanol cannot be used in a meaningful way, except maybe to demonstrate that ethanol was and continues to be used by practicing physicians. Finally, the current state-of-the-art management of AWS comes from studies, many of which were done in the 1960s to 1980s, with similar scientific deficiencies.[106]

Despite ethanol being administered to hospitalized patients, there is no collective knowledge base upon which to determine its efficacy and safety when used in the setting of the acutely ill surgical patient who is alcohol dependent. A brief report demonstrated that intravenous administration to a selected group of trauma patients could be performed safely.[168] The Maryland Institute for Emergency Medical Services Systems has recognized the useful role that ethanol replacement can play in the management of the alcohol dependent-injured patients, stating, "the prophylactic treatment of choice (for AWS) is oral or intravenous alcohol" (1982) and "The prevention of alcohol abstinence syndrome or its rapid resolution, should it occur, is obligatory for an optimal outcome in the seriously injured patient. The most specific and effective antidote is alcohol" (1991).[28] A recent handbook of trauma care recognizes alcohol infusion therapy as an alternative to benzodiazepines in the management AWS.[32] The University of Southern California provides guidelines for the treatment of AWS with ethyl alcohol infusion at: www.usc.edu/hsc/medicine/surgery/trauma/protocols. Finally, a recent review of the management of AWS in the surgical patient lists alcohol replacement as an alternative to benzodiazepine therapy.[153]

ETHANOL REPLACEMENT PROTOCOL Ethyl alcohol (10-20% solution) is administered intravenously according to the following guidelines, based on the patient's clinical status as measured by the CIWA-Ar scoring system. Trained nurses can carry out an evaluation in less than 2 minutes, and the inter-rater reliability is high (r >0.8). The titration of the alcohol drip is based on clinical symptomatology as graded by both the CIWA-Ar score and the OAA/S score (see Fig. 10-2 and Box 10-3).

1. Initiate a continuous intravenous ethanol infusion (1 mL/kg/hr of 10% ethyl alcohol in 0.45% or 0.9% saline or 5% dextrose) via a peripheral or central venous line. If the patient's BAL is not measurable at the time of the initiation of the infusion, a loading dose equal to 0.5–1.0 mL/kg of 10% ethyl alcohol should be given as an intravenous infusion over 5 minutes.

2. **Increase** the ethanol dose according to the patient's clinical condition. Titration of the dose is achieved by giving an initial bolus of 0.5–1.0 mL/kg of 10% ethyl alcohol followed by an increase in drip rate of 10-20 mL/hr. Increases in rate should not be done any more frequently than every 4 hours. One or two additional boluses of 0.5–1.0 mL/kg can be given if the patient's clinical condition warrants additional ethanol prior to the next allowable increase in infusion rate. After the patient has been on a stable infusion for 6 hours, the BAL should be obtained and should be rechecked on a daily basis thereafter *throughout the duration of ethanol administration.* A stable infusion rate is defined as a 4-hour period during which the patient's CIWA-Ar score remains unchanged or improved and there have been no changes in the ethanol dose administered. If there is active titration of the ethanol infusion, then a BAL should be checked at 6 hours following each change in dose. If the patient requires volume

restriction (e.g., cardiopulmonary disease or cerebral edema/intracranial hypertension; CPP <70 mm Hg), a change to 20% solution of ethanol should be undertaken. *The 20% ethyl alcohol solution is cytotoxic (hyperosmolar)[1] and must be administered in D_5W via a central line. No patient should receive a dose in excess of 70 mL/hr of 20% ethanol.* (The measured osmolarity of ethanol solutions in D_5W is 5% ethanol [1160 mOsm], 10% ethanol [4160 mOsm], and 20% ethanol [7820 mOsm]).

3. **Discontinue** the ethanol therapy by stopping treatment after 7 days. At the end of 7 days of therapy, the ethanol infusion is discontinued, without a taper, as the patient is now considered detoxified. All patients are monitored for evidence of withdrawal symptomatology for 72 hours thereafter if they remain hospitalized. If the patient's medical/surgical condition is cleared for discharge *prior* to the 7–10 days (i.e., still potentially alcohol dependent), then subsequent management is dictated by whether the patient has consented to enrollment in an alcohol rehabilitation program. If the patient has consented to further treatment, then arrangements are made for alcohol addiction treatment and rehabilitation through Substance Abuse consultation. Patients who refuse enrollment can be discharged with proper follow-up care for their medical/surgical conditions.

4. Consider transferring patient to an intensive care unit environment when (a) the patient is not responding to treatment (inability to control patient's symptoms within 12–24 hours of initiation of treatment), or (b) if CIWA-Ar score is ≥25 at any time, or (c) OAA/S score is <15.

ADDITIONAL CONSIDERATIONS FOR IMPLEMENTATION OF ALCOHOL REPLACEMENT THERAPY

The intent of ethanol replacement is to attenuate the severity of AWS symptomatology and prevent the development of DTs. Most patients will develop a low-grade fever (101–102 °F) and tachycardia (heart rate 110–120/min), representing mild AWS as the patient is detoxifying. Further increases in ethanol dose, in an attempt to normalize these vital signs, will only lead to reaching toxic blood alcohol levels. Mild pyrexia and tachycardia are accepted as a normal part of the AWS clinical course and are expected to last 48 to 72 hours.

The therapeutic goal of alcohol replacement therapy is to achieve and maintain the patient in a calm but alert state. Generally, the individual's CIWA-Ar score is ≤10 and BAL is <20 mg/dL when this clinical end point is achieved. Once a patient is on an adequate dose, this infusion rate should be continued for 7 days and the BAL obtained daily. It should be emphasized that the use of ethanol in this manner targets a *clinically based therapeutic goal and does not depend on achieving a particular BAL.* Ideally, the BAL should remain at low-to-undetectable levels (i.e., BAL <20 mg/dL); however, rare patients may require a higher BAL for control of their AWS. Patients requiring BALs greater than 40 mg% should have their

infusions reduced once they have responded clinically (i.e., CIWA-Ar score ≤10, or decreased by 5) for 24 hours to achieve a BAL <20 mg% while maintaining the CIWA-Ar ≤10. The purpose of a daily BAL is to ensure the alcohol level remains at a low and stable level. The initiation dose of ethyl alcohol used in this algorithm, 1 mL/kg/min (0.1 g/kg/hr), is just below the level at which the metabolic capacity of the average person becomes saturated. Ethanol is metabolized via a liver enzyme system (following Michaelis-Menton enzyme kinetics, with significant variation depending on the patient's recent alcohol ingestion history); thus, a large increase in the BAL may result from a relatively small increase in the infusion rate, especially at rates >1 mL/kg/hr (i.e., 0.1 g/kg/hr).[169,176] The goal of performing a daily BAL measurement is to prevent a rising BAL during "maintenance" infusion. Individual patient responses may vary and thus require constant clinical and laboratory monitoring throughout the duration of ethanol administration. *No patient should receive a dose in excess of 70 mL/hr of 20 percent ethanol.* If a patient has a detectable BAL and has continued agitation, a prompt reevaluation for other causes of mental status changes must be performed.

Opiates

Opiate withdrawal syndrome is preventable. Management of opiate withdrawal depends on modifying withdrawal symptoms. Temporary substitution with a long-acting opiate reduces symptom severity. The use of short-acting opiates is appropriate for intensive care unit (ICU) and postoperative patients, where frequent monitoring and dosing assessment can be readily accomplished.[72] Long-acting opiates, such as methadone, are currently restricted under U.S. Federal Regulations for the treatment of opiate addiction. They can be used for maintenance therapy or detoxification when an addicted patient is admitted to the hospital for illness other than opiate abuse. It is important to note, however, that patients with non-abuse-related physical pain, who have been treated with methadone for withdrawal prevention, must have their pain needs met by a different opiate rather than by increasing their maintenance methadone dose. Patients treated with opiates for more than 1 to 2 weeks should be instructed to gradually taper their dose, by 25 percent every day or two, to prevent signs and symptoms of withdrawal. If needed, clonidine (0.1–0.2 mg, q4–6hr) can be used to attenuate the autonomic hyperactivity symptoms. Clonidine has been used successfully in suppressing the signs and symptoms of withdrawal within 24 hours, thus shortening the duration of symptoms by 5 to 6 days. Clonidine, an α_2-adrenergic receptor agonist, acts by decreasing catecholamine-associated sympathetic activity and works in synergy with low doses of appropriate opiates. Common side effects of clonidine include dryness of the mouth, orthostatic hypotension, sedation, and constipation. An alternative agent for the management of the opiate addicted individual is buprenorphine. Buprenorphine is considered a partial agonist; unlike methadone, it acts as a pure agonist. It causes fewer withdrawal symptoms and has a reduced risk for respiratory depression with an overdose. Its long half-life allows for daily dosing as well. Some detoxification protocols use buprenorphine on longer regimens ranging up to treatment every 7 weeks.[26] Reported efficacy of buprenorphine is similar to that of methadone and clonidine. Buprenorphine, with high mu receptor affinity, has been used widely in critically ill patients with favorable results. Buprenorphine causes very little sedation, respiratory depression, or hypotension even at supra-therapeutic levels. It is important to note that ongoing substance-abuse counseling, efforts to reduce needle sharing and transmission of viral disease, along with pharmacologic management contribute to patient therapeutic success.[5]

Outpatient use typically involves administration of methadone daily for a maximum of 3 days while the patient awaits acceptance into a licensed methadone treatment clinic. Methadone has also been used successfully for over three decades and is currently the staple of outpatient management. Nalbuphine (Nubain), pentazocine and naloxone (Talwin), and butorphanol (Stadol) are three agents to be avoided by patients on methadone owing to their ability to elicit immediate withdrawal syndromes.

Cocaine

Currently, the clinical efficacy of an agent to prevent cocaine withdrawal has not been identified. The agents that have been most studied in abating cocaine withdrawal are amantadine, bromocriptine, and naltrexone. Agents such as lithium, tricyclic antidepressants, and trazodone have been used in an attempt to manage the later phases of cocaine withdrawal. Current treatment regimens are usually directed at treatment of cocaine intoxication. Benzodiazepines have played a predominant role in preventing hyperthermia, acidosis, seizures, and cardiovascular excitation of acute cocaine intoxication.[149]

Benzodiazepines

The patient who has received continuous infusion of benzodiazepines during the hospital stay should have the dose gradually tapered. Should a patient develop benzodiazepine withdrawal during hospitalization, institution of immediate therapy and subsequent weaning is recommended according to the protocol outlined above for alcohol withdrawal. Once the patient's condition has stabilized, the infusion is decreased by 0.1 mg/hr increments to a minimum of 0.1 mg/hr while the patient's sedation score is assessed. The rate of reduction should not exceed 0.1 mg/hr in 8–12 hours.[102]

Discharge Plans

Following recovery from AWS the patient is now considered detoxified and should be referred to a substance abuse program for follow-up care.[87] Established programs employ a combination of behavioral and pharmacologic therapies.[51]

SUMMARY

Injured and ill patients who come to a general medical hospital frequently carry a secondary substance abuse diagnosis. The physician must remain alert and determine the risk each of these patients has for the development of a medical complication related to substance abuse. Methods to identify patients at moderate-to-high risk for development of alcohol withdrawal syndrome have been presented and reviewed. Risk stratification is the first step. Early recognition of signs and symptoms of acute withdrawal is important. Early signs and symptoms have been reviewed with an emphasis on their time frame of development. Finally, preventive and treatment algorithms have been presented as guidelines that can be applied to the inpatient orthopaedic and pre- and postoperative surgical patient. The need to add substance abuse to the patient's medical record along with appropriate referral to a substance abuse program cannot be overstated in the management of these challenging patient problems.

REFERENCES

1. Agu, O.; Hamilton, G.; Baker, D. Graduated compression stockings in the prevention of venous thromboembolism. Br J Surg 86:992–1004, 1999.
2. Alford, D.P.; Compton, P.; Samet, J.H.; et al. Acute pain management for patients receiving maintenance methadone or buprenorphine therapy. Ann Intern Med 144:127–134, 2006.
3. Al-Sanouri, I.; Dikin, M.; Soubani, A.O. Critical care aspects of alcohol abuse. South Med J 98:372–381, 2005.
4. Argoff, C.E.; Misha-Miroslav, B.; Belgrade, M.J.; et al. Consensus guidelines for diabetic peripheral neuropathic pain: Treatment planning and options. Mayo Clin Proc 81(Suppl 4):S12–S25, 2006.
5. Bailey, K.P. Pharmacological treatment of substance use disorders. J Psych Nurs 42:14–20, 2004.
6. Balaban, N.; Giacometti, A.; Cirioni, O.; et al. Use of the quorum-sensing inhibitor RNAIII-inhibiting peptide to prevent biofilm formation in vivo by drug-resistant *Staphylococcus epidermidis*. J Infect Dis 187:625–630, 2003.
7. Baynard, M.; McIntyre, J.; Hill, K.R.; et al. Alcohol withdrawal syndrome. Am Fam Physician 69:1443–1450, 2004.
8. Blaser, J.; Vergeres, P.; Widmer, A.F.; et al. In vivo verification of in vitro model of antibiotic treatment of device-related infection. Antimicrob Agents Chemother 39:1134–1139, 1995.
9. Blumberg, H.M.; Rimland, D.; Caroll, D.J.; et al. Rapid development of ciprofloxacin resistance in methicillin-susceptible and methicillin-resistant *Staphylococcus aureus*. J Infect Dis 163:1279–1285, 1991.
10. Boscainos, P.J.; McLardy-Smith, P.; Jinnah, R.H. Deep vein thrombosis prophylaxis after total-knee arthroplasty. Curr Opin Orthop 17:60–67, 2006.
11. Bradley, K.A.; Boyd-Wickizer, J.; Powell, S.H.; et al. Alcohol screening questionnaires in women: A critical review. JAMA 280:166–171, 1998.
12. Bramlage, P.; Pittrow, D.; Kirch, W. Current concepts for the prevention of venous thromboembolism. Eur J Clin Invest 35(Suppl 1):4–11, 2005.

13. Bresalier, R.S.; Sandler, R.S.; Quan, H.; et al. Cardiovascular events associated with rofecoxib in a colorectal adenoma chemoprevention trial. N Engl J Med 352:1092–1102, 2005.

14. Broder, K.W.; Moise, P.A.; Schultz, R.O.; et al. Clinical experience with linezolid in conjunction with wound coverage techniques for skin and soft tissue infections and postoperative osteomyelitis. Ann Plast Surg 52:385–390, 2004.

15. Caldwell, B.; Aldington, S.; Weatherall, M.; et al. Risk of cardiovascular events and celecoxib: A systematic review meta-analysis. J R Soc Med 99:132–140, 2006.

16. Cammarano, W.B.; Pittet, J.F.; Weitz, S.; et al. Acute withdrawal syndrome related to the administration of analgesic and sedative medications in adult intensive care unit patients. Crit Care Med 26:676–684, 1998.

17. Camu, F.; Beecher, T.; Recker, D.P.; et al. Valdecoxib, a COX-2 specific inhibitor, is an efficacious, opioid-sparing analgesic in patients undergoing hip arthroplasty. Am J Ther 9:43–51, 2002.

18. Caprini, J.A.; Arcelus, J.I.; Maksimovic, D.; et al. Thrombosis prophylaxis in orthopedic surgery: Current clinical considerations. J South Ortho Assoc 11:190–196, 2002.

19. Carr, D.B.; Jacox, A. Acute Pain Management: Operative or Medical Procedures and Trauma: Clinical Practice Guideline. Rockville, MD: Agency for Healthcare Policy and Research, U.S. Department of Health and Human Services, 1992.

20. Catella-Lawson, F.; Reilly, M.P.; Kapoor, S.C.; et al. Cyclooxygenase inhibitors and the antiplatelet effects of aspirin. N Engl J Med 345:1809–1817, 2001.

21. Chakkalakal, D.A. Alcohol-induced bone loss and deficient bone repair: Alcohol Clin Exp Res 29:2077–2090, 2005.

22. Chang, P.H.; Steinberg, M.B. Alcohol withdrawal. Med Clin North Am 85:1191–1212, 2001.

23. Chen, H.; Lamer, T.J.; Rho, R.H.; et al. Contemporary management of neuropathic pain for the primary care physician. Mayo Clin Proc 79:1533–1545, 2004.

24. Chernik, D.A.; Gillings, D.; Laine, H.; et al. Validity and reliability of the Observer's Assessment of Alertness/Sedation Scale: Study with intravenous midazolam. J Clin Psychopharmacol 10:244, 1990.

25. Cohen, A.T.; Bailey, C.S.; Alikhan, R.; et al. Extended thromboprophylaxis with low-molecular-weight heparin reduces symptomatic venous thromboembolism following lower limb arthroplasty: A meta-analysis. Thromb Haemost 85:940–941, 2001.

26. Collins, E.D.; Kleber, H.D.; Whittington, R.A.; et al. Anesthesia-assisted vs. buprenorphine- or clonidine-assisted heroin detoxification and naltrexone induction: A randomized trial. JAMA 294:903–913, 2005.

27. Colwell, C.; Mouret, P. Ximelagatran for the prevention of venous thromboembolism following elective hip or knee replacement surgery. Semin Vascular Med 5:266–275, 2005.

28. Cowley, R.A.; Dunham, C.M. Shock Trauma/Critical Care Manual. Baltimore, MD, University Park Press, 1982, p. 384.

29. Criscuolo, S.; Auletta, C.; Lippi, S.; et al. Oxcarbazepine monotherapy in postherpetic neuralgia unresponsive to carbamazepine and gabapentin. Acta Neurol Scand 111:229–232, 2005.

30. Dahners, L.E.; Mullis, B.H. Effects of nonsteroidal anti-inflammatory drugs on bone formation and soft-tissue healing. J Am Acad Orthop Surg 12:139–143, 2004.

31. Danielsson, P.E.; Rivara, F.P.; Gentilello, L.M.; et al. Reasons why trauma surgeons fail to screen for alcohol problems. Arch Surgery 134:564–568, 1999.

32. Demetrios, D.; Asensio, J. Trauma Management. Georgetown, TX, Landes Bioscience, 2000, p. 670.

33. Dobesh, P.P. Evidence for extended prophylaxis in the setting of orthopedic surgery. Pharmacotherapy 24:73S–81S, 2004.

34. Douketis, J.D.; Eikelboom, J.W.; Quinlan, D.J.; et al. Short-duration prophylaxis against venous thromboembolism after total hip or knee replacement: A meta-analysis of prospective studies investigating symptomatic outcomes. Arch Intern Med 162:1465–1471, 2002.

35. Drago, L.; Vecchi, E.; Fassina, M.C.; et al. Serum and bone concentrations of teicoplanin and vancomycin: Study in an animal model. Drugs Exp Clin Res 24:185–190, 1998.

36. Drancourt, M.; Stein, A.; Argenson, J.N.; et al. Oral treatment of *Staphylococcus* spp. infected orthopaedic implants with fusidic acid or ofloxacin in combination with rifampicin. J Antimicrob Chemother 39:235–240, 1997.

37. Dunn, C.W.; Donovan, D.M.; Gentilello, L.M. Practical guidelines for performing alcohol interventions in trauma centers. J Trauma 42:299, 1997.

38. Eichinger, S.; Kyrle, P.A. Prevention of deep vein thrombosis in orthopedic surgery. Eur J Med Res 9:112–118, 2004.

39. Ellington, J.K.; Harris, M.; Hudson, M.C.; et al. Intracellular *Staphylococcus aureus* and antibiotic resistance: Implications for treatment of staphylococcal osteomyelitis. J Orthop Res 24:87–93, 2006.

40. Eriksson, B.I.; Wille-Jorgensen, P.; Kalebo, P.; et al. A comparison of recombinant hirudin with a low-molecular-weight heparin to prevent thromboembolic complications after total hip replacement. N Engl J Med 337:1329–1335, 1997.

41. Erstad, B.L.; Grier, D.G.; Scott, M.E.; et al. Recognition and treatment of ethanol abuse in trauma patients. Heart Lung 25:330–336, 1996.

42. Feenstra, J.; Heerdink, E.R.; Grobbee, D.E.; et al. Association of nonsteroidal anti-inflammatory drugs with first occurrence of heart failure and with relapsing heart failure. Arch Intern Med 162:265–270, 2002.

43. Finney, M.S.; Crank, C.W.; Segreti, J. Use of daptomycin to treat drug-resistant gram-positive bone and joint infections. Curr Med Res Opin 21:1923–1926, 2005.

44. Foy, A.; Kay, J.; Taylor, A. The course of alcohol withdrawal in a general hospital. Q J Med 90:253–261, 1997.

45. Freedland, E.S.; McMicken, D.B.; D'Onofrio, G. Alcohol and trauma. Emerg Clin North Am 11:225–239, 1993.

46. Freedman, K.B.; Brookenthal, K.R.; Fitzgerald, R.H.; et al. A meta-analysis of thromboembolic prophylaxis following elective hip arthroplasty. J Bone Joint Surg Am 82:929–938, 2000.

47. Fritsche, T.R.; Sader, H.S.; Stilwell, M.G.; et al. Potency and spectrum of tigecycline tested against an international collection of bacterial pathogens associated with skin and soft tissue infections (2000–2004). Diagn Microbiol Infect Dis 52:195–201, 2005.

48. Gajic, O.; Warner, D.O.; Decker, P.A.; et al. Long-haul air travel before major surgery: A prescription for thromboembolism? Mayo Clin Proc 80(6):728–731, 2005.

49. Gallus, A.S. Applying risk assessment models in orthopedic surgery: Overview of our clinical experience. Blood Coag Fibrinol 10(Suppl 2):S53–S61, 1999.

50. Gannon, R. Pharm. D., Hartford Hospital, August 19, 2002; personal communication.

51. Garbutt, J.C.; West, S.L.; Carey, T.S.; et al. Pharmacologic treatment of alcohol dependence: A review of the evidence. JAMA 281:1318–1325, 1999.

52. Gardell, L.R.; King, T.; Ossipov, M.H.; et al. Opioid receptor–mediated hyperalgesia and antinociceptive tolerance induced by sustained opiate delivery. Neuroscience Letters 396:44–49, 2006.

53. Geerts, W.H.; Pineo, G.F.; Heit, J.A.; et al. Prevention of venous thromboembolism: The seventh ACCP Conference on Antithrombotic and Thrombolytic Therapy. Chest 126:338S–400S, 2004.

54. Gentilello, L.M.; Donovan, D.M.; Dunn, C.W.; et al. Alcohol interventions in trauma centers. JAMA 274:1043–1048, 1995.

55. Gilron, I.; Bailey, J.M.; Dongsheng, T.; et al. Morphine, gabapentin, or their combination for neuropathic pain. N Engl J Med 352:1324–1334, 2005.

56. Glassman, S.D.; Rose, S.M.; Dimar, J.R.; et al. The effect of postoperative nonsteroidal anti-inflammatory drug administration on spinal fusion. Spine 23:834–838, 1998.

57. Goldhaber, S.Z. Pulmonary embolism. Lancet 363:1295–1305, 2004.

58. Goldhaber, S.Z. Venous thromboembolism: An ounce of prevention. Mayo Clin Proc 80:725–726, 2005.

59. Gonzalez, B.E.; Martinez-Aguilar, G.; Hulten, K.G.; et al. Severe staphylococcal sepsis in adolescents in the era of community-acquired methicillin-resistant *Staphylococcus aureus*. Pediatrics 115:642–648, 2005.

60. Gordon, D.B.; Dahl, J.L.; Miaskowski, C.; et al. American Pain Society recommendations for improving the quality of acute and cancer pain management. Arch Intern Med 165:1574–1580, 2005.

61. Gower, W.E.; Kersten, H. Prevention of alcohol withdrawal symptoms in surgical patients. Surg Gynecol Obstet 151:382–384, 1980.

62. Grafenreed, K.M.; Lobo, B.; Sands, C.; et al. Development of alcohol withdrawal delirium prophylaxis protocol in community teaching hospital. Am J Health Syst Pharm 61:1151–1155, 2004.

63. Graninger, W.; Presterl, E.; Wenisch, C.; et al. Management of serious staphylococcal infections in the outpatient setting. Drugs 54(Suppl 6):21–28, 1997.

64. Grass, J.A. Patient-controlled analgesia. Anesth Analg 101(5 Suppl):S44–S61, 2005.

65. Graziani, A.L.; Lawson, L.A.; Gibson, G.E.; et al. Vancomycin concentrations in infected and non-infected human bone. Antimicrob Agents Chemother 32(9):1320–1322, 1988.

66. Greenberg, R.N.; Newman, M.T.; Shariaty, S.; et al. Ciprofloxacin, lomefloxacin, or levofloxacin as treatment for chronic osteomyelitis. Antimicrob Agents Chemother 44:164–166, 2000.

67. Haas, S. Deep vein thrombosis: Beyond the operating table. Orthopedics 23(Suppl 6):S629–S632, 2000.

68. Haines, S.T.; Bussey, H.I. Diagnosis of deep vein thrombosis. Am J Health Syst Pharm 54:66–74, 1997.

69. Haines, S.T.; Bussey, H.I. Thrombosis and the pharmacology of antithrombotic agents. Ann Pharmacother 29:892–905, 1995.

70. Hamed, K.A.; Tam, J.Y.; Prober, C.G. Pharmacokinetic optimization of the treatment of septic arthritis. Clin Pharmacokinet 31:156–163, 1996.

71. Hampton, T. New oral anticoagulants show promise. JAMA 295:743–744, 2006.

72. Hansbrough, J.F.; Zapata-Sirvent, R.L.; Carroll, W.J.; et al. Administration of intravenous alcohol for prevention of withdrawal in alcoholic burn patients. Am J Surg 148:266, 1984.

73. Hantler, C.; Despotis, G.J.; Sinha, R.; et al. Guidelines and alternatives for neuraxial anesthesia and venous thromboembolism prophylaxis in major orthopedic surgery. J Arthroplasty 19:1004–1016, 2004.

74. Harwood, P.J.; Talbot, C.; Dimoutsos, M.; et al. Early experience with linezolid for infections in orthopaedics. Injury 37:818–826, 2006.

75. Howden, B.P.; Ward, P.B.; Charles, P.G.; et al. Treatment options for serious infections caused by methicillin-resistant *Staphylococcus aureus* with reduced vancomycin susceptibility. Clin Infect Dis 38:521–528, 2004.

76. Hull, R.D.; Brant, R.F.; Pineo, G.F.; et al. Preoperative vs postoperative initiation of low-molecular-weight heparin prophylaxis against venous thromboembolism in patients undergoing elective hip replacement. Arch Intern Med 159(2):137–141, 1999.

77. Huo, M.H.; Stuckey, R. Thromboembolism after total hip arthroplasty. Curr Opin Orthop 16:25–28, 2005.

78. Illig, K.A.; Eagleton, M.; Kaufman, D.; et al. Alcohol withdrawal after open aortic surgery. Ann Vasc Surg 15:332–337, 2001.

79. Issioui, T.; Klein, K.W.; White, P.F.; et al. The efficacy of premedication with celecoxib and acetaminophen in preventing pain after otolaryngologic surgery. Anesth Analg 94:1188–1193, 2002.

80. Jacqueline, C.; Caillon, J.; Le Mabecque, V.; et al. In vitro activity of linezolid alone and in combination with gentamicin, vancomycin, or rifampicin against methicillin-resistant *Staphylococcus aureus* by time-kill curve methods. J Antimicrob Chemother 51:857–864, 2003.

81. Jones, J.P., Jr., Peltier, L.F. Alcoholism, hypercortisolism, fat embolism and osseous avascular necrosis. Clin Orthop Rel Res 1:4–12, 2001.

82. Kaplan, S.L.; Mason, E.O.; Feigin, R.D. Clindamycin versus nafcillin or methicillin in the treatment of *Staphylococcus aureus* osteomyelitis in children. South Med J 75:138–142, 1982.

83. Kearon, C. Duration of venous thromboembolism prophylaxis after surgery. Chest 124(6 Suppl): 386S–392S, 2003.

84. Kleinschmidt, K.C. Ethanol. In Delaney, K.A.; et al. (eds.). Ethanol. St. Louis, Mosby, 1998, pp. 475–491.

85. Koch, A.; Ziegler, S.; Breitschwerdt, H.; et al. Low-molecular-weight heparin and unfractionated heparin in thrombosis prophylaxis: Meta-analysis based on original patient data. Thromb Res 102:295–309, 2001.

86. Koo, P. Postoperative pain management with a patient-controlled transdermal delivery system for fentanyl. Am J Health Syst Pharm 62:1171–1176, 2005.

87. Kosten, T.; O'Connor, P. Management of drug and alcohol withdrawal. N Engl J Med 348:1786–1795, 2003.

88. Lange, R.A.; Hillis, L.D. Cardiovascular complications of cocaine use. N Engl J Med 345:351–358, 2001.

89. Lassen, M.R. Comparative efficacy of low-molecular-weight heparins in orthopedic surgery. Semin Thromb Hemost 26(Suppl 1):53–56, 2000.

90. Leese, P.T.; Hubbard, R.C.; Karim, A.; et al. Effects of celecoxib, a novel cyclooxygenase-2 inhibitor, on platelet function in healthy adults: A randomized controlled trial. J Clin Pharmacol 40:124–132, 2000.

91. Leiber, C.S. Medical disorders of alcoholism. N Engl J Med 333:1058–1065, 1995.

92. Litten, R.Z.; Allen, J.; Fertig, J. Pharmacotherapies for alcohol problems: A review of research with focus on developments since 1991. Alcohol Clin Exp Res 20:859–876, 1996.

93. Lobo, B.L. Emerging options for thromboprophylaxis after orthopedic surgery: A review of clinical data. Pharmacotherapy 24(7 Pt 2):66S–72S, 2004.

94. Lovering, A.M.; Zhang, J.; Bannister, G.C.; et al. Penetration of linezolid into bone, fat, muscle and haematoma of patients undergoing routine hip replacement. J Antimicrob Chemother 50:73–77, 2002.

95. Lukan, J.K.; Reed, R.N.; Looney, S.W.; et al. Risk factors for delirium tremens in trauma patients. J Trauma 52:902–906, 2002.

96. Mader, J.T.; Mohan, D.; Calhoun, J. A practical guide to the diagnosis and management of bone and joint infections. Drugs 54:253–264, 1997.

97. Mader, J.T.; Shirtliff, M.E.; Bergquist, S.C.; et al. Antimicrobial treatment of chronic osteomyelitis. Clin Orthop Rel Res 360:47–65, 1999.

98. Mahe, I.; Bertrand, N.; Drouet, L.; et al. Paracetamol: A haemorrhagic risk factor in patients on warfarin. Br J Clin Pharmacol 59:371–374, 2005.

99. Malincarne, L.; Ghebregzabher, M.; Moretti, M.V.; et al. Penetration of moxifloxacin into bone in patients undergoing total knee arthroplasty. J Antimicrob Chemother 57:950–954, 2006.

100. Mayo-Smith, M.F. Pharmacological management of alcohol withdrawal: A meta-analysis and evidence-based practice guideline. JAMA 278:144–151, 1997.

101. Mayo-Smith, M.F.; Beecher, L.H.; Fischer, T.L.; et al. Management of alcohol withdrawal delirium. JAMA 164:1405–1412, 2004.

102. McCaffrey, M.; Pasero, C. American Society of Addiction Medicine Clinical Manual, 2nd ed. St. Louis, Mosby, 2001, pp. 475–491.

103. Milzman, D.P.; Soderstrom, C.A. Substance use disorders in trauma patients. Crit Care Clin 10:595–612, 1994.

104. Mismetti, P.; Laporte, S.; Zufferet, P.; et al. Prevention of venous thromboembolism in orthopedic surgery with vitamin K antagonists: A meta-analysis. J Thromb Haemost 2:1058–1070, 2004.

105. Mitra, S.; Sinatra, R.S. Perioperative management of acute pain in the opioid-dependent patient. Anesthesiology 101:212–227, 2004.

106. Moskowitz, G.; Chalmers, T.C.; Sacks, H.S.; et al. Deficiencies of clinical trials of alcohol assessment: Alcoholism. Clin Exp Res 7:42–46, 1983.

107. National Household Survey on Drug Abuse (NHSDA). Washington, DC: Substance Abuse and Mental Health Services Administration (SAMSHSA), 2006.

108. Nevin, J. Cocaine overdose: What you need to know. Emerg Med Serv 31:87–88, 2002.

109. Neyman, K.M.; Gourin, C.G.; Terris, D.J. Alcohol withdrawal prophylaxis in patients undergoing surgical treatment of head and neck squamous cell carcinoma. Laryngoscope 115:786–790, 2005.

110. Ng, J.; Gosbell, I.B. Successful oral pristinamycin therapy for osteoarticular infections due to methicillin-resistant *Staphylococcus aureus* (MRSA) and other *Staphylococcus* spp. J Antimicrob Chemother 55:1008–1012, 2005.

111. Nicolaides, A.N.; Breddin, H.K.; Fareed, J.; et al. Prevention of venous thromboembolism: International consensus statement: Guidelines, compiled in accordance with the scientific evidence. Int Angiol 20:1–37, 2001.

112. NIH website for alcohol withdrawal syndrome. Available at: http://silk.nih.gov/silk/niaaa1/publications/aao5.htm.

113. Nijkeuter, M.; Huisman, M.V. Pentasaccharides in the prophylaxis and treatment of venous thromboembolism: A systematic review. Curr Opin Pulm Med 10:338–344, 2004.

114. Niv, D.; Gofeld, M.; Devor, M. Causes of pain in degenerative bone and joint disease: A lesson from vertebroplasty. Pain 105:387–392, 2003.

115. Norden, C.W. Experimental chronic staphylococcal osteomyelitis in rabbits: Treatment with rifampin alone and in combination with other antimicrobial agents. Rev Infect Dis 5(Suppl 3):S491–S494, 1983.

116. Norden, C.W.; Fierer, J.; Bryant, R.E. Chronic staphylococcal osteomyelitis: Treatment with regimens containing rifampin. Rev Infect Dis 5(Suppl 3):495–501, 1983.

117. Nussmeier, N.A.; Whelton, A.A.; Brown, M.T.; et al. Complications of the COX-2 inhibitors parecoxib and valdecoxib after cardiac surgery. N Engl J Med 352:1081–1091, 2005.

118. O'Connor, P.G.; Schottenfeld, R.S. Patient with alcohol problems. N Engl J Med 338:592–601, 1998.

119. Ottinger, J.G. Retrospective evaluation of delayed administration of fondaparinux in providing comparable safety and efficacy outcomes in patients undergoing elective-arthroplasty procedures. Hosp Pharm 41:348–353, 2006.

120. Pavoni, G.L.; Falcone, M.; Baiocchi, P.; et al. Conservative medical therapy of infections following osteosynthesis: A retrospective analysis of a six-year experience. J Chemother 14:378–383, 2002.

121. The Physician's Guide to Helping Patients with Alcohol Problems. NIH publication No. 95-3769 Bethesda, MD, National Institute on Alcohol Abuse and Alcoholism, 1995.

122. Planes, A. An equivalency study of two low-molecular-weight heparins in the prevention and treatment of deep-vein thrombosis after total hip replacement. Semin Thromb Hemost 26(Suppl 1):57–60, 2000.

123. Prandoni, P.; Bruchi, O.; Sabbion, P.; et al. Prolonged thromboprophylaxis with oral anticoagulants after total hip arthroplasty. Arch Intern Med 162:1966–1971, 2002.

124. Pulmonary Embolism Prevention (PEP) Trial Collaborative Group: Prevention of pulmonary embolism and deep vein thrombosis with low dose aspirin. Lancet 355:1295–1302, 2000.

125. Raloff, J.; Pruitt, B.A., Jr. The impact of alcohol and other drug problems on trauma care. J Trauma Injury Infect Crit Care 59(3 Suppl):S50–S52; S67–S75, 2005.

126. Rand, K.H.; Houck, H. Daptomycin synergy with rifampicin and ampicillin against vancomycin-resistant enterococci. J Antimicrob Chemother 53:530–532, 2004.

127. Raskob, G.E.; Hish, J. Controversies in timing of the first dose of anticoagulant prophylaxis against venous thromboembolism after major orthopedic surgery. Chest 124:379S–385S, 2003.

128. Recart, A.; Issioui, T.; White, P.; et al. The efficacy of celecoxib premedication on postoperative pain and recovery times after ambulatory surgery: A dose-ranging study. Anesth Analg 96:1631–1635, 2003.

129. Rehm, S.J.; Graham, D.R.; Srinath, L.; et al. Successful administration of quinupristin/dalfopristin in the outpatient setting. J Antimicrob Chemother 47:639–645, 2001.

130. Reuben, S.S.; Ekman, E.F. The effect of cyclooxygenase-2 inhibition on analgesia and spinal fusion. J Bone Joint Surg Am 87:536–542, 2005.

131. Reynolds, L.W.; Hoo, R.K.; Brill, R.J.; et al. The COX-2 specific inhibitor, valdecoxib, is an effective opioid-sparing analgesic in patients undergoing total knee arthroplasty. J Pain Symptom Manage 25:133–141, 2003.

132. Rivara, F.P.; Jurkovich, G.J.; Gurney, J.G.; et al. The magnitude of acute and chronic alcohol abuse in trauma patients. Arch Surg 128:907–913, 1993.

133. Rouse, M.S.; Piper, K.E.; Jacobson, M.; et al. Daptomycin treatment of *Staphylococcus aureus* experimental chronic osteomyelitis. J Antimicrob Chemother 57:301–305, 2006.

134. Rowlingson, J.C.; Hanson, P.B. Neuraxial anesthesia and low-molecular-weight heparin prophylaxis in major orthopedic surgery in the wake of the latest American Society of Regional Anesthesia guidelines. Anesth Analg 100:1482–1488, 2005.

135. Ruhe, J.J.; Monson, T.; Bradsher, R.W.; et al. Use of long-acting tetracyclines for methicillin-resistant *Staphylococcus aureus* infections: Case series and review of the literature. Clin Infect Dis 40:1429–1434, 2005.

136. Saitz, R. Unhealthy alcohol use. N Engl J Med 352:596–607, 2005.

137. Saleh-Mghir, A.; Ameur, N.; Muller-Serieys, C.; et al. Combination of quinupristin-dalfopristin (Synergid) and rifampin is highly synergistic in experimental *Staphylococcus aureus* joint prosthesis infection. Antimicrob Agents Chemother 46:1122–1124, 2002.

138. Schaad, H.J.; Bento, M.; Lew, D.P.; et al. Evaluation of high-dose daptomycin for therapy of experimental *Staphylococcus aureus* foreign body infection. BMC Infect Dis 6:74, 2006.

139. Schad, R.F. Hydroxyzine analgesia: Fact or fantasy? Am J Hosp Pharm 36:1317, 1979.

140. Schaffer, A.; Naranjo, C.A. Recommended drug treatment strategies for the alcoholic patient. Drugs 55:571–585, 1998.

141. Schenker, S.; Bay, M.K. Medical problems associated with alcoholism. Adv Intern Med 43:27–78, 1998.

142. Schiff, R.L.; Kahn, S.R.; Shrier, I.; et al. Identifying orthopedic patients at high risk for venous thromboembolism despite thromboprophylaxis. Chest 128:3364–3371, 2005.

143. Schneekloth, T.D.; Morse, R.; Herrick, L.; et al. Point prevalence of alcoholism in hospitalized patients: Continuing challenges of detection, assessment, and diagnosis. Mayo Clin Proc 76:460–466, 2001.

144. Shanti, C.M.; Luas, C.E. Cocaine and the critical care challenge. Crit Care Med 31:1851–1859, 2003.

145. Silbersack, Y.; Taute, B.M.; Hein, W.; et al. Prevention of deep-vein thrombosis after total hip and knee replacement: Low-molecular-weight heparin in combination with intermittent pneumatic compression. J Bone Joint Surg Br 86:809–812, 2004.

146. Simopoulos, T.T.; Smith, H.S.; Peeters-Asdourian, C.; et al. Use of meperidine in patient-controlled analgesia and the development of a normeperidine toxic reaction. Arch Surg 137:84–88, 2002.

147. Skinner, H.B.; Schulz, M.M. Clinical implication of thromboprophylaxis in the management of total hip and knee arthroplasty. Am J Orthop 31(9S):20–30, 2002.

148. Soderstrom, C.A.; Cole, F.A., Jr., Porter, J.M. Injury in America: The role of alcohol and other drugs—An EAST position paper prepared by the Injury Control and Violence Prevention Committee. J Trauma 50:1–12, 2001.

149. Sofuoglu, M.; Dudish-Poulsen, S.; Poling, J.; et al. The effect of individual cocaine withdrawal symptoms on outcomes in cocaine users. Addict Behav 30:1125–1134, 2005.

150. Spies, C.; Dubisz, N.; Funk, W.; et al. Prophylaxis of alcohol withdrawal syndrome in alcohol dependent patients admitted to the intensive care unit following tumor resection. Br J Anaesth 75:734–739, 1995.

151. Spies, C.D.; Dubisz, N.; Neumann, T.; et al. Therapy of alcohol withdrawal syndrome in intensive care unit patients following trauma: Results of a prospective, randomized trial. Crit Care Med 24:414–422, 1996.

152. Spies, C.D.; Neuner, B.; Neumann, T.; et al. Intercurrent complications in chronic alcoholic men admitted to the intensive care unit following trauma. Intensive Care Med 22:286–293, 1996.

153. Spies, C.D.; Rommelspacher, H. Alcohol withdrawal in the surgical patient: Prevention and treatment. Anesth Analg 88:946–954, 1999.

154. Stengel, D.; Bauwens, K.; Sehouli, J.; et al. Systematic review and meta-analysis of antibiotic therapy for bone and joint infections. Lancet Infect Dis 1:175–188, 2001.

155. Strebel, N.; Prins, M.; Agnelli, G.; et al. Preoperative or postoperative start of prophylaxis for venous thromboembolism with low-molecular-weight heparin in elective hip surgery? Arch Intern Med 162:1451–1456, 2002.

156. Sugarman, B. Osteomyelitis in spinal cord injured people. Am Paraplegia Soc 7:73–75, 1984.

157. Sullivan, J.T.; Sykora, K.; Schneiderman, J.; et al. Assessment of alcohol withdrawal: The revised clinical institute withdrawal assessment for alcohol scale (CIWA-Ar). Br J Addict 84:1353–1357, 1989.

158. Tice, A. The use of outpatient parenteral antimicrobial therapy in the management of osteomyelitis: Data from the Outpatient Parenteral Antimicrobial Therapy Outcomes Registries. Chemotherapy 47 (Suppl 1):5–16, 2001.

159. Tice, A.; Hoaglund, P.A.; Shoultz, P.A. Risk factors and treatment outcomes in osteomyelitis. J Antimicrob Chemother 51:1261–1268, 2003.

160. Tonnesen, H.; Kehlet, H. Preoperative alcoholism and postoperative morbidity. Br J Surg 86:869–875, 1999.

161. Tonnesen, H.; Petersen, K.; Hojgaard, L.; et al. Postoperative morbidity among symptom-free alcohol misusers. Lancet 340:334–340, 1992.

162. Trampuz, A.; Zimmerli, W. New strategies for the treatment of infections associated with prosthetic joints. Cur Opin Invest Drugs 6:185–190, 2005.

163. Turner, R.C.; Lichstein, P.R.; Peden, J.G.; et al. Alcohol withdrawal syndromes: A review of pathophysiology, clinical presentation, and treatment. J Gen Inter Med 4:432–444, 1989.

164. Turpie, A.G.G.; Bauer, K.A.; Eriksson, B.I.; et al. Superiority of fondaparinux over enoxaparin in preventing venous thromboembolism in orthopedic surgery using different efficacy end points. Chest 126:501–508, 2004.

165. Verklin, R.M.; Mandell, G.L. Alteration in effectiveness of antibiotics by anaerobiosis. J Lab Clin Med 89:65–71, 1976.

166. Vila, H.; Smith, R.A.; Augustyniak, M.J.; et al. The efficacy and safety of pain management before and after implementation of hospital-wide pain management standards: Is patient safety compromised by treatment based solely on numerical pain ratings? Anesth Analg 101:474–480, 2005.

167. Viscusi, E.R.; Reynolds, L.; Tait, S.; et al. An iontophoretic fentanyl patient-activated analgesic delivery system for postoperative pain: A double-blind, placebo-controlled trial. Anesth Analg 102:188–194, 2006.

168. Vlessides, M. Alcohol infusions determined safe to treat withdrawal in selected trauma patients. Pharmacy Practice News, September 1999.

169. Wagner, J.G.; Wilkinson, P.K.; Sedman, A.J.; et al. Elimination of alcohol from human blood. J Pharm Sci 65:152–154, 1976.

170. Weigelt, J.; Itani, K.; Stevens, D.; et al. Linezolid versus vancomycin in treatment of complicated skin and soft tissue infections. Antimicrob Agents Chemother 49:2260–2266, 2005.

171. Weisner, C.; Mertens, J.; Parthasarathy, S.; et al. Integrating primary medical care with addiction treatment. JAMA 286:1715–1723, 2001.

172. Westermeyer, J.; Doheny, S.; Stone, B. An assessment of hospital care for the alcoholic patient. Alcohol Clin Exp Res 2:53–57, 1978.

173. Whelton, A. Renal and related cardiovascular effects of conventional and COX-2 specific NSAIDs and non-NSAID analgesics. Am J Ther 7:63–74, 2000.

174. White, R.H.; Romano, P.S.; Zhou, H.; et al. Incidence and time course of thromboembolic outcomes following total hip or knee arthroplasty. Arch Intern Med 158:1525–1531, 1998.

175. Wilkens, L.; Ruschulte, H.; Ruckholdt, H.; et al. Standard calculation of ethanol elimination rate is not sufficient to provide ethanol substitution therapy in the postoperative course of alcohol-dependent patients. Int Care Med 24:459–463, 1998.

176. Wilkinson, P.K. Pharmacokinetics of ethanol: A review. Alcohol Clin Exp Res 4:6–21, 1980.

177. Wille-Jorgenson, P. New therapeutic options in DVT prophylaxis. Orthopedics 23(6S):S639–S642, 2000.

178. Wilson, A.P.R.; Gruneberg, R.N. (eds.). Safety. In Teicoplanin: The First Decade. The Medicine Group (Education), Ltd., Abington, Oxfordshire, U.K., 1997, p. 143.

179. Winawer, N. Postoperative delirium. Med Clin North Am 85(5):1229–1239, 2001.

180. Wunderink, R.G.; Rello, J.; Cammarata, S.K.; et al. Linezolid vs vancomycin: Analysis of two double-blind studies of patients with methicillin-resistant *Staphylococcus aureus* nosocomial pneumonia. Chest 124:1789–1797, 2003.

181. Yin, L.Y.; Lazzarini, L.; Li, F.; et al. Comparative evaluation of tigecycline and vancomycin, with and without rifampicin in the treatment of methicillin-resistant *Staphylococcus aureus* experimental osteomyelitis in a rabbit model. J Antimicrob Chemother 55:995–1002, 2005.

182. Zimmerli, W.; Widmer, A.F.; Blatter, M.; et al. Role of rifampin for treatment of orthopaedic implant-related staphylococcal infections. JAMA 279:1537–1541, 1998.

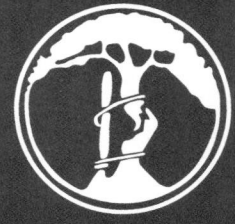

Principles and Complications of External Fixation

Stuart A. Green, M.D.

HISTORICAL BACKGROUND

Early Fixators

The external fixator was invented 12 years before the plaster cast. In 1846, Jean François Malgaigne devised an ingenious mechanism consisting of a clamp that approximated four transcutaneous metal prongs to reduce and maintain patellar fractures[42] (Fig. 11-1). In the 130 years since Malgaigne's invention, many other external fixation systems have been introduced. Among the best known are the Parkhill bone clamp (1897),[51] Lambotte's monolateral external fixator (1902),[38] Roger Anderson's 1934 fixation system,[2] the 1937 Stader apparatus—originally developed for managing fractures in large dogs,[63] and the external fixator of Swiss physician Raoul Hoffmann (1938)[25] (Fig. 11-2).

Several of these devices saw use during the second World War. Toward the end of that cataclysm, however, the high incidence of complications associated with external fixation became apparent. The major disadvantages noted by a military commission that studied the matter included nerve and vessel injuries by pins, the presence of soft tissue infections at the pin sites, the possibility of ring sequestra and osteomyelitis, and the danger of delayed union or nonunion. Other surgeons were distressed by the mechanical difficulty associated with external fixators, as well as by the prospect of converting a closed fracture to an open fracture.[10] As a consequence, by 1950 most American orthopaedic surgeons were not using mechanical fixators although the pins-in-plaster technique was used for special problems, such as unstable wrist fractures[19] and displaced fractures of the tibia and fibula.[1]

In Europe, on the other hand, clinical research on external skeletal fixation continued throughout the years during and following World War II. Raoul Hoffmann improved his device, providing a stronger universal joint and an enlarged pin gripper that held the pins more securely. Charnley, in England, presented his concept of compression arthrodesis of the major joints,[9] utilizing a rather simple skeletal fixator that provided continuous compression of cancellous surfaces of the joint to be fused. In time, the Arbeitsgemeinschaft für Osteosynthesefragen

(AO) group of Switzerland modified Charnley's device to include more pins in his frame configuration.[55]

Also in France during the 1960s, Jacques Vidal and co-workers utilized Hoffmann's equipment but designed a quadrilateral frame to provide rigid stabilization of complex fracture problems and septic pseudarthroses under treatment[70] (Fig. 11-3A).

Fixators for Limb Lengthening

External fixators specifically designed for limb lengthening began to appear after W. V. Anderson developed an apparatus that employed full transcutaneous pins connected to threaded bars.[3] The device permitted gradual distraction of an osteotomized bone. Heinz Wagner,[72] working in Germany, modified Anderson's concept even further, substituting half-pins for Anderson's full pins, while employing a universal distraction bar that the patient could lengthen (Fig. 11-3B). These pioneers have accurately recorded the incidence of complications with their techniques, some of which are unique to limb lengthening.[73]

FIGURE 11-1 *Malgaigne's 1846 external fixator for patellar fractures.*

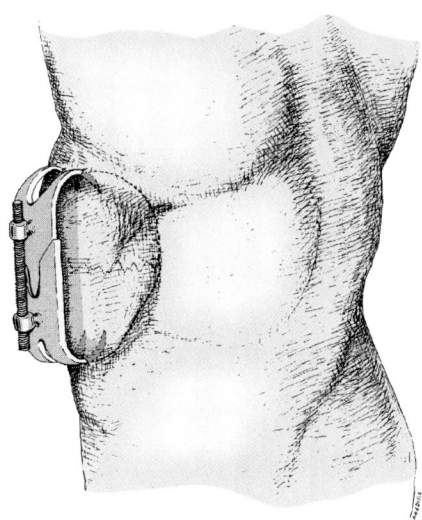

FIGURE 11-2 *Historic external fixators. **A,** Parkhill bone clamp. **B,** Lambotte fixator. **C,** Anderson apparatus. **D,** Stader apparatus. **E,** Hoffmann fixator.*

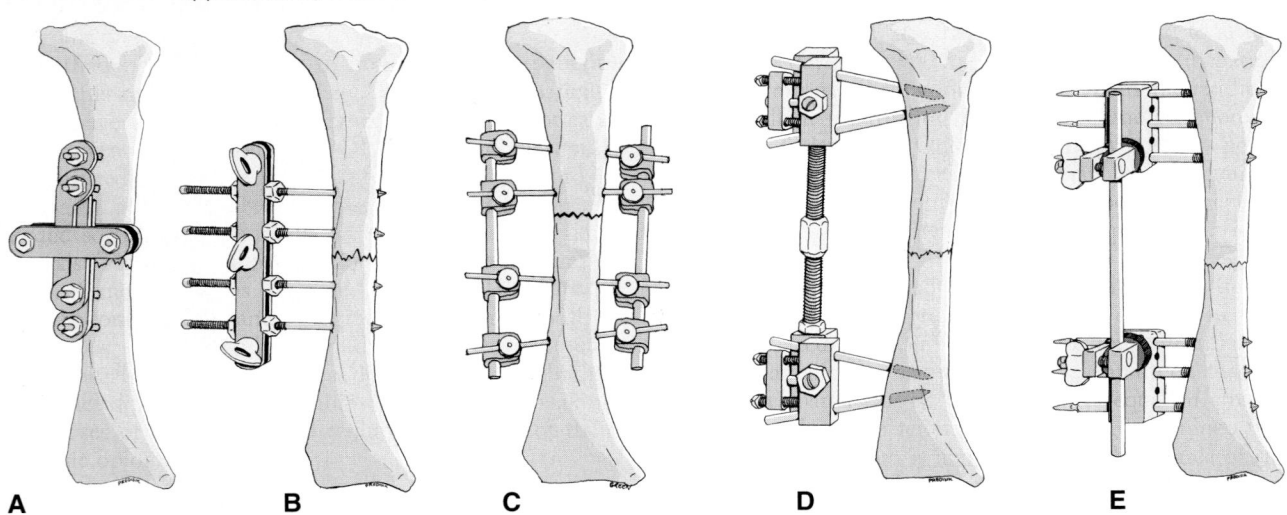

A   **B**   **C**   **D**   **E**

In Russia, external fixation as a modality for fracture treatment remained viable in the period subsequent to World War II. Surgeons in that country focused attention on ring-type fixators that were connected to the bone by thin transfixion wires tensioned by special wire-gripping clamps. Although these fixators are quite cumbersome, some contained ingenious geared articulations that permit precise displacement of the rings in any of three planes independently.

Circular Fixators

In 1951 Dr. Gavriil A. Ilizarov of Kurgan, U.S.S.R., developed the first model of his transfixion-wire circular fixator, which is still used today[28] (Fig. 11-3C). Other Soviet surgeons subsequently designed similar devices,

some with geared couplers that allow gradual repositioning of bone fragments. Within a few years, Ilizarov discovered that bone would form in a widening distraction gap under appropriate conditions of stability, delay, and distraction.[32] His observations and subsequent clinical research have revolutionized deformity correction and limb salvage surgery and contributed to a revived worldwide interest in circular external fixation.[36]

Ilizarov's apparatus consists of separate components that can be assembled into an unlimited number of different configurations that allow a surgeon to perform:

The percutaneous treatment of all closed metaphyseal and diaphyseal fractures as well as many epiphyseal fractures;

FIGURE 11-3 *Modern external fixators. **A,** Vidal quadrilateral frame. **B,** Wagner limb lengthener. **C,** Ilizarov apparatus.*

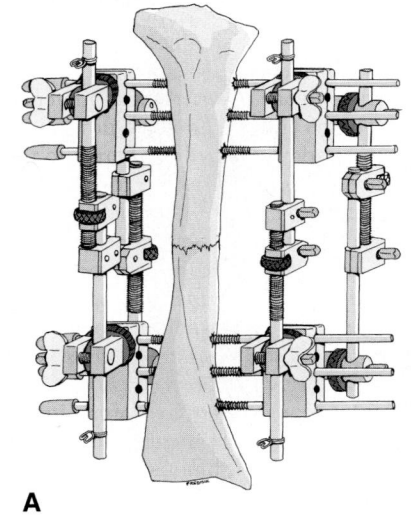 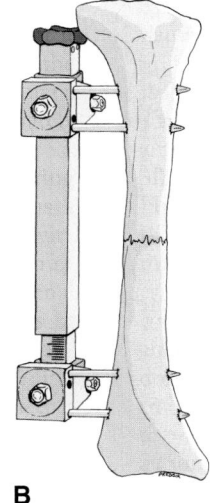 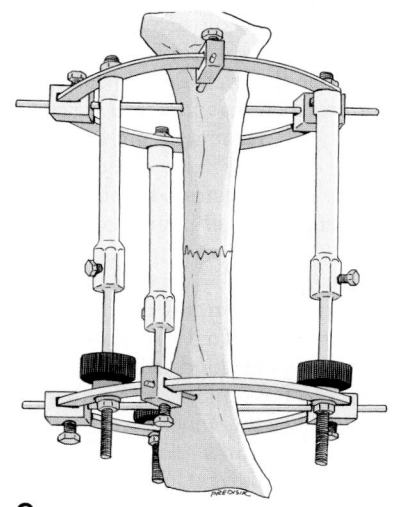

A   **B**   **C**

The repair of extensive defects of bone, nerve, vessel, and soft tissues without the need for grafting, and in one operative stage;

Bone thickening for cosmetic and functional reasons;

The percutaneous one-stage treatment of congenital or traumatic pseudarthroses;

Limb lengthening for growth retardation by distraction epiphysiolysis or other methods;

The correction of long bone and joint deformities, including resistant and relapsed club feet;

The percutaneous elimination of joint contractures;

The treatment of various arthroses by osteotomy and repositioning of the articular surfaces;

Percutaneous joint arthrodesis;

Elongating arthrodesis—a method of fusing major joints without concomitant limb shortening;

The filling in of solitary bone cysts and other such lesions;

The treatment of septic nonunion by the favorable effect on infected bone of stimulating bone healing;

The filling of osteomyelitic cavities by the gradual collapsing of one cavity wall;

The lengthening of amputation stumps;

Management of hypoplasia of the mandible and similar conditions;

The ability to overcome certain occlusive vascular diseases without bypass grafting; and

The correction of achondroplastic and other forms of dwarfism.

An American orthopaedist, David Fischer, visited Moscow in 1975, where he obtained several different Soviet circular external fixators. After applying these frames to his own patients, he became concerned with the problems of frame instability associated with transfixion wires, as well as the perceived weight of the circular frames he tried. Thereafter, Fischer developed a circular fixator, which attached to bone via full and half-pins.[18] The entire system was originally fabricated from titanium—a lightweight, yet strong metal. In general, he noted fewer pin site infections when his device was mounted with titanium pins instead of steel implants. Moreover, when titanium pin site sepsis did occur, the reaction was more benign-appearing, with far less cellulitis and soft tissue reaction than were commonly observed with steel pins.

North American orthopaedic surgeons, exposed to Ilizarov's methods by Italian practitioners in the mid-1980s, modified Ilizarov's technique. Among the most useful of these improvements has been the fabrication of rings and plates of the Ilizarov apparatus from radiolucent carbon fiber. This material, although more expensive than steel, is substantially lighter and thus popular with the patients.

At Rancho Los Amigos Medical Center (Downey, California), the author and his co-workers started using titanium half-pins (in place of steel wires) to secure Ilizarov's circular fixator to long bones requiring either limb lengthening or deformity correction.[21] In this manner, the adaptability of the circular device was retained, but the problem of muscle impalement and transfixion was reduced, especially in bones like the ulna or tibia that have a large subcutaneous surface. In certain anatomic locations, however, wire mounts still appeared superior to pin mountings—especially in the juxta-articular regions where cancellous bone predominates. For more substantial fragments that include both the articular and metaphyseal regions, combinations of pins and wires have proven successful for mounting circular external skeletal fixation.[22]

Several new fixator configurations have been devised specifically for applications that require anchorage in cancellous bone at one end of the frame and cortical bone on the other. These fixators, which are often referred to as hybrid designs, usually combine an Ilizarov-type ring with an AO-type tubular bar. The tensioned wires are secured to the ring (which surrounds the cancellous portion of the bone) while the bar connects to half-pins in the cortical bone.

Ring fixators have a distinct advantage over unilateral or bilateral devices because the apparatus (specially Ilizarov's device) permits a surgeon to gradually reposition fracture fragments (or osseous fragments following osteotomy) with respect to each other in three-dimensional space. To match this capability, several new unilateral fixators incorporate geared articulations that permit the controlled movement of one pin gripper with respect to the others.

Fixators for Severe Trauma

One modern concept of care for severe polytrauma starts with the application of a simple external fixator for preliminary stabilization of each seriously injured limb, followed by more definitive reconstruction later on.[5] The goal of most surgeons who apply a fixator for the temporary stabilization of a limb is to convert from external fixation to internal fixation, usually an intramedullary nail. Unfortunately, there is the potential for medullary osteomyelitis if the microorganisms of the pinhole spread into the bone's medullary cavity during nailing.

A number of protocols have been recommended to reduce the likelihood of such an infection, but one promising concept has been the development of a "pinless" external skeletal fixator by the AO group. With this device, a spring-loaded pair of pins resembling ice tongs grip the cortex but do not penetrate into the endosteal surface, thereby securing bone fragments. In this manner, the medullary canal is (in theory, at least) free of microbial contamination. Time will tell if such an invention reduces the incidence of implant sepsis when an intramedullary nail replaces an external fixator.

A complete understanding of the ideal milieu for rapid fracture healing has yet been ascertained. Around the world, pioneering clinicians and researchers are using fixators to study the influence of stability, distraction, and compression on fracture healing and regeneration of new bone. The results of these studies will certainly advance the clinical applications of both internal and external fixation and improve fracture care in general.

In the mid 1980s when trauma surgeons discovered that open fractures could be safely treated with intramedullary nails, it appeared that external fixation's role in orthopaedic surgery would be greatly diminished. Ilizarov's discovery of distraction osteogenesis, however, has rendered the prediction of external fixation's demise premature indeed. Fixators have become an important part of deformity correction, especially where limb elongation is a concomitant requirement. For this reason, worldwide use of external skeletal fixation is on the rise again, as it was before World War II and again in the 1970s and early 1980s.

Computerized Correction

In the 1990s, Dr. Charles Taylor (co-developer of the Russell-Taylor intramedullary nail) realized that the reduction of a displaced bone fragment (or correction of a deformity) can be accomplished by mathematically defining the path a bone fragment travels as it moves from its displaced position to its corrected position.[65] Using an ingenious design, Taylor connected rings of an Ilizarov-type circular fixator to each other with six struts, each of which can be independently lengthened or shortened (Fig. 11-4). In this

way, the relationship between the rings can be altered in a precise manner, modifying the relationship of the rings—and their attached bone fragments—to each other.[65]

After measuring the precise displacement of the bone fragments and the relationship between the fragments and their respective rings, the data are fed into a computer that has been programmed to determine the pathway to reduction in all planes—angulation, rotation, shortening, and translation. Moreover, the computer program outputs a schedule of strut length changes needed to effect the reduction at whatever predetermined speed is needed for both safety and efficacy. The system, called the Taylor Spatial Frame, is quite popular with surgeons who have become familiar with its use.

A bewildering variety of fixators possessing ingenious articulations and pin-grippers are currently available. Surgical appliance manufacturers continue to introduce new components and fixator frames to the marketplace at a steady pace. The devices vary considerably in configuration and in technique of frame assembly. The feature common to all fixators, however, is that they are attached to the human body with pins or wires that penetrate the skin and affix to bone. The complications associated with transcutaneous pins are thus common to all past, present, and future fixators, regardless of design or construction. Reducing pin site sepsis will, more than any other measure, ensure the continued development of external skeletal fixation.

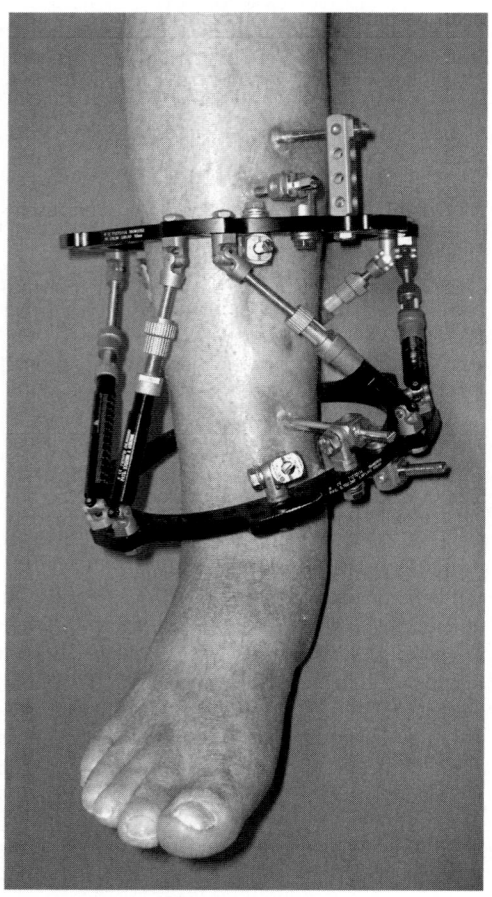

FIGURE 11-4 *The Taylor spatial frame. Six adjustable struts control the relationship between the two rings, one of which must be mounted orthogonal to either the proximal or distal fragment. All deformity and mounting parameters are fed into a computer, which calculates the strut length changes needed to restore the displaced fragment to anatomic alignment.*

FIXATOR TERMINOLOGY

PIN The term *pin* refers to that portion of the fixator that penetrates the skin and soft tissues and attaches to bone. In the European literature pins are sometimes referred to as screws or nails (the distinction resting perhaps on the presence or absence of threads).

FULL PIN A full pin is one that protrudes through the skin and soft tissues on both sides of the limb. Such pins are sometimes referred to as transfixion pins or through-and-through pins.

HALF-PINS A half-pin is one that penetrates the skin and soft tissues on one side of the limb only and that penetrates bone but does not emerge on the other side of the limb. When inserted, such pins are supposed to penetrate both cortices of the bone but not much beyond the second cortex.

WIRE A wire is a thin transosseous implant, usually less than 2 mm in diameter, that is not stiff enough to provide stability to a fixator-bone configuration until tensioned and bolted to the fixator. For this reason, most wires must penetrate the entire limb and be secured to the fixator at both ends.

OLIVE WIRE An olive is a wire with a bead somewhere along its length, which prevents the wire from being pulled through the bone. An olive wire can be employed to pull bone fragments into position or to enhance stability of the bone-fixator configuration.

PIN-GRIPPER This device holds the pin to the rest of the fixator.

BAR The bar is the part of the apparatus that connects the pin-grippers. Bars may be solid or hollow, smooth or threaded, and they may incorporate a compression-distraction apparatus in their structure.

RING The term *ring* refers to a circular bar (or modified bar) that attaches to pin-grippers in a plane that is usually perpendicular to the long axis of the limb. The rings may or may not completely encircle the limb. (Incomplete circles are called half-rings.) The rings must be connected to each other by bars to create a fixator configuration.

ARTICULATIONS A device that connects one bar to another (or a bar to a ring) is an articulation. Some articulations consist of universal joints or hinges, but most do not.

Frame Configuration

Throughout this chapter, we use frame configuration terminology modified from Chao and co-workers[8] (Fig. 11-5).

UNILATERAL The unilateral frame is one that employs one bar connecting two or more pin-gripping clamps, which are attached to half-pins. It is the simplest configuration. This category includes Parkhill's original bone clamp, Lambotte's external fixator, and the apparatuses devised by Stader, Hoffmann, and Wagner.

BILATERAL A bilateral frame is one that employs a rigid bar on both sides of the limb, connected to full pins that transfix the bone. Roger Anderson's external skeletal fixator was of bilateral design.

BIPLANAR OR MULTIPLANAR A bi- or multiplanar frame is one that employs pins in two (or more) planes for increased stability.

RING A ring fixator is one that uses transverse bars that completely encircle the limb. Pins transfix the limb and connect to the rings in various locations. Additional bars, as noted earlier, connect the rings, to each other. Russian investigators have been utilizing these fixators for many years.

HALF-RING A half-ring fixator is one employing bars that incompletely encircle the limb in a manner similar to the ring fixator.

Prefabricated Fixators

External fixation systems in which a manufacturer prefabricates the components can be divided into two broad categories: those with fixed configurations and those with variable configurations.

FIXED CONFIGURATION These external fixation frames are characterized by a relatively fixed, but usually adjustable, spatial configuration that dictates the position, direction, or number of transcutaneous pins.

VARIABLE CONFIGURATION Variable configuration fixator systems are similar to one another in that they consist of many separate components that can be assembled into any spatial configuration as dictated by the nature of the musculoskeletal problem. Precise pin position is generally required only with the individual pins within a cluster (those held by the same pin-gripping clamp).

FIGURE 11-5 *Basic fixator configurations. **A,** Unilateral. **B,** Bilateral. **C,** Multiplanar (quadrilateral). **D,** Multiplanar (delta configuration). **E,** Ring fixator. **F,** Hybrid fixator.*

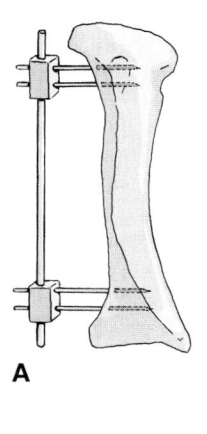
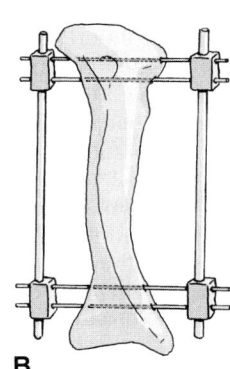

A   B

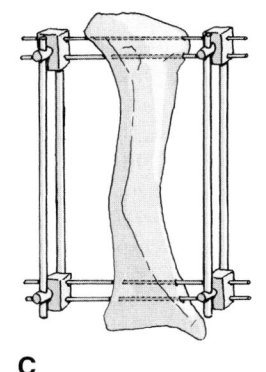
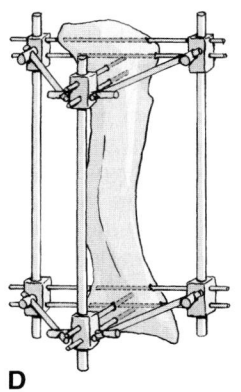

C   D

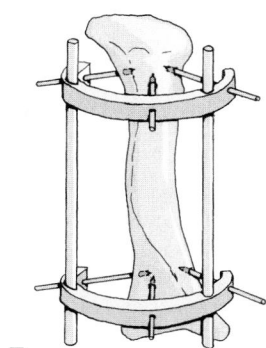
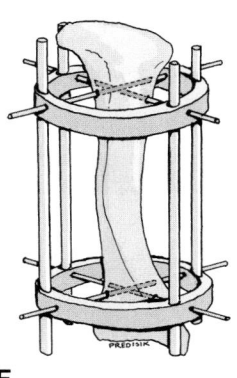

E   F

Improvised Fixators

This category comprises systems of external fracture management in which transcutaneous pins are connected to an unsolidified substance that hardens within a few minutes after being applied. The classic pins-in-plaster technique, methyl methacrylate external pin fixation, and epoxy-filled tube systems belong in this group. These systems permit unlimited pin positions, but they lack adjustability and preclude compression or distraction.

PROBLEMS, OBSTACLES, AND COMPLICATIONS

The application of an external skeletal fixator, especially one that involves the slow repositioning of bone fragments, is different from most other surgical procedures because the "operation" does not end when the patient leaves the operating room. Instead, the procedure stretches out over many months, with many clinic visits needed to follow the progress of the bone fragments. As will be evident from the following discussion, pin tract infections, numbness from nerve stretching, delayed union, deviation of mechanical axis during elongation, and numerous other difficulties occur during a typical case. To call all of these challenging events "complications" leads to the conclusion that external fixator applications have a 500% complication rate. Many practitioners who do large numbers of fixator applications use a scheme of analysis popularized by Paley that includes problems, obstacles, and complications.[49] Problems in this paradigm are those difficulties that are correctable in the clinic, often by either a modification of the mounting parameters or a prescription medication. Obstacles are those difficulties that require a return trip to the operating room for correction, including repeat osteotomy for premature consolidation, pin or wire replacement for sepsis or loosening, or even a bone graft for tardy bone healing. True complications in this scheme are the permanent sequelae of treatment that adversely compromise the outcome. These include permanent nerve injury, persistent infection, failure to obtain union, and so forth. This three-level perspective more correctly describes the entire external fixation encounter and allows comparison with other methods of treatment.

Nerve and Vessel Injury

Reports of serious neurovascular injury from fixator pins and wires are surprisingly uncommon. In fact, workers reporting large series of external skeletal fixator applications usually note the absence of a significant nerve or vascular injury. However, they are not unheard of; descriptions of such injuries do appear from time to time in reports dealing with external skeletal fixation.[4,16,67]

VESSEL INJURIES

When vascular injuries do occur, they sometimes present in a peculiar way.[20] A pin directed at a vessel usually pushes it to the side without transecting it[13] (Fig. 11-6A). As time passes, the pin, resting against the vessel, erodes its wall. As a result, the patient may suddenly experience bleeding from the implant hole quite some time after fixator application[61] (Fig. 11-6B). Alternatively, the pin may create a hole in the side of a vessel, which does not become apparent until the pin is removed. Excessive bleeding through the pinhole may occur[6] (Fig. 11-6C), or a false aneurysm may develop in the soft tissues. If the vessel wall necrosis involves an adjacent artery and vein, an arteriovenous fistula may be created shortly after pin removal.

Reports describing serious distal vascular compromise following pin insertion are also rare, perhaps because collateral circulation is usually adequate to sustain the limb. In those few cases in which a limb has become ischemic after pin or wire insertion, severe trauma usually has preceded fixator application, suggesting loss of collaterals.

One location in particular may be subject to frequent yet undetected neurovascular injury—the distal lateral tibial surface. In that location, Raimbeau and associates[59] analyzed damage to the anterior tibial artery caused by transcutaneous pins. They performed arteriograms on cadaver limbs and

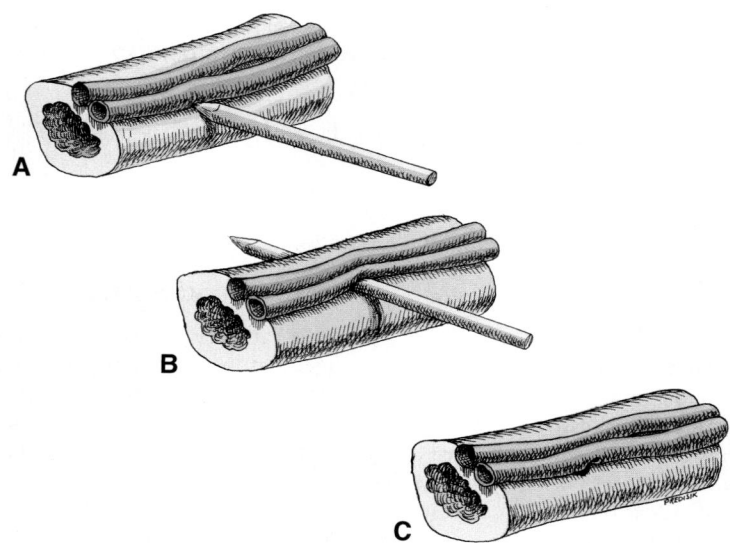

FIGURE 11-6 **A,** *A pin or wire directed at a vessel often pushes the vessel to the side.* **B,** *A vessel resting on an implant may erode and bleed 2 or more weeks after implant insertion.* **C,** *Alternatively, bleeding may occur at the time of implant removal.*

FIGURE 11-7 *The danger zone for implants is one fingerbreadth above and two fingerbreadths below the junction of the third and fourth quarter of the tibia where the anterior artery and deep peroneal nerve lay directly on the bone's lateral surface.*

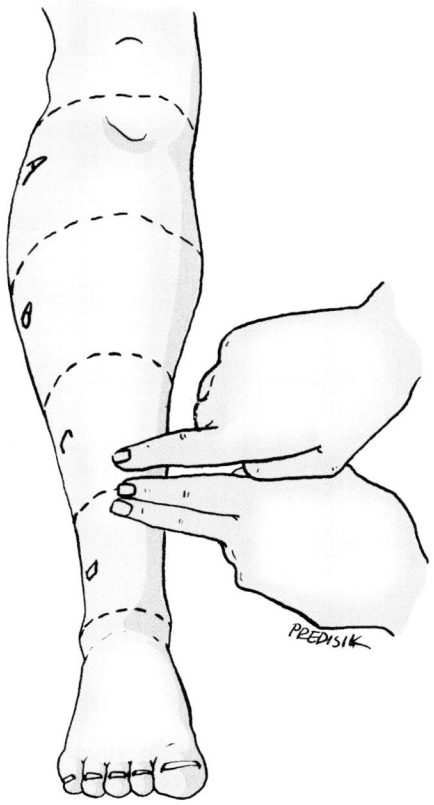

PREDISIK

determined that the region of the tibia between the lower end of the third quarter and the upper end of the fourth quarter is a danger zone for transfixion pin placement because the anterior tibial artery and deep peroneal nerve lay directly on the tibia's periosteum (Fig. 11-7).

COMPARTMENT SYNDROME

On rare occasions, external fixation pins have been blamed for causing anterior tibial compartment syndrome.[13,14,69] Raimbeau and associates also measured tissue pressures in the anterior compartment after insertion of transcutaneous pins.[59] They determined that the intracompartmental pressure was not significantly elevated after insertion of one transfixion pin, but it more than doubled when a second pin was inserted. Insertion of a third pin did not significantly raise the pressure any higher. Thus, they identified two vascular syndromes associated with pin fixation of the lower leg. The first, interference with the distal circulation of the anterior tibial artery, is quite rare because adequate collateral circulation is usually present. The second, anterior compartment syndrome, may also be due to partial occlusion of the anterior tibial artery combined with the increased compartment pressure associated with transfixion pins.

NERVE INJURIES

Acute transection of a major nerve is unlikely with external skeletal fixation. Nerves may, however, be nicked during the course of pin insertion or, more commonly, stretched during limb lengthening or bone transport.[4,67]

In spite of the relative infrequency of reports of serious neurovascular injury, great care is nevertheless required during pin insertion so that major neurovascular structures are not stretched or damaged. I recommend a skin incision, with observation of major neurovascular bundles, when pins are inserted into certain anatomic areas, such as the lateral humerus or proximal radius. Instead of exposing these structures surgically, however, one can select pin placement positions that avoid the possibility of damage to these structures.

Two difficulties are encountered during pin or wire insertion that could lead to nerve or vessel injury. First, the surgeon is occasionally unsure of the precise position of a major nerve or vessel with respect to the bone at the level of the limb selected for implant insertion. This confusion arises from the surgeon's orientation to the local anatomy, which usually considers the position of a nerve or vessel in its *longitudinal* relationship to surgical exposure. Indeed, surgical exposures are purposefully parallel to both the bone and the neurovascular structures in each anatomic region. Second, it is frequently difficult to assess the exact depth to which a pin has penetrated into the bone. This may seem surprising, considering how easy it is to "feel" when a drill bit penetrates the opposite side of a bone during drilling. Nevertheless, because the pin is threaded, there is enough resistance to forward progress to make depth determination difficult.

Implant Placement to Avoid Neurovascular Injury

An atlas showing pin placement positions designed to reduce the likelihood of neurovascular injury from transcutaneous implants appears in this chapter (see Figs. 11-9 through 11-27).[20] By recommending pin or wire placement in certain positions, I do not mean to imply that these are the only acceptably safe positions for insertion. At many points in the limb, pins can be safely inserted in several directions that have not been indicated. The descriptions of these positions were omitted for the sake of simplicity and clarity of illustration.

With experience (and reference to the atlas), surgeons will find additional pin positions to solve specific clinical problems.

In selecting the recommended direction for inserting a pin, I followed several principles designed not only to reduce the incidence of neurovascular injury but also to allow easy, yet solid, pin insertion. First, whenever possible the pins are inserted perpendicular to the bone surfaces. This facilitates the pin insertion process because it reduces the tendency of the pinpoint to "walk" (slide along the bone surface). The tibia, for example, has a triangular cross section. When the patient is supine, the lateral surface is vertical and the medial surface is oblique. Full pins are more easily inserted from lateral to medial because of this anatomic feature.

Second, pin directions should cross the center of the medullary canal to engage both cortices. When widely separated cortices are engaged by a pin, the tendency of the pin to wobble and loosen is reduced and maximum stability of pin fixation is achieved.

Third, pin insertion into dense bony ridges is to be avoided wherever possible. Drilling into very dense cortical bone with hand tools is tedious and frustrating, tempting the surgeon to try to overcome the resistance by pushing harder and drilling faster, which increases thermal injury to bone and consequently the likelihood of pinhole sepsis.

Fourth, pin positions should have a margin of safety on the opposite side of the bone. A pin is considered "safe" if it passes through the bone and emerges from the opposite side of the limb without encountering a major neurovascular structure. Such pins are illustrated as full (through-and-through) pins, although wires or half-pins could, of course, be safely inserted from either direction.

A pin is labeled "caution" if a major nerve or vascular structure is located on the opposite side of the bone at a distance equal to or greater than the diameter of the bone itself. In this respect, the designation refers only to half-pin placement. A full pin may be labeled caution if the direction or angle of pin insertion is critical to avoiding neurovascular injury.

A pin is labeled "danger" if a major neurovascular structure is between one-half and one bone diameter away from the bone on its opposite side. It is wise to insert such pins under radiographic or fluoroscopic control. A pin is also considered a danger pin if it must be inserted adjacent to a neurovascular structure on the near side of the bone. Generally this requires open pin insertion—a longitudinal incision that enables identification of the location of the structure prior to pin insertion.

Pin placement is measured in degrees, rotating around the bone from anterior to posterior, with the center of the bone always presumed to be the center of pin placement. Thus, the direct anterior position is considered to be 0°, and the direct posterior position is considered to be 180°. Pin placement from directly lateral to directly medial is considered to be 90° lateral, and a pin placed from directly medial to directly lateral is considered to be 90° medial. In the forearm where two bones are available for pin placement, the pin position for each is noted separately. The limb must be in the anatomic position during pin insertion if the atlas is to be used correctly. The humerus should be in neutral rotation, and the forearm supinated to correlate with the location of the anatomic structures indicated.

I recommend image intensification fluoroscopy for pin or wire insertion. The correct assessment of the position and depth of the pin can best be determined if the pin is seen in its true lateral projection. (In the true lateral projection of the pin, the central beam of the x-ray tube must be perpendicular to the pin itself.) At times, surgeons have a tendency to judge pin position through use of an oblique projection because a true lateral projection of the pins is difficult to obtain when the patient is supine on a large operating table. The surgeon may have to use considerable ingenuity to position a limb for fluoroscopy with a C-arm image intensifier. It may be necessary, for example, to rotate the limb 45° or more while rotating the C-arm in the opposite direction to obtain a true lateral projection. To determine the exact location of a pin within a bone, it

is necessary to direct the central beam of the x-ray tube along the pin itself. A perfect axial projection of the pin results in a small circular image equal to the diameter of the pin. In this manner, the position of the pin relative to the cortices can be determined. If roentgenograms rather than fluoroscopy are used, the initial evaluation can be obtained after the first pin is inserted to the presumed proper depth. Before the roentgenogram is taken, it is safer to be too shallow than too deep. If a pin is inserted too deeply, there is the obvious danger to neurovascular structures. Also, "backing out" a pin reduces its fixation in bone. When the depth of the first pin is satisfactory, additional pins of the same length can be inserted to the same depth. This strategy for pin insertion can also be employed to reduce x-ray exposure to the operating room personnel when image intensification fluoroscopy is utilized. Only a brief exposure is necessary to determine the position and depth of the first pin. Thereafter, pins can be inserted to the same depth without checking the progress of each pin individually.

The cross-sectional atlas in this chapter was specifically created to aid the surgeon in the operating room. Proper orientation of the cross-sectional diagrams to a patient on the operating table depends on the location of easily palpable landmarks. Each limb section in the atlas is treated in an identical manner. Each anatomic area is divided into four equal zones. Palpable bony landmarks identify the upper and lower limits of each anatomic area under consideration.

- In the thigh, the proximal bony landmark is the lateral prominence of the greater trochanter of the femur; the distal landmark is the lateral prominence of the lateral epicondyle of the femur.
- In the lower leg section, the proximal landmark is the medial tibial joint line; the distal landmark is the medial prominence of the medial malleolus.
- In the upper arm, the proximal landmark is the lateral prominence of the greater tuberosity of the humerus, which is one thumbwidth below the lateral tip of the acromion process. Distally, the landmark is the lateral epicondyle of the humerus.
- In the forearm, the proximal landmark is the lateral prominence of the radial head, which is one thumbwidth distal to the lateral epicondyle of the humerus. The distal landmark is the lateral prominence of the radial styloid process.

TECHNIQUE OF IDENTIFYING LANDMARKS

I have divided each limb segment in the atlas into four zones, labeled A, B, C, and D, with A proximal and D distal (Fig. 11-8). The zones approximate, but are not exactly, the quarters of each limb segment. The atlas illustrates cross-section anatomy in the top, middle, and bottom of each zone. Key diagrams in each figure orient the reader to the zones illustrated. For purposes of clarity, bones, nerves, arteries, and veins have been emphasized in relief. Muscle planes are indicated, but the muscle masses themselves are not labeled. Small cutaneous nerves, veins, and muscular branches of arteries have been omitted. Major arteries are shown with one vein even if they are usually accompanied by two veinae commitantae. In the forearm, deep veins have been omitted completely. I have emphasized some neurovascular structures by making them slightly larger than natural size (Figs. 11-9 through 11-27).

Many structures are labeled only once on each page, rather than on each slice. Mental reconstruction of the zone will fill in labels on the unlabeled slices. Unfortunately, some anatomic features are not easily presented in cross-section views. These are the transverse vessels and nerves that wind around the bone at one level. Furthermore, the atlas figures do not take into account variations in anatomy that can occur at any level. For these reasons, the atlas illustrations must be considered schematic, rather than representational.

FIGURE 11-8   *To mark the zones, stretch a surgical towel between the proximal and distal landmarks described in the text and mark the position of the landmarks on the towel with a surgical pen. Fold the towel so that the marks touch each other and mark the midpoint of the fold. Lay the towel against the limb again and mark the midpoint on the limb using the towel as a guide. In this manner, the limb section is divided in half. Repeat the procedure and find the midpoint of each half, thus dividing the limb segment into four equal zones.*

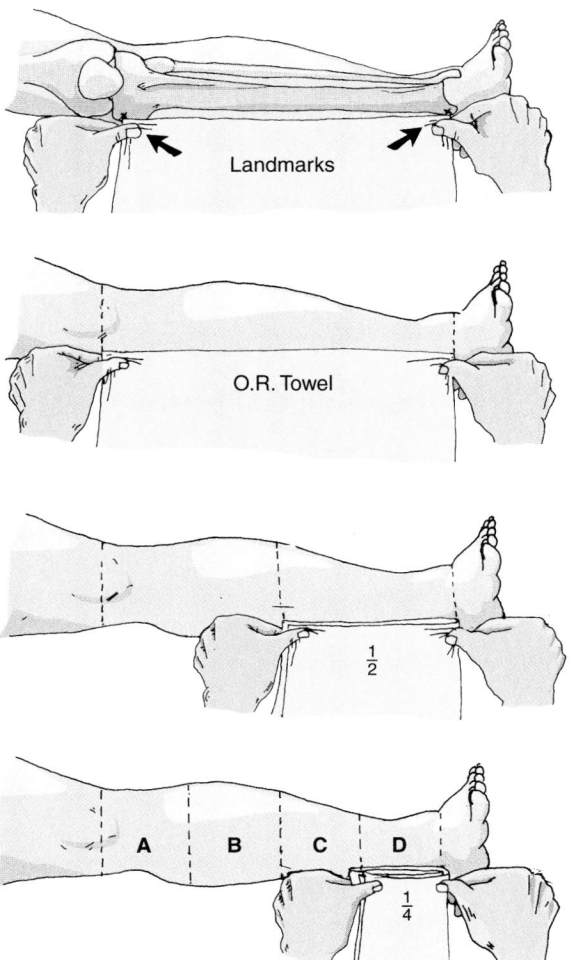

FIGURE 11-9   *Anatomic Considerations*

1. The femoral shaft is quite lateral in the proximal thigh.
2. The sciatic nerve remains posteromedial to the femur throughout zone A.
3. The deep femoral artery comes to lie medial to the femur in the lower end of zone A, separated from it by the origin of the vastus medialis muscle, but only one-half bone width away.
4. The lateral femoral cutaneous nerve is in line with the lateral cortex of the femur.
5. The lateral femoral circumflex artery winds around the lateral cortex of the femur at the base of the greater trochanter.

Pin Placement

1. Half-pin insertion from the 90° lateral position can be done with caution in the upper two thirds of zone A and with extreme caution in lower zone A.
2. With care and image intensification control additional pins can be inserted throughout a range of positions in the upper portion of this zone.

a., artery; br., branch; lat., lateral; n., nerve; post., posterior; v., vein.

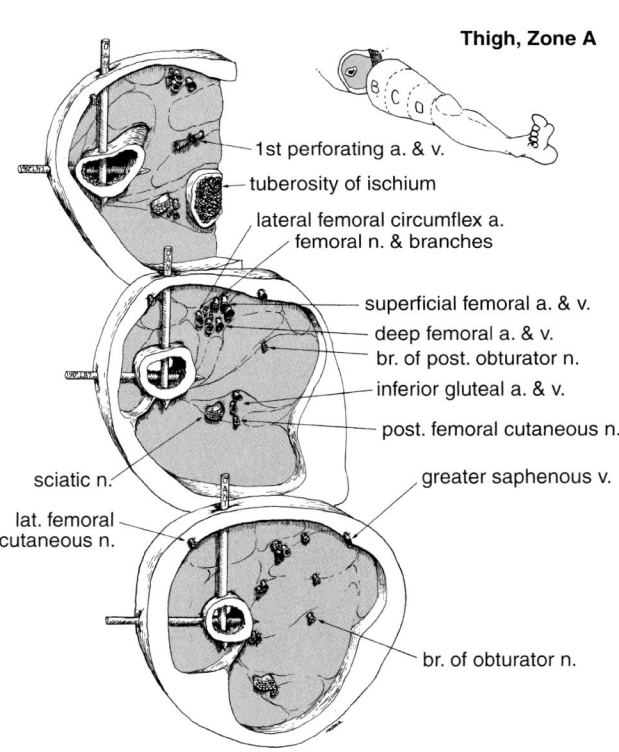

Thigh, Zone A

1st perforating a. & v.
tuberosity of ischium
lateral femoral circumflex a.
femoral n. & branches
superficial femoral a. & v.
deep femoral a. & v.
br. of post. obturator n.
inferior gluteal a. & v.
post. femoral cutaneous n.
greater saphenous v.
sciatic n.
lat. femoral cutaneous n.
br. of obturator n.

(Text continues on p. 307)

FIGURE 11-10 *Anatomic Considerations*

1. The femur is laterally placed throughout zone B.
2. The sciatic nerve is posteromedial to the femur, separated by one bone diameter.
3. The superficial femoral artery crosses the coronal plane of the femur between zone B and zone C.
4. The deep femoral artery and vein are medial to the femur in proximal zone B.
5. The lateral femoral cutaneous nerve is anterior to the femur.

Pin Placement

1. Extreme caution is necessary in proximal zone B with 30° medial placement because the superficial and deep femoral vessels are in a straight line and can both be injured with a pin placed too far medially.
2. Additional half-pins may be placed in other directions, but keep in mind the intimate association of the deep femoral vessels to the shaft of the femur.

a., artery; br., branch; lat., lateral; n., nerve; post., posterior; v., vein.

FIGURE 11-11 *Anatomic Considerations*

1. The femur is more centrally placed on cross section, although anteriorly situated.
2. The sciatic nerve passes from medial to lateral behind the femur, approximately one bone width away.
3. The superficial femoral artery passes the coronal plane of the femur in zone C and is posterior to the bone at the lower end of this zone.
4. The deep femoral artery and vein are adjacent to the posterior surface of the femur, but terminate at the lower end of zone C.

Pin Placement

1. Wires or full or half-pins can be inserted from the 60° medial or 120° lateral position.
2. Half-pins can be cautiously inserted from the 0° anterior position in distal zone C because the deep femoral artery and vein are no longer present (not shown).
3. Wires or full or half-pins can also be inserted 90° medial or 90° lateral in distal zone C.

a., artery; n., nerve; post., posterior; v., vein.

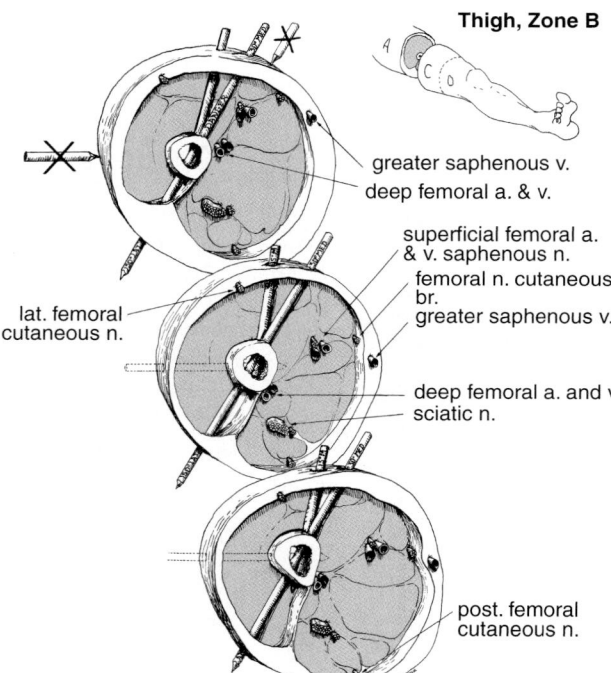

Thigh, Zone B

greater saphenous v.
deep femoral a. & v.

superficial femoral a. & v. saphenous n.
femoral n. cutaneous br.
greater saphenous v.

lat. femoral cutaneous n.

deep femoral a. and v.
sciatic n.

post. femoral cutaneous n.

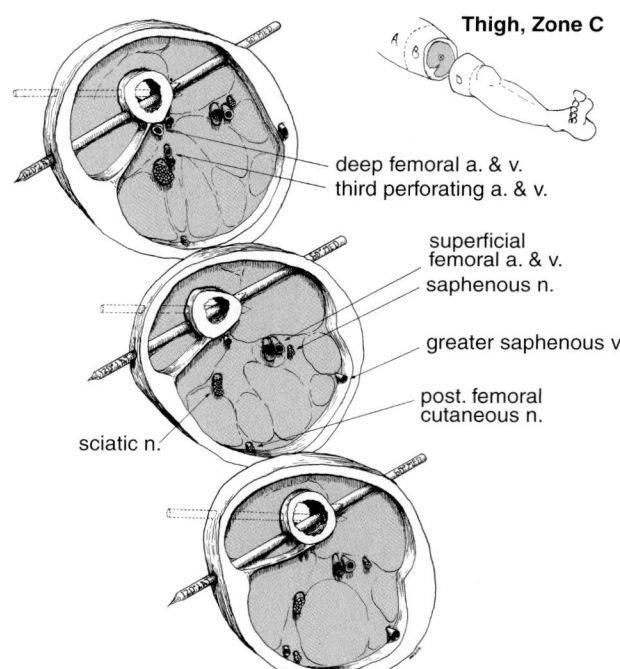

Thigh, Zone C

deep femoral a. & v.
third perforating a. & v.

superficial femoral a. & v.
saphenous n.

greater saphenous v.

post. femoral cutaneous n.

sciatic n.

FIGURE 11-12	*Anatomic Considerations*

1. The femur is an anterior structure until the flare of the condyles.
2. The sciatic nerve is posterior to the femur in proximal zone D, crossing to the lateral side while dividing into the tibial and peroneal divisions.
3. The synovial cavity of the knee joint enlarges to encompass the anterior half of the femur immediately above the joint line.

Pin Placement

1. Wires or full or half-pins from 90° medial or 90° lateral are safe.
2. Half-pins from 90° lateral position have the additional advantage of not transfixing the vastus medialis muscle.
3. At the level of the epicondyles, the synovial cavity is present anteriorly and posteriorly, leaving only 1 inch of extrasynovial bone. Three or four pins may be placed close to one another in a transverse plane through the bone at this level, although if four pins are placed, the most posterior pin may pass through the synovial cavity.

a., artery; br., branch; lat., lateral; n., nerve; post., posterior; v., vein.

FIGURE 11-13	*Anatomic Considerations*

1. The shape of the tibia changes rapidly through this zone.
2. The popliteal artery is posterior to the tibia where it divides into its terminal branches.
3. The superficial and deep peroneal nerves are lateral to the fibula as they wind around the fibular neck.
4. The saphenous nerve and greater saphenous vein are posterior to the tibia on the medial side of the limb.
5. In distal zone A, the anterior tibial artery is on the anterior surface of the interosseous membrane, and the peroneal and posterior tibial arteries, accompanied by their associated veins, are posterior to the tibia.

Pin Placement

1. Wires or full pins (or half-pins) can be placed in the 90° medial to 90° lateral direction throughout zone A.
2. Pins can be placed parallel to the joint line (and to one another) through the condyles of the tibia in proximal zone A.

a., artery; n., nerve; v., vein.

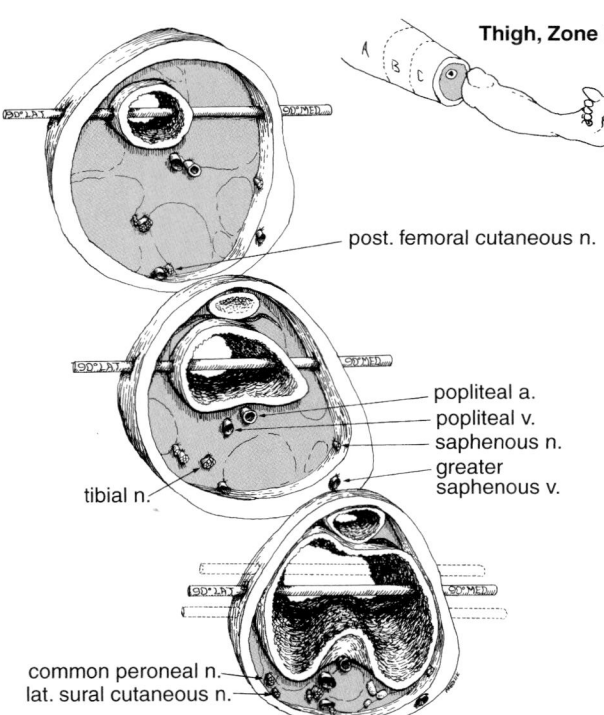

Thigh, Zone D

post. femoral cutaneous n.

popliteal a.
popliteal v.
saphenous n.
greater saphenous v.

tibial n.

common peroneal n.
lat. sural cutaneous n.

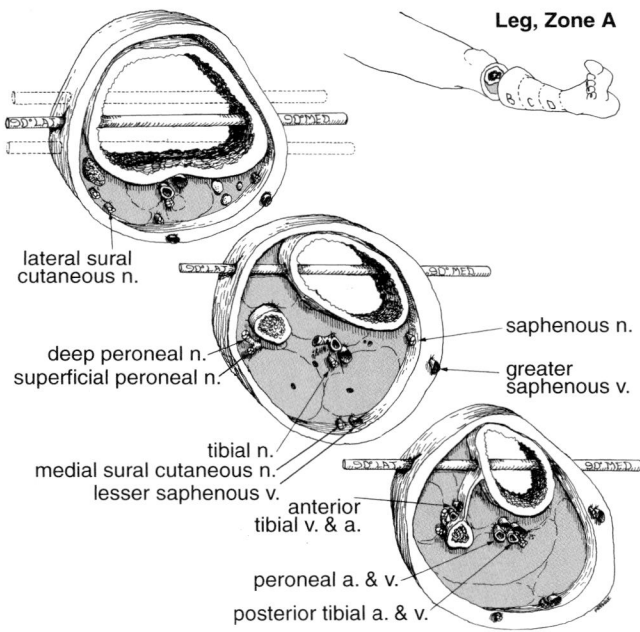

Leg, Zone A

lateral sural cutaneous n.

deep peroneal n.
superficial peroneal n.

saphenous n.

greater saphenous v.

tibial n.
medial sural cutaneous n.
lesser saphenous v.

anterior tibial v. & a.

peroneal a. & v.

posterior tibial a. & v.

FIGURE 11-14 *Anatomic Considerations*

1. The tibia has a triangular cross section throughout zone B, with the lateral surface relatively vertical and the medial surface oblique.
2. The posterior tibial vessels, the tibial nerve, and the peroneal vessels maintain a constant relationship throughout zone B with respect to the posterior surface of the tibia and the medial surface of the fibula.
3. The anterior tibial artery and vein and the deep peroneal nerve lie on the anterior surface of the interosseous membrane in zone B, traversing from the anterior ridge of the fibula toward the lateral ridge of the tibia.

Pin Placement

1. Wires, full pins, or half-pins can be inserted from 90° lateral or 90° medial.
2. Half-pins can be inserted with caution from the 30° medial (or 45° medial) position perpendicular to the oblique medial surface of the tibia. The tip of the pin penetrates the tibialis posterior muscle. Bear in mind the relationship of the peroneal artery and vein, adjacent to the medial corner of the fibula.

a., artery; n., nerve; v., vein.

FIGURE 11-15 *Anatomic Considerations*

1. The tibia retains its distinctive triangular cross section.
2. The posterior tibial artery and vein and the tibial nerve remain posterior to the tibia and the peroneal vessels slightly medial to the fibula.
3. The anterior tibial artery and vein and the deep peroneal nerve have completed their traversal of the interosseous membrane and are adjacent to the posterolateral corner of the tibia throughout zone C.
4. The saphenous nerve and greater saphenous vein are located at the posteromedial corner of the tibia in the subcutaneous tissue.

Pin Placement

1. In the upper part of zone C, wires or full or half-pins can be safely placed from the 90° medial or 90° lateral direction.
2. Half-pins are difficult to place into the oblique medial surface of the tibia in zone C because of the intimate relationship of the anterior tibial vessels to the bone. A 0° half-pin would be safe in distal zone C, but it is technically difficult to place because of the obliquity and thickness of the bone.
3. In distal zone C, pin placement from the 90° lateral or 90° medial position can endanger the anterior tibial artery and deep peroneal nerve.

a., artery; n., nerve; v., vein.

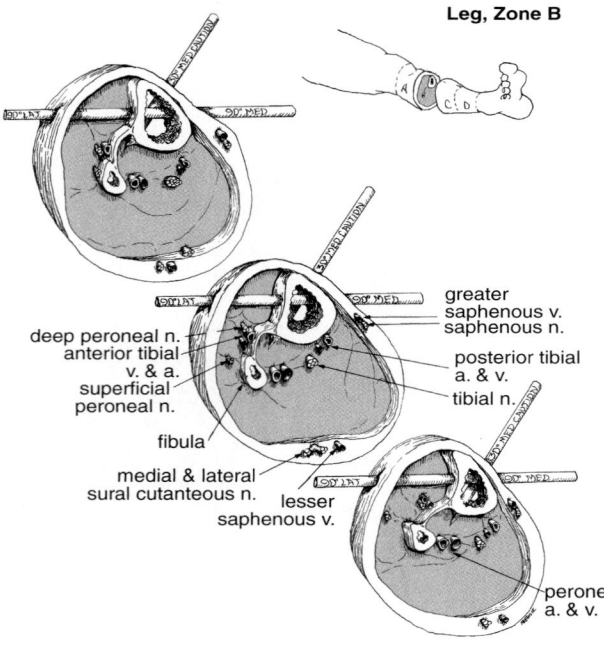

Leg, Zone B

greater saphenous v.
saphenous n.
deep peroneal n.
anterior tibial v. & a.
superficial peroneal n.
posterior tibial a. & v.
tibial n.
fibula
medial & lateral sural cutaneous n.
lesser saphenous v.
peroneal a. & v.

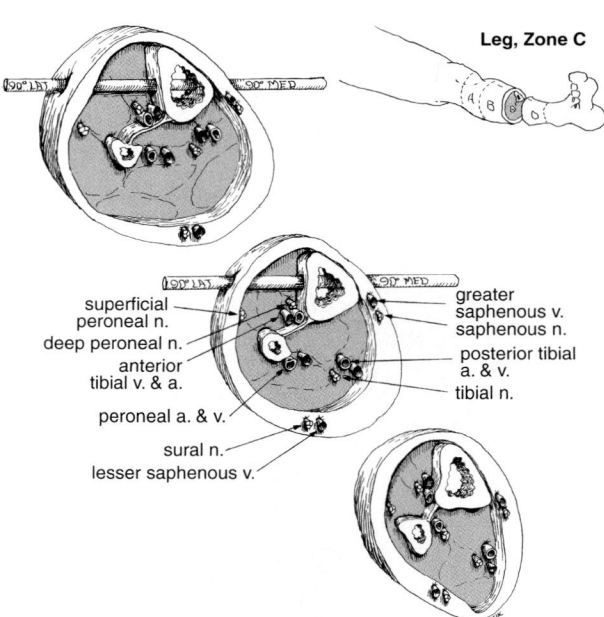

Leg, Zone C

superficial peroneal n.
deep peroneal n.
anterior tibial v. & a.
peroneal a. & v.
sural n.
lesser saphenous v.
greater saphenous v.
saphenous n.
posterior tibial a. & v.
tibial n.

FIGURE 11-16 ***Anatomic Considerations***

1. *The posterior tibial artery and vein and the tibial nerve remain posterior to the tibia, traversing medially as they approach the ankle joint.*
2. *The anterior tibial artery and vein and the deep peroneal nerve are on the lateral surface of the tibia in proximal zone D. They lie on the anterior surface of the tibia in distal zone D.*
3. *The saphenous nerve and greater saphenous vein are on the medial side of the tibia throughout zone D.*
4. *The superficial peroneal nerve has divided into its terminal branches in this zone.*

Pin Placement

1. *Half-pins can be placed from the 30° medial into the subcutaneous portion of the tibia.*
2. *Wire or full pin placement from the 90° medial and 90° lateral directions can be accomplished in the distal two thirds of zone D.*
3. *Wire, full or half-pin placement from 90° medial or 90° lateral can endanger the anterior tibial artery and deep peroneal nerve in the proximal one third of zone D.*

a., artery; n., nerve; v., vein.

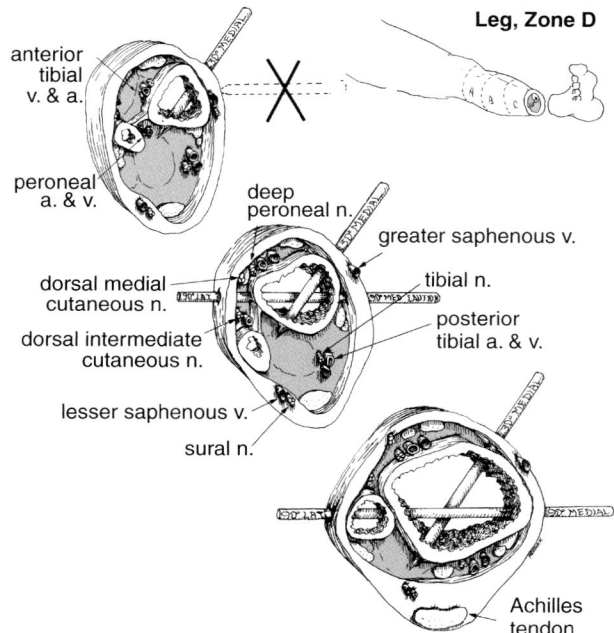

FIGURE 11-17 *Anatomic Considerations*

1. Cross section through the metatarsals demonstrates the curvature of the transverse metatarsal arch.
2. The dorsalis pedis artery is between the first and second metatarsal shafts.
3. The plantar arterial arch crosses beneath the third metatarsal shaft at the level illustrated.
4. The flexor hallucis brevis tendon is adjacent to the lateral inferior surface of the first metatarsal shaft.

Pin Placement

1. A wire or full or half-pin can be inserted from the 90° medial position into the first metatarsal shaft. It penetrates one or perhaps two other metatarsal shafts but cannot transfix them.
2. A 45° medial half-pin can be inserted into the first metatarsal.
3. Other half-pin positions can be safely used into the metatarsal bones, including a 90° lateral pin into the fifth metatarsal shaft (not shown).

a., artery; lat., lateral; n., nerve.

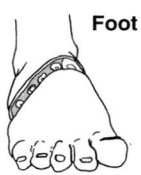

Foot

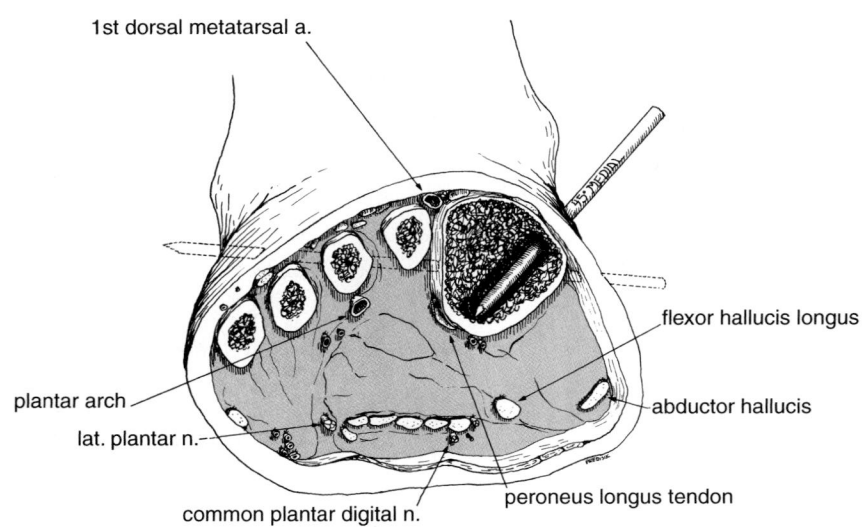

1st dorsal metatarsal a.

flexor hallucis longus

plantar arch

abductor hallucis

lat. plantar n.

peroneus longus tendon

common plantar digital n.

FIGURE 11-18 *Anatomic Considerations*

1. The humeral head is largely intrasynovial, being surrounded by a joint cavity medially and posteriorly and by the subacromial bursa anteriorly.
2. The main neurovascular bundle containing the brachial plexus is medial to the humerus, separated from it by a distance equal to the width of the bone.
3. The anterior and posterior humeral circumflex vessels surround the upper humerus slightly below the surgical neck, accompanied by the axillary nerve.
4. The saphenous nerve and greater saphenous vein are located at the posteromedial corner of the tibia in the subcutaneous tissue.

Pin Placement

1. Half-pins may be cautiously placed in the 90° lateral position.
2. Half-pins can be inserted into the humeral head from 0° anterior around laterally to the 90° lateral position if the tip of the pin does not penetrate the opposite cortex of the humeral head.
3. Below the level of the surgical neck of the humerus, pin placement may endanger the humeral circumflex vessels and the axillary nerve.
4. Below the anatomic neck of the humerus, half-pins can be placed from the 90° lateral position (not shown).

a., artery; ant., anterior; n., nerve; post., posterior; v., vein.

FIGURE 11-19 *Anatomic Considerations*

1. The brachial artery and veins and the brachial plexus remain medial to the humerus in this zone.
2. The radial nerve separates from the main neurovascular bundle and passes posterior to the humerus in zone B, separated from the bone by the medial head of the triceps.
3. The musculocutaneous nerve and cephalic vein are anterior to the humerus in zone B.

Pin Placement

1. Half-pins from 90° lateral must be inserted with caution in mid-zone B because of the position of the radial nerve medial to the humerus.

a., artery; med., medial; n., nerve; v., vein.

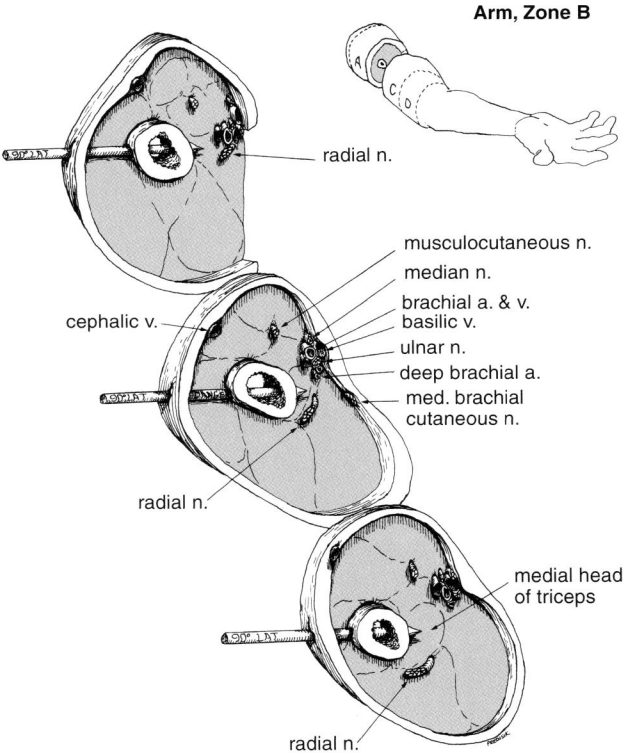

Arm, Zone B

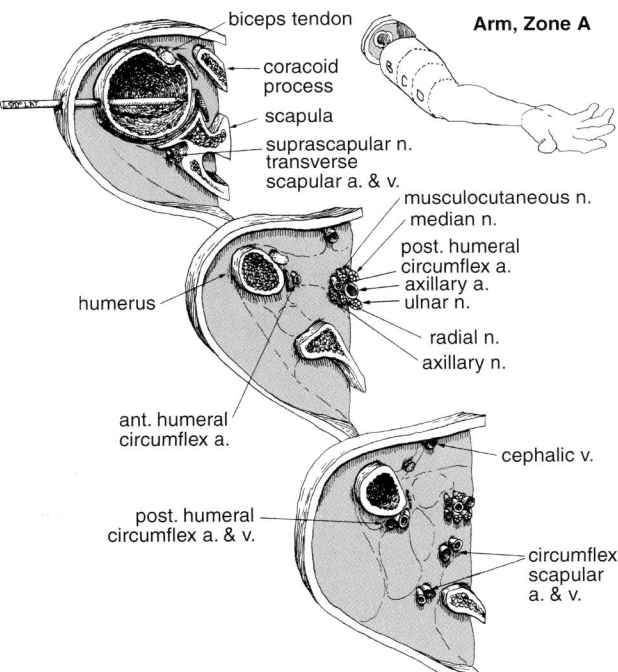

Arm, Zone A

FIGURE 11-20 *Anatomic Considerations*

1. The radial nerve winds around the lateral side of the shaft of the humerus in contact with the bone.
2. The brachial artery and veins and branches of the brachial plexus remain medial to the humeral shaft. The ulnar nerve separates from the main neurovascular bundle in this zone.
3. The musculocutaneous nerve becomes the lateral cutaneous nerve of the forearm and remains anterior to the humerus.

Pin Placement

1. Half-pins should only be placed in the 90° lateral position in the humerus with direct observation of the radial nerve through the surgical exposure.

a., artery; lat., lateral; n., nerve; v., vein.

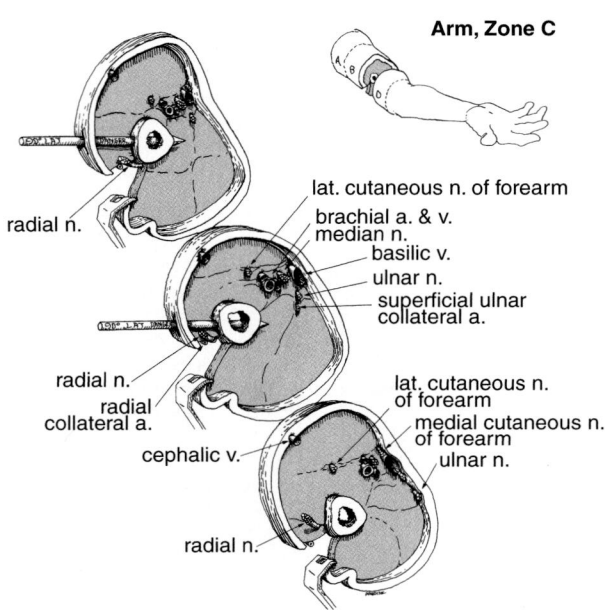

Arm, Zone C

FIGURE 11-21 *Anatomic Considerations*

1. The distal humerus flattens and is rotated with the lateral epicondyle 30° posterior to the medial epicondyle.
2. The radial nerve lies on the lateral side of the radius in proximal zone D but is anterior to it in the distal portion of the zone.
3. The median nerve remains anterior and medial to the bone throughout this zone.
4. The ulnar nerve passes posterior to the plane of the distal humerus and lies in contact with the posteromedial corner of the bone immediately above the elbow.

Pin Placement

1. Half-pins can be placed with caution from the 180° posterior position. The median nerve and brachial artery are separated from the shaft of the humerus by the thickness of the brachialis muscle in zone D. Likewise, half-pins can be placed from the 150° medial position.
2. Half- or full pins or wires can be placed from the lateral epicondyle into the medial epicondyle. Unfortunately, the proximity of the ulnar nerve to the medial epicondyle of the humerus makes pin placement in this position somewhat dangerous. It is recommended that the ulnar nerve be exposed for transepicondylar wire placement.

a., artery; lat., lateral; n., nerve; v., vein.

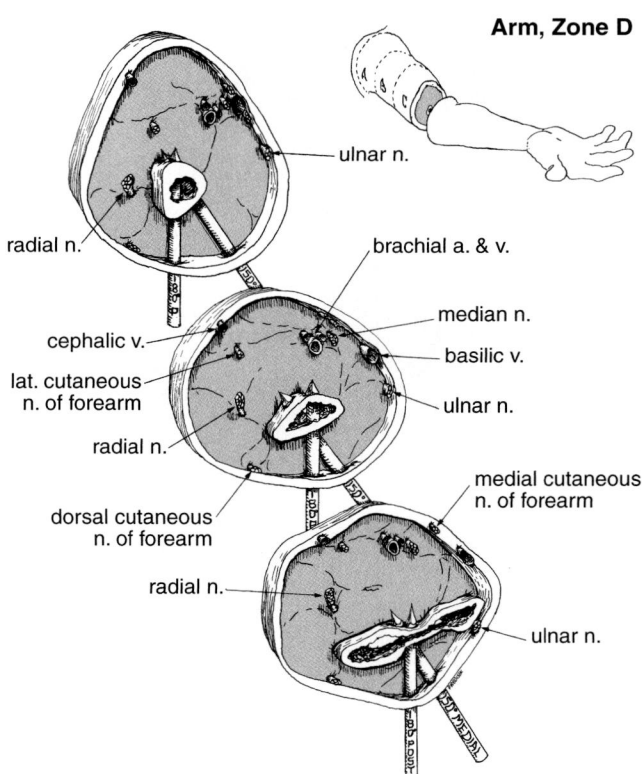

Arm, Zone D

FIGURE 11-22 | *Anatomic Considerations*

1. *The deep branch of the radial nerve winds around the lateral side of the humerus within the substance of the supinator muscle.*
2. *The brachial artery divides into its terminal branches (the common interosseous artery and the ulnar artery) in zone A, which are anterior to the proximal ulna distally.*

Pin Placement

1. *Half-pins can be inserted into the proximal ulna from the 150° medial direction. Image intensification fluoroscopy is recommended. Crossed wires can be placed in the proximal ulna posterior to the ulnar nerve.*
2. *Pin placement into the proximal radius is dangerous because of the location of the deep branch of the radial nerve. If it is necessary to stabilize the proximal radius with external fixation, it is wise to identify this structure before pin insertion.*
3. *In distal zone A, pins may be placed into the ulna from the 150° lateral position (not shown).*

a., artery; br., branch; n., nerve; v., vein.

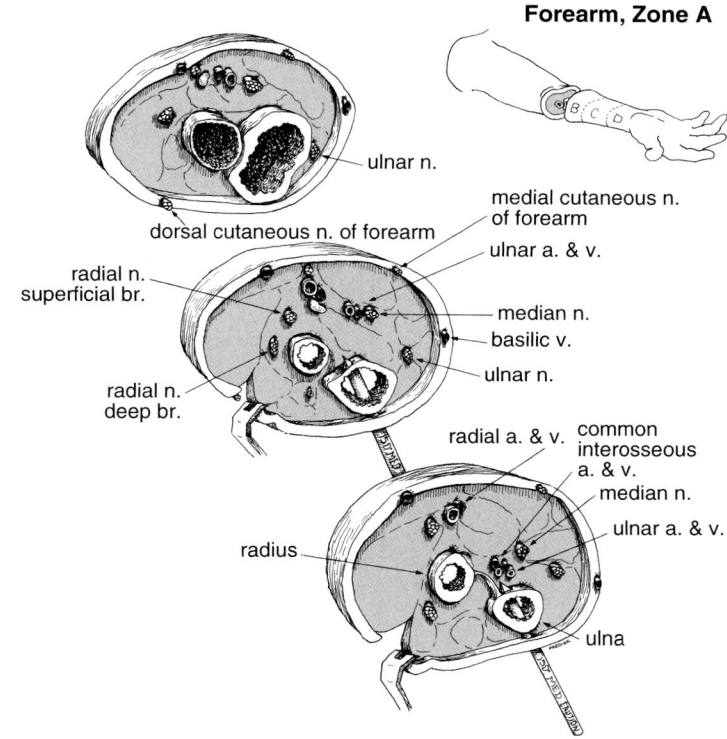

Forearm, Zone A

FIGURE 11-23   *Anatomic Considerations*

1. *The radial, ulnar, and median nerves remain in relatively constant position throughout zone B.*
2. *The anterior interosseous artery and nerve lie on the anterior surface of the interosseous membrane.*
3. *The deep branch of the radial nerve lies adjacent to the posterior interosseous artery, posterior to the interosseous membrane and separated from it by muscle.*

Pin Placement

1. *Half-pins can be inserted into the ulna from the 150° medial position. Depth can be assessed with fluoroscopy.*
2. *Half-pins can be inserted (with considerable caution) into the radius via the 60° lateral position. As with half-pin insertion into the ulna, fluoroscopic control is recommended.*

a., artery; ant., anterior; lat., lateral; med., medial; n., nerve; post., posterior; v., vein.

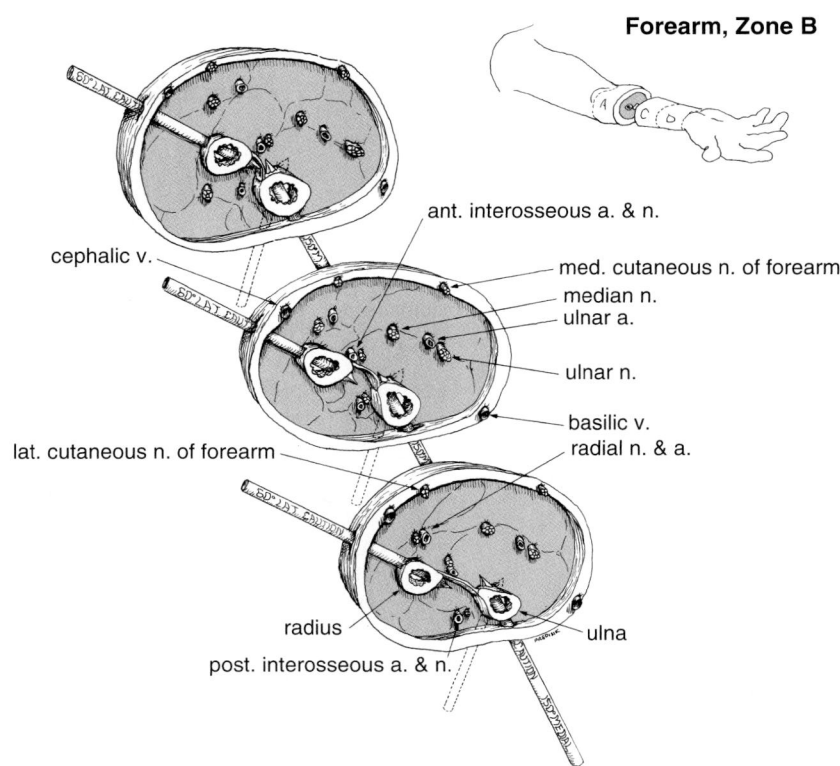

Forearm, Zone B

ant. interosseous a. & n.

cephalic v.

med. cutaneous n. of forearm
median n.
ulnar a.

ulnar n.

basilic v.
radial n. & a.

lat. cutaneous n. of forearm

radius

ulna

post. interosseous a. & n.

FIGURE 11-24   *Anatomic Considerations*

1. The superficial branch of the radial nerve and radial artery are anterior to the radius in zone C, becoming more lateral and superficial in the distal part of this zone.
2. The median nerve remains in the middle of the forearm, surrounded by muscle.
3. The ulnar nerve and ulnar artery remain anteromedial to the ulna throughout zone C.
4. The saphenous nerve and greater saphenous vein are located at the posteromedial corner of the tibia in the subcutaneous tissue.

Pin Placement

1. Half-pins may be placed into the ulna with caution from the 150° medial direction. In fact, half-pins may be inserted into the ulna from the 180° posterior position and the 150° lateral direction as well, as long as the surgeon is mindful of the position of the extensor tendon as illustrated in distal zone C.
2. Half-pins may be placed into the radius from the 150° lateral position. Pins may also be inserted into the radius from the 180° posterior position if care is taken to avoid impalement of the extensor tendons.

a., artery; ant., anterior; ext. carp. rad., extensor carpus radialis; lat., lateral; n., nerve; post., posterior; v., vein.

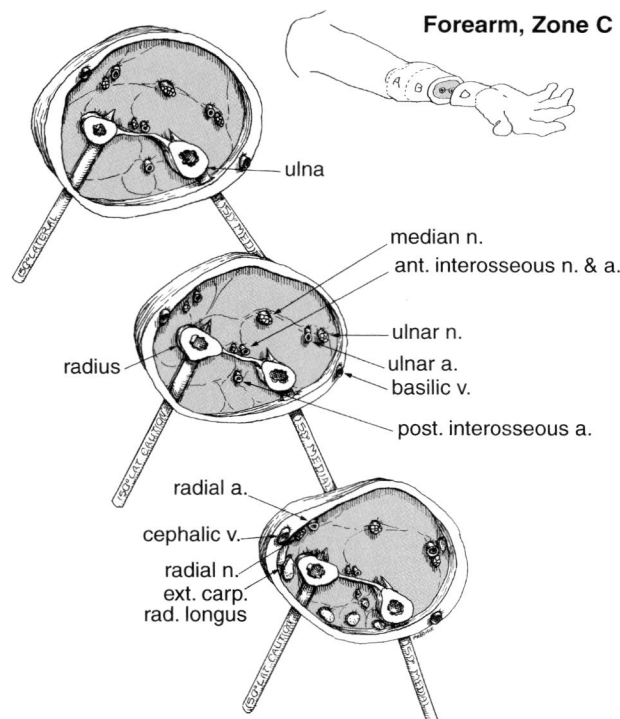

Forearm, Zone C

- ulna
- median n.
- ant. interosseous n. & a.
- ulnar n.
- radius
- ulnar a.
- basilic v.
- post. interosseous a.
- radial a.
- cephalic v.
- radial n.
- ext. carp. rad. longus

FIGURE 11-25   *Anatomic Considerations*

1. The radius and ulna are posteriorly located in the cross section of the forearm.
2. The radial nerve is lateral to the shaft of the radius, dividing into dorsal and volar branches in zone D.
3. The median nerve remains within the volar muscle mass.
4. The ulnar nerve divides into dorsal and volar branches, the dorsal branch passing to the posterior aspect of the distal forearm.
5. The extensor and flexor muscles become tendinous in zone D.

Pin Placement

1. Half-pins may be inserted with caution from the 150° medial direction into the ulna.
2. Half-pins may be placed into the distal radius from the 150° lateral direction. Note the relative position of the extensor tendons.

a., artery; br., branch; n., nerve; v., vein.

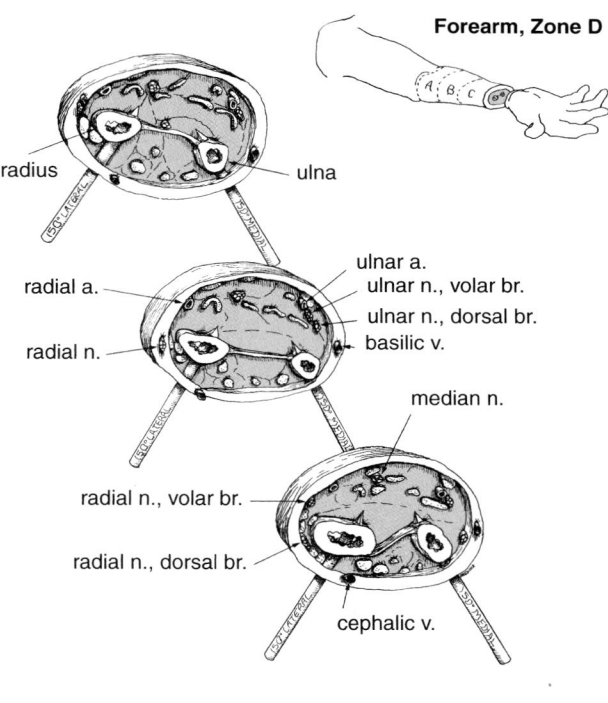

Forearm, Zone D

- radius
- ulna
- radial a.
- ulnar a.
- ulnar n., volar br.
- ulnar n., dorsal br.
- radial n.
- basilic v.
- median n.
- radial n., volar br.
- radial n., dorsal br.
- cephalic v.

FIGURE 11-26 | *Anatomic Considerations*

1. *Cross section through the metacarpal shafts demonstrates the close relationship of the radialis indicis artery to the volar surface of the second metacarpal.*
2. *The palmar metacarpal artery to the second web space is adjacent to the radial volar surface of the third metacarpal shaft.*
3. *The ulnar artery and deep branch of the ulnar nerve are volar to the fourth metacarpal shaft, separated from it by muscle, a distance equal to the width of the bone.*

Pin Placement

1. *Wire or full or half-pin placement from the 90° lateral position can be safely passed through the shafts of the second, third, and fourth metacarpals. Extensor tendon impalement may occur as the pin passes through the skin on the medial side of the dorsum of the hand. The oblique lateral surface of the second metacarpal makes pin insertion difficult because the tip of the pin tends to slide to the bone.*
2. *Half-pin insertion into the second metacarpal from the 150° lateral position can be safely accomplished if done carefully.*
3. *Half-pin placement into the fifth metacarpal shaft from the 120° medial position can be done with caution, although the curved surface of the bone makes pin insertion difficult.*

a., artery; br., branch; n., nerve.

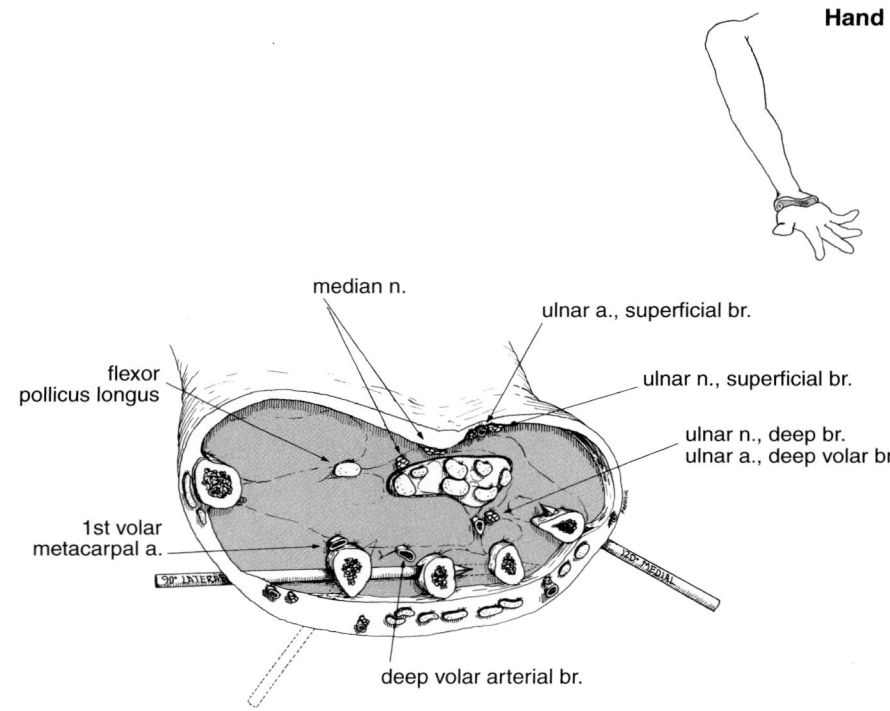

FIGURE 11-27 *Anatomic Considerations*

1. The ilium's inner table is separated from the abdominal contents by the iliacus muscle.
2. The iliac wings are concaved medially.

Pin Placement

1. Half-pins can be inserted along the iliac crest aiming at either the sciatic notch or sacroiliac joint from the 20° lateral position.
2. Full pin placement from the anterior inferior iliac spine to the posterior inferior iliac spine requires a special alignment guide.
3. Pin placement is safer if the tip of the pin penetrates the outer table of the ilium rather than the inner table.

Pelvis

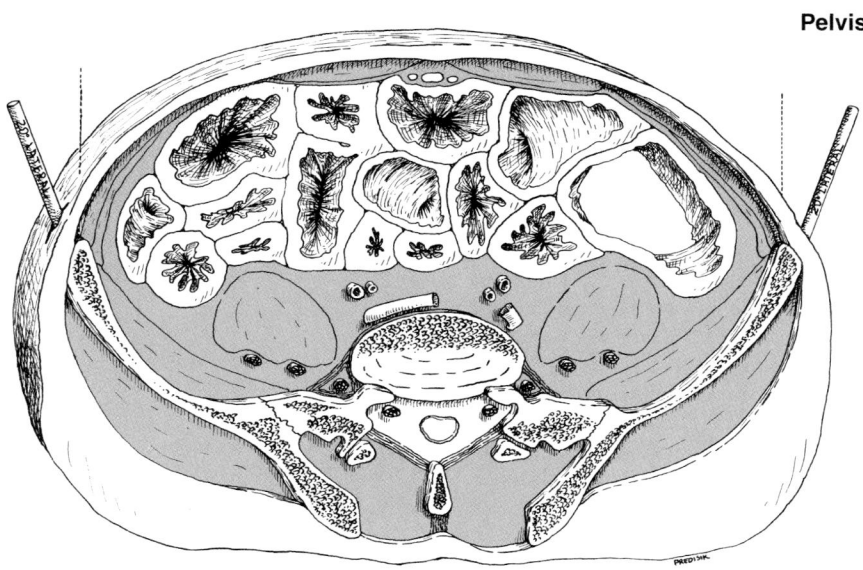

Pin Tract Infection

Pin tract infection has always been the principal drawback to the use of external fixation. Unfortunately, preliminary communications announcing the development of new fixators rarely take note of this complication. Subsequent reports of external fixator applications, however, provide evidence that pin tract infections continue to plague the devices.[23,24,41,45,50] One problem in determining the overall incidence of pin tract infections is that different authors use different sets of criteria to define pin tract infection. This variance is present even within a single institution, making a review of patients' charts an inaccurate procedure for determining the incidence of pin tract sepsis.

For this reason, the concept of "major" and "minor" pin tract infection was introduced, followed by other grading systems using numbers or letters. Using such criteria, just about every patient wearing an external fixator for more than a few weeks can expect at least one implant site infection, something that must be kept in mind when informing a patient about a planned fixator application.

PATHOPHYSIOLOGY OF PIN OR WIRE SITE SEPSIS

FLUID SECRETION A metallic pin (or most hard foreign substances, for that matter) when inserted into the body's tissues provokes the development of a membrane separating the foreign material from the adjacent tissues. If relative motion is present between the foreign material and the local tissues, a bursal membrane usually forms to secrete lubricating fluid. With a transcutaneous pin, however, the bursal fluid becomes contaminated with microorganisms through the pinhole. Nevertheless, the contamination presents no special problem as long as the pinhole drains freely to the outside. Pinholes become infected when the delicate balance between the patient's natural defenses and the bacteria's infective capability changes. This alteration can result from (1) the development of an abscess (closed space) around the pin; (2) the presence of necrotic tissue in the pinhole, which can become the focus of sepsis; and (3) the presence of excessive motion between a pin and adjacent tissues, which increases fluid production.

ABSCESS FORMATION As noted earlier, the fluid formed around the pin by the local tissues drains to the external surface and is contaminated with microorganisms in the process. The amount of fluid may be limited, especially when there is no motion between the soft tissues and the implant, such as over the anterior tibia. The fluid dries on the surface, forming a crust. If this crust restricts free drainage of the contaminated bursal fluid by sealing the pinhole, deep abscess formation may result. Thus, frequent pin care directed toward removal of the crust from the pin-skin interface reduces pin sepsis.

SKIN NECROSIS Necrosis of the skin occurs if the tension (or compression) produced by the pin interferes with the circulation of the local subdermal capillary plexus. Plastic surgeons are mindful of this principle when transposing skin flaps; trauma surgeons utilizing transcutaneous pins for external skeletal fixation must also keep it in mind. Skin tension can occur immediately after implant insertion or whenever a change is made in alignment or length. Skin can also be pinched between pins or wires if they are too close together.

HEAT INJURY Thermal damage to skin and soft tissues occurs when a high-speed drill bit becomes hot while passing through hard cortical bone, burning tissue as it emerges from the opposite side of a bone. Avoid heat build-up by using a start/stop drilling rhythm and irrigating the drill sleeve while drilling (Fig. 11-28).

DEEP SOFT TISSUE NECROSIS

Necrosis of deeper soft tissues develops when tissues are compressed by an implant after it has been inserted. Such tension occurs in the anterior compartment of the lower leg if a pin pushes the anterior compartment musculature posteriorly. (It is far wiser to transfix the muscle by pushing the pin straight in, thereby avoiding undue tension.) Necrosis may also be produced if soft tissue "winds up" around a spinning implant or drill bit. (This can best be prevented by the use of a sleeve for both drilling and pin insertion.) Smooth wires are not likely to wind up soft tissues, although a spinning bayonet point might do so (Fig. 11-29).

BONE NECROSIS

Necrosis of bone can occur with the heat generated from drilling. Damage to osteocytes occurs after exposure to temperatures of 55°C for 1 minute or more. Indeed, the

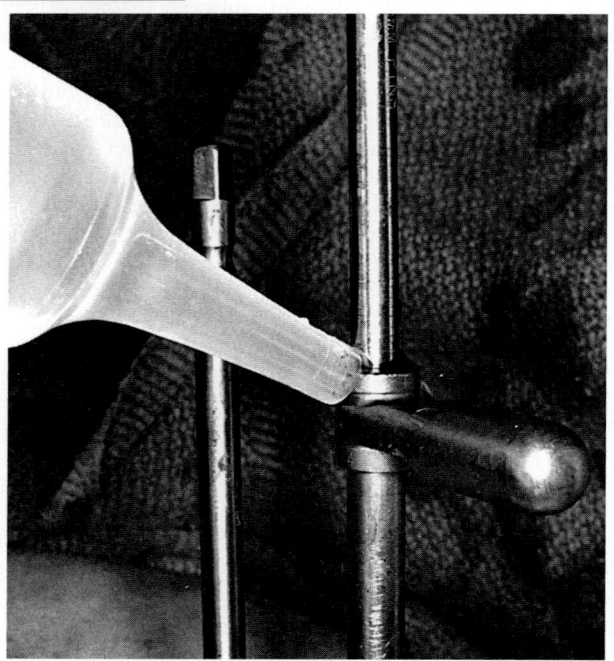

FIGURE 11-29 | *The bayonet point of an Ilizarov wire can wrap up soft tissues, a possible source of deep sepsis. When inserting a wire, push the implant straight through the tissues down to bone before the wire starts to spin.*

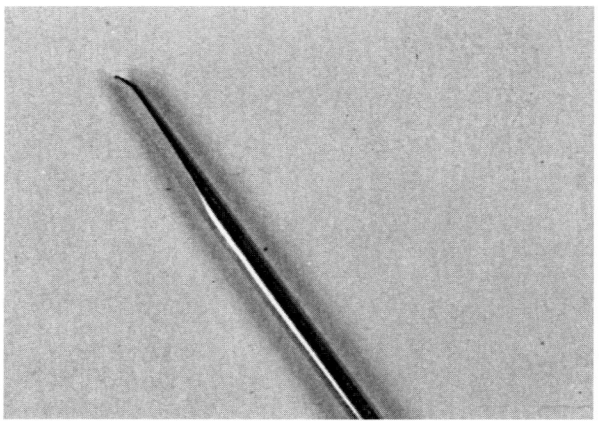

mechanical properties of cortical bone change when exposed to temperatures of 50°C or more.[40,56] The best way to prevent heat build-up is to predrill bone holes with a sharp drill bit, cooled with irrigation fluid, followed by the hand insertion of the implant.

Since each pinhole provides a continuous portal of entry for bacteria into the bone, heat-damaged bone is more likely to become a focus of chronic infection than is normal bone.

Excessive bone pressure—due to compression of a frame—may cause necrosis of osseous tissue at the pin-bone interface. The pressure reduces local bone circulation, resulting in death of osteocytes; necrotic bone may become the focus of a chronic infection.

MOTION

Relative motion between a pin and adjacent tissues contributes to pinhole sepsis. As far as the microenvironment of the pinhole is concerned, it makes little difference whether the pin is moving with respect to the tissue or the tissue is sliding back and forth along the pin. The effect is the same: relative motion between soft tissue and a contaminated foreign body (the pin). Reduction of motion at the pin-tissue interface decreases the incidence of pin tract infections. (The low incidence of pin tract infections in reported series of fractures managed with pins in plaster is due, no doubt, to skin immobilization by the plaster cast.)

THE PIN-SKIN INTERFACE

Wherever possible reduce motion between the pin and soft tissues by selecting areas for pin insertion that avoid muscle transfixion. Further reduction in soft tissue/implant motion can be accomplished by wrapping the pins with a bulky wad of gauze dressing between the skin and the fixator.

Recognizing that implant site sepsis usually starts at the pin-skin interface (rather than the pin-bone interface) has led some researchers and clinicians to try to reduce the infection rate associated with external fixation by coating the shaft of pins and wires with a known bacterial inhibitor, specifically, silver or tobramycin.[11,12,43,71,74]

Silver-based antiseptics are being employed in everything from neonatal eye drops to burn ointments. While initial experimental studies suggested that silver coating of pins could reduce infections in vitro[74] and in a sheep iliac crest model,[12] a subsequent human trial revealed no difference in infection rate.[11] Moreover, the presence of free silver in the serum of patients in the group receiving silver-coated pins caused the researchers to terminate the study and recommend against the continued use of such implants, effectively eliminating further development with such devices.[43]

The effectiveness of the antibiotic tobramycin against both staphylococci and gram-negative rods suggested that local application of the medication might reduce pin site sepsis for transcutaneous implants. Unfortunately, tobramycin cannot be coated directly onto metallic pins with any predictable elution, so tobramycin-impregnated methyl methacrylate pin sleeves were developed,[71] employing the antibiotic-cement combination used for total joint replacement or formed into beads for the treatment of osteomyelitis. As with silver coatings, the tobramycin-acrylic sleeves failed to deliver the expected benefit. Indeed, it seemed to some clinicians that the infection rate increased when tobramycin sleeves were used. A reasonable explanation for this observation is the tobramycin is eluted from the surface of the pins for a very limited amount of time, with antimicrobial levels surrounding tissue dropping off rapidly after a few days following implantation. Although the initial high concentration of tobramycin may sterilize a closed space like a cavitary osteomyelitis or a joint replacement, a pin sleeve constantly exposed to fresh bacteria on the skin surface may function as a contaminated foreign body perpetuating the infection once the antibiotic has leached out of the cement.

THE PIN-BONE INTERFACE

Pin loosening contributes to the development of pin tract infections. Hyldahl and co-workers and Schatzker and colleagues[27,54] and others[39,45] studied the pathophysiology of loosening hardware within bone. They noted that bone resorption and subsequent implant loosening results from cyclic (rather than constant) pressure at the bone-metal interface. Once a pin becomes loose, pin-tissue interface motion will promote sepsis in a manner consistent with mechanisms already described.[45]

Employing only threaded pins can decrease motion at the pin-bone interface. If properly inserted, they do not slip back and forth in the bone as smooth pins do. Threaded pins, especially tapered threaded pins, should not be "backed out" once they are inserted, as they tend to loosen more quickly thereafter.

Another way to reduce cyclic pin motion is to increase the stability (stiffness) of the fixator configuration. Chao and associates[8] and others[15,17,26,37,46,48,60] have determined that fixator stiffness can be increased by (1) increasing the number of pins; (2) increasing the distance between the pins within each pin cluster; (3) applying pins closer to the fracture site; and (4) incorporating pins that are mechanically stiff into the fixator.

The problem of fixator stability becomes critical if one or more loose pins must be removed because of sepsis. Loosening of the remaining pins may occur as the overall stiffness of the frame configuration decreases. These difficulties can be avoided in the first place if a sufficient number of pins are inserted to allow removal of one or more pins without affecting the integrity of the fixation. As Naden puts it, "tis better to add a pin than to have one too few."[47]

Certain recent developments have helped reduce the incidence of pin tract infections caused by loosening, including the use of titanium, rather than steel, pins and hydroxyapatite-coated threads (usually applied to steel pins).

The use of pins made from a titanium alloy rather than stainless steel results in a reduction in implant site sepsis (as observed with other orthopaedic implant systems, including total joint implants and intramedullary nails).[52] The toxic effect of steel on cellular function may be related to the elution of certain metallic ions (perhaps nickel or chromium) from the implant's surface. Titanium pins reduce the incidence of pin tract infections by about 50 percent.[22] Moreover, we have noted that when implant site infections do occur around titanium pins, the problem stays localized to the immediate environment around the implant. Extensive cellulitis that extends for many centimeters around the pinhole (a common phenomenon when stainless steel pins are employed) occurs rarely, if at all, with titanium implants.

The only drawback to the use of titanium pins (aside from their higher cost) is their reduced stiffness compared with stainless steel pins. Although in some situations such flexibility might be desirable, most surgeons prefer stiff fixator-pin-bone configurations, especially when bone fragments must be moved by the fixator to correct deformities. For this reason, researchers and manufacturers searched for a way to retain stainless steel's stiffness yet reduce the likelihood of implant loosening. The result was hydroxyapatite-coated threads on stainless steel pins.[44,57,58]

Hydroxyapatite, the mineral of bone, is applied via an expensive but reliable ion-plasma coating technique to the surface of stainless steel pins to permit osteointegration of the patient's bone with the implant to reduce loosening. In a 1997 prospective randomized study using a sheep model,[44] Italian researchers found that local pin site osseous rarefaction was significantly lower and extraction torque significantly higher when hydroxyapatite-coated pins were compared with uncoated pins. Five years later, German researchers conducted a similar project with human patients, comparing titanium pins and hydroxyapatite-coated pins.[58] They found a four-fold difference in extraction torque in the coated pin group, as well as a marked reduction in pin site sepsis.

On the other hand, Pizà and co-workers in Spain compared hydroxyapatite-coated pins with uncoated pins in a group of patients undergoing limb elongation for stature increase.[57] Although they found a 20-fold decrease in pin loosening in the coated-pin patients, the incidence of pin site sepsis did not differ between the two groups.

Thus, it appears that hydroxyapatite coating on pins, whether studied in animals or humans, significantly reduces implant site loosening but may not decrease pin site sepsis, except perhaps in those situations where the infection is associated with osteolysis and loose pins.

In our own clinical experience, the osteointegration associated with either hydroxyapatite-coated steel pins or biologically inert titanium pins makes it almost impossible to remove threaded external fixation pins from cortical bone in awake patients. Injecting local anesthetic into or around the pin site does not help reduce the intolerable pain associated with trying to break loose an osteointegrated pin; instead, we use general anesthesia for fixator removal when bone ingrowth pins have been used.

Clearly, modern technology has improved the longevity of external fixation with threaded implants, diminishing both late loosening and those infections associated with osteolysis and diminished fixation. However, as mentioned earlier, early soft tissue pin or wire site sepsis has not responded favorably to antibiotic- or antiseptic-coated implants. Instead, surgeons must resort to the time-honored methods of eliminating tissue necrosis at the time of pin or wire insertion, as well as those techniques that stabilize the implant-skin interface once the device is in place.

Strategies to Reduce Implant Site Sepsis

FIXATOR SELECTION

The selection of the appropriate fixator construct is particularly important. In general, the configuration should be quite stiff, which alone will do much to prevent pin sepsis.[45,57] When dealing with a chronic bone infection or an extensively contaminated wound, the fixation frame should be capable of extraordinary rigidity. If the orthopaedic problem is less complex and the application short-term, a less rigid configuration will suffice. If planning a secondary surgery while the fixator is in place, select a frame configuration with the contemplated procedure in mind. If comminution of fracture fragments is present, the frame should permit control of intermediate fragments. Because it is better to insert pins through intact skin, the fixator should permit pin placement to be dictated by the nature of the injury rather than by the configuration of the frame.

PIN SELECTION

SMOOTH PINS Smooth pins should not be used for external skeletal fixation. They create two holes in the bone but do not offer the advantage of "screwed-in" bone fixation. The unfortunate experience with the Stader and Anderson devices in the 1940s was due, I believe, to insufficient fixation with smooth pins.

THREADED PINS Both cylindrical and tapered-thread pins are available, with or without the hydroxyapatite coating.[39] Most knowledgeable surgeons prefer the coated pins, although there is no clear consensus about which thread shape works best. Some pins are both self-drilling and self-tapping, but such implants have fallen out of favor with most surgeons, who prefer to predrill each pin site.

PIN AND WIRE INSERTION CONSIDERATIONS

FRACTURE ALIGNMENT Align the fracture as precisely as possible prior to pin insertion. An unaligned fracture creates undue skin tension (a source of possible necrosis) by the skin on the concave side of the fracture deformity when the fracture is reduced. The pins or wires may also pinch the skin on the convex side of the fracture deformity, creating additional skin necrosis. Moreover, some fixators require precise alignment of rotation at the fracture site before pin insertion because the frame does not permit correction of axial malalignment once the pins are in place.

PREDRILLING Inserting a self-drilling stainless steel pin into the tibia of a young healthy adult male can be an exercise in frustration for the surgeon. After drilling for a while and making no headway, the surgeon tends to push harder and turn the drill faster. Heat (from drilling) increases the microhardness of bone, making progress difficult.[40] To make matters worse, the cuttings (chaff) from the drilling of bone have no place to go because the pin contains no fluting (groove). The chaff also increases friction, making the drilling even more difficult. Friction created by these factors increases the temperature of the pinpoint until it is too hot to touch when it emerges from the opposite side of the limb. It is easier (and safer) if the surgeon predrills cortical bone through a drill sleeve before pin insertion. A sharp drill bit penetrates bone more easily than a pointed pin because the fluting of the drill bit permits the chaff to be carried away from the worksite, reducing friction and also the amount of effort required of the surgeon.

When drilling, stop the drill every few seconds to allow the cutting tip to cool. The heat generated by drilling not only damages the bone, but also "work-hardens" osseous tissue, which then resists further advancement. A worthwhile practice is to irrigate the drill bit to cool it and conduct heat away from the tip.

If much resistance is encountered during drilling, check the drill bit tip between your fingertips for excessive temperature. If the tip cannot be comfortably held for 15 or 20 seconds, do not leave an implant in the bone hole, since necrotic (thermally injured) bone will be in communication with the pin's bacteriologic environment, predisposing to chronic osteomyelitis. Instead, insert the pin (wire) elsewhere. Likewise, the bone in the drill bit's flutes should be white, never black or brown, which are signs of burnt bone (Fig. 11-30).

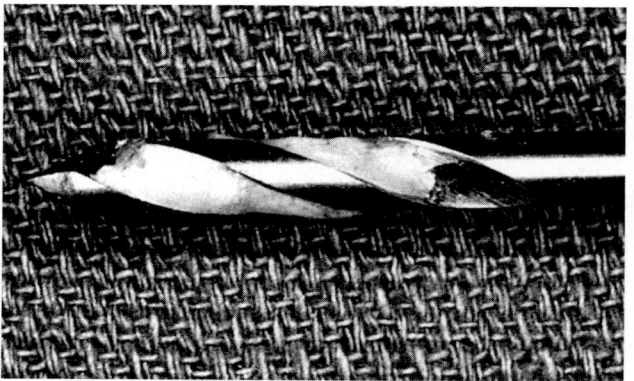

FIGURE 11-30 *The bone in the flutes of a drill bit should be white, never black or brown (a sign of thermal injury to bone).*

PIN INSERTION

Use a manual handle for pin insertion, which should be accomplished through the drill sleeve. Avoid overinsertion.

INSERTING TRANSFIXION WIRES

As with pins, avoid tissue necrosis when inserting wires, which can be caused by wrapping-up of tissues, excessive tension, or thermal injury from heat build-up during drilling.

With transfixion wires, a spinning bayonet point may wind up soft tissues, causing necrosis. Therefore, push transfixion wires straight through the tissue to bone before turning on the drill. If the wire misses the bone, withdraw it completely and reinsert it rather than redirecting it within the limb's tissues.

When inserting transfixion wires into bone with a power drill, the dense cortical bone, by offering substantial resistance to the wire point's progress, may cause heat build-up, which hardens the bone even more, resisting additional progress of the wire point. For this reason, stop the drill every few seconds with a stop/start action to advance a wire slowly through hard osseous tissue.

When inserting a transfixion wire with a motorized chuck, wire flexibility may, at times, cause the wire to bend, reducing accuracy of placement. For this reason, whenever inserting a wire, manually grasp the wire close to its tip to stabilize it. Since a spinning wire can wrap up surgical gloves, hold the wire with a wet gauze pad.

As soon as a transfixion wire's point penetrates a bone's far cortex, stop drilling since the spinning wire tip might damage tissues on the limb's opposite side. Instead, grasp the wire with pliers and hit the pliers with a mallet to drive the wire through (Fig. 11-31).

A most important principle when using any transfixion implant: If the tip of a wire (or pin) emerges from the opposite side of a limb either smoking or too hot to be comfortably held between the surgeon's fingertips, the wire should be withdrawn, cooled, and reinserted elsewhere.

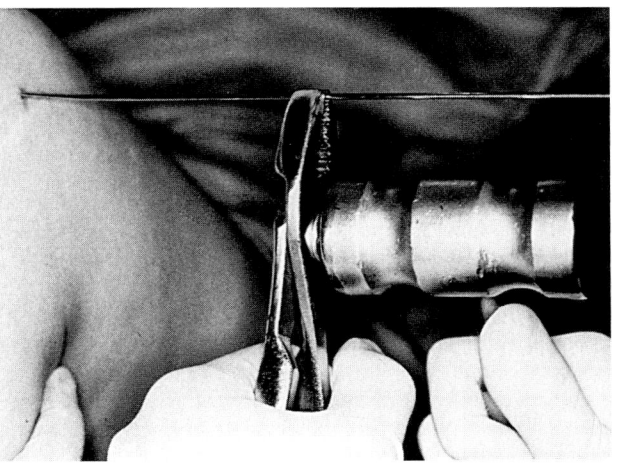

FIGURE 11-31 *After the bone is penetrated with a wire, drive the point of the wire through the skin on the opposite side of the limb with pliers and a mallet.*

IMPLANT-SKIN INTERFACE MANAGEMENT

After inserting a wire or pin, but before attaching it to the frame, check the skin interface for evidence of tissue tension while the limb is in its most functional position, that is, with the knee extended, the ankle at neutral, and so on. Interface tension creates a ridge of skin on one side of a wire or pin. Incise the ridge to enlarge the skin hole around either a transosseous pin or an olive wire. Close the enlarged hole with a nylon suture (if necessary) on the side of the wire opposite the released ridge.

When the ridge of skin is adjacent to a smooth wire, slowly withdraw the wire (with pliers and a mallet) until its tip drops below the skin surface. Allow the skin to shift to a more neutral location and advance the wire again until it passes through the skin in an improved position (Fig. 11-32).

If the interface tension exists on the insertion side of a limb, snap off the wire's blunt end obliquely to create a point and advance the wire to just below the skin surface by the pliers-mallet method on the limb's far side. Tap the wire back through the skin after making a position adjustment.

With either transfixion wires or pins, check the range of motion to make sure that no undue tension occurs during the anticipated movement required while the fixator is on the limb. If necessary, an implant should be reinserted if movement of an adjacent joint causes skin tension.

Certain important techniques of transfixion wire insertion ensure maximum functional limb use and joint mobility:

- Avoid impalement of tendons.
- Avoid (whenever possible) transfixing synovium.
- Penetrate muscles at their maximum functional length.

This last rule, which is critically important for a successful long-term application, means that the position of a nearby joint must change as a pin or wire passes through the flexor and extensor muscle groups. For instance, when inserting a wire into the lower leg, plantarflex the foot when transfixing the anterior compartment, invert the foot when inserting wires into the peroneal muscles, and dorsiflex the foot during triceps surae impalement.

FRAME ASSEMBLY

Frame assembly can be extremely time-consuming if the surgeon is not familiar with the technical details necessary for constructing the proper spatial configuration of the fixator. It is important to practice frame assembly prior to surgery. A piece of wood or synthetic bone can be used. Learn the correct names for the components, asking for them as one would ask for any surgical instrument. The operating room personnel quickly learn the names of the components if they are expected to hand them to the surgeon.

Once the frame is assembled, skeletal alignment should be evaluated with roentgenograms or fluoroscopy. Some projections are difficult to interpret because of the presence of radiopaque components of the fixator. If this occurs, oblique projections can be obtained of both limbs (for purposes of comparison). If alignment is unsatisfactory, the entire frame should be loosened and a manual correction of the limb carried out. The frame should not be used to correct malalignment of a fracture by compressing the convex side and distracting the concave side of the fracture deformity.

FIGURE 11-32   *The wire-skin interface. **A,** Tension on the skin is caused by a transfixion wire. To correct the situation, withdraw the wire to below skin level, allow the skin to shift to a neutral position, and **B,** drive the wire forward. The arrow points to the original wire hole.*

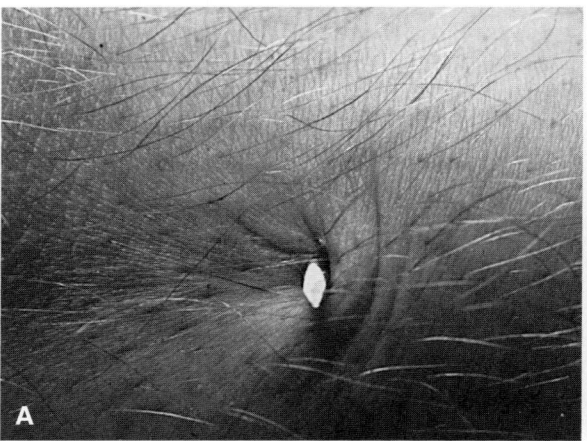 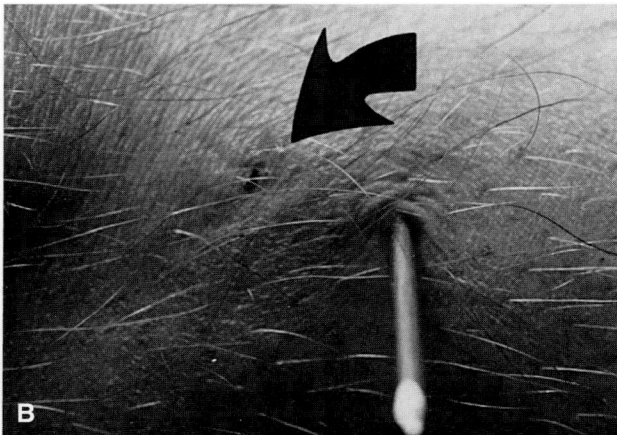

PIN CARE ROUTINE

As noted earlier, it makes little difference to the pinhole microflora whether the pin is moving in the soft tissues or the tissue is sliding along the pin. The effect is the same: relative motion between the tissue and a contaminated foreign body. Reduction of soft tissue motion around the pinhole can be accomplished by forming a bulky wad of gauze dressing wrapped around the pin to completely fill the space between the skin and the fixator. This controls sliding of the skin when the limb swells, following ambulation or activity.

The question of daily pin care stirs much controversy among workers in the field of external skeletal fixation. My routine for pin care consists of daily cleansing of the pins and surrounding skin with a soapy solution, using small swabs or applicator sticks. If the patient is reasonably agile, he or she can wash around the pins with soap and water in the shower. This is followed by application of an antibiotic ointment (Neosporin or Bactroban), and then a bulky wrap (as described earlier) to control the space between the skin and the fixator.

In spite of diligent efforts, however, some pins become septic. Furthermore, pin tract infection, at times, seems to occur when least expected. A most carefully placed, thoroughly released, and well-managed pinhole may become infected and others in the same patient do not. Nevertheless, close adherence to the principles outlined in this chapter will do much to control the factors primarily associated with pinhole sepsis.

AMBULATORY AIDS

Since implant loosening is associated with sepsis, efforts should be focused on reducing cyclic stresses at the implant-bone interface. Such stresses occur with unprotected weight-bearing in lower extremity applications. Therefore, do not permit patients to ambulate with a fixator in place without supplementary ambulatory aids such as crutches (until the bone consolidates). The reason for this is obvious. The external fixator serves as an exterior skeleton when there is no continuity of bone following a fracture. The mechanical stresses of weight-bearing are transferred from the bone to the fixator at the implant-bone interface. The implants, being flexible, transmit cyclic pressure associated with ambulation to the bone. This results in bone resorption and subsequent implant loosening. For this reason, unprotected early weight-bearing with an external skeletal fixator on the lower extremity should be discouraged.

DEALING WITH PINHOLE PROBLEMS

If the patient presents with evidence of pinhole sepsis following application of an external skeletal fixator, the surgeon should make every effort to resolve the problem. Initial management consists of rest with elevation of the affected limb. The frequency of cleansing around the pinhole should be increased. I may enlarge the skin hole by infiltrating the skin around the pin with a local anesthetic and then insert a #11 blade into the skin adjacent to the pin. I also start the patient on oral antistaphylococcal antibiotics. If these measures fail to promptly relieve the problem, the pin clamp should be opened slightly and the pin checked for loosening by wiggling it. If the pin is loose or if the maneuver produces pain, the pin should be removed. If removal of the loose pin affects the stability of the fixator, a new pin must be inserted in another location. The pinhole should be curetted with a small curette after a septic pin is removed. If, however, an infected pin is securely fastened to the bone, the patient should be admitted to the hospital for a brief course of parenteral antibiotics, bed rest, and a deep incision and drainage of the soft tissues around the pinhole. Antibiotic therapy can be guided by cultures of the implant site. If the septic process is not resolved by these actions, the involved pin should be removed and replaced with a new one in a different position. If the infection does not involve the bone, drainage should stop in a few days. If drainage persists, there is a significant probability that the patient has developed a chronic implant hole infection, which requires curettage and perhaps even more extensive care.

Fixator-Associated Problems

Tis a rare individual indeed who happily wears an external skeletal fixator. Patient-related problems caused by the frame are pressure necrosis of the skin and undue or excessive pain. Pin or wire breakage may occur while a fixator is in place, causing distress to the patient and his or her surgeon. The patient's lifestyle may be disrupted, and psychosocial problems associated with external skeletal fixation may arise, generally related to long-term application combined with protracted hospitalization.

PRESSURE NECROSIS

Continuous contact with the frame or one of its components causes intense burning pain for several hours, followed by ischemic necrosis of the tissues being compressed. This usually leads to an infection and a worsening of the fixator experience.

The amount of clearance required between the skin and the fixator varies from region to region. In the upper extremity and in lower extremity applications in which there is bone immediately under the subcutaneous tissues (as in the pretibial region of the leg) two fingerbreadths between the skin and the fixator is sufficient. Three or more fingerbreadths are required over most soft tissue areas in the lower extremity where there is muscle between subcutaneous tissue and bone.

If limb swelling is anticipated, additional clearance is necessary. Often more than three fingerbreadths are required in the lateral aspect of the thigh in an obese patient, because the soft tissues there bulge laterally when the patient is lying down. When applying an external fixator to the pelvis, 10 to 15 cm clearance must be left for the abdomen, so the patient can sit up. It is important to fill the space between the skin and the fixator with a bulky gauze wrap, to prevent excessive motion between the skin and the implants.

BROKEN COMPONENTS

Occasionally, pins break while the fixator is on a patient. Chao and co-workers[8] observed that static stresses on the pins of a fixator applied without compression are 70 times greater than the stresses on the pins of a fixator applied with compression because of the overall fixator stability made by the bone being compressed. Thus, compression of the fracture site should be achieved if at all possible.

DISRUPTION OF LIFESTYLE

When applying an external fixator, the surgeon should consider the logistical problems associated with wearing the frame. Cover the sharp ends of pins and wires with plastic protectors. (Some manufacturers provide protectors with their fixation systems, but they are easy to fabricate from IV tubing.)

Pins and wires should not interfere with the function of the opposite limb. When applying a fixator to the upper extremity, do not inhibit the arm from adducting to the side of the body, if possible. In femoral applications, the frame should not occupy the area medial to the upper thigh for reasons of personal hygiene and comfort. In general, fixators should not be applied around the posterior thigh area, which would force the patient to lie prone for the entire time the fixator frame is in place.

Fixator frames have a tendency to loosen while they are on the patient. At each clinic or office visit, check the patient's frame and tighten if necessary. Loosening tends to occur where the fixator components meet at right angles. Compression or distraction, if necessary, should be carried out in a systematic fashion, that is, symmetrical length adjustments done at each visit. It is important to check for pin loosening, especially if evidence of pin tract sepsis or pain is present when the patient is evaluated.

Pain

Pain following application of an external skeletal fixator is to be expected during the postoperative period and thereafter. The pain is usually well tolerated, but excessive or undue pain requires evaluation and management.

POSTOPERATIVE PAIN

External fixation, like any surgical procedure, can be expected to produce pain postoperatively. The pain is usually appropriate to the nature of the problem for which the fixator was initially applied; for example, one can anticipate as much postoperative pain from the application of a tibial external fixator as would result from the use of internal fixation for the same injury. The patient's personality and pain tolerance threshold also determine the level of pain experienced and, consequently, the quantity of analgesics necessary for pain control. Patients with considerable drug experience seem to require more narcotic medication for relief than do other patients.

Pain around implant sites following surgery, although significant, is usually overshadowed by the operative site symptoms. However, if pain around an implant predominates among the early postoperative complaints, inspect the site. Occasionally, pressure from these dressings against the skin can produce discomfort, not unlike the pressure from a snug-fitting cast. The patient often complains of burning and can usually specify the implant as the cause of the problem.

Skin and soft tissue tension occurs with shifting of a mobile tissue area impaled by transcutaneous implants. As with a too tight bulky wrap, tension on the skin at the implant site produces pain or a burning sensation.

PAIN WHILE THE FIXATOR IS IN PLACE

Ordinarily, the pain associated with a fixator diminishes to a tolerable level within a week after frame application. However, it is not unusual for patients, including those who are quite stoical, to describe a *continuous dull ache* requiring codeine or a similar analgesic medication for control during the entire time the fixator is in place. In some individuals, these symptoms vary with activity levels, being greatest when the patient is ambulatory and relieved by rest.

When the patient is permitted to ambulate in the fixator without supplementary aids (such as crutches), the problem is worse. For this reason (and to prevent pin loosening), supplementary ambulation aids are recommended whenever a lower extremity fixator is applied. The aids should be continued until the fixator is removed.

Excessive or *undue pain* may develop during the time the fixator is in place. This symptom is most distressing to the patient and should be investigated. At times, the patient may describe pain starting at a particular implant and radiating proximally or distally, suggesting nerve compression. The sensation may be continuous or intermittent and may be related to the position of the limb. Any pin that produces significant radiating pain should be removed because the involved pin may be putting pressure on a sensitive nerve.

PAIN ON PIN REMOVAL

Patients who have had a very unpleasant pin removal experience seem to remember the event years later, even when other aspects of the fixator application have long been forgotten. A general anesthetic is usually needed for removal of a modern fixator that is securely integrated into the bone.

PERSISTENT PAIN AFTER FIXATOR REMOVAL

Pain following pin removal usually falls into one of the following categories: (1) bone pain associated with bone hole sepsis; (2) neurogenic pain resulting from persistent nerve irritation; and (3) pain associated with a healing fracture. Other causes of postfixator pain include the usual problems that occur in the post-trauma period. These include joint pain associated with restriction of motion and malalignment of the joint surfaces.

BONE PAIN

Persistent bone pain localized over the pinhole and lasting more than 3 or 4 days after an external fixator is removed is unusual. If it does occur and is associated with persistent inflammation or drainage, expect a chronic implant site infection to develop. Pain at the site can also occur after the hole has sealed over and the limb is quiescent. The patient may describe episodes of recurrent pain, sometimes accompanied by redness and swelling, which may subside spontaneously or after a brief course of oral antibiotics.

NEUROGENIC PAIN

Chronic pain from nerve irritation should subside with the passage of time unless caused by limb lengthening or deformity correction. In such cases (which are rare in post-trauma reconstruction but fairly common is limb elongation to correct congenital deformities) a release of a band of tissue compressing the nerve may be necessary.

PAIN ASSOCIATED WITH FRACTURE HEALING

Pain associated with fracture healing localized to the site of injury is similar to that seen with other modalities of treatment and usually subsides as the fracture consolidates. Solid union in a position of malalignment sometimes causes a dull ache that lasts for many years.

PSYCHOLOGICAL PROBLEMS

Many patients, toward the end of their treatment program, are eager to have the fixator removed, even if no complications or problems had developed while the fixator was in place. Professor Jacques Vidal and his associates found

numerous socioeconomic and psychological effects of long-term treatment in an external skeletal fixator, including a sense of estrangement from their families, concerns about their ability to make a living, and fear of amputation.[68] Their patients were plagued with anxieties, and many had suicidal thoughts at one time or another. Alcohol and drug consumption increased while in fixation. The incidence of these problems reflected the recently described post-trauma stress disorders and depression symptoms that often accompany severe trauma. However, the prolonged nature of an external fixator application usually makes a bad situation worse.

Thus, viewed objectively, patients endure protracted hospitalization, psychological duress, disruption of their personal lives, and significant personality changes for the preservation of a dysfunctional limb. Professional psychological counseling may be helpful.

The surgeon has the responsibility to prepare the patient for fixator application. It is worthwhile to tell the patient that pin tract infections are *likely to* occur. The patient should be told that one or more pins will probably have to be changed during the course of therapy, and that the procedure will probably require general anesthesia. These odds may be a bit higher than the actual likelihood of another anesthetic for pin management, but no harm is done by preparing the patient for the worst and hoping for the best.

PRINCIPLES UNIQUE TO THE ILIZAROV METHOD

In acute traumatology, external fixator applications tend to be static: after application, the surgeon tightens the device's interconnecting hinges, and the apparatus remains unchanged until removal. Once Ilizarov discovered the capacity of bone to form new osseous tissue in a widening distraction gap, however, the indications for external fixation expanded, with limb lengthening and correction of deformities (both congenital and acquired) now being routinely treated with fixator frames.[28-31,33-35] To the familiar complications of external fixation (implant site sepsis, nerve and vessel injury, inhibition of function, failure to obtain union) were added an entirely new set of problems related to moving bone fragments and regenerate bone formation. Moreover, the common complications of fixators tend to become more troublesome when the apparatus is employed for limb lengthening because tension on the soft tissues at the implant-skin interface during elongation increases the likelihood of ischemia and subsequent necrosis of dermal tissues, a setup for infection.

A limb's deep soft tissue structures, especially thick fascial sheets like the interosseous membranes of the forearm and lower leg and the thigh's linea aspera, resist stretching, even when performed slowly over weeks or months. This, in turn, can cause angulation of the lengthening bone segment or contractures of adjacent joints. If the contractures are not addressed while elongation continues, the joints can sublux or even dislocate completely.[64] The author is aware of cases of thigh lengthening for proximal focal femoral deficiency, for example, in which both the hip and knee dislocated during treatment, a worrisome combination that is difficult to correct.

Likewise, along with the typical difficulties encountered while trying to obtain union of fractures treated with external fixation, the creation of a long column of newly formed regenerate bone by the Ilizarov method presents a set of problems unique to that tissue, including failure of ossification, bending while in fixation, and fracture after fixator removal.

Since post-trauma reconstruction usually involves *restoration* of a limb to its original dimensions, one would expect fewer problems than might be encountered when lengthening a congenitally short limb because the injured limb was, after all, once of normal length. This is not always the case: deep muscle trauma and secondary scarring results in tissue as resistant to stretching as natural fascial bands, or even more so. Likewise, protracted unsuccessful trauma care often leads to severe joint contractures before fixator application. Indeed, the equipment may be used solely to overcome post-trauma joint contractures. Needless to say, attempting to restore limb length, even if only a few centimeters, in a limb that already has a stiff post-trauma equinus or knee contracture is a challenging ordeal for both patient and surgeon.

Additionally, our capacity to create a column of new bone of substantial length has enabled surgeons to rebuild limbs that otherwise would have been unsalvageable. The treatment strategy in such cases usually involves intercalary bone transport, a technique that includes internal bone elongation. The moving bone fragment must, of necessity, be secured to a mobile component of the fixator, which slowly pulls the fragment from its original position to its "docked" position on the other side of the original gap (Fig. 11-33). In doing so, the wires securing the fragment to the frame cut through the skin and deeper tissues by a process that involves tissue necrosis and sloughing along the implant's path, with healing, one hopes, on the trailing side. Thus, in spite of advances in pin fixation attributable to hydroxyapatite coating, pin site infections are still a problem, especially when bone fragments are in motion. Therefore, meticulous attention to the principle outlined earlier in this chapter are even more important for fixator applications involving moving bone segments than they are for frames applied for static purposes.

Since this volume deals with trauma to the musculoskeletal system and its consequences, the following considerations apply to situations in which bone fragments move relative to one another, either for restitution of limb length and alignment or for filling in a defect created by traumatic loss of osseous tissue.

FIGURE 11-33 **A,** *Another configuration to provide simultaneous elongation and transverse compression. In this case, bushings slide along threaded rods during lengthening and simultaneously provide a fixation point for transverse compression of the third and fourth rings in the configuration.* **B,** *Pretreatment and post-treatment radiographs of the same patient (a hypertrophic nonunion of the distal tibia 8 months after an open fracture).*

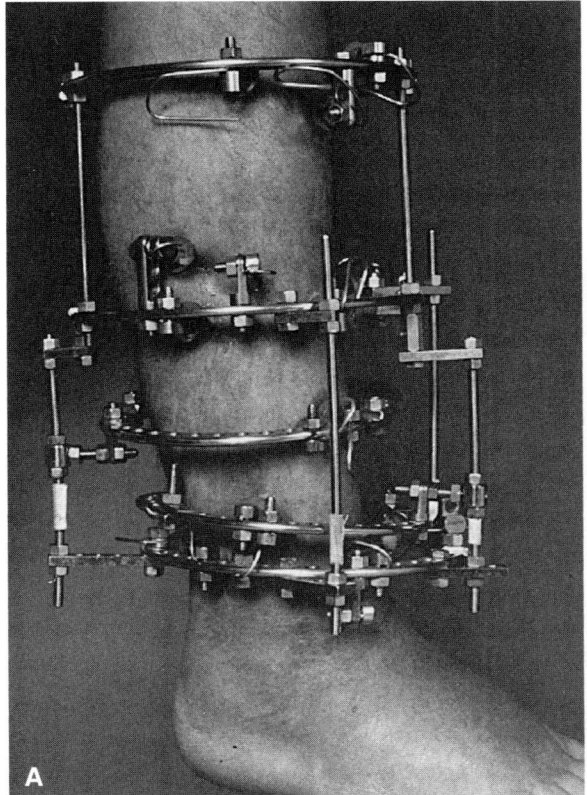

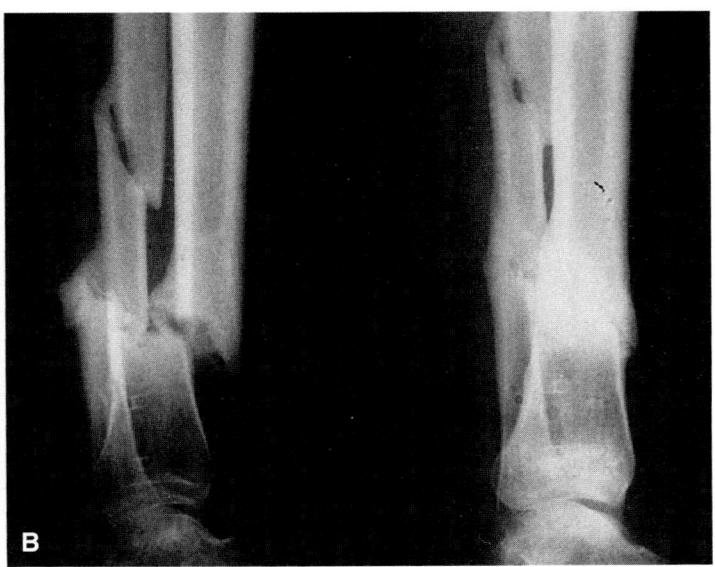

Treatment Principles for Nonunions and Malunions

One fundamental difference between treating a nonunion and a healed malunion is that with a nonunion, the site of any deformity correction (if needed) has been predetermined for the surgeon, since the correction must usually be made through the nonunion site (see Fig. 11-33).

If the nonunion is transverse (perpendicular to the bone's longitudinal axis), compression with either external (or internal) fixation stimulates union. Many nonunions, however, are oblique and often combined with malalignment of the bone fragments in angulation, rotation, displacement (of the mechanical axes), and shortening. When any or all of these deformities are associated with a nonunion, circular external fixation permits the surgeon to gradually correct all deformities, either simultaneously or in succession. With simple angular displacements, a hinged fixator is sufficient to solve the geometric problem, but for more complex malalignment involving multiple planes, the Taylor spatial frame, although rather expensive, has proven invaluable. A surgeon interested in employing this modality should attend a workshop on its use, since many parameters of the deformity and frame configuration must be accurately determined and entered into a proprietary computer program, which produces a prescription for frame adjustment that the patient uses to lengthen or shorten the frame's struts.

When an infection is present at the nonunion site, the surgeon should thoroughly débride the infected bone, while stabilizing the limb in an external fixator, thereby converting the problem of an infected nonunion to an uninfected nonunion. Reconstruction of the limb following débridement usually involves intercalary bone transport if the débridement has resulted in any substantial loss of bone tissue and a segmental skeletal defect.

Segmental Skeletal Defects

Segmental defects may be due to bone loss at the time of trauma, removal of nonviable fragments at initial débridement, or the result of resection of a tumor or necrotic infected bone. When a segmental defect is present, any angulation, rotation, translation, or combination of displacements can easily be corrected through the soft tissues at the level of the defect. For this reason, circular frames designed to deal with segmental defects are usually rather simple; the configuration is tubular, with the connecting rods of the frame parallel to one another and to the bone's biomechanical axis.

A skeletal defect can be overcome by Ilizarov's bone transport method (Fig. 11-34). The bone ends must be matched to fit at final docking of the intercalary fragment with the target fragment. We often graft bone the target site to hasten healing. With very large defects it may be possible to perform two corticotomies and move the resulting bone fragments toward each other.

To eliminate the defect, make a corticotomy through healthy bone at some distance from the defect; thereafter, the intercalary segment between the defect and the corticotomy is pulled through the tissues until the defect is closed and new bone forms in the distraction zone. The fragments should be perfectly aligned with the longitudinal elements of the fixator. If this is not achieved, the transported fragment will not meet up with the target fragment.

If the defect is smaller than 1.5 cm, it is possible to compress the defect acutely (after appropriate débridement) and lengthen the bone through a corticotomy elsewhere.

It is unwise to acutely close a skeletal defect that is more than 1.5 cm, since the redundant soft tissues surrounding the defect tend to bulge out when the fragments are

FIGURE 11-34 *Infected intermedullary ail treated with débridement and bone transport. **A,** Initial presentation. **B,** At surgery, following removal of nail, débridement of nonviable bone, and proximal corticotomy. **C,** During bone transport. Note the widening distraction gap and the narrowing defect. **D,** Oblique view demonstrating cancellous autograft to create a tibiofibular synostosis.*

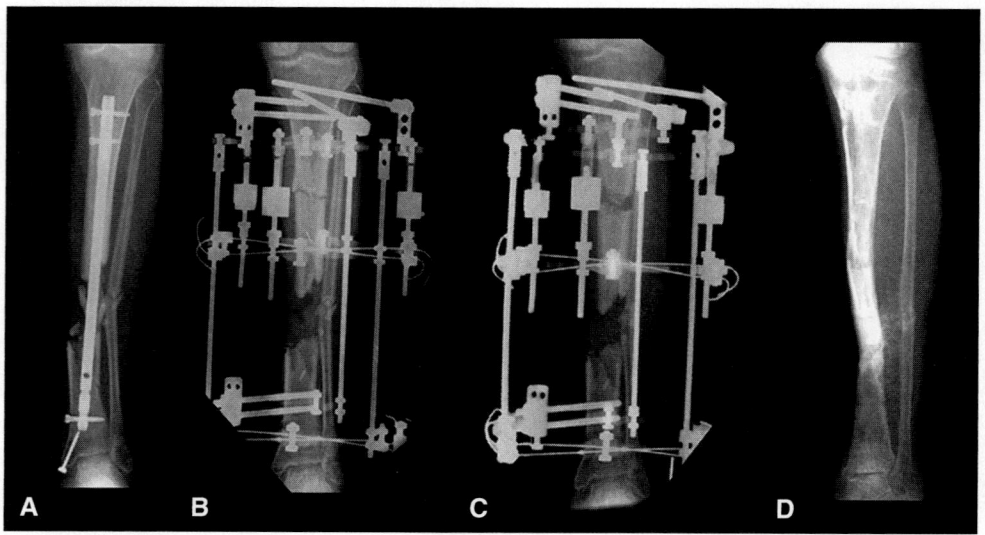

brought together, creating an unsightly appearance to the leg and kinking of both lymphatic and venous drainage. As this redundant skin is trapped between the wires, it cannot contribute to lengthening of the limb through another section of the bone. Therefore, the patient is left with a peculiar-looking limb with bulky redundant tissues at one level and tight, stretched skin at another. With this problem in mind, when dealing with a segmental defect of more than 1.5 cm, it is better to leave the soft tissues at length and eliminate the defect by gradual transport of the intermediate segment. With a large defect, bone fragments may be transported in two directions simultaneously (Fig. 11-35).

A segment of bone can be pulled through a limb with (1) a transport ring and cross wires or pins; or (2) oblique directional wires (Fig. 11-36).

A transport ring and an attached pair of crossed wires or pins is the most stable way to pull a bone fragment through tissue. Unfortunately, the wires cut through the skin and soft tissues as the ring and its attached bone segment move through the limb. At the end of bone transport, however, the crossed transport wires enhance compression at the point of contact between the intermediate fragment and the target fragment.

When oblique directional wires are used to move a bone segment through a limb, there is far less cutting of tissues, since the wires start out nearly parallel to the limb's axis. Unfortunately, such oblique wires often do not provide enough pressure at the end of bone transport to ensure stable interfragmentary compression between the intermediate fragment and the target fragment. For this reason, a surgeon using oblique directional wires must often insert a pair of crossed wires (connected to a ring)

into the intermediate fragment at the end of bone transport to enhance compression at the point of contact. In such a case, the patient requires a second operation to insert the supplementary compression wires.

Joint Mobility

Intensive physiotherapy is also necessary to prevent the joint contractures and subluxations associated with limb elongation and the correction of deformities. Even if the fixator is applied to deal with a fracture or a nonunion—conditions not ordinarily associated with stretching of tissues—irritation of muscles impaled by pins or wires can lead to restriction of joint mobility. Thus, physical therapy has an important place in the treatment of all patients in external fixation.

Whenever bone fragments are moved with respect to one another, soft tissues are placed under tension: the greater the movement, the greater the tension. For this reason, it is important for the surgeon to consider every Ilizarov fixator application that involves movement of bone fragments as a form of limb lengthening, even if the extremity does not end up longer as a result of the procedure.

The important elements of every postoperative physical therapy treatment plan designed to prevent deformities and contractures include elastic splinting, passive stretching, active use of the limb, and appropriate nighttime positioning.

Stretching

Passive muscle stretching is another essential measure designed to prevent contractures. The physical therapist must teach patients and family members how to stretch

---

FIGURE 11-35 *A, With a substantial skeletal defect, it is possible to create two corticotomies in bone, transporting the first intercalary segment at a rate of 2.0 mm/day and the second at a rate of 1.0 mm/day. Each corticotomy gap widens at a rate of 1.0 mm/day with this strategy. B, Another strategy for dealing with a large skeletal defect. Proximal and distal corticotomies are performed, and the two intercalary segments are moved toward each other. The defect closes at the rate of 2.0 mm/day, but each corticotomy site opens at the rate of only 1.0 mm/day.*

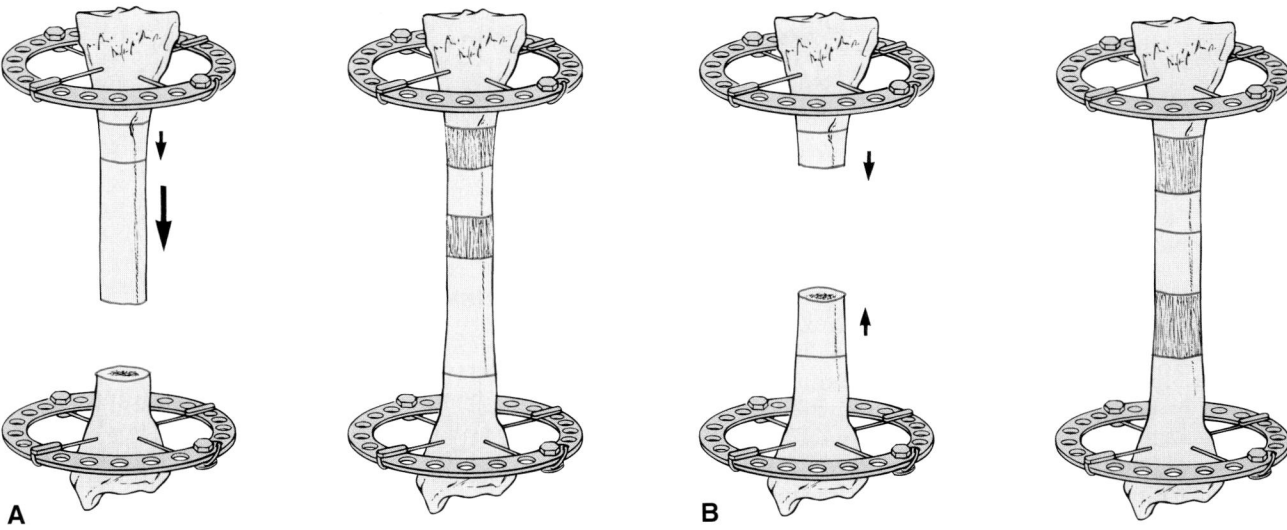

A   B

FIGURE 11-36   *A, A partial skeletal defect can be converted to a complete transverse skeletal defect for reconstruction by the bone transport method. B, With a complete transverse defect, a corticotomy through healthy bone is followed by gradual transport of the intercalary segment toward the target segment. New bone forms in the distraction gap. C, Crossed directional wires can be used in place of a transport ring to move an intercalary bone segment through a limb.*

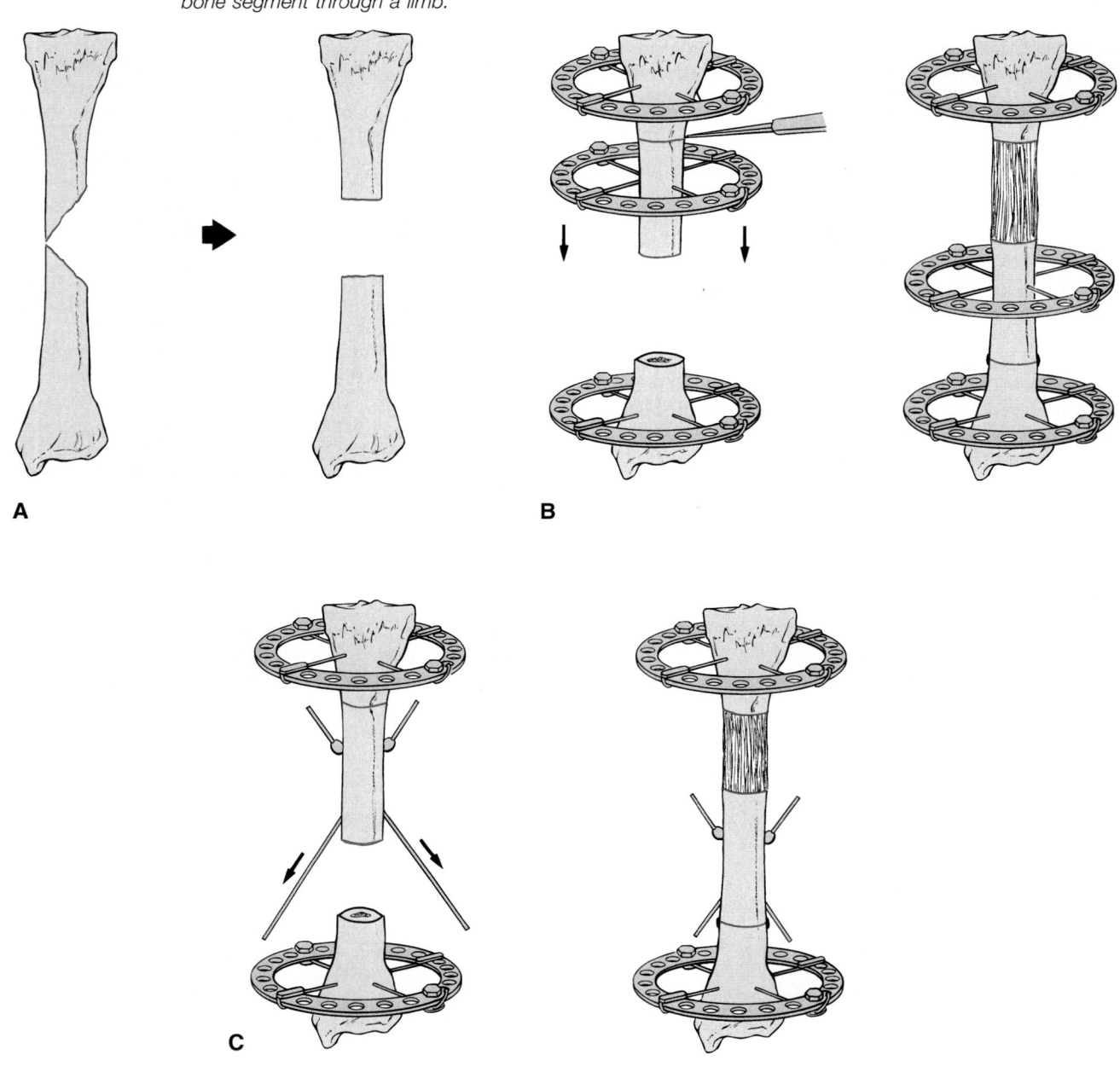

the calf, the hamstrings, and other muscle groups. At least 2 or 3 hours a day should be devoted to this activity, especially in cases involving substantial lengthenings. In fact, the greater the anticipated elongation, the more time per day must be devoted to passive muscle stretching.

Interestingly, active muscle exercises do not help much in preventing contractures. For example, active dorsiflexion of the ankle is not nearly as effective as passive stretching of the calf musculature in limiting equinus contractures.

Contractures

Contractures can occur, of course, whenever a fixator is applied, especially if the movement of muscles and joints is inhibited by the implants, muscle impalement, or pain. The most serious contractures develop, however, when bone segments are moved with respect to one another, especially during limb lengthening. Fortunately for the traumatologist, contractures associated with external fixation for the treatment of acute fracture, nonunions, or malunion almost never proceed to subluxation or frank dislocation. When joint contractures do occur, however, they can prove quite stiff and resistant to correction by simple means (like Achilles tendon lengthening).

Limb Positioning

Proper limb positioning during the night is one of the most important prophylactic measures available during limb elongation or bone fragment movement. The 7 or 8 hours a patient spends in bed may be the most important hours of the day for a patient wearing an external fixator. During that time, joints allowed to fall into suboptimal positions will resist correction during the day. A lower extremity that is permitted to rest with the foot in equinus and the knee flexed is likely to develop a problem at both joints. A support behind the heel (rather than under the knee) forces the knee into neutral position. Likewise, dynamic or static supports of the ankle should be used at all times during bone elongation.

Functional Limb Use

Ambulation and upper extremity use not only promote ossification of the regenerate bone, but also help prevent contractures, subluxations, and dislocations. Weight-bearing, for example, serves as a means of passive calf muscle stretching while maintaining tone and stimulating circulation in the limb. Eating, hair combing, gymnastics, dance therapy, and other similar activities are also useful adjuncts to therapy. The rhythmic movements involved with swimming, cycling, and walking are among the best therapeutic exercises available.

Regenerate Healing and Maturation

Frame stiffness may have to change throughout the course of treatment. Initially, a fixator must be rigid enough to hold the fragments in the proper position, yet flexible enough to allow axial dynamization during loading. Additionally, an overly stiff frame may cause osteoporosis between the proximal and distal mounting clusters as the frame bypasses the bone's weight-bearing function. In the final stages of healing, individual longitudinal elements can be loosened completely or even removed. Likewise, individual pin- or wire-gripping clamps can be released in sequence, permitting greater and greater load on the bone. Before removing the frame, it is wise to allow the patient to walk around for a few days with the transosseous implants in place but with no load sharing by the fixator. Ilizarov calls this final period of consolidation "training the regenerate."[36]

There is evidence that tardy regenerate ossification responds to certain physical stimuli, including ultrasound and electromagnetic stimulation, which speed maturation of the newly forming bone.[7,53,62,66] It is best to use such modalities after reaching the limb's ultimate length or axis correction, lest premature ossification stop the process before reaching the goal. Bone grafting of the regenerated region is rarely necessary. Slow ossification can almost always be traced to limited ambulation or inhibited functional use of the limb.

With bone transport procedures, tardy bone healing frequently occurs at the "docking site," where the moving intercalary fragment of bone meets the target fragment. This happens because the advancing edge of the intercalary fragment becomes progressively dysvascular as it is pulled through the tissues and away from its blood supply. In Russia, Ilizarov's group routinely "freshens" the bone ends about 1 cm before docking by returning the patient to the operating room for curettage of the bone ends about to make contact with each other. In the United States, surgeons often preemptively apply a fresh autogenous bone graft to the docking site shortly after contact between the bones ends is established (see Fig. 11-34D). This may lead to a few too many grafting operations, since some docking without grafting does result in union, especially if the spike of one fragment impales the medullary cavity of the other.

Toward the end of treatment, test the limb manually. The bone should feel quite solid, resisting deflection in any plane. I usually have the patient test the stability of the limb by standing on it. He or she should report no difference in the sense of stability, compared with having the frame secured. I require the patient to walk around for a week with the pins or wires and rings still connected to the limb, but with no longitudinal connecting rods or struts in place. Most often, patients prefer crutches for assisted ambulation during this time.

Management After Frame Removal

After the frame is removed, it should not be necessary to apply a splint, orthosis, or cast to the patient's limb, although this is commonly done by surgeons who remove fixators before x-ray studies show solid cortical bone on three sides of the regenerate. As Ilizarov once told me: "physiotherapy should be finished the day the fixator comes off."

By following the principles outlined in this chapter for both Ilizarov and standard external skeletal fixator applications, a surgeon can reduce the incidence of problems that might lead to an unpleasant experience for both patient and practitioner.

EXTERNAL FIXATORS AS NONUNION MACHINES

External fixators have been condemned as nonunion machines because so many fractures seemingly fail to heal in trauma frames (Fig. 11-37). There are several reasons for this observation: first, fixators are applied to the most severe fractures, those with a natural propensity toward nonunion; second, with so-called spanning external fixators, weight-bearing or functional use is either very difficult or precluded altogether; and third, patients are transferred (often for insurance reasons) to surgeons not familiar with the original treatment plan leaving a patient in a sort of therapeutic limbo.

When applying an external fixator to an acute injury, reduction of bone fragments must be as accurate as with internal plate fixation if the frame is to remain on the limb throughout the entire treatment protocol. Suboptimal reduction might be acceptable with a temporizing fixator when the surgeon plans to soon remove the device and employ internal fixation as the definitive form of

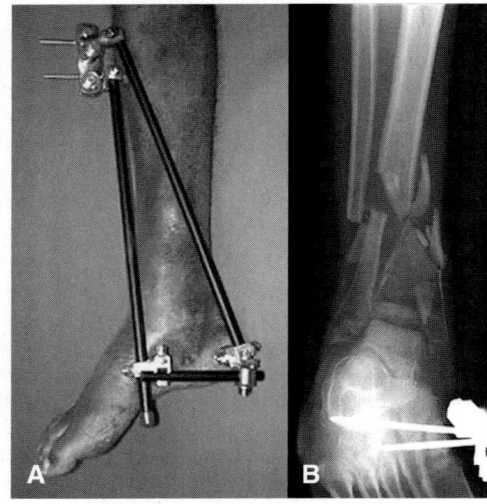

FIGURE 11-37 *Patient placed in external fixator spanning the region of injury.* ***A,*** *The frame was left in place for 6 months without further treatment.* ***B,*** *Established nonunion with severe disuse osteopenia and not a molecule of osteogenesis.*

stabilization. However, such well-laid plans are often not followed. Patients may be transferred after accidents to facilities where a new caregiver may not be comfortable with the plan of the first surgeon and decides to continue the patient in the fixator. The suboptimal alignment then becomes the basis for tardy healing or results in a malnonunion requiring a difficult reconstruction effort. It is far better to strive for optimal alignment when the frame is first applied (unless circumstances preclude the time required to achieve this goal), and then deal with any subsequent tardy union by bone grafting the troublesome region without the need for realignment. Indeed, early bone grafting is the hallmark of a well thought-out treatment plan wherein the surgeon recognizes the worrisome nature of the fracture pattern at the time of injury and prepares to bone graft the limb within the first 6 to 8 weeks after the injury.

REFERENCES

1. Anderson, L.D.; Hutchins, W.C. Fractures of the tibia and fibula treated with casts and transfixing pins. South Med J 59:1026–1032, 1966.
2. Anderson, R. An automatic method of treatment for fractures of the tibia and fibula. Surg Gynecol Obstet 58:639, 1934.
3. Anderson, W.V. Leg lengthening. J Bone Joint Surg [Br] 34:150, 1952.
4. Botte, M.J.; Davis, J.L.; Rose, B.A.; et al. Complications of smooth pin fixation of fractures and dislocations in the hand and wrist. Clin Orthop 276:194–201, 1992.
5. Broos, P.L.; Miserez, M.J.; Rommens, P.M. The monofixator in the primary stabilization of femoral shaft fractures in multiply-injured patients. Injury 23:525–528, 1992.
6. Burny, F. Complications liées a l'utilisation de l'osteotaxis. Acta Orthop Belg 41:103–109, 1975.
7. Ceballos, A.; Pereda, O.; Ortega, R.; et al. Electrically induced osteogenesis in external fixation treatment. Acta Orthop Belg 57:102–108, 1991.
8. Chao, E.Y.S.; Kasman, R.A.; An, K.N. Rigidity and stress analyses of external fracture fixation devices—a theoretical approach. J Biomech 15:971–983, 1982.
9. Charnley, J. Compression Arthrodesis. Edinburgh, Livingstone, 1953.
10. Cleveland, M. The emergency treatment of bone and joint casualties. J Bone Joint Surg [Am] 32:235–279, 1950.
11. Coester, L.M.; Nepola, J.V.; Allen, J.; et al. The effect of silver coated external fixation pins. Iowa Orthop J 26:48–53, 2006.
12. Collinge, C.A.; Goll, G.; Seligson, D.; et al. Pin tract infections: Silver vs uncoated pins. Orthopedics 17:445–448, 1994.
13. Dwyer, N. Preliminary report upon a new fixation device for fractures of long bones. Injury 5:141–144, 1973.
14. Edwards, C.C.; Jaworski, M.; Solana, J.; et al. Management of compound tibia fractures in the multiply injured patient using external fixation. Am Surg 45:190–203, 1979.
15. Egkher, E.; Martinek, H.; Wielke, B. How to increase the stability of external fixation units. Mechanical tests and theoretical studies. Arch Orthop Trauma Surg 96:35–43, 1980.
16. El-Shazly, M.; Saleh, M. Displacement of the common peroneal nerve associated with upper tibial fracture: Implications for fine wire fixation. J Orthop Trauma 16:204–207, 2002.
17. Finlay, J.B.; Moroz, T.K.; Rorabeck, C.H.; et al. Stability of ten configurations of the Hoffmann external-fixation frame. J Bone Joint Surg [Am] 69:734–744, 1987.
18. Fischer, D.A. Skeletal stabilization with a multiplane external fixation device. Clin Orthop 180:50–62, 1983.
19. Frykman, G.K.; Tooma, G.S.; Boyko, K.; et al. Comparison of eleven external fixators for treatment of unstable wrist fractures. J Hand Surg [Am] 14 (2 Pt 1):247–254, 1989.
20. Green, S.A. Complications of External Skeletal Fixation. Springfield, IL, Charles C. Thomas, 1981.
21. Green, S.A. Ilizarov method: Rancho technique. Orthop Clin North Am 22:677–789, 1991.
22. Green, S.A. The Rancho mounting technique for circular external fixation. Adv Orthop Surg 16:191–200, 1992.
23. Green, S.A.; Bergdorff, T. External fixation in chronic bone and joint infections: The Rancho experience. Orthop Trans 4:337, 1980.
24. Herstik, I.; Pelletier, J.P.; Kanat, I.O. Pin tract infections. Incidence and management in foot surgery. J Am Podiatr Med Assoc 80:135–144, 1990.

25. Hoffmann, R. Rotules a os pour la reduction dirigee non sangante de fractures (Osteotaxis). Helv Med Acta 44:1938.

26. Huiskes, R.; Chao, E.Y.S.; Crippen, T.E. Parametric analysis of pin–bone stresses in external fracture fixation devices. J Orthop Res 3:341–349, 1985.

27. Hyldahl, C.; Pearson, S.; Tepic, S.; et al. Induction and prevention of pin loosening in external fixation: An in vivo study on sheep tibiae. J Orthop Trauma 5:485–492, 1991.

28. Ilizarov, G.A. A method of uniting bones in fractures and an apparatus to implement this method. Kurgan U.S.S.R. 1952.

29. Ilizarov, G.A. A new principle of osteosynthesis with the use of crossing pins and rings. In Collected Scientific Works of the Kurgan Regional Scientific Medical Society, pp. 145–160. Kurgan, U.S.S.R., 1954.

30. Ilizarov, G.A. A decade of experience in the application of the author's apparatus for compression osteosynthesis in traumatology and orthopedics. Probl Rehab Surg Traumatol Orthop 8:14, 1962.

31. Ilizarov, G.A. Arthroplasty of the major joints. Invagination Anastomoses. Compression–Distraction Osteosynthesis. Edited, pp. 373–377, Kurgan, U.S.S.R., 1967.

32. Ilizarov, G.A. General principles of transosteal compression and distraction osteosynthesis. In Proceedings of Scientific Session of Institutes of Traumatology and Orthopedics, pp. 35–39. Leningrad, U.S.S.R., 1968.

33. Ilizarov, G.A. Basic principles of transosseous compression and distraction osteosynthesis. Ortop Travmatol Protez 32:7–15, 1971.

34. Ilizarov, G.A. Angular deformities with shortening. In Coombs, R.; Green, S.; Sarmiento, A., eds. External Fixation and Functional Bracing. Frederick, MD, Aspen, 1989.

35. Ilizarov, G.A. Fractures and nonunions. In Coombs, R.; Green, S.; Sarmiento, A., eds. External Fixation and Functional Bracing. Frederick, MD, Aspen, 1989.

36. Ilizarov, G.A. Transosseous Osteosynthesis. Heidelberg, Springer-Verlag, 1991.

37. Knutson, K.; Bodelind, B.; Lidgren, L. Stability of external fixators used for knee arthrodesis after failed knee arthroplasty. Clin Orthop 186:90–95, 1984.

38. Lambotte, A. L'Intervention Operatoire dans les Fractures. Brussels, Lamertin, 1907.

39. Lawes, T.J.; Scott, J.C.R.; Goodship, A.E. Increased insertion torque delays pin–bone interface loosening in external fixation with tapered bone screws. J Orthop Trauma 18:617–622, 2004.

40. Linson, M.A.; Scott, R.A. Thermal burns associated with high speed cortical drilling. Orthopedics 1:394, 1978.

41. Mahan, J.; Seligson, D.; Henry, S.L.; et al. Factors in pin tract infections. Orthopedics 14:305–308, 1991.

42. Malgaigne, J.F. Treatise on Fractures. Edited, Philadelphia, Lippincott, 1859.

43. Masse, A.; Bruno, A.; Bosetti, M.; et al. Prevention of pin track infection in external fixation with silver coated pins: Clinical and microbiological results. J Biomed Mat Res 53:600–604, 2000.

44. Moroni, A.; Caja, V.L.; Maltarello, M.C.; et al. Biomechanical, scanning electron microscopy, and microhardness anaylses of the bone–pin interface in hydroxyapatite coated versus uncoated pins. J Orthop Trauma 11:154–161, 1997.

45. Moroni, A.; Vannini, F.; Mosca, M.; et al. Techniques to avoid pin loosening and infection in external fixation. J Orthop Trauma 16:189–195, 2002.

46. Moroz, T.K.; Finlay, J.B.; Rorabeck, C.H.; et al. External skeletal fixation: Choosing a system based on biomechanical stability. J Orthop Trauma 2:284–296, 1988.

47. Naden, J.R. External skeletal fixation in the treatment of fractures of the tibia. J Bone Joint Surg [Am] 31:586, 1949.

48. Orbay, G.L.; Frankel, V.H.; Kummer, F.J. The effect of wire configuration on the stability of the Ilizarov external fixator. Clin Orthop 279:299–302, 1992.

49. Paley, D. Problems, obstacles and complications of limb lengthening by the Ilizarov technique. Clin Orthop Rel Res 250:81–104, 1990.

50. Parameswaran, A.D.; Roberts, C.S.; Seligson, D.; et al. Pin tract infection with contemporary external fixation, How much of a problem? J Orthop Trauma 17:503–507, 2003.

51. Parkhill, C. A new apparatus for the fixation of bones after resection and in fractures with a tendency to displacement. Trans Am Surg Assoc 15:251, 1897.

52. Pascual, A.; Tsukayama, D.T.; Wicklund, B.H.; et al. The effect of stainless steel, cobalt-chromium, titanium alloy, and titanium on the respiratory burst activity of human polymorphonuclear leukocytes. Clin Orthop 280:281–288, 1992.

53. Paterson, D.C.; Hillier, T.M.; Carter, R.F.; et al. Experimental delayed union of the dog tibia and its use in assessing the effects of an electrical bone growth stimulator. Clin Orthop 128:340–350, 1980.

54. Perren, S.M. Physical and biological aspects of fracture healing with special reference to internal fixation. Clin Orthop 138:175–196, 1979.

55. Perren, S.M.; Huggler, A.; Russenberger, M.; et al. A method of measuring the change in compression applied to living cortical bone. Acta Orthop Scand 125:7–16, 1969.

56. Piska, M.; Yang, L.; Reed, M.; et al. Drilling efficiency and temperature elevation of three types of Kirschner-wire point. J. Bone Joint Surg [Br] 84:137–140, 2002.

57. Pizà, G.; Caja, V.L.; González-Viejo, M.A.; et al. Hydroxyapatite-coated external-fixation pins. The effect on pin loosening and pin-track infection in leg lengthening for short stature. J Bone Joint Surg [Br] 86(6): 892–897, 2004.

58. Pommer, A.; Muhr, G.; David, A. Hydroxyapatite-coated Shanz pins in external fixators used for distraction osteogenesis. J Bone Joint Surg [Am] 84:1162–1166, 2002.

59. Raimbeau, G.; Chevalier, J.M.; Raguin, J. Les risques vasculaires du fixateur en cadre a la jambe. Rev Chir Orthop (Supp 11) 65:77–82, 1979.

60. Reikeras, O. Healing of osteotomies under different degrees of stability in rats. J Orthop Trauma 4:175–178, 1990.

61. Seligson, D.; Harmon, K. Negative experiences with pins in plaster for femoral fractures. Clin Orthop 138:243–246, 1979.

62. Shimazaki, A.; Inui, K.; Azuma, Y.; et al. Low-intensity pulsed ultrasound accelerates bone maturation in distraction osteogenesis. J Bone Joint Surg 82B:1077–1082, 2000.

63. Stader, O. Preliminary announcement of a new method of treating fractures. North Am Vet 37: 1937.

64. Stanitski, D.F.; Bullard, M.; Armstrong, P.F.; et al. Results of femoral lengthening using the Ilizarov technique. J Ped Orthop 15:224–231, 1995.

65. Taylor, J.C. The Taylor Spatial Frame. Memphis, Smith & Nephew Richards, 1997.

66. Uglow, M.G.; Peat, R.A.; Hile, M.S.; et al. Low-intensity ultrasound stimulation in distraction osteogenesis in rabbits. Clin Orthop Relat Res 417:303–312, 2003.

67. Velazquez, R.J.; Bell, D.F.; Armstrong, P.F.; et al. Complications of use of the Ilizarov technique in the correction of limb deformities in children. J Bone Joint Surg [Am] 75:1148–1156, 1993.

68. Vidal, J.; Connes, H.; Buscayret, C.; et al. Complications et incidences socio-professionelles du fixateur externe. In Vidal, J., ed., Proceedings of the 7th International Conference on Hoffmann External Fixation. Geneva, Diffinco, 1979.

69. Vidal, J.; Connes, H.; Buscayret, C.; et al. Treatment of infected non-union by external fixation. In Brooker, A.F., Jr.; Edwards, C.C., eds. External Fixation, The Current State of the Art. Baltimore, Williams and Wilkins, 1979.

70. Vidal, J.M.; Rabischong, P.; Bonnel, F.; et al. Etude biomecanique du fixateur externe d'Hoffmann dans les fractures de jambe. Societe de Chirurgie de Montpellier, 43, 1970.

71. Voos, K.; Rosenberg, B.; Fagrhi, M.; et al. Use of a tobramycin-impregnated polymethylmethacrylate pin sleeve for the prevention of pin-tract infection in goats. J Orthop Trauma 13:98–101, 1999.

72. Wagner, H. Surgical lengthening or shortening of the femur. In Gschwend, N., ed. Progress in Orthopaedic Surgery. New York, Springer-Verlag, 1977.

73. Wagner, H. Operative lengthening of the femur. Clin Orthop Rel Res 136:125–142, 1978.

74. Wassall, M.A.; Santin, M.; Isalberti, C.; et al. Adhesion of bacteria to stainless steel and silver-coated orthopedic external fixation pins. J Biomed Mater Res 36:325–330, 1997.

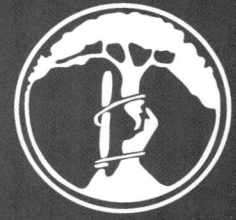

CHAPTER 12

Evaluation and Treatment of Vascular Injuries

David V. Feliciano, M.D.

Recognition of a possible vascular injury is a critical skill for any orthopaedic surgeon. This is true whether the surgeon's primary area of practice is the emergency or urgent procedures associated with orthopaedic trauma or elective reconstruction. When injured patients have fractures of long bones, the pelvis, or spine; dislocations adjacent to major vessels; or severely contused or crushed extremities, loss of limb or life can occur if recognition of the associated vascular trauma is delayed.[14,67] In an elective practice, many orthopaedic operative procedures occur in proximity to major vessels, where an iatrogenic injury may result in loss of limb or life.

HISTORY

Although vascular repairs in the extremities were first performed nearly 250 years ago, progress in this area was limited until the early part of the 20th century. From 1904 to 1906, Alexis Carrel and Charles C. Guthrie at Johns Hopkins Hospital and others developed standard vascular operative techniques, including repair of the lateral arterial wall, end-to-end anastomosis, and insertion of venous interposition grafts.[10,11,46,49,79] Early attempts at operative repair included those by V. Soubbotitch in the Balkan Wars from 1911 to 1913, by the British surgeon George H. Makins and German surgeons in World War I, and by R. Weglowski during the Polish-Russian War of 1920.[83,94,121] Despite the availability of these techniques, it was not until the latter part of World War II that renewed attempts were made to perform peripheral arterial repair rather than ligation.[19] Before that time, the delays in medical care for casualties, lack of antibiotics, and significant incidence of late infection in injured soft tissues of the extremities contributed to an operative approach dominated by ligation.

With the more rapid transfer of casualties to field hospitals, the availability of type-specific blood transfusion, the introduction of antibiotics, and the increased use of the autogenous saphenous vein as a vascular conduit, vascular repairs were performed frequently in the later stages of the Korean War and routinely throughout the Vietnam War.[57,109] More recently, civilian trauma surgeons have treated large numbers of patients with peripheral vascular injuries, many associated with orthopaedic trauma, and they have been able to build on the techniques for repair of traumatic vascular injuries described originally by military surgeons.[6,15,33,35,36,86]

ETIOLOGY

In urban trauma centers, peripheral vascular injuries are most commonly caused by low-velocity missile wounds from handguns. For example, gunshot wounds were a cause of 54.5 percent and 75.5 percent of all vascular injuries in the lower extremities in two retrospective reviews from such centers.[35,85] In contrast, stab wounds account for most of the civilian peripheral vascular injuries in countries in which firearms are more difficult to obtain.[110]

Vascular injures from blunt orthopaedic trauma, such as fractures, dislocations, contusions, crush injuries, and traction (Fig. 12-1), account for only 5 to 30 percent of injuries being treated (Table 12-1).* In particular, vascular injuries associated with long bone fractures in otherwise healthy young trauma patients are rare. The reported incidence of injuries to the superficial femoral artery in association with a fracture of the femur has ranged from 0.4 to 1.9 percent in large series.[4,71] Injuries to the popliteal artery, tibioperoneal trunk, or trifurcation vessels occur in only 1.5 to 2.8 percent of all tibial fractures. When open fractures of the tibia are reviewed separately, the incidence of arterial injuries is approximately 10 percent.[12] With dislocations of the knee joint, the incidence of injuries to the popliteal artery requiring surgical repair has been less than 16 percent in one recent large series.[91]

These figures are significantly lower than those reported in the past for posterior dislocations of the knee and presumably reflect, in part, the current nonoperative approach to nonocclusive lesions (i.e., intimal defect, narrowing) of the popliteal artery.[91]

As previously noted, there are also well-documented associations between certain elective and emergency orthopaedic operative procedures and arterial injuries (Table 12-2 and Fig. 12-2).†

---

*See references 1, 3, 7, 12, 15, 16, 24, 26, 36, 39, 44, 48, 51, 53, 56, 58, 67, 68, 71, 74, 75, 86, 91, 95, 96, 100, 105, 108, 112, 113, 124, 125, 126, 128, 129, 132, 133.
†See references 17, 26, 38, 59, 61, 62, 65, 66, 80, 87, 103, 115, 127, 128, 131.

FIGURE 12-1 | *Pseudoaneurysm of left tibioperoneal trunk in patient with adjacent fracture in the fibula and midshaft fracture of the tibia.*

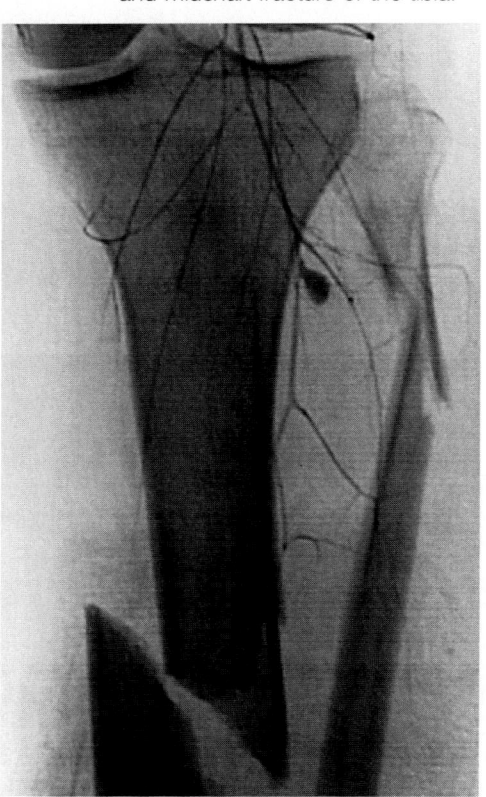

Some of these may be noted during surgery or in the early postoperative period (e.g., occlusion of the iliac artery during total hip arthroplasty), whereas others may appear weeks or months later (e.g., ruptured pseudoaneurysm of a tibial artery).

LOCATIONS AND TYPES OF VASCULAR INJURIES

The brachial artery and vein in the upper extremity and the superficial femoral artery and vein in the lower extremity are the most commonly injured vessels in both civilian and military reports in which penetrating wounds predominate.[86,109] This can be explained by the length of these vessels in the extremities and by the fact that direct compression controls hemorrhage, so that few patients exsanguinate before arrival at the emergency center. Because of the low incidence of injuries to these vessels from blunt trauma, orthopaedic services most commonly encounter occlusions and occasional lacerations of the popliteal, tibioperoneal, tibial, or peroneal arteries from dislocations of the knee or severe fractures of the femur or tibia.[58,96,100]

Intimal injuries (flaps, disruptions, or subintimal hematomas), spasm, complete wall defects with pseudoaneurysms or hemorrhage, complete transections, and arteriovenous fistulas are five recognized types of vascular injuries.

Intimal defects and subintimal hematomas with possible secondary occlusion continue to be most commonly associated with blunt trauma, whereas wall defects, complete transections, and arteriovenous fistulas are usually seen after penetrating wounds. Spasm can occur after either blunt or penetrating trauma to an extremity.

Table 12-1	
Arterial Injuries Associated with Fractures and Dislocations	
Fracture or Dislocation	**Artery Injured**
Upper Extremity	
Fracture of clavicle or first rib	Subclavian artery
Anterior dislocation of shoulder	Axillary artery
Fracture of neck of humerus	Axillary artery
Fracture of shaft or supracondylar area of humerus	Brachial artery
Dislocation of elbow	Brachial artery
Lower Extremity	
Fracture of shaft of femur	Superficial femoral artery
Fracture of supracondylar area of femur	Popliteal artery
Dislocation of the knee	Popliteal artery
Fracture of proximal tibia or fibula	Popliteal artery, tibioperoneal trunk, tibial artery, or peroneal artery
Fracture of distal tibia or fibula	Tibial or peroneal artery
Skull, Face, Cervical Spine	
Basilar skull fracture involving sphenoid or petrous bone	Internal carotid artery
Le Fort II or III fracture	Internal carotid artery
Cervical spine, especially foramen transversarium	Vertebral artery
Thoracic Spine	Descending thoracic aorta
Lumbar Spine	Abdominal aorta
Pelvis	
Anterior-posterior compression	Thoracic aorta
Subtypes of pelvic fractures	Internal iliac, superior gluteal, or inferior gluteal artery
Acetabular fracture	External iliac, superior gluteal, or femoral artery

Table 12-2	
Acute or Delayed Arterial Injuries Associated with Orthopaedic Operative Procedures	
Orthopaedic Procedure	**Artery Injured**
Upper Extremity	
Clavicular compression plate/screw	Subclavian artery
Anterior approach to shoulder	Axillary artery
Closed reduction of humeral fracture	Brachial artery
Lower Extremity	
Total hip arthroplasty	Common or external iliac artery
Nail or nail-plate fixation of intertrochanteric or subtrochanteric hip fracture	Profunda femoris artery
Subtrochanteric osteotomy	Profunda femoris artery
Total knee arthroplasty	Popliteal artery
Anterior or posterior cruciate ligament reconstruction	Popliteal artery
External fixator pin	Superficial femoral, profunda femoris, popliteal, or tibial arteries
Spine	
Anterior spinal fusion	Abdominal aorta
Lumbar spine fixation device	Abdominal aorta
Resection of nucleus pulposus	Right common iliac artery and vein, inferior vena cava
Pelvis	
Posterior internal fixation of pelvic fracture	Superior gluteal artery
Excision of posterior iliac crest for bone graft	Superior gluteal artery

FIGURE 12-2 *Occlusion of the left popliteal artery secondary to injury from orthopaedic drill. A below-knee amputation was necessary because of a delay in diagnosis.*

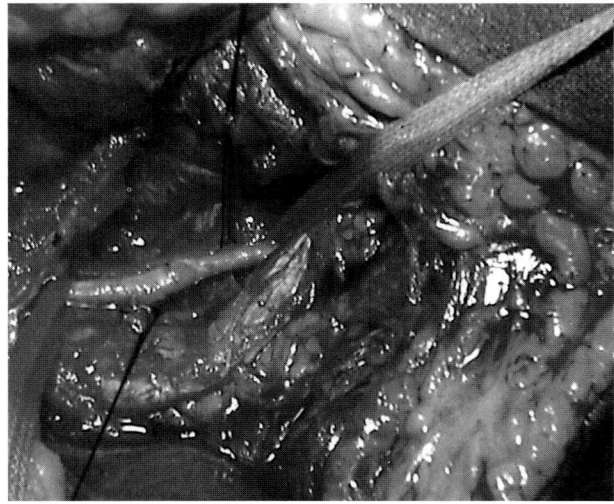

DIAGNOSIS

History and Physical Examination

Patients sustaining peripheral arterial injuries usually have hard or soft signs of injury.[120] Examples of hard signs of arterial injury are any of the classic signs of arterial occlusion (pulselessness, pallor, paresthesias, pain, paralysis, poikilothermy), massive bleeding, a rapidly expanding hematoma, and a palpable thrill or audible bruit over a hematoma. In patients with impending limb loss from arterial occlusion or significant external bleeding from an extremity, immediate surgery without preliminary arteriography of the injured extremity is justified. If a hard sign is present but localization of the defect is necessary before the incision is performed, a rapid duplex ultrasound study, formal arteriogram in a radiology suite, or surgeon-performed arteriogram in the emergency center or operating room should be obtained.[97,98]

Soft signs of arterial injury include a history of arterial bleeding at the scene or in transit; proximity of a penetrating wound or blunt injury to an artery in the extremity; a small, nonpulsatile hematoma over an artery in an extremity; and a neurologic deficit originating in a nerve adjacent to a named artery. These patients still have an arterial pulse at the wrist or foot on physical examination or with use of the Doppler device. The incidence of arterial injuries in such patients ranges from 3 to 25 percent, depending on which soft sign or combination of soft signs is present.[21,22,107] Most, but not all, of these arterial injuries can be managed without surgery because they are small and, by definition, allow for continuing distal perfusion. In some centers, serial physical examinations alone are used to monitor distal pulses, and no arteriogram is performed to document the magnitude of a possible arterial injury. This approach has been safe and accurate in asymptomatic patients with penetrating wounds to an extremity in proximity to a major artery.[21,22,40] Its accuracy with the higher kinetic energy injuries associated with blunt fractures or dislocations, particularly dislocations of the knee, is similar.[91] Observation is appropriate only with complete and continuing out-of-hospital follow-up.[21,22,40] When there is concern about a distal pulse deficit, inability to properly examine for distal arterial pulses, or a combination of soft signs of an arterial injury in an extremity, either duplex ultrasound or some type of arteriography is indicated.

Beyond the obvious hard or soft signs of vascular injury, physical examination of the injured extremity includes observation of the position in which the extremity is held, the presence of any obvious deformity of a long bone or joint, the presence or absence of an open wound or bony crepitus, the skin color of the distal extremity compared with that of the opposite side (in light-skinned persons), the time required for skin capillary refill in the distal digits, and a complete motor and sensory examination. In the lower extremity, the mobility of the knee joint should be carefully assessed as well. Increased laxity of the supporting ligaments suggests that a dislocation of the knee joint from the original trauma has spontaneously reduced (Fig. 12-3). Because of the previously noted association between posterior and other dislocations of the knee and injury to the popliteal artery, immediate arteriography is indicated if pedal pulses are diminished or absent after reduction.[91] Recent studies suggest that routine arteriography is not indicated if normal pulses are present after spontaneous or orthopaedic reduction of a knee dislocation, though not all agree with this approach.[42,91] If the exact vascular

FIGURE 12-3 *Occlusion of the right popliteal artery was missed for 48 hours because spontaneous reduction of a knee dislocation occurred before arrival in the emergency center.*

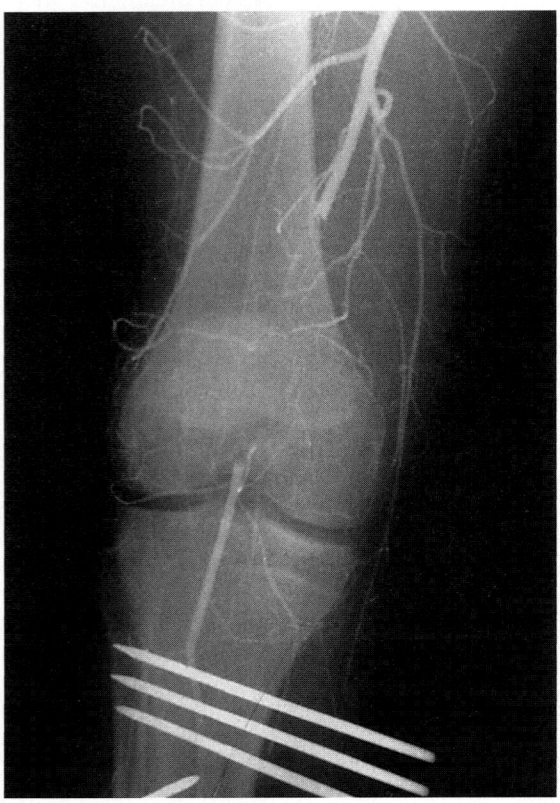

status of the distal extremity is unclear after restoration of reasonable alignment or reduction of a dislocation, a Doppler flow detector should be applied to the area of absent pulses in the distal extremity for audible assessment of blood flow. The Doppler flow detector also can be used to compare systolic blood pressure measurements in an uninjured upper extremity with those in the injured upper or lower extremity.[4] The arterial pressure index (API), defined as the Doppler systolic pressure in the injured extremity divided by that in the uninjured extremity, is then calculated.[64,82] In a study by Lynch and Johansen in which clinical outcome was the standard, an API lower than 0.90 had sensitivity of 95 percent, specificity of 97.5 percent, and accuracy of 97 percent in predicting an arterial injury.[82] An alternative when both lower extremities are injured is to use the ankle branchial index (ABI), which uses branchial artery pressure as the denominator.

Radiologic Studies

A noninvasive diagnosis can be made with use of duplex or color duplex ultrasonography in the emergency center, operating room, or surgical intensive care unit (Table 12-3). Duplex ultrasonography is a combination of real-time B-mode ultrasound imaging and pulsed Doppler flow detection. In recent years, duplex or color duplex ultrasound has been used to evaluate patients with possible or suspected arterial or venous injuries in the extremities.[5,43,70,73,116] Accuracy in detection of arterial injuries, using comparison arteriography as the gold standard, has ranged from 96 to 100 percent in several studies.[5,43]

Percutaneous arteriography performed in the emergency center or in the operating room by the surgical team is infrequently used in most major trauma centers; several urban trauma centers, however, have extensive experience with the technique.[60,97,98] A thin-walled,

Table 12-3
Diagnostic Techniques for Evaluating Possible Vascular Injuries

Cerebrovascular
Duplex ultrasound
Color flow ultrasound
Selective carotid arteriography
CT or MRI arteriography

Thoracic Vascular
Spiral CT
Transesophageal echocardiography
Digital subtraction aortography
Standard aortography

Peripheral Vascular
Arterial pressure index
Duplex ultrasound/color flow ultrasound
Emergency center or operating room arteriography by surgeon
Digital subtraction arteriography
Standard arteriography
CT arteriography

18-gauge Cournand-style disposable needle is inserted either proximal to the area of suspected injury (e.g., in the common femoral artery for evaluation of the superficial femoral artery) or distal to it (e.g., in retrograde evaluation of the axillary or subclavian arteries above a blood pressure cuff inflated to 300 mm Hg). Rapid hand injection of 35 mL of 60 percent diatrizoate meglumine dye is performed, and an anteroposterior radiographic view is taken. The timing for exposure of the x-ray film of the patient's extremity depends on which artery is to be evaluated. Proper evaluation of the tibial and peroneal arteries in the patient with a complex fracture of the tibia mandates that exposure not take place until 4 to 5 seconds after the injection of dye into the common femoral artery. The plane of the film is often changed before the second injection to examine the area in question more thoroughly. False-negative and false-positive results are rare when the technique is performed on a daily basis by experienced practitioners.[97] If a patient has severe combined intracranial or truncal trauma and possible peripheral arterial lesions related to orthopaedic injuries, life-threatening injuries should be treated first, followed by percutaneous intraoperative arteriography of the involved extremity.

Percutaneous intra-arterial digital subtraction arteriography performed in a radiology suite by the interventional radiologist is the most commonly used invasive diagnostic technique in patients with suspected vascular injuries. Multiple sequential views of areas of suspected arterial injury can be obtained at differing intervals after injection of limited amounts of dye. The accuracy of this multiple-view technique has been demonstrated in many studies, although false-negative results have occurred. The disadvantages of the technique are the delays in diagnosis when on-call technicians must return to the hospital, the cost of modern equipment, and the distortion of images when metallic fragments are present (e.g., shotgun wound). At the current time digital subtraction venous arteriography and magnetic resonance arteriography are rarely used because of problems with resolution. In addition, there are obvious disadvantages to placing severely injured patients in the magnetic resonance scanner.

Computed tomographic arteriography (CTA) is slowly replacing intra-arterial digital subtraction arteriography for evaluation of cervical, truncal, and peripheral arteries in many centers. Advantages include rapid evaluation of possible arterial injuries during CT evaluation of body parts, no need to wait for an out-of-hospital team from interventional radiology to return to the hospital, and the possibility of three-dimensional reconstructions of areas of arterial injury.

Venography is rarely performed in major trauma centers because the sequelae of missed peripheral venous injuries such as venous thromboses or pseudoaneurysms are rare. In recent years, color duplex ultrasonography has been used to evaluate veins of the extremities after penetrating trauma.[43] Some centers choose to explore large peripheral hematomas after penetrating wounds without preliminary venography, even if arteriography results are normal, and to observe small, nonexpanding hematomas.

MANAGEMENT OF VASCULAR INJURIES

The Emergency Center

The primary goal of the surgeon in the emergency center is to control hemorrhage in the patient with an extensive injury to the extremity. This is usually accomplished by direct compression with a finger (remembering the aphorism that no vessel outside the human trunk is larger than the human thumb) or by application of a pressure dressing to the area of injury. If neither of these maneuvers controls hemorrhage, a blood pressure cuff is placed proximal to the area of injury and inflated to a pressure greater than the systolic blood pressure. Given the magnitude of the accompanying injuries to soft tissue during the conflict in Iraq, topical hemostatic dressings have been used with great success. It is likely that these dressings will be used by civilian emergency medical services (EMS) units in the near future.[2,69] Once hemorrhage is under temporary control, the patient is transferred to the operating room for definitive vascular repair or ligation.

In a patient with pulses that are questionably palpable or audible by Doppler flow detection distal to a long bone fracture or a dislocation in an extremity, immediate reduction and splinting or application of a traction device should be performed. This relieves compression or kinking, but not spasm, in the adjacent artery. If such a maneuver restores diminished distal pulses in comparison with the uninjured contralateral extremity, the API should be measured if the bony or ligamentous injury is in the proximal extremity. If the API cannot be obtained because of a distal injury, if the API is lower than 0.90, or if distal pulses are absent after reduction, immediate arteriography is mandatory. In children, because examination of the peripheral vascular system is difficult, arteriography should be used liberally whenever fractures are present and distal arterial pulses are questionably palpable.

It is worthwhile to note the significant changes that are occurring in the management of injured patients who come to the emergency center with hypotension secondary to hemorrhage.[81,135] Standard teaching has emphasized the initiation of resuscitation and continuous administration of crystalloid solutions such as lactated Ringer's. The new paradigm emphasizes early and continued resuscitation with fresh whole blood by itself or packed red blood cells—fresh-frozen plasma in a 1:1 ratio rather than the 4:1 ratio taught previously. This "damage control resuscitation" approach has been developed recently by U.S. military physicians in Iraq and is changing the way injured civilian patients are resuscitated as this chapter was being completed.[45,55]

Nonoperative Treatment of Arterial Injuries

If an arteriogram shows occlusion of only one major vessel below the elbow or knee when there is not a severely injured or mangled extremity, viability of the distal extremity is rarely compromised, and some centers choose to observe the patient in this situation. Because there can be retrograde flow into an area of arterial injury beyond the proximal occlusion, a repeat arteriogram should be performed within 3 to 7 days to rule out delayed formation of a traumatic false aneurysm.

Several clinical studies have demonstrated that non-occlusive arterial injuries (e.g., spasm, intimal flap, sub-intimal or intramural hematoma) that often are detected in patients undergoing arteriography for soft signs of injury heal without operation in 87 to 95 percent of cases.[22,41,122] Even small, traumatic false aneurysms have been noted to heal on follow-up arteriograms in some of these patients. Arteriographic follow-up is necessary in patients who develop new symptoms while being observed.

Therapeutic Embolization

Isolated traumatic aneurysms of branches of the axillary, brachial, superficial femoral, or popliteal arteries; of the profunda femoris artery; or of one of the named arteries in the shank can be treated by therapeutic embolization instead of operation.[89,123] Although such an approach has been used primarily in patients with penetrating wounds to the extremities, it is appropriate in selected patients with blunt vascular injuries as well. Patients with injuries to the arteries listed who will especially benefit from therapeutic embolization include those with multisystem injuries, closed fractures, or late diagnosis of a traumatic aneurysm following orthopaedic reconstruction. Contained aneurysms or active hemorrhage from muscular branches is treated with embolization using an absorbable gelatin sponge. When there is a need to occlude a tibial or peroneal artery proximal to a traumatic aneurysm, embolization coils are used.

Endovascular Stents

Balloon-expandable intraluminal arterial stents and stent-grafts are now used routinely in patients with atherosclerotic occlusive disease. An extensive experience has been reported in patients with traumatic arterial injuries over the past 15 years, as well.[84,121] For treatment of an intimal dissection or flap, a angiographic catheter is placed percutaneously across the area of injury via a trans-arterial sheath. This catheter is then exchanged for a separate catheter-mounted balloon inflatable endovascular stent, and the collapsed stent is expanded in place. Should a traumatic aneurysm be present, an endovascular stent-graft is used to occlude the orifice or trans-stent injections of microcoils are used to induce thrombosis of the aneurysmal sac.

The Operating Room

ARTERIAL REPAIR

If the history, physical examination, duplex ultrasound, or arteriogram strongly suggests or documents the presence of an arterial injury that requires operative repair, the patient is given intravenous antibiotics before being moved to the operating room. During the move, all open wounds are covered with sterile gauze soaked in saline or saline-antibiotic solution. In addition, all fractured or dislocated extremities are maintained in a neutral position by splinting or traction.

SKIN PREPARATION AND DRAPING In the operating room, an operative tourniquet can be applied in place of the blood pressure cuff for control of hemorrhage from

injuries in the distal extremity. If the injuries are in the proximal extremity and exsanguinating hemorrhage resumes after removal of finger compression, a compression dressing, or a proximal blood cuff, the surgeon should put on sterile operative gloves immediately. The surgeon then applies direct compression to a large wound with the hands or inserts fingers into an open fracture site or the entrance and exit sites of a penetrating wound to control hemorrhage as preparation of the skin and draping are performed.

Because of the possibility of an associated vascular lesion in all patients with orthopaedic injuries in an extremity, preparation of the skin and draping should encompass all potential areas of proximal and distal vascular control. Also, one or both lower extremities should be prepared and draped to allow for possible retrieval of the greater saphenous vein in case an interposition graft is required for the vascular repair. It is often helpful to have one entire uninjured lower extremity prepared and draped to the toenails, so that the greater saphenous vein may be retrieved from either the groin or the ankle. It is also helpful to drape the hand or foot of the affected extremity in a sterile plastic bag, so that color changes can be noted in light-skinned patients and distal pulses can be palpated under sterile conditions after arterial repair has been completed. The remainder of the extremity, including the area of the incision, is then covered with an orthopaedic-type stockinette.

INCISIONS In patients with peripheral vascular injuries, the skin incision should be generous enough to allow for comfortable proximal and distal vascular control. To this end, it is often best for the inexperienced trauma surgeon to use the most extensive incisions.

There are a number of classic incisions for the management of peripheral vascular injuries. Those used in the upper extremity include the following: (1) supraclavicular incision, with or without division of or resection of the clavicle, for injuries in the second or third portion of the subclavian artery; (2) infraclavicular incision for the first or second portion of the axillary artery; (3) infraclavicular incision curving onto the medial aspect of the upper arm for the third portion of the axillary artery or proximal brachial artery; (4) medial upper arm incision between the biceps and the triceps muscles for the main portion of the brachial artery; and (5) S-shaped incision from medial to lateral across the antecubital crease for the brachial artery proximal to its bifurcation. An injury to the radial or ulnar artery is usually approached by longitudinal incision directly over the site.

In the lower extremity, the preferred incisions for arterial repair are the following: (1) longitudinal groin incision for injury to the common femoral artery, proximal superficial femoral artery, or profunda femoris artery; (2) anteromedial thigh incision for exposure of the superficial femoral artery throughout the thigh; and (3) medial popliteal incision for exposure of the proximal, middle, or distal portions of the popliteal artery. Injuries to the anterior tibial artery are approached directly over the site of injury in the anterior compartment, whereas the posterior tibial artery is approached through a medial incision that often requires transection of the fibers of the soleus muscle.

Finally, the peroneal artery is approached through a medial incision or through a lateral incision that requires excision of a portion of the fibula for proper exposure.

STANDARD TECHNIQUES OF ARTERIAL

REPAIR After the skin incision is made proximally and distally to the bleeding site or area of hematoma, dry skin towels are placed to cover all remaining skin edges if a plastic adherent drape has not been applied. If hemorrhage can be controlled by finger or laparotomy pad compression applied by an assistant, proximal and distal vascular control is usually obtained before the area of injury is entered. Not dissecting far enough proximally and distally from an area of injury is a common error. It is frequently necessary for the inexperienced vascular trauma surgeon to move proximal and distal vascular occlusion clamps or loops repeatedly as débridement of the injured artery is extended back to noninjured arterial intima.

In patients with an extensive hematoma overlying the arterial injury, it can be difficult to obtain proximal and distal vascular control close enough to the injury to prevent backbleeding from collateral vessels. In addition, there are patients in whom external hemorrhage cannot readily be controlled during meticulous dissection. Therefore, if dissection is proceeding extremely slowly through a very large hematoma or the assistant can no longer maintain control of exsanguinating hemorrhage by direct compression, the hematoma or site of hemorrhage should be entered directly. The site of arterial bleeding is visualized, compressed with a finger or vascular forceps, and a proximal vascular clamp or vessel loop is applied. The dissection is then completed starting from the center rather than waiting for proximal and distal control to be obtained at a distance from the hematoma or bleeding site.

After vascular control is obtained in either classic or rapid fashion, vascular occlusion can be maintained by application of small, angled, vascular clamps (such as those found in an angioaccess tray), bulldog vascular clamps, Silastic vessel loops, or umbilical tapes. Occasionally, with complex arterial injuries at bifurcations, vascular control of major branches can be obtained by passage of an intraluminal Fogarty balloon catheter or a calibrated Garrett dilator.

In general, lateral arteriorrhaphy (or venorrhaphy) with 5-0 or 6-0 polypropylene sutures placed transversely is used for small lacerations or for small puncture, pellet, or missile wounds, especially in the smaller vessels of the extremities. If a transverse repair results in significant narrowing of the injured vessel, patch angioplasty is a useful alternative. Any segment of injured vein that has been resected or of autogenous saphenous vein from the ankle or groin of an uninjured lower extremity can be used to create an oval patch to increase the size of the lumen of an injured vessel. The patch is usually sewn in place with 6-0 polypropylene suture.

Resection of injured peripheral vessels is often required in patients with blunt orthopaedic trauma because of the magnitude of the forces applied to cause both bony and vascular injuries. An increasing number of vascular injuries from penetrating wounds also require resection of the injured segment because of the greater wounding power of firearms now available in the United States. Resection

with an end-to-end anastomosis is performed whenever a segment of a vessel has extensive destruction of the wall or a long area of disrupted intima (e.g., from blunt traction injury or through-and-through injury from a penetrating wound). Despite the elasticity of peripheral vessels in the typical young trauma patient, many collateral vessels must be ligated for an end-to-end anastomosis to be performed if more than 2 to 3 cm of the vessel is resected. An end-to-end anastomosis sewn under tension results in an hourglass appearance at the suture line and often leads to thrombosis of the repair in the postoperative period. Although an interrupted suture technique for end-to-end anastomosis is routinely used in growing children, continuous suture techniques with 2-point fixation 180° apart can be used by experienced trauma surgeons for small vessels of the extremities (4–5 mm diameter) in adults.[30,31]

If exposure is difficult, as in the axillary artery near the clavicle or the popliteal artery behind the knee joint, it is often helpful to perform the first third of the posterior anastomosis with an open technique (i.e., one in which no knot is tied). This allows for precise suture bites of the posterior walls, and it prevents leaks after arterial inflow is restored. On completion of the posterior third of the anastomosis, the two ends of the suture are pulled tight, drawing the two ends of the artery together.

Both ends of the artery are then stabilized, and Fogarty embolectomy catheters are passed proximally and distally to remove any thrombotic or embolic material from the arterial tree. The amount of debris distal to an arterial injury can be extensive, especially after a prolonged period of preoperative occlusion. After both ends of the vessel have been cleared, 15 to 20 mL of regional heparin (50 U/mL) is injected into each end and the vascular clamps are reapplied. Injection of a total of 30 to 40 mL of this solution (1500–2000 U or 15–20 mg heparin) provides significantly less anticoagulation than the 1 to 2 mg/kg of heparin used in many elective vascular procedures. More aggressive systemic heparinization is avoided in selected trauma patients because of the risk of hemorrhage from other injuries.

The end-to-end anastomosis is completed by running the two ends of the suture along the two sides of the approximated artery, leaving the last few loops of suture loose to allow for flushing before final tying. The proximal vascular occlusion clamp is first removed and reapplied after completion of flushing. The distal vascular clamp is then removed to allow for flushing from the distal end of the vessel and to clear any residual air underneath the suture line. As blood from the distal arterial tree fills the area that was between the two clamps or loops, the two suture ends are pulled up tightly and tied. The proximal arterial clamp is not released until the first knot is in place. If small suture hole leaks are present at that time, topical hemostatic agents can be applied temporarily.

If an end-to-end anastomosis cannot be performed with minimal tension, a substitute vascular conduit should be inserted into the defect between the two débrided ends of the injured vessel. An autogenous reversed saphenous vein graft from an uninjured lower extremity remains the conduit of choice for most peripheral vascular injuries[35,88,92] (Fig. 12-4). If the vessel to be replaced has a small lumen (4–5 mm), the greater saphenous vein at

FIGURE 12-4   *Saphenous vein graft inserted into left anterior tibial artery in patient with Gustilo IIIC tibial fracture*

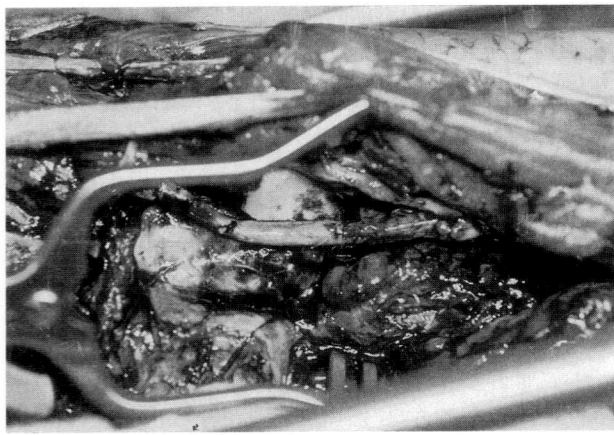

FIGURE 12-5   *Fine points in peripheral arterial repair include use of small vascular clamps or Silastic vessel loops, open anastomosis technique, regional heparinization, passage of a Fogarty catheter proximally and distally, and arteriography on completion. (Courtesy of Baylor College of Medicine, 1981.)*

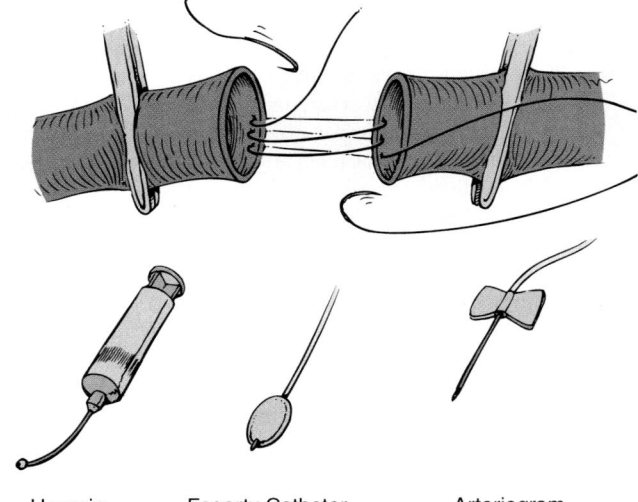

Heparin   Fogarty Catheter   Arteriogram

the medial malleolus is a good choice. If the artery or vein to be replaced has a much larger lumen, the greater saphenous vein in the proximal thigh is a better choice. Major advantages of the autogenous saphenous vein include its ready availability, the superiority of natural tissue in maintaining patency, and a long record of success in vascular and cardiac surgery. The patency of the saphenous vein graft can be improved by using gentle dissection, by avoiding overdistention during flushing, and by using only heparinized autologous blood containing papaverine for flushing.

If a saphenous vein graft is to be inserted, it is often helpful to perform the more difficult distal anastomosis first. Because of the floppy nature of a collapsed saphenous vein graft, it is useful to place two 6-0 polypropylene sutures 180° apart at the two corners of the anastomosis. Another option is to use the classic trifurcation technique originally described by Carrel in 1907.[11] After anastomosis of the graft to the distal end of the artery has been completed, a Garrett dilator can be passed through it to ensure adequate luminal size. The proximal anastomosis is then performed. As with simple end-to-end anastomosis, passage of a Fogarty catheter, injection of heparinized saline solution, and flushing should be performed before completion of the second anastomosis (Fig. 12-5).

If the saphenous vein is surgically absent, injured bilaterally, too small, or of an inappropriate size to fit into the injured vessel, or if the patient is critically injured and the speed of repair is important, many trauma centers use polytetrafluoroethylene (PTFE) grafts for interposition.[36] The early complication and infection rates with the use of PTFE prostheses appear to be the same as those with saphenous vein grafts, but long-term patency is less. If a PTFE graft is to be used, it is best to cut it to an appropriate length with a number 11 scalpel blade rather than a pair of scissors. The rigid, open nature of PTFE allows for rapid performance of an arterial anastomosis, and no fixation sutures are needed. The passage of a Fogarty catheter and regional heparinization are performed as previously described. Laboratory and clinical studies have demonstrated that neointimal

hyperplasia occurs at PTFE-artery suture lines, and patients in whom such a graft is placed are started on aspirin by rectal suppository every 12 hours while in the intensive care unit. Two 81 mg aspirins are taken orally each day for the first 3 postoperative months in the absence of a history of gastric or duodenal ulcers.

Bypass grafting can be applied in selected circumstances of extensive vascular injuries. For example, if ligation around an area of injury is required to prevent exsanguinating hemorrhage, a saphenous vein bypass graft can then be inserted in an end-to-side fashion proximally and distally instead of resection of the injured segment and placement of an interposition graft.

Extra-anatomic bypass grafting is used when extensive injury to soft tissues in the antecubital, groin, or below-knee area is accompanied by injuries to the brachial, femoral, popliteal, or tibioperoneal vessels. In such instances, vigorous débridement of the wound is carried out at the first operation, and the extra-anatomic saphenous vein conduit is inserted around the wound underneath healthy soft tissue, with both end-to-end anastomoses also covered by such tissue[28,32] (Fig. 12-6). The defect in soft tissue is then managed with a vacuum-assisted closure device until delayed primary closure or application of a split-thickness skin graft is performed.[28,32,78] Care of the wound is made easier with this approach, and the danger of suture line blowout is decreased by use of the extra-anatomic bypass through noninjured tissue.

Ligation is reserved for injury to the distal profunda femoris artery in the thigh or to main arteries below the elbow or knee when at least one other named vessel to the hand or foot is still patent and there is not a severely injured or mangled extremity. The technique is used in

FIGURE 12-6   **A,** *The shotgun wound that disrupted the distal femur also avulsed the popliteal artery, as seen on the arteriogram.* **B,** *An extra-anatomic saphenous vein bypass graft inserted around the posterior aspect of the knee joint is shown on the completion arteriogram. (B, from Feliciano, D.V.; Accola, K.D.; Burch, M.J.; et al. Extra-anatomic bypass for peripheral arterial injuries. Am J Surg 158:506, 1989.)*

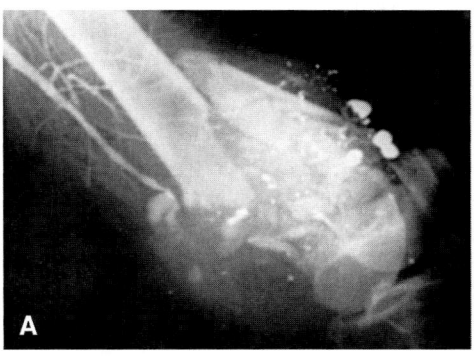
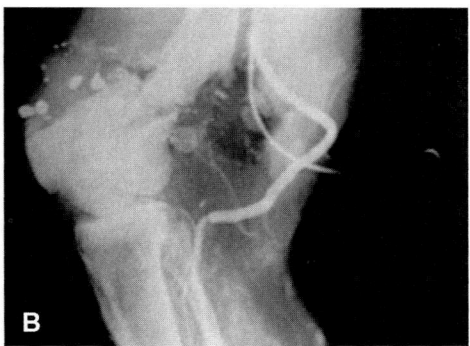

patients with a coagulopathy and in those who are so unstable that the operation must be terminated. See Table 12-4 for a list of all repair techniques.

COMPLETION ARTERIOGRAPHY After arterial in-flow has been restored, distal pulses should be present. In the upper extremity, palpation of normal distal pulses is usually acceptable evidence of a satisfactory arterial repair because distal thrombosis is rare unless a tight arterial tourniquet was in place for several hours preoperatively. Most experienced trauma surgeons, however, use completion arteriography after an end-to-end anastomosis or insertion of an interposition graft of any type in an artery of the lower extremity. This is done to rule out technical mishaps at the one or two suture lines and problems such as distal embolism or in situ thrombosis in the small vessels of the shank. It is helpful to place a small metal tissue clip near any anastomosis, so that it can be localized precisely on the arteriogram. This enables the surgeon to distinguish a narrowed anastomosis from a mark produced by a vascular clamp.

Operative arteriography is easily performed after insertion of a 20-gauge Teflon-over-metal catheter into the artery. Usually, the artery is punctured proximal to the repair, and the Teflon catheter is slipped over the needle

into the lumen of the artery. It is particularly useful to stabilize the artery with vascular forceps as the anterior wall of the artery is entered. This maneuver usually prevents posterior perforation of the artery, which commonly occurs when metal or larger arteriography needles or catheters are inserted into an unstable artery. The Teflon catheter is attached by a short piece of intravenous extension tubing to a 50-mL syringe filled with heparinized saline solution. This is injected through the Teflon catheter before arteriography to ensure proper catheter placement in the lumen. Free return of pulsatile blood into the plastic tubing confirms the position of the catheter. The extremity is aligned in an anteroposterior direction over the film cassette. An excellent operative arteriogram can usually be obtained by exposing the film as the last several milliliters of a 35-mL bolus of 60 percent diatrizoate meglumine dye are injected rapidly[30,31] (Fig. 12-7). If the lower extremity is allowed to rotate externally during arteriography, the overlying bone may obscure the arterial repair in certain areas around and below the knee joint.

After arteriography has been completed, a syringe containing heparinized saline solution is attached to the extension tubing and the artery is flushed with the solution. The Teflon arteriography catheter is not removed until the arteriogram has been returned and is noted to be of satisfactory quality. If the completion arteriogram is satisfactory, a small U-stitch of 6-0 polypropylene suture is placed around the Teflon catheter and tied down tightly as the catheter is removed.

If a technical problem such as an intimal flap, a thrombus at the site of anastomosis, or a distal embolus is present on the completion arteriogram, the arterial repair is opened and the problem is corrected. If distal spasm is present but arterial flow to the foot or hand is adequate, no further therapy is required, because spasm usually resolves within 4 to 6 hours. If the spasm is severe and distal flow is compromised, measurement of the below elbow or knee musculofascial compartment pressures to rule out a compartment syndrome is worthwhile.

VENOUS INJURIES

Venous occlusion or ligation in the groin has a significant adverse effect on femoral arterial inflow.[54] For this reason,

Table 12-4
Techniques of Vascular Repair
Lateral arteriorrhaphy or venorrhaphy
Patch angioplasty
Panel or spiral vein graft
Resection of injured segment
End-to-end anastomosis
Interposition graft
Autogenous vein
Polytetrafluoroethylene
Dacron
Bypass graft
In situ
Extra-anatomic
Ligation

FIGURE 12-7 | *Bilateral occlusions of the superficial femoral arteries associated with fractures of the femur were repaired with autogenous saphenous vein grafts. The left-sided graft* **(A)** *appears too long but was of appropriate length after the fractured femur was realigned* **(B)**. *Arrowheads indicate the proximal and distal anastomoses of the saphenous vein grafts. (From Feliciano, D.V. Managing peripheral vascular trauma. Infect Surg 5:659–669, 682, 1986.)*

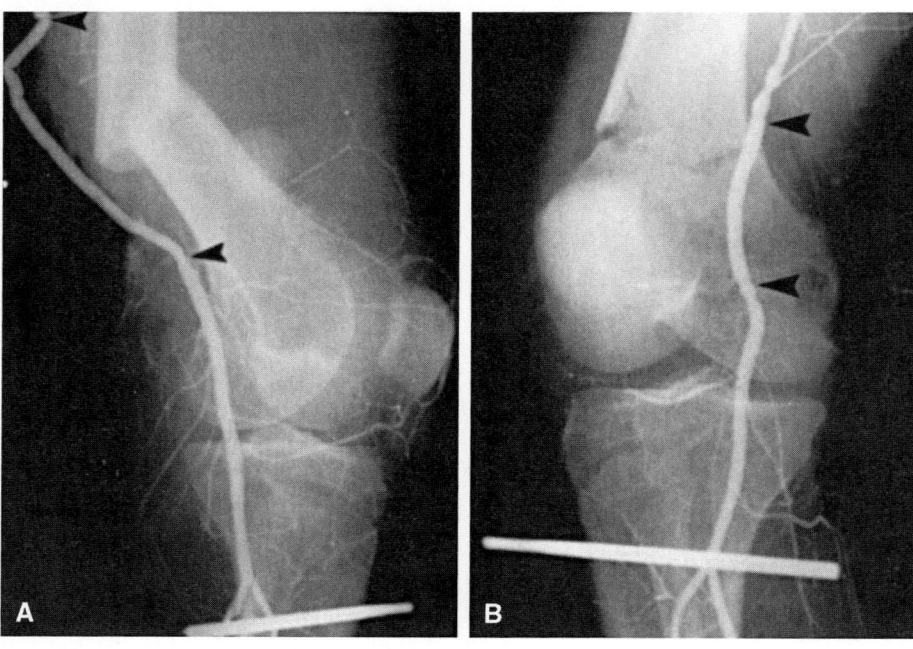

and because of the known adverse effect of popliteal venous ligation on viability of the leg, there is more effort to perform peripheral venous repair rather than ligation in the modern trauma center.[102,119] Of interest, follow-up venography after extremity venorrhaphy has documented that more than 25 percent of simple venous repairs and almost 35 percent of interposition grafts inserted for venous repair are temporarily occluded in the postoperative period. Fortunately, many of these recanalize over time.[119] Therefore, the consensus is that venous injuries in the groin or popliteal area should be repaired if the patient is stable and has no life-threatening intraoperative complications such as hypothermia or a transfusion-induced coagulopathy. If the patient is unstable or has a life-threatening complication that could be aggravated by prolonging general anesthesia, venous ligation or insertion of an intraluminal plastic shunt should be performed. Although this issue is continually debated, the long-term sequelae of venous ligation in young victims of civilian trauma appear to be fewer than originally reported from the Vietnam experience.[6,93,102]

Venous injuries are often difficult to manage because of hemorrhage from the large lumen, the fragile nature of the wall, and the many small branches. Excessive manipulation of the injured vein often leads to further hemorrhage. It is helpful to use finger or sponge-stick compression around the area of perforation for vascular control rather than to attempt application of vascular clamps to all branches feeding the area of injury. After the area of injury has been isolated, lateral venorrhaphy in a transverse direction remains the most common technique of repair for peripheral venous injuries. Occasionally, a more complex repair such as patch venoplasty, resection with end-to-end anastomosis, or resection with insertion of some type of substitute conduit is necessary.[102] The principles of repair for major venous injuries are similar to those for arterial injuries except that Fogarty catheters are not passed and completion venograms are not obtained.

If resection of an injured segment of a peripheral vein is required, ligation of local collateral vessels is necessary to allow for the performance of an end-to-end anastomosis with only modest tension. If a substitute vascular conduit is required to replace a segmental injury in a critical vein (e.g., popliteal, distal superficial femoral), the surgeon must choose from a variety of less satisfactory alternatives. An autogenous saphenous vein graft from an uninjured lower extremity would appear to be an ideal conduit. The diameter of the greater saphenous vein in the groin, however, is often too small to match the size of the proximal superficial femoral or common femoral vein in the lower extremity or the axillary or subclavian vein in the upper extremity. Such a small conduit in a much larger vein would be patent for only a short time.

Two other choices for replacement of an injured vein with autogenous tissue involve the creation of a spiral vein graft or a panel graft. The spiral vein graft is created by opening the harvested autogenous saphenous vein from an uninjured lower extremity over its entire length, wrapping it around a rigid tubular structure such as a thoracostomy tube in a spiral fashion, and sewing the edges together to create a tube of a larger luminal diameter. Construction of a spiral vein graft is time-consuming and cannot be justified for routine use in peripheral venous injuries in light of its 50 percent patency rate.[101] In extraordinary circumstances, such as impending loss of the distal lower extremity from ligation of the popliteal vein, it must be considered. A panel graft is created by longitudinally opening two separate segments of autogenous saphenous vein from an uninjured lower extremity, placing one on top of the other, and sewing the two side edges together to create one tubular structure of a larger luminal diameter. Again, this technique is time-consuming and is rarely justified in the repair of peripheral venous injuries. If the surgeon is willing to insert a "temporary" venous conduit, an externally supported PTFE graft can be placed into large luminal veins of a proximal extremity. These grafts are available in appropriate sizes, but they remain patent for only 2 to 3 weeks if the type without external support is used.[36] If an externally supported PTFE graft is inserted, there is long-term patency for months and possibly years. To encourage dilatation of collateral veins during the period of slow occlusion of an unsupported PTFE graft, it is mandatory to keep the injured extremity elevated and to place elastic wraps around the extremity while the patient is in the hospital.

INDICATIONS FOR FASCIOTOMY

The diagnosis of a compartmental syndrome and techniques of fasciotomy are discussed in Chapter 13.

COMBINED ORTHOPAEDIC-VASCULAR INJURIES

There has been much discussion about the preferred order of repair, that is, orthopaedic stabilization followed by arterial repair or the reverse.[3,4,25,48,56,75,132] A number of authors have emphasized the need for early arterial repair to limit distal ischemia and lessen the risk of in situ thrombosis.[56] Others have noted that early orthopaedic repair stabilizes the extremity and improves exposure of the vascular injury. This approach also lowers the risk of thrombosis in a recently completed vascular repair during subsequent manipulation to reduce a fracture[58] (Fig. 12-8). With either approach, the ultimate amputation rate is substantial (Table 12-5).

In a patient with neither cold ischemia (pulseless without capillary refill) nor a prolonged period of warm ischemia (capillary refill present), the choice of arterial or orthopaedic repair depends primarily on the stability of the fracture site. If the area of the fracture is reasonably stable and the trauma team is experienced in rapid vascular repair, it is appropriate to perform the arterial repair first. If the fracture is comminuted and the extremity cannot be stabilized for proper exposure of the vascular injury, the orthopaedic repair is performed first. In trauma centers with extensive experience in the management of combined injuries in the extremities, consultation among attending surgeons, fellows, or senior residents is mandatory and allows for proper sequencing of repairs.

In a patient with a cold, pulseless hand or foot and little or no capillary refill or in a patient who has undergone a prolonged period of either cold or warm ischemia, restoration of arterial inflow has the highest priority and should be accomplished by formal repair or by the insertion of a

FIGURE 12-8 *Occlusion of distal arterial bed occurred during orthopaedic manipulation following graft repair of the right popliteal artery. The patient eventually needed an above-knee amputation.*

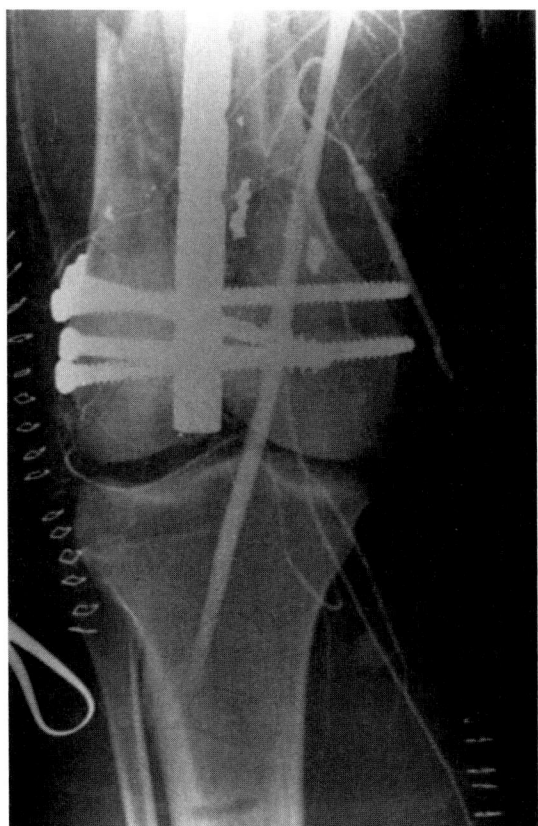

temporary intraluminal vascular shunt. Formal arterial repair is preferred if the extremity is reasonably stable despite the presence of a fracture. If an unstable fracture that precludes appropriate exposure of the vascular injury

Table 12-5		
Amputation Rates with Combined Orthopaedic-Vascular Injuries in an Extremity		
Author, Year	**Fracture or Dislocation**	**Amputation Rate**
Weaver et al. 1984[133]	Femur, knee, tibia	36%
Gustilo et al. 1984[48]	Humerus, femur, knee, tibia	42%
Lange et al. 1985[75]	Tibia	61%
Howe et al. 1987[56]	Femur, tibia	43%
Caudle et al. 1987[12]	Tibia	78%
Drost et al. 1989[25]	Femur, tibia	36%
Alexander et al. 1991[3]	Femur, tibia	28%
		46% (mean)

is present, shunts are inserted to allow for continued arterial inflow and venous outflow during the period of orthopaedic stabilization.

TEMPORARY INTRALUMINAL VASCULAR SHUNTS

A shunt is defined as an intraluminal plastic conduit for temporary maintenance of arterial inflow or venous outflow, or both, to or from a body part. First described for use in peripheral arterial injuries in 1919, there has been a significant increase in the use of these devices in trauma centers over the past 20 years.[18,27,37,63] At this time, suggested indications for the use of shunts include the following: (1) combined orthopaedic-vascular injuries, including mangled extremities; (2) preservation of an amputated upper extremity at the arm, forearm, or wrist level before replantation; (3) rapid restoration of arterial inflow or venous outflow, or both, as part of a life-saving peripheral or truncal "damage control" operation.

As described above, insertion of intraluminal shunts in a patient with a combined orthopaedic-vascular injury promptly restores arterial inflow or venous outflow, or both, and allows for appropriate orthopaedic stabilization, reconstruction, or débridement. A properly fixated shunt will withstand vigorous realignment maneuvers. When the orthopaedic operative procedure is completed, the trauma vascular surgeon can then choose one of two options. In the hemodynamically stable patient without intraoperative hypothermia, metabolic acidosis, or a coagulopathy, the shunts are removed and interposition vascular grafts are inserted under the same general anesthetic. When the injured patient is hemodynamically unstable with a body temperature lower than 35°C, a base deficit less than −10 to −15, or a coagulopathy, the original operative procedure is terminated.[118] Removal of the shunts and vascular repairs are then performed at a reoperation in 24 to 48 hours. In patients with mangled extremities, this time delay will allow for combined consultation by orthopaedic and vascular surgeons and discussions with the patient and family.

The value of temporary intraluminal shunts to maintain viability in amputated parts of the upper extremity is obvious. Identification and tagging of nerves and tendons, débridement of crushed tissue, and orthopaedic stabilization can all be completed while the shunts are in place.

With improvements in prehospital emergency medical services in urban environments, more injured patients with near-exsanguination are admitted to the emergency center than in the past. The insertion of temporary intraluminal shunts in the vessels of the arm, antecubital area, groin, thigh, or knee adjacent to a fracture or dislocation will prevent the need for ligation in the injured patient with profound shock. Indications for peripheral (or truncal) "damage control" shunts are as follows: (1) body temperature lower than 34°C to 35°C (on admission or developing during operation), (2) arterial pH less than 7.2 or base deficit less than −15 in patients younger than 55 years of age or less than −6 in patients older than 55 years of age, and (3) intraoperative international normalized ratio (INR) or partial thromboplastin time (PTT) greater than 50 percent of normal. Any trauma operative procedure is terminated whenever

one of the listed abnormalities is present. Resuscitation including rewarming, hemodynamic monitoring, transfusion, use of inotropes, and correction of coagulopathy is then performed in the surgical intensive care unit rather than the operating room. The third stage of damage control is the return to the operating room for definitive repairs when the patient's previous metabolic failure secondary to hypovolemic shock has been corrected.[116,134]

Intraluminal shunts are readily available in any operating room in which elective surgery on the carotid artery is performed. They range in size from 8-F to 14-F and are held in place with 2-0 silk ties compressing the end of the transected artery or vein onto the shunt. When a large shunt is needed for insertion into the popliteal, superficial femoral, or common femoral veins, standard thoracostomy tubes are used[37] (Fig. 12-9).

THE MANGLED EXTREMITY

A mangled extremity results from high-energy transfer or crushing trauma that causes some combination of injuries to artery, bone, soft tissue, tendon, and nerve. Approximately two thirds of such injuries are caused by motorcycle, motor vehicle, or vehicle-pedestrian accidents, reflecting the significant transfer of energy that occurs during such incidents.[20] Chapman has emphasized that the kinetic energy dissipated in collision with an automobile bumper

FIGURE 12-9 *Patient with open fracture of the left femur from a crush injury had transection of the proximal popliteal artery and vein, also. A 14-F carotid artery shunt was placed into the popliteal artery, while a 24-F thoracostomy tube was placed into the popliteal vein. Because of intraoperative hypothermia, removal of shunts and insertion of interposition grafts was delayed for 18 hours.*

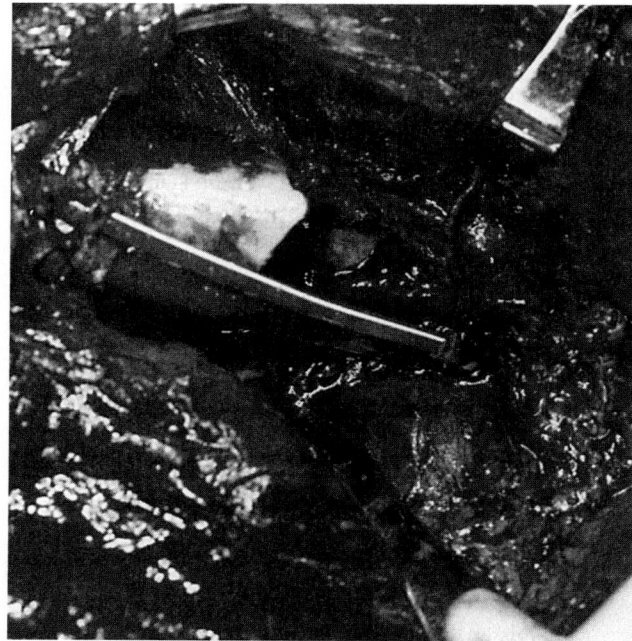

at 20 mph (100,000 ft-lb) is 50 times greater than that from a high-velocity gunshot (2000 ft-lb).[13]

When a patient with a mangled extremity arrives in the emergency center, the trauma team must work its way through the following series of decisions in patient care:

1. If the patient's life is in danger, should the mangled limb be amputated?
2. If the patient is stable, should an attempt be made to salvage the mangled limb?
3. If salvage is to be attempted, what is the sequence of repairs? (See previous section.)
4. If salvage fails, when should amputation be performed?

The most difficult decision is whether to attempt salvage of the limb. Since 1985, at least five separate scoring systems that describe the magnitude of injuries in a mangled extremity have been published[47,56,64,114,117] (Table 12-6). All attempt to predict the need for amputation based on a total score derived from the combination of injuries in the extremity and other factors. Only one system, the Mangled Extremity Severity Score developed by Johansen and co-workers,[53,64] has been studied in a prospective manner. Additionally, the applicability of any of these systems outside the institutions in which they originated has been questioned.[8, 111]

Two major criteria are used most frequently in clinical decisions regarding immediate amputation versus attempted salvage. If either of the following factors is present, amputation is a better choice than prolonged attempts at salvage.[50,74]

1. Loss of arterial inflow for longer than 6 hours, particularly in the presence of a crush injury that disrupts collateral vessels[74,90]
2. Disruption of the posterior tibial nerve[64,74,75]

Lange and associates[74] and Hansen[50] have described relative indications for immediate amputation in patients with Gustilo IIIC tibial fractures as well. These include serious associated polytrauma, severe ipsilateral foot trauma, anticipated protracted course to obtain soft tissue coverage, and tibial reconstruction.[75] If two of these are present, immediate amputation is once again recommended.[50,75]

BLEEDING OR EDEMA IN SOFT TISSUES

In patients with major peripheral vascular injuries and a transfusion-associated coagulopathy, extensive oozing

often occurs in soft tissue as the operation is completed. In such patients, placement of closed or open drains into the blast cavity or area of dissection may be required for several hours postoperatively. The placement of drains prevents formation of a postoperative hematoma that could compress and possibly occlude the vascular repairs.

If a large blast cavity is present in soft tissue near the vascular repairs, some muscle or soft tissue should be sutured in a position that separates the two. A closed or open drain or open packing of the cavity exiting on the opposite side of the extremity from the skin incision and vascular repairs should then be inserted. This allows for drainage of the large blast cavity away from the vascular repairs and helps to avoid the problems of compression by hematoma and of cellulitis and late abscesses near a vascular repair.[31]

Occasionally, primary wound closure is undesirable in patients with extensive muscle hematomas, soft tissue edema, or a severe coagulopathy after a peripheral vascular repair. In such patients, porcine xenografts (pigskin) are placed over the vascular repairs and the wound is packed open with antibiotic-soaked gauze.[76,77] After 24 hours of elevation of the injured extremity, the patient is returned to the operating room for delayed primary closure or closure with a myocutaneous flap performed by the plastic surgery service.[106]

HEROIC TECHNIQUES TO SAVE A LIMB

If vascular repair is satisfactory on the completion arteriogram but the distal extremity has borderline viability because of vascular spasm, extensive destruction of collateral vessels in soft tissue, or prolonged ischemia, various adjuncts for salvage should be considered once a primary or secondary compartment syndrome has been ruled out.[130] Included among these are proximal arterial infusion with a heparin-tolazoline-saline solution (containing 1000 U heparin and 500 mg tolazoline in 1000 mL saline) at a rate of 30 mL/hr,[23,104] and venous infusion with low-molecular-weight dextran at a rate of 500 mL/12 hr.[30]

Postoperative Care

After the patient has been returned to the ward or intensive care unit, the injured extremity should be elevated and wrapped with elastic bandages if venous ligation was performed. Care must be taken to monitor intracompartmental pressure in such a situation, since the combination of venous hypertension and external compression may create an early compartment syndrome. Distal arterial pulses are monitored by palpation or with a portable Doppler unit. Transcutaneous oxygen monitoring has also been used to document revascularization in injured limbs.[72] Intravenous antibiotics are continued for 24 hours if a primary repair or end-to-end anastomosis was performed. If a substitute vascular conduit was inserted, intravenous antibiotics are continued for 72 hours in some centers, much as in elective vascular surgery.

Complications

EARLY OCCLUSION OF ARTERIAL REPAIR

In-hospital occlusion of an arterial repair is almost always related to delayed presentation of the patient after injury, delayed diagnosis of the injury by a physician, a technical mishap in the operating room, or occlusion of venous outflow from the area of injury. In a patient with a delay

Author, Year	Name	Number of Criteria
Gregory et al. 1985[47]	Mangled extremity syndrome index	9
Seiler et al. 1986[117]	—	4
Howe et al. 1987[56]	Predictive salvage index	4
Johansen et al. 1990[64]	Mangled extremity severity score	4
Russell et al. 1991[114]	Limb salvage index	7

Table 12-6 Scoring Systems for Mangled Extremities

FIGURE 12-10 **A,** *Traumatic false aneurysm of the anterior tibial artery related to fractures of the tibia and fibula.* **B,** *Completion arteriogram after operative ligation of the proximal anterior tibial artery.*

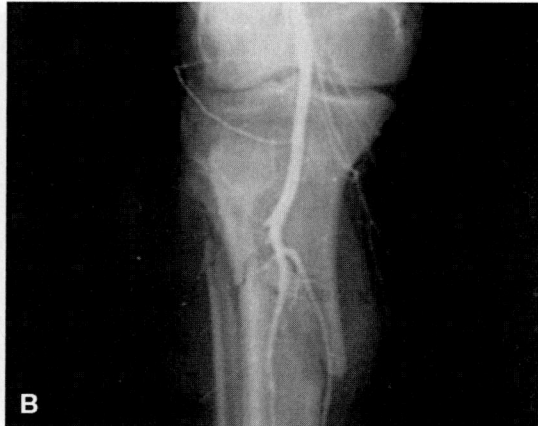

in presentation or diagnosis, in situ distal arterial thrombosis may occur within 6 hours.[90] The passage of a Fogarty embolectomy catheter may not be helpful in such a situation, because it does not remove thrombi from arterial collateral vessels.

Technical mishaps at operation that lead to postoperative thrombosis of a repair include too much tension on an end-to-end anastomosis, failure to remove any thrombi or emboli in the distal arterial tree with a Fogarty embolectomy catheter, narrowing of a circumferential suture line, and failure to flush the proximal and distal arteries before final closure of the repair. Also, ligation or occlusion of a repair in the popliteal vein can lead to occlusion of an arterial repair at the same level.

If distal pulses disappear, the patient is returned immediately to the operating room for thrombectomy or embolectomy and revision of the repair as necessary. If there is not an obvious reason for occlusion of the arterial repair at a reoperation, standard coagulation tests are performed immediately to screen for a thrombotic disorder. Examples include heparin-associated thrombocytopenia, antithrombin III deficiency, deficiency of protein C or S, and the antiphospholipid syndrome.

DELAY IN DIAGNOSIS OF AN ARTERIAL INJURY

Occasionally, a patient has a traumatic false aneurysm or an arteriovenous fistula from a previous arterial injury that was not diagnosed.[34,121] The insertion of an endovascular stent with or without trans-stent angiographic embolization is possible for many of these lesions, and it can be accomplished readily by an experienced interventional radiologist.[99] If a major artery is involved, operative intervention using the principles described previously may be necessary (Fig. 12-10).

SOFT TISSUE INFECTION OVER AN ARTERIAL REPAIR

A dreaded complication of combined orthopaedic-vascular injuries, particularly in the lower extremity, is infection in the soft tissue overlying the arterial repair. If débridement of the soft tissue infection results in exposure of the arterial repair, one option is to attempt coverage of the arterial repair with a porcine xenograft and hope for the gradual growth of granulation tissue over the healthy artery. If the arterial repair starts to leak or suffers a blowout, the patient is returned to the operating room. The exposed portion of the artery is resected, and the aforementioned extra-anatomic saphenous vein bypass graft is placed around the area of soft tissue infection, making sure that both end-to-end anastomoses are covered by healthy soft tissue outside the wound, as described previously.[28,29]

Another option after débridement is for immediate coverage with a local muscle or myocutaneous rotation flap or for coverage with a free flap performed by the plastic surgery service.[106]

LATE OCCLUSION OF ARTERIAL REPAIR

Because saphenous vein grafts placed in peripheral arteries undergo the degenerative changes of atherosclerosis over time, late occlusions of some of these grafts can be expected.

Management is the same as if the patient had occlusion of a primary artery—arteriography is performed based on symptoms, and bypass grafting is chosen if runoff is adequate to support another graft.

SUMMARY

Experience with peripheral arterial injuries in the absence of an associated bony injury documents that limb salvage is possible in almost all such patients without shotgun wounds or near amputations who are treated using the principles outlined in this chapter. These principles include early diagnosis by examination, preoperative arteriography or duplex ultrasonography, frequent use of interposition grafting for arterial repair, completion arteriography, repair of venous injuries in stable patients, and liberal use of fasciotomy.[30,31,35,36,97] If bony injuries accompany arterial injuries, limb salvage is less likely because of delays in diagnosis, a greater magnitude of arterial injury, disruption of vascular collateral vessels in soft tissue, and associated postoperative problems such as infection in adjacent soft tissue or bone.[9,47,52,56,74,75,117] Even so, limb salvage can be accomplished in most properly selected patients in modern trauma centers using the techniques described.[6,35]

REFERENCES

1. Abbott, W.M.; Darling, R.C. Axillary artery aneurysms secondary to crutch trauma. Am J Surg 125:515–519, 1973.

2. Ahuja, N.; Ostomel, T.A.; Rhee, P.; et al. Testing of modified zeolite hemostatic dressings in a large animal model of lethal groin injury. J Trauma 61:1312–1320, 2006.

3. Alexander, J.J.; Piotrowski, J.J.; Graham, D.; et al. Outcome of complex vascular and orthopedic injuries of the lower extremity. Am J Surg 162:111–116, 1991.

4. Alonso, D.T.; Feliciano, D.V.; Rozycki, G.S.; et al. Combined lower extremity arterial and orthopaedic injuries from penetrating trauma: Which to repair first. In press.

5. Bergstein, J.M.; Blair, J.P.; Edwards, J.; et al. Pitfalls in the use of color-flow duplex ultrasound for screening of suspected arterial injuries in penetrated extremities. J Trauma 33:395–402, 1992.

6. Bermudez, K.M.; Knudson, M.M.; Nelken, N.A.; et al. Long-term results of lower extremity venous injuries. Arch Surg 132:963–968, 1997.

7. Biffl, W.L.; Moore, E.E.; Offner, P.J.; et al. Optimizing screening for blunt cerebrovascular injuries. Am J Surg 178:517–522, 1999.

8. Bonanni, P.; Rhodes, M.; Lucke, J.P. The futility of predictive scoring of mangled lower extremities. J Trauma 34:99–104, 1993.

9. Bondurant, P.J.; Cotler, H.B.; Buckle, R.; et al. The medical and economic impact of severely injured lower extremities. J Trauma 28:1270–1273, 1988.

10. Callow, A.D. Development of vascular surgery and medicine. In Callow, A.D.; Ernst, C.B., (eds.). Vascular Surgery: Theory and Practice. Stamford, CT, Appleton & Lange, 1995, pp. xxiii–xxxv.

11. Carrel, A. The surgery of blood vessels. Johns Hopkins Hosp Bull 18:18–28, 1907.

12. Caudle, R.J.; Stern, P.J. Severe open fractures of the tibia. J Bone Joint Surg Am 69:801–807, 1987.

13. Chapman, M.W. Role of bone stability in open fractures. Instr Course Lect 31:75–87, 1982.

14. Cheng, S.L.; Rosati, C.; Waddell, J.P. Fatal hemorrhage caused by vascular injury associated with an acetabular fracture. J Trauma 38:208–209, 1995.

15. Cooper, C.; Rodriguez, A.; Omert, L. Blunt vascular trauma. Curr Probl Surg 29:281–357, 1996.

16. Crawford, D.L.; Yuschak, J.V.; McCombs, P.R. Pseudoaneurysm of the brachial artery from blunt trauma. J Trauma 42:327–329, 1997.

17. Crowley, J.G.; Masterson, R. Popliteal arteriovenous fistula following meniscectomy. J Trauma 24:164–165, 1984.

18. Dawson, D.L.; Putnam, A.T.; Light, J.T.; et al. Temporary arterial shunts to maintain limb perfusion after arterial injury: An animal study. J Trauma 47:64–71, 1999.

19. DeBakey, M.B.; Simeone, F.C. Battle injuries of the arteries in World War II: An analysis of 2,471 cases. Ann Surg 123:534–579, 1946.

20. Dellinger, E.P.; Miller, S.D.; Wertz, M.J.; et al. Risk of infection after open fracture of the arm or leg. Arch Surg 123:1320–1327, 1987.

21. Dennis, J.W.; Frykberg, E.R.; Crump, J.M.; et al. New perspectives on the management of penetrating trauma in proximity to major limb arteries. J Vasc Surg 11:84–93, 1990.

22. Dennis, J.W.; Frykberg, E.R.; Veldenz, H.C.; et al. Validation of nonoperative management of occult vascular injuries and accuracy of physical examination alone in penetrating extremity trauma: Five- to 10-year follow-up. J Trauma 44:243–253, 1998.

23. Dickerman, R.M.; Gewertz, R.L.; Foley, D.W.; et al. Selective intra-arterial tolazoline infusion in peripheral arterial trauma. Surgery 81:605–609, 1977.

24. Dregelid, E.; Jenssen, G.; Jonung, T.; et al. Pseudoaneurysm of the abdominal aorta due to a needle-like osteophyte on the first lumbar vertebra. J Vasc Surg 45:1059–1061, 2007.

25. Drost, T.F.; Rosemurgy, A.S.; Proctor, D.; et al. Outcome of treatment of combined orthopedic and arterial trauma to the lower extremity. J Trauma 29:1331–1334, 1989.

26. Ebong, W.W. False aneurysm of the profunda femoris artery following internal fixation of an intertrochanteric femoral fracture. Injury 9:249–251, 1978.

27. Eger, M.; Golcman, L.; Goldstein, A. The use of a temporary shunt in the management of arterial vascular injuries. Surg Gynecol Obstet 32:67–70, 1971.

28. Feliciano, D.V. Heroic procedures in vascular injury management: The role of extra-anatomic bypasses. Surg Clin North Am 82:115–124, 2002.

29. Feliciano, D.V. Management of infected grafts and graft blowout in vascular trauma patients. In Flanigan, D.P., ed. Civilian Vascular Trauma. Philadelphia, Lea & Febiger, 1992, pp. 447–455.

30. Feliciano, D.V. Managing peripheral vascular trauma. Infect Surg 5:659–669, 1986.

31. Feliciano, D.V. Vascular injuries. Adv Trauma 2:179–206, 1987.

32. Feliciano, D.V.; Accola, K.D.; Burch, M.J.; et al. Extra-anatomic bypass for peripheral arterial injuries. Am J Surg 158:506–510, 1989.

33. Feliciano, D.V.; Bitondo, C.G.; Mattox, K.L.; et al. Civilian trauma in the 1980s: A 1-year experience with 456 vascular and cardiac injuries. Ann Surg 199:717–724, 1984.

34. Feliciano, D.V.; Cruse, P.A.; Burch, J.M.; et al. Delayed diagnosis of arterial injuries. Am J Surg 154:579–584, 1987.

35. Feliciano, D.V.; Herskowitz, K.; O'Gorman, R.B.; et al. Management of vascular injuries in the lower extremities. J Trauma 28:319–328, 1988.

36. Feliciano, D.V.; Mattox, K.L.; Graham, J.M.; et al. Five-year experience with PTFE grafts in vascular wounds. J Trauma 25:71–81, 1985.

37. Subramanian, A.; Vercruysse, G.; Dente, C.; et al. A decade's experience with temporary intravascular shunts at a civilian level I trauma center. J Trauma, Publication pending.

38. Freischlag, J.A.; Sise, M.; Quinones-Baldrich, W.J.; et al. Vascular complications associated with orthopaedic procedures. Surg Gynecol Obstet 169:147–152, 1989.

39. Friedman, R.J.; Jupiter, J.B. Vascular injuries and closed extremity fractures in children. Clin Orthop Relat Res 188:112–119, 1984.

40. Frykberg, E.R.; Dennis, J.W.; Bishop, K.; et al. The reliability of physical examination in the evaluation of penetrating extremity trauma for vascular injury: Results at one year. J Trauma 31:502–511, 1991.

41. Frykberg, E.R.; Vines, F.S.; Alexander, R.H. The natural history of clinically occult arterial injuries: A prospective evaluation. J Trauma 29:577–583, 1989.

42. Gable, D.R.; Allen, J.W.; Richardson, J.D. Blunt popliteal artery injury: Is physical examination alone enough for evaluation? J Trauma 43:541–544, 1997.

43. Gagne, P.J.; Cone, J.B.; McFarland, D.; et al. Proximity penetrating extremity trauma: The role of duplex ultrasound in the detection of occult venous injuries. J Trauma 39:1157–1163, 1995.

44. Gates, J.D.; Knox, J.B. Axillary artery injuries secondary to anterior dislocation of the shoulder. J Trauma 39:581–583, 1995.

45. Gonzalez, E.A.; Moore, F.A.; Holcomb, J.B.; et al. Fresh-frozen plasma should be given earlier to patients requiring massive transfusion. J Trauma 62:112–119, 2007.

46. Goyanes, D.J. Substitution plastica de las arterias por las venas o'arterioplastia venosa, aplicada, como nuevo metodo, al tratamiento de las aneurismas. El Siglo Medico Sept. 1, 1906, p. 346; Sept. 8, 1906, p. 561.

47. Gregory, R.T.; Gould, R.J.; Peclet, M.; et al. The mangled extremity syndrome (M.E.S.): A severity grading system for multisystem injury of the extremity. J Trauma 25:1147–1150, 1985.

48. Gustilo, R.B.; Mendoza, R.M.; Williams, D.N. Problems in the management of type III (severe) open fractures: A new classification of type III open fractures. J Trauma 24:742–746, 1984.

49. Guthrie, C.C. Blood Vessel Surgery. London, Edward Arnold, 1912.

50. Hansen, S.I., Jr. The type IIIC tibial fracture: Salvage or amputation? J Bone Joint Surg Am 69:799–800, 1987.

51. Hayes, J.M.; Van Winkle, G.N. Axillary artery injury with minimally displaced fracture of the neck of the humerus. J Trauma 23:431–433, 1983.

52. Helfet, D.L.; Howey, T.; Sanders, R.; et al. Limb salvage versus amputation: Preliminary results of the Mangled Extremity Severity Score. Clin Orthop Relat Res 256:80–86, 1990.

53. Helfet, D.J.; Schmeling, G.J. Fractures of the acetabulum: Complications. In Tile, M., ed. Fractures of the Pelvis and Acetabulum, 2nd ed. Baltimore, MD, Williams & Wilkins, 1995, pp. 451–467.

54. Hobson, R.W. II; Howard, E.W.; Wright, C.B.; et al. Hemodynamics of canine femoral venous ligation: Significance in combined arterial and venous injuries. Surgery 74:824–829, 1973.

55. Holcomb, J.B.; Jenkins, D.; Rhee, P.; et al. Damage control resuscitation: Directly addressing the early coagulopathy of trauma. J Trauma 62:302–310, 2007.

56. Howe, H.R., Jr.; Poole, G.V., Jr.; Hansen, K.J.; et al. Salvage of lower extremities following combined orthopedic and vascular trauma: A predictive salvage index. Am Surg 53:205–208, 1987.

57. Hughes, C.W. Arterial repair during the Korean War. Ann Surg 147:555–561, 1958.

58. Iannacone, W.M.; Taffet, R.; DeLong, W.G. III; et al. Early exchange intramedullary nailing of distal femoral fractures with vascular injury initially stabilized with external fixation. J Trauma 37:446–451, 1994.

59. Iftikhar, T.R.; Kaminski, R.S.; Silva, I., Jr. Neurovascular complications of the modified Bristow procedure: A case report. J Bone Joint Surg Am 66:951–952, 1984.

60. Itani, K.M.F.; Burch, J.M.; Spjut-Patrinely, V.; et al. Emergency center arteriography. J Trauma 32:302–307, 1992.

61. Jarstfer, B.S.; Rich, N.M. The challenge of arteriovenous fistula formation following disc surgery: A collective review. J Trauma 16:726–733, 1976.

62. Jendrisak, M.D. Spontaneous abdominal aortic rupture from erosion by a lumbar spine fixation device: A case report. Surgery 99:631–633, 1986.

63. Johansen, K.; Bandyk, D.; Thiele, B.; et al. Temporary intraluminal shunts: Resolution of a management dilemma in complex vascular injuries. J Trauma 22:395–402, 1982.

64. Johansen, K.; Daines, M.; Howey, T.; et al. Objective criteria accurately predict amputation following lower extremity trauma. J Trauma 30:568–573, 1990.

65. Johnson, E.E.; Eckardt, J.J.; Letournel, E. Extrinsic femoral artery occlusion following internal fixation of an acetabular fracture: A case report. Clin Orthop Relat Res 217:209–213, 1987.

66. Johnson, R.; Thursby, P. Subclavian artery injury caused by a screw in a clavicular compression plate. Cardiovasc Surg 4:414–416, 1996.

67. Kendall, K.M.; Burton, J.H.; Cushing, R. Fatal subclavian artery transection from isolated clavicle fracture. J Trauma 48:316–318, 2000.

68. Kendall, R.W.; Taylor, D.C.; Salvian, A.J.; et al. The role of arteriography in assessing vascular injuries associated with dislocations of the knee. J Trauma 35:875–878, 1993.

69. Kheirabadi, B.S.; Acheson, E.M.; Deguzman, R.; et al. Hemostatic efficacy of two advanced dressings in an aortic hemorrhage model in swine. J Trauma 59:25–35, 2005.

70. Knudson, M.M.; Lewis, F.R.; Atkinson, K.; et al. The role of duplex ultrasound arterial imaging in patients with penetrating extremity trauma. Arch Surg 128:1033–1038, 1993.

71. Kootstra, G.; Schipper, J.J.; Boontje, A.H.; et al. Femoral shaft fracture with injury of the superficial femoral artery in civilian accidents. Surg Gynecol Obstet 142:399–403, 1976.

72. Kram, H.B.; Wright, J.; Shoemaker, W.C.; et al. Perioperative transcutaneous O_2 monitoring in the management of major peripheral arterial trauma. J Trauma 24:443–445, 1984.

73. Kuzniec, S.; Kauffman, P.; Molnar, L.J.; et al. Diagnosis of limb and neck arterial trauma using duplex ultrasonography. Cardiovasc Surg 6:358–366, 1998.

74. Lange, R.H. Limb reconstruction versus amputation decision making in massive lower extremity trauma. Clin Orthop Relat Res 243:92–99, 1989.

75. Lange, R.H.; Bach, A.W.; Hansen, S.T., Jr.; et al. Open tibial fractures with associated vascular injuries: Prognosis for limb salvage. J Trauma 25:203–208, 1985.

76. Ledgerwood, A.M.; Lucas, C.E. Biological dressings for exposed vascular grafts: A reasonable alternative. J Trauma 15:567–574, 1975.

77. Ledgerwood, A.M.; Lucas, C.E. Split-thickness porcine graft in the treatment of close-range shotgun wounds to extremities with vascular injury. Am J Surg 125:690–695, 1973.

78. Leininger, B.E.; Rasmussen, T.E.; Smith, D.L.; et al. Experience with wound VAC and delayed primary closure of contaminated soft tissue injuries in Iraq. J Trauma 61:1207–1211, 2006.

79. Lexer, E. Die ideale Operation des Arteriellen und des Arteriell-Venosen Aneurysma. Arch Klin Chir 83:459–477, 1907.

80. Lim, E.V.; Lavadia, W.T.; Blebea, J. Vascular impingement by external fixator pins: A case report. J Trauma 38:833–835, 1995.

81. Lipsky, A.M.; Gausche-Hill, M.; Henneman, P.L.; et al. Prehospital hypotension is a predictor of the need for an emergent therapeutic operation in trauma patients with normal systolic blood pressure in the emergency department. J Trauma 61:1228–1233, 2006.

82. Lynch, K.; Johansen, K. Can Doppler pressure measurement replace "exclusion" arteriography in the diagnosis of occult extremity arterial trauma? Ann Surg 214:737–741, 1991.

83. Makins, G.H. On Gunshot Injuries to the Blood Vessels. Bristol, England, John Wright, 1919, pp. 1–251.

84. Marin, M.L.; Veith, F.J.; Cynamon, J.; et al. Initial experience with transluminally placed endovascular grafts for the treatment of complex vascular lesions. Ann Surg 222:449–469, 1995.

85. Martin, L.C.; McKenney, M.G.; Sosa, J.L.; et al. Management of lower extremity arterial trauma. J Trauma 37:591–599, 1994.

86. Mattox, K.L.; Feliciano, D.V.; Burch, J.; et al. Five thousand seven hundred sixty cardiovascular injuries in 4459 patients: Epidemiologic evolution, 1958–1987. Ann Surg 209:698–707, 1989.

87. McAuley, C.E.; Steed, D.L.; Webster, M.W. Arterial complications of total knee replacement. Arch Surg 199:960–962, 1984.

88. McCready, R.A.; Logan, N.M.; Daugherty, M.E.; et al. Long-term results with autogenous tissue repair of traumatic extremity vascular injuries. Ann Surg 206:804–808, 1987.

89. McNeese, S.; Finck, E.; Yellin, A.E. Definitive treatment of selected vascular injuries and post-traumatic arteriovenous fistulas by arteriographic embolization. Am J Surg 140:252–259, 1980.

90. Miller, H.H.; Welch, C.S. Quantitative studies on the time factor in arterial injuries. Ann Surg 130:428–438, 1949.

91. Miranda, F.E.; Dennis, J.W.; Veldenz, H.C.; et al. Confirmation of the safety and accuracy of physical examination in the evaluation of knee dislocation for popliteal artery injury: A prospective study. J Trauma 52:247–252, 2002.

92. Mitchell, F.L. III; Thai, E.R. Results of venous interposition grafts in arterial injuries. J Trauma 30:336–339, 1990.

93. Mullins, R.J.; Lucas, C.E.; Ledgerwood, A.M. The natural history following venous ligation for civilian injuries. J Trauma 20:737–743, 1980.

94. Noszczyk, W.; Witkowski, M.; Weglowski, R. The Zamosc period in the work of Romuald Weglowski. Polski Przegl Chir 1985;57:440–445.

95. Ochsner, M.G., Jr.; Hoffman, A.P.; DiPasquale, D.; et al. Associated aortic rupture–pelvic fracture: An alert for orthopedic and general surgeons. J Trauma 33:429–434, 1992.

96. Odland, M.D.; Gisbert, V.L.; Gustilo, R.B.; et al. Combined orthopedic and vascular injury in the lower extremities: Indications for amputation. Surgery 108:660–666, 1990.

97. O'Gorman, R.B.; Feliciano, D.V. Arteriography performed in the emergency center. Am J Surg 152:323–325, 1986.

98. O'Gorman, R.B.; Feliciano, D.V.; Bitondo, C.G.; et al. Emergency center arteriography in the evaluation of suspected peripheral vascular injuries. Arch Surg 119:568–573, 1984.

99. Pais, S.O. Assessment of vascular trauma. In Mirvis, S.E.; Young, J.W.R., eds. Imaging in Trauma and Critical Care. Baltimore, MD, Williams & Wilkins, 1992, pp. 485–515.

100. Palazzo, J.C.; Ristow, A.V.B.; Schwartz, F.; et al. Traumatic vascular lesions associated with fractures and dislocations. J Cardiovasc Surg 27:688–696, 1986.

101. Pappas, P.J.; Haser, P.B.; Teehan, E.P.; et al. Outcome of complex venous reconstructions in patients with trauma. J Vasc Surg 25:398–404, 1997.

102. Parry, N.G.; Feliciano, D.V.; Burke, R.M.; et al. Management and short-term patency of lower

extremity venous injuries with varied repairs. Am J Surg 186:631–635, 2003.

103. Paul, M.A.; Patka, P.; van Heuzen, E.P.; et al. Vascular injury from external fixation: Case reports. J Trauma 33:917–920, 1992.

104. Peck, J.J.; Fitzgibbons, T.J.; Gaspar, M.R. Devastating distal arterial trauma and continuous intra-arterial infusion of tolazoline. Am J Surg 145:562–566, 1983.

105. Pretre, R.; Bruschweiler, I.; Rossier, J.; et al. Lower limb trauma with injury to the popliteal vessels. J Trauma 40:595–601, 1996.

106. Reath, D.B.; Jeffries, G.E. The mangled lower extremity: Management and long-term results. Adv Trauma Crit Care 6:113–164, 1991.

107. Reid, J.D.S.; Weigelt, J.A.; Thal, E.R.; et al. Assessment of proximity of a wound to major vascular structures as an indication for arteriography. Arch Surg 123:942–946, 1988.

108. Reisman, J.D.; Morgan, A.S. Analysis of 46 intra-abdominal aortic injuries from blunt trauma: Case reports and literature review. J Trauma 30:1294–1297, 1990.

109. Rich, N.M.; Baugh, J.H.; Hughes, C.W. Acute arterial injuries in Vietnam: One thousand cases. J Trauma 10:359–369, 1970.

110. Robbs, J.V.; Baker, L.W. Cardiovascular trauma. Curr Probl Surg 21:1–87, 1984.

111. Roessler, M.S.; Wisner, D.H.; Holcroft, J.W. The mangled extremity: When to amputate? Arch Surg 126:1243–1249, 1991.

112. Ross, S.E.; Ransom, K.J.; Shatney, C.H. The management of venous injuries in blunt extremity trauma. J Trauma 25:150–153, 1985.

113. Roth, S.M.; Wheeler, J.R.; Gregory, R.T.; et al. Blunt injury of the abdominal aorta: A review. J Trauma 42:748–755, 1997.

114. Russell, W.L.; Sailors, D.M.; Whittle, T.B.; et al. Limb salvage versus traumatic amputation: A decision based on a seven-part predictive index. Ann Surg 213:473–481, 1991.

115. Schlosser, V.; Spillner, G.; Breymann, T.H.; et al. Vascular injuries in orthopaedic surgery. J Cardiovasc Surg 23:323–327, 1982.

116. Schwartz, M.; Weaver, F.; Yellin, A.; et al. The utility of color flow Doppler examination in penetrating extremity arterial trauma. Am Surg 59:375–378, 1993.

117. Seiler, J.G. III; Richardson, J.D. Amputation after extremity injury. Am J Surg 152:260–264, 1986.

118. Shapiro, M.B.; Jenkins, D.H.; Schwab, C.W.; et al. Damage control: Collective review. J Trauma 49:969–978, 2000.

119. Sharma, P.V.P.; Shah, P.M.; Vinzons, A.T.; et al. Meticulously restored lumina of injured veins remains patent. Surgery 112:928–932, 1992.

120. Snyder, W.H.; Thal, E.R.; Bridges, R.A.; et al. The validity of normal arteriography in penetrating trauma. Arch Surg 113:424–428, 1978.

121. Soubbotitch, V. Military experiences of traumatic aneurysms. Lancet 2:720–721, 1913.

122. Spirito, R.; Trabattoni, P.; Pompilio, G.; et al. Endovascular treatment of a post-traumatic tibial pseudoaneurysm and arteriovenous fistula: Case report and review of the literature. J Vasc Surg 45:1076–1079, 2007.

123. Stain, S.C.; Yellin, A.E.; Weaver, F.A.; et al. Selective management of nonocclusive arterial injuries. Arch Surg 124:1136–1141, 1989.

124. Stanton, P.E., Jr.; Rosenthal, D.; Clark, M.; et al. Percutaneous transcatheter embolization of injuries to the profunda femoris artery. Angiology 36:650–655, 1985.

125. Starnes, R.W.; Bruce, J.M. Popliteal artery trauma in a forward deployed Mobile Army Surgical Hospital: Lessons learned from the war in Kosovo. J Trauma 48:1144–1147, 2000.

126. Stephen, D.J.G. Pseudoaneurysm of the superior gluteal arterial system: An unusual cause of pain after a pelvic fracture. J Trauma 43:146–149, 1997.

127. Stephen, D.J.G.; Kreder, H.J.; Day, A.C.; et al. Early detection of arterial bleeding in acute pelvic trauma. J Trauma 47:638–642, 1999.

128. Storm, R.K.; Sing, A.K.; de Graaf, E.J.R.; et al. Iatrogenic arterial trauma associated with hip fracture treatment. J Trauma 48:957–959, 2000.

129. Tile, M. Disruption of the pelvic ring: Management. In Tile, M., ed. Fractures of the Pelvis and Acetabulum, 2nd ed. Baltimore, MD, Williams & Wilkins, 1995, pp. 102–134.

130. Tile, M. Fractures of the acetabulum: Management. In Tile, M., ed. Fractures of the Pelvis and Acetabulum, 2nd ed. Baltimore, MD, Williams & Wilkins, 1995, pp. 321–354.

131. Tremblay, L.N.; Feliciano, D.V.; Rozycki, G.S. Secondary extremity compartment syndrome. J Trauma 53:833–837, 2002.

132. Urban, W.P.; Tornetta, P. III. Vascular compromise after intramedullary nailing of the tibia: A case report. J Trauma 36:804–807, 1995.

133. Weaver, F.A.; Rosenthal, R.E.; Waterhouse, G.; et al. Combined skeletal and vascular injuries of the lower extremities. Am Surg 50:189–197, 1984.

134. Weller, S.J.; Rossitch, E., Jr.; Malek, A.M. Detection of vertebral artery injury after cervical spine trauma using magnetic resonance angiography. J Trauma 46:660–666, 1999.

135. Wyrzykowski, A.D.; Feliciano, D.V. Trauma damage control. In Feliciano, D.V.; Mattox, K.L.; Moore, E.E., ed. Trauma, 6th ed. New York, McGraw-Hill, 2008.

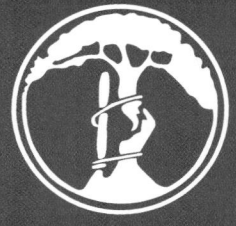

CHAPTER 13

Compartment Syndromes

....

Bruce C. Twaddle, M.D., F.R.A.C.S. and Annunziato Amendola, M.D., F.R.C.S.(C.)

HISTORY

Compartment syndrome is a condition characterized by raised pressure within a closed space with a potential to cause irreversible damage to its contents. Clinical awareness of the condition is attributed to the work of Richard von Volkmann. In 1881, he published an article in which he attempted to relate the state of irreversible contractures of flexor muscles of the hand to ischemic processes occurring in the forearm. Volkmann believed that the pathophysiology of the contracture is related to massive venous stasis associated with simultaneous occurrence of arterial insufficiency. He thought that the condition may be caused by tight bandages, an observation that proved to be accurate.[121]

Other investigators confirmed Volkmann's conclusion[14,105] and Petersen,[91] in 1888, described surgical treatment of a Volkmann contracture, demonstrating some return of function after release of contracted scarred tissue, further supporting the observation that the causative factor is related to an ischemic event. Others at that time theorized that neurologic damage secondary to ischemia was causally related to the Volkmann contracture.[85,120,121]

It was Hildebrand[47] in 1906 who first used the term *Volkmann's ischemic contracture* to describe the end-point of an untreated compartment syndrome and suggested that elevated tissue pressure may be causally related to ischemic contracture. He speculated that the underlying problem was a result of venous obstruction causing increased pressure in muscle and compromising arterial circulation to the muscle itself.

Thomas,[120] in 1909, attempted to review the data concerning the cause of Volkmann's ischemic contracture published up to that time. In his published review of 112 cases, fractures were found to be a causative factor in most end-stage Volkmann ischemic contractures. Other predisposing causes of the condition were noted, however, including arterial injury, embolus, and tight bandaging. Of the 112 cases reported up to that time, 107 had occurred in the upper extremity.

Whereas the early investigators into the cause of compartment syndrome concentrated mainly on the development of the contracture, Rowlands,[105] in 1910, was the first to suggest that reperfusion after a prolonged period of ischemia could result in postischemic congestion and edema of muscle and nerve and could lead to the development of acute compartment syndrome. In 1914, Murphy[85] was the first to suggest that fasciotomy, if done before the development of the contracture, may prevent the contracture from occurring. He was also the first to suggest the relation among tissue pressure, fasciotomy, and the development of a subsequent contracture.

Brooks and colleagues[14] further investigated the cause of acute compartment syndrome. After a series of extensive investigations, they suggested that the late picture of Volkmann's ischemic paralysis could be explained only on the basis of acute venous obstruction causing diminished perfusion of the extremity. After release of the obstruction (bandage or splint), a period of swelling, heat, and "rapidly developing contracture" is likely to occur.

During and after World War II, many cases of Volkmann's contracture were seen as a complication of high-velocity gunshot wounds causing fractures of the upper or lower extremities.[16]

Although the existence of arterial trauma complicating a fracture was well known, the concomitant need for fasciotomy at the time of arterial repair was not generally appreciated. Many surgeons of the day thought that treatment of an impending Volkmann ischemia should be directed toward relief of the arterial spasm. Often, direct arterial injury could not be demonstrated at the time of surgery. In spite of that, however, surgical exploration of the "damaged artery" frequently led to reestablishment of flow distally and, in some cases, to reversal of the acute impending compartment syndrome.[88] It is highly likely that, while exposing the artery, the vascular surgeons were actually performing a limited fasciotomy, and this may have been the reason for the improvement in the patient's symptoms.

In 1970 Patman and Thompson,[88] after an extensive review of 164 patients with peripheral vascular disease in whom fasciotomy had been performed after arterial reconstruction, concluded that fasciotomy has much to offer for limb salvage and implied that it should be performed more often after restoration of arterial inflow to an extremity. Similar observations were made in 1967 during the Vietnam War by Chandler and Knapp,[19] who also suggested that, had more fasciotomies been performed after arterial repair to the extremities, the long-term results might have been better.

Many early cases of compartment syndrome seemed to be confined to the upper extremity. Increased attention focused on the lower extremity, however, after the report by Ellis[26] in 1958 of a 2 percent incidence of ischemic contractures occurring as a complication of tibial fractures. Most early descriptions of compartment syndrome involving the lower extremity were related to the development of the condition in the anterior compartment, but after the reports of Seddon[99] in 1966 and of Kelly and Whitesides[50] in 1967, the existence of four compartments in the leg and hence the need to decompress more than the anterior compartment were pointed out.

Compartment syndrome of the foot has been indirectly alluded to since the description of gangrene as a complication of Lisfranc fracture-dislocations, and increasing reports of this condition have appeared in the literature.[55,86] Similarly, the involvement of thigh and gluteal compartments is now well recognized, particularly as a complication in the multiply traumatized patient.[16,107,108] The anatomy of these various compartments has been documented in the past and has been revisited by several authors in an attempt to define the ideal surgical approaches.[49,86]

The pathophysiology has been elucidated by a number of researchers, who correlated end-stage muscle contracture with such underlying pathophysiologic factors as raised interstitial pressure and muscle and nerve ischemia.[81,87,102,103,110,123] *These investigators also noted that a compartment syndrome can occur in any of the compartments of the leg or arm if the prerequisites for its development are present.*[56]

PATHOPHYSIOLOGY

The prerequisites for the development of a compartment syndrome include a cause of raised pressure within a confined tissue space. Distortions in the relation between volume and pressure interfere with circulation to the compartment leading to the development of an acute compartment syndrome.[56] Any condition that increases the content or reduces the volume of a compartment could be related to the development of an acute compartment syndrome. Excess tissue pressure secondary to increased volume of a compartment has been shown to occur in various conditions, including hemorrhage, fractures, increased capillary permeability after burns, and a temporary period of ischemia resulting in post-ischemic swelling.*

Regardless of the underlying cause, raised tissue pressure ultimately leads to some degree of venous obstruction within a closed space. Pressure continues to rise until the low intramuscular arteriolar pressure is exceeded. At that point, no further blood enters the capillary anastomosis, resulting in shunting within a compartment. If the pressure increase is allowed to continue untreated, muscle and nerve ischemia occurs, leading to irreversible damage to the contents of the compartment.[44,101,102] Using a canine model, it was demonstrated that the extent of tissue injury depends on pressure and time. Rorabeck and colleagues[101,102] found that interference with muscle and nerve function becomes progressively more severe according to the duration of applied pressure. They found that a pressure of 30 mm Hg must be maintained in the anterior

compartment of a dog's leg for 8 hours before changes in conduction velocity can be demonstrated in the peroneal nerve. However, conduction velocity changes can be shown sooner if higher pressures are introduced and maintained.[35,47,61,68,79]

A compartment syndrome occurring as a complication of arterial injury is usually observed after restoration of arterial inflow to the compartment. Diminished arterial inflow caused by the injury results in a period of nerve and muscle ischemia within the compartment. The period of hypoxia experienced by the muscle and nerve allows transudation of fluid through capillary basement membranes and the capillaries of striated muscle.[98] It is also thought that the basement membranes may sustain some anoxic damage secondary to impaired arterial inflow. When arterial inflow to the extremity has been reestablished, fluid continues to leak through the basement membrane into the interstitial spaces. This leakage occurs soon after restoration of arterial inflow and, as a result, the pressure within the compartment continues to increase because of the unyielding fascial walls encasing the compartment. The pressure rise continues until the critical closing pressure of the small arterioles is reached. After that point, no further blood enters the striated muscle of the compartment and shunting occurs. The raised compartment pressure further increases the local venous pressure, thereby reducing the arteriolar-venous gradient. Regardless of the cause of acute compartment syndrome, however, pressure within the compartment never rises sufficiently to obstruct totally the systolic or diastolic pressure in the major vessel traversing the compartment.[98]

Both laboratory and clinical studies have demonstrated that compartment syndrome is not directly comparable to an episode of pure ischemia.[43,44] Heppenstall and associates demonstrated in an animal model the importance of episodes of hypotension in increasing the extent of irreversible muscle ischemia and confirmed the difference between mean arterial pressure and compartment pressures in determining flow and muscle survival. McQueen and Court-Brown[71] demonstrated this distinction clinically, suggesting that a difference between diastolic pressure and compartment pressure of less than 30 mm Hg has a high clinical correlation with development of a compartment syndrome. This difference between diastolic and compartment pressure was labeled Δp and is probably the most important clinical parameter to identify.

Blood flow studies employing technetium 99m and xenon 133 have demonstrated that skeletal muscle blood flow is reduced during acute compartment syndrome in the experimental animal.[102,103] Because of the patchy distribution of muscle necrosis found at the time of fasciotomy, however, variations in muscle blood flow probably occur among areas within the same muscle.

Crush syndrome and crush injury have, at times, been grouped with compartment syndrome in pathophysiology and treatment. This grouping is probably conceptually incorrect. These patients present originally with a history of having been trapped or crushed with pressure on a limb or limbs for an extended period of time. They characteristically have a painless flaccid paralysis initially, followed by the rapid development of swelling and rigid compartments in the affected part of the limb. However, it is now clear

---

*See references 8, 20, 21, 36, 37, 40, 42, 46, 51, 58, 67, 75, 81, 88, 90, 92, 93, 97, 102, 112, and 119.

that the elevation of compartment pressure in crush injury is secondary to intracellular muscle damage rather than being the causative factor and that treatment guidelines are different.[72,94] In particular, fasciotomy is contraindicated in crush syndrome and is associated with higher morbidity and mortality.

The anesthetized or sedated patient is at particular risk for development of a compartment syndrome, which may go unnoticed. Patients who are intubated very early in their initial care need accurate assessment of their injured extremities while in the intensive care unit. Because unrecognized injuries can lead to compartment syndrome in these patients, remembering to perform a secondary survey of all patients involved in high-velocity accidents resulting in ventilatory support is essential. Prolonged positioning of a limb, particularly with the use of a post or traction, or both, such as with hip fracture fixation or femoral nailing, can place the compartments involved at risk,[69] especially if there is ongoing bleeding related to injury. Compartment syndrome may, however, also occur in the uninjured leg if positioning restricts venous return. Hyperextension of the hip to improve imaging of a fractured femur or tibia in the lateral position may result in a risk of compartment syndrome in the well leg. A reperfusion phenomenon, as occurs with vascular repair, may also result in compartment syndrome in the well limb if the positioning of this limb affects arterial flow. Therefore, any patient who undergoes prolonged or unexpectedly protracted surgery, particularly to the lower limb, should have careful clinical assessment of the compartments of both the operated and un-operated limbs several times after surgery.

Considering the underlying pathophysiology, the cause of a compartment syndrome may be related more specifically to conditions that decrease the size or increase the content of a compartment.[58] The most common cause of compartment syndrome associated with decrease in the size of the compartment is the application of a tight cast, constrictive dressings, or pneumatic antishock garments.[20,30,52,70,119]

Closure of fascial defects has been demonstrated to be associated with the development of acute compartment syndrome.[73] This condition most commonly occurs in the anterior compartment of the leg in patients who present with symptomatic muscle hernias and symptoms suggestive of chronic compartment syndrome. Failure to recognize the pitfalls in closing the muscle hernia in this situation can have disastrous consequences for the patient and the surgeon.[73,89,110] Attempts to close the anterior compartment after surgery in this region, such as with a tibial plateau fracture, may also increase the risk of compartment problems. Care should be taken when assessing closure of this layer, taking into consideration the extent of swelling, any sign of ongoing bleeding, and the coagulation status of the patient.

A number of conditions have been shown to increase compartment contents and lead to compartment syndrome. These conditions involve hemorrhage within the compartment or accumulation of fluid (edema) within the compartment. The former is most commonly associated with fractures of the tibia, elbow, forearm, or femur, whereas the latter is most commonly associated with postischemic swelling after arterial injuries or restoration of arterial flow after thrombosis of a major artery.* The compartment syndrome described after arthroscopic treatment of tibial plateau fractures is likely to be related to extravasation of fluid into the compartment through the fracture itself.[9] This event is much more sinister than the fluid extravasation into the superficial soft tissues that can occur during regular arthroscopy because this fluid is generally outside the fascial layer. The use of arthroscopic fluid pumps to increase fluid flow increases the risk of this type of fluid accumulation.

Compartment syndromes have also been reported to occur after other conditions or therapies, including soft tissue injury to an extremity, hereditary bleeding, dialysis, anticoagulant therapy, osteotomy, intraosseous fluid resuscitation in children, and excessive skeletal traction.†

As can be seen, the causes of acute compartment syndrome touch on several medical disciplines, including orthopaedic, general, and vascular surgery and traumatology.‡

DIAGNOSIS: CLINICAL ASSESSMENT

The clinical diagnosis of an acute compartment syndrome is sometimes obvious, but usually the findings are not clear-cut. A review of the literature suggests that there is frequently a delay in reaching a diagnosis of compartment syndrome because the symptoms can be masked by those of other injuries.[30,54,97,98,116]

The presence of an open wound in a compound fracture should not abrogate the possibility of development of a compartment syndrome. Between 6 percent and 9 percent of open tibial fractures are complicated by compartment syndrome, with the incidence being directly proportional to the severity of the soft tissue injury.[12,22]

Assuming the patient is conscious and alert, the most important symptom of an impending compartment syndrome is pain disproportionate to that expected from the known injuries. Frequently, the patient has a relatively pain-free interval (perhaps a few hours) after reduction of the fracture and then develops pain out of proportion to the injury. The degree of pain can usually be assessed by the need for analgesia usually recorded on the drug chart. With the advent of prolongation of regional or epidural analgesia in the peri-operative period, particular attention should be paid to these patients. Often, junior medical staff from several services become involved in managing pain relief in these patients, and increased vigilance is necessary to ensure that the analgesia requirements of the patients are being monitored. There have been various reports of such patients having a delayed diagnosis of compartment syndrome, often beyond the time when intervention can prevent permanent muscle necrosis.[83,113]

The pain felt by the patient is unrelenting and seems to be unrelated to the position of the extremity or to immobilization. It is exacerbated by constricting casts or dressings, and after their release some patients obtain transient but minimal relief of the symptoms. The patient may

---

*See references 5, 12, 29, 33, 34, 37, 45, 64, 69, 77, 87, 98, 104, 108, 111, 117, 125, and 126.

†See references 18, 24, 28, 32, 36, 37, 58, 64, 77, 79, 87, 95, and 125.

‡See references 1, 8, 13, 15, 20, 42, 52, 67, 93, 119.

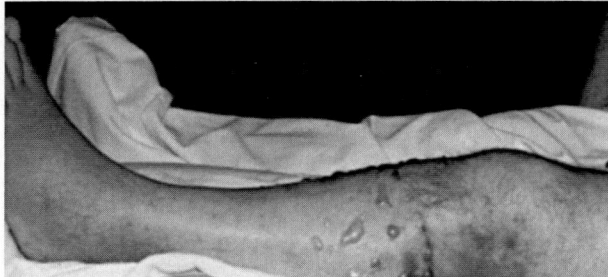

FIGURE 13-1   *Acute compartment syndrome of the leg.*

also complain of feelings of numbness or tingling in the affected extremity. These symptoms are poorly localized and are not to be relied on.

Clinical signs of an impending acute compartment syndrome, irrespective of the underlying cause, include pain on palpation of the swollen compartment, reproduction of symptoms with passive muscle stretch, sensory deficit in the territory of the nerve traversing the compartment, and muscle weakness. The earliest sign of an acute compartment syndrome is a tensely swollen compartment whose palpation reproduces the patient's pain (Fig. 13-1). Because this symptom is frequently associated with a fracture, it can be difficult for the examining physician to be certain how much pain is from the fracture and how much is from the tense, swollen compartment. The compartment feels extremely hard, and the overlying skin can be shiny. Palpation of the compartment at some distance from the level of the fracture may still be extremely painful for the patient. Occasionally, the finding of a tense, swollen compartment is not obvious, particularly in the deep flexor compartment of the forearm and the deep posterior compartment of the leg, where the diagnosis can be missed.

Pain referred to a compartment on passive stretching of the digits is a reliable sign of an impending acute compartment syndrome (Fig. 13-2). Stretch pain per se is *not* a specific sign of acute compartment syndrome but is a sign that

FIGURE 13-2   *Passive extension of the digit causes pain referred to the compartment.*

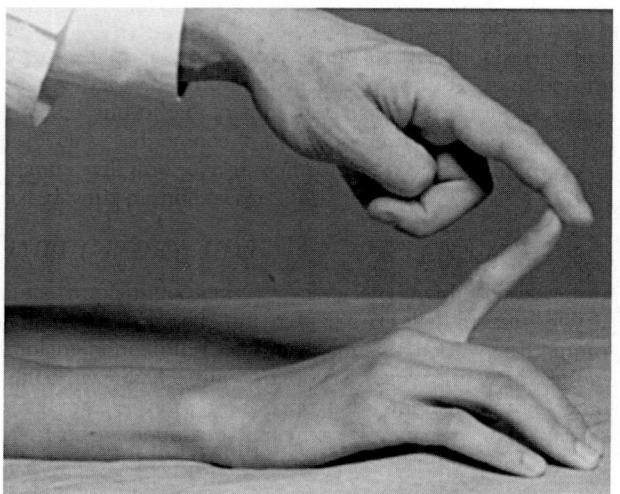

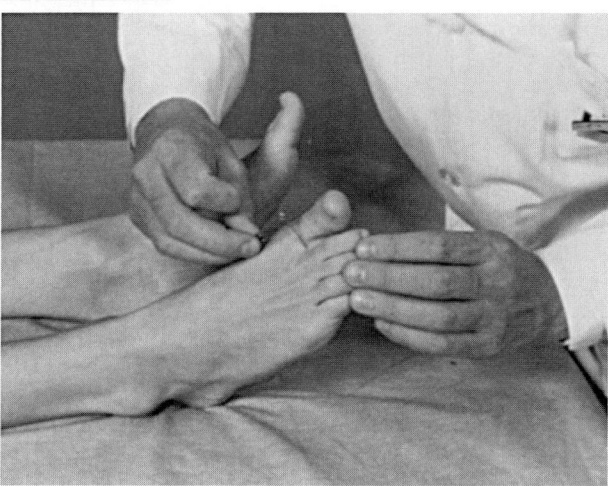

FIGURE 13-3   *Hypesthesia in the first webspace.*

is usually attributed to muscle swelling or ischemia. Therefore, in patients with a fracture and without a compartment syndrome, some degree of stretch pain can be present.

The symptom of pain and the findings of a tense, swollen compartment with some degree of passively induced stretch pain represent the earliest manifestations of an acute compartment syndrome. By the time sensory deficit is obvious, irreversible changes in nerve or muscle may have occurred. The sensory deficit experienced by the patient is usually in the territory of the nerve traversing the compartment. In acute anterior compartment syndrome, the patient may have hypesthesia in the territory of the first webspace (Fig. 13-3). The appearance of a sensory defect in acute compartment syndrome is a reliable sign, assuming there is no superimposed injury to the nerve.

To await the development of frank motor weakness in acute compartment syndrome is to invite disaster. Paresis is a late finding and, if present, requires immediate surgical intervention (Fig. 13-4). Many of the other features of an acute compartment syndrome may be altered by the time such weakness has occurred, making the diagnosis more

FIGURE 13-4   *Weakness of dorsiflexion.*

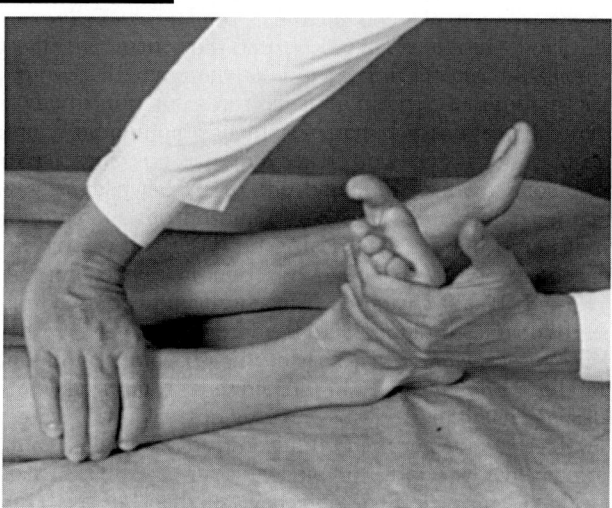

difficult. In particular, pain may become a much less reliable indicator of significant pressure elevation after muscle necrosis has occurred.

Palpable pulses are always present in acute compartment syndrome unless there is an underlying arterial injury. Capillary refill in the digits is often sluggish but may be normal and the peripheral pulses are readily palpable, even with the most florid acute compartment syndrome.

Assuming the patient is normotensive, pressure within the compartment can never rise sufficiently to obstruct systolic pressure totally in the major artery traversing the compartment.[31,53,102] This finding is explained on the basis of the shunting that occurs within the compartment. The presence of pulses and normal capillary filling does not mean that a compartment syndrome is absent.

The differential diagnosis of an acute compartment syndrome includes arterial occlusion, an injury to a peripheral nerve, or crush injury.

Delay in diagnosis of a major arterial injury may occur if poor or absent pulses are attributed to factors such as blood loss, compression by a fracture hematoma, or malalignment of the fracture. In addition, high-velocity trauma with acute limb ischemia can be obscured by shock. The diagnosis of arterial injury should not be difficult, assuming the surgeon has a high index of clinical awareness.

Johansen and colleagues[48] demonstrated the value of measuring the Doppler-assessed arterial pressure index (the systolic arterial pressure in the injured extremity divided by the arterial pressure in the uninvolved arm). A value less than 0.90 necessitates further arterial investigation; 94 percent of patients with an index this low have positive arteriographic findings. No major arterial injuries were missed using these criteria.[48] However, in case of doubt, arteriography is *always* indicated (Fig. 13-5). The risk associated with arteriography is small compared with the problems caused by a delayed or missed diagnosis of arterial injury. Doppler ultrasonography is useful in detection of arterial injury and particularly in monitoring minor arterial injuries treated conservatively. It does not, however, provide any useful information regarding the adequacy of blood flow through a compartment. The diagnosis of a concomitant nerve injury is less difficult because pain is rarely a feature of a nerve injury. Usually, however, the diagnosis of a nerve injury is a diagnosis of exclusion with compartment syndrome, arterial injury, or both.

Crush injury is produced by continuous and prolonged pressure. It can occur in persons who are trapped in one position for a prolonged period or who have collapsed or fallen asleep in one position for an excessive period when under the influence of alcohol or drugs. The patient usually suffers no pain initially and may have no physical complaints. Initially there is flaccid paralysis of the injured limb and a patchy sensory loss. Gross edema takes time to develop, and distal pulses are usually present.

The clinical presentation of these patients is the key to making the diagnosis of crush injury as opposed to compartment syndrome. The patients must have had the limb trapped in one position for a prolonged period. Collapse of a building, being trapped beneath a fallen object, lying in an awkward position after collapse from drug overdose, and failed attempted suicide with carbon monoxide are all clinical scenarios in which crush injury may occur.

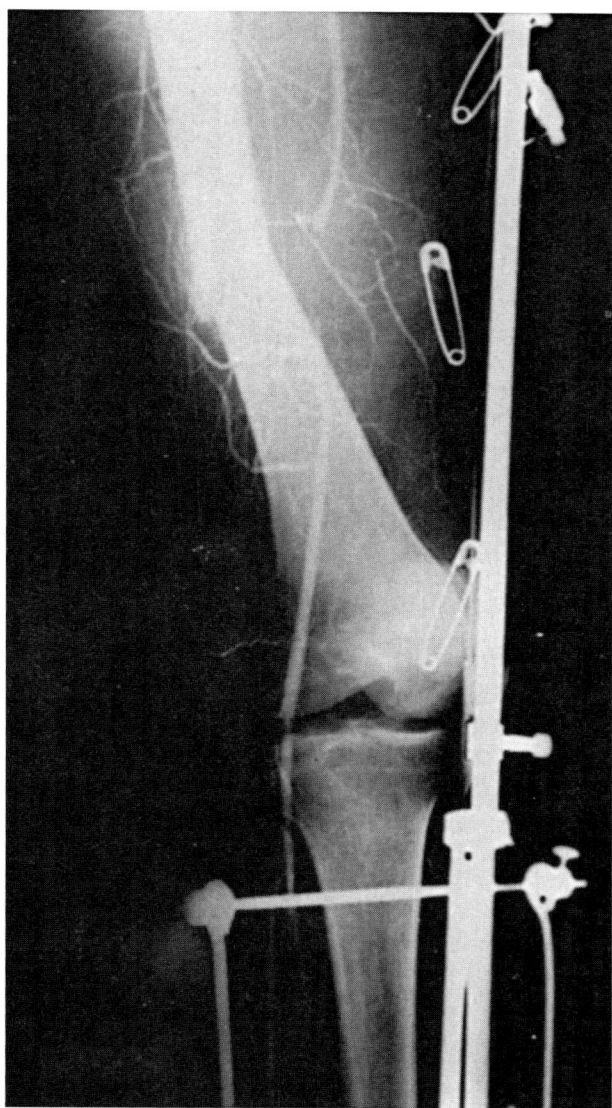

FIGURE 13-5 *An arteriogram showing arterial disruption at the site of a fractured femur. (From Seligson, D., ed. Concepts in Intramedullary Nailing. Orlando, FL, Grune & Stratton, 1985, p. 111.)*

These patients initially have a flaccid paralysis of the limb that is painless. Over the course of hours, swelling rapidly ensues, often far more dramatic than would be seen in compartment syndrome. The swelling is due to rapid release of fluid because of the failure of intracellular mechanisms that allow the cell to retain water. The result is clinical evidence of muscle damage with darkening of the urine related to myoglobinuria and rapid deterioration of renal function. These features again occur more rapidly than would be expected with compartment syndrome, in a day or two after initial presentation. Because the timing of these changes is important in making the diagnosis, particularly as fasciotomy is contraindicated in this condition, it is often necessary to speak to the ambulance or emergency staff who first found the patient if crush syndrome is considered a possibility.

Crush syndrome refers to the systemic manifestations of this type of injury. The hemodynamic status of the injured person deteriorates and the patient becomes severely hypovolemic as edema develops. Acute renal failure secondary to hypovolemia and muscle breakdown ensues unless appropriate treatment is undertaken. Fasciotomy is **not** recommended if the diagnosis of crush injury and crush syndrome can clearly be made, even in the presence of dramatically elevated compartment pressures. Active management of the metabolic complications is the key to treatment.[72,94]

TISSUE PRESSURE MEASUREMENTS

The earliest pathogenic factor in the production of an acute compartment syndrome complicating musculoskeletal trauma is raised tissue pressure. Without an elevation in the tissue pressure, an acute compartment syndrome would not occur. The clinical manifestations of an acute compartment syndrome were discussed in the previous section, but it should be remembered that elevated tissue pressure, by definition, must *precede* the development of the clinical signs and symptoms. With tissue pressure measurements, the physician should be able to diagnose acute compartment syndrome in the incipient rather than in the fulminant stage. A number of techniques are available for diagnosing an incipient compartment syndrome. It is important to have a thorough understanding of the indications for these techniques and to appreciate their benefits and limitations.

Indications

Ideally, it would be helpful to know the underlying tissue pressure that develops after almost every fracture of the upper or lower extremity. However, this is neither feasible nor cost-effective. The surgeon therefore must decide which patients should be monitored.

If a patient with an acute fracture of the tibia begins to have pain disproportionate to what might be expected, stretch pain referred to the compartment with passive dorsi-flexion or plantar flexion of the toes, weakness of the dorsi-flexors of the foot, or hypoesthesia in the territory of the first webspace, tissue pressure measurement is not required but the patient should be taken immediately to the operating room for four-compartment fasciotomy. Conversely, if the same patient seems to require an unusual amount of analgesia and on examination has a tense, painful compartment in the absence of any other physical signs, pressure monitoring should be considered. The indications discussed in the following paragraphs are only guidelines. There are many other situations that are not so clear-cut, in which the surgeon must decide according to knowledge and experience. If one starts to think about tissue pressure measurements, then one should probably be making them (Fig. 13-6).

Polytrauma Patient

The polytrauma patient is at risk for the development of acute compartment syndrome for two reasons. First,

associated head injuries, drug and alcohol intoxication, early endotracheal intubation, and the use of paralyzing drugs interfere with history taking and the assessment of physical signs. Second, in patients with low diastolic pressure, compartment syndrome can occur at relatively low threshold pressures. For various reasons, polytrauma patients may have a lowered diastolic pressure, which again places them at increased risk for acute compartment syndrome.

The approach to this type of patient is to measure pressures in all the compartments at risk and to leave the catheter in place in the compartment with the highest pressure to allow continuous pressure monitoring. This approach can be somewhat cumbersome, and the choice of the compartment may be incorrect. It is extremely important to remain vigilant in the assessment of polytrauma patients and to carry out isolated compartment pressure measurements regularly in the compartments at risk. This monitoring usually involves assessment of the forearm compartments and the compartments of the lower leg. Rarely is continuous pressure monitoring necessary in other compartments, and until more normal baseline data become available, the validity of its use is questionable.

PATIENT WITH CHEMICAL OVERDOSE OR HEAD INJURY AND AN ISOLATED LONG BONE FRACTURE

In these patients it is also difficult to elicit an appropriate history and to assess clinical signs by physical examination. The surgeon must measure compartment pressures in these patients because there is no other way to diagnose the condition.

It is suggested that the pressures in the deep posterior and anterior compartments (for a fracture of the tibia) or in the superficial and deep posterior compartments of the forearm (for a fracture of the forearm) be measured. On the basis of the results, an indwelling catheter is left in the compartment with the highest pressure. Continuous pressure monitoring can be done (see later discussion).

INCONCLUSIVE CLINICAL DIAGNOSIS

Inconclusive diagnosis occurs most commonly with patients in whom, for one reason or another, the symptoms *seem* to be out of proportion to what would be expected given the nature of the injury. Another situation involves the differential diagnosis of a compartment syndrome in a patient with a suspected nerve injury. It is extremely rare to confuse a peripheral nerve injury with an acute compartment syndrome, but occasionally the diagnosis can be confusing. In fact, a nerve injury and a compartment syndrome can coexist, and pressure measurements in this case are valuable adjuncts for interpretation of the physical signs and determination of the timing for fasciotomy.

In other cases, compartment pressure measurements may be of some value but should not be listed as specific indications. For example, with increased reliance on closed intramedullary nailing techniques applied to the tibia (and perhaps the femur), compartment pressure measurements may be required postoperatively. However, in centers experienced in use of intramedullary nails, there has been

FIGURE 13-6 *An algorithm for management for a patient with suspected compartment syndrome. Δp is defined as the difference between the diastolic pressure and the measured compartment pressure in mm Hg as documented by McQueen and Court-Brown.[71]*

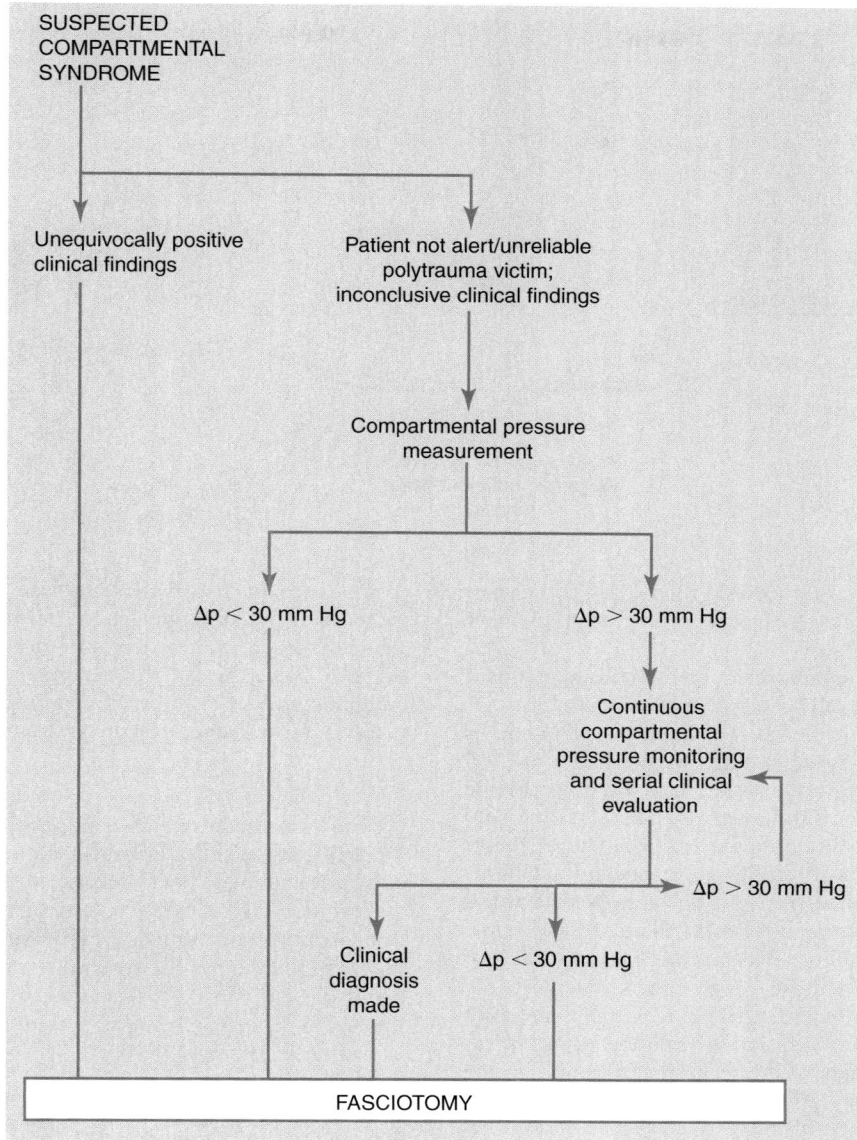

no evidence to support this concern. Some studies have suggested that the problems of compartment syndrome are less with more rapid and rigid stabilization of the fracture. With any active change in management of an acute long bone fracture, however, signs of compartment syndrome should be sought. If this investigation cannot be done clinically, the patient should be considered for compartment pressure measurements.[69,109,119]

Compartment pressure measurements are useful in patients who have undergone successful arterial repair and fasciotomy after a period of limb ischemia. In this situation, if it is difficult to ascertain the efficacy of the fasciotomy, compartment pressure measurement techniques are a valuable adjunct for documenting the adequacy of the decompression.

Measurement Techniques

NEEDLE MANOMETER

The first direct attempt at measurement of interstitial compartment pressure was by Landerer in 1884.[53] Subsequently, French and Price[27] reported on the usefulness of the technique in diagnosis of chronic compartment syndrome. Whitesides and colleagues[123,124] first applied the needle manometer technique to the diagnosis of acute compartment syndrome. In their original description, an 18-gauge needle was connected to a 20-mL syringe by a column of saline and air, and this column was then connected to a standard mercury manometer. After the needle was injected into the compartment, the air pressure within the syringe was raised until the saline-air meniscus

FIGURE 13-7 *The needle injection technique measures compartment pressure by looking for movement of the air-saline meniscus. (Redrawn from Whitesides, T.E., Jr.; Haney, T.C.; Morimoto, K.; Hirada, H. Clin Orthop 113:46, 1975.)*

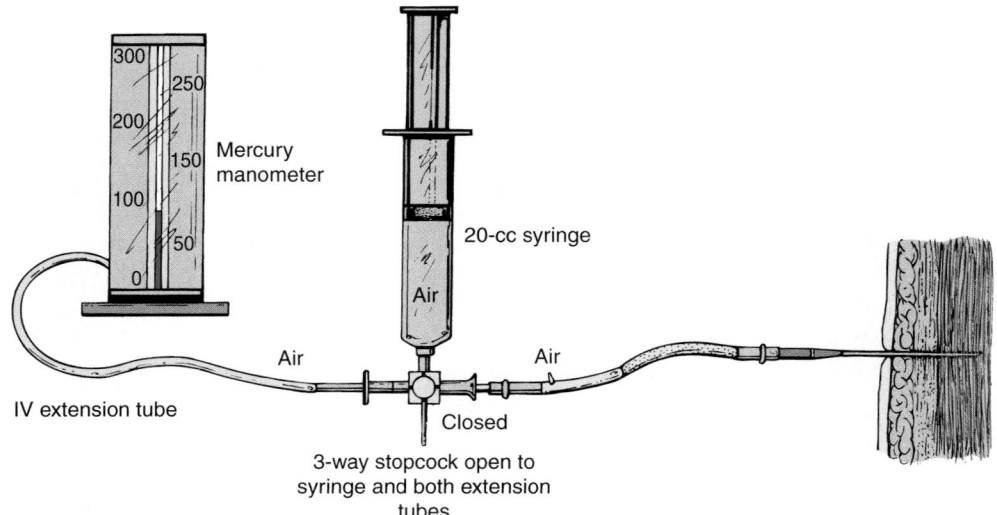

was seen to move. The pressure was then read off the mercury manometer (Fig. 13-7). Details of the technique have been well described.[123,124]

The needle manometer technique employs standard equipment, available in all hospitals. It has the disadvantage of not being as reproducible as other techniques,[101] and it is not suitable for continuous pressure monitoring.[102]

Matsen and co-workers[59,62,64,65,75] modified the needle technique by using a continuous infusion of saline into the compartment. Their technique employed three pieces of equipment attached to an 18-gauge needle and high-pressure tubing. A saline-filled syringe was used to inject the saline through a three-way stopcock transducer dome and high-pressure tubing through the needle and into the compartment (Fig. 13-8). The pressure required to infuse the fluid was recorded. The technique measures the tissue resistance to infusion of saline. According to Mubarak,[76] the accuracy of the technique depends on the compliance of the tissue. Because tissue compliance is reduced at pressures greater than 30 mm Hg, the continuous infusion technique tends to give artificially high readings.[101] Nevertheless, the technique has the advantage of simplicity and allows continuous monitoring of a patient with an acute compartment syndrome.

WICK CATHETER

The wick catheter, which consists of a piece of polyglycolic acid suture pulled into the tip a piece of PE60 polyethylene tubing, was developed by Scholander and colleagues (Fig. 13-9).[106] Originally used to measure tissue pressures in animals, including turtles, snakes, and fish,[104] the technique was subsequently modified for clinical use.[38,39,78,80,83] It was the first technique for measuring intra-compartmental pressure that did not rely on continuous infusion.

The technique requires a catheter placement sleeve and a wick catheter connected to a pressure transducer and recorder. The catheter and tubing are filled by means of a three-way stopcock attached to the transducer. It is calibrated and introduced into the tissues through a large trocar The needle is withdrawn, and the catheter is taped to the skin.

The technique is useful for continuous monitoring of intracompartmental pressure. Its primary disadvantage is that the tip of the catheter may become blocked by a blood clot. In addition, the polyglycolic acid suture can become hydrolyzed.

SLIT CATHETER

The slit catheter technique was originally developed by Rorabeck and associates.[100,101] The slit catheter consists of a piece of PE60 polyethylene tubing with five 3-mm slits in the end of the tube (Fig. 13-10). This design eliminated the risk of leaving the tip of the catheter in the tissues on removal.

FIGURE 13-8 *The continuous infusion technique of compartment pressure measurement. (Redrawn from Matsen, F.A., III; Winquist, R.A.; Krugmire, R.B. J Bone Joint Surg Am 62:286, 1980.)*

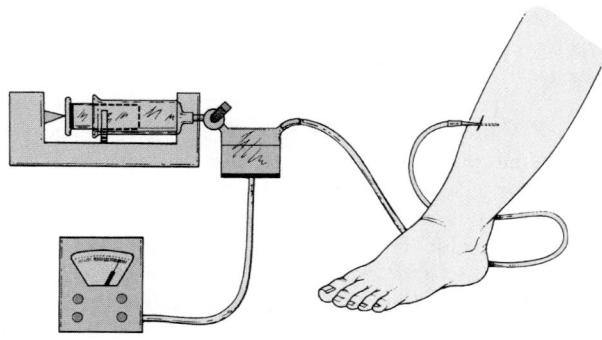

FIGURE 13-9 *A* and *B, The wick catheter.*

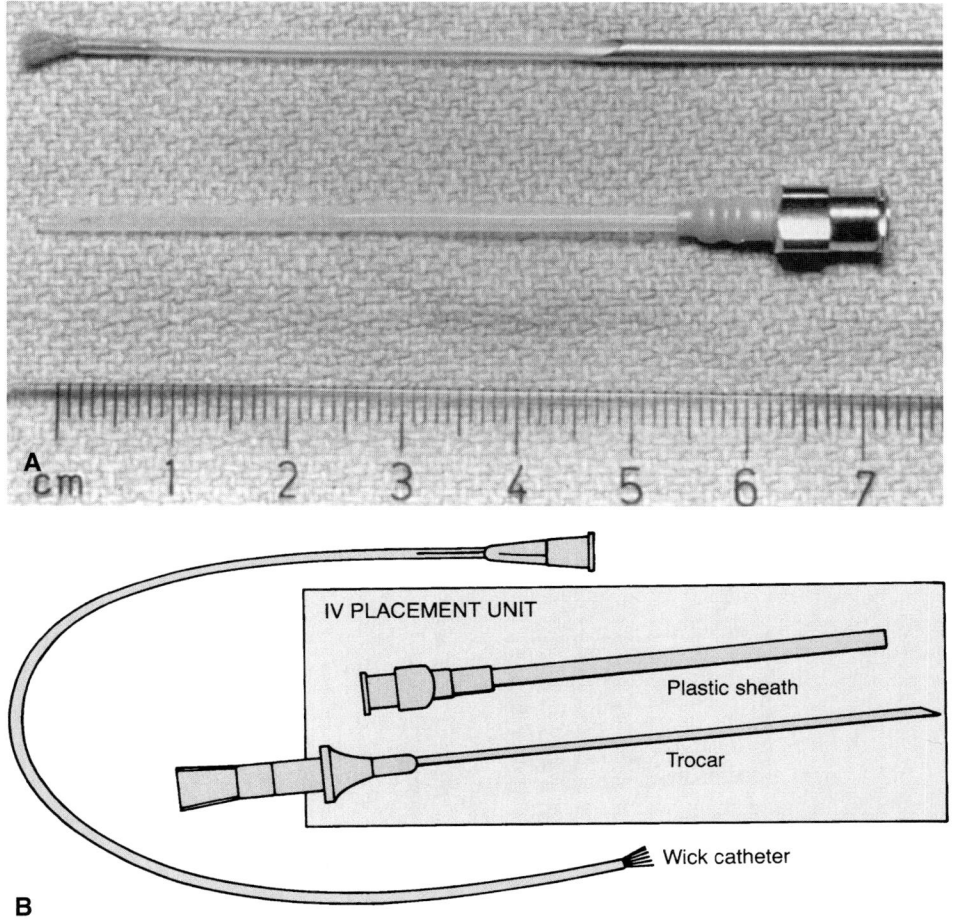

The technique requires a slit catheter, an insertion needle, a pressure transducer connected to a three-way stopcock, and a pressure monitor. The components are connected, and the catheter is filled with sterile saline solution. As with the wick catheter, it is imperative that no air bubbles enter the system. The monitor must be calibrated by placing the tip of the slit catheter level with the transducer dome and adjusting the zero control knob on the monitor until 0.00 appears (Fig. 13-11).

The slit catheter is introduced at an oblique angle to the long axis of the extremity directly into the muscle belly of the compartment to be measured. It is introduced through a 16-gauge needle, which is withdrawn after the catheter has been introduced (Fig. 13-12). The catheter is then taped to the skin. The system can be checked by applying gentle pressure to the skin overlying the catheter. A brisk deflection on the monitor should be noted. Also, if the patient is cooperative, dorsiflexing or plantar flexing of the foot should result in changes on the monitor.

STIC CATHETER SYSTEM

The STIC catheter system manufactured by Stryker is a hand-held device that allows the surgeon to measure acute compartment pressure quickly and simply (Fig. 13-13).

The device is easy to use; it can be carried in the pocket and used in the emergency department without having to search for pieces of equipment. It is potentially as accurate as the slit catheter.

The method of use of this device is relatively simple, which has led to its increase in popularity. The device needs to be adequately "charged" for accurate use. A disposable syringe preloaded with fluid is connected to the measuring instrument, and a disposable needle-catheter that comes as part of the set is then added to the other end. After the system is purged with some fluid, the monitor is zeroed at the level of the compartment to be tested and the needle is then inserted through the fascia. The numbers on the monitor screen fall reasonably rapidly, and as the descent levels off a reading of the compartment pressure can be made. In clinical use of this device, the pressure reading on the monitor may continue to drop slowly with time and some individual variation may occur in determining the pressure at which leveling off has occurred.

MICROCAPILLARY INFUSION

The microcapillary infusion technique described by Styf and Korner[114] was developed primarily to aid in the

FIGURE 13-10 *A* and *B,* The slit catheter monitoring system. Note that the transducer dome is at the same height as the catheter. (*A,* Redrawn from Mubarek, S.J.; Hargens, A.R. Compartment Syndromes and Volkmann's Contracture. Philadelphia, W.B. Saunders, 1980, p. 13. *B,* Reproduced by permission from AAOS Instructional Course Lectures, Vol. 32. St. Louis, C.V. Mosby, 1983, p. 98.)

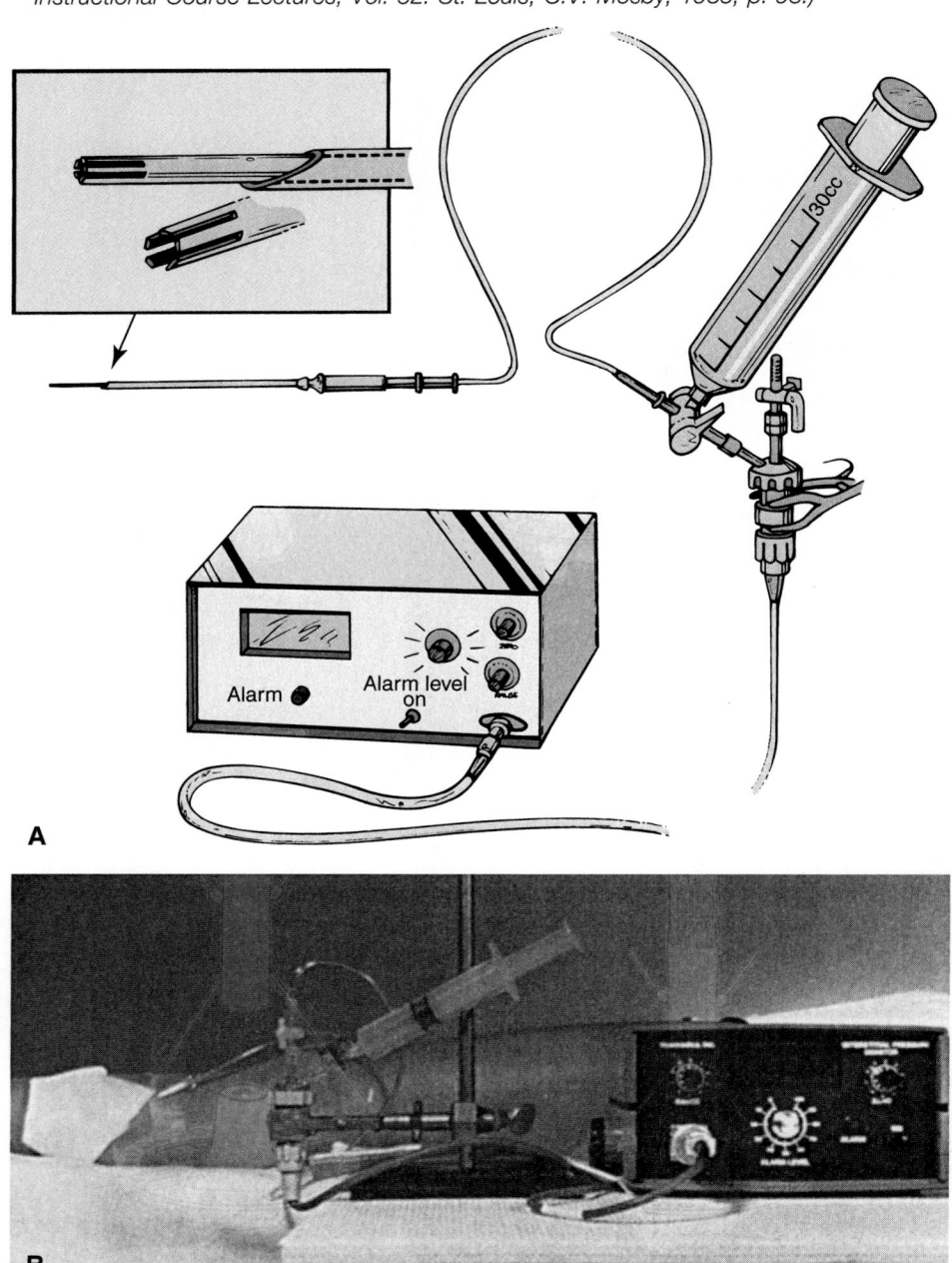

FIGURE 13-11 *The slit catheter technique. **A** (Step 1), Assemble the components, fill the system with normal saline solution, remove all air bubbles, and zero the monitor by placing the catheter level with the transducer dome. Adjust the zero control knob until 0.00 appears. Set the alarm at the desired setting. **B** (Step 2), The transducer dome should be level with the insertion site. Prepare the insertion site and insert a 14-gauge catheter at an acute angle to the long axis of the extremity. (**A, B,** Redrawn by permission from AAOS Instructional Course Lectures, Vol. 32. St. Louis, C.V. Mosby, 1983, pp. 99–101.)*

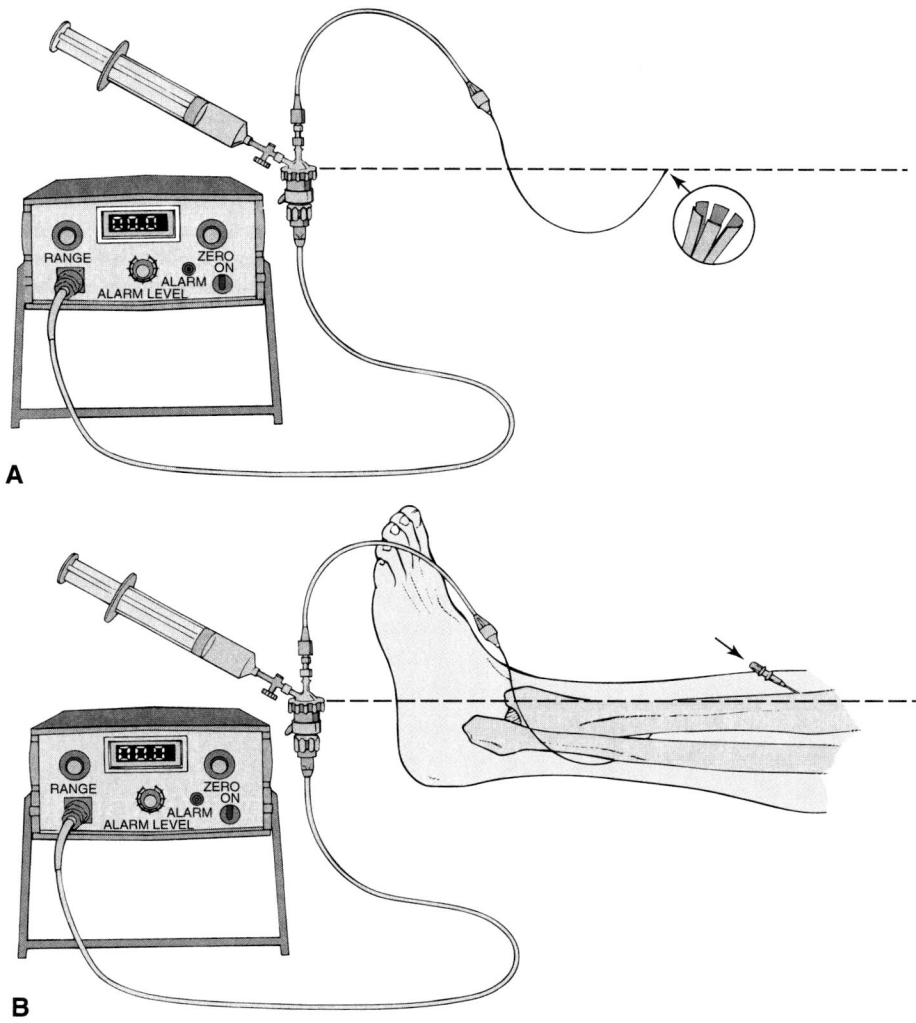

diagnosis of chronic compartment syndrome. It is useful for long-term pressure monitoring and offers excellent dynamic applications.

ARTERIAL TRANSDUCER MEASUREMENT

With advances in technology for arterial pressure monitoring, use of a simple intravenous catheter attached to such pressure transducers has become an alternative for compartment pressure measurement. It is recommended that a catheter of at least 16-gauge diameter be used; the catheter is flushed with saline and connected to the pressure monitor, which is accurately calibrated and set for the level of the compartment being measured. The catheter is placed in the appropriate compartment and the pressure reading taken from an arterial line monitor that is calibrated to the same level as the compartment being measured.

NONINVASIVE TECHNIQUES

Some work has been done on noninvasive techniques of monitoring compartment pressures, mainly in chronic exercise-induced compartment syndrome. These techniques may become more applicable to the investigation of acute compartment syndrome.

Tc 99m-methoxyisobutylisonitrile (Tc 99m-MIBI) scintigraphy was used by Edwards and co-workers[25] to detect regional abnormalities in muscle perfusion with graded treadmill exercise. The method was used as a screening test for invasive pressure monitoring and gave good positive and negative predictive values.

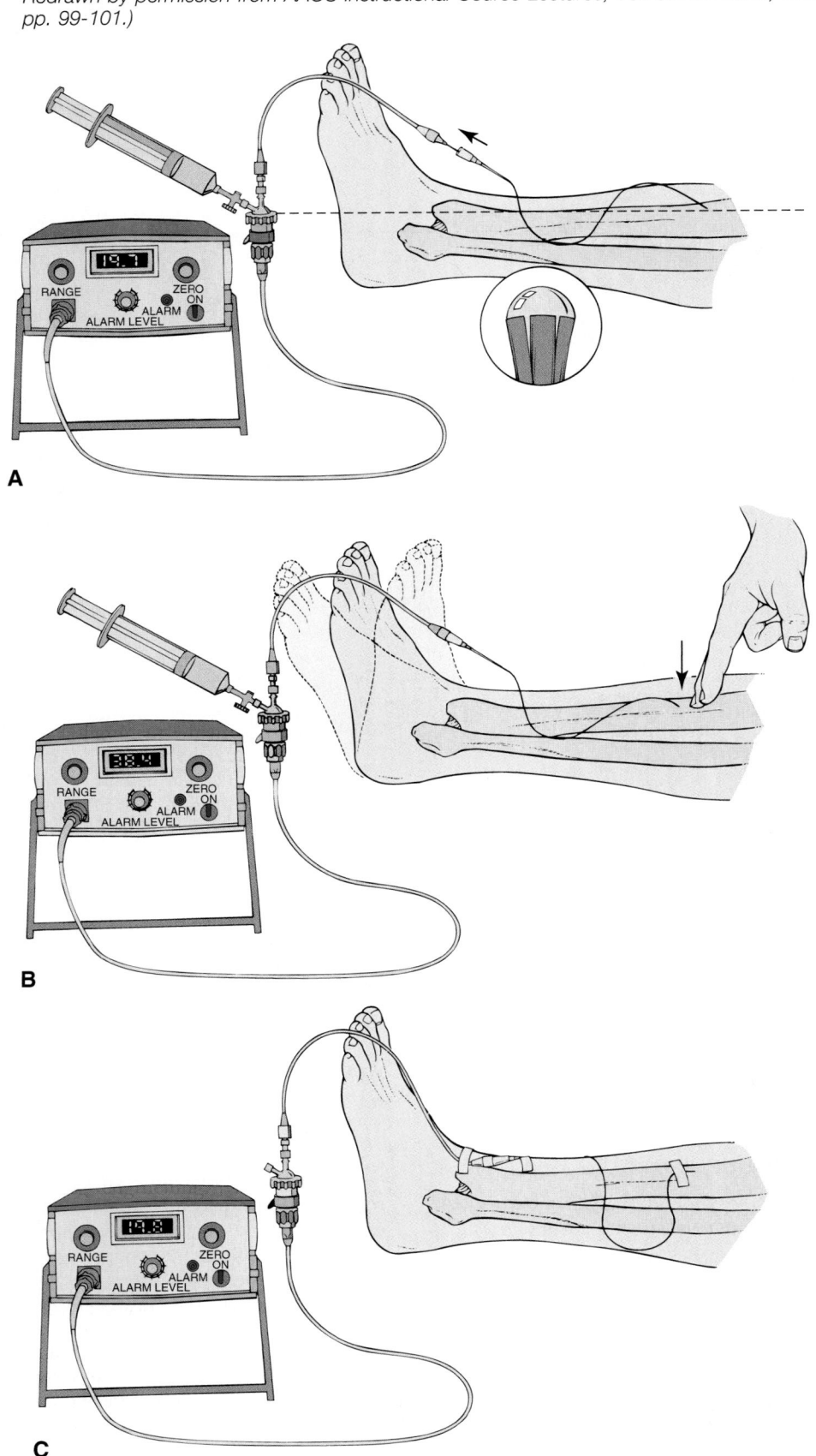

FIGURE 13-12   **A** (Step 3), Raise a drop of saline solution at the tip of the catheter and insert the catheter through the placement sleeve. Withdraw the sleeve. **B** (Step 4), Check the response by plantar flexion and dorsiflexion of the foot and digital pressure to the compartment. The monitor pressure will show a brisk rise in pressure readings. **C,** Remove the syringe, and record intermittent or continuous pressure as required. (**A–C,** Redrawn by permission from AAOS Instructional Course Lectures, Vol. 32. St. Louis, C.V. Mosby, 1983, pp. 99-101.)

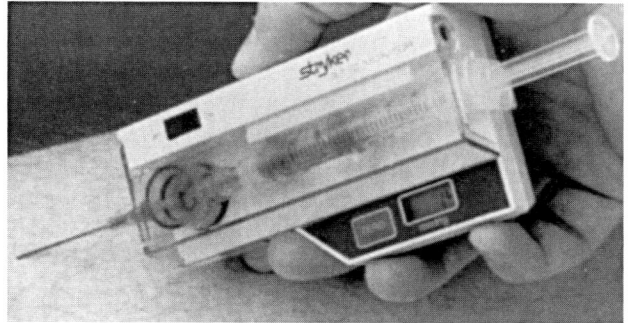

FIGURE 13-13 *The STIC catheter. (Courtesy of Stryker, Mississauga, Ontario, Canada.)*

Abraham and colleagues[2] used laser Doppler flow measurement in a small number of patients with chronic compartment syndrome and a control group and showed clear differences between the control and compartment syndrome groups.

Near-infrared spectroscopy has similarly been used to measure changes in relative oxygenation in a compartment after exercise and was useful in monitoring the rapid return to normal seen in control patients compared with those with chronic compartment syndrome.[35] Establishing normal values for patients with acute compartment syndrome using this technique has some potential application, although there appears to be a range of preoperative measurements in patients with established compartment syndrome with quite a large variation between individuals.[35]

COMPARISON OF TECHNIQUES

Moed and Thorderson[74] compared the slit catheter, the side-ported needle, and the simple needle techniques in an animal model. Use of an 18-gauge needle produced significantly higher values (18 to 19 mm Hg) than the other two techniques, raising some question about its reliability. Wilson and colleagues[127] showed that use of a simple 16-gauge catheter with or without side ports produced measurements within 4 to 5 mm Hg of the slit catheter or STIC catheter readings.

Pressure Threshold for Fasciotomy

Historically, there has been disagreement about the pressure beyond which fasciotomy can be safely performed. Part of the confusion arises because of failure to appreciate the physiologic differences in the various pressure measurement systems. For example, in the needle manometer techniques, with or without continuous infusion, relatively higher values are acceptable, and values vary according to tissue compliance. With the wick, slit, or STIC catheter systems, continuous infusion is not used, and therefore the published values beyond which fasciotomy should be performed are somewhat lower.[78,83,100] Whitesides and colleagues[123] have recommended fasciotomy when compartment pressure rises to within 10 to 30 mm Hg of the patient's diastolic pressure, assuming that the patient has the clinical signs of acute compartment syndrome. Matsen and co-workers[62,64,65] have suggested that, with

the continuous infusion technique, fasciotomy should be performed when the pressure rises above 45 mm Hg.

Another important variable, as outlined by Heckman and associates,[41] is the distance from the fracture at which the compartment pressure is recorded. They concluded that failure to measure tissue pressure within a few centimeters of the fracture (the "zone of peak pressure") can result in serious underestimation of the maximal compartment pressure.

As the indications and sites for compartment pressure monitoring increase with improved techniques, the normal values for various compartments need to be clearly documented. Whether the normal pressure in a small compartment of the hand is the same as that in the gluteal compartment is not known. If any doubt exists, it is safest to rely as much on clinical examination as on the measured compartment pressure.

Others have recommended that decompression be performed when the compartment pressure exceeds 30 to 35 mm Hg.[75,78,101] Although it is tempting to use an absolute value as an indication for decompression, the measurement obtained must be considered with regard to the patient's clinical condition and, more important, the patient's diastolic blood pressure. For example, if a patient is in shock, with a low diastolic blood pressure, an acute compartment syndrome can occur at considerably lower pressure.[44,124] Conversely, when a patient's diastolic pressure is extremely high, an acute compartment syndrome is not likely to occur at the usual pressure threshold. All the compartment pressure measurement techniques are useful, but it is important for the surgeon to understand the pitfalls and limitations of the technique being used.

McQueen and Court-Brown[71] clearly demonstrated that the difference between diastolic pressure and the measured compartment pressure (Δp) is a more reliable clinical indicator of pending compartment syndrome than the absolute compartment pressure. Their recommendation was that a difference of less than 30 mm Hg is surgically significant. Their continued work in this area strongly supports the use of Δp with a threshold of 30 mm or less as the most reliable method of deciding when fasciotomies should be performed. This recommendation is particularly relevant to the monitoring of patients who may have a low diastolic pressure because of blood loss, sedation, or ventilatory support.

Treatment

A major cause of medico-legal problems for surgeons who treat fractures is failure to diagnose and treat a vascular injury or compartment syndrome appropriately. The only effective way to decompress an acute compartment syndrome is by surgical fasciotomy. It cannot be overemphasized how important it is to understand the basic pathophysiology so that the surgeon can recognize the at-risk patient and intervene before the development of irreversible damage to the contents of the compartment.

Incipient Compartment Syndrome

An incipient compartment syndrome is defined as a compartment syndrome that may develop if appropriate steps are not taken to prevent it. An established compartment syndrome obviously must be treated surgically with emergency decompression. With an incipient compartment syndrome, there are some things that the surgeon can do to reduce the chances of the patient's developing a full-blown compartment syndrome.

It is imperative to remove tight dressings and casts in patients complaining of an inordinate amount of pain. Garfin and colleagues,[30] using a canine model, observed that 40 percent less volume was required to raise compartment pressure to equivalent levels in animals with casts than in those without casts. They also demonstrated that the compartment pressure in the hind limb of an animal could be reduced by up to 30 percent by changing to a univalve cast. If a bivalve cast was originally used and the sheet wadding underneath was divided, a 55 percent decrease in compartment pressure occurred. Others have noted that constricting bandages are causative factors in limb ischemia.[9,11,57,68] Implicit in these observations is that removal of casts, tight dressings, or both is an important and simple technique for lowering compartment pressure within the extremity and therefore for maintaining arterial perfusion of muscle and nerve.

Controversy exists about the importance of limb position in a patient with an incipient compartment syndrome. Although it would seem to be a good idea to elevate the swollen extremity, it has been shown experimentally and clinically that limb elevation reduces mean arterial pressure in the arteries of the lower extremity and thereby reduces blood flow to the compartment.[7,66] Elevation can also reduce the arterial venous gradient within the extremity, which increases the susceptibility of the extremity to a compartment syndrome by reducing oxygen perfusion.[60] Therefore, in a patient with an incipient compartment syndrome, the limb should be placed at the level of the heart to promote arterial inflow.

Established Compartment Syndrome

A patient with an established compartment syndrome has the clinical signs and symptoms of nerve and muscle ischemia in conjunction with elevated compartment pressure. A treatment algorithm (see Fig. 13-6) is a useful guide to management for such patients.

Any surgical decompression for acute compartment syndrome must adequately decompress all compartments that are at risk or likely to become at risk. Skin, fat, and fascial layers must all be widely decompressed and left open. Matsen and co-workers[59,64] have shown that each layer contributes to the constriction of the muscle compartment, and attempts at closure of part or all of any one of these layers at the time of fasciotomy risk endangering muscle.

COMPARTMENT SYNDROME OF THE HAND

Compartment syndromes of the hand are rare, and the diagnosis can be difficult to make.[92] The diagnostic triad described by Spinner and associates,[111] stretch pain involving intrinsic muscles and intrinsic paralysis, is a hallmark of the condition. It normally occurs as a result of a crush injury but can also occur in association with fractures of the carpal bone.[3,111] Other causes have been reported.[1,3,40,95]

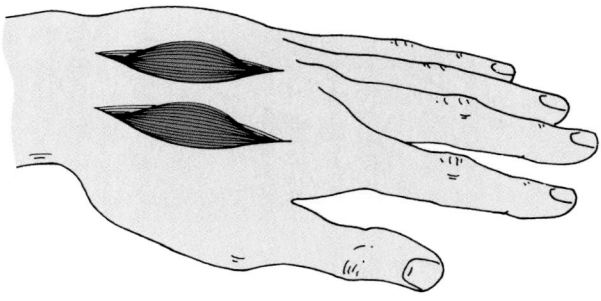

FIGURE 13-14 *Dorsal incisions for decompression of acute compartment syndrome of the hand. (From Mubarak, S.J.; Hargens, A.R. Compartment Syndromes and Volkmann's Contracture. Philadelphia, W.B. Saunders, 1981.)*

The most commonly involved compartments of the hand are the interossei. These can usually be decompressed by longitudinal dorsal incisions (Fig. 13-14).

COMPARTMENT SYNDROME OF THE FOREARM

Compartment syndrome of the forearm is again relatively rare. It is usually associated with a fracture with a direct blow or crushing component of the injury. Court-Brown and McQueen's review of their experience showed that forearm compartment syndrome tended to occur with associated fractures of the distal radius. It has also been seen with inadvertent soft tissue fluid infiltration, grease-gun injuries, and deep infection often associated with intravenous drug abuse. Attempted closure of a tight surgical wound after internal fixation of forearm injuries may also place these compartments at risk.

The forearm consists of three osseofascial compartments—the superficial flexor, the deep flexor, and the extensor compartments.

Fasciotomies of the volar flexor compartments of the forearm are performed through a volar ulnar approach or a volar (Henry) approach. Fasciotomy of the dorsal compartment of the forearm is normally approached through a Thompson exposure. Garber[29] recommended a limited fasciotomy in the forearm, accomplished simply by incising the antecubital aponeurosis, but this did not prove to be effective. Eaton and Green[23] suggested that forearm decompression for an acute compartment syndrome could best be accomplished through a standard Henry approach. Whitesides and colleagues[123] recommended the volar ulnar approach to the forearm. This technique was subsequently adopted by Matsen and co-workers.[63] Gelberman and colleagues[32,33] found that the standard Henry approach and the volar ulnar approach were equally effective for fasciotomy to decompress an acute compartment syndrome of the volar compartment. Regardless of technique, it is mandatory that both the superficial and deep volar compartments be decompressed.

VOLAR (HENRY) APPROACH Decompression of the superficial and deep volar flexor compartments of the

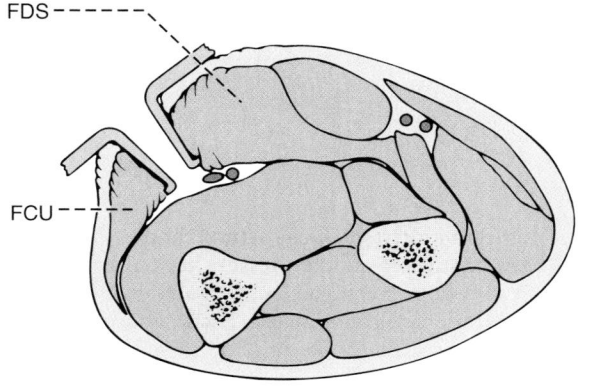

FIGURE 13-15 *The Henry approach to the volar aspects of the forearm. (Modified from Whitesides, T., Jr.; Haney, T.C.; Morimoto, K.; Hirada, H. Clin Orthop 113:46, 1975.)*

FDS

FCU

forearm can be done through a single incision (Fig. 13-15). The skin incision should begin proximal to the antecubital fossa and extend to the palm across the carpal tunnel. Compartmental pressure measurements can be taken intraoperatively to confirm decompression. No tourniquet should be used. The skin incision begins medial to the biceps tendon, crosses the elbow crease, is carried toward the radial side of the forearm, and extends distally along the medial border of the brachioradialis, continuing across the palm along the thenar crease. The fascia overlying the superficial flexor compartment is readily incised, beginning at a point 1 or 2 cm proximal to the elbow and extending distally across the carpal tunnel into the palm. Anything short of this is viewed as an inadequate decompression (Fig. 13-16).

The superficial radial nerve is identified under the brachioradialis, both are retracted to the radial side of the forearm, and the flexor carpi radialis and radial artery are retracted to the ulnar side. This action exposes the flexor digitorum profundus and flexor pollicis longus in the depths, the pronator quadratus distally, and the pronator teres proximally. Because the effects of forearm compartment syndrome most commonly involve the deep flexor compartment in the forearm, it is imperative to decompress the fascia over each of these muscles to ensure that a thorough and complete decompression has been performed. Eaton and Green[23] recommended epimysiotomy in addition to fasciotomy, but this is not usually necessary in the acute case. Muscle viability is difficult to ascertain intraoperatively. Questionably viable muscle should be excised with caution at the time of fasciotomy. The patient should be brought back to the operating room 24 to 48 hours later for a dressing change and further débridement of muscle. The median nerve should be carefully inspected; if it appears excessively swollen, a neurolysis of the nerve should be performed.

VOLAR ULNAR APPROACH The volar ulnar approach is performed in a similar fashion to the Henry approach. The arm is supinated and the incision is begun proximally medial to the biceps tendon, passes the elbow crease, extends distally along the ulnar border of the forearm, and proceeds across the carpal tunnel along the thenar crease (Fig. 13-17). The superficial fascia overlying the flexor carpi ulnaris is incised along with the elbow

FIGURE 13-17 *Ulnar approach to the volar flexor compartment of the forearm. (Modified from Whitesides, T., Jr.; Haney, T.C.; Morimoto, K.; Hirada, H. Clin Orthop 113:46, 1975.)*

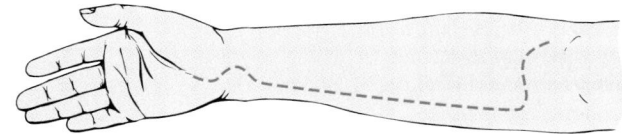

FIGURE 13-16 **A,** *A transverse section through the midforearm illustrating relevant anatomy of the volar flexor compartment. BR, brachioradialis; ECRB, extensor carpi radialis brevis; FCR, flexor carpi radialis; FCU, flexor carpi ulnaris; FDS, flexor digitorum sublimis.* **B,** *The Henry approach to superficial and deep compartments of the forearm. (**A, B,** Modified with permission from AAOS Instructional Course Lectures, Vol. 32. St. Louis, C.V. Mosby, 1983, p. 106.)*

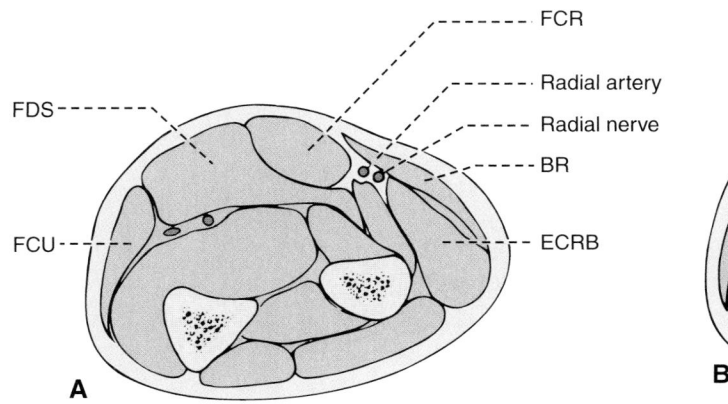

FDS

FCU

- - - - - - FCR
- - - - - - Radial artery
- - - - - - Radial nerve
- - - - - - BR
- - - - - - ECRB

A

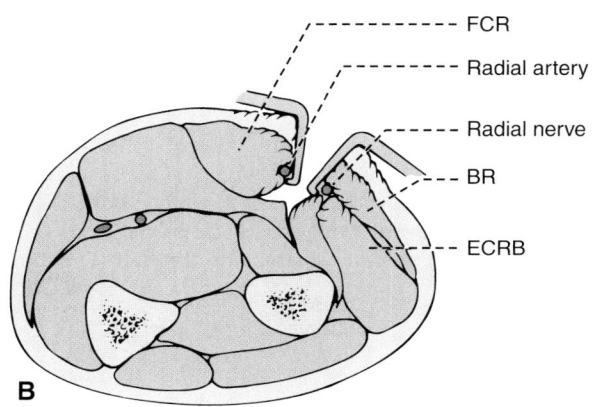

- - - - - - FCR
- - - - - - Radial artery
- - - - - - Radial nerve
- - - - BR
- - - - - - ECRB

B

FIGURE 13-18 | *Ulnar approach to the superficial and deep compartments. Note the ulnar vessels in the depths overlying the deep flexor compartments. FCU, flexor carpi ulnaris; FDS, flexor digitorum sublimis. (Modified with permission from AAOS Instructional Course Lectures, Vol. 32. St. Louis, C.V. Mosby, 1983, p. 105.)*

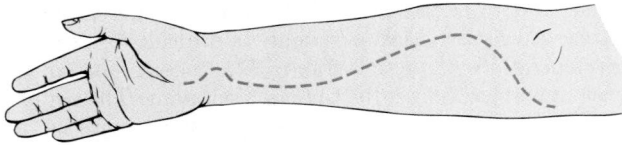

FIGURE 13-20 | *Dorsal approach to the extensor compartment of the forearm. (Redrawn with permission from AAOS Instructional Course Lectures, Vol. 32. St. Louis, C.V. Mosby, 1983, p. 107.)*

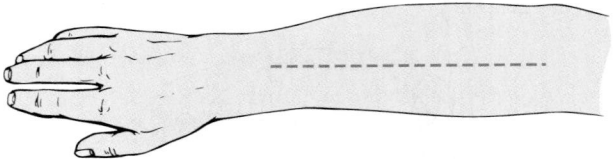

aponeurosis proximally and the carpal tunnel distally. The interval between the flexor carpi ulnaris and flexor digitorum sublimis is identified. Lying deep to the flexor digitorum sublimis and approaching from the radial to the ulnar side are the ulnar nerve and artery, which must be identified and carefully protected (Fig. 13-18). The fascia overlying the deep flexor compartment is now incised. If necessary, the ulnar nerve can be decompressed distally at the level of the wrist and a neurolysis of the median nerve at the level of the carpal tunnel can be performed (Fig. 13-19).

DORSAL APPROACH After the superficial and deep flexor compartments of the forearm have been decompressed, it must be decided whether a fasciotomy of the dorsal (extensor) compartment is necessary. The need is best determined by pressure measurements made in the

operating room after the flexor compartment fasciotomies have been completed. If the pressure continues to be elevated in the dorsal compartment, fasciotomy should be performed with the arm pronated. A straight incision from the lateral epicondyle to the midline of the wrist is used. The interval between the extensor carpi radialis brevis and the extensor digitorum communis is identified, and fasciotomy is performed (Fig. 13-20).

COMPARTMENT SYNDROME OF THE LEG

For an acute compartment syndrome of the lower extremity, three decompression techniques are available. The technique chosen should allow access to all four compartments. The three techniques for the leg are fibulectomy, perifibular fasciotomy, and double-incision fasciotomy. There is no indication for subcutaneous fasciotomy in acute compartment syndrome of the leg.

FIBULECTOMY Although fibulectomy certainly decompresses all four compartments of the leg, this technique,

FIGURE 13-19 | *A and B, Ulnar approach to the forearm between the flexor carpi ulnaris and the flexor digitorum sublimis. (A, B, Modified with permission from AAOS Instructional Course Lectures, Vol. 32. St. Louis, C.V. Mosby, 1983, p. 105.)*

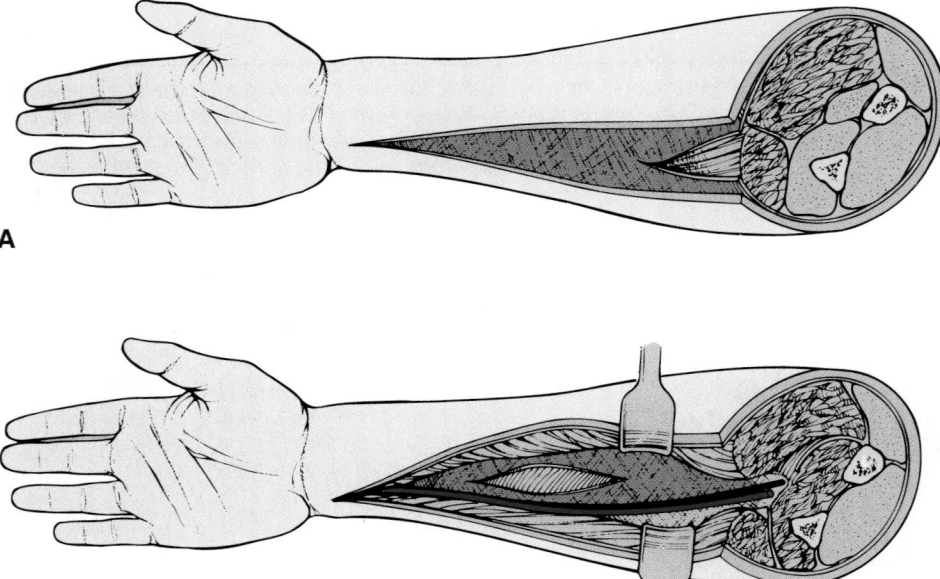

A

B

described by Patman and Thompson[88] and popularized by Kelly and Whitesides,[50] is unnecessary and is too radical a procedure to perform. It is now of only historical interest.

PERIFIBULAR FASCIOTOMY The perifibular fasciotomy, popularized by Matsen and co-workers,[64] allows access to all four compartments of the leg through a single lateral incision that extends proximally from the head of the fibula and distally to the ankle, following the general line of the fibula. The skin incision is made, the skin and subcutaneous tissues are retracted proximally, and the intermuscular septum between the anterior and lateral

compartments is identified. Care must be taken to identify and protect the superficial peroneal nerve. A fasciotomy is performed 1 cm in front of the intermuscular septum (anterior compartment) and 1 cm posterior to the intermuscular septum (lateral compartment) (Fig. 13-21A and B). The superficial posterior compartment is readily identified, and a fasciotomy is performed (Fig. 13-21C). The interval between the peroneal compartment and the superficial posterior compartment is entered by retracting the peroneal compartment anteriorly and the superficial posterior compartment posteriorly to expose the deep posterior compartment. The deep posterior compartment is

FIGURE 13-21   **A,** *A lateral incision is made over the peroneal compartment (2).* **B,** *A skin incision is retracted anteriorly, exposing the anterior compartment (1).* **C,** *The posterior skin incision is retracted posteriorly, and the fascia overlying the superficial posterior compartment (3) is incised.*

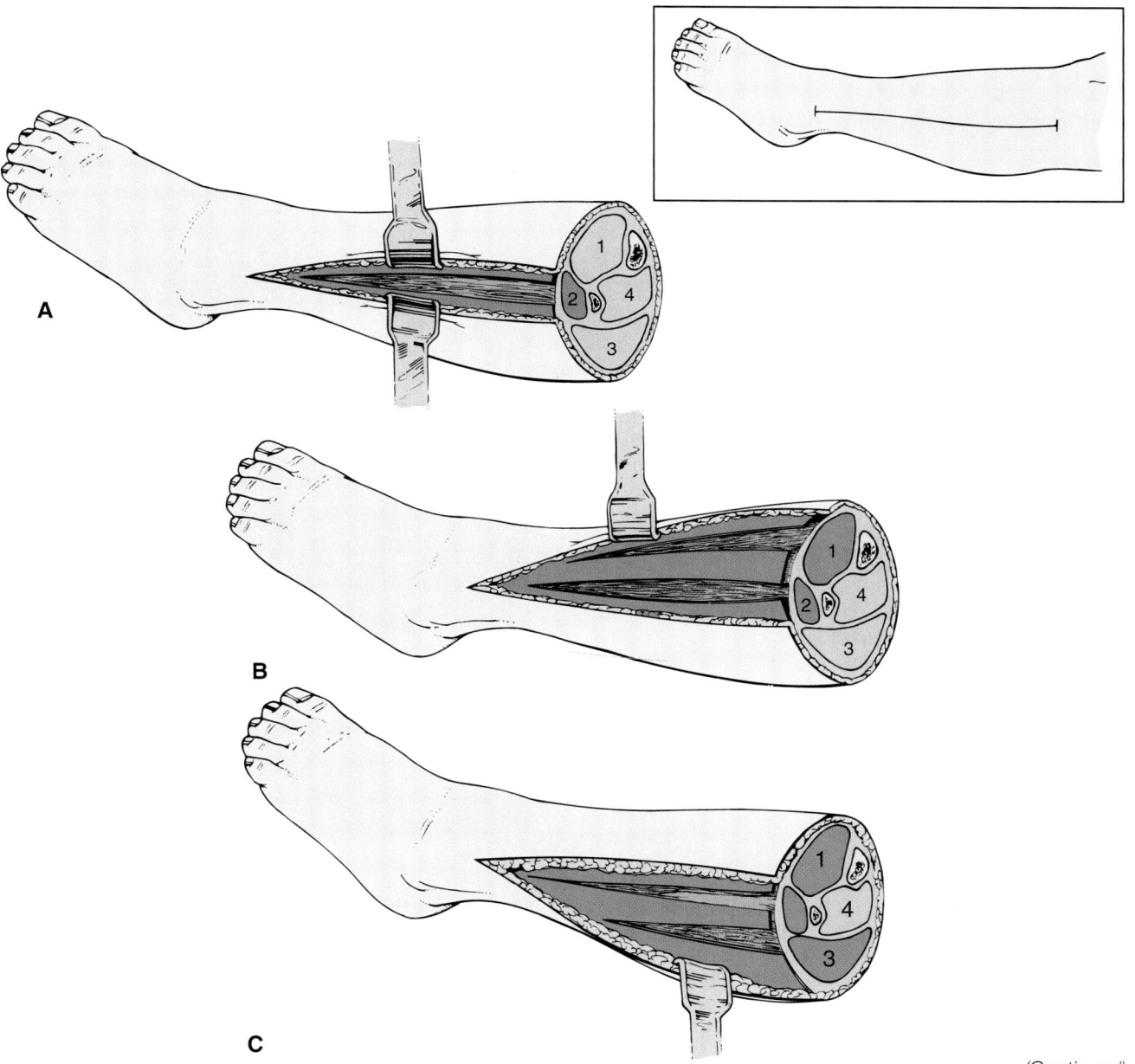

FIGURE 13-21   *(Continued) **D,** The peroneal and superficial posterior compartments are now retracted, and the fascia overlying the deep posterior compartment (4) is incised. (**A–D,** Redrawn from Seligson, D. Concepts in Intramedullary Nailing. Orlando, FL, Grune & Stratton, 1985, pp. 114-115.)*

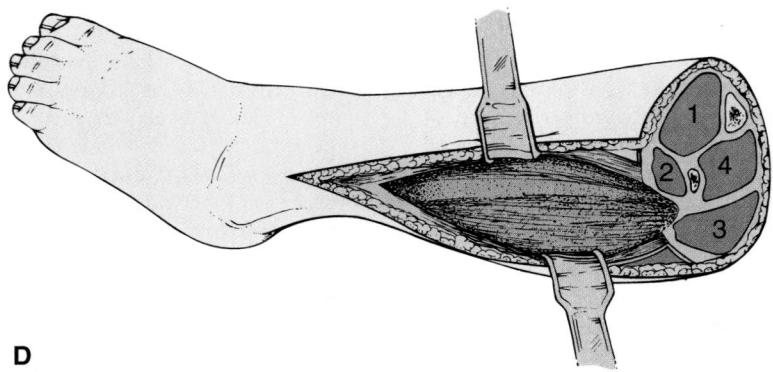

D

reached by following the interosseous membrane from the posterior aspect of the fibula and releasing the compartment from this membrane (Fig. 13-21D). Care must be taken proximally because the peroneal nerve can be injured, particularly in compartment syndrome secondary to trauma, in which the anatomy may be badly distorted. It can also be difficult to be sure of having decompressed all compartments in a badly mangled extremity.

DOUBLE-INCISION TECHNIQUE   The double-incision fasciotomy employs two vertical skin incisions separated by a bridge of skin at least 8 cm wide (Figs. 13-22 and 13-23).[82,99] The first skin incision extends from the knee to the ankle and is centered over the interval between the anterior and lateral compartments. The second incision also extends from the knee to the ankle and is centered 1 to 2 cm behind the posteromedial border of the tibia. The skin

FIGURE 13-22   ***A,*** *The double-incision technique for performing fasciotomies of all four compartments of the lower extremity.* ***B,*** *Cross section of lower extremity showing a position of anterolateral and posteromedial incisions that allows access to the anterior and lateral compartments (1 and 2) and the superficial and deep posterior compartments (3 and 4). (**A, B,** Modified with permission from AAOS Instructional Course Lectures, Vol. 32. St. Louis, C.V. Mosby, 1983, p. 110.)*

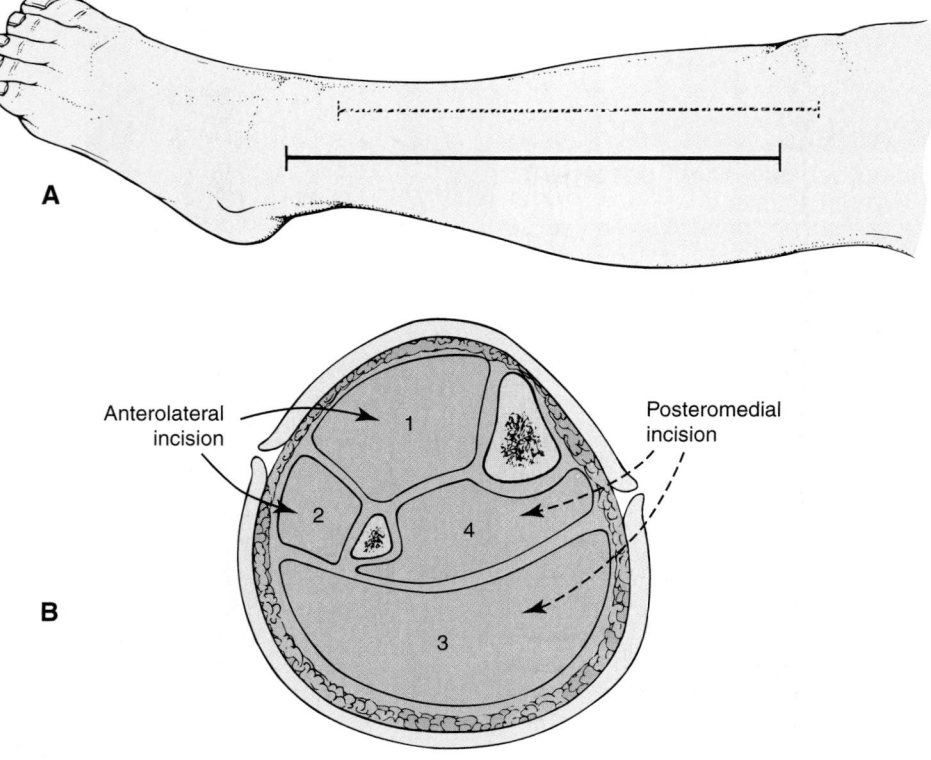

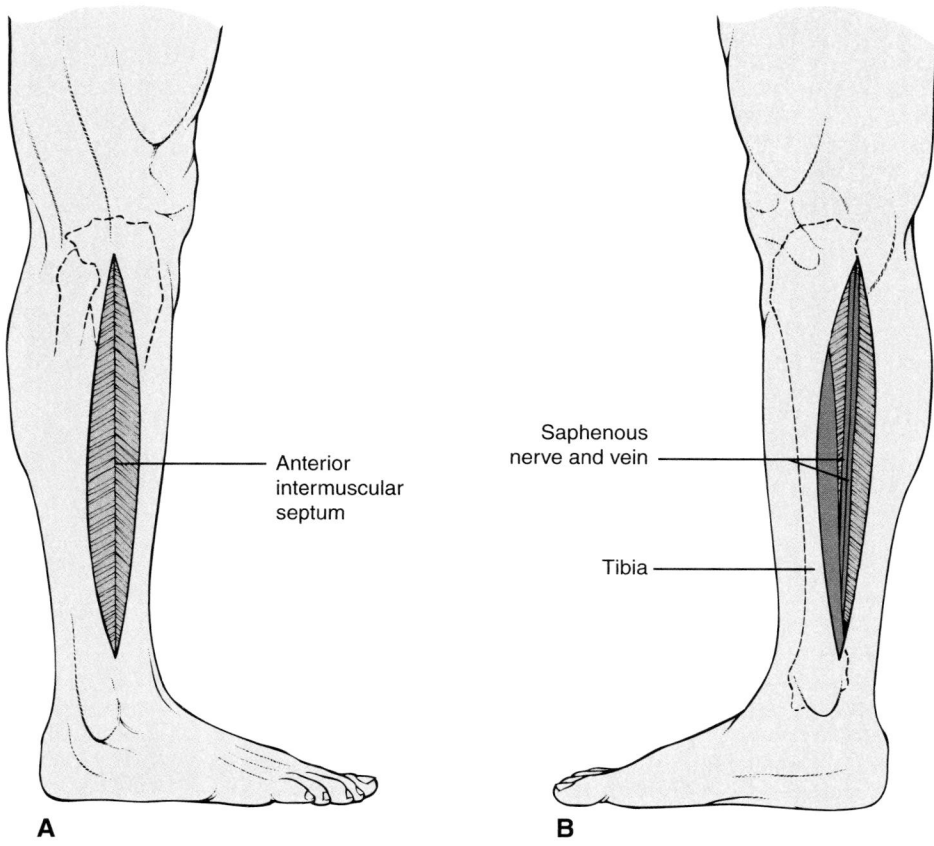

FIGURE 13-23 | **A,** A vertical anterior incision is centered midway between the tibia and the fibula. The anterior intermuscular septum is identified, and two fasciotomy incisions are made, one anterior and one posterior to the septum. **B,** A vertical posteromedial incision is centered 2 cm to the rear of the tibia. Care is taken to avoid injury to the saphenous vein and nerve. (**A, B,** Redrawn with permission from AAOS Instructional Course Lectures, Vol. 32. St. Louis, C.V. Mosby, 1983, pp. 519-520.)

Anterior intermuscular septum

Saphenous nerve and vein

Tibia

A

B

and subcutaneous tissue are separated from the fascia overlying the anterior and lateral compartments after completion of the vertical anterior incision. Care must be taken to identify and protect the superficial peroneal nerve. A fasciotomy of the anterior compartment 1 cm in front of the intermuscular septum is performed, followed by a fasciotomy of the lateral compartment 1 cm behind the intermuscular septum. It is imperative to extend the fasciotomy distally beyond the musculotendinous junction and proximally as far as the origin of the muscle.

The posteromedial incision is made (described previously), with care taken to protect the saphenous vein and nerve. The fascia overlying the gastrocnemius-soleus complex is incised, exposing the deep posterior compartment of the distal third of the leg. To decompress the deep posterior compartment adequately in the proximal direction, it is necessary to detach part of the soleal bridge from the back of the tibia. Doing so exposes the fascia overlying the flexor digitorum longus and the deep posterior compartment, which is then incised, completing the fasciotomy of the deep posterior compartment of the leg (Fig. 13-24). The double-incision technique is relatively

FIGURE 13-24 | Release of the deep posterior compartment through the posterior tibial periosteum.

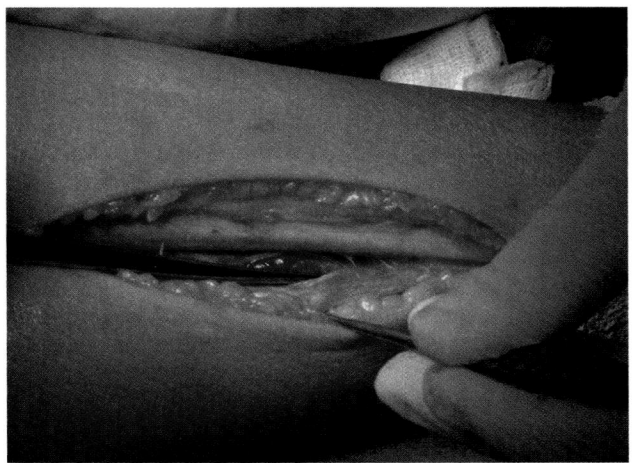

FIGURE 13-25 *A double-incision fasciotomy for acute compartment syndrome.*

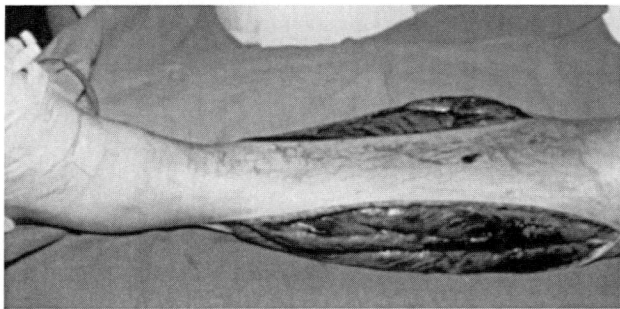

easy to perform. It has the disadvantage of requiring two incisions, which may be inappropriate, particularly in a trauma patient and especially if it results in leaving bone, nerve, or vessel exposed (Fig. 13-25).

COMPARTMENT SYNDROME OF THE THIGH

Compartment syndromes of the thigh, once thought to be rare, are being reported more frequently.[8,69,96,108] According to Schwartz and associates,[108] compartment syndrome can occur in patients undergoing closed intramedullary nailing of the femur; to some extent, its development depends on the Injury Severity Score and the amount of soft tissue damage to the thigh. There is a concern that overdistraction at the time of closed intramedullary nailing, which in effect decreases the compartment volume, can produce a compartment syndrome.

The thigh consists of three muscle compartments—the quadriceps, hamstrings, and adductors. McLaren and co-workers[69] reported an isolated case of adductor compartment syndrome of the thigh, but compartment syndromes

seen as a complication of closed intramedullary nailing usually involve the quadriceps compartment.

The surgical approach recommended depends on the compartment involved, which can be determined by pressure measurements. If the quadriceps compartment is involved, a single anterolateral incision is made along the length of the thigh, splitting the iliotibial band, and the fascia overlying the vastus lateralis is divided along its length (Fig.13-26). The hamstring compartment can then be entered by dividing the intermuscular septum, taking care to avoid further injury to perforating vessels. Release of the adductor compartment, if it is necessary, should be performed through a separate longitudinal incision along its length.

COMPARTMENT SYNDROME OF THE FOOT

Like those of the hand, the interosseous muscles of the foot are bound and contained within compartments. Failure to diagnose an acute compartment syndrome of the intrinsic muscles of the foot can result in myoneural necrosis and subsequent claw-toe deformity.[13] It is seen most commonly after calcaneal fractures, Lisfranc injuries, or significant blunt trauma to the foot.

In our experience, the clinical findings for a patient with acute compartment syndrome of the foot are always equivocal. It is difficult to sort out local pain and tenderness to palpation in this area. Also, stretch pain in the foot is not as reliable a sign as it is in the hand. Therefore, the diagnosis must depend on compartment pressure monitoring. However, because no documentation of the normal compartment pressures in the foot is available, clinical suspicion is required to identify patients requiring fasciotomy.

The compartments of the foot are the medial, central, lateral, and interosseous, all of which must be decompressed (Fig. 13-27). A calcaneal compartment that includes the quadratus plantae muscle has also been

FIGURE 13-26 *Fasciotomy of the thigh (medial compartment).*

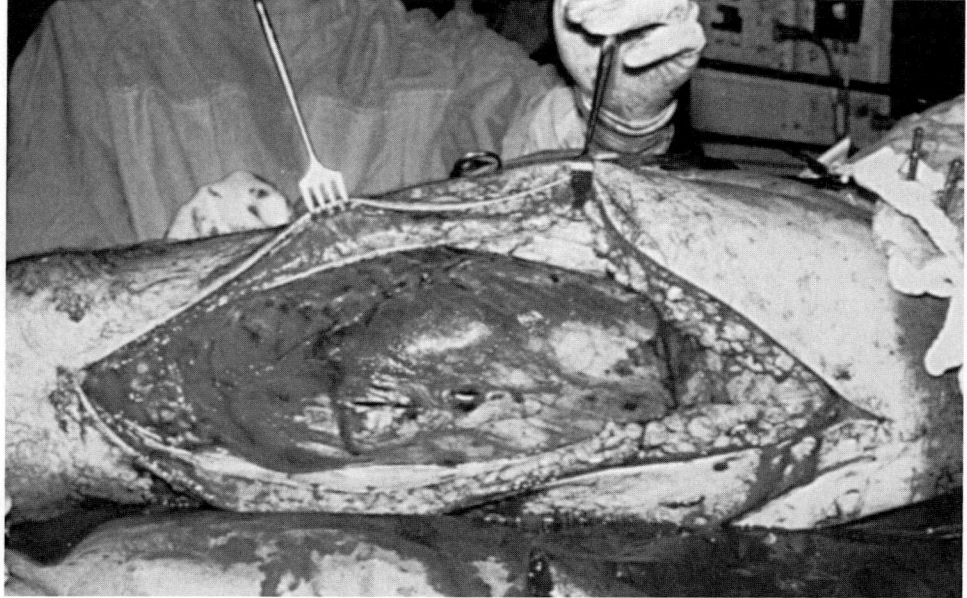

FIGURE 13-27 *Compartments of the foot. Similar detail can be seen with magnetic resonance imaging. (Redrawn with permission from AAOS. Orthopaedic Knowledge Update: Foot and Ankle. Rosemont, IL, American Academy of Orthopaedic Surgeons, 1994, p. 263.)*

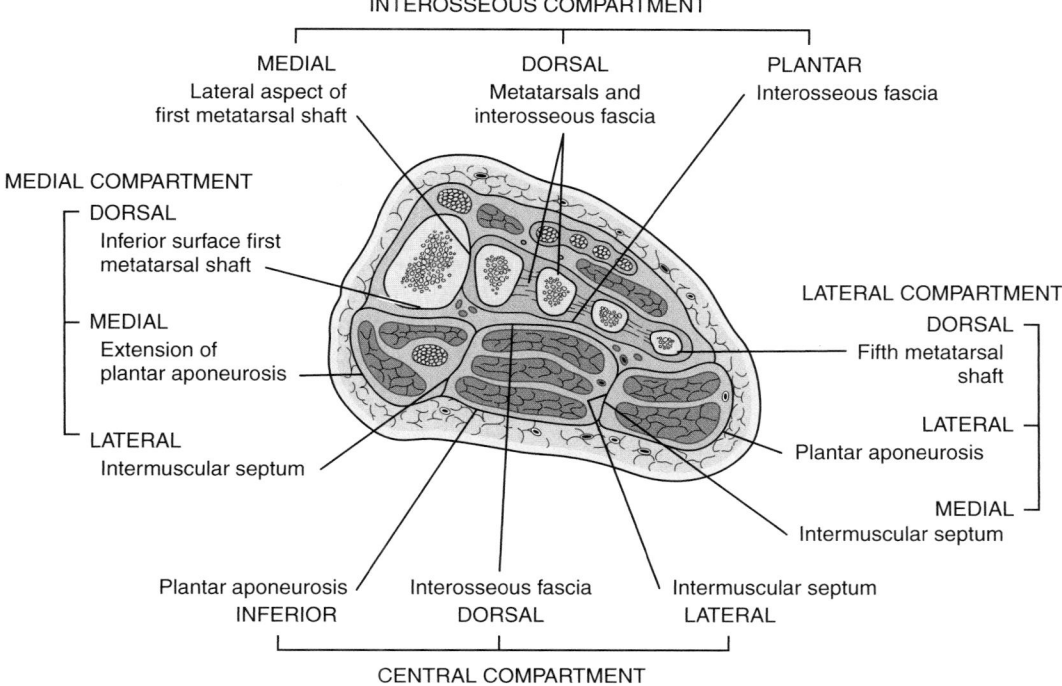

described.[55] After the diagnosis has been made, decompression of the foot can be carried out by a variety of techniques. Two incisions can be used—a dorsal incision that allows exposure of the interossei and a medial incision that allows exposure of the deep flexor muscles. A single medial incision or two dorsal incisions have also been described, and their use is in part determined by the nature of the injury and other treatment objectives (Fig. 13-28).

FIGURE 13-28 *Incisions available for decompression of foot compartment syndromes. (Redrawn with permission from AAOS. Orthopaedic Knowledge Update: Foot and Ankle. Rosemont, IL, American Academy of Orthopaedic Surgeons, 1994, p. 264.)*

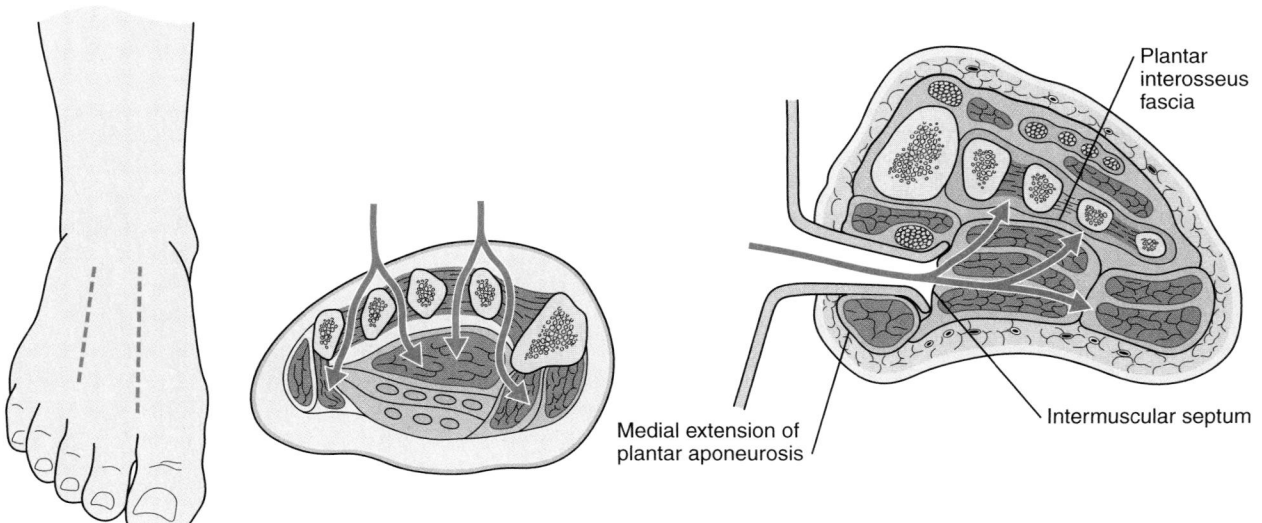

AFTERCARE OF FASCIOTOMY WOUNDS

Fasciotomy wounds are potentially disfiguring, and much dissatisfaction with the end result can occur. Initial dressing using Sofra-Tulle or rayon is applied to the exposed area along with a bulky dressing. After 48 hours, the wound is inspected and any further necrotic tissue is removed.

It is fundamental to the objectives of the procedure to leave the wounds open; the treating surgeon is then left with the need for delayed skin closure, if possible, or for split-skin grafting.

Various methods of mechanical closure of fasciotomy wounds have been published, and each investigator is an enthusiastic supporter of his or her technique.

The Op-Site roller, designed by Bulstrode and associates,[17] offers a solution for closing larger wounds on the leg or forearm without repeated anesthesia. This technique allows serial tightening of an Op-Site sheet spread over the open wound and can be performed easily by nursing staff or by the patient. A randomized study of this device demonstrated its effectiveness in closing most wounds.[118]

The vessel loop bootlace or shoelace technique is another simple, reliable method of improving wound edge apposition and reducing the need for subsequent skin grafting. Vascular loop cord is zigzagged between the skin edges using staples to attach the rubber loop to the skin and so "bootlace" the skin edges together to maintain some tension.[10] This arrangement can be revised at any dressing change if skin tension has diminished or if part of the wound can be closed and the area left open reduced in size. Asgari and Spinelli[6] used this technique to close all fasciotomy wounds in their series successfully by 3 weeks (Fig. 13-29).

Wire sutures and the STAR (suture tension adjustment reel) mechanical method of fasciotomy closure have also been described.[67,125]

MANAGEMENT OF SKELETAL INJURIES

Acute compartment syndrome of the upper or lower extremity is seldom an isolated condition and is almost always seen in association with a long bone fracture. Compartment syndrome occurring as a complication of a number of specific lesions, particularly fractures of the tibia and supracondylar fractures of the humerus, forearm, and femur, has been well documented.* The management of a compartment syndrome in association with any of these fractures deserves special emphasis because two problems coexist—an acute compartment syndrome and the fracture of a long bone. Fasciotomy has to be left open, raising the question of what should be done to the fracture.

Whatever the anatomic location of the injury, the need for fasciotomy is an absolute indication for stabilization of the bone. The technique used depends on the location and character of the fracture and the skill of the surgeon and can involve plating, intramedullary nailing, or external fixation. The technique chosen should be one that minimizes operative trauma to a limb that may already have had its circulation compromised. Therefore, if possible, intramedullary nailing to stabilize the bone (and hence the soft tissues) is recommended. This approach is not always possible, and sometimes the surgeon must resort to a plate or an external fixator. (Fig. 13-30) After the osteosynthesis has been completed, soft tissue coverage over the bone should be attempted. Aftercare of the fasciotomy wounds is similar to that described previously.[34] Gershuni and colleagues[34] have stated that a good functional result is always possible with fasciotomy if the high-risk patient is recognized and the acute compartment syndrome diagnosed early, before the development of irreversible damage to muscle or nerve. On the other hand, if the surgeon procrastinates and fails to recognize the early warning signs and symptoms of an impending compartment syndrome and delays the timing of fasciotomy, irreparable damage can ensue.[34] The most common causes of failure of fasciotomy are delay in the initiation of the operative procedure and an incomplete fasciotomy. Frequently, surgeons do not recognize that adequate decompression for acute compartment syndrome of the leg must involve all four compartments. Similarly, in the arm, both the superficial and deep flexor compartments must be decompressed. The surgeon must have a thorough knowledge of the surgical anatomy of the upper and lower extremities to

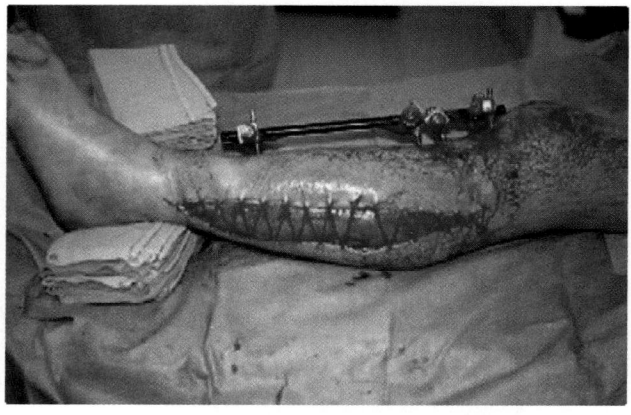

FIGURE 13-30 *Provisional stabilization of fractures associated with compartment syndrome with an external fixator.*

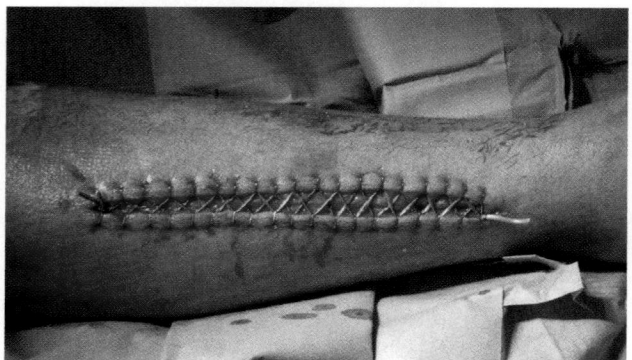

FIGURE 13-29 *Use of the bootlace technique to assist with partial closure a fasciotomy wound.*

*See references 4, 5, 12, 25, 29, 33, 34, 77, 87, 98, 104, 110, 115.

perform an adequate decompression under emergency conditions. If early treatment is better than late treatment, prevention must be better still.

ACKNOWLEDGMENT

We would like to acknowledge the work of Dr. C. H. Rorabeck, M.D., F.R.C.S.(C.), in preparing the original text of this chapter in the first edition and his support in allowing us to revise it for this edition.

REFERENCES

1. Abdul-Hamid, A.K. First dorsal interosseous compartment syndrome. J Hand Surg [Br] 12:269, 1987.
2. Abraham, P.; Leftheriotis, G.; Saumet, J.L. Laser Doppler flowmetry in the diagnosis of chronic compartment syndrome. J Bone Joint Surg Br 80:365, 1998.
3. Ali, M.A. Fracture of the body of the hamate bone associated with compartment syndrome and dorsal decompression of the carpal tunnel. J Hand Surg [Br] 11:207, 1986.
4. Allen, M.J.; Steingold, R.F.; Kotecha, M.; Barnes, M. The importance of the deep volar compartment in crush injuries of the forearm. Injury 16:173, 1985.
5. Allen, M.J.; Stirling, A.J.; Crawshaw, C.V.; Barnes, M.R. Intracompartmental pressure monitoring of leg injuries: An aid to management. J Bone Joint Surg Br 67:53, 1985.
6. Asgari, M.M.; Spinelli, H.M. The vessel loop shoelace technique for closure of fasciotomy wounds. Ann Plast Surg 44:225, 2000.
7. Ashton, H. The effect of increased tissue pressure on blood flow. Clin Orthop 113:15, 1975.
8. Bass, R.R.; Allison, E.J., Jr.; Reines, H.D.; et al. Thigh compartment syndrome without lower extremity trauma following application of pneumatic antishock trousers. Ann Emerg Med 12:382, 1983.
9. Belanger, M.; Fadale, P. Compartment syndrome of the leg after arthroscopic examination of a tibial plateau fracture. Case report and review of the literature. Arthroscopy 13:646, 1997.
10. Bermann, S.S.; Schilling, J.D.; McIntyre, K.E.; et al. Shoelace technique for delayed primary closure of fasciotomies. Am J Surg 16:435, 1994.
11. Bingold, A.C. On splitting plasters: A useful analogy. J Bone Joint Surg Br 61:294, 1979.
12. Blick, S.S.; Brumback, R.J.; Poka, A.; et al. Compartment syndrome in open tibial fractures. J Bone Joint Surg Am 68:1348, 1986.
13. Bonutti, P.M.; Bell, G.R. Compartment syndrome of the foot: A case report. J Bone Joint Surg Am 68:1449, 1986.
14. Brooks, B. Pathologic changes in muscle as a result of disturbances of circulation. Arch Surg 5:188, 1922.
15. Brumback, R.J. Compartment syndrome complicating avulsion of the origin of the triceps muscle: A case report. J Bone Joint Surg Am 69:1445, 1987.
16. Brumback, R.J. Traumatic rupture of the superior gluteal artery, without fracture of the pelvis, causing compartment syndrome of the buttock. J Bone Joint Surg Am 72:134, 1990.
17. Bulstrode, C.K.; King, J.B.; Worpole, R.; Ham, R.J. A simple method for closing fasciotomies. Ann R Coll Surg Engl 67:119, 1985.
18. Bywaters, E.G.L.; Beall, D. Crush injuries with impairment of renal function. Br Med J 1:427, 1941.
19. Chandler, J.G.; Knapp, R.W. Early definitive treatment of vascular injuries in the Viet Nam conflict. JAMA 202:136, 1967.
20. Christensen, K.S. Pneumatic antishock garments (PASG): Do they precipitate lower extremity compartment syndromes? J Trauma 26:1102, 1986.
21. Christensen, K.S.; Klaerke, M. Volkmann's ischemic contracture due to limb compression in drug-induced coma. Injury 16:543, 1985.
22. DeLee, J.C.; Stiehl, J.B. Open tibial fractures with compartment syndrome. Clin Orthop 160:175, 1981.
23. Eaton, R.G.; Green, W.T. Epimysiotomy and fasciotomy in the treatment of Volkmann's ischemic contracture. Orthop Clin North Am 3:175, 1972.
24. Eaton, R.G.; Green, W.T. Volkmann's ischemia: A volar compartment syndrome of the forearm. Clin Orthop 113:58, 1975.
25. Edwards, P.D.; Miles, K.A.; Owens, S.J.; et al. A new non-invasive test for detection of compartment syndromes. Nucl Med Commun 20:215, 1999.
26. Ellis, H. Disabilities after tibial shaft fractures. J Bone Joint Surg Br 40:190, 1958.
27. French, E.B.; Price, W.H. Anterior tibial pain. Br Med J 2:1291, 1962.
28. Galpin, R.D.; Kronick, J.B.; Willis, R.B.; Frewen, T.C. Bilateral lower extremity compartment syndromes secondary to intraosseous fluid resuscitation. J Pediatr Orthop 11:773, 1991.
29. Garber, J.N. Volkmann's contracture of fractures of the forearm and elbow. J Bone Joint Surg 21:154, 1939.
30. Garfin, S.R.; Mubarak, S.J.; Evans, K.L.; et al. Quantification of intracompartmental pressure and volume under plaster casts. J Bone Joint Surg Am 63:449, 1981.
31. Geary, N. Late surgical decompression for compartment syndrome of the forearm. J Bone Joint Surg Br 66:745, 1984.
32. Gelberman, R.H.; Garfin, S.R.; Hergenroeder, P.T.; et al. Compartment syndromes of the forearm: Diagnosis and treatment. Clin Orthop 161:252, 1981.
33. Gelberman, R.H.; Zakaib, G.S.; Mubarak, S.J.; et al. Decompression of forearm compartment syndromes. Clin Orthop 134:225, 1978.
34. Gershuni, D.H.; Mubarak, S.J.; Yaru, N.C.; Lee, Y.F. Fracture of the tibia complicated by acute compartment syndrome. Clin Orthop 217:221, 1987.
35. Giannotti, G.; Cohn, S.M.; Brown, M.; et al. Utility of near-infrared spectroscopy in the diagnosis of lower

extremity compartment syndrome. J Trauma Injury Infect Crit Care 48:396, 2000.

36. Gibson, M.J.; Barnes, M.R.; Allen, M.J.; Chan, R.N. Weakness of foot dorsiflexion and changes in compartment pressures after tibial osteotomy. J Bone Joint Surg Br 68:471, 1986.

37. Graham, B.; Loomer, R.L. Anterior compartment syndrome in a patient with fracture of the tibial plateau treated by continuous passive motion and anticoagulants: Report of a case. Clin Orthop 195:197, 1985.

38. Hargens, A.R.; Akeson, W.H.; Mubarak, S.J.; et al. Tissue fluid states in compartment syndromes. Bibl Anat 15(Pt I):108, 1977.

39. Hargens, A.R.; Romine, J.S.; Sipe, J.C.; et al. Peripheral nerve conduction block by high muscle compartment pressure. J Bone Joint Surg Am 61:192, 1979.

40. Hastings, H.; Misamore, G. Compartment syndrome resulting from intravenous regional anesthesia. J Hand Surg [Am] 12:559, 1987.

41. Heckman, M.M.; Whitesides, T.E., Jr.; Grewe, S.R.; et al. Histologic determination of the ischemic threshold in the canine compartment syndrome model. J Orthop Trauma 7:199, 1993.

42. Heim, M.; Martinowitz, U.; Horoszowski, H. The short foot syndrome: An unfortunate consequence of neglected raised intracompartmental pressure in a severely hemophilic child. A case report. Angiology 37:128, 1986.

43. Heppenstall, R.B.; Sapega, A.A.; Izant, T.; et al. Compartment syndrome: A quantitative study of high-energy phosphorus compounds using ^{31}P-magnetic resonance spectroscopy. J Trauma 29:1113, 1989.

44. Heppenstall, R.B.; Scott, R.; Sapiga, A.; et al. A comparative study of the tolerance of skeletal muscle to ischemia. J Bone Joint Surg Am 68:820, 1986.

45. Hernandez, J., Jr.; Peterson, H.A. Fracture of the distal radial physis complicated by compartment syndrome and premature physeal closure. J Pediatr Orthop 6:627, 1986.

46. Hieb, L.D.; Alexander, A.H. Bilateral anterior and lateral compartment syndromes in a patient with sickle cell trait: Case report and review of the literature. Clin Orthop 228:190, 1988.

47. Hildebrand, O. Die Lehre von den ischamische Muskellahmungen und Kontrakturen. Samml Klin Vortr 122:437, 1906.

48. Johansen, K.; Lynch, K.; Paun, M.; Copass, M. Noninvasive vascular tests reliably exclude occult arterial trauma in injured extremities. J Trauma 31:515, 1991.

49. Kamel, R.; Sakla, F.B. Anatomical compartments of the sole of the human foot. Anat Rec 140:57, 1961.

50. Kelly, R.P.; Whitesides, T.E., Jr. Transfibular route for fasciotomy of the leg. J Bone Joint Surg Am 48:1022, 1967.

51. Khalil, I.M. Bilateral compartment syndrome after prolonged surgery in the lithotomy position. J Vasc Surg 5:879, 1987.

52. Kunkel, J.M. Thigh and leg compartment syndrome in the absence of lower extremity trauma following MAST application. Am J Emerg Med 5:118, 1987.

53. Landerer, A.S. Die Gewebspannung in ihrem Einfluss auf die ortliche Blutbewegung und Lymphbewegung. Leipzig, Vogel, 1884.

54. Lee, B.Y.; Brancato, R.F.; Park, I.H.; Shaw, W.W. Management of compartmental syndrome: Diagnosis and surgical considerations. Am J Surg 148:383, 1984.

55. Manoli, A., II. Compartment syndromes of the foot: Current concepts. Foot Ankle 10:340, 1990.

56. Matsen, F.A., III. Compartmental syndrome: A unified concept. Clin Orthop 113:8, 1975.

57. Matsen, F.A., III. Compartment Syndromes. New York, Grune & Stratton, 1980.

58. Matsen, F.A., III. A practical approach to compartmental syndromes: Part I, definition, theory and pathogenesis. Instr Course Lect 32:88, 1983.

59. Matsen, F.A., III; Hargens, A.R. Compartment Syndromes and Volkmann's Contracture. Philadelphia, W.B. Saunders, 1981, p. 111.

60. Matsen, F.A., III; Krugmire, R.B., Jr. Compartmental syndromes. Surg Gynecol Obstet 147:943, 1979.

61. Matsen, F.A., III; Mayo, K.A.; Krugmire, R.B., Jr.; et al. A model compartment syndrome in man with particular reference to the quantification of nerve function. J Bone Joint Surg Am 59:648, 1977.

62. Matsen, F.A., III; Mayo, K.A.; Sheridan, G.W.; Krugmire, R.B., Jr. Monitoring of intramuscular pressure. Surgery 79:702, 1976.

63. Matsen, F.A., III; Staheli, L.T. Neurovascular complications following tibial osteotomy in children: A case report. Clin Orthop 110:210, 1975.

64. Matsen, F.A., III; Winquist, R.A.; Krugmire, R.B. Diagnosis and management of compartmental syndromes. J Bone Joint Surg Am 62:286, 1980.

65. Matsen, F.A., III; Wyss, C.R.; King R.V. The continuous infusion technique in the assessment of clinical compartment syndromes. In: Hargens, A.R., ed. Tissue Fluid Pressure and Composition. Baltimore, Williams & Wilkins, 1981, p. 255.

66. Matsen, F.A., III; Wyss, C.R.; Krugmire, R.B., Jr.; et al. The effects of limb elevation and dependency on local arteriovenous gradients in normal human limbs with particular reference to limbs with increased tissue pressure. Clin Orthop 150:187, 1980.

67. McKenney, M.G.; Nir, I.; Fee, T.; et al. A simple device for closure of fasciotomy wounds. Am J Surg 172:275, 1996.

68. McLaren, A.; Rorabeck, C.H. The effect of shock on tourniquet-induced nerve injury. Proceedings of the Fifteenth Annual Meeting of the Canadian Orthopaedic Research Society, 1981. Orthop Trans 5:482, 1981.

69. McLaren, A.C.; Ferguson, J.H.; Miniaci, A. Crush syndrome associated with use of the fracture table: A case report. J Bone Joint Surg Am 69:1447, 1987.

70. McLellan, B.A.; Phillips, J.H.; Hunter, G.A.; et al. Bilateral lower extremity amputations after prolonged application of the pneumatic antishock garment: Case report. Can J Surg 30:55, 1987.

71. McQueen, M.M.; Court-Brown, C.M. Compartment monitoring in tibial fractures. J Bone Joint Surg Br 78:99, 1996.

72. Michaelson, M. Crush injury and crush syndrome. World J Surg 16:899, 1992.

73. Miniaci, A.; Rorabeck, C.H. Compartment syndrome: A complication of treatment of muscle hernias. J Bone Joint Surg Am 68:1444, 1968.

74. Moed, B.R.; Thorderson, K. Measurement of intracompartmental pressure: A comparison of the slit catheter, side-ported needle, and simple needle. J Bone Joint Surg Am 75:231, 1993.

75. Mohler, L.R.; Styf, J.R.; Pedowitz, R.A.; et al. Intramuscular deoxygenation during exercise in patients who have chronic anterior compartment syndrome of the leg. J Bone Joint Surg Am 79:844, 1997.

76. Mubarak, S.J. A practical approach to compartmental syndromes: Part II, diagnosis. Instr Course Lect 32:92, 1983.

77. Mubarak, S.J.; Carroll, N.C. Volkmann's contracture in children: Aetiology and prevention. J Bone Joint Surg Br 61:285, 1979.

78. Mubarak, S.J.; Hargens, A.R. Compartment Syndromes and Volkmann's Contracture. Philadelphia, W.B. Saunders, 1981, p. 113.

79. Mubarak, S.J.; Hargens, A.R.; Garfin, S.R.; et al. Loss of nerve function in compartment syndromes: Pressure versus ischemia? Transactions of the Orthopedic Research Society 25th Annual Meeting, San Francisco, February 20, 1979.

80. Mubarak, S.J.; Hargens, A.R.; Owen, C.A.; et al. The wick catheter technique for measurement of intramuscular pressure: A new research and clinical tool. J Bone Joint Surg Am 58:1016, 1976.

81. Mubarak, S.J.; Owen, C.A. Compartment syndrome and its relation to the crush syndrome: A spectrum of disease. Clin Orthop 113:81, 1975.

82. Mubarak, S.J.; Owen, C.A. Double-incision fasciotomy of the leg for decompression in compartment syndromes. J Bone Joint Surg Am 59:184, 1977.

83. Mubarak, S.J.; Owen, C.A.; Hargens, A.R.; et al. Acute compartment syndromes: Diagnosis and treatment with aid of the wick catheter. J Bone Joint Surg Am 60:1091, 1978.

84. Mubarak, S.J.; Wilton, N.C. Compartment syndromes and epidural analgesia. J Pediatr Orthop 17:282, 1997.

85. Murphy, J.B. Myositis. JAMA 63:1249, 1914.

86. Myerson, M.S. Experimental decompression of the fascial compartments of the foot: The basis for fasciotomy in acute compartment syndromes. Foot Ankle 8:308, 1988.

87. Owen, R.; Tsimboukis, B. Ischaemia complicating closed tibial and fibular shaft fractures. J Bone Joint Surg Br 49:268, 1967.

88. Patman, R.D.; Thompson, J.E. Fasciotomy in peripheral vascular surgery. Arch Surg 101:663, 1970.

89. Paton, D.F. The pathogenesis of anterior tibial syndrome. J Bone Joint Surg Br 50:383, 1968.

90. Peck, D.; Nicholls, P.J.; Beard, C.; Allen, J.R. Are there compartment syndromes in some patients with idiopathic back pain? Spine 11:468, 1986.

91. Petersen, F. Uber ischämische Muskellahmungen. Arch Klin Chir 37:675, 1888.

92. Phillips, J.H.; Mackinnon, S.E.; Beatty, S.E.; et al. Vibratory sensory testing in acute compartment syndromes: A clinical and experimental study. Plast Reconstr Surg 79:796, 1987.

93. Reddy, P.K.; Kaye, K.W. Deep posterior compartmental syndrome: A serious complication of the lithotomy position. J Urol 132:144, 1984.

94. Reis, N.D.; Michaelson, M. Crush injury to the lower limbs. J Bone Joint Surg Am 68:414, 1986.

95. Roberts, R.S.; Csencsitz, T.A.; Heard, C.W., Jr. Upper extremity compartment syndromes following pit viper envenomation. Clin Orthop 193:184, 1985.

96. Rooser, B. Quadriceps contusion with compartment syndrome: Evacuation of hematoma in 2 cases. Acta Orthop Scand 58:170, 1987.

97. Rorabeck, C.H. A practical approach to compartmental syndromes: Part III, management. Instr Course Lect 32:102, 1983.

98. Rorabeck, C.H. The treatment of compartment syndromes of the leg. J Bone Joint Surg Br 66:93, 1984.

99. Rorabeck, C.H.; Bourne, R.B.; Fowler, P.J. The surgical treatment of exertional compartment syndrome in athletes. J Bone Joint Surg Am 65:1245, 1983.

100. Rorabeck, C.H.; Castle, G.S.P.; Hardie, R.; Logan, J. The slit catheter: A new device for measuring intracompartmental pressure. Proceedings of the Canadian Orthopedic Research Society, 14th Annual Meeting, Calgary, Alberta, Canada, June 1980, Surg Forum 31:513, 1980.

101. Rorabeck, C.H.; Castle, G.S.P.; Hardie, R.; Logan, J. Compartmental pressure measurements: An experimental investigation using the slit catheter. J Trauma 21:446, 1981.

102. Rorabeck, C.H.; Clarke, K.M. The pathophysiology of the anterior tibial compartment syndrome: An experimental investigation. J Trauma 18:299, 1978.

103. Rorabeck, C.H.; Macnab, I. The pathophysiology of the anterior tibial compartment syndrome. Clin Orthop 113:52, 1975.

104. Rorabeck, C.H.; Macnab, I. Anterior tibial compartment syndrome complicating fractures of the shaft of the tibia. J Bone Joint Surg Am 58:549, 1976.

105. Rowlands, R.P. Volkmann's contracture. Guys Hosp Gaz 24:87, 1910.

106. Scholander, P.F.; Hargens, A.R.; Miller, S.L. Negative pressure in the interstitial fluid of animals. Science 161:321, 1968.

107. Schwartz, J.T., Jr.; Brumback, R.J.; Lakatos, R.; et al. Acute compartment syndrome of the thigh. J Bone Joint Surg Am 71:392, 1989.

108. Schwartz, J.T.; Brumback, R.J.; Poka, A.; et al. Compartment syndrome of the thigh: A review of 13 cases. Proceedings of the 55th Annual Meeting of the American Academy of Orthopaedic Surgeons: Paper 357. Rosemont, IL, American Academy of Orthopaedic Surgeons, 1988, p. 188.

109. Seddon, H.J. Volkmann's ischemia in the lower limb. J Bone Joint Surg Br 48:627, 1966.

110. Sirbu, A.B.; Murphy, M.J.; White, A.S. Soft tissue complications of fractures of the leg. Calif West Med 60:1, 1944.

111. Spinner, M.; Aiache, A.; Silver, L.; Barsky, A. Impending ischemic contracture of the hand. Plast Reconstr Surg 50:341, 1972.

112. Straehley, D.; Jones, W.W. Acute compartment syndrome (anterior, lateral and superficial posterior) following tear of the medial head of the gastrocnemius muscle: A case report. Am J Sports Med 14:96, 1986.

113. Strecker, W.B.; Wood, M.B.; Bieber, E.J. Compartment syndrome masked by epidural anesthesia for postoperative pain. Report of a case. J Bone Joint Surg Am 68:1447, 1986.

114. Styf, J.R.; Korner, L.M. Microcapillary infusion technique for measurement of intramuscular pressure during exercise. Clin Orthop 207:253, 1986.

115. Sundararaj, J.G.D.; Mani, K. Pattern of contracture and recovery following ischaemia of the upper limb. J Hand Surg [Br] 10:155, 1985.

116. Sundararaj, G.D.; Mani, K. Management of Volkmann's ischemic contracture of the upper limb. J Hand Surg [Br] 10:401, 1985.

117. Tarlow, S.D.; Achterman, C.A.; Hayhurst, J.; Ovadia, D.N. Acute compartment syndrome in the thigh complicating fracture of the femur: A report of three cases. J Bone Joint Surg Am 68:1439, 1986.

118. Tasman-Jones, T.C.; Tomlinson, M. Tissue rollers in the closure of fasciotomy wounds. J Bone Joint Surg Br 75:49, 1993.

119. Templeman, D.; Lange, R.; Harms, B. Lower extremity compartment syndromes associated with use of pneumatic antishock garments. J Trauma 27:79, 1987.

120. Thomas, J.J. Nerve involvement in the ischaemic paralysis and contracture of Volkmann. Ann Surg 49:330, 1909.

121. Volkmann, R. Die ischaemischen Muskellahmungen und Kontrakturen. Zentralbl Chir 8:801, 1881.

122. Wallis, F.C. Treatment of paralysis and muscular atrophy after prolonged use of splints or of an Esmarch's cord. Practitioner 67:429, 1901.

123. Whitesides, T.E., Jr.; Haney, T.C.; Morimoto, K.; Hirada, H. Tissue pressure measurements as a determinant for the need of fasciotomy. Clin Orthop 113:43, 1975.

124. Whitesides, T.E., Jr.; Haney, T.C.; Hirada, H.; et al. A simple method for tissue pressure determination. Arch Surg 110:1311, 1975.

125. Wiger, P.; Tkaczuk, P.; Styf, J. Secondary wound closure following fasciotomy for acute compartment syndrome increases intramuscular pressure. J Orthop Trauma 12:117, 1998.

126. Wiggins, H.E. The anterior tibial compartmental syndrome: A complication of the Hauser procedure. Clin Orthop 113:90, 1975.

127. Wilson, S.C.; Vrahas, M.S.; Berson, L.; et al. A simple method to measure compartment pressures using an intravenous catheter. Orthopedics 20:403, 1997.

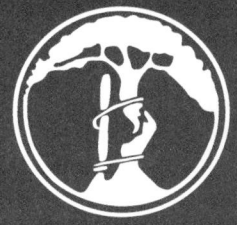

CHAPTER 14

Fractures with Soft Tissue Injuries

Michael Sirkin, M.D., Frank Liporace, M.D., and Fred F. Behrens, M.D. (d)

HISTORICAL PERSPECTIVE AND SCOPE

The serious nature of open fractures has been well understood since antiquity.[178] The Hippocratic physicians[107] recognized that wound size, fracture stability, and the proximity of neurovascular structures all influence the ultimate outcome of these severe injuries. They urged speed, removal of protruding fragments, antiseptic wound dressings (compresses soaked in wine), stable reduction without undue pressure at the injury site, dressing changes every 2 days, and free drainage of pus. Even their final advice sounds modern: "One should especially avoid such cases if one has a respectable excuse, for the favorable chances are few and the risks many. Besides, if a man does not reduce the fracture, he will be thought unskillful. If he does reduce it, he will bring the patient nearer to death than to recovery."[107]

Over the ensuing centuries, an open fracture usually meant death from sepsis within a month. To preserve life was the principal treatment goal, and fire seemed the most effective tool. A red-hot iron and boiling oil of elder were meant to clean the wound, destroy devitalized tissue, and prevent wound sepsis. This practice changed abruptly one day in 1538 when Ambroise Paré (1510 to 1590),[132] a French army surgeon, ran out of hot oil during the siege of Turin. He had only "a digestive made of yolke of egge and oyle of Roses and Turpentine" and was baffled the next morning when all patients "dressed with a digestive oyle"[178] were alive and nearly pain free.

Despite gentler and speedier care, the use of ligatures and tourniquets, and the practice of delayed stump closure, the surgery of open wounds remained, well into the middle of the 19th century, the surgery of amputations. In 1842, Malgaigne[111,178] found that the overall mortality rate for amputations was 30 percent; for major amputations, it was 52 percent, and for thigh amputations, 60 percent.

Although primary amputation was recognized as the safest method to treat open fractures, some surgeons were dissatisfied with this mutilating and life-threatening procedure. This school of thought started with Guy de Chauliac (1546),[44] who first taught the enlargement of open and contaminated wounds to encourage drainage. Paré[178] amputated only when an open fracture was complicated by fever. He advised: "If there bee any strange bodies as peeces of Wood, Irons, Bones, bruised flesh, congealed blood or the like, whether they come from without or from within the body . . . he must take them away for otherwise there is no union to be expected," and "The wound must forthwith be enlarged . . . so there may be free passage for both the pus or matter . . . contained therein."[178] The wounds were held open with a packing of lint or rolls of linen. Just before the beginning of the French Revolution, Pierre Joseph Desault (1738 to 1795)[178] developed the modern concept of débridement, but until World War I the method was used only sporadically because many of the known army surgeons, such as Larrey, continued to favor amputations for combat-related wounds.

Lister's introduction of antisepsis a half-century later seemed another major step toward limb salvage; however, when used alone during the Franco-Prussian War (1870 to 1871),[178] it failed. It was left to Carl Reyher,[177] a young German surgeon in the Russian service, to show in a controlled study carried out during the Russo-Turkish War (1877) that a further reduction in mortality rate was possible only when antisepsis was combined with early débridement. Although his observation was soon confirmed experimentally, it was not until the end of World War I that the Interallied Surgical Conference recommended the resection of all contaminated tissues, the removal of all foreign material, and no primary wound closures unless fewer than 8 hours had elapsed since the open injury was inflicted.[58]

The great medical discoveries of the past 150 years,[178] such as anesthesia, antisepsis, asepsis, the germ theory of infections, advances in prehospital care, fluid and cardiorespiratory resuscitation, and early fracture stabilization,[21,123] brought about a revolution in operative wound care. Although in the past success in treating open fractures was measured by the number of lives lost or limbs amputated, attention is now being focused on reducing wound infections and healing times. Ultimately, we aim to restore our patients with the least delay to as close to their preinjury status as possible. Although the techniques introduced during the past century are important, none was so difficult to learn or so easy to neglect as the art of débridement—and this is still true at the beginning of the 21st century.[178]

Although this chapter emphasizes open fractures and dislocations, it also addresses some closed fractures with associated soft tissue destruction. Pitfalls and complications are common unless these fractures are treated like open lesions.[172,173] Curiously enough, this was well recognized two millennia ago by the Hippocratic physicians: "The same treatment of the wound applies to cases of fractures which are first without wound but where one occurs during treatment either through too great compression of bandages or the pressure of splint or some other cause. In such cases, the occurrence of ulcerations are recognized while pain is dropping …. Treat them for the future in the same manner as cases in which there is a wound from the first. Change the dressing every other day … Correctness of position also contributes to a good result …."[107]

ETIOLOGY, MECHANISMS, AND CHARACTERISTICS

The forceful disruption of skin and underlying tissues is the most obvious expression of an open fracture, but it is only one of many manifestations of a violent encounter between the human body and the environment. The potential damage from such a collision is related to the energy dissipated during the event. According to the equation $KE = \frac{1}{2}mv^2$, the kinetic energy involved (KE) is directly proportional to the mass (m) and the square of the speed (v).[66] Traditionally, warfare or natural catastrophes generated most life- and limb-threatening energies. The ingenious harnessing of natural resources during the past 200 years has not only revolutionized industrial productivity and transportation, it has also progressively exposed the human body to forces that exceed the strength and resilience of its organs and tissues[33] (Table 14-1). Today, more than two thirds of open fractures seen at trauma centers are caused by objects and mechanisms that emerged during the past century[48] (Table 14-2).

The significance of speed, even when small masses are involved, is vividly apparent in the wounds inflicted in military combat, in urban warfare, and in hunting accidents. Although devastating, these wounds usually involve only a limited, well-circumscribed part of the body. In the modern traffic accident, the driver's or passenger's body becomes a high-mass, high-speed projectile that sustains several impacts and thus many superimposed lesions—a polytraumatized patient with axial and appendicular injuries at multiple levels is the consequential and distressing outcome.[32,49,69,147]

Table 14-1	
Energy Dissipated in Injuries	
Injury	**Dissipated Energy (foot-pounds)**
Fall from a curb	100
Skiing injury	300–500
High-velocity gunshot wound	2000
Automobile bumper collision at 20 miles per hour	100,000

Source: Chapman M. Role of stability in open fractures. Instr Course Lect 31:75, 1982.

Table 14-2	
Causes of Open Fractures among Civilians	
Cause	**%**
Motorcycle accident	28
Motor vehicle accident	24
Falls	13
Pedestrian struck by car	12
Crush injuries	8
Firearms	2
Miscellaneous	13

Source: Dellinger, E.; Miller, S.D.; Wertz, M.J.; et al. Risk of infection after open fractures of the arm or leg. Arch Surg 123:1320–1327, 1987.

Injuries caused by a direct force are often thought to be the most serious because they disrupt local soft tissue and contaminate the wound. Yet, all too often the effects of indirect forces are gravely underestimated. A high-energy torsional injury can cause a long bone to explode into sharp fragments that swiftly penetrate the centrally located neurovascular structures and the surrounding soft tissue sleeve, a picture typically seen in injuries caused by farm and other equipment driven by power takeoffs.

As typical high-energy injuries, fractures with major soft tissue disruptions differ radically from simple closed lesions. About 40 to 70 percent are associated with trauma elsewhere,[156] particularly cerebral lesions, cardiothoracic and abdominal disruptions,[156] and fractures or ligamentous injuries involving other extremities.[49] Locally, open fractures usually cause more damage than closed lesions; thus, they are more often associated with soft tissue loss, compartment syndromes,[17,47] neurovascular injuries,[31,42,49,73,96,103,126] and ligamentous disruptions of adjacent joints. In addition to possible bone loss, the fracture patterns associated with open fractures typically have wider initial displacements[124] and greater comminution than closed lesions.[172]

CLASSIFICATIONS

The treatment and prognosis of fractures and dislocations with soft tissue injuries are influenced by many premorbid, injury, and treatment variables; most act independently, and each is expressed by a different severity scale. To calculate summary indices that take all the known injury components into account is tempting but often causes further confusion because it is difficult to assign appropriate weight to different variables that can unduly potentiate or negate each other. For these and other reasons, most accepted classifications of fractures with soft tissue injuries have been simple and pragmatic rather than multifactorial and exhaustive.

Open Fractures

Most classifications of open musculoskeletal injuries follow the initial attempt by Cauchoix and associates,[30] who were mainly interested in the size of the skin defect, the degree of contusion and soft tissue crush, and the complexity of the bony lesion. Rittmann and co-workers[147,148] also maintained three severity groups but focused on direct and indirect injury patterns, amount of dead and foreign material in the wounds, and involvement of neurovascular structures. The classification of Gustilo and Anderson[60] followed the earlier proposals and suggested that farm injuries automatically be considered type III in severity.

Although these classifications have some therapeutic and prognostic implications, all lack sensitivity at the upper end of the severity spectrum. In 1982, Tscherne and Oestern[173] presented a multifactorial classification with four severity types. Each type takes into account the extent of the skin injury, soft tissue damage, fracture severity, and degree of contamination. In 1984, Gustilo and colleagues[72] divided their type III lesions into three subgroups. IIIA fractures are characterized by extensive lacerations yet have sufficient soft tissue to provide adequate bone coverage, IIIB fractures are those with extensive soft tissue loss and much devascularized bone, and IIIC lesions are associated with major vascular disruptions requiring repair (Table 14-3). This revised classification has brought some refinement and enjoys wide popularity. However, as is true for many other classification systems,[23,52,102,164,169] two studies found that interobserver concurrence did not exceed 60 percent.[27,86] Although the classification's reliability has been questioned and modern fixation techniques have allowed primary internal fixation of bone, the soft tissue treatment recommendations continue to be followed virtually unchanged.[71]

Open fractures inflicted by lawn mowers and tornadoes deserve particular consideration. Both generate severe open high-energy injuries either through direct impact (at 3000 revolutions per minute, the blade of a rotary lawn mower generates 2100 foot-pounds of kinetic energy[134]) or through flying debris containing soil and other contaminated material. Post-traumatic infections are common and are usually caused by a mixed flora, mostly gram-negative bacilli.[118] Lawn mower injuries are most common in children younger than 14 years. They are often complicated by compartment syndromes.[134] Tornado and lawn mower injuries should be treated like farm injuries, with broad-spectrum antibiotics including penicillin or an analogue, repeated wide débridement, and possibly extensive soft tissue and reconstructive procedures.

The Mangled Extremity

With continuous improvements in prehospital rescue and resuscitation, more patients with severe extremity injuries involving vascular compromise[31,42,49,73,94,96,103,126] or partial amputation[59,91] are surviving. Traditionally, between 50 and 100 percent of these injuries resulted in amputation.[103] With the development of free flaps,[60,182] temporary intraluminal shunts,[90] and microvascular reconstructions, many of these extremities are now replanted, revascularized, or covered with local or free muscle flaps. The previous felt opinion that many patients may fare better with early amputation followed by vigorous rehabilitation and vocational training[31,59,73] has recently been questioned by the Lower Extremity Assessment Project (LEAP) data.[110]

The difficult choice between sacrificing a potentially useful limb segment and attempting the time-consuming and resource-intensive salvage of a functionally useless extremity has been addressed by several investigators.[66,87,91,103,110] Johansen and colleagues[91] retrospectively analyzed the charts of 25 patients with severe open lower extremity fractures and found that limb salvage was related to energy dissipation, hemodynamic status, degree of limb ischemia, and age of the patient. They scored each of these four variables according to severity and called the sum of the scores the Mangled Extremity Severity Score, or MESS (Table 14-4). Although based on small numbers, the retrospective and subsequent prospective evaluation[77] showed that an MESS of 7 or higher predicted, with a high degree of confidence, the need for initial or delayed amputation, whereas all limbs with a score of 6 or lower remained viable. This scoring system needs further validation in larger field trials. It is also not clear to what extent this classification is applicable to pediatric lesions or fractures other than those affecting the leg.

Although some studies have questioned the sensitivity and reproducibility of the MESS[116] and other similar severity scores that rely on simple, easily obtainable, and quantifiable parameters, such severity scores do facilitate the initial decision-making process because they provide the treating physician with a rational framework to guide an often emotional decision-making process. Possibly the greatest weakness of the MESS is a propensity for false-negative predictions for young patients with intact vessels, minimal blood loss, and major muscle or skeletal destruction.[135,152] Although such injuries can receive a score of less than 7, primary amputation may still be the treatment of choice. None of the current scoring scales helps in making decisions about secondary amputations.

The LEAP study has shown no differences in functional outcomes at 2 and 7 years following either limb salvage or primary amputation.[110] Both involved poor results and significant long-term disabilities. Outcomes were most affected by the patient's economic, social, and personal resources rather than treatment of the injury whether it was by amputation or reconstruction.

Table 14-3	
Classification of Open Fractures	
Fracture Type	**Description**
Type I	Skin opening of 1 cm or less, quite clean. Most likely from inside to outside. Minimal muscle contusion. Simple transverse or short oblique fractures.
Type II	Laceration more than 1 cm long, with extensive soft tissue damage, flaps, or avulsion. Minimal to moderate crushing component. Simple transverse or short oblique fractures with minimal comminution.
Type III	Extensive soft tissue damage including muscles, skin, and neurovascular structures. Often a high-velocity injury with severe crushing component.
Type IIIA	Extensive soft tissue laceration, adequate bone coverage. Segmental fractures, gunshot injuries.
Type IIIB	Extensive soft tissue injury with periosteal stripping and bone exposure. Usually associated with massive contamination.
Type IIIC	Vascular injury requiring repair.

Source: Gustilo, R.B.; Mendoza, R.M.; Williams, D.N. Problems in the management of type III (severe) open fractures: A new classification of type III open fractures. J Trauma 24:742–746, 1984.

Table 14-4	
MESS (Mangled Extremity Severity Score) Variables	
Component	**Points**
Skeletal and Soft Tissue Injury	
Low energy (stab; simple fracture; "civilian gunshot wound")	1
Medium energy (open or multiplex fractures, dislocation)	2
High energy (close-range shotgun or "military" gunshot wound, crush injury)	3
Very high energy (same as above plus gross contamination, soft tissue avulsion)	4
Limb Ischemia (Score Is Doubled for Ischemia >6 hr)	
Pulse reduced or absent but perfusion normal	1
Pulseless; paresthesias, diminished capillary refill	2
Cool, paralyzed, insensate, numb	3
Shock	
Systolic blood pressure always >90 mm Hg	0
Hypotensive transiently	1
Persistent hypotension	2
Age (yr)	
<30	0
30–50	1
>50	2

Source: Johansen, K.; Daines, M.; Harvey, T.; et al. Objective criteria accurately predict amputation following lower extremity trauma. J Trauma 30:568–572, 1990.

Closed Fractures

Not all fractures and joint disruptions caused by violent forces result in open wounds. In fact, the soft tissue destruction in closed injuries may be more extensive and more severe than that seen in open lesions.[107,172,173] Many of these injuries are accompanied by skin contusions, deep abrasions, burns, dermatologic conditions, or frank

Table 14-5	
Classification of Closed Fractures with Soft Tissue Damage	
Fracture Type	**Description**
Type 0	Minimal soft tissue damage. Indirect violence. Simple fracture patterns. Example: Torsion fracture of the tibia in skiers.
Type I	Superficial abrasion or contusion caused by pressure from within. Mild to moderately severe fracture configuration. Example: Pronation fracture-dislocation of the ankle joint with soft tissue lesion over the medial malleolus.
Type II	Deep, contaminated abrasion associated with localized skin or muscle contusion. Impending compartment syndrome. Severe fracture configuration. Example: Segmental "bumper" fracture of the tibia.
Type III	Extensive skin contusion or crush. Underlying muscle damage may be severe. Subcutaneous avulsion. Decompensated compartment syndrome. Associated major vascular injury. Severe or comminuted fracture configuration.

Source: Tscherne, H.; Oestern, H.J. Die Klassifizierung des Weichteilschadens bei offenen und geschlossenen Frakturen. Unfallheilkunde 85:111–115, 1982. Copyright Springer-Verlag.

separation of the cutis from the subcuticular tissues. If hidden under casts or incorporated innocently into a surgical incision, these subtle soft tissue injuries may have catastrophic consequences ranging from delayed wound healing to partial or full tissue slough easily leading to a massively infected open wound.

Tscherne and co-workers[172,173] have classified these closed injuries on a scale from 0 to 3. Although the scale has not been critically validated, it may heighten the physician's awareness of the injury severity and provide some guidance for management[157] (Fig. 14-1 and Table 14-5; see also Fig. 14-28A).

PATHOPHYSIOLOGY OF MUSCULOSKELETAL INJURIES

Violent injuries to the musculoskeletal system typically result in extensive disruptions of the soft and hard tissues. They may introduce foreign material and bacteria and create ischemic and metabolically deprived soft tissue segments,[89] frank tissue necrosis, and dead space. The ensuing hematoma, contaminated with foreign material, invades the injury zone, dissects along disrupted tissue planes, fills empty spaces, and acts as an ideal culture medium for bacteria. Within the first few hours, neutrophils and macrophages enter the wound, but later, monocytes are more common. Simultaneously, the complement and clotting systems are activated. Serotonin, prostaglandins, and kinins released by platelets and the clotting cascade lead to vascular dilatation and, together with histamine released by basophils and mast cells, increase permeability. Massive exudation of plasma proteins and leukocytes follows. The C3b component of the complement system facilitates opsonization of bacteria and foreign material, whereas the C5a component and histamine are the most powerful chemotactic agents. These events set the stage for the phagocytosis of bacteria and necrotic material by neutrophils and macrophages.[35,55,80,151]

FIGURE 14-1 *A closed comminuted tibial plateau fracture with type II soft tissue injury and impending compartment syndrome. Fasciotomy and temporizing external fixation were performed. Definitive reconstruction and internal fixation were delayed for 15 days.*

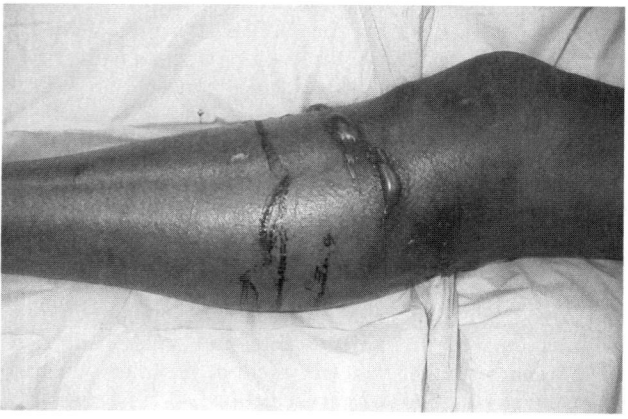

FIGURE 14-2 *Results of the necrotic process: cellular, hematologic, and immunologic responses to injury lead to repair or further tissue destruction.*

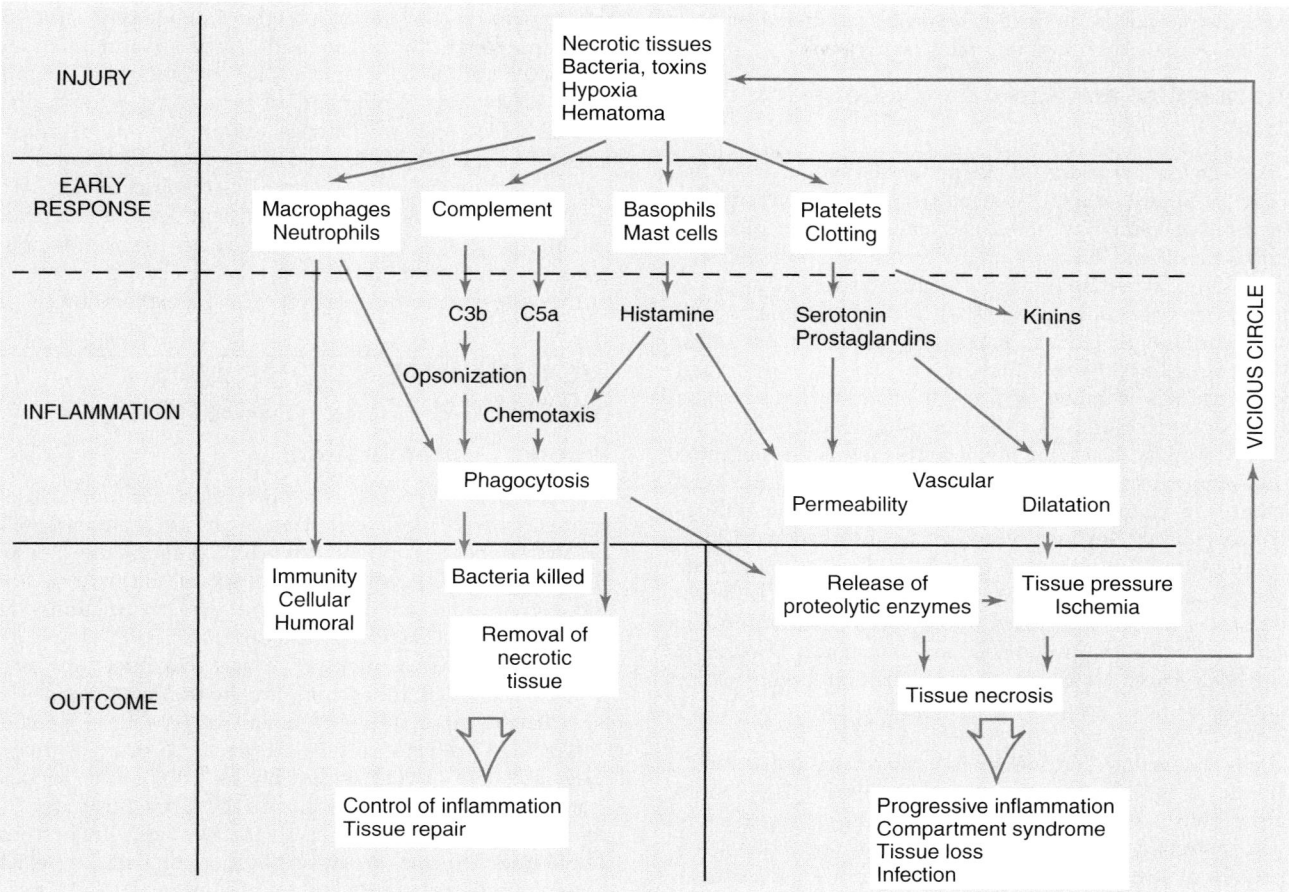

If the injury is minor or if thorough débridement and antibacterial agents have removed most of the necrotic and foreign material, the inflammatory response is controlled and tissue repair ensues. With massive injuries, severe contamination, or timid intervention, however, a different outcome is seen. The macrophages cannot deal with the bacterial load; they die and release lysosomal or other proteolytic enzymes, which cause further necrosis of the surrounding tissues. In concert with increased tissue pressure, this necrotic process propagates a vicious circle leading to progressive inflammation, muscle ischemia, compartment syndromes, tissue loss, and spread of infection[17,47] (Fig. 14-2). A progressive inflammatory response is seen most often after extensive contamination of an open fracture but may also occur in closed fractures and dislocations and after simple crushes of muscle compartments.

TREATMENT PLAN AND EARLY CARE

Overview

Because fractures with major soft tissue disruption often occur in association with injuries to other parts of the body, they must be considered in the context of polytrauma, recognizing the patient as a whole. Care of these patients progresses from an acute to a reconstructive and then to a rehabilitative phase. The *acute* phase includes (1) initial resuscitation and stabilization at the injury site; (2) complete evaluation of all the patient's injuries, including the open fracture, with primary attention to life-threatening lesions; (3) appropriate antimicrobial therapy; (4) extensive wound débridement followed by wound coverage; (5) fracture stabilization; (6) autogenous bone grafting and other measures that facilitate bone union; and (7) early joint motion and mobilization of the patient.[158] The *reconstructive* phase addresses late injury sequelae, such as nonunions, malalignments, and delayed infections. The *rehabilitative* phase focuses on the patient's psychosocial and vocational rehabilitation.

Traditionally, these three phases have been managed sequentially and with little coordination. Reconstructive problems, such as nonunions, were not addressed until 8 to 12 months after the injury, and vocational rehabilitation was considered only after all soft tissue and bone injuries were healed. Not surprisingly, many patients lost self-esteem, some saw their families disintegrate, and few returned to work before 18 to 24 months, if at all.[59] At present, we are striving to see the patient back in the workplace and recreational pursuits before the first anniversary of the injury. To achieve these goals, the patient's course of treatment and recovery must be carefully laid out during the initial hospital stay; the three treatment phases are overlapped, and the patient as a whole, rather than a collection of individual injuries, takes center stage.

Prehospital and Emergency Department Care

Open fractures are surgical emergencies. Any delays at the scene of injury, during transport, or in the emergency department, radiology suite, or operating room jeopardize limb survival and recovery.[158] After resuscitation and stabilization of vital functions, the rescue workers at the accident scene cover open wounds with moist sterile dressings and gently align, reduce, and splint the deformed limbs. Moist dressings prevent desiccation of local soft tissues. Some use sterile saline or povidone-iodine (Betadine) as the hydrating solution for the gauze immediately covering the open injury. Since povidone-iodine has been suggested to have an effect on long-term proliferation and functional activity of bone cells, the authors prefer sterile saline-soaked gauze.[29] Profuse bleeding is controlled with local compression. A tourniquet may be indicated for a traumatic amputation or uncontrollable hemorrhage. Inflation time must be clearly marked. Temporary deflation at regular intervals is warranted for long transports. Pneumatic antishock garments are used with caution because they increase rather than decrease mortality for most injury patterns.[114]

On the patient's arrival in the emergency department, vital functions are reassessed and stabilized. Large-bore intravenous access is established. All organ systems are then systematically evaluated. Dressings and splints are partially removed to check soft tissue conditions and neuromuscular function. Bone fragments or dislocations causing undue skin pressure are reduced gently and the extremities resplinted in proper alignment.

	Table 14-6	
	Schedule of Active Immunization	
Dose	**Age and Intervals**	**Vaccine**
Age <7 yr		
Primary 1	Age 6 wk	DPT
Primary 2	4–8 wk after the first dose	DPT
Primary 3	4–8 wk after the second dose	DPT
Primary 4	About 1 yr after third dose	DPT
Booster	Age 4–6 yr	DPT
Additional boosters	Every 10 yr after last dose	Td
Age ≥7 yr		
Primary 1	First visit	Td
Primary 2	4–6 wk after the first dose	Td
Primary 3	6 mo to 1 yr after last dose	Td
Boosters	Every 10 yr after last dose	Td

Abbreviations: DPT, diphtheria and tetanus toxoids and pertussis vaccine absorbed; Td, tetanus and reduced-dose diphtheria toxoids absorbed (for adult use).
Source: Cates, T.R. In: Mandell, G.L.; Douglas, R.G., Jr.; Bennett, J.E., eds. Principles and Practice of Infectious Diseases. New York, Churchill Livingstone, 1990.

All sterile wound dressings are left in place because redressing of wounds in the emergency department raises the ultimate infection rate by a factor of 3 to 4.[172] Before the patient is transferred to the radiography suite or operating room, the history and physical examination are completed and blood is drawn for a complete blood count, serum electrolytes, typing and crossmatching, and possibly arterial blood gases. Tetanus prophylaxis is administered[165,179] (Table 14-6), and intravenous antibiotics are started. If during the workup a dysvascular limb is suspected, the emergency department stay is curtailed and the patient is quickly transferred to the angiography suite or, preferably, directly to the operating room for further assessment and possible vascular exploration.

WOUND INFECTIONS AND ANTIMICROBIAL AGENTS
Wound Contamination

For practical purposes, all open fractures and closed injuries covered by devitalized skin are contaminated. Severe wound disruption, extensive contamination, associated vascular injuries, advanced age of the patient, and some premorbid conditions (e.g., diabetes mellitus) all predispose to an increased infection rate.

Dellinger and co-workers[40] found that infections were about three times more common in the leg than in the arm. In the same study, 7 percent of type I, 11 percent of type II, 18 percent of type IIIA, and 56 percent of type IIIB and IIIC fractures became infected. The average infection rate for type I, II, and IIIA fractures was 12 percent, and the average for all fractures was 16 percent. These infection rates are typical of modern series, in which systemic antibiotics are used for the initial 1 to 5 days.[48] There has been long-standing concern that a prolonged interval between injury and débridement may increase infection rates. Apparently based on experimental studies carried out by Friedrich in 1898, 6 hours has long been considered the maximal allowable time interval between injury and débridement.[56] The validity of this sacrosanct time interval has rarely been questioned. However, a study by Patzakis and Wilkins[139] documented essentially identical infection rates of 6.8 percent in open fractures débrided within 12 hours and infection rates of 7.1 percent in those débrided after 12 hours.[9,74,97] A recent 12-year retrospective review of open fracture treatment at a tertiary care center could not demonstrate any increased risk of complication with delayed débridement at the 6-, 8-, 12-, 16-, or 24-hour mark although the authors acknowledge the retrospective nature of the study and the need for therapeutic intent to operate as soon as possible.[113] Another retrospective review of 106 open fractures showed no infections occurred in fractures treated within 2 hours of injury. However, there was no significant increase in infection when comparing patients treated after 6 hours versus within 2 to 6 hours of injury.[97]

Test results for culture specimens taken in the emergency department are positive in about 60 to 70 percent of open fractures.[136,138] Most cultures grow saprophytic organisms such as micrococci, diphtheroids, and saprophytic rods.[172] In one study, 40 to 73 percent of the fractures from which pathogenic organisms grew on pre-débridement cultures eventually became infected with one of the pathogens.[172] In another study,[106] 7 percent of the cases with negative pre-débridement cultures became infected. For all the cases that did become infected, pre-débridement cultures included the infective organisms only 22 percent of the time. Post-débridement cultures were more accurate in predicting infection. Yet, of the cases that did become infected, the infecting organism was present only 22 percent of the time. On the basis of these conflicting and inconsistent data and considering their substantial cost, both pre-débridement and post-débridement cultures are at this time deemed to be of little value.

The prevalence of infecting organisms changes over time and with the severity of the injury. Gustilo and colleagues[68,72] found that the percentage of gram-negative organisms in infected fractures rose from 24 to 77 percent over a 20-year period. Dellinger and co-workers[49] noted *Staphylococcus aureus* in 43 percent and aerobic or facultative gram-negative rods in 14 percent of type I, II, and IIIA fractures that became infected. From most type IIIB and IIIC fractures they recovered a mixed flora; *S. aureus* represented only 7 percent and aerobic or facultative gram-negative rods accounted for 67 percent of the recovered organisms.

Clostridial Infections

TETANUS

Tetanus[165,179] is a rare but often fatal disease caused by *Clostridium tetani*, an anaerobic gram-positive rod that produces a neurotoxin. Tetanus spores are found everywhere in nature, particularly in soil, dust, and animal feces and on the skin of humans. Growth of the bacillus is favored under anaerobic conditions and in the presence of necrotic tissue. Only about 100 to 200 cases occur per year in the United States, mostly in persons older than 50 years. The fatality rate is 20 to 40 percent.

The effects of the exotoxin tetanospasmin on various receptor sites cause all clinical manifestations of the disease. Tetanospasmin probably travels along motor nerves and affixes to the gangliocytes of skeletal muscle, spinal cord, and brain. Tetanus occurs in a localized and a generalized form. Generalized tetanus is much more common, and such early findings as cramps in muscles surrounding the wounds, hyperreflexia, neck stiffness, and a change in facial expression occur. Later, contractions of whole muscle groups may follow, causing opisthotonos and acute respiratory failure. Local opisthotonos is rare; it is characterized by muscle rigidity around the site of the injury and usually resolves without sequelae.

Active immunization with tetanus toxoids is the best and most effective method to prevent the disease. For children younger than 7 years tetanus toxoid is available as a combination with 7 to 8 limit flocculating (Lf) units of diphtheria, 5 to 12.5 Lf units of tetanus, and fewer than 16 opacity units of pertussis (DTP) or without pertussis (DT). For adults and older children, tetanus vaccine (Td) contains fewer than 2 Lf units of diphtheria and 2 to 10 Lf units of tetanus. To obtain long-lasting protective levels of antitoxin, three doses of tetanus toxoid should be given at 2 months, 4 months, and 6 months of age followed by boosters at 12 to 18 months and again at 5

years of age. After this initial series, boosters are given every 10 years for life. Any patient who has not completed a series of toxoid immunization or has not received a booster dose in the 5 years before being wounded should receive tetanus toxoid and, if the wound is tetanus prone, passive immunization with human tetanus immune globulin (HTIG). Any patient wounded more than 10 years after the last booster should receive both HTIG and Td. Generally, 250 to 500 IU HTIG are given intramuscularly and concurrently with toxoid but at a separate site. Protection from HTIG lasts about 3 weeks (see Table 14-6).

Patients with suspected immune deficiencies and patients with tetanus-prone injuries who have not received adequate immunization within the past 5 years should receive passive immunization with HTIG (250–500 IU intramuscularly) in addition to active immunization. Wounds that are considered tetanus prone include wounds contaminated with dirt, saliva, or feces; puncture wounds, including nonsterile injections; missile injuries; burns; frostbites; avulsions; and crush injuries.[16]

GAS GANGRENE

Gas gangrene remains a constant threat,[54,62,83] particularly after primary wound closure, in wounds of type IIIB or IIIC severity, in farm- or soil-related injuries, in wounds contaminated by bowel content, and in patients with diabetes mellitus. *Clostridium* spores are found in soil and in the intestinal tract of humans and animals; *Clostridium perfringens* and *Clostridium septicum* are most prevalent in human disease. Clostridia are anaerobic gram-positive bacteria that produce several exotoxins that can be lethal or act as spreading factors. These toxins induce local edema; necrosis of muscle, fat, and fascia; and thrombosis of local vessels. They also generate hydrogen sulfide and carbon dioxide gases. Because these gases easily spread into the surrounding tissues, the process of tissue swelling, necrosis, and vascular thrombosis becomes self-perpetuating and sets the stage for a fulminant spread of the infection. Hemolysis, with a significant drop in hemoglobin followed by tubular necrosis and renal failure, may occur.[83] The body temperature is often initially subnormal. Locally, the wound may drain foul-smelling, serosanguineous fluid. Edema appears early and is often noted at a distance from the site of trauma. Later, gas can be detected in the tissues by crepitation or radiographically as radiolucent streaks along fascial planes. Most patients are unduly apprehensive and some are fearful of dying.

A patient with suspected or established gangrene should receive intravenous penicillin, 20 to 30 million units daily in divided doses. If the patient is allergic to penicillin, intravenous clindamycin, 1.8 to 2.7 g/day, or metronidazole, 2 to 4 g/day, may be used. A cephalosporin and an aminoglycoside are added to cover other organisms. However, the keys to saving life and limb are extensive fasciotomies and repeated radical débridement at short intervals. Transfer to a major trauma center, possibly one with a hyperbaric chamber, deserves serious consideration. Although major clostridial infections remain a serious threat, all but 8 to 10 percent of infected patients can be saved with modern management techniques.

Antimicrobials

SYSTEMIC ANTIBIOTICS

Systemic antibiotics to prevent post-traumatic wound infections in open fractures were controversial until 1974, when Patzakis[136,138] proved their effectiveness in a randomized, double-blind trial. Other studies have since confirmed the findings[49,70,120,135,137,139,167] and established the current routine of using intravenous antibiotics for all open fractures during the first 3 to 5 days.

Optimal antibiotic choice depends on the severity of the soft tissue injury, the contaminating agent, and the local nosocomial flora.[130,161] At present, a first- or second-generation cephalosporin is preferred for types I and II open fractures and closed fractures with soft tissue injuries. These antibiotics are effective against most gram-positive and many gram-negative bacteria except *Pseudomonas*. For example, cefazolin, in an average adult, should be given as a loading dose of 2 g, followed by 1 g every 8 hours intravenously. In type III open fractures, an aminoglycoside (gentamicin or tobramycin) is added. The historical dosage of 3 to 5 mg/kg of lean body weight per 24 hours given in divided doses has been replaced by a single dose of 5.1 mg/kg once daily.

Experimentally, multiple divided dosing has been associated with a higher incidence of nephrotoxicity because it results in a higher trough concentration; conversely, the higher peak values attained with a single dose are more effective in killing *Escherichia coli* and *Pseudomonas*.[184] In a prospective, randomized trial, single-dose gentamycin was shown to be as safe as multiple dosing. There was also a slight decrease in the infection rate.[167] For fractures occurring in a farm environment, vascular compromise, or extensive soft tissue crush, 2 to 4 million units of aqueous penicillin G every 4 hours are added.

Although initial antibiotic coverage is traditionally provided for 1 to 5 days, there is now good evidence that for simple open fractures without major contamination, a first-generation cephalosporin given for 24 hours is as effective as one given for 5 days.[48] More complicated open fractures are usually covered for 48 hours after wound closure.

LOCAL ANTISEPTICS AND ANTIBIOTICS

Although the use of hot liquids and irons by ancient physicians was harmful, soaking wound dressings with vinegar, alcohol, and carbolic acid often had beneficial effects.[178] With the demonstration that many antiseptics have cell-toxic effects, these agents have fallen into disrepute, although the damage they inflict is usually limited to superficial cell layers. Many surgeons[5] soak wound dressings with isotonic saline, iodine-containing solutions with a broad bactericidal and spore-killing spectrum,[18] or such topical antibiotics as neomycin, bacitracin, and polymyxin. There is limited clinical evidence concerning the beneficial or detrimental effects of any of these regimens.

LOCAL ANTIBIOTICS FROM SLOW-RELEASE CARRIERS

In an attempt to increase their local concentration and prolong their action, antibiotics have been mixed with slow-release carriers such as polymethyl methacrylate (PMMA).[78,79,162,175,176] Successful in the management of infected arthroplasties, these carriers have also been used in chronic skeletal infections and, more recently, in high-risk open fractures (Figs. 14-3 through 14-6). In the latter application, polymethyl methacrylate is mixed with the desired antibiotics and molded into beads 5 to 15 mm in diameter to facilitate removal; the beads are then lined up on a thin wire[100] or suture (Fig. 14-7). After the beads are transferred to the wound cavity, the wound is sutured water-tight or covered with an adhesive drape.[78,79] The beads are removed or exchanged at intervals from 3 days

---

FIGURE 14-3 ▌ **A** and **B**, This patient is a middle-aged man with a type IIIB open tibia fracture.

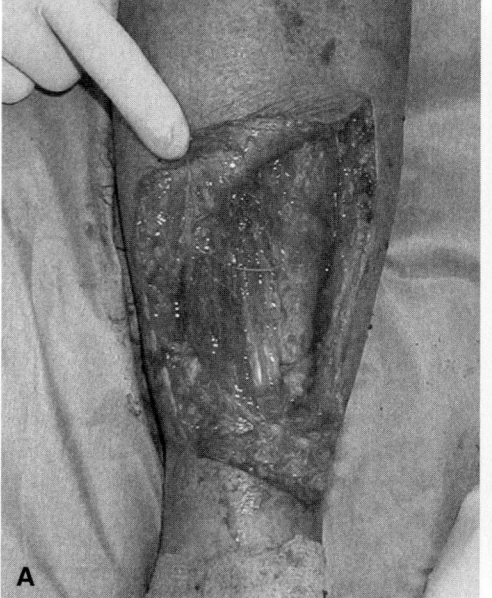 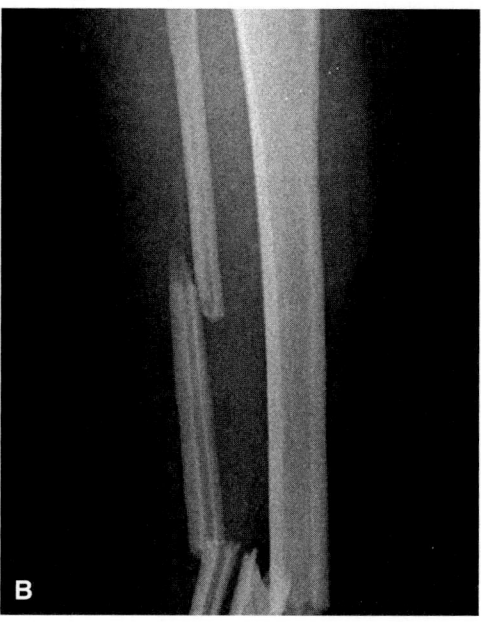

FIGURE 14-4 *Same patient as in Figure 14-3. Irrigation, débridement, and stabilization of the fracture with an external fixator were performed.* **A,** *Antibiotic-impregnated beads on wire.* **B,** *Beads were placed under an adhesive drape to fill the dead space and "sterilize" the wound cavity.*

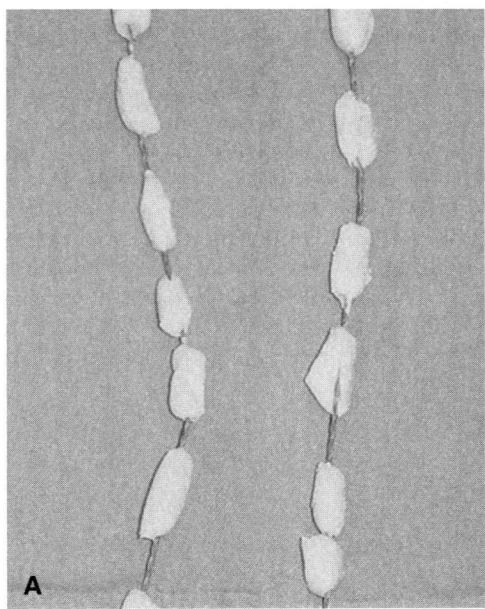

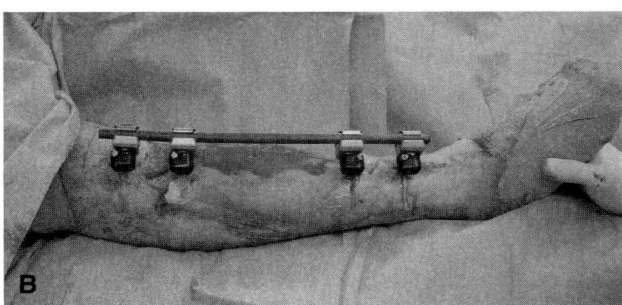

to 6 weeks. If kept in place longer, they are difficult to separate from ingrown soft tissues. Secondary hematogenous infections of beads that were left permanently have been reported.

Although antibiotic concentrations 10 to 30 times higher than those observed after intravenous use are common,[22,108,117,120] little is known about carrier efficiency, optimal bead size and shape, release characteristics, alteration of the antibiotics during the process of polymerization, or antibiotic effectiveness after release.[175] Many different antibiotics have been tried, but much of the scientific work has been limited to aminoglycosides and vancomycin. Compared with high-dose intravenous antibiotics, this form of local application is cheaper, avoids intravenous lines, eases nursing care, is nontoxic to sensitive organs such as the liver, inner ear, and kidney, and may aid in decreasing infection rates in high-grade open fractures.[79,129] Beads also have an advantage when used with ambulatory and noncompliant patients. A study also

indicated that antibiotic beads used alone might be as effective as intravenous antibiotics.[120]

Similar results have been obtained with implantable pumps that deliver antibiotics to the wound at a fixed rate. Although more expensive, this approach appears equally promising.[141] Calcium sulfate can also be used as a delivery vehicle for antibiotics. It has been shown to be as effective

FIGURE 14-6 *Same patient as in Figure 14-3. At 2 weeks, the external fixator and beads were removed. Intramedullary nail placed and appearance at healing.*

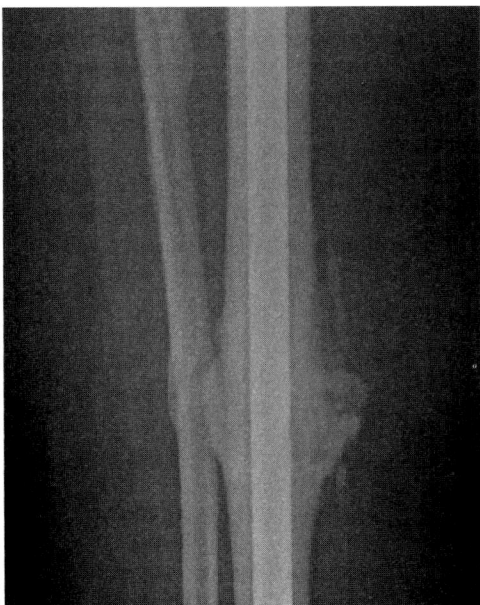

FIGURE 14-5 *Same patient as in Figure 14-3. At 6 days, wound coverage was achieved with a free flap.*

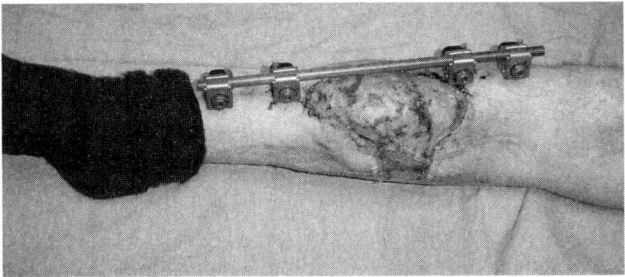

FIGURE 14-7 *Antibiotic beads made with PMMA and tobramycin placed on a No. 1 polypropylene suture.*

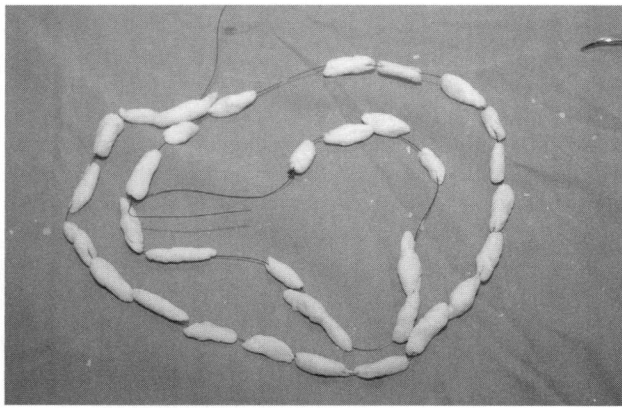

as PMMA–antibiotic–impregnated beads in the treatment of infections in animal models.[8,171] Calcium sulfate offers the potential benefit of being resorbable and not requiring removal, but more clinical series need to be conducted.

WOUND CARE

Irrigation and Débridement

In the operating room and after induction of anesthesia, all splints and bandages are removed, the skin surrounding the wound is shaved, and the injured body part is prepared and draped. A tourniquet is applied but is inflated only in case of massive bleeding. This approach prevents further ischemic damage and makes it easier to assess soft tissue viability. The wound is then cleansed of all dead and foreign material through a dual process of débridement followed by irrigation.

DÉBRIDEMENT

Débridement means the meticulous removal and resection of all foreign and dead material from a wound.[178] Débridement does not remove all bacteria, but it drastically reduces their number and, by leaving only viable tissue behind, greatly diminishes the opportunity for bacterial proliferation. Casual, uninformed, and incomplete débridement has the gravest consequences: remaining bacteria multiply and the surrounding tissues swell, compromising their own blood supply and causing further necrosis. Frank infection ensues along tissue planes and within necrotic muscle bellies, threatening amputation and reamputation at progressively more proximal levels.

Rather than an aimless clipping of necrotic skin edges and muscle strands protruding from the wounds, débridement can be effective only if it is a carefully planned, systematic process. It starts with a thorough exploration of the wound to determine the real size and extent of the injury, which is always substantially larger than what is apparent from the outside (Fig. 14-8). The real extent of the injury has been delineated when all foreign material and necrotic tissue are sharply resected and only the well-perfused walls of a clean wound cavity are left behind.

FIGURE 14-8 **A,** *Type IIIB anterior and medial ankle wounds with multiple tendon lacerations and open lesion of the proximal tibia with extensive tissue loss. Note avulsion of the intervening soft tissue sleeve from the anterior tibia and deep fascia.* **B,** *A simple oblique fracture of the distal tibia and an ankle fracture.*

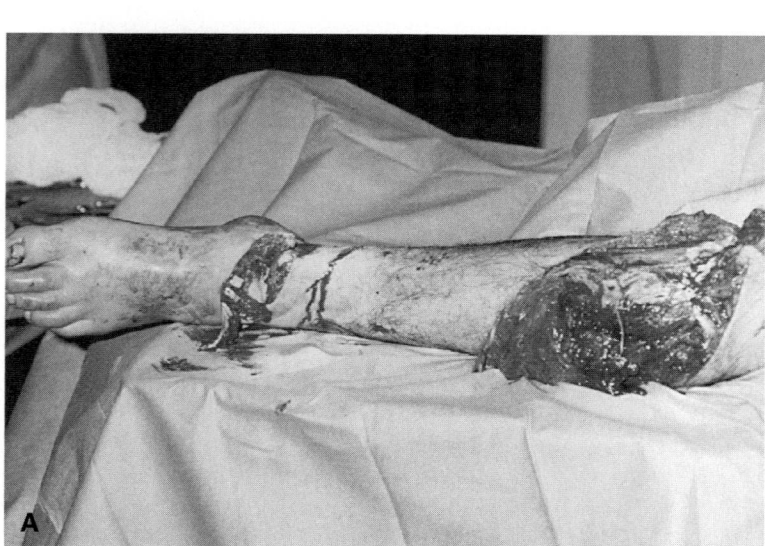

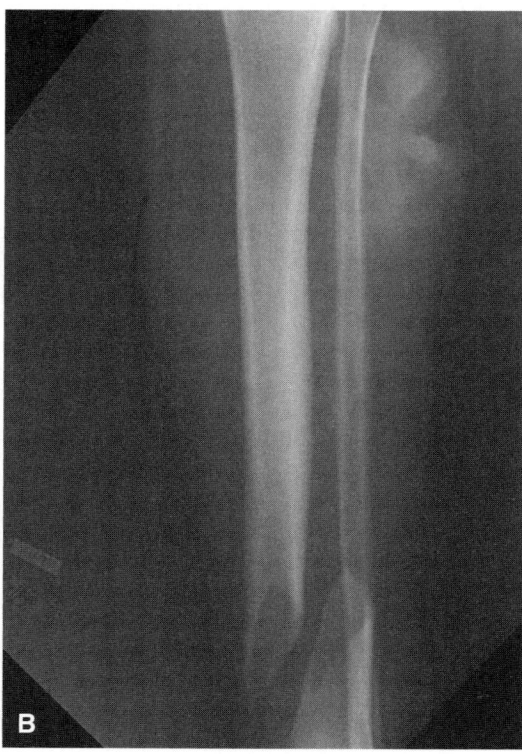

ASSESSING THE EXTENT OF INJURY

In assessing the true extent of the injury zone, information from many different sources is assimilated, including the mechanism of injury; events at the accident site (e.g., whether a protruding fragment was reduced before splinting); examination of the injured extremity (bruises elsewhere; instability of adjacent joints; vascular and neurologic condition; size, location, and contamination of the wound); laboratory findings; and radiographs. In addition to depicting fracture patterns and location, plain radiographs help delineate the extent of the soft tissue destruction by identifying trapped air in different tissue planes, often at a substantial distance from the apparent injury site. The energy causing the injuries is reflected by the multiplicity of fractures, the severity of comminution, and the distance between displaced fragments. Fractures close to points where arteries or nerves are affixed to bone should alert the physician to possible neural and vascular damage. Unless proved otherwise, multiple soft tissue wounds in the same extremity segment are caused by the same injury mechanism, often a bone fragment. Such wounds usually communicate with the fracture site and each other and are telltale signs of a mangled extremity[91] (Figs. 14-8 and 14-9).

The severity of the soft tissue injury is easily misjudged in the proximal extremity segments and in areas in which the bone is covered by a large tissue sleeve, as in the femur or on the posterior aspect of the leg. Because in these areas the external wounds are often small, they easily hide the extent of the underlying muscle disruption, the severity of periosteal stripping, and the degree of contamination at the fracture site.

EXTENDING THE WOUND

Since the cutaneous opening is often just a small peripheral extension of a large underlying injury, the wound must be extended—often by a factor of 3 to 5—until optimal access to all injured tissues is obtained. The enlarging incisions must be extensile, must not create flaps, and must respect neural and vascular territories (Figs. 14-10 through 14-12). They should also facilitate the placement of implants, the transfer of distant soft tissue flaps, and wound closure.

CUTANEOUS TISSUES

Rather than starting with a generous débridement of skin edges, as much of the skin as possible should be preserved during the initial débridement. Obviously, dead and macerated tissues have to be trimmed, but questionable areas become apparent within 24 hours and can easily be removed during a following débridement. Subcutaneous tissue, mainly fat, has a scant blood supply and is freely débrided when contaminated. The skin of amputated parts and large, nonviable, cutaneous flaps can be used as donor sites for the harvest of split-thickness grafts with a dermatome. The resulting skin graft can be used at the end of the procedure or set aside for later needs.

FASCIA

The fascia below the subcutaneous tissue is expendable and can be freely resected if devitalized or contaminated.

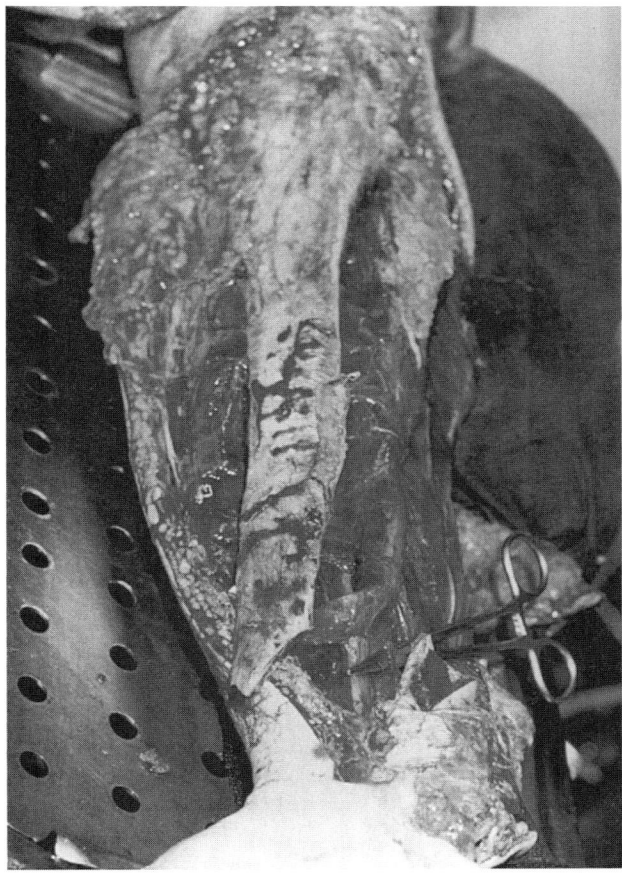

FIGURE 14-9 *Same patient as in Figure 14-8. The true extent of injury is revealed at the end of débridement after both traumatic wounds are connected.*

Contrary to traditional teaching, open fractures do not completely decompress fascial compartments.[72] If constrained spaces remain, the continuing tissue swelling increases the local pressure and interrupts regional blood flow. Further tissue necrosis followed by infection is a common sequela. Prophylactic fasciotomies and epimysiotomies are therefore performed liberally during the initial and subsequent débridement.

MUSCLES AND TENDONS

Because it is a fertile culture medium for bacteria, all muscle of questionable viability should be liberally resected. The "four Cs"—consistency, contractility, color, and capacity to bleed—are not always reliable guides to viability; the capacity to contract after a gentle pinch with a pair of toothed forceps and arterial bleeding are more trustworthy. A contractile reaction to electric cautery may be misleading, since remaining calcium in a nonviable muscle's sarcoplasmic reticulum may be stimulated to respond even though the muscle is nonviable.

Each muscle group that passes through the wound must be individually examined and followed beyond the zone of injury toward its origin and insertion. Disruption or resection of a small blood vessel may lead to ischemic

FIGURE 14-10 | *Clinical (**A**) and radiographic (**B**) appearance of an open fracture in a 12-year-old child struck by an automobile.*

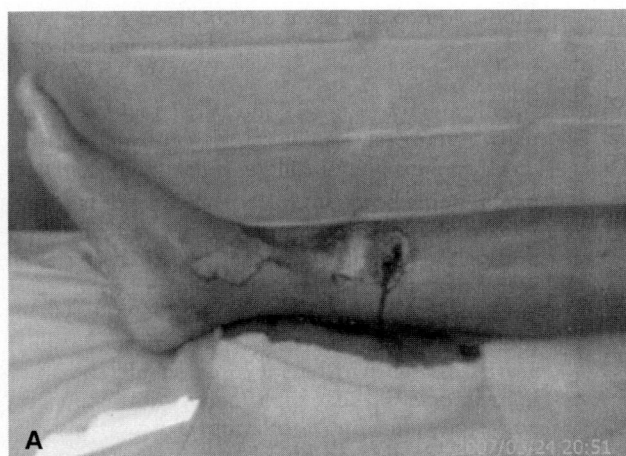 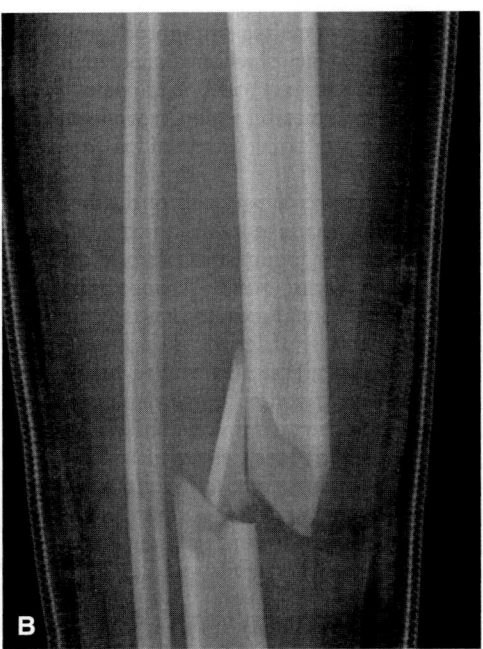

necrosis of a whole muscle segment. Occasionally, a whole muscle group is found to be avascular and must be removed in toto. Contaminated tendons should be cleaned carefully but otherwise can be left intact. They are easily accessible and can be further débrided at a later time.

BONE

When faced with a small outside wound, the physician is tempted just to trim the wound edges and irrigate

FIGURE 14-11 | *Same patient as in Figure 14-10. Wound after extension and débridement. Butterfly fragment was completely devoid of soft tissue attachments and was removed. Notice extent of periosteal stripping not appreciated prior to wound extension.*

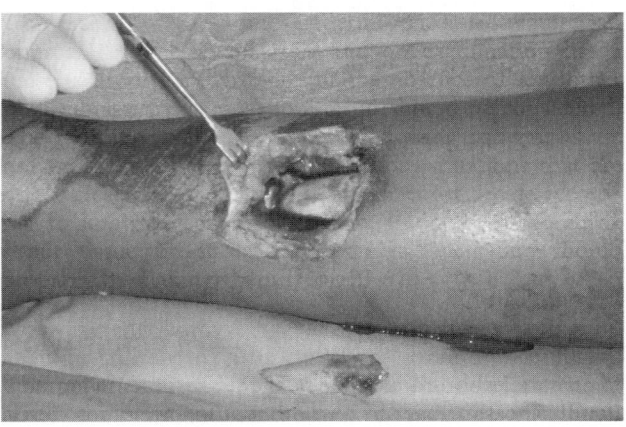

blindly through the wound opening. This casual approach easily misses a foreign body or contaminated bone fragments and thus can lead to a major deep infection followed by an amputation. In most open fractures, at least one bone end penetrates through the wound and makes contact with the surrounding environment, which is never sterile. Therefore, the wound opening must be extended so that the free ends of all principal bone fragments can be delivered into the open and carefully inspected and débrided.

The intramedullary cavity is cleansed of all dirt and other foreign material. All devitalized pieces of cortical bone are removed (see Fig. 14-11). Whenever possible, larger articular fragments should be cleaned and used for joint reconstruction. Severely contaminated fragments are discarded, and the defect is later corrected by a bone graft or distraction osteogenesis.

NEUROVASCULAR STRUCTURES

Major arteries and nerves in the injury zone are often serious obstacles to adequate débridement. They must be carefully identified, mobilized, and separated from surrounding nonviable tissue. Major arteries and nerves that are transected must be repaired.

IRRIGATION

Although irrigation is useful for removing blood clots and debris, particularly from deep interstices, it is simply an adjunct to, and by no means a replacement for, thorough débridement.

Only after a full assessment of the extent of the injury and complete débridement of all nonviable tissue has been performed is the wound ready to be irrigated.

FIGURE 14-12   *Same patient as in Figure 14-10. **A,** Stabilization of fracture with use of external fixator. **B,** Approximation of the wound was accomplished with retention sutures and nylon skin sutures.*

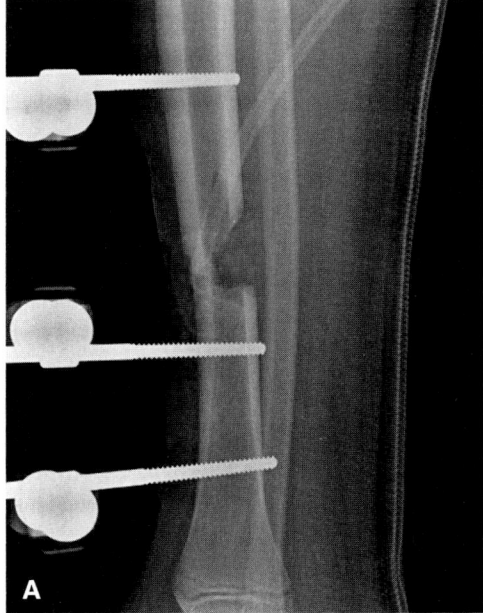

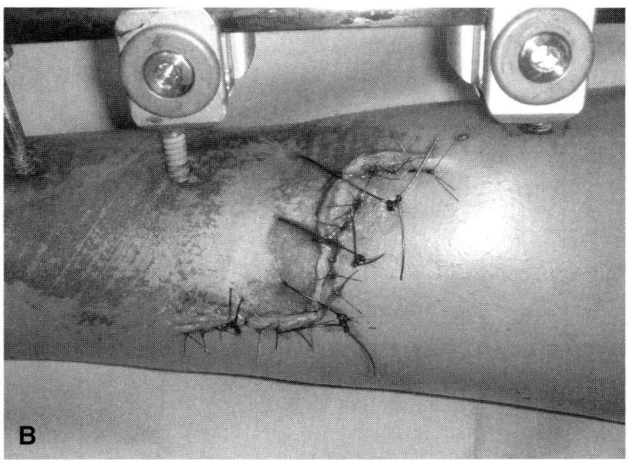

Irrigation with ample amounts of isotonic solution aids in the removal of coagula, fresh blood, foreign material, necrotic tissue, and bacteria. Commonly used delivery methods include gravity feed with arthroscopy tubing, low-pressure (bulb) irrigation, and high-pressure pulsatile lavage. Pulsating irrigation with a sprinkler head appears to be most effective in removing *Staphylococcus*[5] especially after a delay of 3 hours or more.[14] High-pressure lavage damages bone and in the early phases may delay fracture healing, but as healing progresses there seem to be no adverse effects.[1,53] Currently, pulsatile lavage is recommended in open fractures with significant contamination or a delay in treatment, since fracture healing will be delayed only in the early phases. In cases with minimal contamination, bulb syringe is equally effective.[105] However, it must be noted that recent in vitro data suggest that high-pressure lavage causes increased depth of bacterial penetration in soft tissue and the intramedullary canal compared with low-pressure lavage and must be used cautiously.[6,75]

Judging from animal studies, adding antibiotics is not more effective than using saline alone. In fact, the most effective additive to eliminate *Staphylococcus* was benzalkonium chloride.[5,57,170] Although it is nontoxic in rats, its use was accompanied by an increased complication rate.[36] However, with sequential irrigation with benzalkonium chloride followed by castile soap and then saline, these complications were avoided. For *Pseudomonas*, castile soap or sequential irrigation with benzalkonium chloride followed by normal saline was shown to decrease positive cultures when compared with normal saline.[3] Anglen looked at 458 open fractures to compare antibiotic solution irrigation with castile soap. There was no difference in infection rates, but the antibiotic irrigation solution wounds tended to have a higher incidence of wound healing problems.

Vascular Injuries and Compartment Syndromes

VASCULAR INJURIES

When an open fracture is associated with a major vascular injury, particularly in the lower extremity, the prognosis for limb survival remains dismal. Lange and colleagues[103] noted that of 23 open tibial fractures requiring vascular repair, 61 percent were ultimately amputated. Of the patients whose limbs were salvaged by successful vascular repair, more than 50 percent developed chronic problems that interfered with routine daily activities. If the warm ischemia time—the crucial survival parameter—exceeded 4 hours, the amputation rate was 50 percent, and no limbs survived when the warm ischemia time exceeded 6 hours. In another study,[94] the ultimate amputation rate was 58 percent. Although isolated lesions of the anterior tibial and the peroneal artery had a good prognosis, negative outcomes were more common with transection of the popliteal artery or the posterior tibial artery and with injuries involving all three major arteries distal to the trifurcation.

Extremities with major vascular compromise[31,42,49,73,96,103,126] should be cooled at the site of injury and during transport to the nearest trauma center capable of handling the lesion. After stabilization of vital functions, the injured extremity is carefully assessed by both an extremity surgeon and a vascular surgeon. An expedient treatment plan is then established with the goal of having a fully revascularized extremity in less than 6 hours, a grace period that can be extended somewhat with the use of a temporary silicone elastomer arterial shunt.[90] Considering the serious time constraints, initial internal fixation of the fracture is, under most circumstances, too time consuming, and temporary external fixation with immediate vascular repair is safer. It is well to remember that a study carried out during the Vietnam War showed excellent results when vascular care was followed by skeletal traction.[144] Fasciotomies of all compartments in the affected extremity segment are essential, particularly in the lower limb.[17]

COMPARTMENT SYNDROME

There is a widespread assumption that compartment syndromes[153] rarely, if ever, occur with open fractures. Yet in four series, compartment syndromes were diagnosed in 2 to 16 percent of cases of open tibial fracture.[26,38,85,88] The incidence of compartment syndromes is directly proportional to the severity of the injury.[68] They occur most often in polytrauma patients, pedestrians struck by a car, and patients with type III open fractures with major comminution. At risk for a delayed or missed diagnosis are patients with significant injuries and under prolonged anesthesia and those who suffer from a compromised sensorium owing to drugs or handicaps, and patients who are noncommunicative or have a cord transection or a regional nerve lesion. For all patients who are at risk, compartment pressures should be determined before and after the initial operative intervention and at regular intervals thereafter. If the pressure in one of the leg compartments is elevated, it is prudent to decompress all four compartments.[17]

Amputations

Primary amputations in cases of open fractures may be indicated for a severely mangled extremity (type IIIB lesion) or when there is a limb-threatening arterial lesion that is irreparable or has resulted in a failed repair (type IIIC lesion). Whenever possible, the decision to amputate should be made at the time of the initial débridement. Although there are no universally accepted guidelines, information that strongly favors an amputation includes an MESS of 7 or higher,[91,103] a warm ischemia time exceeding 6 hours,[103] and the presence of a serious secondary bone or soft tissue injury involving the same extremity or foot (Fig. 14-13).

In the past, a loss of protective sensation to the foot[19] was an additional indication to amputate. However, if the lesion is due to a neuropraxia of the posterior tibial nerve, it may recover over time. There are also about 20 reports in the world literature detailing the outcomes of direct repairs and grafting of posterior tibial nerve lesions. Most of the grafts were done on a delayed basis about 6 months after the injury. About 70 to 80 percent of the patients showed good results with successful sensory recovery and without trophic ulcerations or the need for ambulatory support.[50,76,82,109,125,180]

The importance of making the proper decision for a primary amputation is difficult to overestimate because primary amputations may lead to better long-term results than either secondary amputations or complex limb reconstructions.[19,59,96] This older view has been recently challenged by longer follow-up in the LEAP study, which shows those patients that have amputation or limb salvage to have significant long-term disability.[110] Early amputation also enhances patients' survival, reduces pain and disability, and shortens hospital stay.

Considering the massive energy that is involved in most limb-threatening injuries, an open amputation at the time of initial débridement is most appropriate. If an amputation is considered, the process is started with a careful débridement of the local wound. As much as possible of the soft tissue sleeve is preserved, and only nonviable tissue is resected. The amputated stump is then dressed open, and the definitive decision about amputation level and type of wound closure is made during a later débridement when the size and function of the remaining soft tissue sleeve have become clear. So-called guillotine amputations, which are transverse transection of all soft tissues and bone proximal to the injury level, may have saved lives on the Napoleonic battlefields, but they are not part of modern trauma care (Fig. 14-14). We currently attempt to salvage as much viable soft and bony tissue as possible to attain the most optimal amputation level. As noted, skin and other viable tissues useful for later reconstructions should be harvested before an amputated limb is sent for pathologic evaluation.

Wound Coverage

At the end of the débridement, the wound cavity should be delineated on all sides by viable bleeding tissue. The remaining soft tissue must not be restricted by encasing fascial layers but should be free to expand with the expected tissue edema. Whenever possible, nerves, vessels, tendons, and denuded bone surfaces are covered with local soft tissue.

FIGURE 14-13 *A* and *B,* Patient with grade III open tibia fracture and mangled foot requiring a below knee amputation.

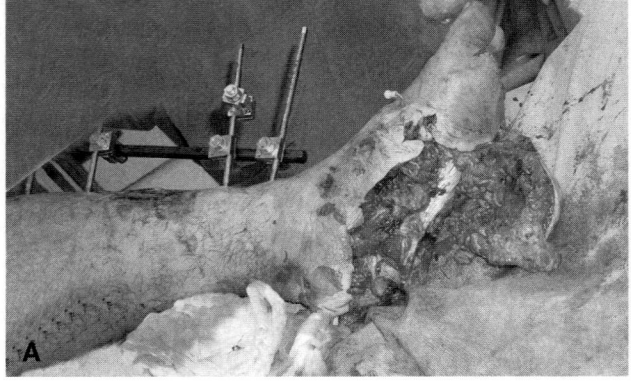
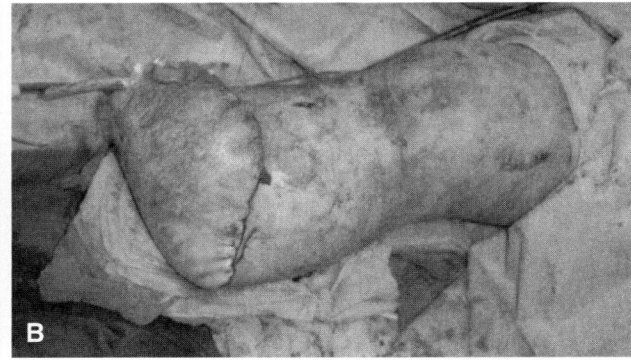

FIGURE 14-14 *Bilateral guillotine amputations after a jackknife trailer accident. Whenever possible, guillotine amputations should be avoided. As much viable soft tissue as possible should be preserved to secure the optimal amputation level.*

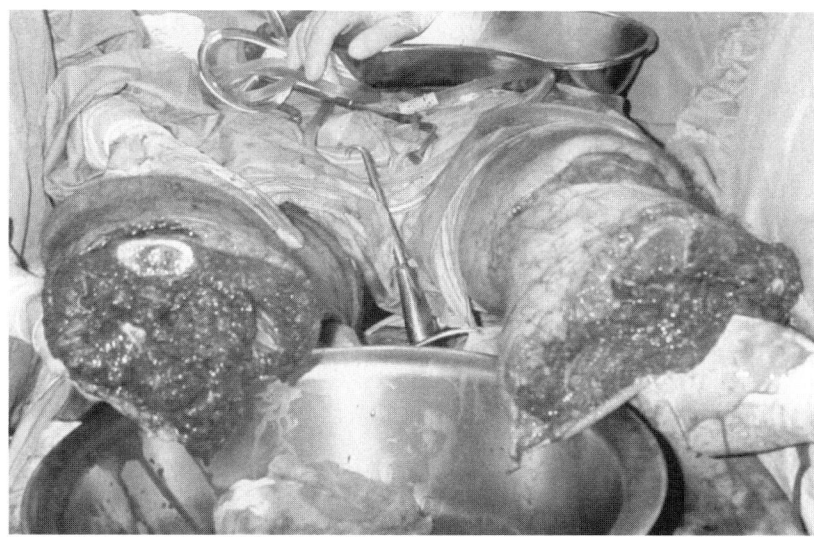

In some earlier studies, primary closures of type I and type II wounds led to significantly higher rates of infection and nonunion.[41,157] It is also noted that primary wound closure could potentially be a contributing factor in the development of gas gangrene.[24,131] Nevertheless, two smaller subsequent studies suggested that low-grade open fracture may be closed primarily without a substantial increase in risk.[51,163] The wound cavity is dressed with a bandage soaked in isotonic saline to which a topical antibiotic or an antiseptic has been added.[18,154] Another option is the creation of an antibiotic bead pouch[78] (see Fig. 14-4B). To prevent undue soft tissue retraction, the skin edges are placed under a moderate amount of traction with the help of retention sutures (see Fig. 14-12B). This technique facilitates secondary wound closure and precludes unnecessary skin grafts or flaps.

In contrast, it has also been shown that multiple débridements may delay fracture healing in an animal model.[133] When reviewing 119 open fractures, those with Gustilo grades I to IIIA treated by immediate primary closure after a thorough débridement did not have a significant increase in infections or problems with union when compared with serially débrided open fractures.[51] After thorough débridement, primary closure can potentially decrease the soft tissue insult of multiple débridements and potential patient morbidity from multiple operating room visits. Surgeon experience and understanding of the injury are quite important in determining whether adequate débridement has been attained and in determining the need for repeated débridement.

Fractures with severe soft tissue involvement may be systematically reexplored and re-débrided in the operating room within 48 to 72 hours. All necrotic tissue that has developed since the initial débridement is resected, and more extensive fasciotomies or epimysiotomies are performed if indicated. If necessary, with severely contaminated wounds, the process of débridement may be repeated every 2 to 3 days until the wound is clean and can be closed or covered.[121]

Timing and method of wound coverage are carefully assessed when the injury is first seen. An expert in soft tissue and microvascular techniques is consulted if the need for a complex soft tissue technique is anticipated (Figs. 14-15 through 14-18). Whenever possible, open fractures should be covered within a week and before the wound is colonized secondarily.[135]

Delayed or primary closure is feasible for most type I, type II, and some type IIIA open wounds as long as retraction of the wound edges is prevented if serial débridement is necessary (see Fig. 14-12B). Healing by secondary intention is a reasonable option for smaller type I wounds not overlying bone surfaces or articulations. Such wounds are often granulated and epithelialized in less than a week. A dense bed of granulation tissue may also be the best initial goal when dealing with an infected wound needing repeated débridement. If the bacterial counts are low, a local or free flap should follow; otherwise, a split-thickness skin graft should be applied as an intermediary step. Split-thickness skin grafts are ideal for covering large skin defects overlying viable tissue such as muscle. They also provide excellent temporary coverage for granulation tissue covering bone and periarticular structures.

Myofascial, local, and free muscle flaps have revolutionized the coverage of large, acute, and chronic soft tissue or bone defects.[28,63,145,183] Local flaps are often ideal, but they are limited in size and are not available in the distal segments of an extremity. Their use is also contraindicated if the muscle has been damaged by the initial injury. Free muscle and composite flaps can deal with almost any defect anywhere in the body (see Fig. 14-17). In addition to giving coverage and possibly structural support, muscle flaps can eliminate low type bacterial contamination in the recipient bed and increase the rate of union in underlying fractures.[145] The placement of a free flap is often the first stage in a complex extremity reconstruction.[63,183] Flaps are rarely applied during the initial débridement because the real extent of injury is often not obvious and the damage to the donor muscle is difficult to assess.

The recent introduction of negative-pressure wound therapy (also known as vacuum-assisted closure, or VAC) has added a tool in treating tenuous wounds. Since "fix-and-flap" coverage in the first 72 hours of injury as

FIGURE 14-15   *A* and *B*, *A type IIIB open pilon (tibial plafond) fracture.*

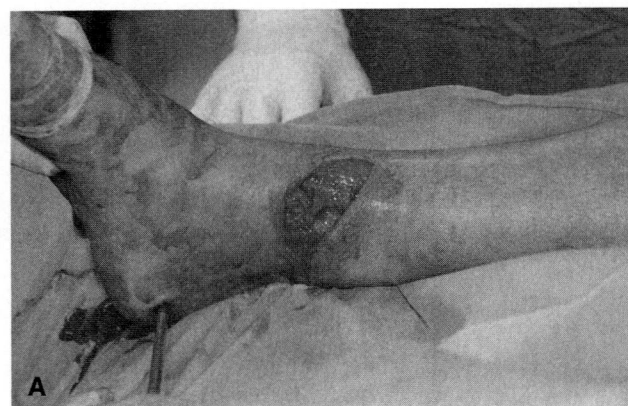

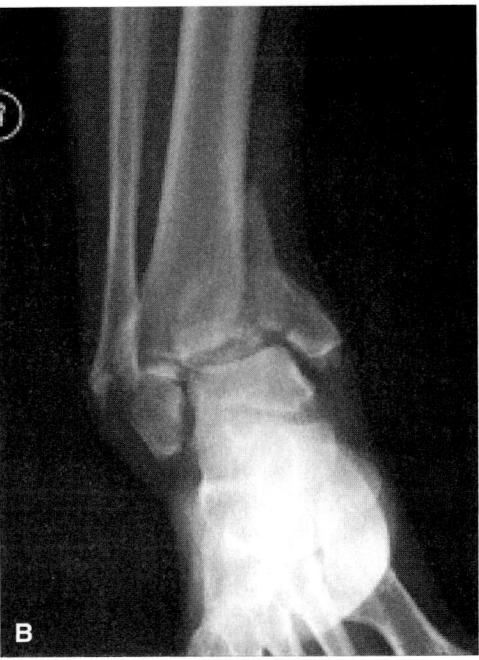

advocated by Gopal et al.[61] is not always possible, VAC is an effective method of temporizing coverage that offers the potential concomitant benefits of decreasing edema, increasing local tissue perfusion, increasing granulation tissue, and decreasing bacterial loads compared with wet-to-dry dressing[6,46,122] (Fig. 14-19). Herscovici et al.[81]

evaluated 21 high-energy soft tissue injuries receiving VAC treatments for an average of 19 days. Only 43 percent needed free tissue transfer. Dedmond et al.[45] had a 45 percent reduction in need of free tissue transfer in 31 suspected grade IIIB tibia fractures when utilizing the VAC system.

FRACTURE FIXATION

Immobilization is crucial for the healing of soft tissue and bone.[128,149] Stabilization of the fracture fragments prevents further injuries to the surrounding soft tissue sleeve, limits the intensity and duration of the inflammatory response, diminishes the spread of bacteria, facilitates tissue perfusion, and encourages early wound repair. Stabilization of the skeletal injury results in decreased pain, greater mobility,[123] fewer respiratory complications such as deaths from adult respiratory distress syndrome,[20,21,92] and greater ease in nursing care and the management of injuries elsewhere.

For centuries, skeletal fixation was possible only indirectly, through pressure on the surrounding soft tissues and prolonged immobilization of adjacent extremity segments.[178] Reduced limb function as a result of shortening, malalignment, nonunion, muscle atrophy, joint contractures, osteopenia, and persistent drainage was the expected sequela of this approach. In contrast, the goal of modern fracture care is a stable, clean injury site that proceeds to union with proper alignment and length and finally regains close to normal function.[123] This goal is achievable only if the methods used to stabilize open fractures provide free wound access for repeated débridement and the placement of local or distant flaps and bone grafts. The methods should not interfere with the blood supply of the fracture fragments and should be sufficiently rigid to allow early joint motion and at least partial weight-bearing.

FIGURE 14-16   *Same patient as in Figure 14-15 after irrigation and débridement, wound extension, and internal fixation.*

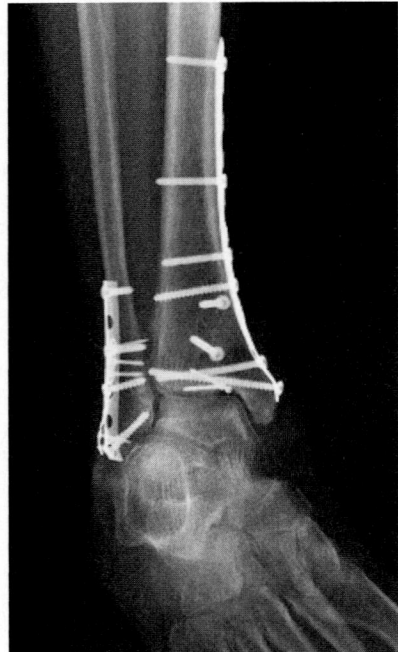

FIGURE 14-17 *Patient with grade IIIB open tibia fracture. It was not possible to close the wound after complete débridement without undue tension. Application of a free flap was performed on day 5.*

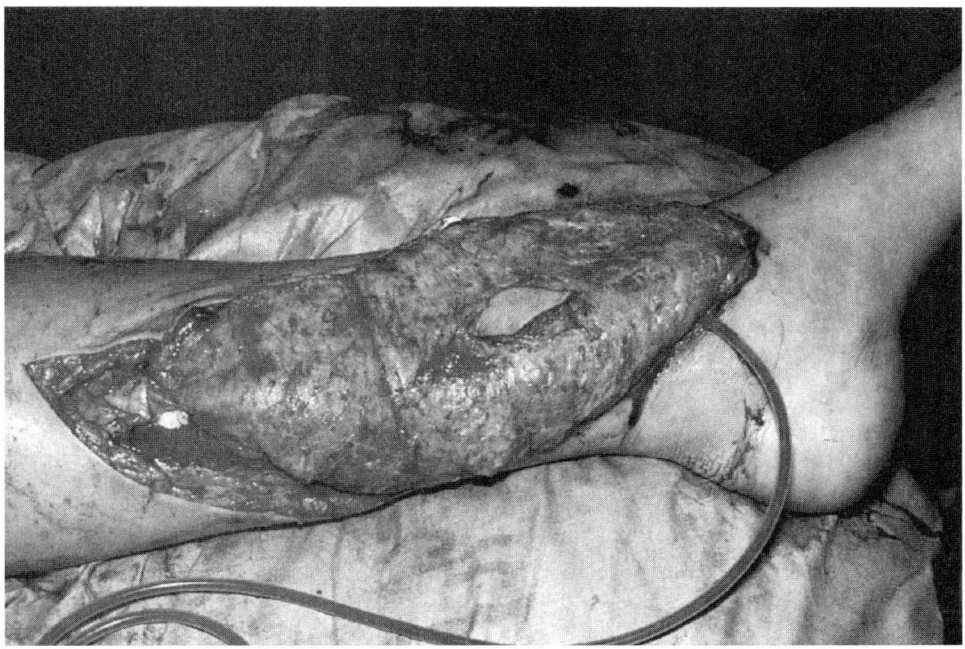

Finally, all of this must be achieved without undue risks and complications.

The rigidity of the fixation determines whether a fracture consolidates through primary or secondary bone healing mechanisms,[119,140] but it does not have a predictable influence on healing times or union rates. Although the literature is replete with reports about the superiority of one method of fracture stabilization over another, most such studies are limited recollections focused on selected populations of patients. They often exclude the most severe injuries, have insufficient follow-up, and are silent about limb length, alignment, and motion in adjacent joints. Rarely do they address functional, occupational,

and recreational outcomes. The optimal fixation method for a particular open fracture depends on numerous variables related to the patient, injury, and treatment, including the surgeon's skill and experience. What constitutes optimal fixation constantly changes with evolving new insights and techniques. Often the best outcome and shortest healing time are achieved when multiple methods are used simultaneously or in sequence (Figs. 14-20 through 14-27).

Slings, Splints, Casts, and Traction

For many centuries, only nonrigid methods, including slings, splints, casts, and traction, were used to stabilize

FIGURE 14-18 *Same patient as in Figure 14-17.* **A** *and* **B,** *Ankle motion, 1 year later.*

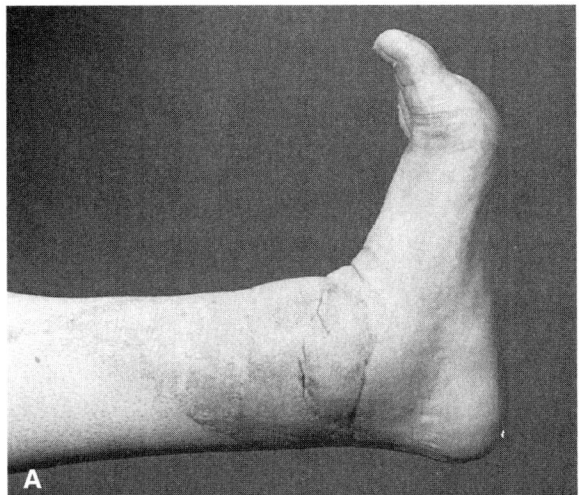
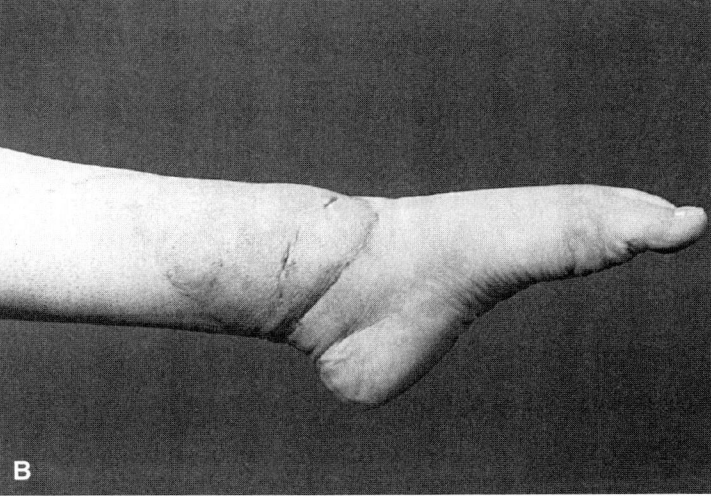

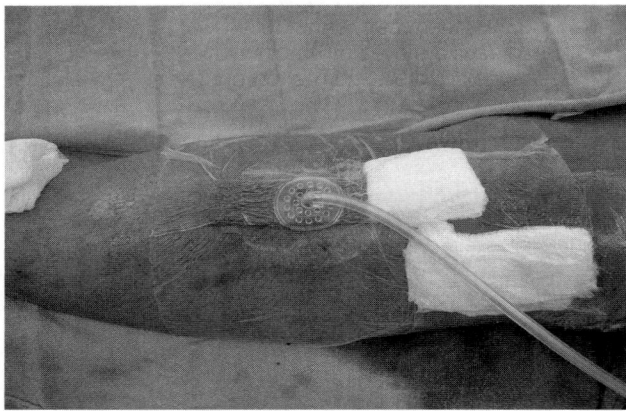

FIGURE 14-19 *Patient with grade III open fracture. Wound VAC in place.*

open fractures.[178] At present, they are used as temporary methods for the initial care of complex fractures.

Slings may be indicated for fractures of the humeral neck and shaft and to provide additional support for internally or externally stabilized forearm lesions. Splints, which can be made of a variety of materials, may provide initial stabilization of open fractures until clear

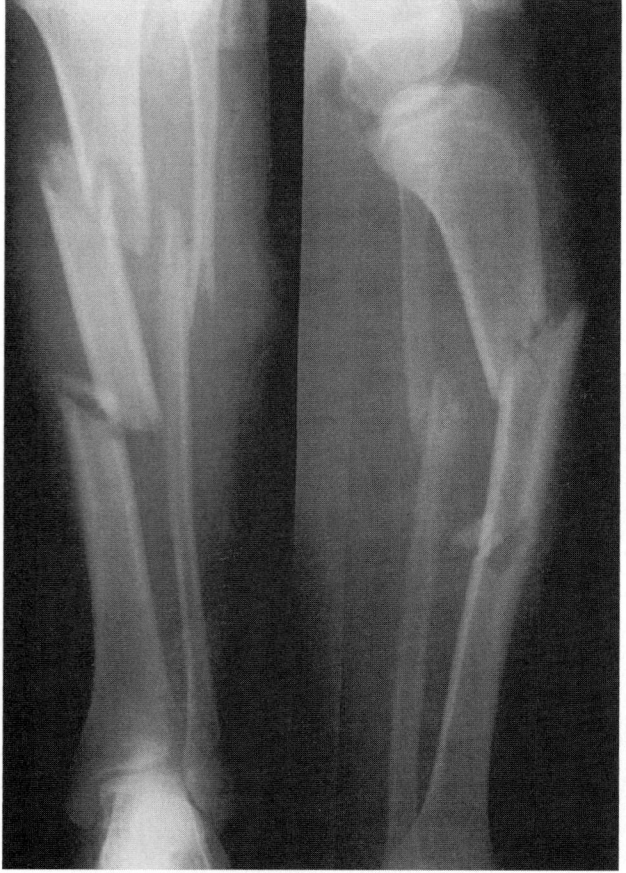

FIGURE 14-20 *A type IIIA open segmental fracture of the tibia.*

decisions can be made about optimal soft tissue coverage or bone fixation.

Circular casts have no place in the early management of open fractures because they cannot accommodate swelling and may prevent the detection of further soft tissue damage, circulatory impairment, or an increase in compartment pressures. They also obstruct the injury site. Casts with openings create window edema and limit the full assessment of the underlying wound. However, in certain circumstances, casts may be ideal for the subsequent care of stable type I and II open tibial fractures after the soft tissue wounds have been closed and swelling has subsided.[25,159] Despite their popularity, casts have a dismal record as a secondary method of immobilization after removal of an external fixator from a fracture that is only partially healed. Under these circumstances, they often permit the development of secondary deformities and later a malunion.[84] The technique of pins and plaster should be reserved for situations in which external fixators are not available.

Skeletal traction is rarely used in the upper extremity but may be indicated for the immobilization of pelvic injuries, acetabular lesions, and open femoral fractures especially prior to fixation.

Internal Fixation

With the development of mechanically and functionally more appropriate implants and safer operating techniques after World War II, internal fixation methods have revolutionized the treatment of many fractures.[123] They provide excellent stabilization of the injury zone, allow for early mobilization of the limb and the patient, and facilitate fracture consolidation while preventing malalignment and loss of length. Most of these methods require additional exposure and can cause partial loss of periosteal, cortical, or intramedullary blood supply, which may increase the rate of nonunion and the risk of infection (see Figs. 14-15 and 14-16). Although there is some evidence that rigid fracture fixation promotes the consolidation of infected fractures,[148,149] metal in contaminated wounds also facilitates the formation of biofilms,[67] which make bacteria inaccessible to antibiotics and host defense mechanisms and thereby promote and maintain a chronic infective process.[142]

WIRES AND SCREWS

When used alone to fix diaphyseal fractures, cerclage, wires, and screws rarely result in stable fixation. Screw fixation is most appropriate for the stabilization of intra-articular and periarticular fractures; it is used alone or in combination with a plate or an external fixator (see Fig. 14-25).

PLATES

Internal fixation with plates is used with utmost caution in all fractures with severe contamination or type IIIB or IIIC soft tissue lesions.[7,34,127] Plates and screws have been particularly successful in the treatment of diaphyseal, periarticular, and intra-articular fractures of the upper extremity.[93,119,150] In the lower extremity, these implants are most useful around joints[181] (see Figs. 14-15 and 14-16) but are rarely

FIGURE 14-21 *Same patient as in Figure 14-20.* **A,** *Irrigation, débridement, and temporary stabilization were accomplished with a two-pin external fixator and Robert Jones dressing. Wound closure at 3 days.* **B,** *Radiographs: the external fixator maintains length; the Robert Jones dressing prevents bending in the frontal plane.*

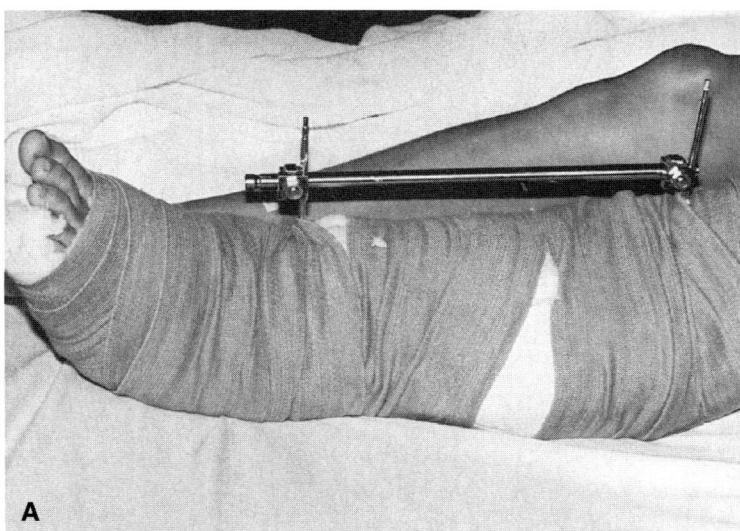
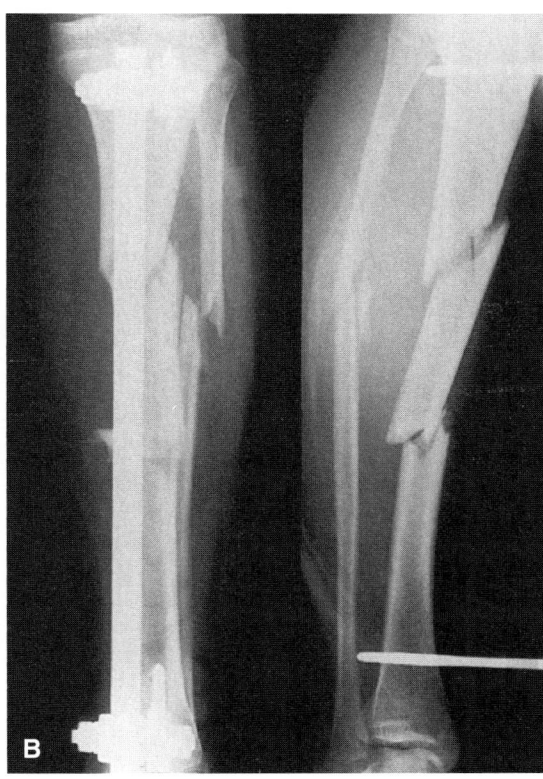

indicated for fractures of the femoral and tibial diaphyses.[7,127] Plates are usually unsuitable for lesions with segmental bone loss,[140] but locked plating may challenge this concept.

Plates should be applied with minimal additional soft tissue and periosteal stripping and must be covered with well-vascularized soft tissues, preferably muscle.[119] Often, this goal is best achieved if the plate is applied not through the wound but through a separate incision.[172] Occasionally, application in a nontraditional location, such as the posterior tibial surface, may be indicated. If delayed primary closure within 3 to 5 days is unlikely, a consultant with soft tissue expertise should be involved promptly, and flap coverage of the wound and implant should be obtained before secondary wound colonization occurs[183] (see Figs. 14-17 and 14-18). A primary bone graft is indicated for fractures of the forearm with extensive soft tissue stripping, comminution, or partial bone loss.[119] Bone grafting in the lower extremity should be performed after flaps and soft tissues have healed, typically in 4 to 6 weeks following wound coverage.

INTRAMEDULLARY NAILS

Because the fragment ends of many diaphyseal fractures are devoid of periosteum, reamed intramedullary nails have been used only cautiously for fear that the additional loss of intramedullary blood supply may increase the chances of infection and nonunion. In fact, animal studies have shown that unreamed nails destroy about 30 percent of the central cortical blood supply. With the addition of reaming, 70 percent of the central blood supply is lost.[99,160] These experimental findings are contrary to the early experience in human tibial fractures, in which reamed nails[37,38] appeared to be associated with shorter healing times and lower complication rates than unreamed nails.[146] A randomized study found that tibial nailing with and without reaming gave equivalent results.[95]

If the fracture configuration permits, intramedullary nails appear safe for types I to IIIA open diaphyseal fractures.[30,95] Although they may also be safe for type IIIB lesions,[31,157] temporary external fixation may represent the more cautious approach.[9,55,58,85,92,122]

External Fixation

Although external fixators long appeared ideal for the management of fractures with soft tissue injuries,[10,11,104,174] only the technical and conceptual advances of the past two decades have allowed us to employ these devices effectively and with acceptable risk.[10,11,13,40,43] Properly applied, external fixators immobilize the fracture at a distance from the injury site without placing foreign material in the wound. They can be applied without additional soft tissue dissection and are easily dismantled if further débridement is necessary. Pin drainage occurs in about 30 percent of all patients, but pin tract infections that require more than local pin care have become rare.

Compared with other methods of fracture stabilization, external fixators provide great versatility and flexibility

FIGURE 14-22 *Same patient as in Figure 14-20. Closed intramedullary nailing at 10 days.*

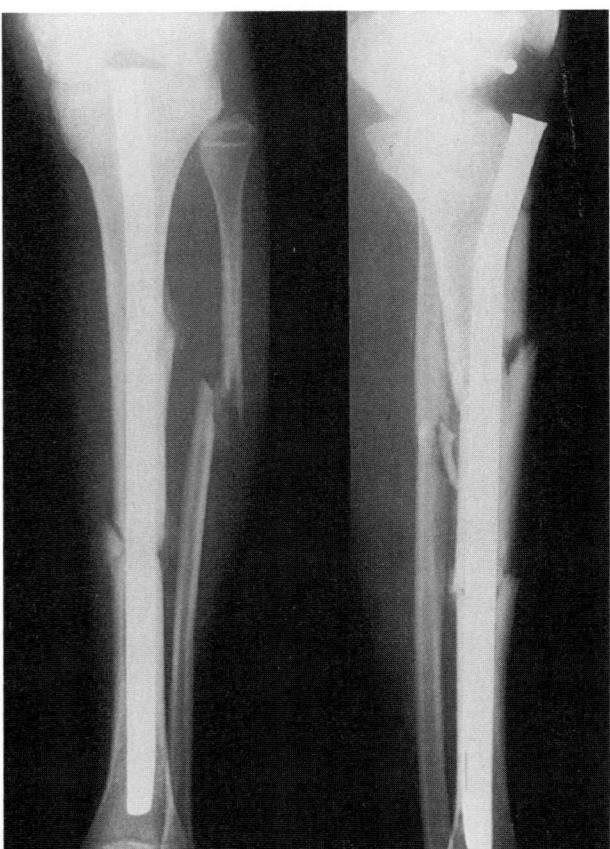

FIGURE 14-23 *Same patient as in Figure 14-20. One year later, after removal of the nail.*

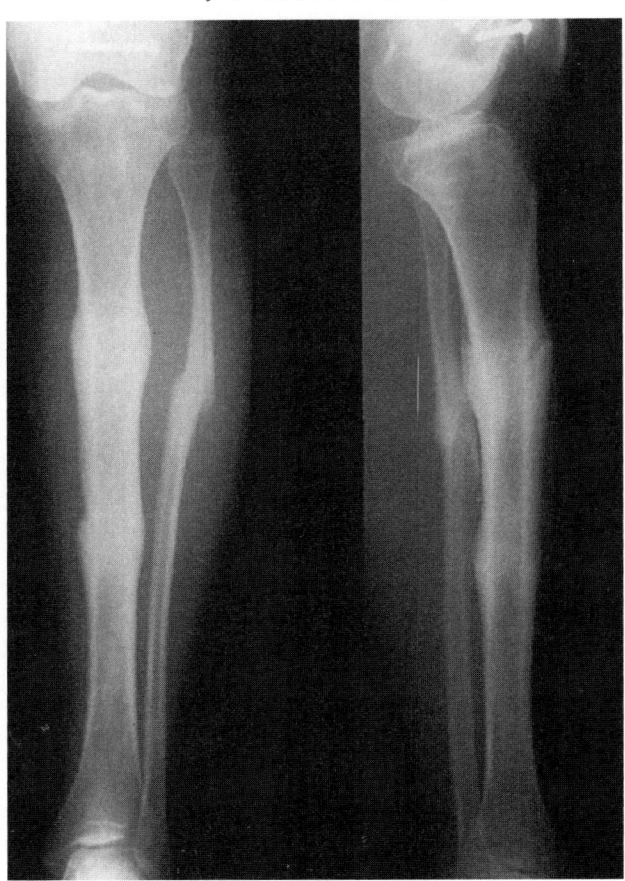

because configurations and rigidity can easily be changed to accommodate many different and newly arising circumstances. They are easily removed, replaced by, or combined with other methods of fixation (see Figs. 14-3 through 14-6 and 14-20 through 14-27).

External fixators are indicated for most contaminated types IIIB and IIIC open fractures and for many closed fractures with severe soft tissue injury.[13,40,43] Transarticular fixators are temporarily applied for some periarticular and intra-articular fractures and joint dislocations[4,166]

FIGURE 14-24 **A,** *Combination of a type IIIA open ulnar fracture and a type II open radial fracture.* **B,** *Radiographs before treatment.*

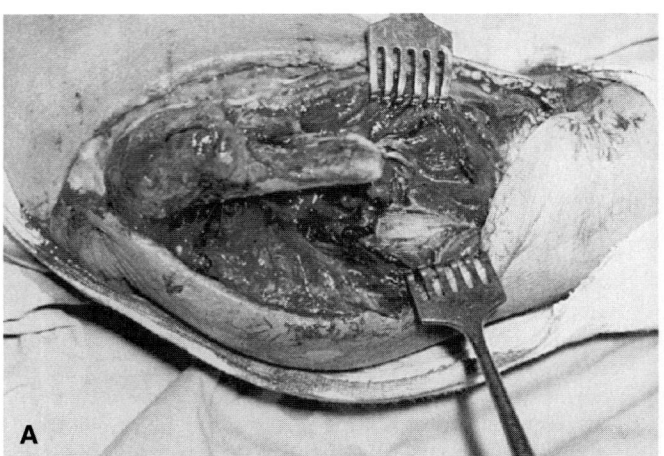

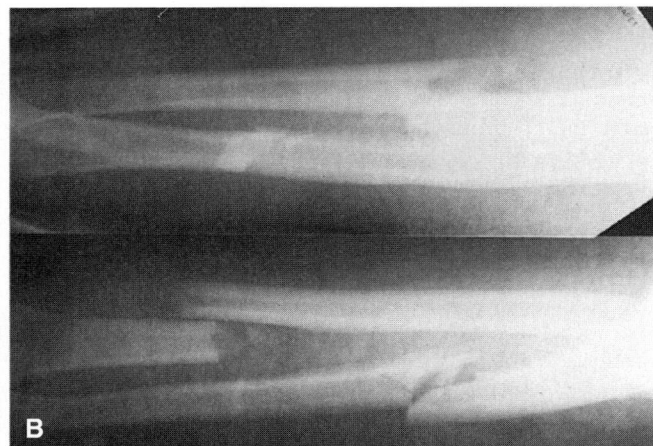

A

B

FIGURE 14-25 *Same patient as in Figure 14-24. On the day of admission, irrigation, débridement, and internal fixation of the radial fracture were performed. The combination of minimal internal fixation and external fixation for the fractured ulna allows delayed tissue healing and early rehabilitation.*

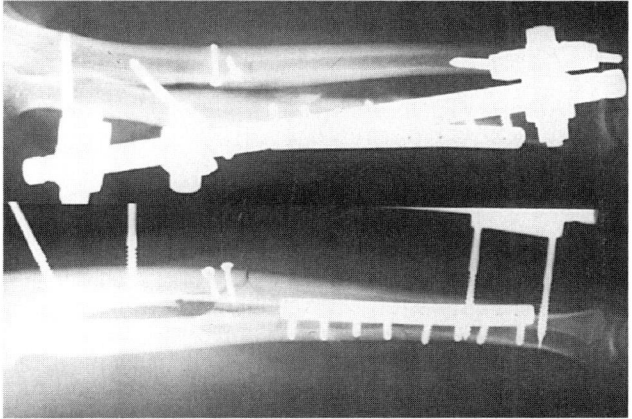

FIGURE 14-27 *Same patient as in Figure 14-24. At 10 weeks, removal of the external fixator and plating and bone grafting of the ulna for impending nonunion were performed.*

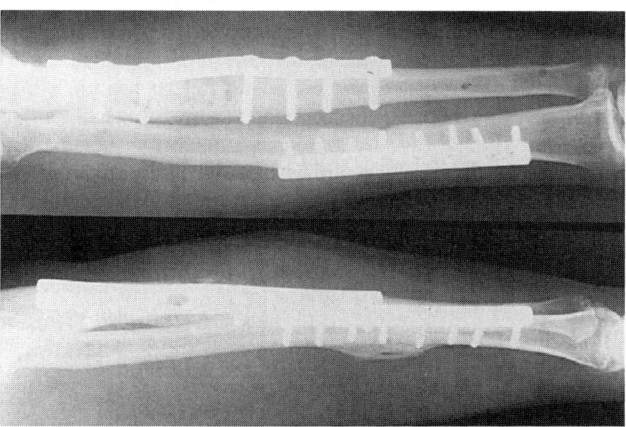

(Figs. 14-28 through 14-33). To prevent permanent joint contractures, they are usually removed or replaced by non-spanning fixators or internal fixation as soon as the soft tissue lesions have healed (see Figs. 14-3 through 14-6 and 14-15 through 14-18). Ring fixators have also been used successfully for the stabilization of open periarticular fractures with and without intra-articular extensions.[168]

External fixators seem to do best if they are applied according to principles that have emerged during the past two decades.[11–13,43,112] Most malunions can be avoided if proper fracture reduction has been obtained at the time of fixator application and if the fixator remains applied until the fracture is healed.[13,43,112] Fixator replacement with a nail is most successful if done within 8 weeks of

fixator application, so long as there have been no fracture site or pin tract infections.[15] However, with suppuration at pin tract and fracture sites, infection rates as high as 70 percent have been noted with secondary nailing.[115] Although the combination of internal and external fixation can be highly successful in metaphyseal fractures,[168] in diaphyseal fractures this practice leads to an increase in healing times and complication rates.[101]

If delayed union of a fracture stabilized with an external fixator is noted and secondary nailing is contraindicated, union should be achieved with the help of a bone graft. To guarantee proper alignment, the external fixator should be kept in place until complete union has been achieved. As noted previously, removal of the external fixator and transfer of a delayed union into a cast lead to serious secondary angulatory deformity in up to 30 percent of cases.

FIGURE 14-26 *Same patient as in Figure 14-24. At 4 weeks, the patient has regained the full range of elbow motion.*

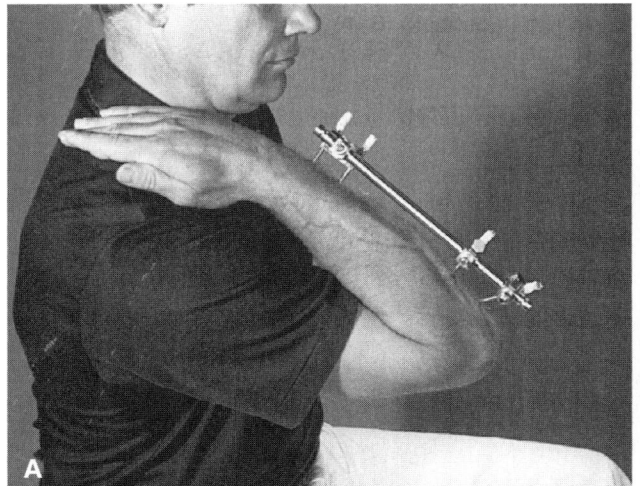

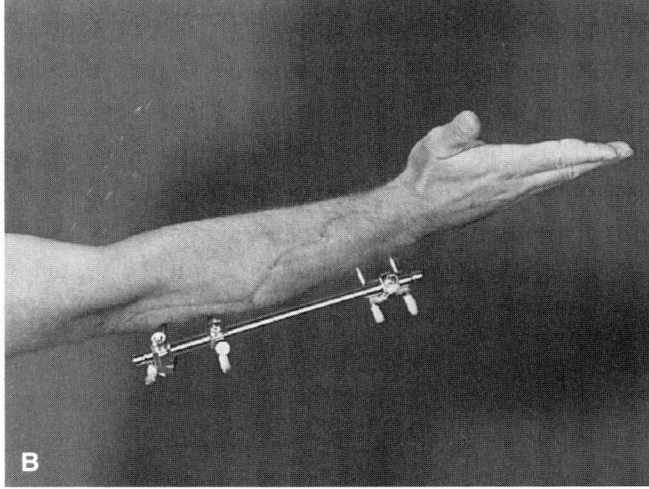

FIGURE 14-28 | *A* and *B*, "Bumper" injury caused a comminuted proximal tibial fracture with intra-articular extension. Closed fracture with Tscherne type II soft tissue compromise.

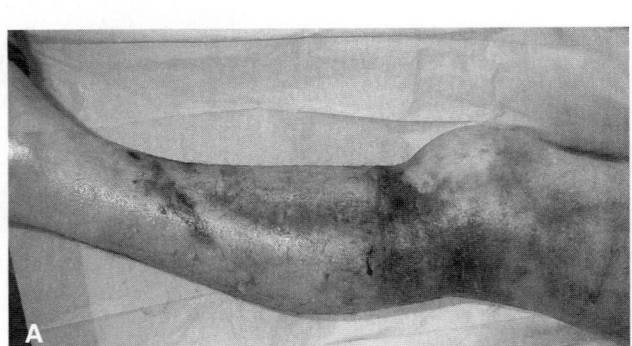
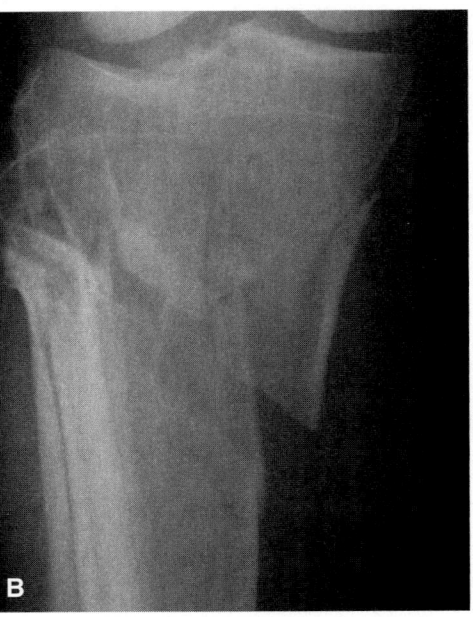

FIGURE 14-29 | *Same patient as in Figure 14-28. **A** and **B**, On the day of admission, stabilization of the articular surface was performed with percutaneous screws. Fracture stability, length, and alignment were maintained with a bridging external fixator.*

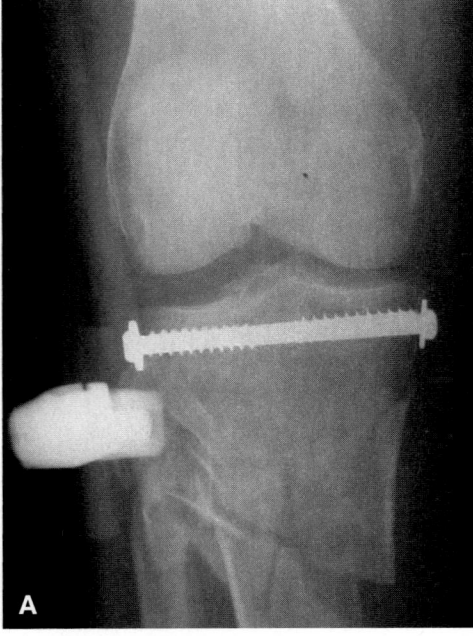
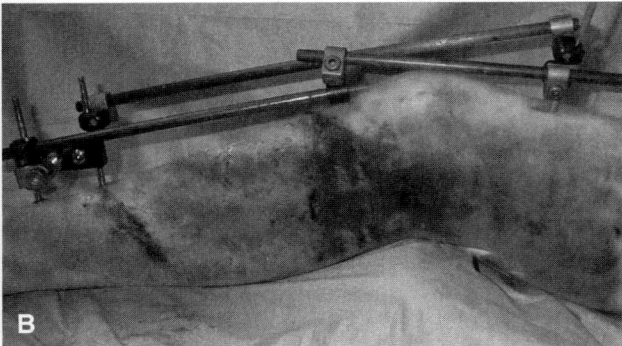

FIGURE 14-30 | *Same patient as in Figure 14-28.* **A** *and* **B,** *At 2 weeks, after soft tissue has stabilized, bridging fixator converted to hybrid fixation.*

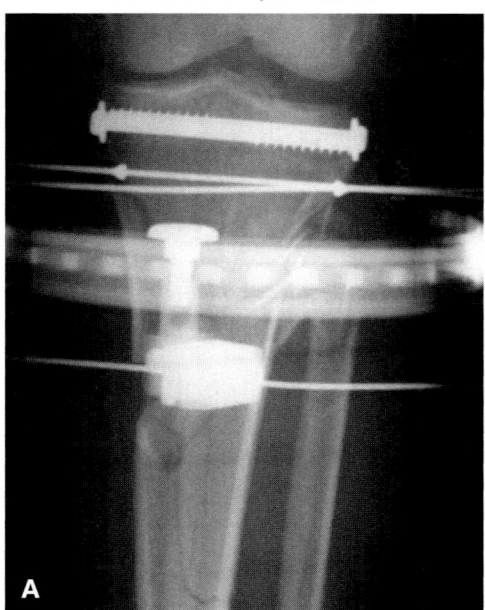

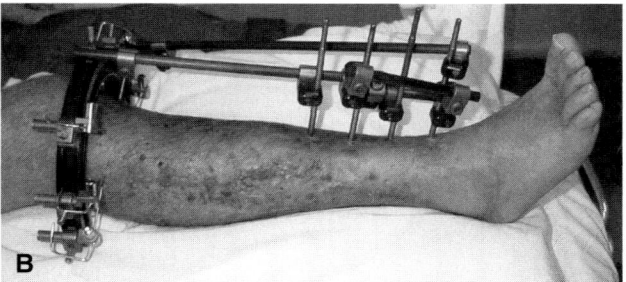

FIGURE 14-31 | *Same patient as in Figure 14-28. Radiograph of healed fracture at 6 months and after frame removal.*

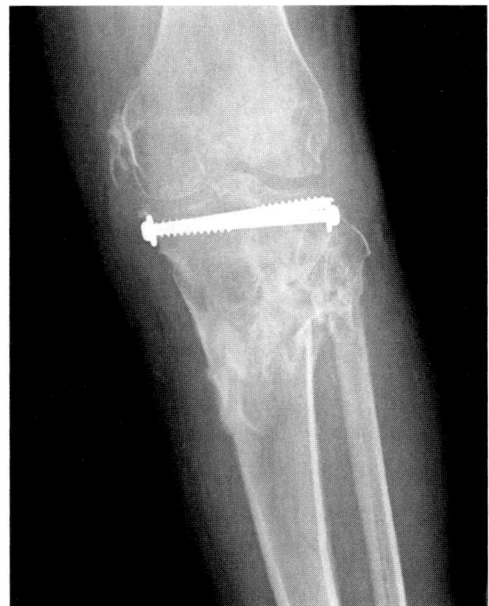

FIGURE 14-32 | *Closed dislocation of the knee with rupture of both collaterals and cruciate ligaments but no vascular compromise.*

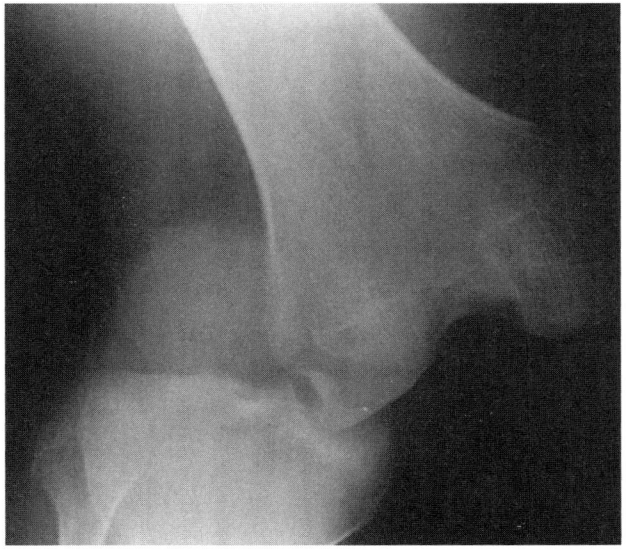

FIGURE 14-33 *Same patient as in Figure 14–32.* **A–C,** *At 3 days, repair and reconstruction of all ligaments were performed. Stabilization of the knee joint with an external fixator for 3 weeks allowed easy assessment of the soft tissue and maintenance of the correct anatomic position.*

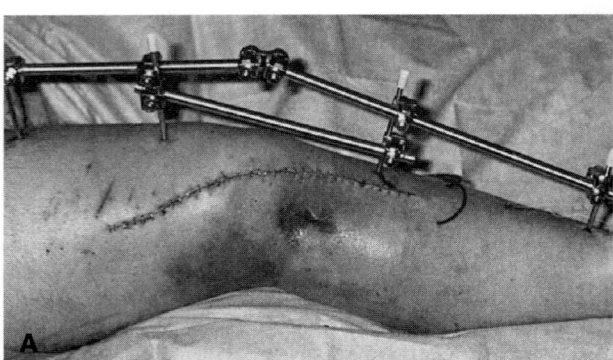
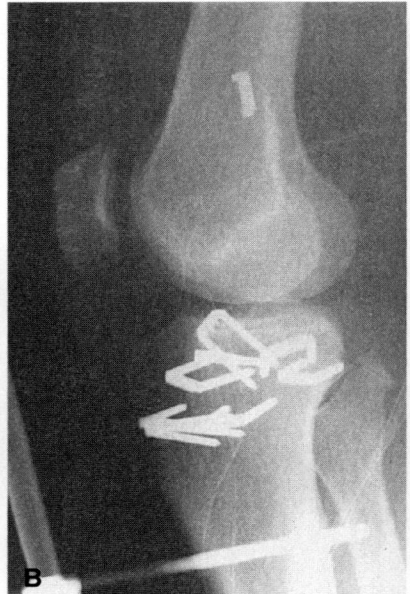
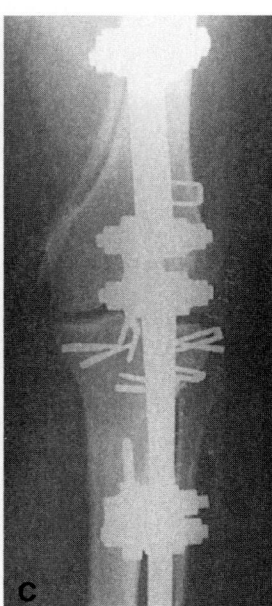

ACHIEVING BONE UNION

Most open diaphyseal fractures have a nonunion rate of 5 to 60 percent.[26,38,124,155] These nonunion rates are directly proportional to the extent of initial displacement, the degree of comminution, the severity of the soft tissue injury, the amount of bone loss, and the presence of infection.[38,98,124,155] Limb function is improved, healing times are reduced, and the likelihood of return to gainful employment is increased if union is achieved before 6 to 8 months, when the formal diagnosis of a nonunion is made.[13]

There are many methods that facilitate bone union, including partial fibulectomy, bone grafting, and secondary internal fixation.[143] Conceptually, fractures of low severity such as type I and type II open fractures, which are most likely to heal without additional intervention, can be observed for 8 to 12 weeks before a decision to intervene is entertained. As soon as soft tissue coverage without drainage has been established, a secondary intervention such as a bone graft[13] is considered for more severe type III lesions.[38,65] In the presence of substantial bone loss, free fibular grafts, free composite grafts, or distraction osteogenesis should be considered as soon as the soft tissue conditions are consolidated.

The use of recombinant human bone morphogenic protein (rhBMP) has recently been evaluated in the treatment of open tibia fractures. In a single-blinded trial of 450 patients with open tibial fractures, a dose-dependent response with the use of rhBMP-2 has been shown. The group receiving 1.50 mg/mL had a significant decrease in the need for secondary invasive intervention, shorter time to union, quicker soft tissue healing, less hardware failure, and fewer infections than the control group.[64] It has been postulated that the up-front cost of rhBMP-2 at the time of initial treatment of open tibia fractures offsets the costs and offers overall monetary savings when the decreased incidence of complications and need for additional procedures are taken into account.[2]

REGAINING FUNCTION

As soon as the patient has recovered from the initial impact of the injuries, he or she should be made aware of the effects these injuries may have on physical well-being, social circumstances, and recreational and occupational aspirations. The patient is made the most important member of the rehabilitation team and must, in conjunction with family and friends, help set the goals for each stage of the rehabilitation process.

After the fractures are stabilized, the patient is encouraged to get into the upright position, move to a chair, and maintain motion and strength in the uninvolved extremities. As soon as the wounds of the injured extremity are covered, assisted active range-of-motion exercises are started (see Figs. 14-18 and 14-26). If large wounds persist, joint motion can be maintained during daily excursions to the whirlpool. Lower extremity injuries stabilized with plates are protected from weight-bearing, but progressive force transmission is allowed across stable injuries held with intramedullary nails or an external fixator.

COORDINATING AND STAGING OF INTERVENTIONS

Fractures with soft tissue injuries present problems of considerable complexity. These injuries not only affect several tissue and organ systems but also require a wide variety of interventions by an often disjointed care team, which ranges from the emergency medical technician applying the initial splint at the scene of an accident to the physical therapist instituting the final work-hardening program. The general trauma surgeon usually handles the resuscitative phase of the patient's care, but it is the extremity surgeon's duty to manage and coordinate the care of the local injury and its effects on the patient's overall well-being.

Whereas some of the local treatment interventions must occur simultaneously (e.g., débridement of a contaminated wound under antibiotic coverage), other procedures are best carried out in sequence after a certain stage of the treatment process has been concluded (e.g., placement of a bone graft after an open wound has been fully débrided or covered with a healthy sleeve of soft tissues). Typical situations in which staging should be considered early in the treatment course include the following:

Wound care. Although one-stage débridement followed by immediate wound closure is almost routine for low-grade open pediatric fractures,[39] a type IIIB open tibial fracture in an adult may involve the following stages: (1) débridement and wound dressing, antibiotic bead pouch, or VAC therapy; (2) repeated débridement and dressing; (3) staged secondary closure or local and free muscle flap.

Stabilization of a diaphyseal fracture. Many adult types I and II open tibial shaft fractures are currently treated with a reamed nail and "loose" primary wound closure. Yet a combined open posterior tibial IIIB and IIIC lesion may require (1) arterial shunt, débridement, restoration of functional arterial and venous flow, antibiotic bead pouch, and external fixation; (2) disassembly of fixator frame, re-débridement of posterior wound, frame reassembly, and bead pouch; (3) flap coverage of wound with fixator in place; (4) removal of fixator and secondary nailing.

Stabilization of closed intra-articular or periarticular fracture. For some of these lesions, particularly in the upper extremity, immediate open reduction followed by early range-of-motion exercises provides the best functional results. Yet the same approach can cause major disasters when applied to tibial plateau and pilon fractures, for which the following sequence is often safer: (1) transarticular external fixation (with or without percutaneous articular fixation); (2) removal of transarticular fixator, limited open articular reduction with periarticular fixator or metaphyseal plating; (3) vigorous joint motion exercises and progressive weight-bearing.

Although different procedures may be involved in staging the treatment of soft and bony tissues, they are often interdependent and mutually beneficial. Thus, a transarticular fixator is as important in preserving length as it is in resolving soft tissue swelling.

As noted earlier, the proper timing of overlapping interventions is equally important in the reconstructive and rehabilitative phases. In choosing the optimal treatment course for a particular patient's injury, the surgeon is forever torn between a desire to complete the task without delay to possibly secure the best outcome and the recognition that a more protracted approach might be safer but not without incurring complexity and possibly a lesser functional result.

REFERENCES

1. Adili, A.; Bhandari, M.; Schemitsch, E.H. The biomechanical effect of high-pressure irrigation on diaphyseal fracture healing in vivo. J Orthop Trauma 16:413–417, 2002.
2. Alt, V.; Heissel, A. Economic considerations for the use of recombinant human bone morphogenetic protein-2 in open tibial fractures in Europe: The German model. Curr Med Res Opin 22(Suppl 1):S19–S22, 2006.
3. Anglen, J.O. Comparison of soap and antibiotic solutions for irrigation of lower-limb open fracture wounds: A prospective, randomized study. J Bone Joint Surg Am 87:1415–1422, 2005.
4. Anglen, J.; Aleto, T. Temporary transarticular external fixation of the knee and ankle. J Orthop Trauma 12:431–434, 1998.
5. Anglen, J.; Apostoles, S.; Christiansen, G.; et al. The efficacy of various irrigation solutions in removing slime-producing *Staphylococcus*. J Orthop Trauma 8:390–396, 1994.
6. Argenta, L.C.; Morykwas, M.J. Vacuum-assisted closure: A new method for wound control and treatment: Clinical experience. Ann Plast Surg 38:563–576; discussion 577, 1997.
7. Bach, A.; Hansen, S. Plates versus external fixation in severe open tibial shaft fractures: A randomized trial. Clin Orthop 241:89–94, 1989.
8. Beardmore, A.A.; Brooks, D.E.; Wenke, J.C.; et al. Effectiveness of local antibiotic delivery with an osteoinductive and osteoconductive bone-graft substitute. J Bone Joint Surg Am 87:107–112, 2005.
9. Bednar, D.; Parikh, J. Effect of time delay from injury to primary management on the incidence of deep infection after open fractures of the lower extremities caused by blunt trauma in adults. J Orthop Trauma 7:532–535, 1993.
10. Behrens, F. External fixation. In Chapman, M., ed. Operative Orthopaedics. Philadelphia, J.B. Lippincott, 1988.
11. Behrens, F. General theory and principles of external fixation. Clin Orthop 241:15–23, 1989.
12. Behrens, F.; Johnson, W. Unilateral external fixation: Methods to increase and reduce frame stiffness. Clin Orthop 241:48–56, 1989.
13. Behrens, F.; Searls, K. External fixation of the tibia. J Bone Joint Surg Br 68:246–254, 1986.

14. Bhandari, M.; Schemitsch, E.H.; Adili, A.; et al. High- and low-pressure pulsatile lavage of contaminated tibial fractures: An in vitro study of bacterial adherence and bone damage. J Orthop Trauma 13:526–533, 1999.

15. Blachut, P.; Meek, R.; O'Brien, P. External fixation and delayed intramedullary nailing of open fractures of the tibial shaft: A sequential protocol. J Bone Joint Surg Am 72:729–735, 1990.

16. Bleck, T. *Clostridium tetani*. In Mandell, G.; Douglas, R.; Bennet, J., eds. Principles and Practice of Infectious Diseases. New York, Churchill-Livingstone, 1995, pp. 2173–2178.

17. Blick, S.; Brumback, R.J.; Poka, A.; et al. Compartment syndrome in open tibial fractures. J Bone Joint Surg Am 68:1348–1353, 1986.

18. Bombelli, R.; Giangrande, A.; Malacrida, V.; et al. The control of infection in orthopaedic surgery. Orthop Rev 10:65–72, 1981.

19. Bondurant, F.; Cotler, H.B.; Buckle, R.; et al. The medical and economic impact of severely injured lower extremities. J Trauma 28:1270–1273, 1988.

20. Bone, L.; Johnson, K. Treatment of tibial fractures by reaming and intramedullary nailing. J Bone Joint Surg Am 68:877–887, 1986.

21. Bone, L.; Johnson, K.D.; Weigelt, J.; et al. Early versus delayed stabilization of femoral fractures: A prospective randomized study. J Bone Joint Surg Am 71:336–340, 1989.

22. Bowyer, G.W.; Cumberland, N. Antibiotic release from impregnated pellets and beads. J Trauma 36:331–335, 1994.

23. Brien, H.; Noftall, F.; MacMaster, S.; et al. Neer's classification system: A critical appraisal. J Trauma 38:257–260, 1995.

24. Brown, P.; Kinman, P. Gas gangrene in a metropolitan community. J Bone Joint Surg Am 56:1145–1451, 1974.

25. Brown, P.; Urban, J. Early weight-bearing treatment of open fractures of the tibia: An end result study of 63 cases. J Bone Joint Surg Am 51:59–75, 1969.

26. Brumback, R.J. Open tibial fractures: Current orthopaedic management. Instr Course Lect 41:101–117, 1992.

27. Brumback, R.; Jones, A. Interobserver agreement in the classification of open fractures of the tibia. J Bone Joint Surg Am 76:1162–1166, 1994.

28. Byrd, H.; Spicer, T.; Cierney, G. Management of open tibial fractures. Plast Reconstr Surg 76:719–728, 1985.

29. Cabral, C.T.; Fernandes, M.H. In vitro comparison of chlorhexidine and povidone-iodine on the long-term proliferation and functional activity of human alveolar bone cells. Clin Oral Investig 11:155–165, 2007.

30. Cauchoix, J.; Duparc, J.; Boulez, P. Traitement des fractures ouvertes de jambe. Med Acta Chir 83: 811–822, 1957.

31. Caudle, R.; Stern, P. Severe open fractures of the tibia. J Bone Joint Surg Am 69:801–807, 1987.

32. Chapman, M. Open fractures. In Chapman, M., ed. Operative Orthopaedics. Philadelphia, J.B. Lippincott, 1988, pp. 173–178.

33. Chapman, M. Role of stability in open fractures. Instr Course Lect 31:75–87, 1982.

34. Chapman, M.; Mahoney, M. The role of internal fixation in the management of open fractures. Clin Orthop 138:120–131, 1979.

35. Clowes, G. Stresses, mediators and responses of survival. In Clowes, G., ed. Trauma, Sepsis and Shock: The Physiological Bases of Therapy. New York, Marcel Dekker, 1988, pp. 1–55.

36. Conroy, B.; Anglen, J.O.; Simpson, W.A.; et al. Comparison of castile soap, benzalkonium chloride, and bacitracin as irrigation solutions for complex contaminated orthopaedic wounds. J Orthop Trauma 13:332–337, 1999.

37. Court-Brown, C.; Christie, J.; McQueen, M. Closed intramedullary tibial nailing: Its use in closed and type I fractures. J Bone Joint Surg Br 73:959–964, 1990.

38. Court-Brown, C.; McQueen, M.M.; Quaba, A.A.; et al. Locked intramedullary nailing of open tibial fractures. J Bone Joint Surg Br 73:959–964, 1991.

39. Cullen, M.; Roy, D.R.; Crawford, A.H.; et al. Open fracture of the tibia in children. J Bone Joint Surg Am 78:1039–1046, 1996.

40. Dabezies, E.J.; D'Ambrosia, R.; Shaji, H.; et al. Fractures of the femoral shaft treated by external fixation with the Wagner device. J Bone Joint Surg Am 66:360–364, 1986.

41. Davis, A. Primary closure of compound fracture wounds. J Bone Joint Surg Am 30:405, 1948.

42. DeBakey, M.; Simeone, F. Battle injuries of the arteries in World War II: An analysis of 2471 cases. Ann Surg 123:534–579, 1946.

43. DeBastiani, G.; Aldegheri, L.; Brivio, L. The treatment of fractures with a dynamic axial fixator. J Bone Joint Surg Br 66:538–545, 1984.

44. DeChauliac, G. Ars Chirurgica. Venice, 1546.

45. Dedmond, B.T.; Kortesis, B.; Punger, K.; et al. The use of negative-pressure wound therapy (NPWT) in the temporary treatment of soft-tissue injuries associated with high-energy open tibial shaft fractures. J Orthop Trauma 21:11–17, 2007.

46. DeFranzo, A.J.; Argenta, L.C.; Marks, M.W.; et al. The use of vacuum-assisted closure therapy for the treatment of lower-extremity wounds with exposed bone. Plast Reconstr Surg 108:1184–1191, 2001.

47. DeLee, J.; Stiehl, J. Open tibia fractures with compartment syndrome. Clin Orthop 160:175–184, 1981.

48. Dellinger, E.P.; Caplan, E.S.; Weaver, L.D.; et al. Duration of preventive antibiotic administration for open extremity fractures. Arch Surg 123:333–339, 1988.

49. Dellinger, E.; Miller, S.D.; Wertz, M.J.; et al. Risk of infection after open fractures of the arm or leg. Arch Surg 123:1320–1327, 1987.

50. Dellon, A.; McKuinnon, S. Results of posterior tibial nerve grafting at the ankle. J Reconstruct Microsurg 7:81–83, 1991.

51. DeLong, W.G., Jr.; Bom, C.T.; Wei, S.Y.; et al. Aggressive treatment of 119 open fracture wounds. J Trauma 46:1049–1054, 1999.

52. Dirschl, D.; Adams, G. A critical assessment of factors influencing reliability in the classification of fractures, using fractures of the tibial plafond as a model. J Orthop Trauma 11:471–476, 1997.

53. Dirschl, D.R.; Duff, G.P.; Dahners, L.E.; et al. High pressure pulsatile lavage irrigation of intra-articular fractures: Effects on fracture healing. J Orthop Trauma 12:460–463, 1988.

54. Drake, S.; King, A.; Slack, W. Gas gangrene and related infections: Classification, clinical features and etiology, management and mortality. Br J Surg 64:104–112, 1977.

55. Farber, J.; Chien, K.; Mittnacht, S. The pathogenesis of irreversible cell injury in ischemia. Am J Pathol 102:271–281, 1981.

56. Friedrich, P. Die aseptische Versorgung frischer Wunden. Arch F Klin Chir 57:288–310, 1898.

57. Gainor, B.; Hockman, D.E.; Anglen, J.O.; et al. Benzalkonium chloride: A potential disinfecting irrigation solution. J Orthop Trauma 11:121–125, 1997.

58. General principles guiding the treatment of wounds of war: Conclusions adopted by the InterAllied Surgical Conference held in Paris, March and May, 1917. London, H. M. Stationery Office, 1917.

59. Georgiadis, G.; Behrens, F.F.; Joyce, M.J.; et al. Open tibia fractures with severe soft tissue loss: Limb salvage with microvascular tissue transfer versus below-knee amputation: Complications, functional results, and quality of life. J Bone Joint Surg Am 75:1431–1441, 1994.

60. Ger, R. The management of open fractures of the tibia with skin loss. J Trauma 10:112–121, 1970.

61. Gopal, S.; Majumder, S.; Batchelor, A.G.; et al. Fix and flap: The radical orthopaedic and plastic treatment of severe open fractures of the tibia. J Bone Joint Surg Br 82:959–966, 2000.

62. Gorbach, S. Other *Clostridium* species (including gas gangrene). In Mandel, G.; Douglas, R.; Bennett, J., eds. Priniciples and Practice of Infectious Diseases. New York, John Wiley, 1985, pp. 1362–1367.

63. Gordon, L.; Chiu, E. Treatment of infected nonunions and segmental defects of the tibia with staged microvascular muscle transplantation and bone grafting. J Bone Joint Surg Am 70:377–386, 1988.

64. Govender, S.; Csimma, C.; Genant, H.K.; et al. Recombinant human bone morphogenetic protein-2 for treatment of open tibial fractures: A prospective, controlled, randomized study of four hundred and fifty patients. J Bone Joint Surg Am 84:2123–2134, 2002.

65. Green, A.; Trafton, P. Early infectious complications in the management of open femur fractures. Clin Orthop 243:36–40, 1989.

66. Gregory, G.; Chapman, M.; Hansen, S. Open fractures. In Rockwood, C.; Green, D., eds. Fractures in Adults. Philadelphia, J.B. Lippincott, 1984, pp. 169–218.

67. Gristina, A.; Costerton, J. Bacterial adherence to biomaterials and tissue: The significance of its role in clinical sepsis. J Bone Joint Surg Am 67:264–273, 1985.

68. Gustilo, R.B. Current concepts in the management of open fractures. Instr Course Lect 36:359–366, 1987.

69. Gustilo, R.B. Management of open fractures and complications. Instr Course Lect 31:64–75, 1982.

70. Gustilo, R.B.; Anderson, J.T. JSBS classics: Prevention of infection in the treatment of one thousand and twenty-five open fractures of long bones: Retrospective and prospective analyses. J Bone Joint Surg Am 84:682, 2002.

71. Gustilo, R.; Anderson, J. Prevention of infection in the treatment of one thousand and twenty-five open fractures of long bones. J Bone Joint Surg Am 58:453, 1976.

72. Gustilo, R.B.; Mendoza, R.M.; Williams, D.N. Problems in the management of type III (severe) open fractures: A new classification of type III open fractures. J Trauma 24:742–746, 1984.

73. Hansen, S. The type IIIC tibial fracture: Salvage or amputation. J Bone Joint Surg Am 69:799–800, 1988.

74. Harley, B.J.; Beaupre, L.A.; Jones, C.A.; et al. The effect of time to definitive treatment on the rate of nonunion and infection in open fractures. J Orthop Trauma 16:484–490, 2002.

75. Hassinger, S.M.; Harding, G.; Wongworawat, M.D. High-pressure pulsatile lavage propagates bacteria into soft tissue. Clin Orthop Relat Res 439:27–31, 2005.

76. Hattrup, S.; Wood, M. Delayed neural reconstruction in the lower extremity: Results of interfascicular nerve grafting. Foot Ankle 7:105–109, 1986.

77. Helfet, D.; Howey, T.; Sanders, R.; et al. Limb salvage versus amputation: Preliminary results of the mangled extremity severity score. Clin Orthop Relat Res 256:80–86, 1990.

78. Henry, S.L.; Ostermann, P.A.; Seligson, D. The antibiotic bead pouch technique: The management of severe compound fractures. Clin Orthop Relat Res 295:54–62, 1993.

79. Henry, S.L.; Ostermann, P.A.; Seligson, D. The prophylactic use of antibiotic impregnated beads in open fractures. J Trauma 30:1231–1238, 1990.

80. Heppenstall, R.; Sapega, A.A.; Scott, R.; et al. The compartment syndrome: An experimental and clinical study of muscular energy metabolism using phosphorus nuclear magnetic resonance spectroscopy. Clin Orthop 226:138–155, 1988.

81. Herscovici, D., Jr.; Saunders, R.W.; Scaduto, J.M.; et al. Vacuum-assisted wound closure (VAC therapy) for the management of patients with high-energy soft tissue injuries. J Orthop Trauma 17:683–688, 2003.

82. Higgins, T.; Deluca, P.; Ariyan, S. Salvage of open tibial fracture with segmental loss of tibial nerve:

A case report and review of the literature. J Orthop Trauma 13:380–390, 1999.

83. Hitchcock, C. Gas gangrene in the injured extremity. In Gustilo, R., ed. Management of Open Fractures and Their Complications. Philadelphia, W.B. Saunders, 1982, pp. 183–201.

84. Holbrook, J.; Swiontowski, M.; Sanders, R. Treatment of open fractures of the tibial shaft: Ender nailing versus external fixation. J Bone Joint Surg Am 71:1231–1238, 1989.

85. Hope, P.; Cole, W. Open fractures of the tibia in children. J Bone Joint Surg Am 74:546–553, 1992.

86. Horn, B.D.; Rettig, M.E. Interobserver reliability in the Gustilo and Anderson classification of open fractures. J Orthop Trauma 7:357–360, 1993.

87. Howe, H.R., Jr.; Poole, C.V., Jr.; Hansen, K.J.; et al. Salvage of lower extremities following combined orthopaedic and vascular trauma: A predictive salvage index. Am Surg 53:205–208, 1987.

88. Irwin, A.; Gibson, P.; Ashcroft, P. Open fractures of the tibia in children. Injury 26:21–24, 1995.

89. Jensen, J.; Jensen, T.G.; Smith, T.K.; et al. Nutrition in orthopaedic surgery. J Bone Joint Surg Am 64:1263–1272, 1982.

90. Johansen, K.; Bandyk, D.; Thiele, B.; et al. Temporary intraluminal shunts: Resolution of a management dilemma in complex vascular injuries. J Trauma 22:395–402, 1982.

91. Johansen, K.; Daines, M.; Harvey, T.; et al. Objective criteria accurately predict amputation following lower extremity trauma. J Trauma 30:568–572, 1990.

92. Johnson, K.; Cadambi, A.; Siebert, G. Incidence of adult respiratory distress syndrome in patients with multiple musculoskeletal injuries: Effect of early operative stabilization of fractures. J Trauma 25:375–384, 1985.

93. Jupiter, J. Complex fractures of the distal part of the humerus and associated complications. J Bone Joint Surg Am 76:1252–1264, 1994.

94. Katzman, S.; Dickson, K. Determining the prognosis for limb salvage in major vascular injuries with associated open tibial fractures. Orthop Rev 21:195–199, 1992.

95. Keating, J.; O'Brien, P.J.; Blachut, P.A.; et al. Locked intramedullary nailing with and without reaming for open fractures of the tibial shaft. J Bone Joint Surg Am 79:334–341, 1997.

96. Keeley, S.; Snyder, W.; Weigelt, J. Arterial injury below the knee: Fifty-one patients with 82 injuries. J Trauma 23:285–290, 1983.

97. Khatod, M.; Botte, M.J.; Hoyt, D.B.; et al. Outcomes in open tibia fractures: Relationship between delay in treatment and infection. J Trauma 55:949–954, 2003.

98. Kindsfater, K.; Johassen, E. Osteomyelitis in grade II and III open tibia fractures with late debridement. J Orthop Trauma 9:121–127, 1995.

99. Klein, M.; Rahn, B.A.; Frigg, R.; et al. Reaming versus non-reaming in medullary nailing: Interference with cortical circulation of the canine tibia. Arch Orthop Trauma Surg 109:314–316, 1990.

100. Klemm, K. Antibiotic bead chains. Clin Orthop 295:63–76, 1993.

101. Krettek, C.; Haas, N.; Tscherne, H. The role of supplemental lag screw fixation for open fractures of the tibial shaft treated with external fixation. J Bone Joint Surg Am 73:893–897, 1991.

102. Kristiansen, B.; Andersen, U.L.; Olsen, C.A.; et al. The Neer classification of fractures of the proximal humerus: An assessment of interobserver variation. Skeletal Radiol 17:420–422, 1988.

103. Lange, R.; Bach, A.W.; Hansen, S.T., Jr.; et al. Open tibial fractures with associated vascular injuries: Prognosis for limb salvage. J Trauma 25:203–207, 1985.

104. Lawyer, R.; Lubbers, L. Use of the Hoffman apparatus in the treatment of unstable tibial fractures. J Bone Joint Surg Am 62:1264–1273, 1980.

105. Lee, E.W.; Dirschl, D.R.; Duff, G.; et al. High-pressure pulsatile lavage irrigation of fresh intra-articular fractures: Effectiveness at removing particulate matter from bone. J Orthop Trauma 16:162–165, 2002.

106. Lee, J. Efficacy of cultures in the management of open fractures. Clin Orthop 339:71–75, 1997.

107. Lloyd, G. Hippocratic Writings. New York, Pelican Books, 1988, pp. 277–314.

108. Lob, G. Lokale antibiotikatherapie bei knochen, gelenk und weichteilinfektionen. Chirurg 56:564–567, 1985.

109. Lusskin, R.; Battista, A.; Lenza, S.; et al. Surgical management of late post-traumatic and ischemic neuropathies involving the lower extremities: Classification and results of therapy. Foot Ankle 7:95–104, 1986.

110. Mackenzie, E.J.; Bosse, M.J. Factors influencing outcome following limb-threatening lower limb trauma: Lessons learned from the Lower Extremity Assessment Project (LEAP). J Am Acad Orthop Surg 14:S205–S210, 2006.

111. Malgaigne, J. Etudes stastiques sur les resultats des grandes operations dans les hopitaux de Paris. Arch Gen Med 13:399, 1842.

112. Marsh, J.; Napola, J.V.; Wuest, T.K.; et al. Unilateral external fixation until healing with the dynamic axial fixator for severe open tibial fractures. J Orthop Trauma 5:341–348, 1991.

113. Mathes, S.; Guy, P.; Brasher, P. Paper No. 64. Orthopaedic Trauma Association, 2006 Annual Meeting, Phoenix, AZ, 2006. Available at: www.ota.org/meetings06_annualmeeting.html.

114. Mattox, K.; Bickell, W.; Pepe, P.E.; et al. Prospective MAST study in 911 patients. J Trauma 29:1104–1111, 1989.

115. Maurer, D.; Merkow, R.; Gustilo, R. Infection after intramedullary nailing of severe open tibial fractures initially treated with external fixation. J Bone Joint Surg Am 71:835–838, 1989.

116. McNamara, M.; Heckman, J.; Corley, F. Severe open fractures of the lower extremity: A retrospective evaluation of the Mangled Extremity Score System (MESS). J Orthop Trauma 8:81–87, 1994.

117. Miclau, T.; Dahners, L.E.; Lindsey, R.W. In vitro pharmacokinetics of antibiotic release from locally implantable materials. J Orthop Res 11:627–632, 1993.

118. Millie, M.; Senkowski, C.; Stuart, L.; et al. Tornado disaster in rural Georgia: Triage response, injury pattern and lessons learned. Am Surg 66:223–228, 2000.

119. Moed, B.R.; Kellam, J.F.; Foster, R.J.; et al. Immediate internal fixation of open fractures of the diaphysis of the forearm. J Bone Joint Surg Am 68:1008–1017, 1986.

120. Moehring, H.D.; Gravel, C.; Chapman, M.W.; et al. Comparison of antibiotic beads and intravenous antibiotics in open fractures. Clin Orthop Relat Res 372:254–261, 2000.

121. Moore, T.; Mauney, C.; Barron, J. The use of quantitative bacterial counts in open fractures. Clin Orthop 248:227–230, 1989.

122. Morykwas, M.J.; Argenta, L.C.; Shelton-Brown, E.I.; et al. Vacuum-assisted closure: A new method for wound control and treatment—Animal studies and basic foundation. Ann Plast Surg 38:553–562, 1997.

123. Muller, M.; Allgower, M.; Schneider, R.; et al. Manual of Internal Fixation, 3rd ed. New York, Springer-Verlag, 1991.

124. Nicoll, E. Fractures of the tibial shaft: A survey of 705 cases. J Bone Joint Surg Br 46:373–387, 1964.

125. Nunley, J.; Gabel, G. Tibial nerve grafting for restoration of plantar sensation. Foot Ankle 14:489–492, 1993.

126. O'Donnell, T.F., Jr.; Brewster, D.C.; Darling, R.C.; et al. Arterial injuries associated with fractures and/or dislocations of the knee. J Trauma 17:775–784, 1977.

127. Olerud, S.; Karlstrom, G. Tibial fractures treated by AO compression osteosynthesis. Acta Orthop Scand 140(Suppl):3, 1972.

128. Orr, H. The treatment of osteomyelitis by drainage and rest. J Bone Joint Surg 9:733, 1927.

129. Ostermann, P.A.; Henry, S.L.; Seligson, D. The role of local antibiotic therapy in the management of compound fractures. Clin Orthop Relat Res 295:102–111, 1993.

130. Pancoast, S.; Neu, H. Antibiotic levels in human bone and synovial fluid. Orthop Rev 10:49–61, 1980.

131. Pappas, A.; Filler, R.M.; Eraklis, A.J.; et al. Clostridial infections (gas gangrene): Diagnosis and early treatment. Clin Orthop Relat Res 76:177–184, 1971.

132. Paré, A. The works of that famous chirurgien Ambrose Paré, ed. T.b.T. Johnson. London, 1634.

133. Park, S.H.; Silva, M.; Bahk, W.J.; et al. Effect of repeated irrigation and debridement on fracture healing in an animal model. J Orthop Res 20:1197–1204, 2002.

134. Park, W.; DeMuth, W. Wounding capacity of rotary lawn mowers. J Trauma 15:36–38, 1975.

135. Patzakis, F.; Wilkins, J.; Moore, T. Considerations in reducing the infection rate of open tibial fractures. Clin Orthop 178:36–41, 1983.

136. Patzakis, M. Management of open fractures. Instr Course Lect 31:62–64, 1982.

137. Patzakis, M.; Harvey, J.; Ivler, D. The role of antibiotics in the management of open fractures. J Bone Joint Surg Am 56:532–541, 1974.

138. Patzakis, M.; Wilkins, J. Factors influencing infection rate in open fracture wounds. Clin Orthop 243:36–40, 1989.

139. Patzakis, M.J.; Bains, R.S.; Lee, J.; et al. Prospective, randomized, double-blind study comparing single-agent antibiotic therapy, ciprofloxacin, to combination antibiotic therapy in open fracture wounds. J Orthop Trauma 14:529–533, 2000.

140. Perren, S. The biomechanics and biology of internal fixation using plates and nails. Orthopedics 12:25–35, 1989.

141. Perry, C.; Rice, S.; Ritterbusch, J.K.; et al. Local administration of antibiotics with an implantable osmotic pump. Clin Orthop Relat Res 192:284–290, 1985.

142. Petty, W.; Spanier, S.; Shuster, J.J.; et al. The influence of skeletal implants on incidence of infection: Experiments in a canine model. J Bone Joint Surg Am 67:1236–1244, 1985.

143. Reckling, F.; Waters, C. Treatment of nonunions of fractures of the tibial diaphysis by posterolateral cortical cancellous bone grafting. J Bone Joint Surg Am 62:863–875, 1980.

144. Rich, N.; Metz, C.W., Jr. Internal versus external fixation of fractures with concomitant vascular injuries in Vietnam. J Trauma 11:463–473, 1971.

145. Richards, R.; Orsin, E.C.; Mahoney, J.L.; et al. The influence of muscle flap coverage on the repair of devascularized tibial cortex: An experimental investigation in the dog. Plast Reconstr Surg 79:946–956, 1987.

146. Riemer, B.; DiChristina, D.G.; Cooper, A.; et al. Nonreamed nailing of tibial diaphyseal fractures in blunt polytrauma patients. J Orthop Trauma 9:66–75, 1995.

147. Rittmann, W.; Matter, P. Die Offene Fraktur. Bern, Switzerland, Hans Huber, 1977.

148. Rittmann, W.; Matter, P.; Allogower, M. Behandlung offener frakturen und infekthaufigkeit. Acta Chir Austriaca 2:18, 1970.

149. Rittmann, W.; Perren, S. Corticale Knochenheilung nach Osteosynthese und Infektion: Biomechanik und Biolgie. Berlin, Springer, 1974.

150. Rittmann, W.; Schibli, M.; Matter, P.; et al. Open fractures: Long-term results in 200 consecutive cases. Clin Orthop Relat Res 138:132–140, 1979.

151. Robbins, S.; Cotran, D.; Kumar, V. Pathologic Basis of Disease, 3rd ed. Philadelphia, W.B. Saunders, 1984, pp. 1–84.

152. Robertson, P. Prediction of amputation after severe lower limb trauma. J Bone Joint Surg Br 73:816–818, 1991.

153. Rorabeck, C. The treatment of compartment syndromes of the leg. J Bone Joint Surg Br 66:93–97, 1984.

154. Rosenstein, B.; Wilson, F.; Funderburk, C. The use of bacitracin irrigation to prevent infection in postoperative skeletal wounds. J Bone Joint Surg Am 71:427–430, 1989.

155. Rosenthal, R.; MacPhail, J.; Ortiz, J. Nonunion in open tibial fractures: Analysis of reasons for failure of treatment. J Bone Joint Surg Am 59:244–248, 1977.

156. Rothenberger, D.; Velasco, R.; Strate, R.; et al. Open pelvic fracture: A lethal injury. J Trauma 18:184–187, 1978.

157. Russel, G.; Henderson, R.; Arnett, G. Primary or delayed closure for open tibial fractures. J Bone Joint Surg Br 72:125–128, 1990.

158. Salter, R.; Simmonds, D.F.; Malcolm, B.W.; et al. The biological effect of continuous passive motion on the healing of full-thickness defects in articular cartilage: An experimental investigation in the rabbit. J Bone Joint Surg Am 62:1232–1251, 1980.

159. Sarmiento, A.; Sobol, P.A.; Sew Hoy, A.L.; et al. Prefabricated functional braces for the treatment of fractures of the tibial diaphysis. J Bone Joint Surg Am 66:1328–1339, 1984.

160. Schemitsch, E.; Kowalski, M.J.; Swiontkowski, M.F.; et al. Cortical bone blood flow in reamed and unreamed locked intramedullary nailing: A fractured tibia model in sheep. J Orthop Trauma 8:373–382, 1994.

161. Schurman, D.; Hirshman, H.; Burton, D. Cephalothin and cefamandole penetration into bone, synovial fluid, and wound drainage fluid. J Bone Joint Surg Am 62:981–985, 1980.

162. Scott, D.; Rotschafer, J.; Behrens, F. Use of vancomycin and tobramycin polymethylmethacrylate impregnated beads in the management of chronic osteomyelitis. Drug Intell Clin Pharm 22:480–483, 1988.

163. Shtarker, H.; David, R.; Stolero, J.; et al. Treatment of open tibial fractures with primary suture and Ilizarov fixation. Clin Orthop 335:268–274, 1997.

164. Sidor, M.; Zuckerman, J.D.; Lyon, T.; et al. The Neer classification system for proximal humeral fractures: An assessment of interobserver reliability and intraobserver reproducibility. J Bone Joint Surg Am 75:1745–1750, 1993.

165. Simon, B. Treatment of wounds. In Rosen, P., ed. Emergency Medicine: Concept in Clinical Practice. St. Louis, MO, Mosby, 1988, p. 371.

166. Sirkin, M.; Sanders, R.; DiPasquales, T.; et al. A staged protocol for soft tissue management in the treatment of complex pilon fractures. J Orthop Trauma 13:78–84, 1999.

167. Sorger, J.I.; Kirk, P.G.; Ruhnke, C.J.; et al. Once daily, high dose versus divided, low dose gentamicin for open fractures. Clin Orthop Relat Res 366:197–204, 1999.

168. Stamer, D.; Schenk, R.; Staggers, B.; et al. Bicondylar tibial plateau fractures treated with a hybrid ring external fixator: A preliminary study. J Orthop Trauma 8:455–461, 1994.

169. Swiontkowski, M.; Sands, A.K.; Agel, J.; et al. Interobserver variation in the AO/OTA fracture classification system for pilon fractures: Is there a problem? J Orthop Trauma 11:467–470, 1997.

170. Tarbox, B.; Conroy, B.P.; Malicky, E.S.; et al. Benzalkonium chloride: A potential disinfecting irrigation solution for orthopaedic wounds. Clin Orthop Relat Res 346:255–261, 1998.

171. Thomas, D.B.; Brooks, D.E.; Bice, T.G.; et al. Tobramycin-impregnated calcium sulfate prevents infection in contaminated wounds. Clin Orthop Relat Res 441:366–371, 2005.

172. Tscherne, H.; Gotzen, L. Fractures with Soft Tissue Injuries. Berlin, Springer-Verlag, 1984.

173. Tscherne, H.; Oestern, H. Die klassifizierung des weichteilschadens bei offenen und geschlossenen frakturen. Unfallheilkunde 83:111–115, 1982.

174. Velazco, A.; Flemin, L. Open fractures of the tibia treated by the Hoffmann external fixator. Clin Orthop 180:125–132, 1983.

175. VonFraunhofer, J.; Polk, H.; Seligson, D. Leaching of tobramycin from PMMA bone cement beads. J Biomed Mater Res 19:751–756, 1985.

176. Wahlig, H.; Dingeldein, E.; Bergmann, R.; et al. The release of gentamicin from polymethylmethacrylate beads. J Bone Joint Surg Br 60:270–275, 1978.

177. Wangensteen, O.; Wangensteen, S. Carl Reyher (1846–1890): Great Russian military surgeon: His demonstration of the role of debridement in gunshot wounds and fractures. Surgery 74:641–649, 1973.

178. Wangensteen, O.; Wangensteen, S. The Rise of Surgery from Empiric Craft to Scientific Discipline. Minneapolis, MN, University of Minnesota Press, 1978, pp. 3–64, 301–325, 407–452, 479–525.

179. Wassilak, S.; Brink, E. Tetanus. In Last, J., ed. Public Health and Preventive Medicine. Norwalk, CT, Appleton-Century-Crofts, 1986.

180. Williams, M. Long-term cost comparison of major limb salvage using Ilizarov method versus amputation. Clin Orthop 335:268–274, 1994.

181. Wiss, D.; Gilbert, P.; Merritt, P.O.; et al. Immediate internal fixation of open ankle fractures. J Orthop Trauma 2:265–271, 1988.

182. Yaremchuk, M.J. Acute management of severe soft-tissue damage accompanying open fractures of the lower extremity. Clin Plast Surg 13:621–632, 1986.

183. Yaremchuk, M.; Brumback, R.J.; Manson, P.N.; et al. Acute and definitive management of traumatic osteocutaneous defects of the lower extremity. Plast Reconstr Surg 80:1–14, 1987.

184. Yourassowsky, E.; Van der Linden, M.P.; Crokaert, F. One shot of high-dose amikacin: A working hypothesis. Chemotherapy 36:1–7, 1990.

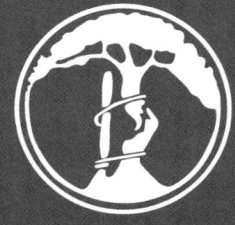

CHAPTER 15

Soft Tissue Coverage
....

Randy Sherman, M.D.

Open fractures resulting from high-velocity trauma develop a zone of soft tissue injury much larger than the ostensible fracture site itself (Fig. 15-1).[12,13,38,89,95,100] As with a burn wound, the traumatic zone of injury includes areas of increasingly severe tissue destruction as the point of impact is approached (Fig. 15-2). A large portion of the soft tissues that are marginally viable at the time of initial injury eventually die or are replaced by scar. The entire area is ultimately characterized by fibrosis, tissue ischemia, lack of normal musculoskeletal architecture, and dead space including nonvascularized sequestrum, clot, foreign bodies, and other debris. Coupled with bone comminution, periosteal stripping, and disruption of the medullary blood supply, these injuries often result in fracture nonunion and post-traumatic chronic osteomyelitis. In open fractures, initial appreciation of the zone of injury is crucial for development of a subsequent strategy for fracture stabilization, débridement, and soft tissue coverage. Successfully designed, a logical and progressive treatment plan will favor success in the patient's orthopaedic outcome. Ignorance or purposefully shortcutting of tried and true principles of wound care more often than not will doom the patient to osteomyelitis, nonunion, and chronic disability.

Aggressive and repeated débridement of not only the fracture site but also the entire zone of injury is paramount to the positive resolution of these complex problems. Neither fracture healing nor soft tissue reconstruction can safely proceed until all necrotic material and foreign bodies have been cleared from the wound. Along with removal of all infected and nonviable tissue, the obliteration of dead space is essential to promote a favorable environment for fracture healing and to avoid development of osteomyelitis.[62] Similarly, radical excision of dead bone, scar, and infected granulation tissue is mandatory in the treatment of established bone infection.

Often, in an attempt to preserve as much bone cortical contact as possible for fracture healing, nonviable bone is left in place, thereby promoting the very complications that the surgeon had intended to avoid. There is no evidence that devascularized bone at the site of an open fracture aids in fracture healing. On the contrary, it is well documented that dead bone harbors bacteria, acts as a foreign body, and plays a central role in the development of osteomyelitis.[37] Historically, orthopaedic surgeons have been reluctant to débride wounds radically in the absence of reliable alternatives for bone reconstruction and soft tissue coverage. However, even without the newer plastic surgical techniques for wound management, there is a clear advantage to radical débridement alone, followed by eventual bone grafting by the Papineau technique or by skin grafting over newly developed granulation tissue.

With both musculoskeletal and head and neck neoplasms, the extent of tumor resection is often limited by the surgeon's ability to close the defect. Recurrence of such tumors depends on the extent of free margins. Prevention or cure of post-traumatic musculoskeletal disease (e.g., osteomyelitis) could be compared with adequate oncologic resection of a malignancy for cure. With the ability to transfer vascularized tissue into the traumatic defect, replacing tissue in kind, both the orthopaedic traumatologist and the oncologic surgeon are free to resect for cure. Godina and Lister[34] have shown the clear advantage of this treatment strategy, and our experience, as well that of many centers, corroborates their data.[79,98]

WOUND PREPARATION

Significant advances have been made over the last several years concerning how to best prepare open wounds for ultimate stable and durable closure. Progress in understanding wound physiology, microbiology, and endocrinology has led to innovations including the antibiotic bead pouch, vacuum-assisted closure (VAC therapy), and manipulation of wound-related growth factors such as vascular endothelial growth factor (VEGF).

Beads

Delivery of pharmacologic doses of bacteriocidal antibiotics used to plague the orthopaedic surgeon during the interval management of open fractures. Dressing changes done several times a day using topical antibacterials were summarily ineffective. The utilization of antibiotic-impregnated methylmethacrylate beads in the wound space contained by an impermeable type of dressing such as OpSite has revolutionized interval wound care in the débridement phase prior to wound closure. It is currently a practice option to place a bead pouch beneath a muscle flap for interval dead space management after vascularized wound coverage and prior to late bone grafting for final osteosynthesis. This practice, aside from more effectively suppressing pathogens, has significantly decreased practitioner workload during hospital stay.

FIGURE 15-1 *Diagrammatic representation of the zone of injury, incorporating an area much greater than the fracture site.*

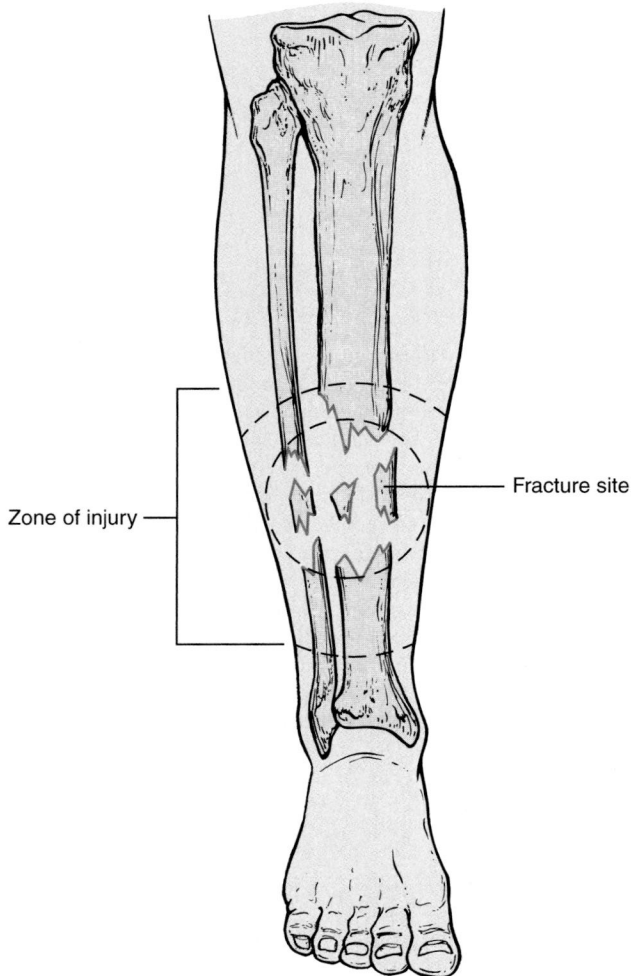

Zone of injury

Fracture site

Wound Vacuum-assisted Closure and Negative-pressure Wound Therapy

Another revolutionary wound care device is the wound VAC, a machine that delivers negative pressure to the closed wound space. First reported on in 1997, this device has gained universal acceptance as an important component of overall wound management in all major surgical subspecialties. The technique is rather simple but the results quite profound. After local cleaning, a sponge is placed over the wound with a fenestrated tube laid over the sponge. Both are secured using a clear plastic, impermeable dressing, making the construct into a closed space. Through a connection of the tube to a suction machine, constant negative pressure is applied to the wound space. This facilitates a series of changes to the wound that result in accelerated deposition of granulation tissue. As use and experience with this device grow, ongoing modifications expand its effectiveness. Different pore size sponges allow for customization of application. Silver-coated sponges seem to be more effective at suppression of bacterial contamination. Irrigation systems are being incorporated to better clear residual unwanted

FIGURE 15-2 *Progressive zones of injury in the burn wound are analogous to the soft tissue zone of injury concept.*

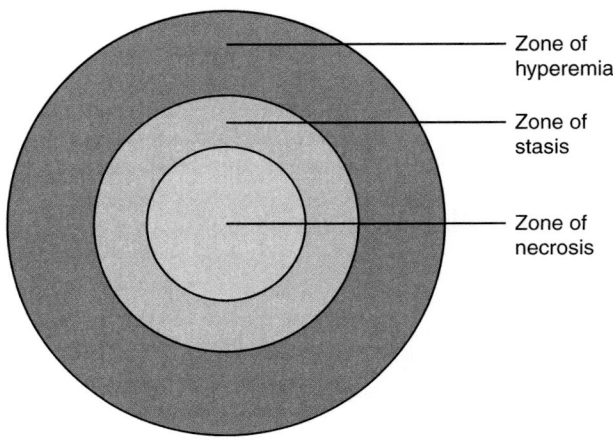

Zone of hyperemia

Zone of stasis

Zone of necrosis

material. Applications in the extremity are wide ranging and include extensive use in trauma where exposed bone and hardware reside. Granulation tissue may cover and close over exposed but intact plate and screw fixation by means of negative-pressure therapy in some cases, allowing for subsequent skin grafting.

Growth Factors

Various cell-derived proteins seem to have a targeted role in facilitating certain stages of wound healing. VEGF appears in hypoxic environments, promoting the growth and deposition of endothelial cells for neovascularization. Platelet-derived growth factor (PDGF), now available as Regranex, is developed from a lyophilized recombinant human derived form. This protein gel, applied directly to certain wounds, appears to significantly improve wound healing and eventual wound closure in certain extremity injuries. Clinical trials demonstrating maximal effectiveness have been limited to patients with diabetic foot ulcers. Research on its effectiveness in broader applications is ongoing.

TIMING

Historically, there has been some controversy about the timing of wound closure, with different centers basing treatment options on the nature and timing of surgical débridement. Early wound closure with the use of vascularized tissue has long been a prerequisite for optimal rehabilitation of function after complex hand injuries.[6,20] In several centers across the United States and in Europe, aggressive débridement and early lower extremity wound closure with muscle flaps have decreased the incidence of osteomyelitis, nonunion, and amputation. Godina and Lister's retrospective historical study[34] evaluating more than 534 free tissue transfers in the treatment of extremity trauma clearly revealed the advantages of radical débridement and early (within 72 hours) wound closure with vascularized tissue (Fig. 15-3). When this technique was used for limb salvage, the percentage of cases of nonunion and osteomyelitis decreased dramatically. In addition, the

FIGURE 15-3 *Graphic compendium of the work of Godina, published by Lister, illustrating the numerous advantages of early wound closure. (Modified from Godina, M.; Lister, G. Early microsurgical reconstruction of complex trauma of the extremities. Plast Reconstr Surg 78:285, 1986.)*

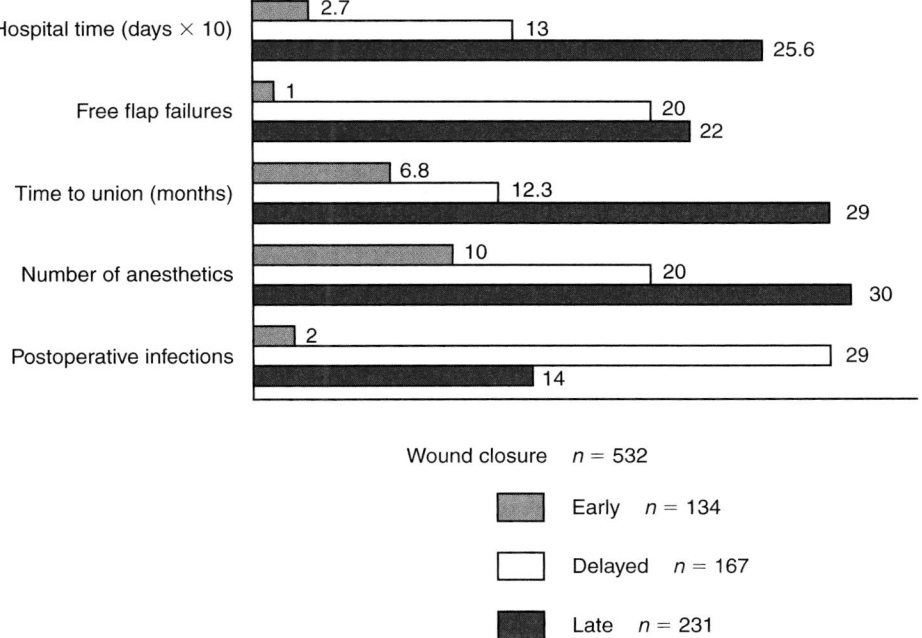

number of hospitalizations, use of anesthesia, and time to fracture healing were all substantially reduced.[34]

Byrd and colleagues[12] at the Parkland Medical Center prospectively compared the classical open wound care of type III tibial fractures with the method of early débridement and wound closure using vascularized muscle. Although the numbers were small, there was a distinct advantage in all the parameters mentioned with the latter approach. Both studies[12,34] found that the number of procedural complications rose markedly if these wounds were not closed in the early phase (defined by Byrd et al. as the first 6 days after injury and by Godina and Lister as the first 72 hours after injury). Subsequent studies have confirmed the numerous advantages of early wound closure with well vascularized tissue. Each study noted that the inflammatory nature of the wound, as it remained open, led to greater chances of continuing infection and an increased rate of thrombotic

complications of free tissue transfer at the time of delayed flap closure.

After aggressively débriding their patients, Yaremchuk and colleagues[100] obtained equivalent results in wound closure to the more favorable groups in the previous studies despite longer periods between initial injury and ultimate closure. The common denominator in these approaches is the dominant role of radical and repeated débridement as the key to success of any subsequent wound closure techniques (Table 15-1).

WOUND COVERAGE TECHNIQUES

In the approach to the treatment of an open wound in the locomotor system, the fundamental principles of the reconstructive ladder should be kept in mind. For injuries in which little or no soft tissue is lost, direct closure can be attempted when all necrotic tissue has been cleared and a lack of tension can be ensured. For injuries in which skin and its supporting elements have been lost but retention of soft tissue is adequate to ensure joint mobility and coverage of all vital structures (i.e., nerve, tendon, vessels, and bone), free grafts of split-thickness or full-thickness skin can be considered. For complex wounds that do not meet these criteria, pedicle or free transfer of vascularized tissue is necessary to restore blood supply, replace lost or devitalized tissues, and provide stable coverage. The biggest danger in early management historically is underappreciation of the soft tissue injury.

Skin Grafts

Split-thickness skin grafts are defined as those that occupy less than the entire depth of the dermis. They can be

Table 15-1
University of Southern California Protocol for the Management of Type III Fractures
Stabilization of patient
Tetanus prophylaxis
Broad-spectrum antibiotics
Fracture reduction with external fixation
Radical débridement of all injured tissues
Redébridement at 24, 48, and 72 hours, if necessary
Early muscle flap wound coverage before 5 days, if possible
Bone grafting at 6 weeks

FIGURE 15-4   *Representative cross-section of the musculoskeletal system and its arterial blood supply.*

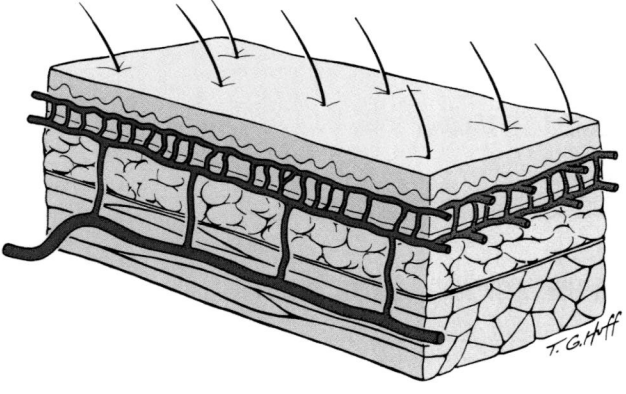

subdivided into thin split-thickness skin grafts, which are smaller than 0.016 inch, and thick split-thickness skin grafts. The advantages of these grafts are their ease of acquisition, their reliable take, and the capability of re-epithelialization of the donor site, which allows large amounts of split-thickness skin graft to be taken to cover sizable wounds. Their corresponding disadvantages are the need to have sophisticated instrumentation for skin graft harvesting (Brown or Padgett dermatome), scarring of the donor site, and variable contraction of the split-thickness skin graft on the recipient bed.

Full-thickness skin grafts are those that incorporate the entire dermal and epidermal structure. These have the

advantages of maintenance of the original texture after transplantation, minimal shrinkage or contraction of the graft, better color match in certain situations, and greater durability. In addition, donor sites can be closed with fine-line scars to minimize unsightly donor site defects. The disadvantages of full-thickness skin grafts are limitations related to their size and greater unreliability of take.

Flap Classification

Unlike a graft, which must derive its blood supply from the recipient bed to ensure adequate survival, a flap is vascularized tissue and contains a blood supply that not only serves to keep the flap alive but also aids in rehabilitation of the recipient defect. Two classification systems must be considered when studying the various flaps available.[16,63]

The flap is classified according to the specific area of skin or muscle from which it is derived (e.g., latissimus dorsi, lateral arm, fibula). The classification should also specify which tissue types are involved in the transfer (e.g., myocutaneous for muscle and skin, osteocutaneous for bone and skin, fasciocutaneous for investing fascia and skin, neural, visceral). In addition, the flap must be classified as to the nature of its blood supply (Fig. 15-4). The major categories include the random skin flap and the axial pattern flap. The latter type can be subclassified into the pedicle flap, the island flap, and the free flap on the basis of how the axial pattern vessels are handled: left attached with surrounding skin, left attached but skeletonized, or detached and revascularized with the use of microsurgical techniques to a distant site, respectively (Fig. 15-5).

The current success in providing alternatives for wound closure and soft tissue reconstruction is based on the work of the physicians who mapped out the anatomic and

FIGURE 15-5   *Flap classification based on the origin of blood supply.* **A,** *Random pattern.* **B,** *Axial pattern.* **C,** *Musculocutaneous.* **D,** *Fasciocutaneous.*

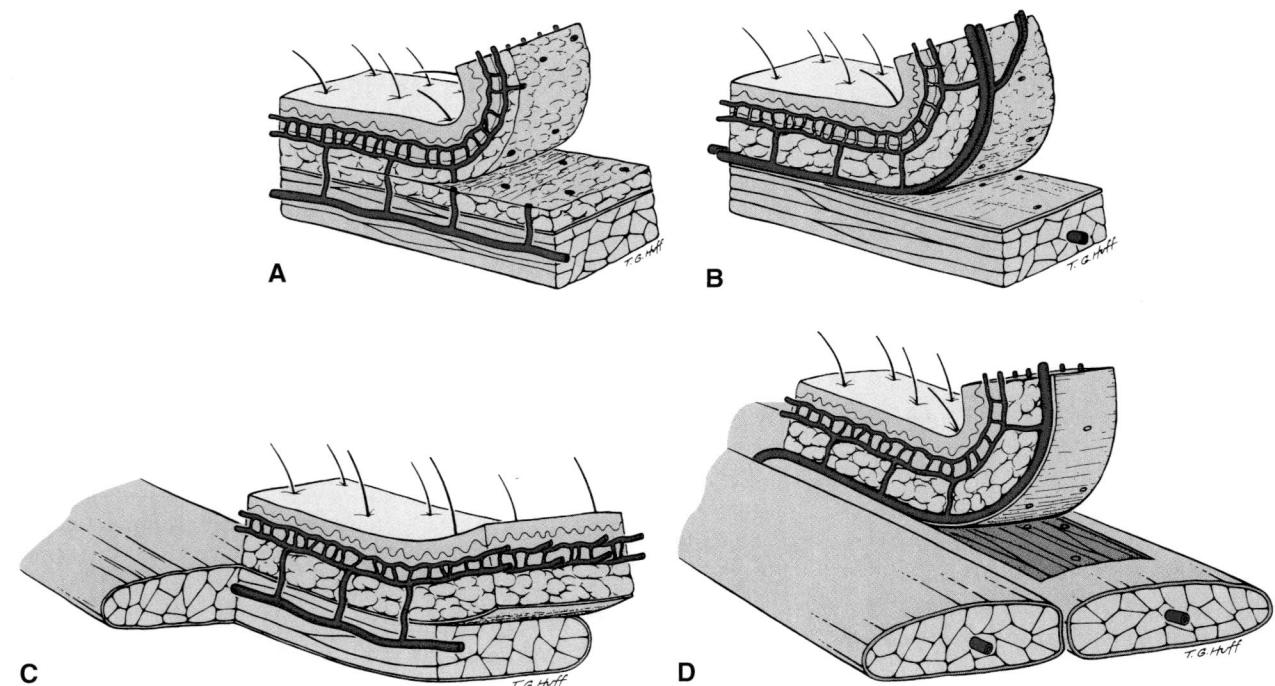

FIGURE 15-6   *Topical atlas of the donor sites most commonly employed for free tissue transfer.*

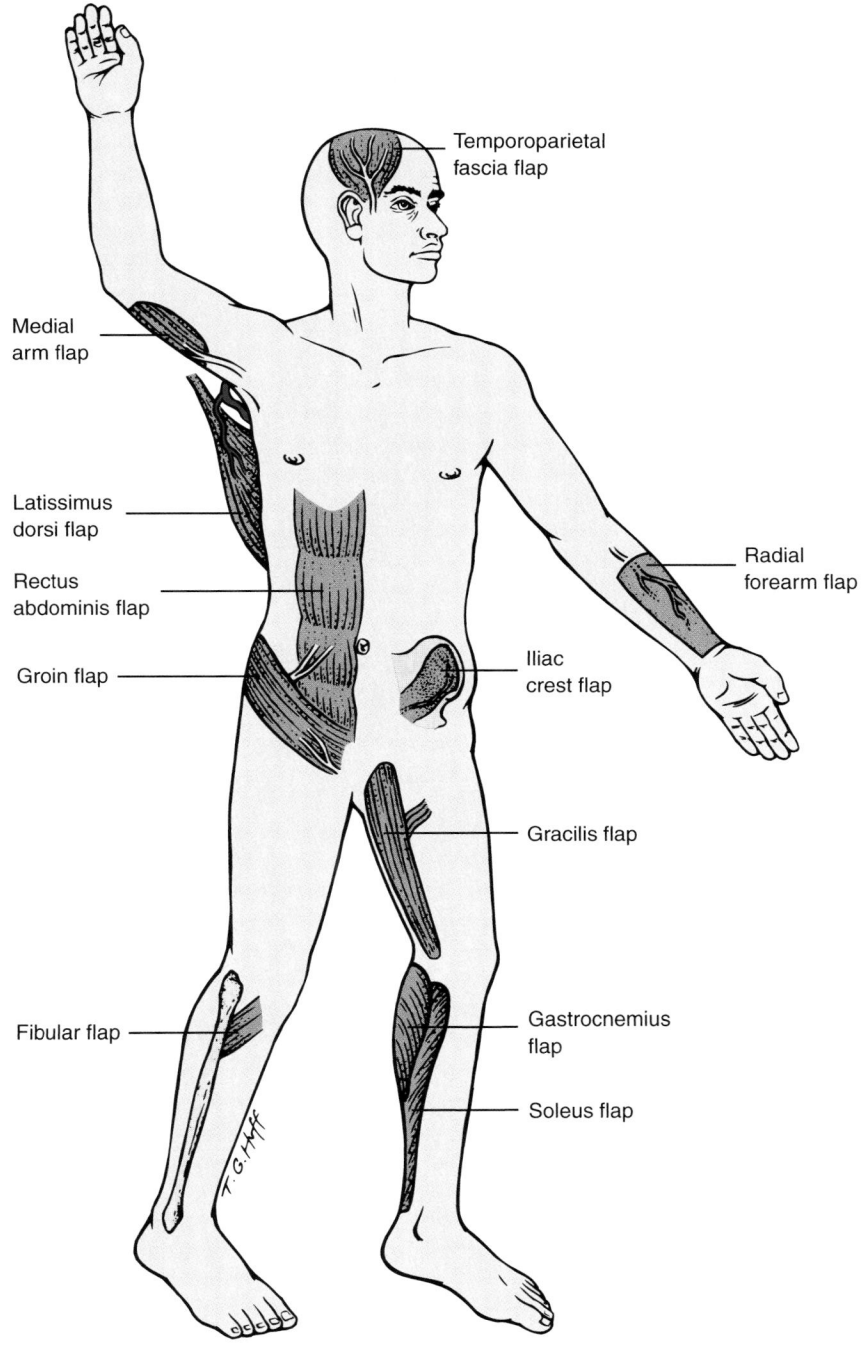

Temporoparietal
fascia flap

Medial
arm flap

Latissimus
dorsi flap

Rectus
abdominis flap

Groin flap

Radial
forearm flap

Iliac
crest flap

Gracilis flap

Gastrocnemius
flap

Fibular flap

Soleus flap

physiologic territories supplied by individual arteriovenous units, using cadaver dissections, barium latex injection radiography, and animal models for physiologic verification. Our understanding of musculoskeletal anatomy has grown to the point that scores of highly tailored composite tissue flaps are now available (Fig. 15-6).[64,69]

RANDOM SKIN FLAPS

Random skin flaps are based on the blood supply that remains at the base of a newly formed pedicle of skin,

where no identifiable inflow or outflow vessels can be found. Traditionally, the principle of maintaining a one-to-one ratio of length to width is applied—that is, the length of the proposed flap should be no longer than the width of the flap at its base. Many reports have documented flap designs that incorporate a length-to-width ratio much greater than this, but there is less certainty of survival of the distal portion of these flaps.

In an effort to transfer longer random skin flaps, delay procedures can be undertaken to exclude contributing blood supply sequentially from all sides of the proposed flap except the base. By creating a state of relative tissue hypoxia, these operations, done at 10- to 14-day intervals, can reorient the blood supply into the base of the flap, allowing more tissue to be transferred.[28,75] This practice, appropriately known as the delay technique, was once the standard method for creation of large flaps of tissue for complex wound coverage. With the development of axial pattern flaps, this tactic is now rarely used. Examples of random flaps include local, rotation, transposition, and advancement flaps used to cover small defects on the dorsum of the hand (see later discussion). The flap derives its blood supply from the subdermal plexus, which lies immediately below the dermal subcutaneous junction.

AXIAL PATTERN SKIN FLAPS

Axial pattern skin flaps, best exemplified by the groin flap, are made up of skin and subcutaneous tissue supplied by an identified arteriovenous pedicle lying superficial to the underlying muscle or its invested fascia. This pedicle supplies the entirety of the defined skin territory through an arborization of the dominant pedicle, connecting with the subdermal plexus previously described. These flaps have the advantage of transferring a much larger amount of tissue on a pedicle base that need be only the width of the arteriovenous unit itself. They can be employed as pedicle flaps or as free tissue transfers.

FASCIOCUTANEOUS FLAPS

Certain areas of the cutaneous anatomy derive their blood supply from perforating vessels that run within the investing muscular fascia. These provide a well-vascularized piece of tissue with an anatomically defined boundary that can be raised solely on the pedicle or transferred as free tissue. Such fasciocutaneous flaps, sometimes also known as septocutaneous flaps, have the advantages of lack of bulk, pliability, and improved match of color and texture. Donor site deformities can often be minimized by primary closure, as with the myocutaneous flap. If a cutaneous nerve is present, sensory innervation can occasionally be restored to the transferred tissue.

MYOCUTANEOUS FLAPS

Since the early to middle 1980s, the myocutaneous flap has become the most commonly used of all axial pattern flaps.[62] This flap derives its blood supply from the major pedicle or one of the predominant minor pedicles that supply the muscle of choice. Through perforating vessels from the muscle, the overlying subcutaneous tissue or skin, or both, can be transferred along with the muscle to provide a flap of sizable bulk and contour.

When taken with the motor nerve in specialized reconstructive situations, these flaps can be used to rehabilitate an otherwise paralyzed or nonfunctional muscle group—for example, the motorized gracilis muscle can be used to restore forearm flexion or to correct facial paralysis.[61] Myocutaneous flaps can be used to cover otherwise nonreconstructible wounds of the extremities because they provide all components necessary for successful healing of the injured tissues.[67] Muscle and myocutaneous flaps also

play an increasingly central role in the treatment of upper and lower extremity osteomyelitis.[97]

PERFORATOR FLAPS

Most recently, the perforator flap has been incorporated into the classification scheme. These flaps are a subgroup of cutaneous flaps that may include the underlying fascia but derive their blood supply from blood vessels that penetrate the subtending muscle. Essentially, they are myocutaneous flaps in which the muscle has been painstakingly left in situ by dissection of the responsible vessels from the muscle proper. The advantage of this construct is the maintenance of muscle function. The cost is borne as a more complicated dissection, longer operative time, and in some cases, diminution of blood supply. The anterolateral thigh flap is one of the more popular examples of this construct. Other popular alternatives include the deep inferior epigastric perforator (DIEP), thoracodorsal artery perforator (TAP), and gluteal artery perforator (GAP). We are sure to see many additional perforator variants in coming years as surgeons grow more comfortable with this type of dissection technique.

SOFT TISSUE COVERAGE BY REGION

Upper Extremity

HAND AND FINGERTIPS

Complex injuries to the fingertip can be particularly devastating because of the crucial role this part of the hand plays in human contact. The fingertip pulp is invested with a greater density and specificity of nerve endings than any other region in the body. Examination must assess the integrity not only of the nail but also of its supporting elements, the eponychium and the underlying nail bed. The treatment of pulp injuries varies according to the size of tissue loss and the exposure of underlying structures. For injuries smaller than 1 cm to the fingertip pulp, several authors have shown the advantage of conservative wound management with sterile dressings, granulation, contraction, and eventual epithelialization or split-thickness skin grafting. In circumstances in which patients have lost a larger amount of tissue or the soft tissue loss is combined with an exposed distal phalangeal bone or flexor tendon, soft tissue transposition has its advantages. Because the finger pulp is the ultimate prehensile surface, durability and sensation are of paramount importance to a successfully rehabilitated fingertip. These prerequisites can be met by the use of various local or regional flaps.[51,82]

ATASOY-KLEINERT FLAP This is a proximally based random skin flap that uses the principle of V-Y advancement to move more proximal volar phalangeal tissue distally to cover the tip loss. The advantage of this flap is its transfer of vascularized sensate skin and supporting elements from an adjacent, normal, uninjured area. Its prerequisites are lack of associated injuries to the phalanx proximal to the tip injury and a realistic limitation on the size of the tip defect (Fig. 15-7).

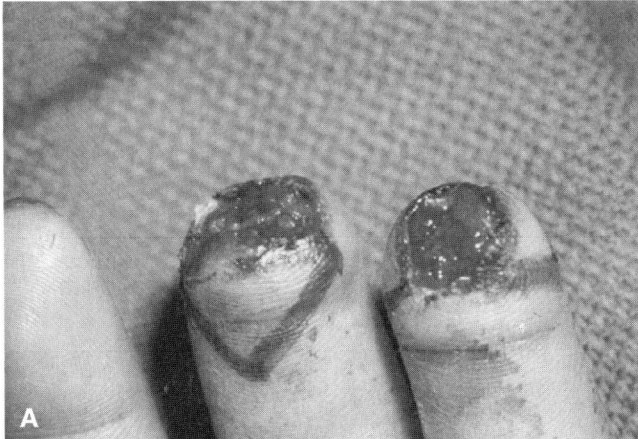

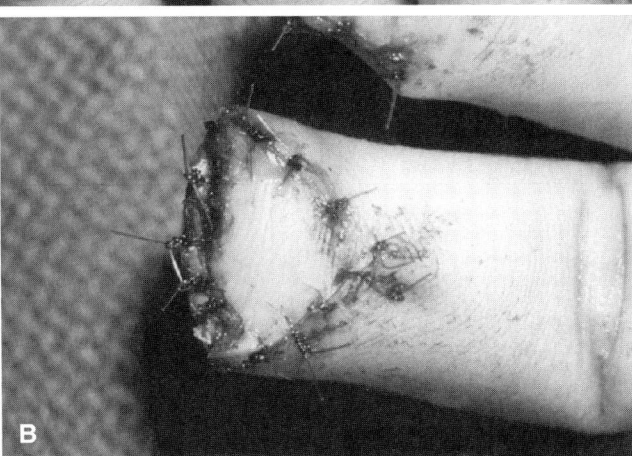

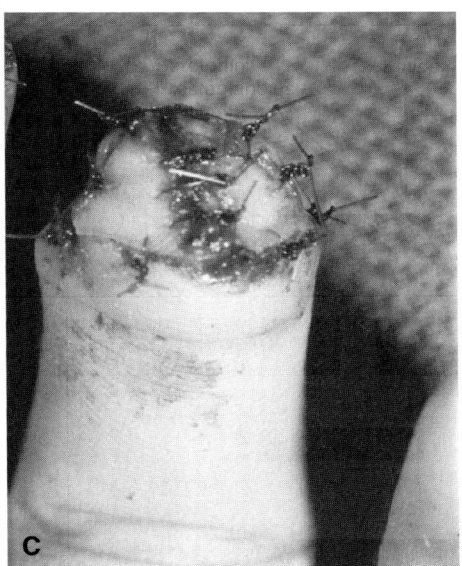

FIGURE 15-7 | **A,** *Complex fingertip injuries to the long and ring digits involving distal phalangeal exposure.* **B,** *The long finger after completion of an Atasoy-Kleinert flap.* **C,** *The ring finger after completion of Cutler flaps.*

CUTLER FLAP Cutler flaps are similar in design and execution to the Atasoy-Kleinert flaps except for their site of origin. These randomly based skin flaps are developed from the lateral soft tissues of the distal phalanx. They can be useful if the geometry of the wound or previous scarring on the volar aspect of the finger mitigates against the use of the Atasoy-Kleinert flap (see Fig. 15-7).[27]

THENAR FLAP This proximally based pedicle flap, well-described by Beasley,[6] employs thenar skin and subcutaneous tissue to cover tip losses of the index and long fingers that require more than local distal phalangeal tissue can provide. The advantages of this flap are good color and texture match, excellent durability, and the ability to reconstruct the contour of the fingertip with revisional surgery. When the flap is properly harvested, the donor site should heal without incident. Because of the digital positioning, however, the recipient finger is at major risk for flexion contracture if the flap is tethered longer than 2 weeks. Early division and aggressive postoperative mobilization are mandatory to prevent this complication (Fig. 15-8).[74]

VOLAR ADVANCEMENT FLAP This alternative for fingertip coverage, first described by Moberg in 1964,[3] employs the volar surface of the involved digit proximal to the metacarpal phalangeal joint of the thumb or to a point immediately proximal to the proximal interphalangeal joint of the remaining fingers.[11,58] The flap is raised by incising along the midaxial line bilaterally and dissecting skin and subcutaneous tissue free along the line of the tendon sheath. The neurovascular bundles are preserved within the flap, and the dorsal branches of these neurovascular bundles are preserved to ensure continued viability of the distal dorsal skin. The finger is slightly flexed at the interphalangeal joint, and the flap is advanced to the distal edge of the tip defect. The flap is then sutured in place and dressed to hold the digit in a position that avoids tension on the advanced tissue. In practice, this procedure is best suited for the thumb and has little clinical value for the remaining digits. Early and aggressive range-of-motion exercises are mandatory to prevent contracture at the interphalangeal joint.

CROSS-FINGER FLAPS This option for fingertip reconstruction also serves amply for coverage of exposed flexor or extensor surfaces throughout the length of the phalanges. The standard cross-finger flap employs the dorsal skin and subcutaneous tissue down to the epitenon of the extensor surface overlying the middle phalanx. The blood supply to this flap is based on the dorsal branch of the digital neurovascular bundle to the donor digit. The flap is raised from the radial to the ulnar side, or vice versa, and then applied to the fingertip or other defect. The donor defect is simultaneously covered with a full-thickness skin graft for optimal aesthetic result (Fig. 15-9). A period of 10 to 14 days is allowed for

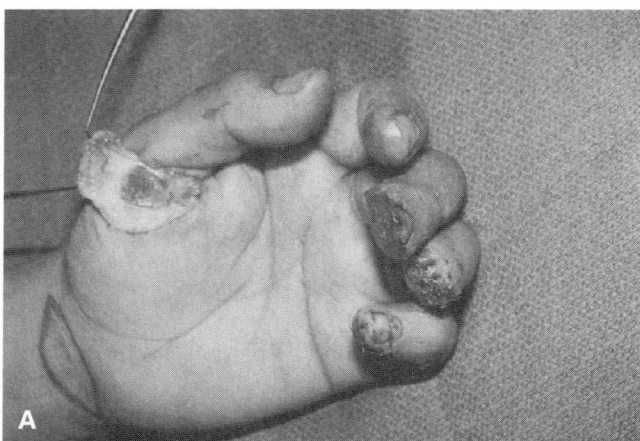

FIGURE 15-8 *A, Thenar flap raised for coverage of a middle fingertip injury with loss of volar pulp tissue and an exposed distal phalanx. B, The flap in place. C, Two months after division.*

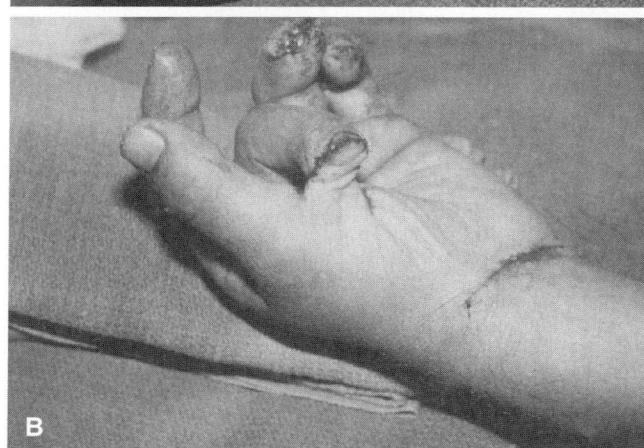

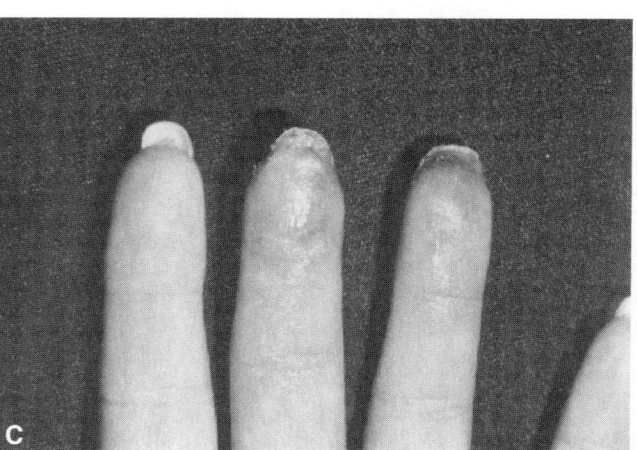

FIGURE 15-9 *A, Gunshot wound to the proximal phalanx of the long finger with exposed, comminuted fracture and tendon loss. Cross-finger flap drawn out. B, Flap transferred and full-thickness skin graft applied to the donor site.*

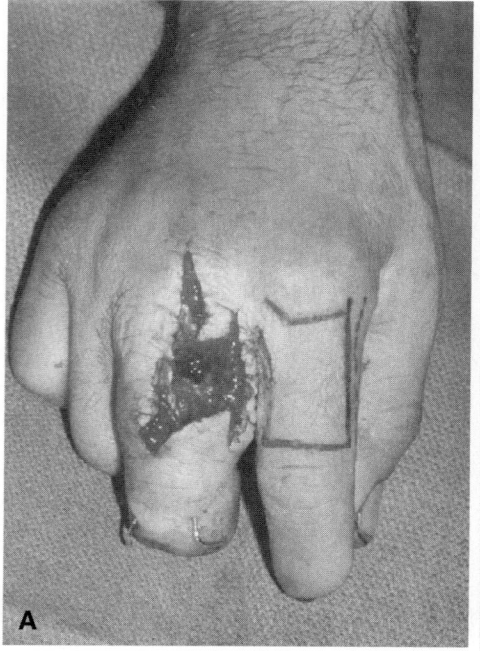

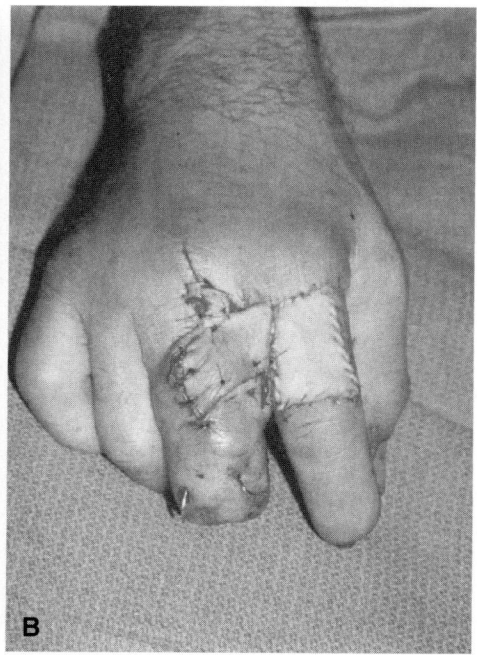

revascularization of the flap from the recipient bed before division is attempted.[19,41,48,49,52,85,96]

NEUROVASCULAR ISLAND FLAP As a modification of the cross-finger flap, numerous varieties of arterialized island flaps based on the digital neurovascular bundles have been described.[84] They have the advantage of a greater transpositional arc than is available with the flaps previously described for injuries to the middle and proximal portions of the phalanges. They provide vascularized tissue with good color and texture match, excellent durability, and in the case of the neurovascular island pedicle flap, proper sensibility, which can sometimes approach that of the native tissue. The major drawback with this type of transfer is the need for cortical reeducation. After intensive occupational therapy, the patient may be able to recognize the afferent stimuli from these flaps as coming from the recipient digit. With any period of disuse or immobilization, however, cortical orientation reverts to that of the donor finger.[11,57,72]

OTHER LOCAL FLAPS For small defects about the dorsum of the hand, wrist, or forearm that cannot be closed directly or repaired with skin grafts, flaps created by local transposition, rotation, or advancement can be used. These are essentially random flaps and consequently are limited by the size of their soft tissue base and their small arc of rotation. Given an understanding of their limitations, however, these flaps can be especially useful to obtain coverage for isolated tendon or bone exposure (Fig. 15-10).[55,71]

FOREARM

Wounds in the forearm region that require more extensive soft tissue coverage include open fractures with major overlying soft tissue loss, degloving injuries, irreversibly exposed tendons or nerves, and osteomyelitic wounds with draining sinuses. As noted previously, large open wounds caused by degloving injuries are adequately treated after débridement by split-thickness skin grafting provided an adequate bed of granulation tissue is present. Many investigators have noted restoration of reasonable tendon function with a split-thickness skin graft applied directly over the intact epitenon. With loss of vascularized tissues covering the tendon substance, nerve, or bone, the importation of vascularized soft tissue becomes mandatory. Quantitative bacteriology can aid in optimizing the timing of closure in these granulating wounds. Counts of less than 10^3 organisms per gram of tissue ensure a much greater chance of skin graft take.[53]

The groin flap, first described by McGregor and Jackson[73] in 1972, continues to be the mainstay for soft tissue replacement in this region.[72] The flap can be raised quickly and easily, with an extremely high degree of reliability. The area of skin that can be taken without fear of distal tip necrosis extends at least 10 cm beyond the anterior superior iliac spine. This area almost always provides adequate tissue for coverage of composite defects of the dorsum, hand, wrist, or distal forearm. Additional advantages of this flap include ease of donor site closure and aesthetic superiority of the donor site scar. As with all pedicle flaps, the main disadvantage is the need for

FIGURE 15-10	*A, Transposition flap. B, Rotation flap. C, Advancement flap.*

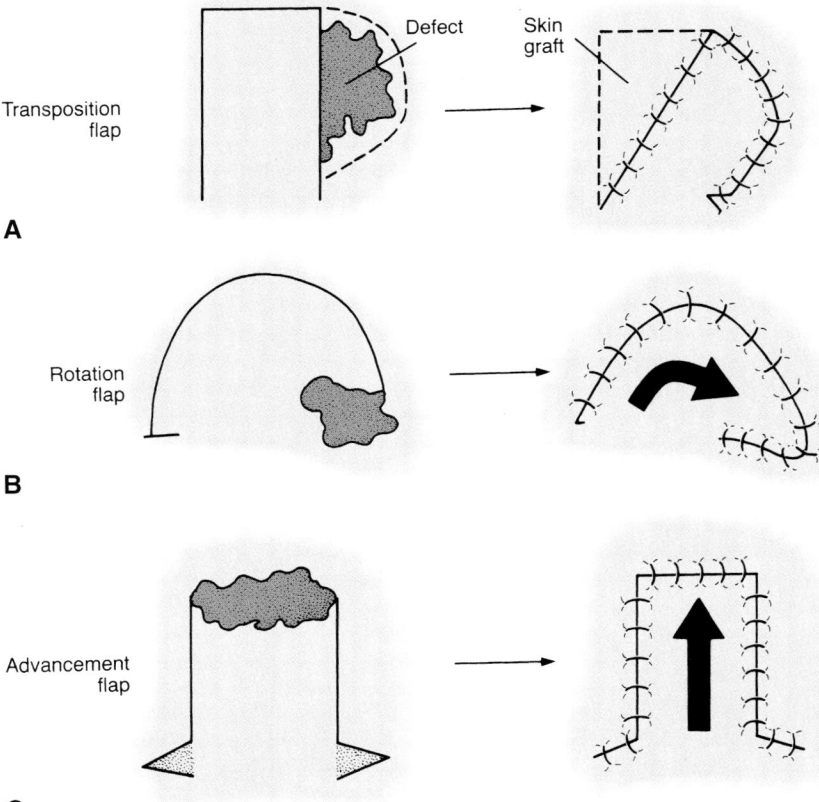

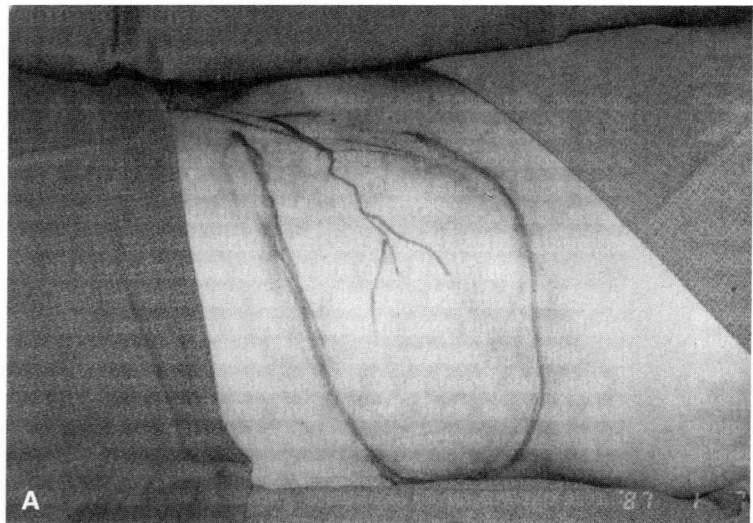

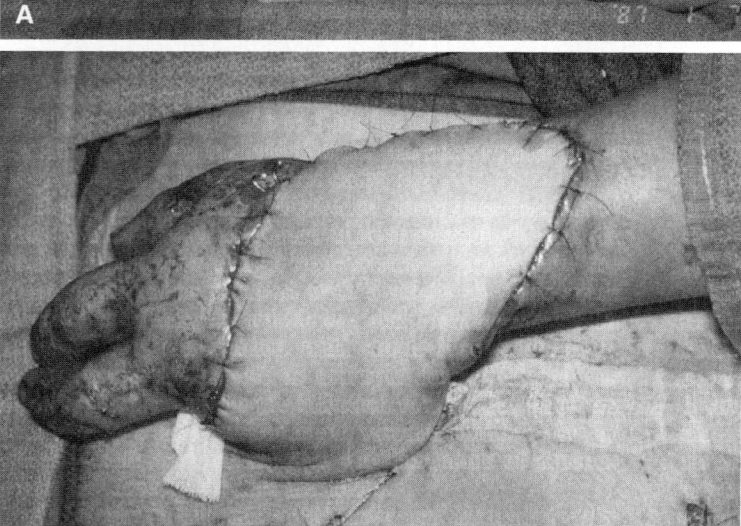

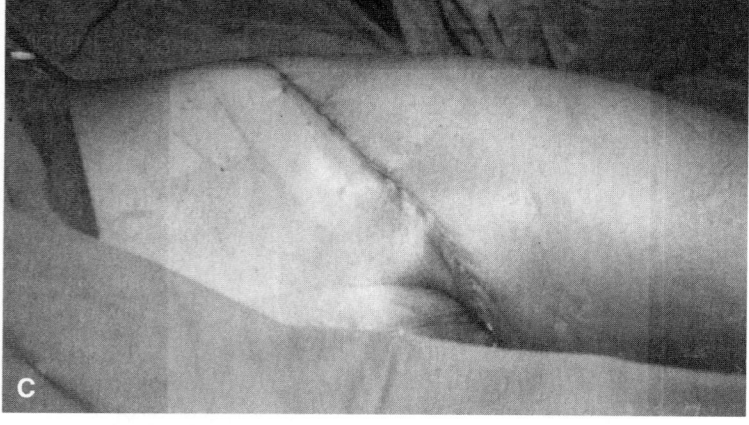

FIGURE 15-11 **A,** *Groin flap donor site with superficial circumflex iliac artery marked.* **B,** *Flap in place over a composite defect of the hand.* **C,** *Donor site scar.*

immobilization of the hand in the groin region for 14 to 21 days before division (Fig. 15-11).[56,73]

The arterial supply of the groin flap arises from the femoral artery, approximately 2.5 cm below the inguinal ligament. This vessel runs parallel to the inguinal ligament and meets it at a point overlying the anterior superior iliac spine. The vessel perforates the sartorius muscle fascia and sends a deep branch below and a superficial branch into the subcutaneous tissue at this point. If the flap is to be elevated medial to the sartorius fascia, the muscle should be included in order to protect both branches of the vessel. The venous drainage to the flap is usually supplied by the venae comitantes of the superficial circumflex iliac vein, but it can also drain predominantly into the superficial

FIGURE 15-12 **A,** *Composite defect of the thumb with exposed extensor pollicis longus and interphalangeal joint.* **B,** *Distally based radial forearm flap.* **C,** *Immediate postoperative result.*

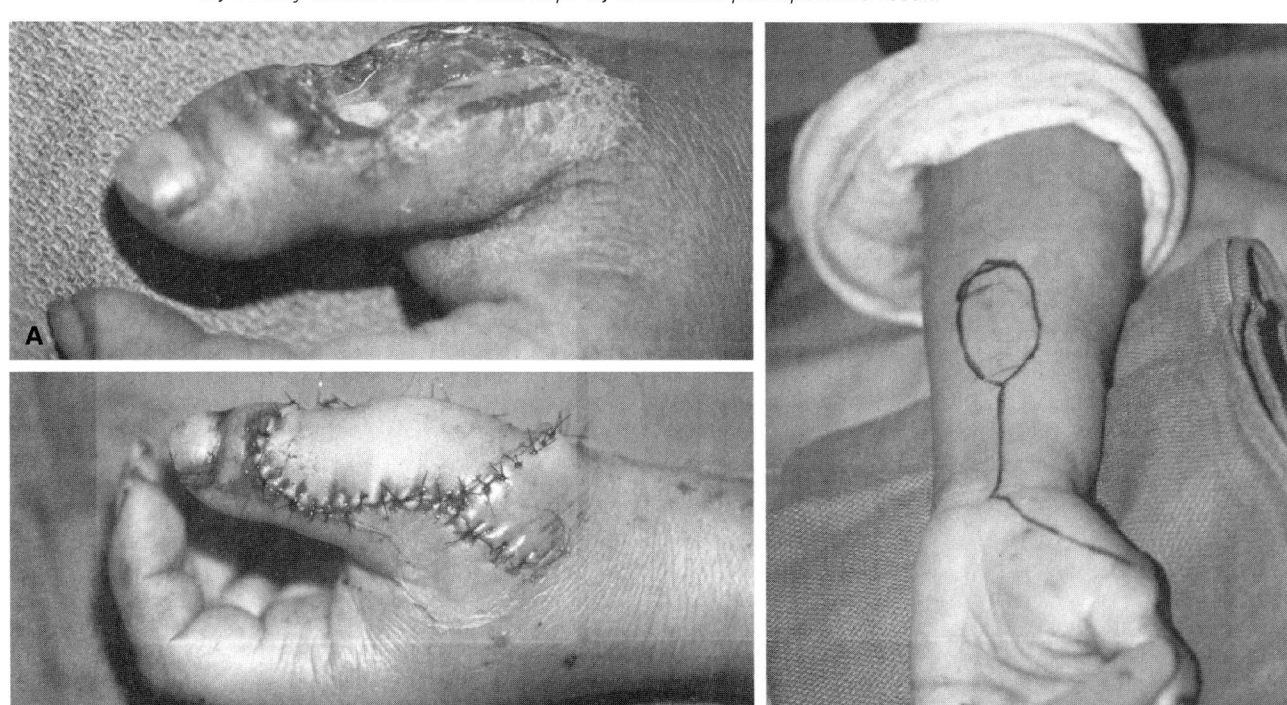

inferior epigastric vein. This variability in venous drainage need not be taken into account when using the flap as a pedicle transfer. The flap can easily be made 10 cm wide while still closing the donor site primarily.

The deltopectoral flap provides tissue that is similar to that of the groin flap. It is taken from an area on the anterolateral chest wall. This medially based skin flap takes its blood supply from perforating vessels of the internal mammary artery. The flap is transversely oriented and raised from the lateral to the medial side at the level of the pectoralis fascia. This tissue provides an excellent color match with the upper extremity. However, donor sites must be closed with the skin graft, which leaves an unsightly donor defect. With the newer alternatives involving free tissue transfer, this type of flap, like other large thoracoabdominal flaps, is of mainly historical interest.

For more extensive wounds of this region, the axial pattern hypogastric or thoracoepigastric flap (based on the superficial inferior epigastric artery and vein) and the rectus abdominis muscle myocutaneous flap can be of use. These flaps are advantageous because of the large quantities of tissue available. As previously described, the disadvantages stem from the need to keep the patient immobilized and relatively dependent for 10 days to 3 weeks. These flaps are in a sense parasitic because they do not bring in new sources of blood supply after division. Rather, they depend exclusively on the wound bed for vascularity and cannot be relied on to enhance the wound environment. In cases of osteomyelitis or other residual infections, additional vascularized tissue is crucial.

A newer flap for the dorsum of the wrist and distal forearm is the pedicle radial artery forearm flap, called the Chinese flap.[26] This fasciocutaneous flap is based on the radial artery and the basilic vein proximally and on the radial artery and cephalic vein distally. The distal flap can be used only if an intact ulnar circulation is ensured by Allen's test and arteriography. The extensive arc of rotation of this flap, given both the proximal and distal pedicles, makes it useful for treatment of wounds of the dorsal and volar surfaces of the forearm, wrist, and hand. However, this soft tissue component cannot be used for complex wounds that involve the flap itself (Fig. 15-12).[23,26,76,92]

The division of pedicle flaps traditionally takes place 14 to 21 days after initial application. This allows time for the skin paddle to become vascularized from the recipient bed. In special circumstances in which the flap has an extremely dominant vascular pedicle or the recipient bed is judged marginal in its ability to revascularize the flap, a delay procedure, with division of only the dominant pedicle on the flap, can be done to augment the development of collateral circulation. Along with Meyers and associates,[75] Furnas and colleagues[28] have documented the ability of intermittent ischemic periods induced by cross-clamping of the flap to augment and speed the formation of collateral circulation from the recipient bed. In a limited clinical study using the progressive intermittent clamping technique, they were able to divide two pedicle flaps only 5 days after initial application.[28] Fluorescein dye studies performed with the clamp applied allow quantification of blood flow from the recipient site before division.

USE OF FREE FLAPS IN THE UPPER EXTREMITY

Although pedicle flaps, such as the groin flap, have worked admirably in many situations for soft tissue coverage, there are increasing indications for the transfer of composite tissues from distant sites using microsurgical techniques, and many such flaps have been developed.[63,64,69,88,91]

INDICATIONS In many complex extremity wounds, the sheer size and complexity of the injury and the loss of structures obviate the use of a local or pedicle flap for adequate replacement. In this situation, several donor sites to fill specific needs can be chosen. Often, the recipient bed cannot support the vascular requirements of the transferred tissue. However rare it may be, osteomyelitis of the upper extremity with overlying tissue loss is best treated by free muscle transfer after débridement. The addition of this highly vascularized tissue increases oxygen tension and decreases bacterial counts in the experimental model.[15,62]

Central to the successful rehabilitation of any hand and upper extremity injury is early mobilization. This need is especially acute in the hand and wrist and can be better accomplished in cases of large soft tissue defects with the use of free tissue transfer. This approach frees the patient from immobilization at the donor site and allows early range-of-motion exercise and prevention of stiffness.

Composite transfers can be undertaken to fulfill the needs of the polytraumatized hand. Often, the combination of tendon and skin or skin and bone is required to complete the reconstruction. With use of the appropriate composite transfer, the reconstruction can frequently be completed in one procedure, allowing more rapid healing and earlier rehabilitation.

Preoperative evaluation requires that the patient be otherwise stable and that more severe injuries be addressed and resolved. Angiography is often advisable to delineate the vascular anatomy of the injured region.[101] Débridement and skeletal stabilization, preferably with external fixation, should be the first order of business at the time of surgery. These procedures must be carried out with an autonomous set of instruments and irrigating tools; after the wound has been cleaned and all remaining tissues are viable, gowns and gloves should be changed and the transfer accomplished. Repeated débridement may be needed, and several procedures may be required before the transfer is complete. Usually, two teams work simultaneously, one at the harvest site and the other at the recipient site. This arrangement shortens the intraoperative interval; reduces pulmonary, vascular, and neurologic complications related to positioning; and helps avoid physician fatigue.

Various free muscle or myocutaneous flaps are available for soft tissue coverage of complex hand and forearm wounds. In our experience, the rectus abdominis muscle transferred as a pure muscle unit alone has worked admirably (Fig. 15-13). The gracilis myocutaneous flap is frequently transferred as a motorized unit for the treatment of Volkmann's ischemic contracture and of associated conditions in which flexor function is lost (Fig. 15-14).[61] The temporoparietal fascial free flap serves well in situations in which bulk must be kept to a minimum and vascularity is

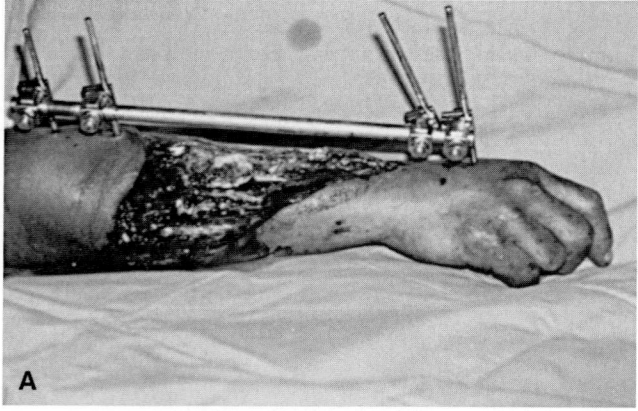

FIGURE 15-13 *A, Proximal forearm defect involving loss of skin, muscle, and bone. B, The injury after radical débridement and transfer of the rectus abdominis muscle. C, Postoperative view 4 months after cancellous bone grafting and subsequent removal of the external fixator.*

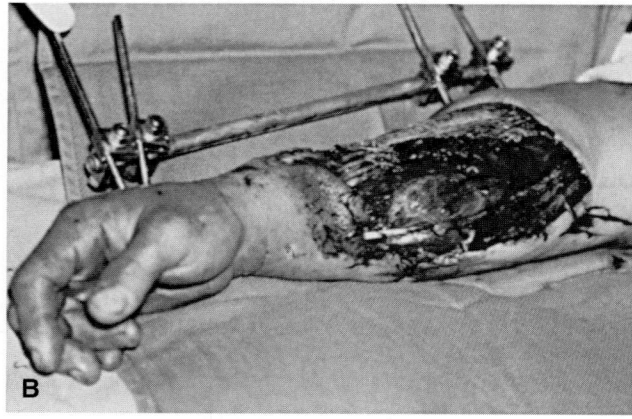

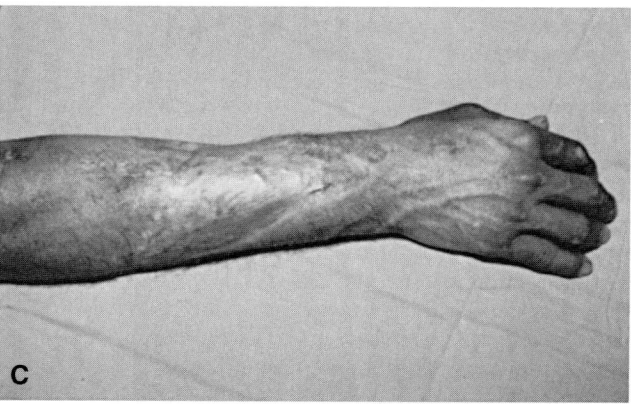

FIGURE 15-14   *A, Loss of volar musculature from machete injury with inability to flex wrist and fingers. B, Motorized gracilis myocutaneous flap outlined. C, Muscle isolated with tracking sutures placed in situ to determine resting muscle fiber length. D, Immediately following transfer. E, Another patient after gracilis transfer—relaxed. F, Fully flexed.*

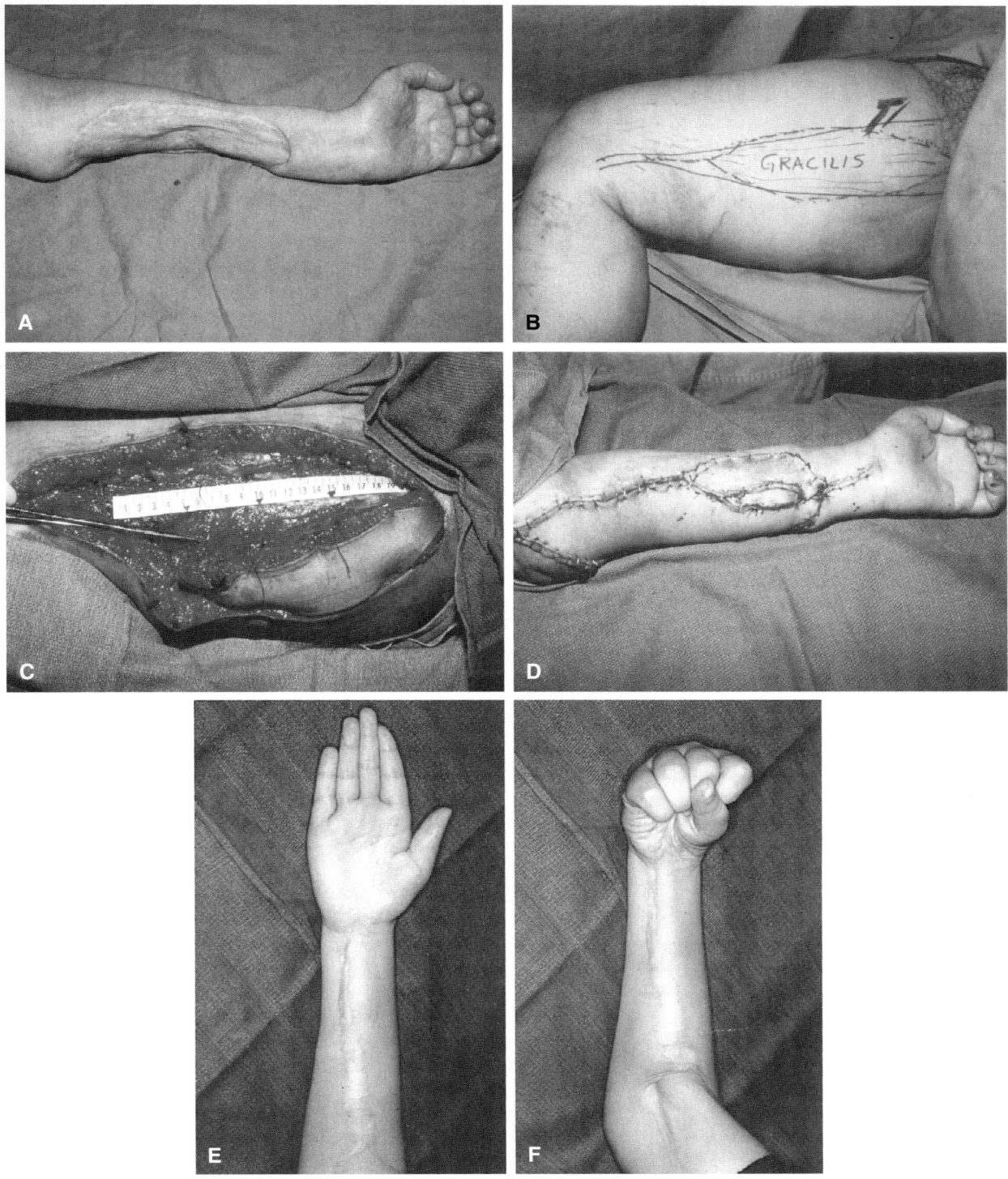

paramount to successful closure of the wound (Fig. 15-15). This is certainly the case in distal forearm osteomyelitis. The latissimus dorsi muscle, the original workhorse of free tissue transfers, always has a place in soft tissue coverage in any area. Donor site seromas occur more frequently with

this muscle than with other donor sites and may necessitate prolonged suction drainage, repeated percutaneous aspiration, or both. The serratus anterior muscle has been used successfully by Buncke and colleagues for coverage of defects over the dorsum and thenar eminence of the

FIGURE 15-15 | **A,** *Composite defect of the hand with loss of skin, avulsion laceration of extensor tendons, and exposure of central metacarpals.* **B,** *Temporoparietal fascia raised and isolated on the superficial temporal artery and vein.* **C,** *Three months after transfer, with simultaneous tendon grafting and split-thickness skin grafting.* **D,** *Invisible donor site defect 2 months after surgery.*

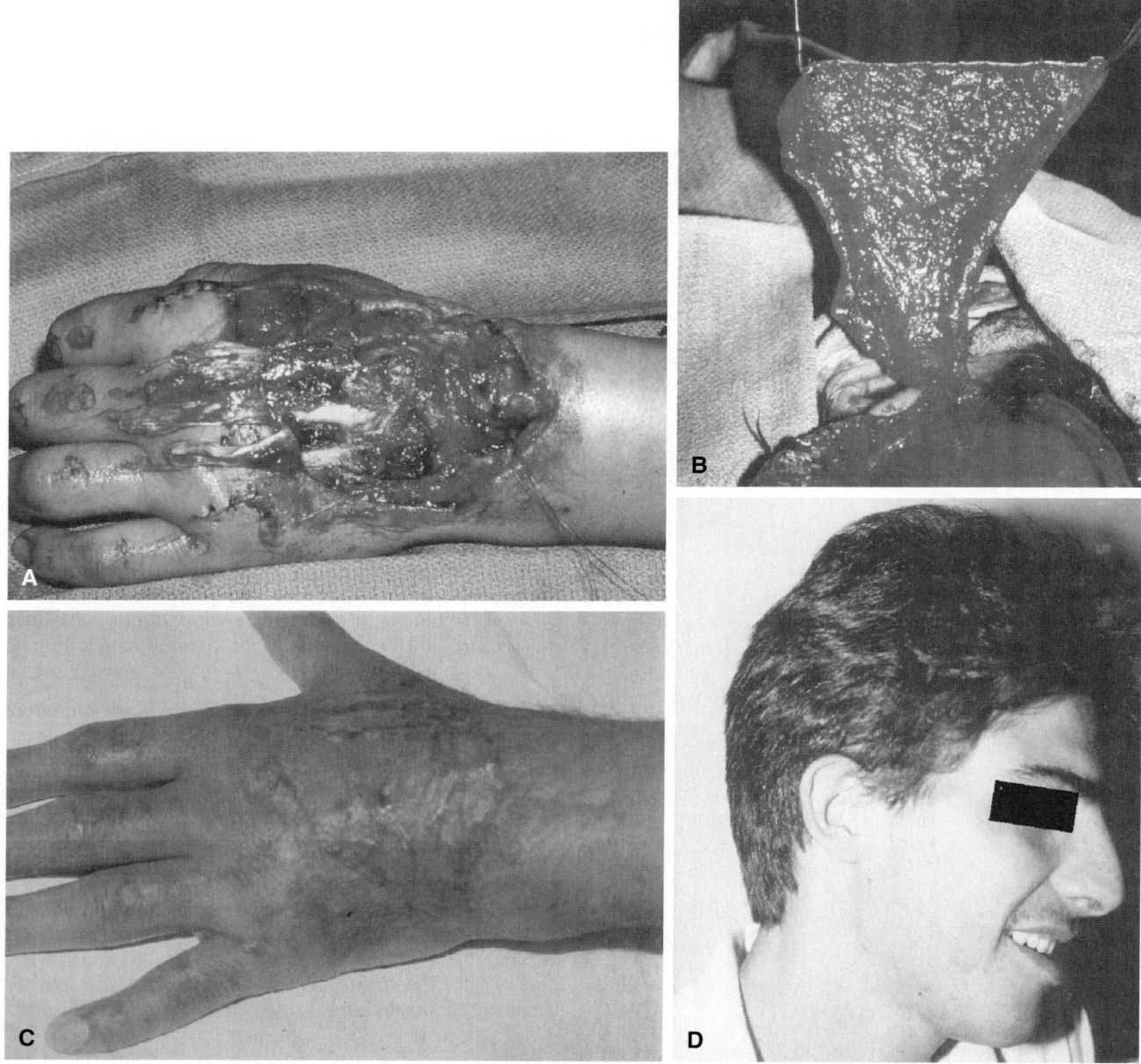

hand. The lower three slips are included, and the remainder of the muscle is left to avoid winging of the scapula.

TYPES OF FLAPS AVAILABLE Free skin and fasciocutaneous flaps useful in the upper extremity include the groin, scapular, lateral arm, dorsalis pedis, and radial forearm flaps (Fig. 15-16).[4,50,59,77,78]

Groin Flap
This flap has gained increasing popularity as a free tissue transfer because of the amount of skin available and the minimal aesthetic deformity of the donor site defect[1,5]

(Fig. 15-17). This was the first skin flap used as a free tissue transfer by Daniel and Taylor in 1973. It soon fell out of favor because of the variability and brevity of the donor site pedicle. These problems remain, but increased familiarity and greater technical confidence have helped overcome them. Although not often employed in hand reconstruction, a modification of this flap used commonly in jaw reconstruction incorporates a segment of the iliac crest along with abdominal wall musculature based on the deep circumflex iliac artery and vein.[93] This allows osteomyocutaneous transfer and can be used if a substantial part

FIGURE 15-16   *A, Distal humeral neoplasm. B, After resection of bone and surrounding soft tissue with transfer of parascapular free flap.*

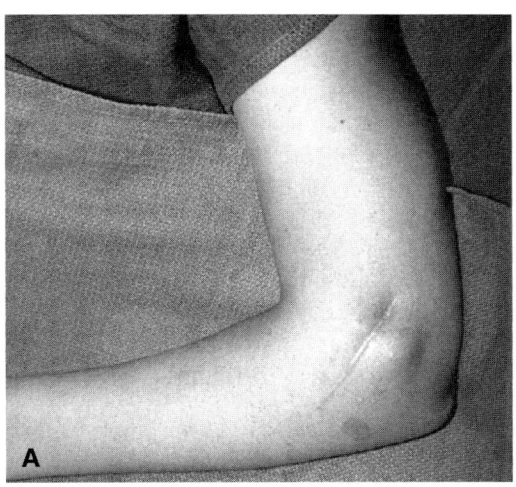
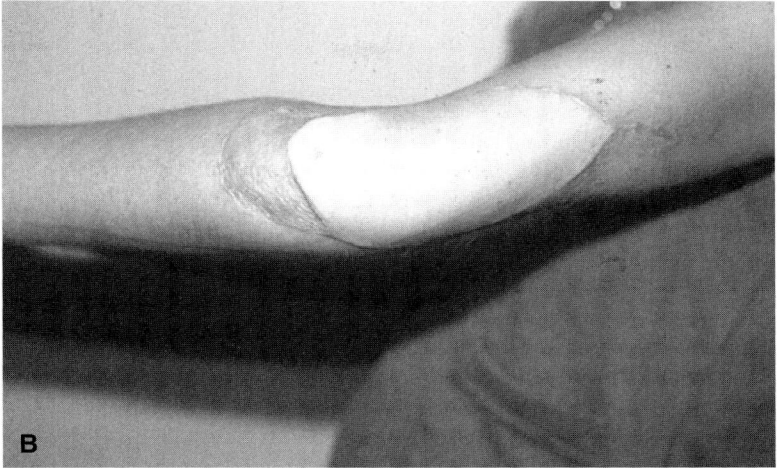

FIGURE 15-17   *A, Composite wound from exiting high-power gunshot blast involving skin, muscle, tendon, and bone. B, One week after free groin flap transfer. Passive range-of-motion exercises were begun shortly after surgery. The patient eventually underwent bone grafting and tendon transfer. C, Combination of internal and external fixation for bone stabilization. D, Closed wound, healed fracture. The patient is now undergoing occupational therapy.*

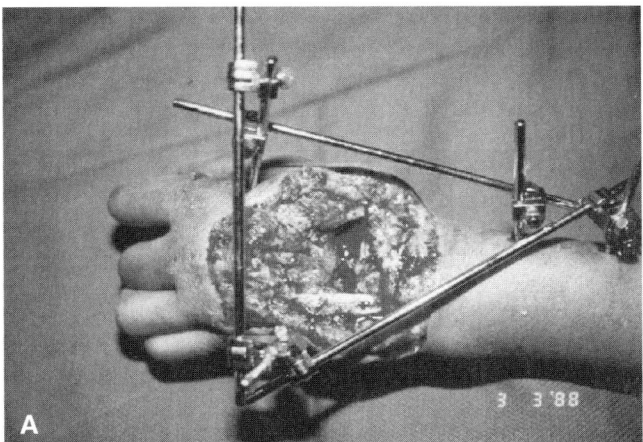
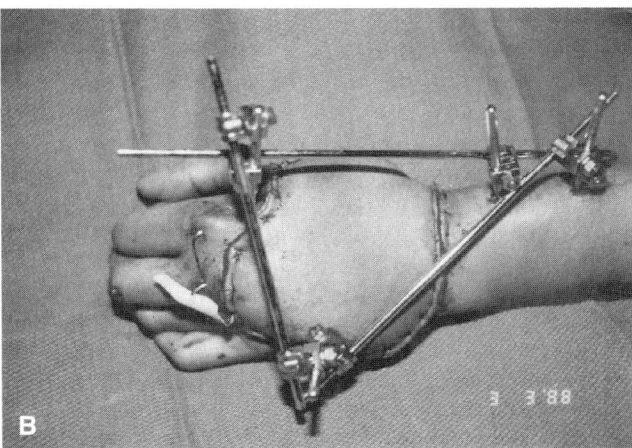
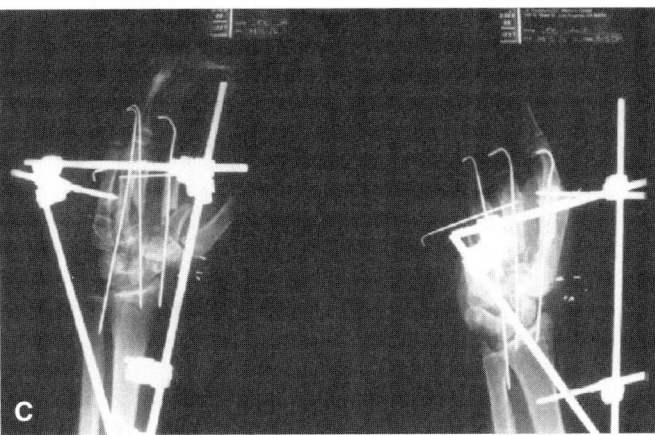
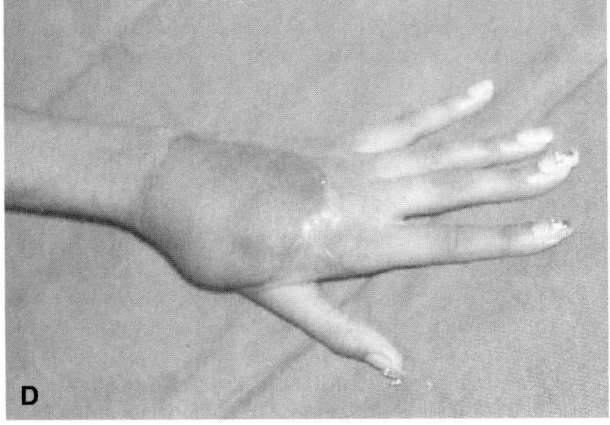

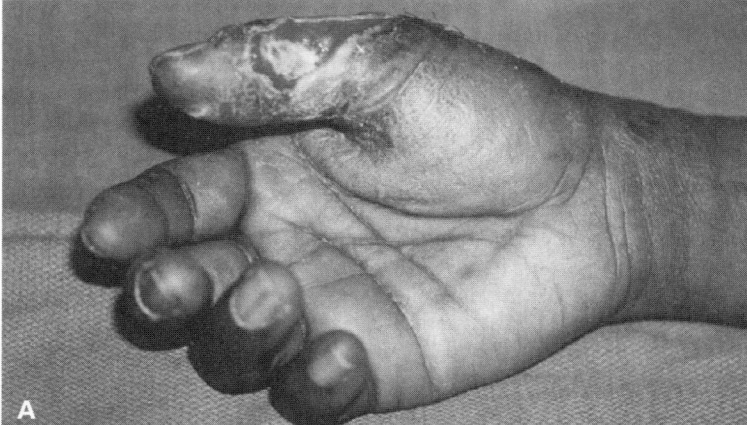

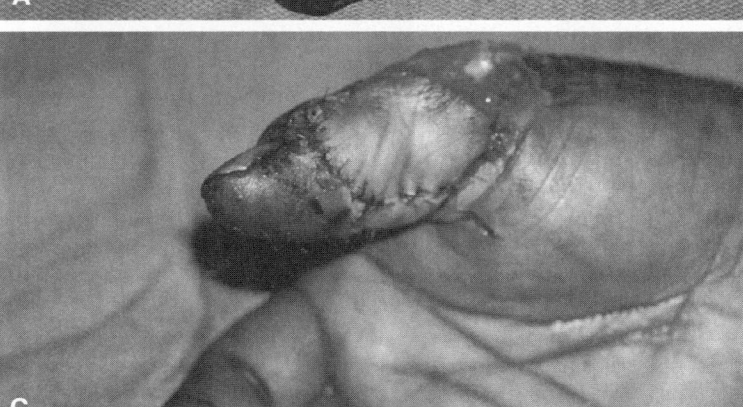

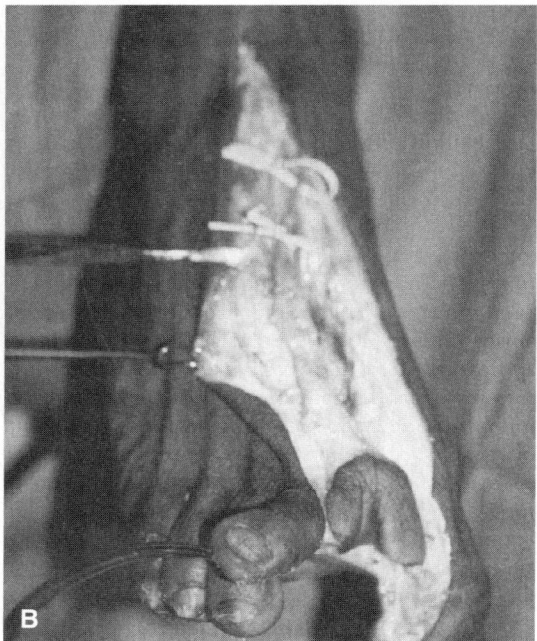

FIGURE 15-18 | *A, Composite defect of the thumb interphalangeal joint with exposed bone. B, Harvesting of the dorsalis pedis first web-space flap. C, Flap in place.*

of the underlying bone architecture has been destroyed along with the overlying soft tissue and skin.[88]

Dorsalis Pedis Flap

This composite flap, based on the dorsalis pedis artery and vein, transfers thin, pliable skin and subcutaneous tissue with a possible addition of vascularized tendon or metatarsal to fit various recipient needs.[59] It is especially useful in the dorsum of the hand, where skin loss and extensor tendon destruction commonly occur together. The main disadvantages of this flap are related to the long and meticulous nature of the dissection and donor site problems. With a successful skin graft take, patients may be bothered by the loss of sensation of the dorsum of the foot and could have difficulties with durability of the skin graft in holding up to the demands of footwear. The flap is also limited by its size, which can be a problem if the entire dorsum of the hand requires coverage (Fig. 15-18).

Scapular and Parascapular Flaps

These newer types of flap allow the harvest of a large area of tissue on the back, either transversely or longitudinally oriented. The blood supply is based on the circumflex scapular artery and vein that arise from the subscapular vessels. Skin up to 20 cm long can be taken with the scapular flap and up to 30 cm long with the parascapular flap. The vessel diameters are 2.5 to 3.5 mm, and the pedicle length is at least 6 cm. The flap can be taken with the underlying latissimus muscle or lateral border of the scapula, or both, and a composite transfer can be built to address complex defects (Fig. 15-19). The disadvantages of this flap are related

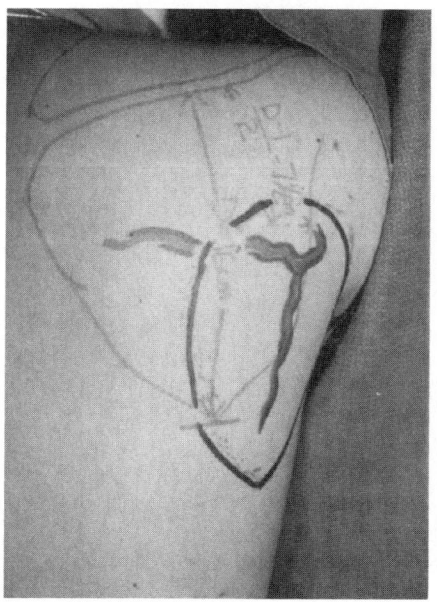

FIGURE 15-19 | *Outline of the parascapular flap, noting its relation to the scapula and the cutaneous branches of the circumflex scapular vessels.*

FIGURE 15-20 *Complex open fracture. **A,** Fracture of the left thumb metacarpal. **B,** Osseous defect of the metacarpal. **C,** Osteocutaneous lateral arm flap dissected. **D,** Flap inset. **E,** Bony reconstruction of the metacarpal. **F,** Appearance at 1-year follow-up.*

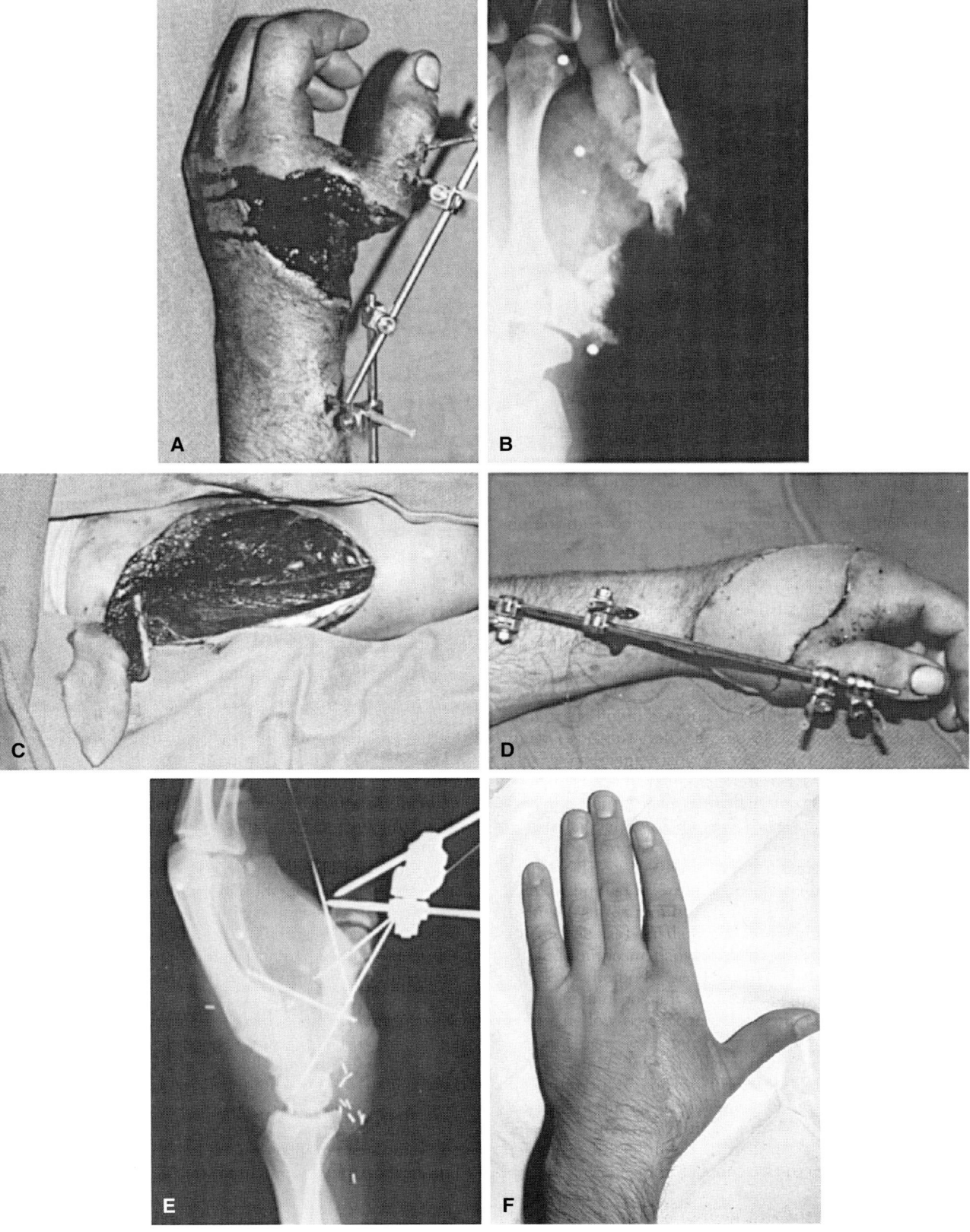

mainly to its composition (thick back skin), which may not match the forearm or hand in color or quality. The donor site is usually closed primarily, but this leaves a wide scar along the posterior axillary line or across the upper posterior torso. These flaps work especially well for repair of the large degloving injuries from machinery that require extensive skin resurfacing.[4,33,77]

Lateral Arm Flap

This septocutaneous flap is based on the posterior radial collateral artery and vein and carries with it a sensory nerve. The vessels are a branch of the profunda brachii artery and supply a pedicle of 2-mm-diameter vessels with a length of 6 to 7 cm. This flap works well for soft tissue defects alone on the hand and wrist area, which can be covered with 6 to 8 cm of tissue (Fig. 15-20). The flap can be taken with a greater width and length, although the donor site then requires a skin graft for closure. One described advantage of this flap is the ability to use the tissue as an innervated flap.[50]

Osseous and Osteocutaneous Fibula Flap

This is primarily a vascularized bone transfer and is best used to reconstruct long segmental cortical defects of the radius, ulna, or humerus. It can be taken as cortical bone alone or with overlying skin and/or soleus muscle through septocutaneous perforators found concentrated mostly in the distal third of the lower leg. It is based on the peroneal artery coming off the tibioperoneal trunk. There are some variations to collateral blood supply to the foot through the posterior tibial and anterior tibial arteries, raising the question as to whether preoperative angiography is uniformly indicated. A modern, noninvasive duplex ultrasonography scan performed preoperatively to outline the anatomy is considered prudent. The pedicle can be easily lengthened by clipping the first few branches going from main pedicle to fibula, allowing the surgeon more versatility of inset without compromising vascularity. Figure 15-21 gives two examples of various uses of this transfer, one for humeral diaphyseal reconstruction and the other for ulnar segmental reconstruction. The head of the fibula can be

FIGURE 15-21 **A,** Long humeral diaphyseal defect. **B,** Harvested fibula osteocutaneous flap. **C,** Transfer in place. **D,** Segmental defect of ulna. **E,** Reconstructed with vascularized fibula transfer.

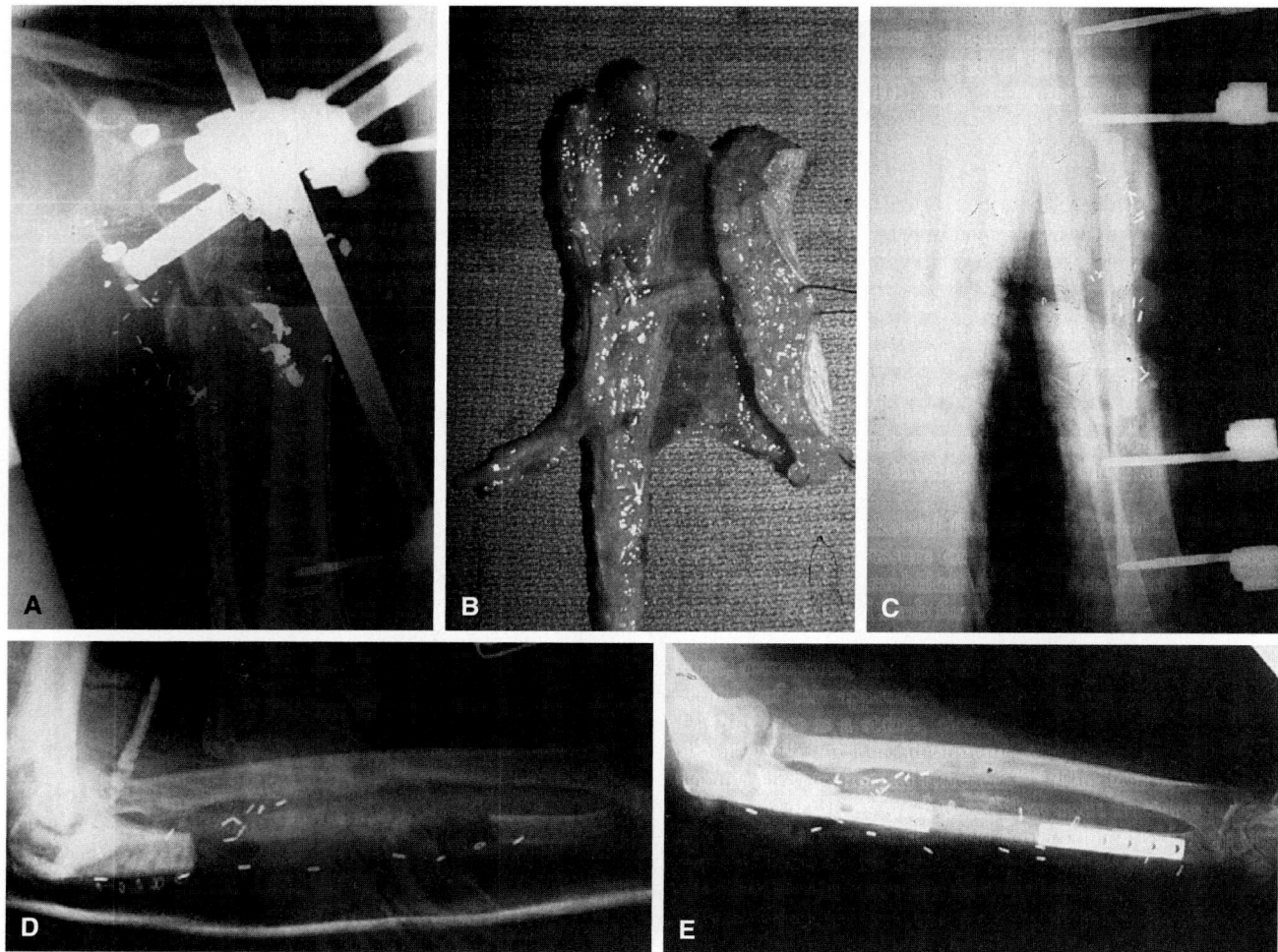

taken as well for attempted joint reconstruction but must be studied angiographically because of vascular supply variations. This type of transfer has met with mixed results at best. Another advantage of the fibula when transferred to the head and neck region for mandible restoration is the ability to accommodate multiple osteotomies.

Radial Forearm Flap

This is a septocutaneous flap based on the radial artery and on the superficial cephalic vein or the deep venae comitantes. It can be harvested as a pedicle flap or free tissue transfer. Because of perforating branches to the periosteum of the radius, a small wedge of radius can be taken to be transferred as part of an osteocutaneous flap. The advantages of this flap stem from the generous amount of tissue on the forearm and the large caliber of the donor vessels. One must be certain that the proximal ulnar artery inflow is intact and able to supply the entire hand; this can be determined by a clinical Allen's test or arteriographic evaluation. The major disadvantage of this flap is the significant donor site deformity. Many authors have suggested modifications for improving the aesthetic results with the use of full-thickness skin grafts and transposition of native tissue proximally and distally.[76,86]

ELBOW

Open wounds about the elbow that are short of soft tissue and that include an exposed fracture or joint require special attention because of the elasticity of the tissues normally found here and the wide range of motion required over the joint. Flaps mentioned previously for the forearm are adaptable to this region, with certain provisos.[20] The thoracoepigastric flap is useful for medial-based or ulnar-based defects requiring coverage (Fig. 15-22). Several free tissue transfers described previously can also be used for coverage of the elbow. In modification, the lateral arm flap turned distalward on its axis can be used to close small defects, especially on the posterior and lateral surfaces.

UPPER ARM AND SHOULDER

Compound fractures of the humerus that require vascularized soft tissue coverage are rare but can be reliably ameliorated with a latissimus dorsi muscle or myocutaneous flap brought from the ipsilateral side[94] (Fig. 15-23). With the flap isolated on its pedicle, incorporating the thoracodorsal artery and vein, release of both the origin and the insertion of the muscle allows coverage of the entire volar or dorsal surface of the upper arm, with extension of the muscle into the proximal forearm. The origin and insertion of the muscle can be reattached and used instead of a ruptured or destroyed biceps muscle to restore elbow flexion. In this situation, preservation of the thoracodorsal nerve along with the arteriovenous pedicle is mandatory. The pectoralis major muscle has also been used for these defects, but it does not have as large an arc of rotation as the latissimus. In addition, this donor site is more unsightly than that on the back.

Lower Extremity

PELVIS

Complex pelvic or acetabular fractures rarely involve marked soft tissue loss. Although many patients with complex pelvic fractures initially have contused ecchymotic skin and subcutaneous tissues, most heal without substantial skin and soft tissue defects. For the few patients who require soft tissue coverage in the pelvic region, the flaps used most often include the rectus abdominis muscle or extended myocutaneous flap, tensor fasciae latae flap, and rectus femoris muscle or myocutaneous flap for anterior and lateral lesions. The gluteus maximus myocutaneous flap is most useful for posterior lesions involving the posterior iliac wing or sacroiliac joints.[80] Of these flaps, the rectus abdominis muscle has gained a preeminent position because of its superior arc of rotation, which extends from the subcostal area to the distal femur and laterally to well past the midaxillary line. Its hardy blood supply based on the deep inferior epigastric artery and vein, its long pedicle, and the relative lack of donor site morbidity have made it

---

FIGURE 15-22 *A, Thoracoepigastric flap in place, covering a large defect of the antecubital region with joint exposure. B, One month after division.*

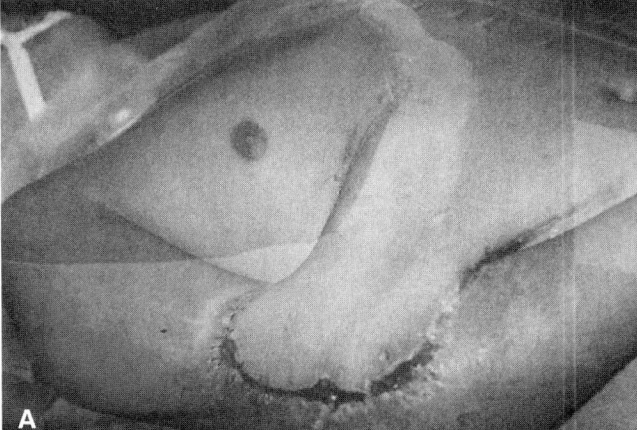
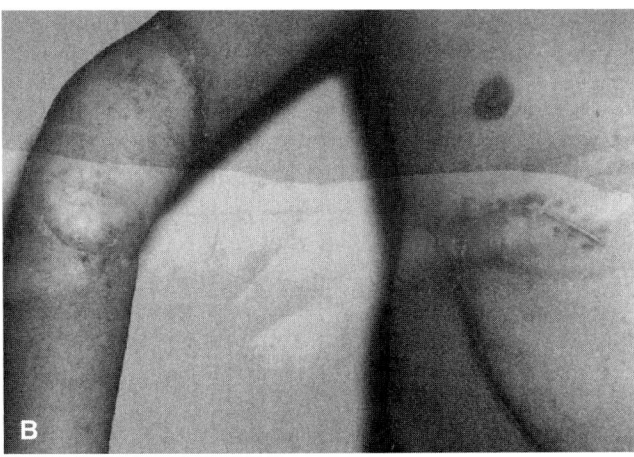

FIGURE 15-23 | **A,** *Type III open elbow fracture with exposed joint.* **B,** *X-ray film revealing the extent of the bone injury.* **C,** *The latissimus dorsi donor site.* **D,** *Myocutaneous flap raised and transferred.* **E,** *Flap and skin grafts in place.*

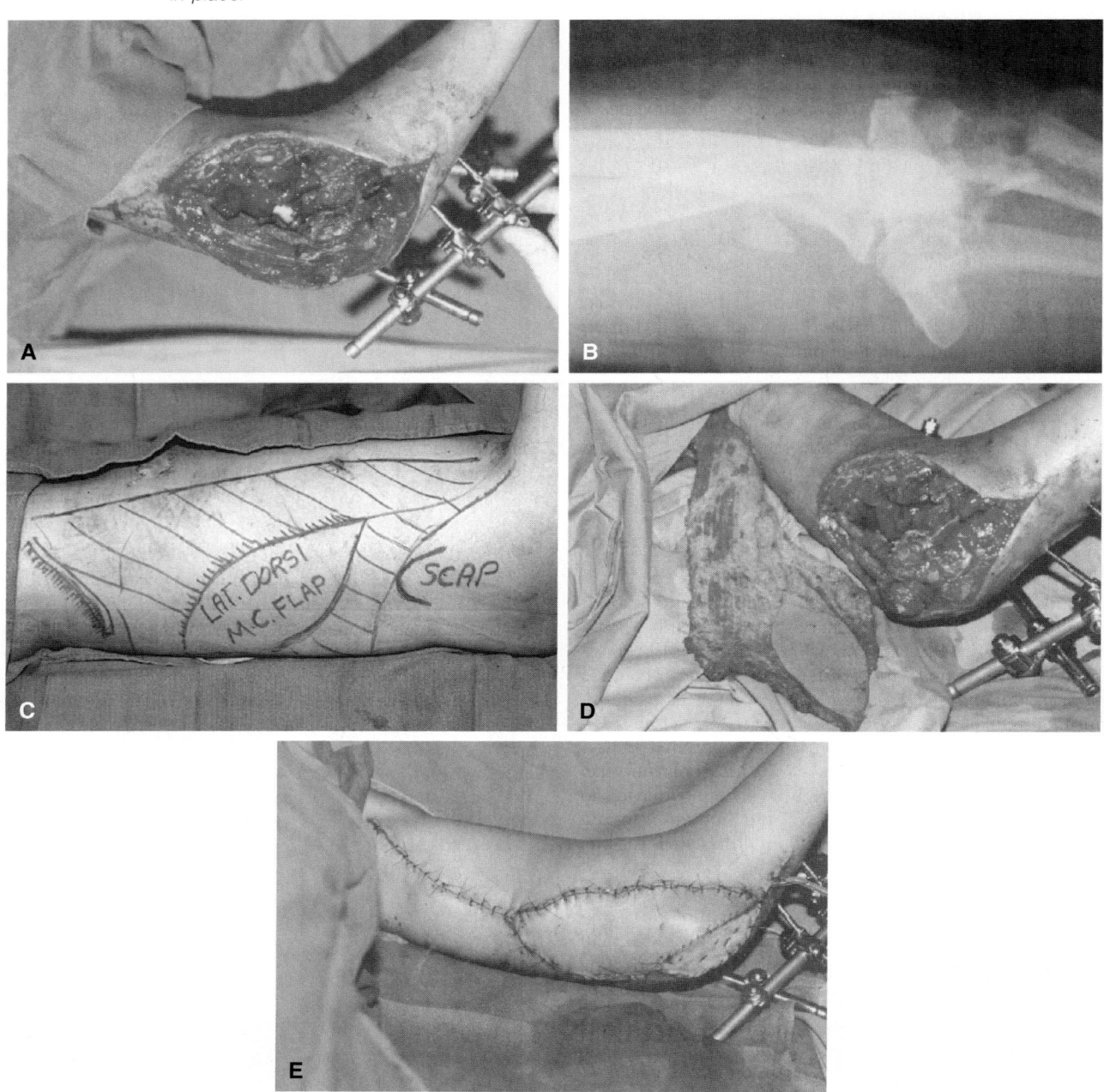

useful in most hip and pelvic reconstructions.[36] Combinations of these flaps can be used to treat areas massively injured by trauma or chronic osteomyelitis (Fig. 15-24).

THIGH

Because of the ample musculature of the thigh, open fractures of the femur, when reduced, rarely involve enough soft tissue loss to require additional placement of distant tissue for soft tissue coverage. In the few patients in whom such requirements exist, injuries of the proximal two thirds of the thigh in the anterior aspect can be treated by an

ipsilateral rotation of the rectus abdominis muscle (described previously). The supracondylar region, both anteriorly and posteriorly, can be treated with the use of one or both gastrocnemius muscles. In cases of massive destruction with marked soft tissue deficits, free tissue transfers remain a reliable alternative for wound coverage over any aspect of the femur.

KNEE AND PROXIMAL TIBIA

The badly displaced tibial plateau fracture with overlying soft tissue loss is a classical example in which internal

FIGURE 15-24 *A,* Traumatic hip disarticulation with exposed ischium and acetabulum. *B,* Extended deep inferior epigastric flap (EDIE). *C,* After transfer of the contralateral rectus abdominis myocutaneous flap based on the deep inferior epigastric artery and veins.

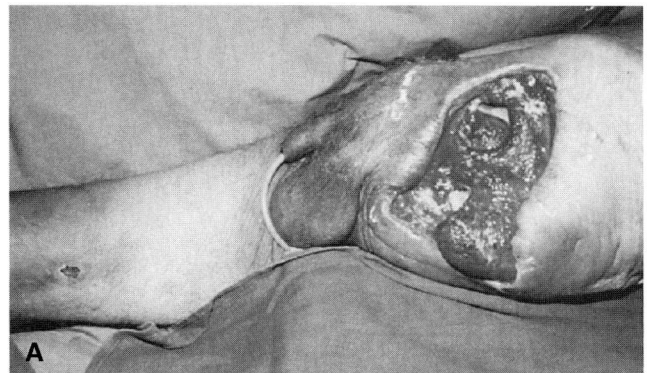
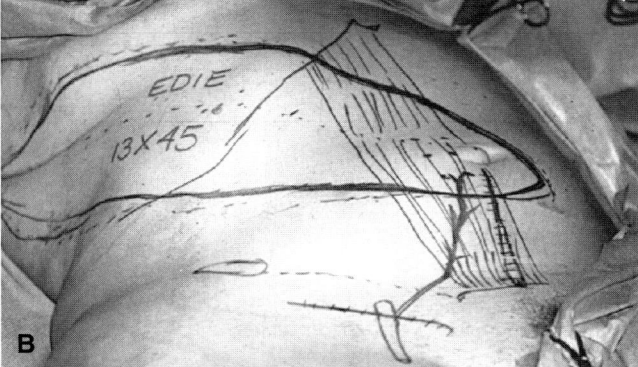
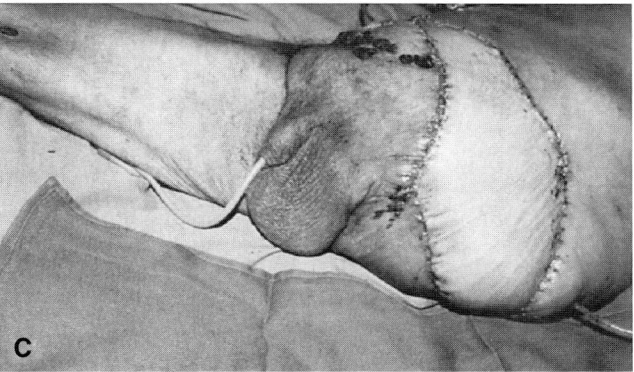

fixation either alone or coupled with cross-knee external fixation provides the patient with the best chance of fracture healing and joint congruity. Often in these open injuries, the additional burden of soft tissue stripping and bilateral plate placement converts a tenuous wound into one with no prospect of primary closure. In such cases, as well as in other cases of type III proximal third tibial fractures, the gastrocnemius muscle is unrivaled in its ability to provide wound closure with minimal donor site deficiencies.[2,24,29,31,32] Based on the sural artery and vein, derived as a direct branch from the popliteal artery in the suprageniculate area, either head of the gastrocnemius muscle can be isolated and transferred to cover the proximal third region (Fig. 15-25).

The muscle can be moved alone, after which it is skin grafted, or it can be transferred with an overlying skin flap, which can measure from 10 to 23 cm. In this situation, the donor site must be skin grafted. To extend its reach, the muscle can be released from its origin on the femoral epicondyle, gaining at least 2 to 3 cm. In addition, serial division of both the posterior and anterior muscular fascia allows the muscle to expand further, providing extended coverage for large, open wounds. When the lateral gastrocnemius muscle is harvested, care must be taken to avoid injury to the peroneal nerve, which lies immediately distal to the head of the fibula and anterior to the gastrocnemius as it descends.

MIDDLE THIRD OF THE TIBIA

Type III tibial fractures in this region can often be covered by transposition of the soleus muscle, which lies deep to the gastrocnemius in the posterior compartment. For smaller defects, the soleus can be split longitudinally because it takes its dual blood supply from the posterior tibial artery for the medial aspect of the muscle and from the peroneal artery for the lateral aspect. Because of the nature of its blood supply, its configuration, and the large area of origin, the arc of rotation of the soleus muscle is relatively limited. Dissection should be performed as distally as possible, carefully freeing the muscle from the overlying Achilles tendon and allowing the gastrocnemius-Achilles unit to remain intact whenever possible. Because of its variability in the distal third of the lower leg, the muscle must be completely exposed through a long longitudinal incision before the final determination to use this flap is made. The use of a distally based soleus muscle flap has been reported but is noted here only to be condemned; it should be rejected rapidly because of its extremely variable distal blood supply. Infrequently, the flexor digitorum longus muscle can be used alone or as a supplement to the soleus for small, selected defects in this region.[68]

Both the tibialis anterior and the extensor digitorum longus muscles have been reported to provide options for muscle flap transfers in small, anterior, mid-third defects.

FIGURE 15-25 | *A, Type III tibial plateau fracture with exposed hardware after débridement of necrotic, infected eschar. B, After transfer of bilateral gastrocnemius muscle rotation flaps. C, Six months after coverage, full weight-bearing in extension. D, Full flexion.*

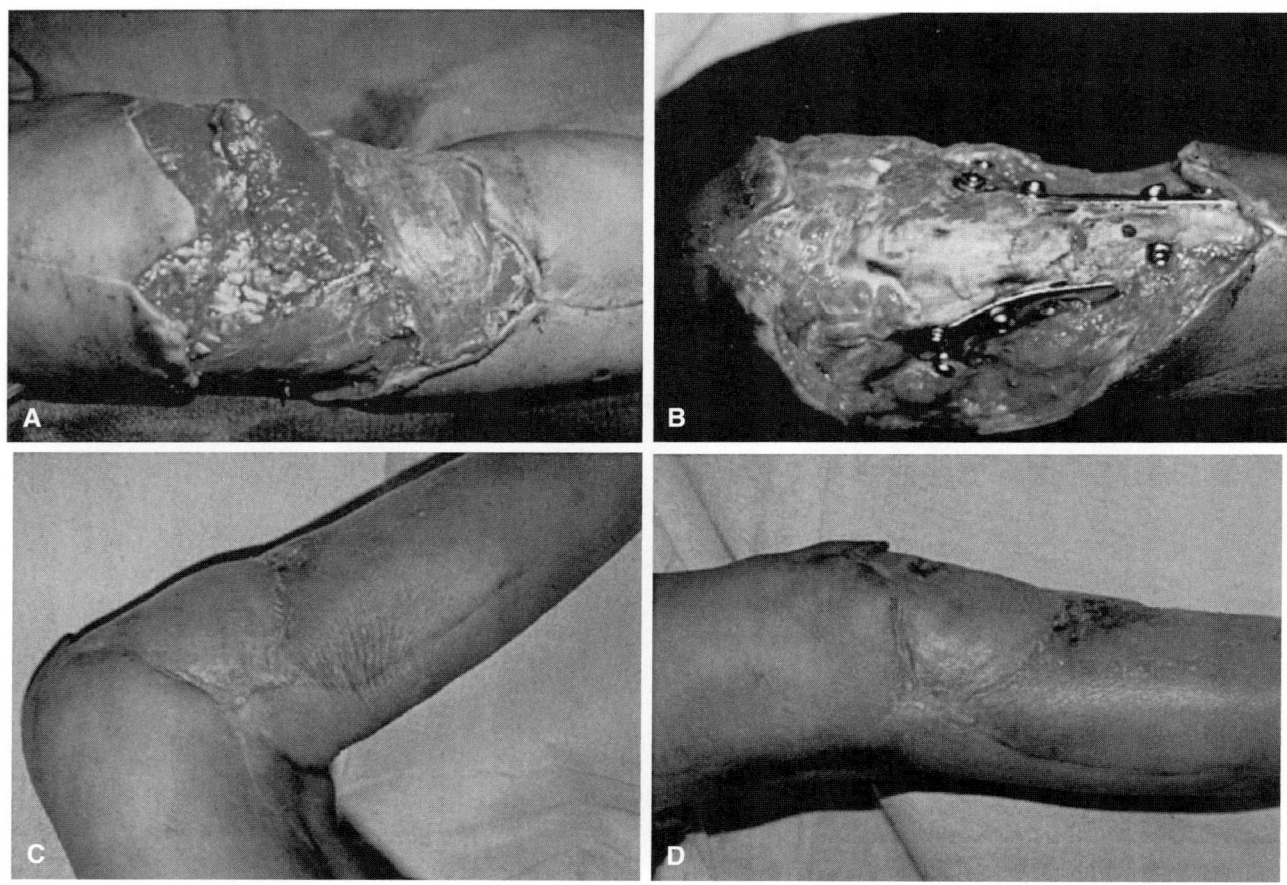

Again, we have found these two muscles to be of little use because of their small muscle bellies, segmental-type blood supply, limited arc of rotation, and donor site disability. Furthermore, we have moved away from local muscle transfer in severe, type III, mid-third tibial fractures, such as those caused by high-velocity projectiles. Often the soleus muscle is damaged acutely or becomes fibrotic in the more chronic wounds, preventing it from acting as an adequate vascularized transfer flap. Therefore, free tissue transfer, using either the latissimus dorsi or the rectus abdominis muscle for larger defects and the gracilis muscle or groin flap for smaller defects, has become more routine (Fig. 15-26).[10,54,65,67,90] This change in strategy has led to a decrease in our complication rate. One-stage composite reconstruction, replacing soft tissue, skin, and bone simultaneously, has been practiced successfully but should be reserved for highly selected cases.[86] Still unknown and under study is the potentially deleterious effect on gait stemming from sacrifice of the soleus.

DISTAL THIRD OF THE TIBIA

As local donor muscles in the distal third of the tibia are almost nonexistent, closure of an open plafond fracture, or of any extensive type IIIb fracture in this area, will usually require free tissue transfer.[22] Again, the primary options are the latissimus dorsi or rectus abdominis muscle for larger defects and the gracilis muscle for smaller wounds (Fig. 15-27).[10,35] Fasciocutaneous flaps also play a role in soft tissue coverage of acute type III injuries (Fig. 15-28). In certain cases, the temporoparietal fascia with an overlying skin graft confers the added advantage of a more normal contour, along with a richly vascularized wound cover (Fig. 15-29). Perforator flaps are again playing a larger role in coverage options in this area, best exemplified by the anterolateral thigh flap. Although the larger muscles initially appear extremely bulky and unaesthetic, they rapidly atrophy as a result of surgical denervation and conform to the contour of the recipient

FIGURE 15-26 ***A,*** *Large middle third type III tibial fracture. Note the retention suture pulling the wound edges together under marked tension.* ***B,*** *After release of the single retention suture. Note the true extent of the soft tissue loss.* ***C,*** *The rectus abdominis donor site diagrammed.* ***D,*** *Immediate postoperative view.* ***E,*** *Six months after operation, full weight-bearing.*

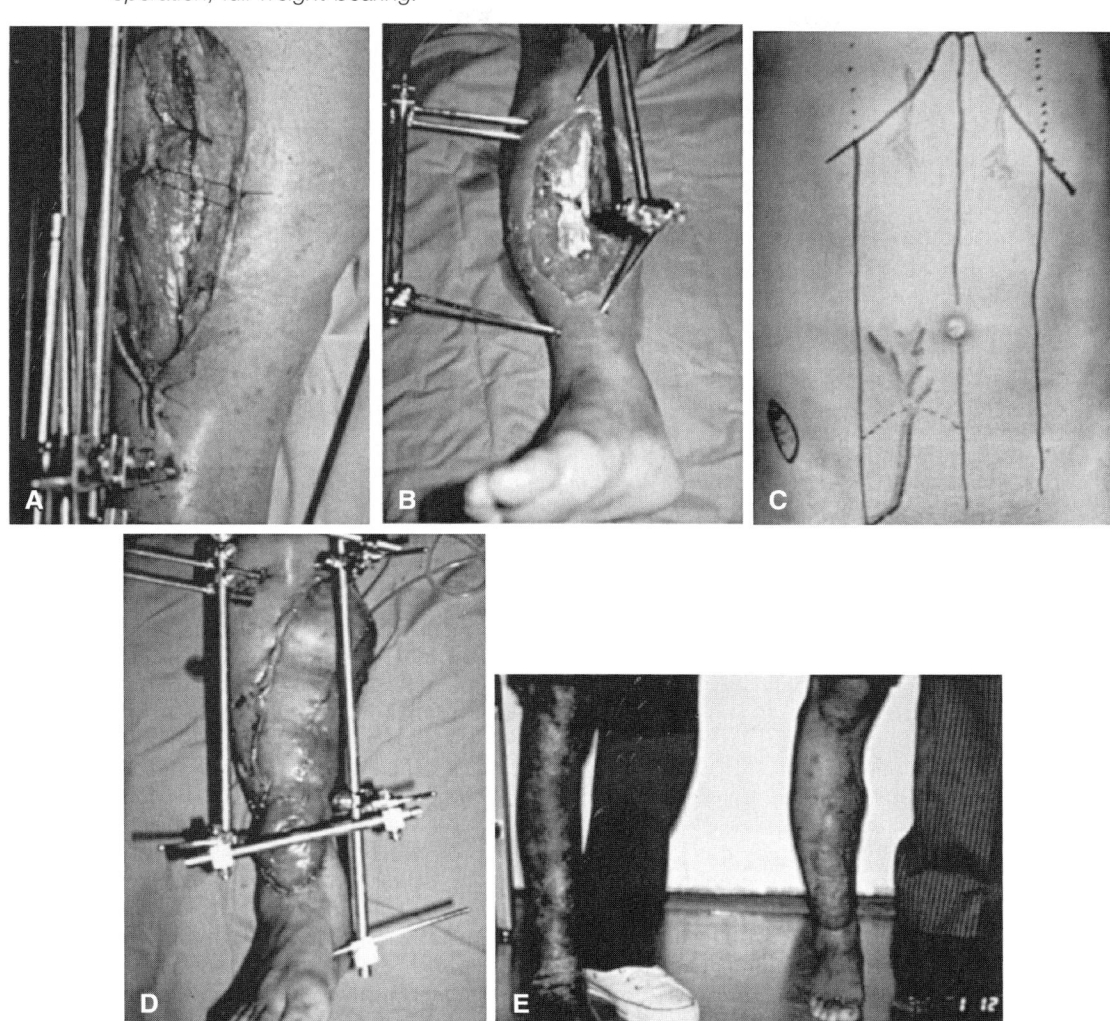

extremity (Fig. 15-30). If the traumatic insult has been severe enough to destroy the normal vascular architecture of the lower leg, vein grafts can be brought from the popliteal fossa to allow more distal vascular access of free tissue transfers (Fig. 15-31).

ANKLE AND FOOT

For the purposes of soft tissue reconstruction in the area of the ankle and foot, the surgeon must first identify the nature of the injuries, the specific regions of the foot requiring reconstruction, and most important, the relative and absolute contraindications to foot and ankle reconstruction.[17] Hidalgo and Shaw[43-45] have developed a classification system for foot injuries that takes into account

the extent of soft tissue destruction and the associated osseous injuries. Type I injuries are those confined to limited soft tissue defects. Type II injuries include major soft tissue loss, with or without distal amputation. The most severe injuries, type III, are those with major soft tissue loss and accompanying open fracture of the ankle, calcaneus, or distal tibia-fibula complex. According to this classification, the foot is divided into four major reconstructive areas: the dorsum, the distal plantar weight-bearing surface, the weight-bearing heel or hindfoot and midplantar area, and the posterior non-weight-bearing heel and Achilles tendon.[43-45]

Although May and co-workers[66] have shown that cutaneous sensibility is not an absolute prerequisite for adequate weight-bearing on the reconstructed foot,

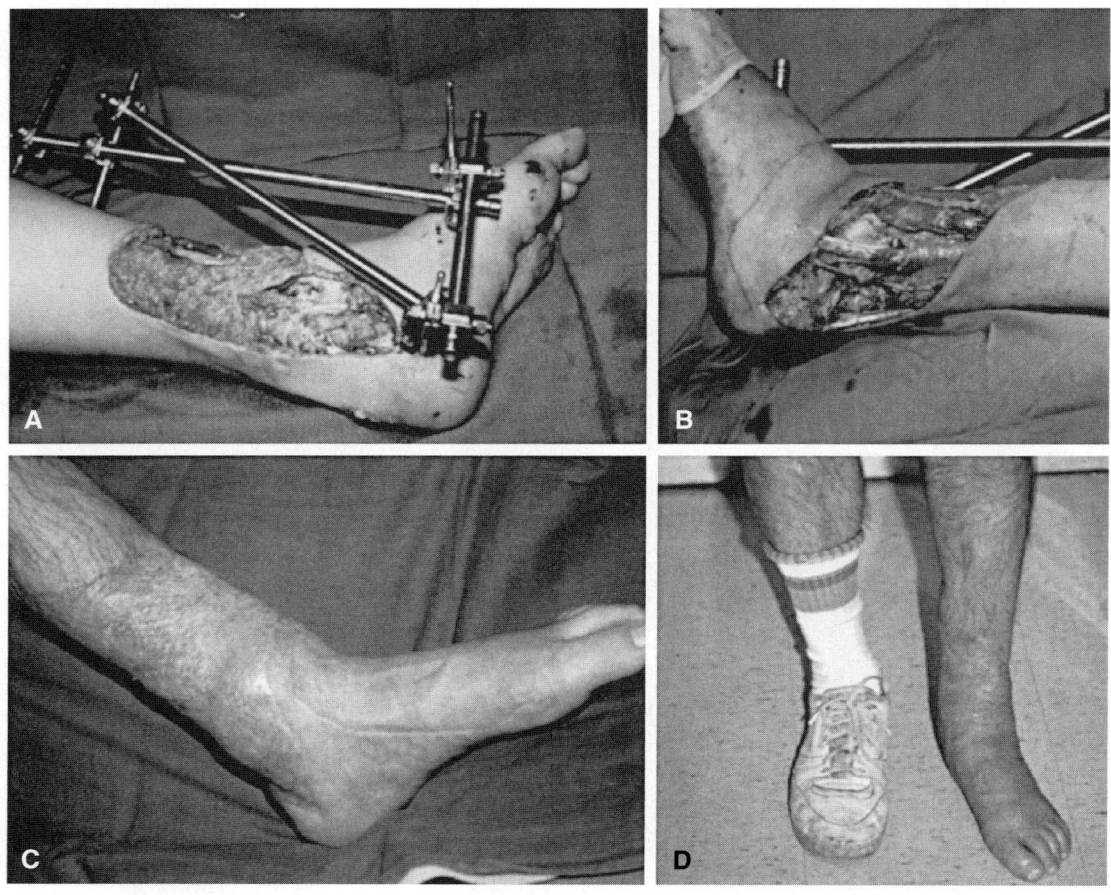

FIGURE 15-27 *A,* Large distal third type III tibia-fibula fracture, medial view. ***B,*** Lateral view with distally based, devascularized skin flap outlined. ***C,*** Eight months after transfer of latissimus dorsi and skin grafting. ***D,*** Full weight-bearing.

complete loss of plantar sensation after avulsion of the posterior tibial nerve in ipsilateral proximal segmental tibial fractures usually serves as a strong contraindication to salvage of the foot in type III injuries.[66] Complete avulsion of the plantar surface of the foot with multiple metatarsal or calcaneal fractures is also best treated with amputation.

After a thorough assessment of the patient's bone, soft tissue, and neurovascular status has been completed and the patient is deemed a candidate for reconstruction, both the size of the defect and the location (as described previously) should be considered in determining the options for coverage. Many limited defects of the dorsum of the foot or the non–weight-bearing plantar surface can be treated adequately with split-thickness skin grafting. The distally based sural fascial or fasciocutaneous flap

has become popular for coverage of composite defects of the malleoli or dorsum of the foot. They require at least 5 to 6 cm of continued contact above the malleoli to ensure sufficient perforators to vascularize the flap adequately. The farther distal one attempts to rotate the flap caudally, the more unreliable it becomes. Figure 15-32 demonstrates one such flap used to close a composite fracture of the lateral ankle. For the limited injuries to the heel and proximal plantar area in which soft tissue padding and retention of sensibility are advantageous, a turnover flexor digitorum brevis muscle flap, dorsalis pedis island flap, or local plantar fascia cutaneous rotation flap based on the proximal plantar subcutaneous plexus may serve well.[7,14,18,21,39,40,46,70,81,99]

As in the case of the type III distal third tibial fracture, extensive injuries to the plantar surface of the foot are by

FIGURE 15-28 **A,** *Distal third type III tibia-fibula fracture.* **B,** *Corresponding soft tissue defect.* **C,** *Placement of parascapular fasciocutaneous flap within 4 days of the injury.* **D,** *Full weight-bearing at 5 months.*

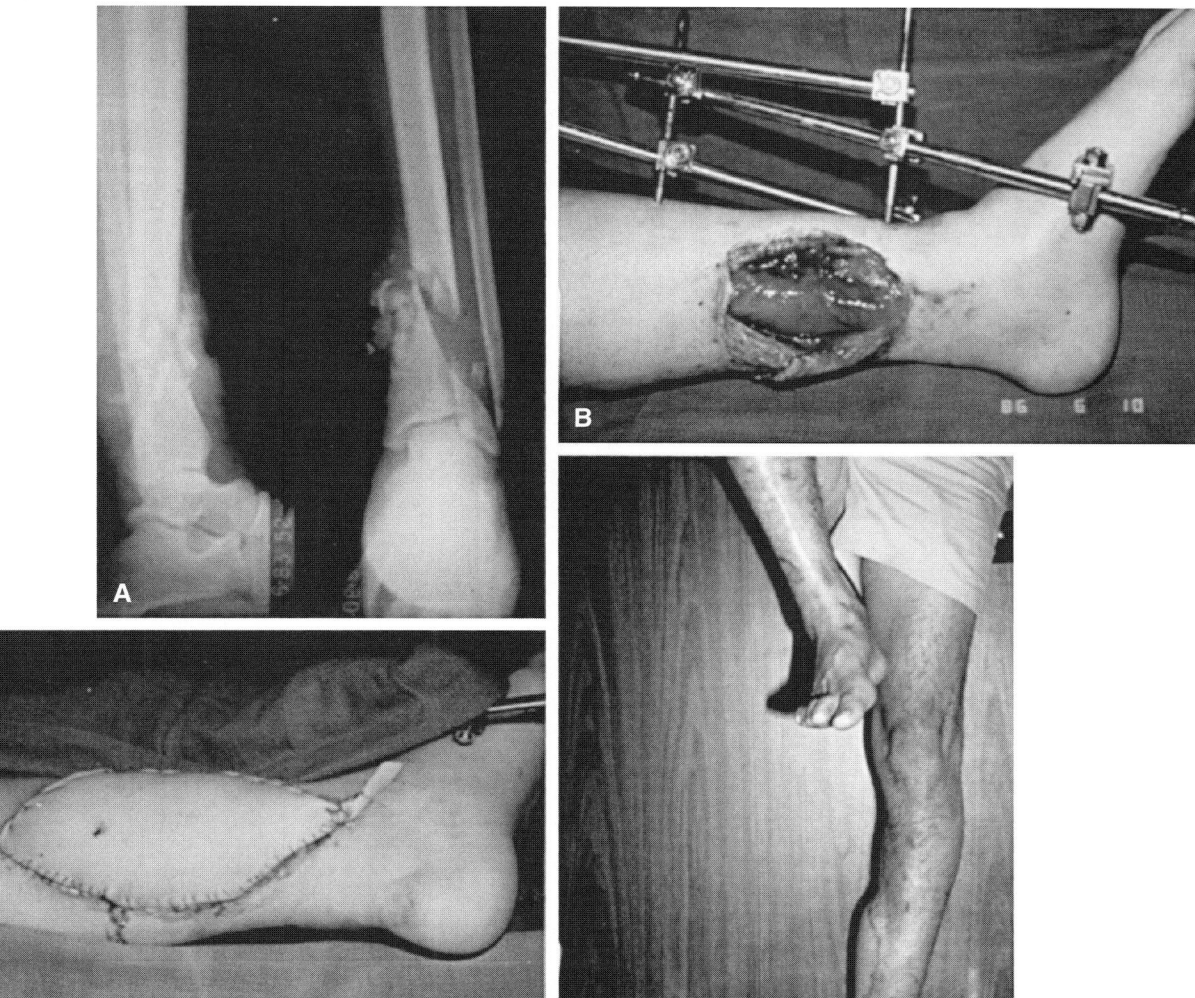

definition not amenable to coverage by local tissue transfer because of the paucity of donor sites. Numerous authors have chronicled the advantage of free muscle transfer with overlying split-thickness skin graft for restoration of an appropriately padded weight-bearing plantar surface, and our experience supports this observation (Fig. 15-33).

May and co-workers[66] have clearly shown that patients who have such reconstructions maintain closed wounds and regain relatively normal gait and weight-bearing profiles. These conclusions were reached after assessment by force vector analysis and Harris mat studies.

(Text continues on p. 425)

FIGURE 15-29 **A,** *Exposed, infected lateral malleolus. Note retention sutures pulling through soft tissue.* **B,** *Temporoparietal fascia harvested with minimal bulk.* **C,** *Flap can be bilaminar. D, After wide débridement, transfer of temporoparietal fascia, and split-thickness skin grafting. Normal contour is maintained.*

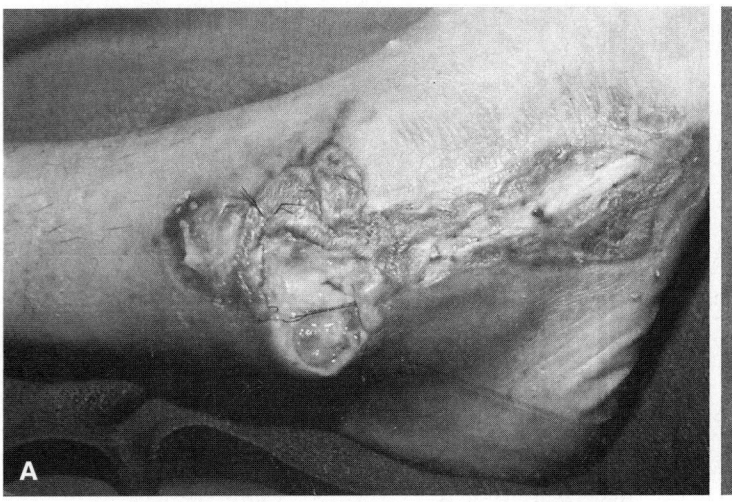

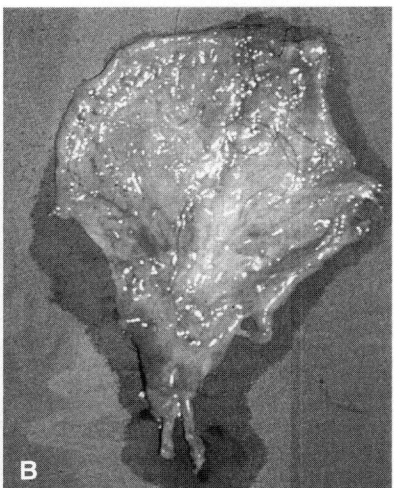

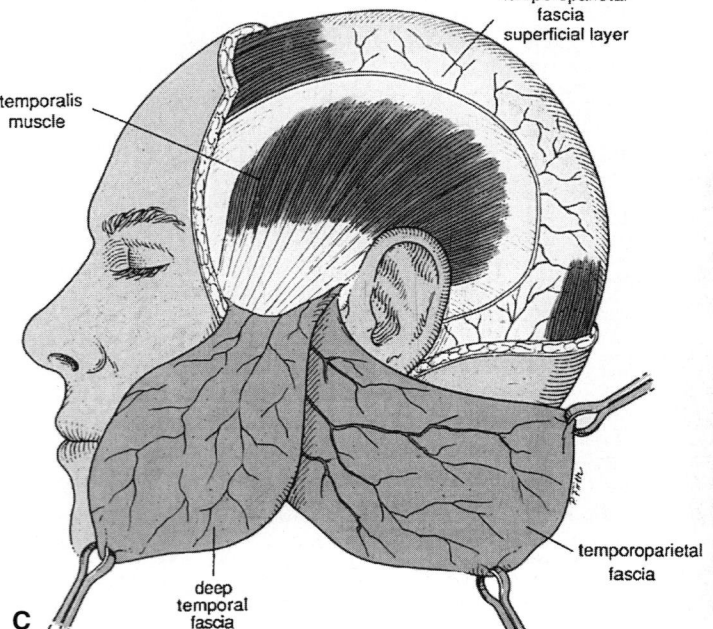

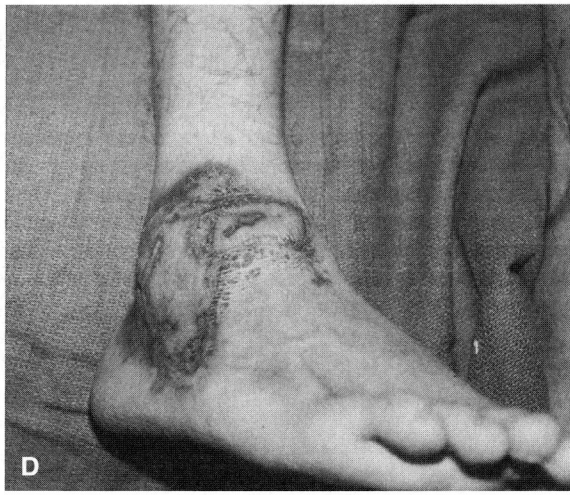

FIGURE 15-30 **A,** *Distal third type III tibia-fibula fracture.* **B,** *Gracilis muscle donor site.* **C,** *The muscle is in place. Note the excess bulk.* **D,** *Two months after transfer and skin grafting, the muscle has atrophied to match the surrounding contour. This phenomenon is a frequent occurrence in free muscle transfer.*

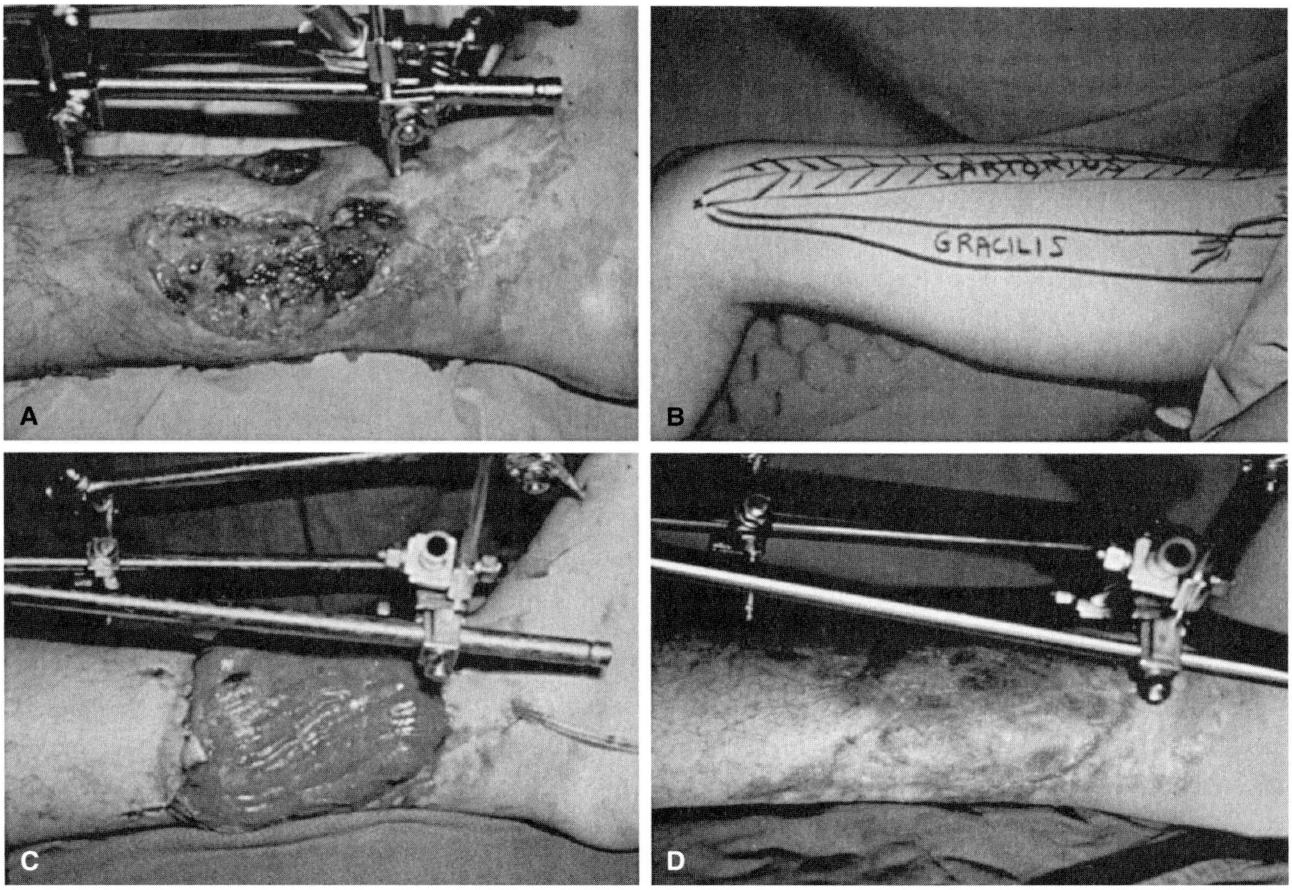

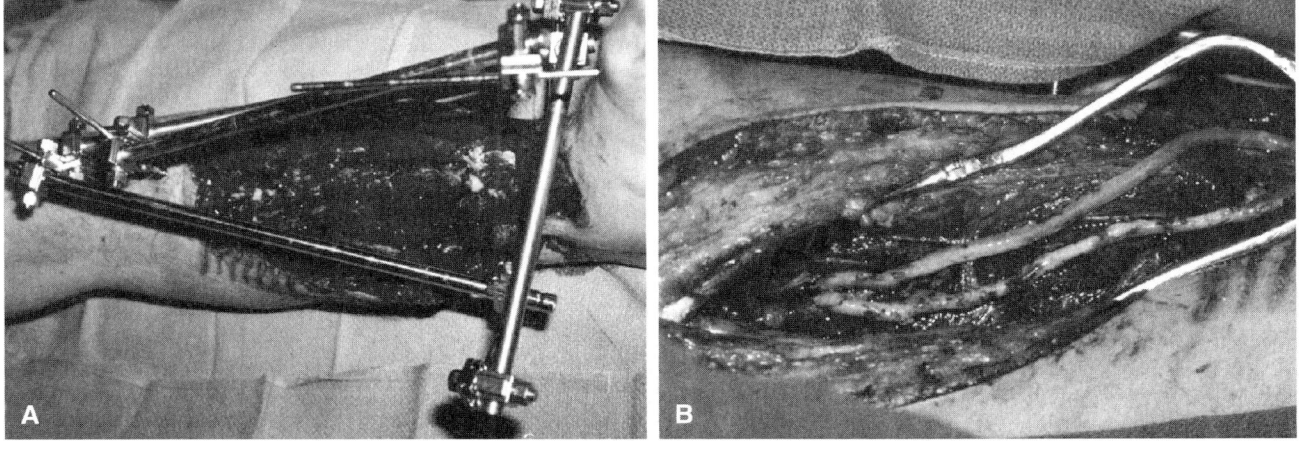

FIGURE 15-31 **A,** *Severe type III tibia-fibula fracture with unsuitable recipient vessels below the trifurcation.* **B,** *Creation of a saphenous vein arteriovenous fistula from the popliteal vessels, which is then used to hook distally into a latissimus dorsi muscle.*

FIGURE 15-32 | **A,** *Open wound—lateral malleolus.* **B,** *Underlying fracture.* **C,** *Sural flap design and rotation point.* **D,** *Flap rotated.* **E,** *Flap in place with skin graft.*

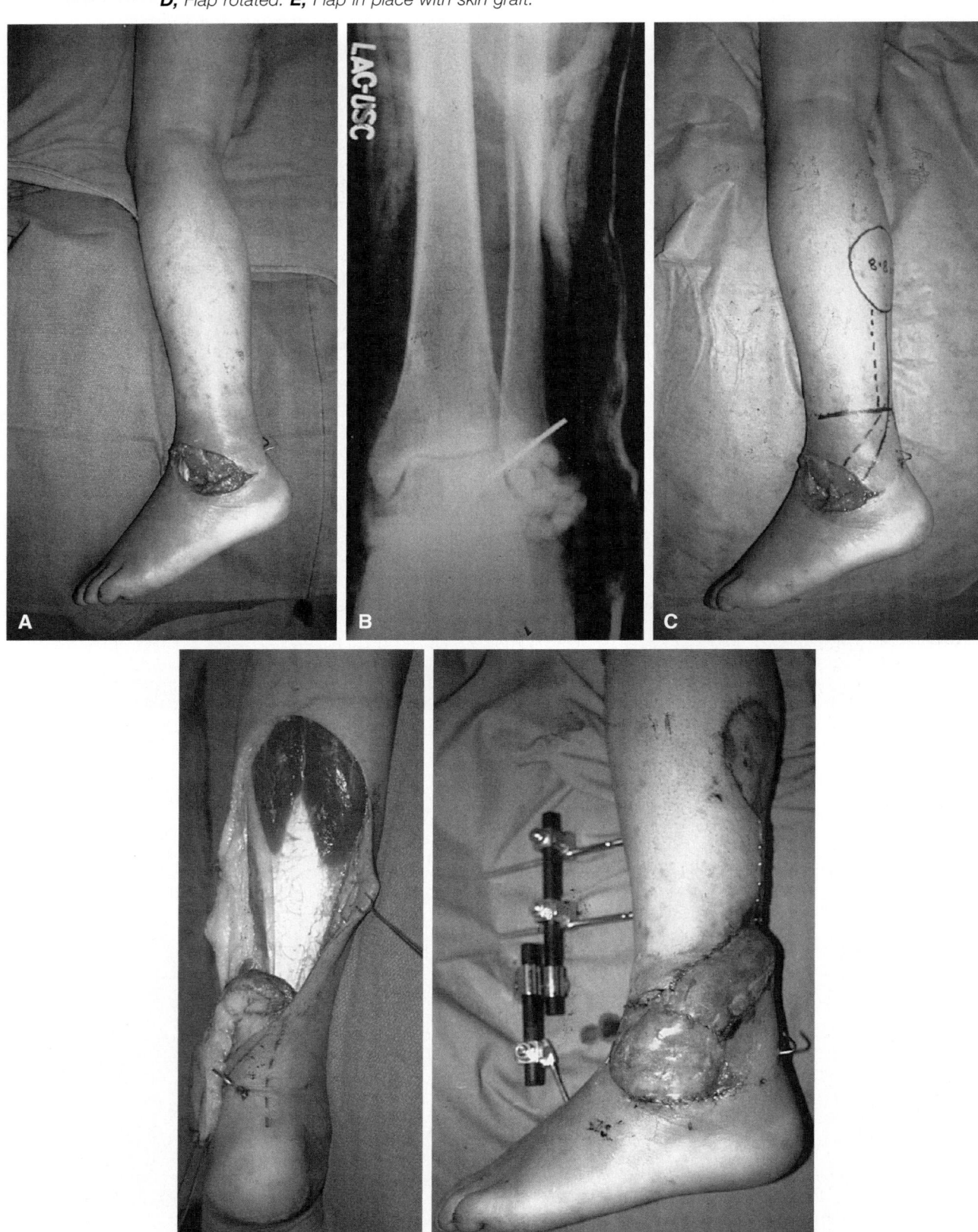

FIGURE 15-33 *A,* Composite heel defect with exposure of the calcaneus. *B,* The latissimus dorsi muscle after transfer. *C,* Immediately after inset. *D,* Six months after surgery, the patient is fully ambulatory without skin graft breakdown.

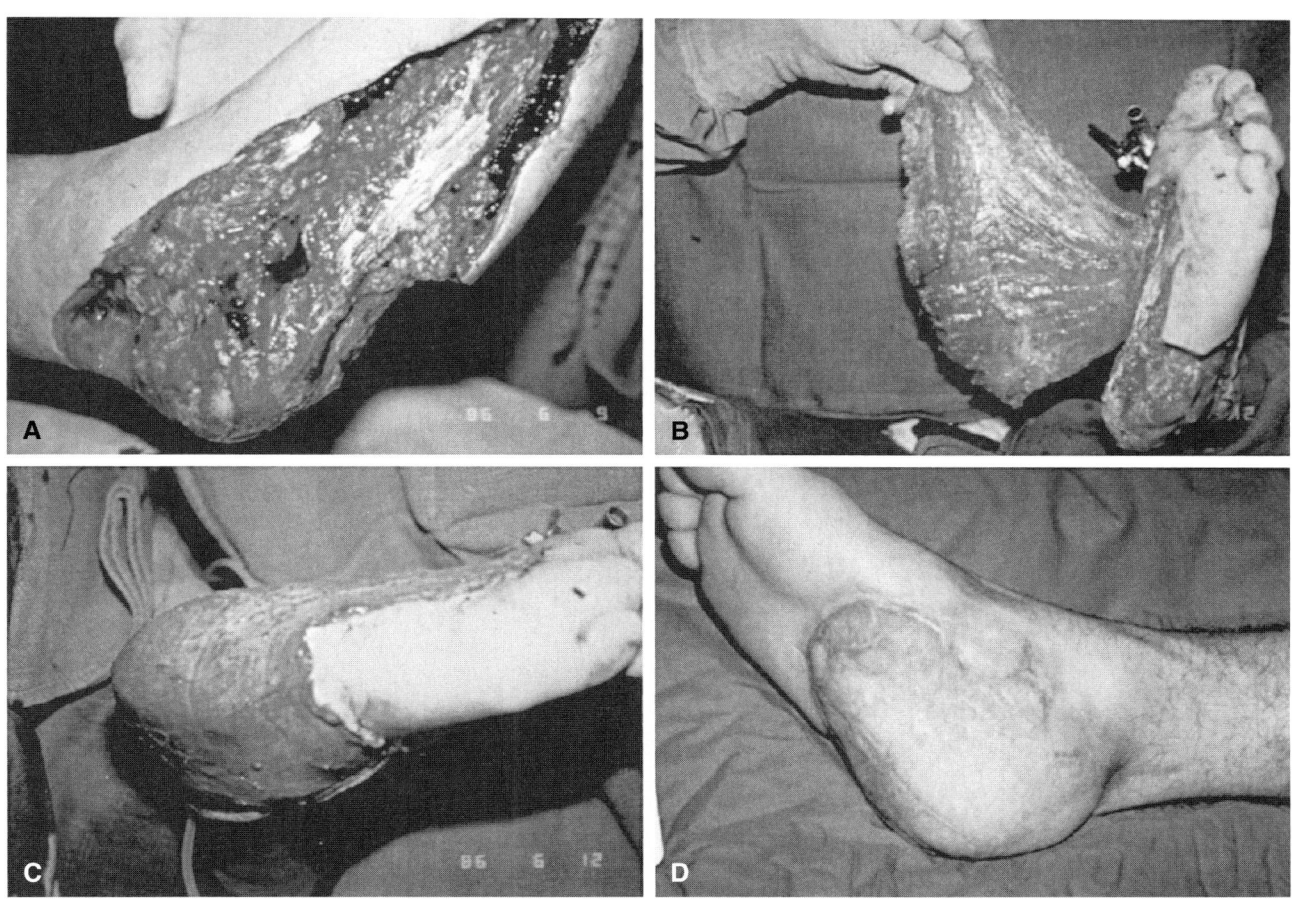

AVULSION INJURIES

The management of avulsion or degloving injuries to the extremities remains problematic. These injuries are usually the result of high-energy shearing forces, which not only separate large areas of skin and subcutaneous tissue from their underlying vascular supply but also disrupt the dermal architecture of the elevated flap. On initial evaluation, much of the avulsed skin is obviously necrotic and can be débrided immediately (Fig. 15-34A). Of greater concern are injuries in which the degloved flaps appear viable and even bleed from their free edges. The tendency in management is to maintain all obviously viable tissue or, worse, to redrape it and close the wounds primarily. However, because of the twofold physiologic insult suffered, these flaps almost always die. After reapproximation, tension further compromises vascularity, sealing the fate of this marginally viable tissue.

Although seemingly radical, aggressive débridement of all degloved tissue with subsequent skin grafting is the treatment of choice (see Fig. 15-34). Previous reports have described the successful use of split-thickness or full-thickness skin grafts harvested from the avulsed flap. In our experience, the take of skin grafts harvested from these flaps is variable. If the possibility presents itself, however, this option should be pursued. Thick split-thickness skin grafts taken from uninvolved donor areas serve well in the coverage of these wounds (see Fig. 15-34C).

In certain cases, with widely based flaps in which there is relatively little undermining and no ostensible skin trauma, it may be prudent to leave all wounds open and monitor the flaps for continued viability. Fluorescein, 15 to 25 mg/kg (according to the patient's pigmentation) given intravenously, can serve as a reliable marker of tissue viability. When the tissue is monitored with a Wood lamp or other ultraviolet light source, a deep purple hue is consistent with

FIGURE 15-34 | *A,* Complex degloving injury of both lower legs. *B,* After thorough débridement of all nonviable tissue. *C,* Shortly after skin grafting. Note the placement of an external fixator for wound care purposes alone.

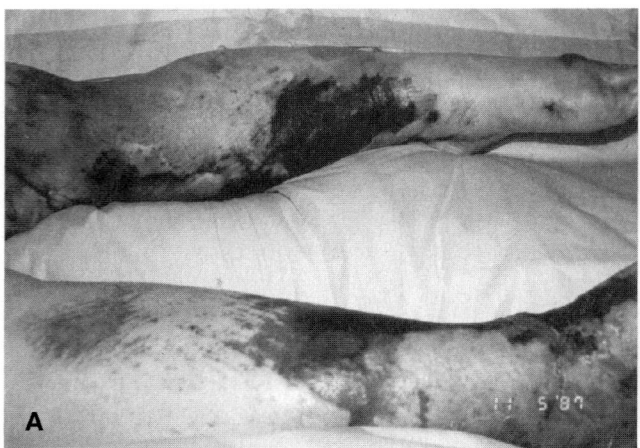
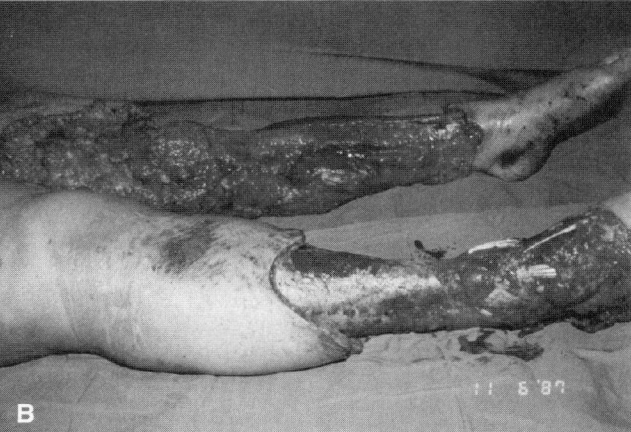
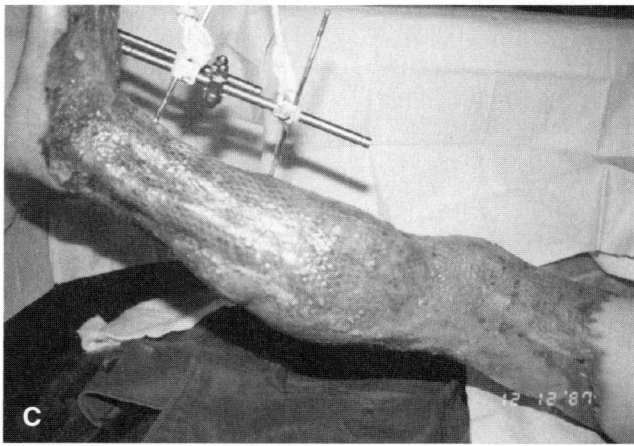

nonviability, whereas an orange-green speckling denotes vascular inflow. Quantitative assessment can be done with a dermofluorometer, and blood flow can be expressed as a percentage of normal.[42,60] Any associated fractures that have a communication with the degloved flaps, even if located well away from the laceration site, must be classified as type II injuries and treated as such. Free tissue transfer can be especially applicable in these situations.[47]

OSTEOMYELITIS: ROLE OF VASCULARIZED MUSCLE FLAP COVERAGE

Stark[87] first reported the efficacy of muscle transposition for coverage of osteomyelitic wounds in 1946. Ger[30] further documented his favorable experience with the use of muscle coverage for the amelioration of tibial osteomyelitis in 1977.

Although a number of centers adopted this therapeutic adjunct in the late 1970s, it was not until the reports of Chang and Mathes[15] and later Feng and co-workers[25] on the wound biology of vascularized muscle and skin that some physiologic basis was established for the positive effects of this procedure. In the wound laboratory, muscle flaps were found to be significantly more effective than random flaps in the rat model in reducing the bacterial count in a standardized wound cylinder. Oxygen tension at the flap-cylinder interface was also found to be markedly higher in the muscle.[15,25] Clearly, aggressive débridement of all necrotic bone, scar, and infected granulation tissue is the cornerstone of the treatment of this most recalcitrant disease. Without this crucial maneuver, no amount of vascularized muscle can resolve the problem.

The classical management of osteomyelitis required multiple 6-week courses of intravenous antibiotics, many of them nephrotoxic, with high rates of failure and recurrence. At best, suppression of the inciting organisms could be expected; because of retained sequestra and persistent dead space, antibiotic delivery to the areas harboring bacteria was unlikely. With our current knowledge of flap physiology, we can now aggressively remove all sequestrum and other nonvascularized tissue, transpose or transplant vascularized muscle to increase blood supply, and more effectively deliver short courses of antibiotics for an increased chance of real cure.[12,13,97]

Several advances have been made in regard to flap harvest and transfer, including use of the endoscope to harvest both pedicle and free tissue transfers. Bostwick and associates[8] presented a thorough approach to these procedures in their textbook. Technique and exposure are similar for both pedicled and free latissimus dorsi transfer, by far the most frequently chosen flap. Other tissues amenable to endoscopic harvest are the rectus abdominis and gracilis muscles and nerve, vein, and fascia lata. Although not universally accepted today, endoscopic harvest is sure to play an increasing role in soft tissue coverage.

REFERENCES

1. Alpert, B.S.; Parry, S.W.; Buncke, H.; et al. The free groin flap. In: Buncke, H.J.; Furnas, D.W., eds. Symposium on Clinical Frontiers in Reconstructive Microsurgery. St. Louis, C.V. Mosby, 1984, pp. 71–83.
2. Arnold, P.G.A.; Mister, R. Making the most of the gastrocnemius muscles. Plast Reconstr Surg 22:4, 1985.
3. Atasoy, E.; Ioakimidis, E.; Kasdem, M.; et al. Reconstruction of the amputated finger tip with a triangular volar flap. J Bone Joint Surg Am 52:921, 1970.
4. Barwick, W.J.; Goodkind, D.J.; Serafin, D. The free scapular flap. Plast Reconstr Surg 69:779, 1982.
5. Baudet, J.; LeMaire, J.M.; Gumberteau, J.C. Ten free groin flaps. Plast Reconstr Surg 57:577, 1976.
6. Beasley, R.W. Hand Injuries. Philadelphia, W.B. Saunders, 1981.
7. Bostwick, J. Reconstruction of the heel pad by muscle transposition and split thickness skin graft. Surg Gynecol Obstet 143:973, 1976.
8. Bostwick, J.; Eaves, F.; Nahai, F. Endoscopic Plastic Surgery. St. Louis, Quality Medical Publishing, 1995.
9. Brent, B.; Upton, J.; Acland, R.D. Experience with the temporoparietal fascia free flap. Plast Reconstr Surg 76:177, 1985.
10. Brownstein, M.C.; Gordon, L.; Buncke, H.J. The use of microvascular free groin flaps for the closure of difficult lower extremity wounds. Surg Clin North Am 57:977, 1977.
11. Buchau, A.C. The neurovascular island flap in reconstruction of the thumb. Hand 1:19, 1969.
12. Byrd, H.S.; Cierny, G.; Tebbets, J.B. The management of open tibial fractures with associated soft tissue loss: External pin fixation with early flap coverage. Plast Reconstr Surg 68:73, 1981.
13. Byrd, H.S.; Spicer, R.E.; Cierny, G. III. The management of open tibial fractures. Plast Reconstr Surg 76:719, 1985.
14. Caffee, H.H.; Hoefflin, S.M. The extended dorsalis pedis flap. Plast Reconstr Surg 64:807, 1979.
15. Chang, N.; Mathes, S.J. Comparison of the effect of bacterial inoculation in musculocutaneous and random pattern flaps. Plast Reconstr Surg 70:1, 1982.
16. Ciresi, K.; Mathes, S. The classification of flaps. Orthop Clin North Am 24:383, 1993.
17. Clark, N.; Sherman, R. Soft tissue reconstruction of the foot and ankle. Orthop Clin North Am 24:489, 1993.
18. Cohn, L.B.; Buncke, H.J. Neurovascular island flaps from the plantar vessels and nerves for foot reconstruction. Ann Plast Surg 12:327, 1984.
19. Curtis, R.M. Cross-finger pedicle flap in hand surgery. Ann Surg 145:650, 1957.
20. Daniel, R.K.; Weiland, A.J. Free tissue transfers for upper extremity reconstruction. J Hand Surg [Am] 7:66, 1982.
21. Duncan, M.J.; Zuker, R.M.; Manktelow, R.T. Resurfacing weight-bearing areas of the heel: The role of the dorsalis pedis innervated free tissue transfer. J Reconstr Microsurg 1:201, 1985.
22. Ecker, J.; Sherman, R. Soft tissue coverage of the distal third of the leg and ankle. Orthop Clin North Am 24:481, 1993.
23. Fatale, M.F.; Davies, D.M. The radial forearm island flap in upper limb reconstruction. J Hand Surg [Br] 9:234, 1984.
24. Feldman, J.J.; Cohen, B.E.; May, J.W. The medial gastrocnemius myocutaneous flap. Plast Reconstr Surg 61:531, 1978.
25. Feng, L.; Price, D.; Hohu, D.; et al. Blood flow changes and leukocyte mobilization in infections: A comparison between ischemic and well-perfused skin. Surg Forum 34:603, 1983.
26. Foucher, G.; van Genecten, F. A compound radial skin forearm flap in hand surgery: An original modification of the Chinese forearm flap. Br J Plast Surg 37:139, 1984.
27. Freiburg, A.; Manktelow, R. The Cutler repair for fingertip amputations. Plast Reconstr Surg 50:371, 1972.
28. Furnas, D.W.; Lamb, R.C.; Achauer, B.M.; et al. A pair of five-day flaps: Early division of distant pedicles after serial cross-clamping and observation with oximetry and fluorometry. Ann Plast Surg 15:262, 1985.
29. Galumbeck, M.; Colen, L. Soft tissue reconstruction—Coverage of the lower leg: Rotational flap. Orthop Clin North Am 24:473, 1993.
30. Ger, R. Muscle transposition for treatment and prevention of chronic posttraumatic osteomyelitis of the tibia. J Bone Joint Surg Am 59:784, 1977.
31. Ger, R. The management of open fractures of the tibia with skin loss. J Trauma 10:112, 1970.
32. Ger, R. The technique of muscle transposition in the operative treatment of traumatic and ulcerative lesions of the leg. J Trauma 11:502, 1971.
33. Gilbert, A.; Teot, L. The free scapular flap. Plast Reconstr Surg 69:601, 1982.
34. Godina, M.; Lister, G. Early microsurgical reconstruction of complex trauma of the extremities. Plast Reconstr Surg 78:285, 1986.
35. Gordon, L.; Buncke, H.J.; Alpert, B.S. Free latissimus dorsi muscle flap with split thickness skin graft cover: A report of 16 cases. Plast Reconstr Surg 70:173, 1982.
36. Gottlieb, M.E.; Chandrasekhar, B.; Terz, J.J.; Sherman, R. Clinical application of the extended deep inferior epigastric flap. Plast Reconstr Surg 78:782, 1986.

37. Gustilo, R.B.; Anderson, J.T. Prevention of infection in the treatment of one thousand and twenty five open fractures of long bones. J Bone Joint Surg Am 58:453, 1976.

38. Gustilo, R.B.; Mendoza, R.M.; Williams, D.N. Problems in the management of type III (severe) open fractures: A new classification of type III open fractures. J Trauma 24:742, 1984.

39. Harrison, D.H.; Morgan, D.G.B. The instep island flap to resurface plantar defects. Br J Plast Surg 34:315, 1981.

40. Hartrampf, C.R.; Scheflan, M.; Bostwick, J. The flexor digitorum brevis muscle island pedicle flap: A new dimension in heel reconstruction. Plast Reconstr Surg 66:264, 1980.

41. Henderson, N.P.; Reid, D.A.C. Long-term follow-up of neurovascular island flaps. Hand 1:21, 1969.

42. Hidalgo, D.A. Lower extremity avulsion injuries. Clin Plast Surg 13:701, 1986.

43. Hidalgo, D.A.; Shaw, W.W. Anatomic basis of plantar flap design. Plast Reconstr Surg 78:627, 1986.

44. Hidalgo, D.A.; Shaw, W.W. Anatomic basis of plantar flap design: Clinical applications. Plast Reconstr Surg 78:637, 1986.

45. Hidalgo, D.A.; Shaw, W.W. Reconstruction of foot injuries. Clin Plast Surg 13:663, 1986.

46. Ikuta, Y.; Murakami, T.; Yoshioka, K.; Tsuge, K. Reconstruction of the heel pad by flexor digitorum brevis musculocutaneous flap transfer. Plast Reconstr Surg 74:86, 1984.

47. Imaya, T.; Harii, K.; Yamada, A. Microvascular free flaps for the treatment of avulsion injuries of the feet in children. J Trauma 22:15, 1982.

48. Iselin, F. The flag flap. Plast Reconstr Surg 52:374, 1973.

49. Johnson, R.K.; Iverson, R.E. Cross finger pedicle flaps in the hand. J Bone Joint Surg Am 53:913, 1971.

50. Katsaros, J.; Schusterman, M.; Beppu, M.; et al. The lateral arm flap: Anatomy and clinical applications. Ann Plast Surg 12:489, 1984.

51. Keitler, W.A. A new method of repair for fingertip amputation. JAMA 133:29, 1947.

52. Kleinert, H.E.; McAlister, C.G.; MacDonald, C.J.; et al. A critical evaluation of cross finger flaps. J Trauma 14:756, 1974.

53. Krizek, T.J.; Robson, M.C. Biology of surgical infection. Surg Clin North Am 55:6, 1975.

54. LaRossa, D.; Mellissinos, E.; Mathews, D.; et al. The use of microvascular free skin-muscle flaps in the management of avulsion injuries of the lower leg. J Trauma 20:545, 1980.

55. Lister, G. Local flaps to the hand. Hand Clin 1:621, 1985.

56. Lister, G.D.; McGregor, L.A.; Jackson, I.T. The groin flap in hand injuries. Injury 4:229, 1973.

57. Littler, J.W. Neurovascular pedicle transfer of tissue in reconstructive surgery of the hand. J Bone Joint Surg Am 38:917, 1956.

58. Macht, S.D.; Watson, H.K. The Moberg volar advancement flap for digital reconstruction. J Hand Surg [Am] 5:372, 1980.

59. Man, D.; Acland, R.D. The microarterial anatomy of the dorsalis pedis flap and its clinical applications. Plast Reconstr Surg 65:419, 1980.

60. Mandel, M.A. The management of lower extremity degloving injuries. Ann Plast Surg 6:1, 1981.

61. Manktelow, R.T.; McKee, N.H. Free muscle transplantation to provide active finger flexion. J Hand Surg [Am] 3:416, 1978.

62. Mathes, S.J.; Alpert, B.S.; Chang, N. Use of the muscle flap in chronic osteomyelitis: Experimental and clinical correlation. Plast Reconstr Surg 69:815, 1982.

63. Mathes, S.J.; Nohai, F. Classification of vascular anatomy of muscles: Experimental and clinical correlation. Plast Reconstr Surg 67:177, 1981.

64. Mathes, S.J.; Nahai, F. Clinical Applications for Muscle and Musculocutaneous Flaps. St. Louis, C.V. Mosby, 1982.

65. Maxwell, G.P.; Manson, P.N.; Hoopes, J.E. Experience with thirteen latissimus dorsi myocutaneous free flaps. Plast Reconstr Surg 64:1, 1979.

66. May, J.W.; Halls, M.J.; Simon, S.R. Free microvascular muscle flaps with skin graft reconstruction of extensive defects of the foot: A clinical and gait analysis study. Plast Reconstr Surg 75:627, 1985.

67. May, J.W., Jr.; Lukash, F.N.; Gallico, G.G. III. Latissimus dorsi free muscle flap in lower extremity reconstruction. Plast Reconstr Surg 68:603, 1981.

68. McCraw, J.B. Selection of alternative local flaps in the leg and foot. Clin Plast Surg 6:227, 1979.

69. McCraw, J.B.; Arnold, P.G. McCraw and Arnold's Atlas of Muscle and Musculocutaneous Flaps. Norfolk, VA, Hampton Press, 1986.

70. McCraw, J.B.; Furlow, L.T. The dorsalis pedis arterialized flap, a clinical study. Plast Reconstr Surg 55:177, 1975.

71. McGregor, I. Flap reconstruction in hand surgery: The evolution of presently used methods. J Hand Surg [Am] 4:1, 1979.

72. McGregor, I.A. Less than satisfactory experiences with neurovascular island flaps. Hand 1:21, 1969.

73. McGregor, L.A.; Jackson, I.T. The groin flap. Br J Plast Surg 25:3, 1972.

74. Melone, C.P.; Beasley, R.W.; Carstens, J.H. The thenar flap. J Hand Surg [Am] 7:291, 1982.

75. Meyers, M.B.; Cherry, G.; Milton, S. Tissue gas levels as an index of the adequacy of circulation: The relation between ischemia and the development of collateral circulation (delay phenomenon). Surgery 71:15, 1972.

76. Muhlbauer, W.; Hernall, E.; Stock, W.; et al. The forearm flap. Plast Reconstr Surg 70:336, 1982.

77. Nassif, T.M.; Vidal, L.; Bovet, J.L.; Baudet, J. The parascapular flap: A new cutaneous microsurgical free flap. Plast Reconstr Surg 69:591, 1982.

78. Ohmori, K.; Harii, K. Free dorsalis pedis sensory flap to the hand with microsurgical anastomosis. Plast Reconstr Surg 58:546, 1976.

79. Patzakis, M.J.; Abdollahi, K.; Sherman, R.; et al. Treatment of chronic osteomyelitis with muscle flaps. Orthop Clin North Am 24:505, 1993.

80. Pederson, W.C. Coverage of hips, pelvis, and femur. Orthop Clin North Am 24:461, 1993.

81. Reading, G. Instep island flaps. Ann Plast Surg 13:488, 1984.

82. Rockwell, W.B.; Lister, G. Coverage of hand injuries. Orthop Clin North Am 24:411, 1993.

83. Russell, R.C.; Zamboni, W.A. Coverage of the elbow and forearm. Orthop Clin North Am 24:425, 1993.

84. Russell, R.C.; Van Beek, A.L.; Warak, P.; et al. Alternative hand flaps for amputations and digital defects. J Hand Surg [Am] 6:399, 1981.

85. Smith, J.R.; Bom, A.F. An evaluation of fingertip reconstruction by cross-finger and palmar pedicle flap. J Plast Reconstr Surg 35:409, 1965.

86. Song, R.; Gao, Y.; Song, Y.; et al. The forearm flap. Clin Plast Surg 9:21, 1982.

87. Stark, W.J. The use of pedicled muscle flaps in the surgical treatment of chronic osteomyelitis resulting from compound fractures. J Bone Joint Surg 28:343, 1946.

88. Swartz, W.M. Immediate reconstruction of the wrist and dorsum of the hand with a free osteocutaneous groin flap. J Hand Surg [Am] 9:18, 1984.

89. Swartz, W.M.; Jones, N.F. Soft tissue coverage of the lower extremity. Curr Probl Surg 22:4, 1985.

90. Swartz, W.M.; Mears, D.C. The role of free tissue transfers in lower extremity reconstruction. Plast Reconstr Surg 76:364, 1985.

91. Takayanagi, S.; Tsukii, T. Free serratus anterior muscle and myocutaneous flaps. Ann Plast Surg 8:277, 1982.

92. Taylor, G.L.; Watson, N. One-stage repair of compound leg defects with free vascularized flaps of groin skin and iliac bone. Plast Reconstr Surg 61:494, 1978.

93. Taylor, T.L.; Townsend, P.; Corlett, R. Superiority of the deep circumflex iliac vessels as a supply for the free groin flap: Clinical work. Plast Reconstr Surg 64:745, 1979.

94. Vasconez, H.C.; Oishi, S. Soft tissue coverage of the shoulder and brachium. Orthop Clin North Am 24:435, 1993.

95. Vasconez, L.O.; Bostwick, J., III; McCraw, J. Coverage of exposed bone by muscle transposition and skin grafting. Plast Reconstr Surg 53:526, 1974.

96. Villian, R. Use of the flag flap for coverage of a small area on a finger or the palm. Plast Reconstr Surg 51:397, 1973.

97. Weiland, A.J.; Moore, J.R.; Daniel, R.K. The efficacy of free tissue transfer in the treatment of osteomyelitis. J Bone Joint Surg Am 66:181, 1984.

98. Wiss, D.; Sherman, R.; Oechsel, M. External skeletal fixation and rectus abdominis free tissue transfer in the management of severe open fractures of the tibia. Orthop Clin North Am 24:549, 1993.

99. Yanai, A.; Park, S.; Iwao, T.; Nakamura, N. Reconstruction of a skin defect of the posterior heel by a lateral calcaneal flap. Plast Reconstr Surg 75:642, 1985.

100. Yaremchuk, M.J.; Brumback, R.J.; Manson, P.N.; et al. Acute and definitive management of traumatic osteocutaneous defects of the lower extremity. Plast Reconstr Surg 80:1, 1987.

101. Yaremchuk, M.J.; Bartlett, A.P.; Sedacca, T.; May, J.W., Jr. The effect of preoperative angiography on experimental free flap survival. Plast Reconstr Surg 68:201, 1981.

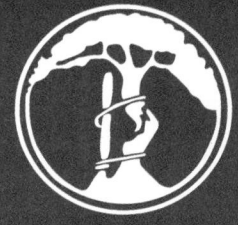

CHAPTER 16

Gunshot Wounds to the Musculoskeletal System

....

Gregory A. Zych, D.O., Steven P. Kalandiak, M.D., and Patrick W. Owens, M.D.

INTRODUCTION

Although violent crime has declined within the last 5 years, approximately 64,000 nonfatal gunshot injuries were reported to the Centers for Disease Control (CDC) in the United States in 2004. Estimates of total cost of injury indicate that firearm/gunshot injuries account for 9 percent or 41.4 billion dollars per year.[25] An unknown but substantial number involved the musculoskeletal system. Gunshot fractures are most common in urban areas and theaters of war but may be encountered in almost any region. The orthopaedic surgeon should therefore become familiar with the various types of gunshot injuries and their treatment.

BALLISTICS

The purpose of a firearm projectile is to crush tissue. Secondary effects are laceration of structures and tissue stretching. When a projectile strikes the body, a permanent cavity, variable in size, is created in the tissues. This cavity is particular to the projectile type and represents the amount of crushed tissue. Some tissue, peripheral to the permanent cavity, will undergo elastic deformation (stretching) and is termed the temporary cavity. The amount of tissue damage is mainly related to the projectile velocity, projectile mass, tissue density, and projectile design.

The kinetic energy of a projectile is defined by $KE = \frac{1}{2}mv^2$. This equation shows that, in general, the velocity is more important than the mass since doubling the velocity quadruples the kinetic energy while doubling the mass only yields twice the kinetic energy. Bullets have been classified, based on muzzle velocity, into low velocity (<2000 fps) and high velocity (≥2000 fps). Much of the previous literature focused on the velocity of the bullet as the most important determinant of tissue damage, but this factor is only one of several that must be considered. What appears to be more important is the degree of kinetic energy transmitted to the body tissues.[6] The human body has many differing tissue densities. Low-density tissues include lung, fat, and muscle and are not so easily damaged by a projectile as the denser tissues of bone and solid organs.

High-velocity bullets may pass through certain low-density tissues such as lung or muscle with minimal damage owing to minimal transfer of the kinetic energy. A low-velocity bullet can produce considerable tissue injury if the majority of the kinetic energy is transmitted to the tissues.

The mass of the projectile also bears importance. An average 9-mm handgun may have a bullet weighing 150 grains, a .44 Magnum 230 grains, and a shotgun load as much as 650 grains. A large increase in mass yields substantially greater kinetic energy and the probability of greater tissue crush.

Design of projectiles has a profound effect on wounding potential. Bullets that deform on impact present a greater cross-sectional area capable of crushing more tissues. This is also true of bullets that fragment, resulting in many secondary "bullets" that scatter throughout the tissues, each creating its own path of destruction. Some bullets will oscillate or yaw before or after encountering the body, increasing the cross-sectional area of tissue contact and leading to more tissue crushing.

Low-velocity handguns cause most civilian gunshot wounds, with minimal soft tissue damage, and these are the most common that the orthopaedic surgeon will encounter. Direct hits onto bone may cause impressive comminution owing to the relatively high density of bone and its physical property of brittleness. The diaphysis is more prone to comminution than the metaphysis. Some types of higher power handguns, such as the .357 Magnum and .44 Magnum have more destructive potential from larger bullet size and more propellant load.

Assault and hunting rifles with higher muzzle velocities and expanding or fragmenting bullets are designed to produce severe internal tissue damage with nearly complete retention of all bullet fragments, a measure of killing potential.

Shotguns can fire loads of either multiple small pellets or single large slugs. The muzzle velocity is classified as low (1200 fps) but the destructive power arises from the multiple or large and heavy projectiles that are utilized. Shotgun loads vary tremendously, but in general the most tissue destruction occurs within a short barrel-to-target distance. At greater distances, the pellets spread out, and tissue damage will be minimized.

Close-range shotgun injuries have extensive wounds. The design of most shot shells incorporates some type of wadding between the lead load and the propellant. This wadding can be either plastic or fiber and will follow the pellets into the tissues. As part of the débridement process, the surgeon should explore for the retained wadding, since this material can become a focus of infection.

DIAGNOSIS

The history of a gunshot injury may yield important clues that will assist in diagnosis and treatment. If possible, the type of weapon, number of rounds, and distance from the weapon to the victim should be elicited from the patient, first responders, or law enforcement officers. High- or intermediate-velocity or shotgun weapons may lead to more tissue injury, but this is not absolutely certain. Most handgun injuries occur within a few feet so the wounding potential of even small-caliber handguns can be significant.

Standard Advanced Trauma Life Support (ATLS) protocol should be followed for the initial physical examination and the treatment. Some special aspects of the physical examination in patients with gunshot wounds should be amplified. The skin should be searched for wounds of entrance and exit, and their location, size, and appearance documented. More than two wounds suggest multiple gunshots. An attempt should be made to match each entrance wound with its corresponding exit wound. Occasionally, bone fragments may be seen within the wound if the gunshot caused a comminuted fracture in a subcutaneous location. Pulsatile bleeding may be an early indication of a major vascular injury.

The gunshot pathway through the patient's body should be determined. All structures that could be violated require close evaluation. Detailed neurologic and vascular examination will detect any deficits. In the absence of obvious fracture, the extremities should be put through a full range of motion. Extremity joints that have been penetrated by the gunshot will typically be painful with an effusion.

After the initial physical examination is completed, the skin wounds should be sterilely dressed. The "time-honored" technique of securely placing a metallic marker (paper clip, coin) on the dressing surface can be helpful in determining the relationship of the skin wounds to the underlying anatomic structures on subsequent imaging studies (Fig. 16-1).

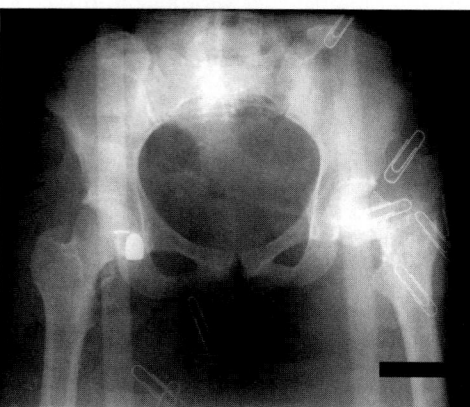

FIGURE 16-1 *Anteroposterior pelvis radiograph in a patient with multiple gunshots to pelvis and thighs. Each paper clip denotes an entrance or exit wound.*

Immobilization via splinting or skeletal traction of all fractures is the next priority.

Plain extremity radiographs, two views at right angles, including the joints above and below, are obtained for all possible involved regions or extremities. Special radiographic views can be taken as needed to assess the pelvis or spine. The imaging studies are scrutinized for the location and number of all metallic gunshot fragments. Certain gunshots will leave an obvious trail of lead particles as they pass through the body tissues. In cases with only an entrance wound, there must be a retained gunshot fragment somewhere in the body. A gunshot fragment that is within the anatomic confines of a joint capsule on the two plain radiographs (perpendicular to each other) must be assumed to be intra-articular. In trauma situations, whole-body multidetector computed tomography (CT) scans will often be done and have been shown to be quite reliable in locating metallic fragments, although less effective at visualizing the path of the gunshot wound.[47] Arthrocentesis and aspiration may reveal occult joint violation in suspicious cases. Standard musculoskeletal imaging studies should be done on the basis of the joint injury or fracture, regardless of the gunshot mechanism.

GENERAL TREATMENT PRINCIPLES

Antibiotic Usage

As early as 1892 Lagarde[41] demonstrated that bullets were not sterile, neither before nor after being fired from a gun. Recently, Grosse Perdekamp and Vennemann[74] have shown that skin particles and the subsequent bacteria adhering to them from the entrance and exit wounds can be found in the bullet tracks within the body. Therefore, it is reasonable to believe that gunshot wounds are contaminated with bacteria and if associated with a fracture, then the fracture should be classified as open. However, the majority of civilian gunshot wounds are small in size with limited tissue damage and would fit the criteria for a type I open fracture according to the classification of Gustilo and Anderson.

Howland and Ritchey[34] studied nonsurgical management and antibiotic prophylaxis in patients with stable low-velocity gunshot fractures, and they concluded that it was not necessary to surgically débride the wounds or administer antibiotics. However, they did stress the importance of distinguishing between civilian and military gunshot fractures.

Dickey[21] treated 73 patients with gunshot fractures that did not require surgical repair and were randomized prospectively into two groups: intravenous antibiotics and no antibiotics. Two infections occurred, one in each group. They concluded that intravenous antibiotic prophylaxis was of no significant benefit.

Knapp[39] reported a series of 190 patients with 222 extra-articular long bone gunshot fractures that did not require operative fixation. They were randomized to both intravenous cephapirin and gentamicin for 72 hours or oral ciprofloxacin for 72 hours. Each group had two infections (2% for each), and it was concluded that these injuries could be treated with oral antibiotics.

Therefore, it appears that the evidence for antibiotic prophylaxis of low-caliber (velocity) gunshot fractures not requiring surgical fixation is weak. Nevertheless, in the urban penetrating trauma population, a brief period, 24 to 48 hours, of antibiotics is often used. This protocol has been thought to be efficacious to treat the wound contamination characteristic of these injuries in these often nutritionally and medically compromised patients. Patients who require surgical fracture fixation should receive standard perioperative antibiotic prophylaxis according to the surgeon's discretion. Shotgun and high-velocity gunshot fractures benefit from intravenous antibiotic treatment for 24 to 48 hours and, in most situations, surgical débridement.

Wound Assessment

One problem facing the surgeon is the assessment of the character of the gunshot injury. The presence of a large wound is an obvious indicator of tissue damage. However, the skin wounds can be deceptive, with many significant injuries presenting with small entrance and exit wounds. In these cases, it is the intercalary tissue appearance and integrity that needs close scrutiny.

Extensive ecchymosis and severe local swelling are potential indications of the need to surgically explore a gunshot wound. Recent authors have stressed the importance of "treating the wound" and not treating the history of the wound mechanism. That is to say, gunshot velocity is only one factor in the decision for surgical exploration.

Close range shotgun injuries require thorough débridement and exploration for the retained wadding, which must be removed. Generally, it is futile to attempt removal of all retained pellets, since normal tissue will be violated in the process. Devitalized bone fragments are best excised unless they are intra-articular and possibly suitable for internal fixation. Longer distance shotgun wounds have multiple pellet entrance wounds without exit wounds. Pellet removal is indicated only if proven to be intra-articular.

High-power handguns, machine pistols, and assault rifles constitute the other end of the spectrum seen in civilian trauma. Some of the wounds associated with these weapons have a completely benign appearance. Large exit wounds are pathognomonic of severe soft tissue crush and laceration and are generally good indications for wound exploration and débridement. Diaphyseal comminution is not uncommon, and judgment must be used if this is the only apparent criterion for exploration.

Upper Extremity

Steven Kalandiak, M.D.

PROXIMAL HUMERUS AND SHOULDER JOINT

Vessel and Nerve Injury

When vascular injury near the shoulder is present, it is often accompanied by nerve injury. Hardin and associates[31] reviewed 99 low-velocity, upper extremity vascular injuries. Eleven (52%) of the 21 patients with axillary artery lesions and 27 (63%) of the 43 limbs with brachial arterial injuries had concomitant nerve injury. At final follow-up, only one patient (9%) had complete return of function. Shotgun injuries produced the most extensive tissue destruction (Fig. 16-2), almost always resulting in permanent functional impairment and often resulting in amputation of all or part of a limb. Borman and co-workers[9] reported numerous successful arterial reconstructions but permanent and severe limitation of function when accompanying nerve or plexus injury was present.

There is no clear consensus about whether and when to explore brachial plexus injuries after a gunshot. Armine and Sugar[2] recommended primary repair of the brachial plexus when there is an associated vascular injury requiring exploration and repair. However, if no vascular or pulmonary injury is present, Leffert[43] recommended that initial management be conservative, with wound and fracture care and physical therapy as needed.

In a study of patients with brachial plexus injury during World War II, Brooks[12] found only 4 of 25 who underwent surgical exploration for plexus lesions to have divided nerves. In an effort to relate the prognosis to the location of the nerve lesion, Brooks suggested three groups: (1) lesions of the roots and trunk of C5 and C6, (2) lesions of the posterior cord, and (3) lesions of C8–T1 of the medial cord. The recovery in the first group was good; in the second, fair;

FIGURE 16-2   *Shotgun blast to shoulder.*

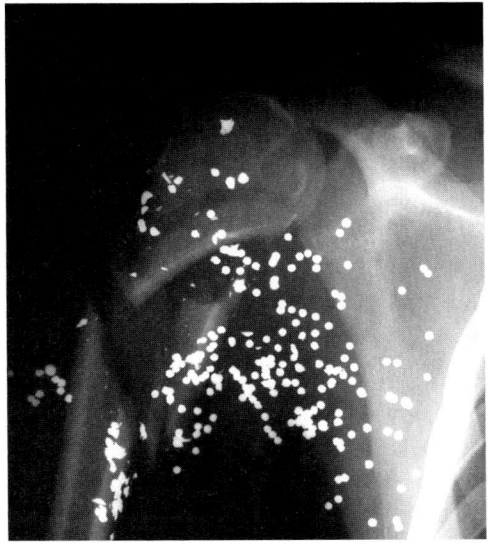

and in the third, poor. Recovery in the small muscles of the hand did not occur if severance of the nerves occurred. Brooks therefore concluded that routine exploration of open wounds of the plexus was rarely indicated.

When managing nerve injuries nonoperatively, we have found that the most useful clinical indication of axonal regeneration in nerve injuries is evidence of an advancing Tinel sign. Percussion over the site of the nerve injury produces the sensation of radiating "electrical shocks" because of stimulation of the free nerve endings. If there is no recovery by 3 months, if the lesion is incomplete with a major area of neurologic deficit, or if a Tinel sign fails to advance for three consecutive monthly examinations, the nerve should be considered for exploration.

When exploration is performed, nerves found transected may be either repaired primarily or grafted. If a neuroma in continuity is found, either it may be resected and repaired or neurolysis may be performed. Whatever the finding at exploration, the outlook for a high nerve injury that fails to recover spontaneously is often poor, and tendon transfers may be an appropriate treatment.

Fracture

Low-energy gunshot injuries are treated with local wound care and intravenous or oral antibiotics. Formal irrigation and débridement are unnecessary; the surgeon should choose nonoperative or operative treatment as if the injury were closed. If surgery is selected, the bullet track remains unexplored unless it lies in the path of the surgical approach. In contrast, high-energy gunshot wounds are treated as grade III open fractures, with prompt irrigation and surgical débridement, frequent use of temporizing external fixation, and definitive fixation only if and when the condition of the soft tissues permits.

With low-energy gunshots, nondisplaced and minimally displaced proximal humeral fractures are treated nonoperatively. The indications for surgery of displaced fractures of the humeral head and neck are the same as those used for closed fractures—displacement of over 1 cm of a "part" of the proximal humerus and angulation greater than 45 degrees are generally considered indications for operative treatment. Plate and screw fixation, closed or open intramedullary nailing, or closed reduction and percutaneous pinning may all be appropriate, according to the experience and preference of the surgeon. Comminution of the surgical neck without bone loss may be bridged with either a locked plate or an intramedullary nail. The proximal humerus is relatively tolerant of shortening, and when bone loss at the surgical neck is present it may often be treated by simply shortening the humerus by a centimeter or two (Figs. 16-2 and 16-3).

Although most low-velocity gunshot injuries to the shoulder girdle can be treated conservatively, if the gunshot wound involves the glenohumeral joint itself, the joint should be explored either arthroscopically or through a formal arthrotomy. The path of the bullet itself can sometimes be a useful portal into the joint.[17] Intra-articular bullets should be removed, since lead may leach out into the joint and deposit within the synovial tissues, causing either periarticular fibrosis or toxic effects to the articular cartilage.[45] Osteochondral fragments that are small and irreparable should be excised, but larger, more significant

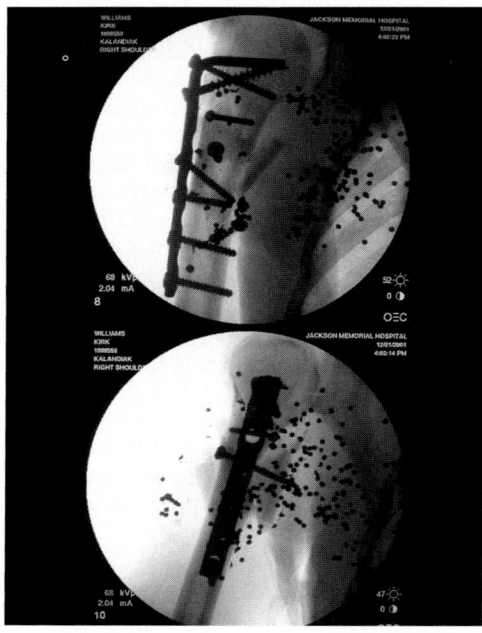

FIGURE 16-3   *Treatment with primary shortening and blade plate fixation.*

pieces of the joint surface should be repaired. Countersunk or headless screws are often useful in these unusual circumstances (Figs. 16-4 and 16-5). In cases of extreme comminution of the articular surfaces, prosthetic replacement or resection arthroplasty may be the only options. Placing either vancomycin or tobramycin in cement used for the prosthesis may decrease the risk of infection.

External fixation is an option for both temporary and definitive treatment of proximal humerus fractures, especially when soft tissue injury or bony comminution is severe (Fig. 16-6). Although we have little experience with it at most American centers, recent war experiences in the Balkans and Middle East have given us a significant literature on the use of external fixation in high-energy gunshot injuries of the upper extremity,[19] reported as external fixation of severe gunshot and blast injuries. Surgeons were able to use the proximal humerus for pin placement in half of their patients but needed to use the scapula and/or clavicle for the most severe injuries. Large soft tissue defects around the shoulder can be covered by rotation of a latissimus dorsi myocutaneous flap on its vascular pedicle. Once a favorable soft tissue environment has been established, the temporizing fixator can be converted to a more elaborate, definitive frame or to internal fixation if desired. Because long-term use of pins or wires in the humeral head can cause soft tissue irritation or infection, if external fixation is to be used until fracture healing has occurred, pin care must be meticulous.

HUMERAL SHAFT AND ARM
Vessel and Nerve Injury

As in the shoulder, gunshot wounds in the upper arm frequently injure arteries and nerves in addition to the bone

FIGURE 16-4 *A* and *B,* Low-velocity gunshot wound to humeral head in a teenaged male.

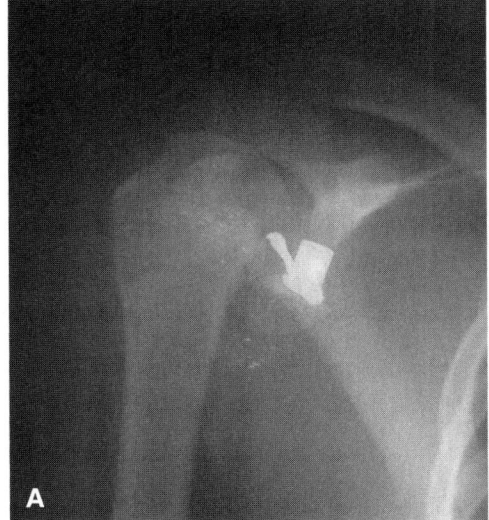
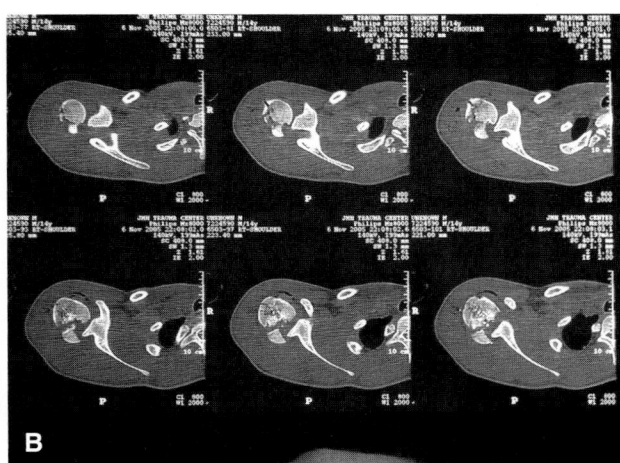

itself. If vascular injuries are treated promptly, critical limb ischemia is rare.[79] Although some[50] have advocated that a fracture be stabilized first if there is an associated vascular injury in order to protect the repair, others have found different results. McHenry et al.[54] reviewed their upper and lower extremity fractures with associated vascular injuries. They definitively repaired 5 fractures first, shunted 13 of the 22 vascular injuries that were addressed before fracture repair, and repaired 9 of 22 vascular injuries definitively first. The need for fasciotomy and the length of hospitalization were both increased when care of the orthopaedic injury preceded the revascularization. Definitive fracture treatment, performed after the revascularization, did not disrupt the shunt or the definitive vascular repair in any case. Despite this, to maximize the safety of the vascular repair, our institution favors shunting of the vascular injury first, followed by either definitive fracture repair if the soft tissues allow or external fixation if not, and then definitive vascular repair.

When fracture and vascular injury are both present, complication rates for the vascular injury may increase. McNamara and co-workers[55] found no amputations in 64 patients without humeral fracture who underwent brachial artery repair, but 10 percent of the 20 patients with humeral fractures had amputations. There was one failure of repair (2.3%) among the 44 patients without fracture, and there were two failures (10%) among those with fracture.

Humeral shaft fractures combined with ipsilateral brachial plexus injuries pose special problems. Of 19 patients with brachial plexus injuries and ipsilateral humeral shaft fractures treated at the Los Angeles County–University of Southern California Medical Center and Rancho Los Amigos Hospital, 3 were treated by compression plate, 4 by intramedullary nail, 2 with external fixation, and 10 with a cast or brace. All fractures treated by compression plating healed, but 4 of the 6 treated with intramedullary

FIGURE 16-5 *A* and *B,* Treatment with open reduction and internally fixed with headless screws.

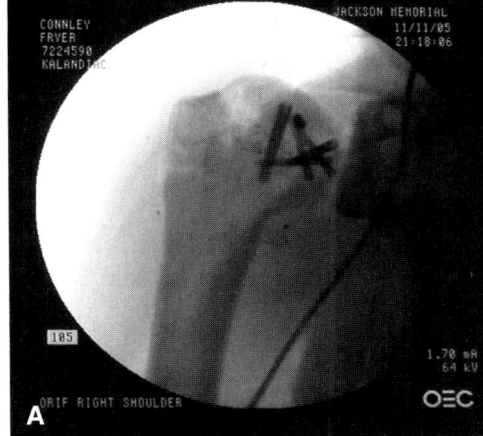
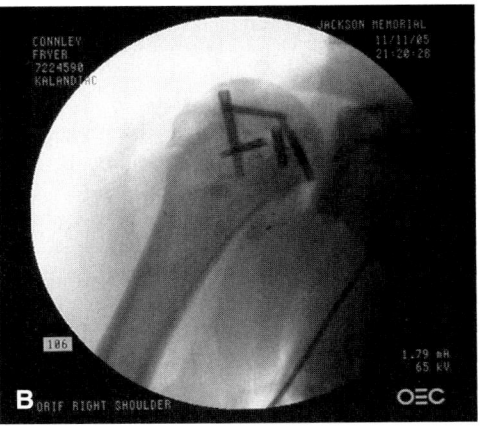

FIGURE 16-6   ***A,*** *A gunshot wound to the proximal humerus resulted in a comminuted fracture with a large soft tissue defect.* ***B,*** *After irrigation and débridement, the fracture was reduced and held with an external fixator.* ***C,*** *The soft tissue defect was constructed with a latissimus dorsi pedicle flap.* ***D,*** *Restoration of the shoulder contour followed flap placement.* ***E,*** *At 1 year, the fracture has healed.*

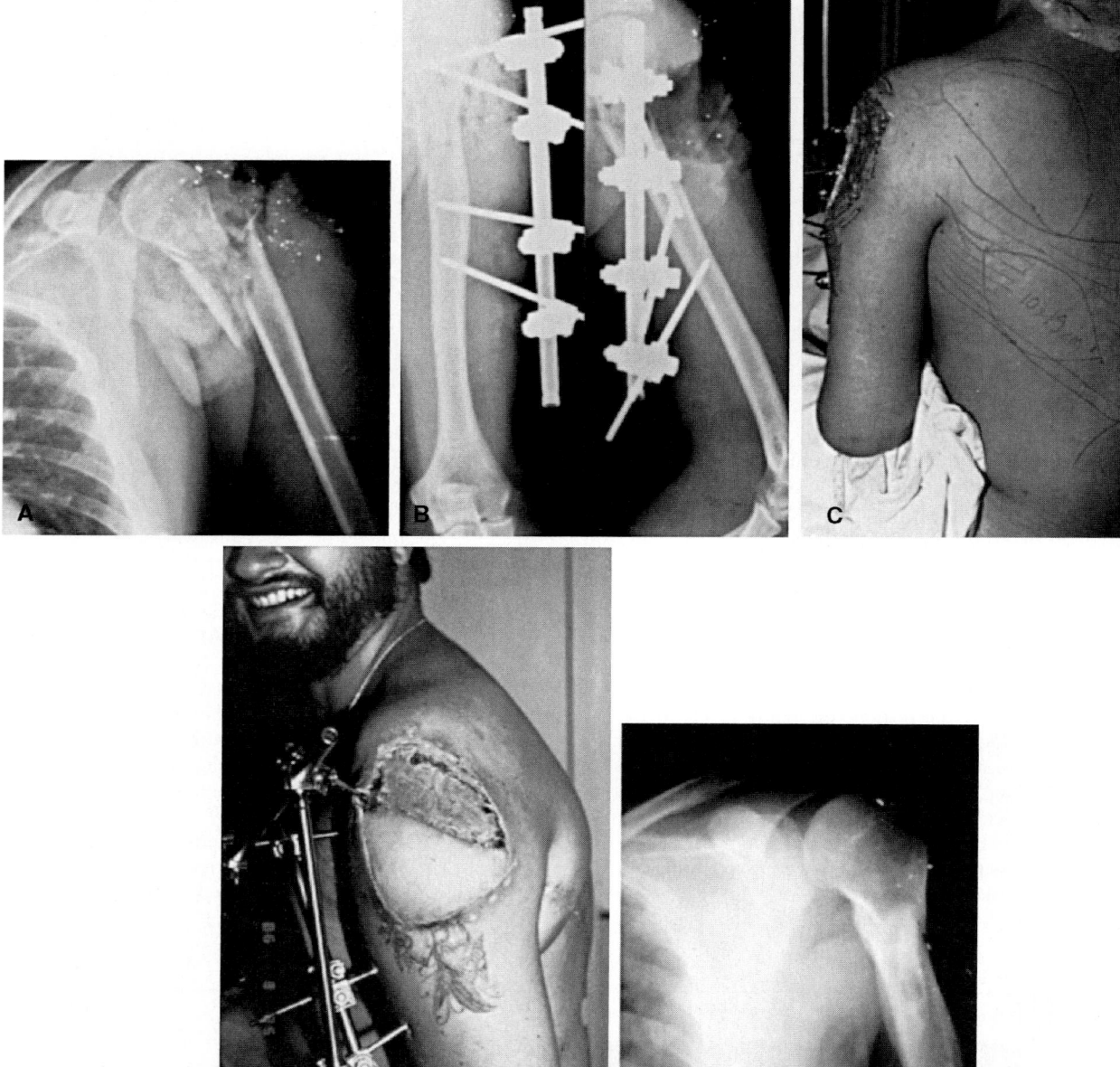

rods or external fixation and 4 of the 10 treated with a cast brace failed to unite.[11] All of the nonunions required open repair with compression plating to achieve union.

If the peripheral nerves traversing a high-energy gunshot wound in the upper arm are not functioning, they should be explored at the time of wound débridement. While repair can sometimes be carried out primarily, the extent of injury to the nerve is typically unclear, so the nerve ends are usually tagged for later repair. When fractures result from lower energy missiles, they can often be treated nonoperatively. In this case, peripheral nerve injuries are usually managed expectantly. Although some have found little benefit to exploration and repair of nerve injury in the upper arm, others have reported large series with better prognosis if the nerve injury is in the arm or more distal.[37,38]

Fracture

Fractures of the humeral shaft, when not complicated by vascular injury, are often best treated with local wound care and plaster or cast brace immobilization. Humeral fracture bracing may be started as soon as the wound permits.

There is no significant difference in the rate of union between closed humeral fractures and uncomplicated humeral fractures caused by a low-velocity gunshot, even if appreciable comminution or displacement is present.[35] When low or even moderate energy soft tissue injury is present, operative stabilization with either a nail or plate may be carried out both promptly and safely if the pattern of fracture merits. In cases of severe soft tissue injury, débridement and external fixation is almost always the initial treatment of choice for the fracture, facilitates subsequent wound and soft tissue care, and may provide definitive fixation. Half-pin frames in the arm often have pin track problems as the patient begins to mobilize the shoulder and elbow, and our preference is to convert to a plate when possible, or to an intramedullary nail, since time required for healing is often prolonged, and the pins may be difficult to maintain for these long periods. However, with careful attention to the frame and appropriate treatment of the anticipated pin track problems, external fixation can certainly be used as definitive treatment.

In centers experienced with their use, Ilizarov type frames can also be utilized with good results.[61] The care of these complex injuries is difficult, and decisions regarding care must be individualized to the patient, the fracture, and the injury (Figs. 16-7 through 16-10).

In addition to neurovascular injury and soft tissue loss, high-energy gunshot wounds can also cause significant loss of diaphyseal bone. Although there are reports of spontaneous reconstitution of humeral bone loss, some type of surgical intervention is generally required to restore bony continuity. Numerous techniques have been proposed to deal with this challenging situation, including wave plating with cancellous grafting,[64] interposition of a titanium mesh cage with bone graft,[5] transposition of composite flap including the lateral border of the scapula,[68] transfer

of a segment of vascularized fibula,[32] and bone transport using an Ilizarov type external fixator.[52]

At present, there is no large series or body of evidence to suggest the superiority of any one method of reconstituting humeral bone loss.

FIGURE 16-8 *Treatment with a plate.*

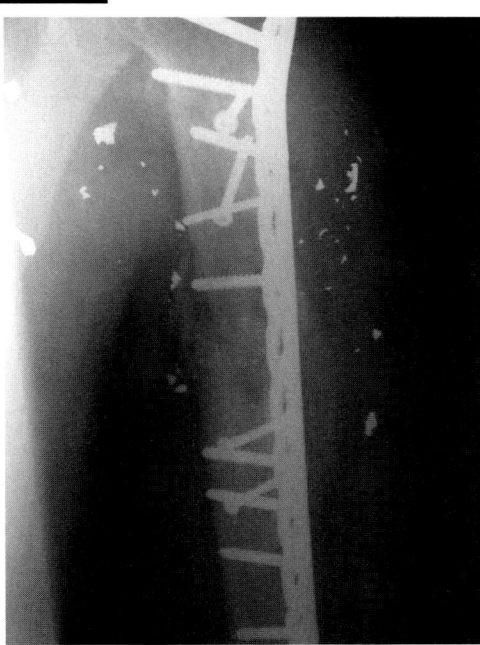

FIGURE 16-7 *Comminuted proximal humeral shaft fracture without significant neurovascular or soft tissue injury.*

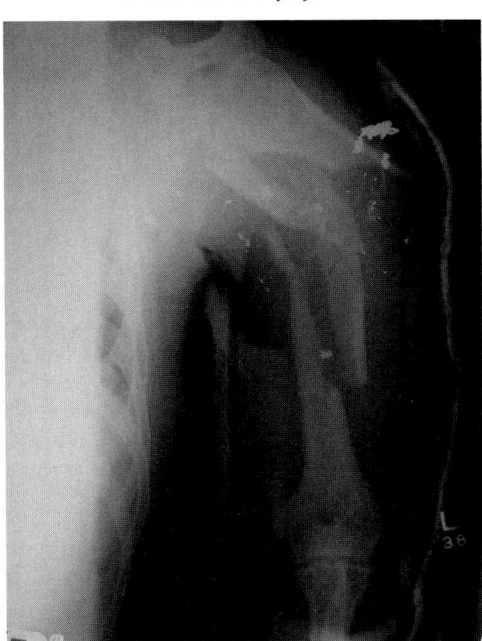

FIGURE 16-9 *Comminuted proximal humeral shaft with vascular injury and delayed revascularization and external fixation. Patient developed infection and compartment syndrome and lost most of the muscle below the deltoid.*

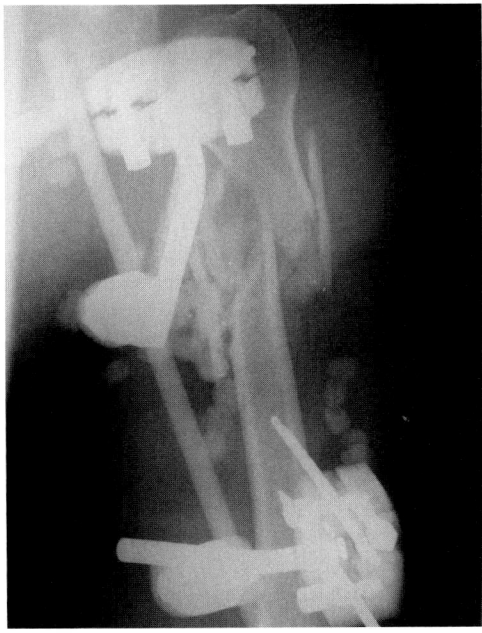

After serial débridement to resolve the infection the patient in Figure 16-10 underwent pedicled latissimus coverage and conversion to an intramedullary nail.

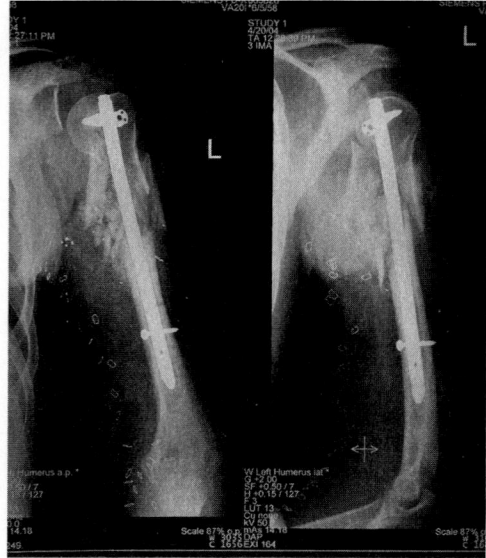

ELBOW

Because of its complex bony anatomy and propensity for stiffness following injury, gunshot wounds about the elbow are particularly difficult. Following severe elbow injuries, the goal of achieving the flexion/extension and forearm rotation required for most activities of daily living is often not realized. Although secondary procedures such as capsular release and resection of heterotopic bone can sometimes help regain lost motion, articular injuries are sometimes so severe that achieving a stable and pain-free elbow with any motion at all may be all that can be hoped for.

The brachial artery at the elbow is particularly vulnerable because of its location. In addition to trauma from the missile itself, displacement of fracture fragments about the elbow can lacerate or completely tear the artery as well. Compression or occlusion of the brachial artery can also result from entrapment between fracture fragments and from the edema that may follow restoration of arterial flow after prolonged ischemia, leading to forearm compartment syndrome.[8] Six compartment syndromes that developed in association with isolated proximal ulna fractures have been reported. Five of the six developed in a delayed fashion; all five were associated with low-velocity gunshots. If a nerve injury is also present at the elbow, pain and paresthesias from forearm compartment syndrome may be absent, and the only reliable way to detect it is with a high degree of suspicion and direct compartment monitoring. In a review of vascular injuries about the elbow, Ashbell and colleagues[3] reported that 86 percent of those who sustained arterial injury also had injury to muscle, nerve, or bone in the same area. Concomitant injuries to one or more major nerves in the arm occurred in 69 percent, with muscle injuries next in frequency (66%). Combined injury to both nerve and muscle was seen in 45 percent.

When there is severe soft tissue and muscle damage, we recommend initial external fixation across the elbow joint. This approach protects arterial repair and allows soft tissue management and recovery. If there is soft tissue loss, an intact soft tissue envelope must be reestablished before further reconstruction can occur. For smaller defects in the surrounding soft tissue, local flaps may be an option. For larger areas of bone and soft tissue loss around the elbow, a composite latissimus flap, such as that described by Evans and Luethke,[24] offers an option for coverage and for osseous reconstruction as well. When soft tissues recover sufficiently to allow it, the surgeon may undertake fixation of the articular injury and reconstruction of any juxta-articular bone loss. Although a significant loss of elbow motion often results if the fixator is left on for more than 4 to 6 weeks, there are times when the severity of the injury allows no other treatment.

DISTAL HUMERUS

Although earlier texts adopted a fairly nihilistic approach toward the reconstruction of these complex articular injuries, techniques and implants have improved to a point where many extremely complex articular injuries can be reconstructed.

For comminuted juxta-articular fractures, external fixation has been described as a means of restoring limb alignment and permitting immediate motion while minimizing dissection in the zone of injury.[71] When the articular surface is comminuted, open reduction of even the most comminuted joint is often possible once the soft tissues have recovered to a point that permits a safe operation.

Triceps splitting or olecranon osteotomy can be used at the surgeon's discretion. Multiple fine, threaded Kirschner-wires or absorbable pins can be used to build small osteochondral fragments onto the epicondyles until the medial and lateral halves of the articular spool can be mated. The repaired articular segment can then be fixed to the humeral shaft, typically with a 3.5 plate on each column. Fixation of a comminuted medial or lateral column may be aided with use of an additional mini-fragment or modular hand plate on the column. Moderate supracondylar bone loss can be addressed with a shortening osteotomy of the supracondylar humerus, with a burr used to recreate the olecranon and coronoid fossae. Columnar bone loss can be grafted with a structural piece of tricortical iliac crest or bridged with a plate and the column grafted with cancellous bone. The goal is to obtain fixation that is sufficiently stable to allow immediate range of motion. When this quality of fixation cannot be obtained, the elbow can be immobilized, although this tends to cause stiffness rapidly and may require secondary release.

Despite improvements in both techniques and implants, some distal humeral injuries remain unreconstructable because of articular loss or comminution or severe soft tissue injury. In these cases, the older technique of skeletal traction applied through a proximal ulnar pin, which allows some early motion and can maintain reasonable alignment of the fracture fragments, can be used.

ULNA

Gunshot wounds of the olecranon and proximal ulna present difficulties for the orthopaedist as well. In simple,

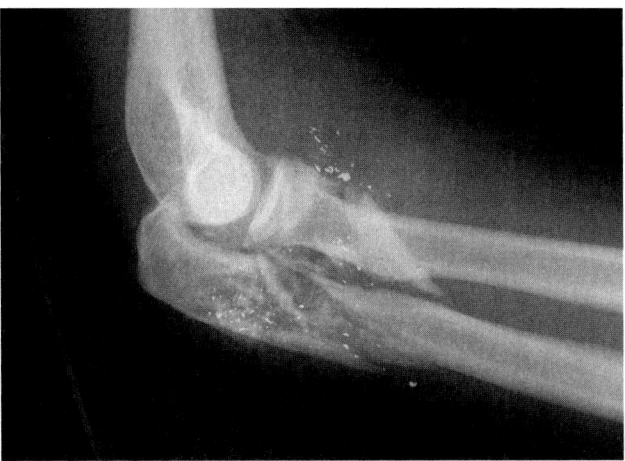

FIGURE 16-11 *Gunshot wound through proximal ulna.*

low-energy injuries with minimal comminution, standard open reduction and internal fixation can be carried out with either a modified tension band or with plate and screw fixation. When olecranon comminution is extensive (75 to 80 percent of the articular surface), it can be managed by excision and the triceps advanced to the remaining bone.[18,51] If the articular surfaces of the olecranon and coronoid can be reconstructed, plates may be used to bridge areas of periarticular comminution. The coronoid is of primary importance in this area, and every effort should be made to preserve it if possible. Figures 16-11 and 16-12 illustrate this point, with use of mini-screws, fine-wire fixation, and an intramedullary mini-plate on the comminuted coronoid to reconstruct the joint surface and plate fixation to bridge the periarticular comminution. Fixation was adequate to begin early motion, and the patient illustrated recovered nearly full range of motion.

Additional techniques are available for salvage of the severely injured elbow. None present ideal solutions for

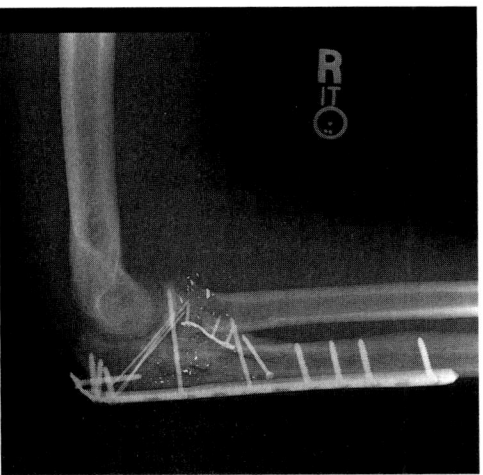

FIGURE 16-12 *Treatment with open reduction and internal fixation.*

these difficult injuries, and the choice of treatment must be individualized according to the injury and the experience of the surgeon. Arthrodesis can relieve pain and provide strength and stability, but the loss of elbow motion is extremely limiting. Techniques of elbow fusion are described using internal,[53] external,[46] and combined[7] methods of fixation, as well as using vascularized free fibulae to make up bony defects.[66]

Hinge distraction can be used to help regain motion after release of contractures or repair of instability or in conjunction with excisional or fascial interposition arthroplasty to obtain motion in stiff elbows with loss of the articular surface of the distal humerus. This technique is particularly helpful in patients who are thought to be too young or too unreliable for total elbow arthroplasty and in those who refuse arthrodesis.

Cadaveric elbow allografts have been used as an alternative to arthrodesis as a final salvage attempt when there is significant bone loss. Dean et al.[20] have reported a 20-year experience with 23 whole elbow allograft reconstructions. Complications were observed in 16 and removal of the allograft was required in 6. Ten of 14 patients followed an average of 7.5 years had satisfactory results. Dean et al. viewed the operation as salvage only and noted that it reestablishes bone stock for future arthrodesis or arthroplasty. Finally, although the indication is rare, total elbow arthroplasty can be done in the older patient who will not place great physical demands on the elbow if adequate bone and soft tissue coverage are present.

FOREARM

Forearm fractures after gunshots have a high incidence of concomitant peripheral nerve injury and resultant loss of hand function. Initial evaluation should include a careful neurologic examination as well as an accurate assessment of swelling in the forearm. Compartment syndromes are common, and a high index of suspicion is essential, especially for fractures in the proximal third of the forearm. Moed and Fakhouri[57] found a 10 percent incidence of compartment syndrome in a series of 131 low-velocity gunshot wounds to the forearm (60 with fractures, 71 without bone injury). Location was the only significant fracture-associated risk factor predicting the development of compartment syndrome; displacement, comminution, and metallic foreign bodies in the wound had no effect. If any doubt exists, intracompartmental pressure measurements are indicated. If there is a possibility of vascular injury, an angiogram should be obtained.

Elstrom and co-workers[23] reviewed 29 extra-articular gunshot fractures of the forearm. Eighty-eight percent of the nondisplaced fractures did well and healed after approximately 7 weeks. Displaced fractures did not do so well, with 77 percent unsatisfactory results. The results in the patients with displaced fractures treated by delayed primary open reduction and internal fixation were superior to those of patients treated by closed methods. Twenty-seven percent had long-term disability secondary to the sequelae of nerve injury or difficulty in obtaining fracture union. Lenihan and associates[44] reviewed 32 patients with gunshot fractures of the forearm. They also found nonoperative treatment to be satisfactory for almost all nondisplaced fractures and unsatisfactory for those that were displaced. Of nine nerve injuries, 55 percent resolved spontaneously. Two patients (7%) underwent fasciotomy for compartment syndrome in the forearm.

Our recommendation for the treatment of uncomplicated, nondisplaced gunshot fractures of the forearm without vascular injury includes local wound care, antibiotics, and cast immobilization. However, displaced fractures of the radius or ulna and injuries involving both bones are best treated by immediate splinting and early open reduction and internal fixation. The patient should be observed for at least 24 hours for signs of ischemia or impending compartment syndrome.

When soft tissue injury is severe, external fixation confers quick and efficient stabilization, facilitates nursing, and aids recovery of both the patient and the injured limb.[33] The fixator may be definitive or may be changed later to plate fixation once soft tissues recover.

Since the majority of nerve injuries recover, they are generally treated expectantly. If open treatment of the fracture is undertaken, the nerve may be explored, but in the acute setting, it can be difficult or impossible to determine the extent of damage. While awaiting recovery from nerve injury, paralyzed joints should be splinted appropriately, and passive range-of-motion exercise should be performed regularly to prevent contracture.

The most useful splints are the lumbrical bar splint for ulnar nerve palsy (to prevent flexion contracture of the proximal interphalangeal joints of the fourth and fifth fingers) and the thumb opposition splint for median nerve injury (to prevent thumb web contracture). Patients with radial nerve palsy often do not need splinting, since contracture can usually be prevented by passive range-of-motion exercise.

When bone loss is present in the forearm, a number of strategies may be utilized to gain union across these gaps. If the soft tissue envelope is compliant, has limited scar, and consists largely of healthy muscle with a good vascular supply, autogenous cancellous bone grafting and stable internal plate fixation results in a high rate of union and improved upper limb function in patients with diaphyseal defects of the radius and/or ulna.[64] For contaminated segmental forearm fractures of up to 6 cm, the use of an antibiotic-impregnated cement spacer followed by delayed cancellous bone grafting has been reported by Georgiadis and DeSilva.[26] To improve stability and decrease the time to fracture union and the possibility of mechanical failure or loosening of the implants, a structural tricortical autogenous iliac crest graft may also be used.[63]

Finally, both Jupiter et al.[36] and Adani et al.[1] have reported on the use of vascularized fibular autograft for forearm defects ranging from 6 to 13 cm.

Gunshot Fractures of the Hand and Wrist

Patrick W. Owens, M.D.

Gunshot wounds of the hand have been more common in recent years as a result of the growing number of civilian injuries in inner city trauma centers. An estimated 20 percent of missile injuries involve the hand. Although these are typically low-velocity injuries, high-velocity injuries do account for a number of civilian injuries. The economic impact of these injuries can be substantial, with one study calculating the average direct hospital costs for hospitalization and operative care at 14,000 dollars per gunshot hand fracture.[16] Treatment of these patients is also challenging because of poor patient compliance. In one study of urban civilian hand gunshot injuries, 85 percent of patients were lost to follow-up before documented fracture healing, and 26 percent were lost to follow-up with removable fixation devices in place.[30]

Gunshot wounds to the wrist and hand can be complicated owing to the multitude of important structures contained within a small area. Frequent involvement of bone, tendons, nerves, and arteries is found with both high- and low-velocity injuries. On presentation to the emergency department, a thorough examination of the patient is crucial. The patient's account of the injury should also be documented for medicolegal reasons. Assessment of the soft tissue envelope, motor, sensory,

and circulation is necessary for treatment planning. Adequate radiographs should be obtained to evaluate the presence and severity of the skeletal injury.

After assessment of the patient and the injury, the wound should be treated with local superficial wound cleansing and local wound care. Simple wounds should be allowed to heal by secondary intention. Prophylactic antibiotics, frequently used because the degree of contamination may not be obvious, may not be necessary.[69] Fracture of the hand may have a higher rate of infection than in other areas of the body. Fracture stability and associated injuries guide further treatment. Stable fractures of the hand can be treated nonoperatively in appropriate casts or splints. A bulky dressing is applied with a dorsal splint maintaining the metacarpophalangeal joints in 70 to 90 degrees of flexion, the interphalangeal joints in extension, and the wrist in 20 degrees of extension.

The majority of civilian gunshot wounds are caused by low-velocity firearms such as handguns. Injuries caused by handguns cause much less damage to the soft tissues and less bony comminution. Thus, many of these fractures can be treated nonoperatively.[16,30]

Gonzalez et al.[29] defined operative indications for gunshot metacarpal fractures as follows: 50 percent or more comminution, angulation greater than 15 degrees, less than 50 percent bony apposition, shortening greater than 5 mm, and multiple fractures. Similar guidelines can be applied to proximal phalangeal fractures[28,29] (Fig. 16-13).

For injuries that require surgical treatment, care should be taken to remove only clearly devitalized tissue. Consideration of the function of structures in the zone of injury is important so that questionable tissue is left because the hand has an amazing capacity to heal. In the hand and wrist, removal of bullet fragments from synovial compartments should be considered (Fig. 16-14). Lead arthropathy and toxicity have been reported with intra-articular bullets and may also occur with retained fragments in tenosynovium.[75]

Tendon injuries are present in 20 to 30 percent of gunshot wounds.[14] Most injuries can be treated with primary repair, but some injuries require single- or two-stage grafting or even late tendon transfers. Tendon repair should be performed if possible at the time of bone reconstruction. In the dorsal aspect of the hand and in the fingers, the tendons are in close proximity to the bone. Even in the absence of direct tendon injury, the tendons can be secondarily affected by entrapment in scar or bony callus. Thus, it is imperative to promptly initiate digital motion to lower the likelihood of tendon adhesion. Bone fixation should be rigid enough to allow for rehabilitation of the tendon injury. Functional results will suffer if appropriate postoperative therapy cannot be instituted in a timely fashion. If there is significant tendon loss, grafting or tendon transfer should be performed.

For the flexor tendons, the A2 and A4 pulleys are crucial for efficient digital flexion, and the tendons should be repaired or reconstructed with local mobilization of tissues.[77] For flexor tendon injuries that cannot be repaired primarily without undue tension, a tendon graft should be employed. For injuries in the pulley region, the graft should extend from the palm to the insertion of the flexor digitorum profundus (FDP) on the distal phalanx. For injuries in the palm or wrist, segmental grafting should be performed to avoid tendon anastomosis within the carpal tunnel. Extensor tendon injuries of the fingers associated with fractures often have poor motion at the proximal interphalangeal (PIP) joint. For extensor damage on the dorsum of the hand or wrist, tendon loss can be treated with segmental grafts, transfer of the extensor indicis proprius (EIP) or extensor digiti quinti (EDQ), or side-to-side repair with the adjacent digital extensor.

Muscle involvement in the hand is not uncommon, mainly injuries to the interosseus muscles. Damage to these muscles can result in loss of grip strength and usually does not require further treatment. Damage to the thenar and hypothenar muscles may result in loss of abduction and opposition of the thumb and small finger and, if severe, may require tendon transfers to restore function.

Compartment syndrome of the hand can occur following gunshot wounds. This may be difficult to diagnose owing to the lack of distal sensory and vascular changes or pain due to the injury itself or in the obtunded patient. The clinician should measure interosseus muscle pressures when the diagnosis is in question. Release of the interosseus muscle fascia is satisfactory to allow room for muscle swelling.

Nerve injuries are commonly found in association with hand gunshot fractures with a frequency of around 30 to 40 percent. Seventy to ninety percent will resolve

---

FIGURE 16-13 *A,* This patient sustained a high-energy gunshot to the hand that resulted in a large soft tissue defect, extensor tendon injury, and highly comminuted fractures of the metacarpal, capitate, and hamate. *B,* One week after initial débridement, the patient underwent bone grafting, tendon repairs, and wound closure.

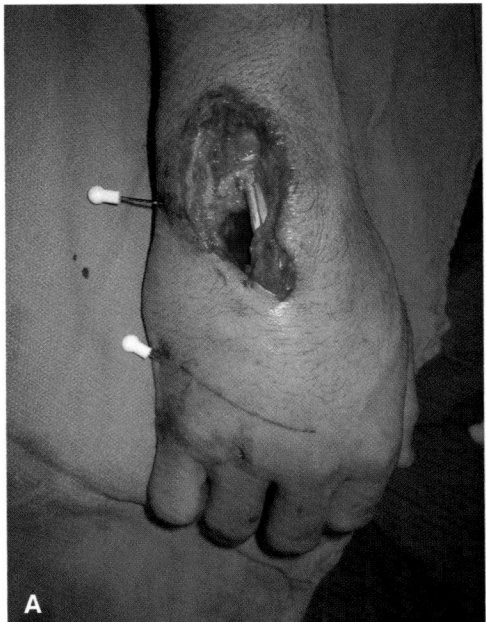
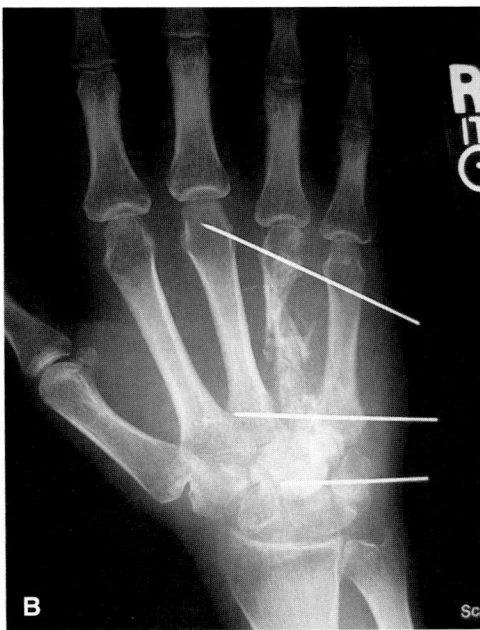

FIGURE 16-14 | **A** and **B,** This patient had a 1-year history of dorsal wrist swelling. Ten years earlier, the patient had sustained a shotgun wound to the wrist. The extensor tenosynovium of the fourth and fifth compartments as well as the distal radioulnar joint are well outlined by the lead from the degraded shot, with one pellet still visible (arrow).

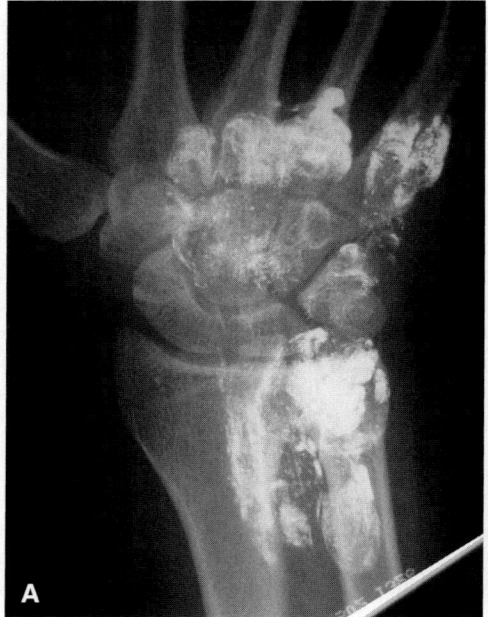
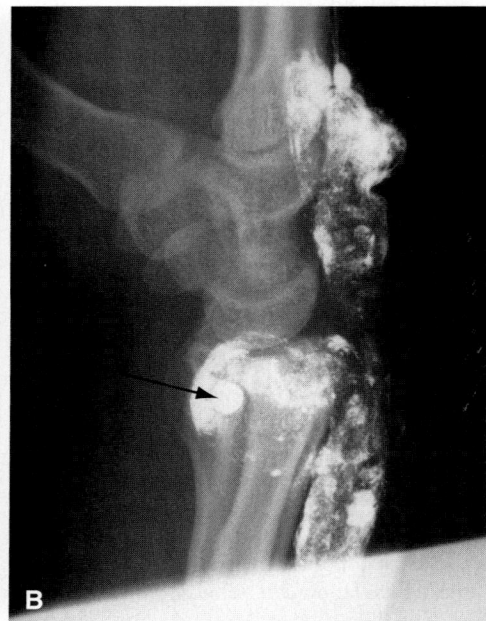

spontaneously.[62] If a complete nerve transection is encountered during surgical exploration, the nerve should be repaired with minimal tension. For high-energy injuries, immediate vein grafting or another nerve conduit can be used with a high rate of satisfactory results.[72]

Damage to the skin and subcutaneous tissues can vary greatly from small, uncomplicated wounds to large areas of soft tissue loss. Treatment for uncomplicated wounds should proceed as described above. For areas of larger soft tissue loss, there are a number of options.[13] Closure by secondary intention, which has a low rate of complications and satisfactory motion for wounds of the hand and fingers, is recommended.[13] Early and intensive hand therapy as well as patient cooperation are necessary for good results. Other options include split-thickness skin grafts, staged coverage with dermal templates with delayed skin grafting, vacuum-assisted closure, and flap coverage. Flaps are preferred in many cases to provide immediate coverage of tendons, nerves, and bone reconstruction, which may facilitate early motion. The groin flap was the workhorse in the past, but pedicled radial forearm, perforator flaps, or posterior interosseus flaps can provide excellent coverage while allowing for elevation of the hand and more effective postoperative therapy.[15]

Fractures of the wrist and hand should be treated with the goal of early rehabilitation. For stable nondisplaced or minimally displaced fractures of the wrist, a short arm cast or splint is satisfactory. For stable fractures of the metacarpals or proximal phalanges, immobilization should be placed dorsally with the metacarpophalangeal (MCP) joints in 70 to 90 degrees and the PIP joints in extension. Flexion exercises can be started in the cast to maintain joint

mobility. Stable fractures of the middle and distal phalanges should be splinted with the next proximal joint free.

Many fractures of the metacarpals and phalanges are unstable owing to comminution or bone loss. Rigid internal fixation with plates, screws, intramedullary rods, or a combination should be attained whenever possible. Bone loss should be treated by grafting with cancellous or corticocancellous bone. Studies of the use of bone graft substitutes in these types of fractures have not been reported. Early bone grafting has a low complication rate and high union rate.[28,29] In cases treated late, bony union and satisfactory motion can still be achieved. Some fractures are not amenable to rigid internal fixation and may require temporary Kirschner-wire spacers, pinning to an adjacent metacarpal, or the use of external fixation. External fixation is especially helpful in patients with complex soft tissue injuries.[27]

Articular fractures in the wrist and hand can be challenging. Essentially all gunshot carpal fractures are articular fractures and may require limited or total wrist arthrodesis. For many injuries, distraction through the use of external fixation can restore articular congruity.[77] If joint congruity can be obtained with traction, PIP joint injuries can potentially be treated with dynamic external fixation that allows for early motion. For nonreconstructable articular injuries of the thumb metacarpophalangeal (MP) or interphalangeal (IP) joint, and for distal interphalangeal (DIP) joints, arthrodesis is preferred. For similar injuries to the MP or IP joints of the fingers, external fixation can be used to maintain length and alignment prior to arthrodesis, arthroplasty, or vascularized free joint transfer.

Lower Extremity

Gregory A. Zych, D.O.

PELVIS

Gunshot wounds of the pelvis are rarely encountered in civilian and military settings. Many different anatomical structures are present within and surrounding the pelvic ring. Thorough assessment of all potentially violated organ systems is indicated. This includes the genitourinary, neurological, vascular, and gastrointestinal systems. The greatest danger zones for injury are central within the true pelvic cavity, in the area bounded by the sacroiliac joints posteriorly and anteriorly, and lateral to the pectineal tubercle/prominence. Four joints—two sacroiliac and two hip—can be penetrated by fragments. Typically, because of the direct nature of the trauma, there is disruption of either the anterior or posterior pelvic ring but rarely both. More central bullet pathways tend to produce more important tissue disruption. The surgeon needs to evaluate all the potential structures within the bullet pathway. Abdominal or peritoneal cavity penetration is possible. Controversy exists over whether patients with gunshots to the abdominopelvic region require acute laparotomy or can be managed expectantly.

All patients with gunshot injuries to the pelvis require consultation by a general trauma surgeon to evaluate for significant abdominal or vascular damage.[80] Patients with hemodynamic instability require appropriate and complete resuscitation, according to ATLS guidelines, a trauma team approach, and often, emergent laparotomy. Intravenous broad-spectrum antibiotics are administered immediately after the diagnosis is made. Stable patients can be evaluated carefully to determine the extent of injury and the necessary imaging studies.

Imaging Studies

Initially a high-quality anteroposterior (AP) pelvis x-ray is obtained to survey the pelvic region and to direct subsequent imaging studies. Bullet location, number of fragments, and obvious fractures are noted. Detailed CT scans with contrast are essential in the determination of (1) bullet trajectory through the pelvis, (2) bone or joint violation, (3) solid or hollow viscus injury, and (4) significant arterial bleeding (Figs. 16-15 through 16-17). Metallic artifacts may preclude precise localization of the fragments. CT reconstructions in the sagittal and coronal planes will reduce some of the metallic artifact effect, especially important in diagnosis of intra-articular fragments. Additional imaging studies should be done as appropriate. MRI of the pelvic area is probably not indicated owing to the possible deleterious effect on ferromagnetic fragments from the bullet.

Intra-articular Bullets

Most bullets that penetrate the pelvic joints will be "stopped" by the relatively dense bones. There may be associated fractures or simply intra-articular penetration by the

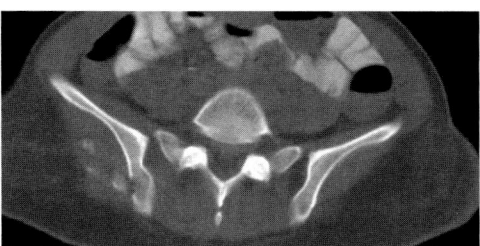

FIGURE 16-15 *CT scan axial image of extra-articular gunshot fracture to posterior ilium.*

bullets. The adverse effects of lead in contact with synovial fluid and the direct mechanical effect of the bullet fragments on the articular cartilage mandate bullet fragment removal. This has been accomplished in several reports utilizing arthrotomy, minimal surgery, or arthroscopy.[48,70,76] Regardless of the method, removal of all bullet fragments and, if possible, joint débridement and thorough joint irrigation are the goals. A brief period (24–48 hours) of antibiotics is indicated. Displaced intra-articular acetabular fractures should be anatomically reduced and stabilized. The surgeon must be aware of the possibility of unrecognized comminution and bone compression and be prepared to handle this intra-operatively.

Intestinal Contamination

Bullets may penetrate the intestinal tract before lodging in the pelvic bones. This information will be known only after a laparotomy has been performed. The question arises as to the proper method of treating a pelvic fracture that is caused by one of these contaminated bullets. It is logical to assume that if a contaminated bullet does violate a pelvic joint, especially the hip, the fracture should be débrided and the joint irrigated. However, a bullet or fragments that penetrate the extra-articular pelvic bones may not pose a serious risk of infection after treatment with a course of prophylactic antibiotics. No specific studies have addressed this problem in the pelvis; however, this has been studied in gunshots to the spine with intestinal perforation. Kumar et al.[40] reviewed patients retrospectively and found no evidence of spinal osteomyelitis without formal surgical débridement. However, a paper by Romanick et al.[67] did show that bullets that passed through the colon were associated with spine infection or meningitis in seven of the eight patients, and they advocated formal débridement for this situation. By consensus, most patients with a spinal fracture and bowel perforation do not receive surgical débridement solely for the gunshot.

Can this information be extrapolated to pelvic gunshots? Perhaps. The bone structures of the spine and pelvis are principally cancellous bone, which has an abundant vascular supply. Antibiotic concentration in this type of bone should

A, Gunshot to supra-acetabular hip region without joint involvement. The plain anteroposterior pelvic radiograph does show radiolucent defect (black arrow) *but does not clearly delineate the bullet pathway.* **B,** Corresponding CT axial image does show the bullet track through the supra-acetabular bone without extension into the hip joint.

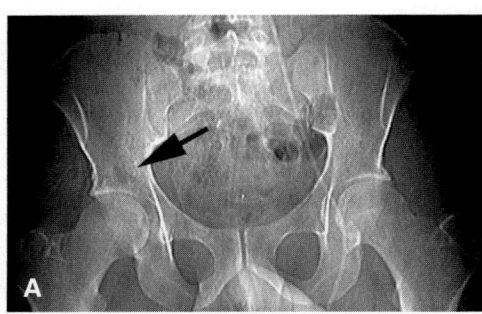 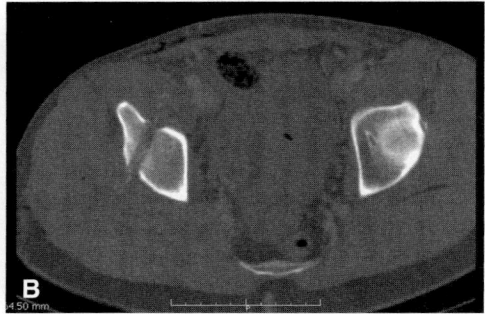

A, Multiple pelvic gunshots with comminuted fracture of femoral neck. **B,** CT scan axial image demonstrating severe fracture comminution and bone loss of femoral neck. Associated profunda femoris arterial injury was treated with primary repair. **C,** Postoperative radiograph showing surgical fixation with compression hip screw implant.

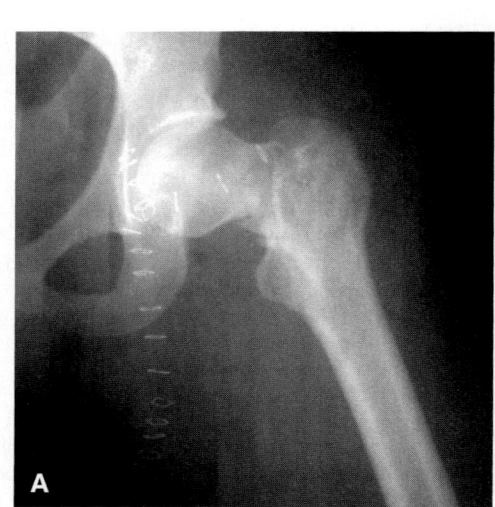 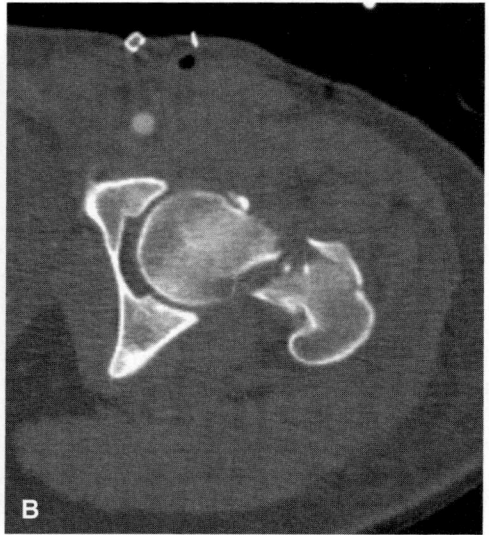

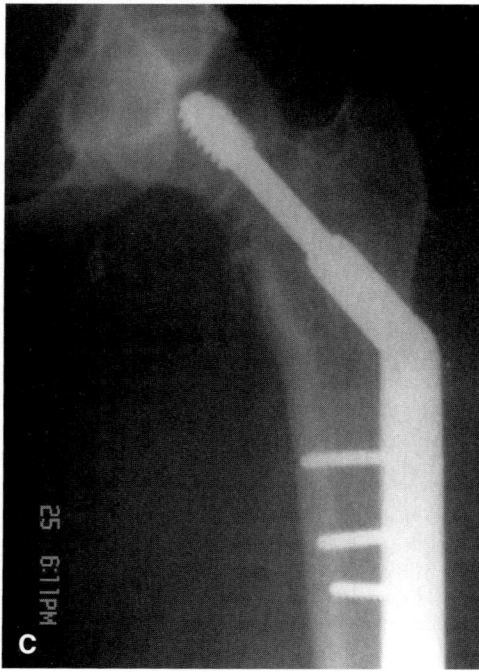

be optimal and the relative therapeutic effect maximized. Formal surgical débridement requires an extensive approach and can be fraught with anatomic hazards. Often, the pelvic cavity is highly contaminated owing to bowel injury, and the pelvic bones will be in constant contact with this bacterial load. A one-time débridement may not accomplish much, given this high level of contamination. With the higher energy (velocity) gunshots, there may be stronger indications for débridement. The surgeon must analyze the risk-benefit ratio to determine the most appropriate treatment strategy for the particular clinical situation.

Fracture Management

Pelvic fractures that are secondary to gunshots should for the most part be managed on the basis of the specific fracture pattern and not the gunshot mechanism. Nondisplaced fractures are treated with protected weight-bearing for several weeks. Disruptions of the pelvic ring are rarely caused by civilian gunshots and, if present, either indicate severe high-velocity/energy projectile injury (e.g., from a shotgun or assault rifle) or are secondary to non-gunshot trauma, which may occur subsequently to the gunshot. A skeletally unstable pelvic ring should be stabilized by one of three methods: skeletal traction, external fixation, or internal fixation. The method chosen depends on the surgeon's expertise and preference and evaluation of the degree of soft tissue and bone damage. Most cases of this magnitude should be referred to a trauma center with orthopaedic traumatologists who specialize in pelvic trauma.

FEMUR

The femur is one of the long bones more frequently affected by gunshots. The thigh is a relatively easy target because of its large size. Inexperienced shooters will attempt to aim for the "kill zone" (the area of the chest and abdomen) and instead will hit the lower extremities, often the thigh. Typical civilian handgun bullets will strike the femur and often fragment upon impact in the diaphysis and pass through the metaphyseal areas. The stress riser created in the bone cortex leads to a secondary extension to a complete fracture from the combination of weight-bearing forces and muscle contraction, especially during an attempt to "flee" from the firearm. Another mechanism occurs when the bullet imparts all the energy to the bone and leads to a fracture with significant comminution.

Long et al.[49] proposed a classification system for gunshot injuries to the femoral diaphysis based on wound size and radiographic appearance. Grade 1 injuries had entrance and exit wounds that were less than 2 cm with minimal radiographic changes. Grade 2 injuries were entrance and exit wounds less than 5 cm with greater radiographic changes. Grade 3 injuries had necrotic muscle by physical examination and extensive soft tissue disruption and segmental bone destruction on radiographs. This classification was used to guide the treatment of 100 femoral diaphyseal gunshot fractures. Although the Grade 3 fractures were treated with repeated surgical débridement and skeletal stabilization, 50 percent developed deep infection, underscoring the severity of these injuries. This classification has not been validated or reported in any other series.

History and Physical Examination

An attempt should be made to obtain as much information as possible from the history and physical examination. The patient will frequently know the type of weapon and the shooting distance. This information may also be available from law enforcement. Usually the patient will be unable to stand or walk although some may actually run a short distance before they fall to the ground.

Emphasis during the physical examination should be placed on neurologic function and vascular status. Soft tissue swelling needs to be evaluated, and the opposite thigh can be used for comparison. The wounds of entrance and exit require inspection for size and character of the wound edges. Large exit wounds greater than the diameter of the suspected bullet strongly suggest higher energy transfer to the bone and soft tissues.

Radiographic Examination

Standard radiographs include anteroposterior and lateral views of the entire femur. Additional views of the hip and knee may be necessary if the fracture is in proximity to these joints. The number of bullets or fragments, location, and distance from the femur should be noted. Fracture comminution per se is not a positive indicator of either the type of bullet or the amount of soft tissue injury. Multiple bone fragments that are displaced away from the femur can be considered a more reliable sign of energy transfer known as "secondary missiles." Bone and bullet fragments that follow the presumed path of the projectile are due to the suction created by the cavity formation and subsequent collapse that accompanies higher velocity or more destructive bullets. A full-length anteroposterior view of the opposite femur will be helpful in estimation of femoral length prior to stabilization of comminuted diaphyseal fractures.

Initial Treatment

An intravenous antibiotic appropriate for open fractures should be administered as soon as the diagnosis of gunshot fracture is made. A first- or second-generation cephalosporin would be a good choice. Displaced fractures are only satisfactorily stabilized by application of skeletal traction via proximal tibial (preferred) or distal femoral pin. An average adult requires a minimum of 15 percent of body weight, approximately 20 lbs for a 70-kg individual. Delayed application of skeletal traction will permit more bleeding within the soft tissue thigh envelope and possibly be a causative agent in development of compartment syndrome of the thigh. Nondisplaced or incomplete fractures are immobilized with splints, or if the fracture is distal, knee orthoses. The entrance and exit wounds should be sterilely dressed. Skin débridement is not indicated for small typical wounds. Hemograms should be followed serially, since it is not uncommon to see substantial drops in blood volume from internal thigh bleeding.

Definitive Treatment

Definitive treatment of the gunshot femoral fracture generally follows the established principles of open fracture management with a few exceptions. Low-energy (velocity) gunshots are treated similarly to closed femoral shaft fractures. High-energy (velocity) gunshots mandate surgical débridement of the soft tissues and bone. Fracture stabilization can be accomplished by the surgeon's choice of either external or internal fixation. Antibiotic coverage should be given as for any open fracture. Soft tissue coverage may be necessary in more severe cases involving tissue loss.

Diaphyseal and Subtrochanteric Fractures

Closed intramedullary nailing has become the treatment of choice for most closed and many open femoral fractures. Functional and clinical outcomes have been highly satisfactory, even in high-energy fractures (Fig. 16-18). Formerly, there was concern that gunshot fractures were a unique kind of open fracture and should be treated with a short course of antibiotics and delayed intramedullary nailing. It has been established through several studies that acute intramedullary nailing of low- to mid-velocity (energy) gunshot femoral fractures produces results that are essentially equivalent to intramedullary nailing of closed fractures.[60] Practical experience in major urban trauma centers has borne out the fact there is no advantage to delayed nailing. The timing of intramedullary nailing of low- to mid-velocity (energy) gunshot femoral fractures is therefore at the discretion of the surgeon and the available resources.

High-velocity (energy) fractures whether caused by handguns, shotguns, or rifles should be considered as serious, or grade III, open fractures because of the significant bone and soft tissue damage that typically occurs. Cavitation and crushing from the projectile produce large amounts of necrotic muscle and devitalized bone fragments that must be débrided. Large entrance or exit wounds are débrided and can be extended in an anatomic manner, as necessary. Thorough pulsatile lavage irrigation assists in removal of loose tissue fragments. The authors prefer to leave the original entrance and exit wounds open for delayed closure and primarily close the surgical extensions only if wound tension permits.

Numerous options exist for fracture stabilization after surgical débridement. Skeletal traction, a time-honored method of femoral immobilization, is useful when the definitive method of fracture fixation has not been determined or there is concern about the status of the soft tissues. Wound care may be difficult in skeletal traction. It will "buy time" but rarely is used for definitive treatment.

External fixation has emerged as an excellent alternative method of fracture stabilization mainly for temporary (and occasionally definitive) purposes. "Damage control" is widely practiced in the management of multiple trauma patients, including those with gunshot injuries. Acute external fixation permits rapid bone fixation, facilitates access to the soft tissues, and eases patient mobilization. Miric and Nikolic[56,59] have reported experience in the use of external fixation with massive war wounds of subtrochanteric and supracondylar femoral fractures. They noted that the final outcome was mainly due not to the skeletal injury but to the soft tissue damage. These studies indicate, at least for severe gunshot wounds, that external fixation generally achieved fracture healing but limitation of joint motion contractures and persistent nerve deficits were a common outcome.

There are some physiologic advantages of external fixation and several options for further fracture care. Occasionally, the initial external fixator can be maintained until complete fracture healing in patients in whom internal fixation is not suitable or possible. A half-pin external frame can be converted to a circular ring system, which will permit distraction osteogenesis in those fractures with large bone defects. However, most common and most appropriate for diaphyseal fractures is conversion to intramedullary nailing, if performed within 2 weeks of the acute injury. Plate fixation can also be performed after external fixation in suitable fracture patterns.

The only series of plate fixation reported for gunshot femoral fractures is the study by Necmioglu et al.[58] They had 17 patients with high-velocity gunshot fractures distributed as subtrochanteric (7), supracondylar (7), and diaphyseal (3). All patients initially had surgical débridement. Seven of the patients underwent minimally invasive percutaneous plate fixation at a mean of 1.3 days, and the remaining ten patients at a mean of 11.5 days. Follow-up averaged 25 months. Fracture union was noted at a mean of 4.4 months in 16 patients. One patient had autogenous bone grafting for a delayed union in the early group, and four in the later group required grafting at the time of plate fixation for bone loss. Eight patients had angulatory malunions (mean, 5 degrees; range, 3–8 degrees). There were two infections—one superficial and one deep. The authors concluded that plate fixation was an alternative method of fracture treatment in high-velocity femoral fractures.

Distal Femoral Fractures

Gunshots to the lower thigh may produce either extra-articular or intra-articular fractures. A series by Tornetta et al.[73] utilized anterograde intramedullary nails for distal shaft and metaphyseal fractures. The distance from the fracture to the distal locking screws was less than 5 cm in all cases, emphasizing the distal fracture location. All 38 patients healed in an average of 8.6 weeks. Many of these fractures would now be treated with a retrograde nail or newer generation distal femoral plate.

Supracondylar fractures with intra-articular extension secondary to gunshots are often deceptive (Fig. 16-19). Fracture comminution may not be appreciated on preoperative radiographs, and limited CT axial, coronal, and sagittal reconstructions are recommended to evaluate all aspects of the fractures. Both retrograde intramedullary nails and precontoured distal femoral plates with some locking capability are effective in achieving stable fixation in these fractures. The method chosen relates to the surgeon's preference and the integrity of the femoral notch region.

TIBIA

The tibia is commonly injured by gunshots. The anteromedial aspect of the leg is quite vulnerable to bullets with dissipation of kinetic energy directly into the tibia not dampened by surrounding muscles. Many gunshot victims are in an upright position at the time of wounding, and the force of body weight acts on the tibia to create more fracture displacement. The diameter of the leg is considerably less than that of the thigh, and the

FIGURE 16-18 | *Possible intermediate velocity (.357 Magnum handgun) gunshot to femoral diaphysis with extensive comminution. **A,** anteroposterior view; **B,** lateral view. Initial treatment was surgical débridement and thigh fasciotomy for an acute compartment syndrome. The fracture was placed in skeletal traction, and surgical fixation was performed 5 days later. Postoperative radiographs, **C,** anteroposterior, and **D,** lateral, at 4 months, demonstrating abundant fracture callus after internal fixation with a cephalomedullary nail.*

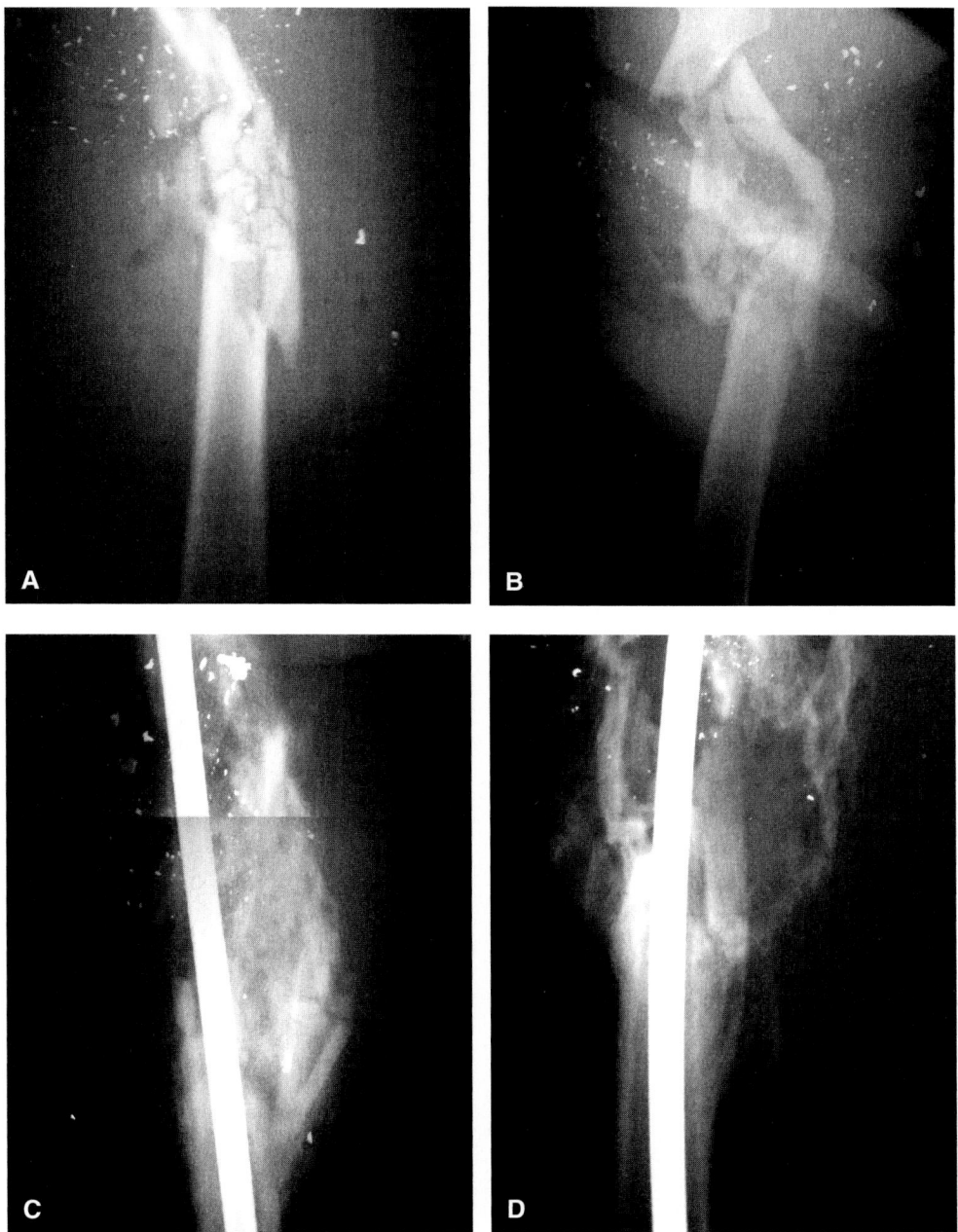

probability of neurologic deficits is greater. Nondisplaced and minimally displaced fractures are clear indications for nonoperative treatment with casting or fracture bracing. Displaced fractures are treated as the surgeon would treat other open tibial fractures. Assessment of the associated soft tissue injury in gunshot tibial fractures can be challenging. Comminuted fracture patterns are frequent and may be indicative of significant soft tissue injury. As with all other gunshots, a large exit wound is highly suggestive

of deep soft tissue disruption. The safest course of action, if there is doubt, is to surgically explore the soft tissue and bone and débride as indicated.

Leffers and Chandler[42] did a retrospective review of 41 tibial gunshot fractures at an urban trauma center. They divided the patients into three groups on the basis of the projectile velocity: low, intermediate, and high. They found that low-velocity gunshots had a characteristic fracture pattern with minimal comminution and that all other gunshots

FIGURE 16-19 | **A,** *Single through-and-through gunshot to the distal femur in an obese patient. Initial radiographs,* **A** *and* **B,** *lateral views, show what appears to be a mildly comminuted supracondylar fracture with intercondylar extension. A CT scan could not be obtained owing to the patient's body weight. At the time of arthrotomy, severe comminution was present with multiple osteochondral fractures. Fracture fixation was performed with a retrograde intramedullary nail supplemented by multiple lag screws and free wires.* **C,** *anteroposterior view;* **D,** *lateral view.*

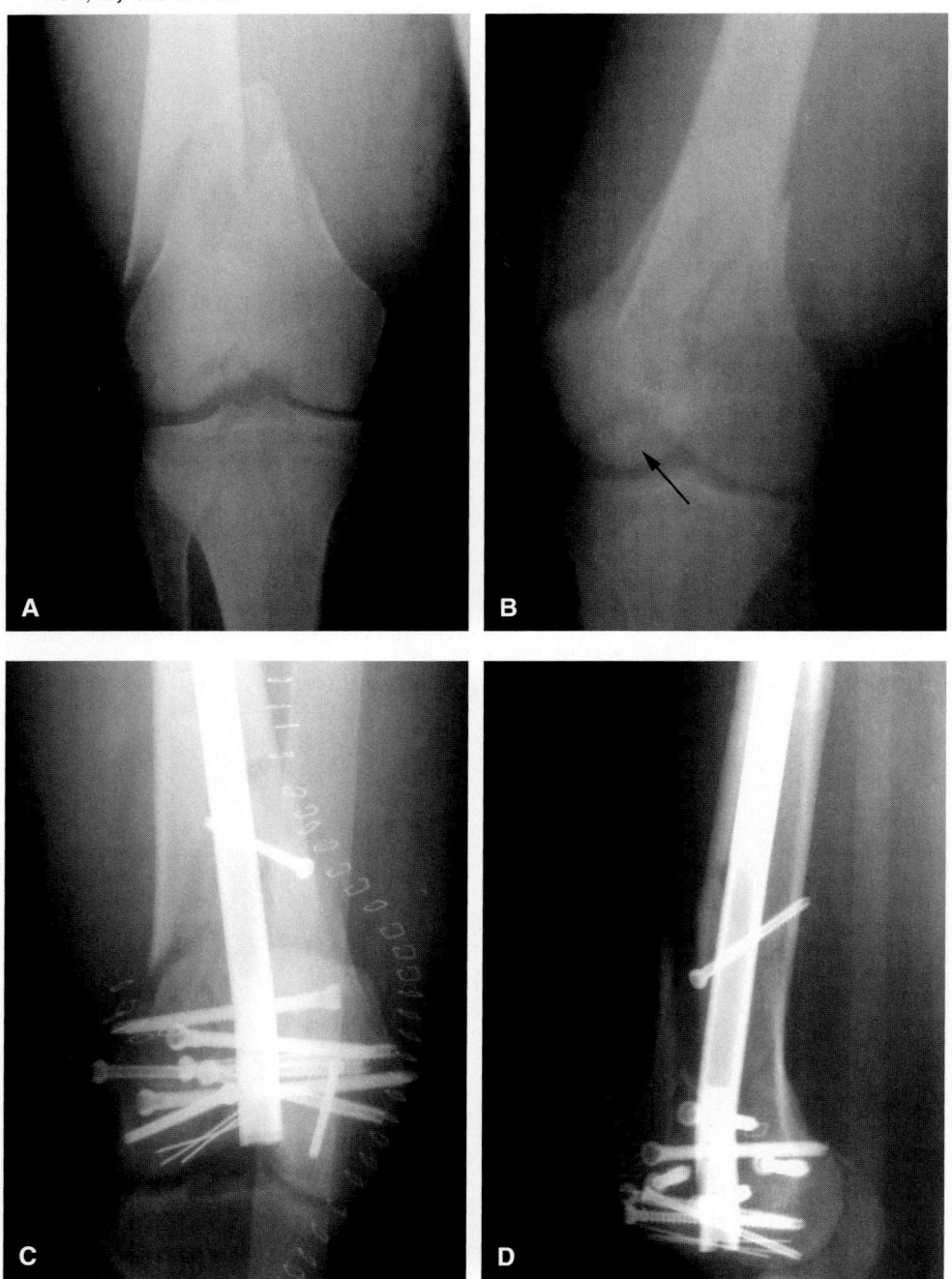

created highly comminuted fractures. Fracture treatment was usually casting, with external fixation used in a minority of patients. Increased length of hospital stay, time to union, and morbidity were associated with the intermediate- and high-velocity groups. Both nonunions in this series occurred in patients with low-velocity fractures.

Displaced gunshot fractures of the tibial diaphysis have been treated with various forms of fixation. There are no specific prospective or retrospective studies of the treatment of gunshot fractures of the tibia with intramedullary fixation. Most major series of tibial intramedullary nailing have included a few cases of gunshots (of low velocity), with no apparent difference in outcome when compared with other open fractures in the series.

Direct evidence in the literature is lacking for the specific results of internal fixation of gunshot tibial fractures. The reported clinical experience with the other mechanisms of injury for open tibial fractures should be a reasonable approximation of the anticipated results with gunshot fractures.

External fixation has been reported recently to be clinically effective in the more severe tibial fractures, especially those involving bone loss. Circular external fixation, flap coverage, and distraction osteogenesis have been utilized to reestablish bone length and continuity with minimal morbidity. Circular external fixation generally permits early weight-bearing with its attendant advantages.

Atesalp et al.[4] reported on seven patients with comminuted gunshot tibial fractures managed with circular external fixation and compression-distraction technique. All fractures united at an average of 3.5 months without infection. These were low-velocity injuries and would be anticipated to unite in this time frame. The major problems associated with circular external fixation are pin track infection and the requirement for additional surgery at the docking site in fractures that have required distraction osteogenesis. It remains a suitable alternative in any displaced fracture.

Intra-articular Fractures

Gunshot fractures of the proximal and distal tibia with intra-articular involvement are unusual. Unfortunately, in the author's experience, there can be a great deal of loss of articular surface and metaphyseal bone. Acute arthrotomy or arthroscopy is indicated for débridement of bone fragments and any lead pieces that are loose or in contact with the joint fluid. However, any fracture fragments with articular cartilage should be retained for definitive joint fixation. Temporary bridging external fixation will maintain fracture length and position. When the soft tissues permit, anatomic restoration of the articular surface is the goal but may not be possible. Bone defects should be filled with either autogenous bone or bone substitutes. Stable internal fixation alone or the combination of limited internal fixation and circular external fixation is recommended. Some degree of early joint motion is preferable for surface lubrication and nutrition. Fracture healing is achieved in the majority of patients, but there is a high incidence of traumatic arthrosis due to irreparable articular cartilage damage and poor functional outcome in the more severe injuries.

Yildiz et al.[78] reported their retrospective results in 13 patients with high-velocity gunshot fractures of the tibial plafond. There were eleven IIIA and two IIIB open fractures. Treatment consisted of débridement, primary wound closure, and Ilizarov fixation. Intra-articular fractures were manipulated indirectly by frame distraction or directly by Kirschner wires; however, no screw or plate fixation was used. Three patients required distraction osteogenesis for bone loss. All fractures healed with an average tibio-talar motion of 30 degrees. Four patients had radiographic arthritis at a mean follow-up of 38.4 months. Pin track infection was seen in the majority of patients. Superficial wound infection occurred in two patients. This group of fractures was probably incorrectly classified in terms of the degree of joint involvement, since it is quite uncommon, in the author's experience, for intra-articular distal tibial fractures to not require some limited internal fixation to restore joint congruity.

FIGURE 16-20 *Low-velocity tangential gunshot to the dorsal foot with severe comminution and bone loss of multiple metatarsals.* **A,** *anteroposterior view;* **B,** *lateral view.*

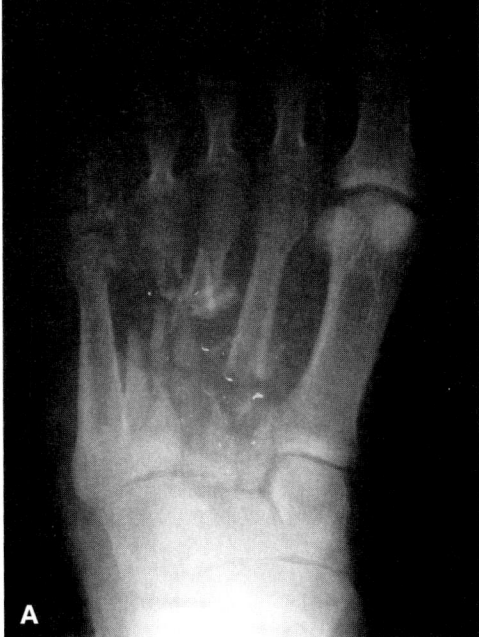
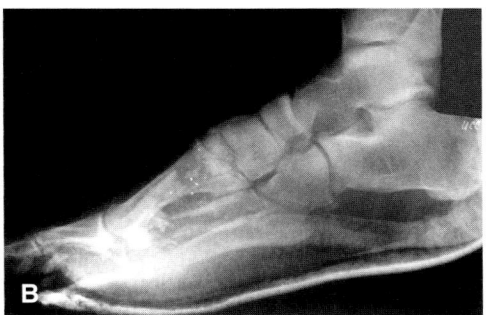

FOOT

Low-velocity gunshot wounds to the foot are often self-inflicted, accidentally or intentionally. Fractures are usually comminuted with minimal displacement. There are many joints within the foot and they are often violated by the gunshot. In most cases the soft tissues do not sustain significant damage. Some gunshots, however, have such a trajectory through the foot that there can be bone loss and severe comminution (Fig. 16-20).

Bullet fragments are not well tolerated in the foot and interfere with weight-bearing and shoe wear. This is one of the few surgical indications to "take the bullet out" especially if the fragment(s) are in a superficial location.

The treatment for most low-velocity gunshot fractures to the foot should follow the principles for closed foot fractures. A variable period of immobilization in a cast, weight-bearing if possible, will achieve fracture healing in a relatively short period of time. Stiffness of the articulations that were violated by the gunshot is fairly common but rarely disabling. Higher grade injuries with bone loss and skeletal deformity require appropriate surgical reconstruction and possibly soft tissue coverage.[22]

Boucree et al.[10] reviewed 101 patients with gunshot wounds of the foot, with 81 fractures. Infection was encountered in approximately 12 percent, equally divided between low-velocity and high-velocity or shotgun injuries. From this experience they recommended a course of intravenous antibiotic for 72 hours for low-velocity gunshot and shotgun injuries. They suggested that high-velocity gunshot and shotgun injuries receive surgical débridement and intravenous antibiotics.

REFERENCES

1. Adani, R.; Delcroix, L.; Innocenti, M.; et al. Reconstruction of large posttraumatic skeletal defects of the forearm by vascularized free fibular graft. Microsurgery 24:423–429, 2004.
2. Armine, A.R.C.; Sugar, O. Repair of severed brachial plexus. JAMA 235:1039, 1976.
3. Ashbell, T.S.; Kleinert, H.E.; Kutz, J.E. Vascular injuries about the elbow. Clin Orthop 50:107, 1967.
4. Atesalp, A.S.; Komurcu, M.; Demiralp, B.; et al. Treatment of close-range, low-velocity gunshot fractures of tibia and femur diaphysis with consecutive compression-distraction technique: A report of 11 cases. J Surg Orthop Adv 13:112–118, 2004.
5. Attias, N.; Lehman, R.E.; Bodell, L.S.; et al. Surgical management of a long segmental defect of the humerus using a cylindrical titanium mesh cage and plates: A case report. J Orthop Trauma 19:211–216, 2005.
6. Bartlett, C.S.; Helfet, D.L.; Hausman, M.R.; et al. Ballistics and gunshot wounds: Effects on musculoskeletal tissues. J Am Acad Orthop Surg 8:21–36, 2000.
7. Bilic, R.; Kolundzic, R.; Bicanic, G.; et al. Elbow arthrodesis after war injuries. Mil Med 170:164–166, 2005.
8. Bleckner, S.A. Proximal ulna shaft fractures and associated compartment syndromes. A J Orthop 30:703–707, 2001.
9. Borman, K.R.; Snyder, W.H.; Weigeit, J.A. Civilian arterial trauma of the upper extremity: An 11-year experience in 267 patients. Am J Surg 148:796, 1984.
10. Boucree, J.B., Jr.; Gabriel, R.A.; Lezine-Hanna, J.T. Gunshot wounds to the foot. Orthop Clin North Am 26:191–197, 1995.
11. Brien, W.; Gellman, H.; Becker, V.; et al. Management of upper extremity fractures in patients with brachial plexus injuries. J Bone Joint Surg Am 72:1208, 1990.
12. Brooks, D.M. Open wounds of the brachial plexus. J Bone Joint Surg Br 31:17, 1949.
13. Burkhalter, W.E.; Butler, B.; Metz, W.; et al. Experiences with delayed primary closure of war wounds of the hand in Vietnam. J Bone Joint Surg Am 50:945, 1968.
14. Burkhalter, W.; Calkins, M.S.; Reyes, F. Traumatic segmental bone defects in the upper extremity: Treatment with exposed grafts of corticocancellous bone. J Bone Joint Surg Am 69:19–27, 1987.
15. Chang, J.; Page, R. Reconstruction of hand soft-tissue defects: Alternatives to the radial forearm fasciocutaneous flap. J Hand Surg 31A:847–856, 2006.
16. Chappell, J.E.; Mitra, A.; Walsh, L.; et al. Gunshot wounds to the hand: Management and economic impact. Ann Plast Surg 42:418–423, 1999.
17. Cho, M.S.; Warme, W.J. Arthroscopic treatment of a transarticular low-velocity gunshot wound using tractoscopy. Arthroscopy 18:532–537, 2002.
18. Compton, R.; Bucknell, A. Resection arthroplasty for comminuted olecranon fractures. Orthop Rev 18:189–192, 1989.
19. Davila, S.; Mikulic, D.; Davila, N.J.; et al. Treatment of war injuries of the shoulder with external fixators. Mil Med 170:414–417, 2005.
20. Dean, G.S.; Holliger, E.H., IV; Urbaniak, J.R. Elbow allograft for reconstruction of the elbow with massive bone loss: Long-term results. Clin Orthop Rel Res 341:12–22, 1997.
21. Dickey, R.L.; Barnes, B.C.; Kearns, R.J.; et al. Efficacy of antibiotics in low-velocity gunshot fractures. J Orthop Trauma 3:6–10, 1989.
22. Durkin, R.C.; Coughlin, R.R. Management of gunshot wounds to the foot. Injury 28:6–10, 1997.
23. Elstrom, J.A.; Pankovich, A.M.; Egwele, R. Extra-articular low-velocity gunshot fractures of the radius and ulna. J Bone Joint Surg Am 60:335, 1978.
24. Evans, G.R.D.; Luethke, R.W. A latissimus/scapula myo-osseous free flap based on the subscapular artery used for elbow reconstruction. Ann Plast Surg 30:175, 1993.
25. Finkelstein, E.A.; Corso, P.S.; Miller, T.R.; et al. Incidence and Economic Burden of Injuries in the United States. New York, Oxford University Press, 2006. [As quoted in The Economic Costs of Injuries. Available at: www.cdc.gov/ncipc/factsheets/Cost_of_Injury.htm.]

26. Georgiadis, G.M.; DeSilva, S.P. Reconstruction of skeletal defects in the forearm after trauma: Treatment with cement spacer and delayed cancellous bone grafting. J Trauma 38:910, 1995.

27. Gomez, W.; Putnam, M.D.; Rosenwasser, M.P.; et al. Management of severe hand trauma with a mini–external fixateur. Orthopedics 10:601–610, 1987.

28. Gonzalez, M.H.; Hall, M.; Hall, R.F. Low-velocity gunshot wounds of the proximal phalanx: Treatment by early stable fixation. J Hand Surg 23A:150–155, 1998.

29. Gonzalez, M.H.; Hall, M.; Hall, R.F. Low-velocity gunshot wounds of the metacarpal: Treatment by early stable fixation and bone grafting. J Hand Surg 18A:267–270, 1993.

30. Gutowski, K.A.; Kiehn, M.W.; Mitra, A. Fracture management of civilian gunshot wounds to the hand. Plast Reconstr Surg 115:478–481, 2005.

31. Hardin, W.D.; O'Connell, R.C.; Adinolfi, M.F.; et al. Traumatic arterial injuries of the upper extremity: Determinants of disability. Am J Surg 150:266, 1985.

32. Heitmann, C.; Erdmann, D.; Levin, L.S. Treatment of segmental defects of the humerus with an osteoseptocutaneous fibular transplant. J Bone Joint Surg Am 84:2216–2223, 2002.

33. Helber, M.U.; Ulrich, C. External fixation in forearm shaft fractures. Injury 31(Suppl 1):45–47, 2000.

34. Howland, W.S., Jr.; Ritchey, S.J. Gunshot fractures in civilian practice: An evaluation of the results of limited surgical treatment. J Bone Joint Surg Am 53:47–55, 1971.

35. Joshi, A.; Labbe, M.; Lindsey, R.W. Humeral fracture secondary to civilian gunshot injury. Injury 29 (Suppl 1):SA13–SA17, 1998.

36. Jupiter, J.B.; Gerhard, H.J.; Guerrero, J.; et al. Treatment of segmental defects of the radius with use of the vascularized osteoseptocutaneous fibular autogenous graft. J Bone Joint Surg Am 79:542–550, 1997.

37. Kim, D.H.; Kam, A.C.; Chandika, P.; et al. Surgical management and outcome in patients with radial nerve lesions. Neurosurg 95:573–583, 2001.

38. Kim, D.H.; Kam, A.C.; Chandika, P.; et al. Surgical management and outcomes in patients with median nerve lesions. J Neurosurg 95:548–594, 2001.

39. Knapp, T.P.; Patzakis, M.J.; Lee, J.; et al. Comparison of intravenous and oral antibiotic therapy in the treatment of fractures caused by low-velocity gunshots: A prospective, randomized study of infection rates. J Bone Joint Surg Am 79:1590, 1997.

40. Kumar, A.; Wood, G.W., II; Whittle, A.P. Low-velocity gunshot injuries of the spine with abdominal viscous injury. J Orthop Trauma 12:514–517, 1998.

41. Lagarde, L.A. Can a septic bullet infect a gunshot wound? N Y Med J 56:458–465, 1892.

42. Leffers, D.; Chandler, R.W. Tibial fractures associated with civilian gunshot injuries. J Trauma 25:1059–1064, 1985.

43. Leffert, R.D. Brachial Plexus Injuries. New York, Churchill-Livingstone, 1985.

44. Lenihan, M.R.; Brien, W.W.; Gellman, H.; et al. Fractures of the forearm resulting from low-velocity gunshot wounds. J Orthop Trauma 6:32, 1992.

45. Leonard, M.H. Solution of lead by synovial fluid. Clin Orthop 64:255, 1969.

46. Lerner, A.; Stein, H.; Calif, E. Unilateral hinged external fixation frame for elbow compression arthrodesis: The stepwise attainment of a stable 90-degree flexion position: A case report. J Orthop Trauma 19:52–55, 2005.

47. Levy, A.D.; Abbott, R.M.; Mallak, C.T.; et al. Virtual autopsy: Preliminary experience in high-velocity gunshot wound victims. Radiology 240:522–528, 2006.

48. Long, W.T.; Brien, E.W.; Boucree, J.B., Jr.; et al. Management of civilian gunshot injuries to the hip. Orthop Clin North Am 26:123–131, 1995.

49. Long, W.T.; Chang, W.; Brien, E.W. Grading system for gunshot injuries to the femoral diaphysis in civilians. Clin Orthop Rel Res 408:92–100, 2003.

50. Luce, E.A.; Griffen, W.O. Shotgun injuries of the upper extremity. J Trauma 18:487, 1978.

51. MacAusland, W.R.; Wyman, E.T. Fractures of the adult elbow. Instr Course Lect 24:169, 1975.

52. Mandrella, B.; Abebaw, T.H.; Hersi, O.N. [Defect fractures of the upper arm and their treatment in difficult circumstances: Three case reports from Ethiopian and Somalian provincial hospitals.] Unfallchirurg 100:154–158, 1997.

53. McAuliffe, J.A.; Burkhalter, W.E.; Ouellette, E.A.; et al. Compression plate arthrodesis of the elbow. J Bone Joint Surg Br 74:300–304, 1992.

54. McHenry, T.P.; Holcomb, J.B.; Aoki, N.; et al. Fractures with major vascular injuries from gunshot wounds: Implications of surgical sequence. J Trauma 53:717–721, 2002.

55. McNamara, J.; Brief, D.K.; Stremple, J.F.; et al. Management of fractures with associated arterial injury in combat casualties. J Trauma 13:17, 1973.

56. Miric, D.M.; Bumbasirevic, M.Z.; Senohradski, K.K.; et al. Pelvifemoral external fixation for the treatment of open fractures of the proximal femur caused by firearms. Acta Orthop Belg 68:37–41, 2002.

57. Moed, B.R.; Fakhouri, A.J. Compartment syndrome after low-velocity gunshot wounds to the forearm. J Orthop Trauma 5:134, 1991.

58. Necmioglu, N.S.; Subasi, M.; Kavikci, C. Minimally invasive plate osteosynthesis in the treatment of femur fractures due to gunshot injuries. Acta Orthop Traumatol Turc 39:142–149, 2005.

59. Nikolic, D.K.; Jovanovic, Z.; Turkovic, G.; et al. Supracondylar missile fractures of the femur. Injury 33:161–166, 2002.

60. Nowotarski, P.; Brumback, R.J. Immediate interlocking nailing of fractures of the femur caused by low- to mid-velocity gunshots. J Orthop Trauma 8:134–141, 1994.

61. Okcu, G.; Aktuglu, K. [Management of shotgun-induced open fractures of the humerus with Ilizarov external fixator.] Ulus Travma Acil Cerrahi Derg 11:23–28, 2005.

62. Omer, G.E. Injuries to the nerves of the upper extremity. J Bone Joint Surg Am 56:1615, 1974.

63. Ouellette, E.A. Gunshot wounds to the upper extremity. Video J Orthop 10: , 1995.

64. Ring, D.; Allende, C.; Jafarnia, K.; et al. Ununited diaphyseal forearm fractures with segmental defects: Plate fixation and autogenous cancellous bone-grafting. J Bone Joint Surg Am 86:2440–2445, 2004.

65. Ring, D.; Jupiter, J.B.; Quintero, J.; et al. Atrophic ununited diaphyseal fractures of the humerus with a bony defect: Treatment by wave-plate osteosynthesis. J Bone Joint Surg Br 82:867–871, 2000.

66. Ring, D.; Jupiter, J.B.; Toh, S. Transarticular bony defects after trauma and sepsis: Arthrodesis using vascularized fibular transfer. Plast Reconstr Surg 104:426–434, 1999.

67. Romanick, P.C.; Smith, T.K.; Kopaniky, D.R.; et al. Infection about the spine associated with low-velocity-missile injury to the abdomen. J Bone Joint Surg Am 67:1195–1201, 1985.

68. Seghrouchni, H.; Martin, D.; Pistre, V.; et al. [Composite scapular flap for reconstruction of complex humeral tissue loss: A case report.] Rev Chir Orthop Reparatrice Appar Mot 89:158–162, 2003.

69. Simpson, B.M.; Wilson, R.H.; Grant, R.E. Antibiotic therapy in gunshot wound injuries. Clin Orthop Rel Res 408:82–85, 2003.

70. Singleton, S.B.; Joshi, A.; Schwartz, M.A.; et al. Arthroscopic bullet removal from the acetabulum. Arthroscopy 21:360–364, 2005.

71. Skaggs, D.L.; Hale, J.M.; Buggay, S.; et al. Use of a hybrid external fixator for a severely comminuted juxta-articular fracture of the distal humerus. J Orthop Trauma 12:439–442, 1998.

72. Stahl, S.; Rosenberg, N. Digital nerve repair by autogenous vein graft in high-velocity gunshot wounds. Mil Med 164:603–604, 1999.

73. Tornetta, P., III; Tiburzi, D. Anterograde interlocked nailing of distal femoral fractures after gunshot wounds. J Orthop Trauma 8:220–227, 1994.

74. Vennemann, B.; Grosse Perdekamp, M.; Kneubuehl, B.P.; et al. Gunshot-related displacement of skin particles and bacteria from the exit region back into the bullet path. Int J Legal Med 121(2):105–111, 2007.

75. Watson, N.; Songcharoen, G.P. Lead synovitis in the hand: A case report. J Hand Surg [Br] 10:423–424, 1985.

76. Williams, M.S.; Hutcheson, R.L.; Miller, A.R. A new technique for removal of intra-articular bullet fragments from the femoral head. Bull Hosp Joint Dis 56:107–110, 1997.

77. Wilson, R.H. Gunshots to the hand and upper extremity. Clin Orthop Rel Res 408:133–144, 2003.

78. Yildiz, C.; Atesalp, A.S.; Demiralp, B.; et al. High-velocity gunshot wounds of the tibial plafond managed with Ilizarov external fixation: A report of 13 cases. J Orthop Trauma 17:421–429, 2003.

79. Zellweger, R.; Hess, F.; Nicol, A.; et al. An analysis of 124 surgically managed brachial artery injuries. Am J Surg 188:240–245, 2004.

80. Zura, R.D.; Bosse, M.J. Current treatment of gunshot wounds to the hip and pelvis. Clin Orthop Rel Res 408:110–114, 2003.

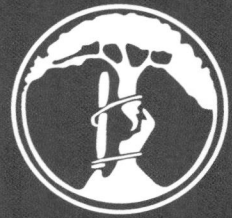

CHAPTER 17

Pathologic Fractures

Alan M. Levine, M.D. and Albert J. Aboulafia, M.D.

Pathologic fractures occur as a result of an underlying process that weakens the mechanical properties of bone. The causes of pathologic fracture include neoplastic and non-neoplastic conditions. The most common non-neoplastic causes of pathologic fracture are osteoporosis and metabolic bone disease.

Primary bone tumors, however, both benign and malignant, may present initially with pathologic fracture. Benign lesions that may present initially with pathologic fracture include solitary bone cysts, aneurysmal bone cysts (ABCs), nonossifying fibromas (NOFs), fibrous dysplasia, and giant-cell tumor (Fig. 17-1). Pathologic fracture may be the initial manifestation in as many as 10 percent of patients with primary malignant bone tumors such as osteogenic sarcoma and chondrosarcoma, although pain (without fracture) is the most common symptom. The treatment of pathologic fractures of long bones resulting from benign tumors depends on the histology and stage of the tumor. In active, nonaggressive lesions such as NOF and unicameral bone cyst (UBC) (stage 2), fracture healing often occurs in a fashion similar to that for nonpathologic conditions even before or certainly after local control of the tumor has been achieved. In most bone cyst cases, local tumor control can be accomplished with intralesional procedures such as curettage. Even in aggressive (stage 3) benign tumors (giant-cell tumor, ABCs), spontaneous fracture healing may occur initially. However, when surgery is performed in order to obtain local control and especially with the use of adjuvant treatments to enhance local control, healing of the large osseous defects usually requires skeletal reconstruction. The treatment of pathologic fractures resulting from primary malignant bone tumors is integrated into the definitive treatment of the tumor, which most commonly requires resection of the bone so fracture healing is not an issue (Fig. 17-2). The focus of this chapter is on the management of pathologic fractures resulting primarily from metastatic tumors and myeloma and not primary tumors. Although myeloma is technically a primary bone tumor, it is a systemic disease, and as such, the orthopaedic management of pathologic fractures resulting from myeloma is more closely related to metastatic lesions than primary bony tumors. This section emphasizes the differences in biologic behavior of pathologic and traumatic fractures. These biologic differences necessitate a treatment approach intended to maximize benefit and minimize complications for the patient with metastatic bone disease.

Neoplastic causes include metastases as well as primary benign and malignant tumors. Skeletal metastases are the most common neoplastic cause of pathologic fracture. They may either occur in the setting of a patient's known cancer diagnosis or as the first manifestation of cancer. Failure to recognize tumor as the underlying cause of fracture can result in either initial inappropriate treatment or failure of the fixation modality (Fig. 17-3).

With the utilization of newer chemotherapeutic regimens and targeted biologic agents resulting in prolonged survival of many patients with solid tumors, the absolute incidence of symptomatic bone metastasis has increased over the last decade. However, the relative incidence of pathologic fractures secondary to metastatic disease has begun to decrease with the use of bisphosphonates.[17,45,133] Initially the data on the use of bisphosphonates in metastatic disease of bone were restricted to patients with breast cancer and myeloma, but more recent studies have extended their use to all tumors, even those with blastic metastases as well as renal cell carcinoma. Fractures that are pathologic and result from the involvement of bone by metastatic tumor are biologically different from fractures resulting from non-neoplastic conditions such as trauma. Therefore the treatment principles for pathologic fractures resulting from metastatic lesions differ from those for fractures that result from trauma (Table 17-1). The assumption that a pathologic fracture resulting from neoplasm can be treated in a similar fashion to nonpathologic fractures often results in a less than satisfactory outcome for the patient with a neoplastic pathologic fracture (Fig. 17-4). Moreover the goal of treating a fracture of traumatic origin is to maximize the potential for fracture healing while minimizing the complications. The goal of treating pathologic fractures is to return the patient as rapidly as possible to maximal function, thus maximizing quality of life. When appropriately treated, many patients may not heal their fracture during their remaining life span but will still function adequately.

The skeleton is the third most common site of involvement by metastatic disease (after lung and liver), in terms of both frequency and the complications arising from metastatic involvement. The incidence of tumors metastatic to bone is far greater than the incidence of primary malignant bone tumors. Therefore, fractures from metastatic lesions are more common than those from primary tumors. Overall, symptomatic skeletal metastases develop in approximately 20 percent of

453

FIGURE 17-1   *This female patient presented with a low-impact fracture to her dominant wrist **(A, B)** and was immobilized until the fracture healed **(C)**. It was thought to be a cyst, and the patient underwent curettage and grafting with allograft **(D)**. At that surgery the diagnosis of giant-cell tumor was made.*

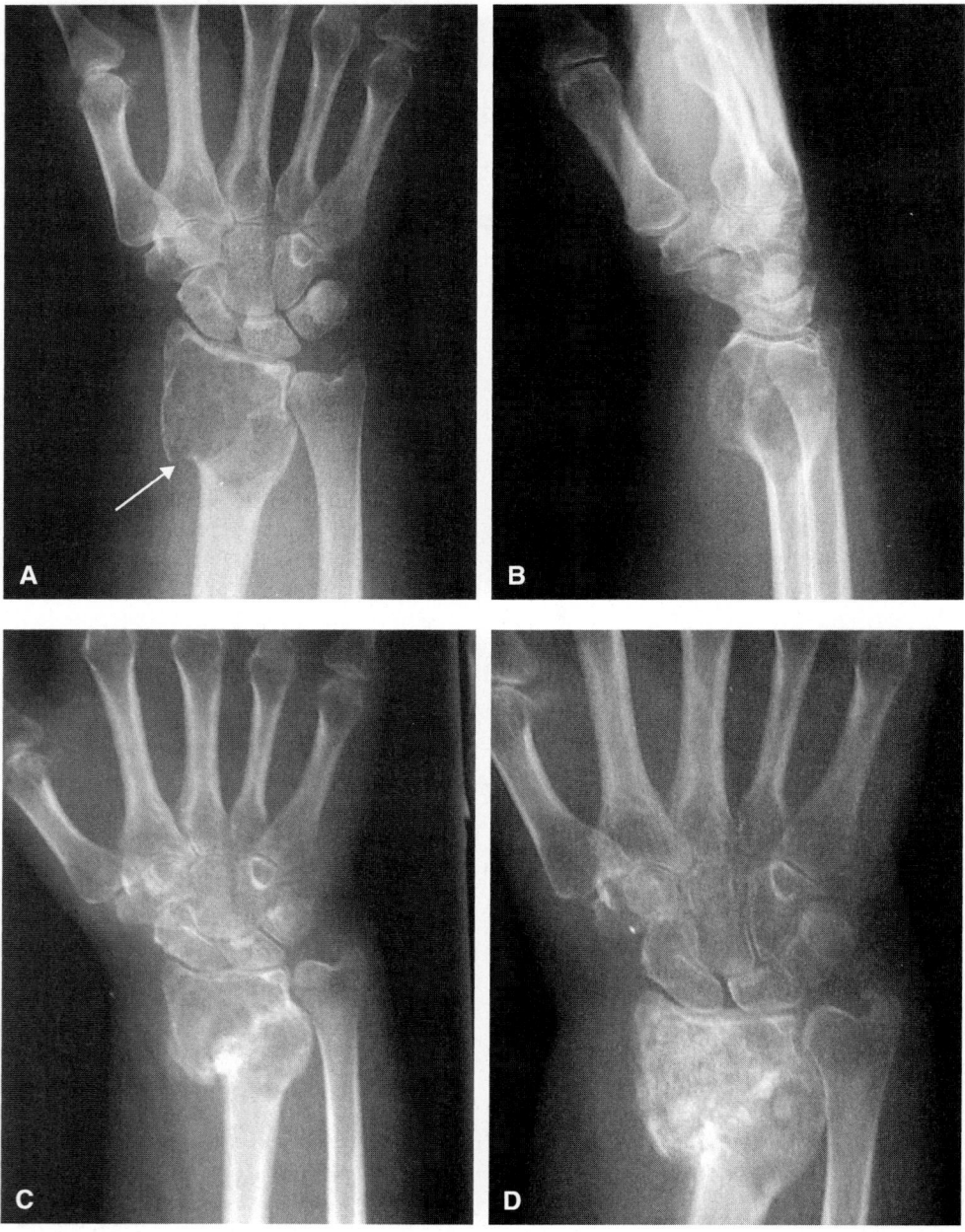

(Continued)

patients with metastatic disease from solid tumors,[59] although autopsy series have suggested that the overall incidence of skeletal metastases in this patient population is closer to 70 percent.[154] Therefore, it is apparent that many patients who die of cancer have skeletal metastases that remain asymptomatic and require no treatment. The incidence of skeletal metastasis varies according to tumor type. The tumors that most commonly develop skeletal metastasis include those from the breast,[47] prostate,[22,24] thyroid, kidney, and lung. Autopsy series have shown rates of bone metastasis may be as high as 80 percent in breast cancer, 85 percent in carcinoma of the prostate, 50 percent in thyroid carcinoma, 44 percent in lung carcinoma, and 30 percent in renal cell carcinoma.[23] Although patients with any type of neoplasm can develop bone metastasis, more than 75 percent of those seen are from breast, prostate, lung, or kidney.[29] However, bone metastases can develop in almost any tumor histology, including gastrointestinal and genitourinary carcinomas, melanoma, and even chordoma.[1,138]

The time from initial diagnosis of the primary tumor to the development of the initial osseous metastasis can vary

FIGURE 17-1 *(Continued)* **(E),** *The patient then had a massive recurrence with both bone and soft tissue infiltration necessitating a resection of the distal radius and soft tissues including the extensors of the thumb. She required tendon transfer and wrist fusion for reconstruction but remains free of disease.*

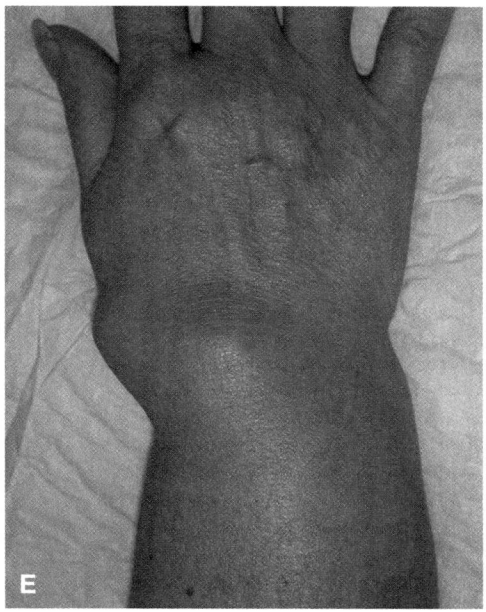

greatly and often has prognostic significance. In some patients bone metastasis may be the first evidence of recurrent disease, even after a prolonged disease-free interval. This is especially true of patients with breast, thyroid cancer, or renal carcinoma whose first sign of relapse may be a symptomatic bone lesion 10 to 15 years after the diagnosis of the primary tumor (Fig. 17-5). Survival rates for patients with osseous metastatic disease depend on several factors including extent of visceral disease, disease-free interval, response to chemotherapy/radiation, and tumor histology.[24,47] Overall median survival span for patients with bone metastasis from follicular thyroid carcinoma is 48 months, prostate 40 months, breast 24 months, and for melanoma and lung 6 months.[30] In patients with breast cancer the mean survival length of those with only bone metastases approaches 30 months but in those who have visceral involvement and osseous metastasis, median survival is only 18 months.[125,136,182] The extent of bone metastasis has prognostic importance as well. Patients may survive for many years who present with a solitary renal metastasis. For those patients, there may be some role for wide excision.[60,172] But survival is shortened with presentation of multiple lesions or pathologic fracture.[58]

The spread of cancer is usually by one of two mechanisms: contiguous extension or hematogenous dissemination. More than 100 years ago Paget recognized that tumor metastasis involved more than simply the random act of deposition of tumor in a site distant from the primary.[132] He proposed the "seed and soil" hypothesis, recognizing

FIGURE 17-2 **A,** *This anteroposterior radiograph demonstrates a pathologic fracture of the proximal humerus in a 62-year-old woman. Needle biopsy was nondiagnostic, demonstrating only hematoma, but the open biopsy was interpreted as a leiomyosarcoma.* **B,** *En bloc resection and prosthetic replacement adequately dealt with the pathologic fracture through this tumor.*

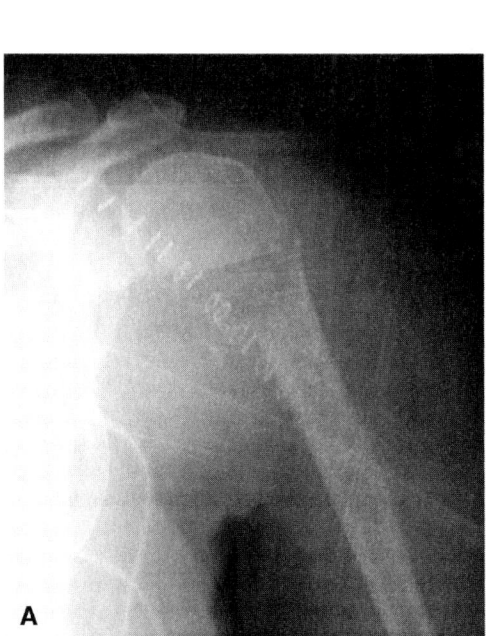
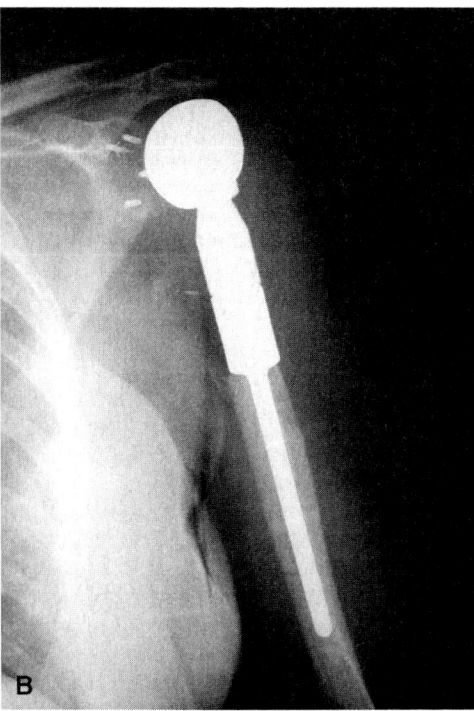

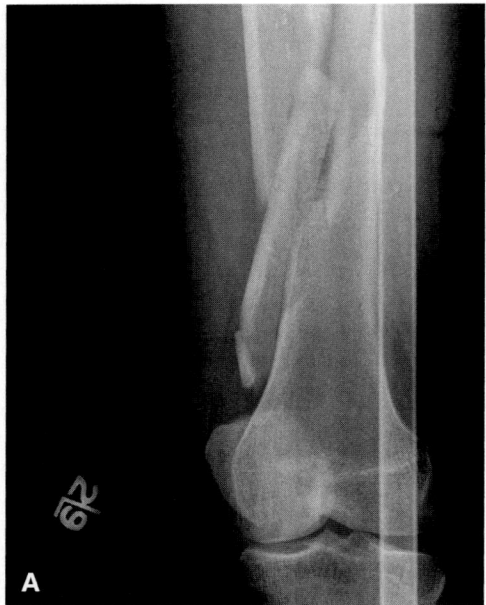

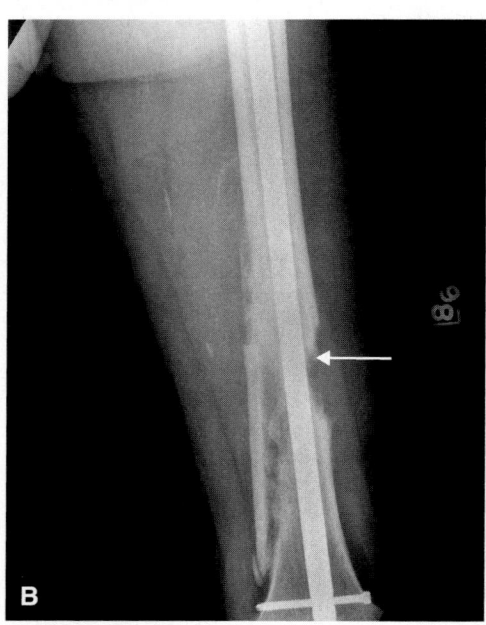

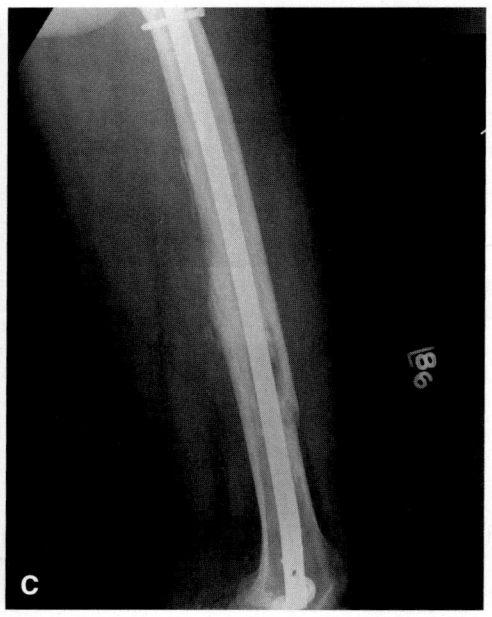

FIGURE 17-3 *Failure to differentiate a pathologic fracture from a traumatic fracture can have marked consequences for the patient. This patient sustained a severely comminuted femoral fracture with relatively low impact* **(A)**, *and a small lesion in his chest was overlooked at the time of admission. At follow-up 1 month after surgery the erosion of the cortex was also not recognized* **(B, C)** (arrow).

(Continued)

that properties inherent to the tumor and the host influenced the development of a metastatic focus. Since then a variety of factors have been identified that influence where bony metastases occur. Three basic but complex processes are involved in the development of skeletal metastasis. The first involves the ability of the tumor cells to leave the primary site and travel to a distant site. The initial steps involved in this process include the loss of cell contact inhibition, and the production of tumor angiogenesis factor and angiogenin. The modulation of cell contact inhibition is regulated by cell adhesion molecules (CAMs).[123,130] CAMs regulate the tumor cells, adhesion properties. For tumor cells to separate from the primary site CAM expression must be down-regulated.[84] Later CAM expression must take place for tumor cells, to accumulate at a distant site.[127] In addition to loss of cell contact inhibition, tumor cells must have a route of gaining access into the vascular or lymphatic system in order to metastasize. With the production of tumor angiogenesis factor and angiogenin by the tumor cells, neovascularization takes place. Tumor cells ultimately cross the vascular basement membrane and gain access to the lymphatic and venous systems. Second, the anatomic properties of the host must favor metastatic deposits at selected sites. The most common sites of skeletal metastasis include the spine, pelvis, proximal femur, and

FIGURE 17-3 *(Continued) By 12 months from the time of surgery the destruction of the cortex was markedly increased **(D, E),** and the mass in the chest was evident. A femoral resection and prosthetic reconstruction were done to decrease pain and restore function **(F, G).***

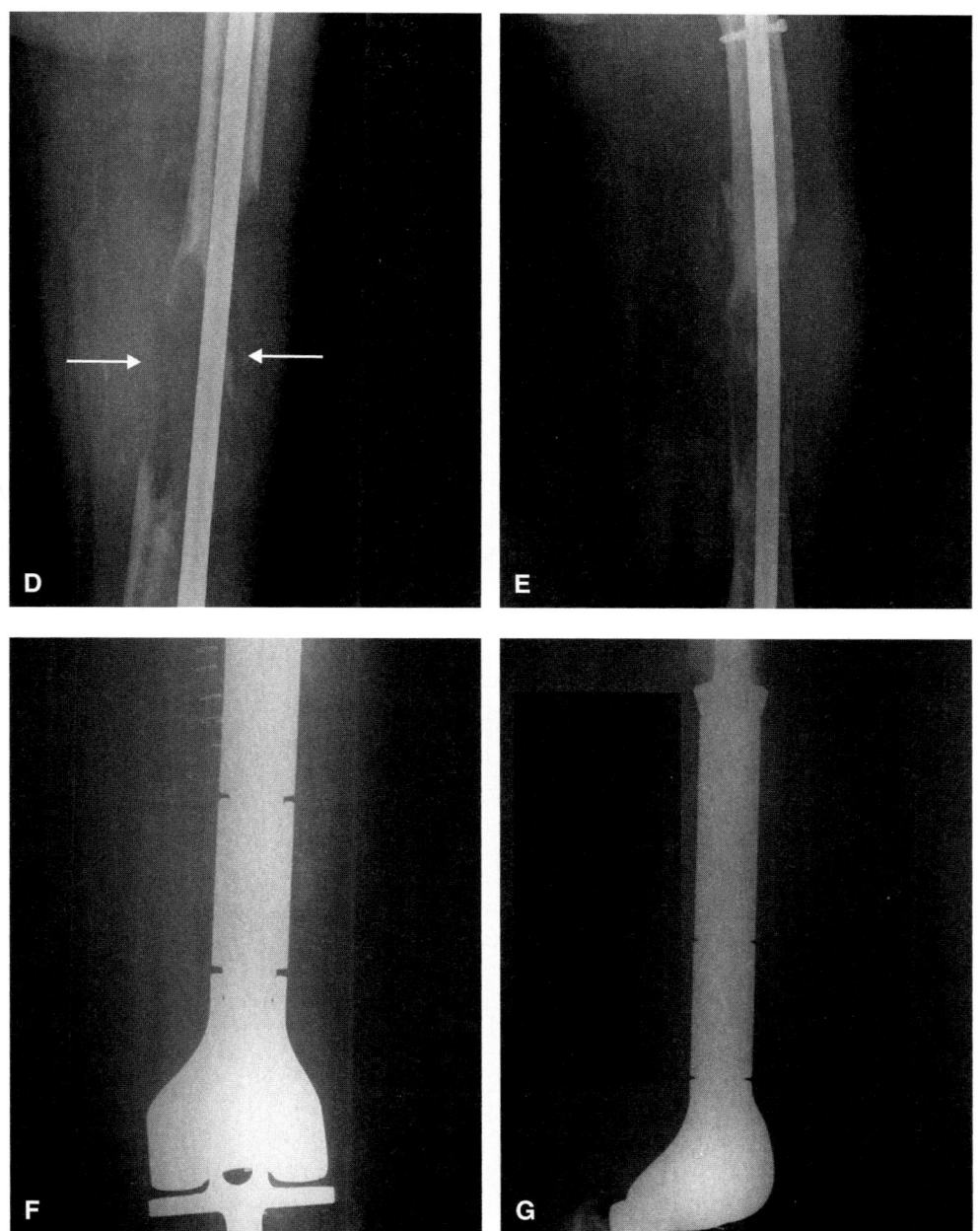

humerus. Metastases distant to the elbow and knee are uncommon and usually associated with a lung primary. These more common sites of skeletal metastasis share the common property of being sites of hematopoietic marrow. These areas are rich in vascular sinuses and allow tumor cells in the circulation access to the marrow.[7] There are regional affinities especially in the spine based on primary tumor location (prostate to lumbar, breast to thoracic). Studies attempting to determine the route of

dissemination of spinal metastasis, either arterial or venous, have not shown differences to suggest a preferred route of metastasis. Batson's plexus[7] probably plays a significant role in the dissemination of tumors to bone (e.g., from prostate or breast).[38] Circulatory distribution alone does not predict metastatic distribution, because the bone receives only about 10 percent of cardiac output but has a significantly higher metastatic prevalence than other sites that have higher blood flow.[96] Early work demonstrated

Table 17-1
Principles of Management

1. Pathologic fractures differ dramatically from traumatic fractures, and therefore the role and methods of fixation are different.
2. Nonoperative treatment is rarely an acceptable modality for treatment of pathologic pelvic and extremity fractures.
3. The method of fixation should allow for immediate mobilization and not require fracture healing to achieve stability.
4. Diagnosis requires two orthogonal radiographic views.
5. Bisphosphonates have decreased the rate of pathologic fractures, especially in patients with breast cancer and myeloma.
6. In determining therapy, the mechanism of pain production is important, especially in the spine.
7. For patients with epidural compression from metastases to the spine and myelopathy, surgical decompression is more effective than radiation, and the approach should allow direct decompression of the spinal cord.

that injection of malignant cells having a preference for lung tissue into animals in which the lung tissue had been transplanted into a subcutaneous location still resulted in metastatic lesions to that tissue. This also has been demonstrated in bone with the Walker carcinosarcoma, which has a propensity to form osseous metastases. Therefore it seems that a third factor must be involved in the development of skeletal metastasis. The third process involved in the development of skeletal metastasis is the response of the host to the tumor cells. Using Paget's terminology this is the "soil" portion of the "seed and soil" hypothesis.[132] For tumor cells to survive within bone, they must have a mechanism to leave the vasculature and gain access to the bone. They do so via the production of proteolytic enzymes, type IV collagenase, and metalloproteinases. Osteocalcin produced by bone protein acts on tumor cells as a chemotactic agent. Other chemotactic substances in bone may be derived from resorbing bone

---

FIGURE 17-4   *This 52-year-old woman had a history of breast carcinoma metastatic to bone. Initially, she had a long-stem cemented hemiarthroplasty on the right for a pathologic femoral neck fracture with an ipsilateral midshaft lesion. One year later she had a pathologic subtrochanteric fracture on the left (**A**) and was treated as if it were a traumatic lesion (**B**), with a sliding hip screw without augmentation in the area of the defect (arrows). The patient was allowed partial weight-bearing on crutches for 6 months but the construct failed and the patient experienced shortening and pain at 9 months (**C**) as a result of delayed healing and poor bone stock. She required a revision by resection of the collapsed segment and reconstruction with a segmental replacement (**D**), which may not have been necessary had the pathologic fracture been treated initially by a method that was rigid enough not to require healing to achieve stability.*

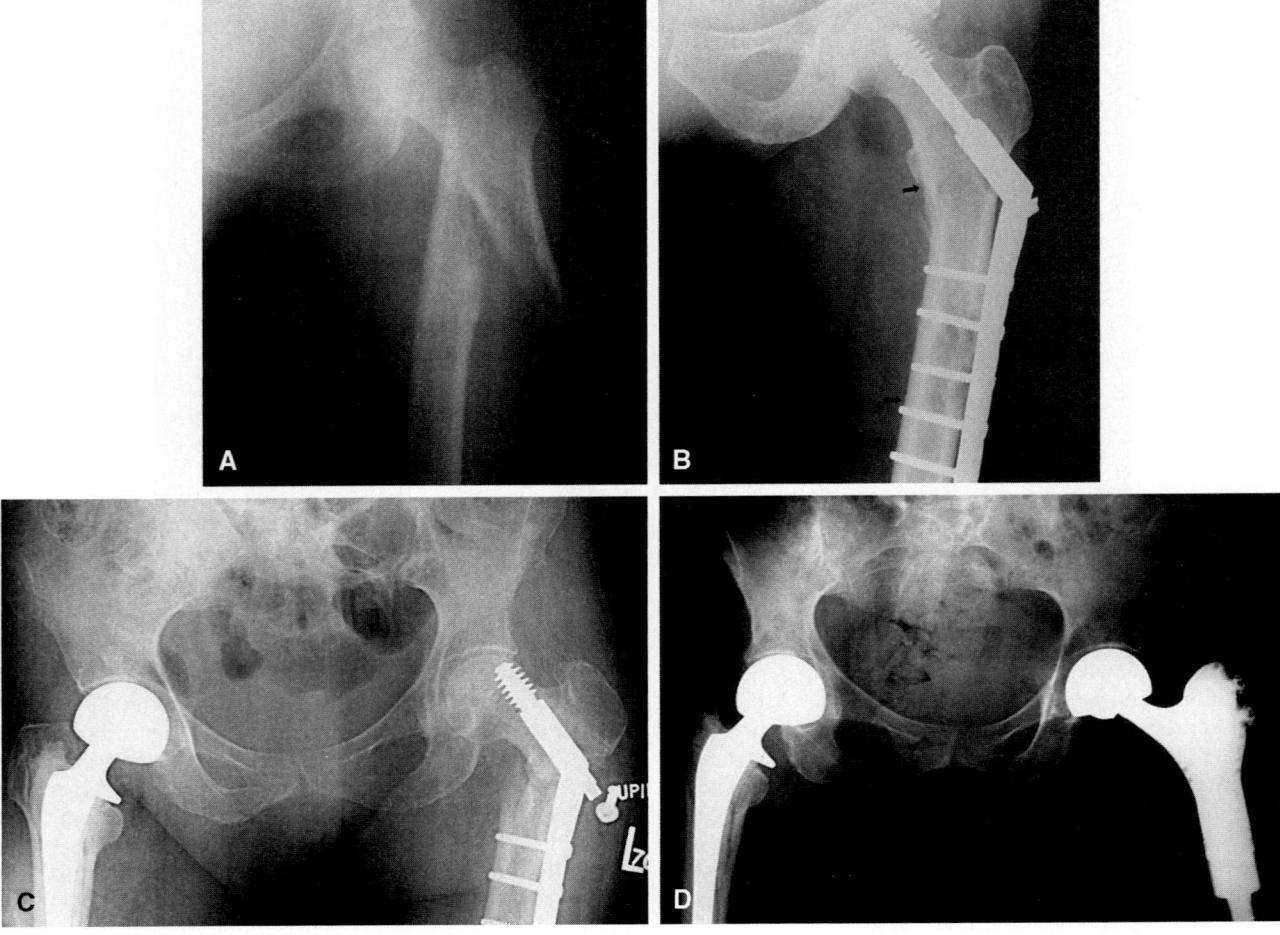

FIGURE 17-5 *Studies for a patient seen approximately 10 years from the time of his nephrectomy for a renal cell carcinoma. He underwent CT scan surveillance of his abdomen on a yearly basis to determine whether an abdominal aneurysm was expanding. A lesion was noted to be slowly growing on the yearly CT (A), but it was thought to be benign and no association was made in any of the reports with his previous nephrectomy for renal cell carcinoma. Finally, after the lesion was present for 2 years, he sustained a fracture and had pain and scoliosis on a standing radiograph (B) as well as mild dural compression on MRI (C). The patient underwent needle biopsy, confirming it was a renal cell carcinoma consistent with his primary. After stereotactic radiosurgery and stabilization he became completely asymptomatic and the lesion regressed in size (D).*

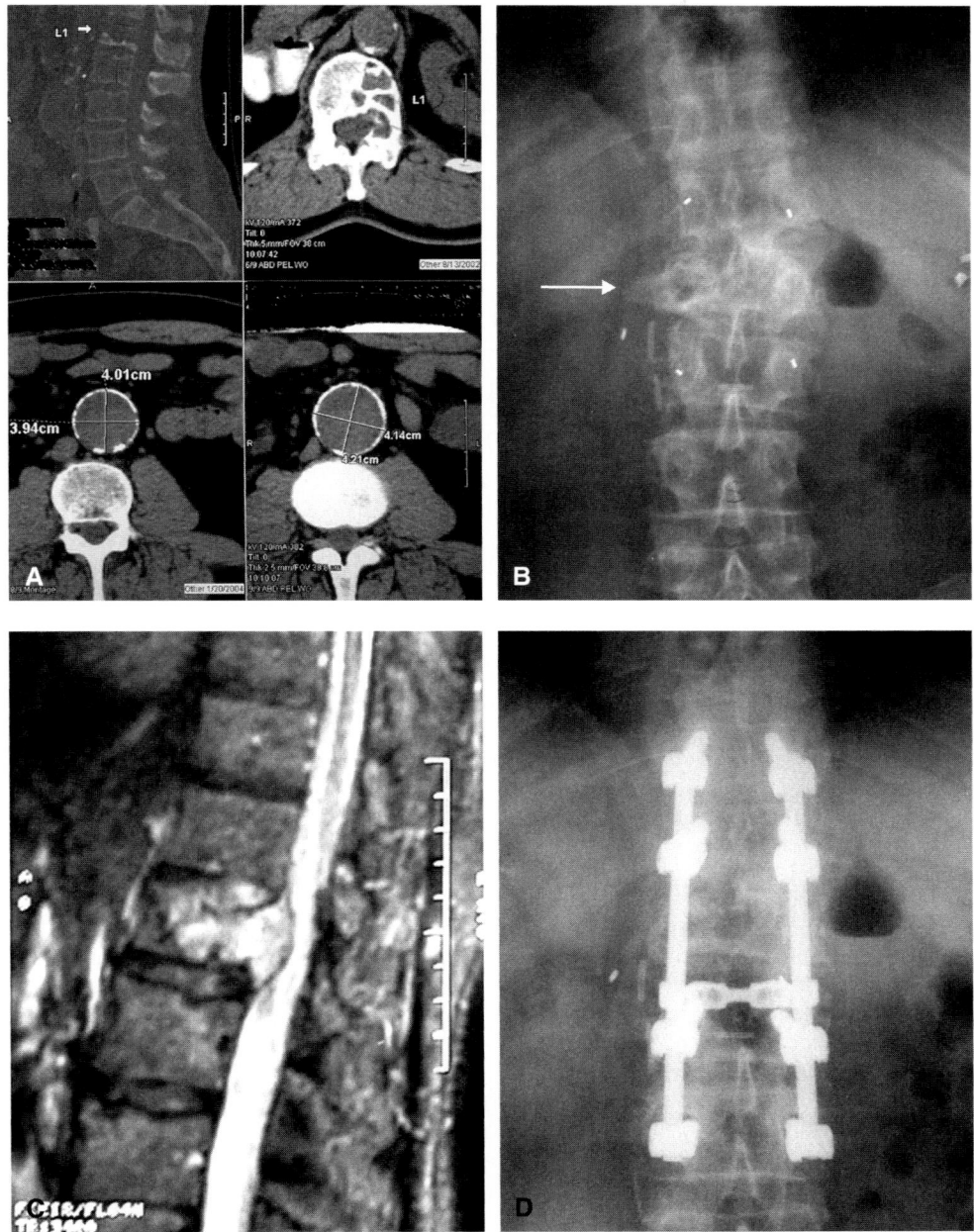

or collagen type I peptides.[10,131] Some authors suggest that this factor may be related to osteoclasts, because any bone resorption is achieved through stimulation of those cells. However, the relation between the bone-resorbing factor and chemotactic activity remains unclear.[109] Without these and other processes taking place, tumor cells lodged in bone cannot survive. Interventions aimed at interrupting these pathways in order to control skeletal metastasis are under investigation (bisphosphonates, receptor activator for nuclear factor κ B ligand [RANKL], denosumab).[17]

Bone metastasis can be lytic, blastic, or mixed.[96] Although some tumor types are typically blastic, lytic, or mixed there is variability within tumor types and even within the same patient. Two main types of new bone formation occur in response to tumor: stromal and reactive.[64] The formation of stromal new bone, in response to tumor invasion, is most likely mediated by humoral factors that stimulate osteoblasts. Reactive new bone formation is somewhat simpler to understand: bone is laid down in response to a stress of weakened bone. Certain tumors (e.g., myelomas, lymphomas, and leukemias) do not seem to stimulate reactive new bone, even though they produce obvious osteoclastic bone destruction. Other tumors, such as prostate cancers, tend to form stromal new bone as part of the process, independent of osteoclastic activity. The osteolysis of bone metastasis can be mediated by two potential mechanisms: the osteoclast, which has been demonstrated in a number of experimental models,[62] and late-stage bone destruction with a disappearance of osteoclasts. The former has become an important mechanism of bone resorption as interference with osteoclastic resorption of bone is the mechanism of action of bisphosphonates in reducing rates of skeletal events. This has been shown to be effective not only in osteolytic metastases but also in osteoblastic lesions as well with the use of zoledronate.[148] In the latter case malignant cells may be responsible for the bone destruction, possibly as a result of their ability to produce lytic enzymes. Human breast cancer has been shown to directly resorb bone.[127] This has also been demonstrated in lung carcinoma, epidermoidomas and adenocarcinomas, and less commonly in small-cell anaplastic and large-cell tumors.[35]

Historically, surgical treatment of skeletal metastasis was directed primarily at lesions involving the femur. This is likely due to the major morbidity and loss of function associated with metastasis in this location. Additionally, the risk of fracture and the ease of prophylactic treatment are greater in the femur than other locations. The incidence of pathologic fractures in patients with bone metastases is only 4 percent, but the incidence in those with breast cancer with lesions in the femur may be as high as 30 percent depending on the location within the femur.[58] However, the relative incidence is decreasing with the use of bisphosphonates. The distribution of skeletal metastasis within a given bone is not random. Proximal femur lesions are more common than are distal lesions. Lesions distal to the elbow and distal to the knee are relatively uncommon and often associated with lung cancer primaries. In the last 20 years improved techniques and equipment have allowed treatment of symptomatic metastases involving not only the femur but also other long bones, the pelvis, and the spine. Metastatic vertebral fractures most commonly occur in patients with breast, myeloma, lung, prostate,[5] and renal cell carcinoma, with the majority occurring in the thoracic and lumbar spine.[101] Symptoms may result from tumor invasion of the body, pathologic fracture, instability, or epidural compression, with either radiculopathy or myelopathy. The application of minimally invasive techniques such as vertebroplasty and kyphoplasty has allowed more effective treatment of some of these patients with pathologic vertebral fractures.[56]

Patients with skeletal metastasis are most commonly identified when they seek medical attention because of pain, although many skeletal metastases currently are found incidentally on computed tomography (CT), magnetic resonance imaging (MRI), or positron emission tomography/computed tomography (PET/CT). The mechanism by which skeletal metastasis causes pain is not completely understood. In cases where osteolysis has taken place and weakened the bone, microscopic or gross fracture is most likely the cause of symptoms. However, in purely blastic lesions, or in lesions without sufficient lysis to mechanically compromise the bone, this explanation is insufficient to account for the patient's symptoms. Direct tumor invasion with the secretion of humoral factors may play a role in this group of patients. In most cases once a metastatic focus becomes symptomatic some degree of resorption usually occurs. Identifying the underlying cause of bone pain in patients with metastatic disease is critical, irrespective of whether the metastases are in the long bones, pelvis, or spine. The pain may be from the tumor volume, compression of adjacent neural structures, or compromised structural integrity of the bone. Depending on the tumor type, those lesions that have not caused significant cortical destruction may respond well to radiation or chemotherapy. Once marked visible osseous destruction has taken place, especially in the femur, pelvis, and spine, the symptoms are less likely to respond to radiation or chemotherapy. In most cases patients usually have mechanical symptoms before pathologic fracture actually occurs. This is especially true for tumors located in the long bones, spine, and pelvis. Pathologic fracture without antecedent symptoms is more common in the clavicles and ribs. The development of neurologic compromise generally does not occur without an antecedent history of pain in that location. Given the increased morbidity associated with the operative treatment of pathologic fractures compared with prophylactic fixation of an impending fracture, it is preferable to attempt to diagnose the lesions at risk before fracture. Patients with spinal metastasis may either be asymptomatic or present with localized pain, mechanical pain, or neurologic symptoms of radiculopathy or myelopathy. In the last case the cause is usually secondary to epidural compression from vertebral metastasis but may also be the result of acute pathologic fracture. Epidural compression resulting in radiculopathy or myelopathy is a more common cause of symptoms than is gross instability, vertebral collapse, and fracture-dislocation. Overt fracture with metastatic lesions should occur infrequently. The symptomatic patient should be evaluated carefully and appropriate patients selected for prophylactic fixation or vertebroplasty before fracture occurs.

DIAGNOSIS OF BONE METASTASES

Patients who are ultimately diagnosed with skeletal metastasis can be divided into three groups. The first group includes those patients with a known history of cancer who seek medical attention because of an area of skeletal symptomology (back, neck, or hip pain). The second group includes patients who have a known cancer diagnosis and for whom staging studies identify an asymptomatic skeletal lesion. The third includes patients who seek medical attention because of a symptomatic osseous lesion and are diagnosed with a skeletal metastasis as the first presentation of an undiagnosed carcinoma. For all three groups the first step in making the diagnosis includes taking a careful history. For the first group of patients it is especially important to have a high degree of suspicion of the possibility of metastatic disease to bone as the cause of the patient's symptoms. Patients commonly seek medical attention due to musculoskeletal pain involving the hip, knee, neck, or back. All too often, the patient's symptoms are evaluated as an isolated problem without obtaining a careful history. In any patient with a prior cancer diagnosis, the possibility of a skeletal metastasis as the cause of the patient's symptoms should be considered. Commonly, the physician does not obtain and the patient does not volunteer the history of prior cancer diagnosis. In some cases the disease-free interval may be so long that the patient or physician may feel that the patient is "cured," and metastasis after so great a time is considered unlikely. Unfortunately, skeletal metastasis after a long disease-free interval is not uncommon, especially for patients with breast, thyroid, or even renal cell carcinomas in which skeletal metastasis may develop more than 10 years after the primary cancer diagnosis (see Fig. 17-5). The cancer history should include all prior surgeries, the histologic diagnosis, and all treatments including radiation and chemotherapy. This is especially true for patients who have had "a skin lesion removed" or "breast surgery" and are uncertain about the

final diagnosis. The history is helpful not only in those patients with skeletal metastasis and a prior cancer diagnosis but also in many without a cancer diagnosis. Additionally, in patients older than age 40 who present with pain and a radiographically destructive bone lesion, the most common diagnosis is still an osseous metastasis. A strong family history or a history of risk factors such as smoking or exposure to carcinogens (i.e., tobacco, asbestos, radiation) may direct the physician to a likely primary site. A complete review of systems emphasizing weight loss, respiratory, endocrine, and genitourinary symptoms may strengthen the suspicion. Flank pain and hematuria should raise the suspicion of an underlying renal cancer, just as a persistent cough and hemoptysis should raise suspicion of an underlying lung carcinoma. Physical examination including the skin lesions, thyroid nodules, and abdominal pain or masses may also aid in suggesting the location of the primary. Serum and urine studies play only a modest role in evaluating patients with a suspected metastasis without a prior cancer diagnosis. Serum and urine protein electrophoresis identify most patients with myeloma, and an elevated prostate-specific antigen (PSA) may identify some patients with metastatic prostate carcinoma. Tumor markers,[11,43] such as carcinoembryonic antigen (CEA), CA 125, and CA 19-9, lack specificity and are most useful

---

FIGURE 17-6 *Anteroposterior (AP) and lateral radiographs of a 70-year-old woman who presented with severe right knee pain. Subsequent positron emission tomography and computed tomography scans demonstrated a large lung mass with a pathologic diagnosis of non–small-cell carcinoma of the lung. These radiographs demonstrate the necessity for obtaining two views of any cylindrical bone to demonstrate a lesion. The patient's AP radiograph (A) does not clearly show the lytic lesion in the distal femur (arrowheads), but the lateral radiograph (B) clearly demonstrates a lytic lesion (arrow).*

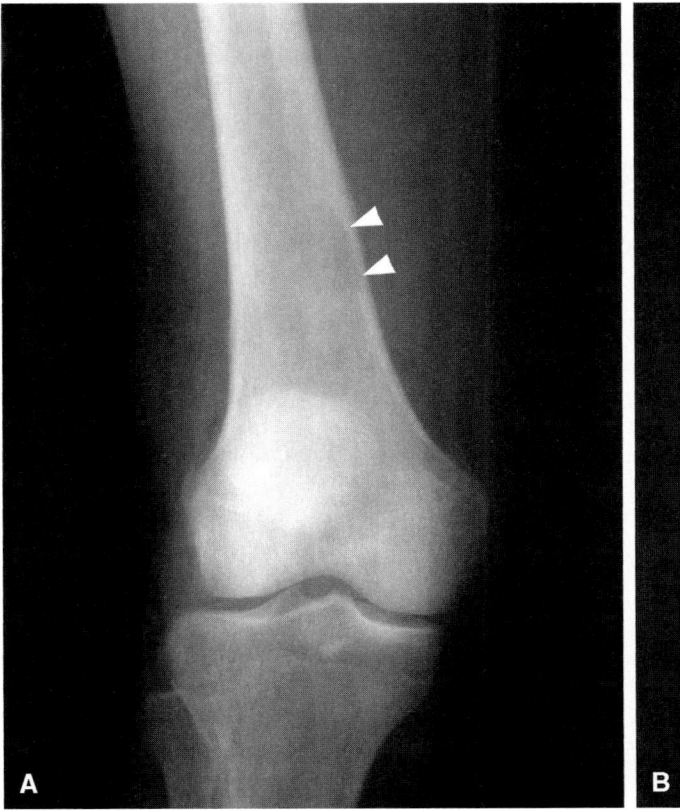
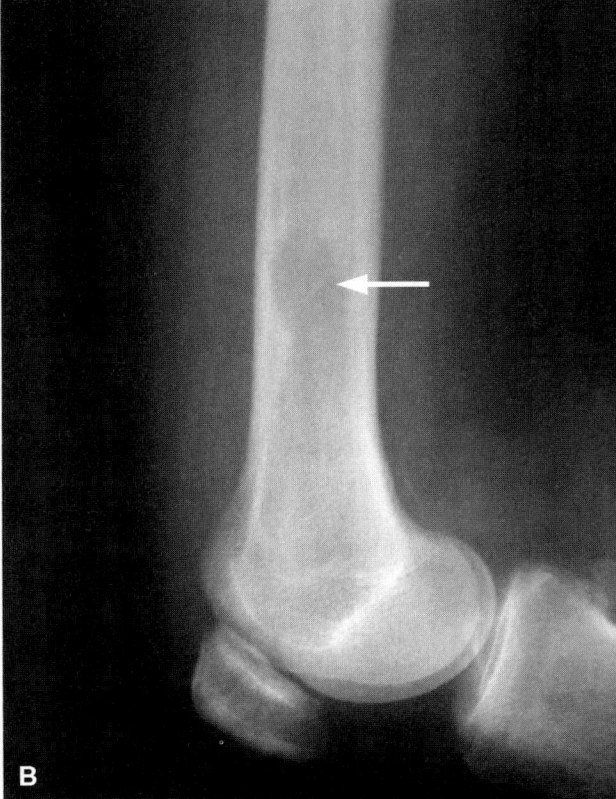

for monitoring response to treatment. A variety of imaging modalities are now available for evaluating suspected or known metastatic disease. These include plain radiographs, CT, technetium bone scan, single-photon emission computed tomography (SPECT), MRI, and PET.[98,152] Plain radiographs of the symptomatic area must include good-quality films in at least two planes, preferably at right angles to each other (Fig. 17-6). Standard anteroposterior (AP) and lateral views are usually sufficient, although in certain instances these two views may not be completely appropriate. Because destruction of at least 50 percent of normal cancellous bone is required to show a lytic defect in a long bone, early detection of metastasis by plain roentgenography is not always sufficiently sensitive. In addition, lesions in certain areas in the pelvis and sacrum such as the supra-acetabular region may not be evident on plain roentgenograms and may require specialized views (e.g., Judet views) (Fig. 17-7). Inadequate plain radiographs may result when the physician does not consider that the patient's symptoms may be secondary to referred pain. A patient with a hip lesion may complain of knee pain, and the lesion may remain unrecognized until radiographs of the hip instead of the knee are obtained. This problem can usually be avoided by performing an appropriate physical exam to include the entire extremity.

If plain roentgenograms do not identify the patient's source of pain and the suspicion of skeletal metastasis remains high, then either a PET scan or whole-body bone scan should be performed depending on the histology of the tumor and the desire to screen only bone or bone and other potential areas of metastases at the same time.

Radiographs are then obtained for follow-up of areas of increased activity on the bone scan or PET scan. Various imaging modalities have a proven utility for the evaluation of patients with skeletal metastasis. The most appropriate sequence for investigating suspected skeletal metastasis depends on the presence or absence of a clinical history of cancer. In some patients with a prior cancer diagnosis (e.g., lung or breast) the primary imaging study to screen for potential osseous metastasis may no longer be the technetium bone (^{99m}Tc) scan. Its timing and application vary depending on the relative risk of skeletal metastasis, presence or absence of pathologic fracture, time during the treatment cycle, and suspected tumor histology. The sensitivity of a ^{99m}Tc bone scan is low with certain histologies such as myeloma and some renal cell carcinomas. It may also be misleading in the woman with osseous metastases from breast carcinomas who has a flare on bone scan with some types of treatment modalities but an improving disease status. Technetium-99m bone scans have a sensitivity of 95 to 97 percent for the detection of skeletal metastases.[16,28,51,68] Despite their sensitivity for diagnosing bone metastases they are not without limitations.[92,97,102,159] One limitation of the bone scan is that it lacks specificity and may yield false positive results in non-neoplastic conditions such as osteoporotic fractures, Paget's disease, or even osteoarthritis. Similarly, some lesions, such as myeloma and extremely aggressive osteolytic tumors, produce extensive destruction without the reparative processes detected on bone scan. In such instances the technetium bone scan may appear normal or even photopenic.[102] The utility of the bone scan includes its role as a staging study at the time

---

FIGURE 17-7 *Radiographs of the hip of a 39-year-old woman with carcinoma of the breast and severe hip pain. The patient initially underwent radiation therapy after a bone scan demonstrated slight activity in the supra-acetabular region and in the proximal femur, but the radiographs were interpreted as negative. **A,** The anteroposterior radiograph of the pelvis suggested the presence of a lytic lesion in the area of the acetabulum. Judet views were necessary to fully demonstrate the extent of the lytic lesion. **B,** As seen on the oblique view of the iliac bone, the lesion occupies the superior aspect and the posterior lip of the acetabulum.*

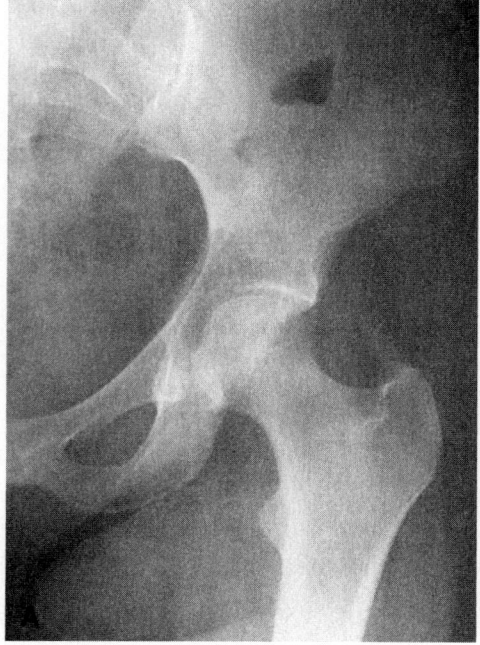
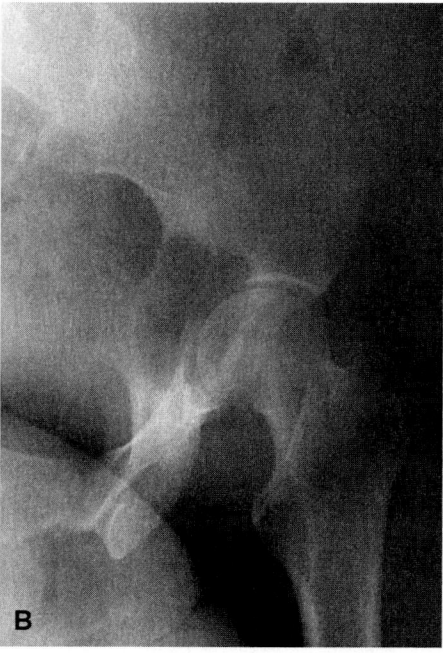

of initial diagnosis for patients with carcinoma that are at high risk for osseous metastases and for those with known bony metastases as follow-up for new areas of involvement.

PET and especially PET/CT scanning have been shown to be useful screening tools in patients with skeletal metastasis from lung, prostate, lymphoma, breast cancer, and other primary lesions. PET has the advantage over bone scan of potentially identifying nonosseous sites of metastases.[52,90,91,98,152,155] PET has been shown to have fewer false positives in the detection of bone metastases than bone scintigraphy.[91] The relative value of whole-body MRI to PET/CT is unclear in terms of sensitivity and specificity. However, PET is also helpful in that a single test can evaluate with extreme sensitivity all sites of metastatic disease (Fig. 17-8). However, it is not uniformly reliable for all tumor histologies. In some patients, such as those with sarcomas, it may identify lesions in some patients reliably and in others be inconsistent, demonstrating some lesions but not others. The concurrent use of CT with PET enhances its utility by increasing specificity especially in the spine. Non-neoplastic conditions can be active on PET scan, and therefore knowing the standardized uptake value (SUV) number of an individual lesion can be important in judging the nature of that lesion but may not be diagnostic.

For lesions of the pelvis, where there is superimposition of structures, plain radiography is often inadequate for determining the presence of a skeletal lesion. CT may be necessary to confirm the presence of a lesion suggested by the bone scan (Fig. 17-9). A Foley catheter should be placed within the bladder prior to bone scan imaging in order to avoid obscuring the sacral area by radiopharmaceutical accumulated in the bladder. MRI is even more

sensitive than bone scintigraphy in the detection of bone metastases.[51,68,92,93] Although it is sensitive to bone marrow abnormalities, MRI remains nonspecific and in many cases cannot differentiate benign from malignant lesions.[118] Nonspecific marrow changes secondary to radiation or chemotherapy treatments may yield false positive readings. In evaluation of metastatic lesions of the extremities and pelvis, it can identify small lesions not seen on plain radiograph or CT and is especially helpful in the assessment of soft tissue masses accompanying bone lesions.

The evaluation of metastatic lesions and fractures of the spine can be complicated and requires a progressive and systematic approach. In the patient who presents with symptomatic spinal metastasis two questions must be answered by the diagnostic tests. The first is the extent of metastatic involvement of the particular spinal level and the presence or absence of instability; the second is the presence or absence of neural compression. Both AP and lateral roentgenograms may give some indication of the extent of metastatic involvement but are notoriously inaccurate (Fig. 17-10). If one half of the vertebra is present and the other side totally absent, the lateral roentgenogram may appear relatively normal. The CT gives the most accurate assessment of vertebral destruction[20] (Fig. 17-11).

Although bone scan has been used as a screening tool for levels of metastases, MRI has essentially replaced it for evaluation of spinal metastatic disease because it is able more accurately to delineate the involved levels and also the presence or absence of cord compression. Midsagittal screening images allow for a rapid evaluation of the entire spine; this is also helpful in patients in whom more than one level may be involved (Fig. 17-12). MRI has been shown to greatly influence treatment planning for patients with spinal metastases,[31] especially for patients with spinal cord compression (Fig. 17-13). Cook and co-workers found that in 25 percent of patients with a sensory level, MRI demonstrated that the site of cord compression was four or more segments distal or three or more segments proximal to the sensory level.[33] Multiple areas of cord compression or impingement were identified in 39 percent of patients. Other studies have confirmed that MRI of the entire spine is the imaging modality of choice for patients with a history of carcinoma and suspected spinal metastases. MRI also has the ability to identify lesions that are extremely destructive, such as myeloma or renal cell carcinoma, which may not be apparent on bone scan. The screening sagittal MRI is also important as a preoperative modality, as it is important to pinpoint areas of asymptomatic spinal involvement prior to performing surgical decompression and stabilization on the index lesion. MRI has two primary shortcomings, however: it lacks specificity (i.e., it cannot accurately differentiate a metastatic fracture from an osteoporotic compression fracture),[118] and it does not allow accurate delineation of the nature of the metastatic involvement and it cannot detail the extent of bone destruction. It also cannot differentiate between viable and nonviable tumor in the spine and cannot be used in patients with cardiac defibrillators and pacemakers. In those patients who have neurologic signs and symptoms and are candidates for surgical intervention, the use of a combination of diagnostic studies is most helpful in identifying the level, extent, nature, and direction of

FIGURE 17-8 *This 34-year-old woman with a known history of breast cancer had a rising carcinoembryonic antigen level with a negative bone scan and computed tomography scan of the chest and abdomen. **A** and **B**, Positron emission tomography showed diffuse bone metastases involving multiple areas of the body (PET scan).*

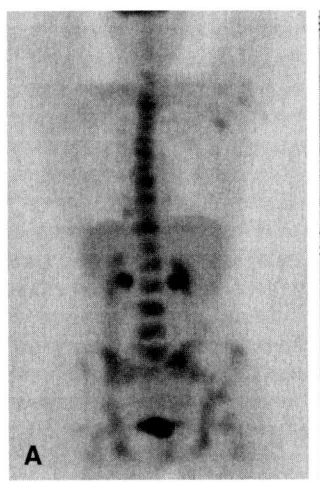

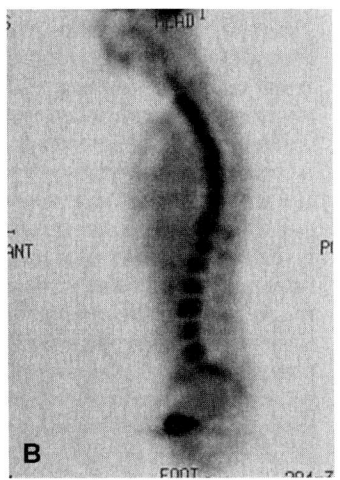

FIGURE 17-9 | *This 53-year-old man had a known history of carcinoma of the lung, which was considered to be in remission until he presented with left leg pain. The patient's workup for metastatic disease of the spine was negative.* **A,** *An anteroposterior view of his pelvis was initially interpreted as negative. However, it demonstrates loss of the subchondral plate of the acetabulum and a large but diffuse-appearing lytic lesion in the supra-acetabular and posterior acetabular regions.* **B,** *A bone scan demonstrated diffuse uptake about the hip on the anterior view.* **C,** *Computed tomography (CT) was necessary for accurate delineation of the lesion. The CT scan demonstrates significant involvement of the posterior lip of the acetabulum and the supra-acetabular region, with partial loss of the subchondral plate.*

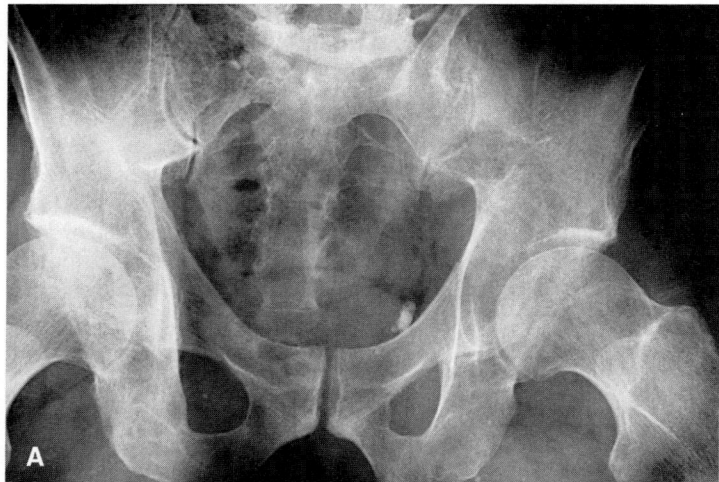
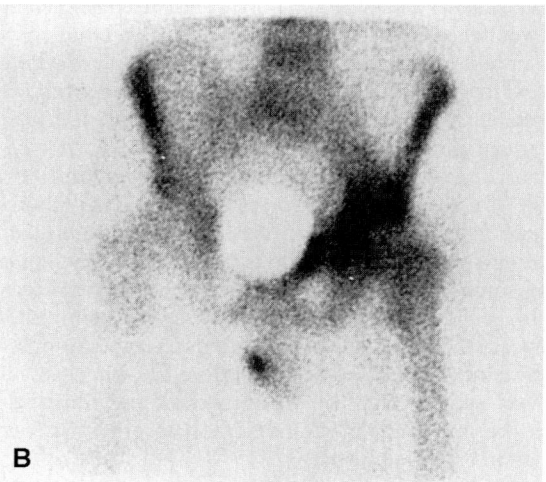
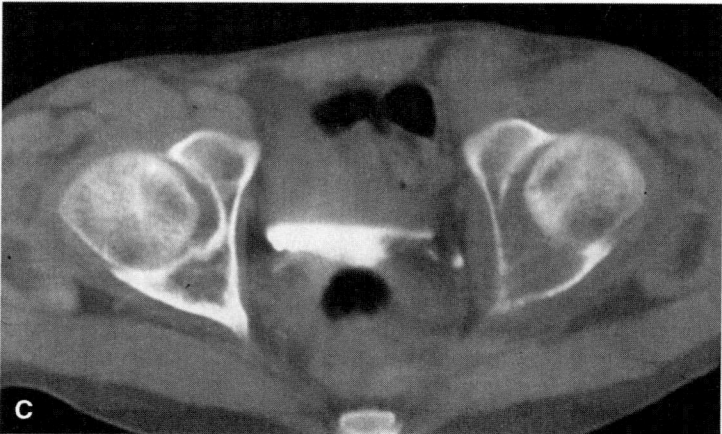

neural compression and identifying additional noncontiguous levels of involvement that may require treatment. MRI can demonstrate the areas of tumor involvement of marrow, the levels and extent of cord compression, and the direction of compression. The addition of a noncontrast CT scan after the MRI further delineates the nature of the compression (retropulsed bone fragment vs. extension of soft tissue mass) and clarifies any structural compromise at the index level as well as the levels above and below, which may be used for instrumentation (Fig. 17-14). The identification of cord compression at two noncontiguous levels by MRI is an indicator of poor prognosis.

TREATMENT

Patients with symptomatic skeletal metastasis who have not sustained a fracture may be treated by nonoperative or surgical methods. Nonoperative treatments include targeted therapies, administration of bisphosphonates, chemotherapy, hormonal therapy, and radiation.[21,34,105,120,144] Many symptomatic metastatic lesions (depending on tumor histology, area, and extent of involvement) respond to nonoperative treatments. In the last 5 years the use of bisphosphonates has become standard in patients with bone metastases, thereby significantly reducing the incidence of skeletally related events (incidence of pathologic fractures, rate of surgery for bone complications, use of radiation for bone lesions, and hypercalcemia) in patients with bone metastases. For patients with osseous metastases from breast cancer, the use of zoledronate reduces the incidence of bony events 20 percent over that for patients given pamidronate and 30 percent over that for patients receiving hormonal therapy.[17,45,105,144,148,162,167] Zoledronate has been approved for use even in managing cancers with blastic metastases, and the use of 4 mg IV every 3 to 4 weeks in patients with breast, myeloma, prostate, and renal

FIGURE 17-10 *This patient with a head and neck carcinoma had interscapular back pain. The anteroposterior radiograph (A) showed an absent pedicle (arrow), which was a relatively minor element of the subtotal destruction of the vertebral body (arrow) best seen on CT scan (B).*

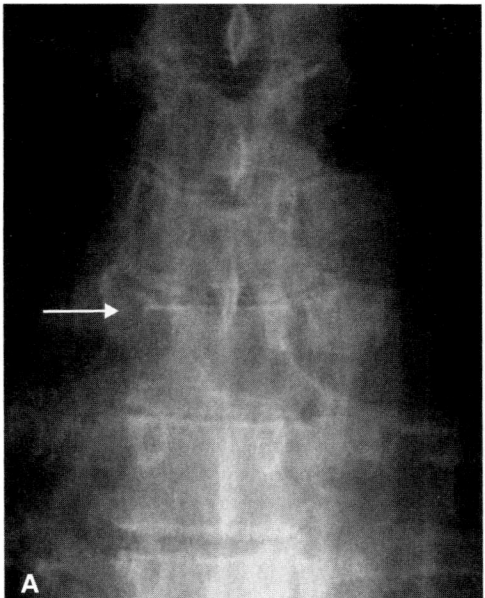

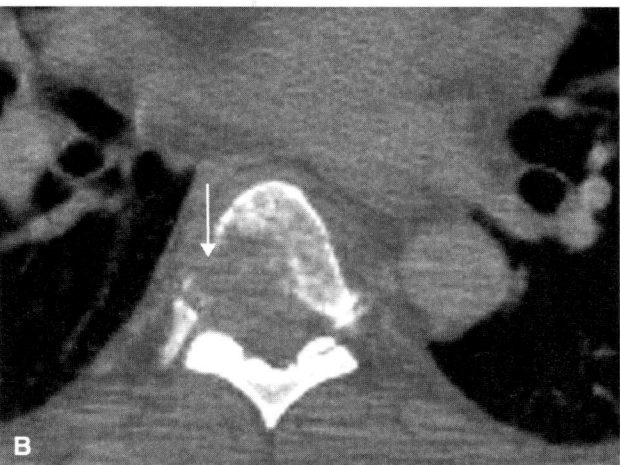

cell carcinoma has been shown to reduce the occurrence of skeletal events approximately 40 percent over placebo during the course of the first year as well as delaying the time to first skeletal event.[105,120,144] The data for vertebral fractures are less clear; however, there seems to be a decrease of about 40 percent in compression fractures and vertebral pain, but the incidence of spinal cord compression has not been shown to decrease with the use of bisphosphonates. This would be expected as compression usually occurs as the result of soft tissue epidural extension and would only be affected if there was a marked antitumor effect as has been suggested in breast cancer and myeloma.

The use of both hormonal and chemotherapeutic agents can have a significant positive effect on bony metastasis and bone healing.[12] Hormonal manipulation in breast cancer and carcinoma of the prostate can result in marked healing of bony lesions. In carcinoma of the prostate, significant pain relief can occur with estrogen therapy. Hormonal therapy with diethylstilbestrol (1 mg/day) or with leuprolide and flutamide[36] can have a response rate of up to 80 percent. Regression is indicated by a reduction in PSA levels. Generally, chemotherapeutic agents are more effective when asymptomatic progression of the tumor has been demonstrated, and they are less effective in those patients who have already become symptomatic. Lesions that remain symptomatic or progress despite systemic therapy usually require surgical stabilization or radiation therapy before returning to chemotherapy.[80,157] The efficiency of radiation in treating a metastatic lesion to bone is probably inversely proportional to the degree of structural impairment; most lytic lesions remain problematic.[94] More than 90 percent of patients who experience pain relief do so within the first 4 weeks of therapy; the average duration of complete relief, however, is only

6 months.[14,67] The durability of this treatment modality depends on a variety of lesional factors including size, location, and histology as well treatment factors (dose, fractionation, a/b ratio). However, radiation may give pain relief without significant bone healing.[99] The repair of metastatic bone lesions after radiation therapy has been described in detail by Matsubayashi and colleagues.[124] They demonstrated that the remineralization of an osteolytic metastatic lesion after radiation therapy is the result of ossification of strands of collagen derived from the proliferative fibrous tissue that has replaced the metastatic cells. This delay or failure of bone healing as a result of the radiation may contribute to the rate of complications, such as vertebral collapse and cord compression or long bone fracture, which occur in most series reporting results of treatment of bony metastases with external beam radiation.[67,83,165]

Radiation therapy is useful for the treatment of metastatic lesions prior to fracture. Once fracture has occurred, however, its role without surgery is limited. The goals of radiation therapy are to relieve pain and obtain local tumor control. Radiotherapy can be administered by a number of different strategies. The number of fractions and the time over which the treatment is delivered can vary. Most recent investigations have compared single-fraction treatment (8 Gy) to multifraction treatment (10 × 3 Gy) and found similar rates of pain relief (60%) with a slightly higher rate of need for retreatment in the single-fraction group (19% vs. 8%).[83,165] In general for patients with spine metastases without pathologic fracture or cord compression, the incidence of pain relief in most series is approximately 60 to 70 percent depending on the radiosensitivity of the tumor, which is similar to that observed in other musculoskeletal metastases outside of the spine. Evaluating the effectiveness and duration of response is difficult as most

FIGURE 17-11 *This 46-year-old man with thyroid carcinoma of long duration began to have back pain. The anteroposterior radiograph was interpreted as normal.* **A,** *The lateral radiograph was thought to show a minor superior end-plate abnormality.* **B,** *However, CT demonstrated that the bulk of the body and all of the posterior wall had been destroyed. There was even a minor degree of canal impingement.* **C,** *Reconstructions showed the extent of destruction. This case demonstrates that a lateral radiograph is a poor tool for screening spinal metastatic disease. The presence of a single cortex, even with complete destruction of the remainder of the body, gives a relatively normal-appearing radiograph.*

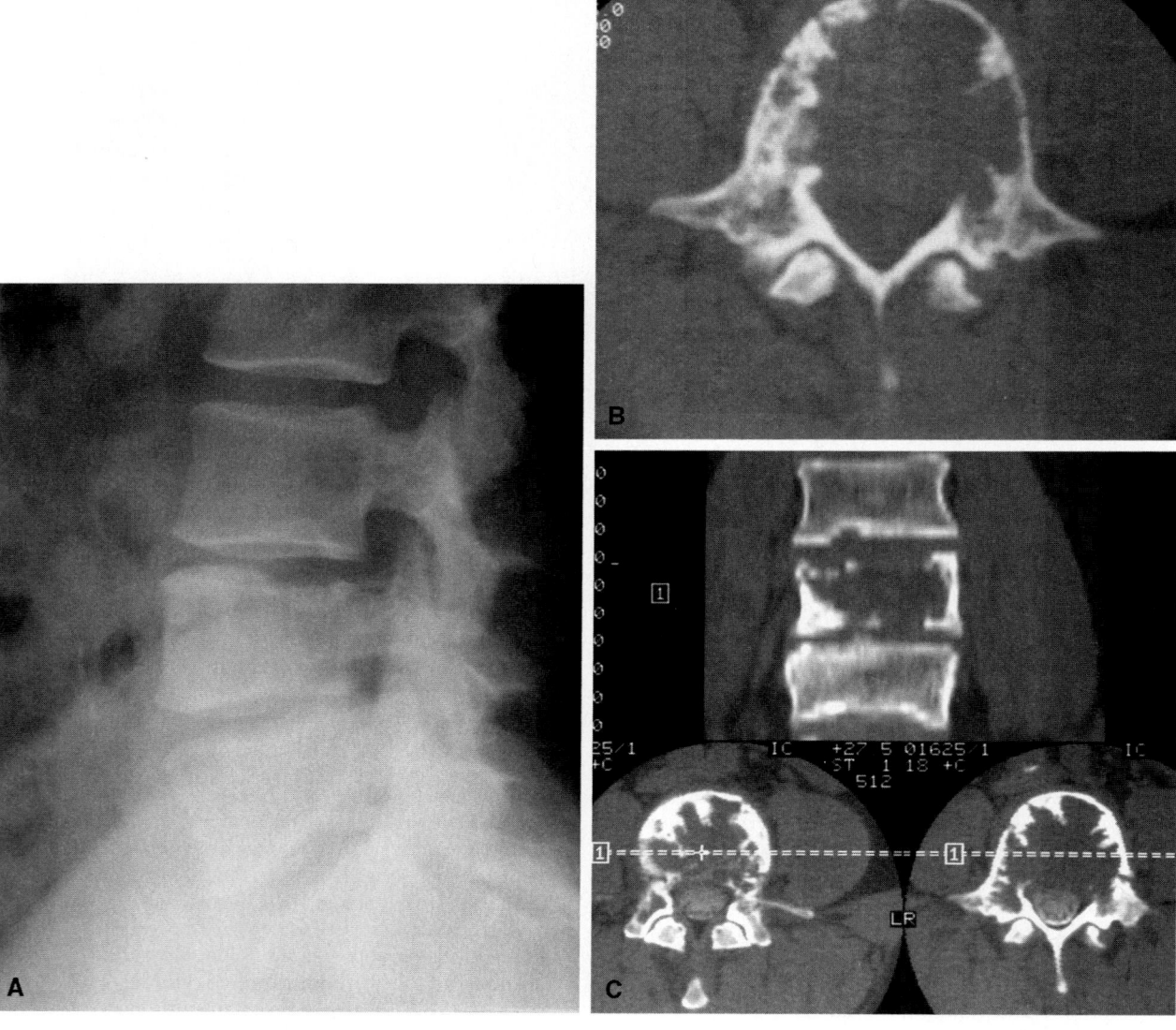

studies fail to document the incidence of pathologic fracture, instability, and tumor sensitivity. Duration of pain response is directly related to tumor histology structural compromise, with more favorable histologies having higher initial response rates and longer durations of response. Response to pain may be independent of dose and fractionation schedule, with the most common regimen being 30 to 35 Gy delivered in 5 to 10 fractions. More recently a single dose of 8 Gy or two consecutive doses of 8 Gy have been used with similar efficacy to the higher dose and fractionation schedules. Doses up to 45 Gy have been used with intensity-modulated radiation therapy (IMRT) technique

in the spine, and doses up to 50 Gy in less-sensitive extremity tumors have been used. However, in a prospective trial of the Trans-Tasman Radiation Oncology Group compared a single fraction of 8 Gy with five fractions totalling 20 Gy. In terms of pain response, 59 percent achieved a complete response and 32 percent a partial response. However, the median time to failure from treatment was only 3.2 months with a mean survival of 5.1 months. New cord compression or fracture occurred in 14 percent.[143] Thus time to pain recurrence can be as short as 2 to 3 months, and other modalities such as stereotactic radiosurgery can currently yield much

FIGURE 17-12 *This elderly female with known osteoporosis and a history of breast cancer without known metastases began to have interscapular back pain and sustained a fracture that was barely evident on plain radiograph as a result of the osteoporosis. Magnetic resonance imaging showed multiple levels of involvement, and a needle biopsy confirmed first evidence of metastatic breast carcinoma.*

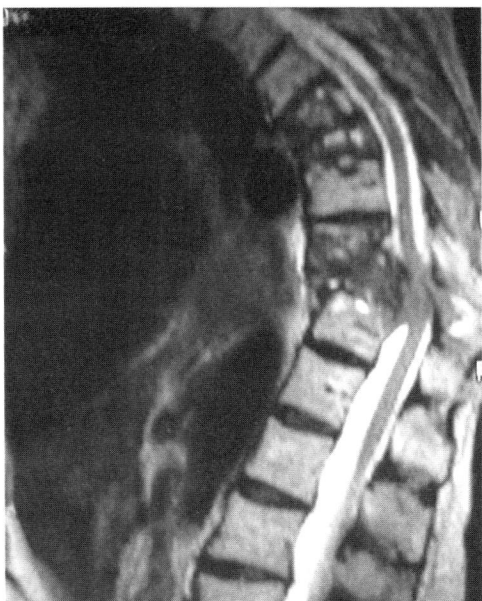

FIGURE 17-13 *This midsagittal magnetic resonance image (MRI) of the thoracic spine of a 56-year-old man with metastatic liposarcoma demonstrates the ability to easily visualize areas of vertebral involvement and epidural compression without significant bony involvement. This patient had previous surgery (asterisk) in the lower thoracic spine for bony destruction and compression, but 6 months later developed severe midthoracic pain without any change in radiographic appearance. A large epidural plaque with dural compression was found on MRI examination (arrow).*

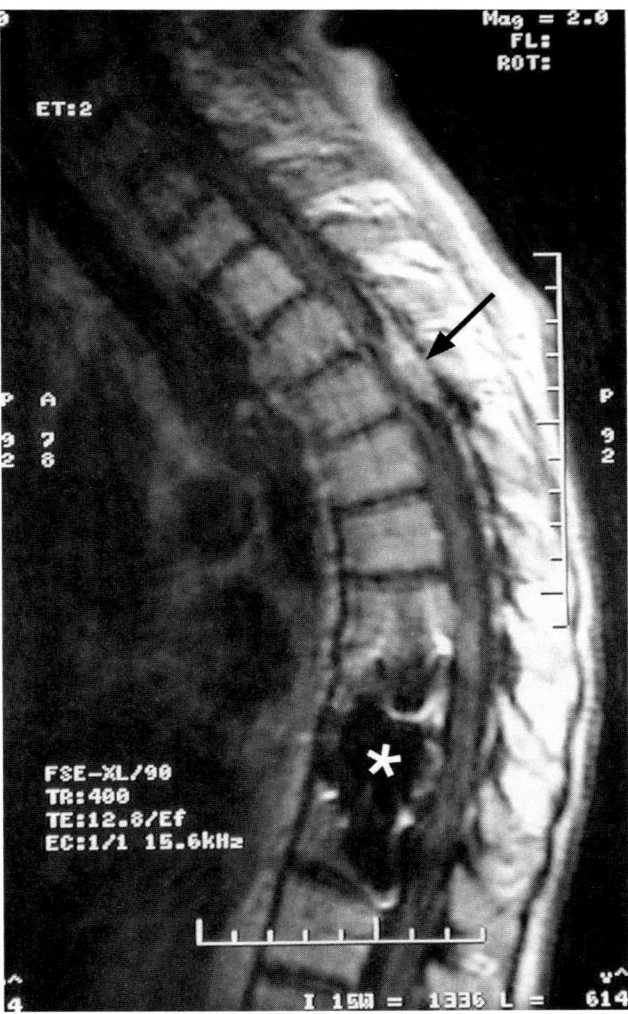

improved duration of pain relief. Radiopharmaceutical treatment with strontium-89 or phosphorus-32 have shown encouraging results for patients with widespread skeletal metastases from primary sites such as breast, prostate, and osteosarcoma.[27,36,44,129,151] Complications of various types do occur, and the incidence of skeletal events during or immediately following radiation varies according to the tumor type—patients with breast cancer having a higher incidence than patients with prostate carcinoma. Similarly, those with lytic lesions have a higher incidence of either cord compression or long bone fracture after radiation therapy than patients with blastic lesions. For patients with a pathologic fracture, radiation is used as an adjuvant following surgical stabilization to help maximize the potential for local tumor control. Despite these advances in nonoperative treatment of skeletal metastases, surgery remains an effective and necessary treatment for the prevention and treatment of pathologic fractures.

Pelvic and Extremity Lesions

The most common sites of skeletal metastasis include the ribs, humerus, and femur. Pathologic fracture in at least one of these locations occurs in approximately 4 percent of all patients with solid tumors.[58] Breast cancer, renal cell carcinoma, myeloma, and lung carcinoma are the most common histologic types of tumors in patients who sustain pathologic fractures. Since most patients survive for a considerable period after the occurrence of a pathologic fracture, the aggressive treatment of these lesions has become increasingly important in maintaining quality of life. The mean survival time after treatment of a pathologic lesion of the humerus is approximately 8 months[113] and after treatment of a femoral lesion is 14 months. A subgroup of patients with expected longer or shorter predicted

FIGURE 17-14   *A, This patient with known metastatic renal cell carcinoma to bone began to have back pain that was severe and radicular in nature. He underwent palliative radiation therapy (3500 rads), which did not relieve his pain. B, Magnetic resonance imaging demonstrated severe dural compression at the T-10 level, with deviation of the dural sac toward the right. C, However, computed tomography allowed better differentiation of the tumor and remaining bone structure, with clear delineation of the degree of posterior element involvement. This necessitated a left-sided approach after appropriate embolization, with preservation of the right cortical wall of the vertebral body. D, E, Frozen section at the time of surgery demonstrated a significant degree of viable tumor despite previous irradiation. The anterior defect was filled with a methylmethacrylate spacer with iodine-125 seeds embedded into the three walls of the cavity not facing the dural sac. The patient remained free of disease in the location 15 months later.*

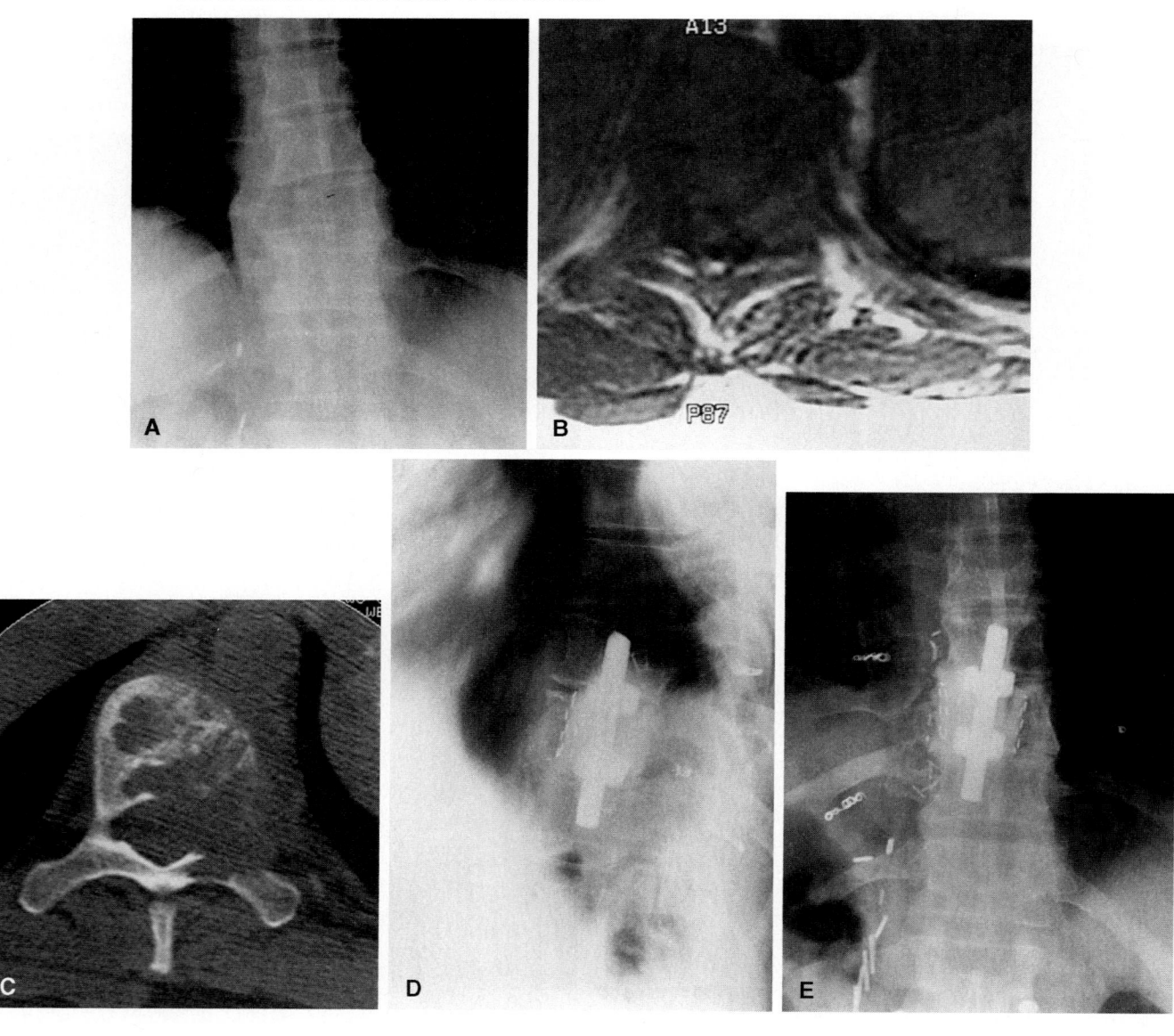

survival can be identified depending on the tumor type, extent of visceral disease, and general health.

Nonoperative management of pathologic fractures involving the pelvis and extremities, either by traction or plaster immobilization, has proven to adversely affect patient function, pain control, and quality of life. The combination of tumor at the fracture site, relatively catabolic state of most patients, and radiation, even in doses as low as 20 Gy, has been shown to significantly inhibit and prolong bone healing in the absence of rigid fixation.[19] Plaster immobilization also diminishes the skin-sparing effect of radiation because electron build-up occurs as the beam traverses the cast. Consequently, radiation through a cast is associated with higher incidence of skin breakdown than in extremities not covered with a cast. Although pathologic fractures can heal in the absence of surgical stabilization, the decision to treat surgically depends not only on the bone involved but the histology of the tumor. Although reports have cited rates of 16 to 35 percent for spontaneous fracture healing in pathologic fractures, a more practical indicator of fracture healing must consider the tumor histology. The incidence of fracture healing within 6 months following pathologic fracture from multiple myeloma is 67 percent, 44 percent for renal cell carcinoma, 37 percent for breast carcinoma, and less than 10 percent for lung carcinoma.[62] Anatomic location of the fracture also determines the likelihood of fracture healing with nonoperative intervention. Displaced pathologic fractures of the femoral neck invariably fail to heal, even with internal fixation. Nonoperative treatment of long bone fractures in the lower extremities or the pelvis may mandate prolonged bedrest. Such treatment increases the risk of complications such as pulmonary embolus, pneumonia, skin breakdown, osteopenia, and hypercalcemia.

As a result of the unacceptably high complication rate, poor pain control, and low union rate associated with nonoperative treatment of pathologic fractures, surgical treatment has assumed an increasingly important role. For pathologic fractures involving long bones, including those of the humerus, radius, ulna, femur, and tibia, operative treatment has become the preferred treatment modality for most patients. Appropriate fixation can reduce pain, improve function, decrease morbidity from immobility, and improve overall quality of life. Patients are not considered candidates for surgery if their life expectancy is very short or their overall condition precludes appropriate anesthesia. A prerequisite for surgery is the presence of adequate bone stock in close proximity to the impending or actual fracture to allow satisfactory fixation. The use of radiation therapy after operative stabilization is necessary in almost all cases to improve local control of the tumor, prevent secondary loss of fixation, and preserve the long-term stability of the construct.[26] When considering surgical stabilization, the size of the soft tissue component and the efficacy of the postoperative radiation must also be considered. In tumors such as renal cell carcinoma, thyroid carcinoma, and others with a high recurrence rate after radiation, the risk of failure of fixation due to local recurrence increases. Additionally in those with a very large soft tissue mass associated with the fracture, the benefit of a resection followed by segmental replacement may exceed that of internal fixation followed by radiation (Fig. 17-15).

Before operative treatment can be considered, certain basic criteria should be met:

1. The magnitude of the surgery should be considered with respect to the patient's general medical condition, life expectancy, recovery time, and expected functional outcome. Previously, it was suggested that surgery should be reserved for patients whose life expectancy was greater than 3 months. This "rule" should not be made without considering the patient's level of pain and functional status. In some cases a relatively short operative procedure (i.e.,

humeral nailing) can be performed that provides immediate pain control and restoration of function without prolonged hospitalization.
2. The planned procedure should in some way improve mobility, decrease pain, and facilitate general care of the patient.
3. The quality of bone proximal and distal to the area of the fracture must be sufficient to support fixation. In cases where bone quality is insufficient, more extensive procedures such as resection and prosthesis replacement may be indicated.
4. Local tumor control must be possible, either by resection of the tumor or use of postoperative adjuvants such as radiation.

Patients with impending fractures (large structural lesions) may also benefit from radiation therapy, surgical intervention, radiofrequency ablation/cementoplasty, or a combination of these in order to relieve pain and prevent fracture. Relative indications for use of these modalities have been suggested, but definitive criteria are still lacking. Symptomatic pain relief with radiation therapy can be expected for lesions that do not significantly compromise the integrity of the bone and are radiosensitive, as predicted by histologic type. Attempts to predict fracture risk in long bones based on radiographic assessment alone have been largely unsuccessful. Harrington used radiographic criteria that included a lesion of 2.5 cm in diameter or greater than 50 percent cortical involvement as predictive of impending pathologic fracture.[74] These recommendations were, however, based on a series of patients with lesions in the subtrochanteric area of the femur only. Others have applied Harrington's criteria to other long bones.[8] However, because of wide variations in the load-bearing capacity of bones, the criteria of a 2.5-cm defect or 50 percent cortical involvement are not universally applicable.[87] Additionally, the recommendations were based on lytic osseous lesions.[8,53] An additional consideration of fracture risk, other than the size and location of the lesion, includes the host bone response to the tumor. Diffuse permeative lesions are harder to assess for their potential for pathologic fractures than are purely lytic lesions.[99] Similarly, the assessment of fracture risk for blastic lesions, such as those from metastatic carcinoma of the prostate or breast, is less predictable than for purely lytic lesions. Experimental data have demonstrated that a hole in the cortex diminishes the ability to resist torsion by 60 percent.[137] Similar studies have shown that the strength of bone is decreased by 60 to 90 percent when a diaphyseal defect involving 50 percent of the cortex is created.[87] Others have suggested that a defect in the cortex of 30 mm is the critical parameter,[173] and a study utilizing finite-element analysis suggests that it is both the size and shape of the lesions.[100] Mirels developed a scoring system to quantify fracture risk in patients with long bone metastases. The scoring system includes factors such as site, pain, radiographic characteristics of the lesion (blastic, mixed, or lytic), and size. These four factors are given a numeric assignment from 1 to 3. The maximum cumulative score is 12, and the minimum is 3. Mirels suggested that a cumulative score of 9 or higher was an indication for prophylactic fixation.[126] The Mirels system has proved to be inaccurate

FIGURE 17-15 *This middle-aged gentleman presented with severe hip and groin pain arising over several months. Plain radiographs **(A, B)** demonstrated a permeative destructive lesion* (arrows) *in the intertrochanteric/subtrochanteric region of his femur.* **C,** *Computed tomography showed an extremely large soft tissue mass extending out of and surrounding the femur. Needle biopsy showed an adenocarcinoma of gastrointestinal origin, but no primary could be found on extensive workup. As a result of the severity of the pain and the permeative nature of the lesion with the very large soft tissue mass, he underwent a proximal femoral resection and prosthetic reconstruction with excellent pain relief and return to function **(D)**.*

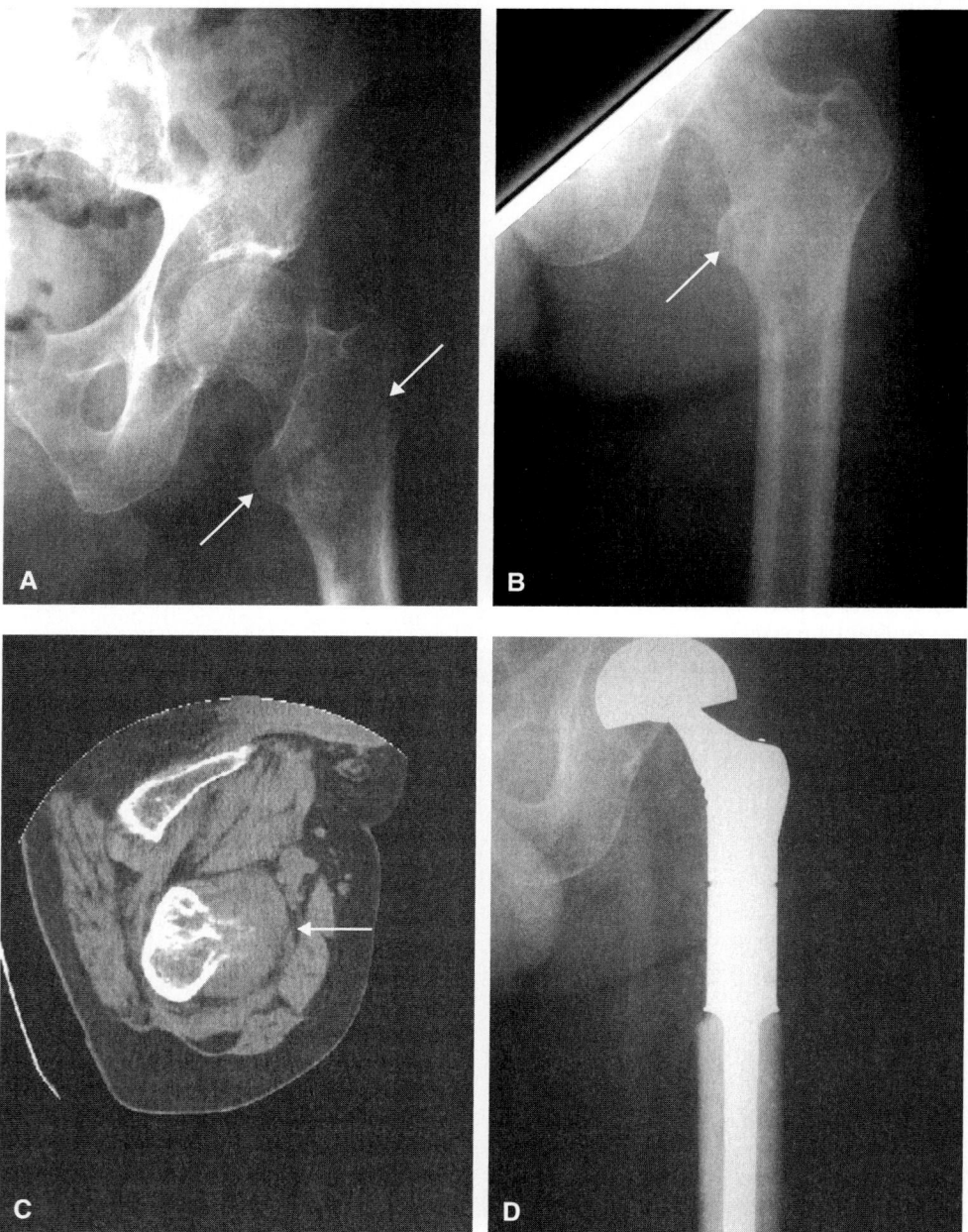

in a number of studies,[40,173] and a recent study suggested that the only effective and reproducible criteria in femoral shafts were axial involvement greater than 30 mm and circumferential cortical involvement greater than 50 percent.[173]

As previously noted, surgical intervention is indicated in most patients with established pathologic fractures and in those patients with large impending lytic lesions of long bones or lesions that are progressively enlarging or who remain symptomatic after other treatment.[150] It has been shown with lesions of the femur that patients who receive prophylactic fixation have a shorter hospitalization and are more likely to be discharged home and to retain aid-free ambulation than those who sustain a completed fracture before undergoing fixation.[176]

Prior to proceeding with surgical treatment of a skeletal metastasis the physician should have a thorough understanding of the anatomic extent of metastatic involvement. In lesions involving long bones, this includes an understanding of the degree of destruction (i.e., a single area of cortex vs. circumferential involvement) that precipitated the fracture as well as the condition of the bone distal or proximal to the lesion. When two or more lesions are located within the same bone, the mode of fixation should allow for protection to both areas. Additionally, an understanding of the biology and natural history of the tumor is critical for minimizing complications related to tumor recurrence or progression with resultant loss of fixation. In tumors such as renal cell carcinoma, thyroid carcinoma, and so on, which are resistant to radiation in normal palliative doses (30–35 Gy in 10 fractions), local tumor recurrence is more likely to occur, and resection with endoprosthetic replacement of the metastatic lesion may be indicated to minimize the risk of local failure (Fig. 17-16). Large contained lesions (e.g., within the pelvis) can also be treated with radiofrequency ablation, which can achieve local control even in patients for whom radiation has previously failed. With tumors that typically involve multiple areas in the same bone (e.g., breast carcinoma, myeloma), isolated fixation of a single area may result in fracture in a more distal location within the same bone. Therefore, prophylactic fixation of the entire bone rather than a single area should be considered (Fig. 17-17). In clinical situations where union is unlikely to occur (and stability depends on union) within the lifespan of the patient, prosthetic replacement is more appropriate than fracture fixation (e.g., pathologic subcapital or femoral neck fractures) to achieve immediate full weight-bearing and return to function. When fracture fixation is indicated the surgeon often cannot rely on the same techniques used for the treatment of nonpathologic fractures. The type of reconstruction and fixation employed must be such that fracture healing is not a necessary component to achieve the full weight-bearing that will allow mobilization of the patient. Load-sharing devices such as compression hip screws that are indicated in non-neoplastic conditions are relatively indicated in neoplastic conditions. In non-neoplastic conditions the internal fixation device maintains fixation until osseous union occurs. In neoplastic conditions, osseous union is usually delayed or may never occur and the race between osseous union and implant failure is lost. Similarly, large defects in the bone further compromise the stability of the fixation, and areas of deficient bone may need to be restored with the use of methylmethacrylate. Therefore, the goals of internal fixation should be directed at achieving immediate rigid rotational and axial stability. If full weight-bearing stability cannot be restored with reconstruction of the remaining bone even with augmentation with methylmethacrylate, then resection and alternative reconstructive techniques such as prosthetic replacement should be considered.

In addition to obtaining immediate rigid internal fixation to restore function and quality of life, the goals of surgery should also include local tumor control. Debulking the tumor by curettage or marginal resection has been used to decrease tumor burden, thereby possibly improving the effects of radiation and decreasing the risk of local recurrence.[50,73] Debulking or use of marginal resection does not usually achieve adequate local control, and postoperative radiation therapy is a critical adjunct. With the increased use of the current generation of locked intramedullary nails more long bone fractures are being treated with closed nailing in lieu of open procedures. Because newer intramedullary nails are stronger and more resistant to failure from repetitive cyclic loading, they can maintain stability for longer times than previously used intramedullary devices. Carefully assess device strength before using it, as the reconstruction nail is stronger than others.[106] However, even these devices may need to be augmented with methylmethacrylate when local bone destruction is extensive, fracture healing does not occur, and longer survival is anticipated.

Upper Extremity Lesions

Often in the past pathologic fractures of the upper extremity were managed with nonoperative techniques. Although humeral and radial fractures, unlike lower extremity fractures, could be managed nonoperatively without hospitalization, management in this fashion often leads to impaired function, decreased independence, and prolonged pain. Only a few reports (most more than 30 years ago) showed satisfactory results in patients treated nonoperatively for humeral fractures,[29,110] whereas utilizing current fixations methods most patients treated with operative stabilization can now achieve excellent pain relief and rapid return to function with a low incidence of complications.[46,49,57,100,107] Thus for actual pathologic fractures, operative stabilization is indicated for almost all cases unless contraindicated by patient condition. Decision making is somewhat more difficult for large impending lesions of the humerus and radius, as neither are weight-bearing bones and fracture is not a catastrophic event in the femur. Additionally many of the criteria for when the lesion is of sufficient size and configuration to warrant fixation were based on mechanical studies of the femur. If radiographic evidence indicates that the lesion of either the humerus or the radius involves 50 percent of the diameter of the bone (and thus destroys the cortex), it should undergo internal fixation as the chance of fracture is relatively high. Decision making about intramedullary lesions that are large and thick but do not penetrate the cortex should be based on whether the lesions occur in the dominant or nondominant extremity, the amount of pain the patient experiences, and the tumor's responsiveness to radiation or chemotherapy. If the lesion causes significant pain and is in the dominant extremity, surgical treatment is indicated, especially if the tumor is not especially responsive such as tumors of the lung, kidneys, or thyroid or melanoma and sarcoma. If the lesion does not cause pain and is of a sensitive histology (myeloma, lymphoma, breast, or prostate), then nonoperative treatment is indicated.

Fixation of pathologic fractures of the humerus has been advocated since the 1960s; at that time, antegrade nailing with Rush rods was the method most commonly used. The technique has been abandoned because of the number of complications and the lack of both rotational and longitundinal stability in a situation where the fracture is unlikely to ever heal during the patient's lifetime. Current advances in instrumentation and surgical technique now allow surgeons to select the most appropriate

FIGURE 17-16 *A, B, This 57-year-old man with renal cell carcinoma sustained a pathologic fracture of the proximal humerus and underwent plating and postoperative radiation therapy. A, At the time of initial surgery, tumor involvement of the soft tissue and the distal fragment was evident. Neither intramedullary fixation to bypass the defect nor resection was considered for this tumor, known to be poorly responsive to radiation therapy and most chemotherapy. C, D, Within 6 months, complete dissolution of the proximal portion of the humerus had occurred, with gross instability and a soft tissue mass. E, F, En bloc resection of the proximal 60% of the humerus was undertaken with reconstruction with a modular prosthesis. One year after resection, the patient continued to function well, having returned to his hobby of fishing.*

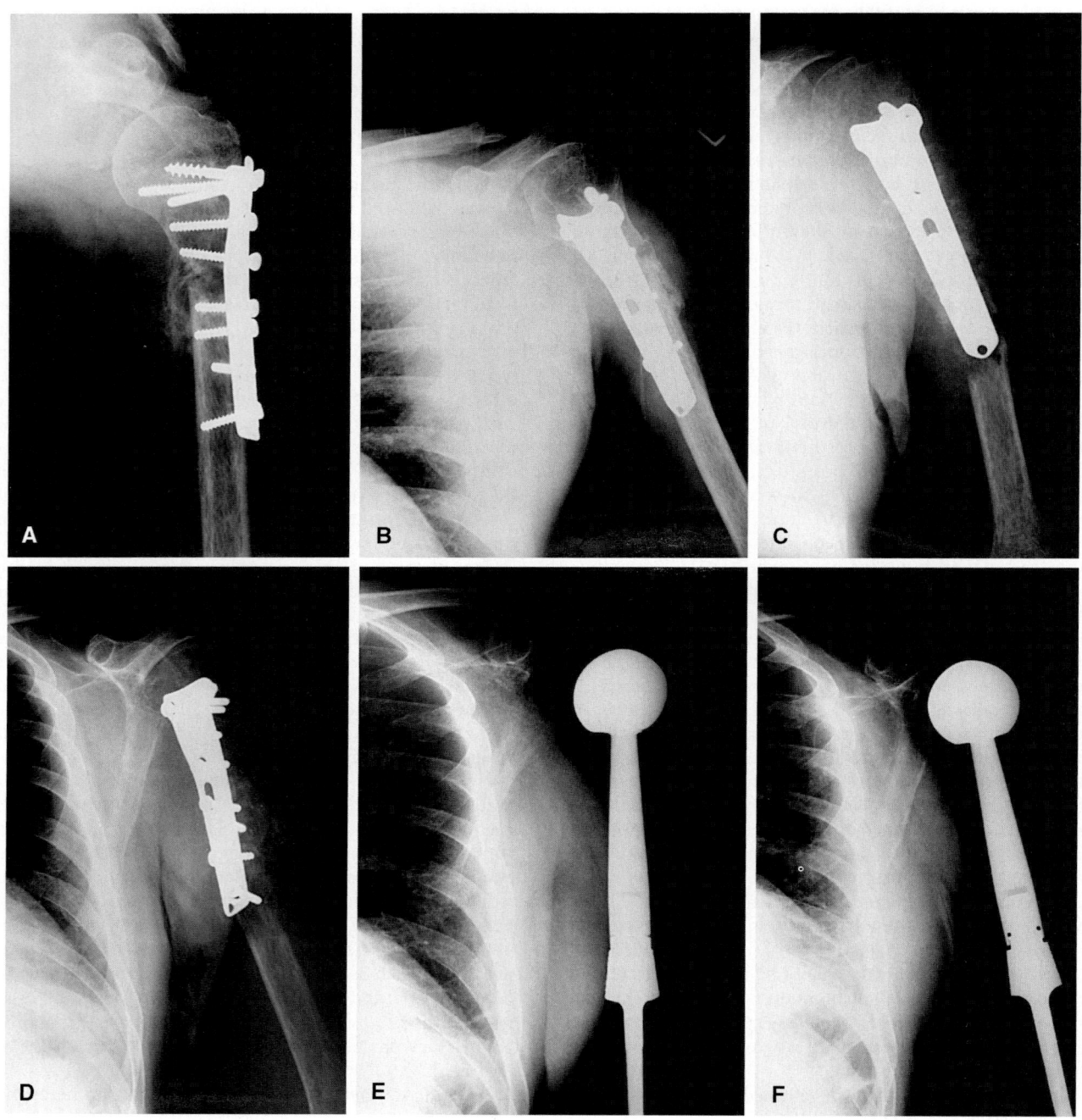

treatment method to fit the clinical situation for either pathologic or impending fractures of the humerus and radius. For the humerus the selection of technique is related to the region of the bone and the extent of tumor destruction.

For proximal humeral lesions with destruction of the head or fracture through the anatomic or even surgical neck of the humerus, endoprosthetic replacement gives the most rapid, reproducible, and stable results.[25,49,61,156] Although function may be somewhat restricted, the results

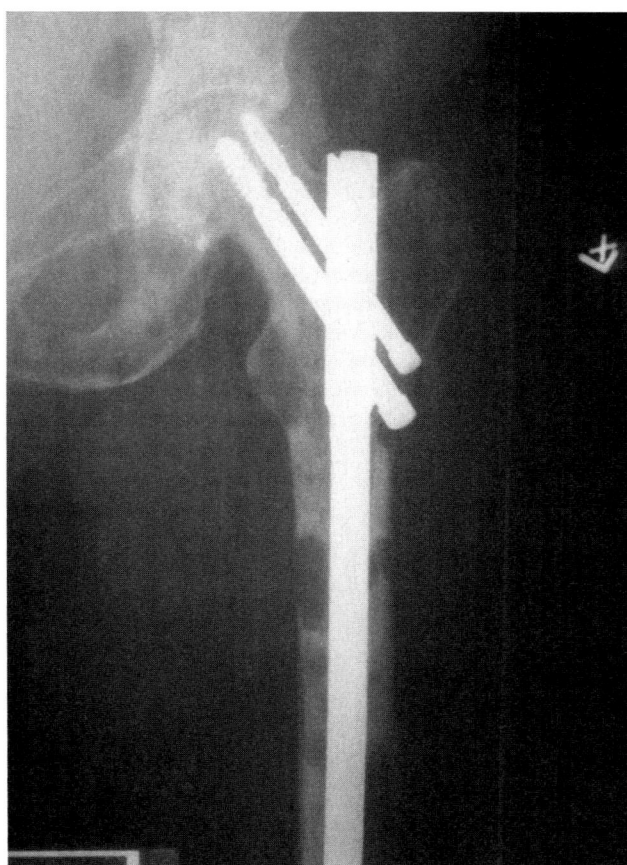

FIGURE 17-17   *Especially in the femur, fixation of the entire bone is critical to prevent subsequent loss of fixation or fracture below or above previous fixation. In this patient with myeloma, the femoral neck intertrochanteric region and distal femur are protected in case the tumor extends proximally or a new lesion arises distally. A standard femoral nail used for this lesion could potentially fail at the proximal end.*

patients with pathologic fractures were minimal, the results were thought to be acceptable.[37,89,95,174] However, in larger series that included patients with both pathologic and nonpathologic fractures treated with an antegrade technique, impaired shoulder function is reported to range from 10 to 37 percent.[86,168,170] Impaired shoulder function resulted from problems associated with the proximal locking screw, impingement from the nail not being adequately seated in bone, and injury to the rotator cuff at the time of surgery[55,86,119](Fig. 17-18). Retrograde closed humeral nailing had been advocated as a method of achieving fixation while avoiding the complications noted with Rush rods and antegrade locked nailing.[88,119,141,142] A retrograde locked technique incorporates the advantages of distal entry portal and a more secure fixation in the wide

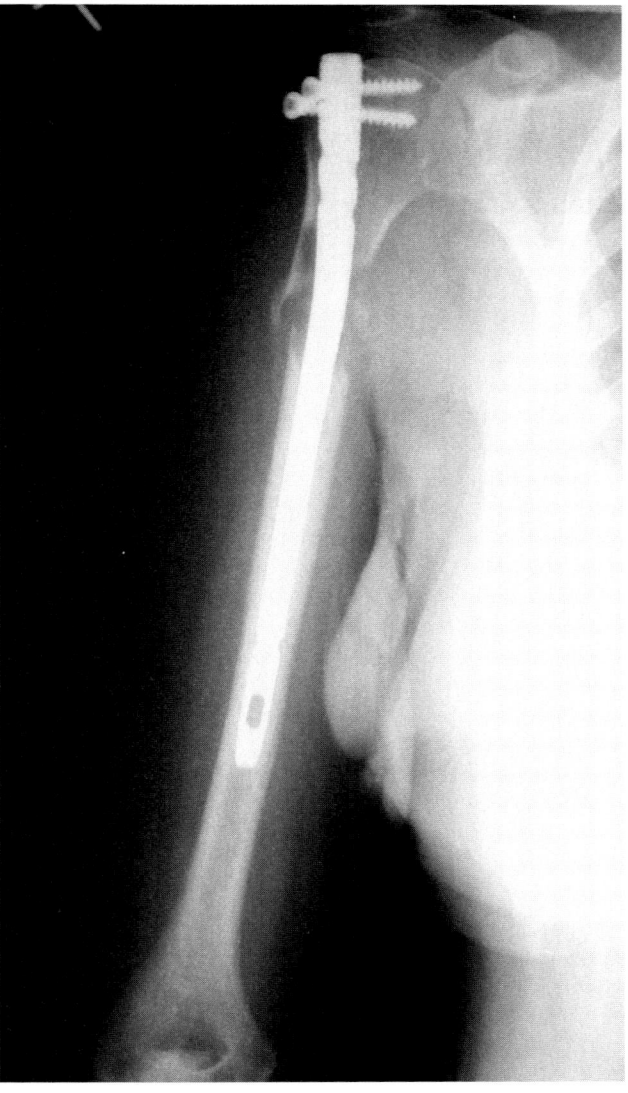

FIGURE 17-18   *This patient sustained a pathologic fracture of the proximal humerus and was stabilized using an antegrade nailing technique. The rod was left prominent and resulted in pain and limited shoulder function.*

are better than attempts at fracture repair with a plate and methylmethacrylate, and the stability and return to function are more immediate.

If sufficient bone proximal and distal to the lesion remains, fixation of humeral lesions with an intramedullary nail can provide immediate and long-lasting pain relief.[117,157] The use of locked intramedullary nails has greatly improved the ability of the surgeon to obtain immediate stability and prevent migration of the implant than was possible with previous implants.[41,46,70,140] Techniques for nail insertion include an antegrade or retrograde approach, with the advantage of the latter being that the entry portal does not violate the rotator cuff.[121] The functional outcomes using an antegrade technique, however, have been mixed in part because of the rotator cuff involvement with the nail insertion site and in part because of the pathology often being in the proximal end of the humerus. Because the functional expectations for

proximal fragment (Fig. 17-19). This technique allows a distal entry portal with proximal fixation extending to just below the subchondral plate of the humeral head (Fig. 17-20). The use of a second surgical incision made directly over the lesion to allow curettage and filling with methylmethacrylate is now rarely necessary with the use of locked nailing. With placement of the tip of the nail up under the subchondral plate of the humeral head, the proximal fragment may be fixed by a freehand technique for interlocking through a small stab wound in the deltoid muscle. This minimizes blood loss as well as allowing for early motion. The potential advantage of this technique is that the shoulder joint is not violated, and therefore problems associated with injury to the rotator cuff are avoided. With this technique, pain relief and stability are achieved in 95 percent of patients. If insufficient bone stock remains in the proximal portion of the humeral shaft, then the head may have to be sacrificed to attain satisfactory fixation, and a long endoprosthetic replacement (with a long stem and polymethylmethacrylate) should be considered[25,61,156] (see Fig. 17-16). Functional reconstruction of the rotator cuff is difficult, especially if there is tumor involvement of the deltoid or the rotator cuff muscles. However, the prosthesis gives satisfactory pain relief and restores some function to the extremity. Distal humeral lesions are uncommon but may be difficult to stabilize when they do occur. Augmentation with methylmethacrylate is almost always necessary to achieve sufficient stability to allow immediate unrestricted activity (Fig. 17-21).

Whereas only 20 percent of all metastatic lesions occur in the upper extremity, only 0.4 percent occur in the radius, and 0.2 percent in the ulna.[157] If sufficient bone is present, the most common treatment is plating and augmentation with methylmethacrylate. Occasionally intramedullary rodding can be employed (Fig. 17-22).

Lower Extremity Lesions

Metastatic lesions to the femur account for approximately 25 percent of all metastatic lesions to bone.[29,80] However, they can be among the most devastating lesions, when the implications of pathologic fracture are considered.[122] Pathologic fractures of the femur most commonly involve the femoral neck, intertrochanteric region, and subtrochanteric region. Midshaft and distal fractures occur less frequently. The goals of treatment include restoration of immediate postoperative full weight-bearing capability and return to function as rapidly as possible. This is important to both maximize quality of life and also minimize any disruption of systemic chemotherapy treatment. For a given fracture pattern, this often requires techniques that are not used in patients with fractures resulting from nonneoplastic causes. Although the mean survival for patients who sustain a pathologic femur fracture is approximately

FIGURE 17-19 *A,* This 45-year-old man was swinging a golf club and sustained a sudden pathologic fracture of his nondominant arm. Subsequent evaluation revealed a large renal mass. *B, C,* He underwent closed, locked intramedullary nailing of the humerus, which restored length and stability while bypassing the defect in the shaft. He began radiation therapy and then chemotherapy within several days of surgery.

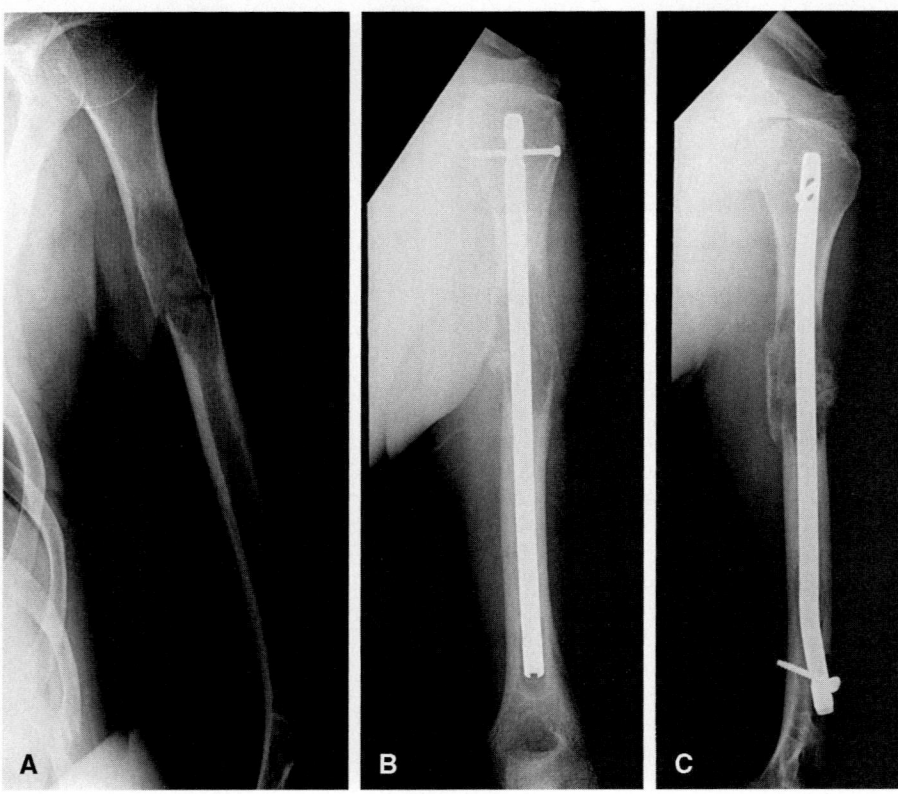

A   B   C

FIGURE 17-20 *Operative technique for retrograde humeral nailing of pathologic lesions. Reamed retrograde humeral nailing for pathologic fractures is done with the patient under general or regional anesthesia, such as supraclavicular block. **A,** The patient is placed supine on a regular operating table with the affected extremity extended over the table's edge. If the patient is positioned so that the scapula of the extremity is at the edge of the table, there is sufficient clearance for the use of an image intensifier to adequately visualize the humeral head. The arm is suspended by use of a finger trap, the head is rotated away from the operative side, and the patient is prepared and draped from the shoulder to the wrist, with the arm free in the field. **B,** The arm is placed across the chest and supported on a towel roll, so that the shoulder and elbow are at 90°. The excision line is made from the tip of the olecranon proximally for about 8 cm. **C,** The incision is carried sharply through the skin and subcutaneous tissue until the triceps tendon is identified. The tendon is carefully visualized, and the entry through the tendon is at its midportion. The tendon is split sharply from the proximal tip of the olecranon. The muscle is then opened bluntly throughout the length of the incision by splitting the fibers of the triceps. Subperiosteal dissection of the posterior humerus is completed. **D,** Hayes retractors are then placed, one on each side of the humerus just proximal to the epicondyles beneath the stripped periosteum, to provide retraction of the posterior aspect of the humerus. Beginning 2 cm above the proximal edge of the olecranon fossa, a 14-inch drill hole is made through the posterior cortex of the humerus. This hole must be directly centered between the medial and the lateral cortices. The second and third drill holes are made just proximal to the first. Using a high-speed bur, an oval hole is made and widened out to the medial and lateral cortices. As indicated in the diagram, the bur is used to form a ramp for subsequent reaming of the humerus, and its distal end is beveled to the olecranon fossa; the posterior cortex on the proximal end is undercut. This allows a flexible reamer to slide easily into the humerus. At this point, a 9-mm end-cutting and side-cutting reamer is placed in the trough to ascertain whether it fits easily and will not bind.*

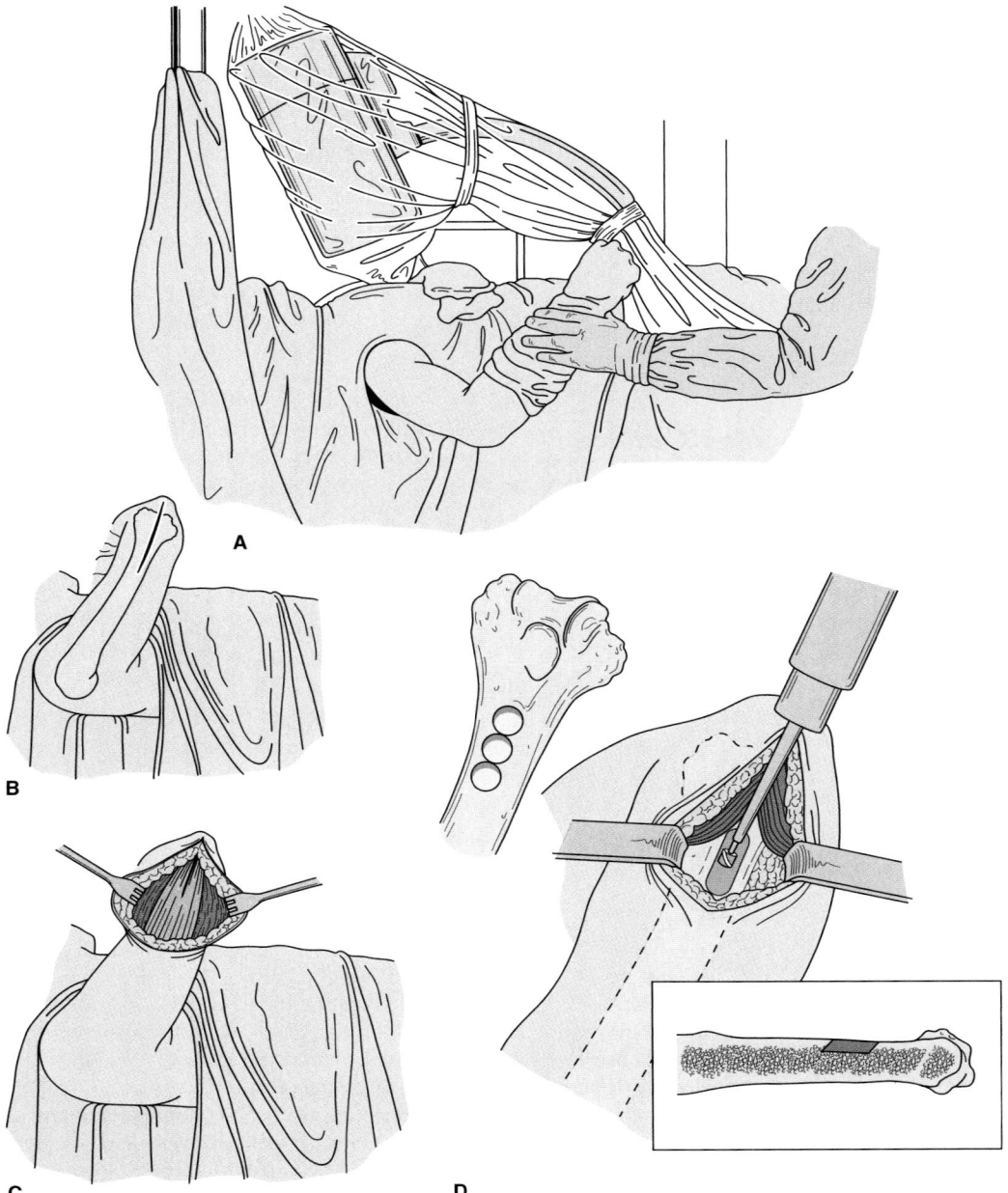

A

B

C

D

(Continued)

FIGURE 17-20 *(Continued)* **E,** *A guide pin is then passed proximally across the fracture site.* **F,** *The guide pin is placed just across the fracture site in a closed fashion. The reamer is then advanced up and over the guide pin. Care is taken so that the reamer passes along the canal and does not ream the anterior cortex.* **G,** *To allow accurate visualization of the humerus with image intensification and to aid in reduction, the arm is positioned at approximately 45° from the side of the table. The humeral shaft is then reamed in 0.5-mm increments. Because most lesions are on the proximal third of the humerus, it is unnecessary to ream this area. All cortical reaming is done at the isthmus, located at the junction of the middle and distal thirds of the humerus. Not reaming the cancellous bone of the proximal third provides more substantial fixation. Care is taken to preserve all cortical bone at the isthmus. Nail sizes are available from 8 mm upward; the smallest possible nail should be used to preserve all cortical bone. Over-reaming by 0.5 to 1 mm is necessary to pass the nail.*

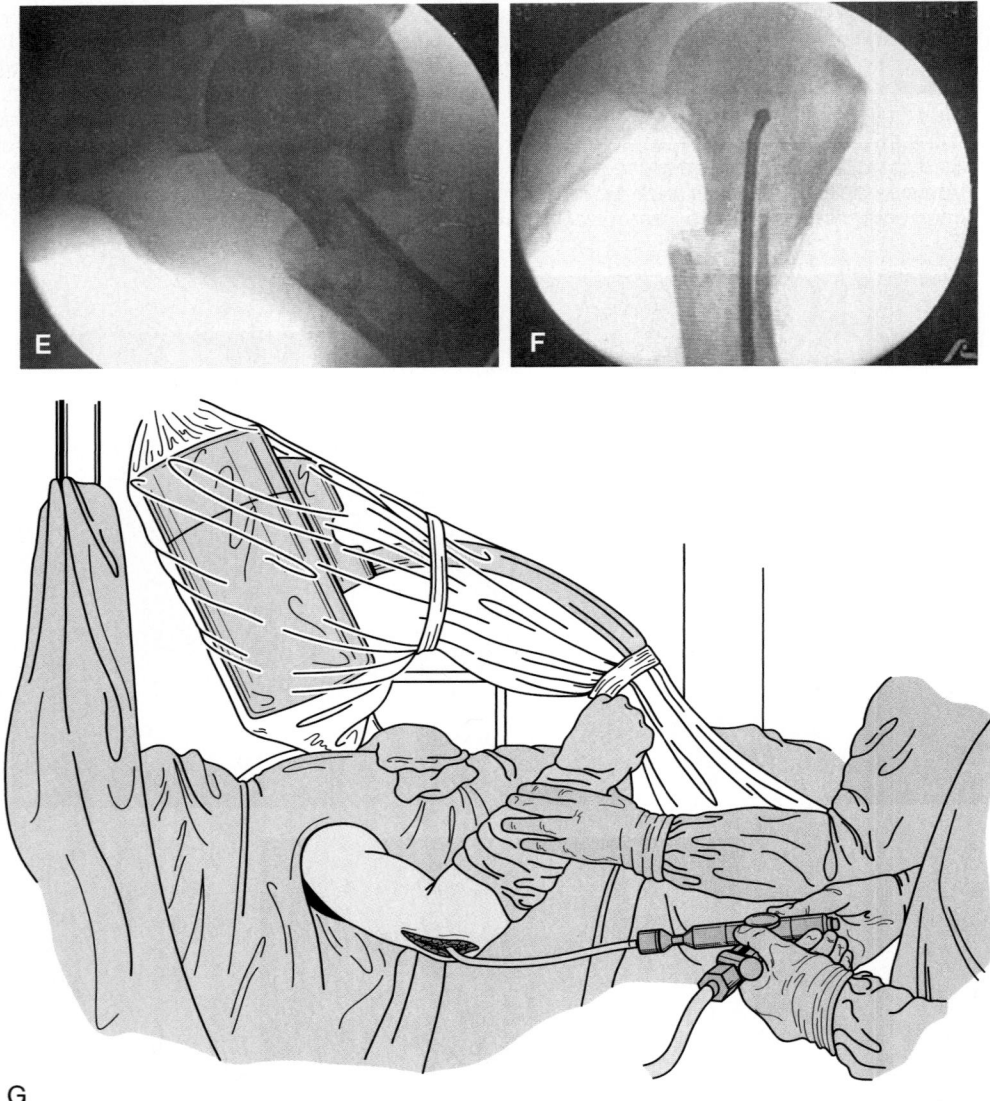

G

(Continued)

14 months, there is a wide range in survival from less than 9 months in a patient with non–small-cell lung cancer (NSCLC) to 10 years or more with patients with myeloma or breast cancer. Therefore, treatment options that allow immediate stability may also need to be durable.

Pathologic fractures of the femoral neck and intertrochanteric region are most commonly managed with endoprosthetic replacement[41,111,116,164] (Fig. 17-23). This method is preferred to standard fixation techniques for three reasons. First, there is a low probability of healing of pathologic femoral neck fractures.[63] Second, endoprosthetic replacement alleviates the necessity for prolonged restricted weight-bearing in a person with a shortened lifespan. Finally, there is often significant bone loss in fractures of the neck and intertrochanteric region, which compromises successful internal fixation.[136] In most series three types of complications are encountered with this technique: dislocation of the endoprosthetic replacement, postoperative abductor insufficiency, and an increased wound complication rate in patients who have received preoperative

FIGURE 17-20 *(Continued)* **H,** *The length of the nail is measured to ensure that the tip comes within 1 cm of the subchondral plate of the humeral head. The distal end sits within the trough after the correct nail size has been selected. The nail is placed over the guide pin and fully inserted. If curettage of the lesion through a second incision is to be done at this point, the nail is inserted only to the distal end of the lesion. The guide pin is left in place across the fracture site. An incision is made on the anterolateral surface of the proximal humerus, and the lesion is thoroughly curetted. The guide pin is used as a marker. After the lesion has been curetted and the proximal humerus has been filled with methylmethacrylate, the nail is impacted into the fully seated position, and the guide pin is removed.* **I,** *If a locking nail is selected, the distal lock is placed first by drilling a unicortical screw placed under direct vision through the screw hole in the distal trough.* **J,** *The proximal lock is placed by a freehand technique with the patient in a supine position and the arm in 90° of internal rotation so that the slot in the proximal end of the nail is fully visualized (top inset). Cannulated 3.5-mm screws are used with a 2.0-mm guide pin. A small incision is made in the skin over the slot, and the guide pin is pushed through the deltoid to the bone. Image intensification is used to orient the guide pin so that it is reduced to a dot, indicating that it is parallel to the slot in the nail. It is then pushed or drilled through the humeral head, depending on the density of the bone, through the nail to the opposite cortex. The position is again checked on image intensification, the arm is carefully rotated 90°, and the position is again checked (bottom inset). Care must be taken not to bend the guide wire, and if it needs to be repositioned, the arm must again be internally rotated to fully visualize the slot before changing the position of the guide wire. The final position of the nail and inspection of the joint are accomplished using image intensification. The final position of the nail in the distal humerus is checked to make sure it is in the trough. Drains are placed in both wounds, and the incisions are closed. The arm is postoperatively immobilized in a sling, and motion begins on the third postoperative day, as soon as the drains are removed. For locked nailings, radiation therapy can begin at the site of the lesion on the third postoperative day.*

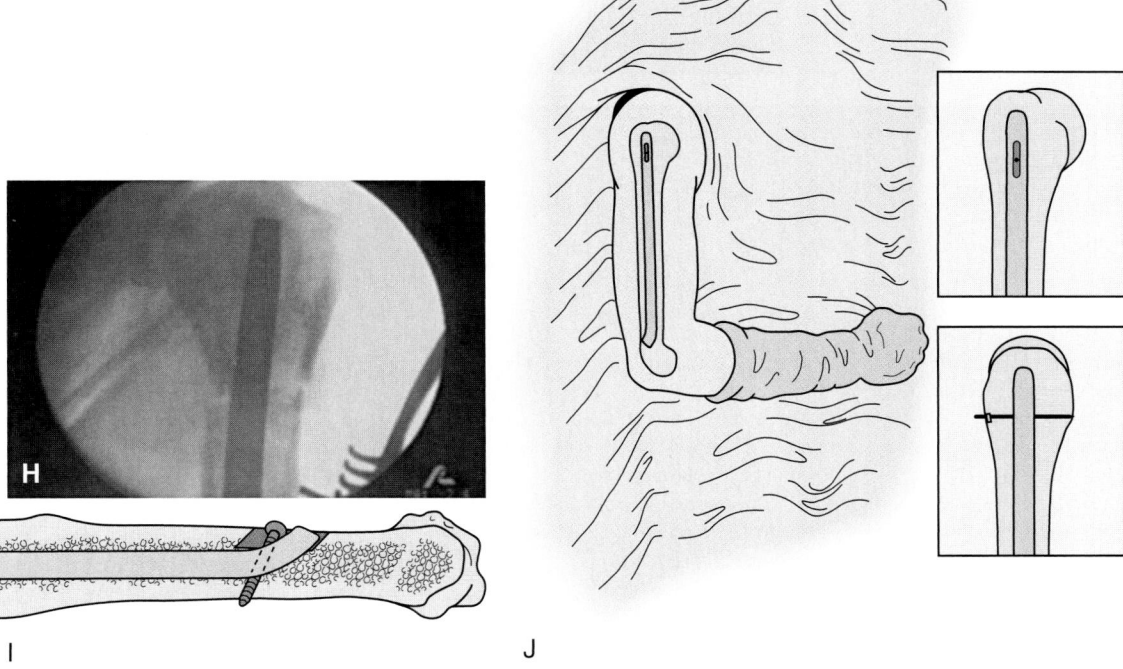

I   J

(Continued)

FIGURE 17-20   *(Continued)* **K,** *This 70-year-old man sustained a pathologic fracture of the proximal humerus from myeloma. He underwent locked retrograde nailing and was removed from his sling on the third postoperative day, regaining full elbow function by 2 weeks.* **L, M,** *At 3 months, the fracture demonstrated a solid union.*

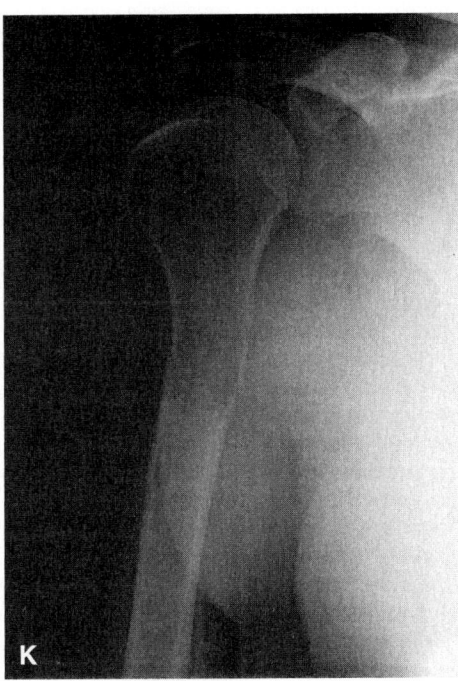

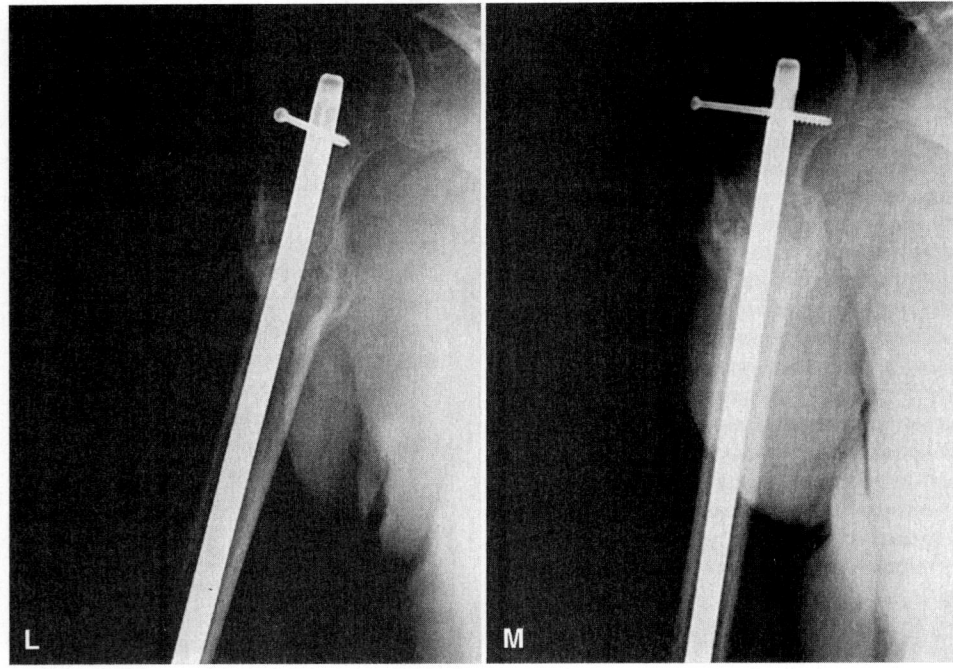

radiation to the area.[177] A series that directly compared reconstruction nails to endoprosthetic replacement in proximal femoral lesions showed fewer complications with the endoprosthetic replacement in lesions in the proximal third of the femur.[177] To achieve an optimal result, several technical features need to be considered, one of which is adequate filling of all defects. When a large area of tumor destruction is present, the region should be thoroughly curetted to remove all visible tumor and then filled completely with methylmethacrylate. In patients in whom the destruction continues below the lesser trochanter, either the defect should be filled with methylmethacrylate or

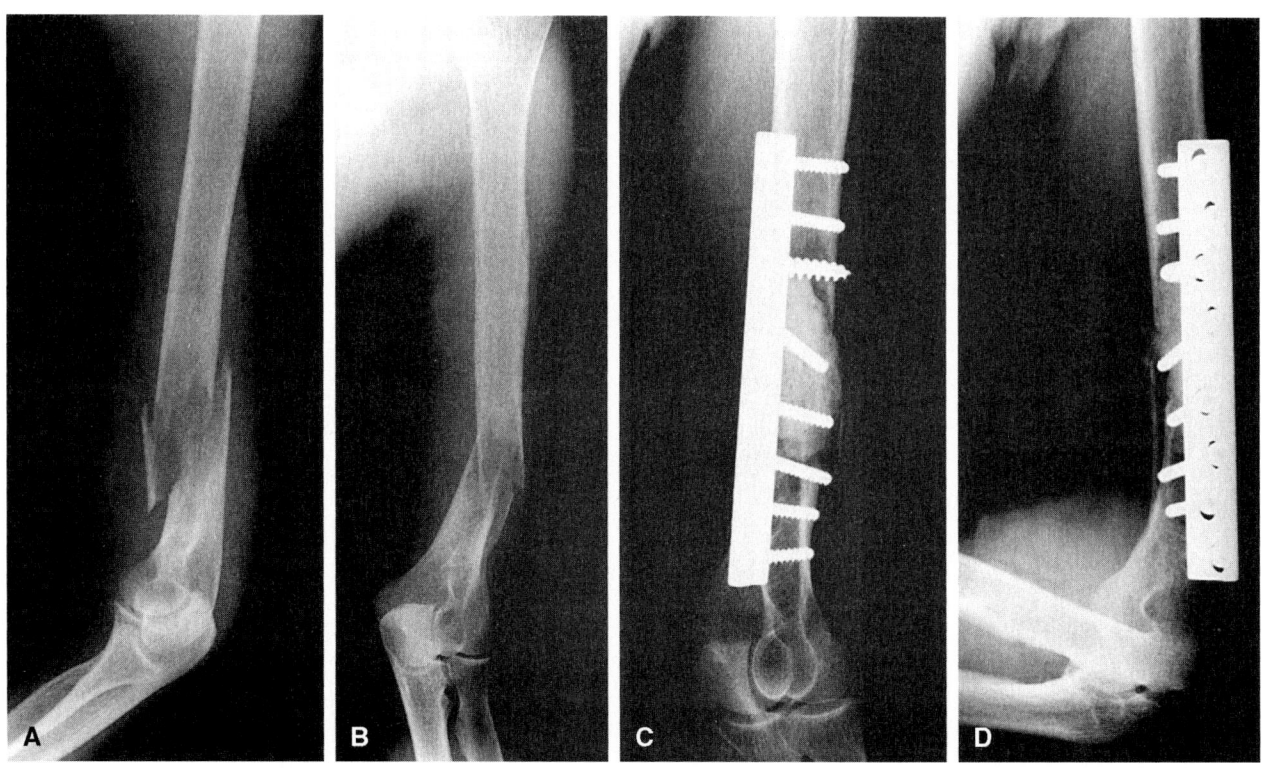

FIGURE 17-21 **A, B,** *This patient with multiple myeloma sustained a comminuted fracture of the distal humerus of his dominant arm.* **C, D,** *Open reduction and internal fixation was done but augmented with methylmethacrylate to enhance fixation and stability. Provisional fixation was obtained by using only three of the screws. The defect was then filled, and the remainder of the screws were placed by drilling and tapping the methacrylate.*

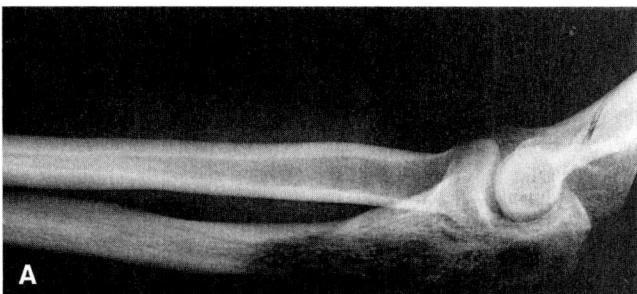

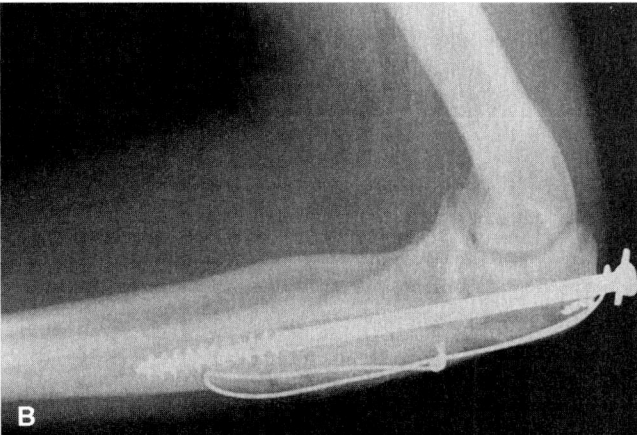

FIGURE 17-22 *This 37-year-old man with carcinoma of the breast sustained a pathologic fracture through the proximal third of his ulna.* **A,** *The lateral radiograph showed a permeative lesion of 3 cm with a pathologic fracture through it. The patient underwent open curettage of the lesion. A 6.5-mm cancellous screw was passed through the lesion and was bound in the normal bone of the distal ulnar canal.* **B, C,** *The defect was filled with methylmethacrylate, and a tension band wire was used to reinforce the repair. The patient had immediate relief of pain and, within 2 weeks, had regained full range of motion of the elbow.*

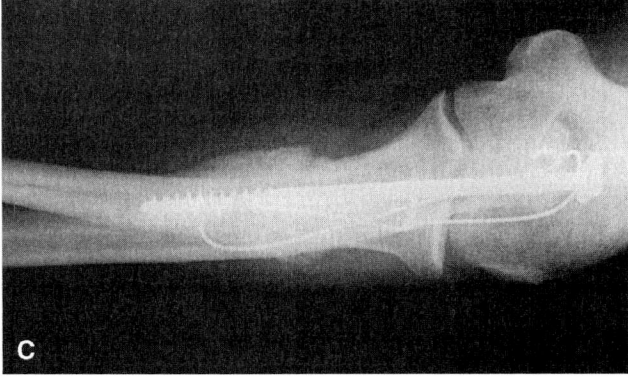

FIGURE 17-23 | *This 55-year-old woman had diffusely metastatic carcinoma of the breast. She presented with bilateral hip pain and incomplete paraplegia resulting from a midthoracic lesion. The patient underwent decompression and stabilization of the thoracic lesion and staged, prophylactic fixation of the left femur with a reconstruction nail. **A,** Because of the displaced subcapital fracture, she underwent bipolar cemented arthroplasty on the right side. **B,** One year after surgery, the patient was ambulatory with a cane.*

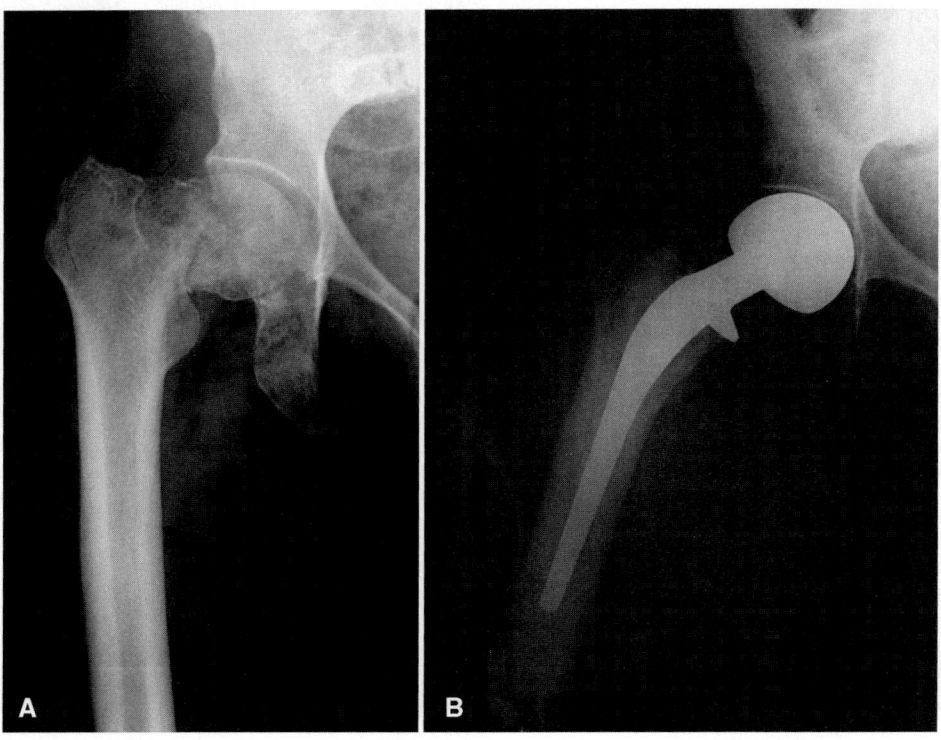

a calcar replacement may be necessary since the methylmethacrylate is not always sufficient to ensure immediate and long-term stability. With an endoprosthetic calcar replacement adequate reattachment of the abductors becomes an issue. In those patients who also have metastases distally within the femoral shaft or who are at risk of developing metastasis within the femoral shaft, a long-stem prosthesis should be chosen to protect those lesions at the same time.[111] It is critical to bypass lesions so that fractures do not occur below the tip of a previously cemented hemiarthroplasty.[104] Therefore, prior to hemiarthroplasy radiographs of the entire femur should be obtained in two planes to assess the need for prophylactic fixation. In patients undergoing elective surgery for an impending fracture of the proximal femur, the entire femur should be assessed not only with plain radiographs but with a bone scan or MRI as well. Noncemented arthroplasties, even in young patients, are discouraged in patients with metastatic tumor because of poor bone stock, compromised healing potential, and the risk of prosthetic loosening associated with tumor progression.

Several methods of treatment are available for impending fractures of the femoral neck and intertrochanteric region (Fig. 17-24). The preferred technique depends on the local extent of tumor, the size of the lesion, tumor histology (responsiveness to radiation), and the presence or absence of concomitant tumor at separate sites within the femur. In those patients in whom the lesion is well confined within the neck, and in whom there is a limited life expectancy (e.g., in adenocarcinoma of the lung, squamous cell carcinoma, or other solid tumors), the probability of additional lesions within the femur developing is limited. In such selected cases, curettage of the lesion and fixation with a compression hip screw may be appropriate but should be augmented with methylmethacrylate and always followed by postoperative radiation.[82] In patients with more than one lesion involving the femur, or with long life expectancy and multiple bone metastases (e.g., adenocarcinoma of the breast, multiple myeloma), prophylactic fixation of the entire femur with a single procedure should be considered. This minimizes the chance that a distal lesion in the same bone may become symptomatic or fracture later. The use of a locked reconstructive nail, with fixation going up into the femoral neck, protects the femoral neck, shaft, and the distal femur and has greatly facilitated the treatment of this patient population.[85,108] Subtrochanteric lesions of the femur are potentially the most devastating and most difficult to manage. Plate-and-screw combinations are generally contraindicated for pathologic subtrochanteric fractures (see Fig. 17-4), as with bone loss, delayed healing, and the need for immediate weight-bearing in the cancer patient, the rate of failure was unacceptable. These were initially supplanted by the Zickel nail, which improved results but

FIGURE 17-24 | *This female with a known history of breast cancer had the gradual onset of pain in her hip. She endured it over several months and gradually decreased her activities until she presented to the emergency room unable to walk. Her admission radiograph showed a severely comminuted intertrochanteric/subtrochanteric fracture (A). Because of her size and the fact that she also had an impending pathologic fracture of the contralateral humerus, she underwent a proximal femoral resection with immediate return to full weight-bearing (B). The humerus was prophylactically fixed as a separate procedure 2 weeks later.*

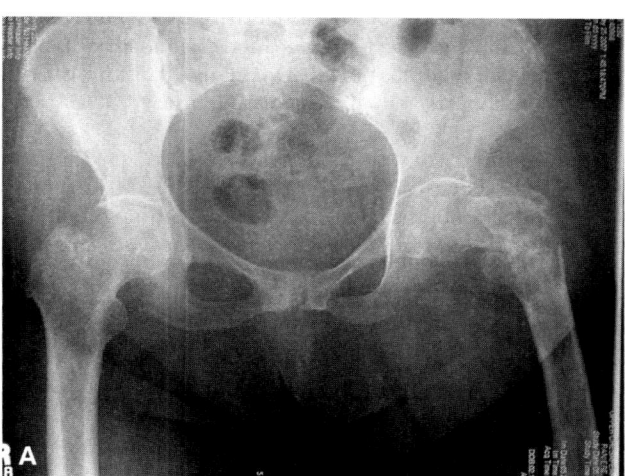
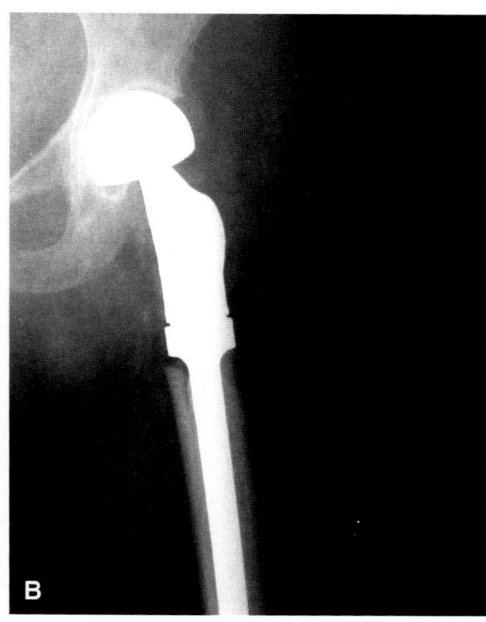

had many technical difficulties.[70] The Zickel nail has been now replaced by newer designs.

The current generation of locked nail devices allows fixation of subtrochanteric lesions with protection of the entire femur. Patients with both subtrochanteric and midshaft or distal femoral lesions and patients who have high potential for additional metastatic deposits during their life span (e.g., those with myeloma or breast or prostate cancer) are best treated with a proximal and distal interlocking nail with proximal fixation up into the femoral neck (Fig. 17-25). The use of a standard femoral nail (nonreconstruction, without fixation into the femoral neck) with a transverse or oblique proximal lock that does not protect the intertrochanteric and femoral neck regions should be discouraged for metastatic lesions.[176] The nail configuration should have at least one large screw directed up into the neck and two screws for distal locking that can support unaided full weight-bearing. The probability of additional lesions proximal to a midshaft or subtrochanteric lesion is significantly high to warrant the use of a device that protects the entire length of the femur in most cases. Augmentation of this type of fixation with methylmethacrylate is not usually necessary unless one or more of the screw entry sites involves or is very close to an area of tumor. Not entering or curetting the tumor decreases the blood loss and morbidity of the procedure. The insertion technique is similar to that used for acute traumatic fractures. Now with nails that allow insertion through the tip of the trochanter, rather than in the piriformis fossa, insertion

is somewhat easier and applies less stress to the femur, perhaps decreasing the rate of inoperative fracture in the patient undergoing prophylactic nailing. Because of bone loss, alignment may have to be adjusted by directing the proximal fragment after screw insertion. There is considerable controversy relating to the need for venting of the femur to decrease pressurization during reaming, which has been shown to be associated with embolization and cardiorespiratory dysfunction in patients undergoing prophylactic nailing for metastatic disease.[6] Although experimentally pressures can be decreased by venting,[146] a recent study showed that most surgeons do not use the technique.[39]

In cases where extensive bone loss is present in the intertrochanteric or subtrochanteric regions, marginal resection and endoprosthetic replacement is indicated. Additionally when a very large soft tissue mass is associated with the bony destruction, resection and reconstruction provide a useful alternative (Fig. 17-15). Since this is a marginal resection and little or no normal muscle needs to be sacrificed, morbidity is relatively low and postoperative function quite satisfactory.[177] For a hemiarthroplasty for a femoral neck or intertrochanteric pathologic fracture as well as for an endoprosthetic replacement after resection, the length of the stem needs to be considered. For those with very short life expectancy, no additional lesions in the femur, and a low probability that one will occur in the future, the intramedullary stem can be relatively short. However, if the patient has multiple femoral

FIGURE 17-25   **A,** *This woman with carcinoma of the breast sustained a pathologic femoral fracture. The fracture was stabilized with a reamed, statically locked, intramedullary reconstruction nail. The fracture site was not opened.* **B,** *Length and rotation of the femur could be maintained with locking screws into the proximal neck and the most distal portion of the femur, despite bone loss. At 12-month follow-up, significant healing of the fracture had occurred, and because of the potentially long survival with this diagnosis, the intertrochanteric region and femoral neck were also protected.*

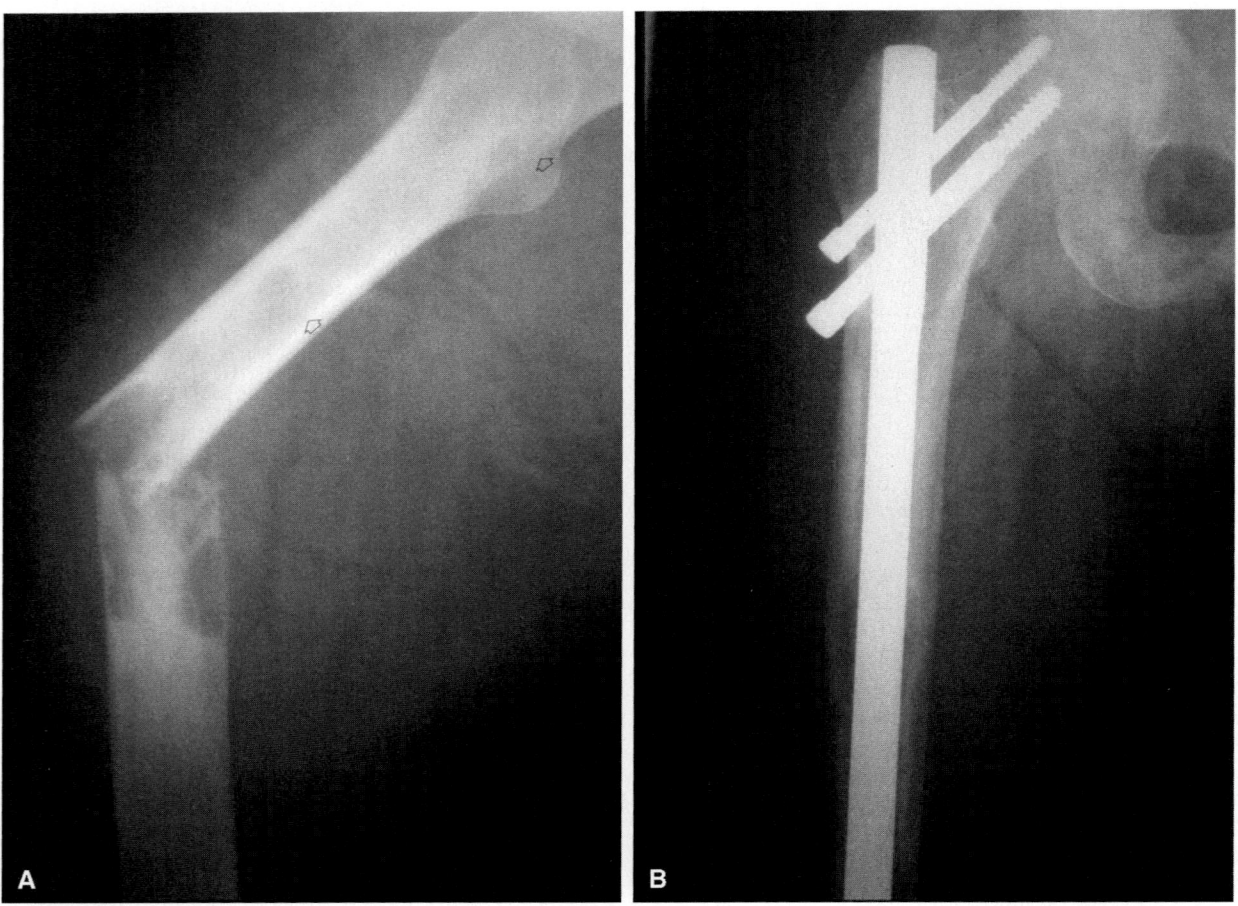

lesions or is expected to live a long time, then the stem should protect the entire length of the femur down to the knee. This adds slight risk of embolization with reaming and cementing, but venting can be considered.

Metastatic lesions distal to the midshaft femur are less common than those proximal to the midshaft, but the principles of treatment are similar. Protection of the femoral neck and intertrochanteric region with an appropriate second-generation nail is advocated. Very distal isolated femoral lesions (within 6 cm of the joint surface) in a patient for whom the life expectancy is limited can be treated effectively by curettage of the lesion, packing with methylmethacrylate, and stabilization with a distal screw-and-plate combination. The use of antegrade intramedullary locked fixation is possible when the lesion is in the distal third of the femur and does not penetrate into the femoral condyles. Retrograde intramedullary nail fixation is also useful and may be technically easier to perform with decreased operative time than is needed for antegrade nailing[85] (see Fig. 17-26). Pain relief with these techniques is immediate, and full weight-bearing can be reinstituted

immediately. It is critical that these femoral lesions are not treated as standard fractures. Because of the significant bone loss, interlocking into good quality proximal and distal bone is necessary, or the fixation should be augmented with methylmethacrylate to restore weight-bearing ability.[3,16,125,161] Both distal locking screws should always be utilized with bicortical purchase to minimize the probability of loosening and failure with weight-bearing without fracture healing or with bone loss. Methylmethacrylate does not interfere with fracture healing unless it is interposed between fracture fragments.[181] As in the proximal humerus and proximal femur, if insufficient bone stock exists to obtain immediate stability, endoprosthetic replacement may be necessary. In rare cases involving extensive bone destruction the use of a custom endoprosthesis may be necessary. These prostheses can be assembled in the operating room to accommodate various amounts of bone loss.[25,156]

Lesions in the tibia are rare but may be treated in a fashion similar to femoral lesions. Small solitary lesions may be treated with curettage and cementation, with or without internal fixation. Alternatively, like in the femur

FIGURE 17-26 *This elderly gentleman with a history of prostate cancer presented with new-onset back pain and distal thigh pain that was very severe with ambulation. His prostate-specific antigen level was low and a permeative destructive lesion (arrows) was evident in the distal femur (**A**) with a large soft tissue mass seen on the lateral radiograph (**B**) (arrow). Because of the very distal location, he underwent a retrograde nailing (**C, D**) and was returned to full weight-bearing status on the first postoperative day.*

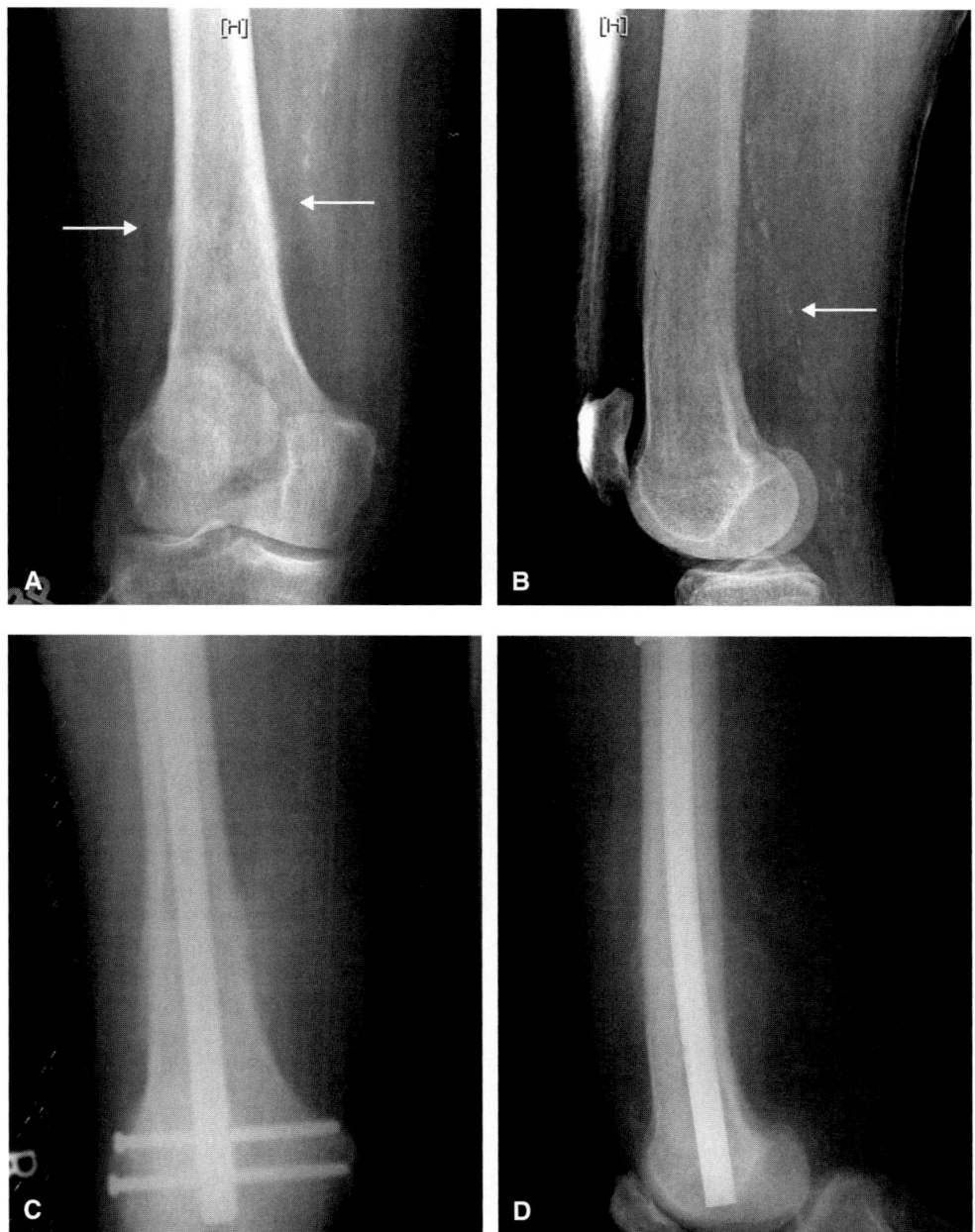

an interlocked tibial nail can provide stability and protect the remainder of the bone (Fig. 17-27). Intercalary or segmental replacement may be indicated for solitary renal or thyroid metastasis.

Pelvic Lesions

Among the most challenging lesions to evaluate and treat are those involving the pelvis. Because the anterior and posterior portions of the pelvis overlap in plain AP roentgenograms, acetabular deficiencies are often difficult to recognize and require specialized views. Often, even when a technetium bone scan reveals activity and is correlated with pain, insufficient attention is given to metastatic lesions about the pelvis until extensive destruction occurs. Harrington proposed a radiographic classification to describe various types of bone loss associated with periacetabular metastasis.[75,77,80,82] He described four classes: in class I, all portions of the wall of the acetabulum are present; in class II, the medial wall is deficient; in class III,

FIGURE 17-27 | *This 56-year-old man with carcinoma of the lung had severe pain in his proximal tibia that, after radiation therapy, was unremitting. **A,** Preoperative radiographs demonstrated a 43-cm lytic lesion (arrowheads) in the proximal tibia. **B,** The patient underwent curettage of the subcutaneous and intramedullary lesions and stabilization with a locked intramedullary nail. He achieved immediate pain relief and full weight-bearing status.*

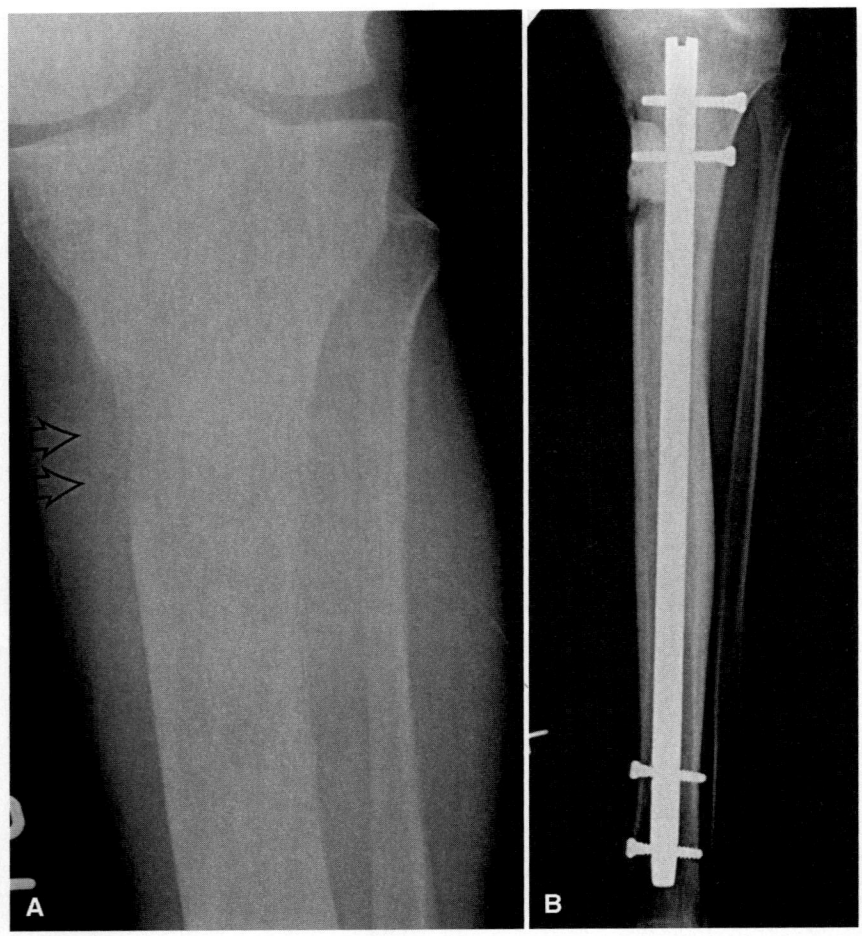

the lateral and superior portions of the acetabulum are deficient; and in class IV, a resection is necessary for cure. A critical feature for treating patients with metastatic disease to the pelvis is the early recognition of periacetabular disease. Early treatment with radiation or by surgical intervention with curettage of the lesion accompanied by either open or percutaneous methylmethacrylate filling of this lesion yields a highly acceptable result with moderate pain relief and good long-term stability of the acetabulum, preventing acetabular collapse and reconstruction by total hip arthroplasty (Fig. 17-28). The use of percutaneous destruction of the tumor with radiofrequency ablation (RFA) followed by filling of the defect with methylmethacrylate obviates the need for radiation and restores stability to the area for lesions up to about 5 cm in diameter (Fig. 17-29).

Metastases to the acetabulum occur primarily in two locations. The first is the medial wall (Fig. 17-30). This may be visualized on plain roentgenograms as destruction

of the lateral aspect of the superior pubic ramus. Because the ramus forms a large portion of the medial wall of the acetabulum, destruction of that area appears as destruction of the medial wall of the acetabulum. Early radiation therapy can prevent further destruction and allow the medial wall of the acetabulum to remain intact. Failure to recognize this situation can lead to pathologic fracture and result in protrusion of the femoral head through a defect in the medial wall.

The other common location for metastatic disease is in the supra-acetabular region and extending to the posterior wall of the acetabulum. Again, this is not well seen on plain roentgenograms and requires Judet views for visualization (see Fig. 17-7). These allow separate visualization of the anterior and posterior columns and bring into perspective large lesions of the superior and posterior aspect that may not be apparent on an AP view of the pelvis. Once a large lytic lesion has come within 1 to 2 mm of the superior dome of the acetabulum, the weight-bearing line of the

FIGURE 17-28 *This diagram shows a modification of the degrees of acetabular insufficiency. Stage 0, a supra-acetabular lesion that does not penetrate the subchondral plate, has been added. In stage 1, there is significant involvement of the superior dome of the acetabulum, but the medial wall is intact. In stage 2, there is significant medial wall involvement. In stage 3, the posterior, superior, and medial walls are involved. In stage 4, total involvement of the acetabulum requires resection for salvage.*

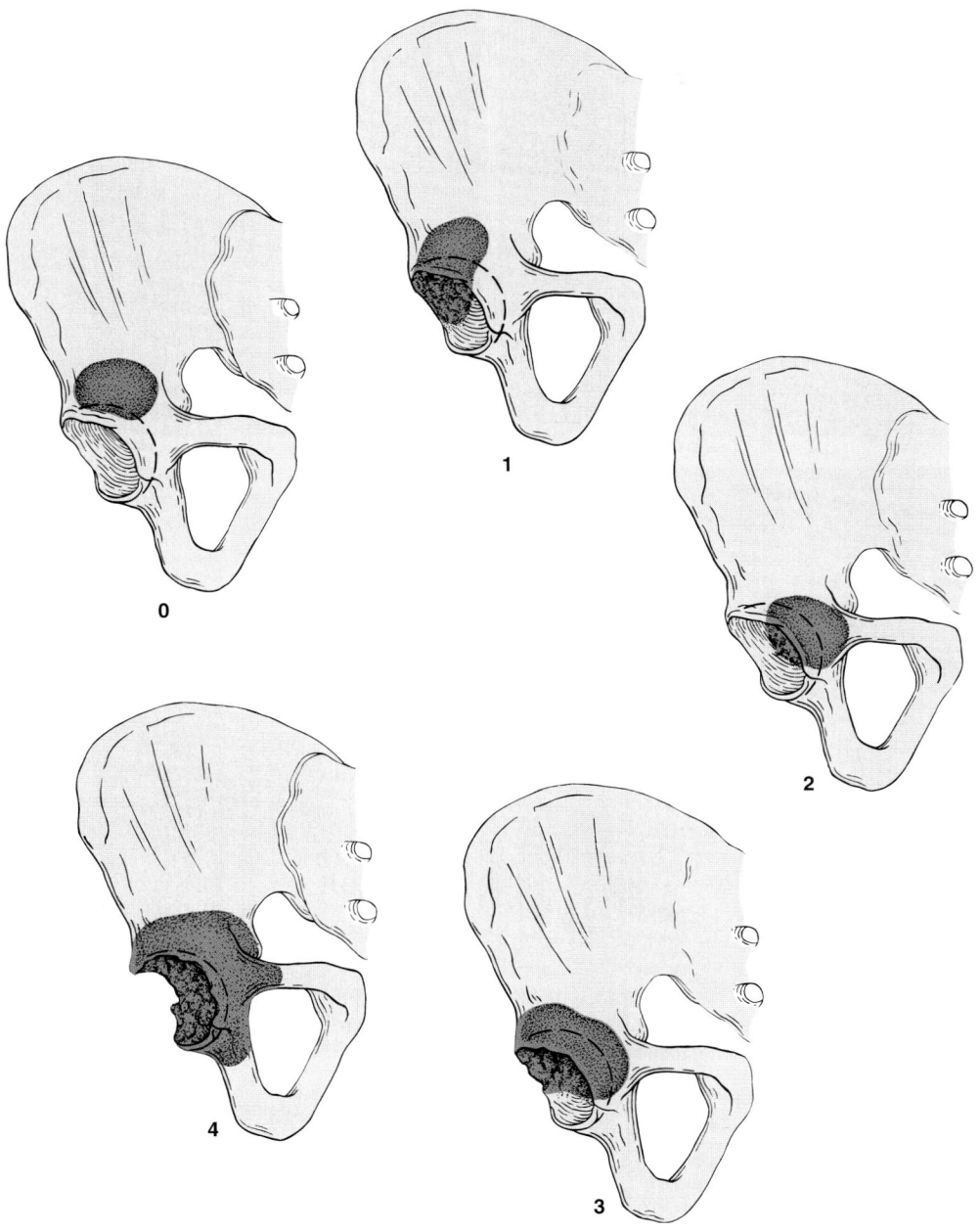

hip joint is severely disturbed. The use of radiation therapy is only infrequently effective in obtaining pain relief for these patients, probably because of the decreased strength of the weight-bearing column and recurrent microfractures, either in the lateral or medial wall, through defects that are not readily apparent. CT better defines the bony architecture and allows visualization of these areas. Curettage of

the lesion through a limited posterior or anterior extra-articular approach and packing with methylmethacrylate lead to long-term relief of pain[114,128] (Fig. 17-31). Usually, unless the subchondral plate of the superior dome of the acetabulum has been disrupted, further reconstruction of the hip is not necessary. In a series of 30 patients who underwent surgery for supra-acetabular metastasis, 28 had

FIGURE 17-29 *This patient with known renal cell metastases to bone developed new pain in his ischium. Plain radiograph **(A)** and computed tomography **(B)** demonstrated a lytic lesion. He underwent radiofrequency ablation (RFA) of the lesion **(C)** with subsequent filling of the lesion with methylmethacrylate at the same sitting **(D)**. The patient remains pain-free and has had no recurrence of the lesion 5 years after RFA **(E)**.*

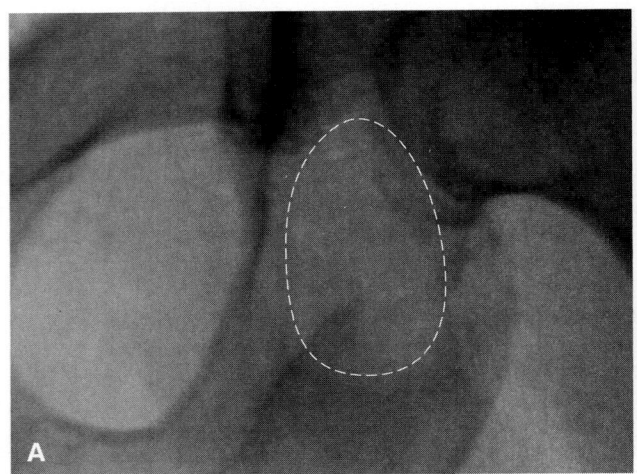

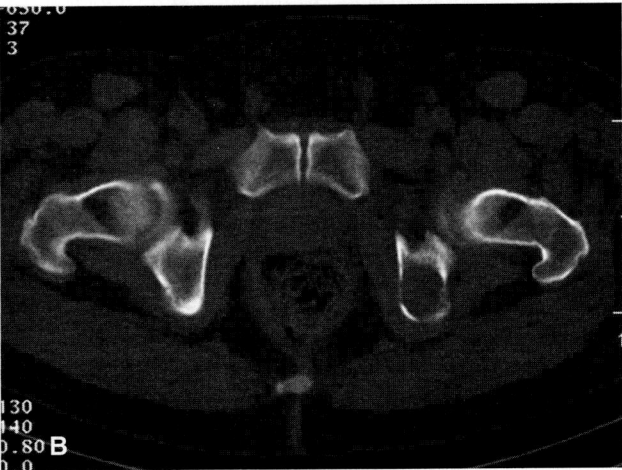

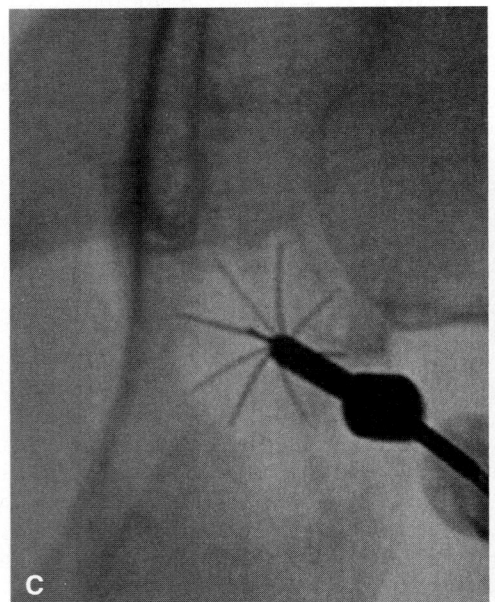

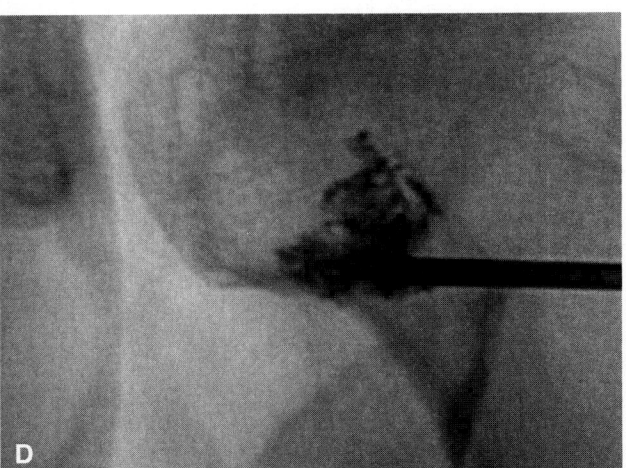

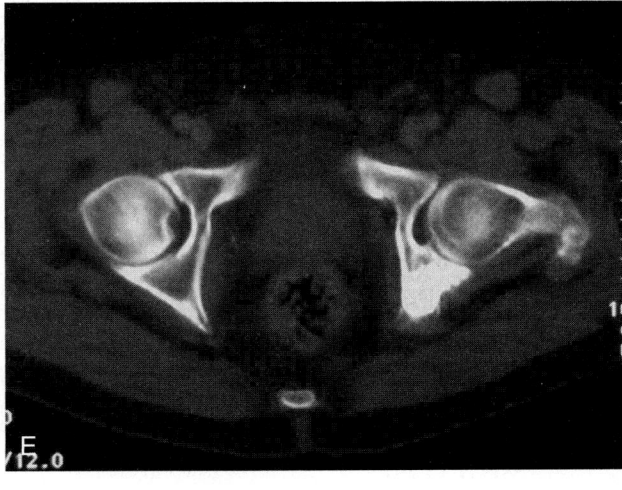

FIGURE 17-30 *A, This 63-year-old man with metastatic squamous cell carcinoma of the larynx experienced severe hip pain, and an anteroposterior radiograph of the pelvis demonstrated complete loss of the superior pubic ramus (arrowheads). The patient received radiation therapy but continued to have severe hip pain. B, Judet views demonstrated that the cause of the hip pain was significant loss of the medial wall of the acetabulum, which is formed by the extension of the superior pubic ramus (arrowheads).*

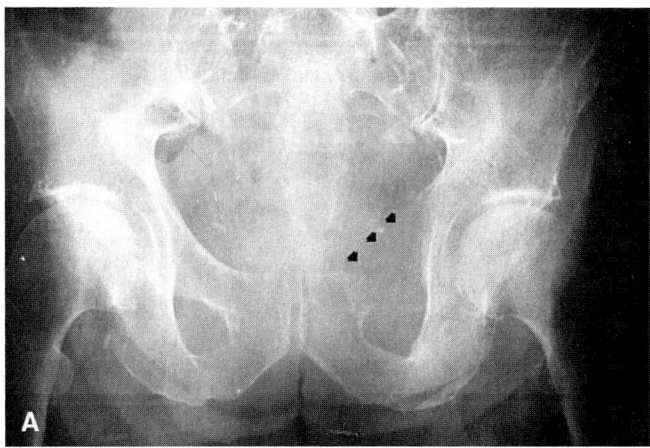
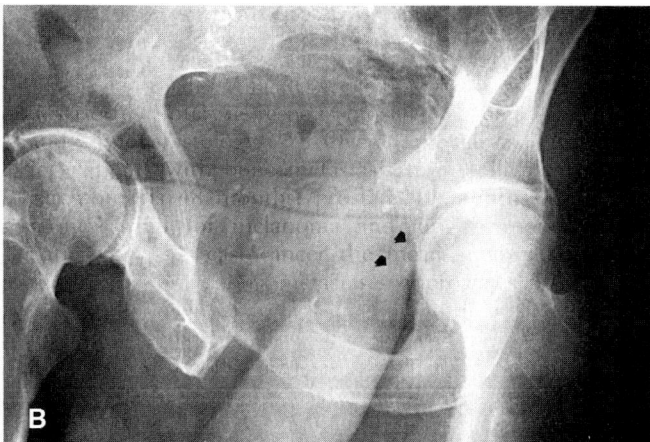

long-term satisfactory results (Fig. 17-32). Even when the lesions are relatively large but the subchondral plate remains intact, a satisfactory result can be obtained with this limited operative approach (Fig. 17-33). For selected lytic lesions without dense tumor, percutaneous filling of the defect with methylmethacrylate may be possible. If early destruction of the hip joint is not recognized, the superior weight-bearing dome will fracture, allowing migration of the femoral head proximally into the defect. Such destruction requires a modified total hip arthroplasty to obtain reasonable reconstruction of the hip, using the more proximal iliac bone to buttress the reconstruction of the large defect in the supra-acetabular region (Fig. 17-34). These more complex reconstructions can give satisfactory long-term results,[175] but the operative and perioperative morbidity is significantly higher than in those patients who are recognized to have defects and are treated primarily with supra-acetabular, extra-articular reconstruction (Fig. 17-35). Occasionally, the destruction of the acetabular bone stock is so great that the joint is unsalvageable and reconstruction by conventional means is impossible. In those very rare instances, resection and reconstruction with a saddle prosthesis provides a more stable alternative to a resection arthroplasty procedure.[2,41,149]

Metastatic Disease of the Spine

Spinal metastases are the most common site of bony metastatic disease. Estimates of the overall incidence of spine metastases in all patients who develop metastatic disease range from 36 to 70 percent, varying with the histology of the tumor from a high of 90 percent in prostate cancer to a low of 30 percent in those with renal cell carcinoma.[149,180] Despite the relatively high incidence of vertebral involvement, only 10 to 20 percent of those with spinal involvement will become symptomatic and only 5 to 10 percent will develop symptomatic epidural compression.

Cord compression can occur with or without pathologic fracture of the vertebra, or simply by replacement of the vertebra by tumor with development of an epidural soft tissue mass causing compression.

Pathologic fractures of the spine are actually more common than initially realized. They basically fall into three different types. The first are compression fractures, which may develop slowly or suddenly and are sometimes confused, both radiographically and clinically, with osteopenic compression fractures. The second is acute vertebral failure, which may radiographically resemble a burst fracture, or fracture dislocation (Fig. 17-36) but is usually accompanied by neurologic deficit either because of the bony displacement or because of the soft tissue component of the tumor involvement. The final type is the most common, with failure of a vertebral element as the result of tumor destruction (often a facet joint, pars, or pedicle), resulting in persistent and sometimes unrecognized pain (Fig. 17-37). This is especially common at the lumbosacral junction but is often characterized by subtle deformity (localized scoliosis or kyphosis) seen only on standing radiographs. Vertebral element failure with subtle instability can be the cause of persistent pain after radiation in what seems to be a relatively limited amount of vertebral metastatic disease. Attempts have been made in a number of different studies to estimate the future incidence of vertebral pathologic fracture from the type and extent of vertebral involvement (as well as other factors). Similarly these studies have attempted to estimate the incidence of epidural compression and the rate of response to various treatment modalities. Taneichi and co-workers examined risk factors for pathologic fracture with lytic vertebral metastases in both the thoracic and lumbar spine.[166] Patients with thoracic spine lesions who had either 50 to 60 percent lytic destruction of the body or costovertebral junction involvement combined with 25 to 30 percent destruction of the body (lateralized

FIGURE 17-31 *Surgical technique for supra-acetabular reconstruction. For reconstruction of lesions of the supra-acetabular region, the patient must have an intact subchondral plate with no apparent destruction visible on computed tomography (CT) of the acetabulum. **A,** The patient is placed in the lateral decubitus position with the affected hip upward. The patient is prepared and draped in the usual sterile fashion, with the leg free in the field. The posterior approach starts just below the greater trochanter, continues over the trochanter, and then curves posteriorly toward the posterior superior iliac crest. **B,** The subcutaneous tissue is dissected, and the fascia of the gluteus is split. The gluteus is split bluntly, in line with its fibers, from the trochanter to the sciatic notch. At the posterior aspect of the incision, the sciatic notch is exposed subperiosteally, and a blunt cobra retractor is placed in the sciatic notch to protect the nerve and superior gluteal vessels. Additional dissection is carried proximally and superiorly, and a thyroid retractor is placed for visualization of the superior margin of the capsule and posterior lip of the acetabulum. **C,** Frequently, a defect is observed in the cortex, and entry into the lesion is through the defect. Otherwise, depending on whether the site of the lesion is predominantly superior or posterior, the entry hole through the cortical bone is made at the superior end of the acetabulum or slightly posterior, so that better curettage of the posterior lip can be obtained. Generally, the bone is soft, and the area of the lesion is easily entered. Otherwise a 14-inch osteotome is used to remove the cortical window. The lesion is then entered and thoroughly curetted posteriorly, into the lip of the acetabulum, and superiorly with an angled curette. All tumor is removed, and the inferior margin (i.e., subchondral plate of the acetabulum) is checked for defects. If a small defect is seen or has been removed during curettage, a piece of fascia lata is removed and is used to cover the defect. **D,** The window for curettage should be large enough to admit at least the index finger for packing the methylmethacrylate, a single package of which is mixed and, in its doughy stage, finger-packed into the lesion. **E,** Packing continues until the entire space is full. A radiograph is then taken to ascertain that no methylmethacrylate has extruded into the acetabulum and that the lesion is completely packed. Ambulation can begin on the first postoperative day.*

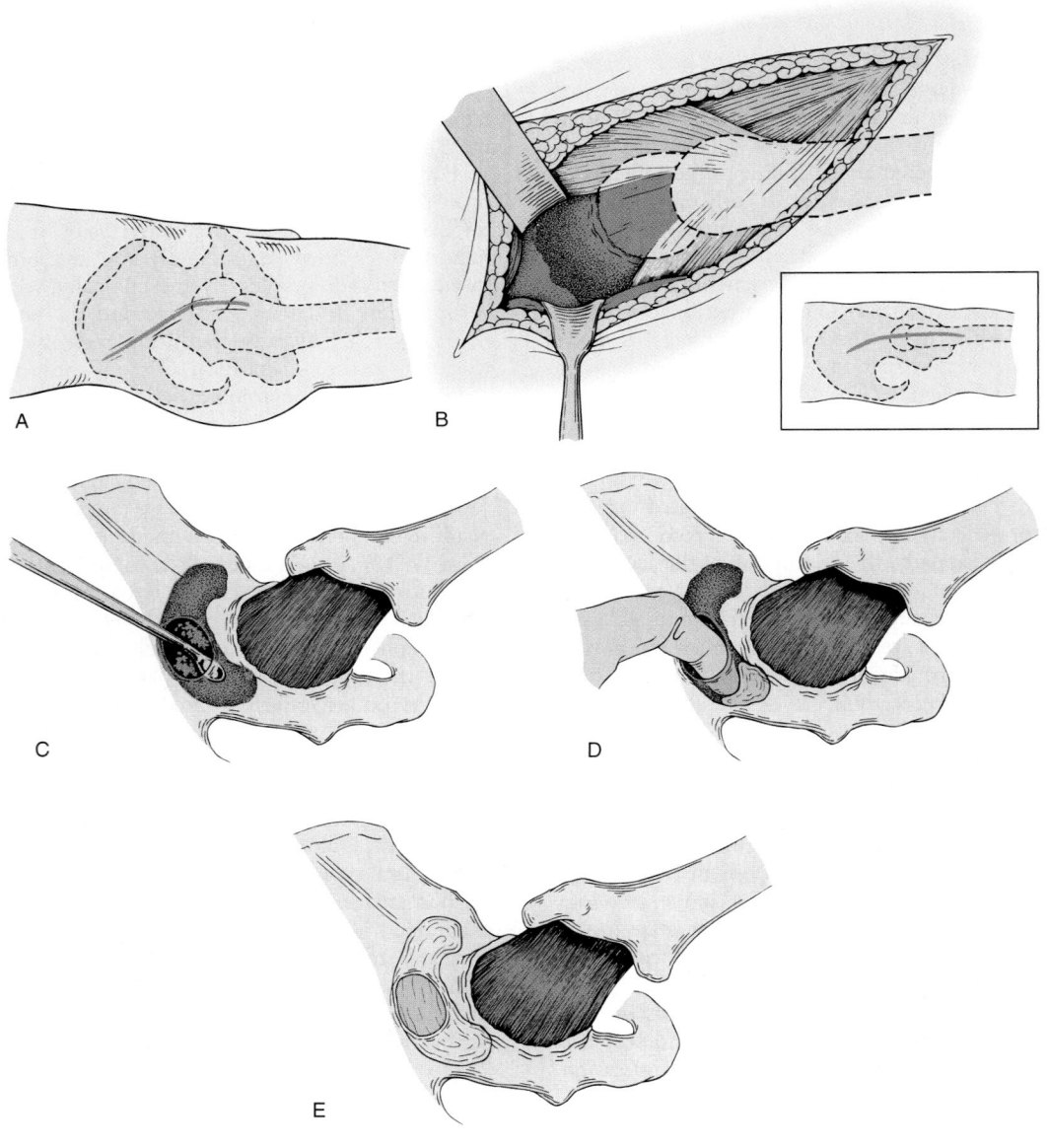

FIGURE 17-32 **A,** *This patient with carcinoma of the breast had a large lesion in the supra-acetabular and posterior acetabular regions. Through a posterior approach, the tumor was completely excised from the posterior and superior aspects of the acetabulum. A small defect in the subchondral plate was covered with graft from the fascia lata, and the defect was filled with methylmethacrylate.* **B,** *At the 3.5-year follow-up, the patient had no degenerative changes about the hip and no hip pain. In the intervening time, a Zickel nail was used for stabilization of a large pathologic lesion in the contralateral femur.*

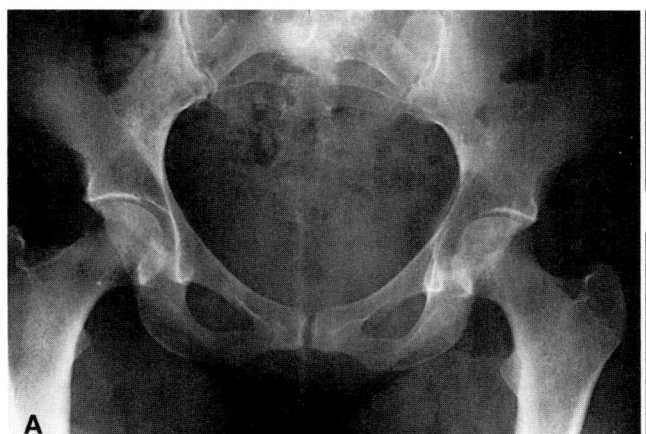
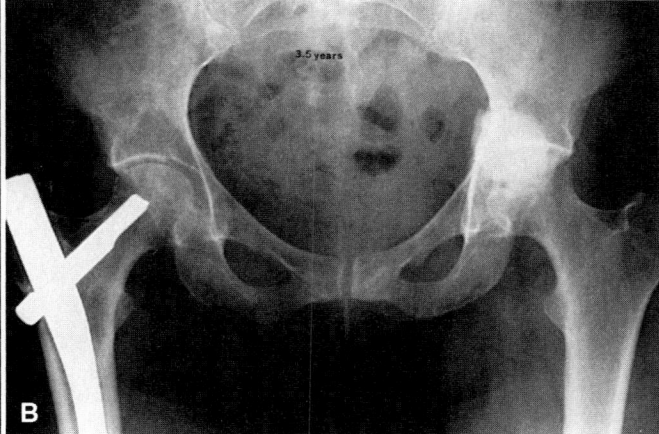

involvement) were more likely to sustain a fracture (Table 17-2). In the lumbar spine, pedicle or posterior element involvement resulted in fracture with only 30 percent tumor destruction in the lumbar spine.[166] In a more general sense, the highest rate of fracture seems to occur in the region of L1-L3 with symmetric vertebral involvement with a poorly undifferentiated tumor (Fig. 17-38). Some authors have suggested that the degree of body involvement needs to be closer to 80 percent to give an increased rate of fracture, although in those studies total tumor involvement included both the lytic and blastic areas, potentially accounting for the difference.[145,153]

No truly reproducible factors have been identified to allow physicians to predict when and how epidural compression will occur. However, the rate of onset of motor deficit in patients with epidural compression seems to be highly significant in terms of response to treatment and prognosis for recovery. Those with slow onset of deficits over more than 14 days are more likely to recover than those with rapid onset of deficit (< 7 days). Similarly those with tumors more responsive to chemotherapy and radiation (breast, lymphoma, etc.) and those with better ambulatory status prior to surgery have a higher statistical probability of a superior outcome after treatment.

Both the cause and the consequences of pathologic fracture of the spine are more complex than with pathologic fractures in the remainder of the axial and appendicular skeleton. Both diagnosis and treatment can sometimes

FIGURE 17-33 *This patient with renal cell carcinoma metastatic to bone had previously undergone a prophylactic nailing for a painful subtrochanteric lesion. Subsequent hip pain necessitated a course of radiation therapy that did not relieve the pain.* **A,** *The large supra-acetabular lesion (dotted area) did not destroy the subchondral plate despite its size.* **B,** *The patient underwent curettage and packing of the lesion through a posterior approach with complete relief of pain. Notice the beginning of a similar lesion on the contralateral side.*

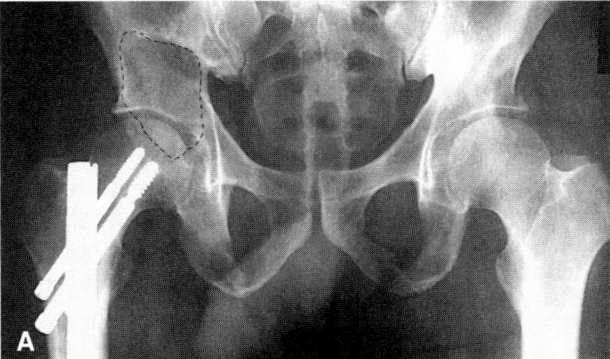
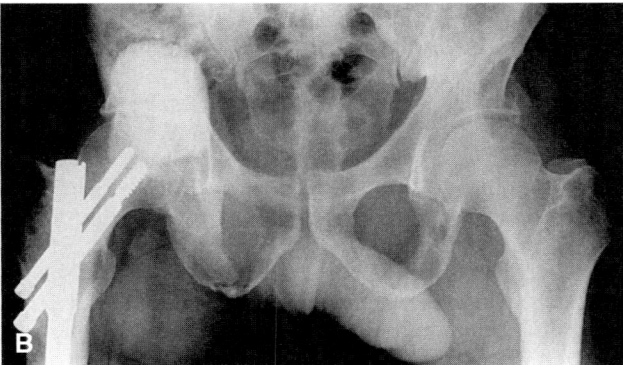

FIGURE 17-34 | *This patient with multiple myeloma experienced insidious onset of hip pain over an approximately 6-month period.* ***A,*** *The patient had significant destruction of the superior and medial walls of the acetabulum (arrowheads) as a result of the myeloma.* ***B,*** *Computed tomography showed destruction of the superior and the medial portions of the acetabulum (i.e., a stage 3 lesion).* ***C,*** *The patient required a complex reconstruction with Steinmann pins through the intact ilium to support reconstruction of the hip. He has had satisfactory pain relief and excellent functional recovery, and his disease is well controlled with chemotherapy.*

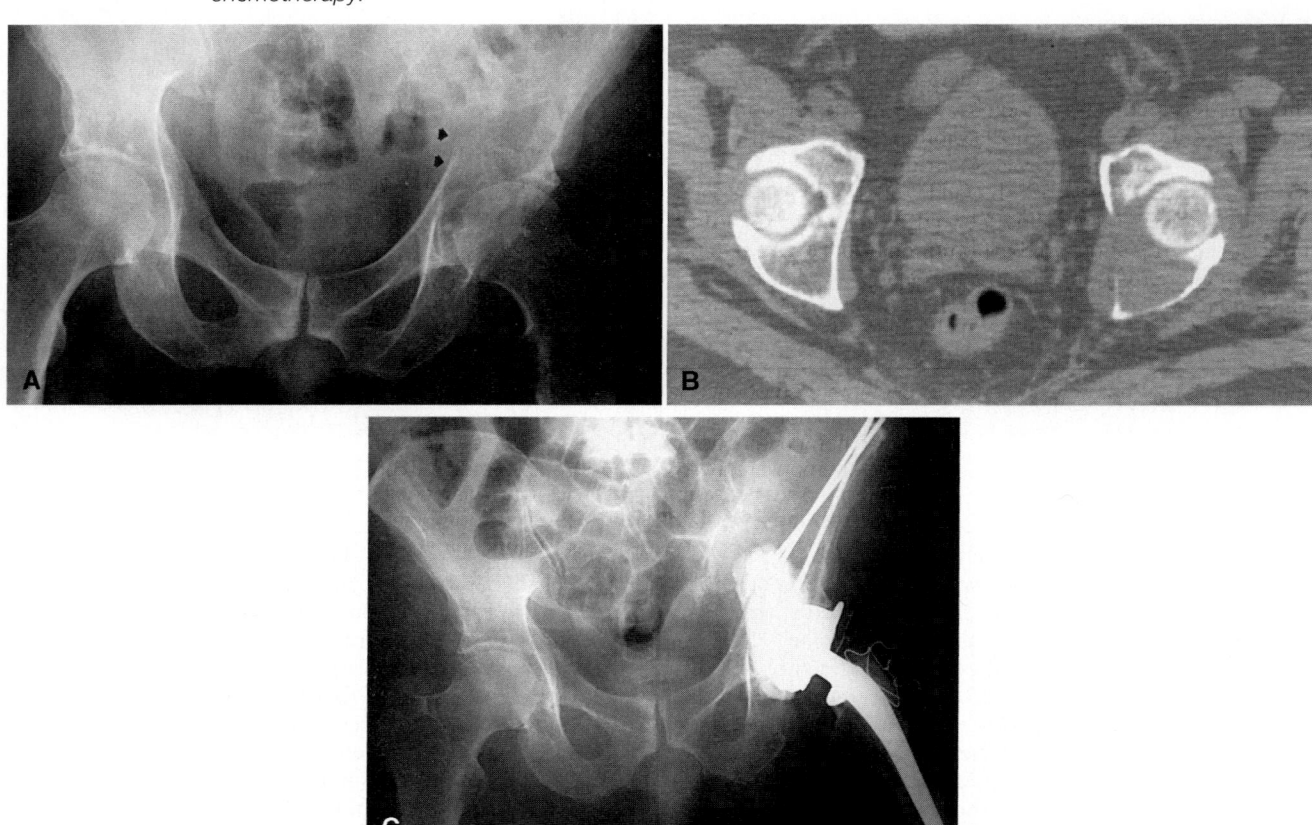

be frustrating because what appears to be perfectly logical and well thought out may not yield the expected results. As will be discussed later, differentiation between osteoporotic and metastatic fractures can be difficult in a population where both can occur. Similarly, myelopathic patients who appear to have had a complete decompression either do not demonstrate neural recovery or continue to deteriorate because of vascular involvement by the tumor. Finally, as in the remainder of pathologic fractures throughout the skeleton, it is critical to remember during treatment that the goals are to give durable palliation of symptoms while returning the patient to full function as rapidly as possible. In most patients with metastatic disease of the spine who undergo radiation for treatment of their vertebral involvement, the mean survival is only 6 months and in those who undergo surgery it is only 12 to 14 months. There are little or no data to support the contention that complete removal of the metastasis improves overall survival. Thus we should attempt to alleviate symptoms with as little interference with future function (no postoperative immobilization or constructs that

require healing to achieve stability) and administration of systemic therapy.

Patients with metastatic spine disease can be grouped into one of three classes (Fig. 17-39). Class 1 includes patients who are asymptomatic, without neurologic symptoms. The spinal lesion has come to the physician's attention because of a finding on an imaging study (bone scan, PET/CT, MRI, or plain radiograph). Patients with positive bone scans, PET/CT, or MRI should have appropriate plain roentgenograms (orthogonal standing views) taken to assess the degree of involvement. At least 50% of cancellous bone must be destroyed before it can be visualized on a plain roentgenogram, but no other study yields as much information about relative stability.[18] On screening radiographs visualization may be possible somewhat earlier in the spine when the pedicle is involved because it is made up predominantly of cortical bone, so when erosion in this area takes place it is more easily seen than in areas of cancellous bone. Therefore the initial radiographic clue of a metastatic lesion involving the body and the pedicle may be seen only in the pedicle, even when quantitatively more extensive disease is located in the body.

FIGURE 17-35 *Surgical technique for reconstruction of a complex acetabular defect. Generally, in patients requiring complex acetabular reconstruction, the superior and medial or the superior and posterior walls of the acetabulum have been destroyed. The patient is placed in a lateral decubitus position and prepared with the leg free in the field. **A,** A straight, lateral incision begins approximately 6 cm above the tip of the greater trochanter and continues down over the midline of the trochanter and femoral shaft. The fascia lata is opened in line with its fibers. A transverse cut is made at the inferior ridge of the greater trochanter, leaving a portion of the fascia of the vastus lateralis for subsequent reattachment. A V-shaped osteotomy in the greater trochanter allows exposure of the superior and posterior portions of the capsule. **B,** The hip is dislocated, and the femoral head and neck are resected in accordance with the configuration of the cemented prosthesis to be used. A large curette is used to remove all tumor from the acetabulum. **C,** Generally, the cartilage remains intact, but with little subchondral bone beneath, it is easily breached to reach the tumor. Curettage is continued until the periosteum is encountered (anteriorly or posteriorly, or both) or a firm cortical margin is encountered on all sides. Because the subchondral plate is totally destroyed, reinforcement must be obtained for the large methylmethacrylate block and acetabular component.*

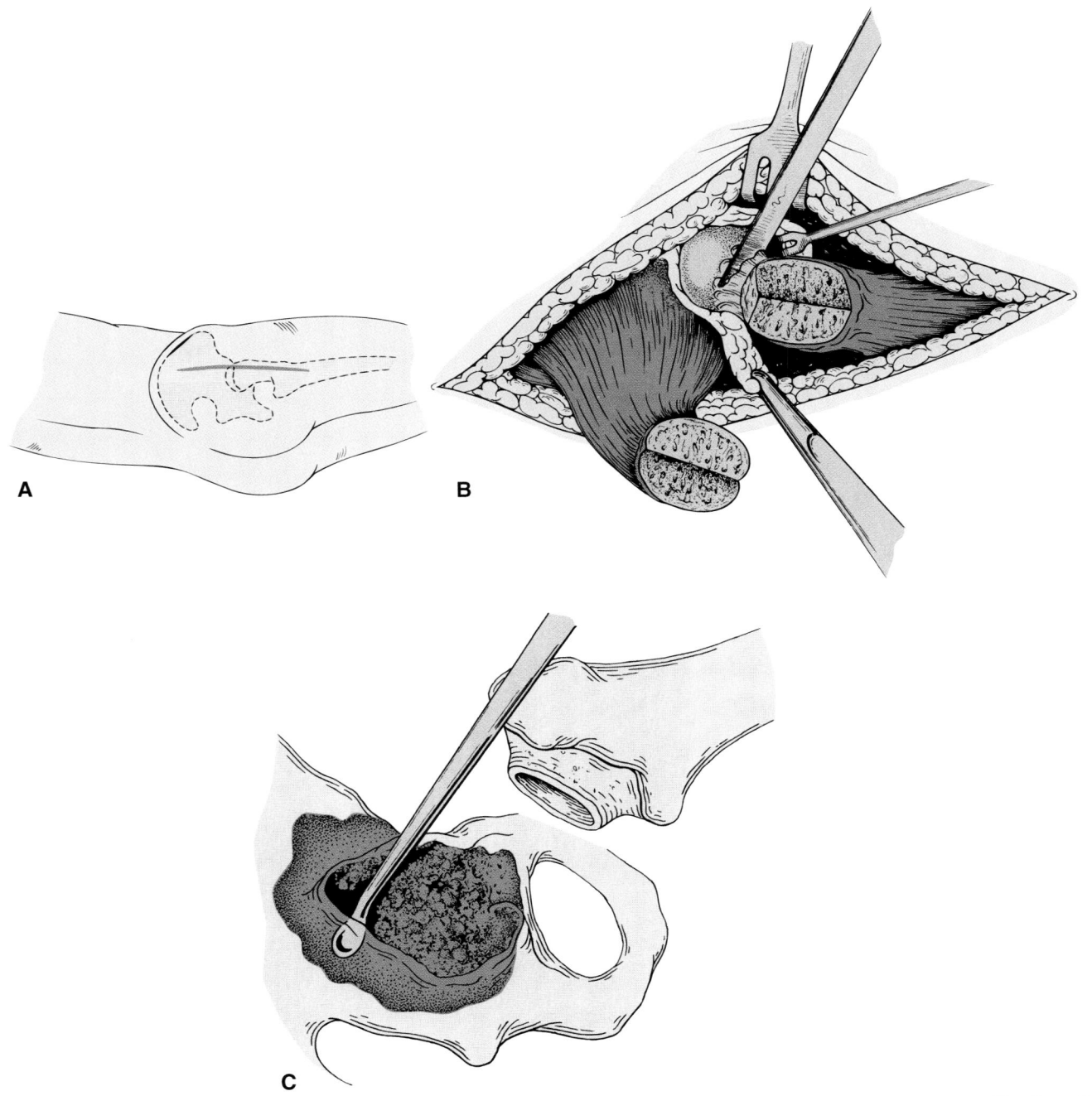

(Continued)

FIGURE 17-35 *(Continued)* **D,** *Using a separate stab incision made directly over the superior iliac crest approximately 3 to 4 cm posterior to the anterior superior crest, threaded Steinmann pins are inserted. It is suggested that a subperiosteal dissection be done on the inner and the outer tables of the ilium, allowing a finger to be used to ascertain the position of the threaded pin as it trasverses the ilium. The threaded pins are aimed into the large defect in the superior dome of the acetabulum. Commonly, three Steinmann pins are placed, fanning out to cover the breadth of the defect for solid attachment of the methylmethacrylate. Care must be taken to ensure that the pins do not protrude so far as to preclude seating of the acetabular component.* **E,** *If the defect is extensive and encompasses the anterior and the posterior portions of the acetabulum, a second set of Steinmann pins may be placed from the acetabulum and aimed at the posterior superior iliac crest. An additional stab incision is not needed in that location. However, if difficulty is encountered in obtaining adequate pin alignment because of the configuration of the hip, a second stab incision can be made along the posterior superior iliac crest, and the pins can be directed from the crest into the defect. In most cases, the Steinmann pins can be directed from the defect toward the iliac crest. Care should be taken that the pins do not traverse the sciatic notch. This can be ascertained by direct palpation or with intraoperative radiographs. Usually, only the pins from the anterior portion of the ilium are necessary.* **F,** *After complete curettage, the pin length is checked, and the pins are cut off flush with the iliac crest.* **G,** *A protrusio cup is sized to fill the defect. The cup allows purchase on the superior or the anterior portion of the acetabular rim (if there is any remaining bone) for better fixation. A high-density polyethylene cup or metal-backed polyethylene cup may then be cemented inside the protrusio cup. Two packages of methylmethacrylate are mixed and, in the doughy stage, are packed in and around the Steinmann pins, filling the entire defect. The protrusio cup is pressed into the doughy methylmethacrylate and is filled with the dough. The acetabular component is placed within it and held in correct orientation until the mixture hardens. The femoral component is inserted in routine fashion after wires are placed in the trochanter for repair of the trochanteric osteotomy. Routine closure is accomplished, and the patient is mobilized with toe-touch weight-bearing until the trochanteric osteotomy heals, followed by full weight-bearing.*

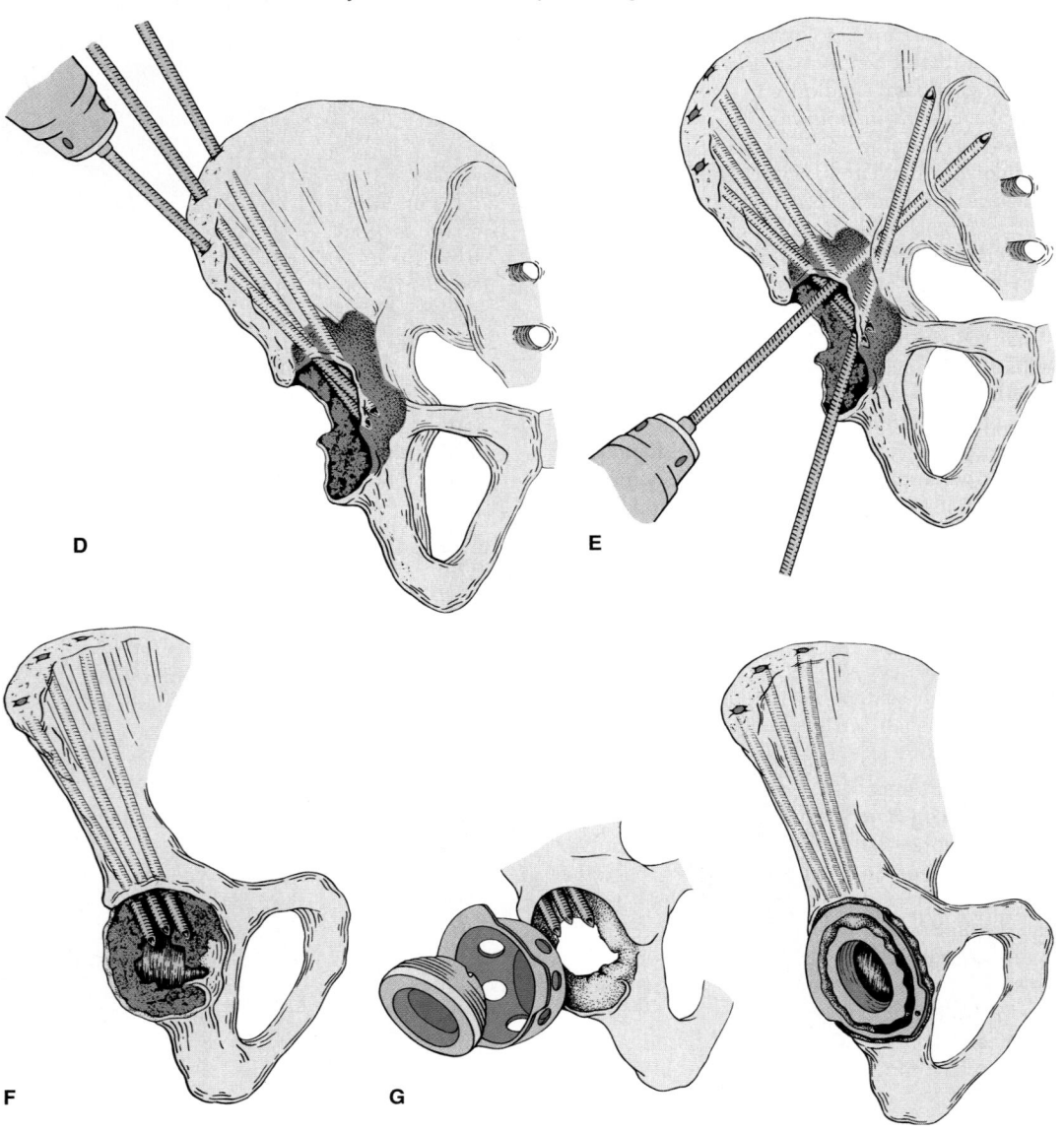

D

E

F

G

FIGURE 17-36 *This patient with metastatic breast carcinoma was thought to have a compression fracture on plain radiograph but suddenly became paraparetic and was found to have a fracture dislocation with translation of T9 over T10 (dashed lines).*

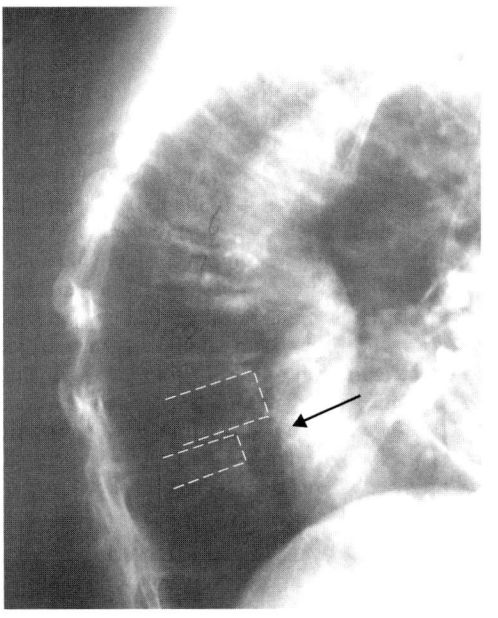

Even if a patient is asymptomatic, if the plain roentgenograms (both AP and lateral) suggest the presence of a destructive process, an MRI should be obtained to better define the extent of involvement of the vertebra and to assess potential epidural compression. Patients with minimal involvement of the vertebral body, who are asymptomatic, and who are not at risk for instability should continue with systemic therapy (i.e., chemotherapy, medical therapy, or hormonal manipulation). However, in patients with radiosensitive tumors with greater than 50 percent destruction of the vertebral body, consideration should be given to the use of radiation therapy even in the absence of symptoms or evidence of instability. Most patients with such extensive involvement of the vertebral body, however, are symptomatic (see Figs. 17-37 and 17-38).

The second class of patients consists of those who present with symptoms.[9] Patients in this class may present with local pain or neurologic signs (or both). In the patient with pain but no neurologic findings, the evaluation must determine whether the pain is related to neural compression or to bone destruction, fracture, and instability. Following a complete history and physical, the initial imaging study should be plain standing radiographs for the thoracic, lumbar, and sacral spine and upright radiographs in the cervical spine. If in question, supine radiographs can be compared with the standing radiographs to assess changes such as localized scoliosis or kyphosis or collapse. Rarely are flexion-extension radiographs necessary but on occasion they can be useful. In the patient with

FIGURE 17-37 *This patient with known metastatic carcinoma of the breast had pain in her sacrum and underwent external beam radiation (30 Gy) without any relief of symptoms. Her pain was worse with standing and better with lying down. A supine radiograph of the lumbosacral junction was not very remarkable **(A)**, but an erect radiograph showed some listing to the side of the tumor destruction (arrow) **(B)**.*

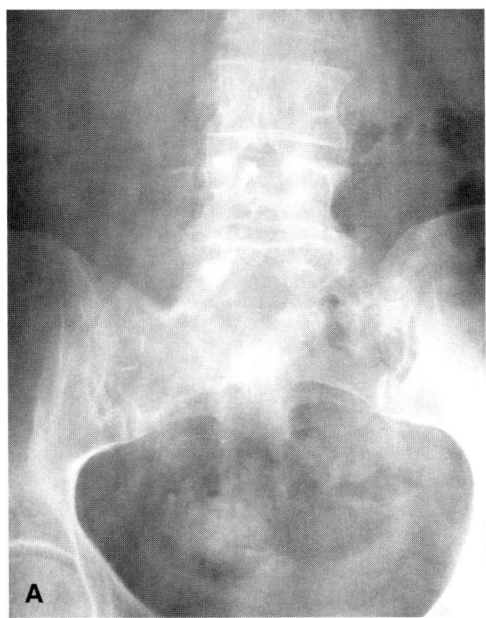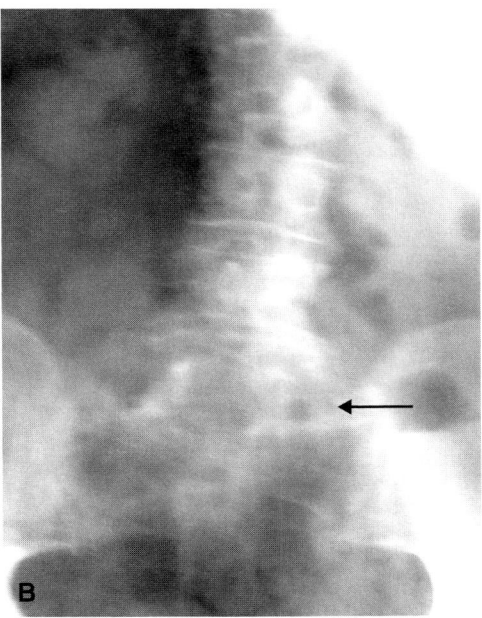

(Continued)

FIGURE 17-37 *(Continued) Magnetic resonance imaging showed complete replacement of the sacral ala with destruction of the L5-S1 facet on that side (C). Stabilization bypassing that area relieved the pain, and the remaining viable tumor in the area was treated with stereotactic radiosurgery (D, E).*

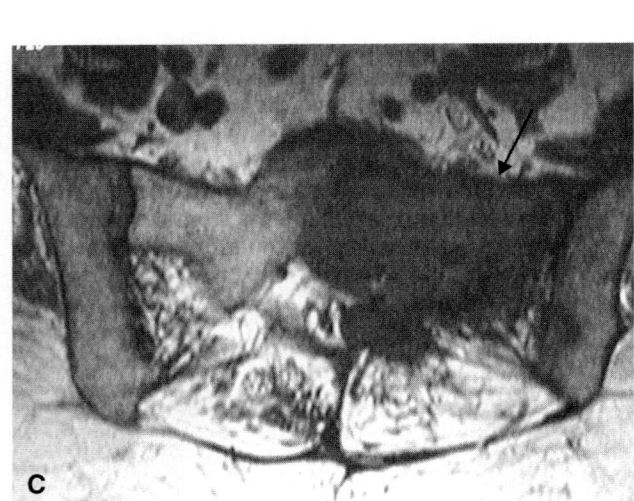

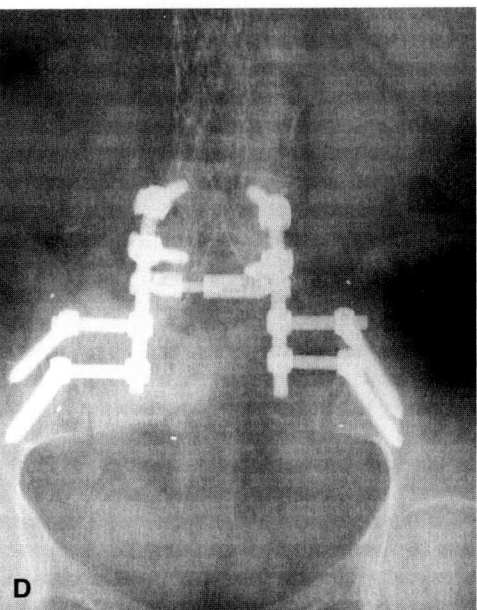

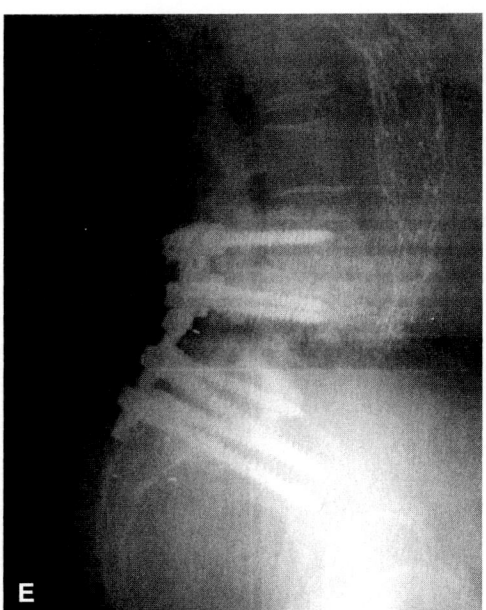

localized scoliosis at the level of the tumor involvement, MRI almost always shows destruction of the facet and pedicle on the side of the concavity. The combination of these findings is prognostic for a poor outcome with radiation alone (see Fig. 17-38A and B). The documentation of collapse of a vertebra over time answers the question of whether the pain is related to fracture or neural compression. Any patient with significant collapse should undergo MRI to assess the degree of canal compromise and neural compression of the roots or dural sac. MRI is limited in not being able to accurately assess the cortical bone structure. Additionally, it is very sensitive to marrow changes but not specific. Therefore, changes within the vertebral body marrow may be related to tumor, osteoporosis, radiation changes, or chemotherapeutic effects (especially associated with growth factors)[118] (Fig. 17-40). Therefore

Table 17-2
Risk Factors for Collapse with Metastatic Disease of the Thoracic and Lumbar Spine

Thoracic Spine

  Risk factors

    Costovertebral joint destruction

    Percent of body involvement

  Criteria for impending collapse

    50% to 60% body involvement alone

    25% to 30% of body with costovertebral involvement

Lumbar Spine

  Risk factors

    Pedicle destruction

    Percent of body involvement

  Criteria for impending collapse

    35% to 40% of body involvement alone

    25% with pedicle and/or posterior element destruction

From Taneichi H, Kaneda K, Takeda N, et al. Risk factors and probability of vertebral body collapse in metastases of the thoracic and lumbar spine. Spine 22:239–245, 1997.

although MRI is very effective in assessing soft tissue and epidural involvement, it is less specific in assessing structural integrity of the vertebrae above and below the index area and may overestimate involvement based on marrow changes, which in fact do not represent tumor. CT is often helpful in preoperative assessment of those patients.

The final group of patients is those who present with neurologic deficit and localized symptomatology. Before any intervention, the degree of spinal involvement must be adequately discerned. In patients who present with neurologic deficit, the combination of plain radiographs with MRI and CT is critical to obtaining the most information from a limited investigation that will allow appropriate treatment planning. The patient who is a candidate for surgical intervention must satisfy a number of criteria before surgery is initiated. First, the patient should have in most cases one level or, at most, two adjacent levels of dural compression. With rare exception, patients with two or more nonadjacent levels of dural compression on the initial MRI have a very limited life expectancy, and their probability for neurologic complications during the procedure is increased. In patients with multiple high-grade lesions, the prognosis for recovery is lower and the overall life span less than for those with a single lesion.[108] Second, the extent, nature, and direction of the impingement on the dural sac must be delineated. The extent and direction can be demonstrated best by MRI, but the nature of the material causing the dural compression may be difficult to determine. In such cases the addition of CT is helpful. Third, the patient must be shown to have adequate bone stability for fixation at levels above and below the pathologic lesion, regardless of whether the intervention is anterior or posterior. Although MRI can obtain data on compression, the quality of the cortical bone necessary for fixation at levels above and below the lesion cannot adequately be ascertained with this method. Although radiologists may suggest that MRI is sufficient to evaluate a pathologic fracture of the spine with neural deficit, additional information significant to planning the surgical intervention can be obtained from CT. Finally the patient should undergo a screening midline sagittal MRI of the spine (unless a PET/CT has been done in appropriate tumors) to rule out a second nonadjacent level of epidural compression. The presence of a second level of

---

FIGURE 17-38 *The patient with metastatic colon carcinoma had a metastasis to L2 (arrow) (**A, B**) and underwent external beam radiation to the lesion without relief of pain. His symptoms were worse with standing or sitting and relieved by lying down.*

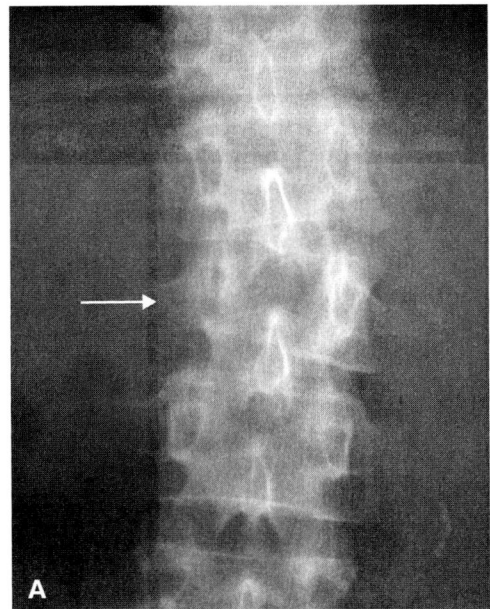
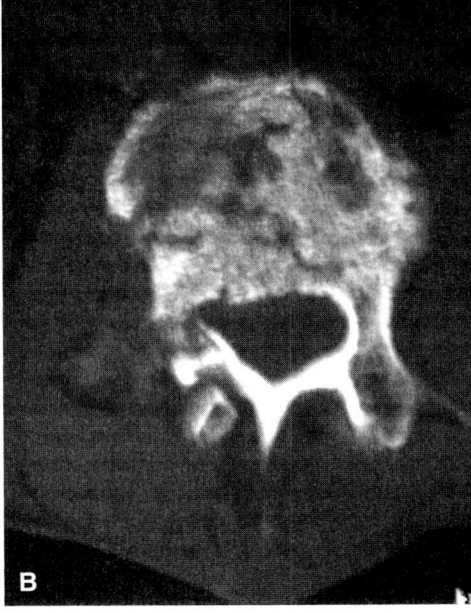

(Continued)

FIGURE 17-38 | *(Continued) Standing anteroposterior radiograph (**C**) demonstrated scoliosis with asymmetric fracture of the vertebral body (arrow) as demonstrated on three-dimensional computed tomographic reconstruction (**D**). After posterior stabilization with supplementary anterior reinforcement with a kyphoplasty, the patient had complete relief of pain (**E, F**).*

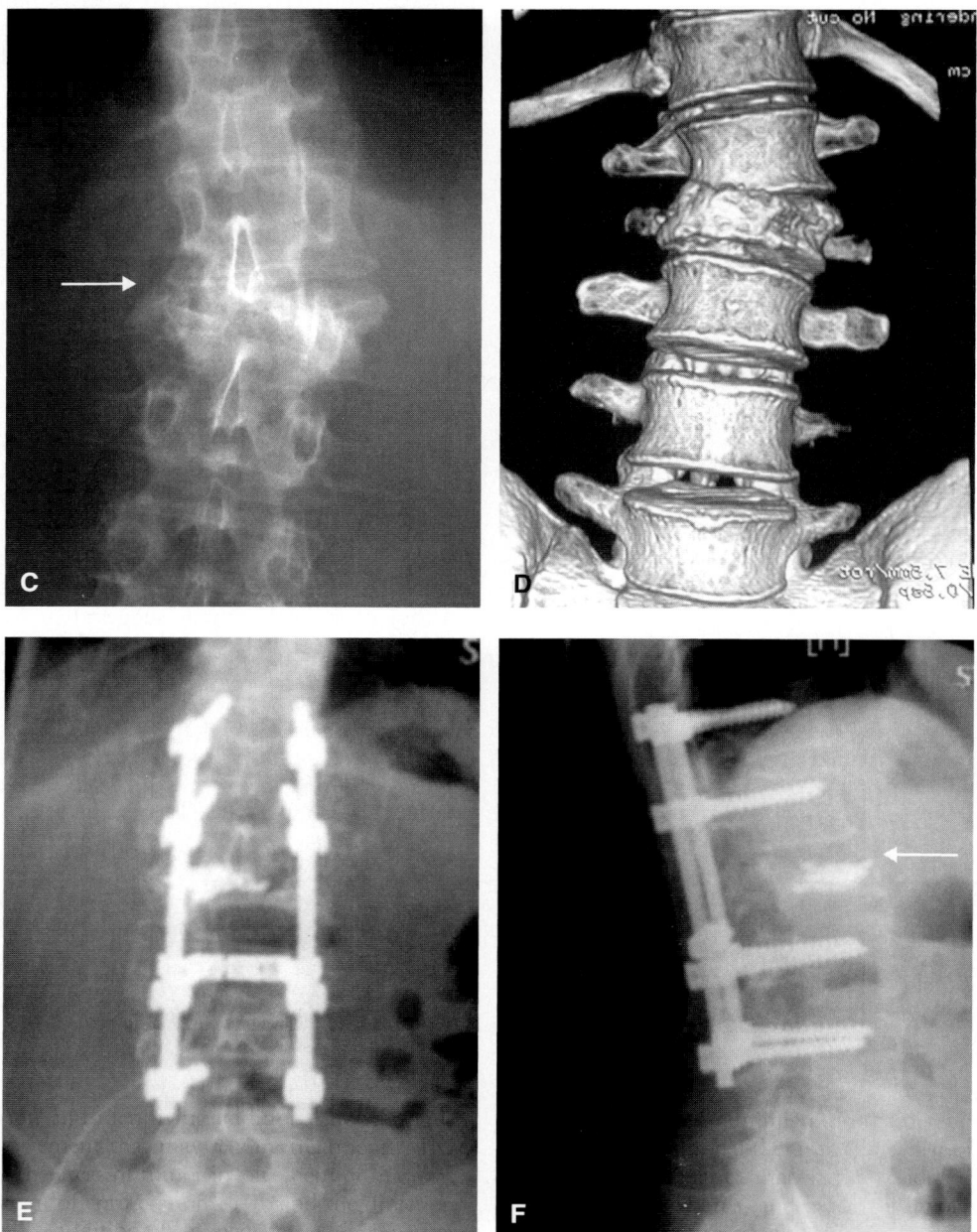

nonadjacent epidural compression predicts a poor outcome and is a relative contraindication to surgery.

Once the anatomic extent of the lesion has been clearly defined, treatment can be instituted. Treatment considerations include general health of the patient, tumor histology, and presence or absence of instability or neurologic deficit. In an effort to identify prognostic factors preoperatively for patients with metastatic spine tumors, Tokuhashi and co-workers developed a scoring system based on six parameters (Table 17-3). These include general performance status,

number of extraspinal metastases, number of vertebrae involved, metastases to internal organs, primary site, and spinal cord palsy. For each parameter a score from 0 to 2 is given. The maximum score is 12. They found that patients with a score of 5 or less survived an average of 3 months or less and patients with a score of 9 or higher survived 12 months or more.[169]

Surgical intervention is appropriate for relief of symptoms in a select group of patients. In those patients with a tumor who are asymptomatic but have significant

FIGURE 17-39 *An algorithm for the evaluation of patients with metastatic disease of the spine.*

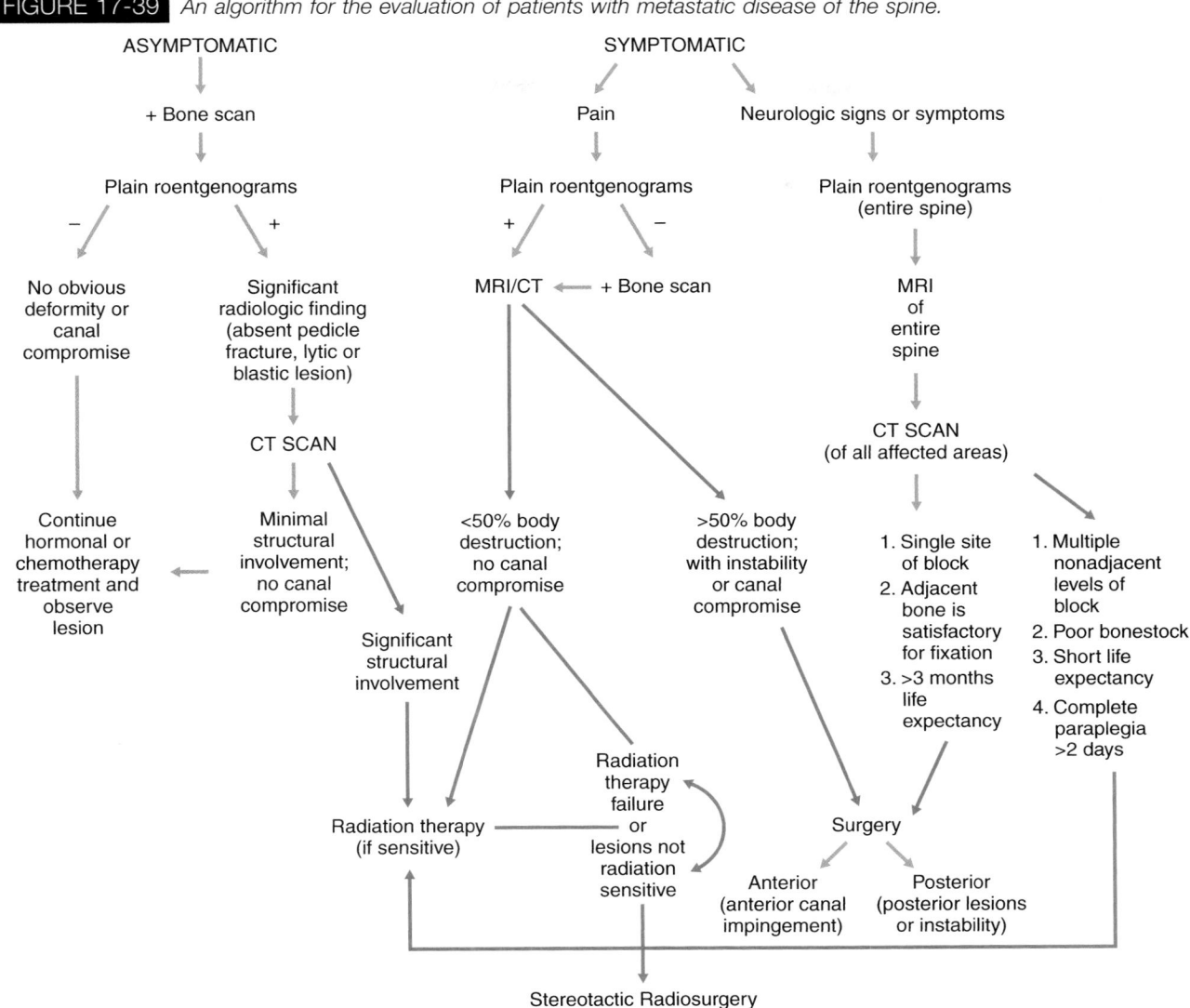

destruction of the vertebral body, radiation therapy should be considered. In patients who present with pain but no neurologic deficit, intervention can be based on the results of the information obtained from the imaging studies including plain radiographs, CT, and MRI. If the imaging studies fail to demonstrate major destruction of the vertebral body (i.e., less than 50% destruction), cord compression, or instability responsible for the pain, radiation therapy with or without chemotherapy or hormonal therapy can be considered. Vertebroplasty-kyphoplasty has been shown to be useful for a select group of patients with painful osseous metastasis.[4,56,178] (Fig. 17-41). This may even be effective in the sacrum.[42] The criteria for patient selection are an intact posterior wall of the vertebra without dural compression. The procedure involves either the percutaneous injection of acrylic surgical cement directly into the vertebral body (vertebroplasty) or insertion of a balloon to create a space and potentially expand the vertebra before placing cement in a less liquid form under less pressure (kyphoplasty), both done under fluoroscopic control. Both procedures have a high rate of success with pain control and have the advantage of being less invasive than surgery but are associated with some complications. The most common complication is extravasation of the cement into the adjacent disk space or soft tissues, and in most instances it is asymptomatic.[4] In those patients who do obtain pain relief, the improvement was stable for greater than 70 percent of patients at 6-month follow-up.

The most common reasons for surgical intervention in the patient with metastatic disease of the spine are epidural compression, myelopathy, radiculopathy, instability, and tumor progression unresponsive to other treatment. The considerations and factors pertinent to the type of surgery and approach are the anatomy of the problem (dural

FIGURE 17-40 **A,** *Magnetic resonance imaging of the spine in this patient with metastatic carcinoma of the breast was markedly abnormal, showing dural compression. At that time, the patient was asymptomatic.* **B, C,** *The radiologists were unable to determine the nature of the block. However, previous radiographs showed this to be an unchanged, healed pathologic fracture of approximately 1.5 years' duration.*

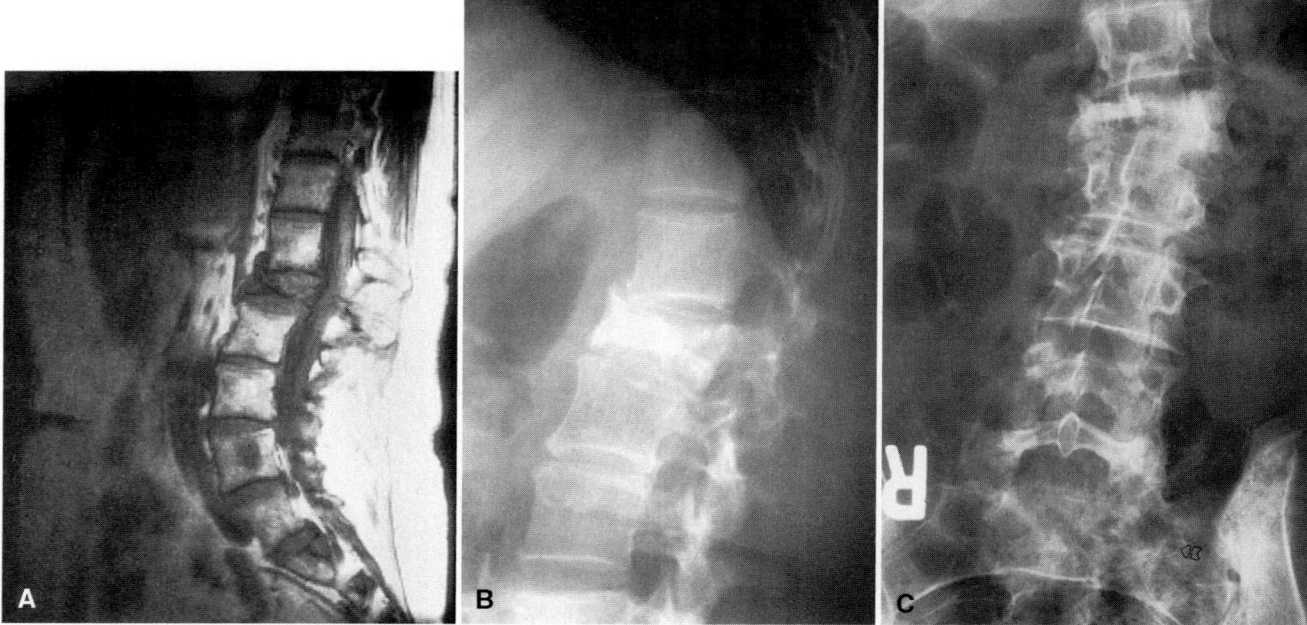

compression from anterior, lateral, or posterior), type and extent of body destruction with collapse and deformity, extent of posterior element and pedicle destruction, patient condition, and the goals of surgery (decompression, stabilization, or both).

In those patients with pain secondary to fracture (not amenable to kyphoplasty) or instability as a result of vertebral element destruction with or without canal compromise, surgical intervention in combination with radiation therapy should be the treatment of choice. Previously it was preferable that the radiation followed the surgical stabilization or decompression, as it was well demonstrated that the rate of wound complications was far higher with preoperative radiation.[66,179] However, with the advent of stereotactic radiosurgery to treat spinal metastases the rate of wound complications in patients treated with that technology preoperatively is less than occurs for those treated with conventional external beam and no different from that for those treated postoperatively. Unless myelopathy from epidural compression is present, surgery in patients with pain from instability or fracture can be limited to posterior pedicle screw fixation without the necessity for tumor debulking. The patient can then have either external beam or stereotactic radiosurgery postoperatively (in histologies relatively resistant to radiation such as lung, renal thyroid, etc.) for control of the tumor

| Table 17-3 |
| Tokuhashi's Evaluation System for Prognosis of Metastatic Spinal Tumors |

Symptoms	Score*		
	0	1	2
General condition (performance status)	Poor (10% to 40%)	Moderate (50% to 70%)	Good (80% to 100%)
Number of extraspinal skeletal metastases	>3	1 to 2	0
Metastases to internal organs	Unremovable	Removable	No metastases
Primary site of tumor	Lung, stomach	Kidney, liver, uterus, unknown	Thyroid, prostate, breast, rectum
Number of metastases to spine	>3	2	1
Spinal cord palsy	Complete	Incomplete	None

*Total score versus survival period:
9 to 12 points: >12 months survival; 0 to 5 points: <3 months survival From Tokuhashi Y, Matsuzaki H, Toriyama S, et al. Scoring system for the preoperative evaluation of metastatic spine tumor prognosis. Spine 15:1110–1113, 1999.

FIGURE 17-41 *Vertebroplasty or kyphoplasty are useful for decreasing symptoms in patients with collapse of the vertebral body without cord compression and with an intact posterior wall. This patient with myeloma has a painful 50% compression **(A)** and underwent percutaneous vertebroplasty **(B),** filling the anterior two thirds with methylmethacrylate **(C)**. Although the posterior wall was intact, a perforation in the superior end-plate permitted extrusion of methylmethacrylate into the disk space **(D),** but the patient had excellent pain relief.*

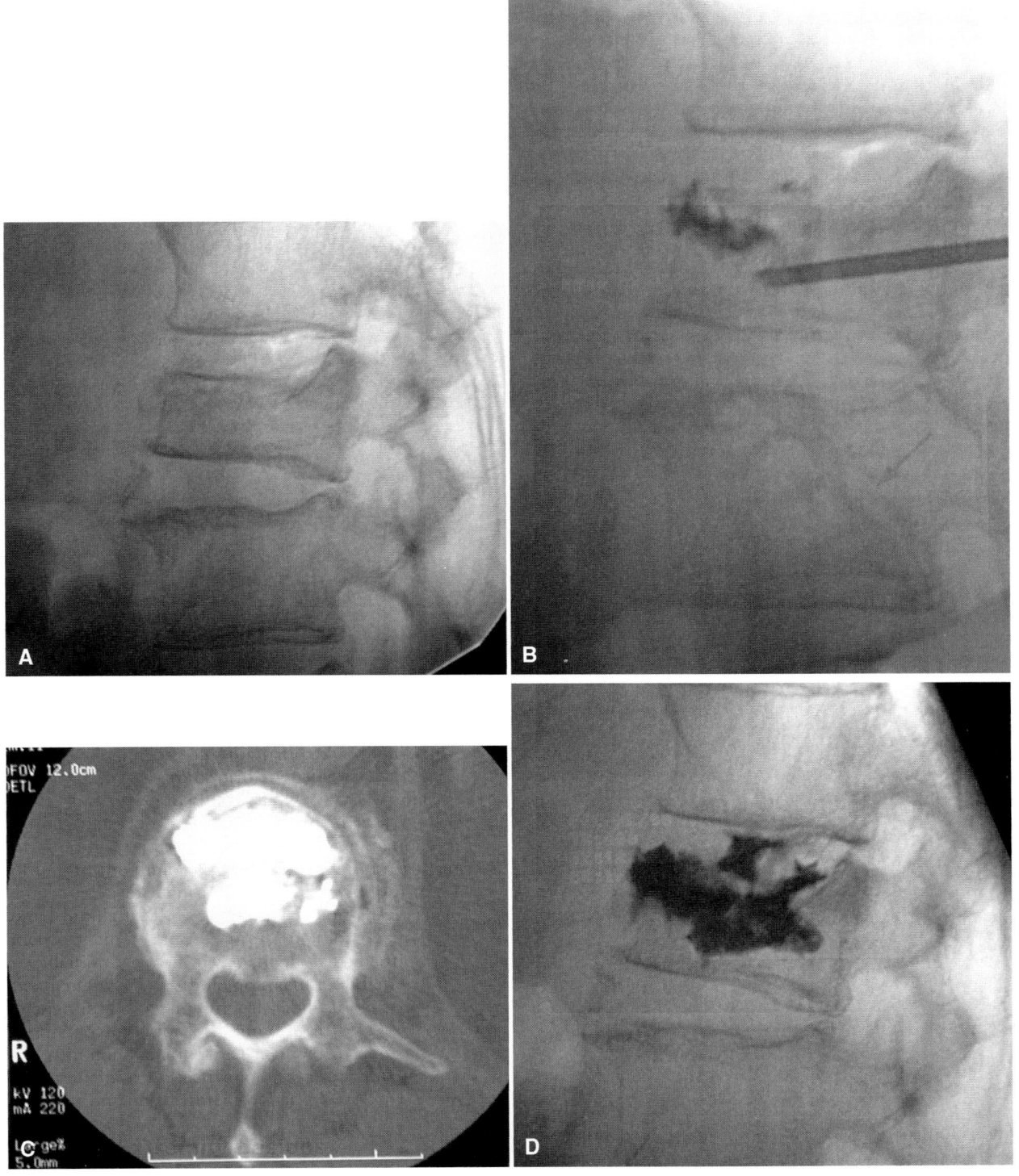

(Fig. 17-42). This limits morbidity, time in the hospital, and delay in system chemotherapy administration but achieves excellent pain relief and tumor control. Anterior surgery or combined anteroposterior surgery is less frequently required today to achieve stability than it was in the past. In patients with vertebral body collapse posterior stabilization can be augmented with an open kyphoplasty with the necessity for a separate anterior procedure, still achieving excellent stability and pain relief (see Fig. 17-38). Anterior corpectomy is infrequently necessary in the absence of epidural cord compression if the posterior elements are completely intact.

Although in the past treatment decisions for patients with myelopathy from metastatic epidural compression were complex because of lack of definitive level I treatment data, new evidence has simplified decision making in these patients. Understanding the patient demographics and the pathophysiology of the cord compression in metastatic disease simplifies the decision making. Approximately 15 percent of the metastatic lesions occur in the cervical spine, 50 percent in the thoracic spine, and 30 percent in the lumbar spine. One of the most important features is the location of the lesion within the vertebral segment and the direction from which the tumor is compressing the dural sac. Compression occurs from anteriorly in 70 percent of patients, predominantly posterolaterally in 20 percent

of patients, and posteriorly in 10 percent of patients. It has been well documented that radiation therapy causes significant improvement in only 50 percent of patients with neurologic impairment resulting from spinal cord compression caused by metastatic disease of the spine.[15,69,135,171] With new emphasis on the quality of the evidence in the literature for decision making, one level I prospective randomized study and several meta-analyses have now dealt with the results of surgical resection for metastatic spinal cord compression. Patchell and associates[134] reported that statistically more patients in the surgery group regained the ability to walk (84% vs. 57% in the radiation group) and retained it longer than those treated with radiation. In addition those for whom radiation failed and who underwent surgery secondarily did not do as well as those who had surgery primarily. A meta-analysis by Klimo and colleagues[103] showed very similar data when comparing the patients from 24 surgical series (1020 patients) and four radiation series (578 patients). In an evidence-based review of the literature, Ryken and co-workers[147] suggested on the basis of four level II studies and a much larger number of level 3 studies that those patients who have undergone surgery for spinal metastases have an improved quality of life. Outcome was also improved for those who underwent surgery prior to radiation. The authors concluded that there was insufficient evidence for absolute conclusions. However, their recommendations based on the literature between 1985 and 2003 was that those patients with incomplete neurologic deficit or severe pain should undergo surgical decompression followed by radiation. Radiation as the primary treatment modality should be reserved for those with radiosensitive tumors, those with little or no pain, and those who present with complete paraplegia. Responses differ depending on tumor type, with those tumors that are radiosensitive responding better than those that are not sensitive to radiation. In addition, those patients who have gross instability as well as collapse of the vertebral body with bone impingement have a lower success rate than those who have pure soft tissue involvement in the absence of gross instability. Laminectomy alone for treatment of epidural cord compression is essentially contraindicated, as it is effective in only 30 percent of patients,[71,158] but it is effective in only approximately 9 percent of patients with anterior compression.[15] Without concomitant posterior stabilization it almost routinely results in instability because of the posterior column insufficiency and thus subsequent collapse and pain. The combination of radiation therapy and laminectomy is no better than laminectomy alone.[32,160] As noted earlier, the most current studies confirmed the findings of many of the older studies that anterior corpectomy (i.e., direct anterior decompression for anterior lesions) has a far higher success rate than does laminectomy.[78,139] In most series, approximately 80 percent of patients improved with anterior corpectomy,[78,79,81] regardless of whether the tumor compression was caused by soft tissue or retropulsed bone. The results are also not affected by the presence of instability because the procedure requires both direct decompression of the anterior portion of the dural sac and stabilization with a variety of different constructs using an anterior spacer (cage, prosthesis, or methylmethacrylate).[48,72] Current data suggest that anterior corpectomy for patients with pure anterior

FIGURE 17-42 *This patient had metastatic chondrosarcoma to the upper thoracic spine. He had undergone decompression for pain and myelopathy secondary to tumor on separate occasions and now had recurrence in the same location with radiculopathy without myelopathy. He underwent stereotactic radiosurgery with complete relief of symptoms and it was a durable result through the last 6 months of his life. He was treated with 3000 cGy in three fractions, which is biologically equivalent to over 8000 Gy given by standard fractionation. Note how the isodose lines bend around the dural sac and spare it from the high radiation dose.*

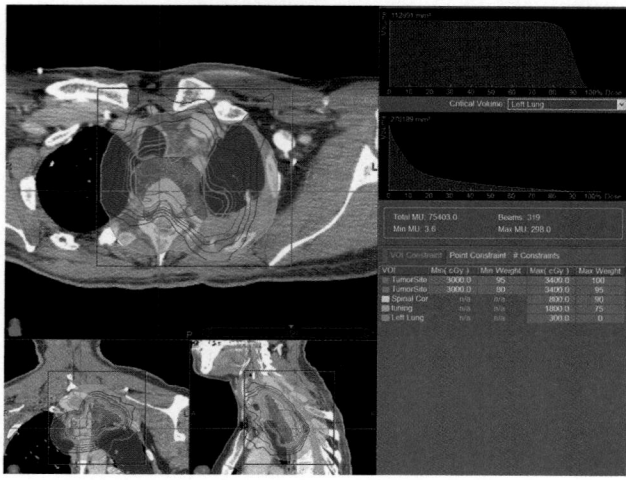

tumor is the most rational treatment and seems to give the best overall results[54] (Fig. 17-45). The posterolateral transpedicular approach may be appropriate in selected cases.[13] However, it is critical to combine the appropriate surgical procedure with postoperative radiation therapy to improve local tumor control. In those tumors that are not radiosensitive, complications related to local recurrence are not uncommon even after effective decompression and recovery.[101] Adjunctive local techniques can be combined with effective surgery to decrease the recurrence rate (Fig. 17-46). Adjuvant therapies such as embolization and brachytherapy[115] are used in an effort to improve local control. The use of stereotactic radiosurgery has decreased the rate of local recurrence after treatment of radioresistant tumors such as renal cell carcinoma.[65] It can also be used to treat local recurrences after conventional external beam radiation. In those patients with pure anterior disease and anterior dural compression, if there is adequate bone stock and the area of dural compression is isolated (extending no more than to adjacent segments), anterior corpectomy and stabilization give adequate results, with pain relief and recovery from neurologic deficits.[75] Although a few preliminary studies support the use of thoracoscopic anterior decompression and stabilization, this technique has not experienced wide adoption. Perhaps due to the vascular nature of many of the tumors and the nature of the required reconstructions, the more extensile thoracotomy remains the standard of care.

There are a variety of options for reconstruction after anterior corpectomy for decompression. The overriding principle to be considered is that any reconstruction method used to restore spinal stability in a tumor patient should not require external immobilization and should allow immediate patient mobilization and return to function. Since most surgical fields either have already been subjected to radiation or will undergo postoperative radiation, the probability of graft healing during the remaining lifetime of the patient (12–14 months) is quite low. Neither autologous graft nor allograft should be used as the primary reconstructive material unless the tumor is low grade, does not require radiation, and the patient has a long life expectancy. In the case of metastatic disease with long life expectancy (bone metastases from breast cancer), bone graft can be used in addition to a primary stabilizer (Fig. 17-44). Thus in most cases a cage, prosthetic device, and methylmethacrylate are the most effective reconstructive materials for treating an anterior corpectomy defect. Early work[76] suggested that methylmethacrylate could be used in the anterior portion of the spine as a vertebral body replacement to form an effective strut that is strongest in compression. It can be augmented by a posterior stabilization and fusion with autologous graft (Fig. 17-43). Its use precludes the use of bone graft anteriorly but allows immediate mobilization (Fig. 17-45). In addition, the combined construct of an anterior methylmethacrylate strut as a vertebral body replacement and a posterior plating with bone graft gives immediate stability and becomes stronger over time if the fusion occurs posteriorly. Use of a methylmethacrylate strut anteriorly plus an anterior plate decreases surgical time and has excellent resultant longevity. Use of

methylmethacrylate in the posterior cervical, thoracic, or lumbar spine to stiffen a construct in extension is absolutely contraindicated. It biomechanically adds little to rod or screw techniques for stabilization and acts as a space-occupying mass prone to an increased rate of infection.

Finally in patients with circumferential disease, the involvement of the vertebral body should be assessed. If the compression is predominantly posterior with gross instability anteriorly, laminectomy combined with posterior stabilization is the treatment of choice.[163] If the disease is predominantly anterior with posterior instability or previous laminectomy, anterior corpectomy and a more rigid stabilization construct are indicated (see Fig. 17-45). In some cases, both anterior and posterior surgery is necessary for adequate decompression. The magnitude of the surgery should be considered in relation to the patient's prognosis, overall health, and potential for recovery.[112]

SUMMARY

The treatment of osseous metastatic disease should be based on several firm principles. Assessment of the area of metastatic disease should be complete. The axial and appendicular skeleton should be evaluated for the presence of tumor and the degree of mechanical impairment and instability before any treatment procedures are instituted. If the primary concern is the presence of tumor and the structural stability of that particular body portion is not significantly compromised, then nonoperative treatment with radiation or chemotherapy (or both) is indicated. If significant mechanical weakness is evident with either fracture or impending fracture, surgical stabilization should be considered. It has been demonstrated that the magnitude of the surgical risk to the patient, time in hospital, and delay in systemic chemotherapy administration are all greater after pathologic fracture than after planned prophylactic fixation. Surgical reconstruction after pathologic fracture follows different principles from those used for management of fractures associated with non-neoplastic causes. Impaired healing potential of fractures resulting from metastases necessitates that more rigid forms of fixation combined with use of materials such as methylmethacrylate at times are needed to regain structural stability. Stabilization of osseous metastases per se may not extend the duration of the patient's life. But among the goals of surgical intervention is to improve quality of life and decrease the incidence of complications associated with metastatic bone disease (i.e., loss of mobility, structural instability, pain, and neurologic dysfunction). These goals should be achieved in the immediate postoperative period. In addition, because local tumor control is necessary for long-term success, postoperative irradiation (which further impairs bone healing) is a critical adjunct to the stabilization of pathologic lesions and fractures. If these principles are adhered to, the orthopaedic surgeon can greatly improve the quality of life of patients with metastatic disease.

FIGURE 17-43 *This 63-year-old woman presented with pain in her neck of 3 months' duration without neurologic symptoms. **A,** The lateral radiograph showed marked destruction of C4, C5, and C6. **B,** Magnetic resonance imaging showed marked cord compression, but the remainder of the workup showed no source. **C,** The computed tomography scan was helpful in demonstrating the degree of vertebral body destruction. **D,** The patient underwent open biopsy, revealing a solitary plasmacytoma, and as a result of the degree of destruction, a partial C4 and complete C5 and C6 corpectomies were reconstructed with a methylmethacrylate strut, followed by posterior plating and an autologous graft before beginning radiation therapy.*

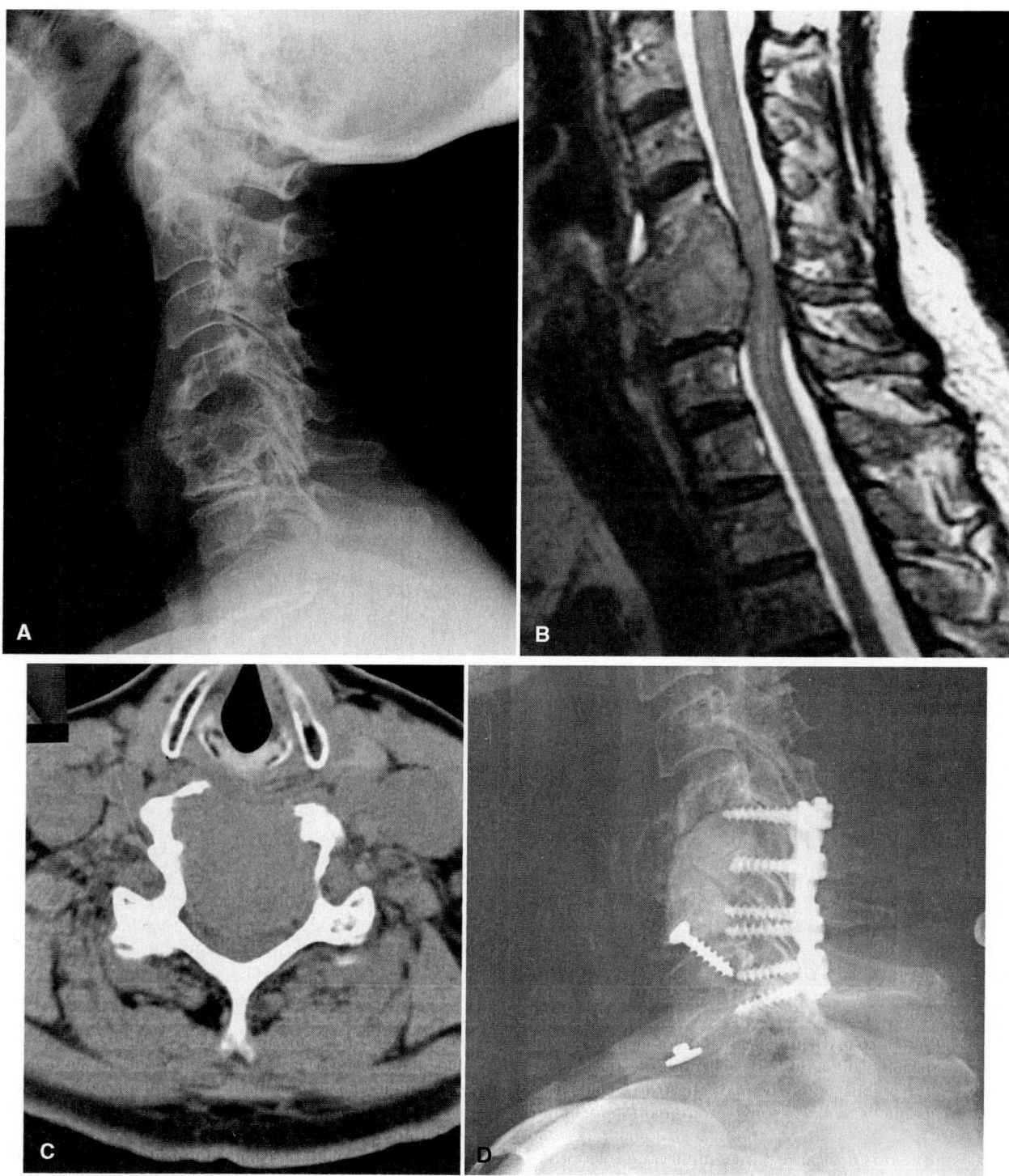

FIGURE 17-44 *This 64-year-old woman with carcinoma of the breast began to have progressive neck pain. She was initially treated with anti-inflammatory drugs.* **A,** *However, a subsequent radiograph demonstrated complete destruction of the C4 body with severe kyphosis and instability. Flexion-extension radiographs did not show significant motion.* **B,** *An anteroposterior radiograph showed the complete destruction of the C4 body.* **C,** *Preoperative computed tomography demonstrated a large soft tissue mass within the canal, with destruction of the vertebrae. The patient was placed in preoperative traction, and the vertebral height was slowly restored. The patient underwent an anterior corpectomy of C4 and C5, because the latter was partially involved. Cancellous screws were placed in the bodies above and below to stabilize methylmethacrylate, which was then inserted into the space in doughy form to fill the defect. The patient was then turned prone on the Stryker frame and underwent interspinous wiring with iliac graft.* **D, E,** *At the 10-year follow-up assessment, the patient was asymptomatic, had returned to all activities, and was neurologically normal.*

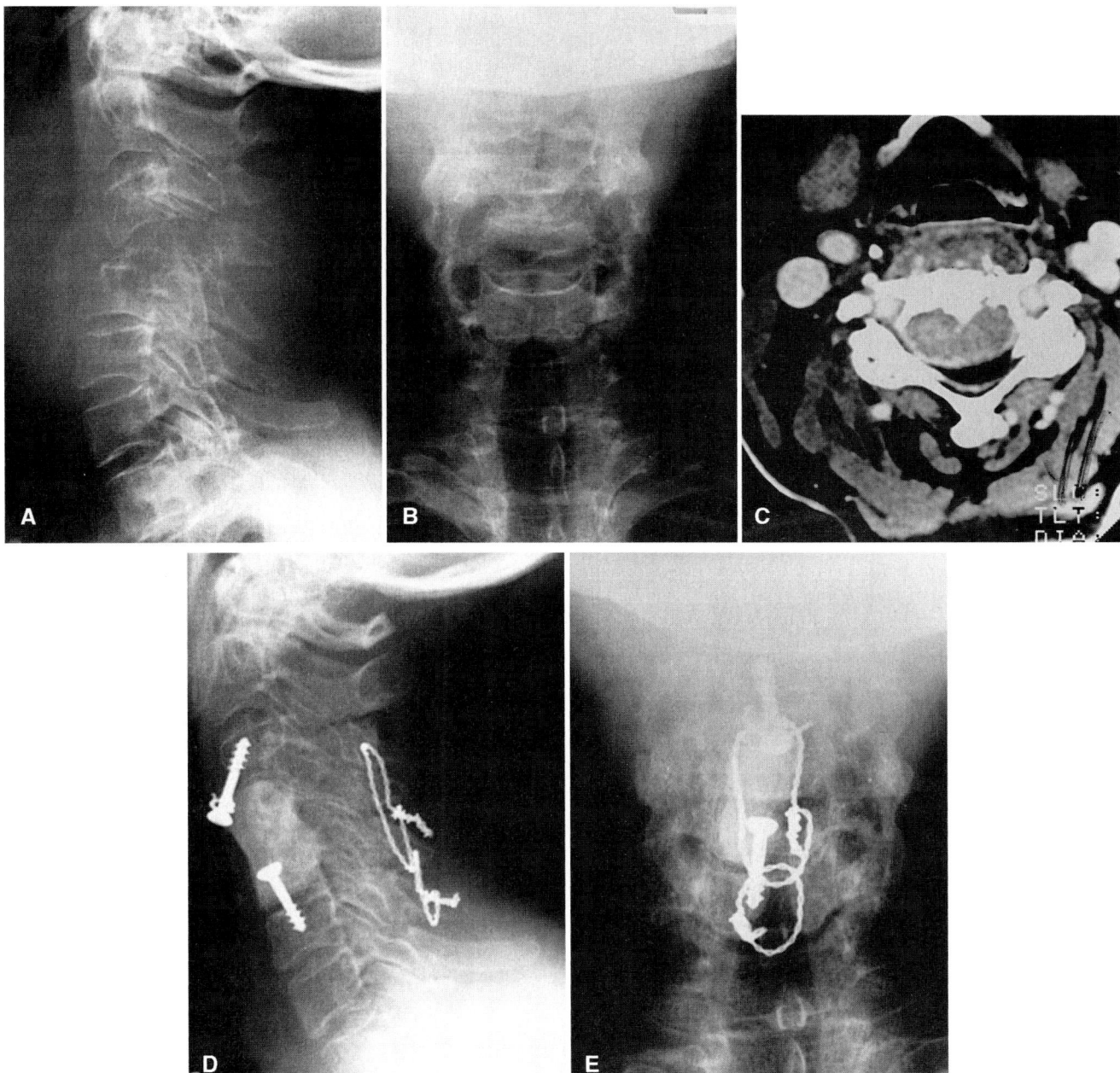

FIGURE 17-45 **A,** *This patient presented with incapacitating pain and a pathologic fracture of the T12 vertebra and a soft tissue tumor anteriorly impinging on a dural sac.* **B,** *The patient underwent anterior corpectomy and excision of the T12 body, with removal of all soft tissue tumor impinging on the dural sac.* **C,** *Stabilization with methylmethacrylate and a plate from T11 to L1 was used to replace the vertebral body. The patient had immediate relief of pain and returned to full functional capacity.* **D, E,** *Intraoperative photographs demonstrate the technique for insertion of the rod spanning the vertebrectomy and application of a plate.*

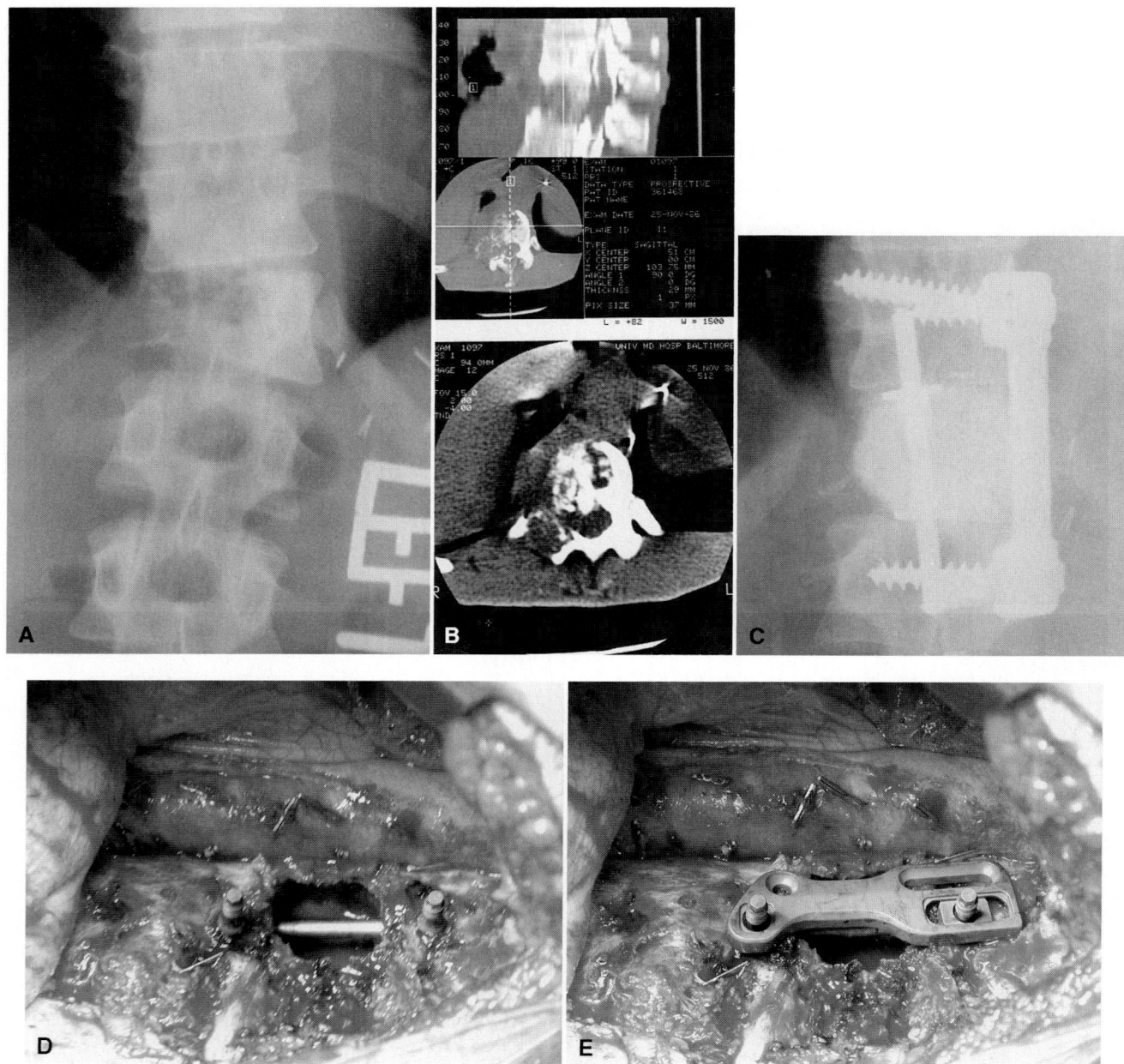

FIGURE 17-46 *A,* This patient with known renal cell carcinoma began to have back pain as a result of an expansile lesion in L4 and underwent radiation therapy with relief of pain for about 3 months. *B,* Preoperatively, he also developed left-sided L3 radiculopathy, and the anteroposterior radiograph showed complete absence of the pedicle on that side (arrow). *C,* Preoperative magnetic resonance imaging showed the degree of compression of the dural sac at L4 and the fact that the L3 lesion was completely separate. Preoperative computed tomography of L4 *(D)* and L3 *(E)* showed the extent of structural compromise and compression in a previously radiated field.

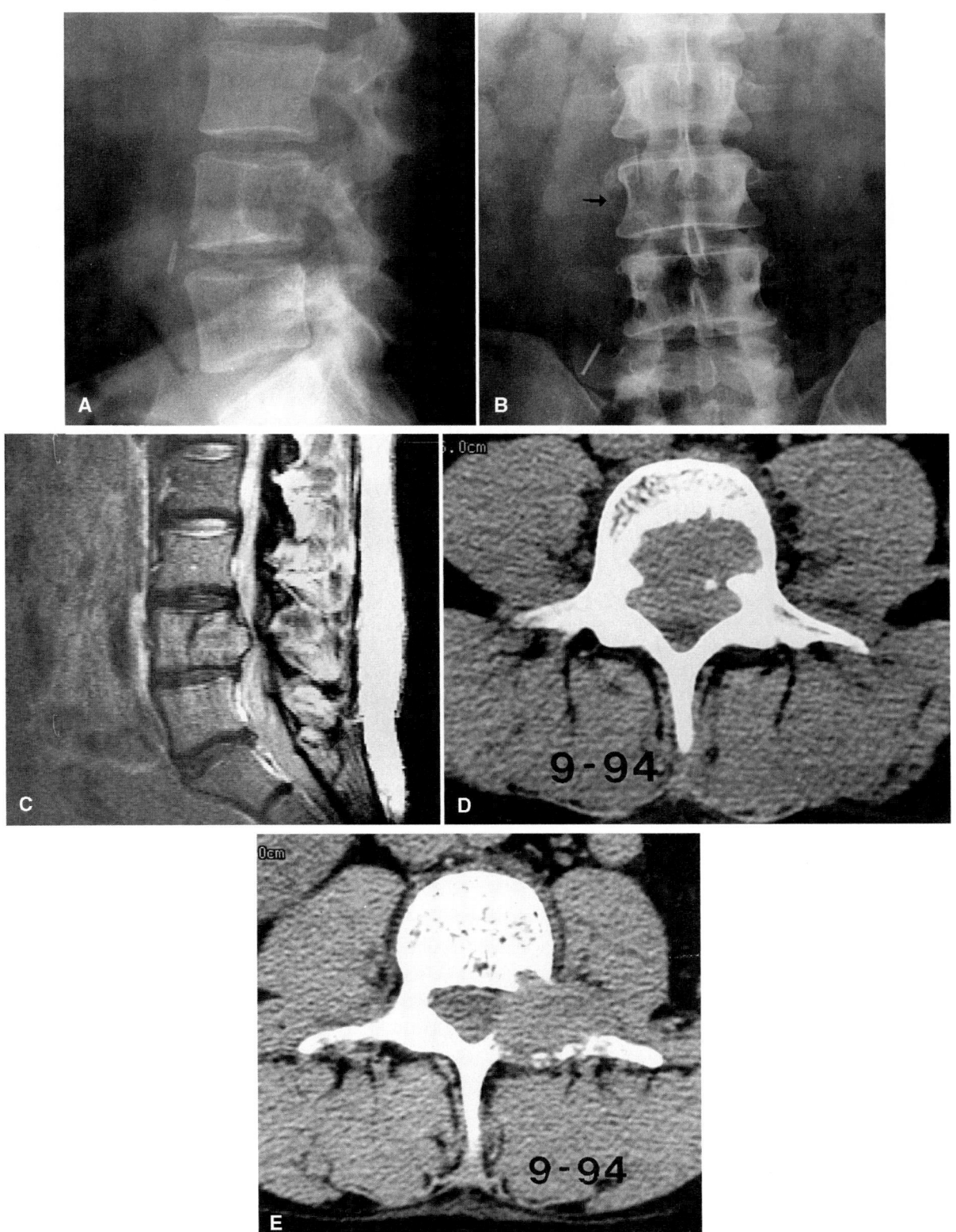

(Continued)

FIGURE 17-46 *(Continued)* ***F, G,*** *The patient underwent an anterior and posterior decompression and stabilization in a single sitting, with implantation of iodine-125 seeds both in the methylmethacrylate block anteriorly and in hemostatic gelatin (Gelfoam) in the defect in the pedicle posteriorly. He remained stable and disease-free in that location 18 months later.*

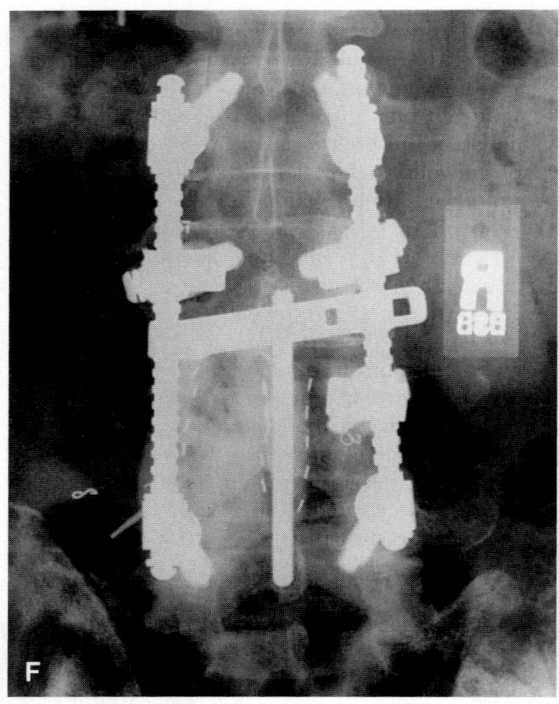
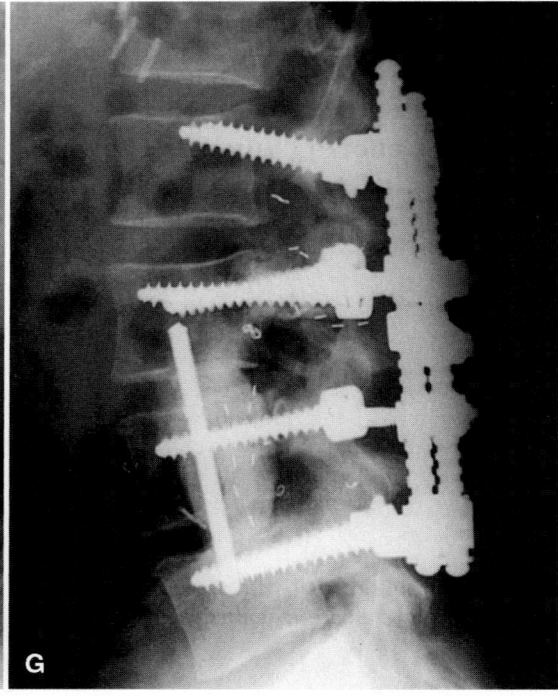

REFERENCES

1. Abdul-Karim, F.W.; Kida, M.; Wentz, W.B.; et al. Bone metastasis from gynecologic carcinomas: A clinicopathologic study. Gynecol Oncol 39:108–114, 1990.

2. Aboulafia, A.J.; Buch, R.; Mathews, J.; et al. Reconstruction using the saddle prosthesis following excision of primary and metastatic periacetabular tumors. Clin Orthop 314:203–213, 1995.

3. Anderson, J.T.; Erickson, J.M.; Thompson, R.C.J.; et al. Pathologic femoral shaft fractures comparing fixation techniques using cement. Clin Orthop Relat Res 131:273–278, 1978.

4. Barragan-Campos, H.M.; Vallee, J.N.; Lo, D.; et al. Percutaneous vertebroplasty for spinal metastases: Complications. Radiology 238:354–362, 2006.

5. Barron, K.D.; Harano, A.; Araki, A.; et al. Experiences with metastatic neoplasms involving the spinal cord. Neurology 9:91–106, 1959.

6. Barwood, S.A.; Wilson, J.L.; Molnar, R.R.; et al. The incidence of acute cardiorespiratory and vascular dysfunction following intramedullary nail fixation of femoral metastasis. Acta Orthop Scand 71:147–152, 2000.

7. Batson, O.V. The function of the vertebral veins and their role in the spread of metastases. Ann Surg 112:138–149, 1940.

8. Beals, R.K.; Lawton, G.D.; Snell, W.E. Prophylactic internal fixation of the femur in metastatic breast cancer. Cancer 28:1350–1354, 1971.

9. Bernat, J.L.; Greenberg, E.R.; Barrett, J. Suspected epidural compression of the spinal cord and cauda equina by metastatic carcinoma. Clinical diagnosis and survival. Cancer 51:1953–1957, 1983.

10. Berrettoni, B.A.; Carter, J.R. Mechanisms of cancer metastasis to bone. J Bone Joint Surg [Am] 68:308–312, 1986.

11. Berruti, A.; Dogliotti, L.; Bitossi, R.; et al. Incidence of skeletal complications in patients with bone metastatic prostate cancer and hormone refractory disease: Predictive role of bone resorption and formation markers evaluated at baseline. J Urol 164:1248–1253, 2000.

12. Bhardwaj, S.; Holland, J.F. Chemotherapy of metastatic cancer in bone. Clin Orthop Relat Res 169:28–37, 1982.

13. Bilsky, M.H.; Boland, P.; Lis, E.; et al. Single-stage posterolateral transpedicle approach for spondylectomy, epidural decompression, and circumferential fusion of spinal metastases. Spine 25:2240–2249, 2000.

14. Blake, D. Radiation treatment of metastatic bone disease. Clin Orthop 73:89–100, 1970.

15. Black, P. Spinal metastasis: Current status and recommended guidelines for management. Neurosurgery 5:726–746, 1979.

16. Blari, R.J.; McAfee, J.G. Radiographic detection of skeletal metastases: Radiographs vs scans. J Radiation Oncol 1:1201, 1976.

17. Boissier, S.; Ferreras, M.; Peyruchaud, O.; et al. Bisphosphonates inhibit breast and prostate carcinoma cell invasion, an early event in the formation of bone metastases. Cancer Res 60:2949–2954, 2000.

18. Boland, P.J.; Lane, J.M.; Sundaresan, N. Metastatic disease of the spine. Clin Orthop Relat Res 169:95–102, 1982.

19. Bonariqo, B.C.; Rubin, P. Nonunion of pathologic fractures after radiation therapy. Radiology 88:889–898, 1967.

20. Braunstein, E.M.; Kuhns, L.R. Computed tomographic demonstration of spinal metastases. Spine 8:912–915, 1983.

21. Bremner, R.A.; Jelliffe, A.M. The management of pathological fractures of the major long bones from metastatic cancer. J Bone Joint Surg [Br] 40B:652–659, 1958.

22. Bubendorf, L.; Schopfer, A.; Wagner, U.; et al. Metastatic patterns of prostate cancer: An autopsy study of 1,589 patients. Hum Pathol 31:578–583, 2000.

23. Cadman, E.; Bertino, J.R. Chemotherapy of skeletal metastases. Int J Radiat Oncol Biol Phys 1:1211–1215, 1976.

24. Carlin, B.I.; Andriole, G.L. The natural history, skeletal complications, and management of bone metastases in patients with prostate carcinoma. Cancer 88:2989–2994, 2000.

25. Chan, D.; Carter, S.R.; Grimer, R.J.; et al. Endoprosthetic replacement for bony metastases. Ann R Coll Surg Engl 74:13–18, 1992.

26. Cheng, D.S.; Seitz, C.B.; Eyre, H.J. Nonoperative management of femoral, humeral, and acetabular metastases in patients with breast carcinoma. Cancer 45:1533–1537, 1980.

27. Ciezki, J.; Macklis, R.M. The palliative role of radiotherapy in the management of the cancer patient. Semin Oncol 22:82–90, 1995.

28. Citrin, D.L.; Bessent, R.G.; Greig, W.R. A comparison of the sensitivity and accuracy of the 99Tcm-phosphate bone scan and skeletal radiograph in the diagnosis of bone metastases. Clin Radiol 28:107–117, 1977.

29. Clain, A. Secondary malignant lesions of bone. Br J Cancer 19:15–29, 1965.

30. Coleman, R. Skeletal complications of malignancy. Cancer 80:1588–1594, 1997.

31. Colletti, P.M.; Siegel, H.J.; Woo, M.Y.; et al. The impact on treatment planning of MRI of the spine in patients suspected of vertebral metastasis: An efficacy study. Comput Med Imaging Graph 20:159–162, 1996.

32. Constans, J.P.; de Divitiis, E.; Donzelli, R.; et al. Spinal metastases with neurological manifestations. Review of 600 cases. J Neurosurg 59:111–118, 1983.

33. Cook, A.M.; Lau, T.N.; Tomlinson, M.J.; et al. Magnetic resonance imaging of the whole spine in suspected malignant spinal cord compression: Impact on management. Clin Oncol (R Coll Radiol) 10:39–43, 1998.

34. Coran, A.G.; Banks, H.H.; Aliapoulios, W.A.; et al. The management of pathologic fractures in patients with metastatic carcinoma of the breast. Surg Gynecol Obstet 132:1225–1230, 1968.

35. Cramer, S.F.; Fried, L.; Carter, K.J. The cellular basis of metastatic bone disease in patients with lung cancer. Cancer 48:2649–2660, 1981.

36. Crawford, E.D.; Allen, J.A. Treatment of newly diagnosed state D2 prostate cancer with leuprolide and flutamide or leuprolide alone, phase III, intergroup study 0036. J Steroid Biochem Molec Biol 37:961–963, 1990.

37. Crolla, R.M.; de Vries, L.S.; Clevers, G.J. Locked intramedullary nailing of humeral fractures. Injury 24:403–406, 1993.

38. Cumming, J.; Hacking, N.; Fairhurst, J.; et al. Distribution of bony metastases in prostatic carcinoma. Br J Urol 66:411–414, 1990.

39. Dalgorf, D.; Borkhoff, C.M.; Stephen, D.J.; et al. Venting during prophylactic nailing for femoral metastases: Current orthopedic practice. Can J Surg 46:427–431, 2003.

40. Damron, T.A.; Morgan, H.; Prakash, D.; et al. Critical evaluation of Mirels' rating system for impending pathologic fractures. Clin Orthop Relat Res 415 (Suppl):S201–S207, 2003.

41. Damron, T.A.; Sim, F.H. [Surgical treatment for metastatic disease of the pelvis and the proximal end of the femur]. Instr Course Lect 49:461–470, 2000.

42. Dehdashti, A.R.; Martin, J.B.; Jean, B.; et al. PMMA cementoplasty in symptomatic metastatic lesions of the S1 vertebral body. Cardiovasc Intervent Radiol 23:235–237, 2000.

43. Demers, L.M.; Costa, L.; Lipton, A. Biochemical markers and skeletal metastases. [Review] [40 refs]. Cancer 88:2919–2926, 2000.

44. Dickie, G.J.; Macfarlane, D. Strontium and samarium therapy for bone metastases from prostate carcinoma. Australas Radiol 43:476–479, 1999.

45. Diel, I.J.; Solomayer, E.F.; Bastert, G. Bisphosphonates and the prevention of metastasis: First evidences from preclinical and clinical studies. [Review] [51 refs]. Cancer 88:3080–3088, 2000.

46. Dijkstra, S.; Stapert, J.; Boxma, H.; et al. Treatment of pathological fractures of the humeral shaft due to bone metastases: A comparison of intramedullary locking nail and plate osteosynthesis with adjunctive bone cement. Eur J Surg Oncol 22:621–626, 1996.

47. Domchek, S.M.; Younger, J.; Finkelstein, D.M.; et al. Predictors of skeletal complications in patients with metastatic breast carcinoma. Cancer 89:363–368, 2000.

48. Dunn, E. The role of methylmethacrylate in the stabilization and replacement of tumors of the cervical spine: A project of the cervical spine research society. Spine 2:15–24, 1977.

49. Eckardt, J.J.; Kabo, J.M.; Kelly, C.M.; et al. Endoprosthetic reconstructions for bone metastases. Clin Orthop Relat Res 415(Suppl):S254–S262, 2003.

50. Eftekhar, N.S.; Thurston, C.W. Effect of irradiation on acrylic cement with special reference to fixation of pathological fractures. J Biomech 8:53–56, 1975.

51. Eil, P.J. Skeletal imaging in metastatic disease. Curr Opin Radiol 3:791–796, 1991.

52. Even-Sapir, E.; Metser, U.; Mishani, E.; et al. The detection of bone metastases in patients with high-risk prostate cancer: 99mTc-MDP planar bone scintigraphy, single- and multi-field-of-view SPECT, 18F-fluoride PET, and 18F-fluoride PET/CT. J Nucl Med 47:287–297, 2006.

53. Fidler, M. Anterior decompression and stablization of metastatic spinal fractures. J Bone Joint Surg [Br] 68:83–90, 1986.

54. Fielding, J.W.; Pyle, R.N.J.; Fietti, V.G., Jr. Anterior cervical vertebral body resection and bone-grafting for benign and malignant tumors. A survey under the auspices of the Cervical Spine Research Society. J Bone Joint Surg [Am] 61:251–253, 1979.

55. Flinkkila, T.; Hyvonen, P.; Lakovaara, M.; et al. Intramedullary nailing of humeral shaft fractures. A retrospective study of 126 cases. Acta Orthop Scand 70:133–136, 1999.

56. Fourney, D.R.; Schomer, D.F.; Nader, R.; et al. Percutaneous vertebroplasty and kyphoplasty for painful vertebral body fractures in cancer patients. J Neurosurg 98:21–30, 2003.

57. Frassica, F.J.; Frassica, D.A. Metastatic bone disease of the humerus. J Am Acad Orthop Surg 11:282–288, 2003.

58. Friedl, W. Indication, management and results of surgical therapy for pathological fractures in patients with bone metastases. Eur J Surg Oncol 16:380–396, 1990.

59. Friedlaender, G.E.; Johnson, R.M.; Brand, R.A.; et al. Treatment of pathological fractures. Conn Med 39:765–772, 1975.

60. Fuchs, B.; Trousdale, R.T.; Rock, M.G. Solitary bony metastasis from renal cell carcinoma: Significance of surgical treatment. Clin Orthop Relat Res 431:187–192, 2005.

61. Fuhrmann, R.A.; Roth, A.; Venbrocks, R.A. Salvage of the upper extremity in cases of tumorous destruction of the proximal humerus. J Cancer Res Clin Oncol 126:337–344, 2000.

62. Gainor, B.J.; Buchert, P. Fracture healing in metastatic bone disease. Clin Orthop Relat Res 178:297–302, 1983.

63. Galasko, C.S. Pathological fractures secondary to metastatic cancer. J R Coll Surg Edinb 19:351–362, 1974.

64. Galasko, C.S. Mechanisms of bone destruction in the development of skeletal metastases: Mechanisms of lytic and blastic metastatic disease of bone. Nature 263:507–508, 1976.

65. Gerszten, P.C.; Burton, S.A.; Ozhasoglu, C.; et al. Stereotactic radiosurgery for spinal metastases from renal cell carcinoma. J Neurosurg Spine 3:288–295, 2005.

66. Ghogawala, Z.; Mansfield, F.L.; Borges, L.F. Spinal radiation before surgical decompression adversely affects outcomes of surgery for symptomatic metastatic spinal cord compression. Spine 26:818–824, 2001.

67. Gilbert, H.A.; Kagan, A.R.; Nussbaum, H.; et al. Evaluation of radiation therapy for bone metastases: Pain relief and quality of life. AJR Am J Roentgenol 129:1095–1096, 1977.

68. Gold, R.I.; Seeger, L.L.; Bassett, L.W.; et al. An integrated approach to the evaluation of metastatic bone disease. [Review] [29 refs]. Radiol Clin North Am 28:471–483, 1990.

69. Greenberg, H.S.; Kim, J.H.; Posner, J.B. Epidural spinal cord compression from metastatic tumor: Results with a new treatment protocol. Ann Neurol 8:361–366, 1980.

70. Habernek, H.; Orthner, E. A locking nail for fractures of the humerus [see comments]. J Bone Joint Surg [Br] 73:651–653, 1991.

71. Hall, A.J.; Mackay, N.N. The results of laminectomy for compression of the cord or cauda equina by extradural malignant tumour. J Bone Joint Surg [Br] 55:497–505, 1973.

72. Harrington, K.D. The use of methylmethacrylate as an adjunct in the internal fixation of malignant neoplastic fractures. J Bone Joint Surg [Am] 54:1665–1676, 1972.

73. Harrington, K.D. Methylmethacrylate as an adjunct in internal fixation of pathological fractures. J Bone Joint Surg [Am] 58:1047–1054, 1976.

74. Harrington, K.D. The role of surgery in the management of pathologic fractures. Orthop Clin North Am 8:841–859, 1977.

75. Harrington, K.D. Management of unstable pathologic fracture dislocations of the spine and acetabulum, secondary to metastatic malignancy. Instr Course Lect 29:51–61, 1980.

76. Harrington, K.D. The management of acetabular insufficiency secondary to metastatic malignant disease. J Bone Joint Surg [Am] 63:653–664, 1981.

77. Harrington, K.D. The use of methylmethacrylate for vertebral body replacement and anterior stabilization of pathological fracture dislocations of the spine due to metastatic malignant disease. J Bone Joint Surg [Am] 63:36–46, 1981.

78. Harrington, K.D. Anterior cord decompression and spinal stabilization for patients with metastatic lesions of the spine. J Neurosurg 561:107–117, 1984.

79. Harrington, K.D. Current concepts review: Metastatic disease of the spine. J Bone Joint Surg [Am] 68:1110–1115, 1986.

80. Harrington, K.D. Impending pathologic fractures from metastatic malignancy: Evaluation and management. Instr Course Lect 35:357–381, 1986.

81. Harrington, K.D. Anterior decompression and stabilization of the spine as a treatment for vertebral collapse and spinal cord compression from metastatic malignancy. Clin Orthop 233:177–197, 1988.

82. Harrington, K.D. Orthopaedic management of extremity and pelvic lesions. Clin Orthop 312:136–147, 1995.

83. Hartsell, W.F.; Scott, C.B.; Bruner, D.W.; et al. Randomized trial of short- versus long-course radiotherapy for palliation of painful bone metastases. J Natl Cancer Inst 97:798–804, 2005.

84. Hashimoto, M.; Hiwa, O.; Niotta, Y.; et al. Unstable expression of E-cadherin adhesion molecules in metastatic ovarian cancer cells. Jpn J Cancer Res 80:459, 1989.

85. Healey, J.H.; Lane, J.M. Treatment of pathologic fractures of the distal femur with the Zickel supracondylar nail. Clin Orthop Relat Res 250:216–220, 1990.

86. Hems, T.E.; Bhullar, T.P. Interlocking nailing of humeral shaft fractures: The Oxford experience 1991 to 1994 [see comments]. Injury 27:485–489, 1996.

87. Hipp, J.A.; Springfield, D.S.; Hayes, W.C. Predicting pathologic fracture risk in the management of metastatic bone defects. [Review] [68 refs]. Clin Orthop Relat Res 312:120–135, 1995.

88. Hyder, N.; Wray, C.C. Treatment of pathological fractures of the humerus with Ender nails. J R Coll Surg Edinb 38:370–372, 1993.

89. Ikpeme, J.O. Intramedullary interlocking nailing for humeral fractures: Experiences with the Russell-Taylor humeral nail. Injury 25:447–455, 1994.

90. Israel, O.; Kuten, A. Early detection of cancer recurrence: 18F-FDG PET/CT can make a difference in diagnosis and patient care. J Nucl Med 48(Suppl 1):28S–35S, 2007.

91. Ito, S.; Kato, K.; Ikeda, M.; et al. Comparison of 18F-FDG PET and bone scintigraphy in detection of bone metastases of thyroid cancer. J Nucl Med 48:889–895, 2007.

92. Jacobson, A.F.; Cronin, E.B.; Stomper, P.C.; et al. Bone scans with one or two new abnormalities in cancer patients with no known metastases: Frequency and serial scintigraphic behavior of benign and malignant lesions. Radiology 175:229–232, 1990.

93. Jacobsson, H.; Goransson, H. Radiological detection of bone and bone marrow metastases. [Review] [54 refs]. Med Oncol Tumor Pharmacother 8:253–260, 1991.

94. Janjan, N.A. Radiation for bone metastases: Conventional techniques and the role of systemic radiopharmaceuticals. [Review] [96 refs]. Cancer 80:1628–1645, 1997.

95. Jensen, C.H.; Hansen, D.; Jorgensen, U. Humeral shaft fractures treated by interlocking nailing: A preliminary report on 16 patients. Injury 23:234–236, 1992.

96. Johnston, A.D. Pathology of metastatic tumors in bone. [Review] [141 refs]. Clin Orthop Relat Res 73:8–32, 1970.

97. Kamby, C.; Vejborg, I.; Daugaard, S.; et al. Clinical and radiologic characteristics of bone metastases in breast cancer. Cancer 60:2524–2531, 1987.

98. Kao, C.H.; Hsieh, J.F.; Tsai, S.C.; et al. Comparison and discrepancy of 18F-2-deoxyglucose positron emission tomography and Tc-99m MDP bone scan to detect bone metastases. Anticancer Res 20:2189–2192, 2000.

99. Keene, J.S.; Sellinger, D.S.; McBeath, A.A.; et al. Metastatic breast cancer in the femur. A search for the lesion at risk of fracture. Clin Orthop Relat Res 203:282–288, 1986.

100. Keyak, J.H.; Kaneko, T.S.; Rossi, S.A.; et al. Predicting the strength of femoral shafts with and without metastatic lesions. Clin Orthop Relat Res 439:161–170, 2005.

101. King, G.J.; Kostuik, J.P.; McBroom, R.J.; et al. Surgical management of metastatic renal carcinoma of the spine. Spine 16:265–271, 1991.

102. Kirchner, P.T.; Simon, M.A. Radioisotopic evaluation of skeletal disease. J Bone Joint Surg [Am] 63:673–681, 1981.

103. Klimo, P., Jr.; Thompson, C.J.; Kestle, J.R.; et al. A meta-analysis of surgery versus conventional radiotherapy for the treatment of metastatic spinal epidural disease. Neurooncology 7:64–76, 2005.

104. Kocialkowski, A.; Wallace, W.A. Reconstruction of the femur with the aid of a combination of a joint replacement and an intramedullary nail. Injury 22:63–65, 1991.

105. Kohno, N.; Aogi, K.; Minami, H.; et al. Zoledronic acid significantly reduces skeletal complications compared with placebo in Japanese women with bone metastases from breast cancer: A randomized, placebo-controlled trial. J Clin Oncol 23:3314–3321, 2005.

106. Kraemer, W.J.; Hearn, T.C.; Powell, J.N.; et al. Fixation of segmental subtrochanteric fractures. A biomechanical study. Clin Orthop Relat Res 332:71–79, 1996.

107. Kunec, J.R.; Lewis, R.J. Closed intramedullary rodding of pathologic fractures with supplemental cement. Clin Orthop Relat Res 188:183–186, 1984.

108. Kurdy, N.M.; Kay, P.R.; Paul, A.S.; et al. The huckstep nail. Stable fixation of mechanically deficient femoral bone. Clin Orthop Relat Res 316:214–220, 1995.

109. Lam, W.C.; Delikatny, E.J.; Orr, F.W.; et al. The chemotactic response of tumor cells. A model for cancer metastasis. Am J Pathol 104:69–76, 1981.

110. Lancaster, J.M.; Koman, L.A.; Gristina, A.G.; et al. Pathologic fractures of the humerus. South Med J 81:52–55, 1988.

111. Lane, J.M.; Sculco, T.P.; Zolan, S. Treatment of pathological fractures of the hip by endoprosthetic replacement. J Bone Joint Surg [Am] 62:954–959, 1980.

112. Lee, C.K.; Rosa, R.; Fernand, R. Surgical treatment of tumors of the spine. Spine 11:201–208, 1986.

113. Levine, A.M. Reamed retrograde intramedullary nailing for metastatic lesions of the humerus. Presented at the ENSOS/AMSTS/ISOLS Meeting 1995.

114. Levine, A.M.; Kenzora, J.E. Management of peri-acetabular metastatic lesions of bone. J Bone Joint Surg 9:1, 1985.

115. Levine, A.M.; Virkus, W.; Amin, P. Brachytherapy in the treatment of spinal neoplasm. Orthop Trans 20:35, 1996.

116. Levy, R.N.; Sherry, H.S.; Siffert, R.S. Surgical management of metastatic disease of bone at the hip. Clin Orthop Relat Res 169:62–69, 1982.

117. Lewallen, R.P.; Pritchard, D.J.; Sim, F.H. Treatment of pathologic fractures or impending fractures of the humerus with Rush rods and methylmethacrylate. Experience with 55 cases in 54 patients, 1968–1977. Clin Orthop Relat Res 166:193–198, 1982.

118. Li, J.; Tio, F.O.; Jinkins, J.R. Contrast-enhanced MRI of healed pathologic vertebral compression fracture mimicking active disease in a patient treated for lymphoma. Neuroradiology 35:506–508, 1993.

119. Lin, J.; Hou, S.M.; Hang, Y.S.; et al. Treatment of humeral shaft fractures by retrograde locked nailing. Clin Orthop Relat Res 342:147–155, 1997.

120. Lipton, A.; Colombo-Berra, A.; Bukowski, R.M.; et al. Skeletal complications in patients with bone metastases from renal cell carcinoma and therapeutic benefits of zoledronic acid. Clin Cancer Res 10:6397S–6403S, 2004.

121. Loitz, D.; Konnecker, H.; Illgner, A.; et al. [Retrograde intramedullary nailing of humeral fractures with new implants. Analysis of 120 consecutive cases]. [German]. Unfallchirurg 101:543–550, 1998.

122. MacAusland, W.R.J.; Wyman, E.T., Jr. Management of metastatic pathological fractures. Clin Orthop Relat Res 73:39–51, 1970.

123. Mareel, M.M.; Behrens, J.; Birchmeier, W.; et al. Down-regulation of E-cadherin expression in Madin Darby canine kidney (MDCK) cells inside tumors of nude mice. Int J Cancer 47:922–928, 1991.

124. Matsubayashi, T.; Koga, H.; Nishiyama, Y.; et al. The reparative process of metastatic bone lesions after radiotherapy. Jpn J Clin Oncol 11(Suppl):253–264, 1981.

125. Miller, F.; Whitehill, R. Carcinoma of the breast metastatic to the skeleton. Clin Orthop Relat Res 184:121–127, 1984.

126. Mirels, H. Metastatic disease in long bones. A proposed scoring system for diagnosing impending pathologic fractures. Clin Orthop Relat Res 249:256–264, 1989.

127. Mundy, G.R.; Eilon, G.; Altman, A.J.; et al. Non-bone cell mediated bone resorption. In Horton, S.E.; Tarpley, T.M.; Davis, W.M.F., eds. Mechanisms of localized bone loss. Washington, D.C.

128. Murray, J.A.; Parrish, F.F. Surgical management of secondary neoplastic fractures about the hip. Orthop Clin North Am 5:887–901, 1974.

129. Needham, P.R.; Mithal, N.P.; Hoskin, P.J. Radiotherapy for bone pain. J R Soc Med 87:503–505, 1994.

130. Oka, J.; Shiozaki, H.; Kobayashi, K.; et al. Expression of E-cadherin cells adhesion molecules in breast cancer tissues and its relationship to metastasis. Jpn J Cancer Res 53:1696, 1993.

131. Orr, W.; Varani, J.; Ward, P.A. Characteristics of the chemotactic response of neoplastic cells to a factor derived from the fifth component of complement. Am J Pathol 93:405–422, 1978.

132. Paget, S. The distribution of secondary growths in cancer of the breast. 1889 [classical article]. Cancer Metastasis Rev 8:98–101, 1989.

133. Papapoulos, S.E.; Hamdy, N.A.; van der Pluijm, G. Bisphosphonates in the management of prostate carcinoma metastatic to the skeleton. Cancer 88:3047–3053, 2000.

134. Patchell, R.A.; Tibbs, P.A.; Regine, W.F.; et al. Direct decompressive surgical resection in the treatment of spinal cord compression caused by metastatic cancer: A randomised trial. Lancet 366:643–648, 2005.

135. Patterson, R.H., Jr. Metastatic disease of the spine: Surgical risk versus radiation therapy. Clinical Neurosurgery 27:641–644, 1980.

136. Poigenfurst, J.; Marcove, R.C.; Miller, T.R. Surgical treatment of fractures through metastases in the proximal femur. J Bone Joint Surg [Br] 50:743–756, 1968.

137. Pugh, J.; Sherry, H.S.; Futterman, B.; et al. Biomechanics of pathologic fractures. Clin Orthop Relat Res 169:109–114, 1982.

138. Ratanatharathorn, V.; Powers, W.E.; Steverson, N.; et al. Bone metastasis from cervical cancer. Cancer 73:2372–2379, 1994.

139. Raycroft, J.F.; Hockman, R.P.; Southwick, W.O. Metastatic tumors involving the cervical vertebrae: Surgical palliation. J Bone Joint Surg [Am] 60:763–768, 1978.

140. Redmond, B.J.; Biermann, J.S.; Blasier, R.B. Interlocking intramedullary nailing of pathological fractures of the shaft of the humerus. J Bone Joint Surg [Am] 78:891–896, 1996.

141. Rommens, P.M.; Blum, J.; Runkel, M. Retrograde nailing of humeral shaft fractures. Clin Orthop Relat Res 350:26–39, 1998.

142. Rommens, P.M.; Verbruggen, J.; Broos, P.L. Retrograde locked nailing of humeral shaft fractures. A review of 39 patients [see comments]. J Bone Joint Surg [Br] 77:84–89, 1995.

143. Roos, D.E.; Davis, S.R.; Turner, S.L.; et al. Quality assurance experience with the randomized neuropathic bone pain trial (Trans-Tasman Radiation Oncology Group, 96.05). Radiother Oncol 67:207–212, 2003.

144. Rosen, L.S. Efficacy and safety of zoledronic acid in the treatment of bone metastases associated with lung cancer and other solid tumors. Semin Oncol 29:28–32, 2002.

145. Roth, S.E.; Mousavi, P.; Finkelstein, J.; et al. Metastatic burst fracture risk prediction using biomechanically based equations. Clin Orthop Relat Res 419:83–90, 2004.

146. Roth, S.E.; Rebello, M.M.; Kreder, H.; et al. Pressurization of the metastatic femur during prophylactic intramedullary nail fixation. J Trauma 57:333–339, 2004.

147. Ryken, T.C.; Eichholz, K.M.; Gerszten, P.C.; et al. Evidence-based review of the surgical management of vertebral column metastatic disease. Neurosurg Focus 15:E11, 2003.

148. Saad, F.; Lipton, A. Zoledronic acid is effective in preventing and delaying skeletal events in patients with bone metastases secondary to genitourinary cancers. BJU Int 96:964–969, 2005.

149. Schaberg, J.; Gainor, B.J. A profile of metastatic carcinoma of the spine. Spine 10:19–20, 1985.

150. Schurman, D.J.; Amstutz, H.C. Orthopedic management of patients with metastatic carcinoma of the breast. Surg Gynecol Obstet 137:831–836, 1973.

151. Serfini, A.N. Current status of systemic intravenous radiopharmaceuticals for the treatment of painful metastatic bone disease. Int J Radiat Oncol Biol Phys 30:1187–1194, 1994.

152. Seto, E.; Segall, G.M.; Terris, M.K. Positron emission tomography detection of osseous metastases of renal cell carcinoma not identified on bone scan. Urology 55:286, 2000.

153. Shah, A.N.; Pietrobon, R.; Richardson, W.J.; et al. Patterns of tumor spread and risk of fracture and epidural impingement in metastatic vertebrae. J Spinal Disord Tech 16:83–89, 2003.

154. Sherry, H.S.; Levy, R.N.; Siffert, R.S. Metastatic disease of bone in orthopedic surgery. Clin Orthop Relat Res 169:44–52, 1982.

155. Shreve, P.D.; Steventon, R.S.; Gross, M.D. Diagnosis of spine metastases by FDG imaging using a gamma camera in the coincidence mode. Clin Nucl Med 23:799–802, 1998.

156. Sim, F.H.; Frassica, F.J.; Chao, E.Y. Orthopaedic management using new devices and prostheses. [Review] [12 refs]. Clin Orthop Relat Res 312:160–172, 1995.

157. Sim, F.H.; Pritchard, D.J. Metastatic disease in the upper extremity. Clin Orthop Relat Res 169:83–94, 1982.

158. Smith, R. An evaluation of surgical treatment for spinal cord compression due to metastatic carcinoma. J Neurol Neurosurg Psychiatry 152–158, 1965.

159. Soloway, M.S.; Hardeman, S.W.; Hickey, D.; et al. Stratification of patients with metastatic prostate cancer based on extent of disease on initial bone scan. Cancer 61:195–202, 1988.

160. Stark, R.J.; Henson, R.A.; Evans, S.J. Spinal metastases. A retrospective survey from a general hospital. Brain 105:189–213, 1982.

161. Stubbs, B.E.; Matthews, L.S.; Sonstegard, D.A. Experimental fixation of fractures of the femur with methylmethacrylate. J Bone Joint Surg [Am] 57:317–321, 1975.

162. Sun, Y.C.; Geldof, A.A.; Newling, D.W.; et al. Progression delay of prostate tumor skeletal metastasis effects by bisphosphonates. J Urol 148:1270–1273, 1992.

163. Sundaresan, N.; Galicich, J.H.; Lane, J.M. Harrington rod stabilization for pathological fractures of the spine. J Neurosurg 60:282–286, 1984.

164. Swanson, K.C.; Pritchard, D.J.; Sim, F.H. Surgical treatment of metastatic disease of the femur. J Am Acad Orthop Surg 8:56–65, 2000.

165. Sze, W.M.; Shelley, M.D.; Held, I.; et al. Palliation of metastatic bone pain: single fraction versus multifraction radiotherapy—a systematic review of randomised trials. Clin Oncol (R Coll Radiol) 15:345–352, 2003.

166. Taneichi, H.; Kaneda, K.; Takeda, N.; et al. Risk factors and probability of vertebral body collapse in metastases of the thoracic and lumbar spine. Spine 22:239–245, 1997.

167. Theriault, R.L.; Lipton, A.; Hortobagyi, G.N.; et al. Pamidronate reduces skeletal morbidity in women with advanced breast cancer and lytic bone lesions: A randomized, placebo-controlled trial. Protocol 18 Aredia Breast Cancer Study Group. J Clin Oncol 17:846–854, 1999.

168. Thomsen, N.O.B.; Mikkelsen, J.B.; Svendsen, R.N.; et al. Interlocking nailing of humeral shaft fractures. J Orthop Sci 3:199–203, 1998.

169. Tokuhashi, Y.; Matsuzaki, H.; Toriyama, S.; et al. Scoring system for the preoperative evaluation of metastatic spine tumor prognosis. Spine 15:1110–1113, 1990.

170. Tome, J.; Carsi, B.; Garcia-Fernandez, C.; et al. Treatment of pathologic fractures of the humerus with Seidel nailing. Clin Orthop Relat Res 350:51–55, 1998.

171. Tong, D.; Gillick, L.; Hendrickson, F.R. The palliation of symptomatic osseous metastases: Final results of the Study by the Radiation Therapy Oncology Group. Cancer 50:893–899, 1982.

172. Tongaonkar, H.B.; Kulkarni, J.N.; Kamat, M.R. Solitary metastases from renal cell carcinoma: A review. J Surg Oncol 49:45–48, 1992.

173. Van der Linden, Y.M.; Dijkstra, P.D.; Kroon, H.M.; et al. Comparative analysis of risk factors for pathological fracture with femoral metastases. J Bone Joint Surg [Br] 86:566–573, 2004.

174. Varley, G.W. The Seidel locking humeral nail: The Nottingham experience. Injury 26:155–157, 1995.

175. Walker, R.H. Pelvic reconstruction/total hip arthroplasty for metastatic acetabular insufficiency. Clin Orthop Relat Res 294:170–175, 1993.

176. Ward, W.G.; Holsenbeck, S.; Dorey, F.J.; et al. Metastatic disease of the femur: Surgical treatment. Clin Orthop Relat Res 415(Suppl):S230–S244, 2003.

177. Wedin, R.; Bauer, H.C. Surgical treatment of skeletal metastatic lesions of the proximal femur:

Endoprosthesis or reconstruction nail? J Bone Joint Surg [Br] 87:1653–1657, 2005.

178. Weill, A.; Chiras, J.; Simon, J.M.; et al. Spinal metastases: Indications for and results of percutaneous injection of acrylic surgical cement. Radiology 199:241–247, 1996.

179. Wise, J.J.; Fischgrund, J.S.; Herkowitz, H.N.; et al. Complication, survival rates, and risk factors of surgery for metastatic disease of the spine. Spine 24:1943–1951, 1999.

180. Wong, D.A.; Fornasier, V.L.; MacNab, I. Spinal metastases: The obvious, the occult, and the impostors. Spine 15:1–4, 1990.

181. Yablon, I.G. The effect of methylmethacrylate on fracture healing. Clin Orthop Relat Res 114: 358–363, 1976.

182. Yamashita, K.; Koyama, H.; Inaji, H. Prognostic significance of bone metastasis from breast cancer. Clin Orthop Relat Res 312:89–94, 1995.

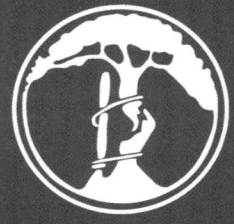

CHAPTER 18

Osteoporotic Fragility Fractures

Joseph M. Lane, M.D. and Charles N. Cornell, M.D.

EPIDEMIOLOGY

Osteoporosis is the most prevalent metabolic bone disease, affecting a large portion of the aging, predominantly female, population in the United States.[112] On the basis of World Health Organization criteria, it is estimated that 15 percent of postmenopausal white women in the United States and 35 percent of women older than 65 years of age have frank osteoporosis.[114] As many as 50 percent of women have some degree of low bone density in the hip. An estimated 1.5 million fractures annually are attributable to osteoporosis, including 700,000 vertebral, 300,000 hip, and 200,000 distal forearm (Colles') fractures.[60,78,101] Increasing age is significantly correlated with the incidence of fractures[82]: fractures in the wrist rise in the sixth decade, vertebral fractures in the seventh decade, and hip fractures in the eighth decade.[111] One of every two white women experiences an osteoporotic fracture at some point in life.[71] Among those who live to the age of 90 years, 32 percent of women and 17 percent of men sustain a hip fracture.[77] Twenty-four percent of patients with hip fracture die within 1 year as a result; 50 percent require long-term nursing care, and only 30 percent ever regain their prefracture ambulatory status.[16,77,83,87] Of patients in nursing homes who sustain a hip fracture, 70 percent do not survive 1 year.[3,50,51,62,65]

The financial burden of osteoporosis is rapidly escalating as the population ages.[99] Patients with fragility fractures create a significant economic burden. Treating osteoporosis is more costly than 400,000 hospital admissions and 2.5 million physician visits per year.[113] Health care expenditures attributable to osteoporotic fractures were estimated as 13.8 billion dollars, of which 10.3 billion dollars was for the treatment of white women.[97] The cost of acute and long-term care for osteoporotic fractures of the proximal femur alone has been estimated to exceed 10 billion dollars annually in the United States.[90] It is estimated that hip fractures alone may cost the United States 240 billion dollars in the next 50 years.[111] These statistics indicate the need for increased physician awareness and diagnosis and, more important, emphasis on prevention of osteoporosis.

BONE AS A METABOLIC ORGAN

The relationship between metabolic bone disease and fracture healing depends on the role of the skeleton as a metabolic resource.[67] Bone consists of a mineral fraction—hydroxyapatite crystals—and an organic fraction—largely (90%) type I collagen.[84] The mineral fraction of bone makes up more than 98 percent of the body calcium.[69] The bone, therefore, is the principal calcium reservoir of the body, and its specific architecture provides both structural support and an extensive bone surface for easy calcium mobilization. Bone is characterized as a composite material in which the collagen provides the tensile strength and hydroxyapatite the compressive strength.[61]

Bone is constantly renewing itself through a process of formation that is under cellular control.[46] It is a dynamic connective tissue, and its responsiveness to mechanical forces and metabolic regulatory signals that accommodate requirements for maintaining the organ and connective tissue functions of bone are operative throughout life.[73] The half-life of bone varies according to structural and metabolic demands. Bone formation is provided by osteoblast activity (measured by alkaline phosphatase and osteocalcin), and bone resorption is under osteoclast control (measured by N-telopeptides).[84]

The remodeling process and bone turnover appear to be coupled to and influenced by local humoral factors, biophysical considerations (Wolff's law: "form follows function"), and systemic demands.[84] Vitamin D, parathyroid hormone (PTH), and estrogen are among the hormones that control bone metabolism. Vitamin D, more specifically 1,25-dihydroxyvitamin D, is responsible for facilitating calcium absorption and osteoclastic resorption.[49] Administration of PTH leads to the release of calcium from bone,[59] and bone mass is directly related to the levels of estrogen in both men and women.[105] Bone is primarily cortical (with a large volume and low surface area) or trabecular (with a large surface area and low volume). Because bone is resorbed and formed on surfaces, mainly the endosteal surface, trabecular bone, with its greater surface-to-volume ratio, is metabolically more active.[56,57,66]

The material properties of bone are, in large part, related to the microdensity of the material.[11] Because the modulus of bone decreases only minimally with age, its primary strength is determined by its mass and structure.[11,58] The importance of structural distribution is evidenced by the greater bending and torsional strength of a tube compared with a rod of equal cross-sectional material area. Maximization of the moment of inertia (distribution of the mass away from the epicenter) in nature enhances the structural strength of bone, particularly when the mass is deficient. A 10 percent shift of bone outward can compensate for a 30 percent loss in bending and torque.

In the aging human, loss of cortical bone mass is partially compensated by expansion of the diameter of the cortex. However, the increase in the diameter of long bones rarely exceeds 2 percent of the original diameter per year.[34,98] Therefore, the actual loss of cortical mass places elderly persons at an increasing risk of fracture. The structural strength is also related to connectivity—the degree of interconnection within bone.[15,98] Lastly, the material properties of a unit volume of bone (modulus) depend on the mineral and collagen state.

MECHANISM OF OSTEOPENIC FRACTURE

The composite structure of bone allows it to withstand compressive and tensile stresses as well as bending and torsional moments.[104] Trabecular bone is often subjected to large impact stresses, whereas cortical bones often handle torque and bending. The vertebral body is largely protected by its trabecular bone, whereas the femoral neck depends on a mixture of cortical and trabecular bone for protection.[11,66]

The hallmarks of osteoporosis are deficient bone density, lack of connectivity, and altered material properties.[37,45,75] The decreased bone mass associated with osteoporosis reduces the load-bearing ability of both cortical and trabecular bone, resulting in an increased risk of fracture. Areas of the skeleton rich in trabecular bone sustain the first consequences of osteoporosis; the trabecular bone is thinner in dimension and shows evidence of osteoclastic resorption, leading to disconnectivity of the trabecular elements.[71] Trabecular bone is resorbed at a higher rate (8% per year) than cortical bone (0.5% per year) after menopause. Riggs and Melton[100] recognized this discrepancy and developed the concept of two forms of osteoporosis with separate fracture patterns.

Type I postmenopausal osteoporosis primarily affects women 55 to 65 years of age, is related to estrogen deficiency, results principally in trabecular bone loss, and is manifested by spinal fractures. Type II senile osteoporosis affects both men and women (1:2 ratio) 65 years of age or older, is related to chronic calcium loss throughout life, results in cortical bone loss, and induces long bone fractures.

Although bone mass is clearly related to fracture risk, a true fracture threshold can only be implied. Structure, fall tendency and type, ability of microfractures to heal before they become macrofractures, quality of bone, and such ill-defined factors as aging all play a role in fracture risk.[1] The overlap of mass determination precludes clearly defining persons at absolute risk. Even at the lowest bone mass

Table 18-2

Spinal Fracture Prevalence in Postmenopausal Women Relative to DEXA

DEXA (g/cm^2)	Percentage with Spinal Fractures
0.8–0.926	26
0.7–0.833	33
0.6–0.751	51
0.5–0.663	63

Abbreviation: DEXA, dual-energy x-ray absorptiometry.

measurements, a percentage of individuals are free of fracture (Tables 18-1 and 18-2).

For patients with hip fractures, Riggs and Melton[93] demonstrated a fourfold increase in fracture rate with a 50 percent decrease in bone mass. The exponential increase in fracture rate with loss of bone mass is in agreement with the laboratory structural data of Carter and Hayes.[11] Bone loss places the aging individual at greater risk of fracture, and fracture treatment therefore should include a bone maintenance strategy (see later discussion). Greenspan and co-workers[43] documented etiologic factors for hip fractures in addition to bone density, including falls to the side, lower body mass index, and a higher potential to fall.[43] Courtney and colleagues[17] showed that the femur of an elderly person has half the strength and half the energy absorption capacity of the femur of a younger person. Falls from standing height exceed femoral breaking strength by 50 percent in elderly people but are below femoral fracture strength by 20 percent in the young.[47]

Cummings and associates[20] included as hip fracture risks, in addition to low bone mass, aging, history of maternal hip fracture, tallness, lack of weight gain with aging, poor health, previously treated hypothyroidism, use of benzodiazepines, use of anticonvulsant drugs, lack of walking for exercise, lack of unsupported standing for 4 hours a day, a resting pulse rate higher than 80 beats per minute, and a history of any fracture after the age of 50 years. If two of these factors are present, 1 in 1000 individuals sustain a hip fracture in a given year. If five or more hip fracture risk factors are present in a patient who also has a low bone mass, the risk rises to 27 in 1000 individuals per year.[21]

Although the fracture risk is greatest for patients with the lowest bone mass, the majority of fractures occur in the osteopenia population. Bone density accounts for only 18 percent of the risk. Issues of bone quality dominate. A prior vertebral or hip fracture profoundly increases the risk of a subsequent fracture.[9]

FRACTURE HEALING AND OSTEOPOROSIS

Normal fracture healing is a specialized process in which structural integrity is restored through the regeneration of bone.[54] Fracture healing traditionally proceeds through the six stages of endochondral bone formation: impact, induction, inflammation, soft tissue callus (chondroid), hard tissue callus (osteoblastic), and remodeling.[67] Although

Table 18-1

DEXA Values in Patients Undergoing Natural Menopause ($P = 0.001$)

Spinal fractures (n=81)	0.80 (0.14 g/cm^2)
No spinal fractures (n=225)	0.89 (0.16 g/cm^2)

Abbreviation: DEXA, dual-energy x-ray absorptiometry.

the stages from fracture through chondrogenesis are unaltered, the final two stages, hard callus and remodeling, are clearly susceptible to alteration in osteoporotic patients.[90]

The synthesis of bone and its mineralization depend on the calcium environment. Osteoporotic patients have a diminished pool of rapidly soluble calcium, inadequate dietary calcium, and a deficient structural calcium bone reserve.[66] Calcium mineralization is subject to delay, and the stage of remodeling is prolonged because of competition for ionized calcium with the rest of the body. Also, substances that may have been mobilized to maintain systemic calcium homeostasis (PTH and vitamin D) may compromise the latter stages of fracture repair. In addition, up to 40 percent of elderly patients are mildly to moderately malnourished, and this condition compromises bone collagen synthesis.[86] Bone scans remain positive (indicating continued metabolic remodeling) well into the third year after fracture in elderly persons, and union cannot be fully ascertained until that time.[28] Studies have demonstrated that osteoporotic rats have delayed healing. It is uncertain whether it is the osteoporosis or the estrogen deficiency that compromises fracture repair.[74,110]

Systemic bone loss occurs in the unaffected skeleton after long bone fractures, even when the patient has adequate calcium intake.[109] Osteoporotic patients, who are typically chronically calcium deficient, may be more affected. Ideally, healing could be stimulated in such patients by physiologic levels of vitamin D (400 to 800 IU/day) and calcium (1500 mg of elemental calcium per day), normal nitrogen balance, and appropriate exercise.[82] Recently a series of animal studies have demonstrated that intermittent PTH can accelerate fracture repair primarily during the chondrogenic stage.[89]

DEFINITION AND DIAGNOSIS OF OSTEOPOROSIS

Osteoporosis is defined as a disease of decreased bone mass and changes in the microarchitecture of the skeleton. The disease may be recognized clinically in one of three ways: acute fracture (most commonly of the wrist, ribs, hip, or spine), asymptomatic thoracic wedge or lumbar compression fracture, or generalized osteopenia on a radiograph. More than 65 percent of individuals presenting with compression fractures are asymptomatic.[40] Critical determinations are the cause and the extent of bone loss. A diagnosis of osteopenia must differentiate among bone marrow disorders, endocrinopathy, osteomalacia, and osteoporosis.[5,84] The workup for osteopenia involves invasive and noninvasive methods.

Operational definitions of osteopenia and osteoporosis are based on bone mass and density. Noninvasive techniques of determining osteopenia are used to quantitate bone mass and evaluate the efficacy of treatment. The simple radiograph is fraught with technical difficulty and may not identify osteopenia until 30 percent of the bone mass has been lost.[55] Current methodology centers on dual-photon absorptiometry, quantitative computed tomography (CT), and ultrasonography. Dual-energy x-ray absorptiometry (DEXA) utilizes two energy levels.[73,63,105] It permits correction for soft tissue and allows direct measurement of total bone mass (cortical and trabecular) within a specified

amount of mineralized tissue of an aerial section of the spine or hip; the measurements are analyzed and expressed as grams per centimeter squared. Radiation is low (5 mrad), and precision (1% in the spine, 3%–4% in the hip) and accuracy (4%–6%) are good. Compression fractures, osteophytes, degenerative changes, and vascular calcifications can elevate local readings. A lumbar lateral radiograph is needed to correct for these artifacts.

After the density has been calculated, comparisons can be made with age-matched peers (z score) and with an adult population with peak bone mass (t test). A bone mass within 1 standard deviation (SD) of peak bone mass is considered healthy. Osteopenia is defined as between 1 and 2.4 SD below peak bone mass. A bone mass 2.5 SD below peak mass is considered frank osteoporosis. Individuals with a bone mass more than 1.5 SD below that of their peers probably have a secondary cause of osteoporosis that must be evaluated.

Alternative methods are also used to determine bone mass. CT is used to measure the mid-portion of the vertebral body and determine trabecular bone mass against a simultaneous phantom; in this way, it can be used to measure trabecular bone mass directly. It uses 20 times as much radiation as and has poorer precision than DEXA.[39] Ultrasonography is used to examine the heel, patella, tibia, and peripheral sites and measure several properties of bone; these measurements have a correlation of 0.75 with central density readings.[107] As discussed previously, these noninvasive methods cannot clearly identify absolute fracture risk, but they can be used as a loose guide for management grouping and as an exacting tool for long-term determination of treatment efficacy.

There are also markers of skeletal metabolic activity. Bone formation markers are bone-specific alkaline phosphatase, osteocalcin, and PNIP (amino-terminal propeptide of procollagen I). Alkaline phosphatase rises within 5 days after a fracture is sustained. If the level is elevated at the time of fracture, it is due to a high-turnover state until proved otherwise. Hyperparathyroidism and osteomalacia must be considered in the workup. Bone collagen breakdown products can be used to measure bone turnover. Collagen molecules in the bone matrix are staggered to form fibrils that are joined by covalent cross-links consisting of hydroxylysyl-pyridinoline (pyridinoline, Pyd) and lysyl-pyridinoline (deoxypyridinoline, Dpd). Dpd has greater specificity because Pyd is present in other connective tissues. Dpd and Pyd are linked to collagen where two amino-telopeptides (N-telopeptides [NTX] and C-telopeptides) are linked to a helical site and are released with Dpd and Pyd during osteoclastic bone resorption. These products are released into the circulation, metabolized by the liver and kidney, and excreted in the urine.

Clinical applications of these markers include monitoring effectiveness of therapy,[36] prediction of fracture risk,[35] and selection of patients for antiresorptive therapy.[13] NTX and DEXA provide highly sensitive, commonly used indices of metabolic activity and bone mass in clinical practice.[75] High-turnover states such as hyperparathyroidism are characterized by high NTX levels. Osteoporosis (as determined by DEXA) can be high turnover (high NTX) related to increased osteoclast activity or low turnover (low NTX) related to low osteoclast activity.[75]

No signs, symptoms, or diagnostic tests are specific for osteoporosis. In one study, 31 percent of osteoporotic women were found to have disorders with possible effects on skeletal health without major risk factors for postmenopausal osteoporosis.[14] An algorithm for the diagnosis of osteopenia has been developed (Table 18-3). When osteopenia has been defined and localized bone disorders have been eliminated, the differential workup commences. First, a hematologic profile, serum protein electrophoresis, and biochemical profile studies are obtained. In common bone marrow disorders, including leukemia and myeloma (which together account for 1%–2% of cases of osteoporosis), the bone marrow screen is usually abnormal (anemia, low white blood cell count, or low platelet count). A biochemical panel provides information on renal and hepatic function, primary hyperparathyroidism (high serum calcium), and possible malnutrition (anemia, low calcium, low phosphorus, or low albumin).

If the bone marrow screen is negative, the diagnostic testing then centers on endocrinopathies. Premature menopause, iatrogenic Cushing's disease, and type I diabetes mellitus are diagnosed by history. Determinations of PTH and thyroid-stimulating hormone identify hyperparathyroidism and hyperthyroidism. The latter may occur as osteoporosis and severe weight loss or as iatrogenic hyperthyroidism, caused by overuse of thyroid replacement hormone medication by obese patients to control weight.[85] Malnutrition is common in osteoporotic patients. Osteomalacia has been reported in 30 to 80 percent of fragility fracture patients and 22 percent of individuals undergoing primary total hip replacement.[41] A relatively common cause of osteomalacia is sprue that occurs in 1/22 individuals.[42] Osteomalacia may be identified by low levels of 25-hydroxyvitamin D, high secondary PTH, high alkaline phosphatase, low urinary calcium, low serum phosphorus, and low to normal serum calcium values. The mild hyperosteoidosis and lag in mineralization are often indistinguishable from those seen in osteoporosis by laboratory studies.

The critical diagnostic study used to differentiate osteomalacia from osteoporosis is the transileal bone biopsy and histomorphometric analysis of the undecalcified bone.[70] These studies permit a definitive diagnosis.

If cost containment were not an issue, bone densitometry would be readily available to almost all postmenopausal women. In the United States, Medicare covers DEXA for estrogen-deficient women older than 65 years. A cost-effectiveness analysis supported by the National Osteoporosis Foundation concluded that it is worthwhile to measure bone density in any woman with a vertebral fracture and in all white women older than 60 to 65 years. In healthy postmenopausal women between 50 and 60 years old, indications for DEXA include a history of low-trauma fracture, weight under 127 pounds, smoking, and a family history of an osteoporotic fracture.[27] Most experts also agree that any patients with secondary causes of known bone loss should have their bone density measured. Males aged 70 years with risk factors also should undergo DEXA evaluation.

MEDICAL TREATMENT AND PREVENTION OF OSTEOPOROSIS

Osteoporosis is a heterogeneous disease of multifactorial causes. The principles of medical management necessitate decisions about whether bone mass should be maintained or augmented. If the patient has crossed his or her fracture threshold, bone augmentation is required. However, if the trauma level was of sufficient magnitude, maintenance may be all that is needed, even after a fracture. A careful history of the cause of the fracture and a noninvasive measurement of bone mass are essential.

Adequate levels of exercise,[1,22,52,64,90] calcium,[43,48] and vitamin D (800 IU/day) maintain both cortical and trabecular bone mass except in the early postmenopausal spine, when the loss is 2 percent per year. Physiologic levels of calcium intake, as determined by a National Institutes of Health

Table 18-3			
Sequence for the Workup of the Most Common Forms of Osteomalacia			
Complete blood count	Abnormal 1%–2% → Bone marrow biopsy		Myeloma
Erythrocyte sedimentation rate	↓ Normal		Leukemia
Serum protein electrophoresis			Benign marrow disorder
Parathyroid hormone	Abnormal 15%–25% →		Hyperparathyroidism
Thyroid-stimulating hormone	↓ Normal		Hyperthyroidism
History of type 1 diabetes			Diabetes mellitus (type 1)
History of steroid use			Cushing's disease
Normal ↓	Abnormal 8% →		Osteomalacia
Calcium (serum-urine)	↓ Normal		
Phosphorus (serum)	Osteoporosis		
Alkaline phosphatase			
Blood urea nitrogen			
25-Hydroxyvitamin D			
Parathyroid hormone			
Transileal bone biopsy (?)			

consensus conference in 1994, are 1200 to 1500 mg/day from age 12 to 24 years, 1000 mg/day from age 25 years until menopause, and 1500 mg/day after menopause.[88] Treatments are antiresorptive agents (bisphosphonates, calcitonin, synthetic estrogen-like modulators [SERMs]) and anabolic agents (PTH). Estrogen is no longer labeled by the U.S. Food and Drug Administration (FDA) for the treatment of osteoporosis.

A treatment program has been approved by the National Osteoporosis Foundation for patients at risk of fragility fracture.[90] Treatment is recommended for any individual with a *t* score of −2.0, or a score of −1.5 with four major risk factors, and prevention is recommended for a patient with osteopenia. If an individual is known to have a low energy fracture, the use of bisphosphonates, calcitonin, SERMs, or PTH is recommended. For a patient without fracture and unwilling to consider treatment, physiologic calcium levels, vitamin D (800 units per day), exercise, and smoking cessation are recommended. Calcium, smoking cessation, and exercise are recommended for postmenopausal patients younger than 65 years without risk factors. These recommendations were made with FDA approval of estrogen for the treatment of osteoporosis; new treatment guidelines need to be established because the new labeled use of estrogen is for the prevention and management of osteoporosis.

Estrogen

Estrogen[2,32,52,74,110] has been the most studied and used drug for the prevention of osteoporosis. Epidemiologic studies, cohort and case-control, indicated that estrogen administration to postmenopausal women decreased skeletal turnover (25%–50%) and the rate of bone loss in women 6 months to 3 years after menopause.[13,76] A large, longitudinal cohort study of 9704 postmenopausal women 65 years of age and older found that estrogen use was associated with a significant decrease in wrist fracture (relative risk [RR], 0.39) and of all nonspinal fractures (RR, 0.66). It appears to reduce risk of hip fractures by 20 to 60 percent[11] (in women). The adverse effects including myocardial infarct, stroke, phlebitis, pulmonary embolism, and breast cancer resulted in removing estrogen as a treatment of osteoporosis.

SERMs

A series of synthetic estrogen-like modulators have been developed. These agents can compete with estrogen-binding sites and seem to function more like an estrogen at bone and work effectively as antiresorptive agents. They are indicated for prevention of osteoporosis and treatment of vertebral fractures. Tamoxifen was used as an antiestrogen, particularly for patients with breast cancer. Bone cells are also responsive to tamoxifen.[95] Individuals taking tamoxifen have 70 percent of the benefit of estrogen in terms of maintaining bone mass.[16] Tamoxifen is not used as an anti-osteoporotic agent, because 70 percent of women have significant postmenopausal symptoms and a high incidence of uterine cancer. Raloxifene, a newer agent, is not associated with an increased incidence of uterine cancer, and early data suggest a decreased risk of breast cancer in patients using raloxifene compared with

control subjects.[24] A trial comparing tamoxifen and raloxifene in preventive action against breast cancer is under way.[19]

Raloxifene is approved for the prevention of osteoporosis. Raloxifene can decrease the risk of vertebral fracture by approximately 40 to 50 percent, but there is no reported protection for the hip.[32] Adverse effects include an 8 percent incidence of leg cramps and an increased risk of thrombophlebitis comparable with that associated with estrogen. It is not recommended in the first 5 years of menopause because it enhances postmenopausal symptoms.

Calcitonin

Calcitonin is a peptide hormone secreted by specialized cells in the thyroid. It may play a role in the skeletal development of the embryo and fetus, but its primary action is on bone to reduce osteoclastic bone resorption by diminution of osteoclasts (shrinkage of cells, loss of ruffled border, reduction in resorptive activity, and increased apoptosis).[12] It has been effectively used in patients with hypercalcemia, Paget's disease, and osteoporosis. It is indicated for the treatment of postmenopausal women more than 5 years after menopause with low bone mass compared with healthy premenopausal women. A nasal form of calcitonin at a dosage of 200 units per day appears to increase bone mass in the spine and decrease spinal fractures by 37 percent. To date, there has been no benefit in hip fracture prevention.[10,92] Calcitonin does have another benefit of providing some analgesia. It has been used in patients with painful osteoporotic fractures and does not interfere with fracture healing.[96] The only established side effect is rhinitis (23% vs. 7% for placebo).[29]

Bisphosphonates

Bisphosphonates are stable, active analgesics of pyrophosphate[73] that inhibit osteoclastic resorption and depress bone turnover[30,55,63,94] by binding to the osteoclast-resorbing surface and acting as a nondegradable shield. When absorbed by the osteoclast, they inhibit osteoclast function. Bisphosphonates have low bioavailability, and less than 1 percent is absorbed orally. Alendronate is the first bisphosphonate approved for the treatment of osteoporosis. Originally, alendronate, 10 mg/day, was approved for prevention of osteoporosis. It has been shown to increase bone mass in the hip and spine. It decreased the risk of all fractures by approximately 50 percent after 1 year of treatment.[6,18,72] Regardless of the degree of bone mass enhancement, all patients treated with alendronate had equal protection against fractures, suggesting an initial improvement in bone quality.

Alendronate has been associated with esophageal irritation, and as many as 30 percent of individuals have had esophagitis; in a carefully controlled study, the rate of esophagitis was comparable to that in the placebo group.[72] Currently, a once weekly dose of 70 mg is as efficacious and produces significantly less indigestion.

Risedronate, 5 mg/day or 35 mg/wk, is the second bisphosphonate approved for both prevention and treatment of osteoporosis. It has a profile similar to that of alendronate and may cause less esophageal irritation. It reduced the risk of new vertebral fractures by 49 percent over 3 years compared with a control group ($P < 0.001$), and the risk of nonvertebral fractures was reduced by 33 percent compared with a control group over 3 years ($P = 0.06$).[103] Risedronate significantly increased bone mineral density at the spine and hip within 6 months. The adverse-event profile of risedronate, including gastrointestinal adverse events, was similar to that of the placebo group.[102] A head-to-head comparison of the two agents has not been performed.

Bisphosphonates have a long-lasting effect on bone. A double-blind, multicenter study of postmenopausal women[108] (at least 2.5 SD below the peak premenopausal mean) compared the efficacy and safety of treatment with oral once-weekly alendronate at 70 mg ($n = 519$), twice-weekly alendronate at 35 mg ($n = 369$), and daily alendronate at 10 mg ($n = 370$) for 1 year. Increases in bone density of the total hip, femoral neck, trochanter, and total body were similar for the three dosing regimens. All three treatment groups similarly showed reduced biochemical markers of bone resorption (urinary N-telopeptides of type I collagen) and bone formation (serum bone-specific alkaline phosphatase) in the middle of the premenopausal reference range. All treatment regimens were well tolerated with a similar incidence of upper gastrointestinal adverse experiences. There were fewer serious upper gastrointestinal adverse experiences and a trend toward a lower incidence of esophageal events in the once-weekly dosing group compared with the daily dosing group. This study suggests that once-weekly dosing of bisphosphonates may provide a more convenient, therapeutically equivalent alternative to daily dosing.

Intravenous forms of bisphosphonates, including zoledronic acid (Reclast) 5 mg/year, pamidronate (Aredia) 30 mg every 3 months, and ibandronate 3 mg every 3 months, all increase bone density. Ibandronate has the approval of the FDA for the treatment of osteoporosis, but there are no fracture trials with the intravenous agents,[31,38,44] except with zoledronic acid.[78a]

Long-term use of the bisphosphonates results in large-scale crystal accumulation with half-lives of 3.5 to 10 years. Animal studies with 10-fold doses of alendronate demonstrate loss of bone toughness. There is an accumulation of microfractures that do not undergo remodeling.[80,81] Odvina[93] reported nine patients with insufficient fractures following 5 years of alendronate. Biopsies of these individuals demonstrated adynamic bone. At this time it is unclear as to how long to remain on bisphosphonates. At the Hospital for Special Surgery we suggest yearly NTX evaluation. After 5 years if the NTX is less than 15 mg/creatinine, we recommend stopping the bisphosphonate until the NTX returns to greater than 25, or we consider intermittent PTH (see below).

A third bisphosphonate, ibandronate, 150 mg/mo, has been introduced. It has the same vertebral fracture prevention profile. Only in the severely osteoporotic patients has it been able to decrease hip fracture. The once-monthly dosing is associated with better compliance and possibly less indigestion, but it is a new agent.[44]

Anabolic Agents (PTH 1–34)

Parathyroid hormone has become the single released anabolic agent for the treatment of osteoporosis.[79] PTH that has 84 amino acids, and in an abbreviated version that has 34 amino acids, has been released for the treatment of osteoporosis. PTH when given continuously is associated with an increased osteoclastic and osteoblastic turnover, leading to a net loss of bone. However, in intermittent administration given once a day in a small subcutaneous dose of 20 µg, PTH has been demonstrated to lead to an active anabolic phase with bone mass increasing up to 13 percent over 2 years in the spine and to a lesser degree within the hip.[8,25,91] Most studies with PTH have been performed on women and have been shown to lead to a significant decrease in fractures in the same range as the bisphosphonates. PTH is recommended for 2 years, after which time its benefit should be locked in place by returning to a bisphosphonate, which can lead to a significant augmentation in bone density. The combination of PTH and bisphosphonate has been shown to be counterproductive,[7] often with no gain whatsoever with either agent and then a slow augmentation over time. Therefore, it is recommended that these drugs be given separately and in sequence. After the PTH is terminated in 2 years, there is a decrease in the bone density back toward the starting point unless locked into place with the bisphosphonates. Further studies have suggested that raloxifene (Evista) or estrogen can function with PTH, and clearly these studies have been performed only in women.[23] Data are much more limited on the use of PTH in men, but it appears to have relatively comparable efficacy.[33] Indications for PTH in both men and women are bone density decline on a bisphosphonate, stabilization on a bisphosphonate at an extremely low level, and development of a subsequent fracture while on bisphosphonate therapy; it is also indicated for patients who initially have a very low turnover rate that clearly warrants an anabolic effect.

Unique for women is the indication for possible use in the premenopausal period. Bisphosphonates have a long half-life of approximately 10 years, and there is concern that in the premenopausal woman of child-bearing age bisphosphonates may interfere with fetal development and growth. Those individuals are ideally suited for treatment with PTH. There is no comparable concern among men regarding their sexual function with these agents. The final indication for PTH is for fractures that are difficult to heal. PTH has been shown in a number of animal studies to augment fracture healing and may be a better agent than the bisphosphonates, particularly when augmentation is needed.[89]

MANAGEMENT OF OSTEOPOROTIC FRACTURES

The impact of skeletal loss becomes most apparent as the skeleton begins to fail in its ability to withstand normal loads. When the skeleton no longer functions structurally, osteoporosis becomes a disease state. The overriding goal of management of fractures in the osteoporotic patient is to achieve early and definitive stabilization of the injured extremity.

At the Hospital for Special Surgery in New York, an osteoporosis treatment center has been established. The experiences derived from a large combined heterogeneous population have given rise to the following treatment principles and protocols:

Elderly patients are best served by rapid, definitive fracture care that allows early mobilization. In the patient with concurrent illnesses or markedly abnormal laboratory results, medical evaluation and stabilization of reversible medical decompensations should be performed before surgery.[40] In most cases, patients are at their respective homeostatic optimum on the day of injury and should ideally be treated with surgery at that time.

Surgical treatment is directed at achieving stable fracture fixation and early return of function. In the lower extremity, this implies early weight-bearing. Anatomic restoration is important in intra-articular fractures, whereas stability is the goal in the treatment of metaphyseal and diaphyseal fractures.

Surgical procedures are designed with an effort to minimize operative time, blood loss, and physiologic stress.

Osteoporotic bone, with its decreased density, lacks the strength to hold screws and plates securely and more often involves comminution.[10] As a result, failure of internal fixation is caused primarily by bone failure rather than by implant failure. Internal fixation devices are chosen that allow impaction of the fracture fragments into stable patterns that minimize the load carried by the implants. In addition, implants that minimize stress shielding are chosen to prevent further skeletal decompensation of the involved bone. For these reasons, sliding nail plate devices and intramedullary devices that are load sharing and allow fracture compression are the devices of choice.

Because most of these fractures are related to underlying metabolic bone disease, a full evaluation of the etiologic condition is performed and an appropriate medical therapeutic program is developed for each patient.

Inadequate calcium intake could result in deficits in callus mineralization or remodeling.[28] Because many elderly patients are malnourished, nutritional assessment should be included in the patient's evaluation.

The specific management of fractures about the knee and of Colles', hip, spine, proximal humeral, and pelvic fractures is discussed in other chapters. This chapter includes a discussion of the femoral neck fracture because of its strong implications for metabolic bone disease. A series of studies from the fracture service at New York Hospital[106] demonstrated that 8 percent of patients with femoral neck fracture had frank osteomalacia. Although 40 percent had marked trabecular bone loss (<15% trabecular bone volume, with normal being >22%), all patients older than 50 years had some reduction of bone mass when compared with younger persons. Twenty-five percent had increased metabolic turnover indices, including a high osteoclast count.

In the series of Scileppi and colleagues,[108] bone histomorphometry appeared to be a good predictor of outcome after treatment for femoral neck fracture.[66] Patients who had trabecular bone volume that was within 60 percent of normal (i.e., volume >15%) had an 85 to 95 percent rate of successful union, whereas for patients who had severe trabecular bone loss (to <15% of bone volume) the rate was lower than 33 percent in women and lower than 50 percent in men. These combined studies at New York Hospital suggest that significant metabolic bone disease, particularly osteoporosis, leads to a high rate of unsuccessful union after femoral neck fracture. Comparable studies

of other fractures commonly associated with osteoporosis are lacking, but presumably osteoporosis per se affects the type, severity, and repair process in these fractures as well.

Application of the outcome studies of femoral neck fractures in relation to osteopenia has resulted in specific protocols at the Hospital for Special Surgery and the New York Presbyterian Hospital. Our current protocol for treatment of a displaced femoral neck fracture in the ambulatory patient who is physiologically younger than 65 years relies on closed reduction and stable internal fixation using the sliding compression screw or cannulated screws as the primary form of treatment. If stability cannot be achieved, the patient is treated with hemiarthroplasty. The ambulatory patient who is physiologically older than 70 years is treated with hemiarthroplasty. Closed reduction and pinning are the methods of choice in caring for the nonambulatory patient. Patients with severe demineralizing bone disease (marked osteoporosis), pathologic fractures secondary to metastasis, or neurologic disorders who require immediate ambulation and patients who cannot comply with physical therapy regimens requiring partial weight-bearing are treated with primary hemiarthroplasty.

Traditionally, treatment of vertebral compression fractures consists of medical pain management. In 1984, vertebroplasty, structural reinforcement of the vertebral body with polymethylmethacrylate cement, was first used in the treatment of osteoporotic vertebral fractures. The primary indication for vertebroplasty is pain relief. The procedure is performed under local or general anesthesia and a transpedicle or extrapedicle approach is used to reach the anteroinferior border of the vertebral body. In vertebroplasty, radiodense polymethylmethacrylate cement is injected into the vertebral body under high pressure using Luer-Lok syringes in 2- to 3-mL allotments. Several cohort studies reported a decrease in pain in 80 to 90 percent of patients, a complication rate of 5 to 6 percent, and no fracture reduction.[4,26,53]

Kyphoplasty is a similar procedure designed to provide significant pain relief, rapid return to activities of daily living, restoration of vertebral body height, and reduction in spinal deformity. In this procedure, a balloon tamp is inserted into the center of the collapsed vertebral body and inflated with radiopaque liquid under fluoroscopic guidance. The patient is continually monitored by sensory evoked potential for neural damage throughout the procedure at the Hospital for Special Surgery. The balloon strikes cancellous bone circumferentially around the tamp and thereby reduces the deformation and restores height to the vertebral body. The balloon is deflated and removed, and the cavity is filled with the surgeon's choice of biomaterial, stabilizing the fracture.

An increasing number of patients have been treated by this technique. A review of 226 kyphoplasty operations in 121 patients[69] found that 96 percent of patients had pain relief as determined using a pain analogue scale. There was 45 percent restoration of height in the anterior plane, 71 percent at the midline, and 54 percent posteriorly. In this series, there was one case of epidural bleeding requiring decompression, one incomplete spinal injury, and one report of transient adult respiratory distress syndrome. No episodes of infection, pulmonary emboli, or myocardial infarction have been reported. In this study, the average age was 73.7 years, and each patient had on average of 3.7 co-morbidities.

A quality-of-life questionnaire (called SF-36) was administered to patients before and after kyphoplasty.[69] The questionnaire is standardized and validated and is designed to assess functional status and well-being. The questions are used to calculate summary measures of physical and mental health such as bodily pain and physical function. The summary measures are then normalized to a scale of 1 to 100, where 1 is the lowest score and 100 is the highest or best score. In these patients, both bodily pain and physical function scores improved significantly ($P < 0.004$ for bodily pain, $P < 0.02$ for physical function) when assessed 1 week after kyphoplasty. These preliminary data suggest that kyphoplasty is an effective, minimally invasive technique for providing pain relief and restoration of vertebral height.

REFERENCES

1. Aloia, J.E.; Cohn, S.H.; Ostuni, J.A.; et al. Prevention of involutional bone loss by exercise. Ann Intern Med 89:356, 1978.
2. American College of Physicians. Guidelines for counseling postmenopausal women about preventive hormone therapy. Ann Intern Med 117:1038, 1992.
3. Avioli, L.V. Postmenopausal osteoporosis: Prevention vs. cure. Fed Proc 40:2418, 1981.
4. Barr, J.D.; Barr, M.S.; Lemley, T.J.; et al. Percutaneous vertebroplasty for pain relief and spinal stabilization. Spine 25:923, 2000.
5. Barth, R.W.; Lane, J.M. Osteoporosis. Orthop Clin North Am 19:845, 1988.
6. Black, D.M.; Cummings, S.R.; Karph, D.B.; et al. Randomized trial of effect of alendronate on risk of fracture in women with existing vertebral fractures. Lancet 348:1535, 1996.
7. Black, D.M.; Greenspan, S.L.; Ensrud, K.E.; et al. PaTH Study Investigators: The effects of parathyroid hormone and alendronate alone or in combination in postmenopausal osteoporosis. N Engl J Med 25 (349):1207–1215, 2003.
8. Body, J.J.; Gaich, G.A.; Scheele, W.H.; et al. A randomized double-blind trial to compare the efficacy of teriparatide recombinant human parathryroid hormone (1-34) with alendronate in postmenopausal women with osteoporosis. J Clin Endocrinol Metab 87:4528–4535, 2002.
9. Bouxsein, M.L.; Kaufman, J.; Tosi, L.; et al. Recommendations for optimal care of the fragility fracture patient to reduce the risk of future fracture. J Am Acad Orthop Surg 12:385–395, 2004.
10. Cardona, J.M.; Pastor, E. Calcitonin versus etidronate for the treatment of postmenopausal osteoporosis: A meta-analysis of published clinical trials. Osteoporos Int 7:165, 1997.
11. Carter, D.R.; Hayes, W.C. The compressive behavior of bone as a two-phase porous structure. J Bone Joint Surg Am 59:954, 1977.
12. Chambers, T.J.; Moore, A. The sensitivity of isolated osteoclasts to morphological transformation by calcitonin. J Clin Endocrinol Metab 57:819, 1983.
13. Chesnut, C.H. III; Bell, N.H.; Clark, G.S.; et al. Hormone replacement therapy in postmenopausal women: Urinary N-telopeptide of type I collagen monitors therapeutic effect and predicts response of bone mineral density. Am J Med 102:29, 1997.
14. Clark, J.; Tannenbaum, C.; Posnett, K.; et al. Laboratory testing in healthy, osteopenic women. J Bone Miner Res 12:S137, 1997.
15. Compston, J.E. Connectivity of cancellous bone: Assessment and mechanical implications. Bone 15:63, 1994.
16. Cosman, F.; Lindsay, R. Selective estrogen receptor modulators: Clinical spectrum. Endocr Rev 20:418, 1999.
17. Courtney, A.C.; Washtel, E.F.; Myers, E.R.; et al. Age-related reductions in the strength of the femur tested in a fall-loading configuration. J Bone Joint Surg Am 77:387, 1995.
18. Cummings, S.R.; Black, D.M.; Thompson, D.E.; et al. Effect of alendronate on risk of fracture in women with low bone density but without vertebral fractures. JAMA 280:2077, 1998.
19. Cummings, S.R.; Eckert, S.; Kreuger, K.A.; et al. The effects of raloxifene on the risk of breast cancer in postmenopausal women: Results from the MORE (Multiple Outcome of Raloxifene Evaluation) randomized trial. JAMA 281:2189, 1999.
20. Cummings, S.R.; Kellsey, J.L.; Nevitt, M.C.; et al. Epidemiology of osteoporosis and osteoporotic fractures. Epidemiol Rev 7:178, 1985.
21. Cummings, S.R.; Nevitt, M.C.; Browner, W.S.; et al. Risk factors for hip fracture in white women: Study of Osteoporotic Fractures Research Group. N Engl J Med 332:767, 1995.
22. Dalsky, G.P.; Stocke, K.S.; Ehsani, A.A.; et al. Weight-bearing exercise training and lumbar bone mineral content in postmenopausal women. Ann Intern Med 108:824, 1988.
23. Deal, C.; Omizo, M.; Schwartz, E.N.; et al. Combination teriparatide and raloxifene therapy for postmenopausal osteoporosis: Results from a 6-month double-blind placebo-controlled trial. J Bone Miner Res 20:1905–1911, 2005.
24. Delmas, P.D.; Bjarnason, N.H.; Mitlak, B.H.; et al. Effects of raloxifene on bone mineral density, serum cholesterol concentrations, and uterine endometrium in postmenopausal women. N Engl J Med 337:1641, 1997.
25. Dempster, D.W.; Cosman, F.; Kurland, E.S.; et al. Effects of daily treatment with parathyroid hormone on bone microarchitecture and turnover in patients with osteoporosis: A paired biopsy study. J Bone Miner Res 16:1846–1853, 2001.
26. Deramond, H.; Darrason, R.; Galibart, P. Percutaneous vertebroplasty with acrylic cement in the treatment of aggressive spinal angiomas. Rachis 1:143, 1989.

27. Eddy, D.M.; Cummings, S.R.; Johnson, C.C.; et al. Osteoporosis: Review of the evidence for prevention, diagnosis, and treatment and cost-effectiveness analysis. Osteoporos Int 8(Suppl 4):S1–S80, 1998.

28. Einhorn, T.A.; Bonnarens, F.; Burstein, A.H. The contributions of dietary protein and mineral to the healing of experimental fractures: A biomechanical study. J Bone Joint Surg Am 68:1389, 1986.

29. Ellerington, M.C.; Hillard, T.C.; Whitcroft, S.I.J.; et al. Intranasal salmon calcitonin for the prevention and treatment of postmenopausal osteoporosis. Calcif Tissue Int 59:6, 1996.

30. Endo, Y.; Nakamora, M.; Kikuchi, T.; et al. Aminoalkylbisphosphonates, potent inhibitors of bone resorption, induce a prolonged stimulation of histamine synthesis and increase macrophages, granulocytes, and osteoclasts in vivo. Calcif Tissue Int 52:248, 1993.

31. Epstein, S. Update of current therapeutic options for the treatment of postmenopausal osteoporosis. Clin Ther 28:151–173, 2006.

32. Ettinger, B.; Black, D.M.; Mitlak, B.H.; et al. Reduction of vertebral fracture risk in postmenopausal women with osteoporosis treated with raloxifene: Results from a three-year randomized clinical trial. JAMA 282:637, 1999.

33. Finkelstein, J.S.; Hayes, A.; Hunzelman, J.L.; et al. The effects of parathyroid hormone, alendronate, or both in men with osteoporosis. N Engl J Med 349:1216–1226, 2003.

34. Frost, H.M. Tetracycline-based histological analysis of bone remodeling. Calcif Tissue Res 3:211, 1969.

35. Garnero, P.; Hausherr, E.; Chapuy, M.C.; et al. Markers of bone resorption predict hip fracture in elderly women: The EPIDOS prospective study. J Bone Miner Res 11:1531, 1996.

36. Garnero, P.; Shih, W.J.; Gineyts, E.; et al. Comparison of new biochemical markers of bone turnover in late postmenopausal osteoporotic women in response to alendronate treatment. J Clin Endocrinol Metab 79:1693, 1994.

37. Genant, H.K.; Boyd, D.P. Quantitative bone mineral analysis using dual energy computed tomography. Invest Radiol 12:545, 1977.

38. Geusens, P.; Reid, D. Newer drug treatments: Their effects on fracture prevention. Best Pract Res Clin Rheumatol 19:983–989, 2005.

39. Glaser, D.L.; Kaplan, F.S. Osteoporosis: Definition and clinical presentation. Spine 22(Suppl 24):12S, 1997.

40. Glimcher, M.A. On the form and structure of bone from molecules to organs: Wolff's law revisited. In Veis, A., ed. The Chemistry and Biology of Mineralized Tissues. New York, Elsevier-North Holland, 1982, p. 613.

41. Glowacki, J.; Hurwitz, S.; Thornhill, T.S.; et al. Osteoporosis and vitamin-D deficiency among postmenopausal women with osteoarthritis undergoing total hip arthroplasty. J Bone Joint Surg Am 85:2371–2377, 2003.

42. Green, P.H. The many faces of celiac disease: Clinical presentation of celiac disease in the adult population. Gastroenterology 128(4 Suppl 1):S74–S78, 2005.

43. Greenspan, S.L.; Myers, E.R.; Maitland, L.A.; et al. Fall severity and mineral density as risk factors for hip fracture in ambulatory elderly. JAMA 271:128, 1994.

44. Guay, D.R. Ibandronate, an experimental intravenous bisphosphonate for osteoporosis, bone metastases, and hypercalcemia of malignancy. Pharmacotherapy 26:655–673, 2006.

45. Hakkinen, K. Force production characteristics of leg extensor, trunk flexor, and extensor muscles in male and female basketball players. J Sports Med Phys Fitness 31:325, 1991.

46. Hansen, M.A.; Overgaard, K.; Riss, B.J.; et al. Role of peak bone mass and bone loss in postmenopausal osteoporosis: Twelve-year study. BMJ 303:1548, 1991.

47. Hayes, W.C.; Myers, E.R.; Morris, J.N.; et al. Impact near the hip dominates fracture risk in elderly nursing home residents who fall. Calcif Tissue Int 52:192, 1993.

48. Heaney, R.P. Effect of calcium on skeletal development, bone loss, and risk of fractures. Am J Med 91 (5B):23S, 1991.

49. Heaney, R.P. Nutrition and Osteoporosis. In Favus, M.J., ed. Primer on the Metabolic Bone Diseases and Disorders of Mineral Metabolism. Philadelphia, Lippincott Williams & Wilkins, 1999, p. 270.

50. Holbrook, T.; Grazier, K.; Kelsey, J.; et al. The Frequency of Occurrence, Impact and Cost of Selected Musculoskeletal Conditions in the United States. Chicago, American Academy of Orthopedic Surgeons, 1984.

51. Horseman, A.; Gallagher, J.C.; Simpson, M.; et al. Prospective trial of oestrogen and calcium in postmenopausal women. BMJ 2:789, 1977.

52. Jacobsen, P.C.; Beaver, W.; Grubb, S.A.; et al. Bone density in women college athletes and older athletic women. J Orthop Res 2:328, 1984.

53. Jansen, M.E.; Evans, A.J.; Mathis, J.M.; et al. Percutaneous polymethylmethacrylate vertebroplasty in the treatment of osteoporotic vertebral body compression fractures: Technical aspects. AJNR 18:1897, 1997.

54. Johnson, T.R.; Tomin, E.; Lane, J.M. Perspectives on growth factors, bone graft substitutes and fracture healing. In Obrant, K., ed. Management of Fractures in Severely Osteoporotic Bone. London, Springer, 2000, p. 111.

55. Johnston, C.C., Jr.; Epstein, S. Clinical, biochemical, epidemiologic, and economic features of osteoporosis. Orthop Clin North Am 12:559, 1981.

56. Jones, B.H.; Bovee, M.W.; Harris, J.M.; et al. Intrinsic risk factors for exercise-related injuries among male and female army trainees. Am J Sports Med 21:705, 1993.

57. Jones, B.H.; Cowan, D.N.; Tomlinson, J.P.; et al. Epidemiology of injuries associated with physical

training among young men in the army. Med Sci Sports Exerc 25:197, 1993.

58. Jowsey, J. Bone morphology: Bone structure. In Sledge, C.B., ed. Metabolic Disease of Bone. Philadelphia, W.B. Saunders, 1977, pp. 41–47.

59. Juppner, H.; Brown, E.M.; Kronenberg, H.M. Parathyroid hormone. In Favus, M.J., ed. Primer on the Metabolic Bone Diseases and Disorders of Mineral Metabolism. Philadelphia, Lippincott Williams & Wilkins, 1999, p. 80.

60. Kelsey, J.F. Osteoporosis: Prevalence and incidence. In Proceedings of the NIH Consensus Development Conference, April 2–4, 1984. Bethesda, MD, National Institutes of Health, 1984, p. 25.

61. Kempson, G. The mechanical properties of articular cartilage and bone. In Owen, R.; Goodfellow, J.; Bullough, P., eds. Scientific Foundations of Orthopaedics and Traumatology. Philadelphia, W.B. Saunders, 1980, p. 49.

62. Kenzora, J.E.; McCarthy, R.E.; Lowell, J.D.; et al. Hip fracture mortality: Relation to age, treatment, preoperative illness, time of surgery, and complications. Clin Orthop 186:45, 1985.

63. Kimmel, P.L. Radiologic methods to evaluate bone mineral content. Ann Intern Med 100:908, 1984.

64. Krolner, B.; Toft, B.; Pors Nielsen, S.; et al. Physical exercise as a prophylaxis against involutional vertebral bone loss: A controlled trial. Clin Sci (Colch) 64:541, 1983.

65. Lane, J.M. Metabolic bone disease and fracture healing. In Heppenstall, R.B., ed. Fracture Treatment and Healing. Philadelphia, W.B. Saunders, 1980, p. 946.

66. Lane, J.M.; Vigorita, V.J. Osteoporosis. Orthop J 1:22, 1985.

67. Lane, J.M.; Werntz, J.R. Biology of fracture healing. In Lane, J., ed. Fracture Healing. New York, Churchill Livingstone, 1987, p. 49.

68. Lane, J.M.; Cornell, C.N.; Healey, J.H. Orthopaedic consequences of osteoporosis. In Riggs, B.L.; Melton, L.J. III, eds. Osteoporosis: Etiology, Diagnosis and Management. New York, Raven Press, 1988, p. 111.

69. Lane, J.M.; Girardi, F.; Parvataneni, H.; et al. Preliminary outcomes of the first 226 consecutive kyphoplasties for the fixation of painful osteoporotic vertebral compression fractures. World Congress on Osteoporosis 2000, Chicago, 2000.

70. Lane, J.M.; Healey, J.H.; Schwartz, E.; et al. The treatment of osteoporosis with sodium fluoride and calcium: Effects on vertebral fracture incidence and bone histomorphometry. Orthop Clin North Am 15:729, 1984.

71. Lane, J.M.; Russell, L.; Khan, S.N. Osteoporosis. Clin Orthop 372:139, 1999.

72. Lane, J.M.; Vigorita, V.J.; Falls, M. Osteoporosis: Current diagnosis and treatment. Geriatrics 39:40, 1984.

73. Leiberman, U.A.; Weiss, S.R.; Broll, J.; et al. Effect of oral alendronate on bone mineral density and the incidence of fracture in postmenopausal osteoporotic women. N Engl J Med 333:1437, 1995.

74. Lindsey, R.; Hart, D.M.; Aitken, J.M.; et al. Long-term prevention of postmenopausal osteoporosis by estrogen. Lancet 1:1038, 1976.

75. Lindsey, R.; Hart, D.M.; Aitken, J.M.; et al. Prevention of spinal osteoporosis in oophorectomised women. Lancet 2:1151, 1980.

76. Lindsey, R.; Hart, D.M.; MacLean, A. Bone response to termination of oestrogen treatment. Lancet 1:1325, 1978.

77. Loucks, A.B.; Motorola, J.F.; Girton, L.; et al. Alterations in the hypothalamic-pituitary-ovarian and the hypothalamic-pituitary-adrenal axis in the athletic woman. J Clin Endocrinol Metab 68:402, 1989.

78. Lufkin, E.G.; Wahner, H.W.; O'Fallon, W.M.; et al. Treatment of postmenopausal osteoporosis with transdermal estrogen. Ann Intern Med 117:1, 1992.

78a. Lyles, K.W.; Colón-Emeric, C.S.; Macaziner, J.S.; et al. Zoledronic acid and clinical fractures and mortality after hip fracture. N Engl J Med 357:1799, 2007.

79. Madore, G.R.; Sherman, P.J.; Lane, J.M. Parathyroid hormone. J Am Acad Orthop Surg 12:67–71, 2004.

80. Mashiba, T.; Hui, S.; Turner, C.H.; et al. Bone remodeling at the iliac crest can predict the changes in remodeling dynamics, microdamage accumulation and mechanical properties in the lumbar vertebrae of dogs. Calcif Tissue Int 77:180–185, 2005.

81. Mashiba, T.; Turner, C.H.; Hirano, T.; et al. Effects of suppressed bone turnover by bisphosphonates on microdamage accumulation and biomechanical properties in clinically relevant skeletal sites in beagles. Bone 28:524–531, 2001.

82. Melton, L.J. III; Riggs, B.L. Epidemiology of age-related fractures. In Avioli, L.V., ed. The Osteoporotic Syndrome. New York, Grune & Stratton, 1987, pp. 1–30.

83. Melton, L.J. III; Riggs, B.L. Epidemiology of age-related fractures. In Avioli, L.V., ed. The Osteoporotic Syndrome: Detection, Prevention and Treatment. Orlando, FL, Grune & Stratton, 1983, p. 45.

84. Melton, L.J.I.; Khosla, S.; Atkinson, E.J.; et al. Relationship of bone turnover to bone density and fractures. J Bone Miner Res 12:1083, 1997.

85. Meunier, P.J. Prevention of hip fractures. Am J Med 95:755, 1993.

86. Mohler, D.G.; Lane, J.M.; Cole, B.J.; et al. Skeletal fracture in osteoporosis. In Lane, J.M.; Healey, J.H., eds. Diagnosis and Management of Pathological Fractures. New York, Raven Press, 1993, p. 13.

87. Mosekilde, L.; Eriksen, E.F.; Charles, P. Effects of thyroid hormone on bone and mineral metabolism. Endocrinol Med Clin North Am 19:35, 1990.

88. Mullen, J.O.; Mullen, N.L. Hip fracture mortality: A prospective multifactorial study to predict and minimize death risk. Clin Orthop 280:214, 1992.

89. Nakazawa, T.; Nakajima, A.; Shiomi, K.; et al. Effects of low-dose, intermittent treatment with recombinant

human parathyroid hormone (1-34) on chondrogenesis in a model of experimental fracture healing. Bone 37:711–719, 2005.

90. National Osteoporosis Foundation. Osteoporosis: Review of the evidence for the prevention, diagnosis, and treatment and cost-effectiveness analysis. Osteoporos Int 8:1, 1998.

91. Neer, R.M.; Arnaud, C.D.; Zanchetta, J.R.; et al. Effect of parathyroid hormone (1-34) on fractures and bone mineral density in postmenopausal women with osteoporosis. N Engl J Med 10:344:1434–1441, 2001.

92. NIH Consensus Conference. Optimal calcium intake. JAMA 272:1942, 1994.

93. Odvina, C.V.; Zerwekh, J.E.; Rao, D.S.; et al. Severely suppressed bone turnover: a potential complication of alendronate therapy. J Clin Endocrinol Metab 90:1294–1301, 2005.

94. Ott, S.M. Clinical effects of bisphosphonates in involutional osteoporosis. J Bone Miner Res 8 (Suppl):597, 1993.

95. Overgaard, K.; Hansen, N.A.; Jensen, S.B.; et al. Effect of calcitonin given intranasally on bone mass and fracture rates in established osteoporosis: A dose response study. Bone Miner 305:556, 1992.

96. The Postmenopausal Estrogen/Progestin Interventions (PEPI) Trial. Effects of estrogen on estrogen/progestin regimens on heart disease risk factors in postmenopausal women. JAMA 273:199, 1995.

97. Powels, T.J.; Hicklish, T.; Kanis, J.A.; et al. Effect of tamoxifen on bone mineral density measured by dual-energy x-ray absorptiometry in healthy premenopausal and postmenopausal women. J Clin Oncol 18:78, 1995.

98. Pun, K.K.; Chan, L.W. Analgesic effect of intranasal salmon calcitonin in the treatment of osteoporotic vertebral fractures. Clin Endocrinol (Oxf) 30:435, 1989.

99. Ray, N.F.; Chan, J.K.; Thamer, M.; et al. Medical expenditures for the treatment of osteoporotic fractures in the United States in 1995: Report from the National Osteoporosis Foundation. J Bone Miner Res 12:24, 1997.

100. Recker, R.R.; Kimmel, D.B.; Parfitt, A.M.; et al. Static and tetracycline-based bone histomorphometric data from 34 normal postmenopausal females. J Bone Miner Res 3:133, 1988.

101. Riggs, B.L.; Melton, L.J. III. Evidence for two distinct syndromes of involutional osteoporosis. Am J Med 75:899, 1983.

102. Riggs, B.L.; Melton, L.J. III. Involutional osteoporosis. N Engl J Med 314:1676, 1986.

103. Riggs, B.L.; Melton, L.J. III. The prevention and treatment of osteoporosis. N Engl J Med 327:620, 1992.

104. Riginster, J.; Minne, H.W.; Sorsenson, O.H.; et al. Randomized trial of the effects of risedronate on vertebral fractures in women with established postmenopausal osteoporosis: Vertebral Efficacy with Risedronate Therapy (VERT) Study Group. Osteoporos Int 11:83, 2000.

105. Rosen, C.J.; Kiel, D.P. The aging skeleton. In Favus, M.J., ed. Primer on the Metabolic Bone Diseases and Disorders of Mineral Metabolism. Philadelphia, Lippincott Williams & Wilkins, 1999.

106. Rubin, C.T.; Rubin, J. Biomechanics of bone. In Favus, M.J., ed. Primer on the Metabolic Bone Diseases and Disorders of Mineral Metabolism. Philadelphia, Lippincott Williams & Wilkins, 1999.

107. Schneider, R.; Math, K. Bone density analysis: An update. Curr Opin Orthop 5:66, 1994.

108. Schnitzer, T.; Bone, H.G.; Crepaldi, G.; et al. Therapeutic equivalence of alendronate 70 mg once-weekly and alendronate 10 mg daily in the treatment of osteoporosis: Alendronate Once Weekly Study Group. Aging 12:1, 2000.

109. Seeger, L.L. Bone density determination. Spine 22 (Suppl 24):49S, 1997.

110. Smith, R.W., Jr.; Walter, R.R. Femoral expansion in aging women: Implications for osteoporosis and fractures. Science 145:156, 1964.

111. Steier, A.; Gegalia, I.; Schwartz, A.; et al. Effect of vitamin D and fluoride on experimental bone fracture healing in rats. J Dent Res 46:675, 1967.

112. Walsh, W.R.; Sherman, P.; Howlett, C.R.; et al. Fracture healing in a rat osteopenia model. Clin Orthop 342:218, 1997.

113. Wasnich, R.D. Epidemiology of Osteoporosis. In Favus, M.J., ed. Primer on the Metabolic Bone Diseases and Disorders of Mineral Metabolism. Philadelphia, Lippincott Williams & Wilkins, 1999, p. 257.

114. Weiss, N.S.; Ure, C.L.; Ballard, J.H.; et al. Decreased risk of fractures of the hip and lower forearm with postmenopausal use of estrogen. N Engl J Med 303:1195, 1980.

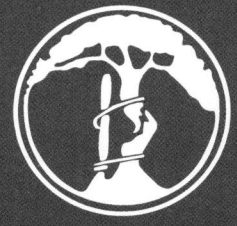

CHAPTER 19

Surgical Site Infection Prevention

Amir Mostofi, M.D., Bruce D. Browner, M.D., M.S., F.A.C.S., Neil Grey, M.D., Jason H. Calhoun, M.D., and Susan MacArthur, R.N., M.P.H., C.I.C.

INTRODUCTION

One of the most prevalent causes of morbidity and mortality continues to be surgical site infections (SSIs). In 2002, there were more than 43 million procedures in the United States of which over 600 thousand included open reduction and internal fixation.[56] Surgical site infections are the second most common cause of nosocomial infections. Significant morbidity is associated with SSI, and the patient is affected both physically and psychologically. Aside from the distress suffered by the patient and the health care provider, there is a significant burden to the national health care cost. Reports indicate that surgical site infections lead to an average of 6.5 additional days in the hospital, resulting in a median excess direct cost of $3,089. Taking readmission into account, total excess hospitalization can be up to 12 days and $5,038 more for each patient. Furthermore, patients suffering from surgical site infections are twice as likely to die, 60 percent more likely to spend time in an intensive care unit (ICU), and more than five times more likely to be readmitted.[54]

National attention has been brought to nosocomial infections and postoperative morbidity and mortality. Public reporting of institutional and physician performance is today's reality. Several states have enacted legislation that requires public reporting of health care-associated infection (HAI). This is largely due to a push by consumers and citizen action groups that believe that information regarding hospital and physician performance should be made public. State regulatory agencies, accrediting bodies such as the Joint Commission on Accreditation of Healthcare Organizations (JCAHO), and insurers support this practice to improve the quality of health care and to hold health care providers more accountable. Currently, an accurate system does not exist to measure physician-specific infection rates. Thus, quality measures and adherence to guidelines are a way of measuring physician and institutional compliance to guidelines intended to reduce nosocomial infections such as SSIs. Once performance measures are made public, the next step would be the practice of pay-for-performance. Pay-for-performance occurs when providers supply data on specified quality measures and purchasers such as Medicare, Medicaid, and insurance companies pay health services differentially based on the outcomes resulting from those preset measures.

The Surgical Care Improvement Project (SCIP) exemplifies the national concern regarding surgical complications. For years the Centers for Disease Control (CDC) has been monitoring infection rates through the National Nosocomial Surveillance System. Through its partnership with the Centers for Medicare & Medicaid Services (CMS) the Surgical Site Infection Project (SSIP) was implemented. With the experience gained through these projects and new partnerships with many organizations, SCIP was founded. SCIP is a partnership of many organizations dedicated to improving surgical care. Table 19-1 lists members of the Steering Committee and Technical Expert Panel who make up the fundamental structure of this organization. The Steering Committee consists of national organizations that have pledged their commitment and full support to SCIP. SCIP's four target areas are advised by a Technical Expert Panel (TEP), which includes the American Academy of Orthopaedic Surgeons (AAOS). The target areas are perioperative cardiac complications, surgery-related infections such as SSI and pneumonia, and deep vein thrombosis. These groups have provided hours of technical expertise and resources to ensure that the SCIP measures are fully supported by evidence-based research. Hospitals can join SCIP and become part of a national movement to reduce surgical complications by 25 percent by year 2010.

Success in reducing surgical site infections requires an organized and consistent surveillance system both nationally and locally. The CDC's National Nosocomial Infections Surveillance system (NNIS), established in 1970, monitors nosocomial infection trends in the United States. Today, this voluntary reporting system includes approximately 300 hospitals. Principles of the NNIS include detection and monitoring of adverse events, assessing risk and protective factors, evaluation of preventive interventions, and providing information to event reporters and stakeholders and partnering with them to implement effective prevention strategies. NNIS provides an annual report of nosocomial infection rates in the country. This system currently is undergoing a major redesign as a Web-based knowledge management and adverse events reporting system called the National Healthcare Safety Network (NHSN). This will allow many hospitals to be a part of the NNIS and compare their infection rates to national averages.

	Table 19-1	
Partners in the Surgical Care Improvement Project (SCIP)		
Steering Commitee	**Panel of Experts**	**Panel of Experts**
Agency for Healthcare Research and Quality	American Society of Colon and Rectal Surgeons	Ascension Health
		Centers for Medicare & Medicaid Services
American College of Surgeons	American Society of Health-Systems Pharmacists	Centers for Disease Control and Prevention
American Hospital Association		American Academy of Orthopaedic Surgeons
American Society of Anesthesiologists	American Society of PeriAnesthesia Nurses	American Association of Critical Care Nurses
Association of periOperative Registered Nurses	Ascension Health	American Association of Nurse Anesthetists
Centers for Disease Control and Prevention	Association of periOperative Registered Nurses	American College of Obstetricians & Gynecologists
Centers for Medicare & Medicaid Services	Association for Professionals in Infection Control and Epidemiology	American College of Surgeons
Institute for Healthcare Improvement		American Geriatrics Society
Joint Commission on Accreditation of Healthcare Organizations	Infectious Diseases Society of America	American Hospital Association
Veterans Health Administration	Joint Commission on Accreditation of Healthcare Organizations	American Society of Anesthesiologists
	The Medical Letter	Society for Health Care Epidemiology of America
	Oklahoma Foundation for Medical Quality	Society of Thoracic Surgeons
		Surgical Infection Society
		VHA, Inc.
		Premier, Inc.
		Qualis Health
		Sanford Guide

With public reporting and pay-for-performance being instituted, hospitals are looking for ways to show their leadership and dedication to detecting and preventing surgical site infections. Effective surveillance requires standardized infection definitions, standardized risk assessment indices, and data feedback. The CDC's NNIS has provided definitions for surgical site infection (Fig. 19-1 and Table 19-2). Use of these definitions will provide a way to accurately record and compare the severity of infections in patients. Adjusting for confounding variables that can affect infection rates is also critical. Standard definitions and risk indices are important for any surveillance system if it is to provide information for comparison between physicians and hospitals. The NNIS has three components to its risk indices stratification scale, and a point is assigned when each component is present. This includes the American Society of Anesthesiologists (ASA) physical status classification of greater than 2 (Table 19-3), either a contaminated or dirty/infected wound classification (Table 19-4), and length of the operation greater than T hours, where T is the approximate 75th percentile of the duration of the specific operation being performed. Patients' scores range from a minimum of 0 to a maximum of 3. Using this scheme, infection rates can be compared between patients with similar risk indices, reducing some of the confounding variables.

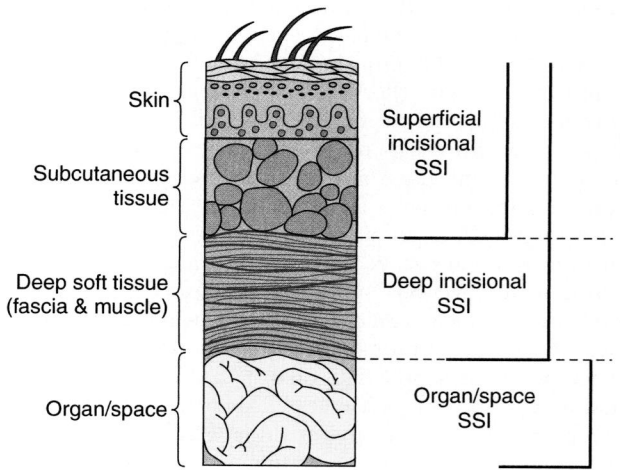

FIGURE 19-1 *Cross-section of the abdominal wall. Wounds are classified as superficial incisional, deep incisional, and organ/space infections. SSI, surgical site infection. (From Mangram, A.J.; Horan, T.C.; Pearson, M.L.; et al. Guideline for Prevention of Surgical Site Infection, 1999. Centers for Disease Control and Prevention (CDC) Hospital Infection Control Practices Advisory Committee. Am J Infect Control 27:97–132, 1999.)*

Table 19-2
Criteria for Defining a Surgical Site Infection (SSI)

Superficial Incisional SSI

Infection occurs within 30 days after the operation *and* infection involves only skin or subcutaneous tissue of the incision *and* at least *one* of the following:

1. Purulent drainage, with or without laboratory confirmation, from the superficial incision.
2. Organisms isolated from an aseptically obtained culture of fluid or tissue from the superficial incision.
3. At least one of the following signs or symptoms of infection: pain or tenderness, localized swelling, redness, or heat *and* superficial incision is deliberately opened by surgeon, *unless* incision is culture-negative.
4. Diagnosis of superficial incisional SSI by the surgeon or attending physician.

Do *not* report the following conditions as SSI:

1. Stitch abscess (minimal inflammation and discharge confined to the points of suture penetration).
2. Infection of an episiotomy or newborn circumcision site.
3. Infected burn wound.
4. Incisional SSI that extends into the fascial and muscle layers (see deep incisional SSI).

Note: Specific criteria are used for identifying infected episiotomy and circumcision sites and burn wounds.

Deep Incisional SSI

Infection occurs within 30 days after the operation if no implant* is left in place or within 1 year if implant is in place and the infection appears to be related to the operation *and* infection involves deep soft tissues (e.g., fascial and muscle layers) of the incision *and* at least *one* of the following:

1. Purulent drainage from the deep incision but not from the organ/space component of the surgical site.
2. A deep incision spontaneously dehisces or is deliberately opened by a surgeon when the patient has at least one of the following signs or symptoms: fever ($>38°C$), localized pain, or tenderness, unless site is culture-negative.
3. An abscess or other evidence of infection involving the deep incision is found on direct examination, during reoperation, or by histopathologic or radiologic examination.
4. Diagnosis of a deep incisional SSI by a surgeon or attending physician.

Notes:

1. Report infection that involves both superficial and deep incision sites as deep incisional SSI.
2. Report an organ/space SSI that drains through the incision as a deep incisional SSI.

Organ/Space SSI

Infection occurs within 30 days after the operation if no implant* is left in place or within 1 year if implant is in place and the infection appears to be related to the operation *and* infection involves any part of the anatomy (e.g., organs or spaces), other than the incision, which was opened or manipulated during an operation *and* at least *one* of the following:

1. Purulent drainage from a drain that is placed through a stab wound† into the organ/space.
2. Organisms isolated from an aseptically obtained culture of fluid or tissue in the organ/space.
3. An abscess or other evidence of infection involving the organ/space that is found on direct examination, during reoperation, or by histopathologic or radiologic examination.
4. Diagnosis of an organ/space SSI by a surgeon or attending physician.

*National Nosocomial Infection Surveillance definition: a nonhuman-derived implantable foreign body (e.g., prosthetic heart valve, nonhuman vascular graft, mechanical heart, or hip prosthesis) that is permanently placed in a patient during surgery.
†If the area around a stab wound becomes infected, it is not an SSI. It is considered a skin or soft tissue infection, depending on its depth.

The definitions and risk indices are the foundation for communication. The next big challenge is accurately and consistently identifying patients with adverse events such as an SSI. The overall concept is that patients need to be followed for inpatient, postdischarge, and outpatient infections. The surveillance can be in the form of direct observation of a surgical site by a surgeon, trained nurse surveyor, or an infection control personnel. Indirect forms of observation include reviewing charts and laboratory data or patient surveys. There is no consensus on this issue, and all methods have their benefits and imperfections. Nevertheless, surgeons need to understand that surveillance will be part of medicine in the future not only to provide accountability for infection rates and medical practices but also to assist in quality assurance initiatives.

Surgical site infections have a great impact on the outcome of medical intervention and significantly influence patient health. This chapter reviews some the important aspects of SSI prevention. Recognizing patient susceptibility and aiding the host through perioperative oxygen supplementation, temperature, and blood glucose regulation are key factors in infection prevention. The operating room setting, hand antisepsis, skin preparation, and perioperative antibiotics are means to reduce the microbial load in a surgical wound. The understanding and application of these concepts will aid the surgeon in the comprehensive treatment of the patient in the operative setting.

SURGICAL ASEPSIS[15]

Skin Preparation

Surgical hand scrubbing is of paramount importance for adherence to aseptic techniques. Since Lister used carbonic acid to clean his hands, many different solutions have been

Table 19-3

Physical Status Classification, from the American Society of Anesthesiologists*

Code	Patient's Preoperative Physical Status
1	Normally healthy patient
2	Patient with mild systemic disease
3	Patient with severe systemic disease that is not incapacitating
4	Patient with an incapacitating systemic disease that is a constant threat to life
5	Moribund patient who is not expected to survive for 24 hours with or without operation

*The above is the version of the ASA Physical Status Classification System that was current at the time of development of, and still is used in, the NNIS Risk Index. Meanwhile, the American Society of Anesthesiologists has revised their classification system; the most recent version is available at http://www.asahq.org/profinfo/physicalstatus.html.
Source: American Society of Anesthesiologists (ASA).

used to reduce the microbial count on the skin of operating room personnel. The skin is usually colonized by transient and resident flora. Resident flora is more adhesive and resides in the deeper layers of the skin, enabling it to be more resistant to removal. Transient flora is found in the superficial layers of the skin and is the main culprit in health care-associated infections. Surgical hand scrubbing is defined as antiseptic hand wash or antiseptic hand rub performed preoperatively by surgical personnel to eliminate transient and reduce resident hand flora. The goal is to use an antiseptic agent having a broad spectrum of activity that quickly reduces microbial counts and maintains a persistent level of activity.[15]

Table 19-4

Surgical Wound Classification

Class I/Clean: An uninfected operative wound in which no inflammation is encountered and the respiratory, alimentary, genital, or uninfected urinary tract is not entered. In addition, clean wounds are primarily closed and, if necessary, drained with closed drainage. Operative incisional wounds that follow nonpenetrating (blunt) trauma should be included in this category if they meet the criteria.

Class II/Clean-Contaminated: An operative wound in which the respiratory, alimentary, genital, or urinary tracts are entered under controlled conditions and without unusual contamination. Specifically, operations involving the biliary tract, appendix, vagina, and oropharynx are included in this category, provided no evidence of infection or major break in technique is encountered.

Class III/Contaminated: Open, fresh, accidental wounds. In addition, operations with major breaks in sterile technique (e.g., open cardiac massage) or gross spillage from the gastrointestinal tract, and incisions in which acute, nonpurulent inflammation is encountered, are included in this category.

Class IV/Dirty-Infected: Old traumatic wounds with retained devitalized tissue and those that involve existing clinical infection or perforated viscera. This definition suggests that the organisms causing postoperative infection were present in the operative field before the operation.

ALCOHOL

Several agents are used for surgical hand antisepsis. The most basic is antimicrobial soap. Although excellent for removing dirt, soil, and loosely adherent transient skin flora through their detergent properties, soaps are ineffective in significantly reducing skin flora counts for the surgical environment. Alcohol, which includes isopropanol, ethanol, n-propanol alcohol, or a combination of these, has been used for many years for antisepsis. Alcohol has been shown to be fast acting with superior antimicrobial activity against most of the organisms encountered. Its antimicrobial activity comes from the ability to denature proteins. The presence of water is also essential to denature proteins; hence, alcohol is used in combination with water and is recorded as a percent by weight or volume in most products. It has good activity against gram-negative, gram-positive, multiresistant bacteria, as well as *Mycobacterium tuberculosis* and various fungi. Alcohol also has good antiseptic strength against most enveloped (lipophilic) viruses, HIV, hepatitis B, and hepatitis C. It lacks strength against bacterial spores, protozoan oocysts, and certain nonenveloped (nonlipophilic) viruses. Alcohol's shortcomings include the lack of persistent activity, flammability, and drying of skin causing irritation. Because of its flammability, complete evaporation of the products containing flammable chemicals must be ensured. Alcohol's lack of persistent activity requires it to be used in combination with other antimicrobial agents as well as skin-conditioning products used to prevent skin breakdown.

CHLORHEXIDINE GLUCONATE

Chlorhexidine gluconate is a water-soluble compound that disrupts cytoplasmic membranes, resulting in both immediate and persistent antimicrobial activity. It has good activity against gram-positive, gram-negative, and enveloped viruses and has been shown to be safe for the use of hand antisepsis.

IODOPHORES

The iodine-based products have been used longer than any other product for surgical skin antisepsis. They function by penetrating organisms and binding amino acids and free fatty acids, thereby affecting protein synthesis and cell wall integrity. Currently, iodine is bound to a polymer carrier (e.g., Povidone) giving it better solubility and sustained release and reducing its most significant negative side effect, skin irritation. Iodine has a broad spectrum of activity against gram-negative bacteria, gram-positive bacteria, mycobacterium, viruses, and fungi. Although its persistent level of activity is variable, iodine has consistently been a reliable compound for safe and effective skin preparation.

OTHER SKIN PREPARATIONS

Other skin preparation compounds include hexachlorophene, chloroxylenol, and triclosan. Triclosan is a safe product that has relatively good, persistent antimicrobial activity. It is mostly bacteriostatic but can be bactericidal at higher concentrations. Currently, its use is in antiseptic hand washes for health care workers and commercial antimicrobial soaps. Hexachlorophene has limited use for hand washes because it does not have so broad a microbial activity as some other agents and it can be absorbed through the skin, causing systemic side effects. Although these products alone are not ideal for surgical hand antiseptics, their use in combination with other agents such as alcohol could prove to be efficacious. Chloroxylenol, also known as parachlorometaxylenol (PCMX), works by altering bacterial enzymes and cell walls, giving it broad, persistent antimicrobial activity. Chloroxylenol is absorbed through the skin but is well tolerated.

Literature to overwhelmingly support one product over another does not currently exist.[30] Alcohol and other alcohol-based products are fastest in reducing resident flora and also are most efficacious at reducing bacterial skin counts. Two to four percent chlorhexidine has the greatest persistent level of activity.[4] Studies in the foot and ankle literature show that combining alcohol with chlorhexidine and using a brush is superior to povidone iodine.[9,53,72] Most of these studies, however, focus on bacterial counts on the skin and not the clinical implication of different skin preparation agents.

Regardless of the product, certain requirements for in vitro and in vivo testing of surgical hand scrubs are needed before approval by the U.S. Food and Drug Administration (FDA). Products intended for use as surgical hand scrubs are evaluated by using a standardized method outlined in the FDA Tentative Final Monograph for Healthcare Antiseptic Drug Products (TFM).

For the clinician, efficacious surgical scrub techniques and adherence to institutional protocols are more critical. Unfortunately because of the different variety of products and the lack of reliable and reproducible evidence, there is no standard scrub technique. Previously a 10-minute surgical scrub (using a brush) was advocated. Now, anatomic scrubbing (without a brush) and shortened scrub times are being proposed. The time required for scrubbing is one of the major obstacles to compliance. Studies have shown that a 5-minute scrub is as efficacious as a 10-minute scrub. There is evidence that even shortened scrub times reduce bacteria counts to acceptable levels. Using a brush has not been shown to make a significant difference and can irritate skin, leading to a further decrease in compliance. Currently a 5-minute anatomic scrub with an antimicrobial soap is the standard.[23] Combining alcohol, which works fast and has a broad spectrum of activity, with antimicrobial agents with a persistent activity may prove to be the best option. Alcohol-based rubs are as efficacious as surgical scrubbing, shorten skin preparation times, and reduce skin irritation.[18,59,74] In this setting, it is important to pre-wash hands and dry completely before the application of the product. Following the manufacturer's recommended technique is advised. Making proper surgical hand scrubbing an institutional priority helps educate everyone involved about the importance of hand hygiene. Regardless of the product, adherence to the recommended instructions is paramount in obtaining true antiseptic techniques. Increasing compliance may require making hand scrubbing stations easy to access, providing health care workers with a sufficient amount of time to scrub, and supplying hand lotions to prevent side effects.

Surgical Attire and Draping

Wearing surgical gloves is important to minimize transmission of microorganisms from the hands of health care workers into sterile wounds. Wearing gloves for prolonged periods of time fosters an environment for bacterial growth. Surgical hand scrubs must have persistent activity to prevent this form of bacterial growth. Double gloving protects against contamination and is recommended in orthopaedic procedures that have a higher risk of puncture wounds from sharp objects.[58,88] Double gloving and changing gloves at regular intervals decreases contamination from inadvertent breaks in asepsis during draping and from unrecognized puncture wounds.[3,66] It is important to remove jewelry before gloving. Artificial nails have been associated with outbreaks. It is recommended for surgical personnel to keep nails short to prevent breaking of gloves.

Sterile gowns and drapes prevent exposure of health care workers to infectious pathogens. They also maintain a sterile environment for surgical procedures. Current testing standards developed by organizations such as the American Society for Testing and Materials categorize gowns and drapes by their protection from liquid penetration. Resistant gowns resist penetration of liquid but their effectiveness declines under hydrostatic pressure. Repellent materials resist wetting by liquids. The most effective barriers are categorized as impervious, which are liquid proof and prevent penetration by liquids and microorganisms. Current testing methods are not infallible, and resistance to liquid penetration does not equate to resistance to microbial penetration. Reusable gowns and drapes are made of polyester sheeting or composite materials made of woven or knitted fabrics. The fabrics are typically woven and laminated or coated with material to enhance protection against strike-through of liquids and microorganisms. Single-use materials are usually nonwoven natural (e.g., wood pulp) or synthetic (e.g., polyester, polypropylene) fabrics that are specially processed and treated with chemicals to improve protective qualities. The superiority of disposable or reusable gowns has not been demonstrated.[81] The performance of gowns and drapes depends on the construction and processing of the fibers, pore size, and repellency.[61] The ideal gown or drape should be low cost, comfortable, conforming, durable, and sterilizable and should prevent the penetration of contaminated liquids and microorganisms.

Body Exhaust Systems

In the early 1970s Sir Charles Charnley introduced the idea of body exhaust systems for decreasing the air contamination of wounds in total joint arthroplasty. Although this system is used by many in joint reconstructive surgery, few have used it in conventional fracture care operations. Multiple variables could affect the rate of surgical site infections including air contamination, skin contamination, patient risk factors, and perioperative antibiotic use. Therefore, it is difficult to assess the true benefit of body exhaust systems. Improper hair coverage and inadvertent breaks in aseptic techniques by health care teams may be reduced by the use of body exhaust systems. Many surgeons use body exhaust systems because the possibility of affecting the rate of infection by even small amounts can have significant clinical implications owing to the large volume of patients seen in practice. At this time, no significant body of knowledge supports or is against the use of body exhaust systems for fracture management.

Operating Room Environment

One of the culprits of wound infection in the operating room theater is airborne contaminants. Controlling traffic patterns and limiting the number of people circulating in the operating room reduce undesirable airflow movements.[2] All surgical operating room suites should maintain positive pressure with respect to the outside environment, thereby affecting airflow pathways and preventing unfiltered air from entering the operating room suite. All hospitals are required to have ventilation systems with two filters in series, increasing the efficiency of the air cleaning system. Air inflow should enter at the ceiling with vents at the floor creating a plenum system. Operating room ventilation systems must produce a minimum of 15 filtered air changes every hour, three of which must come from fresh air.[63] Table 19-5 summarizes the parameters set by the American Institute of Architects in collaboration with the U.S. Department of Health and Human Services.

Sir Charley Charnley provided some of the first studies on laminar flow systems. In laminar airflow systems, filtered "ultra clean" or particle-free air is passed across the surgical field at a uniform velocity of approximately 0.3 to 0.5 μm/sec in a vertical or horizontal direction, preventing contaminated particles from landing on the open surgical field. Charnley and Lidwell provided studies in favor of laminar ultra clean air systems in joint replacement surgery.[22,62] Today, air can be filtered through a high-efficiency particulate air (HEPA) filter, removing any particle larger than 0.3 μm. Studies have shown that reduced air and surface contamination by laminar flow systems can lead to clinically reduced infection rates.[1,42,43,55] Ultraviolet (UV) radiation has also been reported to provide ultra clean air in the operating room theater, although patient and staff safety is a concern with this type of air cleaning system. The efficacy of current ventilation systems has reduced the interest in UV radiation to decrease air contamination. The effect of these ventilation systems in reducing surgical site infections in fracture care surgery is unknown. Most of the knowledge regarding this issue is in the total joint literature, and indeed some fracture care operations involve extensive wounds open for prolonged periods of time, in combination with the

implantation of hardware. Certainly in these cases airborne contamination can be significant, and ventilation systems play an important role in preventing airborne contamination.

PATIENT PREPARATION

Several patient-related factors can affect surgical site infections. In 1999, the CDC placed preoperative showering as a category IB recommendation, thereby strongly recommending it for adoption by all health care facilities.[58] Preoperative bathing or showering with chlorhexidine reduces colony counts of skin flora, but the clinical implication of this activity is not known.[37,45,60,63,96] The CDC also strongly recommended not removing patient's hair unless it interfered with the operation. The use of razors to shave hair leaves cuts that harbor bacteria. If hair removal is necessary, depilatory trimmers must be used.[63]

The same chemicals used for surgical hand scrubbing are also used for patient skin preparation. Table 19-6 reviews some of the most commonly used products, their mechanism of action, and spectrum of activity. Refer to the hand antisepsis section for a detailed discussion of these agents. Products that combine alcohol with chlorhexidine and iodophors are also available. Prior to the surgical scrub, the skin should be cleaned with soap and cleared of any dirt residue or blood. The activity of some products (e.g., povidone iodine) is affected by the presence of organic and inorganic compounds, such as blood and dirt. The skin should be dry prior to application. Apply the scrub in concentric circles starting at the incisional site and expanding outward covering all areas that might need exposure during the operation. Most products require 2 to 5 minutes for maximal bactericidal activity. When alcohol-based products are used, pooling cannot occur and the skin must be completely dry prior to the use of electrocautery.

HOST FACTORS

Infection of a surgical site occurs when the host is unable to eradicate the bacterial load introduced during a procedure. Anything that hinders the host defenses or increases contamination can tip the balance toward infection. Smoking is a preventable risk factor that has been associated with infection. Educating patients and assisting with smoking cessation is an important factor in preventing infection.[85,86] Although malnutrition has not been identified as an independent risk factor for surgical site infection, it certainly affects patient morbidity, and supplemental nutrition should be a part of a comprehensive care plan.[63] Colonization of the nares by *Staphylococcus aureus* has been linked to an increase in nosocomial infections. A relationship between appropriate clinical application of mupirocin ointment and a clear reduction in infection rates has not been established.[76,92] Concern exists regarding perioperative transfusions and infection.[51] The possibility of increased infection due to transfusion-related immunomodulation has resulted in use of white blood cell-reduced blood products.[10,52] The increased risk of infection due to transfusion and the reduction of this risk by filtering leukocytes are still under debate.[50] Withholding transfusion for symptomatic blood loss anemia is not justified, and use of leukocyte-reduced blood can prove

Table 19-5	
Parameters for Operating Room Ventilation	
Temperature	68–73°F, depending on normal ambient temperatures
Relative humidity	30%–60%
Air movement	From "clean to less clean" areas
Air changes	Minimum 15 total air changes per hour
	Minimum 3 air changes of outdoor air per hour

Source: American Institute of Architects, 1996.

		Table 19-6								
Mechanism and Spectrum of Activity of Antiseptic Agents Commonly Used for Preoperative Skin Preparation and Surgical Scrubs										
Agent	**Mechanism of Action**	**Gram-Positive Bacteria**	**Gram-Negative Bacteria**	**Mtb**	**Fungi**	**Virus**	**Rapidity of Action**	**Residual Activity**	**Toxicity**	**Uses**
Alcohol	Denature proteins	E	E	G	G	G	Most rapid	None	Drying, volatile	SP, SS
Chlorhexidine	Disrupt cell membrane	E	G	P	F	G	Intermediate	E	Ototoxicity, keratitis	SP, SS
Iodine/ Iodophors	Oxidation/ substitution by free iodine	E	G	G	G	G	Intermediate	Minimal	Absorption from skin with possible toxicity, skin irritation	SP, SS
PCMX	Disrupt cell wall	G	F*	F	F	F	Intermediate	G	More data needed	SS
Triclosan	Disrupt cell wall	G	G	G	P	U	Intermediate	E	More data needed	SS

Abbreviations: E, excellent; F, fair; G, good; Mtb, *Mycobacterium tuberculosis*; P, poor; PCMX, para-chloro-meta-xylenol; SP, skin preparation; SS, surgical scrubs; U, unknown.
*Fair, except for *Pseudomonas* species; activity improved by addition of chelating agent such as EDTA.
Source: From Mangram, A.J.; Horan, T.C.; Pearson, M.L.; et al. Guideline for Prevention of Surgical Site Infection, 1999. Centers for Disease Control and Prevention (CDC) Hospital Infection Control Practices Advisory Committee. Am J Infect Control 27:97–132, 1999.

costly without added benefit. Finally, of all the patient-related factors that affect infection, hyperglycemia is perhaps the most extensively studied. Glycemic control is paramount in the prevention of surgical site infection.

PERIOPERATIVE GLYCEMIC CONTROL

One of the most important co-morbidities in orthopaedic patients is hyperglycemia. A significant number of patients undergoing elective and urgent orthopaedic intervention suffer from diabetes. In the trauma setting, many patients without diabetes have unrecognized hyperglycemia. Hyperglycemia in the critically ill patient is defined as plasma glucose levels above 200 mg/dL. The incidence of diabetes in hyperglycemic patients treated in the ICU is approximately 13 percent.[41,91] An elevated blood glucose level is extremely common in the multi-trauma patient, occurring in up to 50 percent of patients in the intensive care setting.[34]

The etiology of stress-induced hyperglycemia is multifactorial. The patient is in a catabolic state, and calories supplied by artificial nutrition are high in carbohydrate. There is altered carbohydrate metabolism including enhanced gastrointestinal glucose absorption, increased glucose production from the liver, and increased insulin resistance resulting in hyperglycemia.[67] Hypersecretion of counterregulatory hormones and cytokines provides some of the explanation for the cause of hyperglycemia.[65]

The counterregulatory hormones include epinephrine, growth hormone, and glucocorticoids. Epinephrine affects glucose levels in three ways. Through its α-adrenergic activity, it directly inhibits endogenous insulin secretion. In addition, epinephrine increases hepatic glucose production and secretion by stimulating gluconeogenesis and glycogenolysis. Finally, epinephrine is lipolytic, thus increasing the concentration of free fatty acids, resulting in insulin resistance.[11] These three mechanisms result in

hyperglycemia. Growth hormone and glucocorticoids increase insulin resistance and hepatic glucose output, thereby contributing to hyperglycemia.

Several major cytokines produced as part of the acute stress response have an effect on glucose homeostasis. Tumor necrosis factor alpha (TNF-α) is a proinflammatory cytokine that alters the interaction of insulin with its receptor. Phosphorylation of tyrosine is necessary for the normal interaction of insulin with its receptor. TNF-α interferes with this mechanism by causing serine instead of tyrosine phosphorylation of the receptor, leading to systemic insulin resistance.[49] The combined effects of epinephrine, growth hormone, cortisol, and cytokines such as TNF-α provide an explanation for hyperglycemia seen in nondiabetic critically ill patients as well as the exacerbation of hyperglycemia in previously well controlled diabetic patients.

Hyperglycemia is important in this context because it diminishes the response to infection. High serum glucose levels affect polymorphonuclear function by reducing chemotaxis, phagocytosis, and oxidative bacterial killing (Fig. 19-2).[26,68,70] Furthermore, hyperglycemia results in glycosylation of serum proteins. Glycosylation of complement proteins and immunoglobulin results in an overall state of immunosuppression.[46]

Elevated glucose levels have been shown to have a significant impact on morbidity, mortality, and cost of patient care. Well-controlled clinical trials have documented that these adverse outcomes can be significantly improved by tight glycemic control. The study by van den Burge provided evidence for the benefit of tight glycemic control in critically ill patients. In this prospective randomized trial, patients requiring mechanical ventilation were randomly assigned to intensive versus conventional insulin therapy groups. In the conventional therapy group, patients were started on an insulin infusion only when blood glucose levels exceeded 215 mg/dL and the levels were maintained between 180 and 200 mg/dL. Intensive

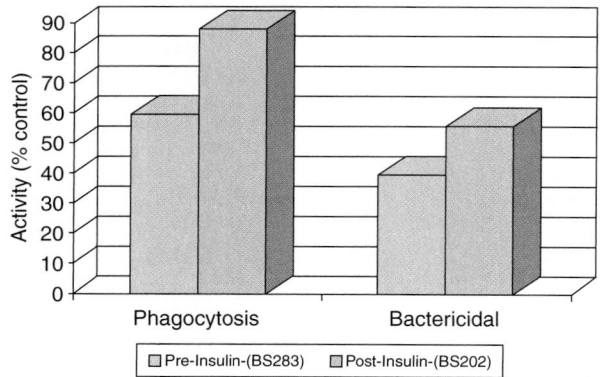

FIGURE 19-2 | *The effects of hyperglycemia on leukocytes obtained before and after implementation of insulin therapy. (From Grey, N.J.; Perdrizet, G.A. Reduction of nosocomial infections in the surgical intensive-care unit by strict glycemic control. Endocr Pract 10(Suppl 2):46–52, 2004.)*

therapy employed an insulin infusion to titrate blood glucose to 80 to 110 mg/dL. There was a significant reduction in sepsis (46%), acute renal failure (41%), and mechanical ventilation requirements. Overall in-hospital mortality (34%) and ICU mortality rates were substantially reduced as well[91] (Fig. 19-3).

Similar benefits of tight glycemic control have been found in other studies. In a study by Grey and Perdrizet, patients in a strict glucose control group had a mean blood glucose level of 125 mg/dL by use of an insulin infusion protocol. These patients had a 5- to 8-fold reduction in the incidence of sepsis, line infection, and surgical site infections compared with patients in the conventional group whose blood sugar was maintained at 180 mg/dL (Fig. 19-4). Hypoglycemia was rare, and there were no major adverse clinical complications such as myocardial infarction, stroke, or arrhythmia.[41]

Reports in the cardiovascular literature clearly document the benefit of glycemic control regarding surgical site infections. Sternal wound infections are a devastating complication in patients undergoing cardiovascular surgery. Studies show that hyperglycemia is a risk factor for sternal wound infections.[79,90] In an attempt to decrease deep sternal wound infection, several investigators use glycemic control protocols to lower blood glucose levels. Furnary and Zerr have used insulin infusion protocols in the last 20 years to achieve glucose readings below 200 mg/dL pre- and postoperatively.[36,97] During the late 1980s and 1990s their institution began an insulin infusion protocol for patients undergoing cardiovascular surgery. They documented a decrease in the incidence of sternal wound infection as glycemic control improved (Fig. 19-5). This study emphasizes the role of hyperglycemia and the importance of tight glycemic control in preventing surgical site infections.

For the multi-trauma patient in the critical care setting, an endocrinologist should play a role in managing the patient's hyperglycemia with an insulin infusion. This therapy is a safe and effective method of achieving euglycemia. There should be a protocol that includes when to start intravenous insulin, what are the target glucose levels, how to adjust the infusion for changes in blood sugar, and how to transition patients to subcutaneous insulin when they leave the ICU. Nurses should be educated about tight glycemic control in critically ill patients and how to utilize the protocol.

Tight glycemic control remains important after the transfer of the patient from the ICU. Transition from intravenous to subcutaneous insulin can be challenging. If the patient has had stable glucose readings over the past

FIGURE 19-3 | *Strict glycemic control reduces the number of days in the intensive care unit (ICU) and lowers hospital mortality rates. (From van den Berghe, G.; Wouters, P.; Weekers, F.; et al. Intensive insulin therapy in the critically ill patient. N Engl J Med 345:1359–1367, 2001.)*

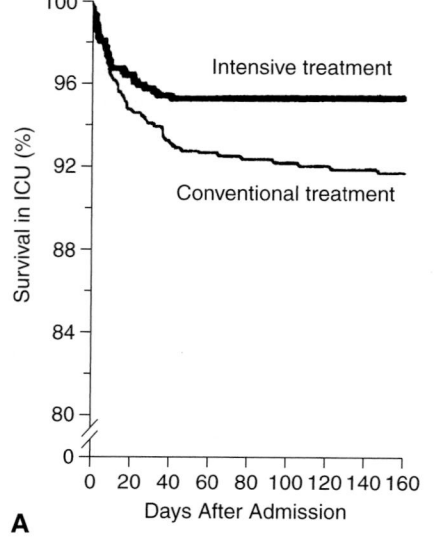

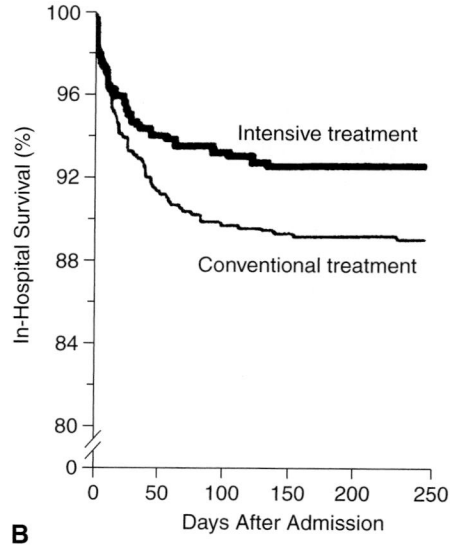

FIGURE 19-4 *Strict glycemic control reduces surgical site infection (SSI) as well as other nosocomial infections including intravenous device infection (IVDI), bloodstream infection (BSI), urinary tract infection (UTI), and nosocomial pneumonia (NP). (From Grey, N.J.; Perdrizet, G.A. Reduction of nosocomial infections in the surgical intensive-care unit by strict glycemic control. Endocr Pract 10(Suppl 2):46–52, 2004.)*

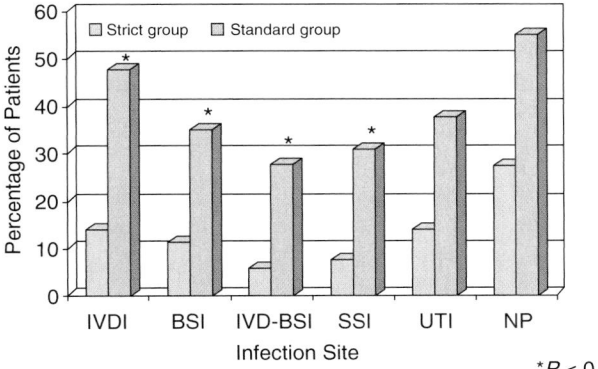

6 hours, the hourly insulin requirement can be extrapolated to 24 hours. Physiologic insulin replacement therapy can be achieved with the combination of basal and prandial insulin. Long-acting basal insulin (e.g., glargine, detemir) can be administered once in a 24-hour period. Basal insulin should constitute 50 percent of the insulin need. The other 50 percent is divided equally and is given before each meal. For example, if a patient requires 3 units of insulin in 1 hour, this is extrapolated to 72 units daily. Half of this, 36 units, would be administered as glargine in a daily dose. The remaining 36 units can be divided equally so that the patient receives 12 units of short-acting

FIGURE 19-5 *Implementation of continuous insulin infusion protocols reduces the rate of deep sternal wound infections (DSWIs). DM, diabetes mellitus. (From Furnary, A.P.; Zerr, K.J.; Grunkemeier, G.L.; et al. Continuous intravenous insulin infusion reduces the incidence of deep sternal wound infection in diabetic patients after cardiac surgical procedures. Ann Thorac Surg 67:352–360, 1999.)*

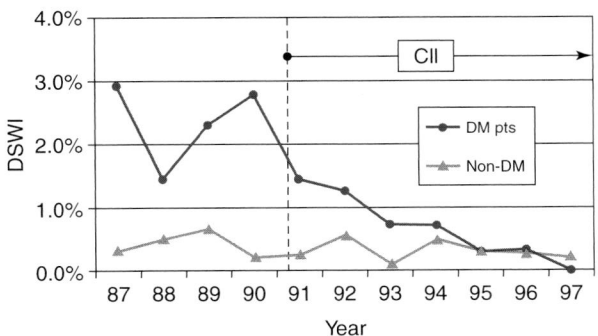

insulin with each meal. As the patient transitions from the ICU and the physiology as well as carbohydrate load changes, readjustment of this dose is necessary. Frequent blood glucose monitoring and a dedication to achieving blood glucose levels below 180 mg/dL are necessary to ensure that the patient is receiving adequate treatment for hyperglycemia during the perioperative period.

Physicians encounter two distinctly separate hyperglycemia scenarios. In the office, diabetic patients present a challenge to the traumatologists. Often patients need subacute care for simple fractures to complex revision work. Regardless of the procedure, diabetics with poor glycemic control are at increased risk for perioperative complications and infection. A thorough history, physical examination, and review of medications is necessary for the surgeon to gain a complete understanding of the patient as a whole. The surgeon needs to be aware of the increased risk of cardiovascular disease in these patients. Diabetic patients often need to be seen by their primary care doctor, cardiologist, or endocrinologist before undergoing fracture care. The surgeon can often be the link between the patient and the appropriate medical specialist. This should be viewed as a valuable time to educate patients regarding their disease and its implications. For elective procedures, dietary consultations and a referral to a primary care physician for diabetes counseling could save the patient and the surgeon from inappropriately selected and timed procedures. Once the patient is admitted to the hospital for a procedure, alterations in diet and metabolic stress in the perioperative period can severely affect blood glucose levels. Frequent pre- and postoperative fingersticks, appropriate insulin therapy, and perhaps a consultation with an endocrinologist are necessary to ensure strict glycemic control.

PERIOPERATIVE OXYGEN SUPPLEMENTATION AND TEMPERATURE REGULATION

When patients are under anesthesia, the fraction of inspired oxygen given is typically 30 to 50 percent. In the postoperative care unit, patients are typically placed on a nasal canula, which provides up to 40 percent Fio_2. The use of high concentrations of inspired oxygen in the operative and postoperative period to reduce surgical site infections has been investigated. For patients to receive a high Fio_2 of 80 percent, the anesthesiologist would have to administer a higher proportion of oxygen versus nitrogen oxide and the postoperative supplementation would require the use of masks with reservoir bags. The molecular basis for this practice is unknown, but enhancement of the NADPH oxygenase system has been implicated.

In 2000 Greif and Sessler presented a prospective double blind study testing the effects of 30 percent versus 80 percent inspired oxygen during the operation and for 2 hours postoperatively. The authors found a 6 percent reduction of postoperative infection in patients receiving 80 percent oxygen.[40] Pryor and co-workers provided evidence to the contrary.[78] In the latter study, the authors found perioperative oxygen to have deleterious effects, resulting in increased infection rates. This study has been the subject of much debate. Critics point to a number of biases and inadequate sample size. Pryor and co-workers did not report important controls such as temperature and fluid regulation. This inconsistency led Belda and co-workers to conduct another study in support of perioperative oxygen supplementation.[8] This double-blind, randomized, controlled study included 300 patients undergoing colorectal surgery. Double-blind investigators screened for the signs of infection for 14 days postoperatively. The risk of infection was 39 percent lower in the 80 percent Fio_2 group than for patients receiving 30 percent Fio_2.

Two of three studies indicate a reduction in surgical site infections with the use of high-concentration perioperative oxygen supplementation. Pooling the data of all three studies shows an absolute risk reduction of 7 percent and a relative risk reduction of 45 percent with 80 percent inspired oxygen during the perioperative period.[27] Oxygen supplementation is a low-cost, low-risk intervention and is supported by two well-conducted studies. Its effects can have major impacts on patient morbidity and health care costs.

Normothermia is best defined as a core temperature ranging from 36°C to 38°C (96.8°F to 100.4°F). Core temperature can be measured in the pulmonary artery and the distal esophagus. Rectal, oral, nasopharygeal, tympanic membrane, and skin temperature are more convenient methods of estimated core temperature values. Vasodilation from the anesthetic, cool ambient temperature, and skin and soft tissue exposed to a colder environment contribute to hypothermia (core temperature <36°C). Conditions that predispose patients to hypothermia must be recognized (Table 19-7). Hypothermia has been associated with an increase in surgical site infections. In the *New England Journal of Medicine*, Kurz presented a study of 200 patients undergoing colorectal surgery.[57] In the control group patients were warmed using traditional warming methods and had a core body temperature of 34.7°C and an infection rate of 19 percent. Conversely, patients who were actively warmed to an average core temperature of 36.6°C had a lower infection rate (6%). Hypothermia can be prevented with passive insulation using warmed cotton blankets, socks, head covering, limited skin exposure, circulating water mattresses, and increase in ambient room temperature. Active warming by warmed intravenous fluids and the use of forced air convection warming systems help achieve and maintain normothermia. Passive and active warming measures to achieve perioperative normothermia are of low cost and can lower infection rates.

PERIOPERATIVE ANTIBIOTICS

Surgical site infections occur from inoculation of bacteria into sterile wounds and inability of the immune system to eradicate the bacterial load. Pharmacologic agents can be used to decrease the bacterial count in wounds, thereby aiding the immune system in preventing infection. Lister, the first surgeon to understand this theory, used carbolic acid in an attempt to reduce infection rates. Before this time, the risk of surgical practice included a much higher rate of death and limb loss from infection. Antibiotics, along with aseptic techniques, radically changed the management of many disease entities. They, however, did not come without a price. Initially, the main concerns of antibiotic use were side effects and allergic responses. Table 19-8 reviews some of the toxicities of the more commonly used antibiotics. With the knowledge of these reactions, greater diversity of choices, and advancement of medical care, physicians have found ways to curtail these negative effects. Today we are faced with the new challenge of antibiotic resistance.

Antibiotics were initially used postoperatively, but their efficacy was questioned owing to their apparent failure to significantly reduce infection rates. In fact, some reports in the 1950s were against the use of antibiotics.[71] To test the ability of antimicrobials to prevent infection, Burke inoculated intradermal wounds of guinea pigs with staphylococci and found a reduction in infection rates when antibiotics were given prior to the inoculation. Burke concluded that an appropriate level of antibiotics must be in the wound prior to inoculation for the antibiotics to have a beneficial effect.[19] In 1976 Stone published a study of 400 patients undergoing gastric, biliary, and colonic operations. In this double-blind study were four treatment arms: patients receiving antibiotics 12 hours preoperatively, just prior to the incision, postoperatively, and no prophylactic antibiotics. The results showed a reduction in infection rates with the *preoperative* administration of antibiotics.[87] It appeared that Burke's work correlated with

Table 19-7
Risk Factors for Hypothermia
Extremes of age
Ambient room temperature
Significant fluid shifts
Use of general anesthesia
Use of regional anesthesia
Preexisting conditions (peripheral vascular disease, endocrine disease, pregnancy, burns, open wounds, etc.)
Female sex
Length and type of surgical procedure
Use of cold irrigates
Cachexia

Table 19-8	
Common Side Effects of Frequently Used Antibiotics	
Antibiotic Class	**Toxicity**
β-Lactams	CNS toxicity, bleeding, nephrotoxicity
Vancomycin	Histamine release
Aminoglycosides	Nephrotoxicity, ototoxicity, neuromuscular toxicity
Tetracyclines	Teeth, bones
Erythromycin	Hepatitis, gastrointestinal toxicity
Clindamycin	Colitis
Chloramphenicol	Gray syndrome, aplastic anemia, excreted in breast milk
Quinolones	CNS toxicity, arthroplasty, QT prolonged
Sulfonamides	Hemolytic anemia
Trimethoprim	Folate antagonism

clinical results. The time of incision must parallel the peak tissue levels of the given antibiotic. Adequate prophylaxis requires effective antibiotics at concentrations above the mean inhibitory concentration (MIC) of the organisms of concern at the time of incision and for the duration of the procedure. Ineffective antibiotic prophylaxis has been attributed to poor antibiotic selection and timing of administration.[77]

The orthopaedic literature provided similar evidence for the benefit of antibiotic prophylaxis. Campbel in 1965 and Fogelberg in 1970 studied the effects of penicillin on surgical site infections in orthopaedic procedures. In Fogelberg's prospective study, patients undergoing spinal fusion and mold arthroplasty benefited from preoperative administration of penicillin. The author attributed the lack of prophylaxis seen in other publications to poorly conducted retrospective studies that combined the results of multiple surgeons who used different antibiotics and administered them at variable times.[32] Shortly after Fogelberg's study, Boyd and Pavel published large double-blinded prospective studies that provided further support for the use of prophylactic antibiotics in orthopaedic procedures.[16,75]

Several years later, the use of antibiotic prophylaxis was still not settled and studies were being conducted concurrently, all attempting to establish the efficacy of antibiotics for surgical site infection prevention. Burnett and Tengve presented studies on antibiotic prophylaxis for hip fractures.[20,89] Both investigations used cephalothin as the agent of choice. Patients received antibiotics prior to the surgical incision and for 2 to 3 days postoperatively. The authors showed a statistically significant increase in infection rates in the placebo groups. Because of the variability in fracture care, Hill studied antibiotic prophylaxis in a more reproducible procedure: total hip arthroplasty. In their large double-blind prospective series of 2137 patients, Hill et al. observed a significant reduction in infections with the use of cefazolin.[48] These studies have provided the foundation for the use of preventative pharmaceuticals to reduce wound infections in orthopaedic surgery.

While most accept the concept that antibiotics are efficacious in orthopaedic surgery, debates continue regarding their exact role. Clinical studies are being conducted to establish the necessity of antibiotics in specific procedures.[73,88] Questions still exist regarding their use in arthroscopy and clean procedures that do not involve hardware placement. Many authors recognize that because of the low incidence of infection, very large trials or combined statistical analysis of previous studies is required to produce results with high statistical power. In an attempt to further support the use of antibiotics in fracture care, Boxma conducted a large, randomized, multicenter, double-blind prospective study of 2195 patients in the Dutch trauma trial. Using ceftriaxone, a significant reduction in superficial and deep wound infections along with an overall reduction in nosocomial infections was shown.[14] Perhaps the most all-encompassing review of the literature has been done by Gillespie and Walenkamp. The authors searched through the Cochrane database for trials that met the following inclusion criterion: any patient undergoing internal fixation or replacement arthroplasty receiving any regimen of systemic antibiotic prophylaxis. They produced a thorough analysis of the data from 22 trials. This review supported the use of antibiotic prophylaxis for patients undergoing surgery for closed fractures.[38] Table 19-9 represents some of the trials that support antibiotic prophylaxis. With this knowledge and the low incidence of complications, the use of antibiotics is advocated by the CDC and the AAOS.

Timing of Administration

The timing of antibiotic administration is of utmost importance. Burke's study was the first to show that antibiotics administered after an incision do little to protect the host.[19] In Stone's study, the group that showed a reduction rate was the arm that received antibiotics *prior* to the surgical incision.[87] The principal idea behind prophylaxis is reducing the bacterial load in the surgical incision and wound and assisting the immune system in eradicating the foreign organisms. The peak concentrations of nafcillin, cefazolin, and gentamicin in serum are within 20 minutes of injection. Although the absolute concentrations in bone are less than in serum, these antibiotics readily penetrated bone tissue with peak levels paralleling serum concentrations.[93] In a large prospective

		Table 19-9		
		Studies Supporting the Use of Preventive Antibiotics		
Study	**Year of Publication**	**Operative Intervention**	**Antibiotic Used**	**Experimental Group vs. Placebo**
Fogelberg et al.[32]	1970	Mold arthroplasty or spinal fusion	Penicillin	1.7% vs. 8.9%
Boyd et al.[16]	1973	Hip fracture	Nafcillin	0.8% vs. 4.8%
Pavel et al.[75]	1974	Clean orthopaedic procedures	Cephaloridine	2.8% vs. 5%
Tengve et al.[89]	1978	Hip fracture	Cephalothin Cephalexin	1.8% vs. 16.9%
Burnett et al.[20]	1980	Proximal femur	Cephalothin	0.7% vs. 4.7%
Hill et al.[48]	1981	Total hip arthroplasty	Cefazolin	0.9% vs. 3.3%
Bodoky et al.[12]	1993	Hip fracture	Cefotiam	1% vs. 5% deep 4% vs. 11% superficial
Boxma et al.[14]	1996	Closed fracture	Ceftriaxone	3.6% vs. 8.3%

study, Classen et al. monitored the timing of antibiotic prophylaxis in 2847 patients. There were four categories of therapy: treatment 2 to 24 hours before the procedure, 2 to 0 hours before the incision, after the start of the case, and 3 to 24 hours after the case was begun. Patients receiving antibiotics 2 hours before the incision had the lowest risk of wound infection (Fig. 19-6).[24]

Vancomycin and clindamycin are the two most popular alternatives for patients with a clear penicillin allergy. Clindamycin 600 mg IV diluted in 50 mL of normal saline given over 30 minutes should be administered for antibiotic prophylaxis. Vancomycin is diluted to at least 5 mg/mL and infused over at least 60 minutes. Fast IV administration of vancomycin can result in "red man" syndrome, which is characterized by sudden and/or profound hypotension during vancomycin IV infusion, with or without a maculopapular skin rash over the face, neck, chest, and extremities. Preoperative administration of antihistamines and prolonged infusions decrease the incidence of red man syndrome. The hypotension and rash usually resolve with the cessation of the infusion. Documented penicillin allergy, high local methicillin-resistant *S. aureus* (MRSA) prevalence, and ICU exposure are three circumstances for which vancomycin use is accepted.

The use of a surgical tourniquet requires administration of the full dose of antibiotics prior to exsanguination and tourniquet inflation. Reports in the literature vary from 2 to 20 minutes as the appropriate time interval needed for soft tissue and bone penetration of the given antibiotic.[6,29,35] We believe that as long as the patient receives the antibiotic prior to the induction of anesthesia in the operating room, adequate time passes while the patient is being sedated, positioned, prepped, and draped. This requires coordination among all staff members responsible for patient preparation prior to the induction of anesthesia. Patients requiring vancomycin or clindamycin that cannot be given as an intravenous bolus need to be identified and

given sufficient time to receive antibiotics prior to entering the operating room.

Although it may appear that most patients receive antibiotics in a timely manner, reports show that only 55.7 percent of patients receive antibiotics 1 hour prior to a procedure (Fig. 19-7).[17] Traditionally writing "on call" to the operating room alerted the nursing staff to start the antibiotics on the floor or in the preoperative holding area. Owing to delays and the vague roles of individuals in this process, this practice has not been effective. Health care workers may assume that another individual has already given the antibiotics. Also, if given too early, antibiotics with a short duration of activity may have low tissue levels during or at the end of the procedure.[28] Assigning the task of antibiotic administration to a specific member of the surgical team increases compliance and accountability. Requiring surgeons to order preoperative antibiotics and flagging patients who may require vancomycin or clindamycin are important for administering these antibiotics in a timely manner. Each facility must have a coordinated system that is reliable. At our institution, all patients must have a preoperative order for antibiotics when indicated. The antibiotics are sent from pharmacy and stored within the patient's chart. The anesthesiologist has been the responsible party for administrating the antibiotic prior to induction. Furthermore, we have begun to add antibiotics to our regular surgical time-out regimen before the start of a case to increase awareness and compliance.

Duration of Administration

The duration of antibiotic use has also been a topic of controversy. The grave consequence of implants seeded with bacteria has led many to place patients on antibiotics for prolonged periods of time postoperatively. This is especially true in the case of joint replacement and hemiarthroplasty where the results of infection lead to higher morbidity and mortality. On the other hand, using the principles introduced by Burke and studies in the last couple of decades, many surgeons have decreased their

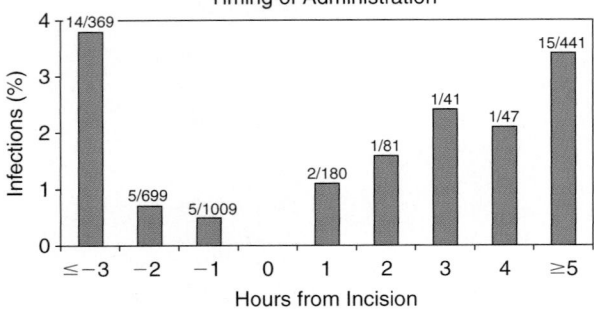

FIGURE 19-6 *Antibiotics given up to 2 hours preoperatively provided the largest reduction in infection rates. (From Classen, D.C.; Evans, R.S.; Pestotnik, S.; et al. The timing of prophylactic administration of antibiotics and the risk of surgical-wound infection. N Engl J Med 326:281–286, 1992.)*

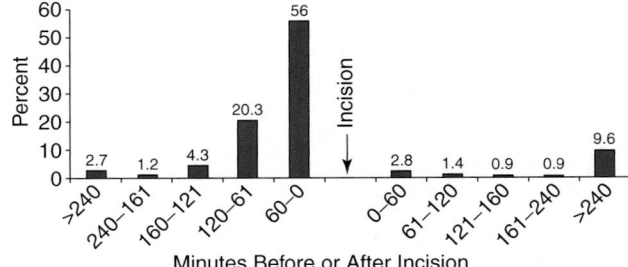

FIGURE 19-7 *Although it may appear that most patients today receive antibiotics at an appropriate time, in this study only 56 percent of patients received antibiotics 1 hour before the incision. (From Bratzler, D.W.; Houck, P.M.; Richards, C.; et al. Use of antimicrobial prophylaxis for major surgery: Baseline results from the National Surgical Infection Prevention Project. Arch Surg 149:174–182, 2005.)*

duration of postoperative antibiotics. This can be seen in the increasing number of patients undergoing outpatient surgery for procedures that in the past required inpatient admission for antibiotic administration. In the early 1980s Nelson recognized that in some of the earlier studies by Pavel, Fogelberg, and Boyde, the duration of antibiotics did not significantly alter the infection rate. Nelson conducted his own study of 358 patients undergoing total hip arthroplasty, total knee arthroplasty, and hip fracture repair and provided support that prolonged antibiotics had no additional benefit.[69] Nelson continued his advocacy of short duration of antibiotics when he and Heydemann published data on 466 patients undergoing joint replacement procedures. There was no difference in infection rates between patients given one intraoperative dose compared to those given 48 hours, 3 days, or 7 days of antibiotics postoperatively.[47]

Williams and Gustillo retrospectively looked at their hip and knee total arthroplasty records between 1975 and 1982. In 1980 they decreased the duration of postoperative antibiotics given in their practice and found no difference in their infection rates.[94] In the early 1990s Mauerhan and Bodoky addressed the same issue with double-blind prospective trials. Mauerhan studied the efficacy of 1 day of cefuroxime compared with 3 days of cefazolin in total joint arthroplasty and also found no statistical difference between the two regimens.[64] Bodoky compared two perioperative doses of cefotiam to placebo in hip fractures. The significant reduction in wound infections with just two doses of antibiotics suggests that longer durations of antibiotics are not justified.[12] Other surgical specialties have come to similar conclusions. Scher looked at 801 consecutive nonorthopaedic procedures and found that 1 g of cefazolin was adequate and administering antibiotics after the completion of the case provided no additional value.[82]

Of even greater importance has been the association of antibiotic selection and duration to microbial resistance. In Burnett's study, aside from a decrease in infection rates in the group receiving cephalothin, these patients showed an increase in bacterial resistance to cephalothin in blood, sputum, and urine cultures.[20] Harbarth studied the effects of prolonged antibiotics on surgical site infections and antibiotic resistance of patients undergoing coronary artery bypass grafting. Longer postoperative courses of antibiotics were associated with an increase in resistant microorganisms (odds ratio, 1.6) without any added benefit for surgical site infections. Despite increasing literature that supports a short duration of antibiotics and the concern of resistance, only 40.7 percent of antibiotics are discontinued within 24 hours of surgery[17] (Fig. 19-8). The current recommendation by the AAOS and SCIP is to discontinue the antimicrobial agent within 24 hours postoperatively.[21]

Antibiotic Selection

The antibiotic selected should have good bone and tissue penetration and provide bactericidal activity against the organisms commonly encountered. Antimicrobial activity above the MIC must be present for the duration of the procedure in bone and soft tissues. The bacteria most

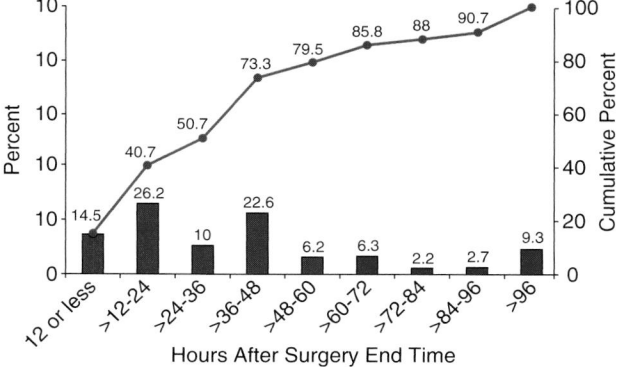

FIGURE 19-8 | *Only 26.2 percent of patients in this study had cessation of their antibiotics at the recommended 12- to 24-hour range despite multiple studies refuting the efficacy of prolonged antibiotics. (From Bratzler, D.W.; Houck, P.M.; Richards, C.; et al. Use of antimicrobial prophylaxis for major surgery: Baseline results from the National Surgical Infection Prevention Project. Arch Surg 149:174–182, 2005.)*

commonly found in orthopaedic surgery are *Staphylococcus* and *Streptococcus* species and occasionally gram-negative organisms. Anti-staphylococcal penicillin antibiotics have good activity against gram-positive organisms but poor activity against most gram-negative organisms. Second- and third-generation cephalosporins provide broad gram-negative coverage but are less efficacious against gram-positive bacteria. The first-generation cephalosporins have excellent bactericidal activity against gram-positive organisms and also provide some coverage for gram-negative and anaerobic organisms. This combined with the relatively few side effects makes cephalosporins an attractive choice for antibiotic prophylaxis in orthopaedic surgery.[31] Cephalosporins also have good tissue and bone penetration. The bone and serum concentrations of five cephalosporins can be seen in Table 19-10.[95] Figure 19-9 presents the serum and bone concentrations of cefazolin and at the same time provides the MIC_{50} and MIC_{90} of cefazolin against common bacterial flora.[95] Cunha et al. showed that 25 to 40 minutes after the injection of cefazolin, cephradine, and cephalothin, the peak bone levels were 60, 6.7, and 15 times the MIC of penicillin-resistant staphylococci, respectively.[25] Cefazolin has superior peak tissue levels and longer half-life than other first-generation cephalosporins, making it an excellent first choice for prophylaxis (Fig. 19-10). Vancomycin and clindamycin also provide good antibiotic activity against gram-positive organisms. Bone concentrations of 5.01 µg/mL are found 1.75 to 3.75 hours after a 300-mg intravenous injection of clindamycin.[5] Organisms sensitive to clindamycin have an MIC less than 1.6 µg/mL. Clindamycin is comparable to methicillin in penetrating bone and exceeding the MIC of gram-positive organisms that cause orthopaedic infections.[84] Vancomycin administered at 15 mg/kg results in cancellous bone concentrations of 2.3 µg/mL.

	1-g Dose, Mean Antibiotic Concentration		2-g Dose, Mean Antibiotic Concentration		Mean Time of Bone Sampling	
Antibiotic	Bone* (µg/g)	Serum† (µg/mL)	Bone* (µg/g)	Serum† (µg/mL)	1-g Dose	2-g Dose
Cephalothin	0.5	5.3	0.9*	31.5	91†	63‡
	(SD = 0.21)		(SD = 0.45)			
Cefazolin	5.9	51.7	14.9	98.3	69	51
Cefamandole	—		6.7	46.7	—	69
Cefoxitin	3.6	17.5	6.3	39.0	74	69
Ceforanide	9.1	67.8	13.4	144.0	62	82

Table 19-10

Bone and Serum Concentrations of Five Cephalosporins

*Statistically significant ($P < 0.01$); 1-g vs. 2-g antibiotic concentration.
†In minutes (after completion of intravenous drug administration).
‡Statistically significant ($P < 0.01$); timing of 1-g vs. 2-g sampling.
Source: From Williams, D.N.; Gustilo, R.B.; Beverly, R.; et al. Bone and serum concentrations of five cephalosporin drugs: Relevance to prophylaxis and treatment in orthopedic surgery. Clin Orthop Rela Res 179:253–265, 1983.

The MIC of vancomycin for *S. aureus* is approximately 1.0 µg/mL for methicillin-susceptible organisms, 1.5 µg/mL for methicillin-resistant strains, and 3.1 µg/mL for coagulase-negative staphylococci.[39] The bone penetration of vancomycin appears to be inferior to that of cephalosporins

and clindamycin. Nevertheless, concentrations do exceed the MIC of most organisms responsible for orthopaedic infections. A comprehensive table of the antibiotics used in surgery, their dosing, and redosing regimens is provided at http://www. and in Table 19-11.

FIGURE 19-9 *The bone and serum concentrations of cefazolin are well above the MIC$_{50}$ and MIC$_{90}$ of the most commonly found infectious organisms. (From Williams, D.N.; Gustilo, R.B.; Beverly, R.; et al. Bone and serum concentrations of five cephalosporin drugs: Relevance to prophylaxis and treatment in orthopedic surgery. Clin Orthop Rela Res 179:253–265, 1983.)*

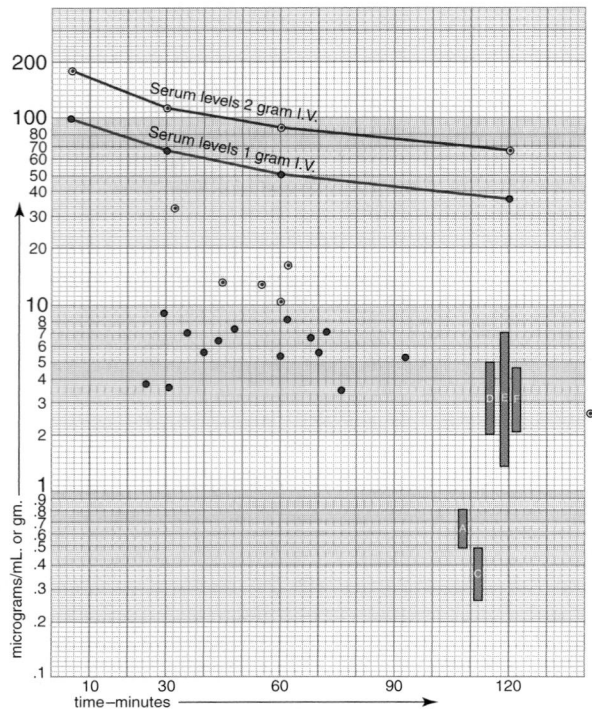

FIGURE 19-10 *Cefazolin is superior to other cephalosporins in the rate of peak serum concentration and duration of action. (From Cunha, B.A.; Gossling, H.R.; Pasternak, H.S.; et al. The penetration characteristics of cefazolin, cephalothin, and cephradine into bone in patients undergoing total hip replacement. J Bone Joint Surg Am 59:856–859, 1977.)*

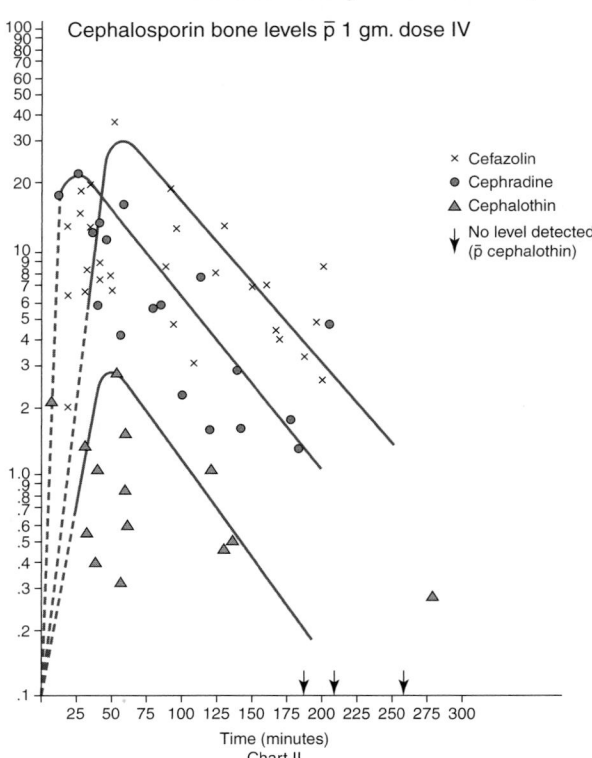

		Table 19-11				
Suggested Initial Dose and Time to Redosing for Antimicrobials Commonly Utilized for Surgical Prophylaxis						
Antimicrobial	**Half-life Normal Renal Function (hr)**	**Half-life End-stage Renal Disease (hr)**	**Recommended Infusion Time (min)**	**Standard Intravenous Dose (g)**	**Weight-based Dose Recommendation* (mg)**	**Recommended Redosing Interval† (hr)**
Aztreonam	1.5–2	6	3–5‡ 20–60§	1–2	Maximum 2 g (adult)	3–5
Ciprofloxacin	3.5–5	5–9	60	400 mg	400 mg	4–10
Cefazolin	1.2–2.5	40–70	3–5‡ 15–60§	1–2	20–30 mg/kg 1 g < 80 kg 2 g ≥ 80 kg	2–5
Cefuroxime	1–2	15–22	3–5‡ 15–60§	1.5	50 mg/kg	3–4
Cefamandole	0.5–2.1	12.3–18‖	3–5‡ 15–60§	1		3–4
Cefoxitin	0.5–1.1	6.5–23	3–5‡ 15–60§	1–2	20–40 mg/kg	2–3
Cefotetan	2.8–4.6	13–25	3–5‡ 20–60§	1–2	20–40 mg/kg	3–6
Clindamycin	2–5.1	3.5–5.0¶	10–60 (do not exceed 30 mg/min)	600–900 mg	< 10 kg: at least 37.5 mg, ≥10 kg: 3–6 mg/kg	3–6
Erythromycin base	0.8–3	5–6	NA	1 g orally 19, 18, 9 hours before surgery	9–13 mg/kg	NA
Gentamicin	2–3	50–70	30–60	1.5 mg/kg#	See footnote ††	3–6
Neomycin	2–3 hr (3% absorbed under normal gastrointestinal conditions)	12–24 or greater	NA	1 g orally 19, 18, 9 hours before surgery	20 mg/kg	NA
Metronidazole	6–14	7–21; no change	30–60	0.5–1	15 mg/kg (adult) 7.5 mg/kg on subsequent doses	6–8
Vancomycin	4–6	44.1–406.4 (Cl$_{cr}$<10 mL/min)	1 g over 60 minutes (use longer infusion time if dose >1 g)	1.0	10–15 mg/kg (adult)	6–12

*Weight-based doses are primarily from published pediatric recommendations.
†For procedures of long duration, antimicrobials should be redosed at intervals of 1–2 times the half-life of the drug. The intervals in the table were calculated for patients with normal renal function.
‡Dose injected directly into vein or running intravenous fluids.
§Intermittent intravenous infusion.
‖In patients with serum creatinine 5–9 mg/dL.
¶The half-life of clindamycin is the same or slightly increased in patients with end-stage renal disease as compared with patients with normal renal function.
#If the patient's weight is more than 30% above ideal body weight (IBW), dosing weight (DW) can be determined as follows: DW = IBW + 0.4(total body weight − IBW).
From MedQIC. Available at: http://www.medqic.org.

Local Antibiotic Delivery

Local antibiotic delivery systems provide higher tissue antibiotic concentrations without systemic side effects. Antibiotic-loaded cement has been used for local delivery of high concentrations of antibiotics for osteomyelitis and infected total joint arthroplasty. High-dose antibiotic-impregnated cement is currently a clinician-directed application to achieve *therapeutic* levels of local antibiotics. This practice appears to adversely impact the biomechanical properties of cement, and thus the application is in the form of spacers and beads.[44] Low-dose antibiotic bone cement is an FDA-approved product available for prophylaxis against deep wound infection. Low doses of antibiotics (<2 g/40 g of cement) do not appear to affect the biomechanical properties of cement.[13] The prophylactic use of this product for all procedures is under debate, and its current use is accepted for patients who are at an increased risk of infection particularly in total joint replacements. Antibiotic resistance and adverse effects on biomechanical properties are the main obstacles to this delivery system, and diligent postmarket surveillance is necessary to confirm preclinical and clinical trials.[13]

Alternative biodegradable delivery products including bone graft substitutes and natural and synthetic polymers are under study for musculoskeletal infections.[44] In 2005, using a goat fracture model, Beardmore et al. showed that tobramycin-impregnated calcium sulfate pellets and demineralized bone matrix were effective in preventing intramedullary *S. aureus* infection in open fractures. Polymer implant coating is an alternative means of delivering local antibiotics. Several in vitro studies have shown the potential of these products.[83] Preliminary results of a clinical trial of open tibia fractures treated with unreamed tibial nails (UTNs) coated with poly(D,L) lactic acid (PDLLA) and gentamicin are promising. Further in vitro and in vivo testing is required before these products can be considered for prophylactic use in orthopaedic procedures.

Coating suture material with antibacterial compounds is another means of reducing surgical site infections. Triclosan-coated suture material inhibits bacterial growth in in vitro studies.[80] Animal studies and early human trials show that triclosan-coated sutures are safe and do not affect the suture characteristics.[7,33] No clinical trials supporting the efficacy of antibacterial sutures exist. If all recommended infection prevention guidelines are followed, a very large clinical study would need to be conducted to show a statistically significant reduction in infection rates using antibacterial sutures.

SUMMARY

Surgical site infections cause significant morbidity and mortality. Infections affect the quality of care and have a major socioeconomic impact. Society and governmental agencies expect physicians to take responsibility in reducing preventable infections by adhering to guidelines set by panels of experts in surgical site infection prevention. Appropriate use of antibiotics, glycemic control, oxygen supplementation, normothermia, and asepsis are actions that are under the control of the treating physician. Surgical planning should include the necessary steps to prevent infection.

REFERENCES

1. Ahl, T.; Dalen, N.; Jorbeck, H.; et al. Air contamination during hip and knee arthroplasties: Horizontal laminar flow randomized vs. conventional ventilation. Acta Orthop Scand 66:17–20, 1995.
2. Allo, M.D.; Tedesco, M. Operating room management: Operative suite considerations, infection control. Surg Clin North Am 85:1291–1297, xii, 2005.
3. Al-Maiyah, M.; Bajwa, A.; Mackenney, P.; et al. Glove perforation and contamination in primary total hip arthroplasty. J Bone Joint Surg Br 87:556–559, 2005.
4. Aly, R.; Maibach, H.I. Comparative antibacterial efficacy of a 2-minute surgical scrub with chlorhexidine gluconate, povidone-iodine, and chloroxylenol spongebrushes. Am J Infect Control 16:173–177, 1988.
5. Baird, P.; Hughes, S.; Sullivan, M.; et al. Penetration into bone and tissues of clindamycin phosphate. Postgrad Med J 54:65–67, 1978.
6. Bannister, G.C.; Auchincloss, J.M.; Johnson, D.P.; et al. The timing of tourniquet application in relation to prophylactic antibiotic administration. J Bone Joint Surg Br 70:322–324, 1988.
7. Barbolt, T.A. Chemistry and safety of triclosan, and its use as an antimicrobial coating on Coated VICRYL* Plus Antibacterial Suture (coated polyglactin 910 suture with triclosan). Surg Infect (Larchmt) 3 (Suppl 1):S45–S53, 2003.
8. Belda, F.J.; Aguilera, L.; Garcia de la Asuncion, J.; et al. Supplemental perioperative oxygen and the risk of surgical wound infection: A randomized controlled trial. JAMA 294:2035–2042, 2005.
9. Bibbo, C.; Patel, D.V.; Gehrmann, R.M.; et al. Chlorhexidine provides superior skin decontamination in foot and ankle surgery: A prospective randomized study. Clin Orthop Relat Res 438:204–208, 2005.
10. Bilgin, Y.M.; van de Watering, L.M.; Eijsman, L.; et al. Double-blind, randomized controlled trial on the effect of leukocyte-depleted erythrocyte transfusions in cardiac valve surgery. Circulation 109:2755–2760, 2004.
11. Boden, G. Free fatty acids, insulin resistance, and type 2 diabetes mellitus. Proc Assoc Am Physicians 111:241–248, 1999.
12. Bodoky, A.; Neff, U.; Heberer, M.; et al. Antibiotic prophylaxis with two doses of cephalosporin in patients managed with internal fixation for a fracture of the hip. J Bone Joint Surg Am 75:61–65, 1993.
13. Bourne, R.B. Prophylactic use of antibiotic bone cement: An emerging standard: In the affirmative. J Arthroplasty 19:69–72, 2004.
14. Boxma, H.; Broekhuizen, T.; Patka, P.; et al. Randomised controlled trial of single-dose antibiotic prophylaxis in surgical treatment of closed fractures: The Dutch Trauma Trial. Lancet 347:1133–1137, 1996.
15. Boyce, J.M.; Pittet, D. Guideline for hand hygiene in health-care settings: Recommendations of the Healthcare Infection Control Practices Advisory Committee and the HIPAC/SHEA/APIC/IDSA Hand Hygiene Task Force. Am J Infect Control 30:S1–S46, 2002.
16. Boyd, R.J.; Burke, J.F.; Colton, T. A double-blind clinical trial of prophylactic antibiotics in hip fractures. J Bone Joint Surg Am 55:1251–1258, 1973.
17. Bratzler, D.W.; Houck, P.M.; Richards, C.; et al. Use of antimicrobial prophylaxis for major surgery: Baseline results from the National Surgical Infection Prevention Project. Arch Surg 149:174–182, 2005.
18. Bryce, E.A.; Spence, D.; Roberts, F.J. An in-use evaluation of an alcohol-based pre-surgical hand disinfectant. Infect Control Hosp Epidemiol 22:635–639, 2001.
19. Burke, J.F. The effective period of preventive antibiotic action in experimental incisions and dermal lesions. Surgery 50:161–168, 1961.
20. Burnett, J.W.; Gustilo, R.B.; Williams, D.N.; et al. Prophylactic antibiotics in hip fractures: A double-blind, prospective study. J Bone Joint Surg Am 62:457–462, 1980.
21. Calhoun, J.H. Use of antibiotic prophylaxis in primary TJA: AAOS Board adopts advisory statement. Available at: http://www2.aaos.org/aaos/archives/bulletin/aug04/fline2.htm.

22. Charnley, J.; Eftekhar, N. Postoperative infection in total prosthetic replacement arthroplasty of the hip-joint: With special reference to the bacterial content of the air of the operating room. Br J Surg 56:641–649, 1969.

23. Cheng, S.M.; Garcia, M.; Espin, S.; et al. Literature review and survey comparing surgical scrub techniques. AORN J 74:218, 221–224, 2001.

24. Classen, D.C.; Evans, R.S.; Pestotnik, S.; et al. The timing of prophylactic administration of antibiotics and the risk of surgical-wound infection. N Engl J Med 326:281–286, 1992.

25. Cunha, B.A.; Gossling, H.R.; Pasternak, H.S.; et al. The penetration characteristics of cefazolin, cephalothin, and cephradine into bone in patients undergoing total hip replacement. J Bone Joint Surg Am 59:856–859, 1977.

26. Delamaire, M.; Maugendre, D.; Moreno, M.; et al. Impaired leukocyte functions in diabetic patients. Diabet Med 14:29–34, 1997.

27. Dellinger, E.P. Increasing inspired oxygen to decrease surgical site infection: Time to shift the quality improvement research paradigm. JAMA 294:2091–2092, 2005.

28. DiPiro, J.T.; Vallner, J.J.; Bowden, T.A., Jr.; et al. Intraoperative serum and tissue activity of cefazolin and cefoxitin. Arch Surg 120:829–832, 1985.

29. Dounis, E.; Tsourvakas, S.; Kalivas, L.; et al. Effect of time interval on tissue concentrations of cephalosporins after tourniquet inflation: Highest levels achieved by administration 20 minutes before inflation. Acta Orthop Scand 66:158–160, 1995.

30. Edwards, P.S.; Lipp, A.; Holmes, A. Preoperative skin antiseptics for preventing surgical wound infections after clean surgery. Cochrane Database Syst Rev 3:CD003949, 2004.

31. Fitzgerald, R.H., Jr.; Thompson, R.L. Cephalosporin antibiotics in the prevention and treatment of musculoskeletal sepsis. J Bone Joint Surg Am 65:1201–1205, 1983.

32. Fogelberg, E.V.; Zitzmann, E.K.; Stinchfield, F.E. Prophylactic penicillin in orthopaedic surgery. J Bone Joint Surg Am 52:95–98, 1970.

33. Ford, H.R.; Jones, P.; Gaines, B.; et al. Intraoperative handling and wound healing: Controlled clinical trial comparing coated VICRYL plus antibacterial suture (coated polyglactin 910 suture with triclosan) with coated VICRYL suture (coated polyglactin 910 suture). Surg Infect (Larchmt) 6:313–321, 2005.

34. Frankenfield, D.C.; Omert, L.A.; Badellino, M.M.; et al. Correlation between measured energy expenditure and clinically obtained variables in trauma and sepsis patients. JPEN J Parenter Enteral Nutr 18:398–403, 1994.

35. Friedman, R.J.; Friedrich, L.V.; White, R.L.; et al. Antibiotic prophylaxis and tourniquet inflation in total knee arthroplasty. Clin Orthop 260:17–23, 1990.

36. Furnary, A.P.; Zerr, K.J.; Grunkemeier, G.L.; et al. Continuous intravenous insulin infusion reduces the incidence of deep sternal wound infection in diabetic patients after cardiac surgical procedures. Ann Thorac Surg 67:352–360, 1999; discussion 67:360–362, 1999.

37. Garibaldi, R.A.; Skolnick, D.; Lerer, T.; et al. The impact of preoperative skin disinfection on preventing intraoperative wound contamination. Infect Control Hosp Epidemiol 9:109–113, 1988.

38. Gillespie, W.J.; Walenkamp, G. Antibiotic prophylaxis for surgery for proximal femoral and other closed long bone fractures. Cochrane Database Syst Rev 1: CD000244, 2001.

39. Graziani, A.L.; Lawson, L.A.; Gibson, G.A.; et al. Vancomycin concentrations in infected and noninfected human bone. Antimicrob Agents Chemother 32:1320–1322, 1988.

40. Greif, R.; Sessler, D.I. Supplemental oxygen and risk of surgical site infection. JAMA 291:1957, 2004; author reply 291:1958–1959, 2004.

41. Grey, N.J.; Perdrizet, G.A. Reduction of nosocomial infections in the surgical intensive-care unit by strict glycemic control. Endocr Pract 10(Suppl 2):46–52, 2004.

42. Gruenberg, M.F.; Campaner, G.L.; Sola, C.A.; et al. Ultraclean air for prevention of postoperative infection after posterior spinal fusion with instrumentation: A comparison between surgeries performed with and without a vertical exponential filtered air-flow system. Spine 29:2330–2334, 2004.

43. Hansen, D.; Krabs, C.; Benner, D.; et al. Laminar air flow provides high air quality in the operating field even during real operating conditions, but personal protection seems to be necessary in operations with tissue combustion. Int J Hyg Environ Health 208:455–460, 2005.

44. Hanssen, A.D. Prophylactic use of antibiotic bone cement: An emerging standard: In opposition. J Arthroplasty 19:73–77, 2004.

45. Hayek, L.J.; Emerson, J.M.; Gardner, A.M. A placebo-controlled trial of the effect of two preoperative baths or showers with chlorhexidine detergent on postoperative wound infection rates. J Hosp Infect 10:165–172, 1987.

46. Hennessey, P.J.; Black, C.T.; Andrassy, R.J. Nonenzymatic glycosylation of immunoglobulin G impairs complement fixation. JPEN J Parenter Enteral Nutr 15:60–64, 1991.

47. Heydemann, J.S.; Nelson, C.L. Short-term preventive antibiotics. Clin Orthop Relat Res 205:84–87, 1986.

48. Hill, C.; Flamant, R.; Mazas, F.; et al. Prophylactic cefazolin versus placebo in total hip replacement: Report of a multicentre double-blind randomised trial. Lancet 1:795–796, 1981.

49. Hotamisligil, G.S.; Spiegelman, B.M. Tumor necrosis factor alpha: A key component of the obesity-diabetes link. Diabetes 43:1271–1278, 1994.

50. Innerhofer, P.; Klingler, A.; Klimmer, C.; et al. Risk for postoperative infection after transfusion of white blood cell–filtered allogeneic or autologous blood

components in orthopedic patients undergoing primary arthroplasty. Transfusion 45:103–110, 2005.

51. Innerhofer, P.; Walleczek, C.; Luz, G.; et al. Transfusion of buffy coat–depleted blood components and risk of postoperative infection in orthopedic patients. Transfusion 39:625–632, 1999.

52. Jensen, L.S.; Kissmeyer-Nielsen, P.; Wolff, B.; et al. Randomised comparison of leukocyte-depleted versus buffy-coat–poor blood transfusion and complications after colorectal surgery. Lancet 348:841–845, 1996.

53. Keblish, D.J.; Zurakowski, D.; Wilson, M.G.; et al. Preoperative skin preparation of the foot and ankle: Bristles and alcohol are better. J Bone Joint Surg Am 87:986–992, 2005.

54. Kirkland, K.B.; Briggs, J.P.; Trivette, S.L.; et al. The impact of surgical-site infections in the 1990s: Attributable mortality, excess length of hospitalization, and extra costs. Infect Control Hosp Epidemiol 20:725–730, 1999.

55. Knobben, B.A.; van Horn, J.R.; van der Mei, H.C.; et al. Evaluation of measures to decrease intraoperative bacterial contamination in orthopaedic implant surgery. J Hosp Infect 62:174–180, 2006.

56. Kozak, L.J.; Owings, M.F.; Hall, M.J. National Hospital Discharge Survey: 2002 annual summary with detailed diagnosis and procedure data. Vital Health Stat 13:1–199, 2005.

57. Kurz, A.; Sessler, D.I.; Lenhardt, R. Perioperative normothermia to reduce the incidence of surgical-wound infection and shorten hospitalization: Study of Wound Infection and Temperature Group. N Engl J Med 334:1209–1215, 1996.

58. Laine, T.; Aarnio, P. Glove perforation in orthopaedic and trauma surgery: A comparison between single, double indicator gloving and double gloving with two regular gloves. J Bone Joint Surg Br 86:898–900, 2004.

59. Larson, E.L.; Butz, A.M.; Gullette, D.L.; et al. Alcohol for surgical scrubbing? Infect Control Hosp Epidemiol 11:139–143, 1990.

60. Leigh, D.A.; Stronge, J.L.; Marriner, J.; et al. Total body bathing with "Hibiscrub" (chlorhexidine) in surgical patients: A controlled trial. J Hosp Infect 4:229–235, 1983.

61. Leonas, K.K.; Jinkins, R.S. The relationship of selected fabric characteristics and the barrier effectiveness of surgical gown fabrics. Am J Infect Control 25:16–23, 1997.

62. Lidwell, O.M.; Elson, R.A.; Lowbury, E.J.; et al. Ultraclean air and antibiotics for prevention of postoperative infection: A multicenter study of 8,052 joint replacement operations. Acta Orthop Scand 58:4–13, 1987.

63. Mangram, A.J.; Horan, T.C.; Pearson, M.L.; et al. Guideline for Prevention of Surgical Site Infection, 1999: Centers for Disease Control and Prevention (CDC) Hospital Infection Control Practices Advisory Committee. Am J Infect Control 27:97–132, 1999.

64. Mauerhan, D.R.; Nelson, C.L.; Smith, D.L.; et al. Prophylaxis against infection in total joint arthroplasty:

One day of cefuroxime compared with three days of cefazolin. J Bone Joint Surg Am 76:39–45, 1994.

65. McCowen, K.C.; Malhotra, A.; Bistrian, B.R. Stress-induced hyperglycemia. Crit Care Clin 17:107–124, 2001.

66. McCue, S.F.; Berg, E.W.; Saunders, E.A. Efficacy of double-gloving as a barrier to microbial contamination during total joint arthroplasty. J Bone Joint Surg Am 63:811–813, 1981.

67. Mizock, B.A. Alterations in carbohydrate metabolism during stress: A review of the literature. Am J Med 98:75–84, 1995.

68. Mowat, A.; Baum, J. Chemotaxis of polymorphonuclear leukocytes from patients with diabetes mellitus. N Engl J Med 284:621–627, 1971.

69. Nelson, C.L.; Green, T.G.; Porter, R.A.; et al. One day versus seven days of preventive antibiotic therapy in orthopedic surgery. Clin Orthop Relat Res 176:258–263, 1983.

70. Nielson, C.P.; Hindson, D.A. Inhibition of polymorphonuclear leukocyte respiratory burst by elevated glucose concentrations in vitro. Diabetes 38:1031–1035, 1989.

71. Oishi, C.S.; Carrion, W.V.; Hoaglund, F.T. Use of parenteral prophylactic antibiotics in clean orthopaedic surgery: A review of the literature. Clin Orthop Relat Res 296:249–255, 1993.

72. Ostrander, R.V.; Botte, M.J.; Brage, M.E. Efficacy of surgical preparation solutions in foot and ankle surgery. J Bone Joint Surg Am 87:980–985, 2005.

73. Paiement, G.D.; Renaud, E.; Dagenais, G.; et al. Double-blind randomized prospective study of the efficacy of antibiotic prophylaxis for open reduction and internal fixation of closed ankle fractures. J Orthop Trauma 8:64–66, 1994.

74. Parienti, J.J.; Thibon, P.; Heller, R.; et al. Hand-rubbing with an aqueous alcoholic solution vs. traditional surgical hand-scrubbing and 30-day surgical site infection rates: A randomized equivalence study. JAMA 288:722–727, 2002.

75. Pavel, A.; Smith, R.L.; Ballard, A.; et al. Prophylactic antibiotics in clean orthopaedic surgery. J Bone Joint Surg Am 56:777–782, 1974.

76. Perl, T.M.; Cullen, J.J.; Wenzel, R.P.; et al. Intranasal mupirocin to prevent postoperative *Staphylococcus aureus* infections. N Engl J Med 346:1871–1877, 2002.

77. Polk, H.C., Jr.; Trachtenberg, L.; Finn, M.P. Antibiotic activity in surgical incisions: The basis of prophylaxis in selected operations. JAMA 244:1353–1354, 1980.

78. Pryor, K.O.; Fahey, T.J., 3rd; Lien, C.A.; et al. Surgical site infection and the routine use of perioperative hyperoxia in a general surgical population: A randomized controlled trial. JAMA 291:79–87, 2004.

79. Ridderstolpe, L.; Gill, H.; Granfeldt, H.; et al. Superficial and deep sternal wound complications: Incidence, risk factors and mortality. Eur J Cardiothorac Surg 20:1168–1175, 2001.

80. Rothenburger, S.; Spangler, D.; Bhende, S.; et al. In vitro antimicrobial evaluation of Coated VICRYL* Plus Antibacterial Suture (coated polyglactin 910 with triclosan) using zone of inhibition assays. Surg Infect (Larchmt) 3(Suppl 1):S79–S87, 2002.

81. Rutala, W.A.; Weber, D.J. A review of single-use and reusable gowns and drapes in health care. Infect Control Hosp Epidemiol 22:248–257, 2001.

82. Scher, K.S. Studies on the duration of antibiotic administration for surgical prophylaxis. Am Surg 63:59–62, 1997.

83. Schmidmaier, G.; Lucke, M.; Wildemann, B.; et al. Prophylaxis and treatment of implant-related infections by antibiotic-coated implants: A review. Injury 37:S105–S112, 2006.

84. Schurman, D.J.; Johnson, B.L., Jr.; Finerman, G.; et al. Antibiotic bone penetration: Concentrations of methicillin and clindamycin phosphate in human bone taken during total hip replacement. Clin Orthop Relat Res 111:142–146, 1975.

85. Silverstein, P. Smoking and wound healing. Am J Med 93:22S–24S, 1992.

86. Sorensen, L.T.; Karlsmark, T.; Gottrup, F. Abstinence from smoking reduces incisional wound infection: A randomized controlled trial. Ann Surg 238:1–5, 2003.

87. Stone, H.H.; Hooper, C.A.; Kolb, L.D.; et al. Antibiotic prophylaxis in gastric, biliary and colonic surgery. Ann Surg 184:443–452, 1976.

88. Tanner, J.; Woodings, D.; Moncaster, K. Preoperative hair removal to reduce surgical site infection. Cochrane Database Syst Rev 3:CD004122, 2006.

89. Tengve, B.; Kjellander, J. Antibiotic prophylaxis in operations on trochanteric femoral fractures. J Bone Joint Surg Am 60:97–99, 1978.

90. Trick, W.E.; Scheckler, W.E.; Tokars, J.I.; et al. Modifiable risk factors associated with deep sternal site infection after coronary artery bypass grafting. J Thorac Cardiovasc Surg 119:108–114, 2000.

91. Van den Berghe, G.; Wouters, P.; Weekers, F.; et al. Intensive insulin therapy in the critically ill patient. N Engl J Med 345:1359–1367, 2001.

92. Wertheim, H.F.; Vos, M.C.; Ott, A.; et al. Mupirocin prophylaxis against nosocomial *Staphylococcus aureus* infections in nonsurgical patients: A randomized study. Ann Intern Med 140:419–425, 2004.

93. Wiggins, C.E.; Nelson, C.L.; Clarke, R.; et al. Concentration of antibiotics in normal bone after intravenous injection. J Bone Joint Surg Am 60:93–96, 1978.

94. Williams, D.N.; Gustilo, R.B. The use of preventive antibiotics in orthopaedic surgery. Clin Orthop Relat Res 190:83–88, 1984.

95. Williams, D.N.; Gustilo, R.B.; Beverly, R.; et al. Bone and serum concentrations of five cephalosporin drugs: Relevance to prophylaxis and treatment in orthopedic surgery. Clin Orthop Relat Res 179:253–265, 1983.

96. Zdeblick, T.A.; Lederman, M.M.; Jacobs, M.R.; et al. Preoperative use of povidone-iodine: A prospective, randomized study. Clin Orthop Relat Res 213:211–215, 1986.

97. Zerr, K.J.; Furnary, A.P.; Grunkemeier, G.L.; et al. Glucose control lowers the risk of wound infection in diabetics after open heart operations. Ann Thorac Surg 63:356–361, 1997.

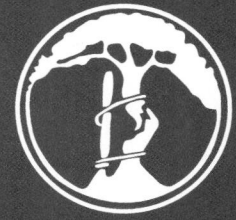

CHAPTER 20

Diagnosis and Treatment of Complications

Craig S. Roberts, M.D., Gregory E. Gleis, M.D., and David Seligson, M.D.

A *complication* is a disease process that occurs in addition to a principal illness. In the lexicon of diagnosis-related groupings, *complications* are co-morbidities. However, a broken bone plate complicating the healing of a radius shaft fracture hardly seems to fit either of these definitions. In orthopaedic trauma terminology, the term *complication* has come to mean an undesired turn of events specific to the care of a particular injury. Complications can be *local* or *systemic* and are caused by, among other things, physiologic processes, errors in judgment, or fate. Codivilla described complications as "inconveniences."[62] A colleague once described a pin tract infection with external fixation as a *problem*, not a complication. Preventing pin tract drainage is indeed a problem that needs a solution, but when it occurs in a patient, it becomes a complication. Additional terminology has been introduced by the Joint Commission on the Accreditation of Healthcare Organizations, such as the "sentinel event," a type of major complication that involves unexpected occurrences such as limb loss, surgery on the wrong body part, and hemolytic transfusion reaction.

Fracture care today demands perfection. These unrealistic expectations lead in part to the current adverse medicolegal situation surrounding the care of broken bones. There are many scales for judging the quality of results but none for complications. As a starter, operative misadventures can be classified as follows: (1) unexpected events that just slow things down—like contaminating a reamer; (2) events that change the operation but have no long-term consequences—like breaking a drill bit, and (3) events that cause long-term harm—like cutting a nerve.

This chapter presents current knowledge about three *systemic* complications (fat embolism syndrome, thromboembolic disorders, and multiple organ system dysfunction and failure) and five *local* complications of fractures (soft tissue damage, vascular problems, post-traumatic arthrosis, peripheral nerve injury, and complex regional pain syndrome [reflex sympathetic dystrophy]).

SYSTEMIC COMPLICATIONS
Fat Embolism Syndrome

Fat embolism syndrome (FES) is the occurrence of hypoxia, confusion, and petechiae a few days after a long bone fracture. FES is distinct from post-traumatic pulmonary insufficiency, shock lung, and adult respiratory distress syndrome (ARDS). When known etiologic factors of post-traumatic pulmonary insufficiency such as pulmonary contusion, inhalation pneumonitis, oxygen toxicity, and transfusion lung are excluded, there remains a group of patients who have FES with unanticipated respiratory compromise several days following a long bone fracture.

Fat embolism was first described by Zenker in 1861 in a railroad worker who sustained a thoracoabdominal crush injury.[383] It was initially hypothesized that the fat from the marrow space embolized to the lungs and caused the pulmonary damage.[323] Fenger and Salisbury believed that fat embolized from fractures to the brain, resulting in death.[96] Von Bergmann first clinically diagnosed fat embolism in a patient with a fractured femur in 1873.[362] The incidence of this now recognized complication of long bone fracture was extensively documented by Talucci and co-workers in 1913 and subsequently studied during World Wars I and II and the Korean conflict.[347] Mullins described the findings in patients who died as "lungs that looked like liver."[234] Wong et al. reported on the use of continuous pulse oximeter monitoring (CPOM) and daily intermittent arterial blood gas (ABG) to define the incidence pattern and severity of long bone fractures compared with controls; they found that long bone fracture patients had more desaturation episodes, longer duration total desaturation, and larger total area under desaturation curves in both the postfracture and the prefracture period.[378]

Although the fat in the lungs comes from bone, other processes are required to produce the physiologic damage to lung, brain, and other tissues. Although the term *fat embolism syndrome* does not describe the pathomechanics of this condition as was originally hypothesized, embolization of active substances and fat from the injured marrow space has traditionally been thought to be the source of embolic fat. Recent studies suggest otherwise. Mudd and associates did not observe any myeloid tissue in any of the lung fields at autopsy in patients with fat embolism syndrome and suggested that the soft tissue injury, rather than fractures, was the primary cause of fat embolism syndrome.[231] Ten Duis in a review of the literature stated

545

that "future attempts to unravel this syndrome...should pay full attention to differences in the extent of accompanying soft tissue injuries that surround a long bone fracture."[348] In a laboratory rabbit model, Aydin et al. found that pulmonary contusion had more deleterious effects than fractures in the formation of cerebral fat embolism.[11]

Although there are many unanswered questions about FES, several issues are apparent. It strikes the young, whereas older patients with significant upper femoral fractures do not seem at risk. It usually occurs after lower, not upper, limb fractures, and is more frequent with closed fractures.[64] Russell and associates reported a case of fat embolism in an isolated humerus fracture.[303] McDermott et al. reported three cases of patients with tibial fractures from football injuries who also had dehydration and developed fat embolism syndrome, and they concluded that adequate preoperative hydration, especially if injuries were sustained during heavy exercise, may reduce the risk of developing fat embolism syndrome.[208] In a prospective study, Chan and associates found an incidence of 8.75 percent of overt FES in all fracture patients, with a mortality rate of 2.5 percent.[56] The incidence rose to 35 percent in patients with multiple fractures. Other investigators reported the incidence of FES between 0.9 and 3.5 percent in patients with long bone fractures.[199,266,349]

Early recognition of the syndrome is crucial to preventing a complex and potentially lethal course.[5] Clinically, FES consists of a triad of hypoxia, confusion, and petechiae appearing in a patient with fractures.[92] The disease characteristically begins 1 to 2 days after fracture, following what has been called the *latent* or *lucid* period.[323] Sixty percent of all cases of FES are seen in the first 24 hours after trauma, and 90 percent of all cases appear within 72 hours.[24] Gurd and Wilson's criteria for fat embolism syndrome are commonly used, with the clinical manifestations grouped into either major or minor signs of FES.[126] The major signs are respiratory insufficiency, cerebral involvement, and petechial rash. The minor signs are fever, tachycardia, retinal changes, jaundice, and renal changes. Petechiae are caused by embolic fat. They are transient and are distributed on the cheek, neck, axillae, palate, and conjunctivae. The fat itself can be visualized on the retina.[1] A fall in hematocrit levels[87] and alterations in blood clotting profile, including a prolongation of the prothrombin time, can be observed. The diagnosis of FES is made when one major and four minor signs are present (Table 20-1) along with the finding of macroglobulinemia.[235] The most productive laboratory test is measurement of arterial oxygenation on room air. When the Po_2 is less than 60 mm Hg, the patient may be in the early stages of FES.

Lindeque and colleagues[193] believe that Gurd and Wilson's criteria are too restrictive and should also include the following:

Pco_2 of more than 55 mg Hg or pH of less than 7.3

Sustained respiratory rate of more than 35 breaths per minute

Dyspnea, tachycardia, and anxiety

If any one of these is present, then the diagnosis of FES is made. Other supportive findings include ST segment

Table 20-1
Major and Minor Criteria for the Diagnosis of Fat Embolism Syndrome*

Major Criteria	Minor Criteria
Hypoxemia (Pao₂ < 60 mm Hg)	Tachycardia >110 bpm
Central nervous system depression	Pyrexia >38.3 °C
Petechial rash	Retinal emboli on fundoscopy
Pulmonary edema	Fat in urine
	Fat in sputum
	Thrombocytopenia
	Decreased hematocrit

*A positive diagnosis requires at least one major and four minor signs.
Source: Gurd, A.R.; Wilson R.I. The fat embolism syndrome. J Bone Joint Surg Br 56:408–416, 1974.

changes on electrocardiography and pulmonary infiltrates on chest radiography.[95]

Neurologic changes have been noted in up to 80 percent of patients.[157] It is important to assess the neurologic status of the patient to differentiate between fat embolization and intracranial mass lesions. Although hypoxia alone can cause confusion, in FES, petechial hemorrhages, particularly in the reticular system, may alter consciousness. These changes persist despite adequate oxygen therapy.[24,97,121] Focal neurologic findings should be investigated to rule out lesions caused by associated head trauma. Persistent alteration of consciousness or seizures are a bad prognostic sign.

Clinically, fat embolism is a diagnosis of exclusion. In the first few days, sudden pulmonary compromise can also result from pulmonary embolism, heart failure, aspiration, and medication reaction. When these possible causes have been excluded along with many other less likely conditions, fat embolism becomes the leading cause of morbidity in the injured patient with a long bone lower limb fracture.

Fat globules are found in blood,[179] sputum, urine, and cerebrospinal fluid. The urine or sputum can be stained for fat using a saturated alcoholic solution of Sudan III. Sudan III stains neutral fat globules yellow or orange. The Gurd test, in which serum is treated with Sudan III and filtered, is also diagnostic. These tests are of historical interest when house staff actually handled specimens.

The specificity of these tests is in question. Fat droplets are normally found in sputum.[238] In addition, Peltier believes that detection of fat droplets in circulating blood and urine is too sensitive a test for the clinical diagnosis of FES.[264] Furthermore, because the embolic phenomena associated with FES are transient and may not be detected on spot testing, these laboratory investigations are of research interest only and are not part of the usual clinical workup.

The experimental study of FES is linked historically to the study of the circulation of blood, the development of intravenous therapy, and transfusion. As early as 1866, Busch experimented with marrow injury in the rabbit tibia and showed that fat in the marrow cavity would embolize to the lungs.[49] Pulmonary symptoms have been produced in the absence of fracture by the intravenous injection of fat from the tibia of one group of rabbits to another.[30]

There are several reasons for uncertainty about the role of bone fat in producing FES. First, researchers have failed to develop an animal model that reproduces the human syndrome. Moreover, injection of human bone marrow fat into the veins of experimental animals has shown that neutral fat is a relatively benign substance, and it is not certain that the bones contain enough fat to cause FES. One hypothesis is that the fat that appears in the lungs originated in soft tissue stores and aggregated in the bloodstream during post-traumatic shock.[143] However, chromatographic analysis of pulmonary vasculature fat in dogs after femoral fracture has shown that the fat most closely resembles marrow fat.[170] In contrast, Mudd and colleagues reported that there was no evidence of myeloid elements on postmortem studies of lung tissue in patients with fat embolism syndrome.[231] Furthermore, extraction of marrow fat from human long bones has shown that sufficient fat is present to account for the observed quantities in the lungs and other tissues.[261] The relative lack of triolein in children's bones may explain why they have a significantly reduced incidence of FES compared with that in adults.[121,129,171]

ETIOLOGY

Although the precise pathomechanics of FES are unclear, Levy found many nontraumatic and traumatic conditions associated with FES.[190] The simplest hypothesis is that broken bones liberate marrow fat that embolizes to the lungs. These fat globules produce mechanical and metabolic effects culminating in FES. The mechanical theory postulates that fat droplets from the marrow enter the venous circulation via torn veins adjacent to the fracture site.

Peltier[262] coined the term *intravasation* to describe the process whereby fat gains access to the circulation. The conditions in the vascular bed that allow intravasation to take place also permit marrow embolization.[228] Indeed, marrow particles are found when fat is found in the lungs (Fig. 20-1).[350]

Mechanical obstruction of the pulmonary vasculature occurs because of the absolute size of the embolized particles. In a dog model, Teng and co-workers[350] found 80 percent of fat droplets to be between 20 and 40 μm. Consequently, vessels in the lung smaller than 20 μm in diameter become obstructed. Fat globules of 10 to 40 μm have been found after human trauma.[190] Systemic embolization occurs either through precapillary shunts into pulmonary veins or through a patent foramen ovale.[260]

The biochemical theory suggests that mediators from the fracture site alter lipid solubility, causing coalescence, because normal chylomicrons are less than 1 μm in diameter. Many of the emboli have a histologic composition consisting of a fatty center with platelets and fibrin adhered.[379] Large amounts of thromboplastin are liberated with the release of bone marrow, leading to activation of the coagulation cascade.

Studies of the physiologic response to the circulatory injection of fats have shown that the unsaponified free fatty acids are much more toxic than the corresponding neutral fats. Peltier hypothesized that elevated serum lipase levels present after the embolization of neutral fat hydrolyzes this neutral fat to free fatty acids and causes local

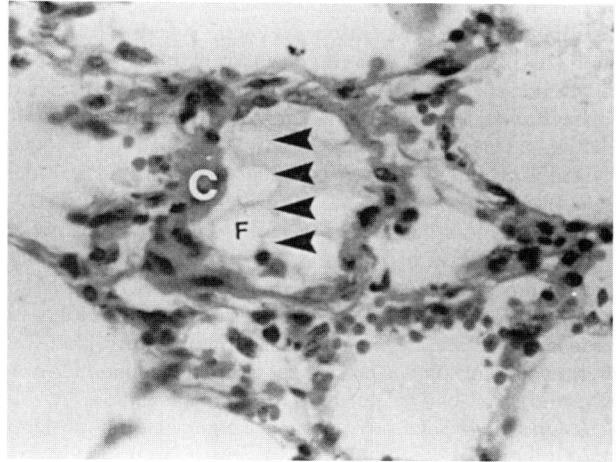

FIGURE 20-1 *Histologic appearance of fat from a pulmonary fat embolism in a vessel of the pulmonary alveoli. C, capillary; F, fat globules (arrowheads). (From Teng, Q.S.; Li, G.; Zhang, B.X. Experimental study of early diagnosis and treatment of fat embolism syndrome. J Orthop Trauma 9:183–189, 1995.)*

endothelial damage in the lungs and other tissues, resulting in FES.[261] This chemical phase might in part explain the latency period seen between the arrival of embolic fat and more severe lung dysfunction. Elevated serum lipase levels have been reported in association with clinically fatal FES.[292,316] Alternative explanations are also possible for the toxic effect of fat on the pulmonary capillary bed. The combination of fat, fibrin, and (possibly) marrow may be sufficient to begin a biochemical cascade that damages the lungs without postulating enzymatic hydrolysis of neutral fat.[121,143,311] Bleeding into the lungs is associated with a fall in the hematocrit level.[82] The resulting hypoxemia from the mechanical and biochemical changes in the lungs can be severe—even to the point of death of the patient.

Pape and associates[258] demonstrated an increase in neutrophil proteases from central venous blood in a group of patients undergoing reamed femoral nailing. In another study, Pape and colleagues[255] demonstrated the release of platelet-derived thromboxane (a potent vasoconstrictor of pulmonary microvasculature) from the marrow cavity. Peltier[263] demonstrated the release of vasoactive platelet amines. These humoral factors can lead to pulmonary vasospasm and bronchospasm, resulting in vascular endothelial injury and increased pulmonary permeability. Indeed, thrombocytopenia is such a consistent finding that it is used as one of the diagnostic criteria of FES. Barie and co-workers[16] associated pulmonary dysfunction with an alteration in the coagulation cascade and an increase in fibrinolytic activity.

Autopsy findings in patients dying of FES do not, however, show a consistent picture.[323] This may not be caused solely by a lack of clear-cut criteria that define patients included in a given series, but may also be because the manifestations of FES depend on a wide number of patient, accident, and treatment variables.[262]

In light of the incidence of fat emboli and FES in trauma patients, it is likely that other precipitating or predisposing factors such as shock, sepsis, or disseminated intravascular coagulation are needed for the phenomenon of embolized fat to cause FES.[115] Müller and associates[233] summarized that "fat embolism syndrome is likely the pathogenetic reaction of lung tissue to shock, hypercoagulability, and lipid mobilization."

Two clinically related treatment questions arise: (1) Is there an association between intramedullary nailing, FES, and other injuries? (2) Is there an effect from different nailing methods on the incidence of FES? Pape and associates[253,254] found that early operative fracture fixation by nailing was associated with an increased risk of ARDS in patients with thoracic injury. These results are in contrast to those of the group without thoracic injury. Thoracic trauma is associated with direct pulmonary injury. The pathogenic mechanisms were examined by Lozman and colleagues.[197] Thus, the timing and the associated injuries are crucial in deciding when and how to use a nail.

In a prospective study, Pape and associates[254] showed a significant impairment of oxygenation in multiple trauma patients who underwent reamed nailing. A group of similar patients who had unreamed nailing did not have the same signs of pulmonary dysfunction. These investigators reasoned that the most likely difference between the two groups was a lower degree of fat embolization in the unreamed group. In sheep, Pape and colleagues[255] demonstrated intravasation of fat associated with reaming of the intramedullary (IM) canal. They concluded that the unreamed procedure caused substantially less severe lung damage than the reamed procedure. However, Heim and associates[139] found that there was a significant increase in IM pressure associated with unreamed nail insertion and that both reamed nailing and unreamed nailing lead to bone marrow intravasation (Fig. 20-2). Thus, the use of an unreamed nail does not solve the problem of bone marrow embolization and resultant pulmonary dysfunction.

What influences the degree of fat embolization? The answer has not been fully elucidated. High IM pressures have been linked with fat embolization and FES.[163] Wozasek and co-workers[379] looked at the degree of fat intravasation during reaming and IM nailing and correlated this with IM pressure changes and echocardiographic findings. They found peak IM pressures in both the tibial and the femoral nailings in the first two reaming steps. Insertion of the nail caused only minimal pressure rises (but this was after reaming). Echocardiography, however, demonstrated that the maximal infiltration of particles occurred when the nail was inserted. They concluded that the phenomenon of fat intravasation did not depend on the rise in IM pressure. Pinney and associates studied 274 patients with isolated femur fractures and found that waiting more than 10 hours after injury was associated with a 2.5-fold increase in fat embolism syndrome.[269] Bulger and co-workers noted that early intramedullary fixation did not seem to increase the incidence or severity of fat embolism syndrome.[47]

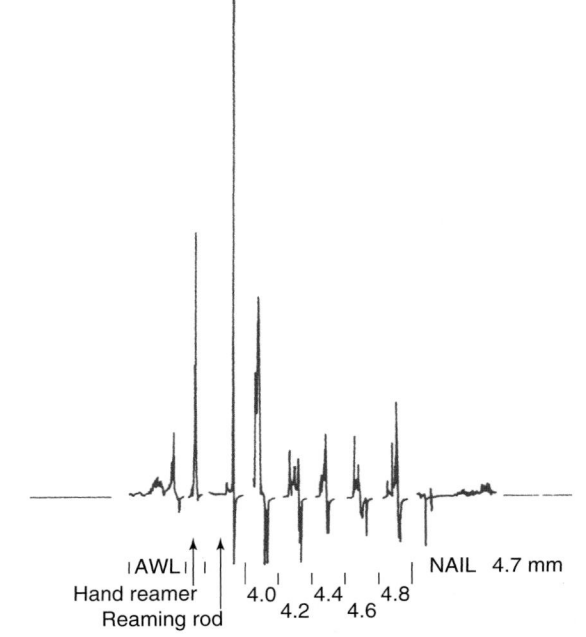

FIGURE 20-2 *Intramedullary pressure during reamed nailing of the femur. (From Heim, D.; Regazzori, P.; Tsakiris, D.A.; et al. Intramedullary nailing and pulmonary embolism: Does unreamed nailing prevent embolization? An in vivo study in rabbits. J Trauma 38:899–906, 1995.)*

PREVENTION AND TREATMENT

The risk of FES can be decreased by several measures. Proper fracture splinting and expeditious transport, use of oxygen therapy in the postinjury period, and early operative stabilization of long bone fractures of the lower extremities are three important measures that can be taken to reduce the incidence of this complication.[7] Blood pressure, urinary output, blood gas values, and—in the more critically injured—pulmonary wedge pressures should be monitored to evaluate fluid status and tissue perfusion more precisely.[190] Dramatic advances in emergency medical transport have resulted in increasing survival of patients with complex polytrauma and high injury severity scores. This has led in some instances to a tendency to "scoop and run" without traction splinting. Unsplinted long bone fractures in patients transported over long distances are a set-up for intravenous fat intravasation. Oxygen therapy by mask or nasal prongs lessens the decrease in arterial oxygenation following fracture and appears to have value in the prevention of FES.

If surgery is delayed, the patient's arterial oxygen on room air is measured daily and supplemental oxygen therapy is continued until the post-traumatic fall in oxygen tension is complete and the Pao_2 on room air returns toward normal. Alternatively, if inspired oxygen tension (Fio_2) can be measured accurately, the shunt equation can be used to monitor pulmonary performance. Teng and co-workers[350] completed preliminary development of a dog model of FES to establish diagnostic criteria sufficiently sensitive and specific enough for diagnosis of FES in the early stages. They correlated blood gas analysis samples with computer image analysis of oil red O-stained pulmonary artery blood samples. Although fracture fixation and particularly medullary nailing cause a transient decrease in oxygenation, the immediate stabilization of fractures before the development of low arterial saturation may prevent the occurrence of FES.[293]

In a prospective randomized study of 178 patients, Bone and associates[32] confirmed that early fracture stabilization, within the initial 24 hours after injury, decreased the incidence of pulmonary complications. Likewise, Lozman and colleagues,[197] in a prospective randomized study, concluded that patients receiving immediate fixation had less pulmonary dysfunction following multiple trauma and long bone fractures than did those patients receiving conservative treatment.

Although current data support primary fracture stabilization over delayed therapy, controversy still exists over the method of stabilization. Böstmann and co-workers found a higher incidence of local infections, delayed bone healing, and decreased stability with plate osteosynthesis compared with a lower incidence of these same complications with IM nailing.[40] In general, IM nailing is the preferred method of stabilization. The timing of nailing, however, is a point of controversy.[47] Among other reasons, this was due to the concern that immediate nailing of long bone fractures early in the postinjury period would increase the incidence of pulmonary complications, including FES. The nonoperative method of treating major long bone fractures has been the use of balanced skeletal traction or delayed rigid fixation, or both. External fixation of long bone fractures is another option that can be used as a temporizing alternative to IM nailing. Earlier studies showed no evidence to support the view that the effect of reaming on intravascular fat is additive or that immediate reamed IM fixation causes pulmonary compromise.[13,347] In fact, the opposite is true, probably because fracture stabilization removes the source of intravascular marrow fat and decreases shunting in the lung, since the patient can be mobilized to an upright position.[204,220,349]

No cases of FES were seen in a retrospective study by Talucci and associates[346] in which 57 patients underwent immediate nailing. Similarly, Behrman and colleagues[25] reported a lower incidence of pulmonary complications for patients undergoing early fixation among 339 trauma patients who underwent either early or late fixation of femoral fractures. In the study by Lozman and colleagues,[197] patients who had delayed fracture fixation had a higher intrapulmonary shunt fraction throughout the study period compared with that in the early fixation group.

Early IM nailing of long bone fractures is not without complications. Pell and co-workers,[260] using intraoperative transesophageal echocardiography, demonstrated varying degrees of embolic showers during reamed IM nailing. FES developed postoperatively in three patients, and one patient died. Other studies showed an increased number of pulmonary complications associated with early, reamed IM nailing of femoral shaft fractures.[236,258,370]

Specific therapy has been used in an attempt to decrease the incidence of FES. No clinical effect on the rate of FES has been found with increased fluid loading, the use of hypertonic glucose, alcohol, heparin, low-molecular-weight dextran, and aspirin. Various studies have looked at the efficacy of corticosteroids in reducing the clinical symptoms of FES. Large doses of steroids immediately after injury do have a beneficial effect.[10,97,193,298,340,350] Corticosteroids most likely decrease the incidence of FES by limiting the endothelial damage caused by free fatty acids. Babalis et al.,[12] in a randomized, prospective study of 87 patients with long bone fractures allocated to either a placebo group or a group treated with intravenous, low-dose methylprednisolone, found that methylprednisolone deceased post-traumatic hypoxemia and probably fat embolism in patients with isolated lower limb long bone fractures, especially when early fracture stabilization is not possible. They concluded that the prophylactic use of methylprednisolone in small doses was useful in preventing post-traumatic hypoxemia and fat embolism syndrome. Although this is encouraging, routine use of steroids is not without significant risk and is not routinely employed. Complications, particularly infection, gastrointestinal bleeding, and avascular necrosis, may outweigh the benefits.

FES is primarily a disease of the respiratory system, and current treatment is therefore mainly with oxygen and meticulous mechanical ventilation.[265] Treatment of FES remains mainly supportive.[47]

Finally, in no way should it be construed that either clinical experience or scientific investigation provides a sure pathway to prevent the appearance of this significant postinjury and potentially lethal problem. Although careful review of the medical record might suggest how things could have been done alternatively, there is no certainty, for example, that waiting another day as the PaO_2 returned toward normal before performing a nailing would have prevented the complication—indeed, it might have invited another one.

Thromboembolic Disorders

PATHOGENESIS

In 1846, Virchow proposed the triad of thrombogenesis: increased coagulability, stasis, and vessel wall damage (Fig. 20-3).[360] These are all factors that are unfavorably affected by trauma. Virchow also linked the presence of deep venous thrombosis (DVT) with pulmonary embolism (PE) and deduced that a clot in the large veins of the thigh embolized to the lungs.[358] Laennec,[184] in 1819, was the first to describe the clinical presentation of an acute pulmonary embolus. The pathogenesis of a proximal DVT was first described by Cruveilhier[77] in 1828. Venous thrombi have been shown to develop near the valve pockets on normal venous endothelium and are not necessarily related to inflammation of the vessel wall.[324]

Trauma creates a hypercoagulable state. Vessel wall injury with endothelial damage exposes blood to tissue factor, collagen, basement membrane, and von Willebrand factor, which induce thrombosis through platelet attraction and the intrinsic and extrinsic coagulation pathway.[167] Antithrombin (AT-III) activity, which decreases the

FIGURE 20-3 *Virchow's triad.*

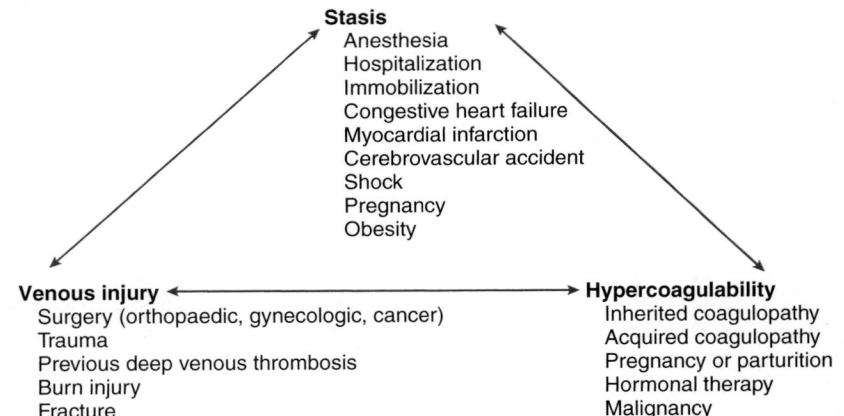

activity of thrombin and factor Xa, was found to be below normal levels in 61 percent of critically injured trauma patients.[249] Also, fibrinolysis is decreased and appears to be from increased levels of PAI-1, which inhibits tissue plasminogen activator and thus decreases the production of plasmin.[130,202]

The presence of heart disease alone increases the risk of pulmonary embolism by 3.5 times, and this is further increased if atrial fibrillation or congestive heart failure is present.[72,73] The risk of DVT is increased during pregnancy and is especially great in the postpartum period. Spinal cord injury is associated with a threefold increase in leg DVT and PE.

A meta-analysis by Velmahos and co-workers[359] looked at DVT and risk factors in trauma patients. Variables studied that did not have a statistically significant effect for increasing the development of DVT were gender, head injury, long bone fracture, pelvic fracture, and units of blood transfused. The variables that were statistically significant were spinal fractures and spinal cord injury, which increased the risk of DVT by twofold and threefold, respectively. They could not confirm that the widely assumed risk factors of pelvic fracture, long bone fracture, and head injury affected the incidence of DVT but did note that the multiple trauma patients may have already been at the highest risk of DVT.

For immobilized trauma patients with no prophylaxis, the incidence of venography-proven thigh and iliofemoral thrombosis is between 60 and 80 percent.[105,181] Even with full prophylaxis, the incidence of DVT is as high as 12 percent.[175] Stannard et al.[334,335] reported a significant rate of deep-vein thrombosis in high-energy skeletal trauma patients despite thromboprophylaxis. They noted in a series of 312 patients with high-energy trauma that 11.5 percent developed venous thromboembolic disease with an incidence of 10 percent in those with non-pelvic trauma and 12.2 percent in the group with pelvic trauma despite thromboprophylaxis. Some investigators have concluded that "there is no adequate prophylaxis against DVT in the trauma patient."[331]

Trauma to the pelvis and lower extremities greatly increases the risk of DVT and PE.[71,147,374] In an autopsy study of 486 trauma fatalities, Sevitt and Gallagher[325] found 95 cases of PE for an incidence of 20 percent. At autopsy, the rate of PE following hip fracture was 52/114 (46%); for tibia fractures, 6/10 (60%); and for femoral fractures, 9/17 (53%). The rate of DVT for hip fractures increased to 39/47 (83%) and for femur fractures to 6/7 (86%) when supplemental special studies of the venous system were done at autopsy.

PE is a significant cause of death following lower extremity injury. Two-thirds of patients having a fatal pulmonary embolus die within 30 minutes of injury (Fig. 20-4).[84] The incidence of fatal pulmonary embolus without prophylaxis after elective hip surgery is from 0.34 to 3.4 percent, whereas the incidence following emergency hip surgery is from 7.5 to 10 percent.[98,128,210,367,376]

Solheim[329] reported a 0.5 percent incidence of fatal PE in a series of tibia and fibula fractures. Similarly, Phillips and co-workers[268] reported 1 of 138 patients (0.7%) with severe ankle fractures developed a nonfatal PE. In a study of 15 patients with tibia fractures, Nylander and Semb[240] found that 70 percent had venographic changes compatible with DVT.

The types of DVT that are at high risk for causing a PE are those that originate at the popliteal fossa or more proximally in the large veins of the thigh or pelvis. Moser and LeMoine[229] found the risk of pulmonary embolization from distal lower extremity DVT to be relatively low. Of DVTs that are first limited to the calf, about 20 to 30 percent extend above the knee.[26,275] Those that extend above the knee carry the same risk as femoral and popliteal thrombi.[306] Kakkar and colleagues[162] speculated that thrombi in the calf are securely attached and resolve rapidly and spontaneously. However, embolization from "calf only" venous thrombi does occur. Calf vein thromboses are responsible for 5 to 35 percent of symptomatic pulmonary emboli,[196,259] 15 to 25 percent of fatal PE,[112,213,324] and 33 percent of "silent" PE.[223,226]

In addition to PE, complications of DVT include recurrent thrombosis and post-thrombotic syndrome. Symptoms of post-thrombotic syndrome are edema, induration, pain, pigmentation, ulceration, cellulitis, and stasis dermatitis.[155,159] Symptoms are present in up to 20 to 40 percent of those having had a DVT.

FIGURE 20-4 *A large embolus in the pulmonary artery, which was the cause of death. (Courtesy of James E. Parker, M.D., University of Louisville, Louisville, KY.)*

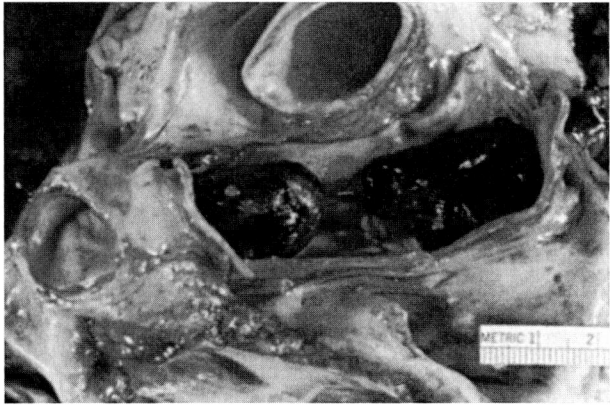

Upper extremity DVT is much less common (2.5%) and can be due to primary or secondary causes. The primary causes are idiopathic and effort thrombosis (Padget-Schroetter syndrome). Effort thrombosis is most common in athletes and laborers who do repetitive shoulder abduction and extension. Predisposing causes of thoracic outlet obstruction should be investigated. Secondary causes are venous catheters, venous trauma, extrinsic compression or malignancy, and hypercoagulable condition.

DIAGNOSIS

The clinical signs and symptoms of DVT are nonspecific. DVT was clinically silent in two-thirds of cases in which thrombosis was found at autopsy or the findings on leg venography were positive.[102,325]

Clinically, the diagnosis of DVT and PE is frequently difficult. With PE, although some patients experience sudden death, many more present with gradual deterioration and symptoms similar to pneumonia, congestive heart failure, or hypotension. Symptoms can be intermittent with episodes of transient pulmonary compromise caused by clusters of small emboli. Because the clinical diagnosis is difficult, diagnostic studies are necessary so that early treatment can be instituted. Various tests are described along with limitations and advantages.

Traditionally, venography has been the diagnostic test of choice for deep venous thromboses, but it is no longer the gold standard. The major drawbacks of venography are that it is usually a one-time test that cannot be done on a serial basis and has been reported to cause phlebitis in about 4 to 24 percent of patients[27,306] and may cause thrombosis.[3] Between 5 and 15 percent of venograms cannot be interpreted because of technical considerations.[373] Patients can have serious allergic reactions to contrast agents.

Radioactive fibrinogen is effective in detecting thrombi in the calf but is less effective in the thigh.[150] Fibrinogen I-125 is incorporated into a forming thrombus and can be detected. DVT in the thigh is poorly detected with this technique, and it is not used as a screening tool for trauma patients.

Impedance plethysmography (IPG) detects the presence of DVT by measuring the increased blood volume in the calf after temporary venous occlusion produced by a thigh tourniquet and the decrease in blood volume within 3 seconds after deflation of the cuff.[152,369,371] IPG is sensitive for diagnosing proximal DVT but is not sensitive for distal DVT.[48,137,149,372] It is a poor screening tool for the trauma patient.

Noninvasive venous Doppler examinations are the current standard for imaging deep venous thromboses. Continuous-wave Doppler (CWD) or Doppler ultrasound examination is easy to do and can be done at bedside, but it requires experience to reduce the false-positive result rate.[17] Venous thrombosis is characterized by the absence of venous flow at an expected site, loss of normal fluctuation in flow associated with respiration, diminished augmentation of flow by distal limb compression, diminished augmentation of flow by release of proximal compression, and lack of change on Valsalva maneuver. Barnes and co-workers[18] found that Doppler ultrasound was 94 percent accurate, and no errors were made in diagnosis above the level of the knee. However, for isolated calf vein thrombosis, CWD is insensitive. An additional disadvantage is that CWD may fail to detect nonobstructive thrombi even in proximal lesions.[63]

Color-flow duplex ultrasonography (CFDU) employs a Doppler component that is color-enhanced and detects blood flow by the shift in frequency from the backscatter of high-frequency sound. The frequency is shifted by an amount proportional to the flow velocity. The color saturation is proportional to the rate of flow. A black image indicates an absence of flow, flow velocities less than 0.3 cm/sec, or flow vectors at a right angle to the second beam.[205] The addition of color allows for the easier and faster detection of vascular structures. Blood flowing away from the transducer appears blue, whereas blood flowing toward the transducer appears red. This has provided improved imaging of the iliac region, the femoral vein in the adductor canal, and the calf veins.[286] CFDU is superior to duplex scanning and B-mode imaging in detecting nonocclusive thrombi because the flow characteristics in the vessels are readily detected.[205] Several studies have reported high sensitivity and specificity in symptomatic patients.[22,41,207,299]

For screening of symptomatic trauma patients, ultrasound is an excellent study, but for asymptomatic patients it is less sensitive at detecting DVT, especially in the calf. Serial ultrasound has been used as surveillance screening to detect DVT in trauma patients, but it was thought not to be cost effective.[132,310] When DVT develops in the calf, about 25 percent extend to the thigh if left untreated. If the initial ultrasound missed the asymptomatic DVT and no treatment is given, approximately 2 percent of cases will have an abnormal proximal scan on testing 1 week later.[165]

Magnetic resonance imaging (MRI) has been recently applied to the detection of deep venous thrombosis in the pelvis. Rubel et al.[300] have reported on the use of MR venography to evaluate deep venous thrombosis in patients with pelvic and acetabular trauma. Stannnard et al.[334,335] reported that ultrasound had a false-negative rate of 77 percent for diagnosing pelvic deep-vein thrombosis compared with MR venography. Stover et al.,[341] in a prospective study of MR venography and contrast-enhanced computed tomography (CT), reported that the false-positive rate for MR venography was 100 percent and the false-positive rate for contrast-enhanced CT was 50 percent. They stated that they cannot recommend the sole use of either CT venography or MR venography to screen and direct the treatment of asymptomatic thrombi in patients with fracture of the pelvic ring because of these high false-positive rates. An additional disadvantage of MR venography is the cost, which is typically 2 to 2.5 times the cost of an ultrasound scan and 1.4 times the cost of venography.[52,188]

PE can be diagnosed with angiography, ventilation perfusion (VQ) scan, or helical CT. Helical CT has largely replaced angiography and VQ scans in most cases. If the VQ scan results are abnormal but not diagnostic of a PE, then depending on the severity of symptoms, either pulmonary angiography or venous ultrasound can be done. Positive findings on venous ultrasound are present in 5 to 10 percent of patients with nondiagnostic lung scans. Of patients with a suspected PE who have a negative venous ultrasound result and a nondiagnostic VQ scan, 80 percent will not have had a PE. The remaining 20 percent will have had a PE, but the residual leg thrombus is too small to be demonstrated or none is present. The risk of recurrent PE and recurrent DVT is highest within 2 weeks and can be monitored with serial venous ultrasounds to determine treatment. With this management approach, there is about a 2 percent incidence of abnormal venous ultrasound on serial testing. The use of serial noninvasive ultrasound scanning has not been evaluated adequately. When there is a high suspicion of PE, pulmonary angiography should be done.[268]

Spiral (helical) CT with intravenous contrast (CT–pulmonary angiography) is being increasingly used as the diagnostic test of choice for PE.[313,354] There is a low risk of PE following negative CT–pulmonary angiography (CT-PA).[267,280] Moores et al.[225] did a meta-analysis and reported a 3-month rate of subsequent venous thromboembolic events of 1.4 percent and a 3-month rate of PE of 0.5 percent following negative CT-PA. These researchers stated that the rate of subsequent venous thromboembolism after negative results on CT-PA was similar to that seen after negative results on conventional pulmonary angiography. These authors concluded that it was safe to withhold anticoagulation after negative CT-PA results. Schoepf et al. have stated that it is safe to withhold anticoagulation on the basis of a negative spiral CT result. Improvements such as the use of multidetector spiral CT have improved visualization of peripheral pulmonary arteries and detection of small emboli.[313] Diagnostic accuracy of CT-PA also can vary from institution to institution.[287] Although CT-PA appears to be becoming the first-line imaging test of choice for negative PE, negative results should be interpreted with caution and skepticism if they are inconsistent with the overall clinical picture.[287] Rathbun et al. cautioned that the safety of withholding anticoagulation treatment in patients with negative results on helical CT is unknown.[287] Therefore, until prospective

randomized study data are available, negative helical CT results in patients with suspected PE ought to be interpreted on a case-by-case basis. If strong suspicion remains of PE after negative helical CT results, it seems prudent that additional workups such as pulmonary angiography ought to be considered. It is likely that multidetector spiral CT will continue to improve and in the future will ultimately supplant other methods of imaging PE.

TREATMENT

If DVT or PE occurs before definitive management of the fracture, the method of treating the fracture may have to be modified because of the use of therapeutic anticoagulants. There are three major approaches to the treatment of DVT: protect the patient from thrombosis (prevention is really a misnomer in trauma), ignore it if it occurs, or treat it. Implicit in each of these approaches is a consideration of (1) the risk of the intervention and (2) the risk if no intervention is taken. For protection of the patient from thrombosis, what is the risk of the agent used versus the risk of DVT and its complications? Once DVT develops, if no treatment is undertaken, what is the risk of PE compared with the complications of therapy?

The concept of venous thromboembolism prophylaxis with orthopaedic traumatic injuries to the musculoskeletal system is a misnomer. The process of clot formation has likely already begun. Prophylaxis is really *ex post facto*.[296] The concept of DVT "protection" rather than prophylaxis is probably more accurate for the orthopaedic trauma patient.

There are four types of patients with orthopaedic trauma who should be considered for VTE (venous thrombosis and pulmonary embolism) protection: the polytrauma patient, the elderly hip fracture patient, the isolated extremity injury patient, and the spinal cord injury patient. It is challenging to generalize about VTE prophylaxis for all four groups together as one. Therefore, VTE prophylaxis/protection for each type of orthopaedic patient is discussed separately.

POLYTRAUMA PATIENT   Without prophylaxis, patients with multisystem or major trauma have a DVT rate that exceeds 50 percent with a fatal pulmonary embolism rate of 0.4 to 2.0 percent. PE is a common cause of death in trauma patients. VTE accounts for about 9 percent of readmissions to the hospital following trauma. Polytrauma patients represent a heterogenous group and present many challenges. These patients are often cared for by multiple services (e.g., general surgery, critical care, orthopaedic trauma surgery) as a team. Many of these polytrauma patients with acidosis, coagulopathy, and hypothermia are initially treated with a damage control orthopaedics approach (e.g., temporary spanning external fixation of long bone fractures).

Although VTE prophylaxis in the treatment of these patients needs to be individualized, several concepts are now becoming fairly standard. The recommendations published by the American College of Chest Physicians (ACCP) every 2 to 3 years as a *Chest* journal supplement are often considered to set the standard.[106] The seventh ACCP recommendations noted, "We recommend that all trauma patients with at least one risk factor for VTE receive prophylaxis."[106] Therefore, any trauma patient (multisystem or major trauma) with a musculoskeletal injury (spine fracture, pelvic or acetabular fracture, or extremity fracture) qualifies. Note, however, that ACCP panelists may have vested economic interests in the agents used for VTE prevention.

The use of low-molecular-weight heparin (LMWH) is recommended in the absence of major contraindications.[106] If LMWH is contraindicated because of major bleeding or hemorrhage, mechanical prophylaxis is recommended (intermittent pneumatic compression [IPC] or graduated compression stockings [GCS]).[106] Doppler screening is recommended for patients who are at high risk of VTE (e.g., spinal cord injury, lower extremity or pelvic fracture, major head trauma, or an indwelling venous line) or who have received suboptimal or no prophylaxis.[106] It has also been recommended that inferior vena cava (IVC) filters not be used as primary prophylaxis in trauma patients.[106] Recommendations have now also been made for the posthospitalization period, including the period of inpatient rehabilitation with continued prophylaxis after discharge with LMWH or vitamin K antagonists (target international normalized ratio [INR] 2.5; INR range, 2.0–3.0) for patients with major impaired mobility. Alternatives to LMWH include heparin and synthetic pentasaccharides.

ELDERLY HIP FRACTURE PATIENT Without prophylaxis, these patients have DVT rates of 50 percent with a proximal DVT rate of 25 percent. Fatal PE is more common in hip fracture patients than in total hip and knee arthroplasty patients. Recommendations for prophylaxis are synthetic pentasaccharides, LMWH, or adjusted-dose vitamin K antagonists (target INR, 2.5; INR range, 2.0–3.0).[106] The use of aspirin was recommended against. If hip fracture fixation will be delayed, it was recommended that low-dose unfractionated heparin or LMWH be used.[106] Mechanical prophylaxis was recommended if anticoagulation was contraindicated.[106] From an ethical standpoint, one might question if over-vigorous anticoagulation is appropriate in every case. Consider, for example, the elderly, demented nursing home patient who falls and has a hip fracture.

ISOLATED EXTREMITY INJURY PATIENT Isolated extremity injuries are probably the most common injuries seen by orthopaedic physicians. The use of thromboprophylaxis routinely in patients with isolated extremity trauma injuries was recommended against.[106] It was stated, "We suggest that clinicians not use thromboprophylaxis routinely in patients with isolated lower extremity injuries."[106] On the other hand, surveillance of patients for VTE and protection/prophylaxis seems prudent. At a minimum, one could consider simple measures (early mobilization, ankle pump exercises, GCS, IPC with or without GCS) or more intensive measures (preoperative and immediate postoperative GCS, followed by a short course of LMWH, synthetic pentasaccharides, or adjusted vitamin K antagonists).

SPINAL CORD INJURY PATIENT Acute spinal cord injury was the risk factor most strongly associated with the development of DVT in major trauma.[105] Rogers et al.[297]

in their meta-analysis noted that spinal cord injuries or spinal fractures are high-risk for venous thromboembolism. It is recommended that "thromboprophylaxis be provided for all patients with acute spinal cord injuries."[106] The use of low-dose unfractionated heparin (LDUH), GCS, or IPC as single prophylaxis modalities was recommended against.[106] Prophylaxis with LMWH once hemostasis is evident is appropriate.[106] As an alternative to LWMH alone, the combined use of IPC and either LDUH or LMWH has been suggested.[106] When chemical anticoagulant prophylaxis is contraindicated early after injury, the use of IPC and/or GCS is recommended.[106] They recommend against the use of an IVC filter as primary prophylaxis.[106] When the spinal cord injury patient is out of the acute phase and in the rehabilitative phase, continuation of LMWH prophylaxis or conversion to an oral vitamin K antagonist (target INR: 2.5; range, 2.0–3.0) is recommended.[106] Variation in clinical practice is wide. There is no convincing evidence that twice daily regimens are more effective than once daily, and no evidence that either low-dose heparin or warfarin to an INR of 1.5 is not as effective as the ACCP recommended doses. Indeed, there is a wide range of mischief particularly in the elderly who may experience significant morbidity—bleeding, stroke, and diagnostic misadventures—as a result of overzealous prophylaxis!

TREATMENT OF EXISTING DEEP VENOUS THROMBOSIS AND PULMONARY EMBOLISM

Once DVT or PE is suspected, the clinical impression should be confirmed by diagnostic testing. Heparin should be started unless contraindicated until diagnostic testing is done. Contraindications include neurologic, spinal cord, or ocular injuries that could be worsened by bleeding. Heparin is started intravenously to reach therapeutic effect rapidly to prevent clot extension and decrease the risk of PE. Subcutaneous LMWH has also been proven to be effective in initial treatment of DVT. However, further documentation of its role in the trauma setting is needed because controlled trials excluded LMWH use if there had been surgery in the prior 5 to 7 days.[150,328] Controlled trials of intravenous heparin versus LMWH in the presence of DVT have shown no difference in rates of symptomatic extension, recurrence, pulmonary embolism, or severe bleeding.[150,176,189,194,276] LMWH has also been used in the treatment of pulmonary embolism.[65,328]

If DVT is present, the patient is continued on heparin until converting to warfarin. The dosage of warfarin is not standardized, and in younger patients the dosage is more difficult to predict. Two studies comparing an initial dose of 5 versus 10 mg suggest that 5 mg is more appropriate.[76,133] Warfarin can also be used without a loading dose. Length of warfarin treatment for DVT and PE is from 3 to 6 months,[51,167] and longer duration of treatment appears to be associated with a lower risk of recurrence. The rate of recurrent DVT and PE is higher when the DVT occurred without an identifiable risk factor than when there was an identifiable transient risk factor.[277,289,314] Longer treatment is indicated for trauma patients with major vein ligation or spinal cord injuries with paralysis. Evidence of re-embolization is an indication for permanent anticoagulation and consideration for an IVC filter.[339]

Thrombolytic drugs are an alternative to heparin, but they are not suitable to the traumatized or postoperative patient for at least 2 weeks because of clot lysis at the surgical site. An advantage of thrombolytic drugs is that the venous system more closely returns to normal when the venous thrombosis is lysed rather than when propagation of the thrombus is simply arrested as is the case with heparin.[66] The Urokinase Pulmonary Embolism Trial (UPET) found a statistically significant lower mortality rate in the patients receiving thrombolytic therapy than in the group receiving heparin anticoagulation.[356] In theory, there should be a lower incidence of post-thrombotic syndrome in patients receiving thrombolytic therapy than in those receiving heparin treatment, but randomized trials are lacking and the beneficial effect of lysis is complicated by increased risk of bleeding.[2,308] IVC filters are used less frequently and are no longer recommended as primary prophylaxis against venous thromboembolism.[106] IVC filters have associated complications such as venous stasis leading to edema, pain, varicose veins, and skin ulcers in a condition known as the *postphlebitic syndrome.*[368] Other complications include bleeding or thrombus formation at the site of insertion, migration of the filter, and perforation of the vena cava.[122,123] Martin and co-workers[205] described a case report of phlegmasia cerulea dolens as a complication of an IVC filter for prophylaxis against PE in a man with a fracture of the acetabulum. In addition, filters are not 100 percent effective.[78]

Vena cava interruption is performed when heparinization is contraindicated, as in patients with a preexisting bleeding disorder; severe hypertension; neurologic injury; or bleeding problems of pulmonary, gastrointestinal, neurologic, or urologic etiology. If anticoagulation fails to stop pulmonary emboli, vena cava interruption is indicated.[161] Also, if patients develop complications with anticoagulation, they can be switched to vena cava interruption. An additional approach is the preoperative use of vena cava interruption in patients who are at extremely high risk for PE. The prophylactic use of vena cava interruption in trauma patients has also been examined.

Surgical thrombectomy is indicated only for patients with massive thrombosis and those who have absolute contraindications for thrombolytic therapy or do not respond to treatment.[20] Pulmonary embolectomy should be considered when thrombolysis is not effective or not feasible in patients with massive pulmonary embolism and hemodynamic instability.[153]

The current literature clearly indicates that certain subsets of trauma patients are at risk for venous thromboembolism and would benefit from some type of prophylaxis or surveillance. Many experts think that prophylaxis for DVT is safer and more cost effective than surveillance tests.[149,218,250,305] In a study of surveillance venous scans for DVT in prophylactically evaluated multiple trauma patients, Meyer and co-workers[218] performed 261 scans, 92 percent of which produced normal results. At their institution, the cost to identify each proximal DVT was $6688. The overall incidence of clinically significant proximal DVT in their patients treated with DVT prophylaxis was 6 percent. They concluded that the routine use of venous surveillance scans should be limited to high-risk or symptomatic patients.

SUMMARY

Deep venous thrombosis and pulmonary embolism are common causes of morbidity, mortality,[57,99,296] and litigation associated with the care of the orthopaedic trauma patient. The complete prevention of thromboembolism in orthopaedic trauma is impossible because trauma cannot be anticipated. One or more components of Virchow's triad are usually present from the time of injury, so the concept of "DVT prophylaxis" is a misnomer for the trauma patient.

Additional experience and data on VTE from Europe may improve the clinical care of the trauma patient. Questions remain such as, "Is there a genetic predisposition to VTE?" Risk stratification is being used in other areas of medicine and is only beginning to be understood in orthopaedic trauma. In addition, combinations of injuries, multiple lower extremity fractures with a spinal cord injury, or a pelvic fracture together with a femur fracture likely exponentially increase the risk of VTE. Nonetheless, our ability to diagnose VTE and protect patients from it is constrained by acute hemorrhage and inability to tolerate anticoagulation, soft tissue contusion, and extremity injuries that prevent the placement of IPC and GCS. Prophylaxis is also impossible, and the best we can do is to try for VTE protection. Nonetheless, there are many methods of DVT surveillance and protection at our disposal, and they ought to be utilized. Although the ideal method of documentation for hospital or outpatient examinations is unknown, we have found that a note such as "no signs or symptoms of PE/DVT" along with the documentation of VTE protection/prophylaxis seems prudent and reasonable. Clinicians are also advised to stay informed of the consensus recommendations that are published every 2 to 3 years in the *Chest* medicine supplement.

Although current prophylactic regimens in trauma patients significantly reduce the relative risk for DVT and PE, no method provides 100 percent protection. Further randomized controlled trials of DVT prophylaxis in trauma patients are needed.

Multiple Organ System Dysfunction and Failure

Multiple organ failure (MOF) can be defined as the sequential failure of two or more organ systems remote from the site of the original insult following injury, operation, or sepsis. The organ failure can be pulmonary, renal, hepatic, gastrointestinal, central nervous, or hematologic.[89,272] These systems can be monitored for objective criteria for failure, but criteria vary from series to series (Tables 20-2 and 20-3).[103,271] The risk of developing MOF and the severity of the MOF can also be graded by measuring the effects on specific organ systems.[120]

MOF is the end result of a transition from the normal metabolic response to injury to persistent hypermetabolism and eventual failure of organs to maintain their physiologic function. A 1991 consensus conference used the term *multiple organ dysfunction syndrome* (MODS) to describe this spectrum of changes.[33] Organ dysfunction is the result of either a direct insult or a systemic inflammatory response, known clinically as the *systemic inflammatory response syndrome* (SIRS),[23] which can be reversible or progress to

Table 20-2

Criteria for Organ Dysfunction and Failure

Organ or System	Dysfunction	Advanced Failure
Pulmonary	Hypoxia requiring intubation for 3–5 days	ARDS requiring PEEP >10 cm H_2O and Fio_2 >0.5
Hepatic	Serum total bilirubin ≥2–3 mg/dL or liver function tests ≥ twice normal	Clinical jaundice with total bilirubin ≥8–10 mg/dL
Renal	Oliguria ≤479 mL/day or creatinine ≥2–3 mg/dL	Dialysis
Gastrointestinal	Ileus with intolerance of enteral feeds >5 days	Stress ulcers, acalculous cholecystitis
Hematologic	PT/PTT >125% normal, platelets <50,000–80,000	DIC
Central nervous system	Confusion, mild disorientation	Progressive coma
Cardiovascular	Decreased ejection fraction or capillary leak syndrome	Refractory cardiogenic shock

Abbreviations: ARDS, adult respiratory distress syndrome; PEEP, positive end-expiratory pressure; Fio_2, fraction of inspired air in oxygen; PT, prothrombin time; PTT, partial thromboplastin time; DIC, disseminated intravascular coagulation.
Source: Deitch, E.A.; Goodman, E.R. Prevention of multiple organ failure. Surg Clin North Am 79(6), 1998; which was adapted from Deitch, E.A. Pathophysiology and potential future therapy. Ann Surg 216:117–134, 1992, with permission.

MODS or MOF. SIRS can be caused by a variety of infectious and noninfectious stimuli[33] (Fig. 20-5). Treatment of the offending source must be undertaken early, because once organ failure has begun, treatment modalities become progressively ineffective.[54] Fry identified the mortality rate for failure of two or more organ systems as about 75 percent. If two organ systems fail and renal failure occurs, then the mortality is 98 percent.[103] Today, MOF is the number one cause of death in surgical intensive care units.[79]

The basic theory behind the development of MOF and the closely related ARDS has undergone modification since the 1970s and mid-1980s. Moore and Moore[224] described the earlier models, which promoted an infectious basis for ARDS/MOF, with two possible scenarios: (1) insult → ARDS → pulmonary sepsis → MOF, or (2) insult → sepsis → ARDS/MOF. Current thinking promotes an inflammatory model of MOF with an inflammatory response from a number of infectious and noninfectious stimuli. Two patterns exist: the one-hit model (massive insult → severe SIRS → early MOF) and the more common two-hit model (moderate insult → moderate SIRS → second insult → late MOF). Research into the pathogenesis of MOF has focused on how the inflammatory response is propagated, independent of infection. Moore and Moore have the global hypothesis that postinjury MOF occurs as the result of a dysfunctional inflammatory response.[224] Deitch created an integrated

Table 20-3

Definition of Organ Failure Based on Fry Criteria

Pulmonary	Need of ventilator support at Fio_2 ≥ 0.4 for 5 consecutive days.
Hepatic	Hyperbilirubinemia >2.0 g/dL and an increase of serum glutamic-oxaloacetic transaminase.
Gastrointestinal	Hemorrhage from documented or presumed stress-induced acute gastric ulceration. This can be documented by endoscopy; if endoscopy is not performed, then the hemorrhage must be sufficient to require two units of blood transfusion.
Renal	Serum creatinine level greater than 2.0 mg/dL. If a patient has preexisting renal disease with elevated serum creatinine level, then doubling of the admission level is defined as failure.

paradigm of the mechanisms of MOF.[79] In general, three broad overlapping hypotheses have been proposed in the pathogenesis of MOF: (1) macrophage cytokine hypothesis, (2) microcirculatory hypothesis, and (3) gut hypothesis. Attempts to understand this highly complex syndrome must extend to the cellular and molecular levels.

Organ injury in MOF is largely due to the host's own endogenously produced mediators and less due to exogenous factors like bacteria or endotoxins (Table 20-4).[79] There is increasing evidence that biologic markers for the risk of development of MOF may be more useful than anatomic descriptions of injuries. Nast-Kolb and associates[236] measured various inflammatory markers in a prospective study of 66 patients with multiple injuries (injury severity score [ISS] >18) and found that the degree of inflammatory response corresponded with the development of post-traumatic organ failure.[236] Specifically, lactate, neutrophil elastase, interleukin-6, and interleukin-8 were found to correlate with organ dysfunction. Strecker and co-workers[342] studied 107 patients prospectively and found that the amount of fracture and soft tissue damage can be estimated early by analysis of serum interleukin-6 and creatine kinase and is of great importance with regard to long-term outcome after trauma. These investigators found significant correlations between fracture and soft tissue trauma and intensive care unit stay, hospital stay, infections, systemic inflammatory response syndrome, multiple organ failure score, and serum concentrations or activities of serum interleukin-6, interleukin-8, and creatine kinase during the first 24 hours after trauma.

Blood transfusions are a frequent part of polytrauma treatment and an independent risk factor for MOF. Zallen and associates have identified the age of packed red blood cells (PRBCs) to be a risk factor, with the number of units over 14 days and 21 days as independent risk factors for MOF.[382] Old but not outdated PRBCs prime the neutrophils for superoxide production and activate the endothelial cells, which are pathogenic mediators for MOF.

Our understanding of the pathogenesis of MOF is constantly increasing. This has led to a hypothesis considering "complex nonlinear systems," which Seely has described.[320] Although recognition and treatment of MOF have improved, there has been little impact on the mortality

FIGURE 20-5 | *The interrelationship among systemic inflammatory response syndrome (SIRS), sepsis, and infection. (From Bone, R.C.; Balk, R.A.; Cerra, F.C.; et al. Definitions for sepsis and organ failure and guidelines for the use of innovative therapies in sepsis. Chest 101:1644–1655, 1992.)*

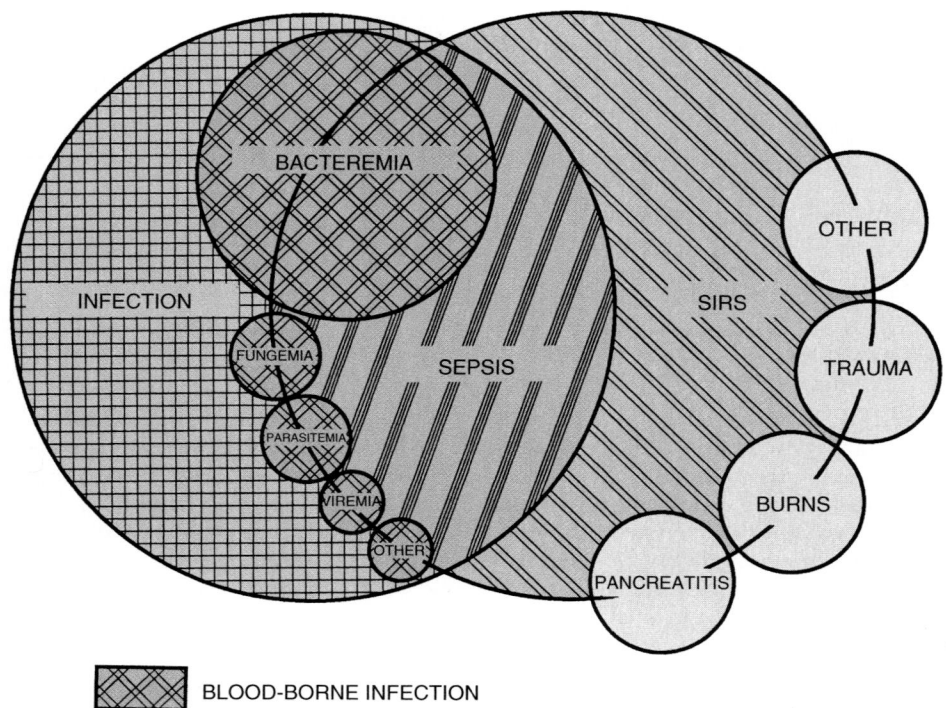

BLOOD-BORNE INFECTION

Table 20-4

Potential Mediators Involved in the Pathogenesis of Multiple Organ Failure

Humoral Mediators

Complement
Products of arachidonic acid metabolism
    Lipoxygenase products
    Cyclooxygenase products
Tumor necrosis factor
Interleukins (1–13)
Growth factors
Adhesion molecules
Platelet activating factor
Procalcitonin
Procoagulants
Fibronectin and opsonins
Toxic oxygen-free radicals
Endogenous opioids-endorphins
Vasoactive polypeptides and amines
Bradykinin and other kinins
Neuroendocrine factors
Myocardial depressant factor
Coagulation factors and their degradation products

Cellular Inflammatory Mediators

Polymorphonuclear leukocytes
Monocytes/macrophages
Platelets
Endothelial cells

Exogenous Mediators

Endotoxin
Exotoxin and other toxins

Source: Adapted with permission from Balk, R.A. Pathogenesis and management of multiple organ dysfunction or failure in severe sepsis and septic shock. Crit Care Clin 16(2):337–352, 2000.

rate in the past 20 years.[80] It has been suggested that future treatment strategies must address multimodality combination therapy aimed at suppressing the inflammatory response while preserving immune competence and antimicrobial defenses.[80]

MOF is a syndrome distinct from respiratory failure, which can complicate airway injury, resuscitation, or anesthesia following an accident. With the development of improved patient categorization, transport, and emergency care, it has become recognized that there is a threshold beyond which the survival from injury is problematic. With simple injuries (e.g., an ankle fracture and laceration from a fall), the physiologic effects are not additive. However, in high-energy blunt trauma, the systemic effects—for example, of a pulmonary contusion, ruptured spleen, and fractured pelvis—become more than additive.

The ISS, used to quantify the extent of trauma,[14] was derived from the abbreviated injury score (AIS) of the American Medical Association Committee on Medical Aspects of Automotive Safety,[67] updated in 1985 as AIS-85. Injuries to six body regions (head and neck, face, chest, abdomen and pelvic viscera, extremities and bony pelvis, and integument) are graded as (1) mild, (2) moderate, (3) severe, (4) critical—outcome usually favorable, and (5) critical—outcome usually lethal. The ISS equals the sum of the squares of the three highest AIS grades. The ISS score has a maximal value of 75.

When the ISS is 25 or greater, the patient is polytraumatized and at risk for MOF. This patient will benefit from specialized trauma center care. The median lethal ISS scores have been determined by age group (in years):

ages 15 to 44, an ISS of 40; ages 45 to 64, an ISS of 29; and ages 65 and older, an ISS of 20.[124] Moore and Moore[224] identified the following variables to be predictive of MOF: age older than 55 years, ISS 25 or greater, more than 6 units of blood in the first 24 hours after admission, high base deficit, and high lactate level. These investigators stratified patients at risk for MOF (Table 20-5).

One of the consequences of MOF is the depletion of body protein reserves. Amino acids are essential components of the energy systems that maintain the body's homeostasis; this deficit cannot be replenished by intravenous glucose or lipids.[37] As MOF progresses, the peripheral metabolic energy source switches from the conventional energy fuels of glucose, fatty acids, and triglycerides to the catabolism of essential branched-chain amino acids. The multiple-injury patient is like a diesel submarine on the bottom of the ocean with a limited air supply. Once the air supply is exhausted, damage control systems can no longer be maintained. Amino acids are lost as muscles are oxidized for energy, and the supply is not replenished.[136,228]

Tscherne emphasized the role of necrotic tissue in the pathogenesis of MOF.[254] It is well known that a gangrenous limb, for example, can provoke a systemic catabolic response. Those with military experience have observed the dramatic reversal of alarming symptoms that occurs when an urgent amputation is undertaken for gangrene. Pape et al. noted the importance of soft tissue injuries (extremities, lung, abdomen, and pelvis), which create a pathophysiologic cascade after blunt trauma.[257]

Dead tissue (e.g., muscle, bone marrow, and skin) provokes an inflammatory autophagocytic response.[118,239] In this setting, consumption of complement and plasma opsonins has been measured.[4,138,227] The complement system is activated with depletion of factors C3 and C5 with elevated levels of C3a and increased metabolism of C5a. C3a and C5a are anaphylatoxins and may cause the pulmonary edema in ARDS by affecting the smooth muscle contraction and vascular permeability.[138] Plasma opsonin activity is decreased with the consumption of the complement system. The opsonins are critical for antibacterial defense, and their consumption may lead to an increased susceptibility to infection.[4] Several investigators identified serum factors that stimulate muscle destruction.[15,61] Multiple mediators and effectors have been implicated in the pathogenesis of MOF, but exactly which

mediator or combination of mediators is responsible for the hypermetabolic response is not known.[135] This response consumes the individual's energy reserve and leads to MOF. Once MOF is established, the sequence of organ failure apparently follows a consistent pattern, with involvement first of the lung, then the liver, gastric mucosa, and kidney.[104]

Positive blood culture results have been documented in 75 percent of patients with MOF, but it is not clear whether infection is the cause or simply accompanies MOF.[104,200] Goris and associates[118] were able to induce MOF in rats by injecting a material that causes an inflammatory response. Sepsis causes tissue destruction and, therefore, like broken bones, releases activators of autophagic systems into the bloodstream.

The immune system's response in polytrauma can be measured. Polk and colleagues[271] defined a scoring system for predicting outcome by combining points for ISS and contamination with a measurement of monocyte function (the surface expression of D-related antigen). This method appears promising in predicting survival.[144]

Because patients with identical injuries can have vastly different inflammatory responses after severe trauma, there may be a genetic predisposition for a compromised immune system after trauma. Hildebrand et al.[145] performed a prospective cohort study of patients with an ISS greater than 16 and noted that the IL-6-174G/C polymorphism was associated with the severity of the posttraumatic systemic inflammatory response. These authors concluded that there may be a genetic predisposition to an enhanced inflammatory response after polytrauma that may be associated with adverse outcome.

A multiple system approach to the multiple-injury patient has proved valuable in preventing the development of MOF (Table 20-6). Avoidance of pulmonary failure, prevention of sepsis, and nutritional support are the keys.[21] Mechanical ventilation is regulated in a special care unit under the supervision of anesthesiologists or traumatologists with experience and training in this area of intensive care. Immediate wound débridement and constant

---

Table 20-5
Risk Stratification for Postinjury Multiple System Organ Failure

Category	Risk Factors	MSOF Probability (%)
I	ISS 15–24	4
II	ISS ≥25	14
III	ISS ≥25 plus >6 U RBCs/first 12 hr	54
IV	ISS ≥25 plus >6 U RBCs/first 12 hr plus lactate ≥2.5 mmol at 12–24 hr	75

Abbreviations: ISS, injury severity score; MSOF, multiple system organ failure; RBCs, red blood cells.
Source: Moore, F.A.; Moore, E.E. Evolving concepts in the pathogenesis of postinjury multiple organ failure. Surg Clin North Am 75:257–277, 1995.

Table 20-6
Prevention of Multiple Organ Failure

Resuscitative Phase

Aggressive volume resuscitation in early stages of treatment

Appropriate monitoring of volume resuscitation with measurement of arterial base deficit and serum lactate level, use of pulmonary artery catheters, calculation of oxygen delivery and consumption, use of gastric tonometry

Operative Phase

Timely operative management of soft tissue injuries with débridement of nonviable and infected tissue

Early fixation of all possible long bone and pelvic fractures

Vigilance in preventing the missed injury

ICU Phase

Early nutritional support

Appropriate use of antibiotics

Specific organ support

Timely reoperative surgery for missed injuries and complications of trauma

attention to the details of wound management, pulmonary toilet, cleanliness of access lines, and urinary tract sterility are required to prevent sepsis. With open fractures, parenteral or local wound antibiotics are therapeutic. An assessment of nutritional reserve, including measurement of triceps skinfold, total lymphocytes, and serum transferrin, is helpful in determining the need for nutritional support. If possible, the gastrointestinal tract should be used, but in patients with extensive intra-abdominal injury and poor nutritional reserves, early total parenteral nutrition with amino acid supplementation is essential. Nutrition has an important role in preventing the translocation of bacteria and toxins from the gut into the splanchnic circulation; once bacteria and toxins are in the circulation, they are transported to the liver, altering liver (Kupffer) cell function and causing progressive hepatocyte hypermetabolism and organ failure.[53,220]

ORTHOPAEDIC MANAGEMENT

Early total care of significant pelvic, spinal, and femoral fractures can have a powerful role in avoiding the cascade of events leading to pulmonary failure, sepsis, and death.[160,195,302] Increased understanding of the metabolic consequences of fracture surgery further clarifies the timing of orthopaedic surgery in the polytrauma patient; specifically, when is early total care of fractures safe, and when is damage control orthopaedics useful? There is a quiet optimism that the damage control orthopaedics approach to the polytrauma patient will decrease the incidence of multisystem organic dysfunction and failure.[256,294] Intramedullary nailing of the femur has been shown to be a "second hit" to the patient.[114] Harwood et al. reported that damage control orthopaedics was associated with a lesser systemic inflammatory response.[134] Despite the fact that damage control orthopaedics is used in many centers for patients with the lethal triad of acidosis, hypercoagulability, and hyperthermia, there is no good scientific evidence (e.g., randomized, prospective studies) that it is effective. There are many studies that support the early fixation of fractures. Demling[83] stressed control of the inflammatory process to prevent further stimulus to MOF by early rapid removal of injured tissue and prevention of further tissue damage by early fracture fixation.

Overall, early fixation has been shown to decrease rates of respiratory, renal, and liver failure.[50] Seibel and associates showed that in the blunt multiple-trauma patient with an ISS ranging from 22 to 57, immediate internal fixation followed by ventilatory respiratory support greatly reduces the incidence of respiratory failure, positive blood culture results, complications of fracture treatment, and MOF.[321] When patients were treated with the same ventilatory support but with 10 days of traction before fracture fixation, pulmonary failure lasted twice as long, positive blood culture results increased 10-fold, and fracture complications increased by a factor of 3.5. If no ventilatory support was used and traction was used for 30 days, pulmonary failure lasted three to five times as long, positive blood culture results increased by a factor of 74, and fracture complications increased by a factor of 17. Carlson and co-workers demonstrated that fixation in less than 24 hours after injury versus nonoperative fracture management decreased the late septic mortality from 13.5 percent

to less than 1 percent.[50] In a series of 56 multiple-injury patients, Goris and colleagues[119] showed that the advantage of controlled ventilation combined with early fracture fixation was greater than that of either ventilation or fracture fixation alone. The greatest advantage was observed in patients with an ISS of more than 50.[119]

Meek and co-workers[212] retrospectively studied 71 multiple-trauma patients with similar age and ISS with respect to timing of fracture stabilization. The group with long bone fractures stabilized within 24 hours had a markedly lower mortality than the group treated with traction and cast methods. In a prospective study, Bone and associates[33] compared the incidence of pulmonary dysfunction in 178 patients with acute femoral fractures who underwent either early (in the first 24 hours after injury) or late (>48 hours after injury) stabilization. The patients were further divided into those who had multiple injuries and those with isolated fracture of the femur. In none of the patients with isolated femoral fractures, whether treated with early or late stabilization, did respiratory insufficiency, required intubation, or needed placement in the intensive care unit occur. In the patients with multiple injuries, those who had delayed stabilization of fractures had a significantly higher incidence of pulmonary dysfunction.

Early femoral fixation may not play as critical a role in the outcome, however, in the aggressively managed surgical intensive care unit. Reynolds and associates studied 424 consecutive patients with femur fractures treated with IM rods, and half of these were done in the first 24 hours.[290] Of these 424 patients, 105 had an ISS of 18 or greater; these patients were studied for the relationship of fracture, fixation, timing, and outcomes. IM fixation was done in the first 24 hours in 35 of 105, between 24 and 48 hours in 12 of 105, and after more than 48 hours in 58 of 105. A few days' delay in fracture fixation did not adversely affect outcome, and pulmonary complications were related to the severity of injury rather than to timing of fracture fixation. Indeed, "fracture fixation" is a generic term for everything from a bloody open attack on a subtrochanteric fracture to the placement of a few large screws through percutaneous incisions for the assembly of a fixator. Only prospective research can identify which variables are truly important—anesthesia, blood loss, narcosis, ventilation, and micromotion, to name a few. The physiologic consequences of medullary nailing of the femur are the best known. Large trials in injured people are needed to compare nailing with other methods.

The type of fixation may play a role in risk consideration. With IM nailing, there is the risk of additional bone marrow emboli and potential associated lung dysfunction. Pape and associates found ARDS in a higher percentage of patients treated with a reamed IM femoral nail acutely performed (8/24, 33%) versus delayed nailing (2/26, 8%) in patients with femur fractures and severe thoracic injuries.[258] Charash and co-workers repeated the Pape study design and reported contradictory findings with favorable results in acute reamed IM nailing versus delayed nailing: pneumonia (14% vs. 48%) and pulmonary complications (16% vs. 56%).[58] Bosse and co-workers studied severe chest-injured patients with femur fracture treated within 24 hours with reamed IM nail or plating.[39] The retrospective study was controlled for group A, femur fracture with thoracic injury; group B, femur fracture with no thoracic injury; and group C, thoracic injury with no femur fracture. The overall ARDS rate in patients with femur fractures was 10 of 453 (2%). There was no significant difference in ARDS or pulmonary complications/MOF whether the femur fracture was treated with rodding or plating. Bosse and associates found no contraindication for reamed femoral nailing in the first 24 hours even if a thoracic injury was present. Pape and associates assessed lung function in two groups of patients undergoing early (≤24 hours) IM femoral nailing.[253] One group had femoral nailing after reaming of the medullary canal (RFN) and the other group had a small-diameter solid nail inserted without reaming (UFN). These investigators found that lung function was stable in UFN patients but deteriorated in RFN patients. They concluded that IM nailing after reaming might potentiate lung dysfunction, particularly in patients with preexisting pulmonary damage such as lung contusion. In contrast, Heim and associates, in a rabbit model, compared reamed versus unreamed nailing of femoral shaft fractures and showed that both techniques resulted in bone marrow intravasation and resulting pulmonary dysfunction.[139] These are examples of the controversies—to ream versus not to ream, rod versus plate, early versus late—in which incisive investigation is needed to guide decision making in a complex patient problem. Recent research regarding central mechanisms of bone regulation suggests that fracture repair depends not only on local but also on central mediators. The response of the organism as a whole to the noxious effects of injury may be needed to optimize repair systems. It may not yet be possible to "have your cake and eat it too"; and as politically correct as freedom from pain is, pain from a physiologic standpoint must be intimately tied to the recovery from injury.

When treating the patient with overt MOF, recognize that a potentially lethal condition is present and that the usual methods to control specific complications (e.g., pneumonia, renal failure, gastrointestinal bleeding) will be ineffective. The patient must be assessed as a whole. Focused intervention is required to turn the situation around. In such conditions, delay in performing operative procedures may be unwise. Significant unstable long bone, pelvic, and spinal fractures can be stabilized. However, long bone stabilization may need to be performed by means of damage control orthopaedics (temporary spanning external fixator) to avoid creating a "second hit" to the patient that would worsen recovery from MOF. Patients often require blood, calories (preferably enteral when feasible), effective antibiotics, controlled ventilation, and dialysis. All of these must be continuously monitored. Keel and Trentz stated that the development of immunomonitoring will help in the selection of the most appropriate treatment for the polytrauma patient.[166] Treatment measures for MOF often require careful balancing of risks and benefits. If anticoagulation prevents the propagation of thrombi, it can also be a cause of bleeding. When a patient dies of a pulmonary embolism, then the "prophylactic" measures can be considered insufficient—but what if the patient had bled to death? For many of these problems, the post-game review reveals how things might have been done differently. The argument when the

patient or family becomes angry changes to how things *should* have been done. No amount of provider education can prevent adverse outcomes from becoming adverse legal proceedings. The system for compensating the injured is broken.

The orthopaedist's role is to assess those fractures that are causing continued recumbency and to locate sources of devitalized tissue and sepsis in the musculoskeletal system. Sacrifice of a crushed but viable limb, loss of fracture reduction, or performance of a quick but not optimal limb stabilization are examples of the difficult choices or procedures that have to be made to save a life. The use of spanning external fixation (traveling traction),[148] so-called damage control orthopaedics,[148,256,294,311] is a good option because of its minimal additional tissue trauma, provisional bony stability, and improved ability to mobilize the patient.

In summary, in the presence of major thoracic and head injuries, there are potential risks of worsening a brain injury or precipitating ARDS from early orthopaedic procedures. Carlson[50] and Velmahos and associates[359] have shown no added morbidity for early fixation when chest or head injuries are present. However, Townsend[353] and Pape report increased risk for secondary brain injury and ARDS associated with early fixation.[253] Reynolds and associates showed modest delay did not affect the outcome.[290] Dunham et al.[86] noted no difference between early and late fracture fixation. Bhandari et al.[28] stated that head injury does not seem to be a contraindication to reamed intramedullary nailing. Giannoudis et al. noted that the literature does not provide clear-cut guidelines for the management of orthopaedic injuries in the head-injured patient. These authors stated that it was best to individualize treatment.[113] Finally, as Deitch and Goodman have noted, the best way to treat multiple organ failure is the prevention of MOF in the first place.[80]

LOCAL COMPLICATIONS OF FRACTURES

Local complications, meaning unwanted therapeutic outcomes, are part of the care of broken bones. Local failures of fracture treatment can manifest as immediate, delayed, or long-term adverse outcomes. Delayed complications include complex regional pain syndromes and disuse atrophy—the "fracture disease." Arthrosis and malunion are examples of the long-term adverse results with permanent impairment and economic importance. Any treatment program, no matter how thoughtfully conceived and carefully performed, has a failure rate that cannot be entirely eliminated. The patient, physician, and system variables inherent in each given clinical situation mean that, in practice, complication rates are usually in excess of those rates published in the literature. With multiple injuries, the rates become more than additive. This is expressed in the ISS by adding the squares of injury components.[14] The purpose of this section is to provide a framework for understanding local complications of fractures.

Soft Tissue and Vascular Problems

An accident, unlike an elective operation, causes the transmission of force of an undetermined magnitude to human tissue. However, through accident reconstruction it is possible to estimate the magnitude of energy transfer. For example, a fall from 30 feet is equivalent to being struck by a car going 30 miles per hour. In the immediate hours, days, and fortnight after injury, it should not be surprising that areas of skin demarcation, skin sloughing, bruising, or thrombosed vessels appear. These areas, if operative interventions are appropriate, are the consequences of injury and not of its treatment. In addition, after an osteosynthesis, there is additional opportunity for the slow accumulation of hematoma from bleeding from bone surfaces. Today's shortened hospitalization with early mobilization has increased the incidence of postoperative hematoma. Postoperative hematoma manifests as swelling, pain, loss of function, and not infrequently, serous drainage either from a wound or from the drain tract. Significant hematomas do not resorb but instead continue to increase in size and cause wound separation, skin sloughing, and infection. Collections of blood or fluid can be detected with ultrasonography. It is usually best to re-explore the wound under adequate anesthesia, evacuate the hematoma, irrigate the fracture site, drain the field, and apply a compression dressing.

Arterial injuries may manifest acutely with signs of hemorrhage and ischemia, or the presentation may be delayed, as in an arteriovenous fistula or a pseudoaneurysm. In civilian injuries with associated fractures or dislocations, the arterial injury rate is from 2 to 6 percent. For isolated fractures or dislocations, the arterial injury rate is less than 1 percent. War-related extremity injuries, a high proportion of which result from high-velocity gunshot wounds, consist of a long bone fracture with associated vascular injury in about one-third of cases.[59] Even if a pulse is present, an arterial injury may still have occurred. The most accurate means of diagnosis is an angiogram, which should be performed if there is evidence of an ischemic extremity, a weak or absent pulse, or a bruit, or if the trajectory of the bullet passes in the vicinity of a major artery. Certain injury patterns such as a knee dislocation, especially a posterior one, have a 30 percent incidence of associated popliteal artery damage. Therefore, with these injuries, an arteriogram is indicated as soon as practical. Today CT-angiography is supplanting contrast arteriography in the evaluation of vascular injury. CT-angiography avoids the hazards of arterial puncture contrast reactions and provides excellent visualization of the vascular tree. Traditional angiography at many centers is being replaced by CT-angiography.

Rieger et al. retrospectively assessed the accuracy of multidetector CT-angiography (MDCT) as the initial diagnostic technique to depict arterial injury in patients with extremity trauma.[291] Prospective sensitivity and specificity were 95 and 87 percent, respectively, and retrospective sensitivity and specificity were 99 and 98 percent, retrospectively. Inaba et al. also studied the ability of multislice helical computed tomography angiography (MCTA) to detect arterial injury in the traumatized.[156] MCTA achieved 100 percent sensitivity and 100 percent specificity in detecting clinically significant arterial injury. No missed injuries were identified during the follow-up period, which was a mean of 48.2 days.[156] Despite these reported accuracies, there are reported concerns about

the limitations of MDCT such as that reported by Portugaller et al. who noted lower sensitivity in the infrapopliteal area due to small vessel diameter.[274]

CT-angiography is clearly the wave of the future for imaging the vascular system. There remain clinical questions and concerns despite its popularity. Improvements in technique and accuracy of interpretation are likely to strengthen the available evidence to support its widespread application.

When femur fractures are associated with femoral artery injury, the results of vascular repair and limb function are characteristically good, although delayed diagnosis of pseudoaneurysm and claudication can be a problem.[100] Cases requiring amputation because of a delay in diagnosis can occur. Popliteal artery injury, even when diagnosed early, may not be amenable to vascular reconstruction. Vascular injuries distal to the popliteal trifurcation are basically not fixable and carry a much worse prognosis. Revascularization is usually not needed if one vessel is patent on angiogram and the distal pressure is 50 percent of the brachial artery pressure. When revascularization is required, a good functional result can be expected in only about 25 percent of cases. In Flint and Richardson's experience, 6 of 16 patients undergoing revascularization distal to the trifurcation required early amputation, and 6 more required late amputation (total, 12/16) for osteomyelitis, nonunion, and persistent neuropathy and its associated complications.[100] Early amputation without revascularization is often appropriate in the patient with loss of vascular inflow, long bone fracture, neurotmesis, or extensive soft tissue damage. The high rate of infection and complications can result in a delayed amputation when revascularization is done.[322]

Post-traumatic Arthrosis

Post-traumatic arthrosis is considered a complication of fractures (Fig. 20-6). However, there is limited insightful research on the actual pathomechanics of post-traumatic arthrosis. Wright, a retired judge, used a questionnaire to determine a consensus view of the factors related to the development of post-traumatic arthrosis after fracture.[43] He found the following: that lower limb joints are more likely to develop arthritis than upper extremity joints, that older patients are at higher risk for the development of post-traumatic arthrosis (although younger patients have a longer time frame to develop post-traumatic arthrosis), and that occupation is a risk factor. Kern and associates also reported the association of osteoarthritis and certain occupations.[169] The potential causes of post-traumatic arthrosis include the following: (1) incongruity of the articular surface, (2) cartilage damage from the load transfer, (3) malalignment, (4) malorientation of the joint, and (5) repetitive loading injury.

JOINT INCONGRUITY

The emphasis on anatomic reduction in fracture surgery focuses on the reestablishment of joint congruity usually at the expense of the soft tissue attachments. Extensive bony comminution of the articular surface, particularly of the knee and the distal tibia, can make a repair of joint congruity a formidable or even an impossible task. Acetabular fractures

FIGURE 20-6 *Radiograph of a hip 18 years after limited internal fixation, an older technique, of a posterior wall acetabular fracture, which demonstrates post-traumatic arthrosis likely secondary to articular cartilage impact and degeneration, and joint incongruity.*

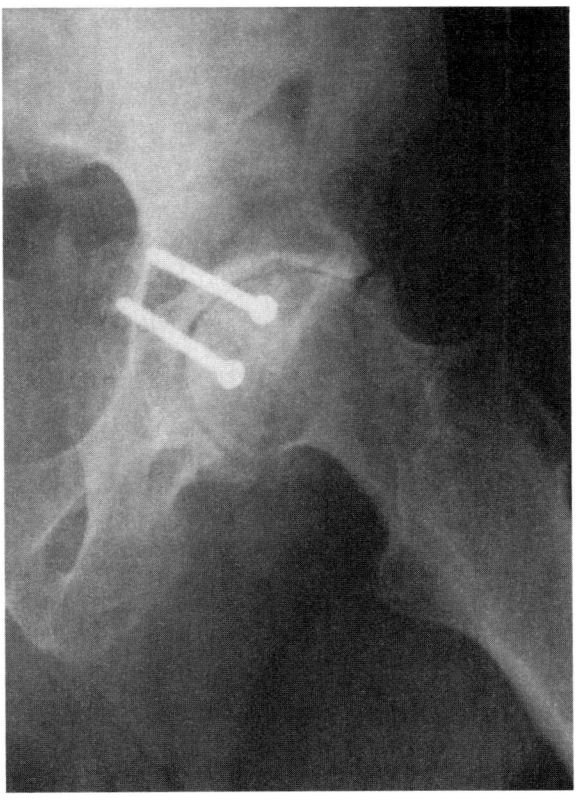

FIGURE 20-7 *Anteroposterior radiograph of a knee with post-traumatic arthrosis secondary to joint incongruity and articular cartilage degeneration 5 years after a high-energy tibial plateau fracture.*

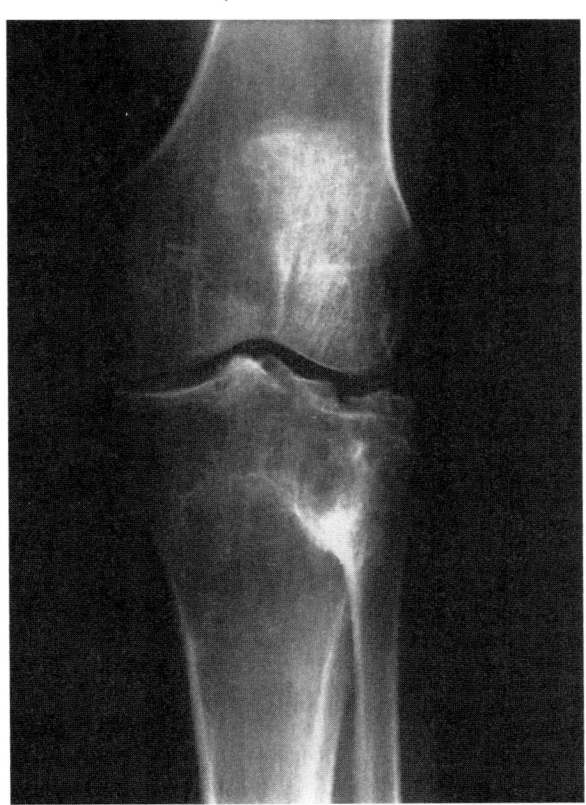

are a good example of articular fractures that are associated with the development of post-traumatic arthrosis[211] largely because of failure to reestablish joint congruity and the articular cartilage injury itself.[206]

ARTICULAR CARTILAGE DAMAGE

The impact to the articular cartilage at the time of injury in high-energy trauma is a likely contributor to the articular cartilage damage and the subsequent development of post-traumatic arthrosis (Figs. 20-7 and 20-8). However, the clinical data are not clear-cut. Volpin and co-workers reported at an average follow-up of 14 years of intra-articular fractures of the knee joint that there were 77 percent good-to-excellent results.[361] Repo and associates stated that the impact loads sufficient to fracture a femoral shaft of an automobile occupant are nearly sufficient to cause significant articular cartilage (chondrocyte death and fissuring).[288]

There is an increasing appreciation of cartilage injury from impact. The advent of MRI of knee injuries has enhanced our appreciation of damage to the articular surfaces (bone bruising) (Fig. 20-9). Spindler and associates studied 54 patients with anterior cruciate ligament tears and found a bone bruise present in 80 percent of cases,

FIGURE 20-8 *Correlative arthroscopic view of the lateral compartment of the knee in Figure 20-7, which demonstrates post-traumatic arthrosis secondary to joint incongruity, articular cartilage degradation, and meniscal degeneration 5 years after a high-energy tibial plateau fracture.*

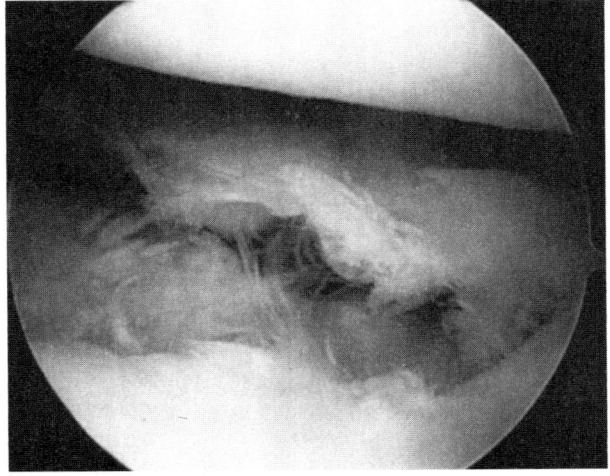

FIGURE 20-9 *Sagittal MR image of the lateral compartment of a knee that demonstrates a bone contusion involving the lateral femoral condyle and the lateral tibial plateau in association with a recent anterior cruciate ligament tear. (Courtesy of Theresa M. Corrigan, M.D.)*

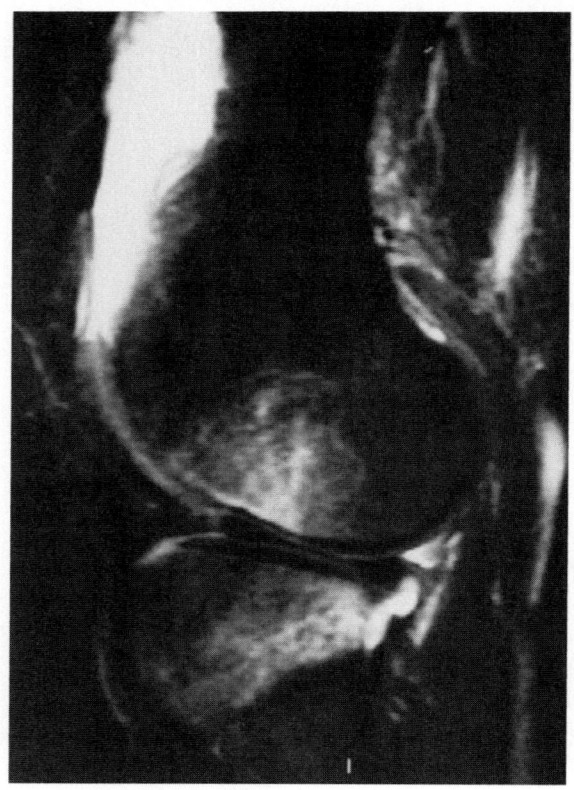

of which 68 percent were in the lateral femoral condyle.[332] Miller and co-workers studied 65 patients who had MRI-detected trabecular microfractures associated with isolated medial collateral ligament injuries.[222] Although these bone bruises were approximately half as common as bone bruises associated with anterior cruciate ligament tears, these investigators stated that medial collateral ligament-associated trabecular microfractures may be a better natural history model.[222] Bone bruises in combination with anterior cruciate ligament tears may be harbingers of future arthritis. Wright and associates noted that isolated bone bruises not associated with ligamentous or meniscal injury may have a better prognosis than bone bruises noted in conjunction with ligamentous and meniscal injury.[380]

The biologic basis for the cartilage degradation is being studied: the pathologic process involves degradation of articular cartilage.[230] It has been theorized that the impact at the time of injury damages the articular cartilage or its blood supply irreversibly and initiates a cascade of post-traumatic arthritis.[288] This etiology of impact arthritis has not been well studied.[288,352,363] Attempts to develop a model have been made. Vrahas and co-workers developed a method of impacting quantifying blows to articular cartilage in a rabbit model.[363] Nonetheless, cartilage

damage, particularly when it is unassociated with bone changes, may not necessarily progress to arthritis.[281] Radin noted that full-thickness cartilage lesions that are less than 1 cm usually will not progress to arthritis.[281]

MALALIGNMENT

Tetsworth and Paley have focused on the relationship between malalignment and degenerative arthropathy.[351] Focusing on degenerative arthritis and changes in the weight-bearing line or mechanical axis (malalignment), changes in the position of each articular surface relative to the axis of the individual segments (malorientation), and changes in joint incongruity, they noted that the joints of the lower extremity are nearly co-linear and that any disturbance in this relationship (malalignment) affects the transmission of load across the joint surfaces.[351]

The hip and shoulder joints, because of their sphericity, tolerate malalignment. The ankle joint is also fairly tolerant of deformity because of compensation through the subtalar joint. However, the knee is most vulnerable to changes in the normal coronal plane relationship of the lower extremity.[351] Malalignment of the knee, which changes the mechanical axis, creates a moment arm, which increases force transmission across either the medial or lateral compartments of the knee joint.[251,252]

Nonetheless, there are conflicting clinical data regarding whether these factors lead to post-traumatic arthrosis. Kettlekamp and associates stated that there are no data to support the position that malalignment always leads to degenerative arthritis.[172] Kristensen and co-workers reported no arthrosis of the ankle 20 years after malaligned tibial fractures.[178] In contrast, Puno and co-workers studied 27 patients with 28 tibial fractures and found that greater degrees of ankle malalignment produced poorer clinical results.[279] Merchant and Dietz stated that they did not find any support in their study for the hypotheses that angulation results in shear rather than compressive forces on articular cartilage and that these forces lead to early arthrosis.[216]

MALORIENTATION

Another postfracture residual deformity that can contribute to post-traumatic arthrosis is malorientation (a change in the orientation of a joint to the mechanical axis). The association of malorientation of the knee and osteoarthritis has been demonstrated.[69,70] Malorientation can result from translation or rotation. When the orientation of the joint is substantially changed in relation to the mechanical axis, the theory is that abnormal loading of the articular cartilage and subchondral plate will occur, which will accelerate joint deterioration and ultimately lead to osteoarthritis. Malorientation is probably more of a problem with weight-bearing joints such as the knee, which are subject to higher and more frequent loading.

REPETITIVE LOADING INJURY

Articular cartilage damage can occur either by sudden impact loading or by repetitive impulsive loading.[81,85,203,282] As a result, portions of the matrix can be fractured, cause cartilage necrosis, and produce subclinical microfractures in the calcified cartilage layer.[110] The effect on cartilage homeostasis appears to lead to changes that are seen in association with osteoarthritis.[81,282,364] Fairbanks' changes,[94] radiographic evidence of knee arthritis after meniscectomy, most likely result from repetitive loading to the articular after changes in load distribution of the knee joint. Deterioration of damaged articular cartilage by repetitive loading may be asymptomatic because cartilage is relatively aneural.[110]

Adult canine articular cartilage after indirect blunt trauma demonstrates significant alterations in its histologic, biomechanical, and ultrastructural characteristics without disruption of the articular surface.[85] Thompson and associates found arthritic-like degeneration of the articular cartilage in an animal model within 6 months after transarticular loads.[352] These investigators also noted that degenerative changes that occur in patients who sustained traumatic insult to the joint may represent a phenomenon similar to their animal model.[94]

Damage to articular cartilage often can occur without perceptible alteration in the macroscopic appearance of the tissue.[110] There is limited potential for cartilage self-repair. Yet there is some evidence that some cartilage repair is possible, which has led to the proliferation of procedures such as autologous cartilage transplantation[44] and microfracture.[338]

SUMMARY

We have tabulated the incidence of post-traumatic arthrosis associated with some common fractures and dislocations (Table 20-7). In addition, post-traumatic arthrosis is discussed elsewhere in the text.

Arthrosis is not necessarily progressive. Letournel studied a small cohort of patients with tibial pilon fractures 5 and 10 years after injury. Results trended toward improvement in time rather than progression. Post-traumatic arthrosis may be an inevitable consequence of musculoskeletal injury. It appears to be related to the magnitude of the original injury. At the present time, fracture surgery techniques cannot fully reverse the articular cartilage injury. Gelber and associates reported that an injury to the knee joint in young adulthood was related to a substantial increased risk for future knee osteoarthritis.[108]

Other confounding factors in determining the relationship between fractures and the development of post-traumatic arthrosis are normal age-related changes. Bonsell and associates reported that age was a significant predictor for degenerative changes observed on radiographs of the shoulder in asymptomatic individuals.[36]

Specific components of the pathomechanics of post-traumatic arthrosis include malalignment, malorientation, joint incongruity, articular cartilage destruction, ligamentous or fibrocartilaginous injury, and repetitive loading injury. Salvage procedures such as joint replacement or osteotomy are less successful for post-traumatic arthrosis than for osteoarthritis.[186] Postinjury counseling and patient education are necessary to convey realistic expectations after fracture surgery. Prospective, multicenter, long-term studies are needed to better understand the natural history of post-traumatic arthrosis and to be able to decipher it from normal age-related osteoarthrosis.

Peripheral Nerve Injuries

Few entities can overshadow the outcome of the treatment of a fracture as much as a peripheral nerve injury. Whether the nerve palsy is diagnosed before or after surgery, it is certain that the patient and other health care providers will be inordinately focused on the nerve palsy itself. Peripheral nerve injuries in orthopaedic trauma are probably underreported because clinical assessment of peripheral lesions is often impossible or impractical. Electrodiagnostic testing is more sensitive than clinical examination alone and can facilitate the diagnosis of traumatic peripheral nerve injuries. A scientific approach to peripheral nerve injury is imperative. Electromyography (EMG) is most useful for localizing entrapment when there are multiple sites that are hard to differentiate clinically. Is the ulnar nerve entrapped in the arm or at the elbow? Otherwise, it is not really better than serial clinical examination *except* it indicates concern on the part of the clinician and buys time while being scheduled and repeated, enough time usually for nerve recovery.

HISTORY OF THE TREATMENT OF NERVE INJURY

George Omer traces the history of the treatment of peripheral nerve injuries to William A. Hammond, Surgeon General of the U.S. Army during the American Civil War.[245] Omer traces the evolution of understanding and treatment of peripheral nerve injuries from the Civil War through the two World Wars, the Vietnam and Korean conflicts, and the development of "The Sunderland Society."[245] The greatest advances have come from the intraoperative microscope and the ingenuity of the surgeon.[333]

CLASSIFICATION OF NERVE INJURY

Historically, Seddon is credited with the scientific classification of peripheral nerve injury into three categories: neurotmesis, axonotmesis, and neurapraxia (Table 20-8).[319] Seddon, however, noted that these three terms were coined by Professor Henry Cohen in 1941.[319] Understanding peripheral nerve injury is predicated on understanding the anatomy of myelinated nerves (Fig. 20-10).

Neurotmesis implies a cutting or separation of related parts in which all essential structures have been "sundered."[319] Seddon noted that although there is not necessarily an obvious anatomic gap in the nerve and the epineural sheath may appear to be in continuity, the effect is as if anatomic continuity has been lost.[319]

Axonotmesis involves a lesion to the peripheral nerve of such severity that wallerian degeneration occurs but the epineurium and supporting structures of the nerve have been "so little disturbed that the internal architecture is fairly well-preserved."[319]

Neurapraxia is described as a lesion in which paralysis occurs in the absence of peripheral degeneration. Seddon noted that "neurapraxia" is preferred to "transient block" because the recovery time can be lengthy and is "invariably complete."[319]

Seddon notes that of the three terms neurotmesis is probably the best understood and that in clinical practice the existence of axonotmesis or neurapraxia could only be

Table 20-7
Incidence of Post-Traumatic Arthritis

Upper Extremity

Shoulder			
	Acromioclavicular joint dislocations		25%–43%
	Scapula fractures	Superior lateral angle	61%
	Anterior shoulder dislocation		7%
Elbow			
	Elbow dislocations—simple	24-yr follow-up	38%
	Elbow dislocations with a radial head fracture		63%
Wrist			
	Colles' fractures		3%–18%
	Colles' fractures	Young adults	57%–65%
	Scapholunate dislocations		58%
	Trans-scaphoid perilunate dislocations; fracture	4.3-yr follow-up	50%

Lower Extremity

Acetabular Fractures			6.5%–56%
Hip Dislocations	Anterior		17%
	Posterior	<6 hr time to reduction	30%
	Posterior	≥6 hr time to reduction	76%
Supracondylar/Intercondylar Femur Fractures			22% (patellofemoral joint)
			5% (tibiofemoral joint)
Patella Fractures			18%
Tibial Plateau Fractures	Fracture patterns	Bicondylar fractures	42%
		Medial plateau fractures	21%
		Lateral plateau fractures valgus	16%
			31%
	Association with alignment after plateau fractures	Normal	13%

Ankle Fractures			20%–40%
Talar Neck	Ankle Joint	Subtalar joint	
Fractures			
Hawkins I	15%	24%	
Hawkins II	36%	66%	
Hawkins III	69%	63%	
Subtalar Joint Dislocations			56%
Taisometatarsal Fracture-Dislocation (Lisfranc Joint Injuries)			78% (15-yr follow-up)

Source: Foy, M.A.; Fagg, P.S. Medicolegal Reporting in Orthopaedic Trauma. New York, Churchill Livingstone, 1996, pp. 2.1-01–4.1-16.

surmised.[319] The advent of electrodiagnostic testing, however, has made the distinction between axonotmesis and neurotmesis much easier. Seddon noted that the most common variety of neurotmesis was from anatomic division. Wallerian nerve degeneration occurs peripherally, and the clinical picture is that of complete interruption of the nerve.

Axonotmesis is characterized by complete interruption of axons but with preservation of the supporting structures of the nerve (Schwann tubes, endoneurium, and perineurium). On a histologic level, there is complete interruption of the axons, preservation of the Schwann tubes and endoneurium, and wallerian degeneration peripherally. Seddon noted that clinically axonotmesis was indistinguishable from neurotmesis until recovery occurs, which in axonotmesis was spontaneous.[319] When exploration is performed, the finding of an intact nerve suggests that the lesion is an axonotmesis.[319] A fusiform neuroma finding suggests that the injury was a mixed lesion of axonotmesis and neurotmesis with the former predominating.[319] A finding of intraneural fibrosis is evidence that the lesion was a neurotmesis.

Table 20-8		
Types of Peripheral Nerve Injuries		
Injury	**Pathophysiology**	**Prognosis**
Neurapraxia	Reversible conduction block characterized by local ischemia and selective demyelination of the axon sheath	Good
Axonotmesis	More severe injury with disruption of the axon and myelin sheath but with an intact epineurium	Fair
Neurotmesis	Complete nerve division with disruption of the endoneurium	Poor

Source: Brinker, M.R.; Lou, E.C. General principles of trauma. In: Brinker M.R., ed. Review of Orthopaedic Trauma. Philadelphia, W.B. Saunders, 2001, p. 8, with permission.

Seddon noted that with neurapraxia, there is no axonal degeneration. There is localized degeneration of the myelin sheaths. Blunt injuries and compression were the most common cause of neurapraxias.[319] He noted that the clinical picture is one of complete motor paralysis and incomplete sensory paralysis.[319] Also, he noted that there was no anatomic "march" to recovery as seen after nerve suture or axonotmesis.[319] Finally, Seddon noted that many nerve injuries were in fact combinations of the three different nerve injuries he described.[319] Of a series of 537 nerve injuries, he noted that there were 96 cases in which a neurotmesis and an axonotmesis were combined.[319]

Sunderland added to the work of Seddon by subdividing peripheral nerve injury into five degrees by basically subdividing the neurotmesis into three types (third-, fourth-, and fifth-degree injuries) while maintaining the concepts of neurapraxia (first-degree injury) and axonotmesis (second-degree injury).[343] He defined five degrees of nerve injury based on changes induced in the normal nerve. Seddon described these injuries in ascending order, which affected successively (1) conduction in the axon, (2) continuity of the axon, (3) the endoneurial tube and its axon, (4) the funiculus and its contents, (5) the entire nerve trunk.[343] The most important part of Sunderland's work is his clarification that nerve injuries previously classified by Seddon as neurotmesis were not all equal.

Sunderland also added to the knowledge of partial and mixed nerve injuries. He noted that some fibers in a nerve may escape injury while others sustain a variable degree of damage.[343] He observed that in partial severance injuries and fourth-degree injuries, it was unlikely that the remaining fibers would escape some injury. This type of injury should be described as a "mixed lesion."[343] However, fourth- and fifth-degree lesions could not coexist either together or in combination with any of the minor types of injuries.[343]

There are difficulties with the classification of peripheral nerve injury. Many nerve injuries are mixed injuries in which various nerve fibers are affected to varying degrees.[187] In addition, the subtypes of Seddon's classification are usually discernible only on histologic examination of the nerve and are seldom possible on the basis of clinical or electromyographic data.

INCIDENCE OF NERVE INJURIES ASSOCIATED WITH FRACTURES

There is a fairly high incidence of nerve injury with some common orthopaedic entities (Table 20-9). Conway and Hubbell reported electromyographic abnormalities associated with pelvic fracture and noted that patients with double vertical pelvic fractures (combined injury to the anterior third of the pelvic ring and the sacroiliac area) were most at risk, with a 46 percent incidence of

---

FIGURE 20-10 *Cross-sectional anatomy of peripheral nerve. Inset at left shows an unmyelinated fiber. Inset at bottom shows a myelinated fiber. (From Lee, S.K.; Wolfe, S.W. Peripheral nerve injury and repair. J Am Acad Orthop Surg 8:243–252, 2000.)*

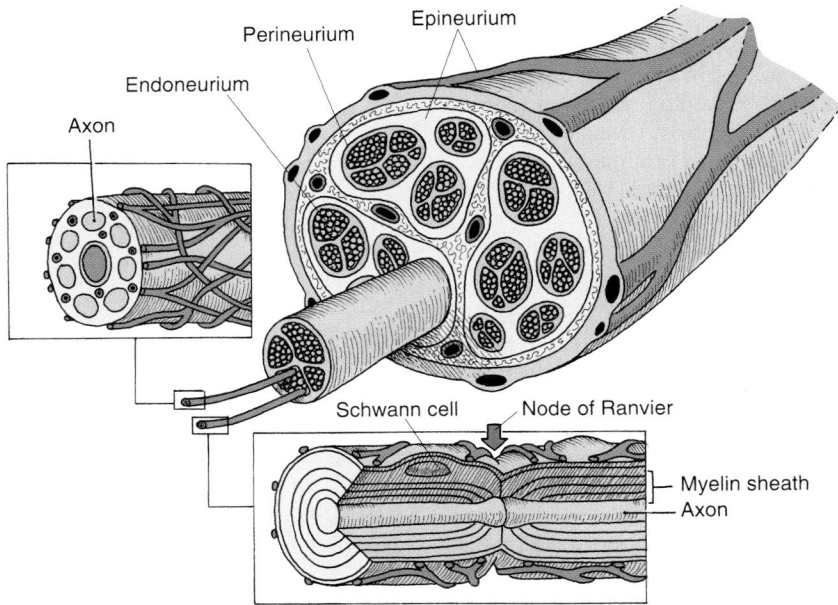

Table 20-9		
Common Orthopaedic Entities Associated with Peripheral Nerve Injuries		
Anatomic Location	**Type of Injury**	**Incidence of Nerve Injury**
Humerus	Midshaft fracture	12%–19% incidence of radial nerve palsy
Pelvis	Double vertical pelvic fracture	46% incidence of neurologic injury
Tibia	Tibia fracture	19%–30% incidence of neurologic findings after intramedullary nailing
Ankle	Ankle eversion	86% incidence of neurologic findings

neurologic injury.[68] Goodall noted that 95 percent of fractures with an associated nerve injury occur in the upper extremity.[116] Of all fracture types, a humerus fracture is the most likely fracture to have an associated nerve injury.[19] Omer reported, based on a collected series,[247] the following distribution of nerve injuries associated with fractures and fracture-dislocations: radial nerve (60%), ulnar nerve (18%), common peroneal nerve (15%), and median nerve (6%).[116,127,191]

EVALUATION OF PERIPHERAL NERVE INJURIES

In the polytrauma patient, the neurologic assessment is incorporated in the initial assessment, which uses the alphabet—ABCD—where D is for disability and neurologic assessment.[345] The Glasgow Coma Scale (GCS), developed by Teasdale and Jennet, specifically assesses eye opening, motor response, and verbal response on a maximum 15-point rating scale.

The assessment of peripheral nerve injury during orthopaedic surgery rounds and emergency department assessments often is reduced to the terms *neurovascularly intact* or *N/V intact*. In our opinion, such terms, although convenient, should not be used unless a complete neurologic examination (cutaneous sensation including light touch, pain, and temperature; vibratory sensation; motor strength in all muscles with grading; deep tendon reflexes; and special tests for clonus, etc.) and a complete vascular examination (pulses, capillary refill, venous examination, tests for thrombosis, auscultation for bruits, etc.) are performed. Formal assessment of peripheral nerve injury is usually performed using electrodiagnostic testing with electromyography (EMG) and nerve conduction velocities (NCVs).

ELECTROMYOGRAPHY AND ELECTRODIAGNOSTICS

In a broad sense, EMG refers to a set of diagnostic tests using neurophysiologic techniques that are performed on muscles and nerves.[344] Strictly speaking, EMG refers to one of these tests, in which a small needle is used to probe selected muscles, recording electrical potentials from the muscle fibers.[344]

Although electrodiagnostic testing has historically been of little interest to the orthopaedic surgeon, there is heightened interest in electrodiagnostics as a result of intraoperative use of sensory-evoked potentials and

motor-evoked potentials in spine surgery, brachial plexus surgery, and acetabular surgery.

It has been said that the best times for electrodiagnostic studies are the day before injury and then about 10 to 14 days after injury. The former is, of course, impossible but nonetheless underscores the importance of baseline studies and changes over time, particularly when one is looking for evidence of reinnervation (which would be consistent with an axonotmesis) or denervation (which would be consistent with a neurotmesis). The latter highlights the fact that reinnervation following Wallerian degeneration takes at least 10 to 14 days to be able to be detected on electrodiagnostic testing.

Basic Science of Electrodiagnostics

To understand EMG, it is necessary to review some basics of nerve structure and function. A motor neuron has a cell body in the spinal cord and extends into the nerve root, an axon that exits the spine, traverses the plexus, travels within a nerve, and then forms many distinct branches.[344] A motor unit consists of one such cell and the several muscle fibers that it innervates.[344] Muscles contain many motor units that are analogous to colored pencils in a bundle.[344] Muscle forces are created by activation of an increasing number of motor units under the command of the brain.[344] When a motor unit fires, a small electrical signal is generated and can be recorded by placing a small needle through the skin and into the muscle near the motor unit fibers acting electronically like an antenna.[344] This signal is amplified, filtered, digitized, and displaced on a computer screen.[344] Single motor unit potentials are sampled first on the oscilloscope. As greater force is generated, there is recruitment of more motor units and an increase in the firing rate.[344] When full muscle force is generated, the oscilloscope screen fills with signals, which has an appearance called the *full interference pattern*.[344] Another important component of EMG interpretation is the sound of the motor potentials, which are amplified and broadcast through a speaker.[344] The experienced electromyographer can recognize characteristic sounds and audible patterns.[344]

The usefulness of EMG for the trauma patient is the ability to localize neurologic lesions anatomically based on a pattern of denervated muscle. EMG is also useful for following nerve recovery over time.

Characteristic Electromyography Patterns

If there is an injury to the axon, as with axonotmesis or neurotmesis, distal degeneration of the nerve (wallerian degeneration) causes it to be electrically irritable.[344] Needle movement generates denervation potentials called fibrillations and positive waves, which have both characteristic appearances on the oscilloscope and sounds on the loudspeaker.[344] These findings are delayed, occurring at least 10 days afterward, even after complete transection.[344] Sprouting and reinnervation that would occur with a recovering axonotmesis create a high amplitude polyphasic motor unit potential (Table 20-10).[344]

NERVE CONDUCTION STUDIES

Distinct from EMG are nerve conduction studies. Nerve conduction studies can be used to test both sensory and motor nerves in skeletal muscle. These studies test only large myelinated

Table 20-10
Electromyographic Findings Related to Trauma

Condition	Insertional Activity	Activity at Rest	Minimal Contraction	Interference
Normal study	Normal	Silence	Biphasic and triphasic potential	Complete
Neurapraxia	Normal	Silence	Reduced number of potentials	Reduced
Axonotmesis (after 2 wk)	Increased	Fibrillations and positive sharp waves	None	None
Neurotmesis (after 2 wk)	Increased	Fibrillations and positive sharp waves	None	None

Source: Adapted with permission from Brinker, M.R.; Lou, E.C. General Principles of Trauma. In Brinker, M.R., ed. Review of Orthopaedic Trauma. Philadelphia, W.B. Saunders, 2001, p. 9, of which the data were adapted with modifications from Jahss, M.H. Disorders of the foot. In Miller, M.D., ed. Review of Orthopaedics, 3rd ed. Philadelphia, W.B. Saunders, 2000.

nerve fiber function. Nerve fibers commonly evaluated include the ulnar, median, radial, and tibial nerves (motor and sensory fibers); the sciatic, femoral, and peroneal fibers (motor fibers only); and the musculocutaneous, superficial peroneal, sural, and saphenous nerves (sensory only). The procedure of nerve conduction testing uses surface electrodes, often silver discs or ring electrodes, to record extracellular electrical activity from muscle or nerve. EMG machines have a nerve stimulator that can apply an electrical shock to the skin surface at accessible points on the nerve.[344] This stimulus depolarizes a segment of the nerve and generates an action potential, which travels in both directions from the point at which it was stimulated.[343] When a sensory nerve is tested, the action potential can be recorded from a distal point (surface electrodes or finger electrodes).[344] By measuring the distance from the stimulus point to the recording site and using the oscilloscope values of the time of latency and action potential amplitude, the examiner can determine the sensory conduction velocity.[344]

Motor nerve conduction velocities (motor NCVs) are recorded from surface electrodes taped over muscles distally in the limb.[343] Normative control values for motor nerve conduction velocities at different ages are used for comparison. This difference is attributable to the degree of myelination, which increases with age over the early developmental years. Although nerve conduction velocities are fairly uniform from age 3 years through adulthood,[344] nerve conduction velocities can vary based on several conditions. Nerve conduction values at birth are about 50 percent of adult values. As surface temperature decreases below 34°C, there is a progressive increase in latency and a decrease in conduction velocity.[31] Upper extremity conduction velocities are generally about 10 to 15 percent faster than those of the lower extremity. Conduction velocities in the proximal segments are usually 5 to 10 percent faster than in the distal segments,[31] which is a function of nerve root diameter.

To study motor conduction, the nerve is supramaximally stimulated at two or more points along its course where it is most superficial. At a distal muscle that is innervated by the nerve, a motor response is recorded.[342] Various parameters measured include latency, conduction velocity, amplitude, and duration. Characteristic nerve conduction study findings for various nerve injuries are shown in Table 20-11.

Sensory nerve conductions are generally unaffected by lesions proximal to the dorsal root ganglion even though there is sensory loss.[31] Sensory testing is good for localizing a lesion relative to the dorsal root ganglia: either proximal (root or spinal cord), in which case the NCV is normal, or distal (plexus or peripheral nerve), abnormal

Table 20-11
Nerve Conduction Study Results Related to Trauma

Condition	Latency	Conduction Velocity	Evoked Response
Normal study	Normal	Upper extremities: >48 m/sec	Biphasic
		Lower extremities: >40 m/sec	
Neurapraxia			
Proximal to lesion	Absent or low voltage (if partial)	Absent or low voltage (if partial)	Absent
Distal to lesion	Normal	Normal	Normal
Axonotmesis			
Proximal to lesion	Absent	Absent	Absent
Distal to lesion (immediate)	Normal	Normal	Normal
Distal to lesion (>7 days)	Absent	Absent	Absent
Neurotmesis			
Proximal to lesion	Absent	Absent	Absent
Distal to lesion (immediate)	Normal	Normal	Normal
Distal to lesion (>7 days)	Absent	Absent	Absent

Source: Adapted with permission from Brinker, M.R.; Lou, E.C. General Principles of Trauma. In: Review of Orthopaedic Trauma. Philadelphia, W.B. Saunders, 2001, p. 8, of which the data were from Jahss, M.S. Disorders of the foot. In: Miller, M.D.; Brinker, M.R., eds. Review of Orthopaedics, 3rd ed. Philadelphia, W.B. Saunders, 2000.

NCV. In addition, sensory nerve potential is lower in amplitude than compound motor action potentials and can be obscured by electrical activity or artifacts. Sensory axons are evaluated in four ways: (1) stimulating and recording from a cutaneous nerve, (2) recording from a cutaneous nerve while stimulating a mixed nerve, (3) recording from a mixed nerve while stimulating a cutaneous nerve, and (4) recording from the spinal column while a cutaneous nerve or mixed nerve is stimulated.[31] Variables measured include onset latency, peak latency, and peak-to-peak amplitude.

Two other parameters that are measured are the F-wave and the H-reflex. The F-wave is a late motor response attributed to a small percentage of fibers firing after the original stimulus impulse reaches the cell body. These F-waves are particularly useful for the evaluation of the proximal segments of peripheral nerves.[31] However, the F-wave is useful only in the assessment of proximal lesions only in the absence of more distal pathology. There is also variability in the F-wave response because different fibers fire each time, making it less quantitative. The H-reflex is an electrically evoked spinal monosynaptic reflex that activates the Ia afferent fibers (large myelinated fibers with the lowest threshold for activation). The Achilles tendon reflex (S1) is the easiest to record and can differentiate between an S1 and an L5 radiculopathy.[31] Again, distal pathology must be ruled out if the latency is prolonged and being used to assess for proximal pathosis.

SOMATOSENSORY-EVOKED POTENTIALS The method of performing somatosensory-evoked potentials (SSEPs) involves an afferent pulse of large nerve fiber sensory activity that travels proximally and enters the spinal cord and then ascends to the brain via the posterior columns in the brainstem after the nerve is stimulated.[344] This postsynaptic activity ultimately reaches the thalamus and the parietal cortex of the brain.[344] A small brain wave occurs following nerve stimulation at a fixed time following nerve stimulation and is recordable from surface electrodes in the scalp.[344] These SSEPs can be recorded simultaneously from various points such as Erb's point, which overlies the brachial plexus, over the cervical spine, and from the scalp overlying the cortex.[344] SSEPs are useful for monitoring the lower extremity in spinal surgery. Upper extremity SSEPs are useful in brachial plexus surgery.

Although the use of somatosensory-evoked potentials was popular[141] for acetabular surgery, SSEPs have been supplanted by spontaneous EMG[140] when monitoring is desired. However, the general use of SSEPs or electromyographic modalities does not seem to be justified.[221]

ASSOCIATION OF PERIPHERAL NERVE INJURY WITH CAUSALGIA

There is a potential after peripheral nerve injury for development of causalgia (type II complex regional pain syndrome). According to Bonica, the incidence of causalgia is 1 to 5 percent of peripheral nerve injuries.[34] Data from the Vietnam War indicate a lower incidence of causalgia than the data from World War II (1.5% vs. 1.8–13.8%). Rothberg and associates and Bonica[34] suggest that this

lower incidence was due to the more rapid transport of the wounded and the higher quality of care.

PROGNOSIS

NERVE INJURIES ASSOCIATED WITH OPEN AND CLOSED FRACTURES AND DISLOCATIONS
Omer noted a spontaneous return of nerve function in 83 percent of nerve injuries associated with fractures.[244] Radial nerve palsy associated with humerus fractures is perhaps a good example in which nerve recovery can be expected in roughly 90 percent of cases.[172,272,326,330] There are further distinctions in prognosis including lower recovery rates of nerve function with open fractures than with closed fractures (17% vs. 83.5% in one series).[318] Omer also reported that nerve injuries associated with a dislocation were less likely to show spontaneous recovery than nerve injuries associated with a fracture.[248] Omer noted that peripheral neuropathy associated with closed fractures is usually neurapraxia lesions, which have an excellent prognosis.[248] Peripheral neuropathy associated with open fractures had a prognosis related to the etiology: lacerations are usually neurotmesis lesions and should be closely examined, explored, and sutured.[248]

NERVE INJURIES ASSOCIATED WITH PROJEC-TILE INJURIES
Data from Vietnam on 595 gunshot wounds studied by Omer had an equal 69 percent spontaneous recovery rate for both low- and high-velocity gunshot wounds.[246] Proximal nerve injuries in extremities take longer to show clinical recovery than more distal extremity injuries because cellular repair occurs from the intact viable cell body distally to the receptor.[246] Civilian peripheral nerve injuries from projectiles with associated vascular injury have a poor prognosis. In one series, only 10 percent of these nerve injuries resolved.[131] Shotgun injuries have a higher incidence of nerve injuries than other types of gunshot injuries, have a worse prognosis (spontaneous recovery rate of about 45%),[198] and have a higher percentage of complete nerve transection (neurotmesis) than even high-velocity missile wounds. High-velocity missiles often create axonotmesis lesions and have a better prognosis than low-velocity missile wounds.[246]

SUMMARY

Peripheral nerve injuries associated with fractures and dislocations are probably underappreciated in the acute trauma setting. The orthopaedic surgeon ought to refrain from using the term *neurovascularly intact* unless a complete neurologic and vascular examination has been performed. Instead, documentation should be limited to what was observed and performed (e.g., "can dorsiflex great toe," "1+ dorsalis pedis pulse"). Heightened surveillance for neurologic injury is protective for the clinician because failure to diagnose nerve injuries may result in patient dissatisfaction, disability, and litigation. The orthopaedic surgeon needs to be familiar with the lexicon of nerve injury (neurapraxia, axonotmesis, and neurotmesis) to communicate with colleagues. From a practical standpoint, evaluation of recovery after a peripheral nerve injury is best performed by serial physical examinations. However, there is a role for electrodiagnostic testing, particularly when there is no sign of recovery of nerve function. Electrodiagnostic studies should be delayed for at least 3 weeks and often need to be repeated serially. Research in nerve regeneration techniques may ultimately hold the key to the treatment of peripheral nerve injuries in the future.

Complex Regional Pain Syndrome

Pain after musculoskeletal injury usually subsides. When patients have peculiar, disagreeable, and persistent painful symptoms several weeks after injury, they may have complex regional pain syndrome (CRPS). CRPS is increasingly recognized as a cause of disability after injury.[365] The index of suspicion in general is not high enough, and many patients are not diagnosed until the later stages when the prognosis is less favorable.[365] Advances have been made in the understanding and treatment of CRPS. Nevertheless, many treatment methods are empirical, and there is a need for research in this area.[365]

MODERN TERMINOLOGY

More than six dozen different terms have been used in the English, French, and German literature over the past two decades to describe CRPS type I, which used to be called reflex sympathetic dystrophy (RSD).[365] A complicated lexicon of RSD has evolved from the more general category of "pain dysfunction syndromes,"[8] to the terminology adopted in 1994 by the International Association for the Study of Pain into "complex regional pain syndromes."[337] CRPS is subdivided into CRPS type I (RSD) and CRPS type II (causalgia).[337] The distinction is based on the absence of a documented nerve injury for type I and a documented nerve injury for type II causalgia (Table 20-12). An additional variant of CRPS, termed complex regional painless syndrome, has been reported.[88] This variant has all the clinical findings of CRPS type I except that pain is not the presenting symptom and is minimal. How common this variant of CRPS type I will prove to be remains to be seen. The focus here is on painful CRPS type I associated with traumatic orthopaedic injuries.

ETIOLOGY AND EPIDEMIOLOGY

Trauma secondary to accidental injury has been described as the most common cause of CRPS type I.[34] These injuries include sprains; dislocations; fractures, usually of the hands, feet, or wrists; traumatic finger amputations; crush injuries of the hands, fingers, or wrists; contusions; and lacerations or punctures of the fingers, hands, toes, or feet.[34] It has been reported that CRPS develops in 1 to 5 percent of patients with peripheral nerve injury, 28 percent of patients with Colles' fracture,[29] and 30 percent of patients with tibial fracture although these percentages are higher than our experience for Colles' and tibia fractures.[309] In a recent series, the three most common inciting events were a sprain or strain in 29 percent, surgery in 24 percent, and a fracture in 16 percent.[290] Interestingly, in this same series, 6 percent of patients could not remember an inciting event.[6] Saphenous neuralgia has been called a *forme fruste* of sympathetically mediated pain around the knee.[270] External fixators appear to be associated with CRPS in the upper extremity, although whether it is a result of the fracture immobilization,

Table 20-12
International Association for the Study of Pain: Diagnostic Criteria for Complex Regional Pain Syndrome

Complex Regional Pain Syndrome Type I (Reflex Sympathetic Dystrophy)

1. The presence of an initiating noxious event or a cause of immobilization.
2. Continuing pain, allodynia, or hyperalgesia with which the pain is disproportionate to the inciting event.
3. Evidence at some time of edema, changes in skin blood flow, or abnormal sudomotor activity in the painful region.
4. The diagnosis is excluded by the existence of conditions that would otherwise account for the degree of pain and dysfunction.

Note: Criteria 2, 3, and 4 are necessary for a diagnosis of complex regional pain syndrome.

Complex Regional Pain Syndrome Type II (Causalgia)

1. The presence of continuing pain, allodynia, or hyperalgesia after a nerve injury, not necessarily limited to the distribution of the injured nerve.
2. Evidence at some time of edema, changes in skin blood flow, or abnormal sudomotor activity in the region of the pain.
3. The diagnosis is excluded by the existence of conditions that would otherwise account for the degree of pain and dysfunction.

Note: All three criteria must be satisfied.

Source: Adapted with permission from Pittman, D.M.; Belgrade, M.J. Complex regional pain syndrome. Am Fam Phys 56:2265–2270, 1997; which was adapted with permission from Merskey, H.; Bodguk, N., eds. Classification of Chronic Pain, Descriptions of Chronic Pain Syndromes and Definitions of Pain Terms, 2nd ed. Seattle, IASP Press, pp. 40–43.

possible traction injury to the nerves, or direct neural trauma from the pins is unclear. CRPS can also be associated with arthroscopic surgical procedures[75] and prolonged usage of extremity tourniquets.

Allen and associates[6] reported on the epidemiologic variables of patients with CRPS. They noted in a series of 134 patients evaluated at a tertiary chronic pain clinic that patients had a history of having seen on average 4.8 different physicians before referral.[6] The average duration of symptoms of CRPS before presentation to the tertiary chronic pain clinic was 30 months.[6] In addition, 54 percent of patients had a workmen's compensation claim and 17 percent of patients had a lawsuit related to the CRPS.[282] Of the 51 of 135 patients who underwent a bone scan, only 53 percent of the studies were interpreted as consistent with the diagnosis of CRPS.[6]

PATHOPHYSIOLOGY

Breivik noted that, as described by the International Association for the Study of Pain, CRPS is a complex neurologic disease involving the somatosensory, somatomotor, and autonomic nervous system in various combinations, with distorted information processing of afferent sensory signals to the spinal cord.[42,217] Autonomic nervous system dysregulation occurs in only 25 to 50 percent of patients with CRPS.[35,94,217] The role of the sympathetic system was further clarified by Ide and associates, who used a noninvasive laser Doppler to assess fingertip blood flow and vasoconstrictor response and found that skin blood flow and vasoconstrictor response returned to normal following successful treatment of the condition.[154] These investigators suggested that the sympathetic nervous system function is altered and is different in the various stages of CRPS type I.

Many CRPS type I patients have a combination of sympathetically maintained pain and sympathetically independent pain. Sympathetically maintained pain (SMP) is defined as pain that is maintained by sympathetic efferent nerve activity or by circulating catecholamines.[35,94,217] SMP is relieved by sympatholytic procedures.[42] Sympathetically maintained pain follows a nonanatomic distribution.[192] Nonetheless, SMP is not essential in the development of CRPS and that is why the term reflex sympathetic dystrophy is no longer in favor.[42] In some patients, sympatholytic procedures will not relieve their pain.[42] Breivik notes that more than half of all patients with CRPS have sympathetically independent pain. In one series, symptoms of increased sympathetic activity occurred in 57 percent of patients, whereas signs of inflammation and muscle dysfunction occurred in 90 percent of patients.[357]

CLINICAL PRESENTATION

Although the differential diagnosis of CRPS type I is extensive (Table 20-13), the diagnosis of florid CRPS type I is not generally difficult.[307] However, recognizing milder cases is challenging because of the changing clinical

Table 20-13
Selected Differential Diagnosis of CRPS Type I

Musculoskeletal
  Bursitis
  Myofascial pain syndrome
  Rotator cuff tear (Buerger's disease)
  Undiagnosed local pathology (e.g., fracture or sprain)
Neurologic
  Poststroke pain syndrome
  Peripheral neuropathy
  Postherpetic neuralgia
  Radiculopathy
Infectious
  Cellulitis
  Infectious arthritis
  Pain of unexplained etiology
Vascular
  Raynaud's disease
  Thromboangiitis obliterans
  Thrombosis
  Traumatic vasospasm
Rheumatic
  Rheumatoid arthritis
  Systemic lupus erythematosus
Psychiatric
  Factitious disorder
  Hysterical conversion reaction

Source: Adapted with permission from Pittman, D.M.; Belgrade, M.J. Complex regional pain syndrome. Am Fam Phys 56:2265–2270, 1997.

features of this syndrome over time (i.e., vasodilatation first, then vasoconstriction, and finally dystrophic changes), dynamic alterations including diurnal fluctuations, and the subjectivity of some complaints.[307] Nonetheless, the importance of early diagnosis is highlighted by the fact that results of treatment are better when treatment is initiated earlier.

Sandroni et al. have prospectively studied whether certain clinical characteristics and laboratory indices correlate with the diagnosis of CRPS type I.[307] They found that both the clinically based CRPS I scoring system, which graded allodynia, vasomotor symptoms, and swelling, and the laboratory-based CRPS I grading system, which incorporated a sudomotor index, vasomotor index, and a resting sweat index, were sensitive and reliable tools and could be combined to provide an improved set of diagnostic criteria for CRPS I. Oerlemans et al. found that bedside evaluation of CRPS type I with Veldman's criteria was in good accord with psychometric or laboratory testing of these criteria.[243] Veldman's criteria are defined as follows: (1) the presence of four or five of the following signs and symptoms: unexplained diffuse pain, difference in skin color relative to the other limb, diffuse edema, difference in skin temperature relative to the other limb, and limited active range of motion; (2) the occurrence or increase of the above signs and symptoms after use; and (3) the presence of the above signs and symptoms in an area larger than the area of primary injury or operation and including the area distal to the primary injury.[357] Schurmann and co-workers studied the incidence of specific clinical features in CRPS type I patients and normal post-trauma patients and assessed the diagnostic value of a bedside test that measures sympathetic nerve function.[315] Sympathetic reactivity was obliterated or diminished in the affected hands of patients with CRPS type I in contrast to age-matched controls with normal fracture patterns.[315]

STAGING

CRPS type I has been separated into three stages: acute, dystrophic (ischemic), and atrophic.[185,273,317] These stages are generally based on chronology, with stage I lasting about 3 months, stage II from 3 to 6 months after the onset of symptoms, and stage III beginning 6 to 9 months after the injury.[74] Stages are also determined based on their symptom complexes. Stage I is characterized by swelling, edema, increased temperature in the extremity, and pain aggravated by movement. Stage I is associated with hyperpathia (delayed overreaction and aftersensation to a painful stimulus, particularly a repetitive one), exaggerated pain response, hyperhidrosis, and allodynia (pain elicited by a normally non-noxious stimulus, particularly if repetitive or prolonged).[74,283] Sympathetic blocks may be curative during this acute stage of CRPS. Stage II occurs typically after about 3 months when the initial edema becomes brawny, trophic changes of the skin appear, the joint may become cyanotic, and joint motion decreases. In the third stage, the pain may begin to decrease, trophic changes are more pronounced, edema is less prominent, the skin becomes cooler and drier with a thinning and glossy appearance, and joint stiffness occurs.[74]

DIAGNOSTIC TESTING

The diagnosis of CRPS type I is usually based on clinical findings. The new criteria for diagnosing CRPS do not include the results of diagnostic testing with sympathetic blocks, and the discerning clinician may disagree on the true presence of CRPS type. Selected diagnostic tests are discussed.

RADIOGRAPHY The early findings of CRPS are patchy demineralization of the epiphyses and short bones of the hands and feet.[283] Genant and associates[109] defined five types of bone resorption that may occur in CRPS type I. These are irregular resorption of trabecular bone in the metaphysis creating the patchy or spotty osteoporosis, subperiosteal bone resorption, intracortical bone resorption, endosteal bone resorption, and surface erosions of subchondral and juxta-articular bone.[109] Radiographic findings such as subperiosteal resorption, striation, and tunneling of the cortex are not diagnostic of CRPS type 1 and may occur with any condition causing disuse.[283] Once patchy osteopenia is present, the patient is usually already in stage II CRPS.[93,377] Osteopenia of the patella is the most common finding of CRPS of the knee.[74]

BONE SCANNING Three-phase bone scanning with technetium has long been used as a diagnostic study for CRPS type I, with the pervasive notion that scans will be hot in all three phases. Although this may often be the case in the acute phase, the bone scan findings in stages II and III are more subtle. There are many false-negative bone scan results in stages II and III.[284] Raj and associates noted that in stage II the first two phases of the bone scan are normal and the delayed images (static phase) of the bone scan demonstrate increased activity.[284] Stage III has decreased activity in phases one and two and normal activity in the third phase (delayed or static phase).[284] In contrast, a study of quantitative analysis of three-phase scintigraphy concluded that scintigraphy should not be considered as the definitive technique for the diagnosis of CRPS type I.[386]

Bone scans have been used to assess the response to treatment and have been found to have no value in monitoring treatment.[385] However, these investigators found that the bone scan had prognostic value: marked hyperfixation of the tracer indicates better final outcome.

THERMOGRAPHY Thermography images temperature distribution of the body surface.[283] Gulevich and associates reported on the use of stress infrared telethermography for the diagnosis of CRPS type I and reported that as a diagnostic technique it was both sensitive and specific.[125] Further study of thermography is needed before global usage can be recommended.

PSYCHOLOGIC OR PSYCHIATRIC ASSESSMENT

Psychologic assessment of patients with CRPS has included structured clinical interviews and personality measures such as the Minnesota Multiphasic Personality Inventory (MMPI) and Hopelessness Index.[283] The MMPI profiles of patients with CRPS resemble those of patients with chronic pain (increasing elevations on the hypochondriasis, depression, and hysteria scales).[283] Patients in stage I have more pessimism than patients in the second and third stages. More pessimism and depression are seen in younger patients than in older patients.[284]

Bruehl and Carlson examined the literature for evidence that psychologic factors predispose certain individuals to development of CRPS.[45] They did find that 15 of 20 studies reported the presence of depression, anxiety, and/or life stress in patients with CRPS[45] and hypothesized a theoretical model in which these factors influenced the development of CRPS through their effects on α-adrenergic activity. They could not determine whether depression, anxiety, and life stress preceded the CRPS and were etiologically related to it.

CURRENT CONCEPTS IN TREATMENT

OVERVIEW The first line of treatment of CRPS type I includes nonsteroidal anti-inflammatory drugs (NSAIDs), topical capsaicin cream, a low-dose antidepressant, and physical therapy (contrast baths, transcutaneous electrical nerve stimulation [TENS] unit treatments, gentle range of motion to prevent joint contractures, and isometric strengthening exercises to prevent atrophy). Treatment at this time can usually be initiated by the orthopaedic surgeon. However, if the patient fails to respond, then referral to a pain specialist, generally an anesthesiologist with a special interest in pain management, should also be considered. The second line of treatment includes possible sympathetic blocks, anticonvulsants (gabapentin), calcium channel blockers (nifedipine), adrenergic blocking agents (phenoxybenzamine), and antidepressants in higher doses. The third line of treatment includes possible sympathectomy (surgical or chemical), implantable spinal cord stimulators, and corticosteroids. Table 20-14 shows the medications commonly used for CRPS type I.

NONSTEROIDAL ANTI-INFLAMMATORY DRUGS The possibility that the inflammatory response is important in the pathophysiology of CRPS[377] highlights the role of NSAIDs in treatment. Veldman and associates[357] suggested that the early symptoms of CRPS are more suggestive of an exaggerated inflammatory response to injury or surgery than a disturbance of the sympathetic nervous system.[357] Nonetheless, Sieweke and associates found no effect of an anti-inflammatory response and hypothesized a noninflammatory pathogenesis in CRPS that is presumably central in origin.[327]

ANTIDEPRESSANTS Antidepressants are useful in treating CRPS primarily by causing sedation, analgesia, and mood elevation. Analgesic action has been attributed to inhibition of serotonin reuptake at nerve terminals of neurons that act to suppress pain transmission, with resulting prolongation of serotonin activity at the receptor.[90]

NARCOTIC ANALGESICS There is a potential for abuse of narcotics in CRPS because of the associated chronic pain. These agents do little to relieve sympathetically mediated pain. However, when narcotics are given epidurally in combination with local anesthetic agents, they are effective. Epidural administration of fentanyl (0.03–0.05 mg/hr) allows maximum effect on the dorsal horn with minimal plasma concentration and minimal side effects.

Table 20-14	
Medications Commonly Used to Treat Reflex Sympathetic Dystrophy	
Medication	**Initial Dosage***
Adrenergic Agents	
Beta-blocker: propranolol (Inderal)	40 mg bid
Alpha-blocker: Phenoxybenzamine (Dibenzyline)	10 mg bid
Alpha- and beta-blocker: guanethidine (Ismelin)	10 mg/day
Alpha-agonist: clonidine (Catapres-TTS)	One 0.1 mg patch/wk
Calcium Channel Blocking Agent	
Nifedipine (Adalat, Procardia)	30 mg/day
Drugs for Neuropathic Pain	
Tricyclic antidepressants:	
Amitriptyline (Elavil)	10 to 25 mg/day
Doxepin (Sinequan)	25 mg/day
Serotonin reuptake inhibitors:	
Fluoxetine (Prozac)	20 mg/day
Anticonvulsant: Gabapentin (Neurontin)	300 mg on the first day, 300 mg bid on the second day, and 300 mg tid there-after
Corticosteroid: Prednisone	60 mg per day, then rapidly taper over 2–3 wk

*The initial dosage may need to be adjusted based on individual circumstances. Consult a drug therapy manual for further information about specific medications.
Source: Adapted with modifications with permission from Pittman, D.M.; Belgrade, M.J. Complex regional pain syndrome. Am Fam Phys 56:2265–2270, 1997.

ANTICONVULSANTS Mellick reported the results of using gabapentin (Neurontin) in patients with severe and refractory CRPS pain.[214] He noted satisfactory pain relief, early evidence of disease reversal, and even one case of a successful treatment of CRPS with gabapentin alone. The specific effects noted included reduced hyperpathia, allodynia, hyperalgesia, and early reversal of skin and soft tissue manifestations.

CALCIUM CHANNEL BLOCKERS (NIFEDIPINE) AND ADRENERGIC BLOCKING AGENTS (PHENOXYBENZAMINE) Nifedipine, a calcium channel blocker, has been used orally to treat CRPS. At a dosage of 10 to 30 mg three times a day, it induces peripheral vasodilatation. Initial treatment is usually at a dosage of 10 mg three times a day for 1 week, which is increased if there is no effect to 20 mg three times a day for 1 week, which is increased to 30 mg three times a day the following week if there is no effect. If partial improvement or relief occurs at any of these doses, then the dosage is continued for 2 weeks and then tapered and discontinued over several days.[279] The most common side effect of nifedipine is headache, which is most likely due to increased cerebral blood flow. Muizelaar and co-workers[232] assessed treatment of both CRPS types I and II with nifedipine or phenoxybenzamine, or both, in 59 patients. They found a higher success rate using phenoxybenzamine in 11 of 12 patients. A lower success rate of 40 percent was found in treating chronic CRPS. Although long-term oral use of phenoxybenzamine has been reported for the treatment of CRPS, there has been a high incidence of orthostatic hypotension (43%).[111] In an attempt to avoid these side effects, intravenous regional phenoxybenzamine has been used to treat CRPS with good results in a small series of patients.[201]

CORTICOSTEROIDS Although the use of corticosteroids in the treatment of CRPS is much less common, Raj and associates note that a trial of steroids might be a reasonable treatment for patients with long-standing pain who have not responded to blocks.[283] It has been reported that the patients who respond to corticosteroids had chronic pain of a mean duration of 25 weeks.[177]

PHYSICAL THERAPY Physical therapy has long been an integral part of treatment of CRPS type I. Oerlemans and associates prospectively studied whether physical therapy or occupational therapy could reduce the ultimate impairment rating in patients with CRPS and found that physical therapy and occupational therapy did not reduce impairment percentages in patients with CRPS.[241] Nonetheless, these same investigators have also reported that adjuvant physical therapy in patients with CRPS results in a more rapid improvement in an impairment level sum score.[242]

ELECTROACUPUNCTURE Chan and Chow reported their results with acupuncture with electrical stimulation in 20 patients with features of CRPS.[55] They found that 70 percent had marked improvement in pain relief and an additional 20 percent had further improvement. In addition, later follow-up reassessment of these patients showed maintenance or continued improvement of their pain relief 3 to 22 months after their course of electroacupuncture.[55] There has been a resurgence of interest in electroacupuncture.[146,285]

REGIONAL INTRAVENOUS AND ARTERIAL BLOCKADE The use of intravenous or intra-arterial infusions of ganglionic blocking agents is becoming increasingly popular in the treatment of CRPS.[283] Guanethidine, bretylium, and reserpine have been used with promising results.[315] Guanethidine has been substituted for reserpine in the intravenous regional block format to lessen side effects.[283]

SYMPATHETIC BLOCKS Sympathetic blockade has historically been useful both as a diagnostic test (placebo injections are included and documented temperature elevation after blockade) and as a basic treatment. Increasing recognition of the presence of nonsympathetically mediated pain in CRPS has contributed to the decreased use of diagnostic sympathetic blockade.

A series of injections are generally performed on an outpatient basis. Alternatively, continuous epidural infusions can be performed on an inpatient basis if the patient is unable or unwilling to have a series of outpatient nerve blocks.[75]

For upper extremity CRPS, the site of blockade is either the stellate ganglion or the brachial plexus. For lower extremity CRPS, the lumbar sympathetic chain or epidural space is the preferred site for sympathetic blockade.

TRANSCUTANEOUS ELECTRICAL STIMULATION

Transcutaneous electrical nerve stimulation (TENS) has been useful in the treatment of CRPS. It most likely works via the gate theory of pain introduced by Melzack and Wall in 1965 in which stimulation of the larger nerve fibers transcutaneously closes the "gate" and may inhibit the transmission of pain.[215]

TOPICAL CAPSAICIN Topical capsaicin cream in concentrations of 0.025 to 0.075 percent, used previously for post–herpetic neuralgia and painful diabetic neuropathy, has been noted to be worth considering for treating localized areas of hyperalgesia.[60,336] The effectiveness of topical capsaicin cream decreases after several weeks of daily usage.

CHEMICAL SYMPATHECTOMY Neurolytic sympathetic block is an alternative for the lower extremity but usually not the upper extremity. The proximity of the cervical sympathetic chain to the brachial plexus makes a cervical neurolytic sympathectomy too hazardous unless placed under fluoroscopic or CT guidance. Neurolytic lumbar sympathetic blockade is considered to be a viable alternative to surgical sympathectomy for lower extremity CRPS.[283] However, there are potential complications with such procedures including dermatologic problems and "sympathalgia" in the second or third postoperative weeks, which is characterized by muscle fatigue, deep pain, and tenderness.[142]

SURGICAL SYMPATHECTOMY Surgical sympathectomy has been advocated for patients who do not get permanent pain relief from blocks and is somewhat of a last resort or end-of-the-road treatment. Criteria have been suggested that should be met before surgical sympathetectomy is selected: patients should have had pain relief from sympathetic blocks on several occasions, pain relief should last as long as the vascular effects of the blocks, placebo injections should produce no pain relief, and secondary gain and psychopathology should be ruled out.[283] Failure of surgical sympathectomy has been attributed to reinnervation from the contralateral sympathetic chain.[173,174] Surgical sympathectomy in our opinion is less effective than chemical sympathectomy.

ELECTRICAL SPINAL CORD STIMULATION Electrical spinal cord stimulation is generally reserved for patients who have severe pain that is unresponsive to conventional treatments. Kemler and associates retrospectively studied the clinical efficacy and possible adverse effects of electrical spinal cord stimulation for the treatment of patients with CRPS.[168] About 78 percent of patients (18 of 23) reported subjective improvement during the test period, and 50 percent had complications related to the device. Prospective studies are needed to assess the efficacy of spinal cord stimulation.

NONTRADITIONAL THERAPIES Certain patients are responsive to nontraditional treatment such as art and music therapy, herbal medicines, and massage therapy. These approaches should be viewed with an open mind because the traditional, evidence-based therapies may not be successful in relieving pain associated with CRPS.

PREVENTION

It has been suggested that optimal pain relief after surgery can reduce the incidence of chronic postoperative pain syndromes, such as those that occur in almost 50 percent of thoracotomies.[164] This hypothesis is based on the concept that an abnormally exaggerated and prolonged hyperalgesia reaction is involved in the development of complex post-traumatic syndromes.[42] Although the potential for dose escalation and dependency has to be considered, perioperative management of pain with appropriate analgesics appears to help prevent CRPS.

PROGNOSIS

The prognosis of CRPS has historically been grim. The assumption has generally been that stage I CRPS will progress in most cases to stage II and then to stage III. In addition, the prognosis has also been linked to the time of diagnosis, with early diagnosis yielding a better prognosis. Zyluk studied the natural history of post-traumatic CRPS without treatment and found that the signs and symptoms of RSD were largely gone in 26 of 27 patients who completed the study at 13 months after diagnosis.[384] Nonetheless, the hands were still functionally impaired, and three patients who withdrew from the study had worsening of the signs and symptoms of CRPS.[384] Geertzen and associates studied 65 patients with CRPS to analyze the relationship between impairment and disability.[108] They found that CRPS patients had impairments and perceived disabilities after a mean interval of 5 years.[107] Furthermore, these investigators found no differences in impairments in patients who were diagnosed within 2 months of the causative event and those diagnosed 2 to 5 months after it. Nonetheless, there is evidence that the effect of treatment for sympathetically mediated pain is better during the first few months after onset.[42] Cooper and DeLee noted that the most favorable prognostic indicator in the management of CRPS of the knee was early diagnosis and early institution of treatment (within 6 months of onset).[74]

SUMMARY

Key for the orthopaedic surgeon is to recognize that the fracture patient may have CRPS, distinct from another condition. Tip-offs to the presence of CRPS are inordinate requests for narcotic medicine, inappropriate emergency department visits, and aggressive contacts with the office staff. CRPS should be considered any time that pain is out of proportion to what is expected. CRPS may take several visits to evaluate before it is obvious. It is important to have heightened awareness to differentiate it from an undetected additional injury; especially in polytrauma patients, making an early presumptive diagnosis of CRPS helps initiate timely, appropriate treatment. The new International Association for the Study of Pain criteria for CRPS type I make the diagnosis easier but less specific.

MANAGEMENT OF COMPLICATIONS

In this chapter, a complication of fracture treatment has been defined as an *undesired turn of events* in the treatment of a fracture. But because patient, doctor, and insurer each bring a different set of values into the assessment of medical outcomes, the question might be asked, "Undesired by whom?" Patient and doctor, for example, may agree to attempt to salvage a difficult compound tibial fracture with contamination and arterial injury. The insurer, facing charges in excess of a quarter of a million dollars for vascular repair, free flap coverage, fracture fixation, bone grafting, and multiple reoperations if infection develops, combined with a prolonged time of total disability before the patient is able to return to work, may regard the outcome as an undesired event when compared with below-the-knee amputation, prosthesis fitting, and early return to work.

An explicit understanding of the *desired* course of events is therefore crucial to recognizing complications. In this respect, fracture treatment is different from many other areas of orthopaedics and, indeed, medicine in general for two reasons. First, the goal of treatment, although often unstated, is generally obvious: secure complete functional healing of a broken bone with return to full activity. Second, the patient did not anticipate the injury; therefore, patient education begins at the perioperative visit, and the choice of physician is largely determined by institutional lines of case referral. Also, the patient must adjust to pain, inconvenience, and an unexpected loss of productivity. To make matters more difficult, some accident victims have associated psychopathology that makes communication difficult.[182] These patients may be stigmatized as "mentally ill," thereby setting the stage for withholding appropriate care.

Many fractures with good results of treatment yield permanent improvement. A difficult supracondylar fracture of the humerus repaired with an open reduction may have a residual loss of 15 degrees of elbow extension. The clinical and radiographic result is excellent in terms of present state-of-the-art treatment despite the presence of measurable permanent impairment. The chain of causation that led to this impairment began when the patient fell and landed on the elbow. It is crucial to maintain this link. When the physician does not acknowledge the presence of impairment and, even worse, fails to recognize that the patient is bothered, for example, by a prominent screw that has backed out of an olecranon osteotomy, there is a risk that the patient, or the patient's lawyer, will attempt to shorten the chain of causation to the operative event. For many patients, an understanding of the loss sustained in injury and the recognition of the complication by the physician are crucial steps. These steps are the only chance of diffusing a potentially explosive situation and allowing the process of controlling and treating complications to put the matter right.

Local complications occurring late in the course of treatment are most often related to disturbances in fracture healing. These may develop insidiously over weeks or months. Often in such cases, the patient is anticipating recovery, and the orthopaedist overlooks a trend toward deformity that, on retrospective viewing of radiographs arranged in sequence, is all too evident.

Each fracture has two complementary problems that must be solved: a biologic one and a mechanical one. The biologic problem consists of providing the setting for fracture healing. In most simple closed fractures, adequate biologic factors are present so that healing will occur. In high-grade compound fractures, the biologic issue is an important one. Only a few strategies are available to improve biology; these include autogenous bone grafting, electrical stimulation, free tissue transfer, and bone morphogenetic proteins. New techniques that harness the power of gene therapy and accelerate future healing will soon be available. Their safety and cost-effectiveness require incisive evidence-based research. The mechanical problem includes the selection of an operative or nonoperative treatment strategy that anticipates the mechanical behavior of a fractured bone and provides an environment that allows biologic processes to heal the fracture. Work by Goodship and associates[117] and by Rubin and Lanyon[301] has begun to define the mechanical circumstances favorable to fracture healing. Although it destroys marrow content, closed reamed IM nailing works well because it does not disturb the soft tissue envelope and the biomechanics of fracture site loading are favorable. When the vitality of the tissues surrounding a fracture site is compromised, the margin of safety is smaller, and adverse outcomes become more prevalent. In this situation, modification of the method (e.g., eliminating reaming and using a mechanically stronger but thinner improved implant) may reduce the incidence of complications to an acceptable level.

New therapies such as absorbable antibiotic implants, biologic bone "glues," implantable proteins that stimulate fracture healing, antibiotic coated implants, absorbable fracture fixation devices, and gene therapy hold promise for improved results.

Database management is at the heart of analyzing complications. Today's information technology explosion provides a tremendous opportunity to improve fracture care information. The data collected must, however, be meaningful. What is put into a database determines what comes out. The standard fracture nomenclature adopted by the Orthopaedic Trauma Association is an attempt to create groupings of similar cases for long-term study.

Because the risk-to-benefit ratio is at the heart of decision making in fracture treatment and in an era of results analysis, new factors will emerge that will have a powerful influence on the expenditure of health care resources for fracture care. The categorization of complications will assume great importance.[375] A model for fracture treatment must be shaped to ensure that equal weight is given to the long-term outcome of a particular treatment pattern and that the focus is shifted away from short-term economic monitors (e.g., days in the hospital, readmission within 2 weeks, implant costs) because these factors do not disclose the true socioeconomic morbidity of this disease and the potential lasting impact of local complications of fracture treatment. The insurance industry has a desire to set practice pattern algorithms to predict and control costs. The problem in trying to standardize treatment routines is that algorithms for care of human conditions are based on faulty assumptions.[304] Despite the appearance of systematization in today's microprocessor-produced output, practice patterns are dependent on human variables, and the treatment of broken limbs remains an art as well as a science.

Risk Management

No discussion about complications would be complete without reviewing the risks and medicolegal implications of complications. Many complications result in a degree of permanence, whether it is pain, decreased range of motion, or muscle weakness. The mere existence of a complication potentially fulfills the criterion that there were damages, one of the triad of criteria for medical malpractice. Malpractice is simply defined as an event in violation of the "standard of care" that causes damages. Rogal noted that a theory of fault can be created for any adverse outcome that occurs while a person is under a physician's care.[295] A bad outcome after surgery itself is associated with the risk of a lawsuit.[43]

There are several reasons why orthopaedic surgeons are near the top of the list in the number of malpractice claims.[295] The work of the orthopaedist is often visible on a radiograph.[295] Because of the emphasis on radiographic cosmesis, fracture surgery is particularly susceptible to scrutiny by anyone. These factors, coupled with the fact that fracture surgery can rarely be performed perfectly, makes fracture surgery a target for malpractice allegations. Rogal also notes that many orthopaedic injuries are "irreconcilable" and cites the example of a decimated articular surface, which is juxtaposed with the public perception that modern technology can return any injury back to normal.[295] He also noted that in many situations time is of the essence (e.g., neurovascular compromise, compartment syndrome), and he noted that lawsuits are often spawned when care is delayed and the outcome is minimally adverse. Related to this last scenario is the unique entity in orthopaedic traumatology of the missed injury.

MISSED INJURIES

Missed injuries are reported in 2 to 9 percent of patients with multiple injuries.[38,46,91,182] The majority of these injuries are musculoskeletal injuries. In one series, Buduhan and McRitchie reported that 54 percent of the injuries were musculoskeletal and 14.3 percent affected the peripheral nerves (14.3%) (Fig. 20-11).[46] They noted that patients with missed injuries tend to be more severely injured and to have initial neurologic compromise. Buduhan and McRitchie reported that in 46 of 567 (8.1%)

missed injuries, 43.8 percent were unavoidable.[46] Born and associates in 1989 reported a delay in diagnosis of musculoskeletal injuries in 26 of 1006 consecutive blunt trauma patients and a total of 39 fractures with a delay in diagnosis.[38] The most common reason for the delay in diagnosis was the lack of radiographs at admission. Enderson and associates in 1990[91] reported that a tertiary survey was able to find additional injuries in patients who had already undergone primary and secondary trauma surveys and that the use of the tertiary survey found a higher percentage of injuries (9%) than the 2 percent incidence in their trauma registry. These investigators noted that the most common reason injuries were missed was altered level of consciousness due to head injury or alcohol. Ward and Nunley in 1991 reported that 6 percent of orthopaedic injuries were not initially diagnosed in 111 multitrauma patients.[365] Seventy percent of occult bony injuries were ultimately diagnosed by physical examination and plain radiographs alone. Risk factors for occult orthopaedic injuries were (1) significant multisystem trauma with another more apparent orthopaedic injury within the same extremity, (2) trauma victim too unstable for full initial orthopaedic evaluation, (3) altered sensorium, (4) hastily applied splint obscuring a less apparent injury, (5) poor quality or inadequate initial radiographs, and (6) inadequate significance assigned to minor signs or symptoms in a major trauma victim. These investigators noted that all orthopaedic injuries cannot be diagnosed on initial patient evaluation.

Spine injuries are a subgroup of injuries that are frequently diagnosed late. In 1996 Anderson and co-workers noted that in 43 of 181 patients with major thoracolumbar spine fractures, there was a delay in diagnosis.[9] This delay in diagnosis was associated with an unstable patient condition necessitating higher priority procedures than emergency department thoracolumbar spine radiographs. Lumbar transverse process fractures have also been reported to be associated with significant lumbar spine fractures in 11 percent of cases and can be easily missed if CT scanning is not used in addition to plain radiographs.[180]

Because many of these patients have a life-threatening condition, the initial evaluations may overlook additional bony injuries that may contribute to the development of MOF. Early missed injuries are frequent even in regional

---

FIGURE 20-11 *Pie diagram of the types of missed injuries in patients with multiple trauma, which demonstrates that the majority of missed injuries are musculoskeletal. (From Buduhan, G.; McRitchie, D.I. Missed injuries in patients with multiple trauma. J Trauma 49:600–605, 2000, with permission.)*

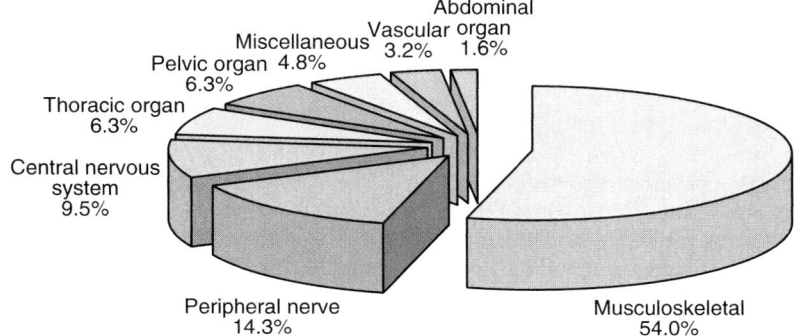

trauma centers. In a series of 206 patients, Janjua and co-workers reported a 39 percent incidence of missed injuries, which included 12 missed thoracoabdominal injuries, 7 missed hemopneumothoraces, and 2 deaths from missed injury complications.[158] A tertiary survey of the patient at 24 to 48 hours and subsequent serial examinations are needed to find these injuries.

DOCUMENTATION OF COMPLICATIONS

Several factors should be considered in documentation. One key point is documenting the precise date that the complication was discussed with the patient. Common sense and tact are critical in these discussions. It may be more difficult to have these discussions in major teaching hospitals, where the patient and family are seeing the resident physicians daily and the attending physician less frequently. Axiomatic in discussing complications with patients and their families is avoidance of self-blame. In a legal context, statements such as "I wish we had done it differently" have the force of a confession and are known as admissions. The complication needs to be disclosed but not adopted. How the recent trend for full disclosure of medical errors will affect the disclosure and discussion of complications remains to be seen. The mere presence of a complication may place the physician at risk for litigation, because the more disabling the outcome of the injury, the higher the chance of an accusation of medical malpractice.[43]

When multiple services are caring for a trauma patient, delineation of responsibility in the medical record is important. It may not be clear to the patient or to the family which service is responsible for which aspect of the patient's care. For example, the patient might assume that the orthopaedic trauma service is responsible for metacarpal fractures when, in fact, there is a separate hand surgery service. Nevertheless, a team approach that presents a "united front" is important when there are multiple services caring for a patient.

Another significant development is the need to satisfy federal compliance issues in the medical record for surgical billing. These rules require the documentation of the presence of the attending physician during surgery for the key and critical parts of the operation. The patient, who subsequently acquires a copy of the medical record, will then know for which part of the surgery the attending physician was present. If any complications arose intraoperatively, particularly if the attending physician was not present for that part of the operation, the situation may become a medicolegal nightmare. A clarifying discussion with the patient and family should include the fact that a team of many hands is needed to treat broken bones.

Documenting systems problems is another potential challenge for the orthopaedic traumatologist. Defining such issues in the medical record, for example, "that the surgery was delayed an additional 2 days because no operating room time was available," can be risky for the physician. Often, from the patient's and the patient's attorney's perspective, the physician and the institution are inextricably linked, even when the physician is an independent contractor. Furthermore, there is tremendous pressure for physicians to support and not to criticize the institution in which they work. The survival of orthopaedic trauma as a field depends on our skill in negotiating a good environment for musculoskeletal care outside of the patient record.

SUMMARY

This chapter has defined complications of fracture treatment and presented specific information about three important systemic disturbances—fat embolism syndrome, thromboembolic disorders, and multiple system organ dysfunction and failure—that can result from broken bones. In addition, a framework for approaching fracture-specific complications—soft tissue and vascular problems, posttraumatic arthrosis, peripheral nerve injury, and complex regional pain syndrome type I—was presented. Lastly, strategies for realistically managing complications were suggested.

Complications, such as missed injuries, are intrinsic to fracture care and are a part of the natural history of fractures rather than markers that something went wrong. In the final analysis, the management of complications begins with understanding the scientific basis for the treatment of injury, listening to what the patient is telling us, and accepting the fact that we as fracture surgeons cannot avoid adverse circumstances.

REFERENCES

1. Adams, C.B. The retinal manifestations of fat embolism. Injury 2:221, 1971.
2. Ageno, W. Treatment of venous thromboembolism. Thromb Res 97:V63–V72, 2000.
3. Albrechtsson, U. Thrombotic side effects of lower limb phlebography. Lancet 1:7234, 1976.
4. Alexander, J.W.; McClellan, M.A.; Ogle, C.K.; et al. Consumptive opsoninopathy: Possible pathogenesis in lethal and opportunistic infection. Ann Surg 184: 672–678, 1976.
5. Alho, A. Fat embolism syndrome: A variant of posttraumatic pulmonary insufficiency. Ann Chir Gynaecol Suppl 186:31–36, 1982.
6. Allen, G.; Galer, B.S.; Schwartz, L. Epidemiology of complex regional pain syndrome: A retrospective chart review of 134 patients. Pain 80:539–544, 1999.
7. Allgower, M.; Durig, M.; Wolff, G. Infection and trauma. Surg Clin North Am 60:133–144, 1980.
8. Amadio, P.C. Current concepts review: Pain dysfunction syndromes. J Bone Joint Surg Am 70:944–949, 1988.
9. Anderson, S.; Biros, M.H.; Reardon, R.F. Delayed diagnosis of thoracolumbar fractures in multiple-trauma patients. Acad Emerg Med 3:832–839, 1996.
10. Ashbaugh, D.G.; Petty, T.L. The use of corticosteroids in the treatment of respiratory failure associated with massive fat embolism. Surg Gynecol Obstet 123:493, 1966.
11. Aydin, M.D.; Akcay, F.; Aydin, N.; et al. Cerebral fat embolism: Pulmonary contusion is a more important

etiology than long bone fractures. Clin Neuropathol 24:86–90, 2005.

12. Babalis, G.A.; Yiannakopoulos, C.K.; Karliaftis, K.; et al. Prevention of posttraumatic hypoxaemia in isolated lower limb long bone fracture with a minimal prophylactic dose of corticosteroids. Injury 35:309–317, 2004.

13. Bach, A.W. Physiologic effects of intramedullary nailing: Fat embolism syndrome. In Seligson, D., ed. Concepts in Intramedullary Nailings. New York, Grune & Stratton, 1985, pp. 91–99.

14. Baker, S.P.; O'Neill, B.; Haddon, W. Jr.; et al. The Injury Severity Score: A method for describing patients with multiple injuries and evaluating emergency care. J Trauma 14:187–196, 1974.

15. Baracos, C.; Rodemann, P.; Dinarello, C.A.; et al. Stimulation of muscle protein degradation and prostaglandin E$_2$ release by leukocytic pyrogen (interleukin-1). N Engl J Med 308:553–558, 1983.

16. Barie, P.S.; Minnear, F.L.; Malik, A.S. Increased pulmonary vascular permeability after bone marrow injection in sheep. Am Rev Respir Dis 123:648–653, 1981.

17. Barnes, R.W. Current status of noninvasive tests in the diagnosis of venous disease. Surg Clin North Am 62:489–500, 1982.

18. Barnes, R.W.; Wu, K.K.; Hoak, J.C. Fallibility of the clinical diagnosis of venous thrombosis. JAMA 234:605–607, 1975.

19. Barton, N.J. Radial nerve lesions. Hand 3:200–208, 1973.

20. Bates, S.M.; Hirsh, J. Treatment of venous thromboembolism. Thromb Hemost 82:870–877, 1999.

21. Baue, A.E.; Chaudry, I.H. Prevention of multiple systems failure. Surg Clin North Am 6:1167–1178, 1980.

22. Baxter, G.M.; McKechnie, S.; Duffy, P. Colour Doppler ultrasound in deep venous thrombosis: A comparison with venography. Clin Radiol 42:32–36, 1990.

23. Beal, A.L.; Cerra, F.B. Multiple organ failure syndrome in the 1990s: Systemic inflammatory response and organ dysfunction. JAMA 271:226–233, 1994.

24. Beck, J.P.; Collins, J.A. Theoretical and clinical aspects of post-traumatic fat embolism syndrome. Instr Course Lect 23:38–87, 1973.

25. Behrman, S.W.; Fabian, T.C.; Kudsk, K.A.; et al. Improved outcome with femur fractures: Early vs. delayed fixation. J Trauma 30:792–797, 1990.

26. Benetar, S.R.; Immelman, E.J.; Jeffery, P. Pulmonary embolism. Br J Dis Chest 80:313–334, 1986.

27. Bettman, M.A.Q.; Paulin, S. Leg phlebography: The incidence, nature and modification of undesirable side effects. Radiology 122:101–104, 1977.

28. Bhandari, M.; Guyatt, G.H.; Khera, V.; et al. Operative management of lower extremity fractures in patients with head injuries. Clin Orthop Relat Res 407:187–198, 2003.

29. Bickerstaff, D.R.; Kanis, J.A. Algodystrophy: An under-recognized complication of minor trauma. Br J Rheumatol 33:240–248, 1994.

30. Bisgard, J.D.; Baker, C. Experimental fat embolism. Am J Surg 47:466–478, 1940.

31. Bodine, S.C.; Lieber, R.L. Peripheral nerve physiology, anatomy, and pathology. In Simon, S.R., ed. Orthopaedic Basic Science. Rosemont, IL, American Academy of Orthopaedic Surgeons, 1994, pp. 325–396.

32. Bone, L.B.; Johnson, K.D.; Weigelt, J.; et al. Early versus delayed stabilization of femoral fractures. J Bone Joint Surg Am 71:336–340, 1989.

33. Bone, R.C.; Balk, R.A.; Cerra, F.C.; et al. Definitions for sepsis and organ failure and guidelines for the use of innovative therapies in sepsis. Chest 101:1644–1655, 1992.

34. Bonica, J.J. Causalgia and other reflex sympathetic dystrophies. In Bonica, J.J., ed. The Management of Pain, 2nd ed. Philadelphia, Lea & Febiger, 1990, pp. 221–222.

35. Bonica, J.J. Causalgia and other sympathetic dystrophies. In Bonica, J.J.; Ventafridda, V., eds. Advances in Pain Research and Therapy. New York, Raven Press, 1979, pp. 141–166.

36. Bonsell, S.; Pearsall, A.W. IV; Heitman, R.J.; et al. The relationship of age, gender, and degenerative changes observed on radiographs of the shoulder in asymptomatic individuals. J Bone Joint Surg Br 82:1135–1139, 2000.

37. Border, J.R.; Chenier, R.; McMenamy, R.H.; et al. Multiple systems organ failure: Muscle fuel deficit with visceral protein malnutrition. Surg Clin North Am 56:1147–1167, 1976.

38. Born, C.T.; Ross, S.E.; Iannacone, W.M.; et al. Delayed identification of skeletal injury in multisystem trauma: The "missed" fracture. J Trauma 29:1643–1646, 1989.

39. Bosse, M.J.; Riemer, B.L.; Brumback, R.J.; et al. Adult respiratory distress syndrome, pneumonia and mortality following thoracic injury and a femoral fracture treated with intramedullary nailing with reaming or with a plate. J Bone Joint Surg Am 79:799–809, 1997.

40. Böstmann, O.; Varjonen, L.; Vainionpaa, S.; et al. Incidence of local complications after intramedullary nailing and after plate fixation of femoral shaft fractures. J Trauma 29:639–645, 1989.

41. Bradley, M.J.; Spencer, P.A.; Alexander, L. Colour flow mapping in the diagnosis of the calf deep vein thrombosis. Clin Radiol 47:399–402, 1993.

42. Breivik, H. Chronic pain and the sympathetic nervous system. Acta Anesthesiologica Scand 1:131–134, 1997.

43. Brennan, T.; Sox, C.M.; Burstin, H.R. Relationship between negligent adverse events and the outcome of medical-malpractice litigation. N Engl J Med 335:1963–1967, 1996.

44. Brittberg, M.; Lindahl, A.; Nilsson, A.; et al. Treatment of deep cartilage defects in the knee with autologous chondrocyte transplantation. N Engl J Med 331:889–895, 1994.

45. Bruehl, S.; Carlson, C.R. Predisposing psychological factors in the development of reflex sympathetic dystrophy: A review of the empirical evidence. Clin J Pain 8:287–299, 1992.

46. Buduhan, G.; McRitchie, D.I. Missed injuries in patients with multiple trauma. J Trauma 49:600–605, 2000.

47. Bulger, E.M.; Smith, D.G.; Maier, R.V.; et al. Fat embolism syndrome: A 10-year review. Arch Surg 132:435–439, 1997.

48. Büller, H.R.; Lensing, A.W.A.; Hirsh, J.; et al. Deep vein thrombosis: New noninvasive tests. Thromb Haemost 66:133–137, 1991.

49. Busch, F. Über feltembolie. Virchows Arch (A) 35:321, 1866.

50. Carlson, D.W.; Rodman, G.H., Jr.; Kaehr, D.; et al. Femur fractures in chest-injured patients: Is reaming contraindicated? J Orthop Trauma 12:164–168, 1998.

51. Carman, T.L.; Fernandez, B.B., Jr. Issues and controversies in venous thromboembolism. Cleve Clin J Med 66:113–123, 1999.

52. Carpenter, J.P.; Holland, G.A.; Baum, R.A.; et al. Magnetic resonance venography for the detection of deep venous thrombosis: Comparison with contrast venography and duplex Doppler ultrasonography. J Vasc Surg 18:734–741, 1993.

53. Carrico, C.J.; Meakins, J.L.; Marshall, J.C.; et al. Multiple organ failure syndrome. Arch Surg 121:196–208, 1986.

54. Cerra, F.B.; West, M.; Keller, G.; et al. Hypermetabolism/organ failure: The role of the activated macrophage as a metabolic regulator. Clin Biol Res 264:27–42, 1988.

55. Chan, C.S.; Chow, S.P. Electroacupuncture in the treatment of post-traumatic sympathetic dystrophy (Sudeck's atrophy). Br J Anaesth 53:899–901, 1981.

56. Chan, K.; Tham, K.T.; Chiu, H.S.; et al. Post-traumatic fat embolism: Its clinical and subclinical presentations. J Trauma 24:45–49, 1984.

57. Channon, G.M.; Wiley, A.M. Aspirin prophylaxis of venous thromboembolic disease following fracture of the upper femur. Can J Surg 22:468–472, 1979.

58. Charash, W.E.; Croce, M.A. Delayed surgical fixation of femur fractures is a risk factor for pulmonary failure independent of thoracic trauma. J Trauma 37:667–672, 1994.

59. Chervu, A.; Quinones-Baldrich, W.J. Vascular complications in orthopaedic surgery. Clin Orthop Relat Res 235:275–288, 1988.

60. Cheshire, W.P.; Snyder, C.R. Treatment of reflex sympathetic dystrophy with topical capsaicin: Case report. Pain 42:307–311, 1990.

61. Clowes, G.H.A., Jr.; George, B.C.; Villee, C.A., Jr.; et al. Muscle proteolysis induced by a circulating peptide in patients with sepsis or trauma. N Engl J Med 308:545–552, 1983.

62. Codivilla, A. On the means of lengthening, in the lower limbs, the muscles and tissues which are shortened through deformity. Am J Orthop Surg 2:353, 1904.

63. Cogo, A.; Lensing, A.W.A.; Prandoni, P.; et al. Comparison of real-time B-mode ultrasonography and Doppler ultrasound with contrast venography in the diagnosis of venous thrombosis in symptomatic outpatients. Thromb Haemost 70:404–407, 1993.

64. Collins, J.A.; Hudson, T.L.; Hamacher, W.R. Systemic fat embolism in four combat casualties. Ann Surg 167:493–499, 1968.

65. The Columbus Investigators. Low-molecular-weight heparin in the treatment of patients with venous thromboembolism. N Engl J Med 337:657–662, 1997.

66. Comerota, A.J. Deep vein thrombosis and pulmonary embolism: Clinical presentation and pathophysiologic consequences. Cardiovasc Intervent Radiol 11:9–14, 1988.

67. Committee on Medical Aspects of Automotive Safety. Rating the severity of tissue damage. I. The abbreviated scale. JAMA 215:277–280, 1971.

68. Conway, R.R.; Hubbell, S.L. Electromyographic abnormalities in neurologic injury associated with pelvic fracture: Case reports and literature review. Arch Phys Med Rehab 69:539–541, 1988.

69. Cooke, T.D.V.; Pichora, D.; Siu, D.; et al. Surgical contributions of varus deformity of the knee with obliquity of joint surfaces. J Bone Joint Surg Br 71:560–565, 1989.

70. Cooke, T.D.V.; Siu, D.; Fisher, B. The use of standardized radiographs to identify the deformities associated with osteoarthritis. In Noble, J.; Galasko, C.S.B., eds. Recent Developments in Orthopaedic Surgery. Manchester, Great Britain, Manchester University Press, 1987, pp. 264–273.

71. Coon, W.W. Risk factors in pulmonary embolism. Surg Gynecol Obstet 143:385–390, 1976.

72. Coon, W.W. Venous thromboembolism: Prevalence, risk factors, and prevention. Clin Chest Med 5:391–401, 1984.

73. Coon, W.W.; Coller, F.A. Some epidemiologic considerations of thromboembolism. Surg Gynecol Obstet 109:487–501, 1959.

74. Cooper, D.E.; DeLee, J.G. Reflex sympathetic dystrophy of the knee. J Am Acad Orthop Surg 2:79–86, 1994.

75. Cooper, D.E.; DeLee, J.C.; Ramamurthy, S. Reflex sympathetic dystrophy of the knee: Treatment using continuous epidural anesthesia. J Bone Joint Surg Am 71:365–369, 1989.

76. Crowther, M.A.; Ginsberg, J.S.; Kearon, C.; et al. A randomized trial comparing 5-mg and 10-mg warfarin loading doses. Arch Intern Med 159:46–48, 1999.

77. Cruveilhier, J. Anatomie pathologique du corps humain. Paris, J.B. Bulligère, 1828.

78. Decousus, H.; Leizorovicz, A.; Parent, F.; et al. A clinical trial of vena cava filters in the prevention of pulmonary embolism in patients with proximal deep-vein thrombosis. N Engl J Med 338:409–415, 1998.

79. Deitch, E.A. Multiple organ failure: Pathophysiology and potential future therapy. Ann Surg 216:117–134, 1992.

80. Deitch, E.A.; Goodman, F.R. Prevention of multiple organ failure. Surg Clin North Am 79:1471–1488, 1998.

81. Dekel, S.; Weissmann, S.L. Joint changes after overuse and peak overloading of rabbit knees in vivo. Acta Orthop Scand 49:519, 1978.

82. Deland, F.H. Bone marrow embolism and associated fat embolism to the lungs. Graduate thesis, University of Minnesota, Minneapolis, MN, June 1956.

83. Demling, R. Wound inflammatory mediators and multisystem organ failure. Prog Clin Biol Res 236A:525–537, 1987.

84. Donaldson, G.A.; Williams, C.; Scannell, J.G.; et al. A reappraisal of the Trendelenburg operation to massive fatal embolism. N Engl J Med 268:171–174, 1963.

85. Donohue, J.M.; Buss, D.; Oegema, T.R.; et al. The effects of indirect blunt trauma on adult canine articular cartilage. J Bone Joint Surg Am 65:948–957, 1983.

86. Dunham, C.M.; Bosse, M.J.; Clancy, T.V.; et al. EAST practice management guidelines work group: Practice guidelines for the optimal timing of long-bone fracture stabilization in polytrauma patients: The EAST practice management guidelines work group. J Trauma 50:958–967, 2001.

87. Dunphy, J.E.; Ilfeld, F.W. Fat embolism. Am J Surg 77:737, 1949.

88. Eisenberg, E.; Melamed, E. Can complex regional pain syndrome be painless? Pain 106:263–267, 2003.

89. Eisman, B.; Beart, R.; Norton, L. Multiple organ failure. Surg Gynecol Obstet 144:323–326, 1977.

90. Elgazzar, A.H.; Abdel-Dayem, H.M.; Clark, J.D. Multimodality imaging of osteomyelitis. Eur J Nucl Med 22:1043–1063, 1995.

91. Enderson, B.L.; Reath, D.B.; Meadors, J.; et al. The tertiary trauma survey: A prospective study of missed injury. J Trauma 30:666–669, 1990.

92. Evarts, C.M. The fat embolism syndrome: A review. Surg Clin North Am 50:493–507, 1970.

93. Fahr, L.M.; Sauser, D.D. Imaging of peripheral nerve lesions. Orthop Clin North Am 19:27–41, 1988.

94. Fairbanks, T.J. Knee joint changes after meniscectomy. J Bone Joint Surg Br 30:665–670, 1948.

95. Feldman, F.; Ellis, K.; Green, W.M. The fat embolism syndrome. Radiology 114:535, 1975.

96. Fenger, C.; Salisbury, J.H. Diffuse multiple capillary fat embolism in the lungs and brain is a fatal complication in common fractures: Illustrated by a case. Chicago Mod J Examin 39:587–595, 1879.

97. Fischer, J.F.; Turner, R.H.; Riseborough, E.J. Massive steroid therapy in severe fat embolism. Surg Gynecol Obstet 132:667, 1971.

98. Fisher, C.G.; Blachut, P.A.; Salvian, A.J.; et al. Effectiveness of pneumatic leg compression devices for the prevention of thromboembolic disease in orthopedic trauma patients: A prospective, randomized study of compression alone versus no prophylaxis. J Orthop Trauma 9:1–7, 1995.

99. Fitts, W.T.; Lehr, H.B.; Bitner, R.L.; et al. An analysis of 950 fatal injuries. Surgery 56:663–668, 1964.

100. Flint, L.M.; Richardson, J.D. Arterial injuries with lower extremity fracture. Surgery 93:5–8, 1983.

101. Foy, M.A.; Fagg, P.S. Medicolegal Reporting in Orthopaedic Trauma. New York, Churchill Livingstone, 1996, pp. 2.1-01–4.1-16.

102. Freeark, R.J.; Bostwick, J.; Fardin, R. Post-traumatic venous thrombosis. Arch Surg 95:567–575, 1967.

103. Fry, D.E. Multiple system organ failure. Surg Clin North Am 68:107–122, 1988.

104. Fry, D.E.; Pearlstein, L.; Fulton, R.L.; et al. Multiple system organ failure: The role of uncontrolled infection. Arch Surg 115:136–140, 1980.

105. Geerts, W.H.; Code, K.I.; Jay, R.M.; et al. A prospective study of venous thromboembolism after major trauma. New Engl J Med 331:1601–1606, 1994.

106. Geerts, W.H.; Pineo, G.F.; Heit, J.A.; et al. Prevention of venous thromboembolism: The seventh ACCP conference of antithrombotic and thrombolytic therapy. Chest 126(3 Suppl):338S–400S, 2004.

107. Geertzen, J.H.B.; Dijkstra, P.U.; Groothoff, J.W.; et al. Reflex sympathetic dystrophy of the upper extremity: A 5.5-year follow-up. Acta Orthop Scand 69(Suppl 279):12–18, 1998.

108. Gelber, A.C.; Hochberg, M.C.; Mead, L.A.; et al. Joint injury in young adults and risk for subsequent knee and hip osteoarthritis. Ann Intern Med 133:321–328, 2000.

109. Genant, H.; Kozin, F.; Bekerman, C.; et al. The reflex sympathetic dystrophy syndrome. Radiology 117:21–32, 1975.

110. Ghivizzanni, S.C.; Oligino, T.J.; Robbins, P.D.; et al. Cartilage injury and repair. Physical Med Rehab Clin North Am 1:289–307, 2000.

111. Ghostine, S.Y.; Comair, Y.G.; Turner, D.M.; et al. Phenoxybenzamine in the treatment of causalgia: Report of 40 cases. J Neurosurg 60:1263–1268, 1984.

112. Giachino, A. Relationship between deep-vein thrombosis in the calf and fatal pulmonary embolism. Can J Surg 31:129–130, 1988.

113. Giannoudis, P.V.; Pape, H.C.; Cohen, A.P.; et al. Review: Systemic effects of femoral nailing: From

Kuntscher to the immune reactivity era. Clin Orthop Relat Res 404:378–386, 2002.

114. Giannoudis, P.V.; Smith, R.M.; Bellamy, M.C.; et al. Stimulation of the inflammatory system by reamed and unreamed nailing of femoral fractures: An analysis of the second hit. J Bone Joint Surg Br 81:356–361, 1999.

115. Gong, H., Jr. Fat embolism syndrome: A puzzling phenomenon. Postgrad Med 62:40, 1977.

116. Goodall, R.J. Nerve injuries in fresh fractures. Tex Med 52:93–94, 1956.

117. Goodship, A.E.; Lanyon, L.E.; McFie, H. Functional adaptation of bone to increased stress. J Bone Joint Surg Am 61:539–546, 1979.

118. Goris, R.J.A.; Boekholtz, T.P.A.; Nuytinck, J.K.S.; et al. Multiple organ failure: Generalized autodestructive inflammation? Arch Surg 120:1109–1115, 1985.

119. Goris, R.J.A.; Gimbrere, J.S.F.; van Niekerk, J.L.M.; et al. Early osteosynthesis and prophylactic mechanical ventilation in the multitrauma patient. J Trauma 22:895–903, 1982.

120. Goris, R.J.A.; Nuytinck, H.K.S.; Redl, H. Scoring system and predictors of ARDS and MOF. Prog Clin Biol Res 236B:3–15, 1987.

121. Gossling, H.R.; Pellegrini, V.D., Jr. Fat embolism syndrome: A review of the pathophysiology and physiological basis of treatment. Clin Orthop Relat Res 165:68–82, 1982.

122. Grassi, C.J. Inferior vena caval filters: Analysis of five currently available devices. Am J Roentgenol 156:813–821, 1991.

123. Greenfield, L.J. Assessment of vena caval filters. J Vasc Interv Radiol 2:425–426, 1991.

124. Greenspan, L.; McLellan, B.A.; Greig, H. Abbreviated Injury Scale and Injury Severity Score: A scoring chart. J Trauma 25:60–64, 1985.

125. Gulevich, S.J.; Conwell, T.D.; Lane, J.; et al. Stress infrared telethermography is useful in the diagnosis of complex regional pain syndrome, type I (formerly reflex sympathetic dystrophy). Clin J Pain 13:50–59, 1997.

126. Gurd, A.R.; Wilson, R.I. The fat embolism syndrome. J Bone Joint Surg Br 56:408–416, 1974.

127. Gurdjian, E.S.; Smathers, H.M. Peripheral nerve injury in fractures and dislocations of long bone. J Neurosurg 2:202–211, 1945.

128. Haake, D.A.; Berkman, S.A. Venous thromboembolic disease after hip surgery: Risk factors, prophylaxis, and diagnosis. Clin Orthop Relat Res 242:212–231, 1989.

129. Haddad, F.S., ed. Fat embolism. In Annual Report. Beirut, Lebanon, The Orient Hospital, 1951, p. 25.

130. Hamsten, A.; Wiman, B.; deFaire, U.; et al. Increased plasma levels of a rapid inhibitor of tissue plasminogen activator in young survivors of myocardial infarction. N Engl J Med 313:1557, 1985.

131. Hardin, W.D.; O'Connell, R.C.; Adinolfi, M.F.; et al. Traumatic arterial injuries of the upper extremity: Determinants of disability. Am J Surg 150:226–270, 1985.

132. Harris, L.M.; Curl, G.R.; Booth, F.V.; et al. Screening for asymptomatic DVT in SICU patients. J Vasc Surg 26:764–769, 1997.

133. Harrison, L.; Johnston, M.; Massicotte, P.; et al. Comparison of 5-mg and 10-mg loading doses in initiation of warfarin therapy. Ann Intern Med 126:133–136, 1997.

134. Harwood, P.J.; Giannoudis, P.V.; van Griensven, M.; et al. Alternations in the systemic inflammatory response after early total care and damage control procedures for femoral shaft fracture in severely injured patients. J Trauma 58:446–454, 2005.

135. Hasselgren, P.O.; Pedersen, P.; Sax, H.C.; et al. Current concepts of protein turnover and amino acid transport in liver and skeletal muscle during sepsis. Arch Surg 123:992–999, 1988.

136. Hasselgren, P.O.; Talamini, M.; James, J.H.; et al. Protein metabolism in different types of skeletal muscle during early and late sepsis in rats. Arch Surg 121:918–923, 1986.

137. Hayt, D.B.; Binkert, B.L. An overview of noninvasive methods of DVT detection. Clin Imaging 14:179–197, 1990.

138. Heideman, M.; Hugli, T.E. Anaphylatoxin generation in multisystem organ failure. J Trauma 24:1038–1043, 1984.

139. Heim, D.; Regazzori, P.; Tsakiris, D.A.; et al. Intramedullary nailing and pulmonary embolism: Does unreamed nailing prevent embolization? An in vivo study in rabbits. J Trauma 38:899–906, 1995.

140. Helfet, D.L.; Anand, N.; Malkani, A.L.; et al. Intraoperative monitoring of motor pathways during operative fixation of acute acetabular fractures. J Orthop Trauma 11:2–6, 1997.

141. Helfet, D.L.; Hissa, E.A.; Sergay, S.; et al. Somatosensory evoked potential monitoring in the surgical treatment of acute acetabular fractures. J Orthop Trauma 5:161–166, 1991.

142. Hermann, L.G.; Reineke, H.G.; Caldwell, J.A. Post-traumatic painful osteoporosis: A clinical and roentgenological entity. Am J Radiol 47:353–361, 1942.

143. Herndon, J.H.; Risenborough, E.J.; Fischer, J.E. Fat embolism: A review of current concepts. J Trauma 11:673, 1971.

144. Hershman, M.J.; Cheadle, W.G.; Kuftinec, D.; et al. An outcome predictive score for sepsis and death following injury. Injury 19:263–266, 1988.

145. Hildebrand, F.; Pape, H.C.; van Griensven, M.; et al. Genetic predisposition for a compromised immune system after multiple trauma. Shock 24:518–522, 2005.

146. Hill, S.D.; Lin, M.S.; Chandler, P.J. Reflex sympathetic dystrophy and electroacupuncture. Tex Med 87:76–81, 1991.

147. Hjeimsiedt, A.; Bergvali, U. Phlebographic study of the incidence of thrombosis in the injured and uninjured limb in 55 cases of tibial fracture. Acta Chir Scand 134:229–234, 1968.

148. Hughes, J.L.; Sauer, W.G. Wagner apparatus: A portable traction device. In Seligson, D.; Pope, M., eds. Concepts in External Fixation. New York, Grune & Stratton, 1982, pp. 203–217.

149. Hull, R.D.; Hirsh, J.; Sackett, D.L.; et al. Replacement of venography in suspected venous thrombosis by impedance plethysmography and 125I fibrinogen leg scanning. Ann Intern Med 94:12–15, 1981.

150. Hull, R.D.; Raskob, G.E.; LeClere, J.R.; et al. The diagnosis of clinically suspected venous thrombosis. Clin Chest Med 5:439–456, 1984.

151. Hull, R.D.; Raskob, G.E.; Pineo, G.F.; et al. Subcutaneous low-molecular-weight heparin compared with continuous intravenous heparin in the treatment of proximal-vein thrombosis. N Engl J Med 326:975–982, 1992.

152. Hull, R.; Van Aken, W.G.; Hirsh, J.; et al. Impedance plethysmography using the occlusive cuff technique in diagnosis of venous thrombosis. Circulation 53:696–700, 1976.

153. Hyers, T.M.; Agnelli, G.; Hull, R.; et al. Antithrombotic therapy for venous thromboembolic disease. Chest 114:561S–578S, 1998.

154. Ide, J.; Yamaga, T.; Kitamura, T.; et al. Quantitative evaluation of sympathetic nervous system dysfunction in patients with reflex sympathetic dystrophy. J Hand Surg Br 22:102–106, 1997.

155. Immelman, E.J.; Jeffery, P.C. The postphlebitic syndrome. Clin Chest Med 5:537–550, 1984.

156. Inaba, K.; Potzman, J.; Munera, F.; et al. Multi-slice CT angiography for arterial evaluation in the injured lower extremity. J Trauma 60:502–506, 2006.

157. Jacobson, D.M.; Terrence, C.F.; Reinmuth, O.M. The neurologic manifestations of fat embolism. Neurology 36:847–851, 1986.

158. Janjua, K.J.; Sugrue, M.; Deanne, S.A. Prospective evaluation of early missed injuries and the role of tertiary trauma survey. J Trauma 44:1000–1007, 1998.

159. Johnson, B.F.; Manzo, R.A.; Bergelin, R.O.; et al. Relationship between changes in deep venous system and the development of the post-thrombotic syndrome after an acute episode of lower limb deep vein thrombosis: A one- to six-year follow-up. J Vasc Surg 21:307–313, 1995.

160. Johnson, K.D.; Cadambi, A.; Seibert, G.B. Incident of adult respiratory distress syndrome in patients with multiple musculoskeletal injuries: Effect of early operative stabilization of fractures. J Trauma 25:375–384, 1985.

161. Jones, T.K.; Barnes, R.W.; Greenfield, L.J. Greenfield vena caval filter: Rationale and current indications. Ann Thorac Surg 42(Suppl):48–55, 1986.

162. Kakkar, V.V.; Howe, C.T.; Flanc, C.; et al. Natural history of deep venous thrombosis. Lancet 2:230, 1969.

163. Kallos, T.; Jerry, E.E.; Golon, F.; et al. Intramedullary pressure and pulmonary embolism of femoral medullary contents in dogs during insertion of bone cement and a prosthesis. J Bone Joint Surg Am 56:1363–1367, 1974.

164. Kaslo, E.; Perttunen, K.; Kaasinen, S. Pain after thoracic surgery. Acta Anaesthesiol Scand 36:96–100, 1992.

165. Kearon, C.; Ginsberg, J.S.; Hirsh, J. The role of venous ultrasonography in the diagnosis of suspected deep venous thrombosis and pulmonary embolism. Ann Intern Med 129:1044–1049, 1998.

166. Keel, M.; Trentz, O. Pathophysiology of polytrauma. Injury 36:691–709, 2005.

167. Kelsey, L.J.; Fry, D.M.; VanderKolk, W.E. Thrombosis risk in the trauma patient. Hematol Oncol Clin North Am 14:417–430, 2000.

168. Kemler, M.A.; Barendse, G.A.M.; Van Kleef, M.; et al. Electrical spinal cord stimulation in reflex sympathetic dystrophy: Retrospective analysis of 23 patients. J Neurosurg 90:79–83, 1999.

169. Kern, D.; Zlatkin, M.B.; Dalinka, M.K. Occupational and post-traumatic arthritis. Radiol Clin North Am 26:1349–1358, 1998.

170. Kerstell, J. Pathogenesis of post-traumatic fat embolism. Am J Surg 121:712, 1971.

171. Kerstell, J.; Hallgren, B.; Rudenstam, C.M.; et al. The chemical composition of the fat emboli in the postabsorptive dog. Acta Med Scand 186(Suppl 499):3, 1969.

172. Kettlekamp, D.B.; Hillberry, B.M.; Murrish, D.E.; et al. Degenerative arthritis of the knee secondary to fracture malunion. Clin Orthop Relat Res 234:159–169, 1988.

173. Kleiman, A. Evidence of the existence of crossed sensory sympathetic fibers. Am J Surg 87:839–841, 1954.

174. Kleinert, H.E.; Cole, N.M.; Wayne, L.; et al. Post-traumatic sympathetic dystrophy. Orthop Clin North Am 4:917–927, 1973.

175. Knudson, M.M.; Morabito, D.; Paiement, G.D.; et al. Use of low molecular weight heparin in preventing thromboembolism in trauma patients. J Trauma 41:446–459, 1996.

176. Koopman, M.M.; Prandoni, P.; Piovella, F.; et al. Treatment of venous thrombosis with intravenous unfractionated heparin administered in the hospital as compared to subcutaneous low-molecular-weight heparin administered at home. N Engl J Med 334:682–687, 1996.

177. Kozin, F.; Ryan, L.M.; Carrera, G.F.; et al. The reflex sympathetic dystrophy syndrome (RSDS). 3. Scintigraphic studies, further evidence for the therapeutic efficacy of systemic corticosteroids, and proposed diagnostic criteria. Am J Med 70:23–30, 1981.

178. Kristensen, K.D.; Kiaer, T.; Blicher, J. No arthrosis of the ankle 20 years after malaligned tibial-shaft fracture. Acta Orthop Scand 60:208–209, 1989.

179. Kroupa, J. Fat globulinemia in early diagnostics of traumatic fat embolism. Czech Med 9:90–108, 1986.

180. Krueger, M.A.; Green, D.A.; Hoyt, D.; et al. Overlooked spine injuries associated with lumbar transverse process fractures. Clin Orthop Relat Res 327:191–195, 1996.

181. Kudsk, K.A.; Fabian, T.; Baum, S.; et al. Silent deep vein thrombosis in immobilized multiple trauma patients. Am J Surg 158:515–519, 1989.

182. Kuhn, W.F.; Lacefield, P.K. Patient, surgeon, nurse: The psychological impact of fracture treatment. In Seligson, D., ed. Concepts in Intramedullary Nailing. New York, Grune & Stratton, 1985, pp. 187–197.

183. Laasonen, E.M.; Kivioj, A. Delayed diagnosis of extremity injuries in patients with multiple injuries. J Trauma 31:257–260, 1991.

184. Laennec, R.T.H. De l'auscultation mediate. Paris, Brossen et Shaude, 1819.

185. Lankford, L.L.; Thompson, J.E. Reflex sympathetic dystrophy, upper and lower extremity: Diagnosis and management. Instr Course Lect 26:163–178, 1977.

186. Laskin, R. Rheumatologic and degenerative disorders of the knee. In Dee, R., ed. Principles of Orthopaedic Practice. New York, McGraw-Hill, 1989, p. 1371.

187. Lee, S.K.; Wolfe, S.W. Peripheral nerve injury and repair. J Am Acad Orthop Surg 8:243–252, 2000.

188. Lensing, A.W.A.; Prins, M.H.; Davidson, B.L. Treatment of deep venous thrombosis with low-molecular-weight heparins. Arch Intern Med 155:601–607, 1995.

189. Levine, M.; Gent, M.; Hirsch, J.; et al. A comparison of low-molecular-weight heparin administered primarily at home with unfractionated heparin administered in the hospital for proximal deep vein thrombosis. N Engl J Med 334:677–681, 1996.

190. Levy, D. The fat embolism syndrome: A review. Clin Orthop Relat Res 261:281–286, 1990.

191. Lewis, D.; Miller, E.M. Peripheral nerve injuries associated with fractures. Ann Surg 76:528–538, 1922.

192. Lindenfeld, T.N.; Bach, B.R.; Wojtys, E.M. Reflex sympathetic dystrophy and pain dysfunction in the lower extremity. J Bone Joint Surg Am 78:1936–1944, 1996.

193. Lindeque, B.G.P.; Schoeman, H.S.; Dommisse, G.F.; et al. Fat embolism and the fat embolism syndrome: A double-blind therapeutic study. J Bone Joint Surg Br 69:128–131, 1987.

194. Lindmarker, P.; Holmstrom, M.; Granqvist, S.; et al. Comparison of once-daily subcutaneous Fragmin with continuous intravenous unfractionated heparin in the treatment of deep vein thrombosis. Thromb Haemost 72:186–190, 1994.

195. Livingston, D.H.; Deitch, E.A. Multiple organ failure: A common problem in surgical intensive care unit patients. Ann Med 27:13–20, 1995.

196. Lohr, J.M.; Kerr, T.M.; Lutter, K.S.; et al. Lower extremity calf thrombosis: To treat or not to treat? J Vasc Surg 14:618–623, 1991.

197. Lozman, J.; Deno, D.C.; Feustel, P.J.; et al. Pulmonary and cardiovascular consequences of immediate fixation or conservative management of long bone fractures. Arch Surg 121:992–999, 1986.

198. Luce, E.A.; Griffin, W.O. Shotgun injuries of the upper extremity. J Trauma 18:487–492, 1978.

199. Magerl, F.; Tscherne, H. Diagnose, therapie und prophylaxe der fettembolic. Langenbecks Arch Klin Chir 314:292, 1966.

200. Malangoni, M.A.; Dillon, L.D.; Klamer, T.W.; et al. Factors influencing the risk of early and late serious infection in adults after splenectomy for trauma. Surgery 96:775–784, 1984.

201. Malik, V.K.; Inchiosa, M.A.; Mustafa, K.; et al. Intravenous regional phenoxybenzamine in the treatment of reflex sympathetic dystrophy. Anesthesiology 88:823–827, 1998.

202. Mammen, E. Pathogenesis of venous thrombosis. Chest 102:641S, 1992.

203. Mankin, H.J. The response of articular cartilage to mechanical injury. J Bone Joint Surg Am 64:460, 1982.

204. Manning, J.B.; Bach, A.W.; Herman, C.M.; et al. Fat release after femur nailing in the dog. J Trauma 23:322–326, 1983.

205. Martin, J.G.; Marsh, J.L.; Kresowik, T. Phlegmasia cerulea dolens: A complication of use of a filter in the vena cava. J Bone Joint Surg Am 77:452–454, 1995.

206. Matta, J.M. Fractures of the acetabulum: Accuracy of reduction and clinical results in patients managed operatively within three weeks after injury. J Bone Joint Surg Am 78:1632–1645, 1996.

207. Mattos, M.A.; Londrey, G.L.; Leutz, D.W.; et al. Color-flow duplex scanning for the surveillance and diagnosis of acute deep venous thrombosis. J Vasc Surg 15:366–375, 1992.

208. McDermott, I.D.; Culpan, P.; Clancy, M.; et al. The role of rehydration in the prevention of fat embolism syndrome. Injury 33:757–759, 2002.

209. McMenamy, R.H.; Birkhahn, R.; Oswald, G.; et al. Multiple systems organ failure. 1. The basal state. J Trauma 21:99–114, 1981.

210. McNally, M.A.; Mollan, R.A.B. Venous thromboembolism and orthopedic surgery. J Bone Joint Surg Br 75:517–519, 1993.

211. Mears, D.C.; Velyvius, J.H. Primary total hip arthroplasty after acetabular fracture. J Bone Joint Surg Am 82:1328–1353, 2000.

212. Meek, R.N.; Vivoda, E.; Crichton, A.; et al. Comparison of mortality with multiple injuries according to method of fracture treatment: Abstract. J Bone Joint Surg Br 63:456, 1981.

213. Meissner, M.H.; Caps, M.T.; Bergelin, R.O.; et al. Propagation, rethrombosis, and new thrombus

formation after acute deep vein thrombosis. J Vasc Surg 22:558–567, 1995.

214. Mellick, G.A.; Mellick, L.B. Reflex sympathetic dystrophy treated with gabapentin. Arch Phys Med Rehabil 78:98–105, 1997.

215. Melzack, R.; Wall, P.D. Pain mechanisms: A new theory. Science 150:971–978, 1965.

216. Merchant, T.C.; Dietz, F.D. Long-term follow-up after fractures of the tibial and fibular shafts. J Bone Joint Surg Am 71:599–606, 1989.

217. Merskey, H.; Bogduk, N., eds. Classification of Chronic Pain. Seattle, WA, IASP Press, 1994, pp. 40–44.

218. Meyer, C.S.; Blebea, J.; Davis, K., Jr.; et al. Surveillance venous scars for deep venous thrombosis in multiple trauma patients. Ann Vasc Surg 9:109–114, 1995.

219. Meyers, J.R.; Lembeck, L.; O'Kane, H.; et al. Changes in functional residual capacity of the lung after operation. Arch Surg 110:576–583, 1975.

220. Michelsen, G.B.; Askanazi, J. The metabolic response to injury: Mechanisms and clinical implications. J Bone Joint Surg Am 68:782–787, 1986.

221. Middlebrooks, E.S.; Sims, S.H.; Kellam, J.F.; et al. Incidence of sciatic nerve monitoring in operatively treated acetabular fractures without somatosensory evoked potential monitoring. J Orthop Trauma 11:327–329, 1997.

222. Miller, M.D.; Osborne, J.R.; Gordon, W.T.; et al. The natural history of bone bruises: A prospective study of magnetic resonance imaging–detected trabecular microfractures in patients with isolated medial collateral ligament injuries. Am J Sports Med 26:15–19, 1998.

223. Mitchell, D.C.; Grasty, M.S.; Stebbings, W.S.C.; et al. Comparison of duplex ultrasonography and venography in the diagnosis of deep venous thrombosis. Br J Surg 78:611–613, 1991.

224. Moore, F.A.; Moore, E.E. Evolving concepts in the pathogenesis of postinjury multiple organ failure. Surg Clin North Am 75:257–277, 1995.

225. Moores, L.K.; Jackson, W.L., Jr.; Shorr, A.F.; et al. Meta-analysis: Outcomes in patients with suspected pulmonary embolism managed with computed tomographic pulmonary angiography. Ann Intern Med 141:866, 2004.

226. Moreno-Cabral, R.; Kistner, R.L.; Nordyke, R.A. Importance of calf vein thrombophlebitis. Surgery 80:735–742, 1976.

227. Morgan, E.L.; Weigle, W.O.; Hugli, T.E. Anaphylatoxin-mediated regulation of the immune response. J Exp Med 155:1412–1426, 1982.

228. Morton, K.S.; Kendall, M.J. Fat embolism: Its production and source of fat. Can J Surg 8:214, 1965.

229. Moser, K.M.; LeMoine, F.R. Is embolic risk conditioned by location of deep venous thrombosis? Ann Intern Med 94:439–444, 1981.

230. Moskowitz, R.W.; Howell, D.S.; Goldberg, V.M.; et al. Osteoarthritis Diagnosis and Management. Philadelphia, W.B. Saunders, 1984.

231. Mudd, K.L.; Hunt, A.; Matherly, R.C.; et al. Analysis of pulmonary fat embolism in blunt force fatalities. J Trauma 48:711–715, 2000.

232. Muizelaar, J.P.; Kleyer, M.; Hertogs, I.A.M.; et al. Complex regional pain syndrome (reflex sympathetic dystrophy and causalgia): Management with the calcium channel blocker nifedipine and/or the alpha-sympathetic blocker phenoxybenzamine in 59 patients. Clin Neurol Neurosurg 99:26–30, 1997.

233. Müller, C.; Rahn, B.A.; Pfister, U.; et al. The incidence, pathogenesis, diagnosis, and treatment of fat embolism. Orthop Rev 23:107–117, 1994.

234. Mullins, M. Personal communication. December 1988.

235. Murray, D.G.; Racz, G.B. Fat embolism syndrome (respiratory insufficiency syndrome): A rationale for treatment. J Bone Joint Surg Am 56:1338–1349, 1973.

236. Nast-Kolb, D.; Waydhas, C.; Jochum, M.; et al. Günstigster operationszeitpunkt für die versorgung von femurschafttrakturen bei polytrauma? Chirurg 61:259–265, 1990.

237. Nowotarski, P.J.; Turen, C.H.; Brumback, R.J.; et al. Conversion of external fixation to intramedullary nailing for fractures of the shaft of the femur in multiply injured patients. J Bone Joint Surg Am 82:781–788, 2000.

238. Nuessle, W.F. The significance of fat in the sputum. Am J Clin Pathol 21:430, 1951.

239. Nuytinek, J.K.S.; Goris, R.J.A.; Heinz, R.; et al. Post-traumatic complications and inflammatory mediators. Arch Surg 121:886–890, 1986.

240. Nylander, G.; Semb, H. Veins of the lower part of the leg after tibial fracture. Surg Gynecol Obstet 134:974–976, 1972.

241. Oerlemans, H.M.; Goris, R.J.A.; de Boo, T.; et al. Do physical therapy and occupational therapy reduce the impairment percentage in reflex sympathetic dystrophy? Am J Phys Med Rehabil 78:533–539, 1999.

242. Oerlemans, H.M.; Oostendorp, R.A.B.; de Boo, T.; et al. Adjuvant physical therapy versus occupational therapy in patients with reflex sympathetic dystrophy/complex regional pain syndrome type I. Arch Phys Med Rehabil 81:49–56, 2000.

243. Oerlemans, H.M.; Oostendorp, R.A.B.; de Boo, T.; et al. Signs and symptoms in complex regional pain syndrome type I/reflex sympathetic dystrophy: Judgment of the physician versus objective measurement. Clin J Pain 15:224–232, 1999.

244. Omer, G.E., Jr. Injuries to nerves of the upper extremity. J Bone Joint Surg Am 56:1615–1624, 1974.

245. Omer, G.E., Jr. Peripheral nerve injuries: 45-year odyssey . . . and the quest continues. In Omer, G.E., Jr.; Spinner, M.; Van Beek, A.L., eds.

Management of Peripheral Nerve Problems. Philadelphia, W.B. Saunders, 1998, pp. 3–6.

246. Omer, G.E., Jr. Peripheral nerve injuries and gunshot wounds. In Omer, G.E., Jr.; Spinner, M.; Van Beek, A.L., eds. Management of Peripheral Nerve Problems. Philadelphia, W.B. Saunders, 1998, pp. 398–405.

247. Omer, G.E., Jr. The prognosis for untreated traumatic injuries. In Omer, G.E., Jr.; Spinner, M.; Van Beek, A.L., eds. Management of Peripheral Nerve Problems. Philadelphia, W.B. Saunders, 1998, pp. 365–370.

248. Omer, G.E., Jr. Results of untreated peripheral nerve injuries. Clin Orthop Relat Res 163:15–19, 1982.

249. Owings, J.; Bagley, M.; Gosselin, R.; et al. Effects of critical injury on antithrombin activity: Low antithrombin levels are associated with thromboembolic complications. J Trauma 41:396, 1996.

250. Paiement, G.D.; Wessinger, S.J.; Harris, W.H. Cost effectiveness of prophylaxis in total hip replacement. Am J Surg 161:519–524, 1991.

251. Paley, D.; Tetsworth, K. Mechanical axis deviation of the lower limbs: Preoperative planning of uniapical angular deformities of the tibia or femur. Clin Orthop Relat Res 280:48–64, 1992.

252. Paley, D.; Tetsworth, K. Mechanical axis deviation of the lower limbs: Preoperative planning of multiapical frontal plane angular and bowing deformities of the femur and tibia. Clin Orthop Relat Res 280:65–71, 1992.

253. Pape, H.C.; Auf'm'Kolk, M.; Paffrath, T.; et al. Primary intramedullary fixation in multiple trauma patients with associated lung contusion: A cause of post-traumatic ARDS. J Trauma 34:540–547, 1993.

254. Pape, H.C.; Dwenger, A.; Grotz, M.; et al. The risk of early intramedullary nailing of long bone fractures in multiple traumatized patients. Contemp Orthop 10:15–23, 1995.

255. Pape, H.C.; Dwenger, A.; Regel, G.; et al. Pulmonary damage after intramedullary femoral nailing in traumatized sheep: Is there an effect from different nailing methods? J Trauma 33:574–581, 1992.

256. Pape, H.C.; Giannoudis, P.V.; Krettek, C.; et al. Timing of fixation of major fractures in blunt polytrauma: Role of conventional indicators in clinical decision making. J Orthop Trauma 19:551–562, 2005.

257. Pape, H.C.; Giannoudis, P.; Krettek, C. The timing of fracture treatment in polytrauma patients: Relevance of damage control orthopedic surgery. Am J Surg 183:622–629, 2002.

258. Pape, H.C.; Regel, G.; Dwenger, A.; et al. Influences of different methods of intramedullary femoral nailing on lung function in patients with multiple trauma. J Trauma 35:709–716, 1993.

259. Passman, M.A.; Moreta, G.L.; Taylor, L.M., Jr. Pulmonary embolism is associated with the combination of isolated calf vein thrombosis and respiratory symptoms. J Vasc Surg 25:39–45, 1997.

260. Pell, A.C.H.; James, C.; Keating, J.F. The detection of fat embolism by transesophageal echocardiography during reamed intramedullary nailing. J Bone Joint Surg Br 75:921–925, 1993.

261. Peltier, L.F. Fat embolism: The amount of fat in human long bones. Surgery 40:657, 1956.

262. Peltier, L.F. Fat embolism: An appraisal of the problem. Clin Orthop Relat Res 187:3–17, 1984.

263. Peltier, L.F. Fat embolism: A current concept. Clin Orthop Relat Res 66:241, 1969.

264. Peltier, L.F. Fat embolism: A perspective. Clin Orthop Relat Res 232:263–270, 1988.

265. Peltier, L.F. Fat embolism: A pulmonary disease. Surgery 62:756–758, 1967.

266. Peltier, L.F.; Collins, J.A.; Evarts, C.M.; et al. Fat embolism. Arch Surg 109:12–16, 1974.

267. Perrier, A.; Roy, P.M.; Sanchez, O.; et al. Multidetector-row computed tomography in suspected pulmonary embolism. N Engl J Med 352:1760, 2005.

268. Phillips, W.A.; Schwartz, H.S.; Keller, C.S.; et al. A prospective, randomized study of the management of severe ankle fractures. J Bone Joint Surg Am 67:67–78, 1985.

269. Pinney, S.J.; Keating, J.F.; Meek, R.N. Fat embolism syndrome in isolated femoral fractures: Does timing of nailing influence incidence? Injury 29:131–133, 1998.

270. Poehling, G.C.; Pollock, F.E., Jr.; Koman, L.A. Reflex sympathetic dystrophy of the knee after sensory nerve injury. Arthroscopy 4:31–35, 1988.

271. Polk, H.C., Jr.; Shields, C.L. Remote organ failure: A valid sign of occult intra-abdominal infection. Surgery 81:310–313, 1977.

272. Pollock, F.H.; Drake, D.; Bovill, E.G.; et al. Treatment of radial neuropathy associated with fractures of the humerus. J Bone Joint Surg Am 63:239–243, 1981.

273. Poplawski, Z.J.; Wiley, A.M.; Murray, J.F. Posttraumatic dystrophy of the extremities. J Bone Joint Surg Am 65:642–655, 1983.

274. Portugaller, H.R.; Schoellnast, H.; Hausegger, K.A.; et al. Multislice spiral CT angiography in peripheral arterial occlusive disease: A valuable tool in detecting significant arterial lumen narrowing? Eur Radiol 14:1681–1687, 2004.

275. Powers, L.R. Distal deep vein thrombosis: What's the best treatment? J Gen Intern Med 3:288–293, 1988.

276. Prandoni, P.; Lensing, A.W.; Buller, H.R.; et al. Comparison of subcutaneous low-molecular-weight heparin with intravenous standard heparin in proximal deep vein thrombosis. Lancet 339:441–445, 1992.

277. Prandoni, P.; Lensing, A.W.A.; Buller, H.R.; et al. Deep vein thrombosis and the incidence of subsequent symptomatic cancer. N Engl J Med 327:1128–1133, 1993.

278. Prough, D.S.; McLeskey, C.H.; Weeks, D.B.; et al. Efficacy of oral nifedipine in the treatment of reflex sympathetic dystrophy. Anesthesiology 61:3A, 1984.

279. Puno, R.M.; Vaughan, J.J.; Stetten, M.L.; et al. Long-term effects of tibial angular malunion on the knee and ankle joints. J Orthop Trauma 5:247–254, 1991.

280. Quiroz, R.; Kucher, N.; Zou, K.H.; et al. Clinical validity of a negative computed tomography scan in patients with suspected pulmonary embolism: A systematic review. JAMA 293:2012, 2005.

281. Radin, E.L. Factors influencing the progression of osteoarthrosis. In Ewing, J., ed. Articular Cartilage and Knee Joint Function: Basic Science and Arthroscopy. New York, Raven Press, 1990, p. 301.

282. Radin, E.L.; Ehrlich, M.G.; Chernack, R.; et al. Effect of repetitive impulsive loading on the knee joints of rabbits. Clin Orthop Relat Res 131:288, 1978.

283. Raj, P.P.; Calodney, A. Complex regional pain syndrome (reflex sympathetic dystrophy). In Browner, B.; Jupiter, J.; Levine, A.; et al., eds. Skeletal Trauma, 2nd ed. Philadelphia, W.B. Saunders, 1998, pp. 589–617.

284. Raj, P.P.; Cannella, J.; Kelly, J.; et al. Management protocol of reflex sympathetic dystrophy. In Stanton-Hicks, M.; Janig, W., eds. Reflex Sympathetic Dystrophy. Boston, Kluwer, 1989.

285. Ramamurthy, S. Electroacupuncture's role in the management of reflex sympathetic dystrophy. Tex Med 87:82, 1991.

286. Ramchandani, P.; Soulen, R.L.; Fedullo, L.M.; et al. Deep venous thrombosis: Significant limitations of noninvasive test. Radiology 156:47–49, 1985.

287. Rathbun, S.W.; Raskob, G.E.; Whitsett, T.L. Sensitivity and specificity of helical computed tomography in the diagnosis of pulmonary embolism: A systematic review. Ann Intern Med 132:227, 2000.

288. Repo, R.U.; Finlat, J.B. Survival of articular cartilage after controlled impact. J Bone Joint Surg Am 59:1068–1076, 1977.

289. Research Committee of the British Thoracic Society. Optimal duration of anticoagulation for deep vein thrombosis and pulmonary embolism. Lancet 340:873–876, 1992.

290. Reynolds, M.A.; Spain, D.A.; Seligson, D.; et al. Is the timing of fracture fixation important for the patient with multiple trauma? Ann Surg 222:470–481, 1995.

291. Rieger, M.; Mallouhi, A.; Tauscher, R.; et al. Traumatic arterial injuries of the extremities: Initial evaluation with MDCT angiography: Comment. Am J Roentgenol 186:656–664, 2006.

292. Riseborough, E.J.; Herndon, J.H. Alterations in pulmonary function, coagulation and fat metabolism in patients with fractures of the lower limbs. Clin Orthop Relat Res 115:248, 1976.

293. Riska, E.B.; Myllynen, P. Fat embolism in patients with multiple injuries. J Trauma 22:891–894, 1982.

294. Roberts, C.S.; Pape, H.C.; Jones, A.L.; et al. Damage control orthopaedics: Evolving concepts in the treatment of patients who have sustained orthopaedic trauma. Instr Course Lect 54:447–462, 2005.

295. Rogal, M.J. Comment: Orthopaedic malpractice: Identifying and managing the high risk of orthopaedic surgery. Pitt Orthop J 11:242–243, 2000.

296. Rogers, F.B. Venous thromboembolism in trauma patients. Surg Clin North Am 75:279–291, 1995.

297. Rogers, F.B.; Cipolle, M.D.; Velmahos, G.; et al. Practice management guidelines for the prevention of venous thromboembolism in trauma patients: The EAST practice management guidelines work group. J Trauma 53:142–164, 2002.

298. Rokkanen, P.; Alho, A.; Avikainen, V.; et al. The efficacy of corticosteroids in severe trauma. Surg Gynecol Obstet 138:69, 1974.

299. Rose, S.D.; Zwiebel, W.J.; Nelson, B.D.; et al. Symptomatic lower extremity deep venous thrombosis: Accuracy, limitations, and role of color duplex flow imaging in diagnosis. Radiology 175:639–644, 1990.

300. Rubel, I.F.; Potter, H.; Barie, P.; et al. Magnetic resonance venography to evaluate deep venous thrombosis in patients with pelvic and acetabular trauma. J Trauma 51:178, 2001.

301. Rubin, C.T.; Lanyon, L.E. Regulation of bone formation by applied dynamic loads. J Bone Joint Surg Am 66:397–402, 1984.

302. Ruedi, T.; Wolff, G. Vermeidung posttraumatischer Komplikationen durch fr'duhe definitive Versorgung von Polytraumatisierten mit Frakturen des Bewegungsapparats. Helv Chir Acta 42:507–512, 1975.

303. Russell, G.V.; Kirk, P.G.; Biddinger, P. Fat embolism syndrome from an isolated humerus fracture. J Orthop Trauma 11:141–144, 1997.

304. Sadler, C. Pitfalls in the use of clinical algorithms. Orthop Clin North Am 17:545–547, 1986.

305. Salzman, E.W.; Davies, G.C. Prophylaxis of venous thromboembolism: Analysis of cost effectiveness. Ann Surg 191:207–218, 1980.

306. Salzman, E.W.; Harris, W.H. Prevention of venous thromboembolism in orthopaedic patients. J Bone Joint Surg Am 58:903–913, 1976.

307. Sandroni, P.; Low, P.A.; Ferrer, T.; et al. Complex regional pain syndrome I (CRPS I): Prospective study and laboratory evaluation. Clin J Pain 14:282–289, 1998.

308. Sanson, B.J. Is there a role for thrombolytic therapy in venous thromboembolism? Haemostasis 29(Suppl 1):81–83, 1999.

309. Sarangi, P.P.; Ward, A.J.; Smith, E.J.; et al. Algodystrophy and osteoporosis after tibial fractures. J Bone Joint Surg Br 75:450–452, 1993.

310. Satiani, B.; Falcone, R.; Shook, L.; et al. Screening for major DVT in seriously injured patients: A prospective study. Ann Vasc Surg 11:626–629, 1997.

311. Scalea, T.M.; Boswell, S.A.; Scott, J.D.; et al. External fixation as a bridge to intramedullary nailing for patients with multiple injuries and with femur fractures: Damage control orthopaedics. J Trauma 48:613–621, 2000.

312. Schnaid, E.; Lamprey, J.M.; Volgoen, M.J.; et al. The early biochemical and hormonal profile of patients with long bone fractures at risk of fat embolism syndrome. J Trauma 27:309–311, 1987.

313. Schoepf, U.J.; Goldhaber, S.Z.; Costello, P. Spiral computed tomography for acute pulmonary embolism. Circulation 109: 2160, 2004.

314. Schulman, S.; Rhedin, A.S.; Lindmarker, P.; et al. A comparison of six weeks with six months of oral anticoagulant therapy after a first episode of venous thromboembolism. N Engl J Med 332:1661–1665, 1995.

315. Schurmann, M.; Gradl, G.; Andress, H.J.; et al. Assessment of peripheral sympathetic nervous function for diagnosing early post-traumatic complex regional pain syndrome type I. Pain 80:149–159, 1999.

316. Schuttemeyer, W. Klinische auswertungen der lipasebestimmungen zur diagnose der fettembolie. Arch Klin Chir 270:50, 1951.

317. Schutzer, S.F.; Gossling, H.R. The treatment of reflex sympathetic dystrophy. J Bone Joint Surg Am 66:625–629, 1984.

318. Seddon, H.J. Nerve lesions complicating certain closed bone injuries. JAMA 135:691–694, 1947.

319. Seddon, H.J. Three types of nerve injuries. Brain 66:238–288, 1943.

320. Seely, A.J. Multiple organ dysfunction syndrome: Exploring the paradigm of complex nonlinear systems. Crit Care Med 28:2193–2200, 2000.

321. Seibel, R.; LaDuca, J.; Hassett, J.M.; et al. Blunt multiple trauma (ISS 36), femur traction, and the pulmonary failure septic state. Ann Surg 202:283–293, 1985.

322. Seiller, J.G.; Richardson, J.D. Amputation after extremity injury. Am J Surg 152:260–264, 1986.

323. Sevitt, S. Fat embolism. London, Butterworths, 1962.

324. Sevitt, S. Pathology and pathogenesis of deep vein thrombi in venous problems. In Bergan, J.J.; Yao, J.S.T., eds. Venous Problems. Chicago, Year Book Medical, 1978, pp. 257–279.

325. Sevitt, S.; Gallagher, N. Venous thrombosis and pulmonary embolism: A clinico-pathological study in injured and burned patients. Br J Surg 48:475–489, 1961.

326. Shah, J.J.; Bhatti, N.A. Radial nerve paralysis associated with fractures of the humerus. Clin Orthop Relat Res 172:171–176, 1983.

327. Sieweke, N.; Birklein, F.; Riedl, B.; et al. Patterns of hyperalgesia in complex regional pain syndrome. Pain 80:171–177, 1999.

328. Simonneau, G.S.; Charbonnier, B.; Page, Y.; et al. A comparison of low-molecular-weight heparin with unfractionated heparin for acute pulmonary embolism. N Engl J Med 337:663–669, 1997.

329. Solheim, K. Fractures of the lower leg: Immediate results of treatment in a series of 500 cases of fractures of the shafts of tibia and fibula treated with plaster, traction plaster and internal fixation, with and without exercise therapy. Acta Chir Scand 119:268–279, 1960.

330. Sonneveld, G.J.; Patka, P.; van Mourik, J.C.; et al. Treatment of fractures of the shaft of the humerus accompanied by paralysis of the radial nerve. Injury 1:404–406, 1987.

331. Spain, D.A.; Richardson, J.D.; Polk, H.C., Jr.; et al. Venous thromboembolism in the high-risk trauma patient: Do risks justify aggressive screening and prophylaxis? J Trauma 42:463–469, 1997.

332. Spindler, K.P.; Schils, J.P.; Bergfeld, J.A.; et al. Prospective study of osseous, articular, and meniscal lesions in recent anterior cruciate ligament tears by magnetic resonance imaging and arthroscopy. Am J Sports Med 21:551–557, 1993.

333. Spinner, M. Peripheral nerve problems: Past, present, and future. In Omer, G.E., Jr.; Spinner, M.; Van Beek, A.L., eds. Management of Peripheral Nerve Problems. Philadelphia, W.B. Saunders, 1998, p. 7.

334. Stannard, J.P.; Lopez-Ben, R.R.; Volgas, D.A.; et al. Prophylaxis against deep-vein thrombosis following trauma: A prospective, randomized comparison of mechanical and pharmacologic prophylaxis. J Bone Joint Surg Am 88:261–266, 2006.

335. Stannard, J.P.; Singhania, A.K.; Lopez-Ben, R.R.; et al. Deep-vein thrombosis in high-energy skeletal trauma despite thromboprophylaxis. J Bone Joint Surg Br 87:965–968, 2005.

336. Stanton-Hicks, M.; Baron, R.; Boas, R.; et al. Complex regional pain syndrome: Guidelines for therapy. Clin J Pain 14:155–166, 1998.

337. Stanton-Hicks, M.; Janig, W.; Hassenbusch, S.; et al. Reflex sympathetic dystrophy: Changing concepts and taxonomy. Pain 63:127–133, 1995.

338. Steadman, J.R.; Rodkey, W.G.; Singleton, S.B.; et al. Micro-fracture technique for full-thickness chondral defects: Technique and clinical results. Oper Tech Orthop 7:300–304, 1997.

339. Stephen, J.M.; Feied, C.F. Venous thrombosis: Lifting the clouds of misunderstanding. Postgrad Med 97:36–47, 1995.

340. Stoltenberg, J.J.; Gustilo, R.B. The use of methylprednisolone and hypertonic glucose in the prophylaxis of fat embolism syndrome. Clin Orthop Relat Res 143:211–221, 1979.

341. Stover, M.D.; Morgan, S.J.; Bosse, M.J.; et al. Prospective comparison of contrast-enhanced computed tomography versus magnetic resonance venography in the detection of occult deep pelvic vein thrombosis in patients with pelvic and acetabular fractures. J Orthop Trauma 16:613–621, 2002.

342. Strecker, W.; Gebhard, F.; Rajer, J.; et al. Early biomedical characterization of soft-tissue trauma and fracture trauma. J Trauma 47:358–364, 1999.

343. Sunderland, S. A classification of peripheral nerve injuries producing loss of function. Brain 74:491–516, 1951.

344. Swenson, M.R.; Villasana, D.R. Neurologic evaluation of the upper extremity. In Kasdan, M.L., ed. Occupational Hand and Upper Extremity Injuries and Diseases. Philadelphia, Hanley & Belfus, 1991, pp. 115–130.

345. Swiontkowski, M.F. The multiply injured patient with musculoskeletal injuries. In Rockwood, C.A., Jr.; Green, D.P.; Bucholz, R.W.; et al., eds. Fractures in Adults, 4th ed. Philadelphia, Lippincott-Raven, 1996, p. 121.

346. Talucci, R.C.; Manning, J.; Lampard, S.; et al. Early intramedullary nailing of femoral shaft fractures: A cause of fat embolism syndrome. Am J Surg 148:107–111, 1983.

347. Talucci, R.C.; Manning, J.; Lampard, S.; et al. Traumatic lipaemia and fatty embolism. Int Clin 4:171, 1913.

348. ten Duis, H.J. The fat embolism syndrome. Injury 28:77–85, 1997.

349. ten Duis, H.J.; Nijsten, M.W.N.; Klasen, H.J.; et al. Fat embolism in patients with an isolated fracture of the femoral shaft. J Trauma 28:383–390, 1988.

350. Teng, Q.S.; Li, G.; Zhang, B.X. Experimental study of early diagnosis and treatment of fat embolism syndrome. J Orthop Trauma 9:183–189, 1995.

351. Tetsworth, K.; Paley, D. Malalignment and degenerative arthropathy. Orthop Clin North Am 25:367–377, 1994.

352. Thompson, R.C.; Oegema, T.R.; Lewis, J.L.; et al. Osteoarthrotic changes after acute transarticular load: An animal model. J Bone Joint Surg Am 73:990–1001, 1991.

353. Townsend, R.H.; Protech, J.; et al. Timing fracture repair in patients with severe brain injury (Glasgow Coma Scale <9). J Trauma 44:977–982, 1998.

354. Trowbridge, R.L.; Araoz, P.A.; Gotway, M.B.; et al. The effect of helical computed tomography on diagnostic and treatment strategies in patients with suspected pulmonary embolism. Am J Med 116:84, 2004.

355. Tscherne, H.A. Keynote Address. Orthopedic Trauma Association Annual Meeting, Dallas, Texas, October 1988.

356. UPET Investigators. The Urokinase Pulmonary Embolism Trial: A national cooperative study. Circulation 47(Suppl 2):1–108, 1973.

357. Veldman, P.H.; Reynen, H.M.; Arntz, I.E.; et al. Signs and symptoms of reflex sympathetic dystrophy: Prospective study of 829 patients. Lancet 342:1012–1016, 1993.

358. Velmahos, G.C.; Nigro, J.; Tatevossian, R.; et al. Inability of an aggressive policy of thromboprophylaxis to prevent deep venous thrombosis in critically injured patients: Are current methods of DVT prophylaxis insufficient? J Am Coll Surg 187:529–533, 1998.

359. Velmahos, G.C.; Ramicone, E.; et al. Timing of fracture fixation in blunt trauma patients with severe head injuries. Am J Surg 176:324–329, 1998.

360. Virchow, R. Cellular Pathology. Translated by F. Chance. New York, R.M. de Witt, 1860.

361. Volpin, G.; Dowd, G.S.E.; Stein, H.; et al. Degenerative arthritis after intra-articular fractures of the knee: Long-term results. J Bone Joint Surg Br 72:634–638, 1990.

362. Von Bergmann, E. Ein fall tödlicher Fettembolie. Berl Klin Wochenschr 10:385, 1873.

363. Vrahas, M.S.; Smith, G.A.; Rosler, D.M.; et al. Method to impact in vivo femoral rabbit cartilage with blows of quantifiable stress. J Orthop Res 15:314–317, 1997.

364. Walker, J.M. Pathomechanics and classification of cartilage lesions, facilitation of repair. J Orthop Sports Phys Ther 28:216, 1998.

365. Ward, W.G.; Nunley, J.A. Occult orthopaedic trauma in the multiply injured patient. J Orthop Trauma 5:308–312, 1991.

366. Ward, W.W. Posttraumatic reflex sympathetic dystrophy. In Foy, M.A.; Fagg, P.S., eds. Medicolegal Reporting in Orthopaedic Trauma. New York, Churchill Livingstone, 1995, pp. 5.5-05–5.5-08.

367. Warkentin, T.E.; Levine, M.N.; Hirsh, J.; et al. Heparin-induced thrombocytopenia in patients treated with low molecular weight or unfractionated heparin. N Engl J Med 332:1330–1335, 1995.

368. Webb, L.X.; Rush, P.T.; Fuller, S.B.; et al. Greenfield filter prophylaxis of pulmonary embolism in patients undergoing surgery for acetabular fracture. J Orthop Trauma 6:139–145, 1992.

369. Wells, P.S.; Ginsberg, J.S.; Anderson, D.R.; et al. Use of a clinical model for safe management of patients with suspected pulmonary embolism. Ann Intern Med 129:997–1005, 1998.

370. Wenda, K.; Ritter, G.; Degreif, J. Zur genese pulmonaler Komplikationen nach Marknagelosteosynthesen. Unfallchirurg 91:432–435, 1988.

371. Wheeler, H.B. Diagnosis of deep venous thrombosis: Review of clinical evaluation and impedance plethysmography. Am J Surg 150(4A):7–13, 1985.

372. Wheeler, H.B.; Anderson, F.A.; Cardullo, P.A.; et al. Suspected deep vein thrombosis. Arch Surg 117:1206–1209, 1982.

373. Wheeler, H.B.; Pearson, D.; O'Connell, D.; et al. Impedance phlebography: Technique, interpretation and results. Arch Surg 104:164–169, 1972.

374. White, R.H.; McGahan, J.P.; Daschbach, M.M.; et al. Diagnosis of deep vein thrombosis using duplex ultrasound. Ann Intern Med 111:297–304, 1989.

375. Wiesel, S.W.; Michelson, L.D. Monitoring orthopedic patients using computerized algorithms. Orthop Clin North Am 17:541–544, 1986.

376. Wiley, A.M. Venous thrombosis in orthopaedic patients: An overview. Orthop Surg 2:388, 1979.

377. Wilson, P. Sympathetically maintained pain. In Stanton-Hicks, M., ed. Sympathetic Pain. Boston, Kluwer, 1989.

378. Wong, M.W.; Tsui, H.F.; Yung, S.H.; et al. Continuous pulse oximeter monitoring for inapparent hypoxemia after long bone fractures. J Trauma 56:356–362, 2004.

379. Wozasek, G.E.; Simon, P.; Redl, H. Intramedullary pressure changes and fat intravasation during intramedullary nailing: An experimental study in sheep. J Trauma 36:202–207, 1994.

380. Wright, R.W.; Phaneuf, M.A.; Limbird, T.J.; et al. Clinical outcome of isolated subcortical trabecular fractures (bone bruise) detected on magnetic resonance imaging in knees. Am J Sports Med 28:663–667, 2000.

381. Wright, V. Posttraumatic osteoarthritis: A medicolegal minefield. Br J Rheumatol 29:474–478, 1990.

382. Zallen, G.; Offner, P.J.; Moore, E.E.; et al. Age of transfused blood is an independent risk factor for postinjury multiple organ failure. Am J Surg 178:570–572, 1999.

383. Zenker, F.A. Beitrage zur Anatomie und Physiologie de Lunge. Dresden, Germany, J. Braunsdorf, 1861.

384. Zyluk, A. The natural history of post-traumatic reflex sympathetic dystrophy. J Hand Surg [Br] 23:20–23, 1998.

385. Zyluk, A. The usefulness of quantitative evaluation of three-phase scintigraphy in the diagnosis of post-traumatic reflex sympathetic dystrophy. J Hand Surg [Br] 24:16–21, 1999.

386. Zyluk, A.; Birkenfeld, B. Quantitative evaluation of three-phase scintigraphy before and after treatment of post-traumatic reflex sympathetic dystrophy. Nucl Med Commun 20:327–333, 1999.

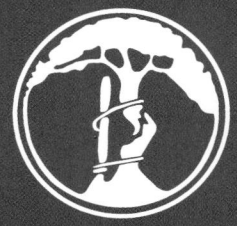

CHAPTER 21

Chronic Osteomyelitis

Craig M. Rodner, M.D., Bruce D. Browner, M.D., M.S., F.A.C.S., and Ed Pesanti, M.D., F.A.C.P.

In adults, bone infections are most commonly seen after direct skeletal trauma or after operative treatment of bone. These infections, usually referred to as post-traumatic, exogenous, or chronic osteomyelitis, are difficult to treat and usually have a protracted clinical course. Surgical débridement constitutes the cornerstone of management with antibiotic therapy playing only an adjunctive role.

TERMINOLOGY

Before embarking on a review of chronic osteomyelitis, it may be wise to begin with a few basic definitions.

The term *osteomyelitis* simply refers to an infection in bone. Such infections are most often caused by pyogenic bacteria (such as *Staphylococcus aureus*), although other microbes, including mycobacteria and fungi, are sometimes responsible. In *hematogenous osteomyelitis,* which most frequently affects children, blood-borne bacteria seed previously healthy bone. In *post-traumatic* or *exogenous osteomyelitis,* the infection is almost always associated with trauma, whether it be of the unplanned variety (e.g., a motor vehicle accident) or planned (e.g., a surgical procedure). The term *acute osteomyelitis* is often used interchangeably with the term hematogenous osteomyelitis; in current usage, both terms reflect a form of osteomyelitis in which osteonecrosis has not yet occurred. At the other end of the spectrum, the term *chronic osteomyelitis* is defined as a bone infection predicated on preexisting osteonecrosis. Note that the difference between *acute* and *chronic* osteomyelitis is not based on the duration of infection, as their names might suggest, but rather on the absence or presence of dead bone. It is precisely the presence of dead bone that makes chronic osteomyelitis a primarily surgical disease.

Although theoretically chronic osteomyelitis can result from an untreated or inadequately treated hematogenous infection, it is most frequently traumatic in origin. It is important to recognize that infection occurring in the setting of skeletal trauma, however *acutely* chronologically, is in fact a *chronic* osteomyelitis from the start. In the post-traumatic milieu, opportunistic bacteria can be thought of as "taking advantage" of bone that has been devitalized by injury (quite the opposite from acute osteomyelitis, wherein microbes seed previously healthy bone). Because of the high congruence between

osteonecrosis and a history of trauma, the terms *chronic* and *post-traumatic* or *exogenous* osteomyelitis are frequently used interchangeably. This is reasonable as long as one understands the subtle differences.

EPIDEMIOLOGY

Bone infection in the adult population is much more likely to be exogenous in origin than hematogenous, in part because of the demographics of high-speed motor vehicle accidents and orthopaedic surgery but also because the predilection for bacterial seeding of bone ceases with closure of the epiphyses. For this reason, hematogenous osteomyelitis is vanishingly rare in people beyond their teens, occurring only in immunocompromised hosts.[32]

Post-traumatic osteomyelitis is one of the few infectious diseases that has become more prevalent in this century, probably because it is one of the few diseases fueled by technology. With the development of bigger and more powerful automobiles, motorcycles, guns, and land mines, the past hundred years have been witness to an ever-increasing potential for devastating soft tissue and skeletal injury. Infection is so closely linked with such injuries for two reasons. First, they provide ubiquitous microbes with an opportunity for breaching host defenses by exposing bone to the contamination of an accident scene. Second, once the microbes have bypassed external defenses, the trauma setting offers an ideal environment for adherence and colonization, namely, devitalized hard and soft tissues. It is not surprising, therefore, that there is a significant incidence of deep infection, of either soft tissue or bone, secondary to open fractures.

A review by Gustilo[54] showed the deep infection rate in the setting of open fractures to be anywhere from 2 to 50 percent. Naturally, not all open fractures carry the same risk of infection. On the basis of the extent of soft tissue injury, the severity of open fractures has traditionally been classified as type I, II, or III according to criteria put forth by Gustilo and Anderson.[55] Not surprisingly, it has been found that the more severe the open fracture, the greater the likelihood of infection: approximately 2 percent for type I and II open fractures and 10 to 50 percent in type III open fractures.[27,54,55,118] Gustilo[27] cited several reasons type III fractures have been shown to be more susceptible to infection, such as lack of bone coverage, massive contamination of the wound, compromised perfusion, and instability of the fracture.

The tibia is the most frequent location of open fractures[37] and, accordingly, is also the most frequently infected. One retrospective[135] study of 948 high-energy open tibial fractures reported a 56 percent post-traumatic infection rate. Although not involved so often as the lower extremity, the upper extremity also is vulnerable to accidental trauma and subsequent infection.[143] In addition to traumatic injury, chronic osteomyelitis can result from surgical implants or, less commonly, from untreated or poorly treated hematogenous infection.

Any discussion of the epidemiology of chronic osteomyelitis should include the role of host factors. Patients with vascular insufficiency, from conditions such as diabetes and peripheral vascular disease, have long been known to be at higher risk for post-traumatic or postoperative osteomyelitis.[154] Even subtle injuries in this population, such as a chronic pressure sore, may lead to the development of exposed bone, surrounding cellulitis, and eventual gangrene of the soft tissues.[123] Diabetic ulcers progress quickly in the setting of co-morbid peripheral vascular disease, neuropathy, and repetitive trauma.[61,91] Additional host factors, such as malnutrition and alcoholism, are said to contribute to the development of post-traumatic osteomyelitis[81] but have not been rigorously studied. Although there are no studies focusing specifically on the correlation between cigarette smoking and the incidence of post-traumatic osteomyelitis, there is evidence supporting significantly faster healing in nonsmokers with tibial infection compared with smokers.[52] Furthermore, there is a vast literature on the detrimental effects of smoking, and nicotine in particular, on wound healing, the survival of muscle flaps and skin grafts, and the rate of fracture union.[154]

Although it is known that a vascular insult predisposes a person to the development of chronic osteomyelitis, this progression should not be viewed solely as an inverse correlation between blood flow and risk of infection. In any acute inflammatory process, the balance between host and microbe is determined in large part by the efficacy of the immune response to the infectious challenge. Patients suffering from a disorder of polymorphonuclear leukocytes, for example, have been shown to be at an increased risk for the development and progression of osteomyelitis. In one series of 42 children with chronic granulomatous disease, the authors identified 13 patients who had osteomyelitis.[134] Other immunocompromised individuals such as organ transplant recipients,[73,154] patients with end-stage renal disease, and those receiving chemotherapy[18] also seem to be at an increased risk. Although human immunodeficiency virus infection has not been identified as an independent risk factor in developing osteomyelitis,[92] skeletal infection in this population is clearly associated with a more severe clinical course with elevated morbidity and mortality.[149]

PATHOGENESIS

Although acute osteomyelitis and chronic osteomyelitis both describe infections of bone, they are fundamentally distinguished by the presence of dead bone in the latter.

Unlike acute osteomyelitis, which usually occurs in the metaphyseal areas of long bones secondary to hematogenous seeding, chronic osteomyelitis is usually localized to the area of traumatic injury, which can be epiphyseal, metaphyseal, or diaphyseal.

Hematogenous Osteomyelitis

In hematogenous infection, microorganisms infiltrate the metaphyseal end-arteries of long bone and replicate, thereby instigating a vigorous inflammatory response from the host. Because bone is a hard and rigid tissue, this influx of inflammatory cells into its canals has the unintended effect of raising intraosseous pressure and occluding its own blood supply.[158] Unless the infection and subsequent inflammation are rapidly controlled by the early administration of antibiotics, an area of devitalized bone begins to form. This fragment of necrotic bone, which is usually cortical and surrounded by inflammatory exudate and granulation tissue, is called a sequestrum. An involucrum (sheath) of reactive bone forms around the sequestrum, effectively sealing it off from the bloodstream much like a walled-off abscess. With the development of dead bone, the infection can properly be referred to as a chronic osteomyelitis. Because it is possible to interrupt this progression with early antibiotics or drainage, acute hematogenous infection rarely evolves into chronic osteomyelitis.[153]

Chronic Osteomyelitis

The adult immune system normally renders bacterial colonization of bone difficult. In a normal host, there are only a few circumstances in which such infection might occur. These include a large inoculum size ($>10^5$ organisms per gram of tissue),[82,119] an environment of ischemic bone and surrounding soft tissue, or the presence of a foreign body.[32,97] Unfortunately for the individual with a contaminated open fracture, virtually all of these conditions are present. In the setting of skeletal trauma and subsequent ischemia, the same bone that is normally quite resistant to bacterial infiltration becomes an ideal target for bacterial adherence and subsequent proliferation.[98]

The first step in the pathogenesis of chronic osteomyelitis is entry of the pathogenic organism through the host's external defenses. Normally a difficult task, breaching the skin and mucous membranes becomes facile in the setting of an open fracture. However, the presence of a foreign microbe at or near bone is not sufficient to produce infection. Indeed, although most open fractures are contaminated by bacteria, only a fraction of these actually progress to osteomyelitis.[144] For osteomyelitis to develop, the microbe must not only penetrate the host's external defenses but actually become adherent to the underlying bone. Whereas the skeleton is normally resistant to bacterial adherence, traumatized tissue is susceptible to attack. This occurs, in part, because pathogenic bacteria have various receptors for host proteins that are laid open by injury to the bone. For example, *S. aureus* has receptors for collagen, which is exposed by skeletal trauma, and fibronectin, which covers injured tissue shortly after the initial insult.[39,51,59,144] Additionally, work is under way to better characterize the fundamental changes in the physiology of bacteria when they are inhabiting biofilms, a key feature of any infection of bone or implanted hardware.[14] Furthermore, external debris (in the case of open fractures) and even the necrotic bone fragments themselves can act as avascular foci for further bacterial adherence. Thus, as the osteonecrotic area expands, the disease is perpetuated by exposure of an increasing number of sites to which opportunistic bacteria can bind. In cases of chronic osteomyelitis secondary to internal fixation, the hardware itself serves as another adherent surface.[35,39,51,62] After bacteria successfully adhere to bone, they are able to aggregate and replicate in the devitalized tissue. Effectively sealed off from the host immune system, as well as from antibiotics, the organisms at the avascular focus of infection proliferate undeterred in a medium of dead bone, clotted blood, and dead space. Eventually, the bacteria disperse to adjacent areas of bone and soft tissue and the infection expands. The rapid growth of bacteria can lead to abscess and sinus tract formation. As pus accumulates and abscesses form within the soft tissues adjacent to the necrotic tissue, the patient experiences cyclic episodes of pain followed by drainage. A chronic course ensues without aggressive surgical débridement of all avascular tissue.

Bacteriology

Gustilo and Anderson[54,55] reported that 70 percent of open fractures had positive wound cultures before the initiation of treatment. Of course, not every contaminated wound leads to frank bone infection. In some circumstances, the combination of host defenses and various treatment modalities is successful in preventing bacteria from reaching some critical threshold necessary for infection. However, as mentioned, there are a few factors that put a person at increased risk for skeletal infection, such as a large inoculum size, an environment of ischemia and devitalized tissue, or the presence of a foreign body.[32,97] Under any of these circumstances, bacteria contaminating an open wound are much more likely to adhere successfully to bone and produce osteomyelitis.

S. aureus is far and away the most common isolate in all types of bone infection and is implicated in 50 to 75 percent of cases of chronic osteomyelitis.[23,28] Although the coagulase-positive staphylococci (*S. aureus*) are often cultured from the wound at the time of initial inspection, superinfection with multiple other organisms, such as coagulase-negative staphylococci (*Staphylococcus epidermidis*) and aerobic gram-negatives (*Escherichia coli* and *Pseudomonas* species), also commonly occurs.[55] One study suggested that *S. epidermidis* and various gram-negative bacilli are each involved in approximately one third of cases of chronic osteomyelitis.[143] Other studies implicated gram-negative rods in 50 percent of cases.[110] Although the exact distribution of microbes may vary from one study to another, a consistent finding has been the much higher incidence of polymicrobial infection in chronic osteomyelitis compared with hematogenous osteomyelitis.[11] This distinction should be recalled when antibiotic coverage is selected for the patient with presumed post-traumatic infection.

Staphylococci are so frequently cultured in open wounds because they are ubiquitous organisms. Both *S. aureus* and *S. epidermidis* are elements of normal skin flora, with *S. aureus* in greater numbers in the nares and anal mucosa and *S. epidermidis* more prevalent on the skin. Any traumatic event gives these bacteria a conduit to internal tissues. As mentioned, in the presence of wounded tissue, *S. aureus* has an increased affinity for host proteins, a phenomenon ascribed to an interaction between its capsular polysaccharide and the exposed collagen and fibronectin on traumatized bone.[39,51,59,144]

Although *S. aureus* produces a variety of enzymes, such as coagulase, the role of these in vivo in blunting the impact of host defenses remains unclear. A surface factor that may be important in its pathogenicity is protein A, which has been shown to bind to immunoglobulin G and thereby inhibit host opsonization and phagocytosis. An additional reason *S. aureus* can lead to such persistent infection may be its ability to alter its structure altogether in surviving without a cell wall. This inactive "L" form allows *S. aureus,* and a variety of other bacteria, to live dormant for years, even in the presence of bactericidal levels of antibiotic.[34,44] Antimicrobial agents that exert their bactericidal activity by disrupting cell wall synthesis, as is the case with the β-lactams (penicillins and cephalosporins), become ineffective when bacteria become cell wall deficient or less metabolically active.[152]

Another way in which staphylococci, in particular *S. epidermidis,* elude antimicrobial action is by secreting biofilm, a polysaccharide "slime" layer that dramatically increases bacterial adherence to virtually any substrate.[16,51,87,128,157] First described by Zobell and Anderson in 1936,[163] biofilm is especially significant[45,69] in the pathogenesis of osteomyelitis because of its adherence to inert substrates, such as osteonecrotic bone, prosthetic devices, and acrylic cement. By establishing tight bonds with the glycoproteins of such substrates, biofilm enables actively dividing staphylococci to form adherent, sessile communities. Like cell wall–deficient strains of *S. aureus,* these communities of dormant bacteria have demonstrated increased antimicrobial resistance.[49,95] In a similar fashion, biofilm has been shown to protect *S. epidermidis* from the host immune response itself.

Like staphylococci, *Pseudomonas aeruginosa* is a ubiquitous organism, with soil and fresh water serving as its primary reservoirs. Puncture wounds of the foot involve *P. aeruginosa* in about 95 percent of cases,[67] probably because of its prevalence in soil and moist, sweaty areas of skin. *Pseudomonas* species are implicated in many opportunistic infections, and thus its presence in the setting of chronic osteomyelitis is not unexpected. However, once *P. aeruginosa* has been introduced into host tissue, its pathogenic properties are less well defined than those of the staphylococci. Because this organism is one of the few obligately aerobic pathogenic bacteria (in contrast to *S. aureus,* a facultative anaerobe), its persistence in areas of hypoxic avascular bone is difficult to understand.

CLASSIFICATION

There are a number of ways to classify a case of osteomyelitis. One way would be to label the osteomyelitis as either *pediatric* or *adult,* distinguishing the infection on the basis of its age of onset. Another possibility is describing it as either *hematogenous* or *exogenous*–post-traumatic, distinguishing the infection on the basis of its pathogenesis. Finally, it could be labeled either *acute* or *chronic*, distinguishing the infection on the basis of whether it requires preexisting osteonecrosis. All these classifications are used more frequently than describing the osteomyelitis by its causative organism, which is of course the standard approach for classifying most other infectious diseases, such as labeling a pneumonia "streptococcal" or a meningitis "meningococcal." The reason that the osteomyelitis literature has not used this nomenclature is probably that it is of little prognostic value. For example, it is of much greater therapeutic and prognostic consequence for the clinician to know whether osteonecrosis is present in a skeletal infection than whether *S. aureus* was one of the several microbes cultured.

Whether the infection has been labeled as adult, post-traumatic, or chronic osteomyelitis, it is helpful to classify it further using the staging system developed by Cierny and colleagues in 1985.[25] This system is currently the one most widely used for the classification of osteomyelitis.[63] The Cierny-Mader staging system classifies bone infection on the basis of two independent factors: (1) the anatomic area of bone involved and (2) the immunocompetence of the host. By combining one of the four anatomic types of osteomyelitis (I, medullary; II, superficial; III, localized; or IV, diffuse) with one of the three classes of host immunocompetence (A, B, or C), this system arrives at 12 clinical stages.[52] Probably more important than memorizing each of these stages is understanding the different anatomic sites that can be involved in osteomyelitis (Fig. 21-1).[25]

As described by Cierny and colleagues, the primary lesion in *medullary osteomyelitis* (type I) is endosteal and confined to the intramedullary surfaces of bone (e.g., a hematogenous osteomyelitis or an infection of an intramedullary rod). *Superficial osteomyelitis* (type II) is a true contiguous focus infection in which the outermost layer of bone becomes infected from an adjacent source, such as a decubitus ulcer or a burn. *Localized osteomyelitis* (type III) produces full-thickness cortical cavitation within a segment of stable bone. It is frequently observed in the setting of fractures or when bone becomes infected from an adjacent implant. When the infected fracture does not heal and there is through-and-through disease of the hard and soft tissue, the condition is called *diffuse osteomyelitis* (type IV). Patients with post-traumatic osteomyelitis almost always have type III or type IV disease.

The immunocompetence portion of the Cierny-Mader classification stratifies patients according to their ability to mount an immune response. A patient with a normal physiologic response is labeled an *A host,* a compromised patient a *B host,* and a patient who is so compromised that surgical intervention poses a greater risk than the infection itself is designated a *C host.* A further stratification is made in *B* hosts on the basis of whether the patient has a local (B^{L}), systemic (B^{S}), or combined ($B^{\mathrm{S,L}}$) deficiency in wound healing. An example of a local deficit in wound healing would be venous stasis at the site of injury, whereas systemic deficits would include malnutrition, renal failure, diabetes, tobacco or alcohol use, or acquired immunodeficiency syndrome.

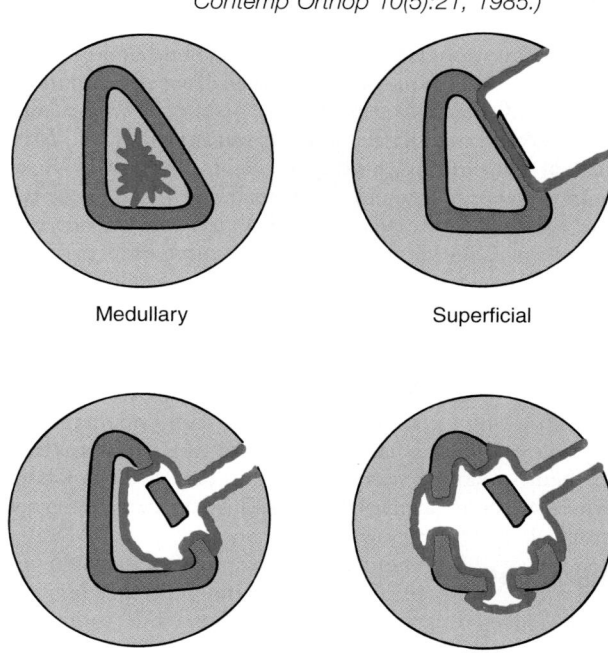

FIGURE 21-1 *Anatomic types of osteomyelitis as they relate to the osseous compartment. (Redrawn from Cierny, G.III; Mader, J.; Penninck, J. Adult osteomyelitis. Contemp Orthop 10(5):21, 1985.)*

Medullary

Superficial

Localized

Diffuse

Other less frequently used classification systems have been developed. One of the older classification systems was created by Kelly and co-workers[70,71] and stratified bone infections on the basis of their etiology: type I described an infection secondary to hematogenous spread, type II referred to an infection with fracture union, type III was an infected nonunion, and type IV meant that there was an exogenous infection without a fracture. A subsequent classification system for post-traumatic tibial osteomyelitis was based on the status of the tibia and fibula after surgical débridement.[86]

Although most of the classification systems developed for osteomyelitis address the extent of the skeletal infection, they do not give a detailed picture of the condition of the bone. Specifically, they do not address issues such as limb length, limb alignment, involvement of adjacent joints, or the presence of bone gaps. Although these are all important, such descriptive features are not necessary in the initial evaluation of osteomyelitis and may only confuse the clinician trying to determine whether surgical intervention is needed.

To make this determination, it is helpful to consult Cierny and Mader's classification system. In their schema, dead space management does not play a large role in any infection deemed to be either a medullary (type I) or superficial (type II) osteomyelitis. However, if an infection is labeled a localized (type III) osteomyelitis, there is usually the need for simple measures to stabilize the bone and dead space management. Any infection classified as diffuse (type IV) osteomyelitis would require extensive skeletal stabilization and extensive dead space management. In this way, the Cierny-Mader classification for osteomyelitis remains the most useful of its kind.

DIAGNOSIS

Initial Assessment

HISTORY

Chronic osteomyelitis is a diagnosis that can potentially be achieved by a thorough history of the patient. It should be suspected in anyone with bone pain who has a past history of trauma or orthopaedic surgery. Complaints include persistent pain, erythema, swelling, and drainage localized to an area of previous trauma, surgery, or wound infection. Walenkamp[155] described a classic history as cyclical pain, increasing to "severe deep tense pain with fever," that often subsides when pus breaks through in a fistula. Although these cyclical episodes are almost pathognomonic for chronic osteomyelitis, they do not occur in everyone with the disease. Most of the time, symptoms are vague and generalized (e.g., "My leg is red and hurts"), making it difficult to differentiate between cellulitis and a true infection of bone.

EXAMINATION

Classically, the cardinal signs of inflammation are rubor (redness), dolor (tenderness), calor (heat), and tumor (swelling). If these signs are noted on physical examination, it is fair to conclude that an infection is present. However, as with the history, signs of an actual osteomyelitis are often difficult to distinguish from those of an overlying soft tissue infection. Suspicion of a bone infection may be confirmed by the presence of exposed necrotic bone, surgical hardware, or draining fistulas (Fig. 21-2). However, such physical examination findings are rare. More commonly, recurrent drainage of small, trivial-appearing sinus tracts is the only sign that infection may be present (Fig. 21-3). The extent of infection and the fact that these tracts communicate with bone are often underappreciated. In addition to the determination of the presence of infection, the involved limb in general should of course be assessed during the physical examination. This assessment includes a thorough evaluation of its neurovascular status, the condition of its soft tissues, its length, alignment, and the presence of any structural deformities.

CULTURES

Culturing drainage fluid, if any is present, is easy to do in the office. Although potentially helpful in identifying causative bacteria and guiding antibiotic choice, these results must be interpreted with caution, because such specimens often yield opportunistic organisms that have simply colonized the nutrient-rich exudate. As a result, these cultures may provide no evidence of the organisms that are actually infecting the damaged bone.[26] Because the results from cultures of sinus tracts and purulent discharge are dubious, the diagnosis of chronic osteomyelitis can be definitively made only by intraoperative biopsy.[81]

PLAIN FILM

Plain radiographs play an important role in the workup of chronic osteomyelitis because they provide the clinician

---

FIGURE 21-2 *The presence of **(A)** exposed bone or **(B)** exposed hardware can be an obvious sign that an underlying skeletal infection is present.*

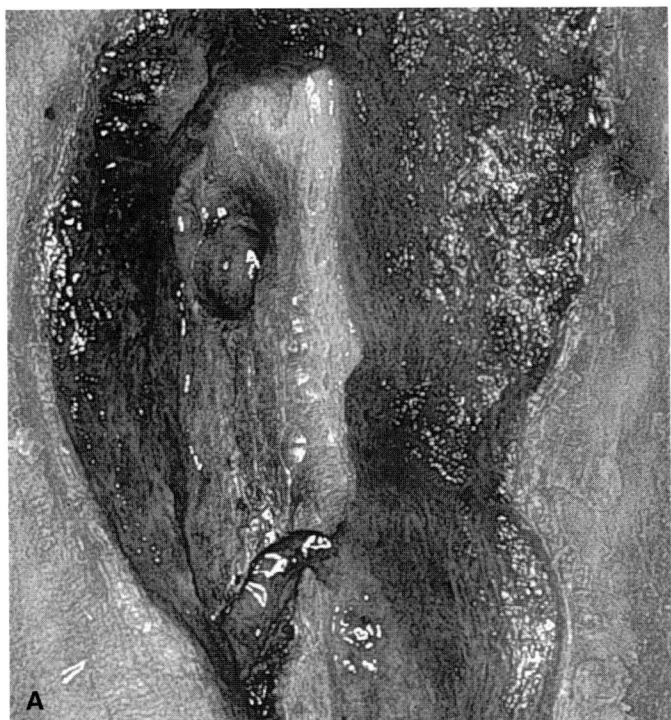

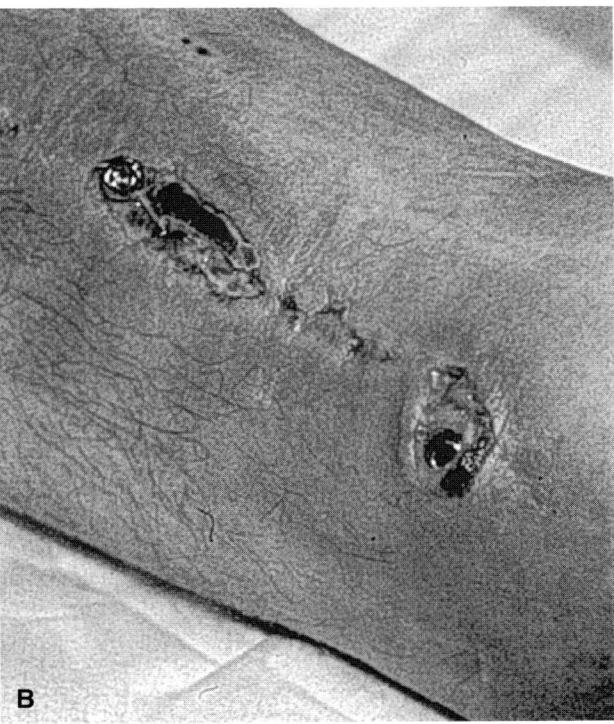

The extent of skeletal infection is often underappreciated by physical examination.

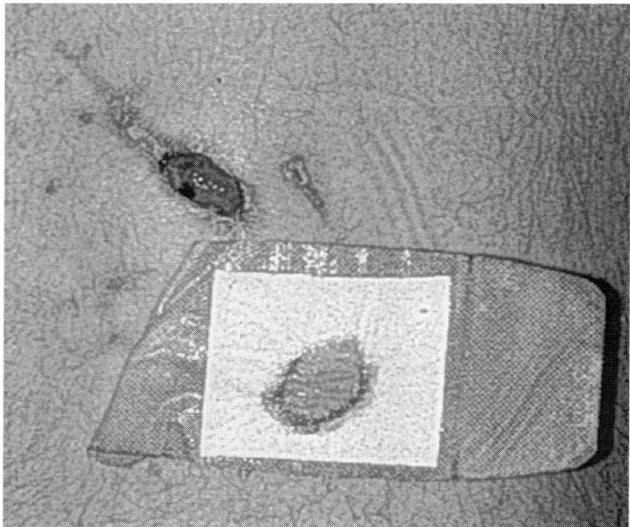

with a sense of the overall bony architecture, limb length and alignment, and presence of orthopaedic implants, as well as any fractures, malunions, or nonunions. Radiographic findings of chronic osteomyelitis can be subtle and include osteopenia, thinning of the cortices, and loss of the trabecular architecture in cancellous bone.[114] Once the bone becomes necrotic and separated from normal bone by an involucrum, it becomes easier to identify on plain film. When isolated in this way, sequestra appear radiodense relative to normal bone.

It is essential to obtain views of the involved bone that include its adjacent joints so that their integrity may be adequately assessed. Furthermore, it is important to include oblique views so as to detect the presence of subtle malunions that may not be seen in the anteroposterior plane alone. Plain films do not play so large a role in the initial workup of acute osteomyelitis, because they typically do not show changes in the bone characteristic of osteomyelitis until 10 to 14 days after the onset of infection.

LABORATORY STUDIES

White blood cell (WBC) counts, erythrocyte sedimentation rate (ESR), and C-reactive protein (CRP) levels have traditionally been part of the workup of any patient with suspected musculoskeletal infection. In an immunocompetent individual, elevated levels of these laboratory values are fairly sensitive indicators of some sort of acute infection, particularly when the WBC count has a so-called left shift (i.e., an elevated ratio of polymorphonuclear leukocytes to other white cells). ESR is a measurement of the rate at which red blood cells sink toward the bottom of a test tube and separate from plasma. ESR is elevated when the erythrocytes clump abnormally well because of an abundance of serum globulins, such as fibrinogen, which are usually produced in response to inflammation. CRP is another acute-phase reactant and a similar marker for systemic inflammation.

There is a paucity of studies showing a correlation between laboratory values and the presence of bone infection, although one group of investigators has shown CRP to be useful in the early detection of sequelae-prone acute osteomyelitis.[120]

Unfortunately, all these values are rather nonspecific to skeletal infection and thus add little to the clinician's ability to distinguish a superficial inflammatory process, such as a cellulitis, from a deeper, osteomyelitic one. Furthermore, although theoretically helpful in screening for an *acute* infection, the WBC count, ESR, and CRP are frequently normal in the setting of *chronic* osteomyelitis and thus are neither sensitive nor specific for it.[155]

To understand why this may be so, it is helpful to reconsider the pathophysiology underlying acute and chronic osteomyelitis. Because acute osteomyelitis is a disease characterized by a vigorous influx of phagocytes and other inflammatory cells into hematogenously seeded bone, it follows that a laboratory test indicating systemic inflammation should be a sensitive marker for infection. However, this should not necessarily be the case in chronic osteomyelitis, which is a disease characterized by devitalized tissues and a muted inflammatory response. It makes sense, therefore, that WBC counts and acute-phase reactants, such as ESR and CRP, are often normal in cases of chronic osteomyelitis. Although Cierny and Mader[26] recommended following all their patients with monthly WBC counts and ESRs for 6 months, there is reason to believe from the vertebral osteomyelitis literature that these values do not always correlate well with response to treatment and may be of limited value.[19]

Nutritional parameters, such as albumin, prealbumin, and transferrin, are helpful to obtain in the workup of a patient with suspected chronic osteomyelitis so that malnutrition can be identified and reversed before taking the patient to the operating room. Orthopaedic surgery patients who are malnourished have significantly higher infection rates than those who have a normal nutritional status.[68] Presumably, it would follow that patients who already have infection present would be more likely to respond to therapy if their nutrition were optimized beforehand.

Advanced Imaging Studies

History, physical examination, plain films, and laboratory work usually establish the diagnosis of infection but do not always define the extent to which the bone is involved and therefore the presence of true osteomyelitis. Additional imaging modalities, such as a variety of nuclear medicine studies, computed tomography (CT), and magnetic resonance imaging (MRI), are frequently useful in determining whether skeletal infection is present and, if so, in evaluating the extent of the disease.

NUCLEAR MEDICINE STUDIES

Traditionally, radionuclide scintigraphy has been the initial advanced imaging study ordered. The three-phase bone scan, as it is better known, is regarded as an excellent screening tool for chronic osteomyelitis, with a sensitivity exceeding 90 percent.[85] Performed in three phases using Tc 99m methylene diphosphonate, the bone scan suggests soft tissue infection when the first two phases (arterial and venous) are positive and the third phase (focal bone uptake) is negative. True skeletal infection should be considered when all three phases are positive, including the delayed (2- to 4-hour) images (Fig. 21-4).[105] However, it is well known that a variety of noninfectious insults to bone, such as the repeated surgeries and hardware implants that are common in this population of patients, also cause the third phase to be positive. As a result, the three-phase bone scan is a notoriously nonspecific test for chronic osteomyelitis (specificity as low as 10%).[127] With a high sensitivity and a poor specificity, three-phase bone scintigraphy should be regarded as a screening tool for patients with suspected bone infection but may not be relied on for providing a definitive diagnosis.

Another radiopharmaceutical that has been classically used in the diagnosis of osteomyelitis is gallium citrate. Gallium scintigraphy, in conjunction with the three-phase technetium scan, was the first dual-tracer technique available for evaluating chronic osteomyelitis.[78] As a calcium and iron analogue, gallium is thought to bind to transferrin as it leaks from the bloodstream to areas of skeletal inflammation. The primary role of gallium scintigraphy currently is in evaluating the patient with suspected vertebral osteomyelitis.[105]

Although gallium provides the best way to detect vertebral osteomyelitis radiographically, labeled leukocyte imaging is the nuclear imaging test of choice for osteomyelitis elsewhere in the body.[105] The principle behind radiolabeled leukocyte imaging, which uses radionuclides such as indium and technetium, is that white blood cells localize around areas of inflammation (Fig. 21-5). What makes this technique so useful in theory is that, unlike the situation in three-phase bone scintigraphy, labeled leukocytes should not accumulate around areas of increased bone mineral turnover unless an infection is present. Results have been variable over the years, with some studies reporting rather poor testing accuracies[161] and others reporting outstanding ones, with sensitivities and specificities exceeding 90 percent for cases of nonvertebral chronic osteomyelitis.[76,89]

On the whole, it can be said that most investigators have found leukocyte labeling to be as sensitive as three-phase bone scintigraphy in detecting chronic osteomyelitis but with dramatically increased specificity. A fairly representative study was conducted by Blume and colleagues[10] in 1997 that showed a nearly 60 percent increase in the specificity of leukocyte labeling (86%) over that of three-phase bone scintigraphy (29%) in the detection of pedal osteomyelitis. Specificity of leukocyte imaging can be increased further when performed in conjunction with a marrow scan. Marrow scans, such as those using sulfur colloid, improve diagnostic accuracy by delineating areas of normal bone marrow activity to compare with the areas of increased radionuclide uptake elsewhere. A congruence between the radionuclide uptake in a leukocyte-labeled image and in a marrow scan suggests that there is not an actual infection present (Fig. 21-6). In contrast, an incongruence between the two is strongly suggestive of infection, with accuracies reported to be as high as 98 percent.[104,105]

COMPUTED TOMOGRAPHY AND MAGNETIC RESONANCE IMAGING

Although nuclear medicine studies are frequently the first radiologic tests used to supplement plain film in the evaluation of bone infection, CT and MRI can be useful as well. CT scans are known to provide excellent resolution of cortical bone and sequestra and may be helpful in the preoperative planning for difficult infections.[131] In the 1990s, MRI began replacing CT at most hospitals for evaluating the extent of osteomyelitis because it provides more detailed imaging of hard and soft tissues (Fig. 21-7). MRI is highly beneficial in surgical planning by providing information regarding the extent of soft tissue edema as well as the location of hidden sinus tracts and abscesses. Initial screening usually consists of T1- and T2-weighted images. On T1-weighted images, there is decreased signal intensity of the marrow in infected areas. On T2-weighted images, infection is signaled by no change or an increased signal. This bright signal is due to the high water content of granulation tissue.[138]

Although there are false positives caused by tumors or healing fractures,[148] the sensitivity and specificity of MRI in the diagnosis of osteomyelitis remain excellent, ranging from 92 to 100 percent and 89 to 100 percent, respectively.[7,138,148] Because a negative MRI study

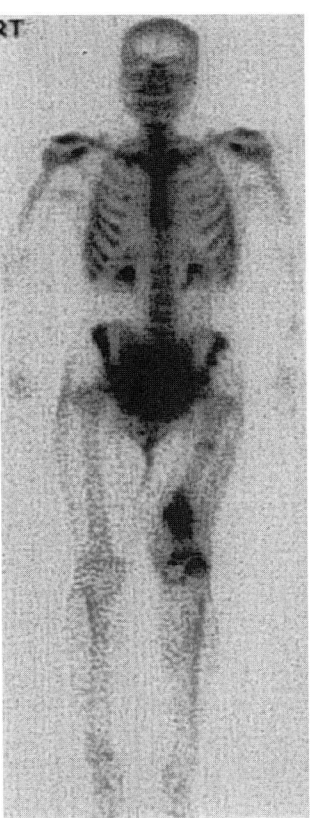

FIGURE 21-4 *With its increased localized activity of the tracer 3 to 4 hours after injection, this three-phase bone scan suggests infection of the patient's distal left femur.*

FIGURE 21-5 These leukocyte-labeled images suggest multiple areas of bilateral pedal osteomyelitis.

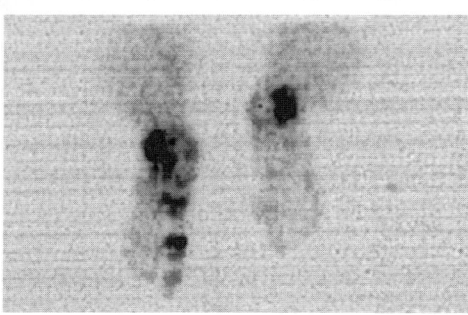 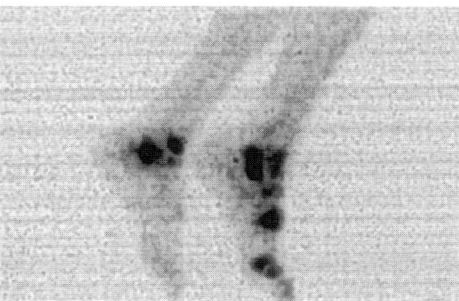

FIGURE 21-6 Sulfur colloid marrow scans can be used in conjunction with other studies to serve as a "control" of normal marrow activity. Congruence between the radionuclide uptake in the leukocyte-labeled image (WBC) and the sulfur colloid marrow scan (marrow) suggests that there is not an infection present in this patient's proximal tibia. Looking at the leukocyte-labeled image alone might lead one to the incorrect diagnosis.

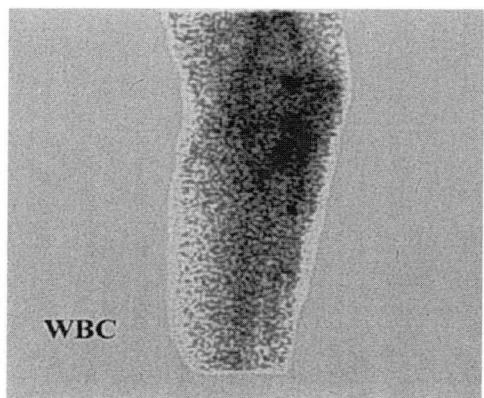 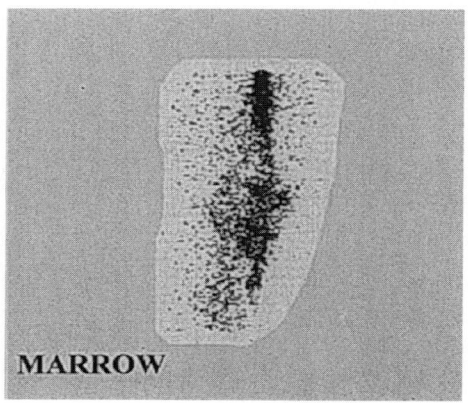

WBC

MARROW

FIGURE 21-7 Magnetic resonance imaging (MRI) provides excellent detail of the hard and soft tissues. This MRI scan demonstrates extensive intramedullary involvement as well as surrounding soft tissue edema in a patient with post-traumatic osteomyelitis of the right femoral diaphysis.

effectively rules out chronic osteomyelitis, it is recommended by some as the most appropriate step after a nondiagnostic radiograph in determining whether to treat.[151] Although MRI has extremely high sensitivity and specificity for chronic osteomyelitis, it is often not possible to obtain this study because of the presence of metal at the site of infection, as is frequently the case in patients with a history of skeletal trauma.

MANAGEMENT
Overview of Decision Making

The definitive treatment of chronic osteomyelitis includes the surgical elimination of all devitalized hard and soft tissues. Only by completely excising all avascular tissue is it possible to arrest this self-perpetuating infection. Filling in the dead space created by débridement, providing adequate soft tissue coverage, stabilizing the fracture or nonunion (if present), and administering antibiotics are important adjuncts in management.

The excision of necrotic tissue represents the key step in arresting infection in patients with chronic osteomyelitis. In certain cases in which the area of osteonecrosis is limited, only a modest excision may be required. In other instances, however, the extent of osteonecrosis may be so great that adequate débridement necessitates a limb amputation. The first question to be asked, then, when dealing with a patient with chronic osteomyelitis is precisely whether the limb can be salvaged. If limb salvage is deemed possible, the second question to ask is whether the patient can tolerate the procedure (or, as is so often the case, multiple procedures) required for complete débridement. The answer to this question depends on the patient's systemic and local capabilities for wound healing. For example, limb salvage procedures that may be feasible for a healthy teenager may be life-threatening for an elderly individual with cancer.

These differences in host immunocompetence hearken back to the Cierny-Mader classification, which introduced the concept of *C hosts* as those in whom the risks of surgery outweigh the risks of infection.[25] In such individuals, an alternative course of action to *arresting* the infection would be to retain the dead bone and *suppress* bacterial activity with long-term antimicrobial therapy. If limb salvage is deemed feasible and the patient is thought to be able tolerate the surgery, a third question to ask is whether the patient wishes to go down a path that frequently involves multiple surgical procedures and months, if not years, of physical and emotional hardship. Answering this question requires a thoughtful dialogue between doctor and patient as well as with the patient's family.

Finally, the patient and family should understand that, despite embarking down the path of limb salvage surgery, the end result may still be an amputation. A study that reviewed 31 patients with long bone chronic osteomyelitis treated with combined débridement, antibiotic bead placement, and bone grafting showed that four patients (13%) had received amputations at an average follow-up of 4 years.[22] In our series, 6 percent of the patients we initially treated with an intent to salvage the involved limb underwent amputation.[124] These figures are not insignificant and suggest that there is a select group of patients who would benefit from early amputation. Because of the tremendous amount of resources allocated to ultimately failed limb salvage procedures, society at large may also benefit from identification of this group.[12]

Although not specifically directed at the population with chronic osteomyelitis, several classification systems have been described over the past few decades that attempt to sort out which post-traumatic injuries would most likely end in amputation. In 1976, Gustilo and Anderson[55] demonstrated that type III open fractures had the worst prognosis for subsequent amputation. A decade later, they created a subclassification for type III fractures (IIIC, defined as those involving arterial injury requiring repair) that predicted even poorer outcomes.[56] Amputation rates for type IIIC fractures have been reported to exceed 50 percent.[58,77] The Mangled Extremity Severity Index[48] and Mangled Extremity Severity Score[58] have also traditionally been used as guides for prognosis. Despite all the classification systems that have been developed, the decision regarding amputation remains highly subjective based on the experience of the surgeon and the desires of the patient. Unless obvious criteria for amputation are met, this decision truly remains more of an art than a science.[33]

Amputation

As mentioned, at the beginning of every treatment algorithm for chronic osteomyelitis is the question of whether the limb is, in fact, salvageable. In circumstances in which patients have such extensive infection and osteonecrosis that segmental resection and limb reconstruction are not possible, amputation may be necessary to arrest the disease. Early amputation may give such an individual with extensive infection the best chance to be symptom-free and to return to his or her level of functioning as soon as possible.

Once amputation is selected as a treatment modality, the level of amputation must be chosen. In the 1930s, most amputations for tibial osteomyelitis were done above the level of the knee to ensure that there was enough blood supply for adequate healing. With the experience of large numbers of below-knee amputees in World War II, this approach grew out of favor as it was learned that amputating across the femur put the patient at a disadvantage for future prosthetic use and ambulation.[93]

Although it has been shown that the energy expenditure required for ambulation is much greater in above-knee than below-knee amputees,[43] studies comparing energy expenditure for different levels of transtibial amputees indicate that there is no ideal level at which to perform a below-knee amputation (BKA). A reasonable empirical guideline that adjusts for differences in patients' height is to select the level at which the calf muscle belly flattens out into the aponeurosis. The most proximal level of a BKA that still allows proper knee function is just distal to the tibial tubercle where the extensor mechanism inserts. Using 15 cm below the knee joint line or 3 to 4 fingerbreadths distal to the tibial tubercle as landmarks has been shown to provide safe markers.[5,15] Although the surgical technique for performing amputations varies among surgeons, most would agree that the key to this operation is identifying and ligating all major neurovascular structures. Unlike amputations done for dry gangrene, amputations in the setting of infection (wet gangrene) are usually staged with initial open amputation followed by delayed closure (Fig. 21-8).

TECHNIQUE

During BKA, the surgeon should proceed systematically through each compartment of the lower leg, first dissecting the soft tissues of the anterior compartment (anterior to the interosseus membrane) and isolating and clamping the anterior tibial vessels and deep peroneal nerve. Using a periosteal elevator, the periosteum of the tibia should be stripped distally from the level of transection. This process should continue posteriorly, carefully avoiding damage to the tibial vessels of the deep posterior compartment. The fibula is then cleared of soft tissue a few centimeters proximal to the level of the tibial transection. Both the tibia and fibula are transected, usually with an oscillating or Gigli saw. The posterior tibial and peroneal vessels, as well as the tibial nerve, are then isolated and clamped.

The soleus muscle in the superficial posterior compartment is then dissected away from the medial and lateral heads of the gastrocnemius to the level of the tibial stump and transected just distal to the clamped neurovascular structures. The posterior flap, which consists of the remaining gastrocnemius muscle, receives its blood supply from sural arteries coursing off the popliteal artery. The muscles of the lateral compartment are excised and the superficial peroneal nerve is clamped. All vessels are ligated and all nerves are ligated in traction, transected distally, and allowed to withdraw from the stump. To avoid

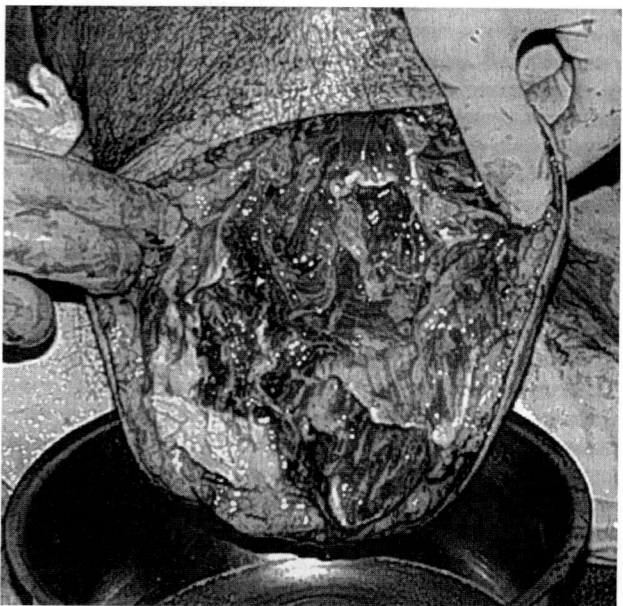

FIGURE 21-8   *Below-knee amputations in the setting of osteomyelitis are usually left open and closed in delayed fashion to minimize the chance of recurrent infection.*

dislodgement of ligatures, pulsatile arteries should be suture-ligated. The end of the tibia, especially the anterior portion that lies subcutaneously, should be beveled and the sharp edges smoothed with a rasp.

After the stump is closed, whether it be in primary or delayed fashion, immediate compressive dressings such as shrink wraps or Ace bandages become important in protecting the wound, promoting wound healing, and minimizing edema. These dressings are usually kept on for a few days unless signs or symptoms of infection develop.

POSTOPERATIVE CARE

During the first few postoperative days, physical therapy should be initiated to aid in transfers and in-bed range-of-motion and strengthening exercises. Non-weight-bearing ambulation with the aid of parallel bars, walkers, or crutches should begin soon thereafter. The patient is ready to be fitted for a temporary prosthesis when the suture line is healed, usually 6 to 8 weeks postoperatively.[5] Some prosthetists favor fitting patients even before the suture line has healed, 10 to 14 days after surgery. Prostheses are of great practical value, because they require a considerably lower energy expenditure than ambulation with crutches.[90]

An important and often overlooked aspect of postoperative care is teaching the patient how to put on the prosthesis so that there is total contact between stump and prosthetic socket. Training can take 2 to 3 weeks for unilateral below-knee amputees. After the first several postoperative weeks, physical and occupational therapists should focus their efforts on goals of increasing mobility and functional independence, especially as they relate to activities of daily living. The patient is usually fitted for a permanent prosthesis at about 3 to 6 months, after the greatest amount of stump shrinkage has occurred.

The preceding discussion has focused on BKA simply because of the prevalence of post-traumatic osteomyelitis of the tibia. Of course, above-knee or through-knee amputations become necessary when the area of osteonecrosis and subsequent infection has expanded more proximally. The principles of these procedures, as well as amputations elsewhere in the body, are basically the same as those outlined for the BKA. Dissection should proceed compartment by compartment, with major neurovascular structures being identified and ligated. At approximately 6 to 8 weeks, the above-knee amputee who is a candidate for a prosthetic limb may be fitted and begin gait training.[5]

Limb Salvage

In circumstances in which there is documented progressive destruction of bone, limb salvage is deemed feasible, and the patient is thought to be able to tolerate surgery, radical débridement should be thought of as the most fundamental intervention. Even if the patient is asymptomatic, symptoms such as fever and pain are likely to return as long as the area of osteonecrosis remains. If the preceding criteria are met and the patient feels that the benefits of limb salvage surgery (surgeries) outweigh its risks and hardships, treatment should be initiated along the following path:[24–26,54,139,155]

Thorough débridement of necrotic tissue and bone

Stabilization of bone

Culture of intraoperative tissue

Dead space management

Soft tissue coverage

Limb reconstruction

Systemic antibiotic therapy

We discuss each of these treatment principles in turn.

DÉBRIDEMENT

"Make an incision or opening that will thoroughly uncover (saucerize) the infected area... Remove as much foreign material and dead or dying tissue as possible... do not remove bony or soft parts that may contribute to repair... Fill entire cavity..."[103]

Although this may look like the most recent guidelines for the treatment of chronic osteomyelitis, these excerpts were in fact taken from an article written by H. Winnett Orr in 1930. Although some of his recommendations on the management of bone infection are now outdated, his emphases on thorough débridement and filling in of subsequent dead space are as relevant today as they were 75 years ago. Despite all the advances in medical technology over this time period, the quality of the surgical débridement remains the most critical factor in successfully managing chronic osteomyelitis.[139]

Even with detailed imaging techniques such as MRI, it is often difficult to assess the extent of osteonecrosis and infection preoperatively. Before making an incision, Walenkamp[155] supported the practice of injecting an obvious fistula with methylene blue dye to localize the focus of infection. This, he said, should cause the patient to feel the same or similar pain as during the stowing of pus. Cierny and colleagues[25] have not found the use of dyes to be helpful, however.

Once the area of necrosis is localized, débridement proceeds using a variety of instruments, such as curettes, rongeurs, and high-speed power burs. Stated simply, the goal of surgery is the complete excision of all dead or ischemic hard and soft tissues (Fig. 21-9). If not removed, they would serve as a nidus for recurrent infection and cure would be impossible. If adequate débridement is the key to treatment, the question arises: how does the surgeon know when all of the necrotic bone has been removed? Classically, punctate haversian bleeding, referred to as the paprika sign,[25] has been used as a sign of healthy bone and helps establish the limits of débridement. However, this sign may not always be relied on, such as during débridement of dense cortical bone or operations in which a tourniquet is used. In such cases where there is less bleeding, the use of a laser Doppler probe may be helpful in establishing skeletal viability.[136] However, in general, this practice can be rather cumbersome and is not currently regarded as the standard of care.[139]

In addition to surgical excision of all necrotic tissues, the infected areas should be copiously irrigated. Authors from Patzakis and colleagues[110] to Gustilo and Anderson[55] have recommended from 10 to 14 L of normal saline to wash out the contaminated material. The efficacy of débridement has been shown to be optimized by high-pressure pulsatile lavage using fluid

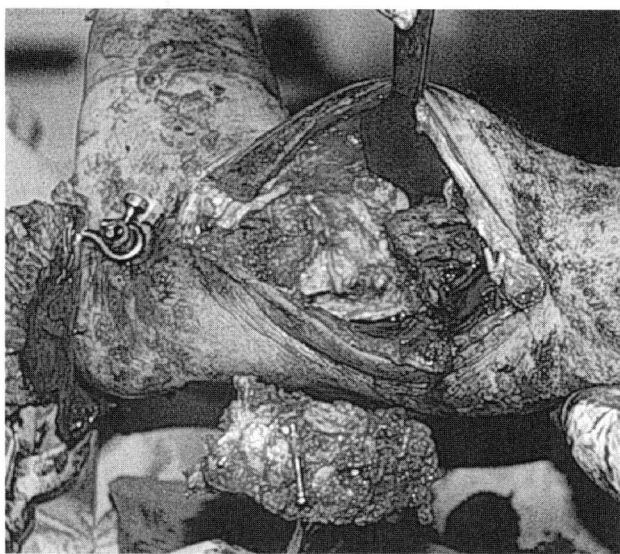

FIGURE 21-9 *Thorough excision of all devitalized tissues constitutes the cornerstone of management in chronic osteomyelitis. Although adequate débridement may sometimes require limb amputation, at other times, as shown here, the removal of a solitary mass of necrotic tissue and hardware is sufficient.*

pressures of 50 to 70 pounds per square inch and 800 pulses per minute.[9] Although adding various antibiotic solutions to the process of irrigation has become common practice for many surgeons, such practices have not been supported by the literature. The work of Anglen and associates[1,2] has, in fact, shown soap solution to be the only mixture more effective than normal saline irrigation in reducing bacterial counts.

Although thorough débridement is necessary for eliminating all pathogenic bacteria, it is frequently not sufficient. Because of antimicrobial resistance factors, such as bacterial secretion of biofilm, persistent infection is unfortunately a fairly common occurrence. In a study of 53 patients who had positive cultures at the time of their initial débridement for chronic osteomyelitis of the tibia, 26 percent still did at the time of their second débridement.[162] To arrest this disease, therefore, several trips to the operating room for repeated débridement and a variety of reconstructive procedures are often necessary.

In a study reviewing 189 patients with chronic osteomyelitis, Cierny and colleagues[25] found that the average number of operations for a patient undergoing limb salvage was 3.8. In his approach to chronic osteomyelitis, Cierny's focus during the first operation is on a thorough débridement of all necrotic tissues, fracture stabilization, and the acquisition of tissue biopsies. He then takes patients back to the operating room approximately 5 to 7 days after this initial surgery for a repeated débridement. Cierny uses this second look both to make sure that the wound is viable and to address the issue of dead space management (usually with the placement of antibiotic beads or a cancellous bone graft, or both).

STABILIZATION OF BONE

In 1974, Rittman and Perren[117] conducted a study that showed that rigid stabilization of bone facilitated union in the setting of chronic osteomyelitis. In this study, tibial osteotomies were performed on sheep and stabilized by plates of varying rigidities. Pathogenic bacteria were injected into the osteotomy site 1 week after surgery, which produced changes equivalent to those seen in chronic osteomyelitis. After 8 weeks of follow-up, it was shown that bone union of these infected sites was correlated with the degree of skeletal stabilization. One reason for this may be that skeletal stability promotes revascularization, thus enhancing perfusion at the fracture site.[98] This enhanced perfusion may maximize the host's immune response, which allows it to resist infection at the fracture site more effectively.[21]

The method by which fracture stability is obtained is not inconsequential. Although several studies support primary intramedullary nailing of open tibial fractures over external fixation, citing superior postoperative outcomes,[125,126,140] this technique is usually not recommended when the trauma is more than 12 hours old, when there is extensive soft tissue damage, or in the presence of osteomyelitis.[113] In such cases, bacteria are more likely to gain access to the intramedullary canal and potentially infect the entire diaphysis.

There are data to support the use of external fixation in the presence of infection. After stabilizing experimental osteotomies with either an external fixator or an intramedullary rod and then contaminating these sites with *S. aureus,* a group of investigators in 1995 found the sites stabilized with external fixators to have fewer and less severe infections than those stabilized internally.[30] Gustilo[54] claimed that primary intramedullary nailing should be avoided altogether in all type III open fractures, arguing that they already have compromised periosteal and extraperiosteal circulations (i.e., from surrounding muscle) secondary to injury. In such cases, he recommended achieving skeletal stabilization through plating or external fixation (Fig. 21-10).[54]

INTRAOPERATIVE CULTURES

The definitive diagnosis of post-traumatic osteomyelitis is made by isolating bacteria from the intraoperative biopsy specimen of the involved bone.[81] Although the best specimens are generally thought to be tissue fragments directly from the center of infection,[155] there is evidence to suggest that copious intraoperative cultures from a variety of sources may be beneficial. Comparing the results of bacterial cultures from various sites in long bone chronic osteomyelitis, Patzakis and co-workers[111] found the culture of bone biopsy specimens to be inadequate for identifying *all* organisms present. As a result, they recommended that intraoperative culture specimens be taken from the sinus tract, samples of purulent material, and samples of soft tissue, in addition, of course, to the involved bone.

To avoid false-negative culture results, patients might be encouraged to stop taking antibiotics at least 1 week before surgery. Unfortunately, doing so may have the unintended effect of instigating a cellulitis in the soft tissues. If this occurs and becomes very uncomfortable

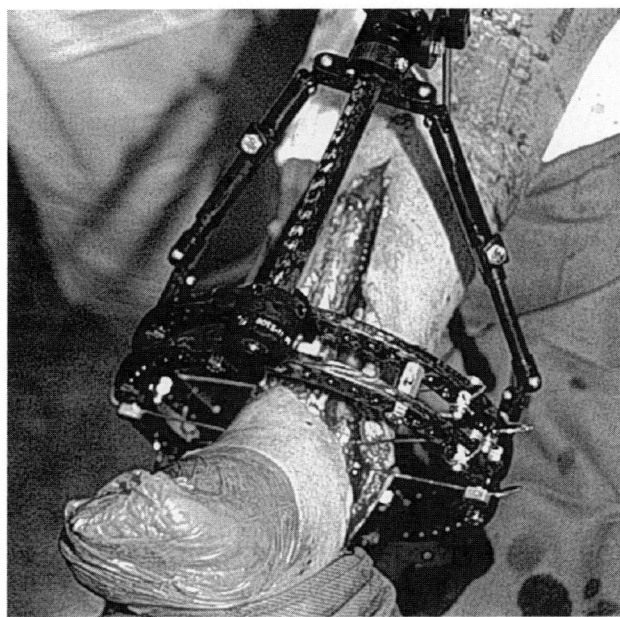

FIGURE 21-10 *External fixators are frequently used to achieve fracture stabilization in the presence of infection or massive soft tissue injury.*

for the patient, the clinician may wish to restart antibiotics. If the symptoms of the cellulitis are manageable, it is in the patient's best interest to remain without antibiotics before surgery. After deep cultures have been obtained in the operating room, broad-spectrum intravenous antibiotics are started if the causative organism is unknown. Coverage is narrowed when culture and sensitivity results return from the laboratory.

DEAD SPACE MANAGEMENT

When the bone and tissues deemed devitalized have been removed, the focus shifts toward managing the dead space that is left behind. Healing with secondary intention is discouraged, because the scar tissue that would fill the defect is avascular and may lead to persistent drainage.[25]

ANTIBIOTIC BEADS Since the 1980s, many surgeons have favored filling this space, at least initially, with polymethylmethacrylate beads impregnated with antibiotic, usually an aminoglycoside (such as gentamicin) or vancomycin (Fig. 21-11). Although polymethylmethacrylate is the most widely used drug delivery system, calcium hydroxyapatite implants that become incorporated into host bone have also been shown to be effective.[162] More recently, calcium sulfate (Osteoset) beads impregnated with antibiotics have shown effectiveness,[42] and methacrylate has been used to form permeable capsules for local antibiotic delivery.[13] Whatever the material, the antibiotic-laden beads are placed directly in the operative wound, which is then primarily closed. Unless the depot material is biodegradable, almost all antibiotic bead chains are intended for removal at a later date. Generally, they remain in the wound for approximately 4 weeks. Beads placed within the intramedullary canal, however, should

FIGURE 21-11 *Antibiotic beads serve a dual role as a local depot of antibiotic in the débridement site as well as a temporary filler of dead space. Polymethylmethacrylate (PMMA) beads connected together in a chain are the most widely used drug delivery system.*

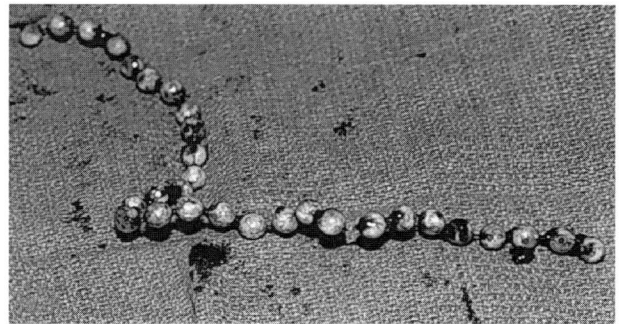

FIGURE 21-11

be removed sooner (within 2 weeks) before the layer of granulation tissue has formed, which would make removal difficult.[139] The beads should be oriented in layers from deepest to most superficial. Adequate concentrations of antibiotic can be achieved only when it diffuses from the beads into the postoperative wound hematoma, which serves as a transport medium. Thus, open wound treatment or irrigation-suction drainage is incompatible with this mode of therapy.[74]

Several clinical trials have supported the efficacy of local antibiotic bead implantation.[20,74,156] Even though the gentamicin concentration remains at sufficient levels for approximately 30 days after implantation, some skeptics may claim that beads are beneficial only insofar as they are able to fill dead space. Animal studies have demonstrated the efficacy of antibiotic beads in eradicating osteomyelitis above and beyond placebo beads that have no antibiotic.[96] Thus, it appears that bead chains are helpful not only by serving as a temporary filler of dead space before reconstruction but also as an effective depot for the local administration of antibiotic.

CANCELLOUS BONE GRAFT After antibiotic beads are placed, dressings are applied to the wound and changed frequently to promote the growth of a healthy layer of granulation tissue, a process that can take 2 to 4 weeks. After this time period, the wound is usually suitable for the second stage of dead space management, namely, reentry and bone reconstruction. Bone reconstruction is usually achieved with an autogenous cancellous bone graft. Bone chips are typically taken from the iliac crests, greater trochanter, or proximal tibia. Grafting involves taking small strips of cancellous bone from these areas and packing them down over a fresh granulation bed in the débrided area.

Papineau and colleagues[108] pioneered this technique and recommended taking the grafts in strips 3 to 6 cm long by 3 mm thick by 4 mm wide and placing them in concentric and overlapping layers to fill in the defect completely.[30] Cancellous grafts have the benefit of being able to become rapidly revascularized and incorporated in the final bone structure. Open cancellous grafting has produced some excellent outcomes, with clinical success rates ranging from 89 percent in 1979[108] to 92 percent in 1984[122] and 100 percent in 1995.[37]

SOFT TISSUE COVERAGE

The soft tissues covering the area of skeletal injury must be allowed to heal or the patient will be at a very high risk for persistent or recurrent infection. After the necrotic tissues are excised, the débrided (and possibly bone-grafted) area can conceivably be covered in one of three ways: (1) simply by letting the tissues heal by secondary intention, (2) by split-thickness skin grafting, or (3) by muscle transfer (Fig. 21-12). The last two techniques are favored in almost all cases of post-traumatic osteomyelitis and should be performed after a layer of granulation tissue has formed.

Covering the débrided site with a well-vascularized tissue graft offers the healing bone a new blood supply and thus decreases the chance of deep infection.[83,160] Delayed coverage is associated with a higher chronic infection rate.[120] Local muscle flaps, which have the advantage of keeping vascular supply intact, are almost always used if an adjacent muscle is available. Although local muscle flaps work well for the proximal two thirds of the tibia, the more distal one third requires the use of transplanted flaps to provide a sufficient soft tissue envelope for healing. These so-called free flaps were developed in the early

FIGURE 21-12 *The use of muscle transfers, with or without overlying skin grafts, guards against persistent or recurrent infection by filling the dead space created by surgical débridement with well-vascularized tissue.*

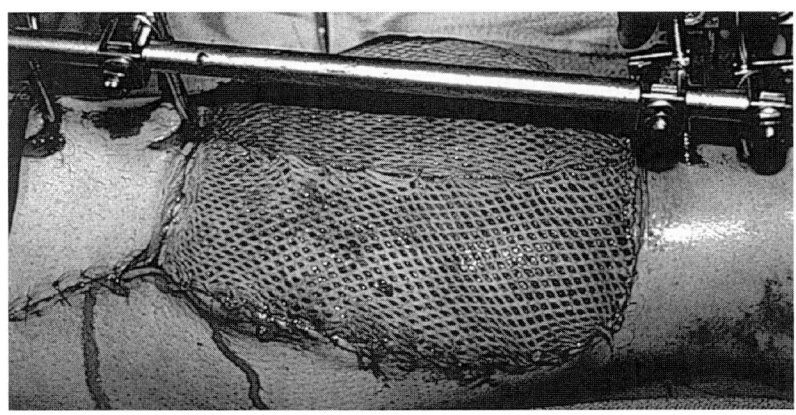

1980s and are usually from such donor muscles as rectus abdominis, latissimus dorsi, gracilis, and tensor fasciae latae.[3]

It is difficult to study the isolated effect that the use of muscle transfers has had on clinical outcome. After all, this technique is almost always used in combination with several other therapeutic modalities, such as bone grafting, antibiotics, and of course débridement. Nonetheless, there is certainly a large amount of evidence that supports the use of muscle flaps as part of the therapeutic regimen.[3,4,40,88] Fitzgerald and colleagues,[40] using either local or free flaps combined with thorough débridement and antibiotics, reported a 93 percent success rate in treating a sample of 42 patients with chronic osteomyelitis. These results demonstrated a significant improvement over previous treatment regimens that did not employ the use of muscle flap coverage. In another study, which retrospectively reviewed 34 patients with chronic osteomyelitis of the tibia, it was found that those who had received free muscle flap transfers as part of their surgical treatment were more likely to be drainage-free after more than 7 years of follow-up than patients who had received débridement alone.[88]

Although the primary purpose of local or free muscle transfer is to revascularize the débrided area, it also serves a purpose akin to bone grafting by simply filling in the dead space created by surgery. This notion is supported by studies that have found the recurrence of infection in patients with lower leg osteomyelitis to be significantly reduced when the muscle flaps completely pack the cavity left by surgical débridement.[130,146]

LIMB RECONSTRUCTION

Sometimes the segmental defects in bone left from débridement or from the injury itself cannot be corrected with antibiotic beads, bone graft, and muscle flaps alone. The technique used for the reconstruction of such defects (and the malunion and angulation deformities so common in the setting of infected open fractures) depends on the patient and the type of deformity.[113] Long-term cast therapy, for instance, is an option for the management of relatively minor nonunions. Other possibilities include open reduction and plate fixation, intramedullary nailing, and electrical stimulation. Electrical stimulation is discussed in "Complementary Therapies" later in the chapter. One of the more recent developments in the management of more severe nonunions and infected nonunions has been the dynamic external fixation technique described by Ilizarov.

In the Ilizarov method,[66] an area of noninfected bone is corticotomized and allowed to begin the healing process with a normal fracture callus. This area of callus is then distracted progressively over small increments using an external fixator device. In this way, Ilizarov external fixation gradually stimulates skeletal regeneration, which can be of obvious value in correcting the segmental, rotational, translational, and angular deformities frequently seen in patients with post-traumatic osteomyelitis. This method of so-called *distraction osteogenesis,* wherein bone is lengthened at one quarter of a millimeter every 6 hours, should be distinguished from *compression osteogenesis,* which can be described as pressing the bone ends together

in a fracture or delayed union until they are stable enough to heal by themselves. In both distraction and compression techniques, bone transport may serve as an adjunct to facilitate osteogenesis across segmental defects. Although there are many drawbacks to the Ilizarov method, such as pain from the external fixator, frequent pin infections, and a long period of time spent in the device (almost 9 months on average),[17,31] it has produced excellent outcomes in several studies.[31,47,106,116,147] What makes this mode of treatment even more valuable to patients is that it allows them to remain ambulatory throughout its duration.[17,46,53,66]

Although the method of distraction osteogenesis has been shown time and again to aid in limb reconstruction, it should be remembered that it is not a cure-all. As emphasized earlier in the chapter, some extremities are so severely compromised by traumatic injury, infection, or the extent of surgical débridement that amputation may be the inevitable outcome. These patients should be identified early and spared futile reconstructive attempts. However, even in patients who have salvageable limbs, Ilizarov limb relengthening is not a panacea. In part, its success depends on the preoperative planning of the orthopaedic surgeon, who must determine how to employ the principles of distraction osteogenesis during the course of reconstruction.

Generally speaking, the surgeon may wish to proceed down one of two reconstructive paths: (1) acutely shortening the extremity via resection of a diseased or malunited segment of bone with compression at that site, followed by limb relengthening, or (2) holding the extremity out to length and using bone transport to fill in the gap. In patients who have only a short segment of diseased bone (i.e., on the order of 4 cm or less), the first technique is probably the better option. However, if the length of the necrotic bone exceeds 4 cm, this technique becomes less favorable because of both the greater distance through which the limb must be shortened and the potential danger of kinking blood vessels when the excess soft tissue envelope is compressed together. In instances in which a large bone gap exists, it probably makes more sense to hold the limb out to length and transport bone into the defect.

To elucidate the application of these two approaches, we describe how each was used in the care of patients seen in our bone infection clinic at the University of Connecticut Health Center.

ILLUSTRATIVE CASES OF RECONSTRUCTIVE STRATEGIES
Case 1
Acute Shortening and Relengthening The reconstructive strategy of acute shortening and limb relengthening consists of the following steps: (1) excising the necrotic bone and avascular scar, (2) applying the Ilizarov external fixator, (3) acutely shortening the limb by compression at the excision site, (4) making a corticotomy proximal or distal to the excision site, (5) providing soft tissue coverage if necessary, and finally (6) relengthening through the corticotomy site.

This technique, most effectively employed if the length of the necrotic bone is less than or equal to 4 cm, is illustrated by the case of Mr. J.S., a 27-year-old man who was referred to our clinic with chronic osteomyelitis and nonunion of his right tibia. Three years before, he had sustained a grade IIIB open fracture of his right tibial diaphysis in a motorcycle accident. At the time of the accident, he was initially treated with external fixation, which was later converted to an intramedullary nail. Unfortunately, because Mr. J.S. went on to have a diaphyseal osteomyelitis, this nail had to be removed and a second external fixator was applied (Fig. 21-13). In addition to the massive comminution and displacement of the fracture, his right leg sustained significant soft tissue damage secondary to the accident that required both a gastrocnemius muscle flap and a split-thickness skin graft to cover the exposed bone adequately (Fig. 21-14).

When the patient arrived at our clinic, he had no external fixator in place and the skin grafts were healing quite well (Fig. 21-15) He complained of pain with walking. On physical examination, the patient's right leg was in obvious varus. There was no erythema, fluctuance, or sinus tracts visible on the overlying skin. The gastrocnemius flap was pink, and the leg was neurovascularly intact with nearly full range of motion at the knee and ankle. Radiographic examination revealed a nonunion of the right tibia with approximately 25 degrees of varus and 30 degrees of

dorsal angulation (Fig. 21-16). A bone scan was negative for active infection. At this point, a lengthy conversation was held with the patient and limb salvage was decided on. Mr. J.S. was instructed to stop the oral antibiotics he had previously been prescribed (to optimize the yield of intraoperative cultures), and surgery was scheduled for a few weeks after this visit.

In the operating room, it was first important to determine how much tibial bone was involved in the disease process. To visualize the area in question, an incision was made lateral to the anterior muscle flap and dissection was continued down to the periosteum of the previous fracture site. Using a periosteal elevator to identify its cortices, the bone was found to be very sclerotic about 1.5 cm on either side of the nonunion. There was no evidence of frank pus. At this point, intraoperative biopsy specimens were obtained and sent for culture. Given the fact that the area of necrosis was limited, the decision was made to pursue a course of acute shortening followed by limb relengthening.

The next aspect of the surgery was thorough débridement of the sclerotic bone at and around the nonunion site. Using an oscillating saw, a 4-cm portion of the tibia that included the nonunion site was resected. The diaphyseal bone both proximal and distal to the débridement area

FIGURE 21-13 *Sequential radiographs of Mr. J.S. showing, from left to right, his leg after he had his initial injury (with external fixator in place); his leg after the external fixator was replaced with an intramedullary nail; and, lastly, his leg after the nail became infected and was removed in favor of a second external fixator.*

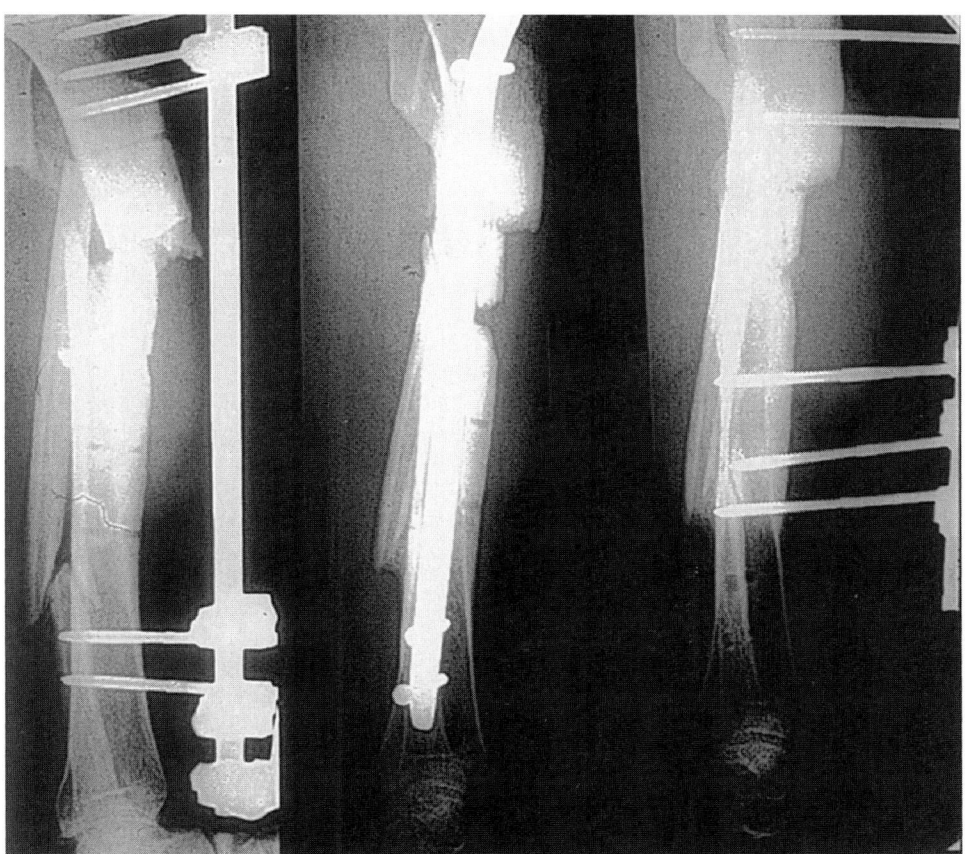

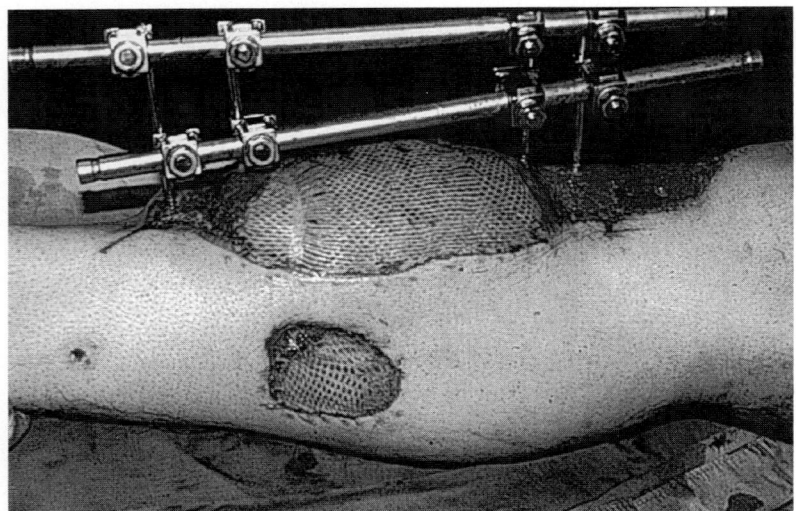

FIGURE 21-14 | *The massive soft tissue loss Mr. J.S. suffered from his initial injury necessitated a gastrocnemius muscle flap and split-thickness skin graft over the open area.*

was curetted to bleeding bone. The area was irrigated with several liters of soap and saline by pulsatile lavage. Drill holes were made both proximally and distally to allow adequate purchase of the reduction forceps that would compress the diaphyseal shaft. Before compression, a fibular

osteotomy was also done at this level, approximately at the junction of the middle and distal thirds of the fibula. As the two ends of the tibia were compressed together, proper alignment was verified with anteroposterior and lateral fluoroscopic imaging.

After an adequate reduction was achieved, the focus of the operation turned toward application of the Ilizarov

FIGURE 21-15 | *On our initial physical examination, Mr. J.S. demonstrated well-healed soft tissues of his leg.*

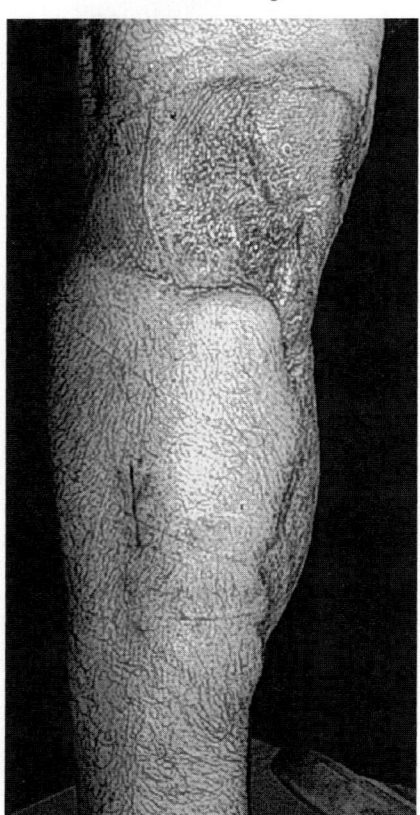

FIGURE 21-16 | *Initial radiographs of Mr. J.S. at our clinic revealed a nonunion of the right tibia with approximately 25 degrees of varus and 30 degrees of dorsal angulation.*

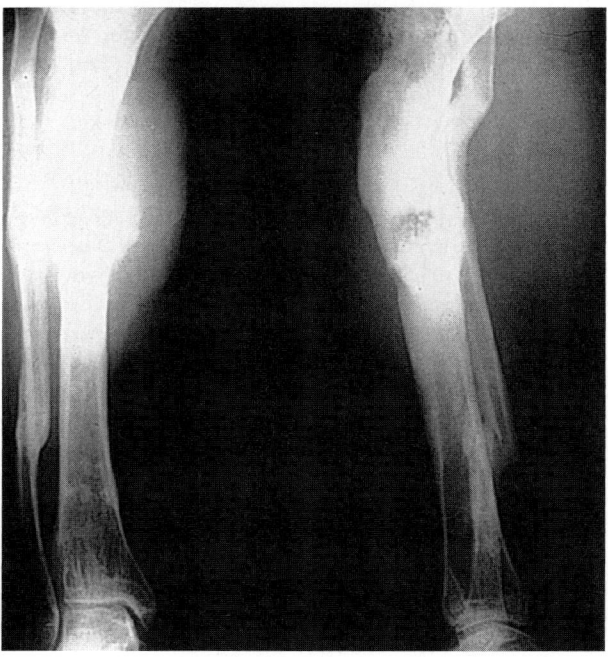

external fixator frame. When the fixator was pinned to the proximal and distal portions of the tibia, rotational alignment was verified under fluoroscopy and the frame was secured. The excision site was then placed under forceful compression. The final part of this operation was to make a more distal metaphyseal corticotomy to allow subsequent limb relengthening. Although proximal corticotomies are often employed in this technique, a distal site was chosen in this patient simply because skin graft lay adherent to the bone more proximally. If the corticotomy were performed through the skin graft site, there would not have been the pliability and elasticity in the remaining soft tissue envelope necessary for adequate closure. Thus, the corticotomy that would serve as the regenerate zone for future limb relengthening was made distal to the excision site.

The immediate postoperative course for Mr. J.S. was unremarkable. He received early mobilization from physical therapy with weight-bearing as tolerated on the right lower extremity. Before discharge from the hospital on postoperative day 3, the patient was instructed in how to lengthen the Ilizarov apparatus by approximately one quarter of a millimeter four times a day starting 1 week after the operation. Although he was maintained with intravenous antibiotics during his brief hospital stay, Mr. J.S. was discharged home with oral antibiotics (a first-generation cephalosporin and rifampin) to which his intraoperative culture (*S. aureus)* would prove to be sensitive.

Radiographs 2 weeks after his operation revealed excellent alignment and distraction at the distal corticotomy but unfortunately some distraction at the more proximal compression site. This area was compressed further in the office by tightening the Ilizarov rings closer together. Three weeks postoperatively, the patient was ambulating on crutches without difficulty. Although the right leg was measured and found to be fully out to length approximately 4 months after the surgery, adequate fusion at the compression site remained problematic and the decision was made to augment the area with multiple half-pins and cancellous bone graft from the posterior iliac crest. After bone grafting, the patient did very well, and follow-up radiographs over the next several months showed increasing incorporation of the bone graft at the compression site as well as progressive lengthening and bone formation in the regenerate zone (Fig. 21-17).

Because Ilizarov external fixation allows early weight-bearing, Mr. J.S. remained active during the course of his treatment and continued to enjoy many of his favorite activities, including bow hunting (Fig. 21-18). Seven months after visiting our clinic, with radiographic evidence of excellent bone formation at both the proximal compression site and the distal regenerate zone, Mr. J.S. was brought back to the operating room to have the external fixator removed. He did extremely well in the months to follow, using only a right leg orthosis for support. One year after the initial operation, Mr. J.S. was found to have no leg length disparity and to be enjoying an extremely active life. Radiographic examination showed excellent leg alignment, with further callus formation at both the proximal and distal sites (Fig. 21-19).

Case 2

Bone Transport If the segment of necrotic bone and tissue to be resected is large, employing a strategy of acute shortening and limb relengthening may be difficult. Although it is certainly possible, compressing together two diaphyseal ends over a distance much greater than 4 cm risks buckling the remaining soft tissue envelope and compromising its vascular supply. In such circumstances, a more favorable reconstructive strategy is not to shorten the limb at all but to hold it out to length and subsequently fill in segmental gaps with bone transport. This technique consists of the following steps: (1) excising the

FIGURE 21-17 *Sequential radiographs of Mr. J.S.'s leg over several months show, from left to right, increasing incorporation of the bone graft at the more proximal compression site as well as progressive lengthening, though in the more distal regenerate zone.*

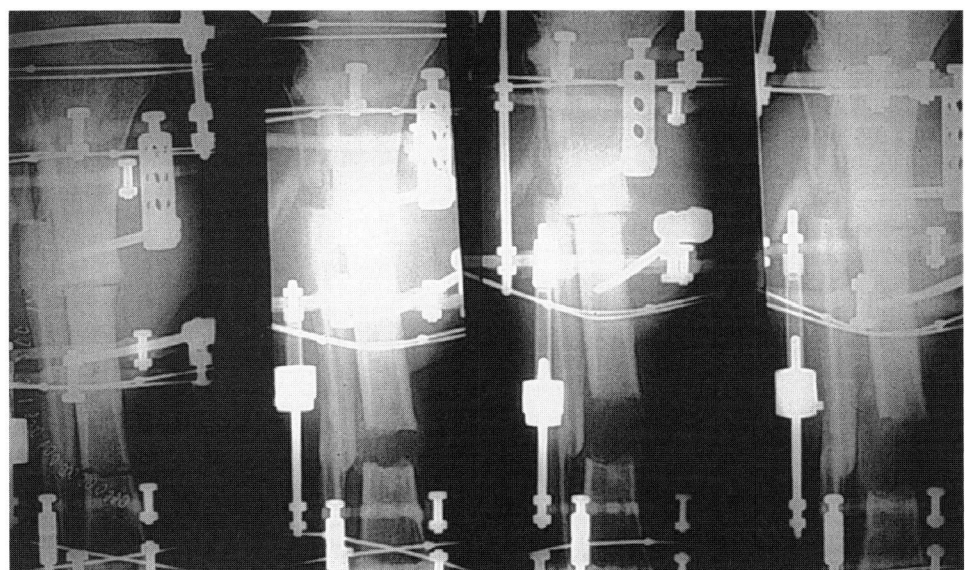

FIGURE 21-18   *This picture of Mr. J.S. bow hunting with his Ilizarov external fixator frame in place illustrates that patients are able to remain active during their treatment.*

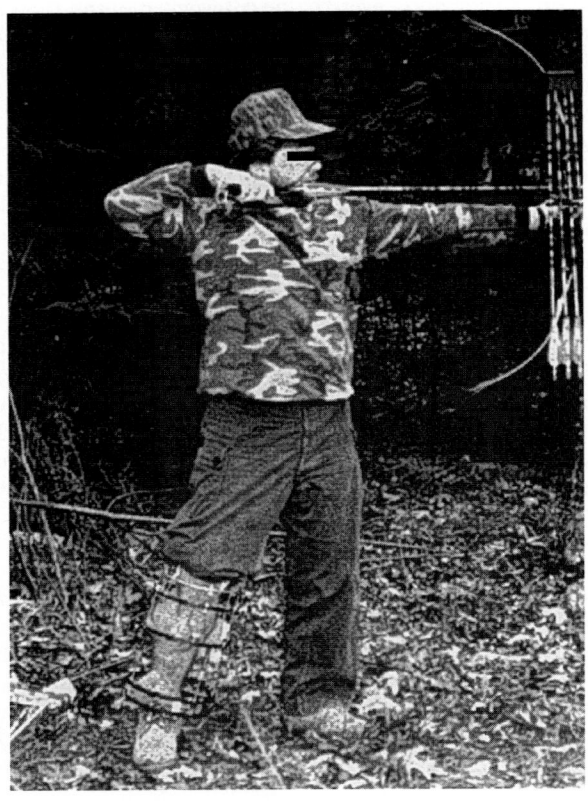

necrotic bone and avascular scar, (2) applying the Ilizarov external fixator, (3) holding the limb at length, (4) making a corticotomy proximal or distal to the excision site, (5) providing soft tissue coverage if necessary, (6) lengthening through the corticotomy site, and (7) transporting bone to the excision site.

This strategy can be used to fill large gaps within bone, to fuse diseased joints, or sometimes both, which happened to be the case with Mr. J.L., a 39-year-old man who came to our clinic 15 months after sustaining a grade IIIB open fracture of his left distal tibia in a motorcycle accident. His past medical history was significant for insulin-dependent diabetes mellitus, intravenous drug abuse, and smoking two packs of cigarettes a day for over 20 years. Previous intraoperative cultures had been positive for methicillin-resistant *S. aureus,* for which Mr. J.L. had been treated with several months of intravenous vancomycin therapy. Surgically, he was initially treated with external fixation, bone grafting, and free flap coverage. He had been doing fairly well until 1 year after his injury, when he suffered a fracture through his bone graft site. At that point he had a repair of his nonunion, followed by repeated bone grafting. Since that time, from about 12 to 15 months after the initial trauma, he had been complaining of intermittent fevers and persistent drainage from his wounds.

On initial physical examination, the patient's left lower extremity was remarkable for a draining wound on both the medial and lateral aspects of his ankle. He had a free flap over the dorsum of his ankle that appeared to be healthy. His leg was neurovascularly intact distally with fair range of motion at the ankle joint. Plain films revealed a nonunion of his left distal tibia and fibula with

FIGURE 21-19   *Sequential radiographs demonstrating, from left to right, progressive bone formation at both the proximal compression site and distal regenerate zone. The last film was taken 1 year after Mr. J.S.'s initial operation, approximately 5 months after his external fixator was removed. It shows abundant callus formation at both the proximal and distal sites.*

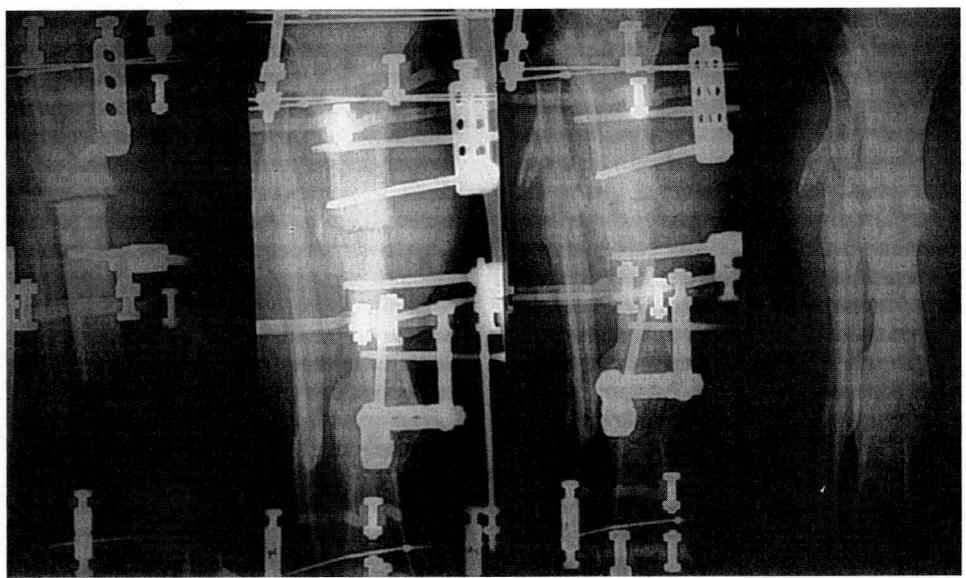

posterior and medial angulation of the distal fragment (Fig. 21-20A). The presumptive diagnosis of an infected distal tibial metaphysis with articular involvement was made. At this point, a lengthy discussion was conducted with the patient and his family regarding therapeutic options. In particular, given the patient's multiple co-morbidities and his treatment failure over a 15-month period with several previous surgeries and a prolonged vancomycin trial, amputation was given a great deal of consideration.

Mr. J.L. understood that amputation would most likely return him to work sooner than if he embarked on a course of limb salvage surgery. Furthermore, he was made aware that proceeding down the path of attempted limb salvage would probably require an additional year in an external fixator. The importance of ceasing all substance and tobacco use was emphasized. Finally, it was discussed that, despite everyone's best efforts, embarking on a course of limb salvage might ultimately result in a below-knee amputation. In the end, Mr. J.L. was firm in his decision to try to save his leg. As a result, all antibiotics were stopped and surgery was scheduled. Because the amount of diseased bone appeared to be extensive (affecting the distal tibia and ankle joint), the planned approach was to resect all of the necrotic areas, hold the limb out to length,

and use bone transport to achieve a fusion between the remaining tibia and the talus.

Three weeks after his initial visit, Mr. J.L. was brought to the operating room and underwent a radical excision of approximately 7 cm of necrotic distal tibia. The area was irrigated copiously with pulsatile lavage. In addition, antibiotic beads were placed, an Ilizarov external fixator applied, and a corticotomy performed proximal to the area of resection. Antibiotic beads were used in this case and not in that of Mr. J.S. because the site of disease here was being held out to length rather than being compressed. As a result, a vast potential space was created in which residual bacteria could proliferate. Before filling this dead space with antibiotic beads, intraoperative biopsy specimens were obtained and sent for culture.

In the months that followed his surgery, Mr. J.L. did very well with oral antibiotics (trimethoprim-sulfamethoxazole and metronidazole) to which his intraoperative culture (methicillin-resistant *S. aureus)* was sensitive, remaining afebrile and without drainage. Radiographs showed increasing distraction at the proximal corticotomy site (see Fig. 21-20B). The antibiotic beads were exchanged approximately 3 months after their placement and again at 5 months. Exchanging beads is important not only to maintain an adequate depot of local antibiotic but also to adjust to

FIGURE 21-20 | *A, Plain radiograph of Mr. J.L.'s left leg at the time of his initial visit reveals nonunion of his left distal tibia and fibula with medial angulation of the distal fragment, in which there are five screws. **B,** Plain film 3 months postoperatively shows increasing distraction at the proximal corticotomy site. **C,** Radiograph 10 months after the initial surgery reveals a 9-cm distraction zone at the proximal corticotomy site, allowing the tibia nearly to reach the talus. **D,** At 14 months after the initial placement of the external fixator, plain film demonstrates bone fusion at the tibiotalar docking site and adequate bone growth in the regenerate zone.*

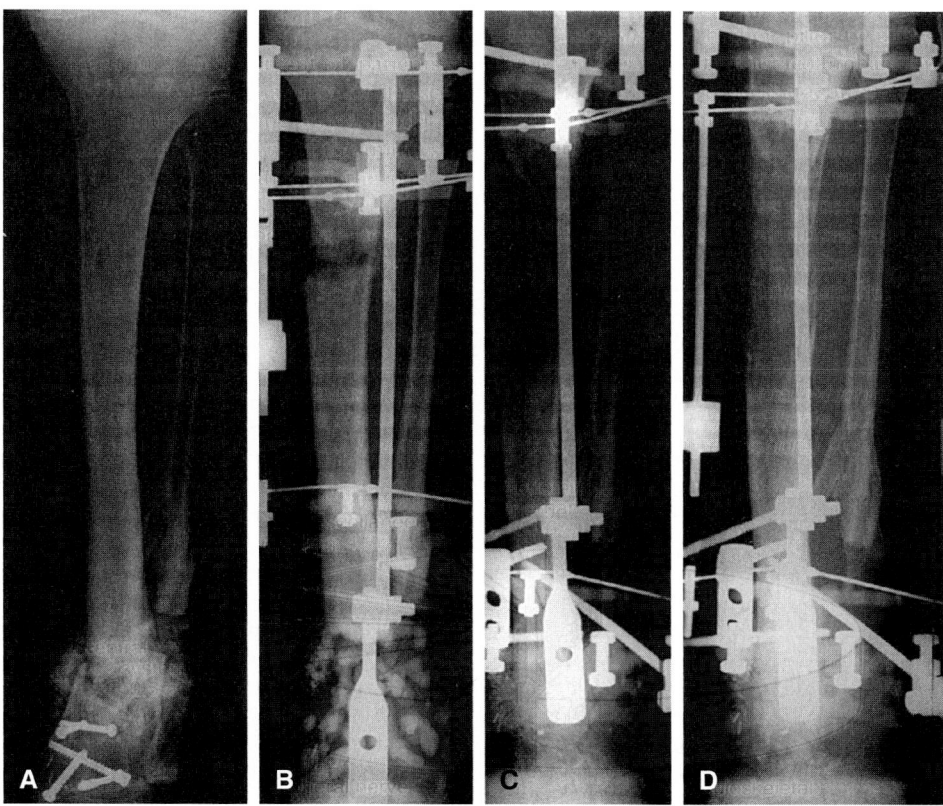

the decreasing size of the resection site. Ten months after the initial surgery, radiographs revealed a 9-cm distraction zone at the proximal corticotomy, allowing the tibia nearly to reach the talus (see Fig. 21-20C). Proper alignment continued to be maintained.

Because the limb was determined to be nearly out to length, Mr. J.L. was brought back to the operating room for the bone transport phase of the reconstruction. The antibiotic beads, having fulfilled their role as temporary fillers of dead space, were removed to create room for the graft. The leading edges of the tibia and talus were redébrided to healthy, bleeding bone, and cancellous graft from the posterior iliac crest was transported to augment the fusion site. Although the patient did well immediately after the surgery, he returned 1 month postoperatively complaining of foul-smelling drainage from his medial and lateral ankle wounds. For this, the patient was soon brought back to the operating room for an incision and drainage. Cultures at that time revealed *Xanthomonas* and *Enterococcus* species sensitive to doxycycline. The patient did well with a regimen of doxycycline, trimethoprim-sulfamethoxazole, and metronidazole and his wounds closed secondarily over the next several months.

Approximately 14 months after the initial placement of the external fixator, all drainage had cleared. Radiographically, the bone fusion at the tibiotalar docking site and the bone growth in the regenerate zone appeared sufficiently strong (see Fig. 21-20D). With the fusion site and regenerate zone no longer needing protection, the decision was made to bring the patient back to the operating room to have the external fixator removed. This procedure went smoothly, and 6 months later Mr. J.L. was symptom-free and ambulatory. Radiographs at this time and 1 year later confirmed successful tibiotalar fusion and continued cortical re-formation of the regenerate zone (Fig. 21-21).

SYSTEMIC ANTIBIOTIC THERAPY

As mentioned from the outset, systemic antibiotic therapy is the most appropriate therapy for acute osteomyelitis, in which bone is still well vascularized. The treatment of vertebral osteomyelitis is also primarily with antibiotics,[72] although there is a role for surgery in cases of severe vertebral destruction.[84]

In contrast, of course, the role for systemic antibiotics in the management of chronic osteomyelitis is mostly adjunctive, helping to keep the surrounding, viable tissues infection-free after débridement. Much attention has been given in the past to the ability of various antibiotics to penetrate bone and to the role of high blood levels of antibiotics in promoting that penetration. In our view, this is problematic because the site of infection that is of fundamental concern is dead bone, usually surrounded by inflammatory cells or frank pus. The focus of disease therefore is not only avascular but also surrounded by an acidic and hypoxic environment, precisely the conditions that render penicillins and cephalosporins unstable and aminoglycosides inactive.[45,115,141,150] Furthermore, in the necrotic bone, it is likely that the bacteria are not very metabolically active, rendering the action of any antibiotic much less potent.[50,94] It is clear that, in the setting of chronic osteomyelitis, systemic antibiotics should

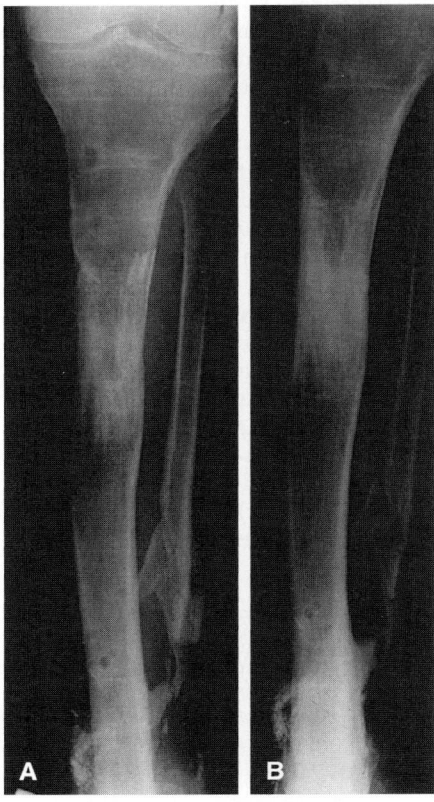

FIGURE 21-21   *Radiographs of Mr. J.L.'s leg at* **(A)** *2 years and* **(B)** *3 years after his initial operation confirm successful tibiotalar fusion and continued cortical re-formation of the regenerate zone.*

be thought of as adjuncts in the management of what is a primarily surgical illness.

Antibiotic administration is helpful in this setting only insofar as it allows optimal healing of the operative site and decreases the risk of infection in surrounding and distant sites.[142] After intraoperative culture specimens are taken from the infected bone, the patient should be restarted with broad-spectrum intravenous antibiotics to cover the common offending agents, such as *S. aureus* and *P. aeruginosa*.[55] When culture results are available, the antibiotic choice should be tailored to the patient's specific organisms and their sensitivities. For *S. aureus*, a penicillinase-resistant penicillin or first-generation cephalosporin has traditionally been the first choice. If the *S. aureus* is oxacillin resistant (as is now the case in the large majority of patients in our practice), other agents must be used. It is our practice to use vancomycin for the initial empiric coverage, changing to dicloxacillin if we isolate oxacillin-sensitive *S. aureus* or to trimethoprim-sulfamethoxazole, doxycycline or minocycline, or linezolid depending on the sensitivity pattern of the isolate. We often supplement any agent used in treatment with 1 to 2 months of rifampin on the basis of animal studies[101,102,133] as well as clinical data.[99,100] Since rifampin is a potent inducer of cytochrome activity, initiation of treatment with that agent should be delayed until postoperative pain is no longer a problem, since it dramatically increases elimination of narcotics and can make dosing difficult.

The approach is similar for other staphylococci and gram-negative organisms: choose an antibiotic on the basis of in vitro sensitivities and, with laboratory confirmation of rifampin sensitivity, supplement with rifampin. Although commonly used for therapy of tuberculosis and of difficult to treat staphylococcal infections, rifampin is truly a broad-spectrum antibiotic, inhibiting the majority of bacteria of any genus. Although a very active agent, it cannot be used as sole therapy because of a high spontaneous mutation rate in *Staphylococcus, Mycobacterium,* and presumably other species of bacteria. Patients treated with rifampin monotherapy for pyogenic infections can be expected to have active infections and rifampin-resistant bacteria within 1 to 2 weeks.

The appropriate duration of systemic antibiotic therapy is not currently known. Interestingly, some of the best results reported in the literature are from a group who used antibiotics only perioperatively, coupled with aggressive débridement.[36] Recalling the pathophysiology of chronic osteomyelitis, this approach seems to be entirely logical but one that requires incredible fortitude on the part of both patient and surgeon. Many of the patients in this study were taken to the operating room several times during the first week. At the University of Connecticut Health Center, we generally have our patients continue antibiotics until the operative site has healed completely (approximately 3 to 4 months).

As long as antibiotics are chosen that have been shown to be active against the infecting microbes in vitro, the route of antibiotic delivery (i.e., oral or intravenous) is probably inconsequential.[137] Although intravenous therapy has long been the norm in the treatment of post-traumatic osteomyelitis, there is evidence to suggest that switching to an oral route of administration earlier in the postoperative course may yield a similar outcome. Swiontkowski and co-workers[137] conducted a study in which they treated 93 patients with chronic osteomyelitis with combined surgical débridement, soft tissue coverage, and an antibiotic regimen of 5 to 7 days of intravenous therapy followed by oral antibiotics for 6 weeks. They compared the outcomes of these patients with those of a group of 22 patients treated previously with the same surgical management but 6 weeks of culture-specific intravenous antibiotics. Interestingly, there were no differences in the outcomes of the two groups. Our data[124] and a recent study of the use of linezolid in the treatment of staphylococcal osteomyelitis certainly support the view that well-absorbed oral agents are efficacious as adjuncts to surgical treatment of osteomyelitis. The advantages of oral therapy (enhanced comfort of the patient, elimination of the chance of intravenous line complications, and improved cost-efficiency) are such that it is likely that regimens based on primarily oral administration of antibiotics will soon supplant prolonged parenteral regimens.

COMPLEMENTARY THERAPIES

Several so-called complementary therapies have been used with some regularity in the treatment of chronic osteomyelitis and deserve mention in this chapter. Such therapies have as their goal either improvement of the host response to infection or promotion of healing of the bone. Hyperbaric oxygen has long been proposed as an adjunctive measure that would improve host defenses at the site of infection. The principle behind this treatment is that low oxygen tensions in infected bone inhibit the normal activity of immune mediators, such as macrophages and polymorphonuclear leukocytes. In in vitro studies, for example, *S. aureus* is not killed by polymorphonuclear leukocytes incubated in either severely hypoxic or anaerobic environments, with intermediate levels of hypoxia causing lesser reductions in killing efficiency. Furthermore, as we have discussed, the activity of many antibiotics is greatest in aerobic environments. Hyperbaric oxygen therapy, which increases oxygen tension above 250 mm Hg, is theorized to augment the host's immune system, create a hostile environment for anaerobes, allow the formation of peroxides that kill bacteria, and promote wound healing.[79,80] Although the use of hyperbaric oxygenation has shown some promise in several studies,[60,65,79,80] there has not yet been a single controlled study to our knowledge that demonstrates its utility in the treatment of chronic osteomyelitis.

Other complementary modalities are used in an attempt to enhance skeletal healing after the infection has been controlled. One such modality is electrical stimulation. That electrical stimulation may have a role in inducing the healing of delayed unions and nonunions is based on findings that fractures in bone have a negative charge and manipulating that potential can lead to alterations in fracture healing.[6,41] Three different types of electrical stimulation delivery are commonly described (direct current, inductive coupling, and capacitive coupling),[112] and each has data supporting its efficacy. One study from 1990 demonstrated healing in 12 of 20 patients with delayed tibial unions treated with inductive coupling compared with 1 of 20 who were in a randomized, blinded placebo group.[132] A 1994 study reported equally impressive results in cases of long bone nonunions: 6 of 10 in the capacitive coupling group were healed versus 0 of 10 who received treatment with placebo.[129] The indication for this mode of therapy is having a nonunion that is in acceptable alignment. Contraindications for electrical stimulation include an unacceptable malalignment, the presence of septic pseudarthrosis, and a gap of greater than half the diameter of the bone.[29]

Another means of stimulating bone healing is ultrasound. In a multicenter, prospective, randomized, double-blind, placebo-controlled study, using low-intensity ultrasound was shown to decrease the amount of time to radiographic union in the treatment of displaced distal radius fractures.[75] Although the reasons behind this finding are currently unclear, it is theorized that ultrasound waves act as a mechanical deforming force that acts as an impetus for accelerated bone formation.[121] The role of ultrasound in treating chronic osteomyelitis is not well defined.

SUMMARY

Chronic osteomyelitis is most often due to trauma and generally has a protracted, indolent clinical course. It should be acknowledged as a *concrete absce*ss and treated with a combined approach of surgical débridement, skeletal stabilization, dead space management, soft tissue coverage, and antibiotic therapy. Although these principles are the cornerstone of management, it is important to recognize the formidable physical and psychologic challenges facing patients with chronic osteomyelitis and foster a multidisciplinary approach in their care. The entire staff of health care professionals, from physicians and nurses to physical therapists and social workers, must work together to communicate effectively and compassionately with the patient and family to establish a dynamic, ongoing dialogue. In so doing, we may be able not only to treat disease but also to educate people about their condition, from the practical importance of dressing changes or quitting smoking to a more global understanding of its frequently unrelenting nature.

REFERENCES

1. Anglen; J.O.; Apostles; P.S.; Christensen, G.; et al. Removal of surface bacteria by irrigation. J Orthop Res 14:251, 1996.
2. Anglen, J.O.; Apostles, P.S.; Christensen, G.; et al. The efficacy of various irrigation solutions in removing slime-producing Staphylococcus. J Orthop Trauma 8:390, 1994.
3. Anthony, J.P.; Mathes, S.J.; Alpert, B.S. The muscle flap in the treatment of chronic lower extremity osteomyelitis: Results in patients over 5 years after treatment. Plast Reconstr Surg 88:311, 1991.
4. Arnold, P.G.; Yugueros, O.; Hanssen, A.D. Muscle flaps in osteomyelitis of the lower extremity: A 20-year account. Plast Reconstr Surg 104:107, 1999.
5. Barnes, R.W. Amputations: An Illustrated Manual. Philadelphia, Hanley & Belfus, 2000.
6. Becker, R.O. The bioelectric factors in amphibian limb regeneration. J Bone Joint Surg Am 43:643, 1961.
7. Beltran, J.; Noto, A.M.; McGhee, R.B.; et al. Infection of the musculoskeletal system: High field strength MR imaging. Radiology 164:449, 1987.
8. Bergman, B.R. Antibiotic prophylaxis in open and closed fractures—A controlled clinical trial. Acta Orthop Scand 53:57, 1982.
9. Bhaskar, S.N.; Cutright, D.; Hunsuck, E.E.; et al. Pulsating water jet devices in the débridement of combat wounds. Mil Med 136:264, 1971.
10. Blume, P.A.; Dey, H.M.; Daley, L.J.; et al. Diagnosis of pedal osteomyelitis with Tc-99m HMPAO labeled leukocytes. J Foot Ankle Surg 36:120, 1997.
11. Bohm, E.; Josten, C. What's new in exogenous osteomyelitis? Pathol Res Pract 1888:254, 1992.
12. Bondurant, F.J.; Cotler, H.B.; Buckle, R.; et al. The medical and economic impact of severely injured lower extremities. J Trauma 28:1270, 1988.
13. Borzsei, L.; Mintal, T.; Koos, Z.; et al. Examination of a novel, specified local antibiotic therapy through polymethylmethacrylate capsules in a rabbit osteomyelitis model. Chemotherapy 52:73–79, 2006.
14. Brady, R.A.; Leid, J.G.; Camper, A.K.; et al. Identification of Staphylococcus aureus proteins recognized by the antibody-mediated immune response to a biofilm infection. Infect Immun 74:3415–3426, 2006.
15. Burgess, E.M. The below-knee amputation. Bull Prosthet Res 10:19, 1968.
16. Buxton, T.B.; Horner, J.; Hinton, A.; et al. In vivo glycocalyx expression by Staphylococcus aureus phage type 52/52A/80 in S. aureus osteomyelitis. Infect Dis 156:942, 1987.
17. Calhoun, J.H.; Anger, D.M.; Mader, J.; et al. The Ilizarov technique in the treatment of osteomyelitis. Tex Med 87:56, 1991.
18. Carragee, E.J. Pyogenic vertebral osteomyelitis. J Bone Joint Surg Am 79:874, 1997.
19. Carragee, E.J.; Kim, D.; Van Der Vlugt, T.; et al. The clinical use of erythrocyte sedimentation rate in pyogenic vertebral osteomyelitis. Spine 22:2089, 1997.
20. Chan, Y.S.; Ueng, S.W.; Wang, C.J.; et al. Management of small infected tibial defects with antibiotic-impregnated autogenic cancellous bone grafting. J Trauma 45:758, 1998.
21. Chapman, M.W. Role of bone stability in open fractures. Instr Course Lect 31:75, 1982.
22. Cho, S.H.; Song, H.R.; Koo, K.H.; et al. Antibiotic-impregnated cement beads in the treatment of chronic osteomyelitis. Bull Hosp Joint Dis 56:140, 1997.
23. Cierny, G. III. Classification and treatment of adult osteomyelitis. In Evarts, C.M., ed. Surgery of the Musculoskeletal System, 2nd ed. London, Churchill Livingstone, 1990, p. 4337.
24. Cierny, G. III. Infected tibial nonunions (1981–1995): The evolution of change. Clin Orthop 360:97, 1999.
25. Cierny, G. III; Mader; J.; Penninck, J. A clinical staging system for adult osteomyelitis. Contemp Orthop 10:5, 1985.
26. Cierny, G. III; Mader, J.T. Approach to adult osteomyelitis. Orthop Rev 16:259, 1987.
27. Clansey, B.J.; Hansen, S.T. Open fractures of the tibia: A review of 102 cases. J Bone Joint Surg Am 60:118, 1978.
28. Clawson, D.K.; Dunn, A.W. Management of common bacterial infections of bones and joints. J Bone Joint Surg Am 49:165, 1974.
29. Connolly, J.F. Selection, evaluation and indications for electrical stimulation of ununited fractures. Clin Orthop 161:39, 1981.
30. Curtis, M.J.; Brown, P.R.; Dick, J.D.; et al. Contaminated fractures of the tibia: A comparison of treatment modalities in an animal model. J Orthop Res 13:286, 1995.
31. Dendrinos, G.K.; Kontos, S.; Lyritisis, E. Use of the Ilizarov technique for treatment of non-union of the tibia associated with infection. J Bone Joint Surg Am 77:835, 1995.
32. Dirschl, D.R.; Almekinders, L.C. Osteomyelitis: Common causes and treatment recommendations. Drugs 45:29, 1993.

33. Dirschl, D.R.; Dahners, L.E. The mangled extremity: When should it be amputated? J Am Acad Orthop Surg 4:182, 1996.

34. Domingue, G.J.; Woody, H.B. Bacterial persistence and expression of disease. Clin Microbiol Rev 10:320, 1997.

35. Dougherty, S.L.T.; Simmens, R.L. Infections in bionic man: The pathology of infections in prosthetic devices. Curr Probl Surg 19:265, 1982.

36. Eckardt, J.J.; Wirganowicz, P.Z.; Mar, T. An aggressive surgical approach to the management of chronic osteomyelitis. Clin Orthop 298:229, 1994.

37. Emami, A.; Mjoberg, B.; Larson, S. Infected tibial nonunion: Good results after open cancellous bone grafting in 37 cases. Acta Orthop Scand 66:447, 1995.

38. Emami, A.; Mjoberg, B.; Ragnarsson, B.; et al. Changing epidemiology of tibial shaft fractures: 513 cases compared between 1971–1975 and 1986–1990. Acta Orthop Scand 67:557, 1996.

39. Fischer, B.; Vaudaux, P.; Magnin, M.; et al. Novel animal model for studying the molecular mechanisms of bacterial adhesion to bone-implanted metallic devices: Role of fibronectin in *Staphylococcus aureus* adhesion. J Orthop Res 14:914, 1996.

40. Fitzgerald, R.H., Jr.; Ruttle, P.E.; Arnold, P.G.; et al. Local muscle flaps in the treatment of chronic osteomyelitis. J Bone Joint Surg Am 67:175, 1985.

41. Friedenberg, Z.B.; Brighton, C.T. Bioelectric potentials in bone. J Bone Joint Surg Am 48:915, 1966.

42. Gitelis, S.; Brebach, G.T. The treatment of chronic osteomyelitis with a biodegradable antibiotic-impregnated implant. J Orthop Surg (Hong Kong):10:53–60, 2002.

43. Gonzalez, E.G.; Corcoran, P.J.; Reyes, R.L. Energy expenditure in below-knee amputees: Correlation with stump length. Arch Phys Med Rehabil 55:111, 1974.

44. Gordon, S.L.; Greer, R.B.; Craig, C.P. Report of four cases culturing L-form variants of staphylococci. J Bone Joint Surg Am 53:1150, 1971.

45. Gray, E.D.; Peters, G.; Verstegen, M.; et al. Effect of extracellular slime substance from *Staphylococcus epidermidis* on human cellular immune response. Lancet 1:365, 1984.

46. Green, S.A. Osteomyelitis: The Ilizarov perspective. Orthop Clin North Am 22:515, 1991.

47. Green, S.A. Skeletal defects: A comparison of bone grafting and bone transport for skeletal defects. Clin Orthop 301:111, 1994.

48. Gregory, R.T.; Gould, R.J.; Peclet, M.; et al. The mangled extremity syndrome (M.E.S.): A severity grading system for multi-system injury of the extremity. J Trauma 25:1147, 1985.

49. Gristina, A.B.; Jennings, R.A.; Naylor, P.T.; et al. Comparative in vitro antibiotic resistance of surface colonizing coagulase-negative staphylococci. Antimicrob Agents Chemother 33:813, 1989.

50. Gristina, A.G.; Naylor, P.T.; Myrvik, Q.N. Mechanisms of musculoskeletal sepsis. Orthop Clin North Am 22:363, 1991.

51. Gristina, A.G.; Oga, M.; Webb, L.X.; et al. Adherent bacterial colonization in the pathogenesis of osteomyelitis. Science 228:990, 1985.

52. Gualdrini, G.; Zati, A.; Degli Esposti, S. The effects of cigarette smoke on the progression of septic pseudoarthrosis of the tibia treated by Ilizarov external fixator. Chir Organi Mov 81:395, 1996.

53. Gugenheim, J.J., Jr. The Ilizarov method: Orthopedic and soft tissue applications. Clin Plast Surg 25:567, 1998.

54. Gustilo, R.B. Management of infected non-union. In Evarts, C.M., ed. Surgery of the Musculoskeletal System, 2nd ed. London, Churchill Livingstone, 1990, pp. 4429, 4455.

55. Gustilo, R.B.; Anderson, J.T. Prevention of infection in the treatment of one thousand and twenty-five open fractures of long bones. J Bone Joint Surg Am 58:453, 1976.

56. Gustilo, R.B.; Mendoza, R.M.; Williams, D.N. Problems in the management of type III (severe) open fractures: A classification of type III open fractures. J Trauma 24:742, 1984.

57. Harwood, P.J.; Talbot, C.; Dimoutsos, M.; et al. Early experience with linezolid for infections in orthopaedics. Injury 37:818–826, 2006.

58. Helfet, D.L.; Howery, T.; Sanders, R.; et al. Limb salvage versus manipulation: Preliminary results of the mangled extremity severity score. Clin Orthop 256:80, 1990.

59. Hermann, M.; Vaudaux, P.E.; Pittet, D.; et al. Fibronectin, fibrinogen and laminin act as mediators of adherence of clinical staphylococcal isolates to foreign material. J Infect Dis 158:693, 1988.

60. Hill, G.B.; Osterhout, S. Experimental effects of hyperbaric oxygen on selected clostridial species: In vitro studies. J Infect Dis 125:17, 1972.

61. Hill, S.L.; Holtzman, G.I.; Buse, R. The effects of peripheral vascular disease with osteomyelitis in the diabetic foot. Am J Surg 177:282, 1999.

62. Hogt, A.; Dankert, J.; Feijen, J. Adhesion of coagulase-negative staphylococci to methacrylate polymers and copolymers. J Biomed Mater Res 20:533, 1986.

63. Holtom, P.D.; Smith, A.M. Introduction to adult posttraumatic osteomyelitis of the tibia. Clin Orthop 360:6, 1999.

64. Hong, S.W.; Seah, C.S.; Kuek, L.B.; et al. Soft tissue coverage in compound and complicated tibial fractures using microvascular flaps. Ann Acad Med Singapore 27:182, 1998.

65. Hunt, T.K.; Pai, M.P. The effect of varying ambient oxygen tensions on wound metabolism and collagen synthesis. Surg Gynecol Obstet 135:756, 1972.

66. Ilizarov, G.A. Transosseous Osteosynthesis: Theoretical and Clinical Aspects of the Regeneration and Growth of Tissue. Berlin, Springer-Verlag, 1992.

67. Jacobs, R.F.; McCarthy, R.E.; Elser, J.M. Pseudomonas osteochondritis complicating puncture wounds of the foot in children: A 10-year evaluation. J Infect Dis 160:657, 1989.

68. Jensen, J.E.; Jensen, T.G.; Smith, T.K.; et al. Nutrition in orthopaedic surgery. J Bone Joint Surg Am 64:1263, 1982.

69. Johnson, G.M.; Regelmann, W.E.; Gray, E.D.; et al. Interference with granulocyte function by *Staphylococcus epidermidis* slime. Infect Immun 54:13, 1986.

70. Kelly, P.J. Infections of bones and joints in adult patients. Instr Course Lect 26:3, 1977.

71. Kelly, P.J.; William, W.J.; Coventry, M.B. Chronic osteomyelitis: Treatment with closed irrigation and suction. JAMA 213:1843, 1970.

72. Khan, I.A.; Vaccaro, A.R.; Zlotolow, D.A. Management of vertebral diskitis and osteomyelitis. Orthopedics 22:758, 1999.

73. Klein, M.B.; Chang, J. Management of hand and upper-extremity infections in heart transplant recipients. Plast Reconstr Surg 106:598, 2000.

74. Klemm, K. Antibiotic bead chains. Clin Orthop 295:63, 1993.

75. Kristiansen, T.K.; Ryaby, J.P.; McCabe, J.; et al. Accelerated healing of distal radial fractures with the use of specific low-intensity ultrasound. J Bone Joint Surg Am 79:961, 1997.

76. Krznaric, E.; DeRoo, M.; Verbruggen, A.; et al. Chronic osteomyelitis: Diagnosis with technetium-99m-D, l-hexamethylpropylene amine oxime labeled leukocytes. Eur J Nucl Med 23:792, 1996.

77. Lange, R.H. Limb reconstruction versus amputation decision making in massive lower extremity trauma. Clin Orthop 243:92, 1989.

78. Lisbona, R.; Rosenthall, L. Observations on the sequential use of 99mTc-phosphate complex and 67Ga imaging in osteomyelitis, cellulitis, and septic arthritis. Radiology 123:123, 1977.

79. Mader, J.T.; Adams, R.K.; Wallace, W.R.; et al. Hyperbaric oxygen as adjunctive therapy for osteomyelitis. Infect Dis Clin North Am 4:433, 1990.

80. Mader, J.T.; Brown, G.L.; Guckian, J.C.; et al. A mechanism for the amelioration by hyperbaric oxygen of experimental staphylococcal osteomyelitis in rabbits. J Infect Dis 142:915, 1980.

81. Mader, J.T.; Cripps, M.W.; Calhoun, J.H. Adult posttraumatic osteomyelitis of the tibia. Clin Orthop 360:14, 1999.

82. Marshall, K.A.; Edgerton, M.T.; Rodeheaver, G.T.; et al. Quantitative microbiology: Its application to hand injuries. Am J Surg 131:730, 1976.

83. Mathes, S.J.; Alpert, B.S.; Chang, N. Use of the muscle flap in chronic osteomyelitis: Experimental and clinical correlation. Plast Reconstr Surg 69:815, 1982.

84. Matsui, H.; Hirano, N.; Sakaguchi, Y. Vertebral osteomyelitis: An analysis of 38 surgically treated cases. Eur Spine J 7:50, 1998.

85. Maurer, A.H.; Chen, D.C.P.; Camargo, E.E. Utility of three-phase scintigraphy in suspected osteomyelitis: Concise communication. J Nucl Med 22:941, 1981.

86. May, J.W.; Jupiter, J.B.; Weiland, A.J.; et al. Clinical classification of post-traumatic tibial osteomyelitis. J Bone Joint Surg Am 71:1422, 1989.

87. Mayberry-Carson, K.J.; Tober-Meyer, B.; Smith, J.K.; et al. Bacterial adherence and glycocalyx formation in osteomyelitis experimentally induced with *Staphylococcus aureus*. Infect Immun 43:825, 1984.

88. Maynor, M.L.; Moon, R.E.; Camporesi, E.M.; et al. Chronic osteomyelitis of the tibia: Treatment with hyperbaric oxygen and autogenous microsurgical muscle transplantation. J South Orthop Assoc 7:43, 1998.

89. McCarthy, K.; Velchik, M.G.; Alavi, A.; et al. Indium-111-labeled white blood cells in the detection of osteomyelitis complicated by a pre-existing condition. J Nucl Med 29:1015, 1988.

90. Moshirfar, A.; Showers, D.; Logan, P.; et al. Prosthetic options for below knee amputations and nonunion of the tibia. Clin Orthop 360:110, 1999.

91. Muha, J. Local wound care in diabetic foot complications: Aggressive risk management and ulcer treatment to avoid amputation. Postgrad Med 106:97, 1999.

92. Munoz-Fernandez, S.; Macia, M.A.; Pantoja, L.; et al. Osteoarticular infection in intravenous drug abusers: Influence of HIV infection and differences with non drug abusers. Ann Rheum Dis 52:570–574, 1993.

93. Murdoch, G. Levels of amputation and limiting factors. Ann R Coll Surg Engl 40:204, 1967.

94. Musher, D.M.; Lamm, N.; Darouiche, R.O.; et al. The current spectrum of *Staphylococcus aureus* infection in a tertiary care hospital. Medicine (Baltimore) 73:186, 1994.

95. Naylor, P.T.; Myrvik, Q.N.; Gristina, A.B. Antibiotic resistance of biomaterial-adherent coagulase-negative and coagulase-positive staphylococci. Clin Orthop 26:126, 1990.

96. Nelson, C.L.; Hickmon, S.G.; Skinner, R.A. Treatment of experimental osteomyelitis by surgical débridement and the implantation of bioerodable, polyanhydride-gentamicin beads. J Orthop Res 15:249, 1997.

97. Norden, C.W. Experimental osteomyelitis: A description of the model. J Infect Dis 122:410, 1970.

98. Norden, C.W. Lessons learned from animal models of osteomyelitis. Rev Infect Dis 10:103, 1988.

99. Norden, C.W.; Bryant, R.; Palmer, D.; et al. Chronic osteomyelitis caused by *Staphylococcus aureus*: Controlled clinical trial of nafcillin therapy and nafcillin-rifampin therapy. South Med J 79:947, 1986.

100. Norden, C.W.; Fierer, J.; Bryant, R. Chronic staphylococcal osteomyelitis: Treatment with regimens containing rifampin. Rev Infect Dis 5(Suppl 3): S495, 1983.

101. Norden, C.W.; Shaffer, M. Treatment of experimental chronic osteomyelitis due to *Staphylococcus*

aureus with vancomycin and rifampin. J Infect Dis 147:352, 1983.

102. O'Reilly, T.; Kunz, S.; Sande, E.; et al. Relationship between antibiotic concentration in bone and efficacy of treatment of staphylococcal osteomyelitis in rats: Azithromycin compared with clindamycin and rifampin. Antimicrob Agents Chemother 36:2693–2697, 1992.

103. Orr, H.W. A New Era of Treatment for Osteomyelitis and Other Infections. St. Paul, MN, Bruce Publishing, 1930, p. 48.

104. Palestro, C.J.; Roumanas, P.; Swyer, A.J.; et al. Diagnosis of musculoskeletal infection using combined In-111 labeled leukocyte and Tc-99m SC marrow imaging. Clin Nucl Med 17:269, 1992.

105. Palestro, C.J.; Torres, M.A. Radionuclide imaging in orthopedic infections. Semin Nucl Med 27:334, 1997.

106. Paley, D.; Catagni, M.A.; Argnani, F.; et al. Ilizarov treatment of tibial nonunions with bone loss. Clin Orthop 241:146, 1989.

107. Panda, M.; Ntungila, N.; Kalunda, M.; et al. Treatment of chronic osteomyelitis using the Papineau technique. Int Orthop 22:37, 1998.

108. Papineau, L.J.; Alfageme, A.; Dalcourt, J.P.; et al. Ostéomyélite chronique: Excision et greffe de spongieux a l'air libre après mises a plat extensives. Int Orthop 3:165, 1979.

109. Patzakis, M.J.; Greene, N.; Holtom, P.; et al. Culture results in open wound treatment with muscle transfer for tibial osteomyelitis. Clin Orthop 360:66, 1999.

110. Patzakis, M.J.; Harrey, J.P.; Ivler, D. The role of antibiotics in the management of open fractures. J Bone Joint Surg 56:532, 1974.

111. Patzakis, M.J.; Wilkins, J.; Kumar, J.; et al. Comparison of the results of bacterial cultures from multiple sites in chronic osteomyelitis of long bones. J Bone Joint Surg Am 76:664, 1994.

112. Perry, C.R. Bone repair techniques, bone graft, and bone graft substitutes. Clin Orthop 360:71, 1999.

113. Perry, C.R.; Rames, R.D.; Pearson, R.L. Treatment of septic tibial nonunions with local antibiotics and intramedullary nail. Orthop Trans 12:657, 1989.

114. Peters, K.M.; Adam, G.; Biedermann, M.; et al. Osteomyelitis today: Diagnostic imaging and therapy. Zentralbl Chir 118:637, 1993.

115. Reynolds, A.V.; Hamilton-Miller, J.M.T.; Brumfitt, W. Diminished effect of gentamicin under anaerobic and hypercapnic conditions. Lancet 1:447, 1976.

116. Ring, D.; Jupiter, J.B.; Toh, S. Salvage of contaminated fractures of the distal humerus with thin wire external fixation. Clin Orthop 359:203, 1999.

117. Rittman, W.W.; Perren, S.M. Cortical Bone Healing after Internal Fixation and Infection. New York, Springer-Verlag, 1974.

118. Rittmann, W.W.; Schibili, M.; Matter, P.; et al. Open fractures: Long-term results in 200 consecutive cases. Clin Orthop 138:132, 1979.

119. Robson, M.C.; Duke, W.F.; Krizek, T.J. Rapid bacterial screening in the treatment of civilian wounds. J Surg Res 14:426, 1973.

120. Roine, I.; Arguedas, A.; Faingezicht, I.; et al. Early detection of sequelae-prone osteomyelitis in children with use of simple clinical and laboratory criteria. Clin Infect Dis 24:849, 1997.

121. Rubin, J.; McLeod, K.J.; Titus, L.; et al. Formation of osteoclast-like cells is suppressed by low frequency, low intensity electric fields. J Orthop Res 14:7, 1996.

122. Sachs, B.L.; Shaffer, J.W. A staged Papineau protocol for chronic osteomyelitis. Clin Orthop 184:256, 1984.

123. Saltzman, C.L.; Pedowitz, W.J. Diabetic foot infections. Instr Course Lect 48:317, 1999.

124. Salvana, J.; Rodner, C.; Browner, B.D.; et al. Chronic osteomyelitis: Results obtained by an integrated team approach to management. Conn Med 69:195–202, 2005.

125. Santoro, V.; Henley, M.; Benirschke, S.; et al. Prospective comparison of unreamed interlocking IM nails versus half-pin external fixation in open tibial fractures. J Orthop Trauma 5:238, 1991.

126. Schandelmaier, P.; Krettek, C.; Rudolf, J.; Tscherne, H. Outcome of tibial shaft fractures with severe soft tissue injury treated by unreamed nailing versus external fixation. J Trauma 39:707, 1995.

127. Schauwecker, D.S. The scintigraphic diagnosis of osteomyelitis. AJR Am J Roentgenol 158:9, 1992.

128. Schurman, D.J.; Smith, R.L. Bacterial biofilm and infected biomaterials, prostheses and artificial organs. In Esterhai, J.L.; Gristina, A.G.; Poss, R., eds. Musculoskeletal Infection. Park Ridge, IL, American Academy of Orthopaedic Surgeons, 1992, p. 133.

129. Scott, G.; King, J.B. A prospective, double-blind trial of electrical capacitative coupling in the treatment of non-union of long bones. J Bone Joint Surg Am 76:820, 1994.

130. Sekiguchi, J.; Haramoto, U.; Kobayashi, S.; et al. Free flap transfers for the treatment of osteomyelitis of the lower leg. Scand J Plast Reconstr Surg Hand Surg 32:171, 1998.

131. Seltzer, S.E. Value of computed tomography in planning medical and surgical treatment of chronic osteomyelitis. J Comput Assist Tomogr 8:482, 1984.

132. Sharrard, W.J. A double-blind trial of pulsed electromagnetic fields for delayed union of tibial fractures. J Bone Joint Surg Br 72:347, 1990.

133. Shirtliff, M.E.; Mader, J.T.; Calhoun, J. Oral rifampin plus azithromycin or clarithromycin to treat osteomyelitis in rabbits. Clin Orthop 359:229, 1999.

134. Sponseller, P.D.; Malech, H.L.; McCarthy, E.F.; et al. Skeletal involvement in children who have chronic granulomatous disease. J Bone Joint Surg Am 73:37, 1991.

135. Sudekamp, N.; Barbey, N.; Veuskens, A.; et al. The incidence of osteitis in open fractures: An analysis of 948 open fractures. J Orthop Trauma 7:473, 1993.

136. Swiontkowski, M.F. Surgical approaches in osteomyelitis: Use of laser Doppler flowmetry to determine non-viable bone. Infect Dis Clin North Am 4:501, 1990.

137. Swiontkowski, M.F.; Hanel, D.P.; Vedder, N.B.; et al. A comparison of short- and long-term intravenous antibiotic therapy in the postoperative management of adult osteomyelitis. J Bone Joint Surg Br 81:1046, 1999.

138. Tang, J.S.H.; Gold, R.H.; Bassett, L.W.; et al. Musculoskeletal infection of the extremities: Evaluation with MR imaging. Radiology 166:205, 1988.

139. Tetsworth, K.; Cierny, G. III. Osteomyelitis débridement techniques. Clin Orthop 360:87, 1999.

140. Tornetta, P.; Bergman, M.; Watnik, N.; et al. Treatment of grade IIIB open tibial fractures. J Bone Joint Surg Br 76:13, 1994.

141. Tresse, O.; Jouenne, T.; Junter, G.A. The role of oxygen limitation in the resistance of agar-entrapped, sessile-like *Escherichia coli* to aminoglycoside and beta-lactam antibiotics. J Antimicrob Chemother 36:521, 1995.

142. Trueta, J.; Morgan, J.D. Late results in the treatment of one hundred cases of acute haematogenous osteomyelitis. Br J Surg 41:449–457, 1954.

143. Tsai, E.; Failla, J.M. Hand infections in the trauma patient. Hand Clin 15:373, 1999.

144. Tsukayama, D.T. Pathophysiology of posttraumatic osteomyelitis. Clin Orthop 360:22, 1999.

145. Tsukayama, D.T.; Guay, D.R.; Gustilo, R.B.; et al. The effect of anaerobiosis on antistaphylococcal antibiotics. Orthopedics 11:1285, 1988.

146. Tvrdek, M.; Nejedly, A.; Kletensky, J.; Kufa, R. Treatment of chronic osteomyelitis of the lower extremity using free flap transfer. Acta Chir Plast 41:46, 1999.

147. Ueng, S.W.; Wei, F.C.; Shih, C.H. Management of femoral diaphyseal infected nonunion with antibiotic beads, local therapy, external skeletal fixation, and staged bone grafting. J Trauma 46:97, 1999.

148. Unger, E.; Moldofsky, P.; Gatenby, R.; et al. Diagnosis of osteomyelitis by MR imaging. AJR Am J Roentgenol 150:605, 1988.

149. Vassilopoulos, D.; Chalasani, P.; Jurado, R.L.; et al. Musculoskeletal infections in patients with human immunodeficiency virus infection. Medicine (Baltimore) 76:284, 1997.

150. Verkin, R.M.; Mandell, G.M. Alteration of effectiveness of antibiotics by anaerobiosis. J Lab Clin Med 89:65, 1977.

151. Vesco, L.; Boulahdour, H.; Hamissa, S.; et al. The value of combined radionuclide and magnetic resonance imaging in the diagnosis and conservative management of minimal or localized osteomyelitis of the foot in diabetic patients. Metabolism 48:922, 1999.

152. Von Eiff, C.; Bettin, D.; Proctor, R.A.; et al. Recovery of small colony variants of *Staphylococcus aureus* following gentamicin bead placement for osteomyelitis. Clin Infect Dis 25:1250, 1997.

153. Waldvogel, F.A.; Medoff, G.; Swartz, M.N. Osteomyelitis: A review of clinical features, therapeutic considerations, and unusual aspects. Pt. 1. N Engl J Med 282:198, 1970.

154. Waldvogel, F.A.; Medoff, G.; Swartz, M.N. Osteomyelitis: A review of clinical features, therapeutic considerations, and unusual aspects. Pt. 3. N Engl J Med 282:316, 1970.

155. Walenkamp, G.H. Chronic osteomyelitis. Acta Orthop Scand 68:497, 1997.

156. Walenkamp, G.H.; Kleijn, L.L.; de Leeuw, M. Osteomyelitis treated with gentamicin-PMMA beads: 100 patients followed for 1–12 years. Acta Orthop Scand 69:518, 1998.

157. Webb, L.X.; Holman, J.; de Araujo, B.; et al. Antibiotic resistance in staphylococci adherent to cortical bone. J Orthop Trauma 8:28, 1994.

158. Weiss, S.J. Tissue destruction by neutrophils. N Engl J Med 320:365, 1989.

159. Williams, R.L.; Fukui, M.B.; Meltzer, C.C.; et al. Fungal spinal osteomyelitis in the immunocompromised patient: MR findings in three cases. AJNR Am J Neuroradiol 20:381, 1999.

160. Wood, M.B.; Cooney, W.P.; Irons, G.B. Lower extremity salvage and reconstruction by free-tissue transfer. Clin Orthop 201:151, 1985.

161. Wukich, D.K.; Abreu, S.H.; Callaghan, J.J.; et al. Diagnosis of infection by preoperative scintigraphy with indium-labeled white blood cells. J Bone Joint Surg Am 69:1353, 1987.

162. Yamashita, Y.; Uchida, A.; Yamakawa, T.; et al. Treatment of chronic osteomyelitis using calcium hydroxyapatite ceramic implants impregnated with antibiotic. Int Orthop 22:247, 1998.

163. Zobell, C.E.; Anderson, D.Q. Observations on the multiplication of bacteria in different volumes of stored seawater and the influence of oxygen tension and solid surfaces. Biol Bull 71:324, 1936.

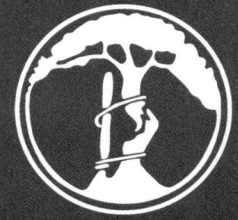

CHAPTER 22

Nonunions: Evaluation and Treatment

....

Mark R. Brinker, M.D. and Daniel P. O'Connor, Ph.D.

INTRODUCTION

While fracture nonunions may represent a small percentage of the traumatologist's case load, they can account for a high percentage of a surgeon's stress, anxiety, and frustration. Arrival of a fracture nonunion may be anticipated following a severe traumatic injury, such as an open fracture with segmental bone loss, but may also appear following a low-energy fracture that seemed destined to heal.

Fracture nonunion is a chronic medical condition associated with pain and functional and psychosocial disability.[180] Because of the wide variation in patient responses to various stresses[177] and the impact that may have on the patient's family (relationships, income, etc.), these cases are often difficult to manage.

Some 90 to 95 percent of all fractures heal without problems.[87,245] Nonunions are that small percentage of cases in which the biological process of fracture repair cannot overcome the local biology and mechanics of the bony injury.

DEFINITIONS

A fracture is said to have "gone on to nonunion" when the normal biologic healing processes cease to the extent that solid healing will not occur without further treatment intervention. The definition is subjective, with criteria that result in high interobserver variability.

The literature reveals a myriad of definitions of nonunion. For the purposes of clinical investigations, the U.S. Food and Drug Administration (FDA) defines a nonunion as a fracture that is at least 9 months old and has not shown any signs of healing for 3 consecutive months.[125,307] Müller's[209] definition is failure of a (tibia) fracture to unite after 8 months of nonoperative treatment. These two definitions are widely utilized, but their arbitrary use of a temporal limit is flawed.[113] For example, several months of observation should not be required to declare a tibial shaft fracture with 10 cm of segmental bone loss a nonunion. Conversely, how does one define a fracture that continues to consolidate but requires 12 months to heal?[264]

We define nonunion as a fracture that, in the opinion of the treating physician, has no possibility of healing without further intervention. We define delayed union as a fracture that, in the opinion of the treating physician, shows slower progression to healing than anticipated and is at risk of nonunion without further intervention.

To understand the biological processes and clinical implications of fracture nonunion, an understanding of the normal fracture healing process is required. The following section reviews the local biology of fracture healing, requirements for fracture union, and types of normal fracture repair.

FRACTURE REPAIR

Fracture repair is an astonishing process that involves spontaneous, structured regeneration of bony tissue and restores mechanical stability. The process begins at the moment of bony injury, initiating a proliferation of tissues that ultimately leads to healing.

The early biological response at the fracture site is an inflammatory response with bleeding and the formation of a fracture hematoma. The repair response occurs rapidly in the presence of osteoprogenitor cells from the periosteum and endosteum and hematopoietic cells that are capable of secreting growth factors. Following fracture healing, bony remodeling progresses according to Wolff's law.[20,21,238,272,328]

The repair process, involving both intramembranous and enchondral bone formation, requires mechanical stability, an adequate blood supply, good bony contact, and the appropriate endocrine and metabolic responses. The biological response is related to the type and extent of injury and the type of treatment (Table 22-1).

Healing via Callus

In the absence of rigid fixation (e.g., cast immobilization), stabilization of bony fragments occurs by periosteal and endosteal callus formation. If the fracture site has an adequate blood supply, callus formation proceeds and results in an increase in the cross-sectional area at the fracture surface. This increased cross-sectional area enhances fracture stability. Fracture stability is also provided by the formation of fibrocartilage, which replaces granulation tissue at the fracture site. Enchondral bone formation, in which bone replaces cartilage, occurs only after calcification of the fibrocartilage.

Table 22-1
Type of Fracture Healing Based on Type of Stabilization

Type of Stabilization	Predominant Type of Healing
Cast (closed treatment)	Periosteal bridging callus and interfragmentary enchondral ossification
Compression plate	Primary cortical healing (cutting cone-type remodeling)
Intramedullary nail	Early: periosteal bridging callus Late: medullary callus
External fixator	Depends on extent of rigidity Less rigid: periosteal bridging callus More rigid: primary cortical healing
Inadequate immobilization	
With adequate blood supply	Hypertrophic nonunion (failed enchondral ossification)
Without adequate blood supply	Atrophic nonunion
Inadequate reduction with displacement at the fracture site	Oligotrophic nonunion

Direct Bone (Osteonal) Healing

Direct osteonal healing occurs without formation of external callus and is characterized by gradual disappearance of the fracture line. This process requires an adequate blood supply and absolute rigidity at the fracture site, most commonly accomplished via compression plating. In areas of direct bone-to-bone contact, fracture repair resembles cutting-cone type remodeling. In areas where small gaps exist between fracture fragments, "gap healing" occurs via appositional bone formation.

Indirect Bone Healing

Indirect bone healing occurs in fractures that have been stabilized with less than absolute rigidity, including intramedullary nail fixation, tension band wire techniques, cerclage wiring, external fixation, and plate-and-screw fixation (applied suboptimally). Indirect healing involves coupled bone resorption and bone formation at the fracture site. Healing occurs via a combination of external callus formation and enchondral ossification.

ETIOLOGY OF NONUNIONS

Predisposing Factors—Instability, Inadequate Vascularity, Poor Contact

The most basic requirements for fracture healing include (1) mechanical stability, (2) an adequate blood supply (i.e., bone vascularity), and (3) bone-to-bone contact. The absence of one or more of these factors predisposes the fracture to the development of a nonunion. The factors may be negatively affected by the severity of the injury, suboptimal surgical fixation resulting from either a poor plan or a good plan carried out poorly, or a combination of injury severity and suboptimal surgical fixation.

INSTABILITY

Mechanical instability, excessive motion at the fracture site, can follow internal or external fixation. Factors producing mechanical instability include inadequate fixation (implants too small or too few), distraction of the fracture surfaces (hardware is as capable of holding bone apart as holding bone together), bone loss, and poor bone quality (i.e., poor purchase) (Fig. 22-1). If an adequate blood supply exists, excessive motion at the fracture site results in abundant callus formation, widening of the fracture line, failure of fibrocartilage to mineralize, and ultimately failure to unite.

INADEQUATE VASCULARITY

Loss of blood supply to the fracture surfaces may arise because of the severity of the injury or because of surgical dissection. Several studies have shown a relationship between the extent of soft tissue injury and the rate of fracture nonunion.[50,62,124] Open fractures and high-energy closed injuries may strip soft tissues, damage the periosteal blood supply, and disrupt the nutrient vessels, impairing the endosteal blood supply.

Injury of certain vessels, such as the posterior tibial artery, may also increase risk of nonunion.[34] Vascularity may also be compromised by excess stripping of the periosteum as well as damage to bone and the soft tissues during open reduction and hardware insertion. Whatever the cause, inadequate vascularity results in necrotic bone at the ends of the fracture fragments. These necrotic surfaces inhibit fracture healing and often result in fracture nonunion.

POOR BONE CONTACT

Poor bone-to-bone contact at the fracture site may result from soft tissue interposition, malposition or malalignment of the fracture fragments, bone loss, and distraction of the fracture fragments (see Fig. 22-1). Whatever the cause, poor bone-to-bone contact compromises mechanical stability and creates a defect. The probability of fracture union decreases as defects increase in size. The threshold value for rapid bridging of cortical defects via direct osteonal healing, the so-called osteoblastic jumping distance, is approximately 1 mm in rabbits[291] but varies from species to species. Larger cortical defects may also heal, but at a much slower rate and bridge via woven bone. The "critical defect" represents the distance between fracture surfaces that will not be bridged by bone without intervention. The critical defect size depends on a variety of injury-related factors and varies considerably among species.

Other Contributing Factors

In addition to mechanical instability, inadequate vascularity, and poor bone contact, other factors may contribute to development of nonunion (Table 22-2). These factors, however, are not direct causes of nonunion per se.

INFECTION

Infection in the zone of fracture increases the risk of nonunion.[124] Infection of the bone or the surrounding soft tissues can create the same local environment that predisposes noninfected fractures to fail to unite. Infection may result in instability at the fracture site as implants loosen in infected bone. Avascular, necrotic bone at the fracture site (sequestrum), common with infection, discourages bony union. Infection also produces poor bony contact as osteolysis at the fracture site results from ingrowth of infected granulation tissue.

NICOTINE/CIGARETTE SMOKING

Cigarette smoking adversely affects fracture healing. Nicotine inhibits vascular ingrowth and early revascularization of bone[65,256] and diminishes osteoblast function.[76,96,248] In rabbit models, cigarette smoking and nicotine impair bone healing in fractures,[247] in spinal fusion,[298,337] and during tibial lengthening.[315,316]

Delayed fracture healing and higher nonunion rates have been reported in patients who smoke. In 146 closed and type I open tibial shaft fractures, Schmitz et al.[293] reported a significant delay of fracture healing in smokers. Similarly, Kyrö et al.[171] and Adams et al.[4] reported higher rates of delayed union and nonunion in smokers with tibia fractures. Hak et al.[122] reported a markedly higher rate of persistent femoral nonunion in smokers. Cobb et al.[58] reported an extremely high risk of nonunion of ankle arthrodesis in smokers. Cigarette smoking is also associated with osteoporosis and generalized bone loss,[244] so mechanical instability due to poor bone quality for purchase may play a role.

CERTAIN MEDICATIONS

Some animal studies have shown that nonsteroidal anti-inflammatory drugs (NSAIDs) negatively affect the healing of experimentally induced fractures and osteotomies.[8,9,38,92,134,157,181,265,305] Other animal studies have reported no significant effect.[138,204]

Delayed long-bone fracture healing has been documented in humans taking oral NSAIDs.[39,110,161] Giannoudis et al.[110] reported a marked association between NSAID use and delayed fracture healing and nonunion in fractures of the femoral diaphysis. Butcher and Marsh[39] reported similar findings for tibia fractures, as did Khan[161] for clavicle fractures. While a body of literature suggests that NSAIDs are a factor in delayed fracture healing, no consensus exists. Furthermore, the mechanism of action (direct action at the fracture site vs. indirect hormonal actions) remains obscure. Finally, whether all NSAIDs display similar effects and the dose-response characteristics

---

FIGURE 22-1 *Mechanical instability at the fracture site can lead to nonunion. Mechanical instability can be caused by the following.* **A, Inadequate fixation**. *A 33-year-old man had a femoral shaft nonunion 8 months following inadequate fixation with flexible intramedullary nails.* **B, Distraction**. *A 19-year-old man with a tibia fracture treated with plate-and-screw fixation; this patient is at risk for nonunion because of distraction at the fracture site.*

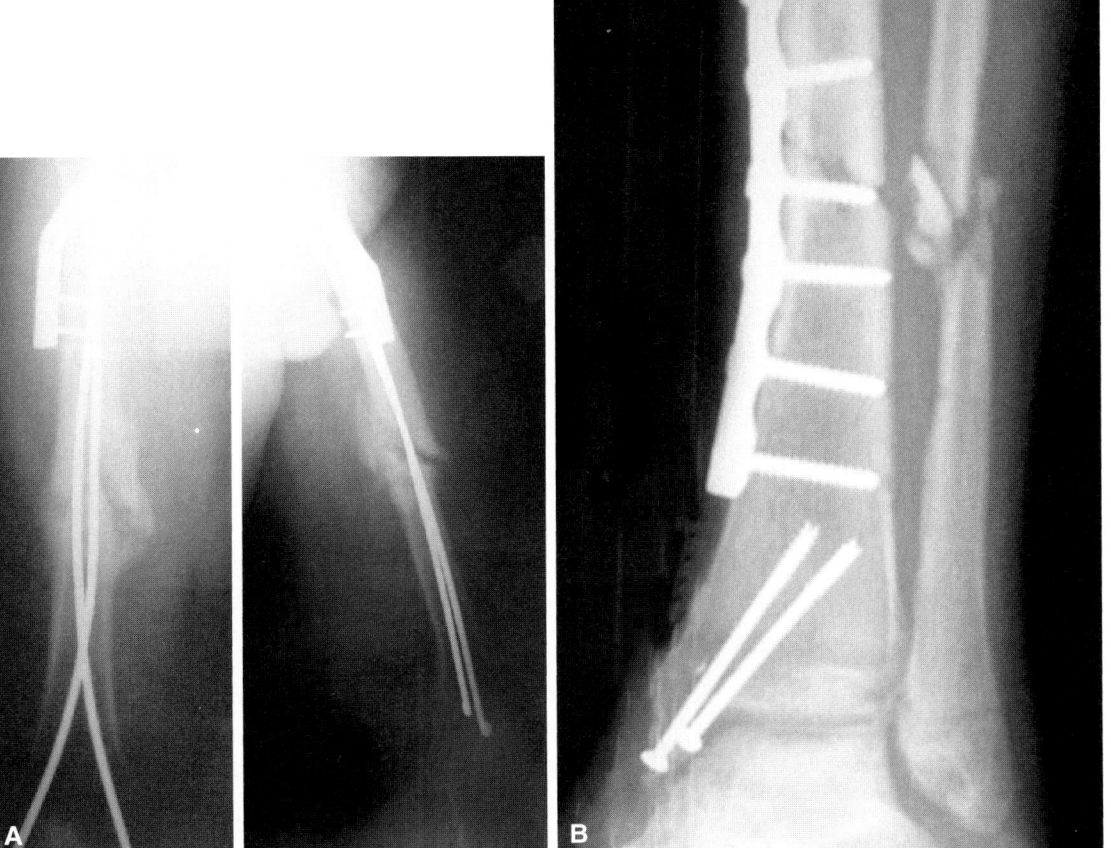

(Continued)

FIGURE 22-1   *(Continued)* **C, Bone loss**. *A 57-year-old man had segmental bone loss following débridement of a high-energy open tibia fracture.* **D, Poor bone quality**. *A 31-year-old woman 2 years following open reduction internal fixation for an ulna shaft fracture; loss of fixation proved to be due to poor bone from chronic osteomyelitis.*

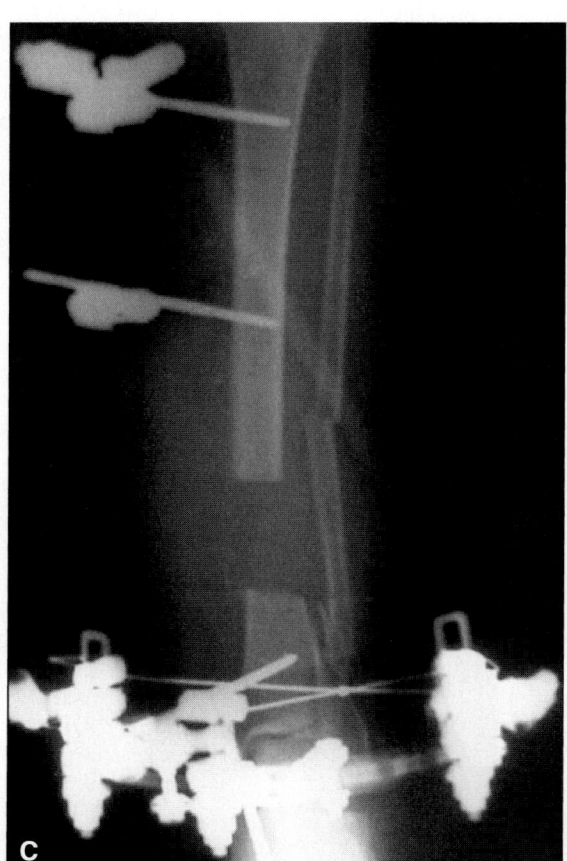

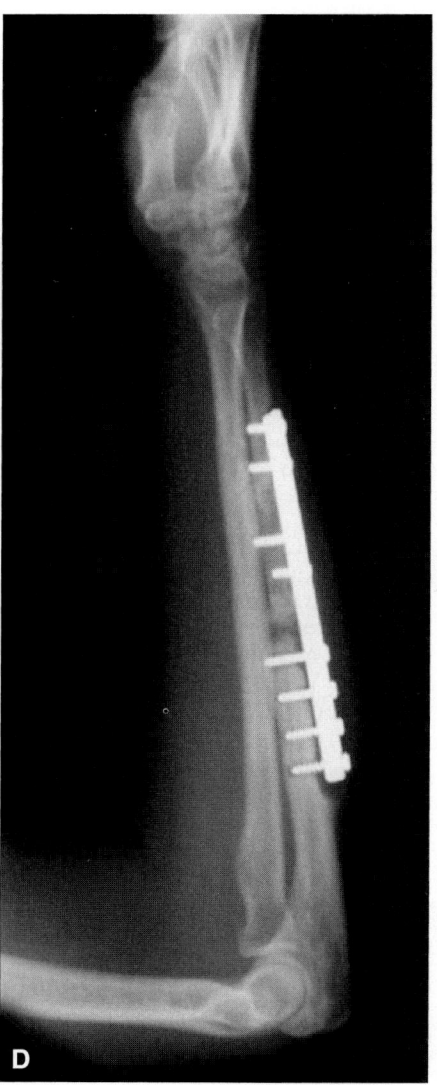

of specific NSAIDs relative to delayed union or nonunion remain unknown.

Other medications have been postulated to affect fracture healing adversely, including phenytoin,[125] ciprofloxacin,[136] corticosteroids, anticoagulants, and others.

OTHER CONTRIBUTING FACTORS

Other factors that may retard fracture healing or contribute to fracture nonunion include advanced age,[125,171,271] systemic medical conditions (such as diabetes),[104,236] poor functional level with inability to bear weight, venous stasis, burns, irradiation, obesity,[102] alcohol abuse,[102,104,236] metabolic bone disease, malnutrition and cachexia, and vitamin deficiencies.[78]

Animal studies (in rats) have shown that albumin deficiency produces a fracture callus with reduced strength and stiffness,[242] although early fracture healing proceeds normally.[88] Dietary supplementation of protein during fracture repair reverses these effects and augments fracture healing.[73,88] Protein intake in excess of normal daily requirements is not beneficial.[117,242] Inadequate caloric intake, such as occurs among the elderly, also contributes to failure of fracture union.[303]

EVALUATION OF NONUNIONS

No two patients with fracture nonunion are identical. The evaluation process is perhaps the most critical step in the patient's treatment pathway and is when the surgeon begins to form opinions about how to heal the nonunion. The goals of the evaluation are to discover the etiology of the nonunion and form a plan for healing the nonunion.

Table 22-2
Causes of Nonunions

Predisposing Factors

Mechanical instability
  Inadequate fixation
  Distraction
  Bone loss
  Poor bone quality

Inadequate vascularity
  Severe injury
  Excessive soft tissue stripping
  Vascular injury

Poor bone contact
  Soft tissue interposition
  Malposition or malalignment
  Bone loss
  Distraction

Contributing Factors

Infection

Nicotine/cigarette smoking

Certain medications

Advanced age

Systemic medical conditions

Poor functional level

Venous stasis

Burns

Irradiation

Obesity

Alcohol abuse

Metabolic bone disease

Malnutrition

Vitamin deficiencies

Without an understanding of the etiology, the treatment strategy cannot be based on knowledge of fracture biology. A worksheet is an excellent method of assimilating the various data (Fig. 22-2).

Patient History

Evaluation begins with a thorough history, including the date and mechanism of injury of the initial fracture. Preinjury medical problems, disabilities, or associated injuries should be noted. The patient should be questioned regarding pain and functional limitations related to the nonunion. The specific details of each prior surgical procedure to treat the fracture and fracture nonunion must be obtained through the patient and family, the prior treating surgeons, and a review of all medical records since the time of the initial fracture.

Knowledge of prior operative procedures is empowering and critical for designing the right treatment plan. Conversely, ignorance of any prior surgical procedure can lead to needlessly repeating surgical procedures that have failed to promote bony union in the past. Worse yet, ignorance of prior surgical procedures can lead to avoidable complications. For example, awareness of the prior use of external fixation is important when the use of intramedullary nail fixation is contemplated because of the increased risk of infection.[27,148,189,192,198,257,338]

The hospital records and operative reports from the time of the initial fracture may also be used to determine the condition of the tissues in the zone of the injury (open wounds, contamination, crush injuries, periosteal stripping, devitalized bone fragments, etc.) and the history of prior soft tissue coverage procedures.

The history should also include details regarding prior wound infections. Culture reports should be sought in the medical records. Intravenous and oral antibiotic use should be documented, particularly if the patient remains on antibiotics at the time of presentation. Problems with wound healing and episodes of soft tissue breakdown should be documented. Other perioperative complications (venous thrombosis, nerve or vessel injuries, etc.) should also be documented. The use of adjuvant nonsurgical therapies, such as electromagnetic field and ultrasound therapy, should be documented.

Finally, the patient should be questioned regarding other possible contributing factors for nonunion (see Table 22-2). A history of NSAID use should be obtained and its use discontinued. The pack-year history of cigarette smoking should be documented, and active smokers should be offered a program to halt the addiction. From a practical standpoint, however, it is unrealistic to delay treatment of a symptomatic nonunion until the patient stops smoking.

Physical Examination

Following the history, a physical examination is performed. The general health and nutritional status of the patient should be assessed, since malnutrition and cachexia diminish fracture repair.[90,117,242,303] Arm muscle circumference is the best indicator of nutritional status. Obese patients with nonunions have unique management problems related to achieving mechanical stability in the presence of high loads and large soft tissue envelopes.[152]

The skin and soft tissues in the fracture zone should be inspected. The presence of active drainage, sinus formation, and deformity should be noted.

The nonunion site should be manually stressed to evaluate motion and pain. Generally, nonunions that display little or no clinically apparent motion have some callus formation and good vascularity at the fracture surfaces. Nonunions that display motion typically have poor callus formation but may have vascular or avascular fracture surfaces. Assessment of motion at a nonunion site is difficult in limbs with paired bones where one of the bones remains intact.

A neurovascular examination should be performed to document vascular insufficiency and motor or sensory dysfunction. Active and passive motion of the joints adjacent to the nonunion, both proximal and distal, should be performed. Not uncommonly, motion at the nonunion site diminishes motion at an adjacent joint. For example, patients with a long-standing distal tibial nonunion often have a fixed equinus contracture and limited ankle motion (Fig. 22-3). Similarly, patients with supracondylar humeral nonunions commonly have fibrous ankylosis of the elbow joint (Fig. 22-4). Such problems may alter both the treatment plan and the expectations for the ultimate functional outcome.

FIGURE 22-2 *Worksheet for patients with nonunions.*

GENERAL INFORMATION

Patient Name: _____   Age: _____   Gender: _____

Referring Physician: _____   Height: _____   Weight: _____

Injury (description): _____

Date of Injury: _____

Mechanism of Injury: _____   Pain (0 to 10 VAS): _____

Occupation: _____   Was Injury Work Related?: Y   N

PAST HISTORY

Initial Fracture Treatment (Date): _____

Total # of Surgeries for Nonunion: _____

    Surgery #1 (Date): _____

    Surgery #2 (Date): _____

    Surgery #3 (Date): _____

    Surgery #4 (Date): _____

    Surgery #5 (Date): _____

    Surgery #6 (Date): _____

    (Use backside of this sheet for other prior surgeries)

Use of Electromagnetic or Ultrasound Stimulation? _____

Cigarette Smoking   # of packs per day _____   # of years smoking _____

History of Infection? (include culture results) _____

History of Soft Tissue Problems? _____

Medical Conditions: _____

Medications: _____

NSAID Use: _____

Narcotic Use: _____

Allergies: _____

PHYSICAL EXAMINATION

General: _____

Extremity:

    Nonunion: _____ Stiff   _____ Lax

    Adjacent Joints (ROM, compensatory deformities): _____

    Soft Tissues (defects, drainage): _____

    Neurovascular Exam: _____

RADIOLOGIC EXAMINATION

    Comments _____

OTHER PERTINENT INFORMATION _____

_____

_____

NONUNION TYPE

    _____ Hypertrophic

    _____ Oligotrophic

    _____ Atrophic

    _____ Infected

    _____ Synovial Pseudarthrosis

An interesting situation worth noting is the stiff nonunion with an angular deformity. These patients may already have developed a compensatory fixed deformity at an adjacent joint. The fixed deformity at the joint must be recognized preoperatively, and the treatment plan must include its correction. Realigning a stiff nonunion with a deformity without addressing an adjacent compensatory joint deformity results in a straight bone with a deformed joint, thus producing a disabled limb. For example, patients who have a stiff distal tibial nonunion with a varus deformity often develop a compensatory valgus deformity at the subtalar joint to achieve a plantigrade foot for gait. Upon visual inspection, the distal limb segment appears aligned, but radiographs show the distal tibial varus deformity. To determine whether the subtalar joint deformity is fixed or mobile (reducible), the patient is asked to position the subtalar joint in varus (i.e., invert the foot). If the patient cannot invert the subtalar joint, and the examiner cannot passively invert the subtalar joint, the joint deformity is fixed. Deformity correction will therefore be required at both the nonunion site and the subtalar joint. On the other hand, if the patient can achieve subtalar inversion, the deformity at the joint will resolve with deformity correction at the nonunion. In summary, if the patient cannot place the joint into the position that parallels the deformity at the nonunion site, the joint deformity is fixed and requires correction. If the patient can achieve the position, the joint deformity will resolve with realignment of the long bone deformity (Fig. 22-5).

FIGURE 22-3 *A 20-year-old woman had a distal tibial nonunion 22 months following a high-energy open fracture.* **A,** *Clinical photograph.* **B,** *Lateral radiograph showing apex anterior angulation at the fracture site resulting in the clinical equivalent of a severe equinus contracture.*

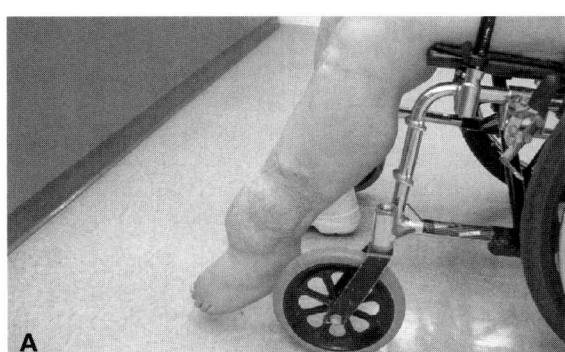

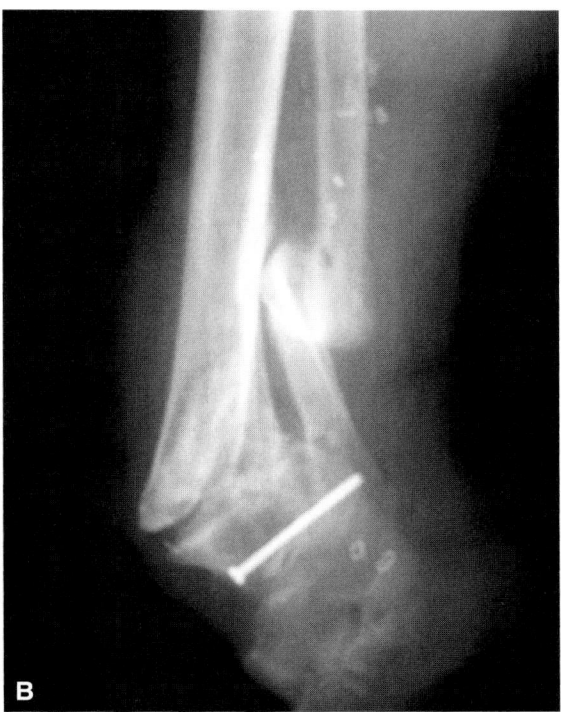

If bone grafting is contemplated, the anterior and posterior iliac crests should be examined for evidence (e.g., incisions) of prior surgical harvesting. In a patient who has had prior spinal surgery with a midline posterior incision, determining which posterior crest has already been harvested may be difficult. In such a case, the posterior iliac crests may be evaluated via plain radiographs or computed tomography (CT) scan.

Radiologic Examination

PLAIN RADIOGRAPHS

A review of the original fracture films reveals the character and severity of the initial bony injury. They can also show the progress or lack of progress toward healing when compared with the most recent plain radiographs.

Subsequent radiographs of the salient aspects of previous treatments will always tell the story of the nonunion. The story, however, may reveal itself only to the astute observer. The prior plain films should be carefully examined for the status of orthopaedic hardware (e.g., loose, broken, inadequate in size or number of implants), including removal or insertion, on subsequent films. The evolution of deformity at the nonunion site—whether a gradual process or single event, for instance—should be evaluated via the prior radiographs. The presence of healed or unhealed articular, butterfly, and wedge fragments should also be noted. The time course of missing or removed bony fragments, added bone graft, and implanted bone stimulators should be reconstructed so that the subsequent fracture repair response can be evaluated.

The nonunion is next evaluated with current radiographs, including an anteroposterior (AP) and lateral radiograph of the involved bone, including the proximal and distal joints; AP, lateral, and two oblique views of the nonunion site on small cassette films, which improve magnification and resolution (Fig. 22-6); bilateral AP and lateral 51-in. alignment radiographs for lower extremity nonunions (for assessing length discrepancies and deformities) (Fig. 22-7); and flexion/extension lateral radiographs to determine the arc of motion and to assess the relative contributions of the joint and the nonunion site to that arc of motion.

The current plain films are used to evaluate the following radiographic characteristics of a nonunion: anatomic location, healing effort, bone quality, surface characteristics, status of previously implanted hardware, and deformities.

ANATOMIC LOCATION Diaphyseal nonunions involve primarily cortical bone, whereas metaphyseal and epiphyseal nonunions largely involve cancellous bone. The presence or absence of intra-articular extension of the nonunion should also be evaluated.

HEALING EFFORT AND BONE QUALITY The radiographic healing effort and bone quality help define the biological and mechanical etiologies of the nonunion. The assessment of healing includes evaluating radiolucent lines, gaps, and callus formation. The assessment of bone quality includes observing sclerosis, atrophy, osteopenia, and bony defects.

Radiolucent lines seen along fracture surfaces suggest regions that are devoid of bony healing. The simple

FIGURE 22-4 | *A, Anteroposterior (AP) radiograph of a 32-year-old man with a supracondylar humeral nonunion. On physical examination it can be difficult to differentiate motion at the nonunion site and the elbow joint. This patient had very limited range of motion at the elbow but gross motion at the nonunion site. Cineradiography can be useful for evaluating the contribution of the adjacent joint and the nonunion site to the arc of motion. B and C, Cineradiographs showing flexion and extension of the elbow, respectively, reveal that most of the motion is occurring through the nonunion site, not the elbow joint. This patient should be counseled preoperatively regarding elbow stiffness following stabilization of the nonunion.*

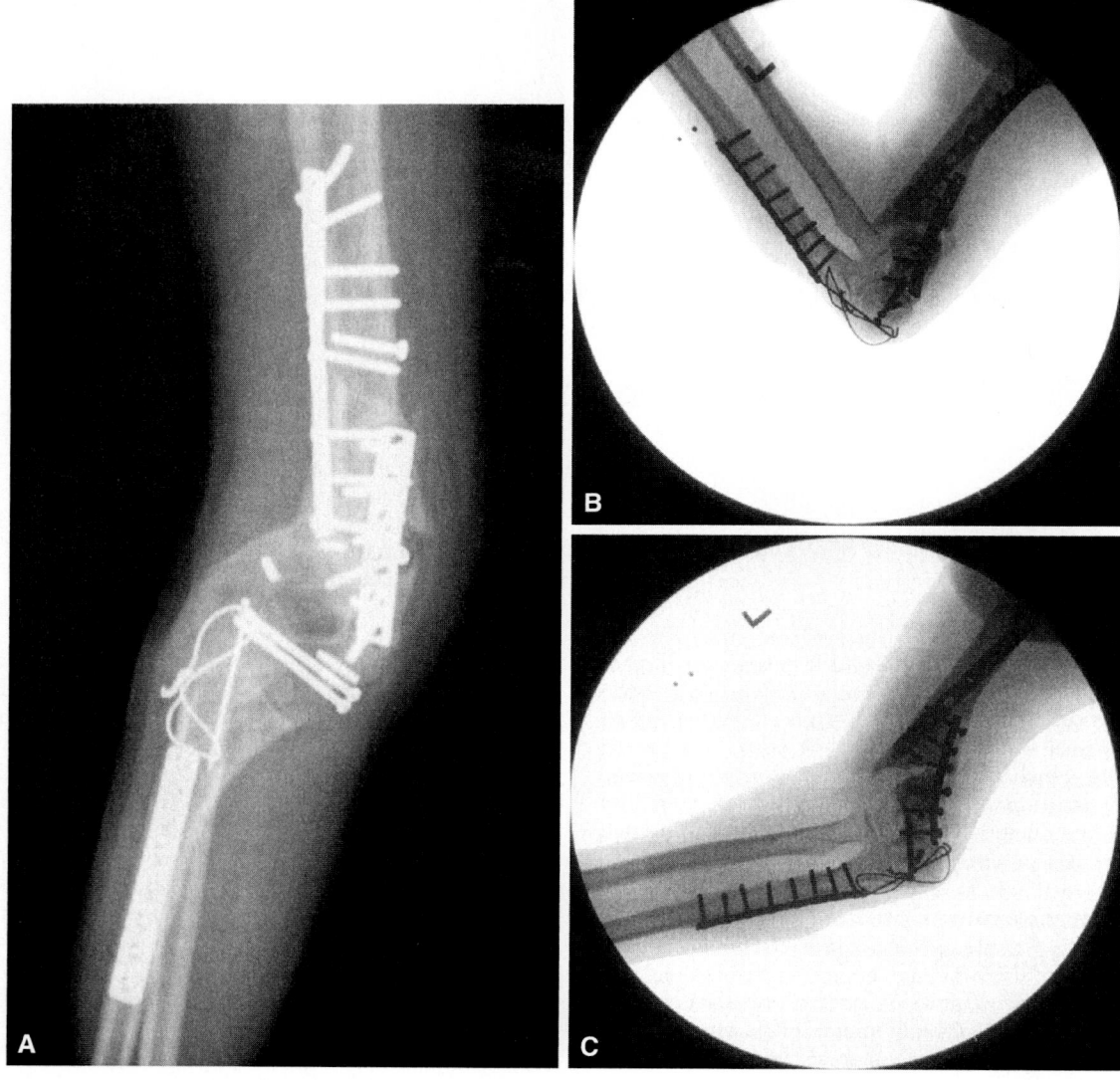

presence of radiolucent lines seen on plain radiographs is not synonymous with fracture nonunion. Conversely, the lack of a clear radiolucent line does not confer fracture union (Fig. 22-8).

Callus formation occurs in fractures and nonunions with an adequate blood supply but does not necessarily imply the bone is solidly uniting. AP, lateral, and oblique radiographs should be assessed for callus bridging the zone of injury. The radiographs should be carefully checked for radiolucent lines so that a nonunion with abundant callus is not mistaken for a solidly united fracture (see Fig. 22-8).

Weber and Cech[329] classify nonunions based on radiographic healing effort and bone quality as *viable nonunions*, which are capable of biological activity, and *nonviable nonunions*, which are incapable of biological activity.

Viable nonunions include *hypertrophic nonunions* and *oligotrophic nonunions*. Hypertrophic nonunions possess adequate vascularity and display callus formation. They arise as a result of inadequate mechanical stability with persistent motion at the fracture surfaces. The fracture site is progressively resorbed with accumulation of unmineralized fibrocartilage and displays a progressively widening

FIGURE 22-5   *Angular deformity at a nonunion site that is near a joint can result in a compensatory deformity through a neighboring joint. For example, coronal plane deformities of the distal tibia can result in a compensatory coronal plane deformity of the subtalar joint. A deformity of the subtalar joint is fixed if the patient's foot cannot be positioned into the deformity of the distal tibia (A) or flexible if it can be positioned into the deformity of the distal tibia (B). Sagittal plane deformities of the distal tibia can result in a sagittal plane deformity of the ankle joint. A deformity of the ankle joint is fixed if the patient's foot cannot be positioned into the deformity of the distal tibia (C) or flexible if it can be positioned into the deformity of the distal tibia (D).*

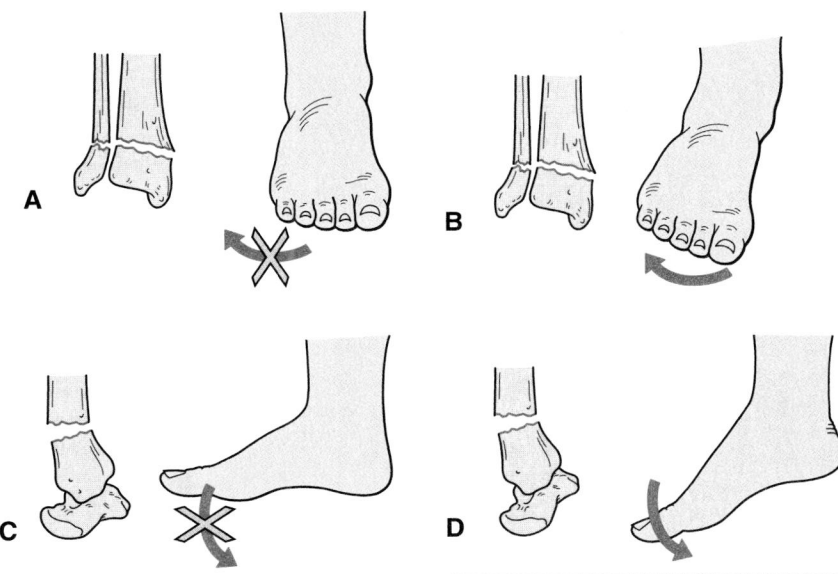

FIGURE 22-7   *A 60-year-old man with a tibial nonunion and an oblique plane angular deformity as seen on the 51-in. AP alignment view (A) and 51-in. lateral alignment view (B).*

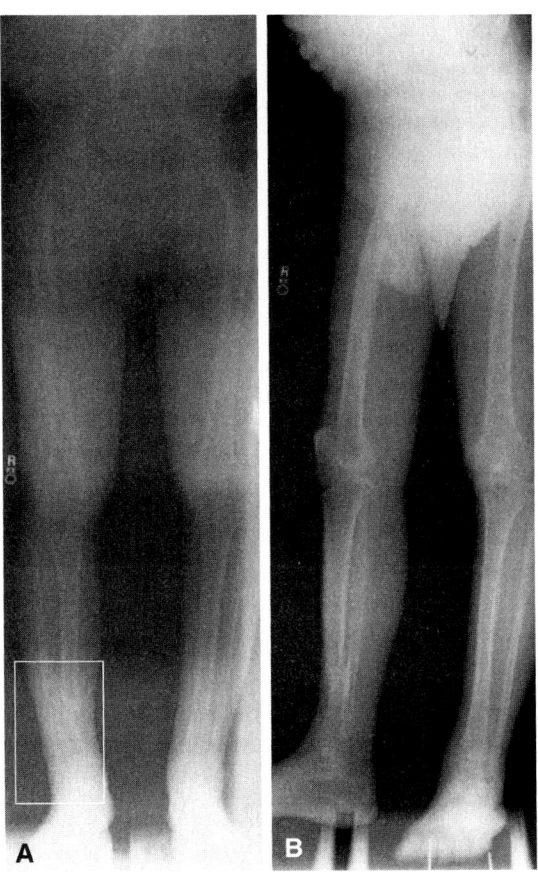

FIGURE 22-6   *A nonunion is visualized better on small cassette views than on large cassette views (see Fig. 22-7 for comparison).*

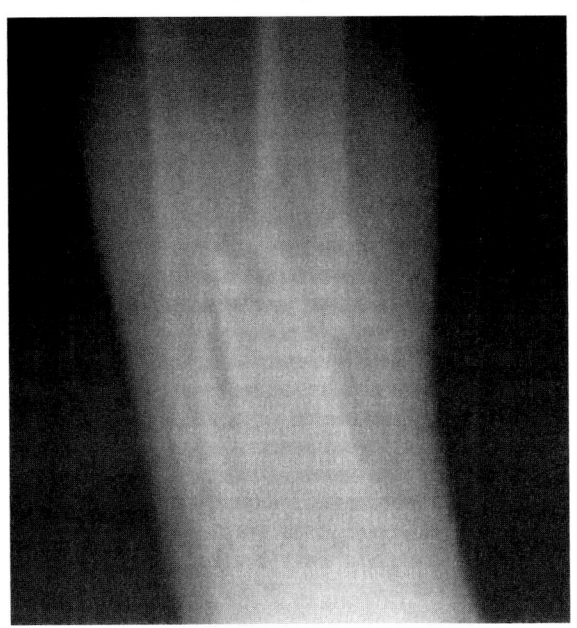

FIGURE 22-8 | *A definitive decision cannot always be made about bony union based on plain radiographs.* **A,** *An 88-year-old woman 14 months following a distal tibial fracture treated with external fixation. AP and lateral radiographs are shown. Is this fracture healed, or is there a nonunion? (See Fig. 22-17.)* **B,** *A 49-year-old man 13 months after open reduction internal fixation of a distal tibia fracture. AP and lateral radiographs are shown. Is this fracture healed or is there a nonunion? (See Fig. 22-17.)*

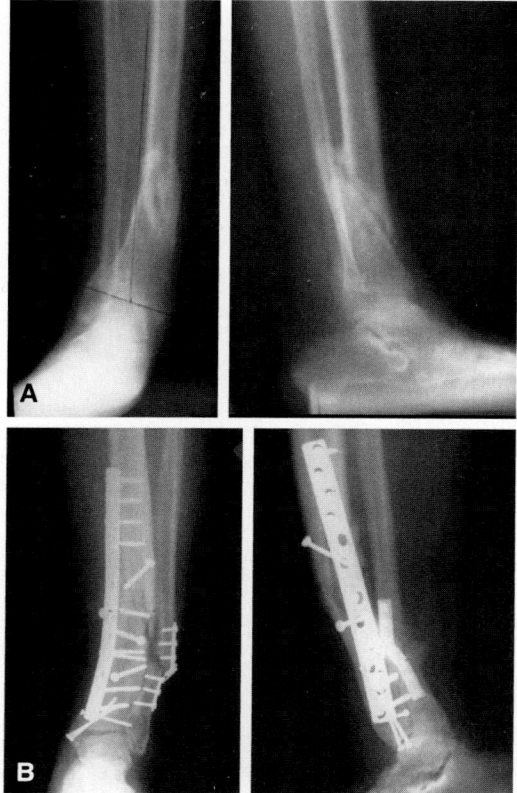

FIGURE 22-9 | *Microangiogram of a hypertrophic delayed union of a canine radius. Note the tremendous increase in local vascularity. The capillaries, however, are unable to penetrate the interposed fibrocartilage (arrows). (From Rhinelander, F.W. The normal microcirculation of diaphyseal cortex and its response to fracture. J Bone Joint Surg Am 50:784–800, 1968.)*

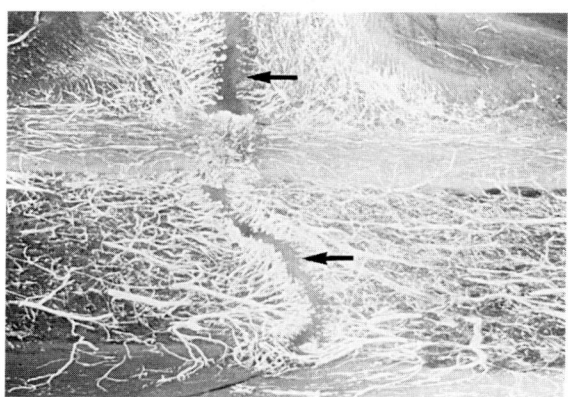

radiolucent line with sclerotic edges. The reason that persistent motion inhibits calcification of fibrocartilage remains obscure.[237] Capillaries and blood vessels invade both sides of the nonunion but do not penetrate the fibrocartilaginous tissue (Fig. 22-9).[252] Since motion persists at the nonunion site, endosteal callus may accumulate and seal off the medullary canal, increasing production of hypertrophic periosteal callus. Hypertrophic nonunions may be classified as *elephant foot type*, with abundant callus formation, or *horse hoof type*, which are still hypertrophic but with less abundant callus formation.

Oligotrophic nonunions have an adequate blood supply but little or no callus formation. Oligotrophic nonunions arise from inadequate reduction with displacement at the fracture site.

Nonviable nonunions do not display callus formation and are incapable of biological activity. Their inadequate vascularity precludes the formation of periosteal and endosteal callus. The radiolucent gap observable on plain radiographs is bridged by fibrous tissue that has no osteogenic capacity. An *atrophic nonunion* is the most advanced type of nonviable nonunion. Classically, the ends of the bony surfaces have been thought to be avascular, although a recent study has questioned this conventional wisdom.[37,249] Radiographically, the fracture surfaces appear partially absorbed and osteopenic. Severe cases may show large sclerotic avascular bone segments or segmental bone loss.

SURFACE CHARACTERISTICS A nonunion's surface characteristics (Fig. 22-10) are prognostic in regard to its resistance to healing with various treatment strategies. Surface characteristics that should be evaluated on plain radiographs include the surface area of adjacent fragments, extent of current bony contact, orientation of the fracture lines (shape of the bone fragments), and stability to axial compression (a function of fracture surface orientation and comminution). The nonunions that are generally the easiest to treat have good bony contact and large, transversely oriented surfaces that are stable to axial compression.

STATUS OF PREVIOUSLY IMPLANTED HARDWARE Plain radiographs reveal the status of previously implanted hardware and thus the stability of the mechanical construct used to fixate the bone. Loose or broken implants denote instability at the nonunion site (i.e., the race between bony union and hardware failure has been lost),[209,226,267–270,273,275] which requires further stabilization before union can occur. Radiographs are also useful in terms of planning which hardware will need to be removed to carry out the next treatment plan.

DEFORMITIES After assessment is performed for clinical deformity via physical examination, plain radiographs are used to further and more fully characterize all other deformities associated with the fracture nonunion. Deformities are characterized by location (diaphyseal, metaphyseal,

FIGURE 22-10 *Surface characteristics at the site of nonunion.* **A,** *Surface area.* **B,** *Bone contact.* **C,** *Fracture line orientation.* **D,** *Stability to axial compression.*

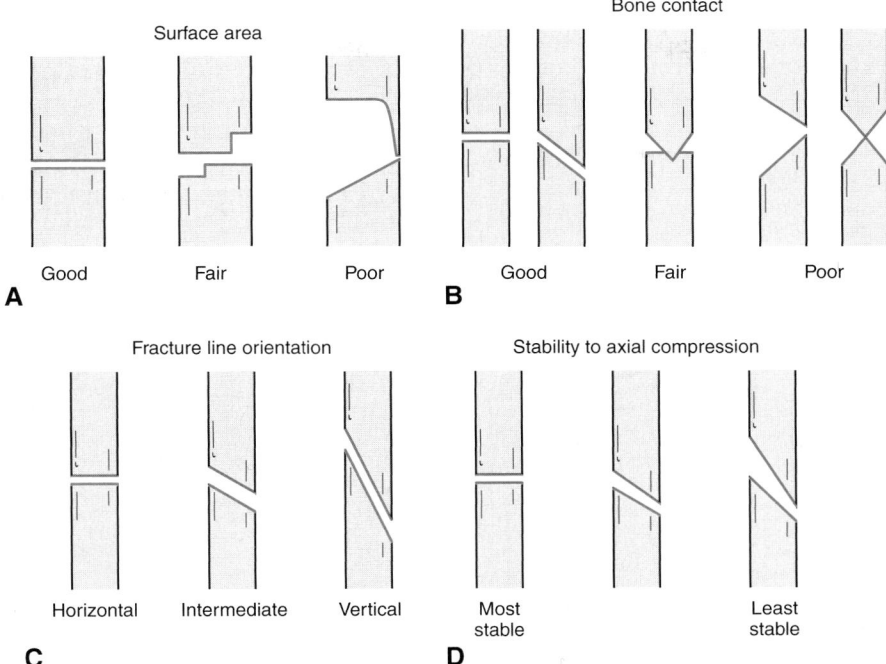

Surface area

Good   Fair   Poor

A

Bone contact

Good   Fair   Poor

B

Fracture line orientation

Horizontal   Intermediate   Vertical

C

Stability to axial compression

Most   Least
stable   stable

D

epiphyseal), magnitude, and direction and are described in terms of length, angulation, rotation, and translation.[219]

Deformities involving length include shortening and overdistraction. They are measured in centimeters on plain radiographs by comparison to the contralateral normal extremity, using an x-ray marker to correct for magnification. Shortening may result from bone loss (from the injury or débridement) or overriding fracture fragments (malreduction). Overdistraction may result from a traction injury or improper positioning at the time of surgical fixation.

Deformities involving angulation are characterized by magnitude and direction of the apex of angulation. Pure sagittal or coronal plane deformities are simple to characterize. When coronal plane angulation is present in the lower extremity, it commonly results in an abnormality to the mechanical axis of the extremity (mechanical axis deviation) (Fig. 22-11). Varus deformities result in medial mechanical axis deviation, and valgus deformities in lateral mechanical axis deviation.

Oblique plane angular deformities occur in a single plane that is neither the sagittal nor the coronal plane. Oblique plane angular deformities can be characterized using either the trigonometric method or the graphic method (see Fig. 22-11).[33,133,221–223]

Angulation at a diaphyseal nonunion is usually obvious on plain radiographs. The angulation results in divergence of the anatomic axes (mid-diaphyseal lines) of the proximal and distal fragments (see Fig. 22-11). The magnitude and direction of angulation can be measured by drawing the anatomic axes of the proximal and distal segments (see Fig. 22-11).

Angular deformities associated with nonunions of the metaphysis and epiphysis (juxta-articular deformities) may not be so obvious and are not so simple to evaluate as diaphyseal deformities. The mid-diaphyseal line method will not characterize a juxta-articular deformity. Recognition and characterization of a juxta-articular deformity require using the angle formed by the intersection of a joint orientation line and the anatomic or mechanical axis of the deformed bone (Fig. 22-12). When the angle formed differs markedly from the contralateral normal extremity, a juxta-articular deformity is present. If the contralateral extremity is also abnormal (e.g., bilateral injuries), the normal values described for the lower extremity are used (Table 22-3).[35,223]

The center of rotation of angulation (CORA) is the point at which the axis of the proximal segment intersects the axis of the distal segment (Fig. 22-13).[219] For diaphyseal deformities, the anatomic axes are convenient to use. For juxta-articular deformities, the axis line of the short segment is constructed using one of three methods: extending the segment axis from the adjacent, intact bone if its anatomy is normal; comparing the joint orientation angle of the abnormal side to the opposite side if the latter is normal; or drawing a line that creates the population normal angle formed by the intersection with the joint orientation line.

The bisector is a line that passes through the CORA and bisects the angle formed by the proximal and distal axes (see Fig. 22-13).[219] Angular correction along the bisector results in complete deformity correction without the introduction of a translational deformity.[33,221–223]

Rotational deformities associated with a nonunion may be missed on physical and radiologic examination because attention is focused on more obvious problems (un-united bone, pain, infection, etc). Accurate clinical assessment of the magnitude of a rotational deformity is difficult, and plain x-rays offer little assistance. The best method of radiographic assessment of malrotation is described below in the CT scanning section.

FIGURE 22-11   *A, Nonunion of the diaphysis of the tibia with a varus deformity resulting in medial mechanical axis deviation (MAD). Note the divergence of the anatomic axis of the proximal and distal fragments of the tibia. B, Close-up view of a section of an AP 51-in. alignment radiograph of a 37-year-old woman with an 18-year history of a tibial nonunion. Note the medial mechanical axis deviation of 26 mm. C, AP and lateral radiographs show a 25° varus deformity and a 21° apex anterior angulation deformity, respectively. D, Characterization of the oblique plane angular deformity using the trigonometric method. E, Characterization of the oblique plane angular deformity using the graphic method.*

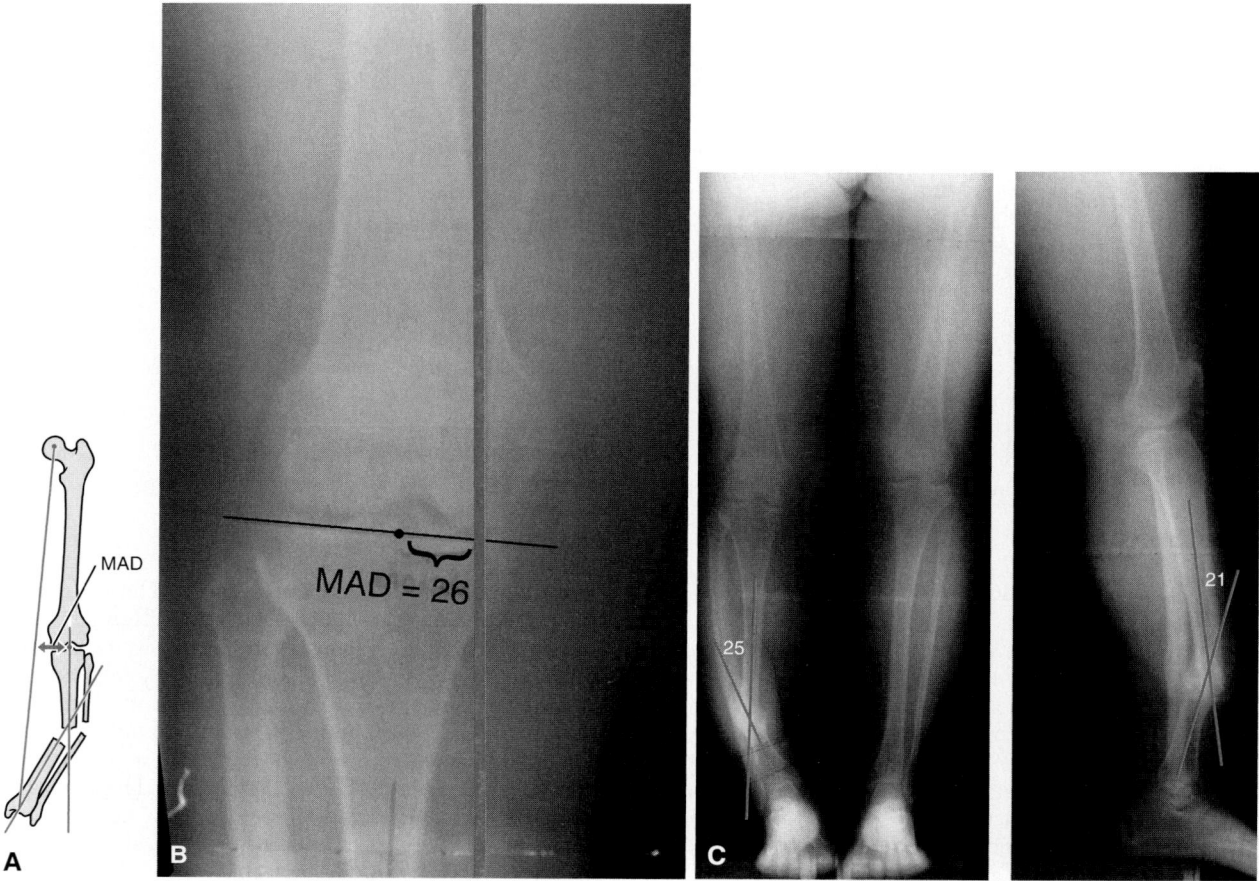

Trigonometric Method

Magnitude of oblique plane deformity =

$$\tan^{-1}\sqrt{\tan^2 \text{ coronal deformity} + \tan^2 \text{ sagittal deformity}}$$

$$\tan^{-1}\sqrt{\tan^2\ 25° + \tan^2\ 21°}$$

Solution = 31°

Orientation of oblique plane deformity =

$$\tan^{-1}\frac{\tan \text{ sagittal deformity}}{\tan \text{ coronal deformity}}$$

$$\tan^{-1}\frac{\tan\ 21°}{\tan\ 25°}$$

Solution = 39°

Graphic Method

Magnitude of oblique plane deformity =

$$\sqrt{\text{Coronal deformity}^2 + \text{Sagittal deformity}^2}$$

$$\sqrt{25^2 + 21^2}$$

Solution = 33°

Orientation of oblique plane deformity =

$$\tan^{-1}\frac{\text{Sagittal deformity}}{\text{Coronal deformity}}$$

$$\tan^{-1}\frac{21°}{25°}$$

Solution = 40°

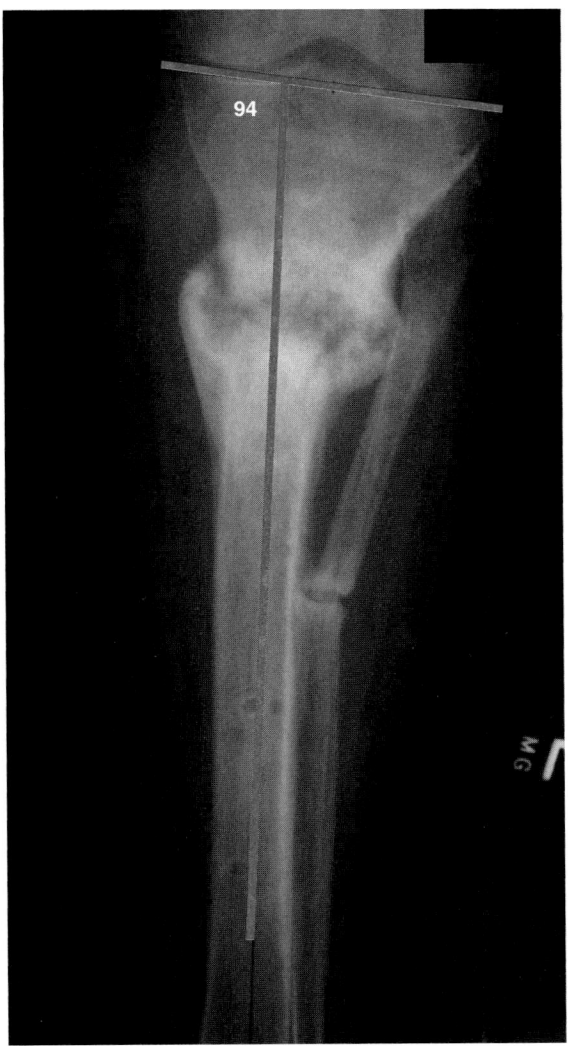

FIGURE 22-12 *Nonunion of the proximal tibia with a valgus deformity resulting in lateral mechanical axis deviation. The proximal medial tibial angle of 94° is abnormally high compared to both the contralateral normal extremity and the population normal values (see Table 22-3).*

deformities of the joints adjacent to the nonunion. In some cases, these compensatory deformities are clinically apparent, but not always. As previously stated, failure to recognize and correct the compensatory joint deformity leads to a healed and straight bone with suboptimal functional improvement.

Radiographic analysis should therefore be performed at adjacent joints when a deformity is present at the site of a nonunion. This is particularly important for a tibial nonunion with a coronal plane angular deformity because a compensatory deformity at the subtalar joint is not only common but commonly missed. Varus tibial deformities result in compensatory subtalar valgus deformities, and valgus tibial deformities result in compensatory subtalar varus deformities. Compensatory subtalar joint deformities are evaluated using the extended Harris view of both lower extremities, which allows measurement of the orientation of the calcaneus relative to the tibial shaft in the coronal plane (Fig. 22-16).

COMPUTED AND PLAIN TOMOGRAPHY

Plain radiographs are not always sufficient regarding the status of fracture healing. Sclerotic bone and orthopaedic hardware may obscure the fracture site, particularly in stiff nonunions or those well-stabilized by hardware.[26] CT scans and tomography are useful in such cases (Fig. 22-17). CT scans can be used to estimate the percentage of the cross-sectional area that shows bridging bone (Fig. 22-18). Nonunions typically show bone bridging of less than 5 percent of the cross-sectional area at the fracture surfaces (see Fig. 22-18). Healed or healing fracture nonunions typically show bone bridging of greater than 25 percent of the cross-sectional area. Serial CT scans may be followed to evaluate the progression of fracture consolidation (see Fig. 22-18). CT scans are also useful for assessing intra-articular nonunions for articular step-off and joint incongruence.

Plain tomography helps evaluate the extent of bony union when hardware artifact compromises CT images.

Rotational deformities may be accurately quantified using CT by comparing the relative orientations of the proximal and distal segments of the involved bone to the contralateral normal bone. This technique has been mostly used for femoral malrotation[129,135,184] but may be used for any long bone.

NUCLEAR IMAGING

Several nuclear imaging studies are useful for assessing bone vascularity at the nonunion site, the presence of a synovial pseudarthrosis, and infection.

Technetium-99m–pyrophosphate ("bone scan") complexes reflect increased blood flow and bone metabolism and are absorbed onto hydroxyapatite crystals in areas of trauma, infection, and neoplasia. The bone scan will show increased uptake in viable nonunions because there is a good vascular supply and osteoblastic activity (Fig. 22-19).

A *synovial pseudarthrosis* (nearthrosis) is distinguished from a nonunion by the presence of a synovium-like fixed pseudocapsule surrounding a fluid-filled cavity. The medullary canals are sealed off, and motion occurs at this "false joint."[274,329] Synovial pseudarthrosis may arise in sites

Like angular deformities, translational deformities associated with a nonunion are characterized by magnitude and direction. The magnitude of translation is measured as the perpendicular distance from the axis line of the proximal fragment to the axis line of the distal fragment. With combined angulation and translation (where the fragments are not parallel), translation is measured at the level of the proximal end of the distal fragment (Fig. 22-14).

When both angular and translational deformities are present at a nonunion site, the CORA will be at different levels on AP and lateral radiographs (Fig. 22-15). When the deformity involves pure angulation (without translation), the CORA will be at the same level on both radiographs.

In addition to assessing bony deformities, the radiographic evaluation should identify any compensatory

			Table 22-3	
Normal Values[222,223] Used to Assess Lower Extremity Metaphyseal and Epiphyseal Deformities (Juxta-articular Deformities) Associated with Nonunions				
Anatomic Site of Deformity	**Plane**	**Angle**	**Description***	**Normal Values**
Proximal femur	Coronal	Neck shaft angle	Defines the relationship between the orientation of the femoral neck and the anatomic axis of the femur	130° (range, 124°–136°)
		Anatomic medial proximal femoral angle	Defines the relationship between the anatomic axis of the femur and a line drawn from the tip of the greater trochanter to the center of the femoral head	84° (range, 80°–89°)
		Mechanical lateral proximal femoral angle	Defines the relationship between the mechanical axis of the femur and a line drawn from the tip of the greater trochanter to the center of the femoral head	90° (range, 85°–95°)
Distal femur	Coronal	Anatomic lateral distal femoral angle	Defines the relationship between the distal femoral joint orientation line and the anatomic axis of the femur	81° (range, 79°–83°)
		Mechanical lateral distal femoral angle	Defines the relationship between the distal femoral joint orientation line and the mechanical axis of the femur	88° (range, 85°–90°)
	Sagittal	Anatomic posterior distal femoral angle	Defines the relationship between the sagittal distal femoral joint orientation line and the mid-diaphyseal line of the distal femur	83° (range, 79°–87°)
Proximal tibia	Coronal	Mechanical medial proximal tibial angle	Defines the relationship between the proximal tibial joint orientation line and the mechanical axis of the tibia	87° (range, 85°–90°)
	Sagittal	Anatomic posterior proximal tibial angle	Defines the relationship between the sagittal proximal tibial joint orientation line and the mid-diaphyseal line of the tibia	81° (range, 77°–84°)
Distal tibia	Coronal	Mechanical lateral distal tibial angle	Defines the relationship between the distal tibial joint orientation line and the mechanical axis of the tibia	89° (range, 88°–92°)
	Sagittal	Anatomic anterior distal tibial angle	Defines the relationship between the sagittal distal tibial joint orientation line and the mid-diaphyseal line of the tibia	80° (range, 78°–82°)

*Anatomic axes: femur, mid-diaphyseal line; tibia, mid-diaphyseal line. Mechanical axes: femur, defined by a line from the center of the femoral head to the center of the knee joint; tibia, defined by a line from the center of the knee joint to the center of the ankle joint; lower extremity, defined by a line from the center of the femoral head to the center of the ankle joint.

with hypertrophic vascular callus formation or in sites with poor callus formation and poor vascularity. The diagnosis of synovial pseudarthrosis is made when technetium-99m–pyrophosphate bone scans show a "cold cleft" at the nearthrosis between hot ends of un-united bone (see Fig. 22-19).[32,93,94,274]

Radiolabeled white blood cell scans (such as with indium-111 or technetium-99m-HMPAO [hexamethyl-propylene amine oxime]) are used for evaluating acute bone infection. Labeled polymorphonuclear leukocytes (PMNs) accumulate in areas of acute infections.

Gallium scans are useful in the evaluation of chronic bone infections. Gallium-67 citrate localizes to sites of chronic inflammation. The combination of gallium-67 citrate and technetium-99m sulfa colloid bone marrow scans can clarify the diagnosis of a chronically infected nonunion.

OTHER RADIOLOGIC STUDIES

Fluoroscopy and cineradiography (see Fig. 22-4) may be needed to determine the relative contribution of a joint and an adjacent nonunion to the overall arc of motion. Fluoroscopy is also helpful for guided needle aspiration of a nonunion site.

Ultrasonography is useful for assessing the status of the bony regenerate (distraction osteogenesis) during bone transport or lengthening. Fluid-filled cysts in the regenerate can be visualized and aspirated using ultrasound technology, thereby shortening the time of regenerate maturation (Fig. 22-20). Ultrasonography can also confirm the presence of a fluid-filled pseudocapsule when synovial pseudarthrosis is suspected.

Magnetic resonance imaging (MRI) is occasionally used to evaluate the soft tissues at the nonunion site or the cartilaginous and ligamentous structures of the adjacent joints.

Sinograms may be used to image the course of sinus tracts in infected nonunions.

Angiography provides anatomic detail of vessels as they course through a scarred and deformed limb. This study is unnecessary in most patients with a fracture nonunion but is indicated if the viability of the limb is in question.[114]

Preoperative venous Doppler studies should be used to rule out deep venous thrombosis in patients with a lower extremity nonunion who have been confined to a wheelchair or bedridden for an extended period. Intraoperative or postoperative recognition of a venous thrombus or an embolus in a patient who has not been screened preoperatively does not make for a happy patient, family, or orthopaedic surgeon.

Laboratory Studies

Routine laboratory work, including electrolytes and a complete blood count (CBC), are useful for screening general health. The sedimentation rate and C-reactive protein are useful in regard to the course of infection. If necessary, the nutritional status of the patient can be assessed via anergy panels, albumin levels, and transferrin levels. If wound-healing potential is in question, an albumin level (3.0 g/dL or more is preferred) and a total lymphocyte count (>1500 cells/mm^3 is preferred) can be obtained.

FIGURE 22-13 *The same case shown in Figure 22-11 with a diaphyseal nonunion with deformity. The center of rotation of angulation (CORA) and bisector are shown.*

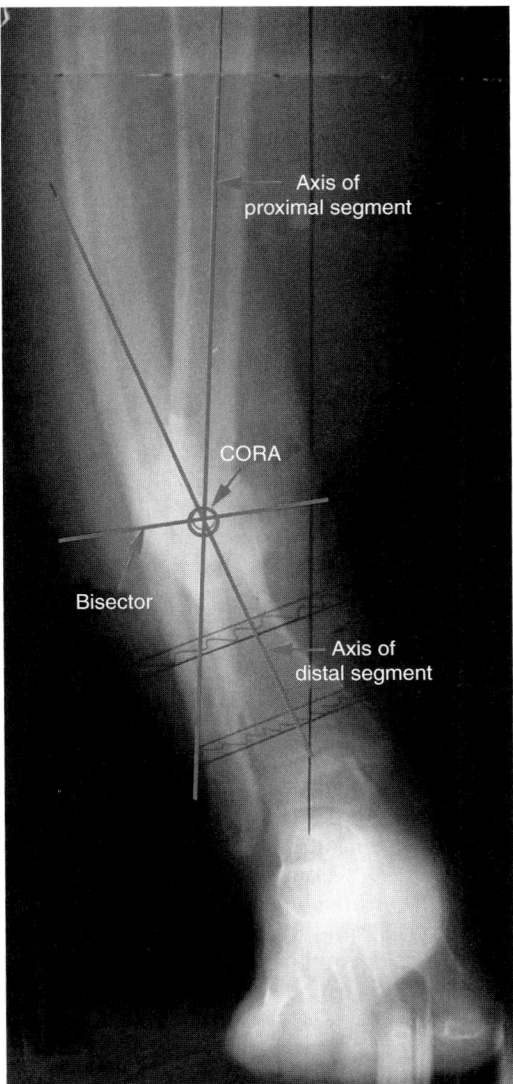

FIGURE 22-14 *Method for measuring translational deformities. The magnitude of translation is measured at the level of the proximal end of the distal fragment.*

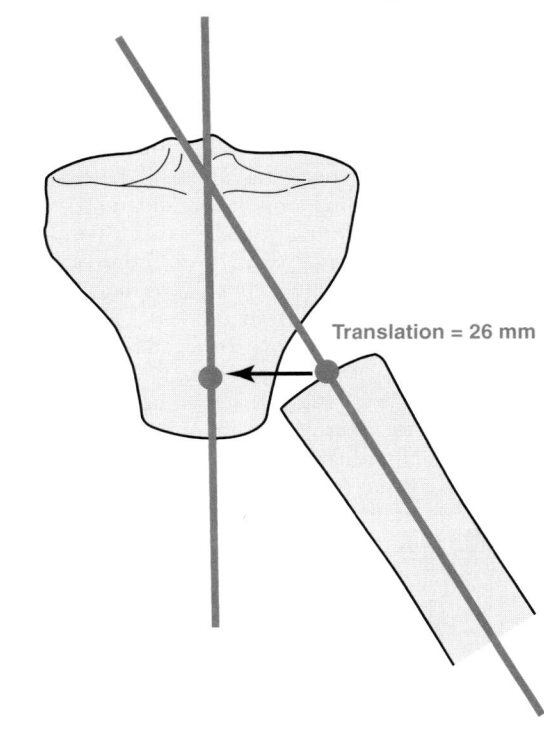

Translation = 26 mm

FIGURE 22-15 *A, When the deformity at the nonunion site involves angulation without translation, the center of rotation of angulation (CORA) will be seen at the same level on both AP and lateral radiographs. B, When the deformity at the nonunion site involves both angulation and translation, the CORA will be seen at a different level on AP and lateral radiographs.*

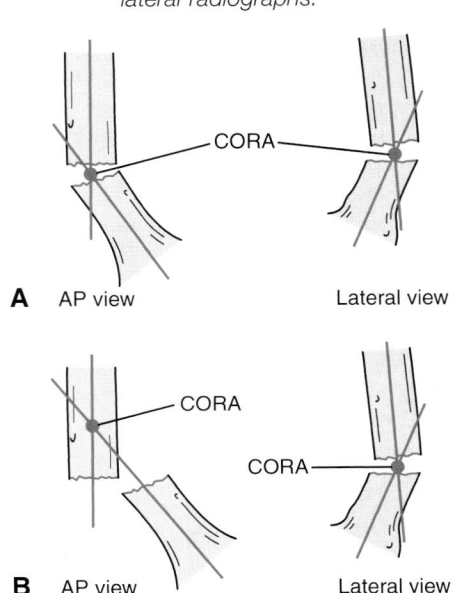

For patients with a history of multiple blood transfusions, a hepatitis panel and an HIV test may also be useful.

When infection is suspected, the nonunion site may be aspirated or biopsied under fluoroscopic guidance. The aspirated or biopsied material is sent for a cell count and gram staining, and cultures are done for aerobic, anaerobic, fungal, and acid-fast bacillus organisms. To encourage the highest yield possible, all antibiotics should be discontinued at least 2 weeks prior to aspiration.

Consultations

Many issues commonly accompany nonunion, including soft tissue problems, infection, chronic pain, depression, motor or sensory dysfunction, joint stiffness, and unrelated medical problems. A team of subspecialists usually is

FIGURE 22-16 | *The extended Harris view is performed to image the orientation of the hindfoot to the tibial shaft in the coronal plane.* **A,** *The patient is positioned lying supine on the x-ray table with the knee in full extension and the foot and ankle in maximal dorsiflexion. The x-ray tube is aimed at the calcaneus at a 45° angle with a tube distance of 60 in.* **B,** *AP radiograph of the tibia shows a distal tibial nonunion with a valgus deformity. This patient had been treated with an external fixator. In an effort to correct the distal tibial deformity, the hindfoot had been fixed in varus through the subtalar joint.* **C,** *On clinical inspection, this situation is not always obvious and can be missed.* **D,** *The extended Harris view of the normal left side as compared with the abnormal right side. Note the profound subtalar varus deformity of the right lower extremity. Both the distal tibial valgus deformity and the subtalar varus deformity must be corrected.*

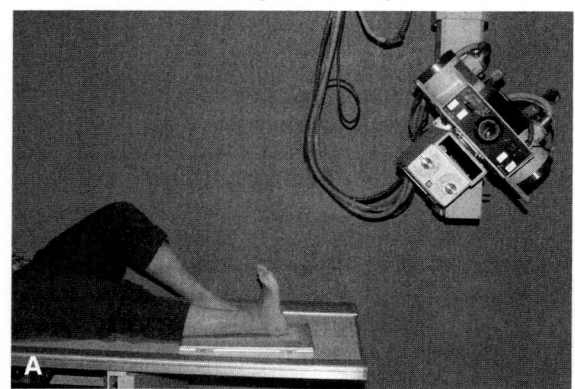

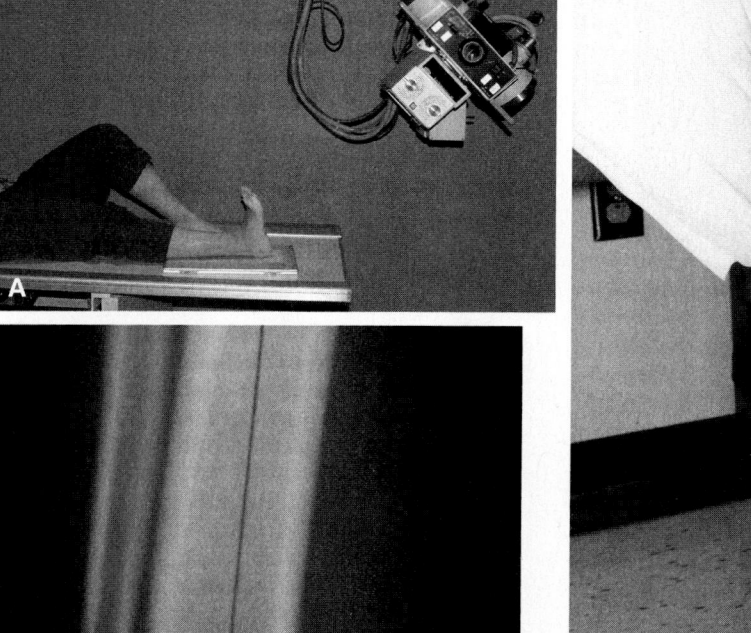

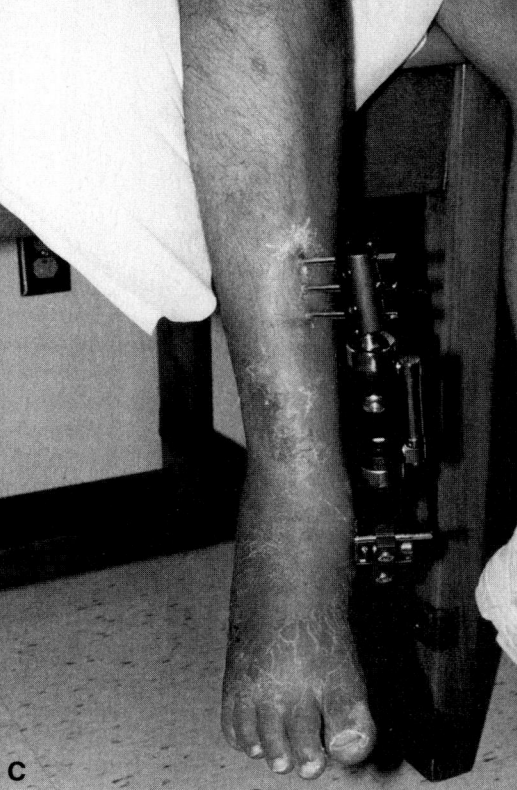

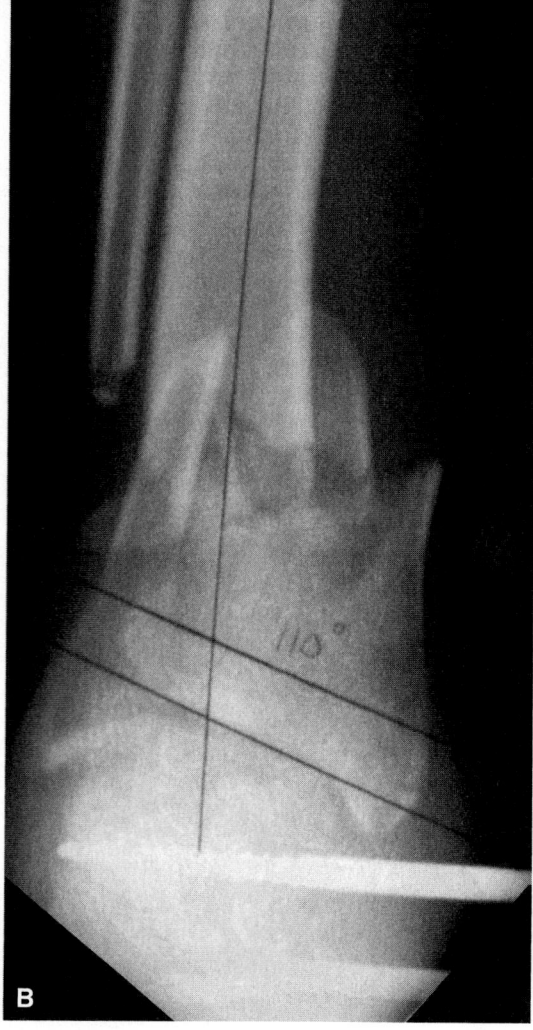

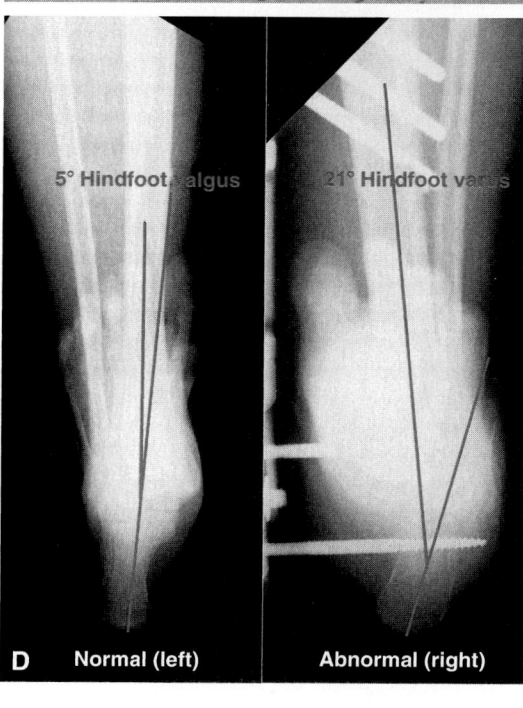

5° Hindfoot valgus   21° Hindfoot varus

D   **Normal (left)**   **Abnormal (right)**

FIGURE 22-17   ***A,*** *CT scan of the 88-year-old woman shown in Figure 22-8A shows that this fracture is healed.* ***B,*** *CT scan of the 49-year-old man shown in Figure 22-8B shows that this fracture has gone on to nonunion.*

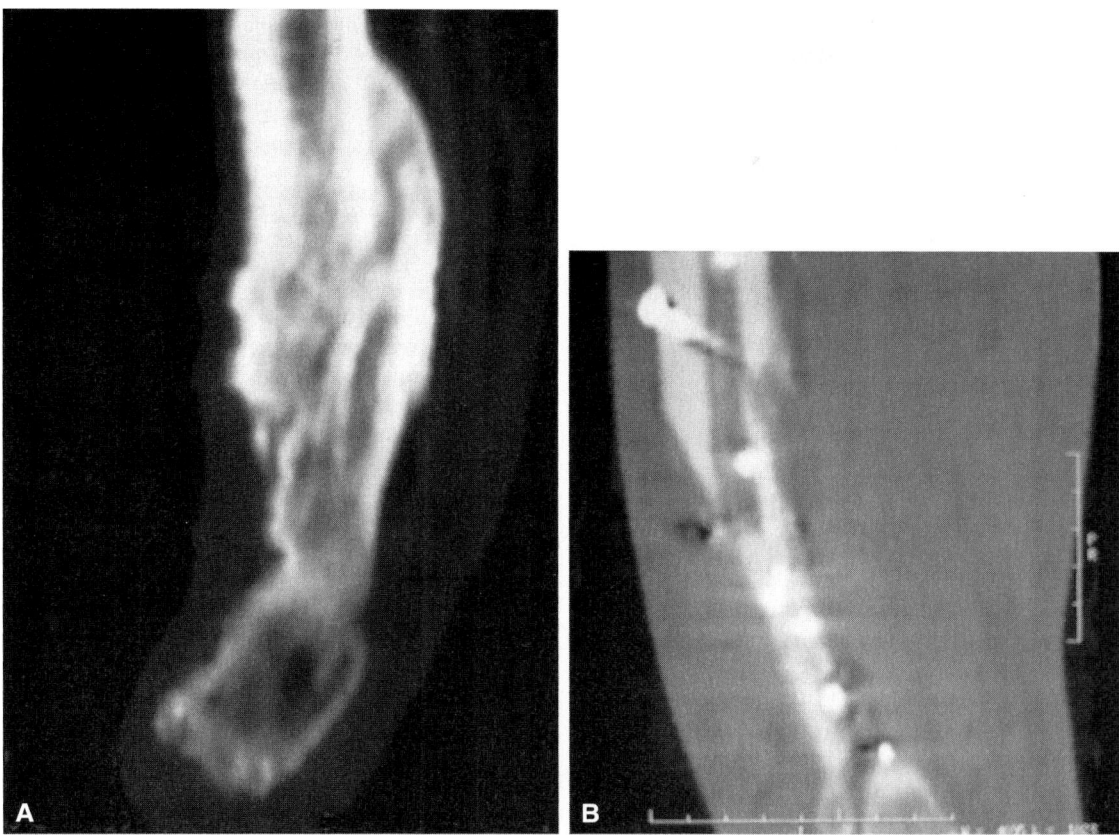

needed to assist in the care of the patient with a nonunion. The consultants participate in the initial evaluation and throughout the course of treatment.

A plastic reconstructive surgeon may be consulted preoperatively to assess the status of the soft tissues, particularly when the need for coverage is anticipated following serial débridement of an infected nonunion. Consultation with a vascular surgeon may be necessary if the viability (vascularity) of the limb is in question.

An infectious disease specialist can prescribe an antibiotic regimen preoperatively, intraoperatively, and postoperatively, particularly for the patient with a long-standing, infected nonunion.

Many patients with nonunions have dependency on oral narcotic pain medication. Referral to a pain management specialist is helpful both during the course of treatment and ultimately in detoxifying and weaning the patient off all narcotic pain medications.[111,286,309]

Depression is common in patients with chronic medical conditions.[79,155,156,170] Patients with nonunions often have signs of clinical depression. Referral to a psychiatrist for treatment can be of great benefit.

A neurologist should evaluate patients with motor or sensory dysfunction. Electromyography and nerve conduction studies can document the location and extent of neural compromise and determine the need for nerve exploration and repair.

A physical therapist should be consulted for preoperative and postoperative training with respect to postoperative activity expectations and the use of assistive or adaptive devices. The goals of immediate postoperative (inpatient) rehabilitation include independent transfer and ambulation, when possible. Outpatient physical therapy primarily addresses strength and range of motion of the surrounding joints but may also include sterile or medicated whirlpool treatments to treat or prevent minor infections (e.g., pin site irritation in patients treated with external fixation).

Occupational therapy is useful for activities of daily living and job-related tasks, particularly those involving fine motor skills such as grooming, dressing, and use of hand tools. Occupational therapy may also provide adaptive devices for activities of daily living during nonunion treatment.

A nutritionist may be consulted for patients who are malnourished or obese. Poor dietary intake of protein (albumin) or vitamins may contribute to delayed fracture union and nonunion.[73,88–90,117,242,303] A nutritionist may also counsel severely obese patients to reduce body weight. Obesity increases the technical demands of nonunion treatment, and a higher complication rate should be anticipated.[152]

Anesthesiologists and internists should be consulted for the elderly or patients with serious medical conditions.

FIGURE 22-18 | *In addition to helping determine whether a fracture has united or has gone on to nonunion, CT scans are a useful method for estimating the cross-sectional area of healing. In this case of an infected mid-shaft tibial nonunion, CT scanning is a useful method of estimating the progression of the cross-sectional area of healing over time.* ***A,*** *Radiograph of the tibia 4 months following injury. It is difficult to definitively say whether this fracture is healing.* ***B,*** *CT scan shows a clear gap without bony contact or bridging bone (0% cross-sectional area of healing).* ***C,*** *Radiograph 6 months later following gradual compression across the nonunion site.* ***D,*** *CT scan shows solid bony union (cross-sectional area of healing >50% in this case).*

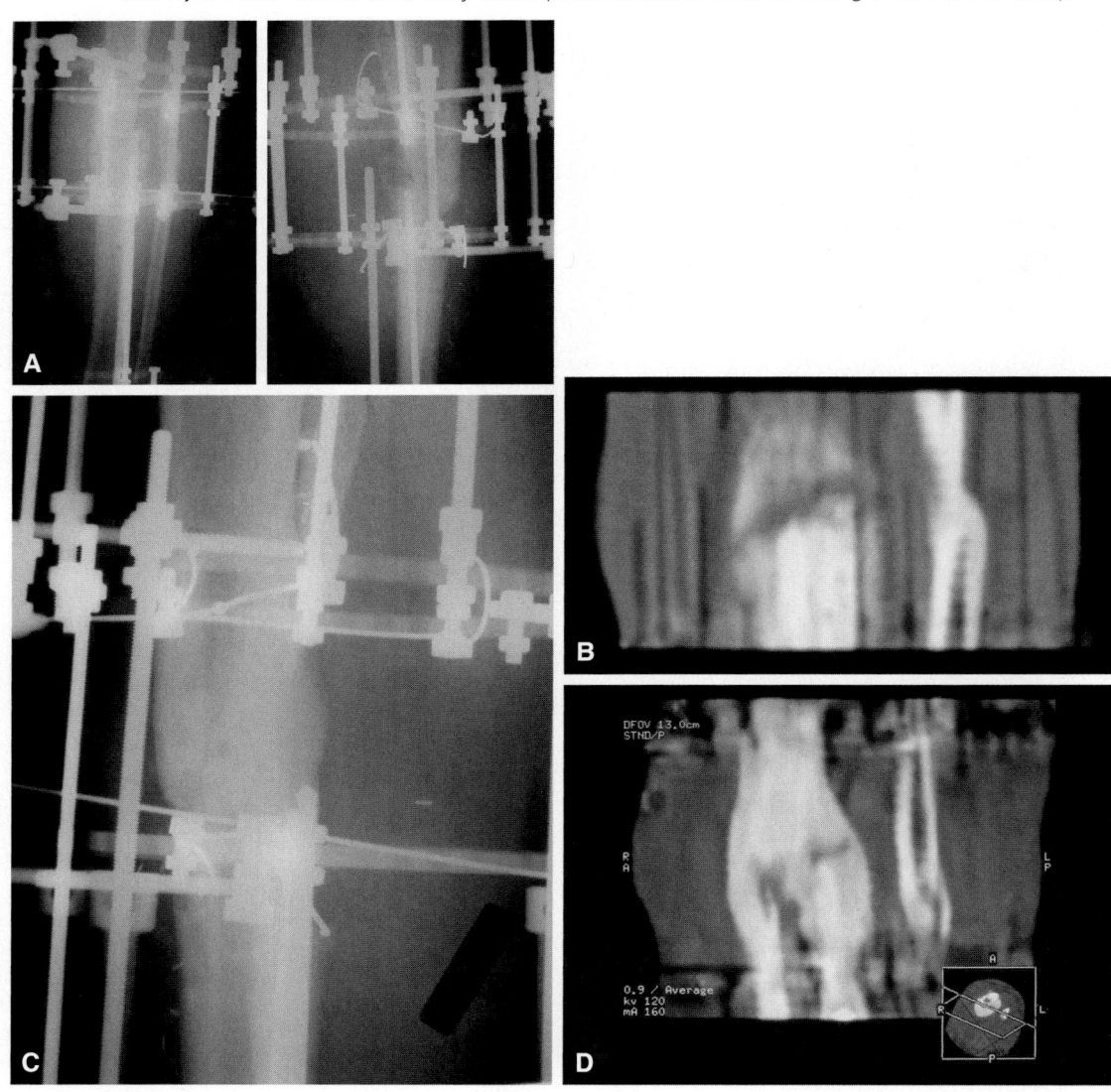

Preoperative planning of special anesthetic and medical needs diminishes the likelihood of intraoperative and postoperative medical complications.

TREATMENT

Objectives

Obviously, treatment is directed at healing the fracture. This, however, is not the only objective, since a nonfunctional, infected, deformed limb with pain and stiffness of the adjacent joints will be an unsatisfactory outcome for most patients even if the bone heals solidly. Emphasis is thus placed on returning the extremity and the patient to the fullest function possible during and after the treatment process.

Treating a nonunion can be likened to playing a game of chess; it is difficult to predict the course until the process is under way. Some nonunions heal rapidly with a single intervention. Others require multiple surgeries. Unfortunately, the most benign-appearing nonunion occasionally mounts a terrific battle against healing. The treatment must therefore be planned so that each step anticipates the possibility of failure and allows for further treatment options.

The patient's motivation, disability, social problems, legal involvements, mental status, and desires should be considered before treatment begins. Are the patient's expectations realistic? Informed consent prior to any treatment is essential. The patient needs to understand the

FIGURE 22-19 *Technetium bone scanning of three different cases showing a viable nonunion **(A)**, a nonviable nonunion **(B)**, and a synovial pseudarthrosis **(C)**.*

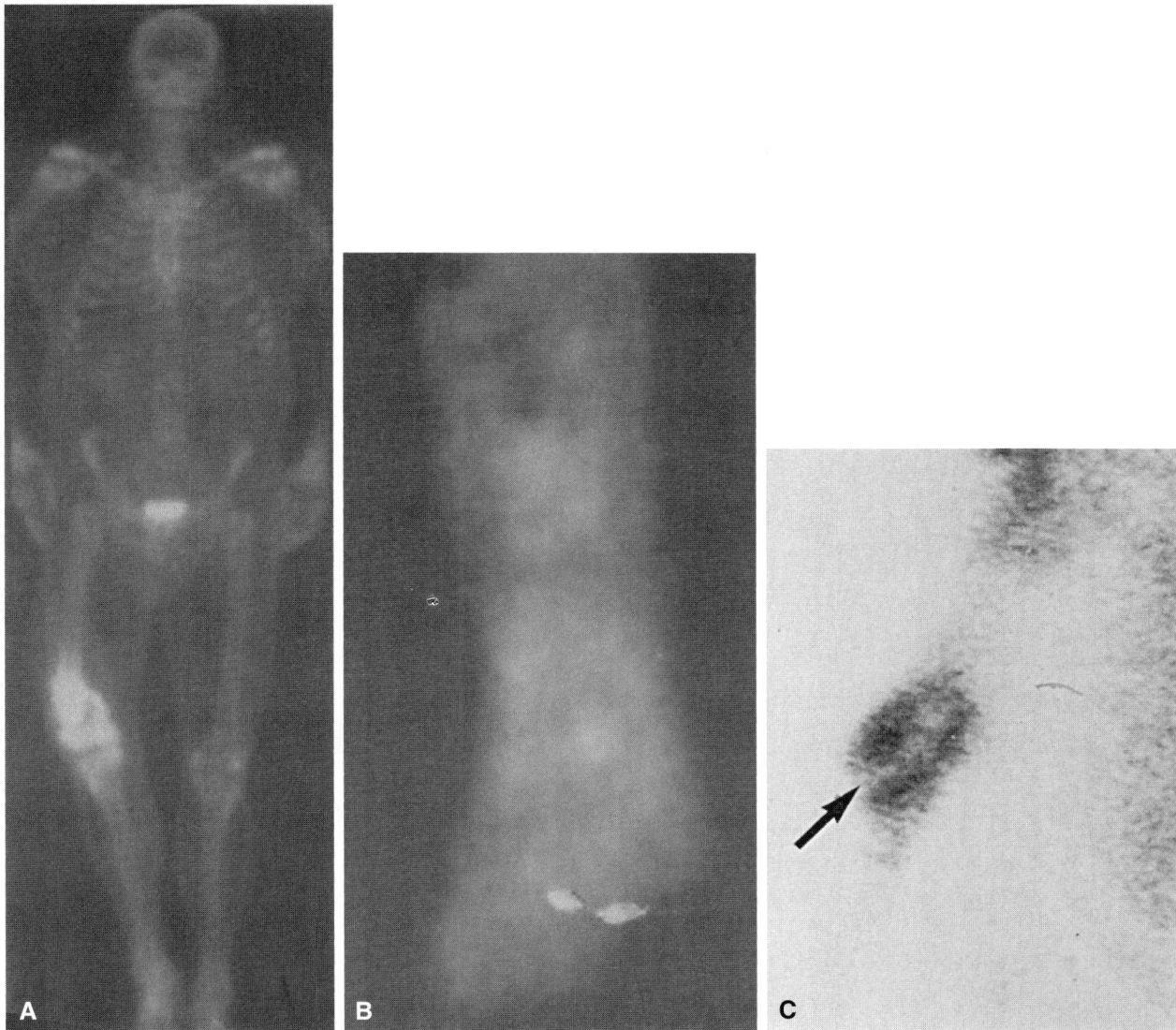

uncertainties of nonunion healing, time course of treatment, and number of surgeries required. No guarantees or warranties should be given to the patient. If the patient is unable to tolerate a potentially lengthy treatment course or the uncertainties associated with the treatment and outcome, the option of amputation should be discussed. While amputation has obvious drawbacks, it does resolve the medical problem rapidly and may therefore be preferred by certain patients.[29,57,132,276,306] It is unwise to talk a patient into or out of any treatment, particularly amputation.

When feasible, eradication of infection and correction of unacceptable deformities are performed at the time of nonunion treatment. When this is not practical or possible, the treatment plan is broken up into stages. The priorities of treatment are to

1. Heal the bone.
2. Eradicate infection.

3. Correct deformities.
4. Maximize joint motion and muscle strength.

These priorities do not necessarily denote the temporal sequencing of surgical procedures. For example, in an infected nonunion with a deformity, the first priority is to heal the bone. The treatment, however, may begin with débridement in an effort to eliminate infection, but the overriding priority remains to heal the bone.

Strategies

The in-depth evaluation using the history and physical examination, radiologic examinations, laboratory studies, and consulting physicians provides for assessment of the overall situation. This assessment culminates in a treatment strategy specific to the patient's particular circumstances.

The choice of treatment strategy is based on accurate classification of the nonunion (Table 22-4). Classification

FIGURE 22-20 | **A,** *Radiograph of a slowly maturing proximal tibial regenerate.* **B,** *Ultrasonography shows a fluid-filled cyst (arrow).*

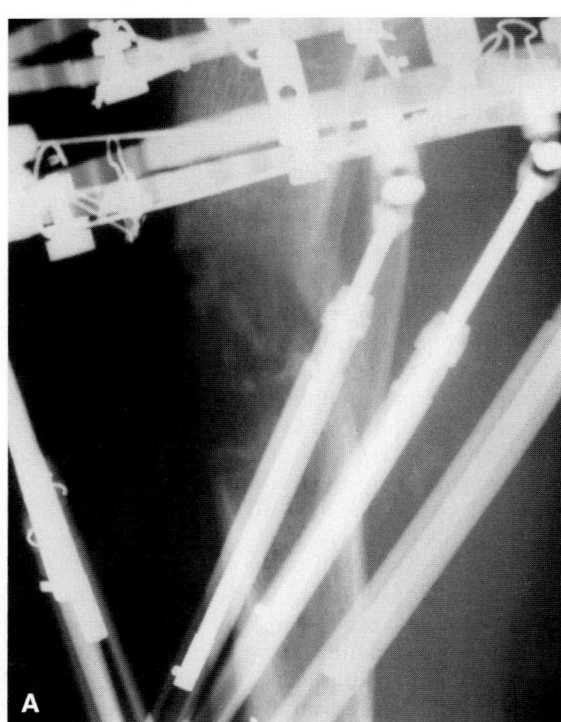

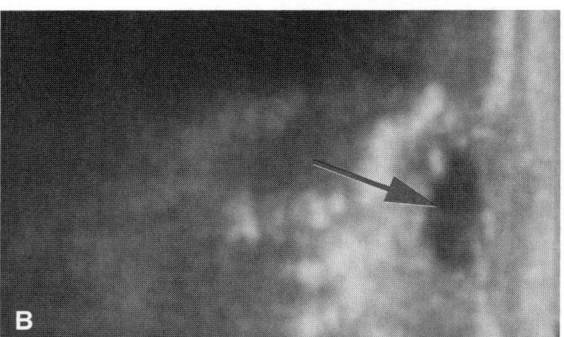

Table 22-4

Nonunion Types and Their Characteristics

Nonunion Type	Physical Examination	Plain Radiographs	Nuclear Imaging	Laboratory Studies
Hypertrophic	Typically does not display gross motion; pain elicited on manual stress testing	Abundant callus formation; radiolucent line (unmineralized fibrocartilage) at the nonunion site	Increased uptake at the nonunion site on technetium bone scan	Unremarkable
Oligotrophic	Variable (depends on the stability of the current hardware)	Little or no callus formation; diastasis at the fracture site	Increased uptake at the bone surfaces at the nonunion site on technetium bone scan	Unremarkable
Atrophic	Variable (depends on the stability of the current hardware)	Bony surfaces partially resorbed; no callus formation; osteopenia; sclerotic avascular bone segments; segmental bone loss	Avascular segments appear cold (decreased uptake) on technetium bone scan	Unremarkable
Infected	Depends on the specific nature of the infection: Active purulent drainage Active nondraining—no drainage but the area is warm, erythematous, and painful Quiescent—no drainage or local signs or symptoms of infection	Osteolysis; osteopenia; sclerotic avascular bone segments; segmental bone loss	Increased uptake on technetium bone scan; increased uptake on indium scan for acute infections; increased uptake on gallium scan for chronic infections	Elevated erythrocyte sedimentation rate and C-reactive protein; white blood cell count may be elevated in more severe and acute cases; blood cultures should be obtained in febrile patients; aspiration of fluid from the nonunion site may be useful in the workup for infection
Synovial pseudarthrosis	Variable	Variable appearance (hypertrophic, oligotrophic, or atrophic)	Technetium bone scan shows a "cold cleft" at the nonunion site surrounded by increased uptake at the ends of the united bone	Unremarkable

is based on the nonunion type and 13 treatment modifiers (Table 22-5).

Nonunion Type

The primary consideration for designing the treatment strategy is nonunion type (Fig. 22-21). Categorizing the nonunion identifies the mechanical and biological requirements of fracture healing that have not been met. The surgeon can then design a strategy to meet the healing requirements.

HYPERTROPHIC NONUNIONS

Hypertrophic nonunions are viable, possess an adequate blood supply,[252] and display abundant callus formation[207] but lack mechanical stability. Providing mechanical stability to a hypertrophic nonunion results in chondrocyte-mediated mineralization of fibrocartilage at the interfragmentary gap (Fig. 22-22). Mineralization of fibrocartilage may occur as early as 6 weeks following rigid stabilization and is accompanied by vascular ingrowth into the mineralized fibrocartilage[207,290] (see Fig. 22-22). By 8 weeks following stabilization, there is resorption of calcified fibrocartilage, which is then arranged in columns and acts as a template for deposition of woven bone. Woven bone is subsequently remodeled into mature lamellar bone (see Fig. 22-22).[290]

Hypertrophic nonunions require no bone grafting.[68,142,207,208,268,270,273,275,327–329] The nonunion site tissue should not be resected. Hypertrophic nonunions simply need a little "push" in the right direction (Fig. 22-23). If the method of rigid stabilization involves exposing the nonunion site (e.g., compression plate stabilization), decortication of the nonunion site may accelerate the consolidation of bone. If the method of rigid stabilization does not involve exposure of the nonunion

	Table 22-5	
	Treatment Strategies for Nonunions Based on Classification	
	Treatment Strategy	
Classification	**Biological**	**Mechanical**
Primary Consideration (Nonunion Type)		
Hypertrophic		Augment stability
Oligotrophic	Bone grafting for cases that have poor surface characteristics and no callus formation	Improve reduction (bone contact)
Atrophic	Biological stimulation via bone grafting or bone transport	Augment stability, compression
Infected Draining, active Nondraining, active Nondraining, quiescent	Débridement, antibiotic beads, dead space management, systemic antibiotic therapy, biological stimulation for bone healing (bone grafting or bone transport)	Provide mechanical stability, compression
Synovial pseudarthrosis	Resect synovium and pseudarthrosis tissue, open medullary canals with drilling and reaming, bone grafting	Compression
Treatment Modifiers		
Anatomic location Epiphyseal Metaphyseal Diaphyseal	Treatment modifiers are described in the text.	
Segmental bone defects		
Prior failed treatments		
Deformities Length Angulation Rotation Translation		
Surface characteristics		
Pain and function		
Osteopenia		
Mobility of the nonunion Stiff Lax		
Status of hardware		
Motor/sensory dysfunction		
Patient's health and age		
Problems at adjacent joints		
Soft tissue problems		

FIGURE 22-21 | *Classification of nonunions (nonunion types).*

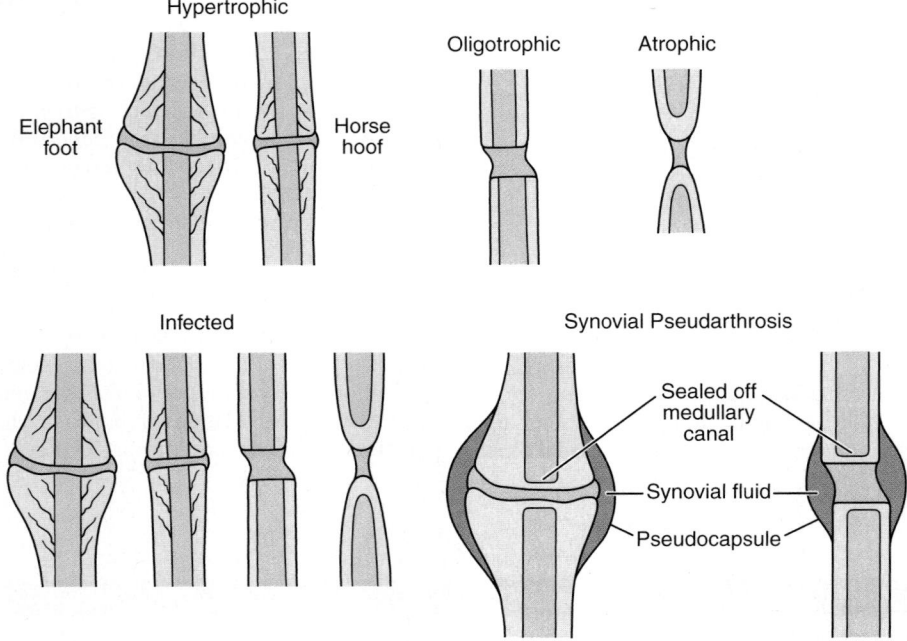

site (e.g., intramedullary nail fixation or external fixation), surgical dissection to prepare the nonunion site is unnecessary.

OLIGOTROPHIC NONUNIONS

Oligotrophic nonunions also are viable and possess an adequate blood supply but display little or no callus formation, typically as a result of inadequate reduction with little or no contact at the bony surfaces (Fig. 22-24). Therefore, treatment methods for oligotrophic nonunions include reduction of the bony fragments to improve bone contact, bone grafting to stimulate the local biology, or a combination of the two. Reduction of the bony fragments to improve bony contact can be performed with either internal or external fixation. Reduction is appropriate for oligotrophic nonunions with large surface areas without comminution across which compression can be applied. Bone grafting is appropriate for oligotrophic nonunions that have poor surface characteristics and no callus formation.

ATROPHIC NONUNIONS

Atrophic nonunions are nonviable. Their blood supply is poor and they are incapable of purposeful biological activity (Fig. 22-25). While the primary problem is biological, the atrophic nonunion requires a treatment strategy that employs both biological and mechanical techniques. Biological stimulation is most commonly provided by an autogenous cancellous graft laid onto a widely decorticated area at the nonunion site. Small free necrotic fragments are excised and the resulting defect is bridged with bone graft; treatment of large bony defects is discussed later in this chapter. Mechanical stability can be achieved using either internal or external fixation, and the fixation method must provide adequate purchase in poor quality (osteopenic) bone.

When stabilized and stimulated, an atrophic nonunion is revascularized slowly over the course of several months, as visualized radiographically by observing the progression of osteopenia as it moves through sclerotic, nonviable fragments.[267,329]

No consensus exists regarding whether large segments of sclerotic bone should be excised from uninfected atrophic nonunions. Those who favor plate-and-screw fixation tend to leave large sclerotic fragments that revascularize over several months following rigid plate stabilization, decortication, and bone grafting. Those who favor other treatment methods tend to excise large sclerotic fragments and reconstruct the resulting segmental bony defect using one of several available methods. Both of these treatment strategies result in successful union in a high percentage of cases. Our decision largely depends on the treatment modifiers, discussed in the next section.

INFECTED NONUNIONS

Infected nonunions pose a dual challenge. The condition is often further complicated by incapacitating pain (often with narcotic dependency), soft tissue problems, deformities, joint problems (contractures, deformities, limited range of motion), motor and sensory dysfunction, osteopenia, poor general health, depression, and a myriad of other problems. Infected nonunions are the most difficult type of nonunion to treat.

The goals are to obtain solid bony union, eradicate the infection, and maximize function of the extremity and the patient. Before a particular course of treatment is begun, the length of time required, the number of operative procedures anticipated, and the intensity of the treatment plan must be discussed with the patient and the family. The course of treatment for infected nonunions is especially difficult to predict. The possibility of persistent infection and nonunion despite

FIGURE 22-22   *A, Photomicrograph of unmineralized fibrocartilage in a canine hypertrophic nonunion (von Kossa stain). B, Six weeks following plate stabilization, chondrocyte-mediated mineralization of fibrocartilage is observed in this hypertrophic nonunion. C, This will go on to form woven bone, and will ultimately remodel to compact cortical bone 16 to 24 weeks following stabilization (D). (From Schenk, R.K. History of fracture repair and nonunion. Bull Swiss ASIF, October, 1978).*

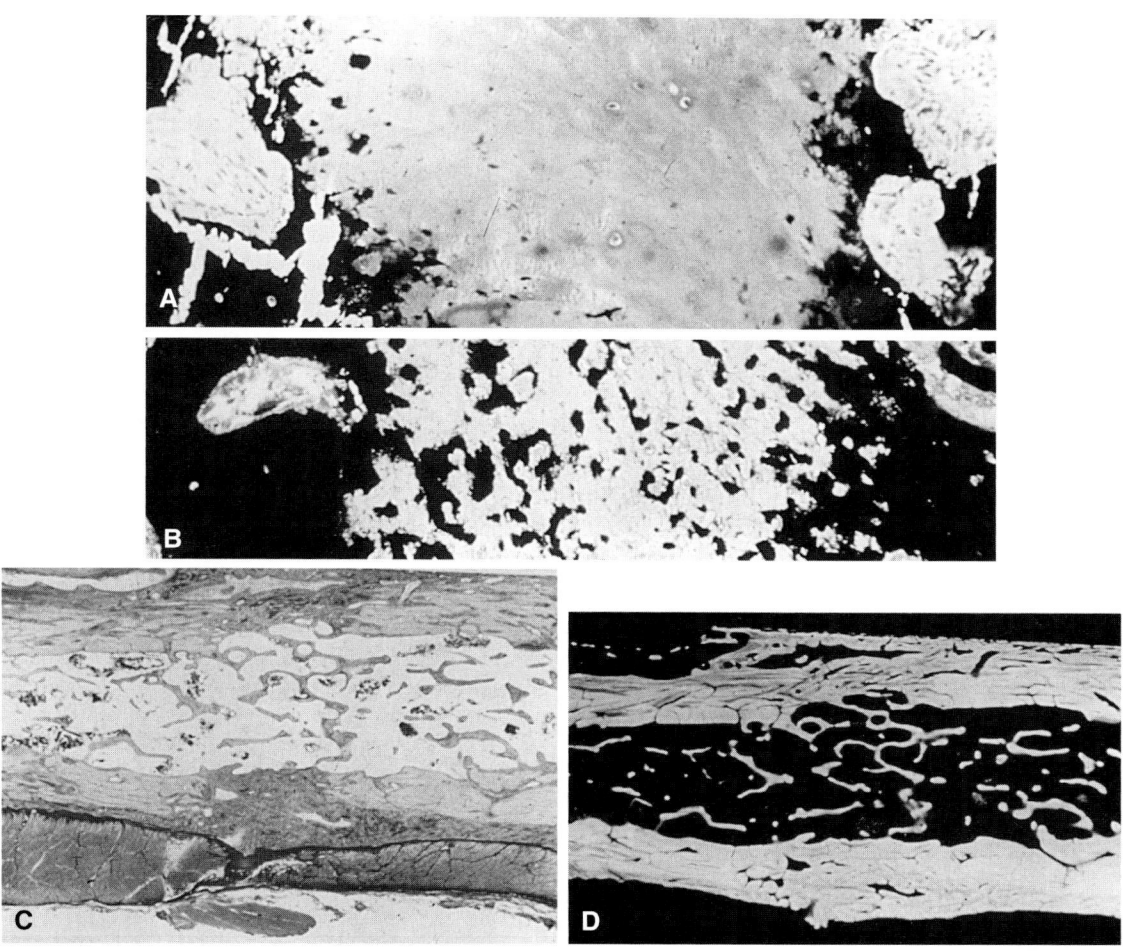

appropriate treatment should be discussed, and the possibility of future amputation should be considered.

The treatment strategy depends on the nature of the infection (draining, nondraining-active, nondraining-quiescent)[271] and involves both a biological and a mechanical approach.

PURULENT, DRAINING INFECTION When purulent drainage is ongoing, the nonunion takes longer and is more difficult to heal (Fig. 22-26). An actively draining infection requires serial débridement. The first débridement should include obtaining deep culture specimens, including soft tissues and bone. No perioperative antibiotics should be given at least 2 weeks prior to obtaining deep intraoperative culture specimens. All necrotic soft tissues (e.g., fascia, muscle, abscess cavities, and sinus tracts), necrotic bone, and foreign bodies (e.g., loose orthopaedic hardware, shrapnel) should be excised.[147,233] The sinus tract should be sent for pathologic study to rule out carcinoma.[233] Pulsatile irrigation with antibiotic solution is effective in washing out the open cavity.

A dead space is commonly present following débridement. Initially, antibiotic-impregnated polymethylmethacrylate (PMMA) beads are inserted,[233] and a bead exchange is performed at each serial débridement. The dead space can subsequently be managed in a number of ways. Currently, the most widely utilized method involves filling the dead space with a rotational vascularized muscle pedicle flap (e.g., gastrocnemius, soleus[233,238]) or a microvascularized free flap (e.g., latissimus dorsi, rectus[331,332]). Another method involves open wound care with moist dressings, as in the Papineau technique,[226] until granulation occurs and skin grafting can be performed.

Bony defects present following débridement can be reconstructed using a variety of bone grafting techniques, as discussed in the section on Segmental Bone Defects.

FIGURE 22-23 *Plate-and-screw fixation of this hypertrophic clavicle nonunion led to rapid bony union. **A,** Radiograph shows a hypertrophic nonunion 8 months following injury. **B,** X-ray taken 15 weeks following open reduction internal fixation (without bone grafting) shows complete and solid bony union.*

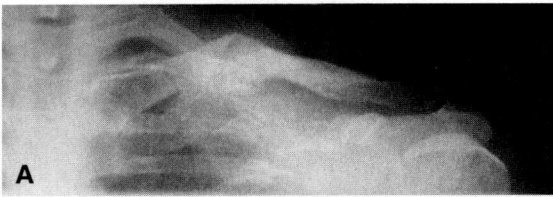
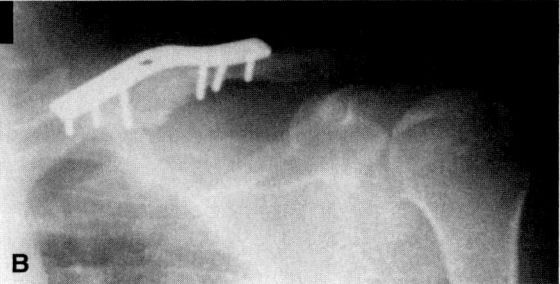

FIGURE 22-24 *Oligotrophic nonunion of the femoral shaft 21 months following failed treatment of the initial fracture with plate-and-screw fixation. Note the absence of callus formation and poor contact at the bony surfaces.*

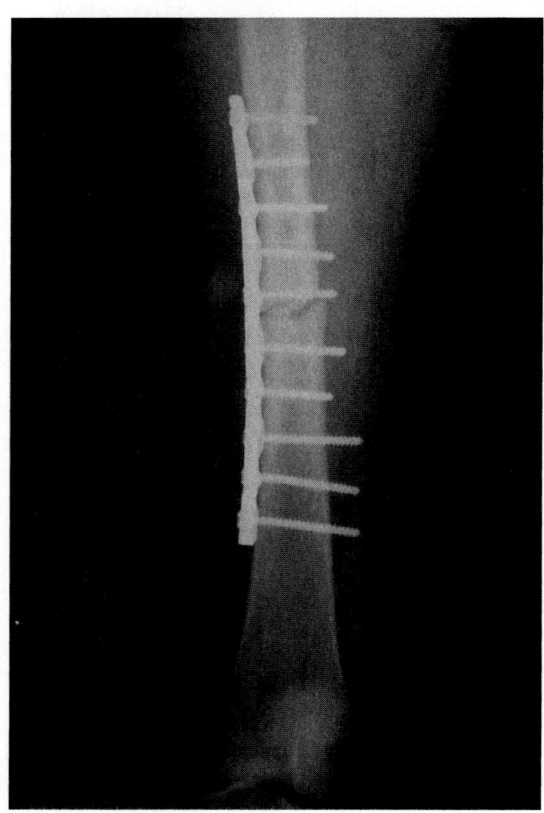

FIGURE 22-25 *Atrophic nonunion of the proximal humerus. Note the lack of callus formation, the bony defect, and the avascular-appearing bony surfaces.*

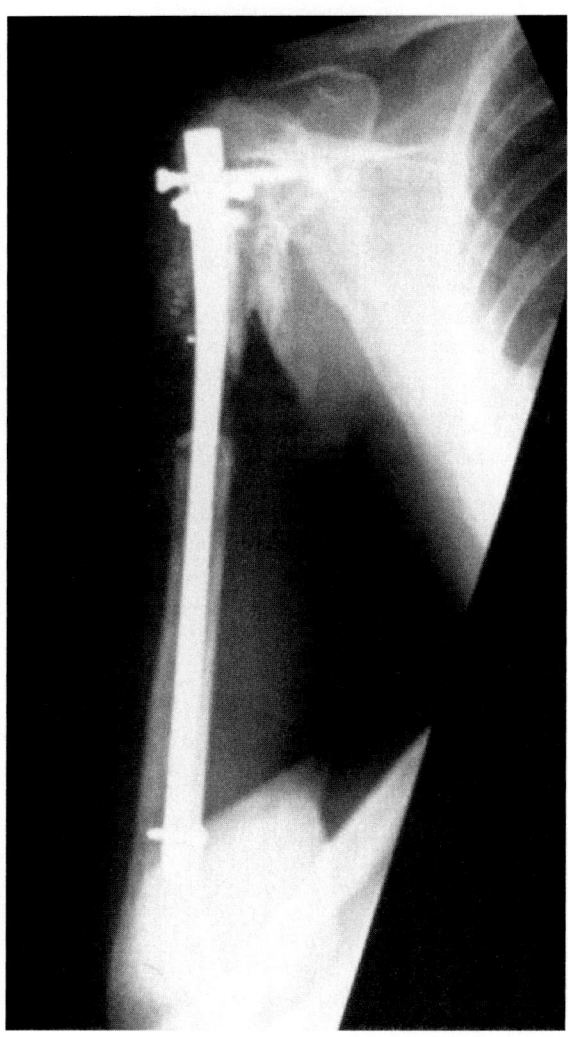

The consulting infectious disease specialist generally directs systemic antibiotic therapy. Following procurement of deep surgical cultures, the patient is placed on broad-spectrum intravenous antibiotics. When the culture results are available, antibiotic coverage is directed at the infecting organisms.

ACTIVE, NONDRAINING INFECTION Nondraining infected nonunions present with swelling, tenderness, and local erythema (see Fig. 22-26). The history often includes episodes of fever. Treatment principles are similar to those described for actively draining infected nonunions: débridement, intraoperative cultures, soft tissue management, stabilization, stimulation of bone healing, and systemic antibiotic therapy. These cases typically require incision and drainage of an abscess and excision of only small amounts of bone and soft tissues. Nondraining infected nonunion cases may be managed with primary

FIGURE 22-26 ▪ *A, Clinical photograph of an actively draining infected tibial nonunion. **B,** Clinical photograph of a nondraining infected tibial nonunion. Note the presence of local swelling (there is also erythema) without purulent drainage. **C,** Radiograph of a nondraining, quiescent, infected tibial nonunion (this patient had a history of multiple episodes of purulent drainage, and the gallium scan was positive).*

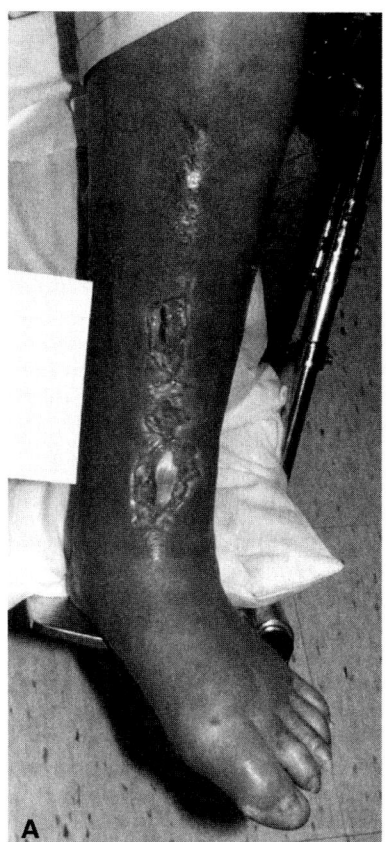
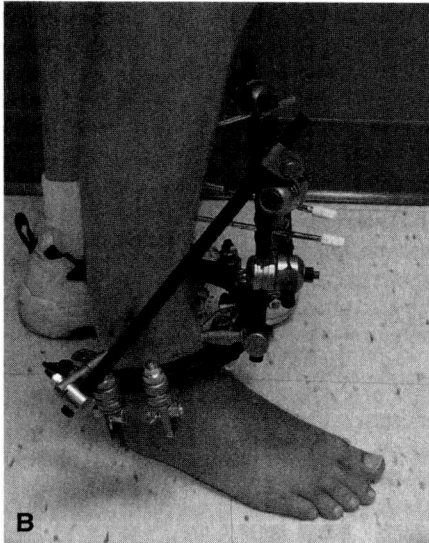
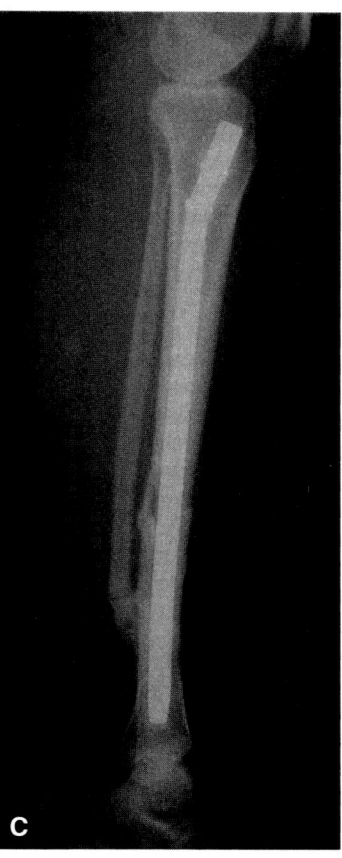

closure following incision and drainage or with a closed suction-irrigation drainage system until the infection becomes quiescent.

QUIESCENT INFECTION Nondraining quiescent infected nonunions occur in patients with a history of infection but without drainage or symptoms for 3 or more months[271] or without a history of infection but with a positive indium or gallium scan (see Fig. 22-26). These cases may be treated like atrophic nonunions. With plate-and-screw stabilization, the residual necrotic bone may be débrided at the time of surgical exposure. The bone is decorticated and stabilized, and bone grafting may also be performed. If external fixation is used, the infection and nonunion may be treated with compression without open débridement or bone grafting.[294]

SYNOVIAL PSEUDARTHROSIS

Synovial pseudarthroses are characterized by fluid bounded by sealed medullary canals and a fixed synovium-like pseudocapsule (Fig. 22-27). Treatment entails both biological stimulation and augmentation of mechanical stability. The synovium and pseudarthrosis

tissue are excised, and the medullary canals of the proximal and distal fragments are drilled and reamed. The ends of the major fragments are fashioned to allow for interfragmentary compression with either internal or external fixation. Bone grafting and decortication encourage more rapid healing.

According to Professor Ilizarov, gradual compression across a synovial pseudarthrosis results in local necrosis and inflammation, ultimately stimulating the healing process.[143,294] We have had mixed results with this method and have found that resection at the nonunion followed by monofocal compression or bone transport more reliably achieves good results.

Treatment Modifiers

The treatment modifiers (see Table 22-5) provide a more specific classification of the nonunion and thus help "fine-tune" the treatment plan.

ANATOMIC LOCATION

The bone involved and the specific region or regions (e.g., epiphysis, metaphysis, diaphysis) define the anatomic location of a nonunion. A bone-by-bone discussion is beyond

FIGURE 22-27 *Plain radiograph of a tibial nonunion with a synovial pseudarthrosis.*

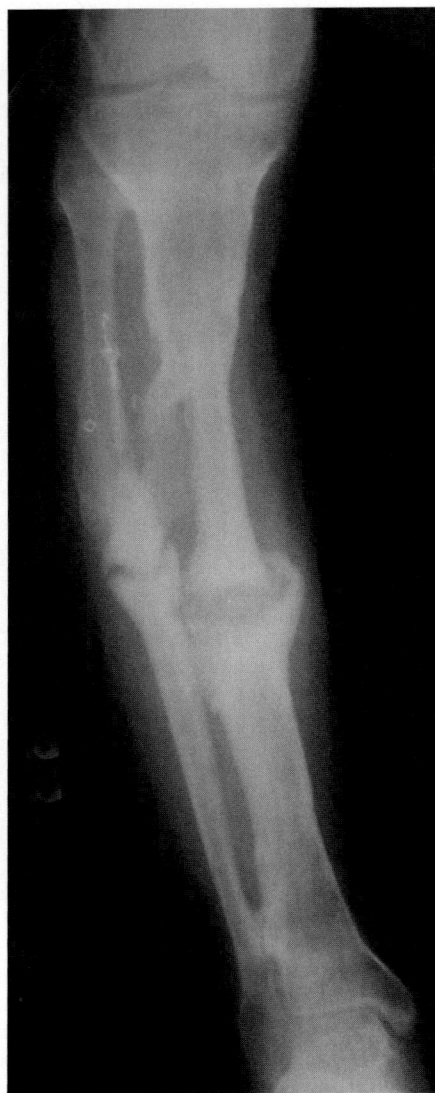

the scope of this chapter; we address the influence of anatomic region on the treatment of nonunions in general terms.

EPIPHYSEAL NONUNIONS Epiphyseal nonunions are relatively uncommon. The most common etiology is inadequate reduction that leaves a gap at the fracture site. These nonunions therefore commonly present with oligotrophic characteristics. The important considerations when evaluating epiphyseal nonunions are reduction of the intra-articular components (eliminate step-off at the articular surface), juxta-articular deformities (e.g., length, angulation, rotation, translation), motion at the joint (typically limited due to arthrofibrosis), and compensatory deformities at adjacent joints.

Epiphyseal nonunions are typically treated with interfragmentary compression using screw fixation, best achieved by a cannulated lag screw technique (overdrilling a glide hole) with a washer beneath the screw head. Previously placed screws holding the nonunion site in a distracted position should be removed. Arthroscopy is a useful adjunctive treatment for epiphyseal nonunions (Fig. 22-28). The articular step-off can be evaluated and reduced under arthroscopic visualization, and the cannulated lag screws can be placed percutaneously using fluoroscopy. The intra-articular component of the nonunion may be freshened up using an arthroscopic burr if necessary (it is typically not). Arthroscopy also facilitates lysis of intra-articular adhesions to improve joint range of motion. Occasionally open reduction is required to reduce an intra-articular or juxta-articular deformity. In such cases, the surgical approach may include arthrotomy for lysis of adhesions.

METAPHYSEAL NONUNIONS Metaphyseal nonunions are relatively common. In general, the nonunion type determines the treatment strategy. Unstable metaphyseal nonunions may be treated with internal or external fixation.

Plate-and-screw stabilization provides rigid fixation and is performed in conjunction with bone grafting, except for hypertrophic nonunions (Fig. 22-29). Screw fixation alone (without plating) should never be used for metaphyseal nonunions.

Intramedullary nail fixation is another option (see Fig. 22-29). Because the medullary canal is larger at the metaphysis than at the diaphysis, this method of fixation is predisposed to instability. Treatment of metaphyseal nonunions with nail fixation therefore requires good bone-to-bone contact at the nonunion site, a minimum of two interlocking screws in the short segment (custom-designed nails can provide for multiple interlocking screws), placement of blocking (Poller) screws[168,169] to provide added stability (see Fig. 22-29), and intraoperative manual stress testing under fluoroscopy to ensure stable fixation.

External fixation may also be used to treat metaphyseal nonunions. Ilizarov external fixation is the preferred method because it offers not only enhanced stability and early weight-bearing (for lower extremity nonunions) but also gradual compression at the nonunion site (see Fig. 20-29). Metaphyseal nonunions are particularly well suited for thin-wire external fixation because of the predominance of cancellous bone. However, internal fixation is generally preferable to external fixation for nonunions in the proximal humeral and proximal femoral metaphyses because the proximity of the trunk makes Ilizarov frame application technically difficult.

Stable metaphyseal nonunions are frequently oligotrophic and typically unite rapidly when stimulated by means of conventional cancellous bone grafting or a percutaneous bone marrow injection. While both methods have a high rate of success, percutaneous marrow injection provides the benefits of minimally invasive surgery.[131]

The special considerations for metaphyseal nonunions are similar to those for epiphyseal nonunions and include juxta-articular deformities, motion at the adjacent joint, and compensatory deformities at the adjacent joints. These issues are addressed in greater detail below.

FIGURE 22-28 | *Epiphyseal nonunion (oligotrophic) of the distal femur in an 18-year-old 5 months following injury.* ***A,*** *Preoperative radiograph.* ***B,*** *Preoperative CT scan.* ***C,*** *Final result following arthroscopically assisted closed reduction and percutaneous cannulated screw fixation shows solid bony union.*

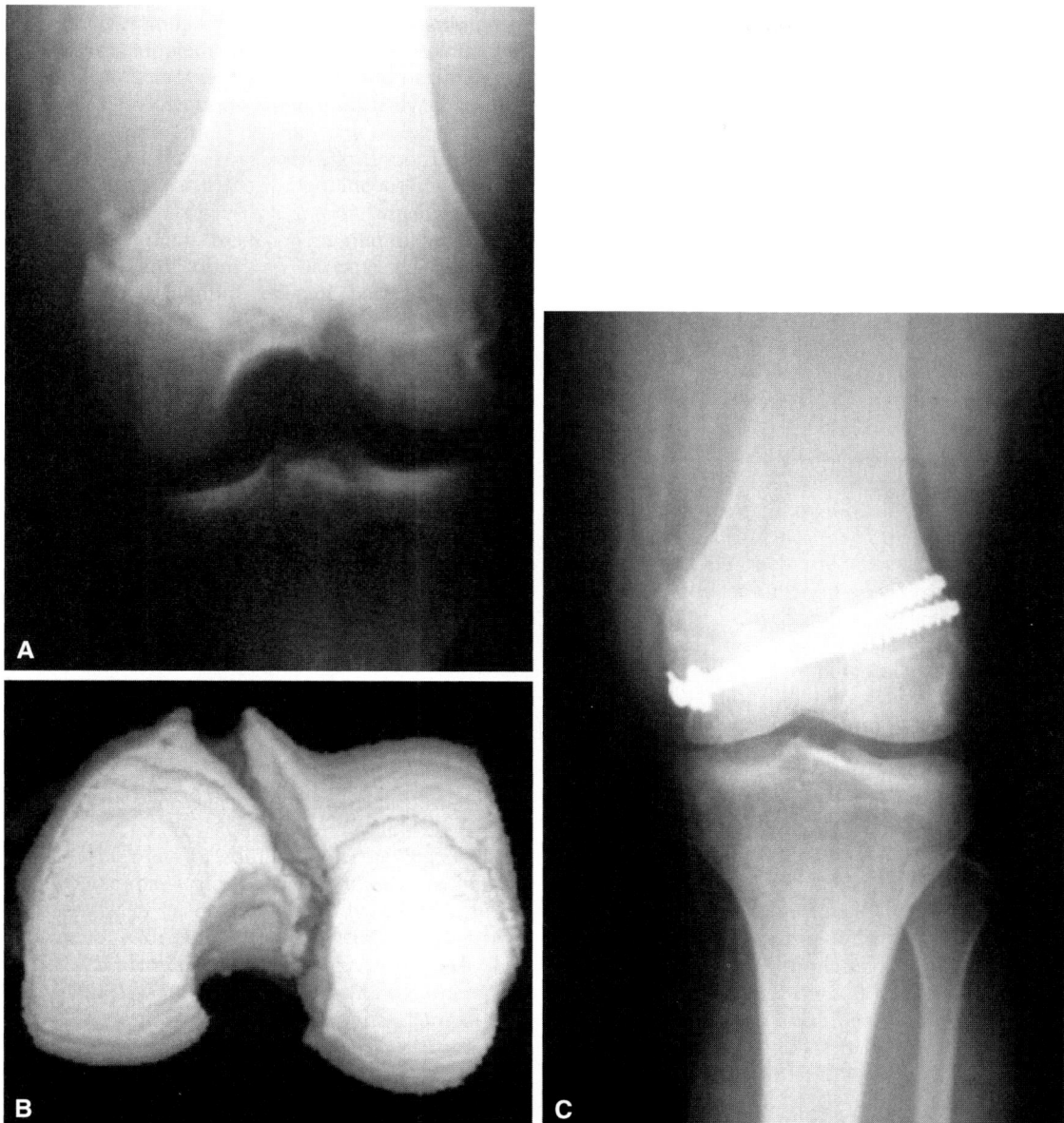

DIAPHYSEAL NONUNIONS Diaphyseal nonunions traverse cortical bone and may be more resistant to union than metaphyseal and epiphyseal nonunions, which traverse primarily cancellous bone. By virtue of their more central location, however, diaphyseal nonunions are amenable to the widest array of fixation methods (Fig. 22-30).

NONUNIONS THAT TRAVERSE MORE THAN ONE ANATOMIC REGION Nonunions that traverse more than one anatomic region require a strategy plan for each region. In some cases, the treatment can be performed using the same strategy for each region, whereas in others several strategies must be used. For example, a nonunion of the proximal humeral metaphysis with

diaphyseal extension could be treated with a reamed intramedullary nail with proximal and distal interlocking screws. This single strategy provides mechanical stability and biological stimulation (reaming) to both nonunions. By contrast, a nonunion of the distal tibial epiphysis with extension into the metaphysis and diaphysis could be treated using several strategies: cannulated screw fixation of the epiphysis, percutaneous marrow injection of the metaphysis, and Ilizarov external fixation stabilizing all three anatomic regions.

SEGMENTAL BONE DEFECTS

Segmental bone defects associated with nonunions may be a result of high-energy open fractures with bone lost at the

FIGURE 22-29 | *Metaphyseal nonunions can be treated with a variety of methods.* ***A,*** *Preoperative and final radiographs of an atrophic distal tibial nonunion treated with plate-and-screw fixation and autologous cancellous bone grafting.* ***B,*** *Preoperative and final radiographs of an oligotrophic distal tibial nonunion treated with exchange nailing. Note the use of Poller screws in the short distal fragment to enhance stability.* ***C,*** *Preoperative and final radiographs and final clinical photograph of a proximal metaphyseal humeral nonunion treated with intramedullary nail stabilization and autogenous bone grafting.* ***D,*** *Preoperative, during treatment, and final radiographs of a distal tibial nonunion treated using Ilizarov external fixation.*

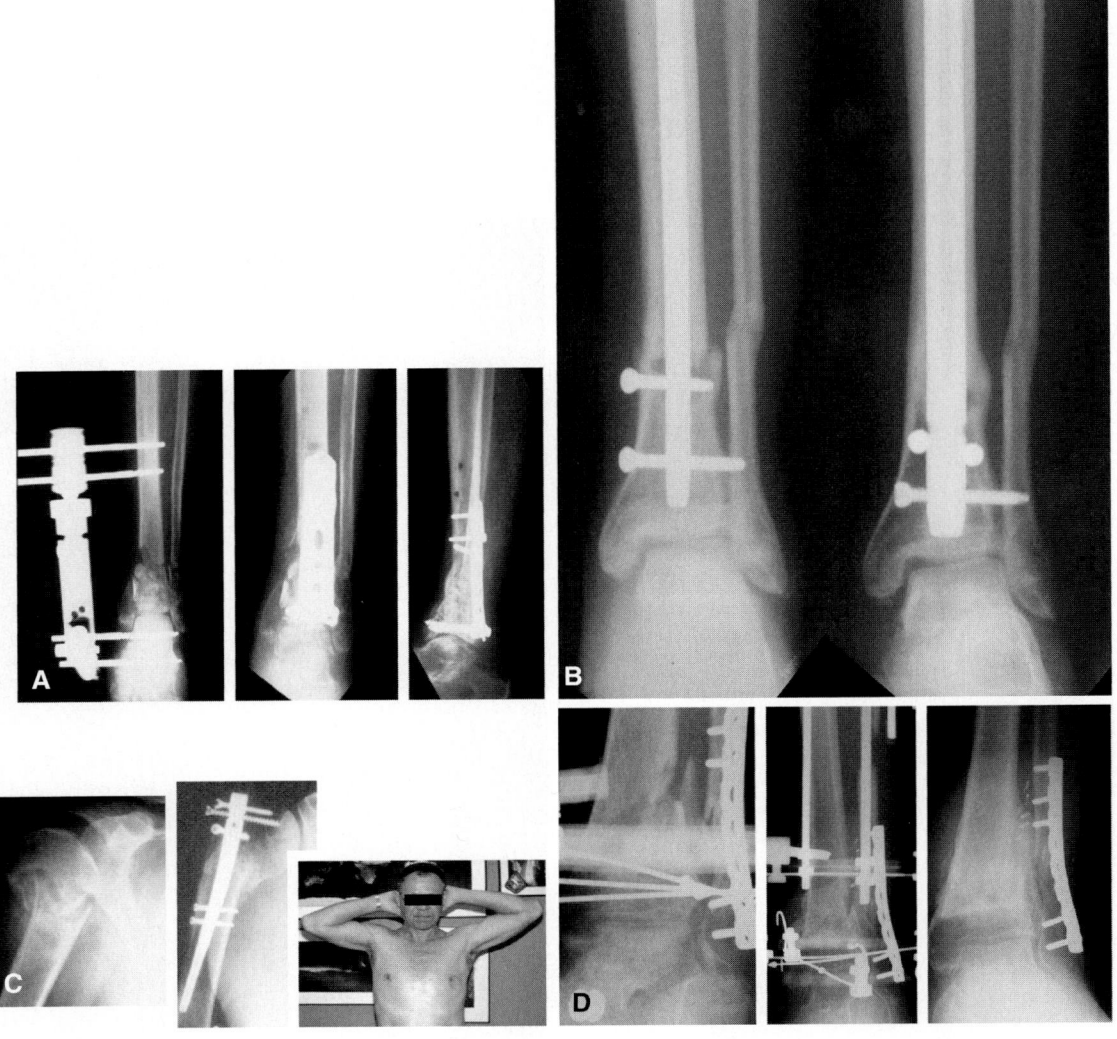

accident, surgical débridement of devitalized bone fragments following a high-energy open fracture, surgical débridement of an infected nonunion, surgical excision of necrotic bone associated with an atrophic nonunion, or surgical trimming at a nonunion site to improve surface characteristics.

Segmental bone defects may have partial (incomplete) bone loss or circumferential (complete) bone loss (Fig. 22-31). Treatment methods for these defects fit into three broad categories: static, acute compression, and gradual compression.

STATIC TREATMENT METHODS Static treatment methods fill the defect between the bone ends. In static methods, the proximal and distal ends of the nonunion are fixed using internal or external fixation. Thus, it is important to ensure that the bone is not foreshortened or overdistracted. Static methods for treating bone defects include autogenous cancellous bone graft, autogenous cortical bone graft, vascularized autograft, bulk cortical allograft, strut cortical allograft, mesh cage–bone graft constructs, and synostosis techniques.

Autogenous cancellous bone graft may be used to treat either partial or circumferential defects. The other methods are typically used to treat circumferential segmental defects. These methods are discussed in detail in the Treatment Methods section.

ACUTE COMPRESSION METHODS Acute compression methods obtain immediate bone-to-bone contact at the nonunion site by acutely shortening the extremity. Soft tissue compliance, surgical or open wounds, and neurovascular structures limit the extent of acute shortening that is possible. Some authors[115,144,294] have suggested

*Diaphyseal nonunions can be treated with a variety of methods. **A,** Preoperative and final radiographs of a left humeral shaft nonunion treated with plate-and-screw fixation and autologous cancellous bone grafting. **B,** Preoperative and final radiographs of a left humeral shaft nonunion treated with intramedullary nail fixation. **C,** Preoperative, during treatment, and final radiographs of an infected humeral shaft nonunion treated using Ilizarov external fixation.*

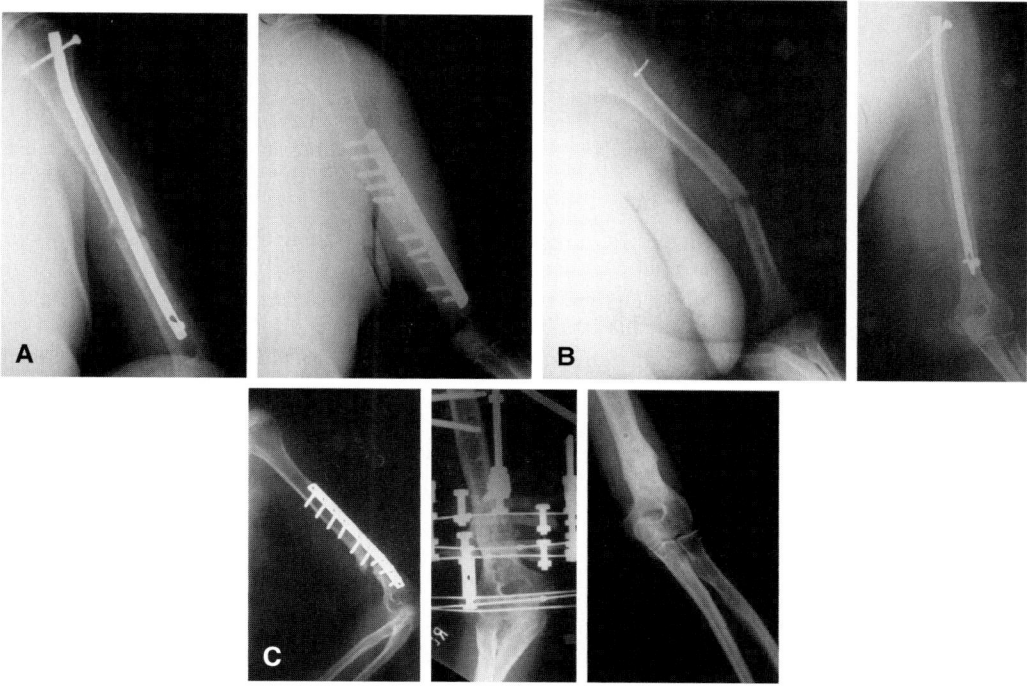

that greater than 2 to 2.5 cm of acute shortening may lead to wound closure difficulties or kinking of blood vessels and lymphatic channels. In our experience, up to 4 to 5 cm of acute shortening is well tolerated in many patients (Fig. 22-32). Acute shortening is appropriate for defects up to 7 cm in length. Longitudinal incisions tend to bunch up when acute shortening is performed. An experienced plastic reconstructive surgeon is invaluable for the closure of these wounds. Transverse incisions are less difficult to

close because they bunch up less when acute shortening is performed.

In the leg and forearm, the unaffected bone (e.g., fibula) must be partially excised to allow for acute compression of the un-united bone (e.g., tibia).

Acute compression methods provide immediate bone-to-bone contact and compression at the nonunion site, beginning the process of healing as early as possible. The bone ends should be fashioned to create opposing surfaces that are as parallel as possible. Flat cuts with an oscillating saw improve bone-to-bone contact but likely damage the bony tissues. Osteotomes, rasps, and rongeurs create less damage to the bony tissues but are less effective in creating flat cuts. No consensus exists regarding which method is best. We prefer to use a wide, flat oscillating saw and intermittent short bursts of cutting under constant irrigation. Acute compression with shortening also allows concomitant cancellous bone grafting of the decorticated bone at the nonunion site and promotes bony healing.

A disadvantage of acute compression of segmental defects is the functional consequence of foreshortening the extremity. In the upper extremity, up to 3 to 4 cm of foreshortening is well tolerated. In the lower extremity, up to 2 cm of foreshortening may be treated with a shoe lift. Many patients poorly tolerate a shoe lift for 2 to 4 cm of shortening, and most do not tolerate greater than 4 cm of foreshortening. Therefore, many patients undergoing acute compression concurrently or subsequently undergo a lengthening procedure of the ipsilateral extremity or a foreshortening procedure of the contralateral extremity (see Fig. 22-32).

Segmental bone defects may be associated with either partial (incomplete) bone loss or circumferential (complete) bone loss.

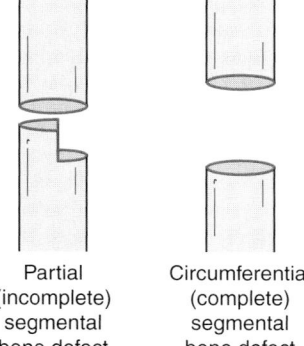

Partial (incomplete) segmental bone defect

Circumferential (complete) segmental bone defect

FIGURE 22-32 | *A, Circumferential (complete) segmental bone defect in a 66-year-old woman with an infected distal tibial nonunion who was taking high-dose corticosteroids for severe rheumatoid arthritis. B, Radiograph during treatment following acute compression (2.5 cm) using an Ilizarov external fixator and bone grafting at the nonunion site. C, Final radiograph shows a healed distal tibial nonunion and restoration of length from concomitant lengthening at a proximal tibial corticotomy site.*

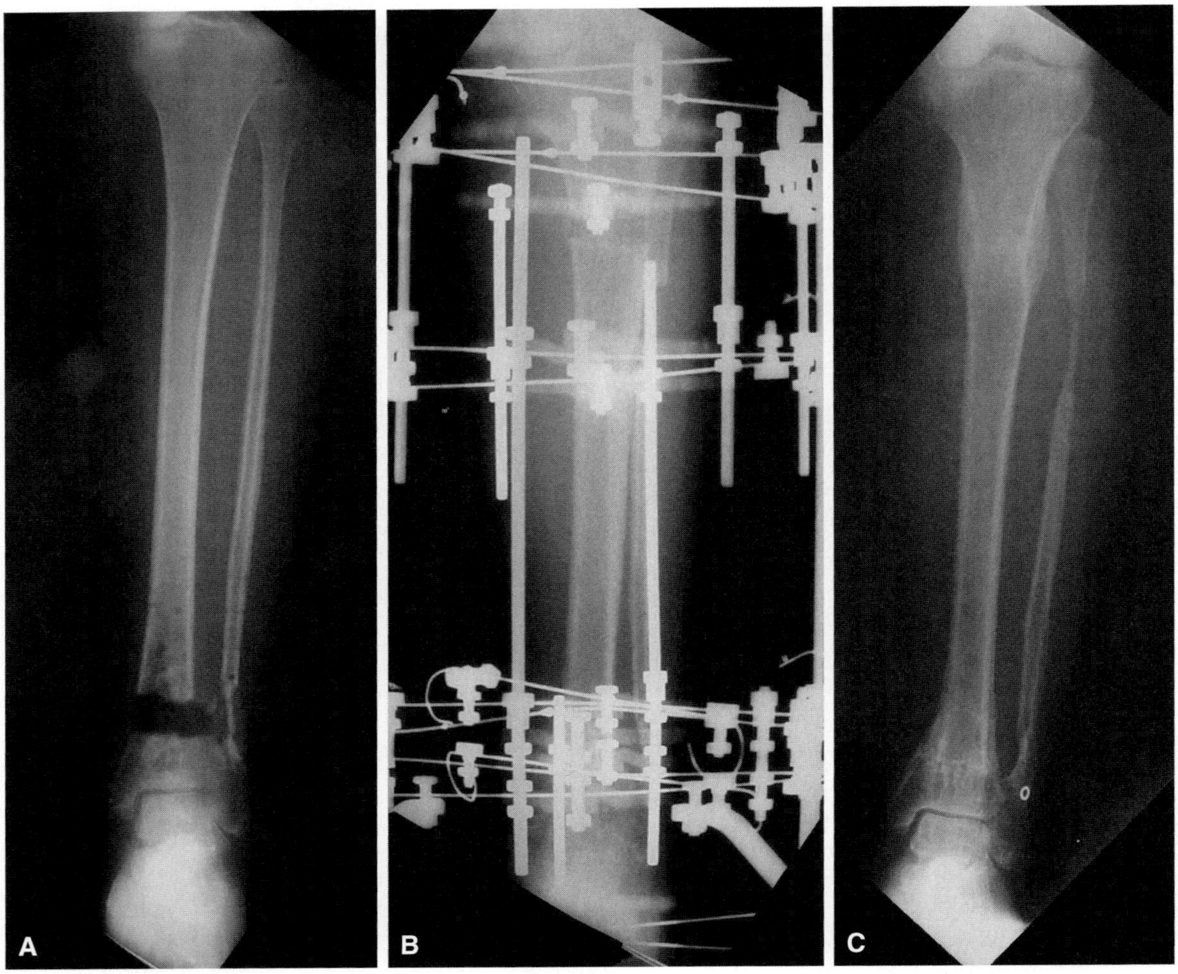

Acute compression across the nonunion site is typically used to treat circumferential segmental defects. When internal fixation devices are employed, acute compression is most effectively applied by the intraoperative use of a femoral distractor or a spanning external fixator. When plate-and-screw fixation is employed, an articulating tension device may be used to gain further interfragmentary compression. Dynamic compression plates (DCP; Synthes, Paoli, PA) may be used to provide further interfragmentary compression and rigid fixation. Oblique parallel flat cuts allow for enhanced interfragmentary compression via lag screws (Fig. 22-33). With intramedullary nail fixation, acute compression across the segmental defect can also be applied intraoperatively by means of a femoral distractor or a spanning external fixator (Fig. 22-34). Compression can be applied using these temporary devices before or after

FIGURE 22-33 | *Oblique parallel flat cuts allow for enhanced interfragmentary compression via lag screw fixation when a segmental defect is treated with acute compression and plate stabilization.*

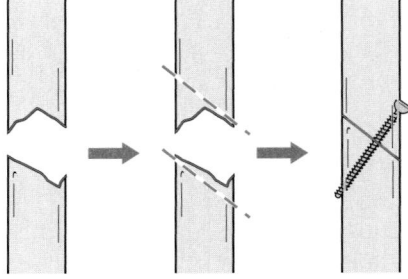

FIGURE 22-34 *Acute compression of a tibial nonunion with a segmental defect using a temporary (intraoperative use only) external fixator. Definitive fixation was achieved with an intramedullary nail. Note the use of Poller screws in the proximal fragment for enhanced stability.* **A,** *Radiograph on presentation.* **B,** *Intraoperative radiographs.* **C,** *Final result.*

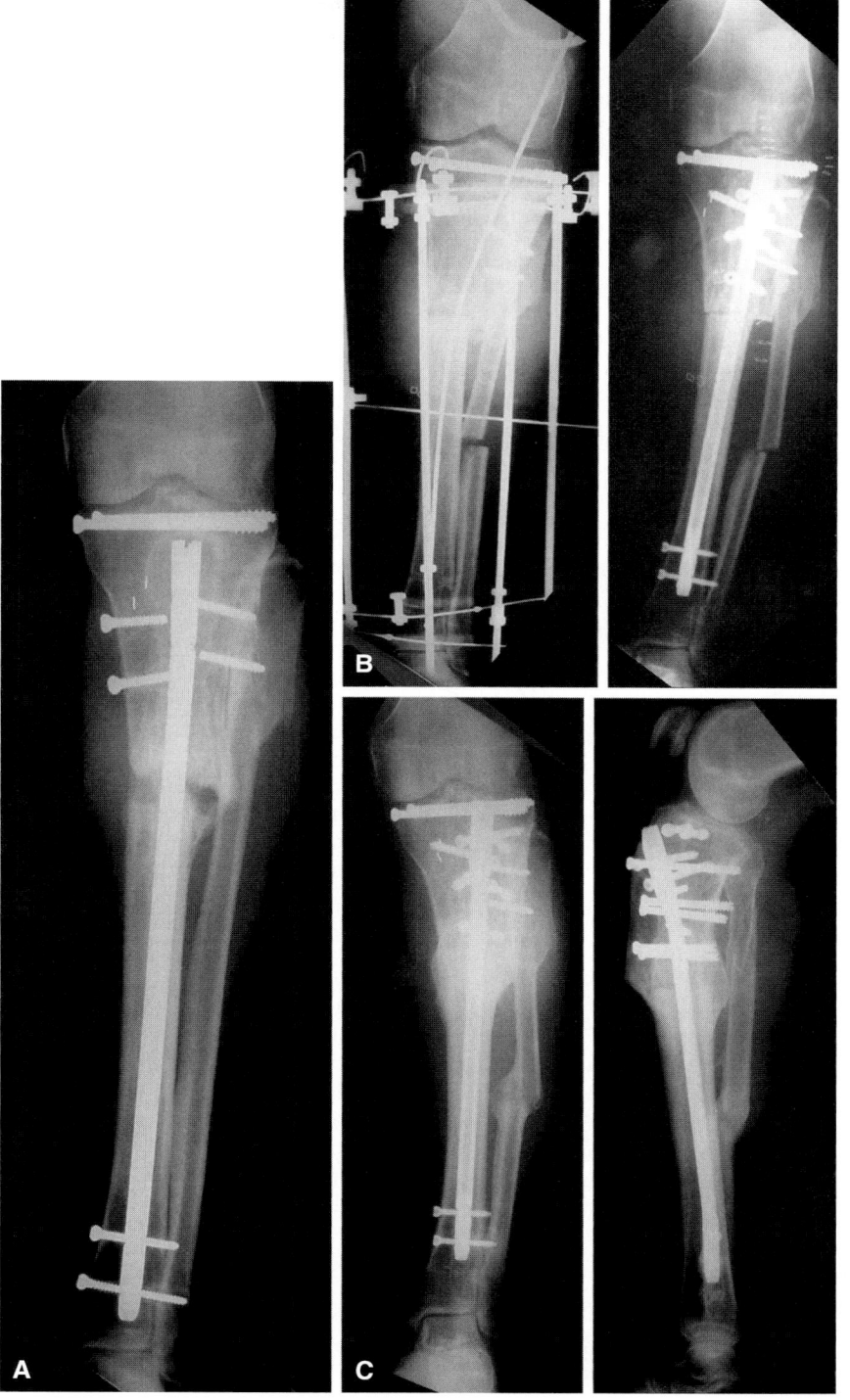

nail insertion but prior to static interlocking. In either case, the medullary canal should be over-reamed to at least 1.5 mm larger than the nail diameter. When the nail is placed after compression (shortening), over-reaming permits nail passage without distraction at the nonunion site. When the nail is placed before compression, over-reaming allows the proximal and distal fragments to slide over the nail and compress without jamming on the nail. Prior to removal of the intraoperative compression device, the nail must be statically locked both proximal and distal to the nonunion site. Some intramedullary devices, such as the Ankle Arthrodesis Nail (Biomet, Warsaw, IN), allow for acute compression across the fracture or nonunion site during the operative procedure (Fig. 22-35). In our experience, nails that allow for acute compression, when available, are preferable to conventional nails for this specific type of treatment.

Acute compression can also be applied by the use of an external fixator as the definitive mode of treatment. Transverse parallel flat cuts accommodate axial compression and minimize shear moments at the nonunion site.

FIGURE 22-35   *Some intramedullary nails allow for acute compression across a fracture site or a nonunion site. An example of such a nail is shown here. The Biomet Ankle Arthrodesis Nail (Warsaw, IN) is designed to allow for acute compression at the time of the operative procedure.* **A,** *Prior to compression.* **B,** *Acute compression being applied across the ankle joint using the compression device.*

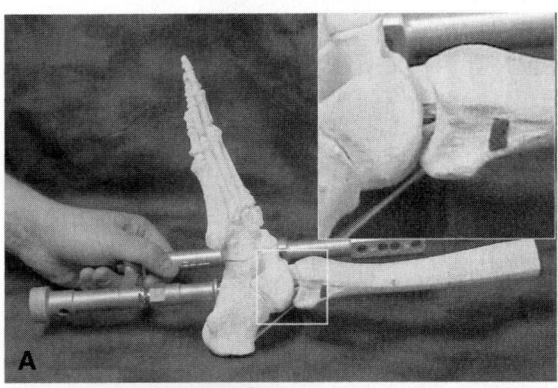
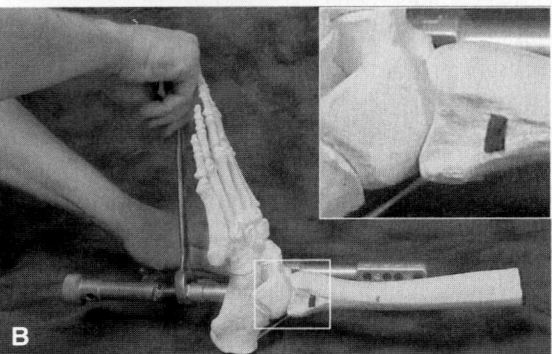

We favor the Ilizarov device when using external fixation for acute compression across a segmental defect. The Ilizarov frame can also be used for restoring length via corticotomy with lengthening at another site of the same bone (bifocal treatment).

GRADUAL COMPRESSION METHODS Gradual compression methods to treat a nonunion with a circumferential segmental defect include simple monofocal gradual compression (shortening) and bone transport. Both methods are most commonly accomplished via external fixation; again, we favor the Ilizarov device. Neither method is associated with the soft tissue and wound problems associated with acute compression. Monofocal compression and bone transport, however, are both associated with malalignment at the docking site, whereas acute compression is not.

For monofocal gradual compression, the external fixator frame is constructed to allow for compression in increments of 0.25 mm (Fig. 22-36). Slow compression at a rate of 0.25 mm to 1.0 mm per day is applied in one or four increments, respectively. When a large defect exists, compression is applied at a rate of 1.0 mm per day; at or near bony touchdown, the rate is slowed to 0.25 mm to 0.5 mm per day. Compression in limbs with paired bones requires partial excision of the intact, unaffected bone.

For bone transport, the frame is constructed to allow a transport rate ranging from 0.25 mm every other day to 1.5 mm per day (Fig. 22-37). The transport is typically started at the rate of 0.5 mm to 0.75 mm per day in two or three increments, respectively. The rate can be increased or decreased based on the quality of the bony regenerate.

When poor surface characteristics are present, open trimming of the nonunion site is recommended to improve the chances of rapid healing following docking. When trimming is performed during the initial procedure, the docking site can be bone-grafted if the anticipated time to docking is approximately 2 months or less (e.g., 6-cm defect compressed at a rate of 1.0 mm/day). If the time to docking will be significantly greater than 2 months (for larger defects), two options exist. First, gradual compression or transport can be continued at a rate ranging from 0.25 mm per week to 0.25 mm per day after bony touchdown is seen on plain radiographs. Continued compression at the docking site is seen clinically and radiographically as bending of the fixation wires, indicating that the rings are moving more than the proximal and distal bone fragments. Second, the docking site can be opened when the defect is approximately 1 to 2 cm to freshen the proximal and distal surfaces and bone-graft the defect. Gradual compression or transport then proceeds into the graft material.

In our experience, continued compression without open bone grafting and surface freshening leads to successful bony union in many patients. Others believe that bone-grafting the docking site significantly decreases the time to healing. The literature is not helpful in clarifying this issue. A useful alternative to open bone grafting is percutaneous marrow injection at the docking site. We use this

FIGURE 22-36 | *Example of a nonunion treated with gradual monofocal compression. **A,** Presenting radiograph of a proximal tibial nonunion in a 79-year-old woman with a history of multiple failed procedures and chronic osteomyelitis. **B,** Intraoperative radiographs following bone excision and Ilizarov application shows a segmental defect. **C,** Radiographs showing gradual compression at the nonunion site over the course of several weeks. **D,** Radiograph showing final result with solid bony union.*

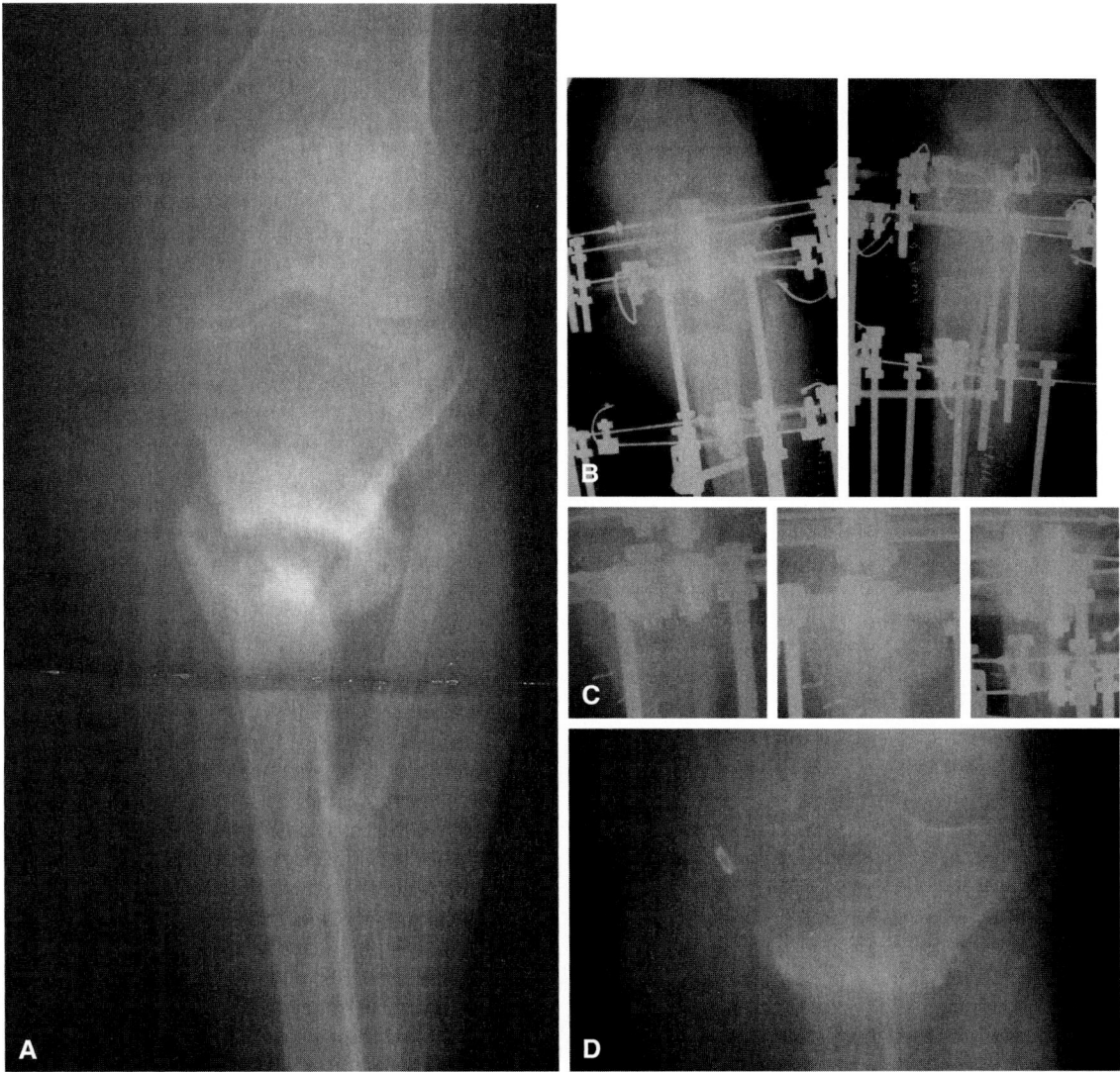

technique in patients who have one or two "contributing factors" (see Table 22-2) and are thus at increased risk for persistent nonunion. We reserve open bone grafting of the docking site for one or more of the following scenarios: patients with no radiographic evidence of progression to healing despite 4 months of continued compression after bony touchdown, patients with three or more "contributing factors" for nonunion who are therefore at very high risk for persistent nonunion at the docking site, and patients who require trimming of the bone ends to improve contact at the docking site.

Nonunions with partial segmental defects are not amenable to many of the treatment strategies that have been

discussed. These defects are most commonly treated with a static method, such as autologous cancellous bone grafting and internal or external fixation. As the partial bone loss segment increases in length, the likelihood of bony union using conventional bone-grafting techniques decreases. In cases of nonunion with a large (>6 cm) segment of partial (incomplete) bone loss, the treatment options are "splinter (sliver) bone transport" (Fig. 22-38); surgical trimming of the bone ends to enhance surface characteristics, followed by an acute or gradual compression method; or strut cortical allogenic bone grafting.

The diverse nature of nonunions with segmental bone defects makes synthesis of the literature quite difficult.

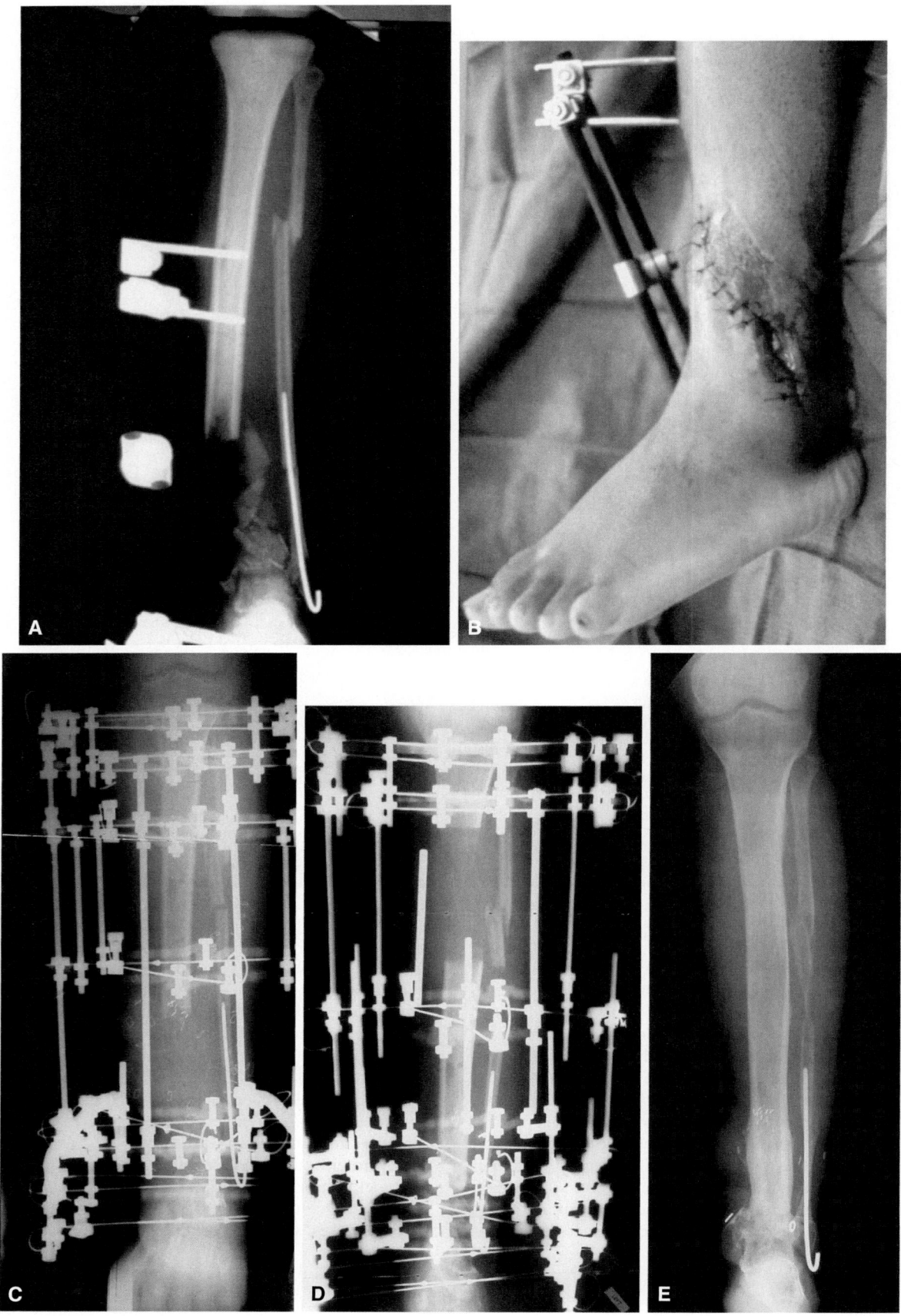

FIGURE 22-37 **A,** *Radiograph on presentation 8 months after a high-energy open tibia fracture treated with an external fixator.* **B,** *Clinical photograph on presentation.* **C** and **D,** *Bone transport in progress at a rate of 1.0 mm per day (0.25 mm four times per day).* **E,** *Final radiographic result shows solid union at the docking site (slow, gradual compression without bone grafting resulted in solid bony union) with mature bony regenerate at the proximal corticotomy site.*

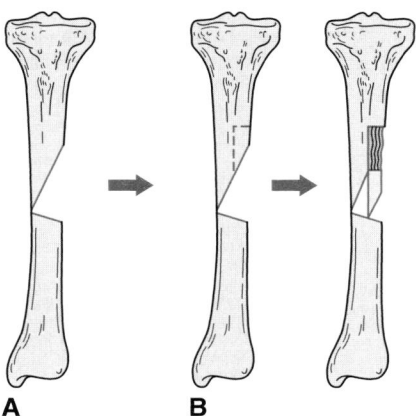

FIGURE 22-38 **A,** *Nonunion with a partial (incomplete) segmental defect.* **B,** *Splinter (sliver) bone transport can be used to span this defect.*

A review of recommendations for treatment of complete segmental bone defects is shown in Table 22-6. Our preferred methods are shown in Table 22-7.

PRIOR FAILED TREATMENTS

The response of a nonunion (or lack thereof) to various treatment modalities will provide insight into its character. Why did the prior treatments fail? Were the treatments appropriate? Were there any technical problems with the treatments? Were there any positive biological responses to any prior treatment? Did mechanical instability contribute to the prior failures? Did any treatment improve the patient's pain and function?

A prior treatment that has provided no clinical or radiographic evidence of progression to healing should not be repeated unless the treating physician believes that technical improvements will lead to bony union. Repeating a prior failed procedure may also be considered if the prior procedure produced a measurable clinical or radiographic

Table 22-6
Review of Literature on Segmental Bone Defects

Author	Patient Population	Findings/Conclusions
May et al., 1989[190]	Current Concepts review based on the authors' experience treating more than 250 patients with post-traumatic osteomyelitis of the tibia.	The authors' recommended treatment options for segmental bone defects are as follows: *Tibial defects 6 cm or less with an intact fibula*—open bone grafting vs. Ilizarov reconstruction *Tibial defects greater than 6 cm with an intact fibula*—tibiofibula synostosis techniques vs. free vascularized bone graft vs. nonvascularized autogenous cortical bone graft vs. cortical allograft vs. Ilizarov reconstruction *Tibial defects greater than 6 cm without a usable intact fibula*—contralateral vascularized fibula vs. Ilizarov reconstruction
Esterhai et al., 1990[95]	42 patients with infected tibial nonunions and segmental defects. The average tibial defect was 2.5 cm (range, 0–10 cm); three treatment strategies were employed. All patients underwent débridement and stabilization and received parenteral antibiotics; following this protocol 23 underwent open cancellous bone grafting (Papineau technique), 10 underwent posterolateral bone grafting, and 9 underwent a soft tissue transfer prior to cancellous bone grafting.	Bony union rates for the three groups were as follows: Papineau technique = 49% Posterolateral bone grafting = 78% Soft tissue transfer = 70%
Cierny and Zorn, 1994[55]	44 patients with segmental infected tibial defects; 23 patients were treated with conventional methods (massive cancellous bone grafts, tissue transfers, and combinations of internal and external fixation); 21 patients were treated using the methods of Ilizarov.	The final results in the two treatment groups were similar. The Ilizarov method was faster, safer in B-host (compromised) patients, less expensive, and easier to perform. Conventional therapy is recommended when any one distraction site is anticipated to exceed 6 cm in length in a patient with poor physiologic or support group status. When conditions permit either conventional or Ilizarov treatment methods, the authors recommend Ilizarov reconstruction for defects of 2 to 12 cm.
Green, 1994[116]	32 patients with segmental skeletal defects; 15 were treated with an open bone graft technique; 17 were treated with Ilizarov bone transport.	The authors' recommendations are as follows: *Defects up to 5 cm*—cancellous bone grafting vs. bone transport *Defects greater than 5 cm*—bone transport vs. free composite tissue transfer
Marsh et al., 1994[185]	25 infected tibial nonunions with segmental bone loss greater than or equal to 2.5 cm; 15 patients were treated with débridement, external fixation, bone grafting, and soft tissue coverage; 10 were treated with resection and bone transport using a monolateral external fixator.	The two treatment groups were equivalent in terms of rate of healing, eradication of infection, treatment time, number of complications, total number of operative procedures, and angular deformities after treatment. Limb-length discrepancy was significantly less in the group treated with bone transport.

(Continued)

	Table 22-6	
	Review of Literature on Segmental Bone Defects—Cont'd	
Author	**Patient Population**	**Findings/Conclusions**
Emami et al., 1995[91]	37 cases of infected nonunion of the tibial shaft treated with open cancellous bone grafting (Papineau technique) stabilized via external fixation; 15 nonunions had partial contact at the nonunion site, 22 had a complete segmental defect ranging from 1.5 to 3 cm in length.	All nonunions united at an average of 11 months following bone grafting. The authors recommend cancellous bone grafting for complete segmental defects up to 3 cm in length.
Patzakis et al., 1995[232]	32 patients with infected tibial nonunions with bone defects less than 3 cm; all were stabilized with external fixation and were grafted with autogenous iliac crest bone at a mean of 8 weeks following soft tissue coverage.	Union was reported in 91% of patients (29 of 32) at a mean of 5.5 months following the bone graft procedure; union was achieved in the remaining 3 patients following posterolateral bone grafting.
Moroni et al., 1995[205]	24 patients with nonunions with bone defects averaging 3.6 cm; 15 ulnar and 9 radial; all were treated with débridement, intercalary bone graft, and internal fixation with a cortical bone graft fixed opposite to a plate.	Union was reported in 96% of patients (23 of 24) at a mean of 3 months following surgery.
Polyzois et al., 1997[243]	42 patients with 25 tibial and 17 femoral nonunions with bone defects averaging 6 cm; 19 (45%) patients had an active infection, and 9 had a history of previous infection; all were treated with Ilizarov bone transport.	Union was reported in all patients (100%), although 4 (10%) patients required bone grafting of the docking site; all cases of infection resolved without further surgery; final leg length discrepancy was less than 1.5 cm in all cases.
Song et al., 1998[304]	27 patients with tibial bone defects averaging 8.3 cm; 13 (48%) patients had an active infection; all were treated with Ilizarov bone transport.	Union was reported in all patients (100%), although 25 (96%) patients required bone grafting of the docking site; all cases of infection resolved without further surgery.
Atkins et al., 1999[15]	5 patients with massive tibial bone defects; all were treated with Ilizarov transport of the fibula into the defect.	Union at the proximal and distal graft sites and hypertrophy of the graft were reported in all patients (100%).
McKee et al., 2002[195]	25 patients with infected nonunions (15 tibia, 6 femur, 3 ulna, 1 humerus) and associated bone defects averaging 30.5 cm were treated with tobramycin-impregnated bone graft substitute (calcium sulfate alpha-hemihydrate pellets).	Union and elimination of infection were reported in 23 of 25 (92%) patients, although 9 (39%) patients required autogenous bone grafting; three (12%) patients had refractured, infection recurred in two (8%) patients, and nonunion persisted in 2 (8%) patients.
Ring et al., 2004[259]	35 patients with nonunions of the forearm (11 ulna, 16 radius, 8 ulna and radius) with defects averaging 2.2 cm; 11 patients had a history of previous infection; all were treated with plate-and-screw fixation and autogenous cancellous bone grafting.	Union was reported in all patients (100%) within 6 months of surgery; 11 (31%) patients had unsatisfactory functional results due to elbow or wrist stiffness; one (3%) patient had a poor result owing to deformity following bony union.

improvement in the nonunion. For example, repeat exchange nailing of the femur can be effective in certain groups of patients[122] but relatively ineffective in others.[335] Those who heal following serial exchange nailings tend to show improvement following each successive procedure. Those whose nonunions persist tend to show little or no clinical and radiographic response after each nail exchange (Fig. 22-39).

The nonunion specialist must be part surgeon, part detective, and part historian. History has a way of repeating itself. Without a clear understanding and appreciation of why prior treatments have failed, the learning curve becomes a circle.

DEFORMITIES

The priority in patients who have a fracture nonunion with deformity is healing the bone. Healing the bone and correcting the deformity at the same time is not always possible. Will the effort to correct the deformity significantly increase the risk of persistent nonunion? If so, then treatment is planned to first address the nonunion and later address the deformity (sequential approach). If not, then both problems are treated concurrently.

In our experience, the majority of nonunions with deformity benefit from the concurrent treatment approach. Deformity correction often improves bone contact at the nonunion site and thereby promotes bony union. Certain cases, however, are better treated with a sequential approach. The sequential approach is preferred if the deformity is unlikely to limit function after successful bony union, if adequate bony contact is best achieved by leaving the fragments in the deformed position, or if soft tissue restrictions make the concurrent approach too complex.

Deformity correction can be performed acutely or gradually. Acute correction is generally performed in lax nonunions, particularly those with a segmental bone defect. Acute correction allows the treating physician to focus on healing the bone, now without deformity.

Table 22-7

Authors' Recommendations for Treatment Options for Complete Segmental Bone Defects

Bone	Host	Segmental Defect	Recommended Treatment Options
Clavicle	Healthy or compromised	<1.5 cm	Cancellous autograft bone grafting; skeletal stabilization
Clavicle	Healthy or compromised	≥1.5 cm	Tricortical autogenous iliac crest bone grafting; skeletal stabilization
Humerus	Healthy	<3 cm	Cancellous autograft bone grafting vs. shortening; skeletal stabilization
Humerus	Healthy	≥3 cm	Bulk cortical allograft vs. vascularized cortical autograft vs. bone transport; skeletal stabilization
Humerus	Compromised	<3 cm	Cancellous autograft bone grafting vs. shortening; skeletal stabilization
Humerus	Compromised	3–6 cm	Bulk cortical allograft vs. vascularized cortical autograft vs. bone transport; skeletal stabilization
Humerus	Compromised	>6 cm	Bulk cortical allograft vs. vascularized cortical autograft; skeletal stabilization
Radius or ulna	Healthy	<3 cm	Cancellous autograft bone grafting vs. tricortical autogenous iliac crest bone grafting vs. shortening; skeletal stabilization
Radius or ulna	Healthy	≥3 cm	Bulk cortical allograft vs. vascularized cortical autograft vs. bone transport vs. synostosis; skeletal stabilization
Radius or ulna	Compromised	<3 cm	Cancellous autograft bone grafting vs. tricortical autogenous iliac crest bone grafting vs. shortening; skeletal stabilization
Radius or ulna	Compromised	3–6 cm	Bulk cortical allograft vs. vascularized cortical autograft vs. bone transport vs. synostosis; skeletal stabilization
Radius or ulna	Compromised	>6 cm	Bulk cortical allograft vs. vascularized cortical autograft vs. synostosis; skeletal stabilization
Femur	Healthy	<3 cm	Cancellous autograft bone grafting vs. bone transport vs. bifocal shortening and lengthening; skeletal stabilization
Femur	Healthy	3–6 cm	Bone transport vs. bifocal shortening and lengthening; skeletal stabilization
Femur	Healthy	6–15 cm	Bone transport vs. bulk cortical allograft; skeletal stabilization
Femur	Healthy	>15 cm	Bulk cortical allograft; skeletal stabilization
Femur	Compromised	<3 cm	Cancellous autograft bone grafting vs. bone transport vs. bifocal shortening and lengthening; skeletal stabilization
Femur	Compromised	3–6 cm	Bone transport vs. bifocal shortening and lengthening vs. bulk cortical allograft; skeletal stabilization
Femur	Compromised	>6 cm	Bulk cortical allograft with skeletal stabilization vs. bracing vs. amputation
Tibia	Healthy	<3 cm	Cancellous autograft bone grafting vs. bone transport vs. bifocal shortening and lengthening; skeletal stabilization
Tibia	Healthy	3–6 cm	Bone transport vs. bifocal shortening and lengthening; skeletal stabilization
Tibia	Healthy	6–15 cm	Bone transport vs. bulk cortical allograft; skeletal stabilization
Tibia	Healthy	>15 cm	Bone transport vs. bulk cortical allograft vs. synostosis; skeletal stabilization
Tibia	Compromised	<3 cm	Cancellous autograft bone grafting vs. bone transport vs. bifocal shortening and lengthening; skeletal stabilization
Tibia	Compromised	3–6 cm	Bone transport vs. bifocal shortening and lengthening; skeletal stabilization
Tibia	Compromised	6–15 cm	Bone transport vs. bulk cortical allograft vs. synostosis; skeletal stabilization
Tibia	Compromised	>15 cm	Bulk cortical allograft with skeletal stabilization vs. synostosis with skeletal stabilization vs. bracing vs. amputation

Deformity correction in a stiff nonunion is more challenging. Acute correction typically requires surgical takedown of the nonunion site or an osteotomy at the nonunion site. Both effectively correct the deformity but damage the nonunion site and may impair bony healing. With a large deformity, the ultimate fate of the neighboring soft tissues and neurovascular structures must be considered when acute deformity correction is contemplated. Gradual correction of a deformity in a stiff nonunion may be accomplished using Ilizarov external

fixation. Correction of length, angulation, rotation, and translation may be performed in conjunction with compression or distraction at the nonunion site. The Taylor Spatial Frame (Smith & Nephew, Memphis, TN) has simplified frame preconstruction and expanded the combinations of deformity components that can be treated simultaneously (Figs. 22-40 through 22-43).[97]

The extent of deformity that can be tolerated without correction varies by anatomic location and from patient to patient. Generally, if the deformity is anticipated to

FIGURE 22-39 *Example of a femoral nonunion that has failed multiple exchange nailings. This 51-year-old woman had three failed prior exchange nailing procedures.*

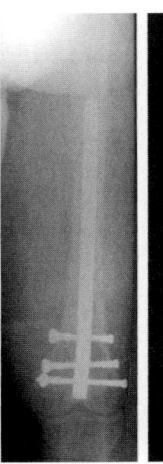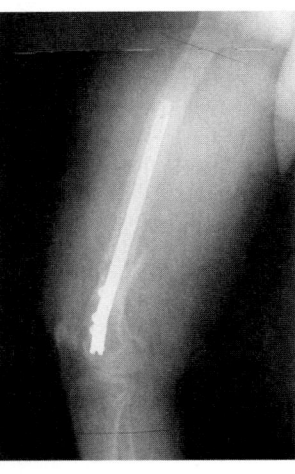

limit function following successful bony union, correction should be considered.

SURFACE CHARACTERISTICS

Nonunions that have large, transversely oriented adjacent surfaces with good bony contact are generally stable to axial compression and relatively easy to bring to successful bony union. By contrast, nonunions with small, vertically oriented surfaces and poor bony contact are generally more difficult to bring to bony union (Fig. 22-44).

Compression generally leads to bony union in nonunions when the opposing fragments have a large surface area. When the surface area is small, trimming of the ends of the bone may be necessary to improve the surface area for bony contact (Fig. 22-45). Similarly, transversely oriented nonunions respond well to compression. Oblique or vertically oriented nonunions have some component of shear, with the bones sliding past each other when subjected to axial compression. Use of interfragmentary screws with plate-and-screw fixation or steerage pins with external fixation minimizes these shear moments (Figs. 22-33 and 22-46).

FIGURE 22-40 *The Taylor Spatial Frame (Smith & Nephew, Memphis, TN) allows for simultaneous correction of deformities involving length, angulation, rotation, and translation. **A,** Saw bone demonstration of a tibial nonunion with a profound deformity. Note how the Taylor Spatial Frame mimics the deformity. **B,** Following deformity correction accomplished by adjusting the Spatial Frame struts. The strut lengths are calculated with a computer software program provided by the manufacturer.*

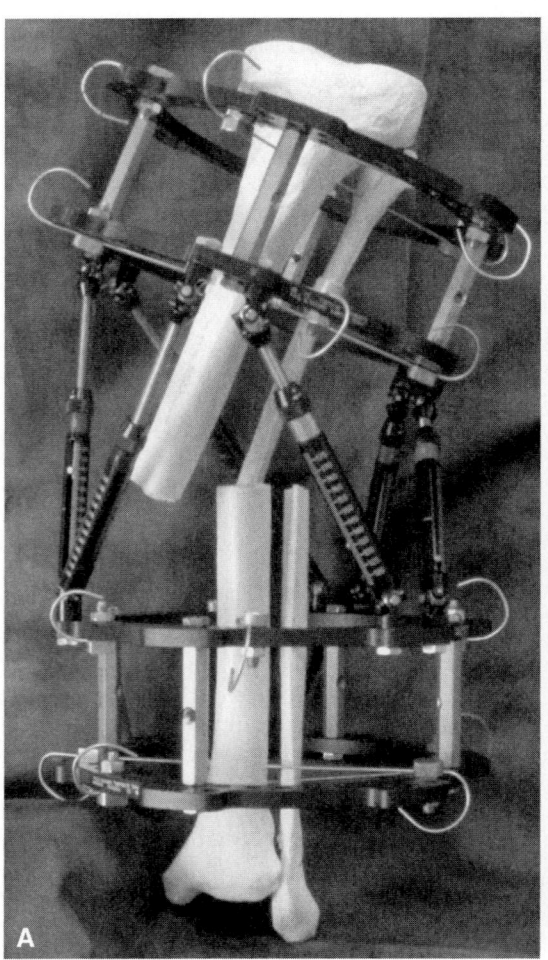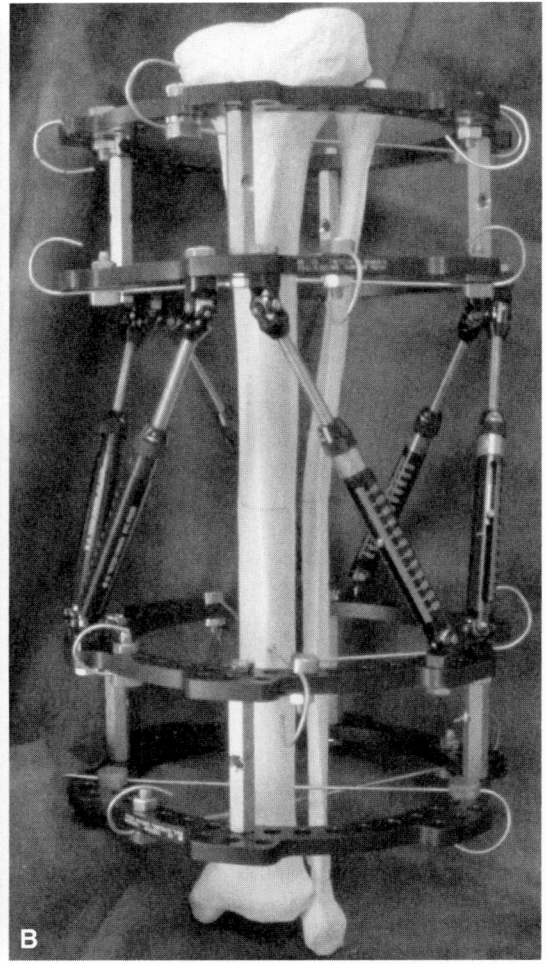

FIGURE 22-41 *A, Preoperative clinical photograph showing frame fitting in the office, AP and lateral radiograph of a 58-year-old woman with a distal tibial nonunion with deformity 14 months following a high-energy open fracture. B, Clinical photograph and AP radiograph during correction using the Taylor Spatial Frame. C, Final radiographic result.*

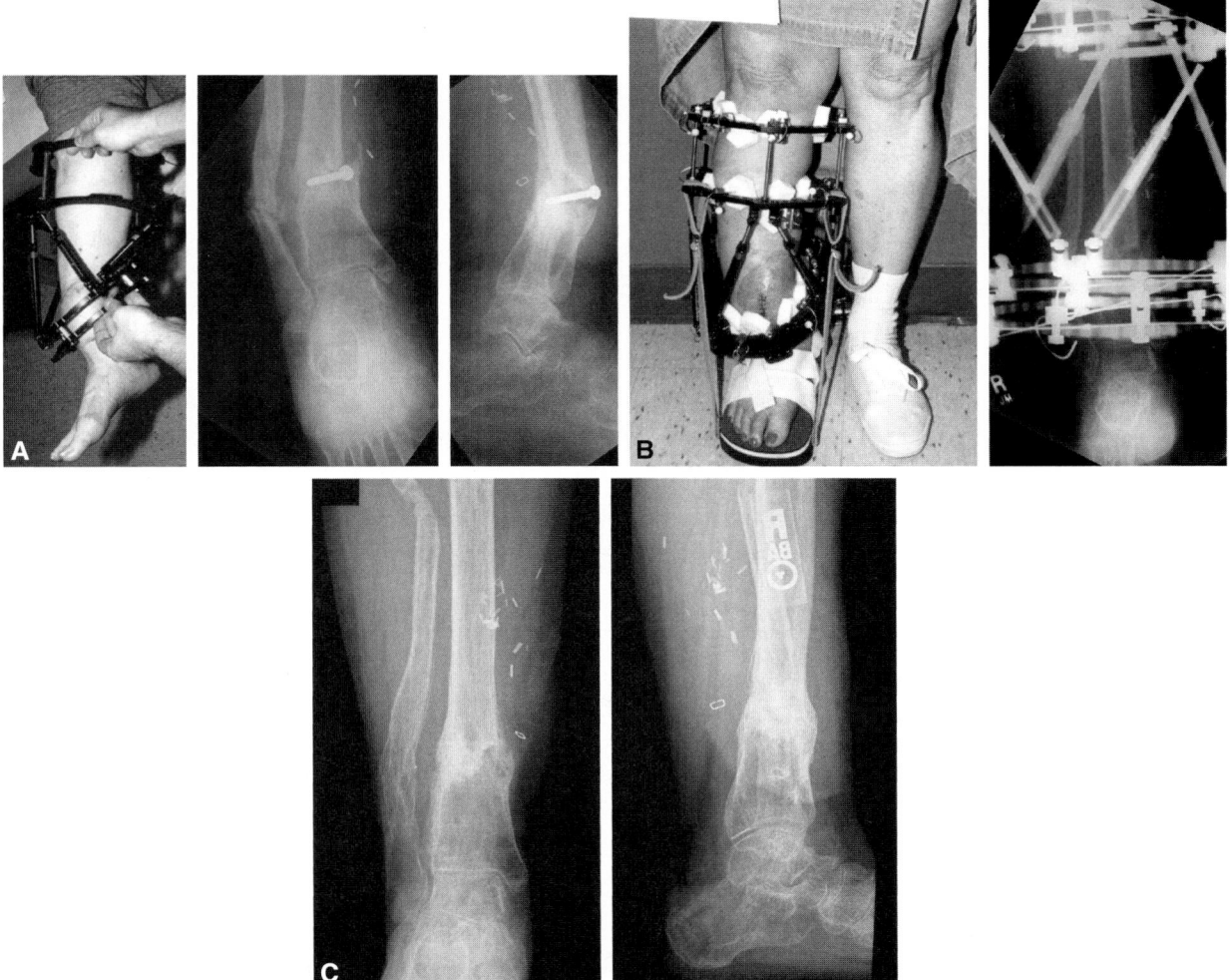

PAIN AND FUNCTION

The "painless" nonunion is seen in three specific instances: hypertrophic nonunions, elderly patients, and Charcot neuropathy.

Some hypertrophic nonunions have relative stability and therefore may not cause symptoms during normal daily activities unless the fracture nonunion site is stressed (e.g., running, jumping, lifting, or pushing). Painless hypertrophic nonunions occur mostly in the clavicle, humerus, ulna, tibia, and fibula. They are identified by a fine line of cartilage at a hypertrophic fracture site visible only on an overexposed radiograph. Subsequent tomograms or a CT scan confirms the nonunion (Fig. 22-47).

Painless nonunions are also seen in the elderly, most typically involving the humerus, but occasionally in the proximal ulna, and less frequently in the femur, tibia, and fibula. Nonoperative treatment can be acceptable as long as day-to-day function is not affected. Nonoperative treatment should be considered in the elderly patient with multiple medical comorbidities that increase the risk of perioperative complications. In such cases, immobilization in a brace or cast (Fig. 22-48), possibly including ultrasonic or electrical stimulation of the nonunion site, may be warranted.[246] Operative stabilization may be necessary if the patient's routine daily activities are impaired or if there is concern about the overlying soft tissues (Fig. 22-49).

Fracture nonunion in the presence of Charcot neuropathy can produce severely deformed and injured bones and joints that are relatively painless. These cases are usually treated with bracing and without surgery unless the overlying soft tissues are jeopardized (see Fig. 22-49).

In all cases of painless fracture nonunion, the medical history, physical examination, and imaging studies should all be carefully considered when determining the treatment strategy. Operative intervention does not always improve the patient's condition and can result in serious problems. Simple, nonoperative treatment may control the patient's symptoms and maintain or restore function, thus providing a satisfactory outcome.

FIGURE 22-42 | ***A,*** *Preoperative radiograph of a 60-year-old man with a distal femoral nonunion with deformity 6 months following open reduction internal fixation.* ***B,*** *Radiograph during correction using the Taylor Spatial Frame.* ***C,*** *Final radiographic result.*

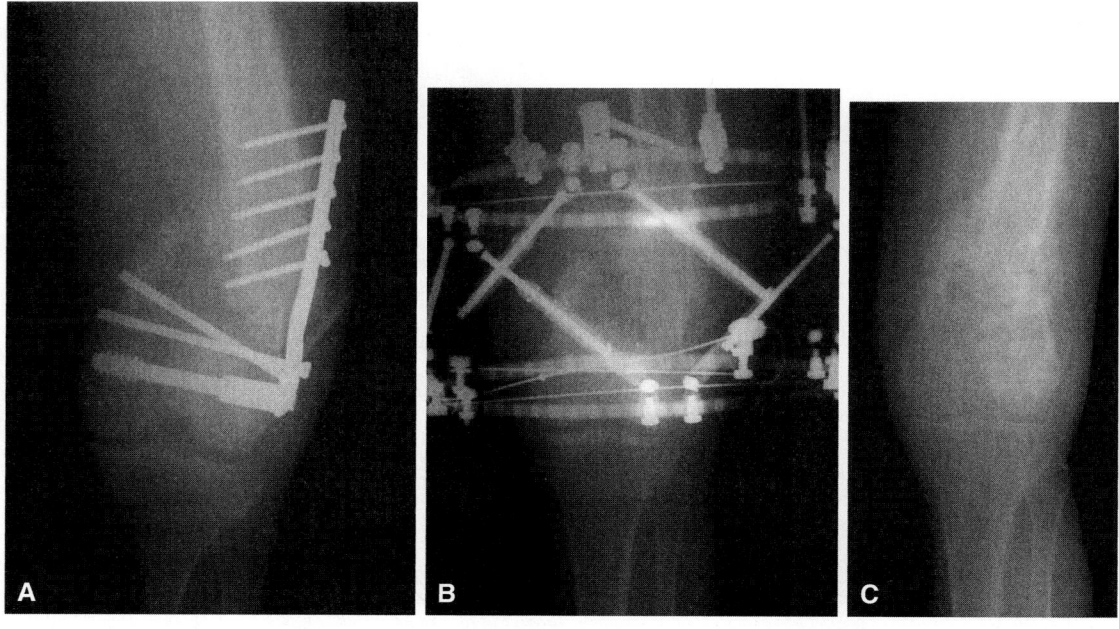

FIGURE 22-43 | ***A,*** *Preoperative AP radiograph of a 73-year-old woman with a distal radius nonunion with a fixed (irreducible) deformity 9 months following injury.* ***B,*** *AP radiograph during deformity correction using the Taylor Spatial Frame.* ***C,*** *Early postoperative radiograph following deformity correction and plate-and-screw fixation with bone grafting for a wrist arthrodesis.*

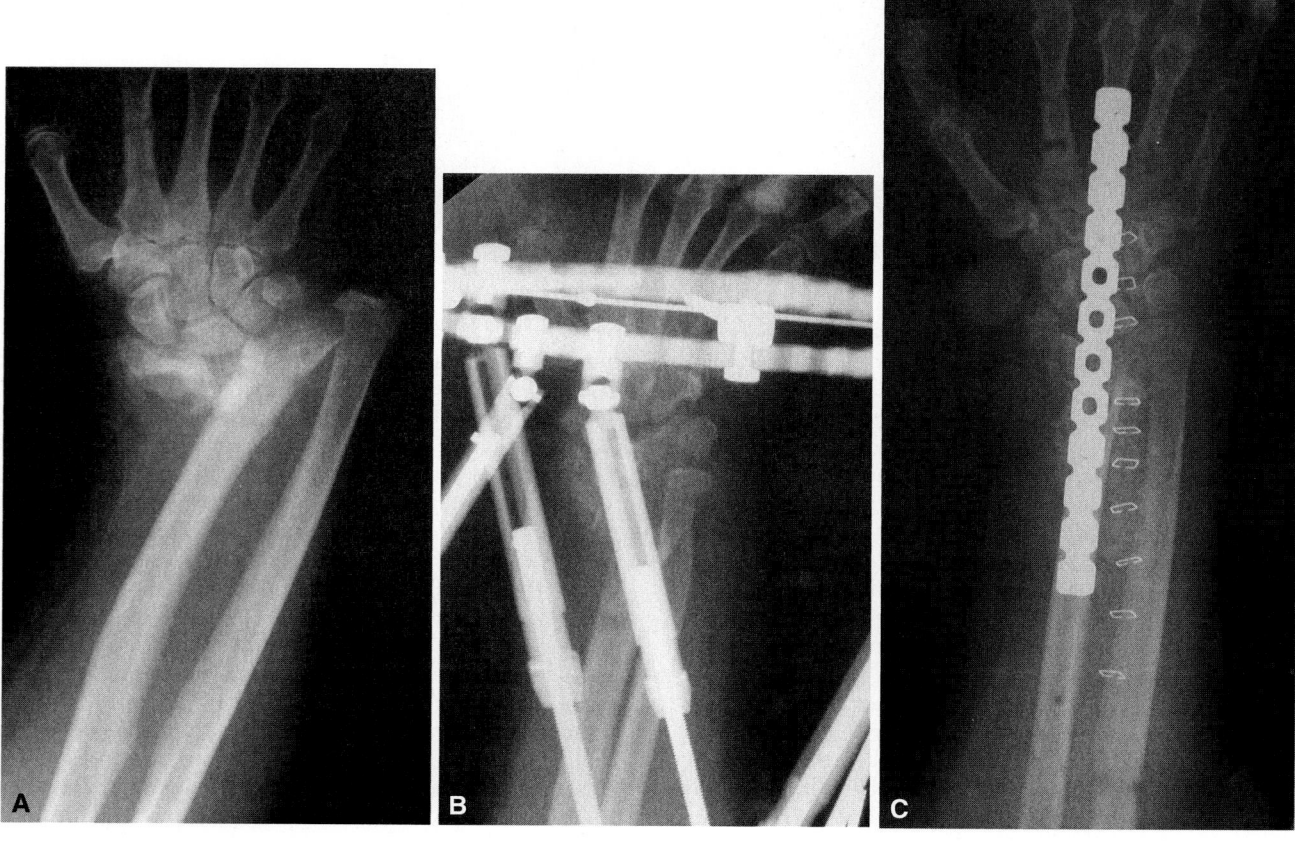

FIGURE 22-44 *Lateral radiograph of tibial nonunion in a 59-year-old man 6 months following fracture. Nonunions such as this with vertically oriented surfaces and poor bony contact can be challenging.*

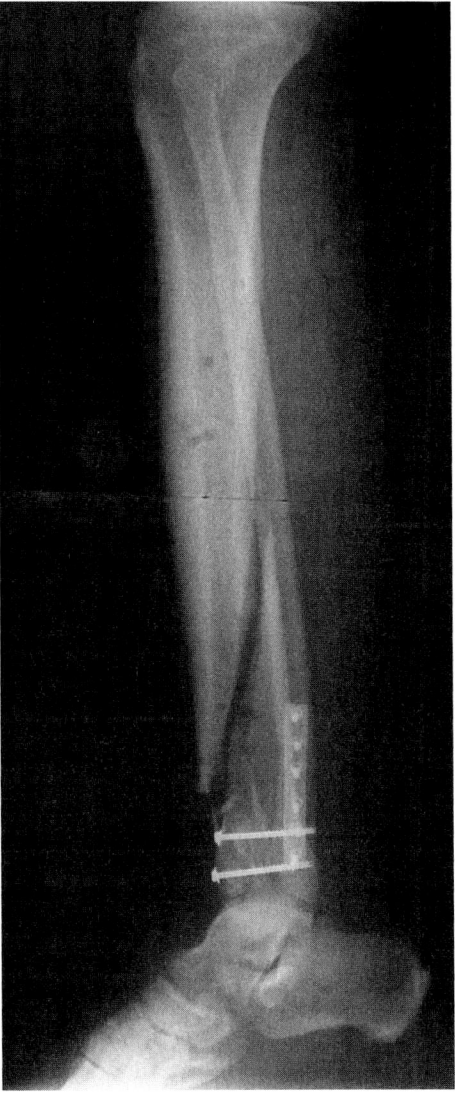

FIGURE 22-46 *Steerage pins (arrow) enhance skeletal stabilization.*

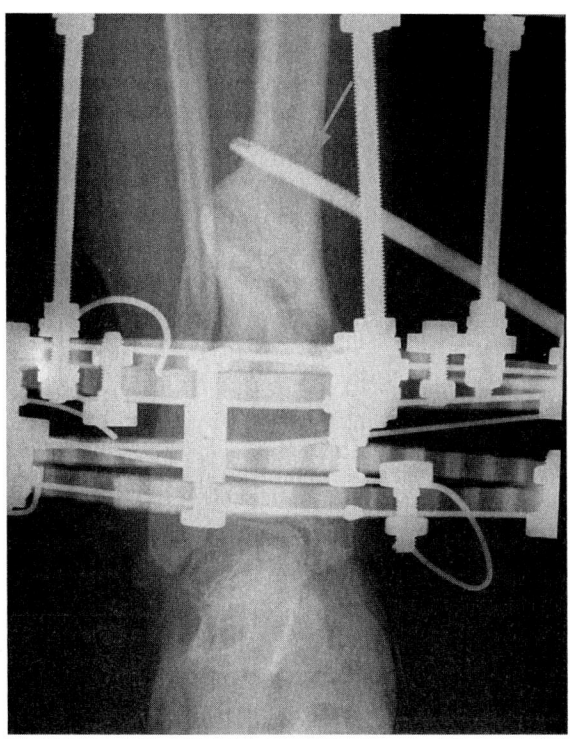

FIGURE 22-47 ***A,*** *AP radiograph of a 17-year-old male 6 months following a clavicle fracture. He had been told by his prior treating physician that his clavicle was solidly healed. He had no complaints of pain. He was brought in by his mother, who was concerned about the bump on his collarbone.* ***B,*** *CT scan confirms the diagnosis of nonunion.*

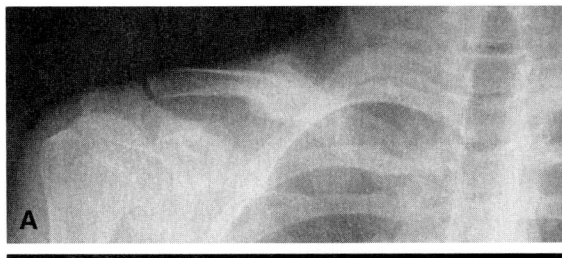

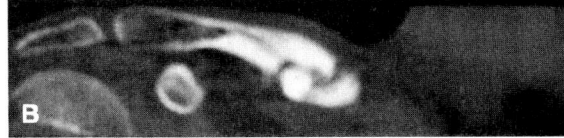

FIGURE 22-45 *Trimming of the ends of the bone at a nonunion site may improve the surface area for bony contact.*

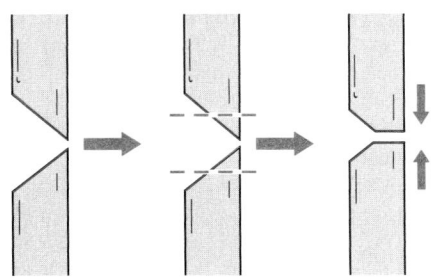

FIGURE 22-48 | **A,** *AP radiograph of a 71-year-old right-hand-dominant woman with multiple medical problems 27 months after a left humeral shaft fracture.* **B,** *Clinical examination is consistent with a lax (flail) nonunion that is not associated with pain. This patient is an excellent candidate for nonoperative treatment with functional bracing.*

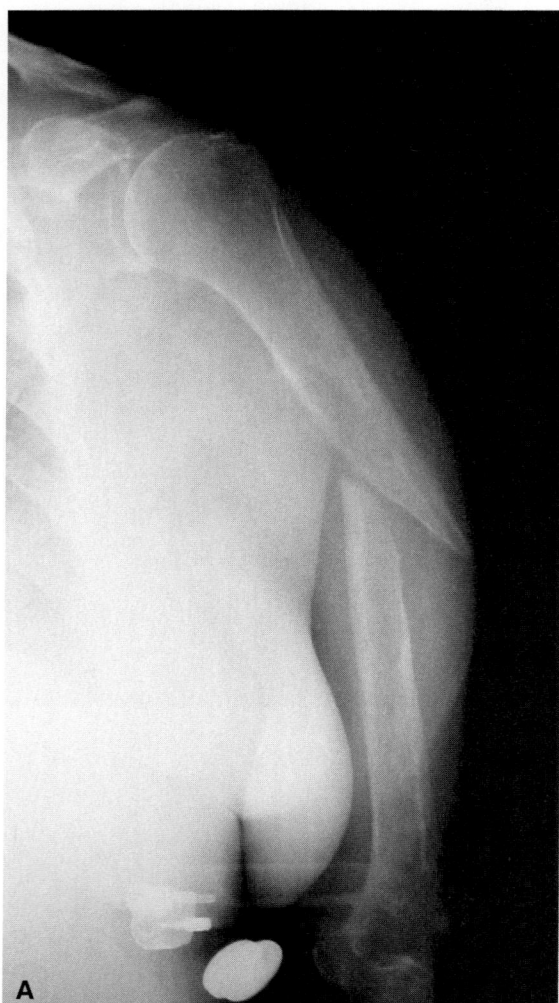

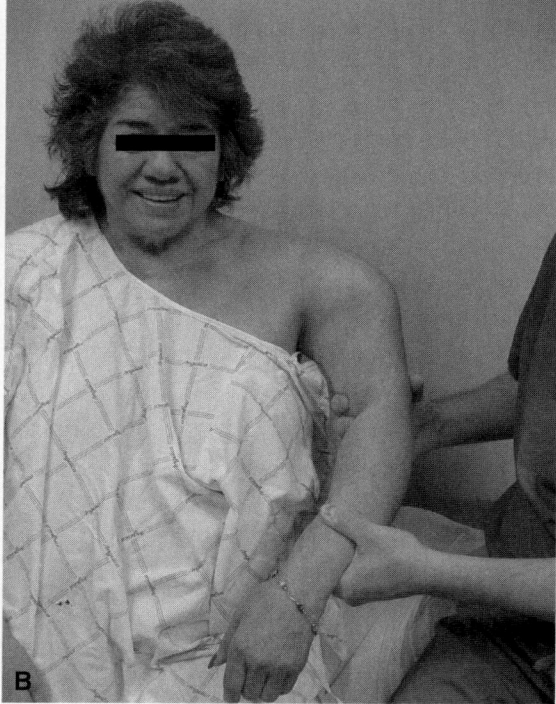

OSTEOPENIA

Nonunions in patients with osteopenic bone are especially challenging. Osteopenia may be isolated to one bone, as with an atrophic or infected nonunion, or it may involve many areas of the skeleton, as in osteoporosis or metabolic bone disease. Metabolic bone disease should be suspected in patients with nonunions in locations that do not typically have healing problems (Fig. 22-50), in long-standing cases that have failed to unite despite adequate treatment, or in cases with loss of hardware fixation but without technical deficiencies.

Intramedullary nailing is a good technique for osteopenic bone. Intramedullary nails function as internal splints and have beneficial load-sharing characteristics. Proximal and distal interlocking screws help maintain rotational and axial stability. Specially designed interlocking screws for purchase in poor bone stock are available. In cases requiring rigid fixation, an "intramedullary plate" construct can be achieved with a custom intramedullary nail and multiple interlocking screws (Fig. 22-51).

Plate-and-screw devices are prone to loosening in osteopenic bone where purchase at the screw-bone junction may be poor. Fixation may have to be augmented in such cases. Van Houwelingen and McKee described the use of cortical allograft struts and bone grafting to augment fixation of a standard compression plate in the treatment of osteopenic humeral nonunions.[320] Weber and Cech[329] described the reinforcement of the screw holes with PMMA bone cement (Fig. 22-52), which is especially useful for nonunion of an osteopenic metaphysis. Locking plates greatly enhance fixation in osteopenic bone. Each screw acts as a fixed-angle device and distributes loads evenly across all screw-bone interfaces. Fixation is particularly enhanced with the use of diverging and converging locking screws.

The thin wires in Ilizarov external fixation provide surprisingly good purchase in osteopenic bone. Olive wires increase stability by discouraging translational moments at the wire-bone interface. A washer at the olive wire–bone interface distributes the load to prevent erosion of the olive into the bone.

FIGURE 22-49 ***A,*** *Radiograph of an asymptomatic humeral shaft nonunion in an 82-year-old woman with Charcot neuropathy (and a Charcot shoulder) of the left upper extremity from a large syrinx. The patient had been managed nonoperatively with a functional brace by her initial treating physician.* ***B,*** *The patient was referred for skeletal stabilization when a bony spike at her nonunion site eroded through her tenuous soft tissue envelope.* ***C,*** *Definitive plate-and-screw stabilization following irrigation and débridement led to bony union.*

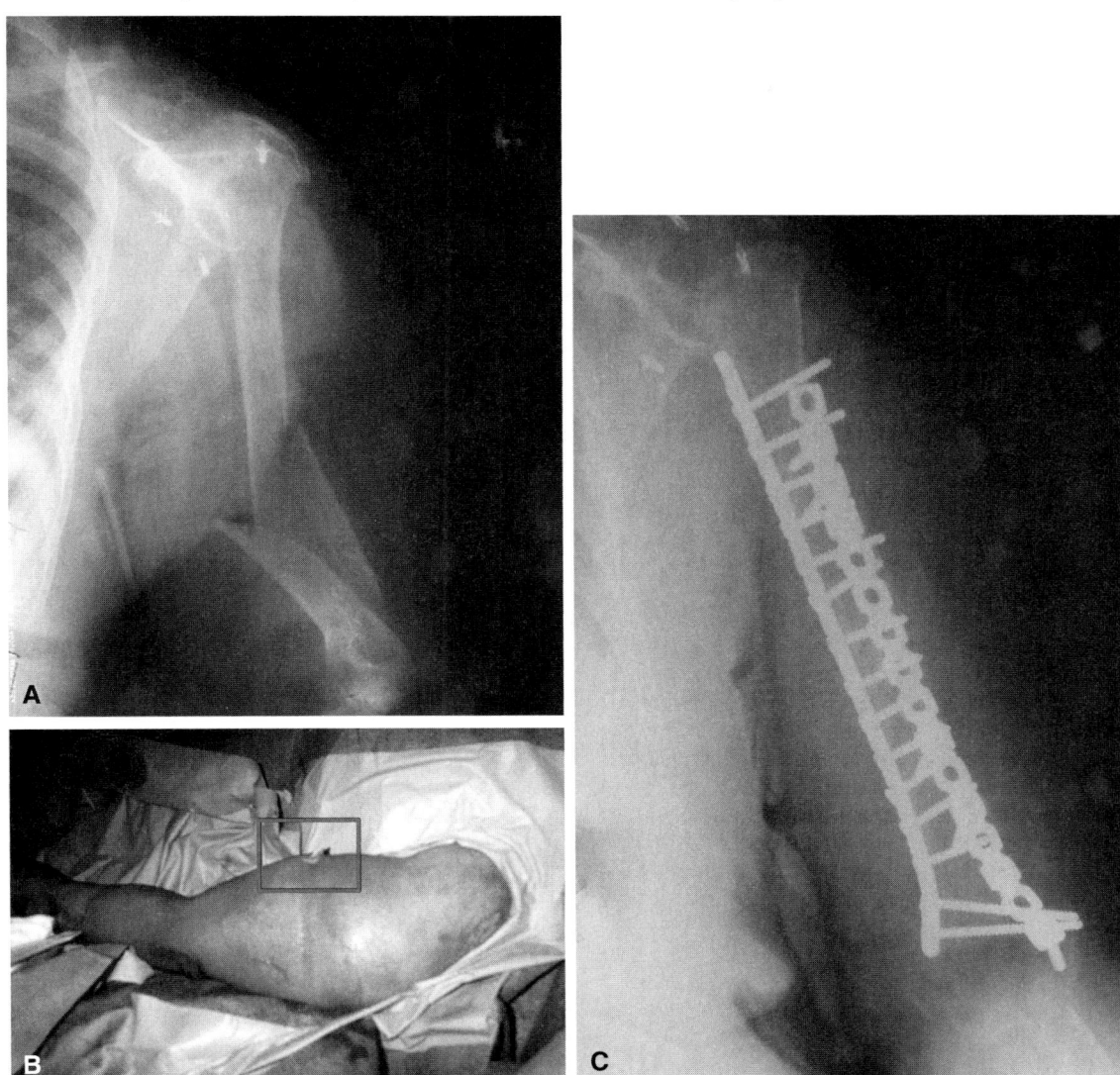

MOBILITY OF THE NONUNION

A nonunion may be described as stiff or lax, based on the results of manual stress testing. A stiff nonunion has an arc of mobility of 7° or less, whereas a lax nonunion has an arc greater than 7°.[144,294] These terms are most applicable when treatment involves Ilizarov external fixation.

Stiff hypertrophic nonunions may be treated using compression, distraction, or sequential monofocal compression-distraction. Lax hypertrophic and oligotrophic nonunions may be treated with gradual compression. Some authors[294] recommend 2 to 3 weeks of compression followed by gradual distraction, but we have found distraction unnecessary in most cases (Fig. 22-53). Others[220] have recommended sequential monofocal distraction-compression in the treatment of hypertrophic nonunions. Lax infected nonunions and synovial pseudarthrosis are treated as described previously. The specifics of the Ilizarov methods are covered later in this chapter.

STATUS OF HARDWARE

Previously placed hardware affects nonunion treatment strategy. One consideration is whether removal of the existing hardware is required. Removal of previously placed hardware is recommended when it is associated with an infected nonunion, it interferes with the contemplated treatment plan, or it is broken or loose and causing symptoms. Previously placed hardware may be retained when it augments the contemplated treatment plan or when surgical dissection to remove the hardware might not be desirable (e.g., obesity, previous infection, or multiple prior soft tissue reconstructions) and the hardware does not interfere with the contemplated treatment plan.

FIGURE 22-50 *AP radiograph of the pelvis of a 50-year-old woman 16 months following a superior and inferior pubic ramus fracture. The endocrinology workup in this patient with a nonunion in an unusual location revealed an underlying metabolic bone disease.*

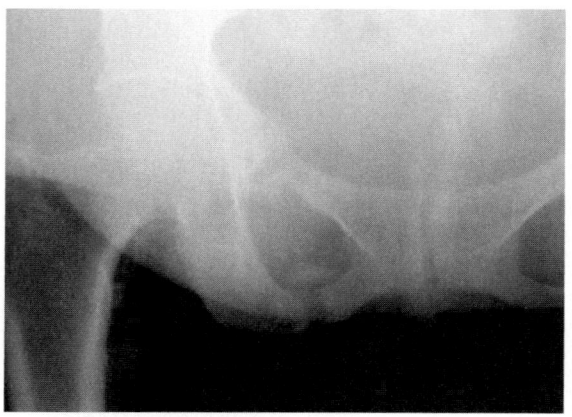

The previously placed hardware can sometimes be used in the definitive treatment. For example, if a statically locked nail is holding the bone fragments of an oligotrophic nonunion in distraction, the interlocking screws may be removed proximally or distally to compress the nonunion site acutely using an external device.

MOTOR AND SENSORY DYSFUNCTION

Many compensatory and adaptive strategies are available to address motor or sensory deficits associated with a nonunion. Bracing, strengthening of intact muscles in the region, and the use of assistive devices may preserve or restore function and thus allow retention of the limb. For example, if anterior compartment motor function of the leg is impaired following successful nonunion treatment, ambulation can be improved by applying an ankle-foot orthosis or by performing a tendon transfer.

There are several factors to consider when designing a treatment plan in a patient with a nonunion associated with neural dysfunction (Table 22-8). If neural reconstruction cannot restore purposeful limb function, and techniques such as tendon transfers or bracing are not likely to be

FIGURE 22-51 *Custom-manufactured intramedullary nails with multiple interlocking screw capability augment the rigidity of fixation and function as an "intramedullary plate." We have used this type of construct with great success in elderly patients with symptomatic humeral shaft nonunions with large medullary canals and osteopenic bone.* **A,** *Preoperative radiograph of an 80-year-old woman with a painful humeral nonunion 14 months after fracture.* **B,** *Early postoperative radiograph following percutaneously performed "intramedullary plating" using a custom-made humeral nail.*

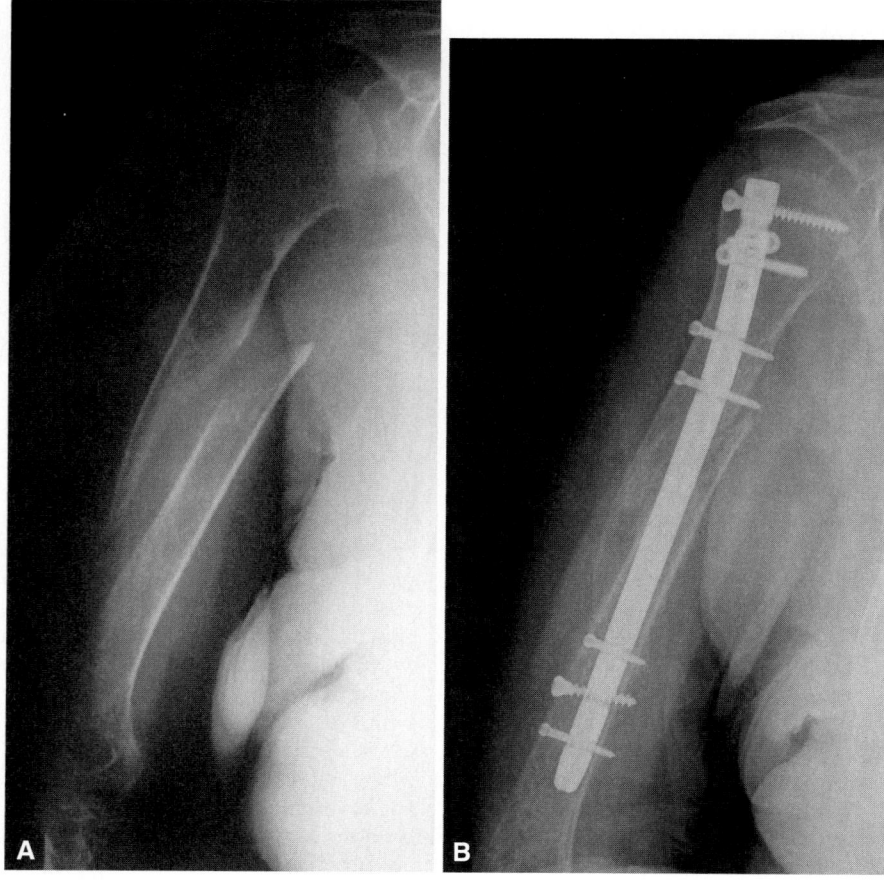

FIGURE 22-52 *Polymethylmethacrylate (PMMA) cement is an effective method for obtaining screw purchase in osteoporotic bone.* ***A,*** *The loose screws are removed, except for those adjacent to or crossing the nonunion and those at the proximal and distal ends of the plate.* ***B,*** *Slow-setting PMMA is mixed for 1 minute and then poured into a 20-mL syringe. The liquid cement is injected into the screw holes.* ***C,*** *The screws are rapidly reinserted into the cement in the holes. The cement should not be allowed to enter the fracture site or go around the bone. After approximately 10 minutes to allow cement hardening, the screws are tightened and checked for stability. If the end screws are essential for fixation and are also loose, they are removed, another batch of cement is mixed and injected, and the end screws are reinserted. (Redrawn from Weber, B.G; Cech, O. Pseudarthrosis. Bern, Hans Huber, 1976.)*

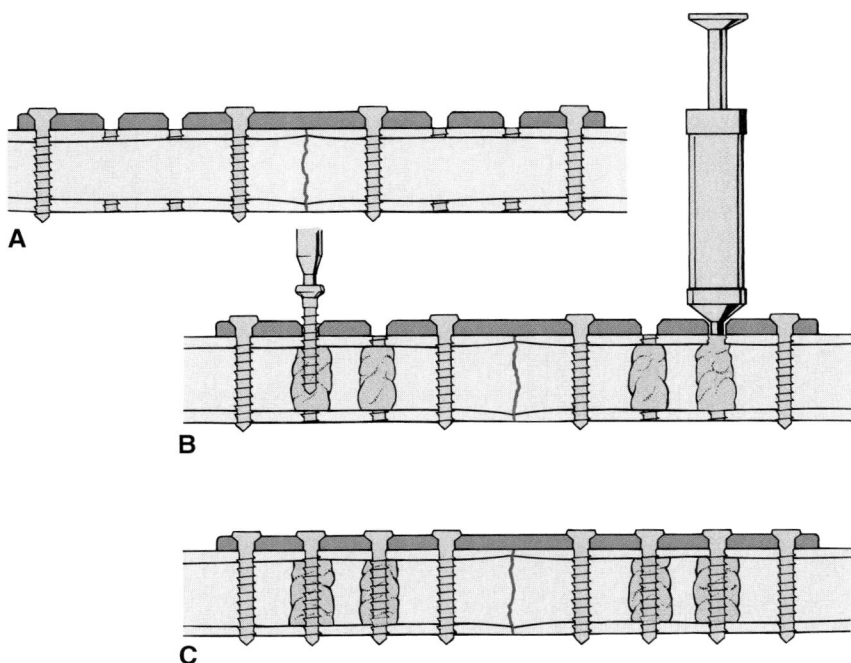

of benefit, amputation may be considered. While limb ablation has obvious disadvantages, it is less prolonged, less costly, and less traumatizing than multiple reconstructions that may not improve an insensate or flaccid limb or improve the patient's quality of life.

PATIENT HEALTH AND AGE

Patients who have serious medical conditions may be poor surgical candidates, and elderly patients are more likely to have such medical conditions. In addition, elderly patients who have been nonambulatory for an extended period, are cognitively impaired, or are confined to a long-term care facility may not benefit from reconstructive surgery for nonunions. The functional status of these patients is unlikely to improve with surgery, and noncompliance with postoperative instructions may produce further complications. In such cases, nonoperative treatment such as bracing is appropriate and engenders greater compliance.

When health is such that survival takes precedence over healing the nonunion, amputation may be considered. On the other hand, elderly patients often benefit from treatment that allows immediate weight-bearing and functional activity, which may decrease the risk of complications such as pneumonia and thromboembolism (Fig. 22-54).

PROBLEMS AT ADJACENT JOINTS

Stiffness or deformity of the joints adjacent to the non-union can limit outcome. Nonoperative therapies, such as joint mobilization and range-of-motion exercises, are commonly prescribed either preoperatively, to prepare for postoperative activity, or postoperatively, to restore limb function following successful nonunion treatment. Alternatively, joint stiffness or deformity can be treated with arthrotomy or arthroscopy either concomitantly with the procedure for the nonunion or as a subsequent, staged surgical procedure. Several treatment options for a compensatory joint deformity adjacent to a nonunion with an angular or rotational deformity exist: joint mobilization via physical therapy, surgical lysis of adhesions at the time of surgery for the fracture nonunion, surgical lysis of adhesions after the nonunion has solidly united in a reduced anatomic position, arthrodesis of the involved joint with acute correction of the compensatory deformity at the time of surgery for the fracture nonunion, and arthrodesis of the involved joint with acute correction of the compensatory deformity after the nonunion has solidly united in a reduced anatomic position.

SOFT TISSUE PROBLEMS

Patients with nonunion often have substantial overlying soft tissue damage resulting from the initial injury or multiple surgical procedures, or both. Whether to approach a nonunion through previous incisions or by elevating a soft tissue flap or through virgin tissues is a difficult decision made on a case-by-case basis. Consulting a plastic reconstructive surgeon is advisable.

FIGURE 22-53   **A,** *Radiograph of a mid-shaft oligotrophic tibial nonunion in a 53-year-old man 10 months following unilateral external fixator stabilization for an open tibia fracture. Because of a history of recurrent pin tract infections and because the external fixator had been removed 3 weeks prior to presentation, intramedullary nail fixation was not believed to be an entirely safe treatment option. The patient was treated with gradual compression using an Ilizarov external fixator.* **B,** *Radiograph during treatment shows gradual dissolution of the nonunion site with gradual compression.* **C,** *Final radiographic result.*

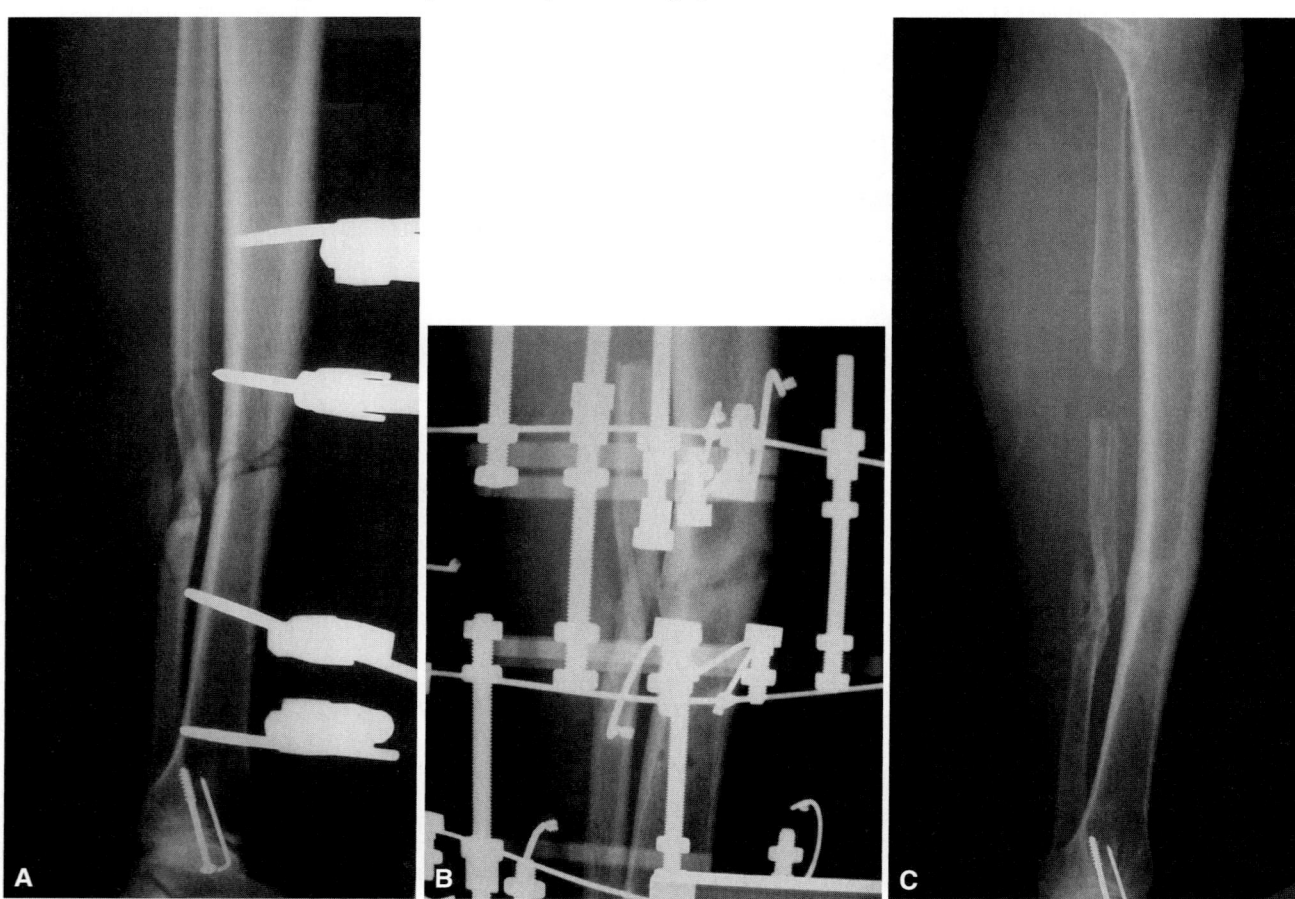

Extremities with extensive soft tissue problems may benefit from less invasive methods such as Ilizarov external fixation and percutaneous marrow grafting. Nonunions associated with soft tissue defects, open wounds, or infection may require a rotational or free flap coverage procedure.

Occasionally, wound closure is facilitated by creating a deformity at the nonunion site to approximate the edges of the soft tissue defect (Fig. 22-55). Three to four weeks following wound closure, the deformity at the nonunion

site is gradually corrected, typically using Ilizarov fixation. This technique is useful for patients who are poor candidates for extensive soft tissue reconstructions, such as those who are elderly, are immunocompromised, or have significant vascular disease or medical problems.

Treatment Methods

Treatment methods that can be used in the care of patients with fracture nonunions include those that augment mechanical stability, those that provide biological stimulation, and those that both augment mechanical stability and provide biological stimulation (Table 22-9). Depending on the nonunion type and associated problems, nonunion treatment may require only a single method or several methods used in concert.

MECHANICAL METHODS

Mechanical methods promote bony union by providing stability and, in some cases, bone-to-bone contact. They may be used alone or in concert with other methods.

Table 22-8

Considerations Affecting Treatment Strategy for a Nonunion with Neural Dysfunction

Quality and extent of plantar or palmar sensation

Location and extent of other sensory deficits

Magnitude, location, and extent of motor loss

Potential for improvement following reconstructive procedures

FIGURE 22-54 *A, Presenting radiograph of a 73-year-old woman with a distal tibial nonunion 14 months following her initial injury. B, Ilizarov external fixation allows immediate weight-bearing and improvement in functional activities, which is important in elderly patients to decrease the risk of medical complications. C, Final radiographic result.*

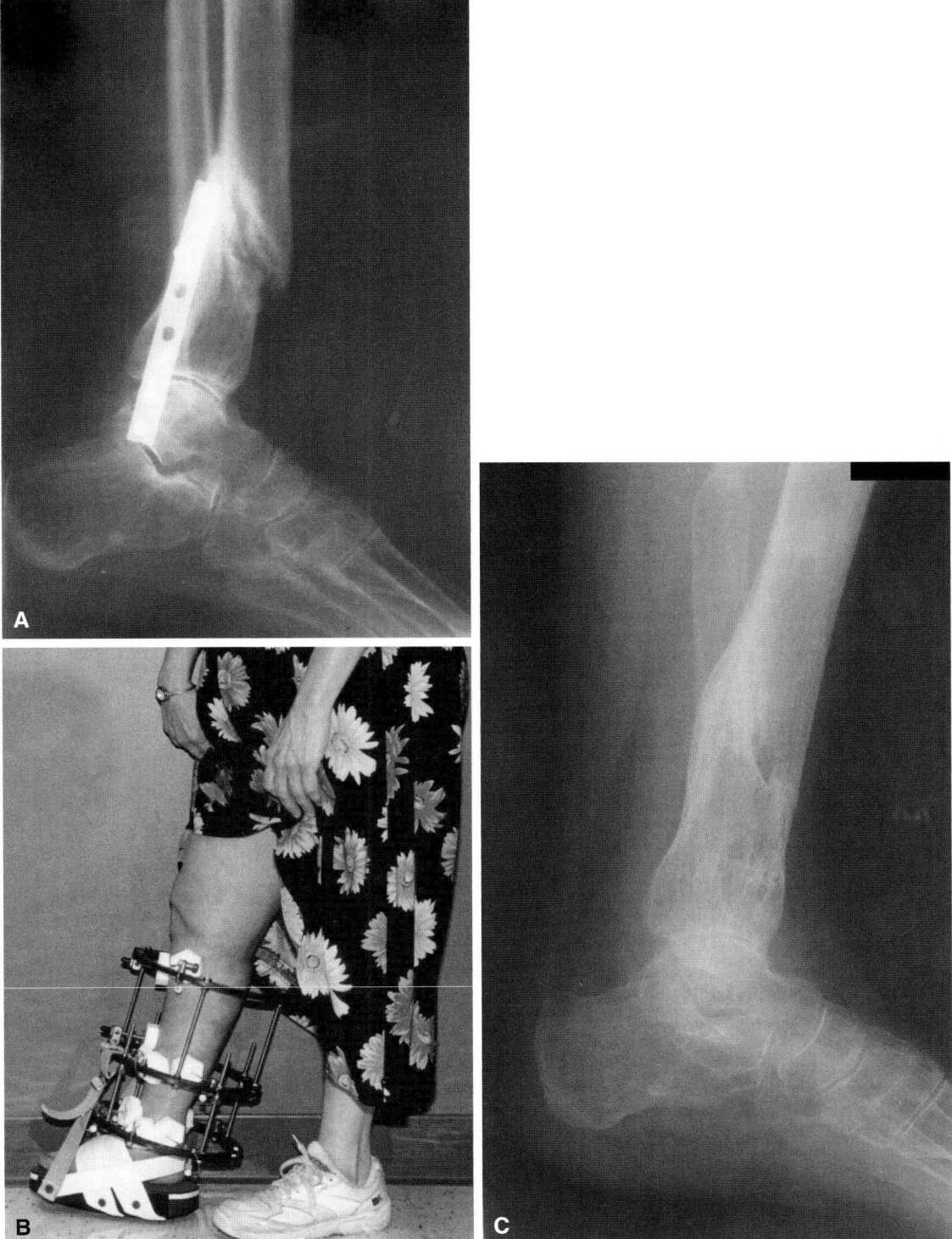

FIGURE 22-55   *In certain cases, creating a deformity at the site of a nonunion facilitates wound closure. This is a particularly useful technique in elderly patients, immunocompromised patients, those with significant vascular disease, and those with severe medical problems who are not good candidates for extensive operative soft tissue reconstructions.* **A,** *In this example, there is a distal tibial nonunion with an open medial wound that cannot be closed primarily because of retraction of the soft tissues.* **B,** *Creating a varus deformity at the nonunion site places the soft tissue edges in approximation and allows for primary closure. The deformity at the nonunion site may be corrected later following healing of the soft tissues.*

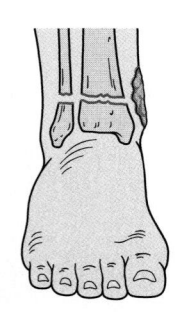
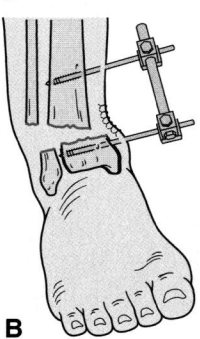

A   **B**

WEIGHT-BEARING Weight-bearing is used for nonunions of the lower extremity, primarily the tibia. Weight-bearing is usually used in conjunction with an external supportive device, dynamization, or excision of bone (Fig. 22-56).

EXTERNAL SUPPORTIVE DEVICES Casting, bracing, and cast bracing can augment mechanical stability at the site of nonunion. In certain instances, especially hypertrophic nonunions, the increase in stability from these devices may result in bony union. External supportive devices are most effective when used with weight-bearing for lower extremity nonunions. Functional cast bracing with weight-bearing as a treatment for tibial nonunion has been advocated by Sarmiento.[285] The advantages of casting, bracing, and cast bracing are that they are noninvasive and useful for patients who are poor candidates for operative reconstruction. Disadvantages of these methods are that they do not provide the same degree of stability as operative methods of fixation, do not allow for concurrent deformity correction, may create or worsen deformities, and may break down the soft tissues in lax nonunions (see Fig. 22-49).

External supportive devices are most effective for stiff hypertrophic nonunions of the lower extremity. Oligotrophic nonunions that are not rigidly fixed in a distracted position may also benefit from casting or bracing and weight-bearing. Unless surgery is absolutely contraindicated, external supportive devices have no proven role in the treatment of atrophic nonunions, infected nonunions, or synovial pseudarthrosis.

DYNAMIZATION Dynamization entails creating a construct that allows axial loading of bone fragments, ideally while discouraging rotational, translational, and shear moments. Dynamization is most commonly used as an adjunctive treatment method for nonunions of the lower extremity that are being treated by intramedullary nail fixation or external fixation.

Removing the interlocking screws of a statically locked intramedullary nail allows the bone fragments to slide toward one another over the nail during weight-bearing. This results in improved bone contact and compression at the nonunion site. In most cases, the interlocking screws on one side of the nonunion (proximal or distal) are removed, typically those at the greatest distance from the nonunion site (Fig. 22-57). When dynamization of an intramedullary nail is contemplated, axial stability and anticipated shortening must be considered. If shortening is anticipated to the extent that the intramedullary nail will penetrate the joint proximal or distal to the nonunion, treatment methods other than dynamization should be employed.

The advantages of nail dynamization are that it is minimally invasive and allows for immediate weight-bearing.

Table 22-9		
Treatment Methods for Nonunions		
Mechanical Methods	**Biological Methods**	**Methods That Are Both Mechanical and Biological**
Weight-bearing	Nonstructural bone grafts	Structural bone grafts
External supportive devices	Decortication	Exchange nailing
Dynamization	Electromagnetic, ultrasound, and shock wave stimulation	Synostosis techniques
Excision of bone		Ilizarov method
Screws		Arthroplasty
Cables and wires		Arthrodesis
Plate-and-screw fixation		Amputation
Intramedullary nail fixation		
Osteotomy		
External fixation		

FIGURE 22-56 | *A, Presenting radiograph of a 44-year-old man 8 months following a tibial shaft fracture. The patient did not desire any operative intervention and was treated with weight-bearing in a functional brace. **B,** Final radiograph 5 months following presentation shows solid bony union.*

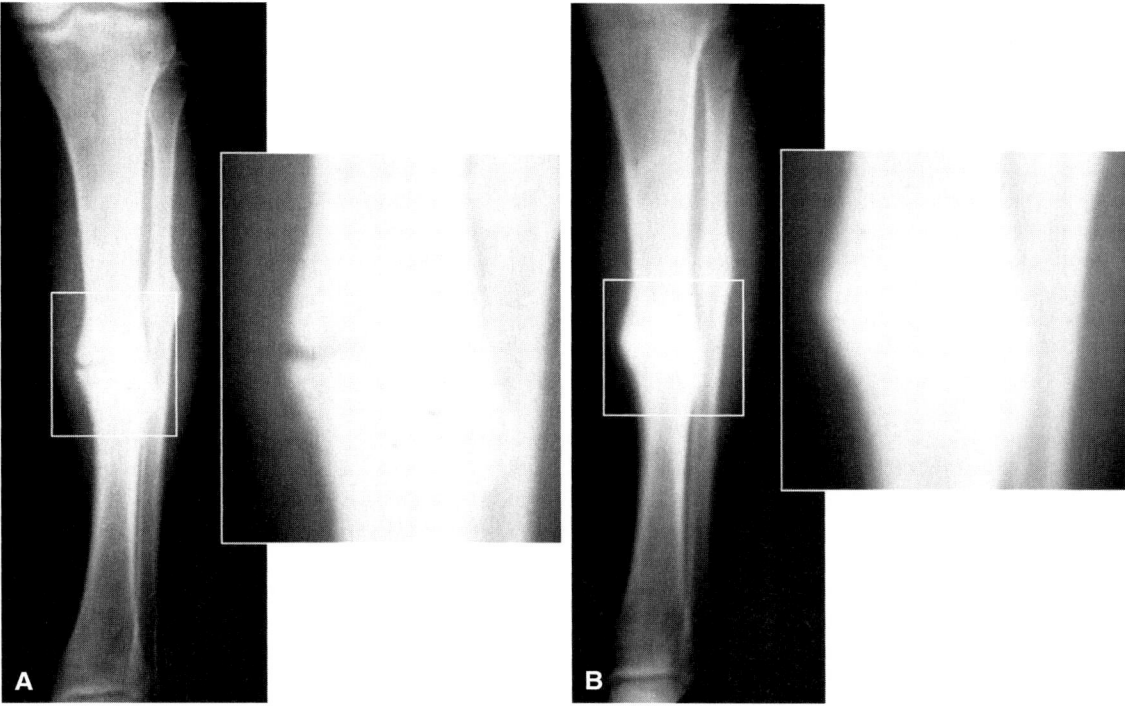

Disadvantages are that it results in axial instability with possible shortening[341] and in rotational instability, although some intramedullary nails have oblong interlocking screw holes that prevent rotational instability (see Fig. 22-57). The technique may be useful for hypertrophic and oligotrophic nonunions of the lower extremity. Atrophic and infected nonunions and synovial pseudarthroses are best treated by other methods.

Dynamization of an external fixator involves removal, loosening, or exchange of the external struts spanning the nonunion. The method is most effective for lower extremity cases and is commonly used only after bony incorporation at the nonunion site is believed to be under way. Dynamizing an external fixator is therapeutic because axial loading at the nonunion site promotes further bony union. It is also diagnostic because an increase in pain at the nonunion site following dynamization suggests motion, indicating that bony union has not progressed to the extent presumed.

EXCISION OF BONE Excision of bone in the treatment of a nonunion is performed by three distinct methods. The first involves excision of one or more bone fragments to alleviate pain associated with the rubbing of the fragments at the nonunion site. Injection of local anesthetic into the nonunion site may suggest the extent of pain relief anticipated following bone excision (Fig. 22-58). Excision of bone will alleviate pain without impairing function at the fibula shaft (assuming the syndesmotic tissues are competent) and the ulna styloid. Partial excision of un-united fragments of the olecranon and patella may be indicated

in certain cases. Partial excision of the clavicle as a treatment for nonunion has been reported by Middleton et al.[200] and Patel and Adenwalla,[229] although we do not advocate this treatment option.

In the second method, excision of bone is performed on an intact bone to allow for compression across an un-united bone in limbs with paired bones. Most commonly, partial excision of the fibula allows compression across an un-united tibia in conjunction with external fixation or intramedullary nail fixation (Fig. 22-59).

The third method of bone excision is trimming and débriding to improve the surface characteristics (surface area, bone contact, and bone quality) at the nonunion site. This technique may be used for atrophic and infected nonunions and synovial pseudarthroses.

SCREWS Interfragmentary lag screw fixation is an effective treatment for epiphyseal nonunions (see Fig. 22-28), patella nonunions[163] (Fig. 22-60), and olecranon nonunions.[225] Interfragmentary lag screw fixation may also be used with other forms of internal or external fixation for metaphyseal nonunions. Screw fixation alone is not recommended for nonunions of the metaphysis or diaphysis.

CABLES AND WIRES Cables or a cable-plate system can be used to stabilize a periprosthetic bone fragment that contains an intramedullary implant, thus eliminating the need for implants traversing the occupied medullary canal. This type of reconstruction is commonly performed with autogenous cancellous bone grafting, either with or without structural allograft bone struts (Fig. 22-61).

FIGURE 22-57   *A, Presenting radiographs of a 40-year-old man 31 months following a closed femur fracture. This patient had unsuccessful multiple prior procedures including exchange nailing and open bone grafting. The patient refused to have any type of major surgical reconstruction and was treated with nail dynamization by removal of the proximal interlocking screws. B, Final radiographs showing solid bony union 14 months following dynamization. C, Intramedullary nails designed with oblong interlocking screw holes allow for dynamization without loss of rotational stability.*

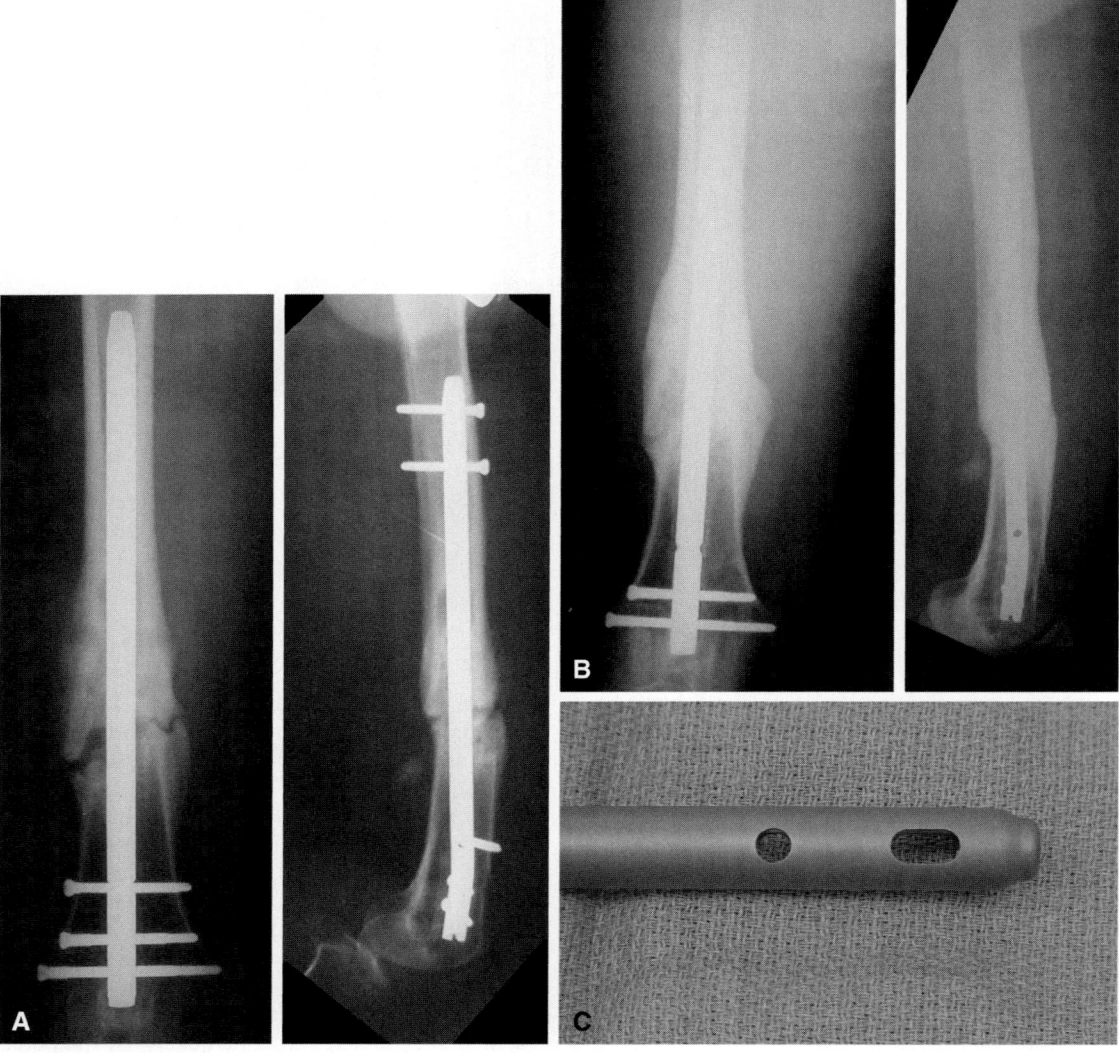

Tension band and cerclage wire techniques may also be used to treat nonunions of the olecranon and patella,[163] although we prefer more rigid fixation techniques.

PLATE-AND-SCREW FIXATION The modern era of nonunion management with internal fixation can be traced to the establishment of the Swiss AO (Arbeitsgemeineschaft für Osteosynthesefragen) by Müller, Allgöwer, Willenegger, and Schneider in 1958. Building from the foundation of the pioneers that had preceded them[49,68,83,150,151,160,172,173,234] and utilizing the metallurgic skills of Swiss industries and a research institute in Davos, the AO Group developed a system of implants and instruments that remain in use today. The AO Group developed the most widely utilized modern concepts of nonunion treatment (Table 22-10).

Advantages of plate-and-screw fixation include rigidity of fixation; versatility for various anatomic locations (Fig. 22-62) (e.g., periarticular and intra-articular nonunions) and situations (e.g., periprosthetic nonunions); correction of angular, rotational, and translational deformities (under direct visualization); and safety following failed or temporary external fixation. Disadvantages of the method include extensive soft tissue dissection, limitation of early weight-bearing for lower extremity applications, and inability to correct significant foreshortening from bone loss. Plate-and-screw fixation is applicable for all types of nonunions. In cases with large segmental defects, other methods of skeletal stabilization should be considered.

Many reports have documented success using plate-and-screw fixation for nonunions of the intertrochanteric

FIGURE 22-58 **A,** *Presenting radiograph of a 70-year-old man 28 months following a high-energy pilon fracture. The patient's primary complaint was pain over the fibula nonunion. Injection in this area with local anesthetic resulted in complete relief of the patient's pain.* **B,** *Final radiograph following treatment of the fibula nonunion via partial excision. The procedure resulted in complete pain relief.*

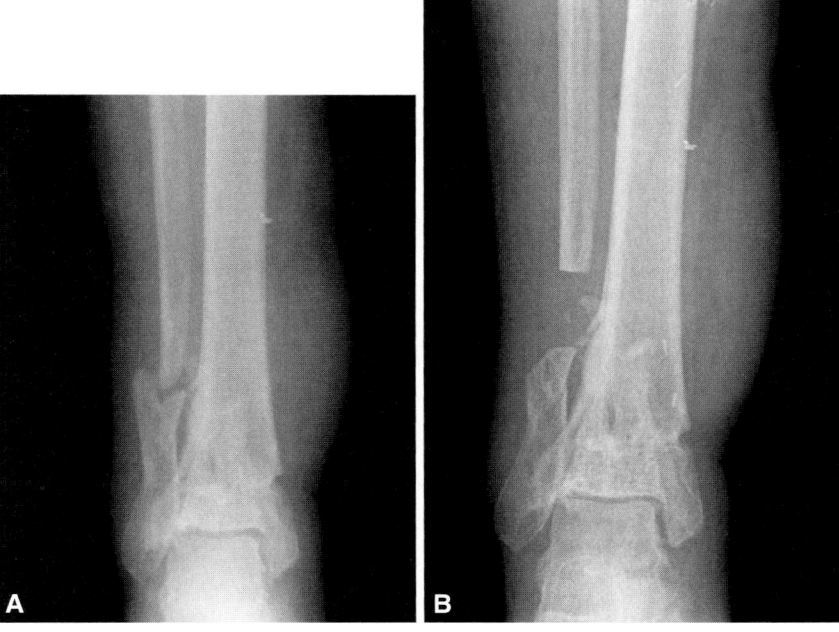

FIGURE 22-59 **A,** *Presenting radiograph of a 42-year-old man 5 months following a distal tibia fracture.* **B,** *The patient was treated with deformity correction and slow, gradual compression using an Ilizarov external fixator. This required partial excision of the fibula (arrow).* **C,** *Final radiographic result.*

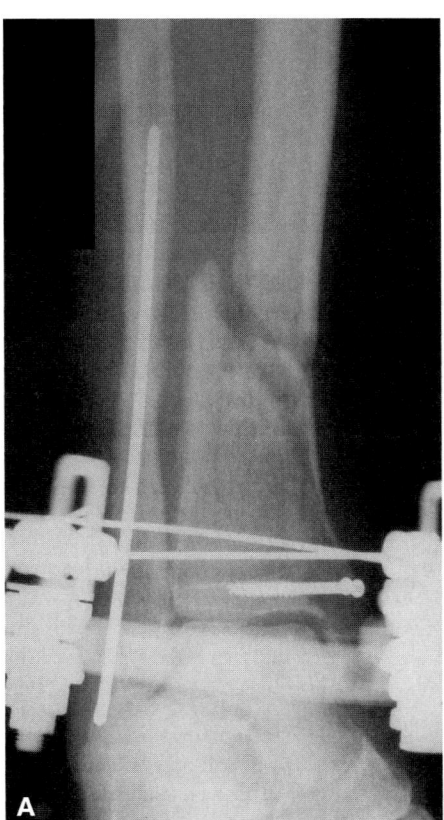
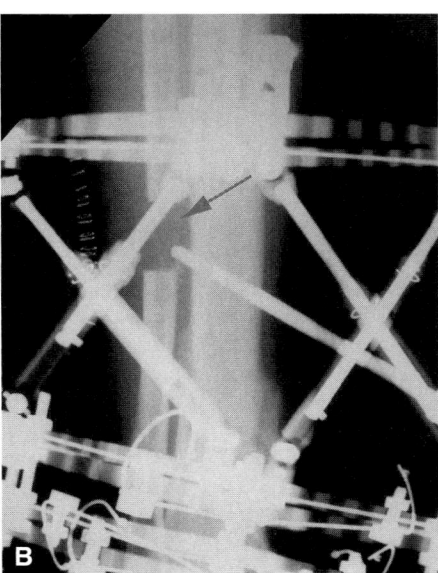
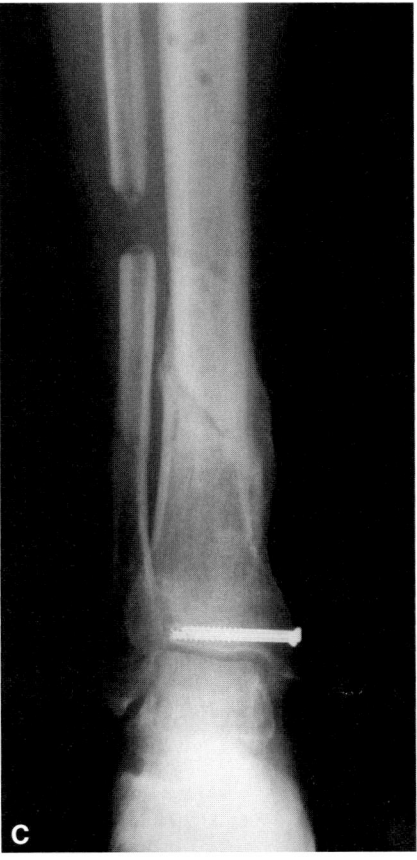

FIGURE 22-60 **A,** *Presenting radiograph of a 55-year-old woman with a patella nonunion who had had four prior failed reconstructions. The patient was treated with open reduction and interfragmentary lag screw fixation.* **B,** *Final radiographic result shows solid bony union.*

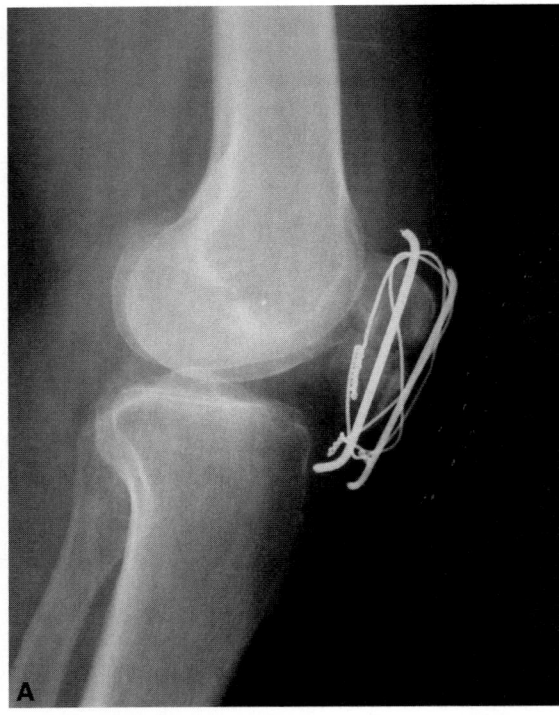

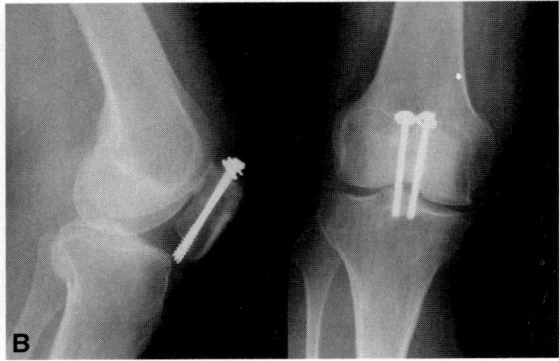

femoral region,[284] femur,[23,314,317] proximal tibia,[40,43,339] tibial diaphysis,[127,240] distal tibial metaphysis,[52,250] fibula,[321] clavicle,[31,71,80,153,218,348] scapula,[47,99,199] proximal humerus,[107,126] humeral shaft,[109,186,274,310,345] distal humerus,[24,128,193,260,283,299] olecranon,[69] proximal ulna,[262] ulnar and radial diaphysis,[259] and distal radius.[88,98] A variety of plate types and techniques are available and are presented in the chapters covering specific anatomic regions.

Locking plates use screws with threaded heads that lock into threaded screw holes on the corresponding plate. The locking of the screws creates a fixed-angle device, or "single-beam" construct, because no motion is allowed between the screws and the plate (Fig. 22-63).[42,85,121] The locked screws resist bending moments and thus resist progressive deformity during bony healing. A locking plate construct distributes axial load across all screw-bone interfaces, in contrast to traditional plate-and-screw constructs in which axial load is distributed unevenly across the screws.[85,121]

The bone fragments must be reduced prior to locking the plate, although newer designs include various adjunctive devices to assist in fracture reduction.[42,121] Care must also be taken to avoid leaving gaps at the nonunion site, because the rigidity of the locking plate construct will maintain distraction at the site.[121] In addition, locking plates are considerably more expensive than traditional plates, and they should therefore be reserved for use in cases that are not amenable to traditional plate-and-screw fixation.[42]

The use of locking plates has been reported to be successful in the treatment of nonunions of the clavicle,[165] humerus,[263,334] femur,[2] and distal femur[23] as well as in the treatment of periprosthetic femoral nonunions.[253]

INTRAMEDULLARY NAIL FIXATION Intramedullary (IM) nailing is an excellent method of providing mechanical stability to a fracture nonunion of a long bone whose injuries have previously been treated by another method (removal of a previously placed nail followed by placement of a new nail is exchange nailing, a distinctly different technique discussed below).

IM nail fixation is particularly useful for lower extremity nonunions because of the strength and load-sharing characteristics of IM nails. IM implants are an excellent treatment option for osteopenic bone where purchase may be poor.

IM nail fixation as a treatment for nonunion is commonly combined with a biological method such as open bone grafting, IM bone grafting, or IM reaming. These techniques stimulate biological activity at the nonunion site, but IM nailing itself is strictly a mechanical method.

Hypertrophic, oligotrophic, and atrophic nonunions, as well as synovial pseudarthroses, may be treated with IM nailing. IM nailing in cases with active infection has been reported[164,167,196,296] but remains controversial. Because of the potential risk of seeding the medullary canal, and because safer options exist, we and others[191] generally recommend against IM nailing in cases of active or prior deep infection. Exchange nailing in the face of infection is a different situation because the medullary canal has likely already been seeded and can therefore be appropriate in selected patients.

Differing opinions also exist regarding IM nailing in patients who have previously been treated with external fixation.[27,148,189,192,198,257,338] The risk of infection following IM nailing in a patient with prior external fixation

FIGURE 22-61 ┃ **A,** *Presenting radiograph of an 83-year-old man with a periprosthetic fracture nonunion of the femur. The patient was treated with intramedullary nail stabilization with allograft strut bone graft with circumferential cable fixation.* **B,** *Final radiographic result shows solid bony union and incorporation of the allograft struts.* **C,** *Presenting radiographs of an 80-year-old woman with multiple failed attempts at surgical reconstruction of a periprosthetic femoral nonunion. The patient was treated with plate stabilization with allograft strut bone graft with circumferential cable fixation.* **D,** *Final radiograph shows solid bony union.*

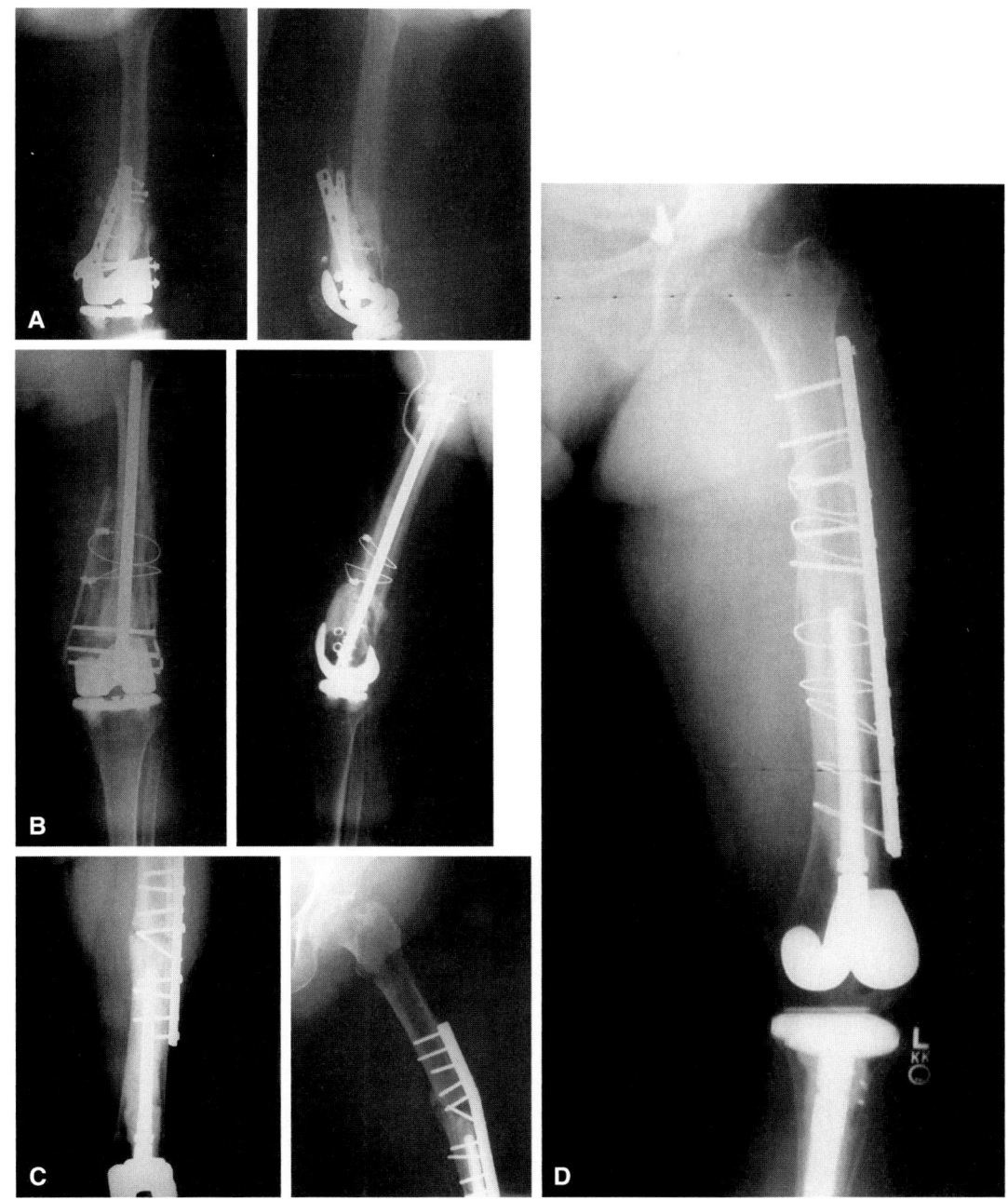

Table 22-10
AO Concepts for Nonunion Treatment
Stable internal fixation under compression
Decortication
Bone grafting in nonunions associated with gaps or poor vascularity
Leaving the nonunion tissue undisturbed for hypertrophic nonunions
Early return to function

is related to a long duration (months) of external fixation, a short time span (days to weeks) from removal of external fixation to IM nailing, and a history of pin site infection (pin site sequestra on current radiographs).

Other factors that likely are related to the risk of infection are related to the application of the external fixator: implant type (tensioned wires vs. half pins), surgical technique (intermittent low-speed drilling under constant irrigation decreases thermal necrosis of bone when placing half pins

FIGURE 22-62 | **A,** *Presenting and final radiographs of a proximal ulna nonunion in a 60-year-old man who had three prior failed attempts at reconstruction. Blade plate fixation provided absolute rigid stabilization and in conjunction with autogenous bone grafting led to rapid bony union.* **B,** *Presenting and final radiographs of a tibial shaft nonunion that had failed treatment with an external fixator. Plate-and-screw fixation with autogenous bone grafting led to successful bony union.* **C,** *Presenting and final radiograph of a humeral shaft fracture that had failed nonoperative treatment and had gone on to nonunion. Plate-and-screw fixation with autogenous bone grafting led to successful bony union.*

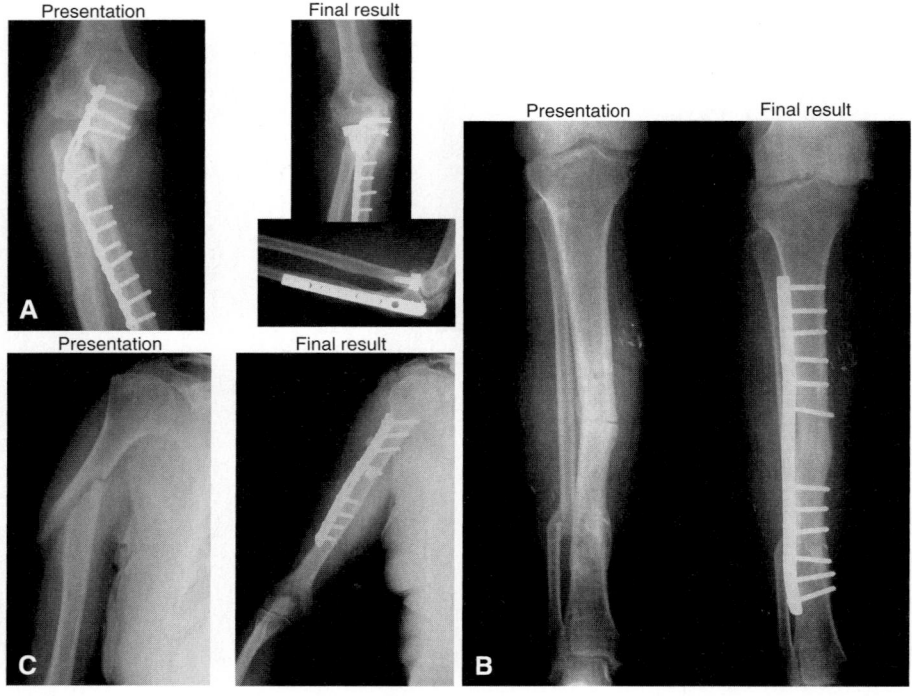

FIGURE 22-63 | **A and B,** *Presenting radiographs of a 41-year-old man 4 months after a high-energy femoral fracture treated at the time of injury by intramedullary nailing.* **C and D,** *The patient was treated with open reduction internal fixation with locking plates, which led to successful bony union.*

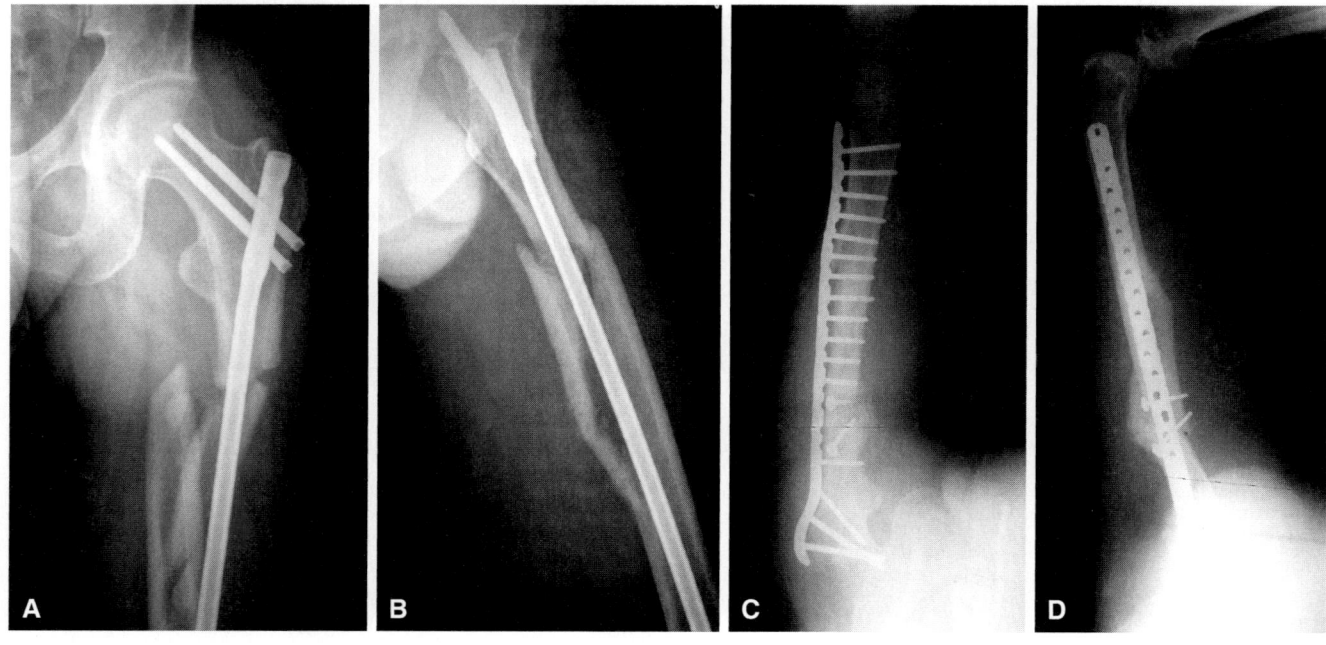

and wires), and implant location (implants that traverse less soft tissue create less local irritation).

A variety of other factors must be considered when treating long bone nonunions with IM nail fixation. First, the alignment of the proximal and distal fragments should be assessed on AP and lateral radiographs to determine whether closed passage of a guide wire will be possible. Second, plain radiographs and, when necessary, CT scans should be studied to determine whether the medullary canal is open or sealed at the nonunion site and whether it will allow passage of a guide wire and reamers. Use of T-handle reamers or a pseudoarthrosis chisel for closed recanalization is effective only when the proximal and distal fragments are relatively well aligned. If these methods fail, a percutaneously performed osteotomy (without wide exposure of the nonunion site), or percutaneous drilling of the medullary canals of both fragments, or both (using fluoroscopic imaging), may facilitate passage of the guide wire and nail (Fig. 22-64). Following the percutaneously performed osteotomy, deformity correction may be facilitated by the use of a femoral distractor or a temporary external fixator. Third, the fixation strategy using interlocking screws must be considered; the choices include static interlocking, dynamic interlocking, and no interlocking. This decision is based on a number of factors: nonunion type, the surface characteristics of the nonunion, the location and geometry of the nonunion, the importance of rotational stability, and others. Fourth, loading and bone contact at the nonunion site can be optimized by a few special techniques. When static locking is to be performed, distal locking followed by "backslapping" the nail (as if extracting it) followed by proximal locking may improve contact at the nonunion site. Some IM nails allow acute compression at the nonunion site during the operative procedure. In addition, a femoral distractor or a temporary external fixator may aid in compression or deformity correction, or both, at a nonunion site being stabilized with IM nail fixation (see Fig. 22-34). For tibial nonunions, partial excision of the fibula facilitates acute correction of tibial deformities as well as compression at the nonunion site during nail insertion and later during weight-bearing ambulation.

Some authors advocate exposure and open bone grafting for all nonunions being treated with IM nail fixation.[227,296,342,343] Other authors recommend exposure of the nonunion site only in cases requiring hardware removal,[196,198] deformity correction,[196,198,277] "nonunion takedown,"[167] open recanalization of the medullary canal,[191] and soft tissue release.[196] Still others,[7,191,340] as do we, discourage routine open bone grafting of nonunion sites being treated with IM nail fixation. Closed nailing without exposure of the nonunion site has the following advantages: no damage to the periosteal blood supply, lower infection rate, and no disruption of the tissues at the nonunion site that have osteogenic potential.

In cases requiring a wide exposure of the nonunion site for open bone grafting, resection of bone, deformity correction, or hardware removal, we use other methods of fixation, such as plate and screws or external fixation to avoid impairing both the endosteal (IM nailing) and periosteal (open exposure of the nonunion site) blood supplies. Exceptions for which we may somewhat reluctantly combine these methods include the following:

1. Nonviable nonunions in patients with poor bone quality, where bone grafting is needed to stimulate the local biology and nail fixation is mechanically advantageous
2. Segmental nonunions with bone defects when we do not believe reaming will result in union and believe nailing is the best method to stabilize the segmental bone fragments
3. Nonunions associated with deformities in noncompliant or cognitively impaired individuals where the biomechanical advantages of IM nail fixation are required (over plate fixation) and external fixation is a poor option
4. Nonunions with large segmental defects where bulk cortical allograft and IM nail fixation are the chosen treatment (Fig. 22-65)

Closed intramedullary bone grafting, as described by Chapman,[46] may be used in conjunction with nail fixation to treat diaphyseal defects. We have used this technique to treat nonunions of the femur and tibia with excellent results (Fig. 22-66). Grafting by means of IM reaming is another excellent method (discussed below with Exchange Nailing).

IM nail fixation as a treatment for tibial nonunions has healing rates reported to range from 92 to 100 percent.* With the availability of specialized and custom-designed nails, the anatomic zone of the tibia that can be treated with IM nail fixation has expanded from that recommended by Mayo and Benirschke[193] in 1990. Each tibial nonunion should be evaluated on a case-by-case basis with templating performed when nail fixation is contemplated for proximal or distal diametaphyseal or metaphyseal nonunions.

A situation worth noting is the slow or arrested proximal tibial regenerate following an Ilizarov lengthening or bone transport procedure. In a very few patients, we have treated this problem with external fixator removal; 6 to 8 weeks of casting and bracing (to allow healing of the pin sites); and reamed, statically locked IM nailing.

This protocol has been used only in patients who were poor candidates for open techniques (bone grafting, plate-and-screw fixation) because of soft tissue concerns (morbid obesity, multiple prior soft tissue reconstructions). Most regenerates fully mature 3 to 6 months following reamed nailing without development of infection (Fig. 22-67).

The clinical results of nail fixation for femoral nonunions have generally been favorable.[19,48,100,158,196,326,343,344,346] Koval et al.,[167] however, reported a high rate of failure for distal femoral nonunions treated with retrograde IM nailing.

IM nail fixation as a treatment for nonunion has also been reported in the clavicle,[28] proximal humerus,[213] humeral shaft,[187,342] distal humerus,[227] olecranon,[66] and fibula.[3]

OSTEOTOMY An osteotomy is used to reorient the plane of the nonunion. Reorienting the angle of inclination of a nonunion from a vertical to a more horizontal position encourages healing by promoting compressive

---

*See references 7, 158, 191, 196, 198, 203, 240, 255, 277, 296, 302, 325, 338.

FIGURE 22-64	*Procedure for recannulating a sealed off medullary canal associated with a nonunion to be treated with intramedullary nail insertion.* **A,** *Without significant deformity (proximal and distal canals aligned). Step 1: Manual T-handle reaming. Step 2: Pseudarthrosis chiseling. Step 3: Passage of a bulb tip guide rod. Step 4: Flexible reaming.* **B,** *With significant deformity (proximal and distal canals are not aligned). Step 1: Percutaneous osteotomy. Step 2: Percutaneous guide wire placement (fluoroscopically guided) into the proximal and distal canals. Step 3: Cannulated drilling of the proximal and distal canals. Step 4: Manual T-handle reaming. Step 5: Pseudarthrosis chiseling. Step 6: Passage of a bulb tip guide rod. Step 7: Flexible reaming.*

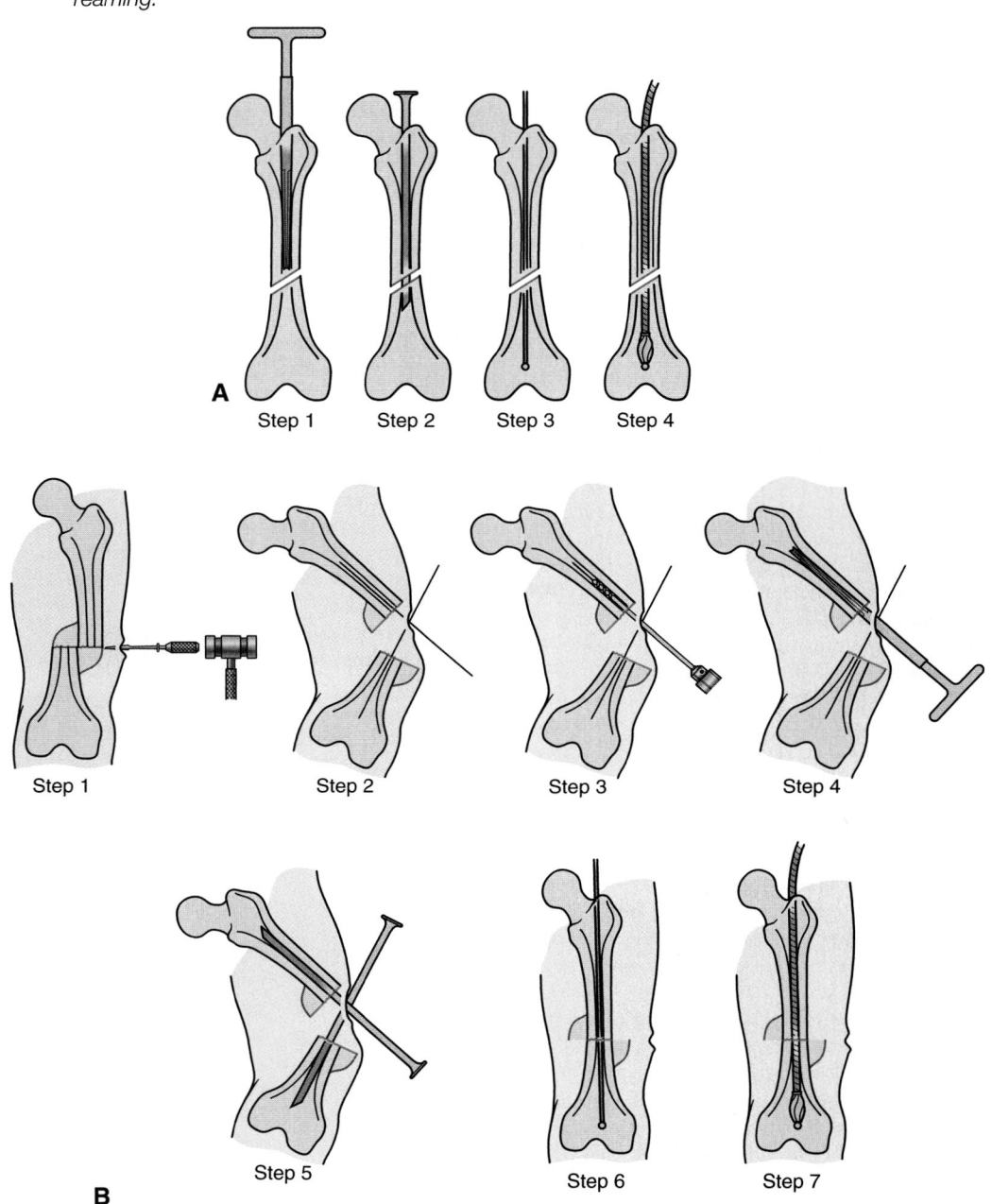

forces across the nonunion site. The osteotomy can be performed either through the nonunion site, such as by trimming the bone ends to decrease the inclination, or adjacent to the nonunion site, such as with Pauwels' osteotomy, for a femoral neck nonunion,[16,188,235] or a dome osteotomy for cubitus valgus deformity associated with lateral humeral condylar nonunion.[312]

EXTERNAL FIXATION External fixation has primarily been used to treat infected nonunions of the femur,[318] tibia,[50,91,232] and humerus.[51,176,240] The method is commonly combined with serial débridement, antibiotic beads, soft tissue coverage procedures, and bone grafting. The Ilizarov method of external fixation is discussed below in Methods That Are Both Mechanical and Biological.

BIOLOGICAL METHODS

Biological methods stimulate the local biology at the non-union site. These methods may be used alone but typically are combined with a mechanical method.

NONSTRUCTURAL BONE GRAFTS

Autogenous Cancellous Graft

Autogenous cancellous bone grafting remains an important weapon in the trauma surgeon's armamentarium. Successful treatment of oligotrophic, atrophic, and infected nonunions, as well as synovial pseudarthroses, often depends on copious autologous cancellous bone grafting.

Cancellous autograft is osteogenic, osteoconductive, and osteoinductive. The graft stimulates the local biology in viable nonunions that have poor callus formation and in nonviable nonunions. The graft's initially poor structural integrity improves rapidly during osseointegration.

Cancellous autograft is not necessary in the treatment of hypertrophic nonunions, which are viable and often have abundant callus formation.

Oligotrophic nonunions are viable and typically arise as a result of poor bone-to-bone contact. Cancellous autograft bone promotes bridging of un-united bone gaps. The decision about whether to bone-graft an oligotrophic nonunion is determined by the treatment strategy. If the strategy involves operative exposure of the nonunion site (e.g., plate-and-screw fixation), then decortication and autogenous bone grafting are recommended. If the strategy does not involve exposure of the nonunion site (e.g., compression via external fixation), we do not routinely bone-graft.

FIGURE 22-65 ***A,*** *Presenting radiograph of an infected femoral nonunion resulting from an open femur fracture 32 years earlier. This 51-year-old man had undergone more than 20 prior attempts at surgical reconstruction, the most recent being external fixation and bone grafting performed at an outside facility.* ***B,*** *Clinical photograph at the time of presentation.* ***C,*** *Clinical photograph showing antibiotic beads in situ.*

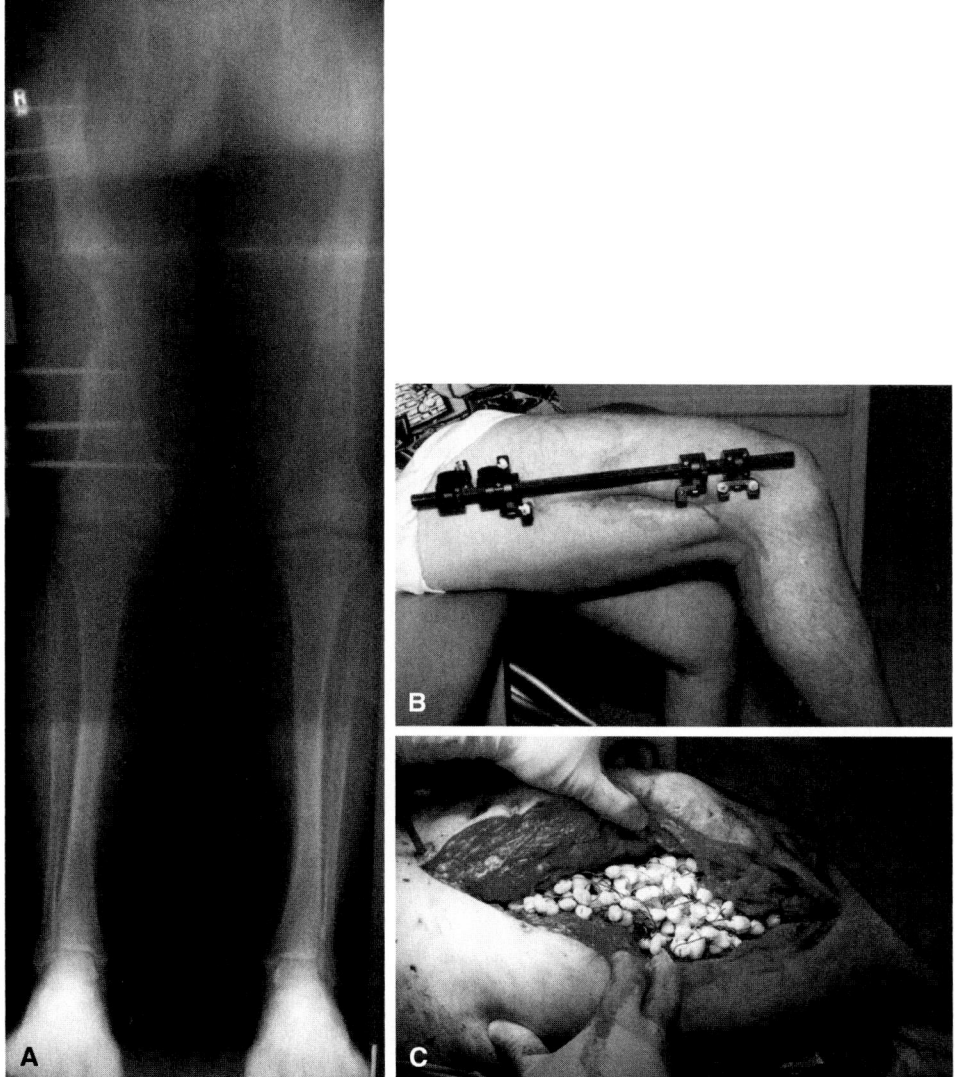

(Continued)

FIGURE 22-65 *(Continued)* **D,** Gross specimen. **E,** Radiograph following radical resection shows a bulk antibiotic spacer that remained in situ for 3 months. **F,** Radiographs 7 months following reconstruction using a bulk femoral allograft and a custom two-piece femoral nail (the proximal portion of the nail is an antegrade reconstruction nail; the distal portion of the nail is a retrograde supracondylar nail). **G,** Clinical photograph 7 months following reconstruction.

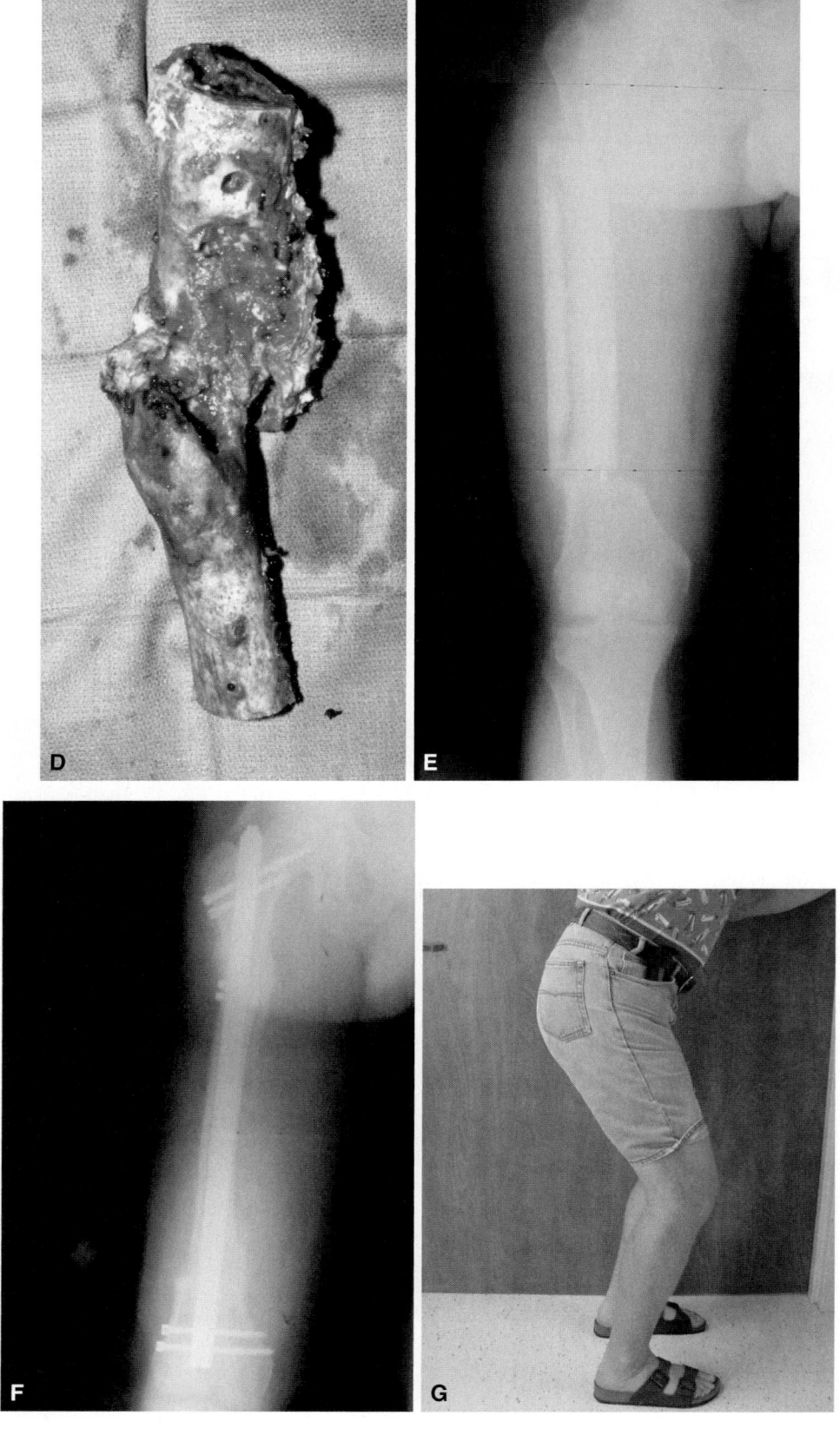

FIGURE 22-66 | *Closed intramedullary autogenous cancellous bone grafting can be used to treat diaphyseal bony defects. Autogenous cancellous bone harvested from the iliac crest is delivered to the defect via a tube positioned in the medullary canal.*

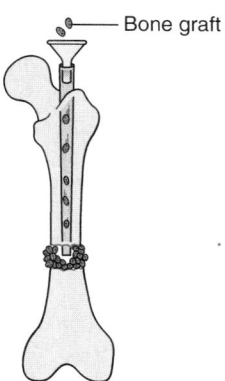

Bone graft

Atrophic and infected nonunions are nonviable and incapable of callus formation. They are typically associated with segmental bone defects. Recommendations vary regarding the maximum size of a complete segmental defect that will unite following autogenous cancellous bone grafting (see Table 22-6).[55,91,95,116,185,190,232] Our recommendations for segmental bone defects are shown in Table 22-7.

Synovial pseudarthrosis is typically treated with excision of the pseudarthrosis tissue and opening of the medullary canal. Decortication and autogenous cancellous bone grafting are recommended to encourage healing.

Cancellous autogenous bone graft may be harvested from the iliac crest, the distal femur, the greater trochanter, the proximal tibia, and the distal radius. The iliac crest yields the most osseous tissue. The posterior iliac crest yields dramatically more bone, less postoperative pain, and a lower risk of postoperative complications in comparison to the anterior iliac crest.[6] The posterior iliac crest bone of intramembranous origin (ilium) appears to be

FIGURE 22-67 | ***A,*** *Radiograph of the proximal tibial regenerate in a 54-year-old woman who had undergone bone transport for an infected distal tibial nonunion. Although the technique led to solid bony union of the distal tibial nonunion site, her bony regenerate failed to mature and was mechanically unstable. This patient was treated with removal of her external fixator and 8 weeks of bracing. Following complete healing of the pin sites, a reamed, statically locked, custom (short) intramedullary nail was placed. **B,** Follow-up radiograph at 8 months after intramedullary nailing shows solid healing and maturation of the proximal tibial regenerate.*

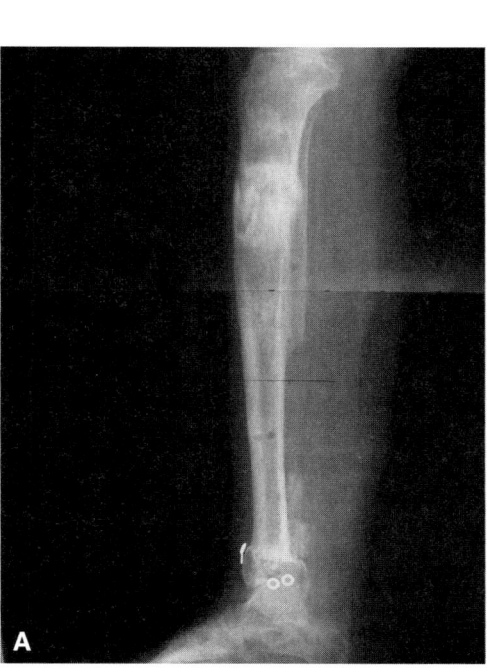

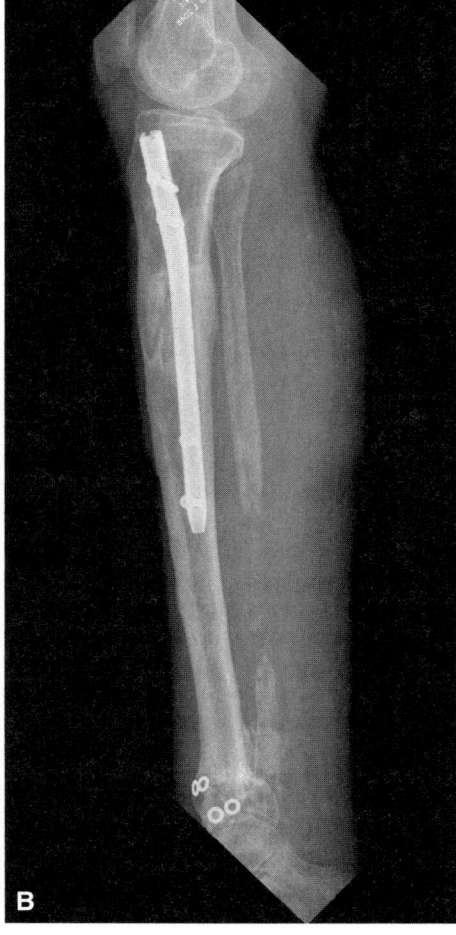

A

B

more osteoconductive than bone of enchondral origin (tibia, femur, radius).[241]

Autogenous cancellous autograft techniques for the treatment of nonunions include the following:

Papineau technique (open cancellous bone grafting)[226]

Posterolateral grafting of the tibia

Anterior grafting of the tibia (following soft tissue coverage)

Intramedullary grafting[46]

Intramedullary reaming

Endoscopic bone grafting[162]

Percutaneous bone grafting[25,130,131,159]

Furthermore, various protocols for the timing of bone grafting exist. These include

Early bone grafting without prior bony débridement or excision

Early open bone grafting following débridement and skeletal stabilization

Delayed bone grafting following débridement, skeletal stabilization, and soft tissue reconstruction

The disadvantages of autogenous bone grafting are the limited quantity of bone available for harvesting and donor site morbidity and complications.

Allogenic Cancellous Graft

In the treatment of nonunions, allogenic cancellous bone is commonly mixed with autogenous cancellous bone graft or bone marrow. Since allogenic cancellous bone functions primarily as an osteoconductive graft, mixing it with autograft enhances the graft's osteoinductive and osteogenic capacity. Combining cancellous allograft and autograft also increases the volume of graft available to fill a large skeletal defect. Little is known about using allograft cancellous bone alone to treat nonunions. We do not recommend using allogenic cancellous bone (alone or mixed with cancellous autograft) in patients with any history of recent or past infection associated with their nonunion.

Allogenic bone can be prepared in three ways: fresh, fresh-frozen, and freeze-dried. Fresh grafts have the highest antigenicity. Fresh-frozen grafts are less immunogenic than fresh grafts and preserve the graft's bone morphogenetic proteins (BMPs). Freeze-dried grafts are the least immunogenic, have the lowest likelihood of viral transmission, are purely osteoconductive, and have the least mechanical integrity.

Bone Marrow

Bone marrow contains osteoprogenitor cells capable of forming bone.[130,131] Animal models of fracture and nonunion have shown enhanced healing with bone marrow grafting,[224,311] especially when demineralized bone matrix (DBM) is mixed with bone marrow.[311] Injection of marrow-derived mesenchymal progenitor cells also showed enhanced bone formation during distraction osteogenesis in a rat model.[254]

Percutaneous bone marrow injection as a clinical treatment for fracture nonunion has been reported with favorable results.[60,61,295] Percutaneous bone marrow grafting involves harvesting autogenous bone marrow from the anterior or posterior iliac crest with a trochar needle.[131]

We prefer the posterior iliac crest, an 11-gauge, 4-in. Lee-Lok needle (Lee Medical Ltd., Minneapolis, MN), and a 20-mL heparinized syringe (Fig. 22-68). Small aliquots are harvested to increase the concentration of osteoblast progenitor cells. The preferred volume of bone marrow aspirated from each site is 2 mL to 4 mL.[212] We harvest marrow in 4-mL aliquots, changing the position of the trochar needle in the posterior iliac crest between aspirations. Depending on the size and location of the nonunion site, we harvest 40 to 80 mL of marrow. Marrow is injected into the nonunion site percutaneously under fluoroscopic imaging using an 18-gauge spinal needle. The technique is minimally invasive, has low morbidity, and can be performed on an outpatient basis.[131] The technique works well for nonunions with small defects (<5 mm) that have excellent mechanical stability (see Fig. 22-68). Percutaneous marrow injection also enhances healing at the docking site in cases of Ilizarov bone transport.

Bone Graft Substitutes

Bone graft substitutes, such as calcium phosphate, calcium sulfate, hydroxyapatite, and other calcium-based ceramics, may have a future role in the treatment of nonunions. Some of these materials may be impregnated with antibiotic and used in the treatment of infected nonunions.[22,195] Some may be combined with autogenous bone graft to expand the volume of graft material.[30,282] To date, the efficiency of and indications for these substitutes in the treatment of nonunions remain unclear.

Growth Factors

Ongoing research in the area of growth factors holds promise for rapid advancement in the treatment of fracture nonunions.[75,77,81,82,86,106]

DECORTICATION Shingling, as described by Judet et al.[150,151] and Phemister[239] (Fig. 22-69), entails the raising of osteoperiosteal fragments from the outer cortex or callus from both sides of the nonunion using a sharp osteotome or chisel. Using an osteotome, thin (2 to 3 mm) fragments of cortex each measuring approximately 2 cm in length are elevated. The resulting decorticated region measures approximately 3 to 4 cm in length on either side of the nonunion and involves approximately two thirds of the bone circumference. The periosteum and muscle, which remain attached and viable, are then retracted with a Hohmann retractor. This increases the surface area between the elevated shingles and the decorticated cortex into which cancellous bone graft can be inserted to stimulate bony healing.

If the bone is osteoporotic, shingling may weaken the thin cortex and should therefore be avoided. In addition, shingling should not be performed over the area of the bone fragments where a plate is to be applied. Petaling,[210] or "fish scaling" (see Fig. 22-69), is performed with a tiny gouge. Once elevated, the osteoperiosteal flakes resemble the petals of a flower or scales of a fish. Alternatively, a small drill bit cooled with irrigation can be used to drill multiple holes. Petaling or drilling is performed over a region 3 to 4 cm on either side of the nonunion. These techniques promote revascularization of the cortex, especially when combined with cancellous bone grafting.

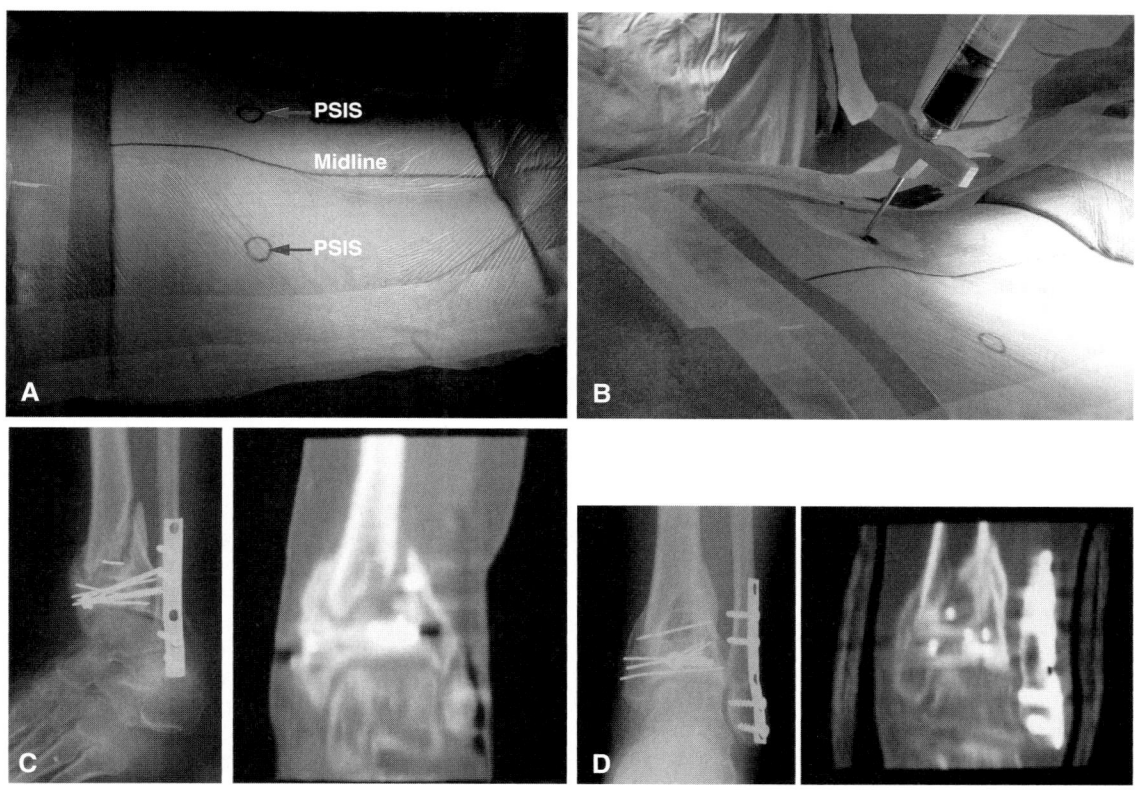

FIGURE 22-68 *A, Clinical photograph showing the bony landmarks for harvesting bone marrow from the posterior iliac crest. The patient has been positioned prone. B, Marrow being harvested in 4-mL aliquots. C, Presenting radiograph and CT scan of a 39-year-old woman with a stable oligotrophic distal tibial nonunion. D, Radiograph and CT scan 4 months following percutaneous marrow injection show solid bony union.*

ELECTROMAGNETIC, ULTRASOUND, AND SHOCK-WAVE STIMULATION

Electrical stimulation of non-unions by invasive and noninvasive methods has gained popularity since the 1970s,[231] with some practitioners reporting success in a high percentage of cases.[300] We have been delighted by successes in a number of cases (Fig. 22-70).

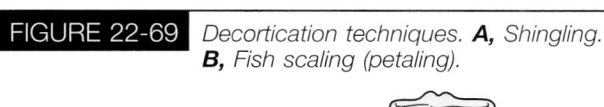

FIGURE 22-69 *Decortication techniques. A, Shingling. B, Fish scaling (petaling).*

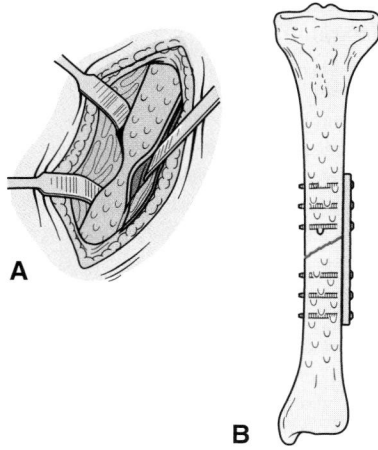

Devices available to treat nonunions via electrical stimulation are of three varieties: constant direct current, time-varying inductive coupling (including pulsed electromagnetic fields), and capacitive coupling.[1,56,118,214] Direct current lowers the partial pressure of oxygen and increases proteoglycan and collagen synthesis.[214] Time-varying inductive coupling affects the synthesis and function of growth factors and other cytokines, particularly TGF-β, that modulate chondrocytes and osteoblasts.[56,214] Pulsed electromagnetic fields also induce mRNA expression of bone morphogenetic proteins, producing an osteoinductive effect.[56] Capacitive coupling induces a proliferation of bone cells that is thought to be related to the activation of voltage-gated calcium channels increasing prostaglandin E_2, cytosolic calcium, and calmodulin.[214]

Electrical stimulation does not correct deformities and usually requires a long period (3 to 9 months) of non-weight-bearing and cast immobilization, which may give rise to muscle and bone atrophy and joint stiffness. Electrical stimulation may be used to treat stiff nonunions without significant deformity or bone defect. The method is seldom effective for atrophic nonunions, infected non-unions, synovial pseudarthroses, nonunions with gaps of more than 1 cm, or lax nonunions.[214]

Ultrasound stimulates bone healing by activating potassium ions, calcium incorporation in differentiating cartilage and bone cells, adenylate cyclase activity, and various

FIGURE 22-70 *A, Presenting radiograph of a 40-year-old woman 26 months following open reduction internal fixation of a distal clavicle fracture. This patient did not wish any type of surgical intervention and therefore was treated with external electrical stimulation. B, Radiograph following 8 months of electrical stimulation shows solid bony union.*

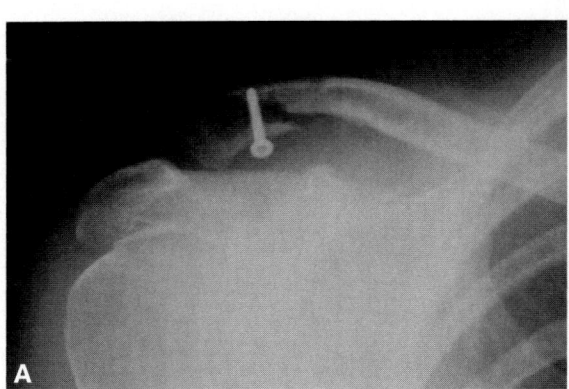
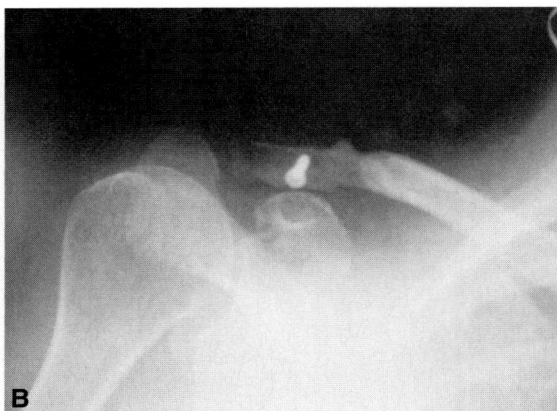

cytokines.[214,228,278] Ultrasound therapy has been an FDA-approved treatment for fracture healing since 1994 and for the stimulation of healing of established nonunions since February 2000.[214] Several studies of ultrasound therapy in the treatment of nonunion have reported bony union rates ranging from 85 to 91 percent.[108,215,278] According to Parvizi and Vegari, ultrasound may be used to treat stiff atrophic, oligotrophic, or hypertrophic nonunions that have no significant deformity.[228] It is inappropriate for infected nonunions, nonunions with a large segmental defect, and lax nonunions.

High-energy extracorporeal shock wave therapy for nonunions has been reported by a number of investigators, with union rates exceeding 75 percent.[289,292,319,322] The technique may be more effective in pseudarthroses or nonunions showing uptake on technetium bone scan.[266] Atrophic nonunions may show no signs of healing until more than 6 months after the initial shock wave application.[322] It should not be used when the gap at the nonunion site is greater than 5 mm; when open physes, alveolar tissue, brain or spine, or malignant tumor are in the shock wave field; or in patients with coagulopathy or pregnancy.[289]

METHODS THAT ARE BOTH MECHANICAL AND BIOLOGICAL

STRUCTURAL BONE GRAFTS Several types of structural bone grafts are available. Each type has specific advantages and disadvantages (Table 22-11).

Vascularized autogenous cortical bone grafts provide structural integrity and living osseous tissue to the site of bony defects. Some vascularized grafts respond to functional loading via hypertrophy,[45,139] thus increasing in strength over time. Vascularized bone grafts may be obtained from several sites for the treatment of nonunions of various bones,[64,70,281,287,330,340,349] but the vascularized fibula is currently preferred because of its shape, strength, size, and versatility.[112,137,149,178,279]

Nonvascularized autogenous cortical bone grafts provide structural integrity using the patient's own tissue to the site of bony defects.

Bulk cortical allografts may be used to reconstruct large post-traumatic skeletal defects[53] (see Figs. 22-64 and 22-70). Bone of virtually every shape and size from the bone bank is available, permitting reconstruction in most anatomic locations. Graft fixation may be achieved using a variety of methods; we prefer intramedullary fixation when possible because of its ultimate strength, load-sharing characteristics, and protection of the graft. Bulk allografts can be used in four ways: intercalary, alloarthrodetic (Fig. 22-71), osteoarticular, and alloprosthetic.

Infected nonunions may be treated with bulk allograft after the infected cavity has been débrided and sterilized. For infected nonunions with massive defects, we perform serial débridement with antibiotic bead exchanges until the cavity is culture negative. A custom-fabricated antibiotic-impregnated PMMA spacer is then implanted, and the soft tissue envelope is closed or reconstructed. At a minimum of 3 months, the spacer is removed and the defect is reconstructed using bulk cortical allograft (Figs. 22-64 and 22-72). Active infection is an absolute contraindication to bulk cortical allograft.

Strut cortical allografts may be used to reconstruct partial (incomplete) segmental defects, reconstruct complete segmental defects in certain cases, augment fixation and stability in osteopenic bone,[323] and augment stability in periprosthetic nonunions (see Fig. 22-61).

Intramedullary cortical allografts are typically used for long bone nonunions associated with osteopenia where the method of treatment is plate-and-screw fixation with cancellous autografting. The technique is particularly useful for humeral nonunions in elderly patients with osteopenic bone who have had multiple prior unsuccessful treatments (Fig. 22-73).

Mesh cage–bone graft constructs are a relatively new technique for treating segmental long bone defects.[59] The segmental defect is spanned using a titanium mesh cage (DuPuy Motech, Warsaw, IN) of slightly larger diameter than the adjacent bone. The cage is packed with allogenic cancellous bone chips and demineralized bone matrix. This construct is reinforced by an IM nail traversing the mesh cage–bone graft construct.

Table 22-11
Types of Structural Bone Graft

Type of Bone Graft	Potential Harvest Site	Advantages	Disadvantages
Vascularized autogenous cortical bone graft	Fibula[330,340,349]	Immediate structural integrity	Technically demanding
	Iliac crest[281]	One-stage procedure	Propensity for fracture fatigue, particularly in lower extremity applications
	Ribs[330]	Potential for graft hypertrophy	Prolonged non-weight-bearing
		Ability to span massive segmental defects	Poorer results in patients with a history of infection[123]
			Donor site morbidity: pain, neurovascular injury, joint instability or limited motion
			Fixation problems when the defect is periarticular
			Contraindicated for children
Nonvascularized autogenous cortical bone graft	Fibula Tibia	Can be used to reconstruct large defects	Prolonged non-weight-bearing
			Prolonged support required in upper extremity applications
	Iliac crest		Donor site morbidity, including fracture for grafts from the tibia
			Graft weakening during revascularization (years)
			Propensity for fatigue fracture
Bulk cortical allograft	Virtually unlimited	Less technically demanding than vascularized grafts	Infection
		No donor site morbidity	Fatigue fracture
		Can be used in four ways: intercalary, alloarthrodetic, osteoarticular, and alloprosthetic	Nonunion at the host-graft junction
			Disease transmission from donor to recipient
Strut cortical allograft	Virtually unlimited	Versatility; may be used to treat partial (incomplete) segmental defects and complete segmental defects, augment fixation and stability in osteopenic bone, and augment stability in periprosthetic nonunions	Infection
			Fatigue fracture
			Nonunion at the host-graft junction
			Disease transmission from donor to recipient
Intramedullary cortical allograft	Virtually unlimited	Used in long bone nonunions with osteopenia	Infection
		Augments stability by acting like an intramedullary nail	Fatigue fracture
		Improves screw purchase; screws each traverse four cortices	Nonunion at the host-graft junction
			Disease transmission from donor to recipient

EXCHANGE NAILING IM nail fixation, a purely mechanical treatment method, is distinguished from exchange nailing in that the latter is a method that is both mechanical and biological.

Technique

By definition, exchange nailing requires the removal of a previously placed IM nail. With a nail already spanning the nonunion site, the problem of a sealed-off medullary canal is not an issue. Additionally, the medullary canal is already known to accept passage of an IM nail, unless the nail has broken and there has been progressive deformity over time. Such a case may require extensive bony and soft tissue dissection at the nonunion site, so other treatment options may need to be considered.

Once the previously placed nail has been removed, the medullary canal is reamed with progressively larger reamer tips in 0.5-mm increments until bone is observed in the

FIGURE 22-71 ▐ *A, Presenting radiograph of a 25-year-old man treated with open reduction internal fixation of an open femur fracture taken 16 months following the injury. Clinical examination revealed gross purulence and exposed bone at the nonunion site with global knee joint instability and an arc of knee flexion/extension of approximately 20°. Aspiration of the knee yielded frank pus. **B,** Radiographs following radical débridement with placement of antibiotic beads and later an antibiotic spacer. **C,** Follow-up radiograph 6 years after alloarthrodesis using a bulk cortical allograft and a knee fusion nail shows solid bony incorporation. The patient is fully ambulatory, is without pain, and has no evidence of infection.*

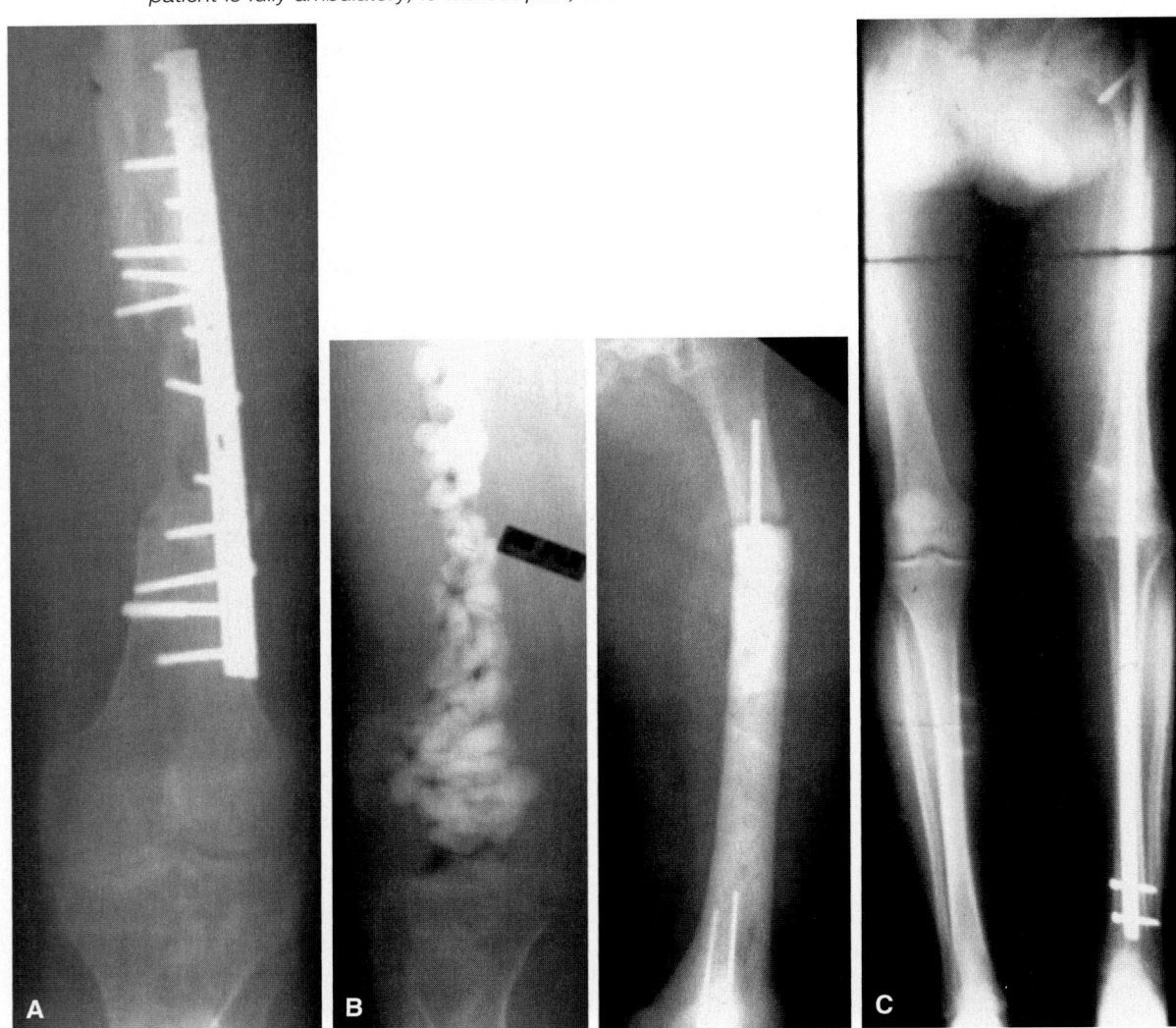

flutes of the reamers. As a general rule, we try to use an exchange nail that is 2 to 4 mm in diameter larger than the previous nail, and we over-ream 1 mm larger than the new nail. Reaming, therefore, typically proceeds to a reamer tip size 3 to 5 mm larger than the removed nail.

Following reaming, a larger diameter nail is inserted. We prefer to use a closed technique to preserve the periosteal blood supply. Closed nailing likely also lessens the risk of infection. Provided that good bony contact exists at the nonunion site, we statically lock exchange nails, although many authors do not.[62,122,308,335,346] In most instances, we do not favor partial excision of the fibula with exchange nailing of the tibia because it diminishes stability of the construct.

Modes of Healing

Exchange nailing stimulates healing of nonunions by improving the local mechanical environment in two ways and by improving the local biological environment in two ways (Fig. 22-74).

The first mechanical benefit is that reaming to enlarge the medullary canal allows a larger diameter nail, which is stronger and stiffer. The stronger, stiffer nail augments stability, which promotes bony union. The second mechanical benefit is that reaming widens and lengthens the isthmic portion of the medullary canal, which increases the endosteal cortical contact area of the nail.

The first biological benefit is that the reaming products act as local bone graft at the nonunion site to stimulate

FIGURE 22-72 **A,** *Presenting radiograph of a 45-year-old man 7 months following open reduction internal fixation of a both-bone forearm fracture. This patient had an open wound draining purulent material over the radius. The patient was treated with serial débridement and antibiotic beads. Following serial débridement, the patient was left with a segmental defect of the radius.* **B,** *Radiograph following placement of a bulk cortical allograft over an intramedullary nail and plate-and-screw fixation of the ulna.* **C,** *Follow-up radiograph at 11 months after reconstruction shows solid union of the proximal host-graft junction but a hypertrophic nonunion of the distal host-graft junction of the radius. The hypertrophic nonunion was treated with compression plating (without bone grafting).* **D,** *Final radiograph 14 months following compression plating shows solid bony union.*

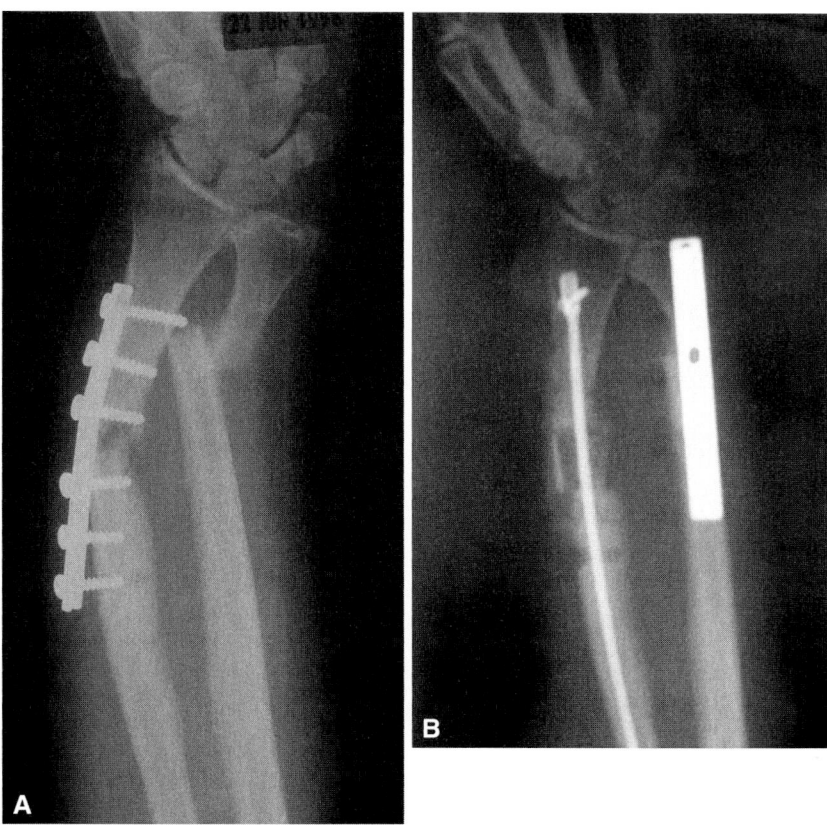

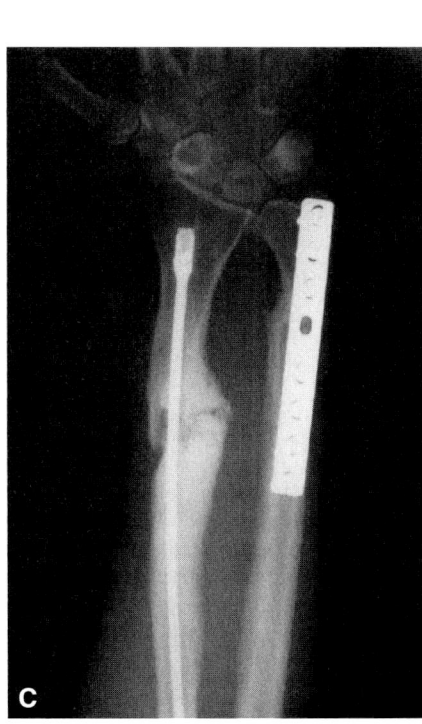

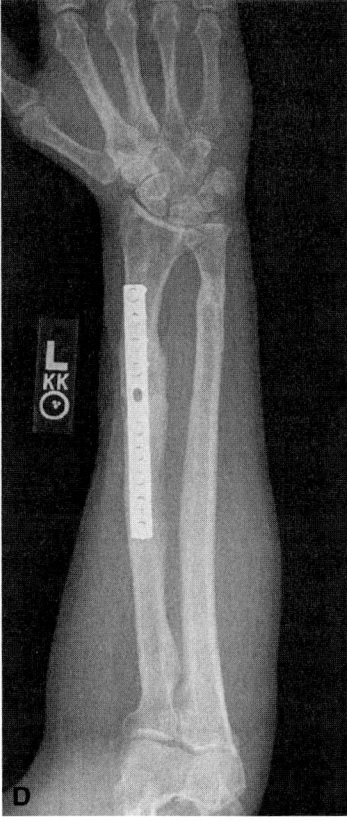

FIGURE 22-73 | *A, Presenting radiograph of an 83-year-old woman 15 months following a humeral shaft fracture. The patient found this humeral nonunion painful and debilitating. Because of the patient's profound osteopenia, she was treated with an intramedullary cortical fibular allograft and plate-and-screw fixation. B, Intraoperative fluoroscopic image showing positioning of the intramedullary fibula. C, Final radiograph 7 months following reconstruction shows bony incorporation without evidence of hardware loosening or failure. At follow-up, the patient was without pain and had marked improvement in function.*

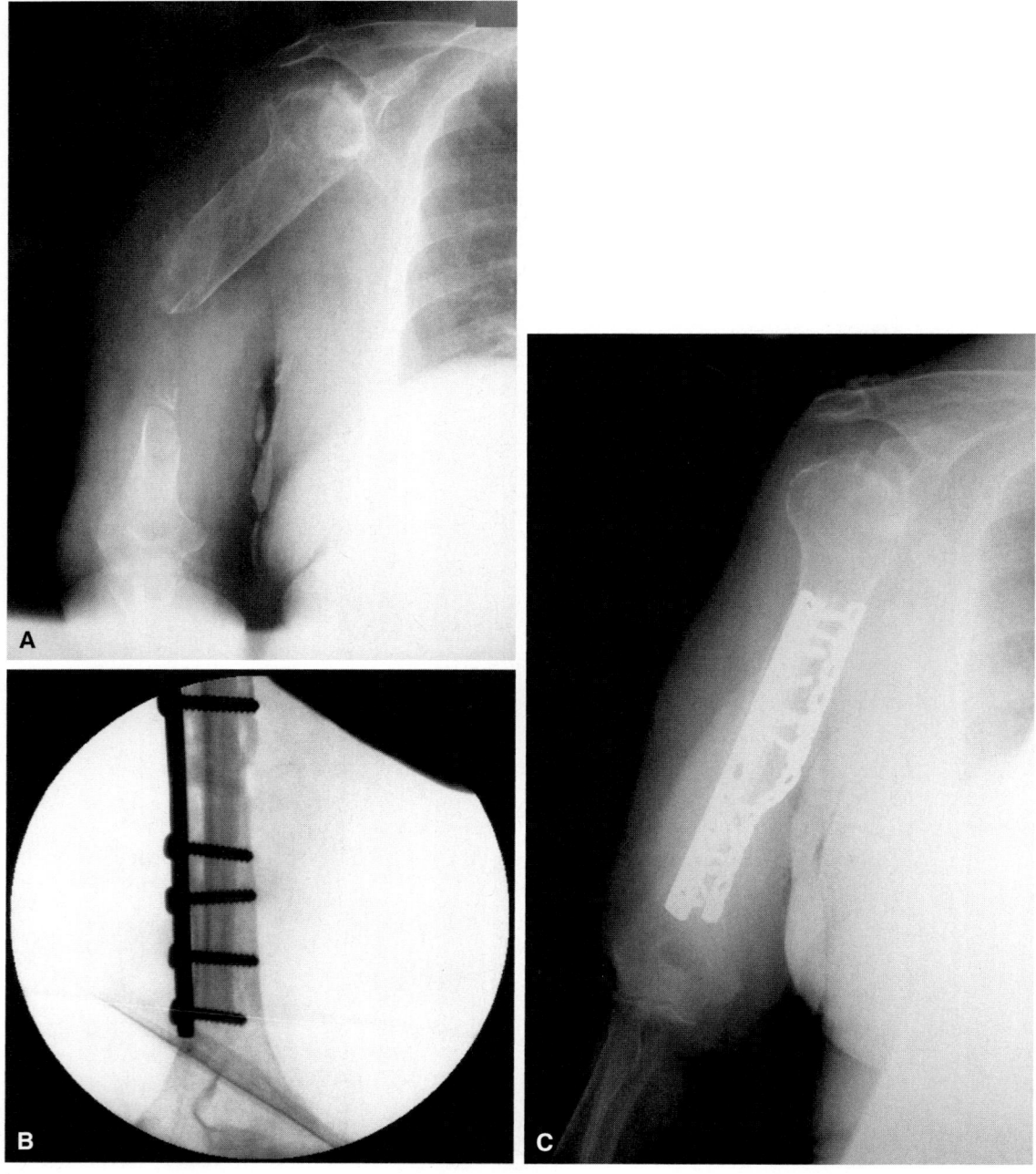

FIGURE 22-74 *A, Presenting radiograph of a 51-year-old woman 29 months following intramedullary nail fixation of an open tibia fracture. B, Five months following exchange nailing, the tibia is solidly united.*

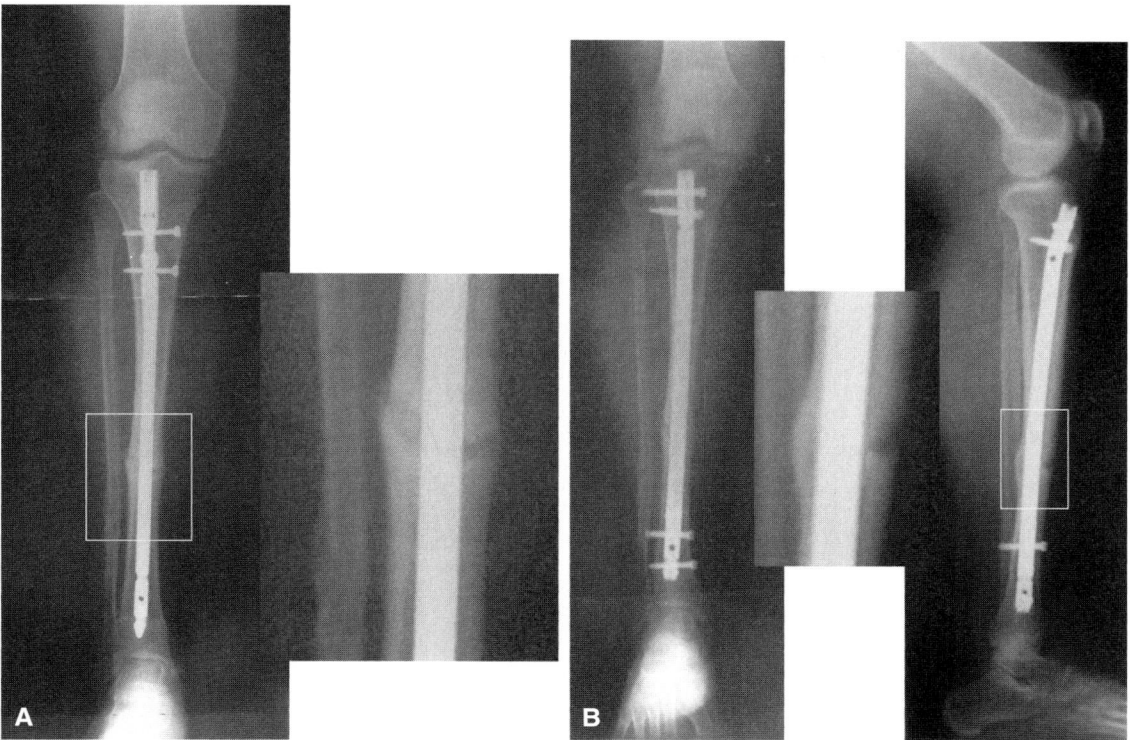

medullary healing. The second biological benefit is that medullary reaming results in a substantial decrease in endosteal blood flow.[35,119,146,217,301] This loss of endosteal blood flow stimulates a dramatic increase in both periosteal flow[251] and periosteal new bone formation.[67]

These mechanical and biological effects of exchange nailing make it applicable for both viable and nonviable nonunions.

Other Issues
Three noteworthy circumstances relative to exchange nailing are nonunions with incomplete bony contact, nonunions associated with deformity, and infected nonunions.

Bone Contact Exchange nailing is excellent when good bone-to-bone contact is present, but not when large partial or complete segmental bone defects exist. Because healing of nonunions with defects depends on many factors (as discussed above), it is difficult to determine which defects will unite with exchange nailing. Templeman and coauthors[308] advocate exchange nailing in the tibia when there is 30 percent or less circumferential bone loss. Court-Brown and coauthors[62] reported failures for exchange nailing in tibial nonunions when bone loss exceeded 2 cm in length and involved more than 50 percent circumferential bone loss. We have used intramedullary bone grafting[46] with excellent results during exchange nailing of long

bones with defects, although the indications for this technique for nonunions are still evolving.

Deformity We are astonished by how a straight nail can result in a very crooked bone (Fig. 22-75). Deformities that will ultimately limit the patient's function require correction. In a previously nailed long bone, clinically significant deformities may include length, angulation, and rotation. Translational deformities are somewhat limited by the nail (if unbroken) and are uncommonly clinically significant.

Deformity correction can be acute or gradual and can be performed during or after treatment of the nonunion. If deformity correction is to follow successful bony union, exchange nailing may be undertaken as described above. If the decision is to address the nonunion and the deformity concurrently, then it must be decided whether to correct the deformity gradually or acutely. If acute deformity correction is felt to be safe, exchange nailing with acute deformity correction simplifies the overall treatment strategy. Acute deformity correction is relatively simple for lax nonunions. Stiff nonunions may require a percutaneously performed osteotomy and the intraoperative use of a femoral distractor or a temporary external fixator to achieve acute deformity correction. If the status of the soft tissues or bone favors gradual correction, then exchange nailing is rejected and the Ilizarov method is used.

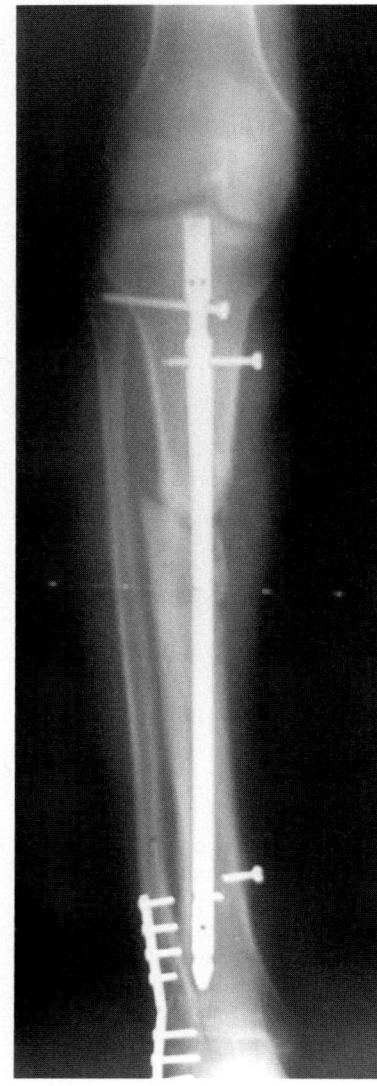

FIGURE 22-75 *Presenting radiograph of a 22-year-old man following multiple failed treatments of a tibial nonunion. Note that a crooked bone can result despite the use of a straight nail.*

Infection Numerous authors have reported the use of intramedullary nail fixation for infected nonunions.[7,122,164,167,196,296,343] There is no consensus in the literature regarding the use of exchange nailing as a treatment for infected nonunions. For cases in which the injury has been previously treated with a method other than nailing, placement of an intramedullary nail can seed the entire medullary canal. The case of exchange nailing is entirely different. With an in situ intramedullary nail, the intramedullary canal is likely already infected, to some degree, along its entire length, and we are therefore not strictly opposed to exchange nailing of an infected nonunion (Fig. 22-76).

Exchange nailing for infected nonunions is best suited to the lower extremity in patients who are poor candidates for plate-and-screw fixation (osteopenia, multiple soft tissue reconstructions, segmental nonunions) or external fixation (poor compliance or cognitive impairment), where the load-sharing characteristics of a nail may be of great benefit. When exchange nailing is utilized for infected nonunions, aggressive reaming of the medullary canal is a means of débridement. Reaming should use progressively larger reamer tips in 0.5-mm increments until the reamer flutes contain what appears to be viable healthy bone. All reamings should be sent for culture and sensitivity in cases of known or suspected infection. The medullary canal is irrigated copiously with antibiotic solution, and the larger diameter nail is placed. Serial débridement can be performed with an antibiotic-eluting nail being placed down the medullary canal at each operative session.

Literature Review

The reported results for exchange nailing of uninfected tibial nonunions have been excellent. Court-Brown and coauthors[62] reported an 88 percent rate of union (29 of 33 cases) following a single exchange nailing of the tibia; the four remaining cases united following a second exchange nailing. Templeman and coauthors[308] reported a 93 percent rate of union (25 of 27 cases), and Wu and coauthors[347] reported a 96 percent rate of union (24 of 25 cases) with exchange nailing of the tibia.

The reported results for exchange nailing of femoral nonunions have been less consistent. Oh and co-workers[216] and Christensen[54] both reported a 100 percent union rate for aseptic femoral nonunions treated with exchange nailing, whereas Hak and coauthors[122] reported a union rate of only 78 percent (18 of 23 cases). Weresh and coauthors[335] reported a union rate of only 53 percent (10 of 19 cases) and Banaszkiewicz and coauthors of only 58 percent (11 of 19 cases) for exchange nailing of nonunions of the femoral shaft.[17] Both sets of authors pointed out that recent technological advances have allowed IM nailing to be used in the treatment of more comminuted and complex femoral fractures than had previously been possible. When these types of fracture go on to nonunion, they may not be appropriate for exchange nailing.[17,335]

The results of exchange nailing for humeral shaft nonunions have been suboptimal. McKee and co-workers[194] reported a 40 percent union rate (4 of 10 cases) for exchange nailing of humeral nonunions. Flinkkilä and coauthors[101] reported union in only 23 percent (3 of 13 cases) of humeral shaft nonunions treated with antegrade exchange nailing.

Summary

Based on the literature and our own experience, the following comments and recommendations are offered:

1. Tibia—Exchange nailing achieves healing in 90 to 95 percent of tibial nonunions.
2. Femoral shaft—Exchange nailing remains the treatment of choice for aseptic, noncomminuted nonunions of the femoral shaft, but the success rate is lower than for tibial nonunions when nonunion follows IM nailing of a comminuted or complex femoral shaft fracture.
3. Supracondylar femur—The supracondylar femur is poorly suited for stabilization of a nonunion with

FIGURE 22-76 *A, Radiograph of a 23-year-old man with an actively draining infected femoral nonunion resulting from a gunshot blast. This patient was treated with serial débridement followed by exchange nailing (with intramedullary autogenous iliac crest bone grafting) of the femoral nonunion. B, Follow-up radiograph 13 months after treatment shows solid bony healing. This patient has no clinical evidence of infection.*

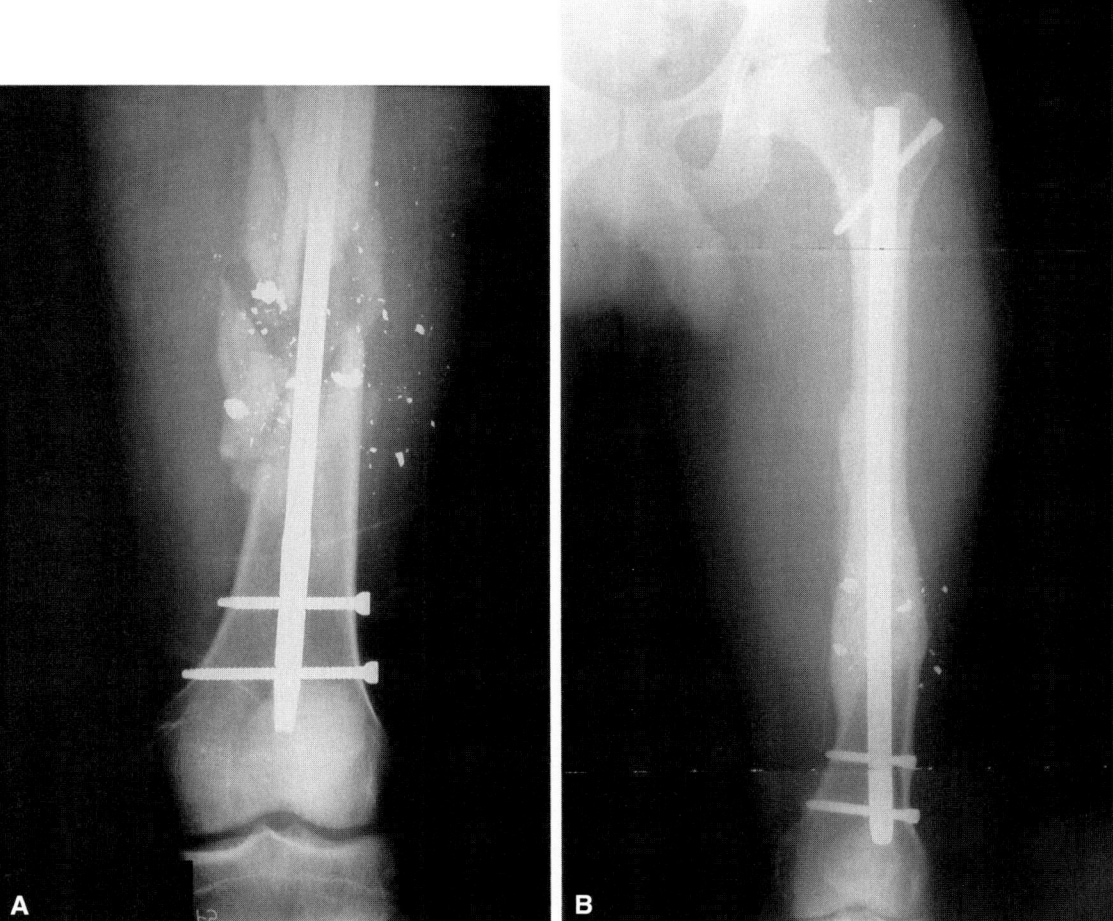

an IM nail; dismal results have been reported by Koval et al.[167] The medullary canal is flared in this region, resulting in poor cortical bone contact with the nail. Reaming during exchange nailing for nonunions of the supracondylar region may not increase periosteal blood flow or induce new bone formation. Other treatment methods should be utilized for supracondylar nonunion of the femur (Fig. 22-77).

4. Humeral shaft—Poor results have been reported for exchange nailing of humeral shaft nonunions.[101,194] Nail removal and plate-and-screw fixation with autogenous cancellous bone grafting is more effective. Ilizarov methods may be required for complex cases.

SYNOSTOSIS TECHNIQUES The leg and forearm benefit from structural integrity provided by paired bones, which permits the use of unique treatment methods for nonunions with bone defects. The literature regarding these methods is fraught with inconsistent and contradictory terms: fibula-pro-tibia, fibula transfer, fibula transference, fibula transposition, fibular bypass, fibulazation,

medialization of the fibula, medial-ward bone transport of the fibula, posterolateral bone grafting, synostosis, tibialization of the fibula, transtibiofibular grafting, and vascularized fibula transposition.

All of these techniques can be distinguished as either a synostosis technique or local grafting from the adjacent bone (Fig. 22-78).

Synostosis techniques entail the creation of bone continuity between paired bones above and below the nonunion site. The bone neighboring the un-united bone unites to the proximal and distal fragments of the un-united bone such that the neighboring bone transmits forces across the nonunion site. From a functional standpoint, the limb becomes a one-bone extremity. Synostosis techniques do not necessarily rely on union of the original nonunion fragments to one another.

Many techniques have been described to create a tibiofibular synostosis for the treatment of tibial nonunions. Milch[201,202] described a tibiofibular synostosis technique for nonunion using a splintered bone created by longitudinally splitting the fibula, which could be augmented

FIGURE 22-77 *Radiograph of a 57-year-old man with a supracondylar femoral nonunion and two prior failed exchange nailing procedures. Exchange nailing is a poor treatment method for nonunions in this region.*

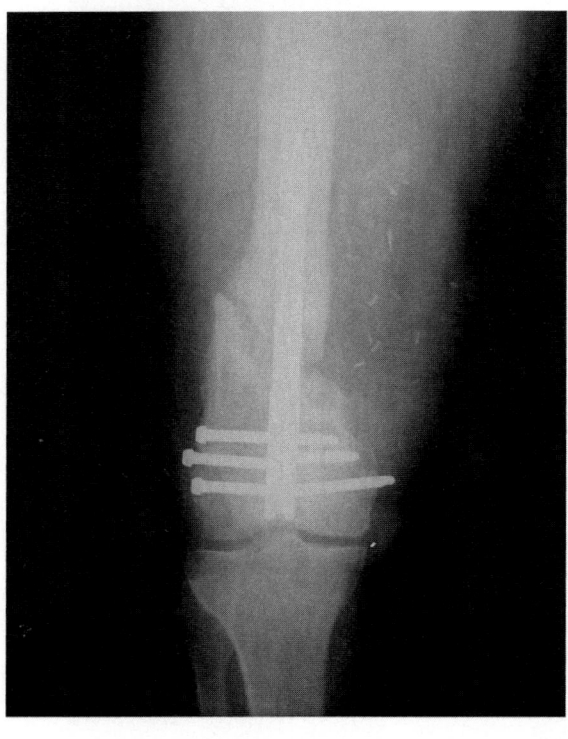

with autogenous iliac bone graft. McMaster and Hohl[197] used allograft cortical bone as tibiofibular cross-pegs to create a tibiofibular synostosis for tibial nonunion. Rijnberg and van Linge[258] described a technique to treat tibial shaft nonunions by creating a synostosis with autogenous iliac crest bone graft through a lateral approach anterior to the fibula.

Ilizarov[141] described the medial-ward (horizontal) bone transport of the fibula to create a tibiofibular synostosis for the treatment of tibial nonunions with massive segmental defects (see Fig. 22-78).

Weinberg and colleagues[333] described a two-stage technique for cases with massive bone loss. In the first stage, a distal tibiofibular synostosis was created; at least 1 month later the second stage created a proximal tibiofibular synostosis.

The term fibula-pro-tibia sometimes describes a synostosis technique, but it is used inconsistently in the literature. Campanacci and Zanoli[41] described a fibula-pro-tibia tibiofibular synostosis technique using internal fixation to stabilize the proximal and distal tibiofibular articulations for tibial nonunions without large defects. Banic and Hertel[18] described a "double vascularized fibula" fibula-pro-tibia technique for large tibial defects in which the laterally grafted fibula with its intact blood supply creates a synostosis proximal and distal to the defect. By contrast, others[190,324] have described transference of a vascularized fibula graft into a tibial defect as a fibula-pro-tibia technique; transference does not create a synostosis. None of the techniques in the literature described as fibular transference, fibular transfer, fibular transposition, and tibialization refer to synostosis procedures.[5,15,45,137,154,297,313]

FIGURE 22-78 *Synostosis techniques for the tibia compared with local bone grafting from the fibula for bony defects of the tibia.*

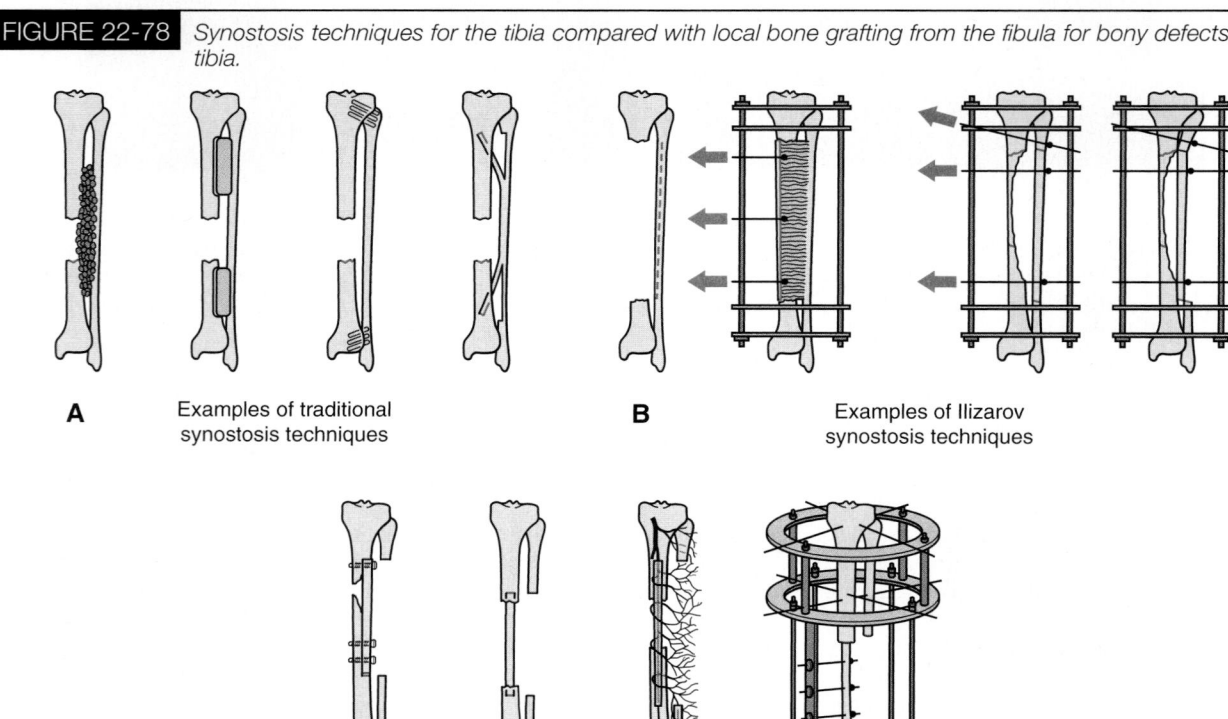

A Examples of traditional synostosis techniques

B Examples of Ilizarov synostosis techniques

C Examples of local grafting techniques

The synostosis method may also be used to treat segmental defects or persistent nonunions of the forearm (Fig. 22-79). This technique is most commonly used for forearm nonunions when there is massive bone loss to both radius and ulna.

ILIZAROV METHOD Ilizarov techniques for treatment of nonunions have many advantages (Table 22-12). The Ilizarov construct resists shear and rotational forces. The tensioned wires allow for the somewhat unique "trampoline effect" during weight-bearing activities. The Ilizarov method allows augmentation of the treatment as needed

through frame modification. Frame modification generally is not associated with pain, does not require anesthesia, and can be performed in the office. Frame modification is not treatment failure; it is continued treatment. Modifying other treatment methods, such as IM nailing, requires repeat surgical intervention and is therefore considered treatment failure.

The Ilizarov method is applicable for all types of nonunions, particularly those associated with infection, segmental bone defects, deformities, and multiple prior failed treatments. A variety of modes of treatment can be employed using the Ilizarov external fixator, including

FIGURE 22-79 Two cases of forearm nonunions treated with synostosis. **A,** Presenting radiograph and clinical photograph of 32-year-old man with segmental bone loss from a gunshot blast to the forearm. **B,** Radiograph and clinical photograph of the forearm during bone transport of the proximal ulna into the distal radius to create a one-bone forearm (synostosis). **C,** Final radiograph and clinical photographs. **D,** Presenting radiograph of a 48-year-old man with multiple failed attempts at a synostosis procedure of the forearm.

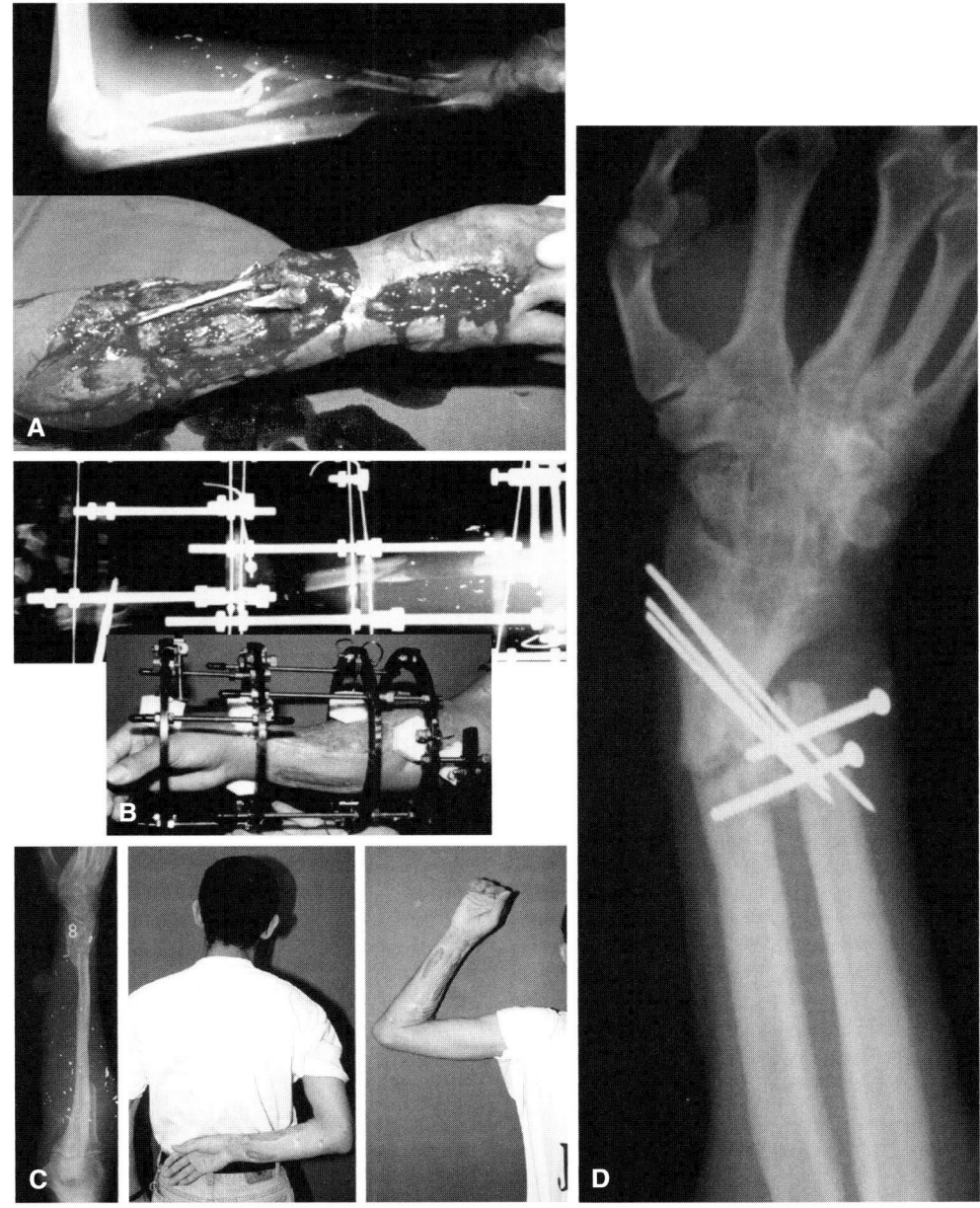

(Continued)

FIGURE 22-79 | *(Continued)* **E,** *Radiograph of the forearm during Ilizarov treatment with slow, gradual compression.* **F,** *Final radiographic result shows solid bony union.*

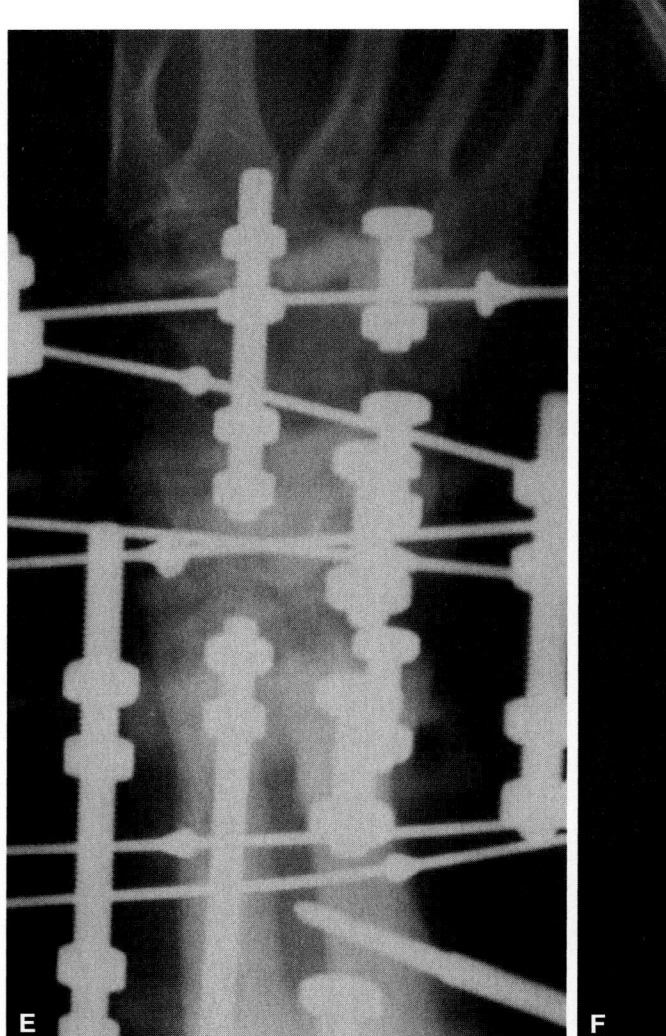

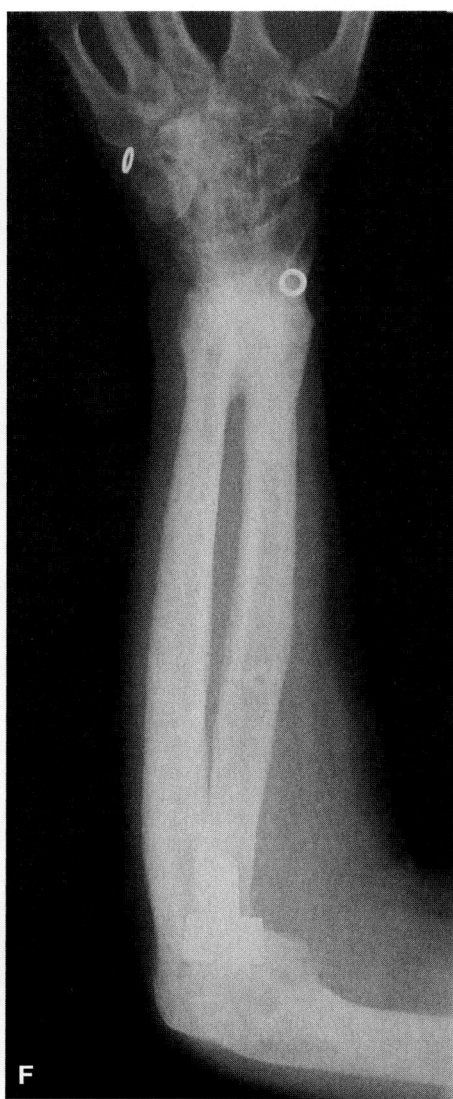

compression, distraction, lengthening, and bone transport. Monofocal treatment involves simple compression or distraction across the nonunion site. Bifocal treatment denotes that two healing sites exist, such as a bone transport where healing must occur at both the distraction site (regenerate bone formation) and the docking (nonunion) site. Trifocal treatment denotes that three healing sites exist, such as in a double-level bone transport (Table 22-13).

Compression (monofocal) osteosynthesis allows both simple compression and differential compression, which is used in deformity correction. The technique is applicable for hypertrophic nonunions (although distraction is classically used) (Fig. 22-80), oligotrophic nonunions (Figs. 22-80 through 22-83), and, according to Professor

Table 22-12
Advantages of Ilizarov Techniques
Minimally invasive
Can promote bony tissue generation
Often require only minimal soft tissue dissection
Versatile
Can be used in the face of acute or chronic infection
Allow for stabilization of small intraarticular or periarticular bone fragments
Allow for simultaneous bony healing and deformity correction
Allow for immediate weight-bearing
Allow for early joint mobilization

Table 22-13
Ilizarov Treatment Modes

Monofocal
   Compression
   Sequential distraction-compression
   Distraction
   Sequential compression-distraction
Bifocal
   Compression-distraction lengthening
   Distraction-compression transport (bone transport)
Trifocal
   Various combinations

Ilizarov, synovial pseudarthroses.[144,294] Gradual compression is generally applied at a rate of 0.25 to 0.5 mm per day for a period of 2 to 4 weeks. As the rings spanning the nonunion site move closer together after the bone ends are in contact, the thin wires bow (see Figs. 22-79 and 22-80). Compression stimulates healing for most hypertrophic and oligotrophic nonunions. Compression is usually unsuccessful for infected nonunions with purulent drainage and intervening segments of necrotic bone. There is disagreement regarding compression as a treatment for atrophic nonunions.[174,220]

Slow compression over a nail using external fixation (SCONE) is a useful method for certain patients in whom IM nailing has failed.[36,145,230] We have used this technique

---

FIGURE 22-80 *Ilizarov treatment of a hypertrophic distal humeral nonunion using gradual monofocal compression.* **A,** *Presenting radiograph.* **B,** *Radiograph during treatment using slow compression. Note the bending of the wires proximal and distal to the nonunion site, indicating good bony contact.* **C,** *Final radiographic result shows solid bony union.*

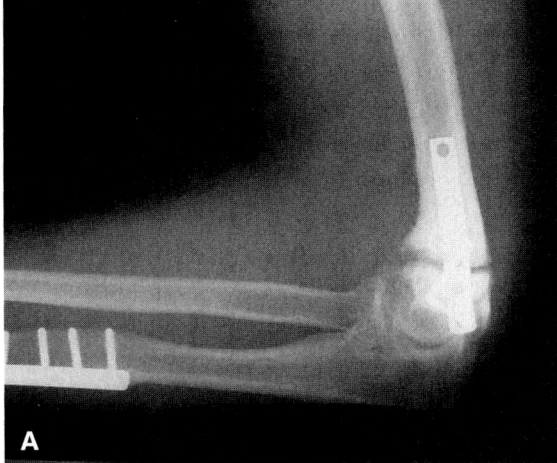
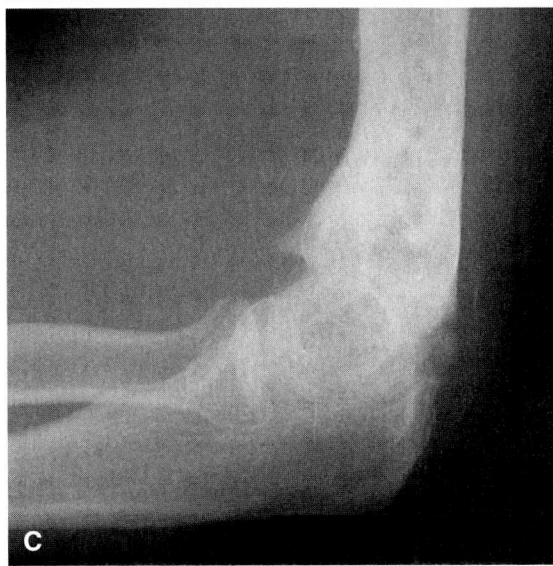
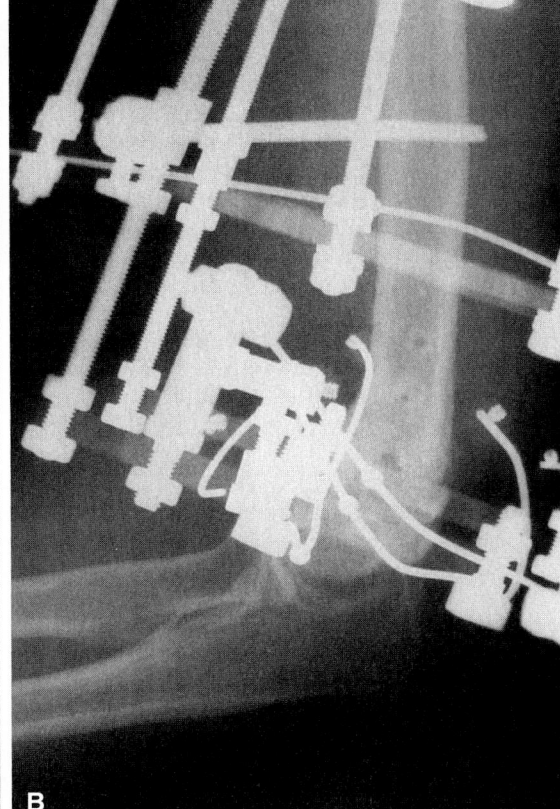

FIGURE 22-81   *Example of an oligotrophic nonunion of the distal humerus treated with slow, gradual compression using Ilizarov external fixation. **A,** Presenting radiographs. **B,** Radiograph during treatment using slow, gradual compression. Note the bending of the wires, indicating good bony contact. **C,** Final radiographic result shows solid bony union.*

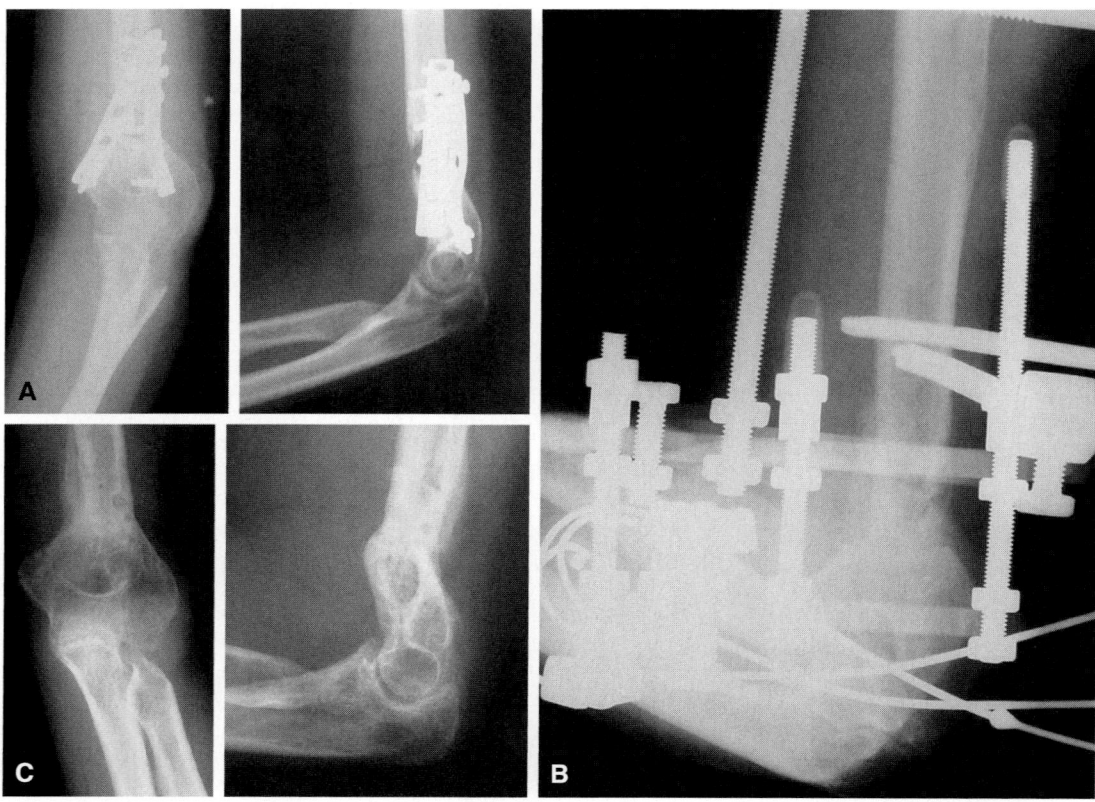

with great success in two distinct patient populations: patients in whom multiple exchange femoral nailings have failed (Fig. 22-84) and morbidly obese patients with distal femoral nonunions in whom primary retrograde nail fracture fixation has failed (Fig. 22-85).[36] The SCONE method is performed with percutaneous application of the Ilizarov external fixator. The method augments stability and allows for monofocal compression at the nonunion site once the nail is dynamized. The presence of the nail in the medullary canal encourages compressive forces while discouraging translational and shear moments.

Sequential monofocal distraction-compression has been recommended as a treatment for lax hypertrophic nonunions and atrophic nonunions. According to Paley,[220] "distraction disrupts the tissue at the nonunion site, frequently leading to some poor bone regeneration. This poor bone regeneration is stimulated to consolidate when the two bone ends are brought back together again."

Distraction is the treatment method of choice for stiff hypertrophic nonunions, particularly those with deformity (Fig. 22-86). Distraction of the abundant fibrocartilaginous tissue at the nonunion site stimulates new bone formation[44,141,220,280] and results in a high rate of healing.[44,166,280]

Sequential monofocal compression-distraction involves an initial interval of compression followed by gradual distraction for lengthening or deformity correction. This technique is applicable for stiff hypertrophic and oligotrophic nonunions but is not recommended for atrophic, infected, and lax nonunions.[120,220]

Bifocal compression-distraction lengthening involves acute or gradual compression across the nonunion site with lengthening through an adjacent corticotomy (Fig. 22-87). This method is applicable for nonunions associated with foreshortening and nonunions with segmental defects. Segmental defects may also be treated with bifocal distraction-compression transport (bone transport) (Fig. 22-88). This method involves the creation of a corticotomy (usually metaphyseal) at a site distant from the nonunion. The bone segment produced by the corticotomy is then gradually transported toward the nonunion site (into the bony defect). As the transported segment arrives at the docking site, compression is successful in many cases in obtaining union. Occasionally bone grafting with marrow or open bone graft is required.

Corticotomy and bone transport result in profound biological stimulation, similar to bone grafting. In a study of dogs undergoing distraction osteogenesis, Aronson[12] reported that blood flow at the distraction site increased nearly ten-fold relative to the control limb, peaking about 2 weeks after surgery. The distal tibia, remote from the distraction site, showed a similar pattern of increased blood flow. Consequently, bone transport can be useful in the treatment of atrophic nonunions.

FIGURE 22-82 *Example of an oligotrophic nonunion of the distal tibia treated with gradual deformity correction followed by slow, gradual compression using Ilizarov external fixation.* **A,** *Presenting radiograph.* **B,** *Radiograph during treatment.* **C,** *Final radiographic result shows solid bony union with complete deformity correction.*

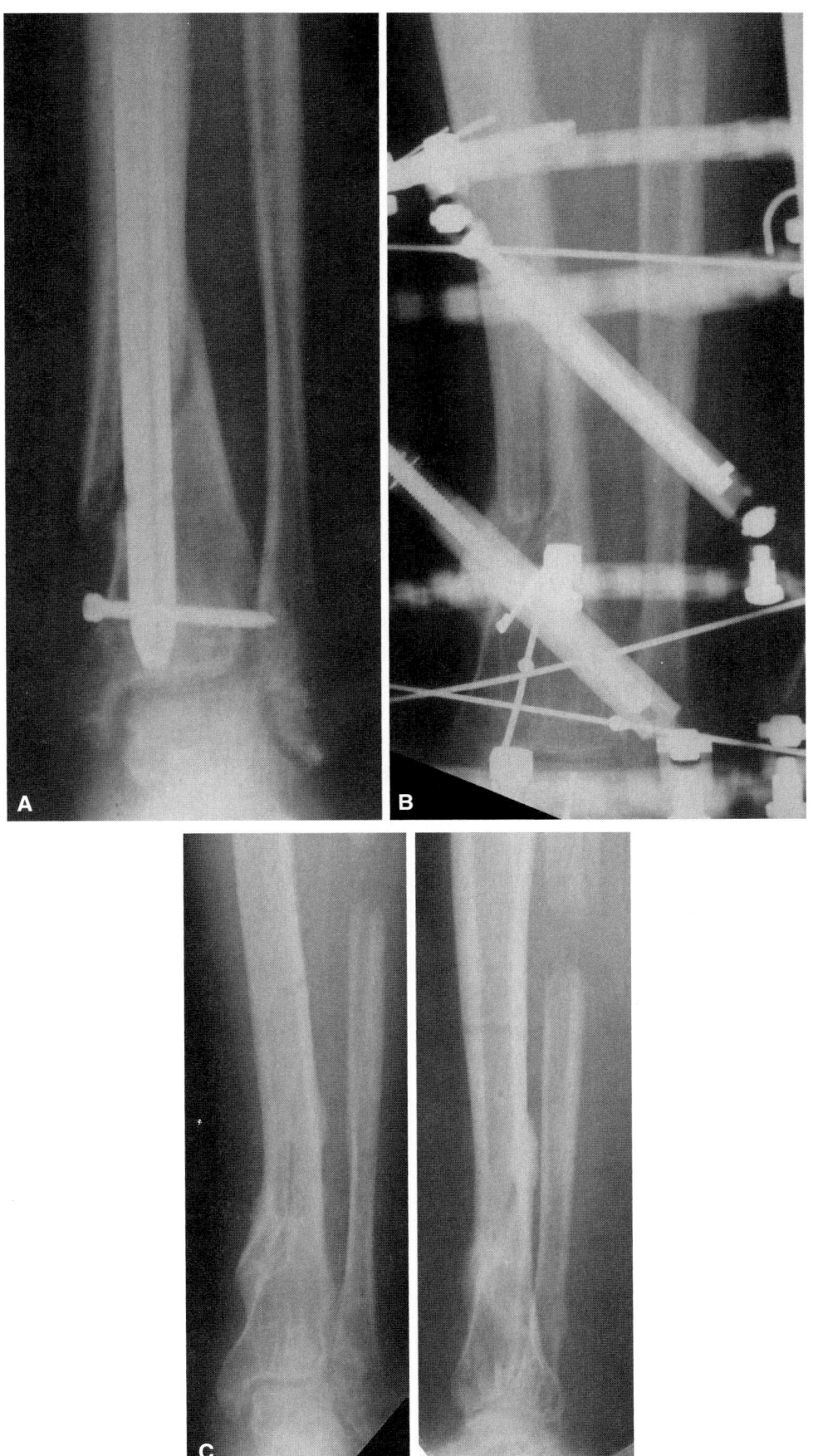

FIGURE 22-83 *Example of an oligotrophic nonunion of the proximal tibia treated with slow, gradual compression using Ilizarov external fixation.* **A,** *Presenting radiograph.* **B,** *Radiograph during treatment using slow, gradual compression.* **C,** *Final radiographic result shows solid bony union.*

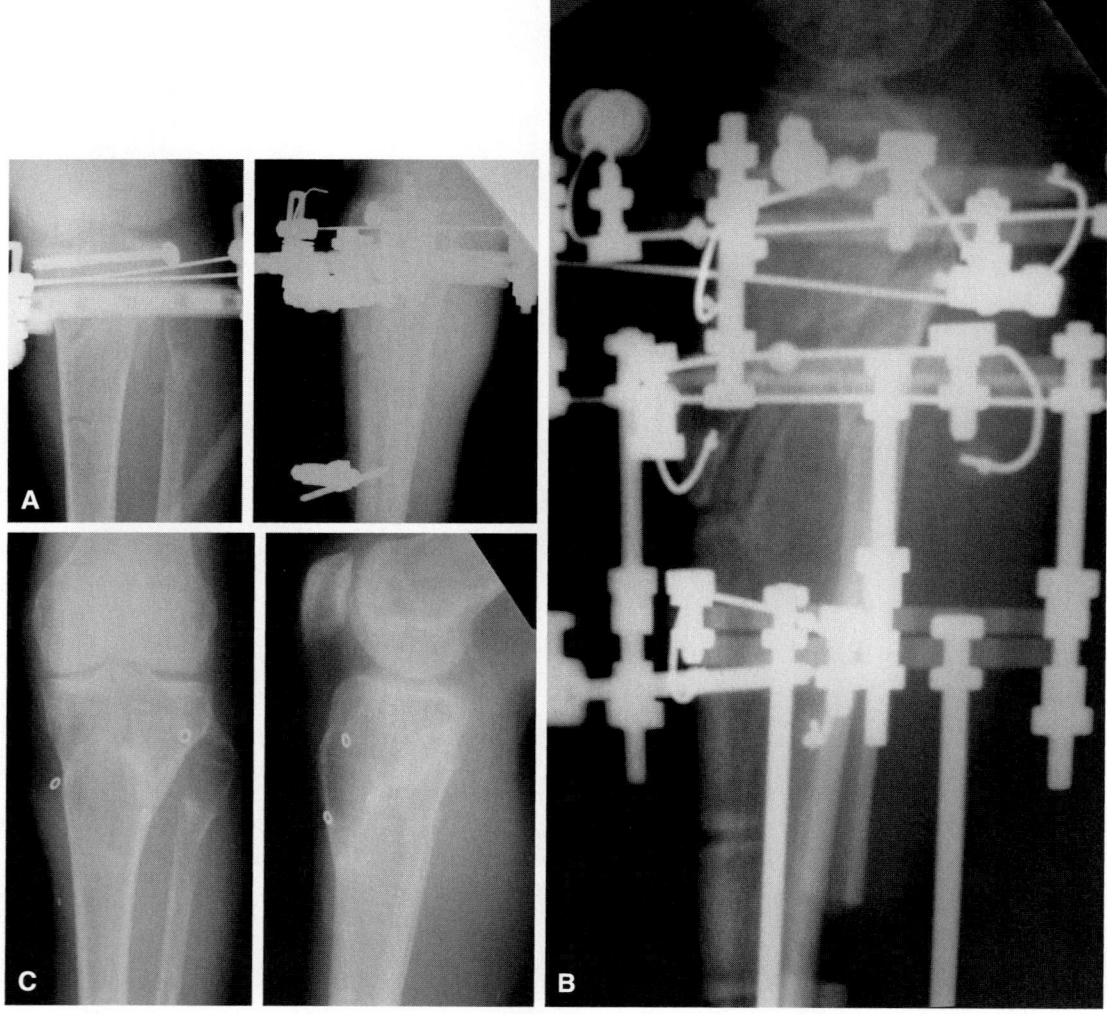

The bone formed at the corticotomy site in lengthening and bone transport is formed under gradual distraction (distraction osteogenesis).[13,14,74,140,211] The tension-stress effect of distraction causes neovascularity and cellular proliferation. The method of bone regeneration is primarily via intramembranous bone formation.

Distraction osteogenesis depends on a variety of mechanical and biological requirements. The corticotomy/osteotomy must be performed using a low-energy technique. Corticotomy/osteotomy in the metaphyseal or metadiaphyseal region is preferred over diaphyseal sites. Stable external fixation promotes good bony regenerate. A latency period prior to distraction of 7 to 14 days is recommended. The rate and rhythm of distraction are controlled by the treating physician, who monitors the progression of the regenerate on x-rays. The distraction phase classically is performed at a rate of 1.0 mm per day in a rhythm of 0.25 mm of distraction performed 4 times per day, although we typically begin distraction at 0.75 mm per day because some patients make bony regenerate more slowly. Following distraction, maturation and hypertrophy of the bony regenerate occur during the consolidation phase. The consolidation phase is generally two to three times as long as the distraction phase, but this varies widely.

Using Ilizarov methods, two different strategies can be employed for infected nonunions and nonunions associated with segmental defects: bifocal compression-distraction (lengthening) or bifocal distraction-compression transport (bone transport). The treatment strategy for these challenging problems depends on many factors (bone, soft tissue, and medical health characteristics). No clear consensus exists. Treatment options include conventional methods (resection, soft tissue coverage, massive cancellous bone grafting, and skeletal stabilization) and Ilizarov methods.

(Text continues on p. 694)

FIGURE 22-84 *Successful treatment of a resistant femoral nonunion with slow compression over a nail using external fixation (SCONE technique).* ***A,*** *Presenting radiograph shows a femoral nonunion. The patient is a 67-year-old man with two failed exchange nailings and two open bone graft procedures.* ***B,*** *Radiograph during treatment with slow compression over a nail using external fixation.* ***C,*** *Clinical photograph during treatment.* ***D,*** *Final radiographs show solid bony union.*

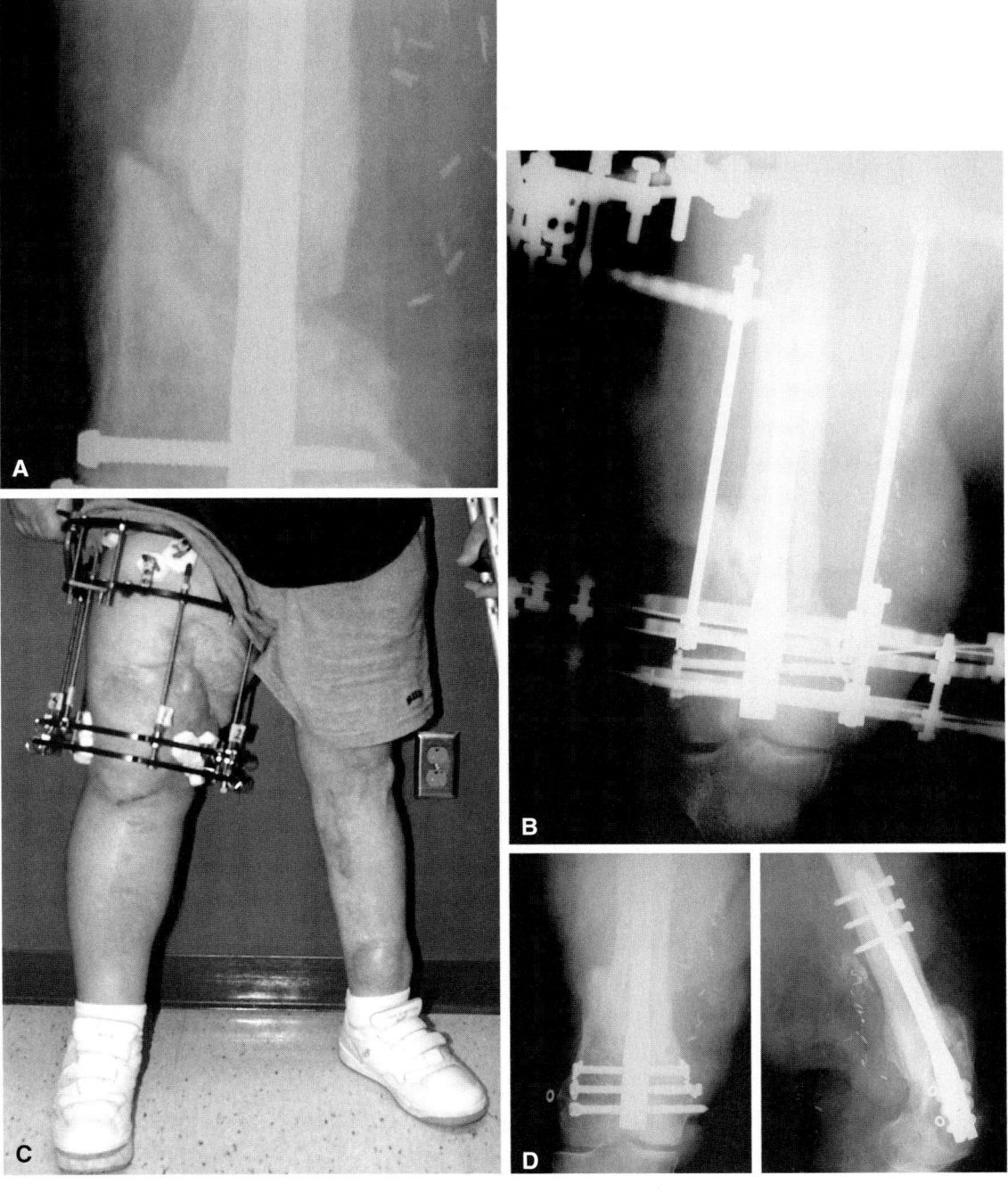

FIGURE 22-85 *Successful treatment of a distal femoral nonunion in a morbidly obese elderly diabetic woman 10 months after retrograde intramedullary nailing for a fracture. **A,** Presenting radiographs show a distal femoral nonunion. **B,** Radiograph during treatment with slow compression over a nail using external fixation (SCONE technique). **C,** Final radiographs show solid bony union. **D,** Clinical photograph following successful treatment.*

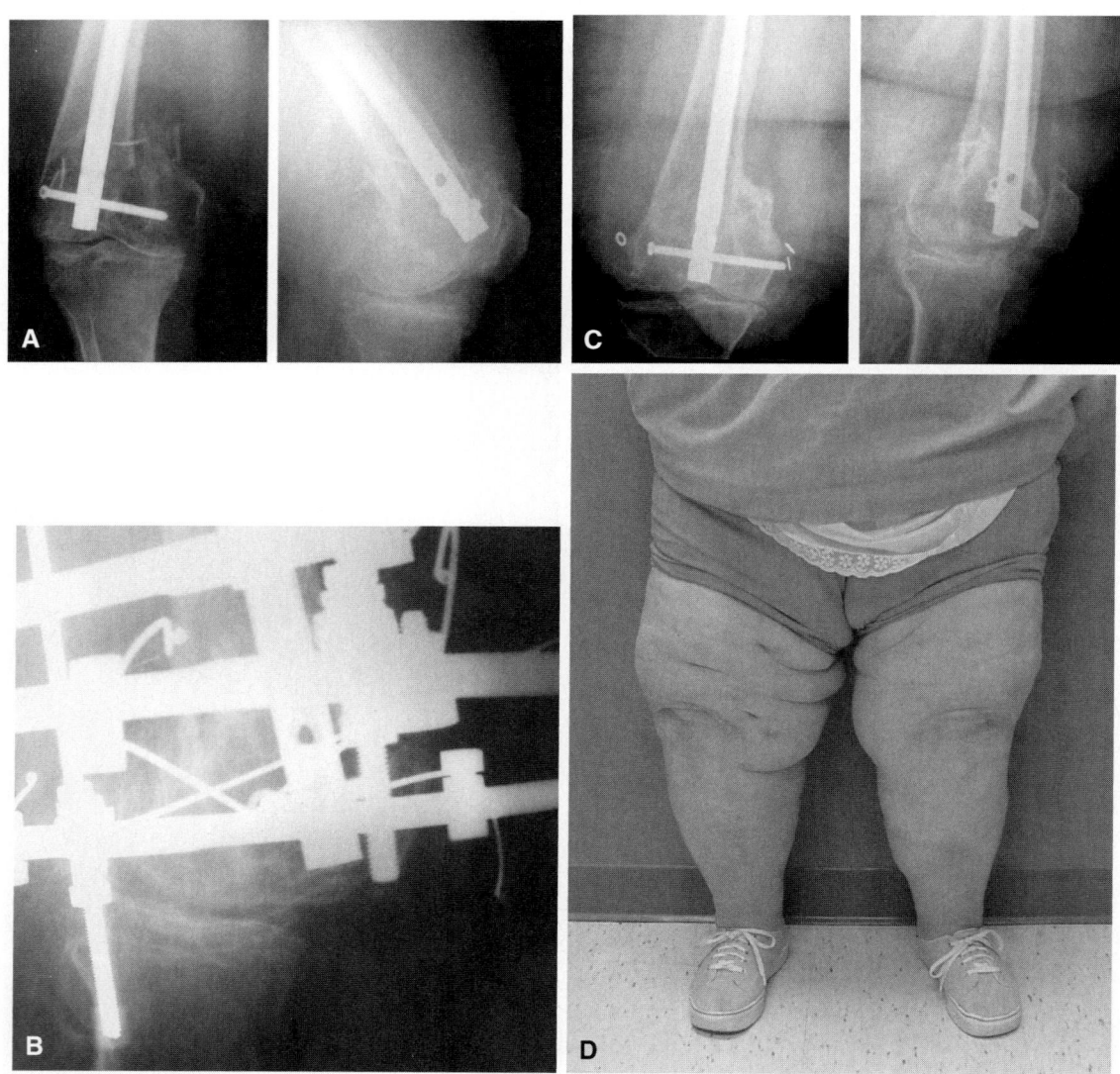

FIGURE 22-86   *Treatment of a stiff hypertrophic nonunion of the femoral shaft using distraction.* **A,** *Presenting radiographs.* **B,** *Radiograph during treatment via distraction using the Ilizarov external fixator. Note that differential distraction also results in deformity correction.* **C,** *Final radiographic result shows solid bony union and deformity correction.*

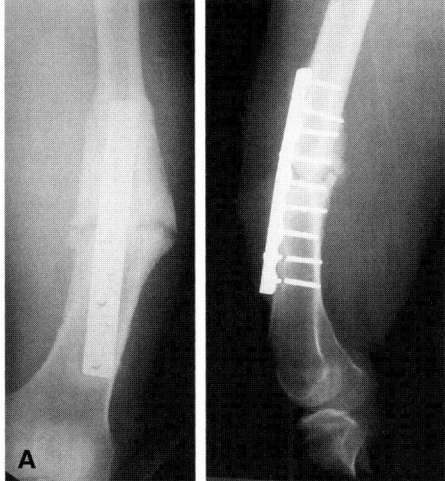

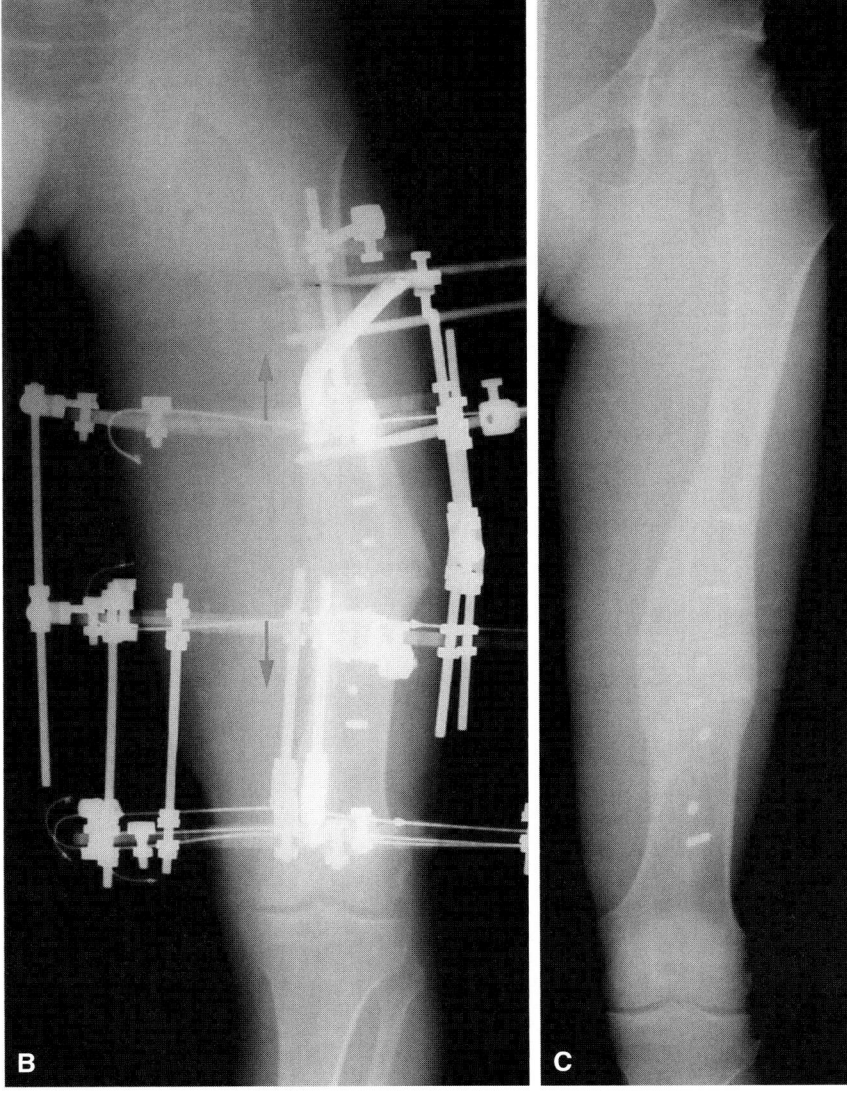

FIGURE 22-87   *Compression-distraction lengthening.*

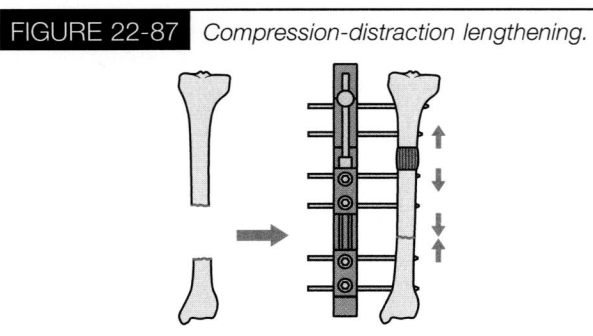

Bone loss   Early contact/ lengthening

A number of studies have compared these various methods. Green[116] compared bone grafting and bone transport in the treatment of segmental skeletal defects. For defects of 5 cm or less, he recommended the use of either technique, but he recommended bone transport or free composite tissue transfer for larger defects. In a similar study, Marsh and co-workers[185] compared resection and bone transport to treatment with less extensive débridement, external fixation, bone grafting, and soft tissue coverage and found that the groups were similar in terms of healing rate, healing and treatment time, eradication of infection, final deformity, complications, and total number of operative procedures. The final limb length discrepancy was significantly less in the group treated with bone transport. Cierny and Zorn[55] compared conventional (massive cancellous bone grafts and tissue transfers) versus Ilizarov methods in the treatment of segmental tibial defects. The Ilizarov group averaged 9 fewer hours in the operating room, 23 fewer days of hospitalization, 5 months less of disability, and a savings of nearly $30,000 per case. Ring and coauthors[261] compared autogenous cancellous bone grafting versus Ilizarov treatment for infected tibial nonunions and concluded that the Ilizarov methods may best be utilized for large limb length discrepancy or for very proximal or distal metaphyseal nonunions. Acute shortening with subsequent relengthening has a significantly lower complication rate and requires less time in

FIGURE 22-88   *Distraction-compression transport (bone transport).*

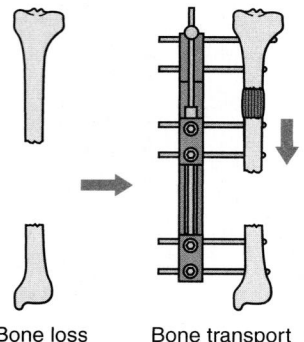

Bone loss   Bone transport

the external fixator than does bone transport for tibial defects, although both techniques provide excellent overall results. Mahaluxmivala and colleagues also recommended acute shortening with subsequent relengthening over bone transport because of shorter treatment time and fewer additional treatments (e.g., bone grafting) needed to achieve bony union.[183]

ARTHROPLASTY In certain situations, joint replacement arthroplasty may be the chosen treatment method for a fracture nonunion. The advantages are early return to function with immediate weight-bearing and joint mobilization. The main disadvantage is the excision of native anatomic structures (bone, cartilage, ligaments, etc.). Arthroplasty as a treatment of nonunion is indicated in older patients with severe medical problems; long-standing, resistant periarticular nonunions; periarticular nonunions associated with small osteopenic fragments; nonunions associated with painful post-traumatic or degenerative arthritis; and periprosthetic nonunions that either cannot be readily stabilized by conventional methods or have failed conventional treatment methods (Fig. 20-89).

Arthroplasty as a method of treatment for nonunion has been reported in a variety of anatomic locations including the hip,[63,182,188] knee,[10,72,103,288,336] shoulder,[11,105,126,213] and elbow.[206,225]

ARTHRODESIS Arthrodesis as a treatment method for nonunion is indicated for patients with previously failed (un-united) arthrodesis procedures (Fig. 22-90); infected periarticular nonunions; unreconstructable periarticular nonunions in locations that are not believed to have good long-term result with arthroplasty (e.g., the ankle); unreconstructable periarticular nonunions in young patients who are not long-term candidates for arthroplasty; infected nonunions in which débridement necessitates removal of important articular structures (see Fig. 22-71); and nonunions associated with unreconstructable joint instability, contracture, or pain that are not amenable to arthroplasty (see Fig. 22-71).

An alloarthrodesis procedure may be performed when a segmental bone defect extends to the epiphyseal region in a patient in whom an alloprosthesis is contraindicated (see Fig. 22-71).

AMPUTATION Lange et al.[175] published indications for amputation in the patient with an acute open fracture of the tibia associated with a vascular injury. Delay in amputation of a severely injured limb may lead to serious systemic complications, including death, so rapid, resolute decision-making in the acute setting is important.

The decision whether to amputate or reconstruct a nonunion is a different matter. The patient is not in extremis and has typically been living with the problem for a long time. In a study of quality of life in 109 patients with post-traumatic sequelae of the long bones, Lerner et al.[179] described the choice determinants in patients undergoing amputation:

1. Patients decided to discontinue medical and surgical treatment.
2. Amputation was recommended by a doctor.
3. Patients believed that they would never be cured.

FIGURE 22-89 **A,** *Presenting radiograph of an 82-year-old woman with a distal femoral periprosthetic nonunion. This patient had been wheelchair-bound for 2 years and had three prior failed attempts at nonunion treatment.* **B,** *Radiograph following joint replacement arthroplasty. The patient has had excellent pain relief and has resumed ambulation without the need for walking aids.*

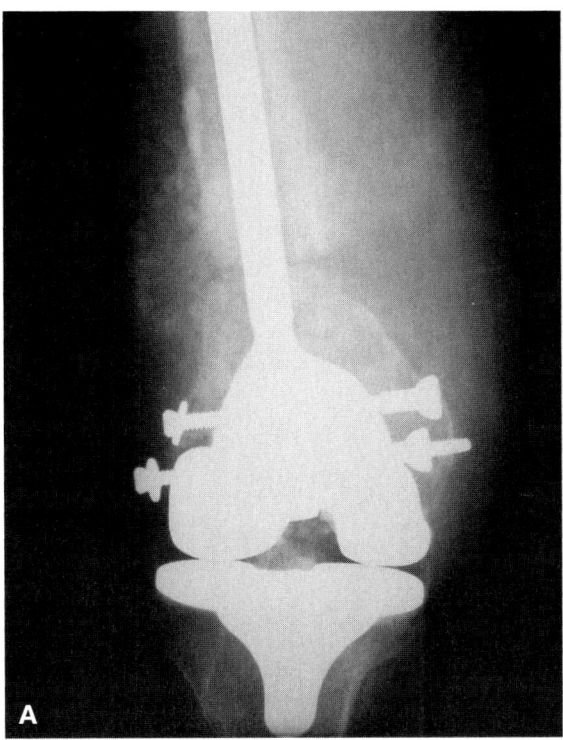
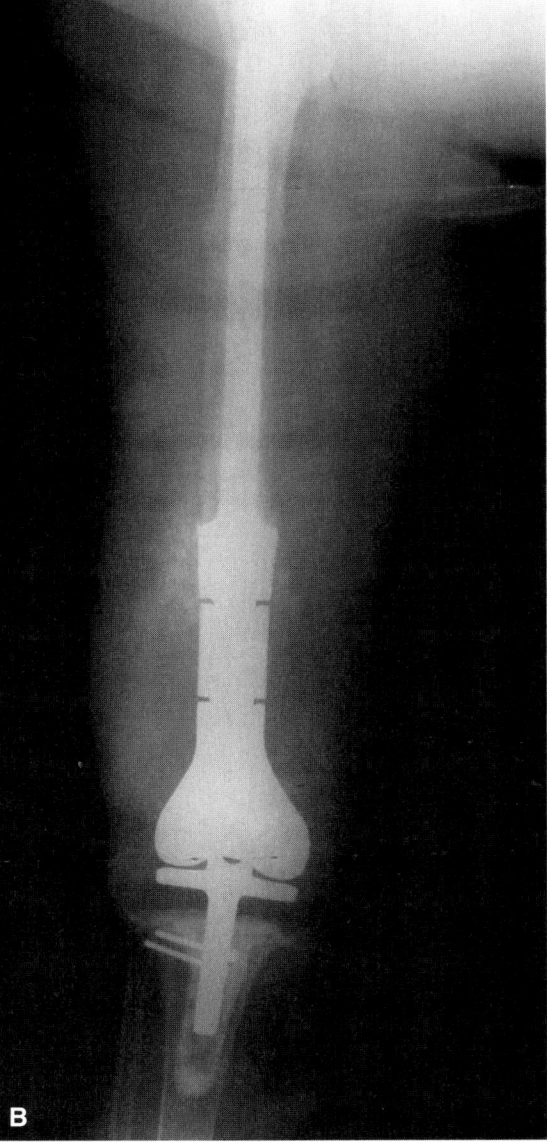

There are no absolute indications for amputation of a chronic un-united limb. Each case is unique and includes multiple complex issues, and treatment algorithms are usually not helpful.

Amputation of an un-united limb should be considered in several situations:

Sepsis arises in a frail, elderly, or medically compromised patient with an infected nonunion, and there is concern about the patient's survival.

Loss of neurologic function (motor or sensory or both) is unreconstructable and precludes restoration of purposeful limb function.

Chronic osteomyelitis associated with the nonunion is in an anatomic area that precludes reconstruction (e.g., the calcaneus).

The patient wishes to discontinue medical and surgical treatment of the nonunion and desires to have an amputation.

All patients considering amputation for a nonunion should seek a minimum of two opinions from orthopaedic surgeons specializing in nonunion reconstruction techniques. Amputation should not be undertaken because the treating physician has run out of ideas, treatment recommendations, or stamina. The motivated patient who has

FIGURE 22-90   *A, Presenting radiographs of a 25-year-old man who had had a total of 18 prior ankle operations and five failed prior attempts at ankle arthrodesis. **B,** The patient was treated with percutaneous hardware removal and gradual compression using an Ilizarov external fixator. The ankle joint was not operatively approached and no bone grafting was performed. **C,** Final radiographic result following simple gradual compression shows solid fusion of the ankle.*

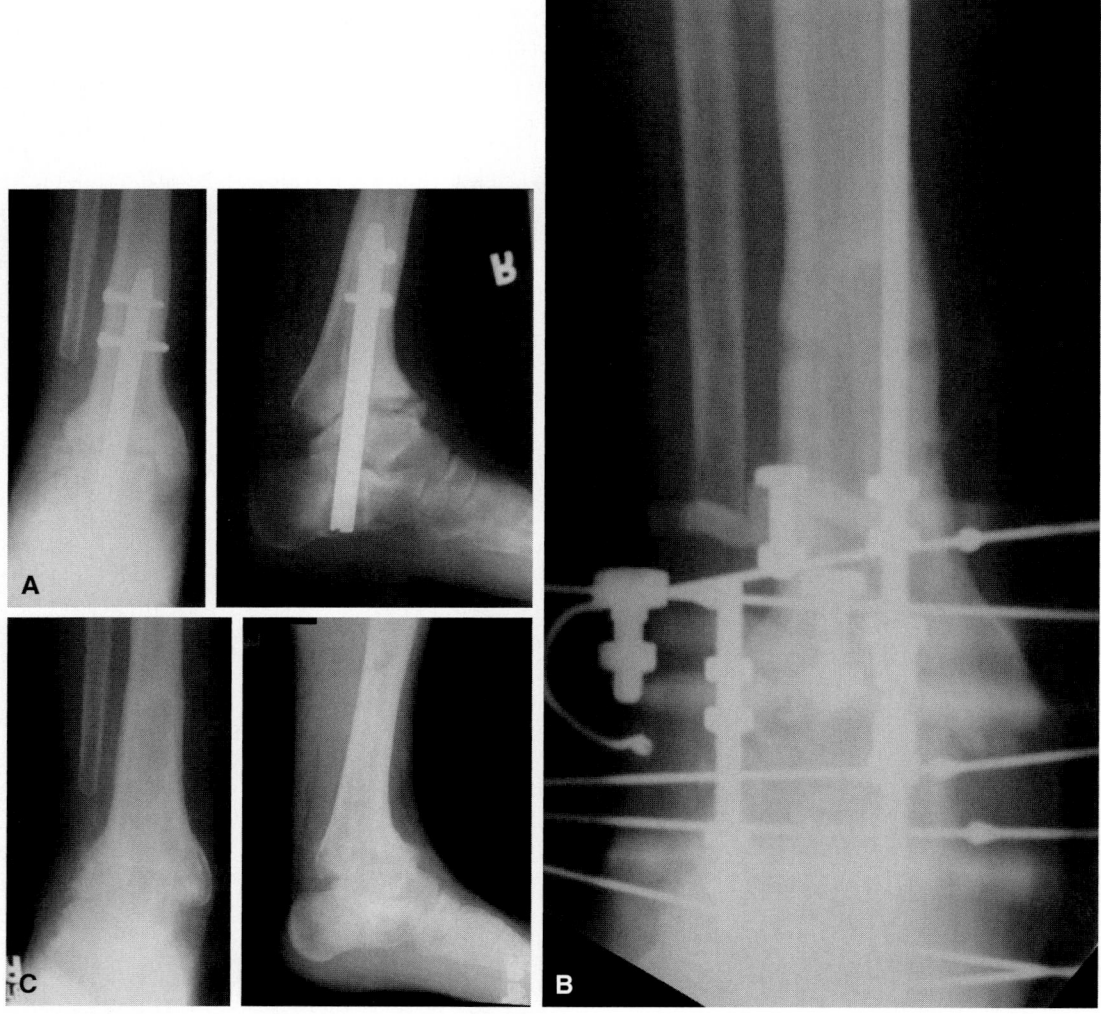

a recalcitrant nonunion but wishes to retain the limb can be referred to a colleague. Once a limb has been cut off, it cannot be reattached.

SUMMARY

The care of the patient who has a nonunion is always challenging and sometimes troubling. Because of the various nonunion types and the constellation of possible problems related to the bone, soft tissues, prior treatments, patient's health, and other factors, no simple treatment algorithms are possible. The care of these patients requires patience with the ultimate goal of bony union, restoration of function, and limited impairment and disability. An approach

to the evaluation and treatment of these patients has been provided. A few simple axioms bear further emphasis.

The 10 Commandments of Nonunion Treatment

Thou shalt

1. Examine thy patient, and carefully consider all available information.
2. Learn about the personality of the nonunion from the prior failed treatments.
3. Not repeat failed prior procedures (those which have not yielded any evidence of healing effort) over and over and over again.

4. Base thy treatment plan on the nonunion type and the treatment modifiers, and not upon false prophecies.
5. Forsake the use of the same hammer for every single nail (the treatment of nonunions requires surgical expertise in a wide variety of internal and external fixation techniques).
6. Honor the soft tissues, and keep them whole.
7. Consider minimally invasive techniques (Ilizarov method, bone marrow injection, etc.) where extensive surgical exposures have failed.
8. Not take the previous treating physician's name or treatment method or results in vain, particularly in the presence of the patient. Honor thy referring physician, and keep him or her informed of the patient's progress.
9. Burn no bridges, and leave thyself the option of a "next treatment plan."
10. Covet stability, vascularity, and bone-to-bone contact.

ACKNOWLEDGMENTS

The authors thank Joseph J. Gugenheim, M.D., Jeffrey C. London, M.D., Ebrahim Delpassand, M.D., and Michele Clowers for editorial assistance with the manuscript, and Rodney K. Baker for assistance with the figures.

REFERENCES

1. Aaron, R.K.; Ciombor, D.M.; Simon, B.J. Treatment of nonunions with electric and electromagnetic fields. Clin Orthop Relat Res 419:21–29, 2004.
2. Abdel-Aa, A.M.; Farouk, O.A.; Elsayed, A.; et al. The use of a locked plate in the treatment of ununited femoral shaft fractures. J Trauma 57:832–836, 2004.
3. Abhaykumar, S.; Elliott, D.S. Closed interlocking nailing for fibular nonunion. Injury 29:793–797, 1998.
4. Adams, C.I.; Keating, J.F.; Court-Brown, C.M. Cigarette smoking and open tibial fractures. Injury 32:61–65, 2001.
5. Agiza, A.R. Treatment of tibial osteomyelitic defects and infected pseudarthroses by the Huntington fibular transference operation. J Bone Joint Surg Am 63:814–849, 1981.
6. Ahlmann, E.; Patzakis, M.; Roidis, N.; et al. Comparison of anterior and posterior iliac crest bone grafts in terms of harvest-site morbidity and functional outcomes. J Bone Joint Surg Am 84:716–720, 2002.
7. Alho, A.; Ekeland, A.; Stromsoe, K.; et al. Nonunion of tibial shaft fractures treated with locked intramedullary nailing without bone grafting. J Trauma 34:62–67, 1993.
8. Allen, H.L.; Wase, A.; Bear, W.T. Indomethacin and aspirin: Effect of nonsteroidal anti-inflammatory agents on the rate of fracture repair in the rat. Acta Orthop Scand 51:595–600, 1980.
9. Altman, R.D.; Latta, L.L.; Keer, R.; et al. Effect of nonsteroidal anti-inflammatory drugs on fracture healing: A laboratory study in rats. J Orthop Trauma 9:392–400, 1995.
10. Anderson, S.P.; Matthews, L.S.; Kaufer, H. Treatment of juxta-articular nonunion fractures at the knee with long-stem total knee arthroplasty. Clin Orthop Relat Res 260:104–109, 1990.
11. Antuña, S.A.; Sperling, J.W.; Sanchez-Sotelo, J.; et al. Shoulder arthroplasty for proximal humeral nonunions. J Shoulder Elbow Surg 11:114–121, 2002.
12. Aronson, J. Temporal and spatial increases in blood flow during distraction osteogenesis. Clin Orthop Relat Res 301:124–131, 1994.
13. Aronson, J.; Good, B.; Stewart, C.; et al. Preliminary studies of mineralization during distraction osteogenesis. Clin Orthop Relat Res 250:43–49, 1990.
14. Aronson, J.; Harrison, B.; Boyd, C.M.; et al. Mechanical induction of osteogenesis: Preliminary studies. Ann Clin Lab Sci 18:195–203, 1988.
15. Atkins, R.M.; Madhavan, P.; Sudhakar, J.; et al. Ipsilateral vascularised fibular transport for massive defects of the tibia. J Bone Joint Surg Br 81:1035–1040, 1999.
16. Ballmer, F.T.; Ballmer, P.M.; Baumgaertel, F.; et al. Pauwels osteotomy for nonunions of the femoral neck. Orthop Clin North Am 21:759–767, 1990.
17. Banaszkiewicz, P.A.; Sabboubeh, A.; McLeod, I.; et al. Femoral exchange nailing for aseptic non-union: Not the end to all problems. Injury 34:349–356, 2003.
18. Banic, A.; Hertel, R. Double vascularized fibulas for reconstruction of large tibial defects. J Reconstr Microsurg 9:421–428, 1993.
19. Barquet, A.; Mayora, G.; Fregeiro, J.; et al. The treatment of subtrochanteric nonunions with the long gamma nail: Twenty-six patients with a minimum 2-year follow-up. J Orthop Trauma 18:346–353, 2004.
20. Bassett, C.A.L. Current concepts of bone formation. J Bone Joint Surg Am 44:1217–1244, 1962.
21. Bassett, C.A.L.; Pilla, A.A.; Pawluk, R.J. A nonoperative salvage of surgically resistant pseudoarthroses and nonunions by pulsing electromagnetic fields. Clin Orthop Relat Res 124:128–143, 1977.
22. Beardmore, A.A.; Brooks, D.E.; Wenke, J.C.; et al. Effectiveness of local antibiotic delivery with an osteoinductive and osteoconductive bone-graft substitute. J Bone Joint Surg Am 87:107–112, 2005.
23. Bellabarba, C.; Ricci, W.M.; Bolhofner, B.R. Results of indirect reduction and plating of femoral shaft nonunions after intramedullary nailing. J Orthop Trauma 15:254–263, 2001.
24. Beredjiklian, P.K.; Hotchkiss, R.N.; Athanasian, E.A.; et al. Recalcitrant nonunion of the distal humerus: Treatment with free vascularized bone grafting. Clin Orthop Relat Res 435:134–139, 2005.
25. Bhan, S.; Mehara, A.K. Percutaneous bone grafting for nonunion and delayed union of fractures of the tibial shaft. Int Orthop 17:310–312, 1993.
26. Bhattacharyya, T.; Bouchard, K.A.; Phadke, A.; et al. The accuracy of computed tomography for the diagnosis of tibial nonunion. J Bone Joint Surg Am 88:692–697, 2006.

27. Blachut, P.A.; Meek, R.N.; O'Brien, P.J. External fixation and delayed intramedullary nailing of open fractures of the tibial shaft: A sequential protocol. J Bone Joint Surg Am 72:729–735, 1990.

28. Boehme, D.; Curtis, R.J., Jr.; DeHaan, J.T.; et al. The treatment of nonunion fractures of the midshaft of the clavicle with an intramedullary Hagie pin and autogenous bone graft. Instr Course Lect 42:283–290, 1993.

29. Bondurant, F.J.; Cotler, H.B.; Buckle, R.; et al. The medical and economic impact of severely injured lower extremities. J Trauma 28:1270–1273, 1988.

30. Borrelli, J., Jr.; Prickett, W.D.; Ricci, W.M. Treatment of nonunions and osseous defects with bone graft and calcium sulfate. Clin Orthop Relat Res 411:245–254, 2003.

31. Bradbury, N.; Hutchinson, J.; Hahn, D.; et al. Clavicular nonunion: 31/32 healed after plate fixation and bone grafting. Acta Orthop Scand 67:367–370, 1996.

32. Brighton, C.T.; Esterhai, J.L., Jr.; Katz, M.; et al. Synovial pseudoarthrosis: A clinical, roentgenographic-scintigraphic, and pathologic study. J Trauma 27:463–470, 1987.

33. Brinker, M.R. Principles of fractures. In Brinker, M.R., ed. Review of Orthopaedic Trauma. Philadelphia, W.B. Saunders, 2001.

34. Brinker, M.R.; Bailey, D.E. Fracture healing in tibia fractures with an associated vascular injury. J Trauma 42:11–19, 1997.

35. Brinker, M.; Cook, S.; Dunlap, J.; et al. Early changes in nutrient artery blood flow following tibial nailing with and without reaming: A preliminary study. J Orthop Trauma 13:129–133, 1999.

36. Brinker, M.R.; O'Connor, D.P. Ilizarov compression over a nail for aseptic femoral nonunions that have failed exchange nailing: A report of five cases. J Orthop Trauma 17:668–676, 2003.

37. Brownlow, H.C.; Reed, A.; Simpson, A.H. The vascularity of atrophic non-unions. Injury 33:145–150, 2002.

38. Burd, T.A.; Hughes, M.S.; Anglen, J.O. Heterotopic ossification prophylaxis with indomethacin increases the risk of long-bone nonunion. J Bone Joint Surg Br 85:700–705, 2003.

39. Butcher, C.K.; Marsh, D.R. Nonsteroidal anti-inflammatory drugs delay tibial fracture union [abstract]. Injury 27:375, 1996.

40. Cameron, H.U.; Welsh, R.P.; Jung, Y.B.; et al. Repair of nonunion of tibial osteotomy. Clin Orthop Relat Res 287:167–169, 1993.

41. Campanacci, M.; Zanoli, S. Double tibiofibular synostosis (fibula pro tibia) for non-union and delayed union of the tibia. J Bone Joint Surg Am 48:44–56, 1966.

42. Cantu, R.V.; Koval, K.J. The use of locking plates in fracture care. J Am Acad Orthop Surg 14:183–190, 2006.

43. Carpenter, C.A.; Jupiter, J.B. Blade plate reconstruction of metaphyseal nonunion of the tibia. Clin Orthop Relat Res 332:23–28, 1996.

44. Catagni, M.A.; Guerreschi, F.; Holman, J.A.; et al. Distraction osteogenesis in the treatment of stiff hypertrophic nonunions using the Ilizarov apparatus. Clin Orthop Relat Res 301:159–163, 1994.

45. Chacha, P.B.; Ahmed, M.; Daruwalla, J.S. Vascular pedicle graft of the ipsilateral fibula for non-union of the tibia with a large defect: An experimental and clinical study. J Bone Joint Surg Br 63:244–253, 1981.

46. Chapman, M.W. Closed intramedullary bone grafting for diaphyseal defects of the femur. Instr Course Lect 32:317–324, 1983.

47. Charlton, W.P.; Kharazzi, D.; Alpert, S.; et al. Unstable nonunion of the scapula: A case report. J Shoulder Elbow Surg 12:517–519, 2003.

48. Charnley, G.J.; Ward, A.J. Reconstruction femoral nailing for nonunion of subtrochanteric fracture: A revision technique following dynamic condylar screw failure. Int Orthop 20:55–57, 1996.

49. Charnley, J. Compression Arthrodesis. Edinburgh and London, E. and S. Livingstone, 1953.

50. Chatziyiannakis, A.A.; Verettas, D.A.; Raptis, V.K.; et al. Nonunion of tibial fractures treated with external fixation: Contributing factors studied in 71 fractures. Acta Orthop Scand Suppl 275:77–79, 1997.

51. Chen, C.Y.; Ueng, S.W.; Shih, C.H. Staged management of infected humeral nonunion. J Trauma 43:793–798, 1997.

52. Chin, K.R.; Nagarkatti, D.G.; Miranda, M.A.; et al. Salvage of distal tibia metaphyseal nonunions with the 90-degree cannulated blade plate. Clin Orthop Relat Res 409:241–249, 2003.

53. Chmell, M.J.; McAndrew, M.P.; Thomas, R.; et al. Structural allografts for reconstruction of lower extremity open fractures with 10 centimeters or more of acute segmental defects. J Orthop Trauma 9:222–226, 1995.

54. Christensen, N.O. Kuntscher intramedullary reaming and nail fixation for non-union of fracture of the femur and the tibia. J Bone Joint Surg Br 55:312–318, 1973.

55. Cierny, G. III; Zorn, K.E. Segmental tibial defects: Comparing conventional and Ilizarov methodologies. Clin Orthop Relat Res 301:118–123, 1994.

56. Ciombor, D.M.; Aaron, R.K. The role of electrical stimulation in bone repair. Foot Ankle Clin 10:579–593, vii, 2005.

57. Clarke, P.; Mollan, R.A. The criteria for amputation in severe lower limb injury. Injury 25:139–143, 1994.

58. Cobb, T.K.; Gabrielsen, T.A.; Campbell, D.C. II; et al. Cigarette smoking and nonunion after ankle arthrodesis. Foot Ankle Int 15:64–67, 1994.

59. Cobos, J.A.; Lindsey, R.W.; Gugala, Z. The cylindrical titanium mesh cage for treatment of a long bone segmental defect: Description of a new technique and report of two cases. J Orthop Trauma 14:54–59, 2000.

60. Connolly, J.F. Injectable bone marrow preparations to stimulate osteogenic repair. Clin Orthop Relat Res 313:8–18, 1995.

61. Connolly, J.F.; Shindell, R. Percutaneous marrow injection for an ununited tibia. Nebr Med J 71:105–107, 1986.

62. Court-Brown, C.M.; Keating, J.F.; Christie, J.; et al. Exchange intramedullary nailing: Its use in aseptic tibial nonunion. J Bone Joint Surg Br 77:407–411, 1995.

63. Crockarell, J.R., Jr.; Berry, D.J.; Lewallen, D.G. Nonunion after periprosthetic femoral fracture associated with total hip arthroplasty. J Bone Joint Surg Am 81:1073–1079, 1999.

64. Crow, S.A.; Chen, L.; Lee, J.H.; et al. Vascularized bone grafting from the base of the second metacarpal for persistent distal radius nonunion: A case report. J Orthop Trauma 19:483–486, 2005.

65. Daftari, T.K.; Whitesides, T.E., Jr.; Heller, J.G.; et al. Nicotine on the revascularization of bone graft: An experimental study in rabbits. Spine 19:904–911, 1994.

66. Dalal, S.; Stanley, D. Locked intramedullary nailing in the treatment of olecranon nonunion: A new method of treatment. J Shoulder Elbow Surg 13:366–368, 2004.

67. Danckwardt-Lilliestrom, G. Reaming of the medullary cavity and its effect on diaphyseal bone: A fluorochromic, microangiographic and histologic study on the rabbit tibia and dog femur. Acta Orthop Scand Suppl 128:1–153, 1969.

68. Danis, R. Theorie et Pratique de l'Osteosynthese. Paris, Masson, 1949.

69. Danziger, M.B.; Healy, W.L. Operative treatment of olecranon nonunion. J Orthop Trauma 6:290–293, 1992.

70. Davey, P.A.; Simonis, R.B. Modification of the Nicoll bone-grafting technique for nonunion of the radius and/or ulna. J Bone Joint Surg Br 84:30–33, 2002.

71. Davids, P.H.; Luitse, J.S.; Strating, R.P.; et al. Operative treatment for delayed union and nonunion of midshaft clavicular fractures: AO reconstruction plate fixation and early mobilization. J Trauma 40:985–986, 1996.

72. Davila, J.; Malkani, A.; Paiso, J.M. Supracondylar distal femoral nonunions treated with a megaprosthesis in elderly patients: A report of two cases. J Orthop Trauma 15:574–578, 2001.

73. Day, S.M.; DeHeer, D.H. Reversal of the detrimental effects of chronic protein malnutrition on long bone fracture healing. J Orthop Trauma 15:47–53, 2001.

74. Delloye, C.; Delefortrie, G.; Coutelier, L.; et al. Bone regenerate formation in cortical bone during distraction lengthening: An experimental study. Clin Orthop Relat Res 250:34–42, 1990.

75. Delloye, C.; Suratwala, S.J.; Cornu, O.; et al. Treatment of allograft nonunions with recombinant human bone morphogenetic proteins (rhBMP). Acta Orthop Belg 70:591–597, 2004.

76. de Vernejoul, M.C.; Bielakoff, J.; Herve, M.; et al. Evidence for defective osteoblastic function: A role for alcohol and tobacco consumption in osteoporosis in middle-aged men. Clin Orthop Relat Res 179:107–115, 1983.

77. Dimitriou, R.; Dahabreh, Z.; Katsoulis, E.; et al. Application of recombinant BMP-7 on persistent upper and lower limb non-unions. Injury 36(Suppl 4):S51–S59, 2005.

78. Dodds, R.A.; Catterall, A.; Bitensky, L.; et al. Abnormalities in fracture healing induced by vitamin B6 deficiency in rats. Bone 7:489–495, 1986.

79. Dworkin, S.F.; Von Korff, M.; LeResche, L. Multiple pains and psychiatric disturbance: An epidemiologic investigation. Arch Gen Psychiatry 47:239–244, 1990.

80. Ebraheim, N.A.; Mekhail, A.O.; Darwich, M. Open reduction and internal fixation with bone grafting of clavicular nonunion. J Trauma 42:701–704, 1997.

81. Eckardt, H.; Christensen, K.S.; Lind, M.; et al. Recombinant human bone morphogenetic protein 2 enhances bone healing in an experimental model of fractures at risk of non-union. Injury 36:489–494, 2005.

82. Eckardt, H.; Ding, M.; Lind, M.; et al. Recombinant human vascular endothelial growth factor enhances bone healing in an experimental nonunion model. J Bone Joint Surg Br 87:1434–1438, 2005.

83. Eggers, G.W.N. Internal contact splint. J Bone Joint Surg Am 31:40–52, 1949.

84. Eglseder, W.A., Jr.; Elliott, M.J. Nonunions of the distal radius. Am J Orthop 31:259–262, 2002.

85. Egol, K.A.; Kubiak, E.N.; Fulkerson, E.; et al. Biomechanics of locked plates and screws. J Orthop Trauma 18:488–493, 2004.

86. Einhorn, T.A. Clinical applications of recombinant human BMPs: Early experience and future development. J Bone Joint Surg Am 85(Suppl 3):82–88, 2003.

87. Einhorn, T.A. Enhancement of fracture healing. Instr Course Lect 45:401–416, 1996.

88. Einhorn, T.A.; Bonnarens, F.; Burstein, A.H. The contributions of dietary protein and mineral to the healing of experimental fractures: A biomechanical study. J Bone Joint Surg Am 68:1389–1395, 1986.

89. Einhorn, T.A.; Gundberg, C.M.; Devlin, V.J.; et al. Fracture healing and osteocalcin metabolism in vitamin K deficiency. Clin Orthop Relat Res 237:219–225, 1988.

90. Einhorn, T.A.; Levine, B.; Michel, P. Nutrition and bone. Orthop Clin North Am 21:43–50, 1990.

91. Emami, A.; Mjoberg, B.; Larsson, S. Infected tibial nonunion: Good results after open cancellous bone grafting in 37 cases. Acta Orthop Scand 66:447–451, 1995.

92. Engesaeter, L.B.; Sudmann, B.; Sudmann, E. Fracture healing in rats inhibited by locally administered indomethacin. Acta Orthop Scand 63:330–333, 1992.

93. Esterhai, J.L., Jr.; Brighton, C.T.; Heppenstall, R.B. Nonunion of the humerus: Clinical, roentgenographic, scintigraphic, and response characteristics to

treatment with constant direct current stimulation of osteogenesis. Clin Orthop Relat Res 211:228–234, 1986.

94. Esterhai, J.L., Jr.; Brighton, C.T.; Heppenstall, R. B.; et al. Detection of synovial pseudarthrosis by 99mTc scintigraphy: Application to treatment of traumatic nonunion with constant direct current. Clin Orthop Relat Res 161:15–23, 1981.

95. Esterhai, J.L., Jr.; Sennett, B.; Gelb, H.; et al. Treatment of chronic osteomyelitis complicating nonunion and segmental defects of the tibia with open cancellous bone graft, posterolateral bone graft, and soft-tissue transfer. J Trauma 30:49–54, 1990.

96. Fang, M.; Frost, P.; Iida-Klein, A.; et al. Effects of nicotine on cellular function in UMR 106-01 osteoblast-like cells. Bone 12:283–286, 1991.

97. Feldman, D.S.; Shin, S.S.; Madan, S.; et al. Correction of tibial malunion and nonunion with six-axis analysis deformity correction using the Taylor Spatial Frame. J Orthop Trauma 17:549–554, 2003.

98. Fernandez, D.L.; Ring, D.; Jupiter, J.B. Surgical management of delayed union and nonunion of distal radius fractures. J Hand Surg [Am] 26:201–209, 2001.

99. Ferraz, I.C.; Papadimitriou, N.G.; Sotereanos, D.G. Scapular body nonunion: A case report. J Shoulder Elbow Surg 11:98–100, 2002.

100. Finkemeier, C.G.; Chapman, M.W. Treatment of femoral diaphyseal nonunions. Clin Orthop Relat Res 398:223–234, 2002.

101. Flinkkilä, T.; Ristiniemi, J.; Hämäläinen, M. Nonunion after intramedullary nailing of humeral shaft fractures. J Trauma 50:540–544, 2001.

102. Foulk, D.A.; Szabo, R.M. Diaphyseal humerus fractures: Natural history and occurrence of nonunion. Orthopedics 18:333–335, 1995.

103. Freedman, E.L.; Hak, D.J.; Johnson, E.E.; et al. Total knee replacement including a modular distal femoral component in elderly patients with acute fracture or nonunion. J Orthop Trauma 9:231–237, 1995.

104. Frey, C.; Halikus, N.M.; Vu-Rose, T.; et al. A review of ankle arthrodesis: Predisposing factors to nonunion. Foot Ankle Int 15:581–584, 1994.

105. Frich, L.H.; Sojbjerg, J.O.; Sneppen, O. Shoulder arthroplasty in complex acute and chronic proximal humeral fractures. Orthopedics 14:949–954, 1991.

106. Friedlaender, G.E.; Perry, C.R.; Cole, J.D.; et al. Osteogenic protein-1 (bone morphogenetic protein-7) in the treatment of tibial nonunions. J Bone Joint Surg Am 83(Suppl 1):S151–S158, 2001.

107. Galatz, L.M.; Williams, G.R., Jr.; Fenlin, J.M., Jr.; et al. Outcome of open reduction and internal fixation of surgical neck nonunions of the humerus. J Orthop Trauma 18:63–67, 2004.

108. Gebauer, D.; Mayr, E.; Orthner, E.; et al. Low-intensity pulsed ultrasound: Effects on nonunions. Ultrasound Med Biol 31:1391–1402, 2005.

109. Gerber, A.; Marti, R.; Jupiter, J. Surgical management of diaphyseal humeral nonunion after intramedullary nailing: Wave-plate fixation and autologous bone grafting without nail removal. J Shoulder Elbow Surg 12:309–313, 2003.

110. Giannoudis, P.V.; MacDonald, D.A.; Matthews, S.J.; et al. Nonunion of the femoral diaphysis: The influence of reaming and non-steroidal anti-inflammatory drugs. J Bone Joint Surg Br 82:655–658, 2000.

111. Goldman, B. Use and abuse of opioid analgesics in chronic pain. Can Fam Physician 39:571–576, 1993.

112. Gonzalez del Pino, J.; Bartolome del Valle, E.; Grana, G.L.; et al. Free vascularized fibular grafts have a high union rate in atrophic nonunions. Clin Orthop Relat Res 419:38–45, 2004.

113. Goulet, J.A.; Templeman, D. Delayed union and nonunion of tibial shaft fractures. Instr Course Lect 46:281–291, 1997.

114. Graves, M.L.; Ryan, J.E.; Mast, J.W. Supracondylar femur nonunion associated with previous vascular repair: Importance of vascular exam in preoperative planning of nonunion repair. J Orthop Trauma 19:574–577, 2005.

115. Green, S.A. The Ilizarov method. In Browner, B.D.; Levine, A.M.; Jupiter, J.B., eds. Skeletal Trauma: Fractures, Dislocations, Ligamentous Injuries, 2nd ed. Philadelphia, W.B. Saunders, 1998, pp. 661–701.

116. Green, S.A. Skeletal defects: A comparison of bone grafting and bone transport for segmental skeletal defects. Clin Orthop Relat Res 301:111–117, 1994.

117. Guarniero, R.; de Barros Filho, T.E.; Tannuri, U.; et al. Study of fracture healing in protein malnutrition. Rev Paul Med 110:63–68, 1992.

118. Guerkov, H.H.; Lohmann, C.H.; Liu, Y.; et al. Pulsed electromagnetic fields increase growth factor release by nonunion cells. Clin Orthop Relat Res 384:265–279, 2001.

119. Gustilo, R.B.; Nelson, G.E.; Hamel, A.; et al. The effect of intramedullary nailing on the blood supply of the diaphysis of long bones in mature dogs. J Bone Joint Surg Am 46:1362–1363, 1964.

120. Gyul'nazarova, S.V.; Shtin, V.P. Reparative bone tissue regeneration in treating pseudarthroses with simultaneous lengthening in the area of the pathological focus (an experimental study). Ortop Travmatol Protez 4:10–15, 1983.

121. Haidukewych, G.J. Innovations in locking plate technology. J Am Acad Orthop Surg 12:205–212, 2004.

122. Hak, D.J.; Lee, S.S.; Goulet, J.A. Success of exchange reamed intramedullary nailing for femoral shaft nonunion or delayed union. J Orthop Trauma 14:178–182, 2000.

123. Han, C.S.; Wood, M.B.; Bishop, A.T.; et al. Vascularized bone transfer. J Bone Joint Surg Am 74:1441–1449, 1992.

124. Harley, B.J.; Beaupre, L.A.; Jones, C.A.; et al. The effect of time to definitive treatment on the rate of

nonunion and infection in open fractures. J Orthop Trauma 16:484–490, 2002.

125. Haverstock, B.D.; Mandracchia, V.J. Cigarette smoking and bone healing: Implications in foot and ankle surgery. J Foot Ankle Surg 37:69–74, 1998.

126. Healy, W.L.; Jupiter, J.B.; Kristiansen, T.K.; et al. Nonunion of the proximal humerus: A review of 25 cases. J Orthop Trauma 4:424–431, 1990.

127. Helfet, D.L.; Jupiter, J.B.; Gasser, S. Indirect reduction and tension-band plating of tibial non-union with deformity. J Bone Joint Surg Am 74:1286–1297, 1992.

128. Helfet, D.L.; Kloen, P.; Anand, N.; et al. Open reduction and internal fixation of delayed unions and nonunions of fractures of the distal part of the humerus. J Bone Joint Surg Am 85:33–40, 2003.

129. Hernandez, R.J.; Tachdjian, M.O.; Poznanski, A.K.; et al. CT determination of femoral torsion. Am J Roentgenol 137:97–101, 1981.

130. Hernigou, P.; Poignard, A.; Beaujean, F.; et al. Percutaneous autologous bone-marrow grafting for nonunions: Influence of the number and concentration of progenitor cells. J Bone Joint Surg Am 87:1430–1437, 2005.

131. Hernigou, P.; Poignard, A.; Manicom, O.; et al. The use of percutaneous autologous bone marrow transplantation in nonunion and avascular necrosis of bone. J Bone Joint Surg Br 87:896–902, 2005.

132. Herve, C.; Gaillard, M.; Andrivet, P.; et al. Treatment in serious lower limb injuries: Amputation versus preservation. Injury 18:21–23, 1987.

133. Herzenberg, J.E.; Smith, J.D.; Paley, D. Correcting tibial deformities with Ilizarov's apparatus. Clin Orthop Relat Res 302:36–41, 1994.

134. Hogevold, H.E.; Grogaard, B.; Reikeras, O. Effects of short-term treatment with corticosteroids and indomethacin on bone healing: A mechanical study of osteotomies in rats. Acta Orthop Scand 63:607–611, 1992.

135. Horstmann, H.; Mahboubi, S. The use of computed tomography scan in unstable hip reconstruction. J Comput Tomogr 11:364–369, 1987.

136. Huddleston, P.M.; Steckelberg, J.M.; Hanssen, A.D.; et al. Ciprofloxacin inhibition of experimental fracture healing. J Bone Joint Surg Am 82:161–173, 2000.

137. Huntington, T.W. Case of bone transference: Use of a segment of fibula to supply a defect in the tibia. Ann Surg 41:249–251, 1905.

138. Huo, M.H.; Troiano, N.W.; Pelker, R.R.; et al. The influence of ibuprofen on fracture repair: Biomechanical, biochemical, histologic, and histomorphometric parameters in rats. J Orthop Res 9:383–390, 1991.

139. Ikeda, K.; Tomita, K.; Hashimoto, F.; et al. Long-term follow-up of vascularized bone grafts for the reconstruction of tibial nonunion: Evaluation with computed tomographic scanning. J Trauma 32:693–697, 1992.

140. Ilizarov, G.A. Clinical application of the tension-stress effect for limb lengthening. Clin Orthop Relat Res 250:8–26, 1990.

141. Ilizarov, G.A. Transosseous Osteosynthesis: Theoretical and Clinical Aspects of the Regeneration and Growth of Tissue. Berlin, Springer-Verlag, 1992.

142. Ilizarov, G.A.; Devyatov, A.A.; Kamerin, V.K. Plastic reconstruction of longitudinal bone defects by means of compression and subsequent distraction. Acta Chir Plast 22:32–41, 1980.

143. Ilizarov, G.A.; Kaplunov, A.G.; Degtiarev, V.E.; et al. Treatment of pseudarthroses and ununited fractures, complicated by purulent infection, by the method of compression-distraction osteosynthesis. Ortop Travmatol Protez 33:10–14, 1972.

144. Ilizarov, G.A.; Kaplunov, A.G.; Grachova, V.I.; et al. Close Compression-Distraction Osteosynthesis of the Tibial Pseudoarthroses with Ilizarov Method (Metodicheskoe Posobie). Kurgan, USSR, Kniiekot Institute, 1971.

145. Inan, M.; Karaoglu, S.; Cilli, F.; et al. Treatment of femoral nonunions by using cyclic compression and distraction. Clin Orthop Relat Res 436:222–228, 2005.

146. Indrekvam, K.; Lekven, J.; Engesaeter, L.B.; et al. Effects of intramedullary reaming and nailing on blood flow in rat femora. Acta Orthop Scand 63:61–65, 1992.

147. Jain, A.K.; Sinha, S. Infected nonunion of the long bones. Clin Orthop Relat Res 431:57–65, 2005.

148. Johnson, E.E.; Simpson, L.A.; Helfet, D.L. Delayed intramedullary nailing after failed external fixation of the tibia. Clin Orthop Relat Res 253:251–257, 1990.

149. Jones, N.F.; Swartz, W.M.; Mears, D.C.; et al. The "double barrel" free vascularized fibular bone graft. Plast Reconstr Surg 81:378–385, 1988.

150. Judet, R. La Decortication: Actualites de Chirurgie Orthopedique. Paris, Masson, 1965.

151. Judet, R.; Judet, J.; Roy-Camille, R. La vascularisation des pseudoarthroses des os longs d'après une étude clinique et experimental. Rev Chir Orthop 44:5, 1958.

152. Jupiter, J.B.; Ring, D.; Rosen, H. The complications and difficulties of management of nonunion in the severely obese. J Orthop Trauma 9:363–370, 1995.

153. Kabak, S.; Halici, M.; Tuncel, M.; et al. Treatment of midclavicular nonunion: Comparison of dynamic compression plating and low-contact dynamic compression plating techniques. J Shoulder Elbow Surg 13:396–403, 2004.

154. Kassab, M.; Samaha, C.; Saillant, G. Ipsilateral fibular transposition in tibial nonunion using Huntington procedure: A 12-year follow-up study. Injury 34:770–775, 2003.

155. Katon, W. The impact of major depression on chronic medical illness. Gen Hosp Psychiatry 18:215–219, 1996.

156. Katon, W.; Sullivan, M.D. Depression and chronic medical illness. J Clin Psychiatry 51:3–11, 1990.

157. Keller, J.; Bunger, C.; Andereassen, T.T.; et al. Bone repair inhibited by indomethacin. Acta Orthop Scand 58:379–383, 1987.

158. Kempf, I.; Grosse, A.; Rigaut, P. The treatment of noninfected pseudarthrosis of the femur and tibia with locked intramedullary nailing. Clin Orthop Relat Res 212:142–154, 1986.

159. Kettunen, J.; Makela, E.A.; Turunen, V.; et al. Percutaneous bone grafting in the treatment of the delayed union and non-union of tibial fractures. Injury 33:239–245, 2002.

160. Key, J. Positive pressure in arthrodesis for tuberculosis of the knee joint. South Med J 25:909, 1932.

161. Khan, I.M. Fracture healing: Role of NSAIDs [abstract]. Am J Orthop 26:413, 1997.

162. Kim, S.J.; Yang, K.H.; Moon, S.H.; et al. Endoscopic bone graft for delayed union and nonunion. Arthroscopy 15:324–329, 1999.

163. Klassen, J.F.; Trousdale, R.T. Treatment of delayed and nonunion of the patella. J Orthop Trauma 11:188–194, 1997.

164. Klemm, K.W. Treatment of infected pseudarthrosis of the femur and tibia with an interlocking nail. Clin Orthop Relat Res 212:174–181, 1986.

165. Kloen, P. Bilateral clavicle non-unions treated with anteroinferior locking compression plating (LCP): A case report. Acta Orthop Belg 70:609–611, 2004.

166. Kocaoğlu, M.; Eralp, L.; Sen, C.; et al. Management of stiff hypertrophic nonunions by distraction osteogenesis: A report of 16 cases. J Orthop Trauma 17:543–548, 2003.

167. Koval, K.J.; Seligson, D.; Rosen, H.; et al. Distal femoral nonunion: Treatment with a retrograde inserted locked intramedullary nail. J Orthop Trauma 9:285–291, 1995.

168. Krettek, C.; Miclau, T.; Schandelmaier, P.; et al. The mechanical effect of blocking screws (Poller screws) in stabilizing tibia fractures with short proximal or distal fragments after insertion of small-diameter intramedullary nails. J Orthop Trauma 13:550–553, 1999.

169. Krettek, C.; Stephan, C.; Schandelmaier, P.; et al. The use of Poller screws as blocking screws in stabilising tibial fractures treated with small diameter intramedullary nails. J Bone Joint Surg Br 81:963–968, 1999.

170. Krishnan, K.R.; France, R.D. Chronic pain and depression. South Med J 80:558–561, 1987.

171. Kyrö, A.; Usenius, J.P.; Aarnio, M.; et al. Are smokers a risk group for delayed healing of tibial shaft fractures? Ann Chir Gynaecol 82:254–262, 1993.

172. Lambotte, A. L'Intervention Operatoire Dans les Fractures. Paris, A. Maloine, 1907.

173. Lambotte, A. Le Traitement des Fractures. Paris, Masson, 1907.

174. Lammens, J.; Bauduin, G.; Driesen, R.; et al. Treatment of nonunion of the humerus using the Ilizarov external fixator. Clin Orthop Relat Res 353:223–230, 1998.

175. Lange, R.H. Limb reconstruction versus amputation decision making in massive lower extremity trauma. Clin Orthop Relat Res 243:92–99, 1989.

176. Lavini, F.; Renzi Brivio, L.; Pizzoli, A.; et al. Treatment of non-union of the humerus using the Orthofix external fixator. Injury 32(Suppl 4):SD35–SD40, 2001.

177. Lawlis, G.F.; McCoy, C.E. Psychological evaluation: Patients with chronic pain. Orthop Clin North Am 14:527–538, 1983.

178. LeCroy, C.M.; Rizzo, M.; Gunneson, E.E.; et al. Free vascularized fibular bone grafting in the management of femoral neck nonunion in patients younger than fifty years. J Orthop Trauma 16:464–472, 2002.

179. Lerner, R.K.; Esterhai, J.L., Jr.; Polomono, R.C.; et al. Psychosocial, functional, and quality of life assessment of patients with posttraumatic fracture nonunion, chronic refractory osteomyelitis, and lower extremity amputation. Arch Phys Med Rehabil 72:122–126, 1991.

180. Lerner, R.K.; Esterhai, J.L., Jr.; Polomano, R.C.; et al. Quality of life assessment of patients with posttraumatic fracture nonunion, chronic refractory osteomyelitis, and lower-extremity amputation. Clin Orthop Relat Res 295:28–36, 1993.

181. Lindholm, T.S.; Tornkvist, H. Inhibitory effect on bone formation and calcification exerted by the anti-inflammatory drug ibuprofen: An experimental study on adult rat with fracture. Scand J Rheumatol 10:38–42, 1981.

182. Mabry, T.M.; Prpa, B.; Haidukewych, G.J.; et al. Long-term results of total hip arthroplasty for femoral neck fracture nonunion. J Bone Joint Surg Am 86:2263–2267, 2004.

183. Mahaluxmivala, J.; Nadarajah, R.; Allen, P.W.; et al. Ilizarov external fixator: Acute shortening and lengthening versus bone transport in the management of tibial non-unions. Injury 36:662–668, 2005.

184. Mahboubi, S.; Horstmann, H. Femoral torsion: CT measurement. Radiology 160:843–844, 1986.

185. Marsh, J.L.; Prokuski, L.; Biermann, J.S. Chronic infected tibial nonunions with bone loss: Conventional techniques versus bone transport. Clin Orthop Relat Res 301:139–146, 1994.

186. Marti, R.K.; Verheyen, C.C.; Besselaar, P.P. Humeral shaft nonunion: Evaluation of uniform surgical repair in fifty-one patients. J Orthop Trauma 16:108–115, 2002.

187. Martinez, A.A.; Herrera, A.; Cuenca, J. Marchetti nailing of humeral shaft delayed unions. Injury 35:257–263, 2004.

188. Mathews, V.; Cabanela, M.E. Femoral neck nonunion treatment. Clin Orthop Relat Res 419:57–64, 2004.

189. Maurer, D.J.; Merkow, R.L.; Gustilo, R.B. Infection after intramedullary nailing of severe open tibial fractures initially treated with external fixation. J Bone Joint Surg Am 71:835–838, 1989.

190. May, J.W., Jr.; Jupiter, J.B.; Weiland, A.J.; et al. Clinical classification of post-traumatic tibial osteomyelitis. J Bone Joint Surg Am 71:1422–1428, 1989.

191. Mayo, K.A.; Benirschke, S.K. Treatment of tibial malunions and nonunions with reamed intramedullary nails. Orthop Clin North Am 21:715–724, 1990.

192. McGraw, J.M.; Lim, E.V.A. Treatment of open tibial-shaft fractures: External fixation and secondary intramedullary nailing. J Bone Joint Surg Am 70:900–911, 1988.

193. McKee, M.; Jupiter, J.; Toh, C.L.; et al. Reconstruction after malunion and nonunion of intra-articular fractures of the distal humerus: Methods and results in 13 adults. J Bone Joint Surg Br 76:614–621, 1994.

194. McKee, M.D.; Miranda, M.A.; Riemer, B.L.; et al. Management of humeral nonunion after the failure of locking intramedullary nails. J Orthop Trauma 10:492–499, 1996.

195. McKee, M.D.; Wild, L.M.; Schemitsch, E.H.; et al. The use of an antibiotic-impregnated, osteoconductive, bioabsorbable bone substitute in the treatment of infected long bone defects: Early results of a prospective trial. J Orthop Trauma 16:622–627, 2002.

196. McLaren, A.C.; Blokker, C.P. Locked intramedullary fixation for metaphyseal malunion and nonunion. Clin Orthop Relat Res 265:253–260, 1991.

197. McMaster, P.E.; Hohl, M. Tibiofibular crosspeg grafting: A salvage procedure for complicated ununited tibial fractures. J Bone Joint Surg Am 57:720–721, 1975.

198. Megas, P.; Panagiotopoulos, E.; Skriviliotakis, S.; et al. Intramedullary nailing in the treatment of aseptic tibial nonunion. Injury 32:233–239, 2001.

199. Michael, D.; Fazal, M.A.; Cohen, B. Nonunion of a fracture of the body of the scapula: Case report and literature review. J Shoulder Elbow Surg 10:385–386, 2001.

200. Middleton, S.B.; Foley, S.J.; Foy, M.A. Partial excision of the clavicle for nonunion in National Hunt Jockeys. J Bone Joint Surg Br 77:778–780, 1995.

201. Milch, H. Synostosis operation for persistent nonunion of the tibia: A case report. J Bone Joint Surg Am 21:409–413, 1939.

202. Milch, H. Tibiofibular synostosis for non-union of the tibia. Surgery 27:770–779, 1950.

203. Moed, B.R.; Watson, J.T. Intramedullary nailing of aseptic tibial nonunions without the use of the fracture table. J Orthop Trauma 9:128–134, 1995.

204. More, R.C.; Kody, M.H.; Kabo, J.M.; et al. The effects of two nonsteroidal anti-inflammatory drugs on limb swelling, joint stiffness, and bone torsional strength following fracture in a rabbit model. Clin Orthop Relat Res 247:306–312, 1989.

205. Moroni, A.; Caja, V.L.; Sabato, C.; Rollo, G.; Zinghi, G. Composite bone grafting and plate fixation for the treatment of nonunions of the forearm with segmental bone loss: a report of eight cases. J Orthop Trauma 9:419–426, 1995.

206. Morrey, B.F.; Adams, R.A. Semiconstrained elbow replacement for distal humeral nonunion. J Bone Joint Surg Br 77:67–72, 1995.

207. Müller, J.; Schenk, R.; Willenegger, H. Experimentelle untersuchungen uber die entstehung reaktiver pseudoarthrosen am hunderadius. Helv Chir Acta 35:301–308, 1968.

208. Müller, M.E. Treatment of nonunions by compression. Clin Orthop Relat Res 43:83–92, 1965.

209. Müller, M.E.; Allgöwer, M.; Schneider, R. Manual of Internal Fixation: Techniques Recommended by the AO Group. Berlin, Springer-Verlag, 1979.

210. Müller, M.E.; Allgöwer, M.; Willenegger, H. Technique of Internal Fixation of Fractures. New York, Springer-Verlag, 1965.

211. Murray, J.H.; Fitch, R.D. Distraction histiogenesis: Principles and indications. J Am Acad Orthop Surg 4:317–327, 1996.

212. Muschler, G.F.; Boehm, C.; Easley, K. Aspiration to obtain osteoblast progenitor cells from human bone marrow: The influence of aspiration volume. J Bone Joint Surg Am 79:1699–1709, 1997.

213. Nayak, N.K.; Schickendantz, M.S.; Regan, W.D.; et al. Operative treatment of nonunion of surgical neck fractures of the humerus. Clin Orthop Relat Res 313:200–205, 1995.

214. Nelson, F.R.; Brighton, C.T.; Ryaby, J.; et al. Use of physical forces in bone healing. J Am Acad Orthop Surg 11:344–354, 2003.

215. Nolte, P.A.; van der Krans, A.; Patka, P.; et al. Low-intensity pulsed ultrasound in the treatment of nonunions. J Trauma 51:693–702, 2001.

216. Oh, I.; Nahigian, S.H.; Rascher, J.J.; et al. Closed intramedullary nailing for ununited femoral shaft fractures. Clin Orthop Relat Res 106:206–215, 1975.

217. Olerud, S. The effects of intramedullary reaming. In Browner, B.D.; Edwards, C.C., eds. The Science and Practice of Intramedullary Nailing. Philadelphia, Lea & Febiger, 1987, pp. 61–66.

218. Olsen, B.S.; Vaesel, M.T.; Sojbjerg, J.O. Treatment of midshaft clavicular nonunion with plate fixation and autologous bone grafting. J Shoulder Elbow Surg 4:337–344, 1995.

219. Paley, D. Principles of Deformity Correction. Berlin, Springer-Verlag, 2002.

220. Paley, D. Treatment of tibial nonunion and bone loss with the Ilizarov technique. Instr Course Lect 39:185–197, 1990.

221. Paley, D.; Chaudray, M.; Pirone, A.M.; et al. Treatment of malunions and mal-nonunions of the femur and tibia by detailed preoperative planning and the Ilizarov techniques. Orthop Clin North Am 21:667–691, 1990.

222. Paley, D.; Tetsworth, K. Mechanical axis deviation of the lower limbs: Preoperative planning of multiapical frontal plane angular and bowing deformities of the femur and tibia. Clin Orthop Relat Res 280:65–71, 1992.

223. Paley, D.; Tetsworth, K. Mechanical axis deviation of the lower limbs: Preoperative planning of uniapical angular deformities of the tibia or femur. Clin Orthop Relat Res 280:48–64, 1992.

224. Paley, D.; Young, M.C.; Wiley, A.M.; et al. Percutaneous bone marrow grafting of fractures and bony defects: An experimental study in rabbits. Clin Orthop Relat Res 208:300–312, 1986.

225. Papagelopoulos, P.J.; Morrey, B.F. Treatment of nonunion of olecranon fractures. J Bone Joint Surg Br 76:627–635, 1994.

226. Papineau, L.J.; Alfageme, A.; Dalcourt, J.P.; et al. Osteomyelite chronique: Excision et greffe de spongieux à l'air libre après mises à plat extensives. Int Orthop 3:165–176, 1979.

227. Paramasivan, O.N.; Younge, D.A.; Pant, R. Treatment of nonunion around the olecranon fossa of the humerus by intramedullary locked nailing. J Bone Joint Surg Br 82:332–335, 2000.

228. Parvizi, J.; Vegari, D. Pulsed low-intensity ultrasound for fracture healing. Foot Ankle Clin 10:595–608, vii, 2005.

229. Patel, C.V.; Adenwalla, H.S. Treatment of fractured clavicle by immediate partial subperiosteal resection. J Postgrad Med 18:32–34, 1972.

230. Patel, V.R.; Menon, D.K.; Pool, R.D.; et al. Nonunion of the humerus after failure of surgical treatment: Management using the Ilizarov circular fixator. J Bone Joint Surg Br 82:977–983, 2000.

231. Paterson, D.C.; Lewis, G.N.; Cass, C.A. Treatment of delayed union and nonunion with an implanted direct current stimulator. Clin Orthop Relat Res 148:117–128, 1980.

232. Patzakis, M.J.; Scilaris, T.A.; Chon, J.; et al. Results of bone grafting for infected tibial nonunion. Clin Orthop Relat Res 315:192–198, 1995.

233. Patzakis, M.J.; Zalavras, C.G. Chronic posttraumatic osteomyelitis and infected nonunion of the tibia: Current management concepts. J Am Acad Orthop Surg 13:417–427, 2005.

234. Pauwels, F. Grundriss liner biomechanik der fracturheilung. In Verh Dtsch Orthop Ges, 34 Kongress, 1940, pp. 62–108.

235. Pauwels, F. Schenkelhalsbruch ein mechanisches Problem: Grundlagen des Heilungsvorganges, Prognose und kausale Therapie. Stuttgart, Germany, Ferdinand Enke Verlag, 1935.

236. Perlman, M.H.; Thordarson, D.B. Ankle fusion in a high risk population: An assessment of nonunion risk factors. Foot Ankle Int 20:491–496, 1999.

237. Perren, S.M.; Cordey, J. The concepts of interfragmentary strains. In Uhthoff, H.K., ed. Current Concepts of Internal Fixation of Fractures. New York, Springer-Verlag, 1980.

238. Pers, M.; Medgyesi, S. Pedicle muscle flaps and their applications in the surgery repair. Br J Plast Surg 26:313–321, 1977.

239. Phemister, D.B. Treatment of ununited fractures by onlay bone grafts without screw or tie fixation and without breaking down of the fibrous union. J Bone Joint Surg Am 29:946–960, 1947.

240. Phieffer, L.S.; Goulet, J.A. Delayed unions of the tibia. J Bone Joint Surg Am 88:206–216, 2006.

241. Phillips, J.H.; Rahn, B.A. Fixation effects on membranous and endochondral onlay bone-graft resorption. Plast Reconstr Surg 82:872–877, 1988.

242. Pollak, D.; Floman, Y.; Simkin, A.; et al. The effect of protein malnutrition and nutritional support on the mechanical properties of fracture healing in the injured rat. J Parenter Enteral Nutr 10:564–567, 1986.

243. Polyzois, D.; Papachristou, G.; Kotsiopoulos, K.; et al. Treatment of tibial and femoral bone loss by distraction osteogenesis: Experience in 28 infected and 14 clean cases. Acta Orthop Scand Suppl 275:84–88, 1997.

244. Porter, S.E.; Hanley, E.N., Jr. The musculoskeletal effects of smoking. J Am Acad Orthop Surg 9:9–17, 2001.

245. Praemer, A.; Furner, S.; Rice, D.P. Musculoskeletal Conditions in the United States. Park Ridge, IL, American Academy of Orthopaedic Surgeons, 1992, pp. 83–124.

246. Pugh, D.M.; McKee, M.D. Advances in the management of humeral nonunion. J Am Acad Orthop Surg 11:48–59, 2003.

247. Raikin, S.M.; Landsman, J.C.; Alexander, V.A.; et al. Effect of nicotine on the rate and strength of long bone fracture healing. Clin Orthop Relat Res 353:231–237, 1998.

248. Ramp, W.; Lenz, L.; Galvin, R. Nicotine inhibits collagen synthesis and alkaline phosphatase activity, but stimulates DNA synthesis in osteoblast-like cells. Exp Biol Med 197:36–43, 1991.

249. Reed, A.A.; Joyner, C.J.; Brownlow, H.C.; et al. Human atrophic fracture non-unions are not avascular. J Orthop Res 20:593–599, 2002.

250. Reed, L.K.; Mormino, M.A. Functional outcome after blade plate reconstruction of distal tibia metaphyseal nonunions: A study of 11 cases. J Orthop Trauma 18:81–86, 2004.

251. Reichert, I.L.H.; McCarthy, I.D.; Hughes, S.P.F. The acute vascular response to intramedullary reaming: Microsphere estimation of blood flow in the intact ovine tibia. J Bone Joint Surg Br 77:490–493, 1995.

252. Rhinelander, F.W. The normal microcirculation of diaphyseal cortex and its response to fracture. J Bone Joint Surg Am 50:784–800, 1968.

253. Ricci, W.M.; Loftus, T.; Cox, C.; et al. Locked plates combined with minimally invasive insertion technique for the treatment of periprosthetic supracondylar femur fractures above a total knee arthroplasty. J Orthop Trauma 20:190–196, 2006.

254. Richards, M.; Huibregtse, B.A.; Caplan, A.I.; et al. Marrow-derived progenitor cell injections enhance new bone formation during distraction. J Orthop Res 17:900–908, 1999.

255. Richmond, J.; Colleran, K.; Borens, O.; et al. Nonunions of the distal tibia treated by reamed intramedullary nailing. J Orthop Trauma 18:603–610, 2004.

256. Riebel, G.D.; Boden, S.D.; Whitesides, T.E.; et al. The effect of nicotine on incorporation of cancellous bone graft in an animal model. Spine 20:2198–2202, 1995.

257. Riemer, B.L.; Butterfield, S.L. Comparison of reamed and nonreamed solid core nailing of the tibial diaphysis after external fixation: A preliminary report. J Orthop Trauma 7:279–285, 1993.

258. Rijnberg, W.J.; van Linge, B. Central grafting for persistent nonunion of the tibia: A lateral approach to the tibia, creating a central compartment. J Bone Joint Surg Br 75:926–931, 1993.

259. Ring, D.; Allende, C.; Jafarnia, K.; et al. Ununited diaphyseal forearm fractures with segmental defects: Plate fixation and autogenous cancellous bone-grafting. J Bone Joint Surg Am 86:2440–2445, 2004.

260. Ring, D.; Gulotta, L.; Jupiter, J.B. Unstable nonunions of the distal part of the humerus. J Bone Joint Surg Am 85:1040–1046, 2003.

261. Ring, D.; Jupiter, J.B.; Gan, B.S.; et al. Infected nonunion of the tibia. Clin Orthop Relat Res 369:302–311, 1999.

262. Ring, D.; Jupiter, J.B.; Gulotta, L. Atrophic nonunions of the proximal ulna. Clin Orthop Relat Res 409:268–274, 2003.

263. Ring, D.; Kloen, P.; Kadzielski, J.; et al. Locking compression plates for osteoporotic nonunions of the diaphyseal humerus. Clin Orthop Relat Res 425:50–54, 2004.

264. Ring, D.; Psychoyios, V.N.; Chin, K.R.; et al. Nonunion of nonoperatively treated fractures of the radial head. Clin Orthop Relat Res 398:235–238, 2002.

265. Ro, J.; Sudmann, E.; Marton, P.F. Effect of indomethacin on fracture healing in rats. Acta Orthop Scand 47:588–599, 1976.

266. Rompe, J.D.; Rosendahl, T.; Schollner, C.; et al. High-energy extracorporeal shock wave treatment of nonunions. Clin Orthop Relat Res 387:102–111, 2001.

267. Rosen, H. Fracture healing and pseudarthrosis. In Taveras, J.M., ed. Radiology: Diagnosis-Imaging-Intervention. Philadelphia, J.B. Lippincott, 1986.

268. Rosen, H. Internal fixation of nonunions after previously unsuccessful electromagnetic stimulation. In Siegel, P.G., ed. Techniques in Orthopedics: Topics in Orthopedic Trauma. Baltimore, MD, University Park Press, 1984.

269. Rosen, H. (Late) reconstructive procedures about the ankle joint. In Jahss, M.H., ed. Disorders of the Foot and Ankle: Medical and Surgical Management. Philadelphia, W.B. Saunders, 1991.

270. Rosen, H. The management of nonunions and malunions in long bone fractures in the elderly. In Zuckerman, J.D., ed. Comprehensive Care of Orthopedic Injuries in the Elderly. Baltimore, MD, Urban and Schwarzenberg, 1990.

271. Rosen, H. Nonunion and malunion. In Browner, B.D.; Levine, A.M.; Jupiter, J.B., eds. Skeletal Trauma: Fractures, Dislocations, Ligamentous Injuries, 2nd ed. Philadelphia, W.B. Saunders, 1998, pp. 501–541.

272. Rosen, H. Operative treatment of nonunions of long bone fractures. J Contin Educ Orthop 7:13–39, 1979.

273. Rosen, H. Treatment of nonunions: General principles. In Chapman, M.W.; Madison, M., eds. Operative Orthopaedics. Philadelphia, J.B. Lippincott, 1988.

274. Rosen, H. The treatment of nonunions and pseudarthroses of the humeral shaft. Orthop Clin North Am 21:725–742, 1990.

275. Rosen, H.; Stempler, E.S. A simplified method of closed suction irrigation for treating orthopedic infections. Orthopaedic Digest 5:21, 1978.

276. Rosenberg, G.A.; Patterson, B.M. Limb salvage versus amputation for severe open fractures of the tibia. Orthopedics 21:343–349, 1998.

277. Rosson, J.W.; Simonis, R.B. Locked nailing for nonunion of the tibia. J Bone Joint Surg Br 74:358–361, 1992.

278. Rubin, C.; Bolander, M.; Ryaby, J.P.; et al. The use of low-intensity ultrasound to accelerate the healing of fractures. J Bone Joint Surg Am 83:259–270, 2001.

279. Safoury, Y. Use of a reversed-flow vascularized pedicle fibular graft for treatment of nonunion of the tibia. J Reconstr Microsurg 15:23–28, 1999.

280. Saleh, M.; Royston, S. Management of nonunion of fractures by distraction with correction of angulation and shortening. J Bone Joint Surg Br 78:105–109, 1996.

281. Salibian, A.H.; Anzel, S.H.; Salyer, W.A. Transfer of vascularized grafts of iliac bone to the extremities. J Bone Joint Surg Am 69:1319–1327, 1987.

282. Sammarco, V.J.; Chang, L. Modern issues in bone graft substitutes and advances in bone tissue technology. Foot Ankle Clin 7:19–41, 2002.

283. Sanders, R.A.; Sackett, J.R. Open reduction and internal fixation of delayed union and nonunion of the distal humerus. J Orthop Trauma 4:254–259, 1990.

284. Sarathy, M.P.; Madhavan, P.; Ravichandran, K.M. Nonunion of intertrochanteric fractures of the femur: Treatment by modified medial displacement and valgus osteotomy. J Bone Joint Surg Br 77:90–92, 1995.

285. Sarmiento, A.; Burkhalter, W.E.; Latta, L.L. Functional bracing in the treatment of delayed union and nonunion of the tibia. Int Orthop 27:26–29, 2003.

286. Savage, S.R. Opioid use in the management of chronic pain. Med Clin North Am 83:761–786, 1999.

287. Sawaizumi, T.; Nanno, M.; Nanbu, A.; et al. Vascularised bone graft from the base of the second metacarpal for refractory nonunion of the scaphoid. J Bone Joint Surg Br 86:1007–1012, 2004.

288. Sawant, M.R.; Bendall, S.P.; Kavanagh, T.G.; et al. Nonunion of tibial stress fractures in patients with deformed arthritic knees: Treatment using modular total knee arthroplasty. J Bone Joint Surg Br 81:663–666, 1999.

289. Schaden, W.; Fischer, A.; Sailler, A. Extracorporeal shock wave therapy of nonunion or delayed osseous union. Clin Orthop Relat Res 387:90–94, 2001.

290. Schenk, R.K. Histology of fracture repair and nonunion. Bulletin of the Swiss Association for Study of Internal Fixation. Bern, Switzerland, Swiss Association for Study of Internal Fixation, 1978.

291. Schenk, R.; Willenegger, H. Zur Histologie der primären Knochenheilung: Modifikationen und grenzen der Spaltheilung in Abhängigkeit von der Defektgrösse. Unfallheilkunde 81:219–227, 1977.

292. Schleberger, R.; Sengem, T. Non-invasive treatment of long-bone pseudarthrosis by shock waves (ESWL). Arch Orthop Trauma Surg 111:224–227, 1992.

293. Schmitz, M.A.; Finnegan, M.; Natarajan, R.; et al. Effect of smoking on tibial shaft fracture healing. Clin Orthop Relat Res 365:184–200, 1999.

294. Schwartsman, V.; Choi, S.H.; Schwartsman, R. Tibial nonunions: Treatment tactics with the Ilizarov method. Orthop Clin North Am 21:639–653, 1990.

295. Seitz, W.H., Jr.; Froimson, A.I.; Leb, R.B. Autogenous bone marrow and allograft replacement of bone defects in the hand and upper extremities. J Orthop Trauma 6:36–42, 1992.

296. Shahcheraghi, G.H.; Bayatpoor, A. Infected tibial nonunion. Can J Surg 37:209–213, 1994.

297. Shapiro, M.S.; Endrizzi, D.P.; Cannon, R.M.; et al. Treatment of tibial defects and nonunions using ipsilateral vascularized fibular transposition. Clin Orthop Relat Res 296:207–212, 1993.

298. Silcox, D.H. III; Daftari, T.; Boden, S.D.; et al. The effect of nicotine on spinal fusion. Spine 20:1549–1553, 1995.

299. Simonis, R.B.; Nunez, V.A.; Khaleel, A. Use of the Coventry infant hip screw in the treatment of nonunion of fractures of the distal humerus. J Bone Joint Surg Br 85:74–77, 2003.

300. Simonis, R.B.; Parnell, E.J.; Ray, P.S.; et al. Electrical treatment of tibial non-union: A prospective, randomised, double-blind trial. Injury 34:357–362, 2003.

301. Sitter, T.; Wilson, J.; Browner, B. The effect of reamed versus unreamed nailing on intramedullary blood supply and cortical viability [abstract]. J Orthop Trauma 4:232, 1990.

302. Sledge, S.L.; Johnson, K.D.; Henley, M.B.; et al. Intramedullary nailing with reaming to treat nonunion of the tibia. J Bone Joint Surg Am 71:1004–1019, 1989.

303. Smith, T.K. Prevention of complications in orthopedic surgery secondary to nutritional depletion. Clin Orthop Relat Res 222:91–97, 1987.

304. Song, H.R.; Cho, S.H.; Koo, K.H.; et al. Tibial bone defects treated by internal bone transport using the Ilizarov method. Int Orthop 22:293–297, 1998.

305. Sudmann, E.; Dregelid, E.; Bessesen, A.; et al. Inhibition of fracture healing by indomethacin in rats. Eur J Clin Invest 9:333–339, 1979.

306. Swartz, W.M.; Mears, D.C. Management of difficult lower extremity fractures and nonunions. Clin Plast Surg 13:633–644, 1986.

307. Taylor, J.C. Delayed union and nonunion of fractures. In Crenshaw, A.H., ed. Campbell's Operative Orthopaedics, 8th ed. St. Louis, MO, Mosby, 1992, pp. 1287–1345.

308. Templeman, D.; Thomas, M.; Varecka, T.; et al. Exchange reamed intramedullary nailing for delayed union and nonunion of the tibia. Clin Orthop Relat Res 315:169–175, 1995.

309. Tennant, F.S., Jr.; Rawson, R.A. Outpatient treatment of prescription opioid dependence: Comparison of two methods. Arch Intern Med 142:1845–1847, 1982.

310. te Velde, E.A.; van der Werken, C. Plate osteosynthesis for pseudarthrosis of the humeral shaft. Injury 32:621–624, 2001.

311. Tiedeman, J.J.; Connolly, J.F.; Strates, B.S.; et al. Treatment of nonunion by percutaneous injection of bone marrow and demineralized bone matrix: An experimental study in dogs. Clin Orthop Relat Res 268:294–302, 1991.

312. Tien, Y.C.; Chen, J.C.; Fu, Y.C.; et al. Supracondylar dome osteotomy for cubitus valgus deformity associated with a lateral condylar nonunion in children. J Bone Joint Surg Am 87:1456–1463, 2005.

313. Tuli, S.M. Tibialization of the fibula: A viable option to salvage limbs with extensive scarring and gap nonunions of the tibia. Clin Orthop Relat Res 431:80–84, 2005.

314. Ueng, S.W.; Chao, E.K.; Lee, S.S.; et al. Augmentative plate fixation for the management of femoral nonunion after intramedullary nailing. J Trauma 43:640–644, 1997.

315. Ueng, S.W.; Lee, M.Y.; Li, A.F.; et al. Effect of intermittent cigarette smoke inhalation on tibial lengthening: Experimental study on rabbits. J Trauma 42:231–238, 1997.

316. Ueng, S.W.; Lee, S.S.; Lin, S.S.; et al. Hyperbaric oxygen therapy mitigates the adverse effect of cigarette smoking on the bone healing of tibial lengthening: An experimental study on rabbits. J Trauma 47:752–759, 1999.

317. Ueng, S.W.; Shih, C.H. Augmentative plate fixation for the management of femoral nonunion with broken interlocking nail. J Trauma 45:747–752, 1998.

318. Ueng, S.W.; Wei, F.C.; Shih, C.H. Management of femoral diaphyseal infected nonunion with antibiotic beads local therapy, external skeletal fixation, and staged bone grafting. J Trauma 46:97–103, 1999.

319. Valchanou, V.D.; Michailov, P. High energy shock waves in the treatment of delay and nonunion of fractures. Int Orthop 15:181–184, 1991.

320. Van Houwelingen, A.P.; McKee, M.D. Treatment of osteopenic humeral shaft nonunion with compression plating, humeral cortical allograft struts, and bone grafting. J Orthop Trauma 19:36–42, 2005.

321. Walsh, E.F.; DiGiovanni, C. Fibular nonunion after closed rotational ankle fracture. Foot Ankle Int 25:488–495, 2004.

322. Wang, C.J.; Chen, H.S.; Chen, C.E.; et al. Treatment of nonunions of long bone fractures with shock waves. Clin Orthop Relat Res 387:95–101, 2001.

323. Wang, J.W.; Weng, L.H. Treatment of distal femoral nonunion with internal fixation, cortical allograft struts, and autogenous bone-grafting. J Bone Joint Surg Am 85:436–440, 2003.

324. Ward, W.G.; Goldner, R.D.; Nunley, J.A. Reconstruction of tibial bone defects in tibial nonunion. Microsurgery 11:63–73, 1990.

325. Warren, S.B.; Brooker, A.F., Jr. Intramedullary nailing of tibial nonunions. Clin Orthop Relat Res 285:236–243, 1992.

326. Webb, L.X.; Winquist, R.A.; Hansen, S.T. Intramedullary nailing and reaming for delayed union or nonunion of the femoral shaft: A report of 105 consecutive cases. Clin Orthop Relat Res 212:133–141, 1986.

327. Weber, B.G. Lengthening osteotomy of the fibula to correct a widened mortice of the ankle after fracture. Int Orthop 4:289–293, 1981.

328. Weber, B.G.; Brunner, C. The treatment of nonunions without electrical stimulation. Clin Orthop Relat Res 161:24–32, 1981.

329. Weber, B.G.; Cech, O. Pseudarthrosis. Bern, Switzerland, Hans Huber, 1976.

330. Weiland, A.J. Current concepts review: Vascularized free bone transplants. J Bone Joint Surg Am 63:166–169, 1981.

331. Weiland, A.J.; Daniel, R.K. Microvascular anastomoses for bone grafts in the treatment of massive defects in bone. J Bone Joint Surg Am 61:98–104, 1979.

332. Weiland, A.J.; Moore, J.R.; Daniel, R.K. Vascularized bone autografts: Experience with 41 cases. Clin Orthop Relat Res 174:87–95, 1983.

333. Weinberg, H.; Roth, V.G.; Robin, G.C.; et al. Early fibular bypass procedures (tibiofibular synostosis) for massive bone loss in war injuries. J Trauma 19:177–181, 1979.

334. Wenzl, M.E.; Porte, T.; Fuchs, S.; et al. Delayed and non-union of the humeral diaphysis: Compression plate or internal plate fixator? Injury 35:55–60, 2004.

335. Weresh, M.J.; Hakanson, R.; Stover, M.D.; et al. Failure of exchange reamed intramedullary nails for ununited femoral shaft fractures. J Orthop Trauma 14:335–338, 2000.

336. Wilkes, R.A.; Thomas, W.G.; Ruddle, A. Fracture and nonunion of the proximal tibia below an osteoarthritic knee: Treatment by long-stemmed total knee replacement. J Trauma 36:356–357, 1994.

337. Wing, K.J.; Fisher, C.G.; O'Connell, J.X.; et al. Stopping nicotine exposure before surgery: The effect on spinal fusion in a rabbit model. Spine 25:30–34, 2000.

338. Wiss, D.A.; Stetson, W.B. Nonunion of the tibia treated with a reamed intramedullary nail. J Orthop Trauma 8:189–194, 1994.

339. Wolff, A.M.; Krackow, K.A. The treatment of nonunion of proximal tibial osteotomy with internal fixation. Clin Orthop Relat Res 250:207–215, 1990.

340. Wood, M.B.; Cooney, W.P. III. Vascularized bone segment transfers for management of chronic osteomyelitis. Orthop Clin North Am 15:461–472, 1984.

341. Wu, C.C. The effect of dynamization on slowing the healing of femur shaft fractures after interlocking nailing. J Trauma 43:263–267, 1997.

342. Wu, C.C. Humeral shaft nonunion treated by a Seidel interlocking nail with a supplementary staple. Clin Orthop Relat Res 326:203–208, 1996.

343. Wu, C.C.; Shih, C.H. Distal femoral nonunion treated with interlocking nailing. J Trauma 31:1659–1662, 1991.

344. Wu, C.C.; Shih, C.H. Treatment of 84 cases of femoral nonunion. Acta Orthop Scand 63:57–60, 1992.

345. Wu, C.C.; Shih, C.H. Treatment for nonunion of the shaft of the humerus: Comparison of plates and Seidel interlocking nails. Can J Surg 35:661–665, 1992.

346. Wu, C.C.; Shih, C.H.; Chen, W.J. Nonunion and shortening after femoral fracture treated with one-stage lengthening using locked nailing technique: Good results in 48/51 patients. Acta Orthop Scand 70:33–36, 1999.

347. Wu, C.C.; Shih, C.H.; Chen, W.J.; et al. High success rate with exchange nailing to treat a tibial shaft aseptic nonunion. J Orthop Trauma 13:33–38, 1999.

348. Wu, C.C.; Shih, C.H.; Chen, W.J.; et al. Treatment of clavicular aseptic nonunion: Comparison of plating and intramedullary nailing techniques. J Trauma 45:512–516, 1998.

349. Yajima, H.; Tamai, S.; Mizumoto, S.; et al. Vascularized fibular grafts in the treatment of osteomyelitis and infected nonunion. Clin Orthop Relat Res 293:256–264, 1993.

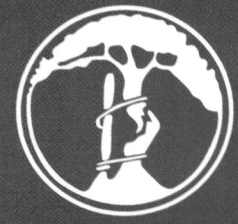

CHAPTER 23

Physical Impairment Ratings for Fractures

Brent B. Wiesel, M.D., Richard A. Saunders, M.D., and Sam W. Wiesel, M.D.

Fractures account for only about 10 percent of all musculoskeletal traumatic injuries, but they cause a disproportionate amount of medical impairment. The costs of fracture care, including lost productivity, medical expenses, and disability payments, make this class of injury a significant burden both to employers and to society in general.

The role of physicians in the medical care of fractures is well established, but their job does not end when union has been achieved and rehabilitation is complete. Physician participation is equally vital in the impairment evaluation process. Many state and federal laws limit physician discretion in assigning permanent impairment ratings, and the physician is often caught between a desire to benefit the patient and the need to comply with these laws. This chapter presents some generic issues of impairment, reviews the epidemiology of fractures in the United States, and comments on commonly used existing impairment guides.

GENERIC ISSUES OF DISABILITY AND IMPAIRMENT

Definitions

There is a certain amount of confusion about the role of the physician in determination of permanent disability and about the difference between impairment and disability. According to *Guides to the Evaluation of Permanent Impairment,* Fifth Edition, published by the American Medical Association (AMA), the following definitions apply.[3]

Impairment is a loss, loss of use, or derangement of any body part, organ system, or organ function. A permanent impairment exists when the patient has reached maximal medical improvement but such a loss or derangement persists. Maximal medical improvement has been achieved when the injury or illness has stabilized and no material improvement or deterioration is expected in the next year, with or without treatment. Many jurisdictions require that a year elapse after the injury or most recent surgery related to the injury before determining that maximal medical improvement has been attained.

Disability, which is assessed by nonmedical means, is an alteration of an individual's capacity to meet personal, social, or occupational demands because of an impairment. The determination of permanent disability is dependent on a number of nonmedical factors, among them a patient's level of education, work training and work history, residual access to the workplace, and socioeconomic background. Disability is context specific, not inherent to the individual, in that it depends on the interaction between the individual and each specific work environment. If adaptations can be made to the work environment or task in question, a particular impairment may not limit an individual from performing the task. Physicians, in general, are considered expert only in the determination of impairment.

Role of the Physician

According to the AMA guidelines, determining whether an injury or illness results in a permanent impairment requires a medical assessment performed by a physician. The functions evaluated in determining permanent impairment are those that allow the individual to perform common activities of daily living, excluding work. These include self-care, communication, physical activity (including sitting, standing, reclining, walking, and stair climbing), sensory functions, nonspecialized hand activities, travel, sexual function, and sleep. Because musculoskeletal injuries account for the majority of impairment determinations, orthopaedists are frequently involved in this process.

Depending on local regulations, the physician determining impairment may be the treating physician with whom the patient has an established doctor-patient relationship or an independent physician who examines the patient only for the purposes of determining impairment and is not otherwise involved in the patient's care. In general, physicians acting as independent consultants for determination of impairment ratings do not establish a doctor-patient relationship with the patient being examined. If new diagnoses are uncovered during the course of an impairment evaluation, the physician has a medical obligation to inform the requesting party and the individual about the condition and advise the individual to seek appropriate medical treatment.

Third-Party Payers

Impairment evaluations are most frequently requested by a third-party payer before settlement of a claim. The largest third-party payers are state workmen's compensation boards, private insurance companies, the Social Security Administration, and the Department of Veterans Affairs.[12] Each of these groups has its own requirements for and definitions of impairment. Workmen's compensation laws vary widely from state to state, and federal agency regulations are amended yearly. The agency requesting the impairment evaluation should specify which rules apply in the specific case, and the reviewing physician should abide by the specified rules. In some cases, older editions of the AMA guides have been incorporated in state laws, in which case the appropriate edition must be consulted. Tort law (civil litigation or lawsuits) in some states does not specify any particular body of rules; in these cases, the evaluating physician has considerably greater freedom to describe and quantify a given impairment.

Correspondence is between the physician and the third-party payer. Updates should be in the form of letters mailed directly to the representative of the third-party payer. The patient should not act as an intermediary, although the patient's right to review his or her chart in the presence of the attending physician should always be honored.

Work Restrictions

In addition to assigning a rating of permanent partial impairment, the physician is often called on to give an estimate of residual work capacity. In this role, the physician is responsible for determining the level of physical activity that the patient can safely tolerate. The most widely accepted physical exertion requirement guidelines are those published by the Social Security Administration:

Very heavy work is that which involves lifting objects weighing more than 100 pounds at a time, with frequent lifting or carrying of objects weighing 50 pounds or more.

Heavy work involves lifting of no more than 100 pounds at a time, with frequent lifting or carrying of objects weighing up to 50 pounds.

Medium work involves the lifting of no more than 50 pounds at a time, with frequent lifting or carrying of objects weighing up to 25 pounds.

Light work involves lifting of no more than 20 pounds at a time, with frequent lifting or carrying of objects weighing up to 10 pounds.

Sedentary work involves the lifting of no more than 10 pounds at a time and occasional lifting or carrying of articles such as docket files, ledgers, or small tools.

TEMPORARY TOTAL DISABILITY

In general, a patient is judged temporarily totally disabled if, in the opinion of the treating physician, the patient is incapable of performing any job, for any reasonable period of time, during the course of a workday. Note that, by this definition, a patient's inability to perform his or her own job is not the primary issue. For example, a construction worker in a short arm cast for a Colles fracture may well be incapable of his or her usual work but capable of sedentary or one-handed light work, so the worker is not totally disabled. Temporary total disability is also granted for patients whose pain is great enough to warrant regular narcotic use, whose mobility is so severely compromised as to make getting from home to the workplace unreasonably difficult, or who are hospitalized in an inpatient unit.

Patients are temporarily totally disabled from the moment of occurrence of a skeletal injury until they achieve a reasonable degree of mobility and independence, are able to perform their own activities of daily living to a reasonable degree, and are no longer dependent on narcotic analgesics. Obviously, patients who are hospitalized, are inpatients in a rehabilitation facility, or are homebound and require skilled nursing care are temporarily totally disabled. Patients who are dependent on crutches for ambulation are not necessarily totally disabled at all times unless they meet the other definitions of temporary total disability.

Periodic evaluation in the physician's office is necessary during the period of temporary total disability. Most state workmen's compensation laws mandate at least monthly visits during the period of temporary total disability, during which further documentation for ongoing temporary total disability status must be entered in the patient's record.

TEMPORARY PARTIAL DISABILITY

Temporary partial disability begins with the termination of temporary total disability and continues until rehabilitation is complete and the patient is back to full activities with no restrictions or until a permanent impairment is assigned. During the period of temporary partial disability, the patient is allowed to return to the workplace with certain restrictions judged appropriate by the treating physician.

Once the period of temporary total disability is lifted, appropriate restrictions must be instituted by the physician. These may allow the patient to return to work in a light duty situation in which the physical requirements of the job do not compromise healing or cause unacceptable discomfort. The physician is responsible for identifying the level of safe activity, which may be limited to sedentary work during the early recovery phase of an injury.

Patients recovering from back and neck injuries may benefit from a restriction on bending, twisting, stooping, lifting, and heavy overhead work. Upper extremity injury restrictions often include avoidance of heavy or repetitive use of the involved extremity. Restrictions after lower extremity injuries frequently include prohibitions against excessive walking, climbing, stooping, kneeling, running, and carrying.

Many employers and third-party payers publish and distribute forms with a listing of possible activities for the physician to check off. To the extent that the listed activities are of concern to the physician, these forms may be used, but it is often more useful for the physician to attach a note on letterhead stationery outlining the restrictions rather than to try to make his or her best judgment about appropriate restrictions fit within the confines of existing forms and classifications.

Periodic reevaluations of the patient's clinical status are made, usually at 2- to 6-week intervals. State law varies considerably on the issue of mandatory frequency of reevaluations during a period of temporary partial disability. In general, state laws permit somewhat longer intervals between clinic visits for patients with temporary partial disability than for those with temporary total disability, often between 4 and 8 weeks. Again, documentation in the record of the reason for ongoing temporary partial disability is important. Physician records and occasionally physician testimony are required for insurance payments for disability determination. It is worthwhile periodically to record range of motion, functional restrictions, medication use, and degree of autonomy with activities of daily living; these data can be used later to document the patient's degree of disability during any given period.

Temporary partial impairment restrictions should be modified as the patient's symptoms warrant. This modification may require instituting greater restrictions and moving the patient back toward more sedentary activities if symptoms become excessive, or gradual liberalization of activities as clinical status permits. Occasional periods of temporary total disability may be warranted, particularly after surgical procedures or operative manipulations of fractures.

PERMANENT PARTIAL DISABILITY

After maximal medical recovery has been achieved, the physician, possibly in cooperation with other occupational specialists, may be asked to recommend a permanent restricted activity level if the patient is unable to return to his or her original job. There are no widely accepted guidelines for determining the level of job restriction, but, in general, a patient who has any permanent partial impairment secondary to skeletal injury is unable to perform very heavy or heavy work safely.[16,17] If the permanent partial impairment is greater than 25 percent, most patients are unlikely to perform successfully in any but part-time or home-based occupations at the sedentary level. Between these two extremes, the physician must decide what is a reasonable expectation for the patient, taking into consideration the type of injury and impairment and the sorts of activities that are likely to exacerbate persistent pain. The physician may utilize functional capacity evaluations performed in conjunction with a physical therapist as an objective measure of particular activities that an individual patient is capable of tolerating.

As an example, a well-healed 10 percent compression fracture of the lumbar spine with some chronic back pain may result in a 5 percent permanent partial impairment. The patient is likely to have exacerbation of pain with bending, twisting, stooping, lifting of more than 20 pounds, or prolonged overhead work. He or she would be qualified for a job involving light work, with the restrictions specified previously.

The physician assigns impairment and specifies work restrictions, but the responsibility for finding an appropriate job lies with the patient or the third-party payer. With more aggressive job retraining and work hardening programs, patients with significant impairment are now returning to the workplace. When an injured individual is declared disabled from injury it is almost always economically unfavorable both for the individual and for society as a whole.[10] If the physician performing the impairment evaluation is also the patient's treating physician, it is often worthwhile for the physician to work with the social worker, nurse, or occupational therapist representing the third-party payer to find an acceptable job for the patient or to encourage occupational retraining when appropriate.

EPIDEMIOLOGY OF FRACTURES IN THE UNITED STATES

Given the vast array of health care providers for musculoskeletal injuries in the United States it is extremely difficult to accurately estimate the epidemiology of fractures. Using data compiled by the National Center for Health Statistics, the American Academy of Orthopaedic Surgeons estimates that in 2003 there were 3,148,000 emergency room visits for fractures of the extremities, 7,310,000 physician visits for fractures of the extremities, and 867,000 hospitalizations for fractures of the extremities.[2] These numbers remained relatively stable from 1999 through 2003 (Fig. 23-1).

The United States Bureau of Labor Statistics tracks work-related injuries and resulting time away from work. In 2004, there were 1,259,320 occupational injuries involving days away from work.[15] Ninety-four thousand

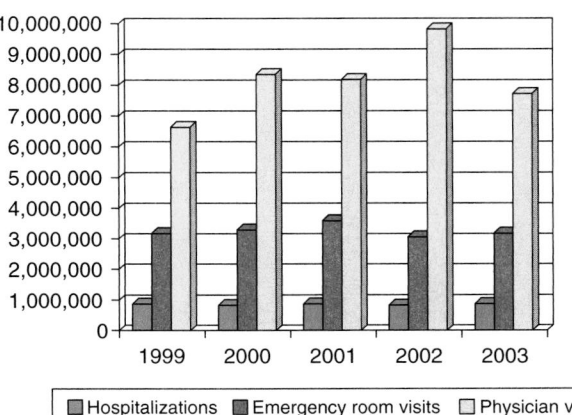

FIGURE 23-1 *Hospitalizations, emergency room visits, and physician visits for extremity fractures in the United States from 1999 to 2003. (Source: American Academy of Orthopaedic Surgeons, 2006.)*

FIGURE 23-2 | *Percentage distribution of nonfatal occupational injuries and illnesses involving days away from work in the United States in 2004. (Source: U.S. Bureau of Labor Statistics, 2005.)*

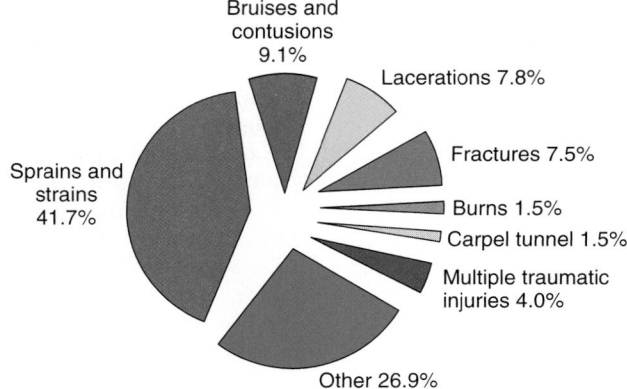

Bruises and contusions 9.1%
Lacerations 7.8%
Fractures 7.5%
Burns 1.5%
Carpel tunnel 1.5%
Multiple traumatic injuries 4.0%
Sprains and strains 41.7%
Other 26.9%

forty (7.5%) of these injuries involved fractures, while 525,390 (41.7%) were classified as sprains and strains (Fig. 23-2). These figures translate to 10.6 fractures per 10,000 full-time workers and 59 sprains and strains per 10,000 full-time workers. Workers in construction, manufacturing, transportation, and health services were most likely to experience a work-related fracture. On average, a fracture led to 28 missed days of work with 46.4 percent of fractures leading to 31 or more missed days of work (Fig. 23-3).

GUIDES TO IMPAIRMENT DETERMINATION

Historical Perspective

Before the 1930s, in both the United States and Europe, arbitrary disability values were assigned for individual injuries. The entire disability determination process was performed by physicians, despite their lack of special training in social, economic, and occupational evaluation. This practice may have simplified rendering a judgment of disability, but it led to the awarding of the same compensation to individuals with markedly different degrees of residual disability.[4,12] Beginning in the 1930s, new systems of classifying residual deficits were introduced in the United States by individual authors in an effort to make the system of disability evaluation more equitable and objective.

Kessler described evaluation based on objective criteria such as range of motion in degrees and motor strength measured in foot-pounds.[4,5,6] McBride published a 10-point scale based on five anatomic and five functional criteria that, taken together, gave an estimate of overall impairment.[7,8] In an effort to reduce the influence of subjective and potentially biased data, Thurber published impairment scales based on range of motion alone.[14]

Development of the modern system for rating of permanent partial impairment by physicians began in 1956 with the introduction by the AMA of a series of guides designed to provide objective, reproducible impairment ratings.[1,3] These guides were intended to standardize evaluation of the result of industrial accidents for determining workmen's compensation claims. The AMA series is now complete and is updated regularly. In addition to the guides for the spine and extremities, the AMA provides guides to the evaluation of other organ systems (e.g., neurologic, hematopoietic), but the evaluation of these systems is outside the area of training of orthopaedic surgery.

Numerous impairment guides are in use in the United States. Most states mandate the use of one particular set of guidelines for workmen's compensation impairment determination. Some states create their own unique guidelines, which are based on a variety of practical, idiosyncratic, or occasionally political considerations. Increasingly, most states and the District of Columbia have adopted the guidelines published by the AMA. Most federal agencies concerned with impairment determination also use the AMA guides. More widespread use of the AMA guides seems to be leading to increasingly uniform and probably fairer impairment determinations across most jurisdictions.

Modern Impairment Scales

The AMA guides rate impairment by a "whole person" concept. In this system, each part of the body is assigned

FIGURE 23-3 | *Percentage distribution of days away from work secondary to fractures in United States workers in 2004. (Source: U.S. Bureau of Labor Statistics, 2005.)*

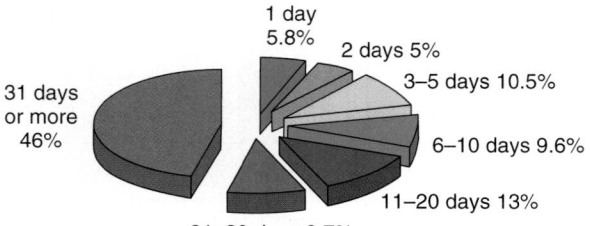

1 day 5.8%
2 days 5%
3–5 days 10.5%
6–10 days 9.6%
11–20 days 13%
21–30 days 9.7%
31 days or more 46%

a value reflecting the contribution of that part to the patient as a whole. The percentage each part contributes to the whole is based on the notion of function. Loss of function of the extremity is expressed as a percentage of the value of the extremity as a whole, and impairment to the whole person is calculated from this value. The upper extremities are valued at 60 percent of the whole person, the lower extremities at 40 percent. As an example, amputation at the wrist results in a 90 percent loss of function of the arm and a 54 percent impairment of the whole person.

The AMA guides historically relied solely on range-of-motion measurements for the determination of partial impairments of the spine and extremities, offering no consideration of pain, atrophy, shortening, and other subjective and objective data. The fourth and fifth editions of the guides incorporated a much broader range of evaluation criteria and also introduced the concept of diagnosis-related impairment estimates.

Traditional range-of-motion–based estimates ignore causal issues and focus solely on measurable outcomes, specifically, motion of local joints or spine segments. Diagnosis-related impairment estimates attempt to overcome the inherent limitations of a one-dimensional motion-based estimating tool by focusing on the underlying diagnosis. For example, all patients with multiple operations for a herniated lumbar disc with residual, verifiable neurologic deficits might be grouped together for the purpose of impairment determination, leading to a more uniform and ultimately fairer determination than would be possible using range-of-motion measures alone. Another advantage of diagnosis-based impairment determinations is the reduced dependence on subjective or difficult to measure variables such as range of motion, pain, weakness, or clumsiness.

The validity of the AMA guides in assessing impairment after lower extremity fractures was validated in a study by McCarthy et al.[9] They evaluated 302 patients 1 year after an isolated lower extremity fracture and found a mean residual impairment of 27 percent. The impairment rating calculated using the AMA guide correlated strongly with the performance of functional tasks. Interestingly, the correlation was highest when the impairment rating was based on strength evaluation instead of range-of-motion or diagnosis-related ratings.

Impairment and Fractures

Fractures cause several kinds of permanent changes, any of which may lead to a degree of partial impairment. Each element of fracture healing must be considered separately in determining the overall level of impairment caused by a given injury. Existing impairment scales address some but not all of these factors. Traditionally, some incremental percentage of increased impairment is assigned for sequelae of fracture healing such as limb length discrepancy, loss of joint motion, or ankylosis. Some complications, including nonunion, infection, and secondary soft tissue injury, are not addressed explicitly in the literature, and the practitioner is left to his or her own discretion in assessing permanent impairment.

HANDEDNESS

The AMA does not allow for handedness or side dominance in the determination of impairment, the contention being that activities of daily living, the functional standard by which medical impairment is judged, are not affected by handedness. Therefore, no increased impairment value is allowed for impairments in the dominant upper extremity. Obviously, disability determination must take handedness into consideration. Traditionally, 5 percent extremity impairment is added for impairments of 1 to 50 percent of the dominant extremity and 10 percent for impairments greater than 50 percent of the dominant upper extremity.

NONUNION

Occasionally, a fracture fails to unite despite optimal medical and surgical intervention, or a patient may legitimately choose not to accept the risks associated with surgical intervention for treatment of a nonunion. Because joint motion above and below the nonunion is compromised, the AMA system recognizes increased impairment in this situation. The impairment resulting from nonunion can be more profound than simple loss of joint motion. Pain, motion at the fracture site, and weakness may complicate nonunion. It is reasonable to add 5 percent to the limb impairment for an asymptomatic nonunion and 10 percent for a nonunion that causes significant compromise beyond loss of joint motion.

LIMB LENGTH

Limb length discrepancy after fracture is of much greater significance in the leg than in the arm. One convention for dealing with leg length discrepancy is to allow 5 percent permanent impairment for each half inch of shortening in excess of the half inch generally considered to be normal.[11] Thus, a leg length discrepancy of 2 inches after fracture would result in a 15 percent limb impairment on the basis of this factor alone.

MALUNION

A fracture healing with angulation may result in loss of motion at the joint above or below it, in which case the AMA guide pertaining to motion deficit provides a correct estimate of impairment.[3] If symptoms other than loss of motion are present, some additional degree of impairment should be allowed. If the malunion causes significant symptoms, such as weakness, skin breakdown, altered gait, or rotational deformity, an additional 10 percent impairment should be allowed.

INFECTION

If chronic osteomyelitis occurs, some additional level of impairment should be assigned to compensate for the well-recognized potential complications and daily inconvenience of this disease. If symptomatic osteomyelitis exists at the time permanent impairment is determined, an additional impairment of 10 percent of the limb value is assigned. If the infection is minimally symptomatic or quiescent at the time of determination, an additional impairment of 5 percent is assigned.

INTRA-ARTICULAR INVOLVEMENT

Long-term sequelae of fractures may not be apparent at the time of determination of impairment. Degenerative changes are far more likely to develop in a joint that has sustained an intra-articular fracture, especially in the presence of residual articular displacement. The determination of permanent impairment after a fracture must therefore include an allowance for the occasional development of post-traumatic arthritis. As an example, a well-healed, nonpainful fracture of the medial malleolus with no residual intra-articular displacement warrants a finding of 5 percent impairment of the limb because of the anticipated future problems such an injury could cause. A similar fracture with intra-articular displacement would merit a 10 percent impairment of the limb.

PREEXISTING CONDITIONS AND APPORTIONMENT

Preexisting medical conditions need to be apportioned before assignment of a scheduled loss-of-use rating. Apportionment is the process of dividing the degree of impairment detected at the time of examination between current and prior injuries or conditions. Apportionment generally implies a preexisting condition that has been made materially or substantially worse by a second injury or illness. Numerous methods can be used to assess apportionment, and no universal standard seems to have been adopted. The AMA guides recommend subtracting the whole person impairment established for the preexisting condition from the current impairment rating. This recommendation clearly assumes that perfect, incontrovertible data exist about the preexisting condition, a circumstance rarely encountered. In most cases, a somewhat more arbitrary division is needed.

A reasonable starting place is a 50 percent to 50 percent apportionment between preexisting and current causes unless objective new data show a worsening of the condition after onset of the current injury or illness. For example, a patient with a preexisting arthritic knee and a subsequent tibial plateau fracture on the affected side with subjective complaints of worsening symptoms after the fracture warrants an apportionment of 75 percent to the current injury and 25 percent to the preexisting condition. A patient with chronic low back pain made subjectively worse after a lifting injury warrants a 50 percent to 50 percent apportionment in the absence of magnetic resonance imaging, electromyographic, or radiographic evidence of a new condition. If new test findings cannot be reliably assigned to the new or old injury or illness, the 50 percent to 50 percent apportionment rule should be applied.

NEUROLOGIC INJURIES

The AMA guides outline appropriate standards for evaluating combined skeletal and neurologic injuries. In general, impairment secondary to joint stiffness after fracture is considered separately from nerve injuries caused by the same injury. Loss of motion related to nerve injury, such as limited shoulder abduction following axillary nerve injury, is not considered separately, as the neurologic injury is solely responsible for the motion deficit. Neurologic loss resulting from spine fractures should be evaluated with the diagnosis-related estimates because of the difficulty of evaluating spine range of motion in the paralyzed patient.

PREEXISTING OSTEOARTHRITIS

Some fractures inevitably occur in individuals already suffering from musculoskeletal disease, most often osteoarthritis. Injuries are slower to heal and residual loss of joint motion may be greater in such patients.[5,17] Symptoms caused by the osteoarthritis are often perceived to be more disabling after a fracture.

Assuming that radiographs taken at the time of injury show degenerative changes or that late films show changes in excess of what might reasonably be expected to develop in the elapsed time, an allowance for exacerbation of the preexisting disease should be made. To compensate fairly for the contribution of the injury to preexisting arthritis, a 5 percent additional impairment should be added to the limb impairment for patients who are subjectively worse and a 10 percent additional impairment to those who are both subjectively and objectively worse after their injury.[17]

SPINE FRACTURES

Individual investigators have offered various schemes for determining impairment related to spinal fracture. Miller, for instance, allowed 5 percent whole person impairment for lumbar compression fractures up to 25 percent, 10 percent impairment for compression of 25 percent to 50 percent, and 20 percent impairment for lumbar compression fractures greater than 50 percent. He halved these values for fractures of the thoracic spine and allowed no impairment assignment for healed compression fractures of the cervical spine unless some other factor such as nerve injury is present.[11,13]

In an effort to provide a fair and uniform assignment of impairment for spine injuries, Wiesel and colleagues[16,17] collected data from 75 members of the International Society for Study of the Lumbar Spine and from 53 American members of the Cervical Spine Research Society. The objective was to establish diagnosis-related impairment ratings for a variety of common spinal disorders. The results as applied to spinal fractures are presented in Table 23-1.

The AMA offers the most widely used spine impairment guidelines. Again, the AMA guides are used in more than three out of four states and most federal agencies. Starting with the third edition and extending through the fifth, the AMA algorithm has included diagnosis-related impairment estimates, with range of motion-based estimates used only in a few situations where diagnosis-related categories fit the situation poorly. Spine fractures are generally amenable to diagnosis-related grouping, the major exception being multiple fractures within an anatomic region, for example, two compression fractures occurring simultaneously in the lumbar spine. In the case of poor applicability of diagnosis-related categories, the AMA allows impairment determination on the basis of range-of-motion measures.

SUMMARY

Establishing a fair level of permanent partial disability after fracture requires the expertise of many professionals, including the orthopaedist, social worker, and vocational and rehabilitation therapists, as well as input from the

Table 23-1

Permanent Partial Impairment and Work Restriction after Fractures of the Cervical and Lumbar Spine

Fracture Type	Percent Impairment	Work Allowed
Cervical Spine		
Odontoid, external fixation	10	Medium
Odontoid, surgical fusion	20	Light
Hangman's, external fixation	10	Medium
Hangman's, surgical fusion	15	Light
Burst or compression, lower cervical spine, external fixation, no neurologic deficit	15	Light
Burst or compression, lower cervical spine, surgical fusion, no neurologic deficit	15	Light
Lumbar Spine		
Acute spondylolysis or spondylolisthesis, conservative care, complete recovery	0	Heavy
Acute spondylolysis or spondylolisthesis, conservative care, residual discomfort	10	Light
Spondylolysis or spondylolisthesis, laminectomy and/or fusion, complete recovery	10	Light
Spondylolysis or spondylolisthesis, laminectomy and/or fusion, residual discomfort	20	Sedentary
Compression fracture, healed, with		
10% compression	5	Medium
25% compression	10	Light
50% compression	20	Sedentary
75% compression	20	Sedentary
Transverse process fracture, no displacement or malunion	0	Heavy

patient and third-party payer. The evaluation of permanent partial impairment is the sole responsibility of the physician; this chapter is intended to evaluate some of the factors involved in making impairment determinations. By considering all the factors that contribute to the outcome of fracture care, a level of permanent impairment can be established that is fair to the patient. This impairment rating can then be used as one factor in determining a disability rating that is fair to the patient, the third-party payer, and society in general.

REFERENCES

1. American Academy of Orthopaedic Surgeons. Manual for Orthopaedic Surgeons in Evaluating Permanent Physical Impairment. Chicago, American Academy of Orthopaedic Surgeons, 1962.
2. American Academy of Orthopaedic Surgeons. Hospitalizations, Physician Visits, and Emergency Room Visits for Fractures: 1999 to 2003. Available at: http://www.aaos.org/wordhtml/research/stats/fracture_all.htm.
3. American Medical Association. Guides to the Evaluation of Permanent Impairment, 5th ed. Chicago, American Medical Association, 2001.
4. Kessler, E.D. The determination of physical fitness. JAMA 115:1591, 1940.
5. Kessler, H. Low Back Pain in Industry. New York, Commerce and Industry Association of New York, 1955.
6. Kessler, H.H. Disability—Determination and Evaluation. Philadelphia, Lea & Febiger, 1970.
7. McBride, E.D. Disability Evaluation. Philadelphia, J.B. Lippincott, 1942.
8. McBride, E.D. Disability evaluation. J Int Coll Surg 24:341, 1955.
9. McCarthy, M.L.; McAndrew, M.P.; MacKenzie, E.J.; et al. Correlation between the measures of impairment, according to the modified system of the American Medical Association, and function. J Bone Joint Surg Am 80:1034–1042, 1998.
10. Melhorn, J.M. Impairment and disability evaluations: Understanding the process. J Bone Joint Surg Am 83:1905–1911, 2001.
11. Miller, T.R. Evaluating Orthopedic Disability, 2nd ed. Oradell, NJ, Medical Economics Books, 1987.
12. Mooney, V. Impairment, disability, and handicap. Clin Orthop 221:14, 1987.
13. Nordby, E.J. Disability evaluation of the neck and back: The McBride system. Clin Orthop 221:131, 1987.
14. Thurber, P. Evaluation of Industrial Disability. New York, Oxford University Press, 1960.
15. U.S. Bureau of Labor Statistics. Lost-Worktime Injuries and Illnesses: Characteristics and Resulting Time Away from Work, 2004. United States Department of Labor, Washington, DC, 2005.
16. Wiesel, S.W.; Feffer, H.L.; Rothman, R.H. Industrial Low Back Pain: A Comprehensive Approach. Charlottesville, VA, The Michie Company Law Publishers, 1985.
17. Wiesel, S.W.; Feffer, H.L.; Rothman, R.H. Neck Pain. Charlottesville, VA, The Michie Company Law Publishers, 1986.

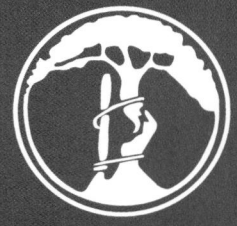

CHAPTER 24

Outcomes Research in Orthopaedics

William T. Obremskey, M.D., M.P.H., Rebecca Bauer, M.D., M.P.H., and Marc F. Swiontkowski, M.D.

OUTCOMES ASSESSMENT

Outcomes research has rapidly become the focus of clinical researchers, insurance companies, and health care delivery corporations. As described by the Agency for Healthcare Research and Quality, "Outcomes research seeks to understand the *end results* of particular health care practices and interventions. *End results* include effects that people experience and care about, such as change in the ability to function. By linking the care people get to the outcomes they experience, outcomes research has become the key to developing better ways to monitor and improve the quality of care." Recently published data indicate that approximately 30 percent of surgical treatment is questionably effective.[20] The implications of such data regarding patient care are profound, but considering that health care accounted for 15 percent of the 2003 gross national product (GNP) of the United States, the financial implications are significant as well. Innovative treatments are often questioned by insurance companies and government payers, driving the production of evidence that correlates treatments with the ideal end result, as represented by patients' overall physical function and quality of life. Health-related quality of life outcomes, in addition to classical clinical outcomes, can both improve care to patients as well as indicate appropriate utilization of health care resources.

Consistency in care follows established, or standard, quality of care. By way of *small area analysis,* Wennberg and co-workers noted that health care interventions varied widely in terms of population-based rates.[78,79] For instance, they noted that residents of the New Haven, Connecticut, region were twice as likely to undergo spinal surgery for disc disease than their age- and sex-matched counterparts in Boston, Massachusetts. In contrast, the residents of Boston were twice as likely to undergo total hip replacement as their New Haven counterparts.[38,40] Elective procedures have a large (3–5 times) variation in incidence in a given population[3,42] while urgent/emergent conditions are less variable—the incidence of hip fracture surgery and both-bone forearm fracture surgery is fairly constant in all regions in the United States.[41,42] Similarly, the range of operative fixation incidence ran from 5.1 percent in Greenville, North Carolina, to 50.7 percent in Casper, Wyoming, independent of fracture severity.[3] The

explanation for these phenomena is not clear. Two possibilities are physician uncertainty regarding the best way to treat patients, and a paucity of data regarding which treatments work best for patients.

Interestingly, the term *end result* was coined in 1914 by Ernest Codman, M.D., the Massachusetts orthopaedic surgeon best known for his work in shoulder diseases. Codman proposed that knowledge of the end result for patient management in hospitals be the fundamental yardstick by which medical/surgical treatment be judged as worthy to be loosed on the public.[17,18] Although his concept fell on deaf ears at the time, it served as a catalyst for further evolution of the concept of assessing the result of treatment.

CLINICAL VERSUS PATIENT-ORIENTED OUTCOMES

The types of patient-related outcomes include clinical outcomes, functional outcomes, health-related outcomes, and satisfaction with the process of care. Clinical outcomes (such as range of motion, radiographic union, implant loosening, and infection) have been the focus of clinical research in orthopaedic surgery.[27,30] A significant amount of literature supports the observation that good clinical outcomes do not necessarily indicate good functional outcomes.[63] Functional outcomes primarily involve patient function at the most complete level, not as a joint or condition but as an individual in society.[38,40,41] Health-related quality of life involves patients' perception of how they are functioning as affected by their overall health. The areas of individual function covered include mental health, social function, role function (i.e., worker, spouse, parent), physical function, and activities of daily living.[31,61]

The published clinical literature regarding management of musculoskeletal injury is generally retrospective in design, with rare exception, and is focused on traditional clinical outcomes, such as range of motion, alignment, stability, and radiographic assessments.[73] The relative lack of controlled trials in orthopaedics has complicated the definition of optimal management strategies. Even the most frequently investigated areas of the field, such as joint replacement, demonstrate significant deficiencies.[27,30] Both Gartland[27] and Gross[30] have confirmed that research regarding hip arthroplasty is "process based," meaning that it is focused on elements important to the technical aspects of the procedure (i.e., cement lucency, dislocation rates) or to the delivery of care, and not on the effect of the procedure on patient function. This paucity of patient-oriented functional outcome data is seen in literature regarding critically ill patients as well. Examples of frequently reported, process-based data related to injured patients include length of intensive care unit (ICU) stay, ventilator days, wound infection and other complications, and knee range of motion, but patient-oriented functional outcome data traditionally have not been investigated.

Objective clinical outcomes can have significant weaknesses. Intra- and interobserver reliability have been studied thoroughly and shown to be problematic throughout orthopaedic literature with objective outcomes.[22,66,67] In fact, Pynsent recently stated, "a well-designed patient-reported questionnaire that has undergone rigorous testing may be more objective."[62] Many researchers believe that the lack of patient-reported "end-result" information is responsible for the previously mentioned variations in medical/orthopaedic practice that have become apparent.[41,78] However, quality study of musculoskeletal injury, both objective and subjective, often is limited by low incidence of a particular injury and therefore insufficient power for statistical significance. Improvement in the quality of orthopaedic research specifically that relates to musculoskeletal injury requires emphasis on quality clinical trial methodology and statistical preparation, and when this is not feasible because of low incidence conditions, the use of standardized outcome assessment via multi-center studies whenever appropriate.[64] Standardized outcomes questionnaires facilitate uniform data collection within and among multiple sites, and scoring formulas for each questionnaire prevent intra- or interobserver error.[38,43]

Retrospective clinical reports in orthopaedics often use nonvalidated scales to arbitrarily divide patient results into good, fair, or poor. Such scales are surgeon-derived, rarely used in more than one retrospective review, and internally weighted for scoring determined by the author and not by patient input (i.e., relative value of pain to that of range of motion, alignment).[23,69] This lack of use of validated scales has undermined the utility of the literature for assessment of efficacy of injury treatment strategies. A current example of clinical debate is that of the effect of early stabilization of long bone fractures in the multiple injury patient. Although the sense of the literature would push us to a more aggressive clinical protocol, we are limited by the existence of only one published controlled trial on the subject.[13,14,26,35,56,65] The lack of adequate numbers of randomized trials for most topics in trauma surgery makes the technique of meta-analysis difficult for addressing effectiveness issues.[13,15,28,44,45,49,55,72] All these factors contribute to the current inadequate knowledge on which to base treatment decisions and recommendations.

INSTRUMENT DEVELOPMENT

The creation of an instrument to detect significant differences in patient responses relative to the general population is a detailed process. Questions that are reflective of patient function cannot be developed solely on the basis of clinical experience, as physicians' perceptions of functional issues are often inaccurate. Guyatt and associates[32] have described the following steps in the development of a functional assessment questionnaire:

Item Development. The patient population to be evaluated must be identified and described. Functional issues of concern to this group must be selected from interviewing both patients and clinicians or, alternatively, from a literature search and validated questionnaire review.

Item Reduction. Item reduction is determined by the frequency and importance of item endorsement in a sample patient cohort. The significance of specific items may also be derived from statistical methods such as factor analysis.

Format Selection. Format selection includes the choice of scaled responses or endorsed statements. Scaled responses (e.g., "on a scale of 1 to 10") provide better discrimination between responses but are more difficult for patients, while the endorsed statements format (responses include "strongly agree," "agree," to "strongly disagree") tends to be easier for patients, and dichotomous endorsable questions (yes/no) are easiest for patients to discern, especially for older patients.

Pretesting. Pretesting consists of administration of the questionnaire to a sample population to discover poorly worded or confusing items.

Reproducibility and Responsiveness. In short, reproducibility and responsiveness ask, "Does this instrument measure what it is intended to measure?" *Reproducibility* is evaluated by reviewing the variability in responses in relation to the variability in clinical status. This is addressed by a "test-retest" exercise in which the same patients complete the questionnaire twice within several days to 1 week during which no clinical change has taken place. *Responsiveness* is the measure of the questionnaire's ability to detect clinically important changes, even if they are small. Responsiveness is assessed by administering the questionnaire at a minimum of 3 months after a clinical intervention of known efficacy.

Validity. *Face validity* is determined by clinician evaluation of correlation between instrument and clinical assessment. *Construct validity* is assessed by developing hypotheses about how the scores should change between and within subjects and comparing results with already validated instruments. *Criterion validity* is addressed by comparing scores of the same group of patients with objective tests (e.g. range of motion, self-selected walking speed), clinician evaluations, or the particular current "gold standard" of outcome assessment.

ORTHOPAEDIC FUNCTIONAL OUTCOME INSTRUMENTS

Patient-based outcome instruments can be categorized broadly as generic, disease-specific, region-specific, joint- and injury-specific, and patient-specific measures. In addition, a number of instruments have been designed specifically to assess pain and therefore are applicable to multiple categories. Several well-validated health status instruments have been developed and are available for use in assessing patient function following musculoskeletal injury (Table 24-1), and some are discussed below. In fact, the use of patient-based measures in orthopaedic literature increased from 8 percent overall in 1991 to 18 percent in 2001.[5]

Pain

The Visual Analog Scale (VAS) is a simple, yet elegant, instrument that is commonly used to evaluate pain. Patients are shown a 10 cm line and asked to rate their pain along the line, with 0 being no pain, and 10 being worst pain. Quantitative responses are obtained by measuring patients' responses along the line. The VAS has been validated for pain assessment and is very commonly reported in literature from many specialties.[10,17] The VAS, however, has limitations. VAS responses may not correlate between patients, because other factors, such as self-reported health status and the experience surrounding pain, can affect patient responses.[37] Recently, a method of standardization of the VAS between patients by scoring specifically described pains, thereby allowing comparisons of VAS responses between different patient populations, has been implemented.[38]

Generic Instruments

Generic instruments measure general health status, including physical and emotional symptoms and function, also

				Table 24-1			
				HRQOL Instruments and Scoring Resources			
Instrument	**Method**	**Time to Complete**	**Target Population/ Conditions**	**Scientifically Developed?**	**Validated?**	**Source**	
SF-36	Self or interviewer	5–10 min	General health status/quality of life measures	Yes	Yes	http://www.sf-36.org/	
QWB	Trained interviewer	12 min	General health status/quality of life measures	Yes	Yes	http://medicine.ucsd. edu/fpm/hoap/qwb.htm	
SIP	Self or interviewer	30 min	General health status/quality of life measures	Yes	Yes	http://www.outcomes-trust.org/instruments. htm	
EQ-5D	Self	10 min	General health status	Yes	Yes	http://gs1.q4matics. com/ EuroqolPublishWeb/	
MFA	Self or interviewer	15 min	HRQOL measure applied to musculoskeletal disease	Yes	Yes	http://www.med.umn. edu/ortho/research.html	
SMFA	Self or interviewer	10 min	HRQOL measure applied to patients with musculoskeletal disease	Yes	Yes	http://www.med.umn. edu/ortho/research.html	
WOMAC	Self	10 min	Arthritis	Yes	Yes	http://www.womac.org/ womac/	
Brigham CTS instrument	Self	10 min	Carpal tunnel	Yes	Yes	Levine, D.W.; Simmons, B.P.; Koris, M.J.; et al. J Bone Joint Surg Am 75:1585–1592, 1993	
DASH	Self	10 min	Upper extremity injury or disease	Yes	Yes	http://www.dash.iwh.on. ca/	
AAOS Lower Limb Questionnaire	Self	10 min	Lower limb dysfunction	Yes	Yes	http://www.aaos.org/ research/outcomes/ outcomes.asp	
AAOS Foot and Ankle Questionnaire	Self	15 min	Foot and ankle dysfunction	Yes	Yes	http://www.aaos.org/ research/outcomes/ outcomes.asp	
AAOS Hip/Knee Questionnaire	Self	10 min	Hip and knee dysfunction	Yes	Yes	http://www.aaos.org/ research/outcomes.asp	
Toronto Salvage Score (TESS)	Self or Interviewer	20 min	Function after limb salvage surgery	Yes	Yes	Davis, A.M.; Wright, J.G.; Williams, A.I.; et al. Qual Life Res 5:508–516, 1996	
Simple Shoulder Test	Self	10 min	Shoulder dysfunction	Yes	No	Matsen, F.A.; Ziegler, D.W.; DeBartolo, S.E. J Shoulder Elbow Surg 4:345–351, 1995	
ASES Shoulder Evaluation System	Self	5 min	Shoulder dysfunction	Yes	Yes	Michener, L.; McClure, P.; Sennett, B. J Shoulder Elbow Surg 11:587–594, 2002	

(Continued)

Table 24-1
HRQOL Instruments and Scoring Resources—Cont'd

Instrument	Method	Time to Complete	Target Population/ Conditions	Scientifically Developed?	Validated?	Source
UCLA Shoulder Rating Scale	Interviewer	15 min	Shoulder pain and dysfunction	No	No	Ellman, H.; Hanker, G.; Bayer, M. J Bone Joint Surg Am 68:1136–1142, 1986
Constant Score – Shoulder	Interviewer	15 min	Shoulder pain and dysfunction	No	No	Constant, C.R.; Murley, A.H.G. Clin Orthop Relat Res 214:160–164, 1987
Western Ontario Shoulder Index	Self	20 min	Shoulder pain and dysfunction	Yes	No	Kirkley, A.; Griffin, S.; McLintock, H.; et al. Am J Sports Med 26:764–772, 1998.
Morrey/Mayo Clinic Performance Index for the Elbow	Interviewer	15 min	Elbow pain and dysfunction	No	No	Morrey, B.F.; Adams, R.A. J Bone Joint Surg Am 74:479–490, 1992.
Harris Hip Score	Interviewer	30 min	Hip pain and dysfunction	No	No	http://exper.ural.ru/ trauma/harris_e.phtml
Knee Society Knee Score	Examiner	20 min	Knee function	Yes		http://www.kneesociety. org/index.asp/ fuseaction/site.rationale
International Knee Documentation Committee Ligament Evaluation Form	Self	10 min	Knee injury/pain	Yes	Yes	http://www.esska.org/ pdf/IKDCeng.pdf
Iowa Knee Score	Interviewer/ examiner	15 min	Knee function	No	No	Merchant, T.C.; Dietz, F.R. J Bone Joint Surg Am 71:599–606, 1989
Iowa Ankle Score	Interviewer/ examiner	15 min	Ankle function	No	No	Merchant, T.C.; Dietz, F.R. J Bone Joint Surg Am 71:599–606, 1989
Foot and Ankle Score (AAFAOS)	Self	10 min	Foot and ankle dysfunction, specifically lateral ankle instability, Achilles tendinosis, and plantar fasciitis	Yes	Yes	http://www.koos.nu
Foot Function Index	Self	30 min	Foot dysfunction	Yes	Yes	Budiman-Mak, E.; Conrad, K.J.; Roach, K.E. J Clin Epidemiol 44:561–570, 1991

Abbreviations: AAOS, American Academy of Orthopaedic Surgeons; MFA, Musculoskeletal Functional Assessment; QWB, Quality of Well-being Scale; SF-36, Short Form–36; SIP, Sickness Impact Profile; WOMAC, Western Ontario and McMaster University Osteoarthritis Index.

known as health-related quality of life (HRQOL). Generic instruments are not designed to detect subtle differences among patients with the same disease process or changes in individuals over time—to evaluate these differences would require a more specific questionnaire to minimize ceiling and floor effects. The Medical Outcomes Study Short Form–36 Item Health Survey (SF-36), the Quality of Well-being Scale (QWB), the Sickness Impact Profile (SIP), and the EuroQol (EQ-5D) are used often in orthopaedic outcomes research. These four instruments are widely used in all areas of outcomes research, and all are appropriate for use in evaluating musculoskeletal disease and injury. The use of generic instruments to obtain functional outcome data has become so commonplace that some granting institutions require the incorporation of a generic questionnaire to the design of clinical projects. Each of these instruments assesses domains of human activity,

including physical, psychological, social, and role functioning. The ultimate effect is a global evaluation of the patient as a whole being, rather than a disease, an injury, or an organ system. They are reproducible, are responsive, and have been validated in many patient populations. Of note, none are physician administered, which increases reliability. Scores from all these instruments are affected by a patient's co-morbidities, age, and gender, best described in the SF-36.[75,82] Specifically, arthritic back pain and depression each have a significant impact on altering an HRQOL score. The effect that these variables have on patient-reported function must be recognized when data analysis is performed, since the patients in question may not be appropriate comparisons to population norms.

The SF-36 was developed by Ware and colleagues and the Rand Corporation as a part of the Medical Outcomes Study.[68,70,76,77] The SF-36 is the most widely applied general health status instrument and has certain features that make it particularly appealing for studying musculoskeletal injury. The SF-36 consists of 36 *scaled-response* questions (0 = poor, 100 = best) concerning eight different functional subscales: bodily pain, role function–physical, role function–emotional, social function, physical function, energy/fatigue, mental health, and general health perceptions. Each scale is scored separately. Scores cannot be combined into a single aggregate scale, but the subscales can be combined into the Physical Component Score and the Mental Component Score. The SF-36 has been validated as a reliable and reproducible questionnaire, and it can be administered by the patient or an interviewer, either in person, over the phone, or by mail. The entire questionnaire takes approximately 10 to 15 minutes to complete, making it appealing for the office or clinic setting. The SF-36 has been published with normative values for the U.S. population, which vary with age and gender, as well as values for patients with multiple comorbidities, which impact the physical function, role function (physical), bodily pain, general health, and vitality subscales.[74] The SF-36 is thought to be limited with regard to musculoskeletal conditions in that it may have a "ceiling effect" (scores are concentrated at best function). Therefore, the SF-36 may inadequately characterize clinically important functional problems because the disability is too minimal to be detected by the questions. Patients with mild to moderate dysfunction (such as overuse injuries and minor fractures) may score near the highest possible scores and further improvement is not able to be measured. The SF-36 may be limited in detecting upper extremity dysfunction as well.

The QWB is a 78-item *scaled-response* questionnaire that requires a trained interviewer for administration, which takes approximately 25 to 30 minutes. Patients are questioned on physical activity, social activity, and mobility. The QWB is thought to be more sensitive than the SF-36 at detecting small changes in functional status, although the QWB physical function scale also likely suffers from "ceiling effects." The QWB forms the backbone of the Quality Adjusted Life Years (QALYs) methodology, popularly used to determine the cost-effectiveness of medical interventions, and is therefore a "utility instrument."[80] Multiplying QWB data from large populations times years of life expectancy and cost per intervention yields the QALY—cost of a given intervention per year of well life expectancy. QALYs provide a methodology for making difficult decisions regarding resource allocation. Orthopaedic interventions such as hip arthroplasty and hip fracture fixation have fared well with this methodology.[58,80]

The SIP, a 136-question *endorsable statement* (yes/no) questionnaire, requires trained interviewers for administration, which takes 25 to 35 minutes to complete.[7–9] The SIP inquires about 12 different domains, which are first scored independently, then combined into physical and psychosocial subscales, as well as one aggregate score. The scale is 0 to 100 points—the higher the score, the worse the disability. Patients with scores in excess of the mid-30s have significantly diminished quality of life. The SIP has been used in patients with multiple health conditions and allows for comparisons of impact of disease on health. The SIP has been used in musculoskeletal

trauma with good success.[50,51] Lesser degrees of musculoskeletal dysfunction are not identified, and therefore the SIP also suffers from the ceiling effect. Because of the difficulty and length of its administration, the SIP may be most useful for well-funded outcome studies or controlled trials.

The EQ-5D is so named because it assesses five dimensions of health status—mobility, self-care, usual activities, pain/discomfort, and anxiety/depression. The first three dimensions reflect physical functioning. For pain level estimation, patients are asked to choose between three responses for level of pain and discomfort (none, moderate, or extreme). However, if chronic pain is well controlled, the patient's best response may be most appropriately described as "mild," which is not an option. The answers within each dimension are then weighted, based on preferences from 0 to 1 that correlate to worst versus best health, and then used to calculate a final score. The EQ-5D is also a "utility instrument" in that scores can be used in cost-effectiveness analyses.

Interestingly, the Musculoskeletal Functional Assessment (MFA) and the Short Musculoskeletal Functional Assessment (SMFA) questionnaires collect both general health information and musculoskeletal function information with fewer floor and ceiling effects than the SF-36.[57] In response to the need for an instrument to measure functional outcomes of patients with musculoskeletal disease or injury (extremity trauma, overuse syndromes, osteoarthritis, or rheumatoid arthritis), the MFA was developed under National Institutes of Health/National Institute of Child Health and Human Development sponsorship.[25,53] The MFA is a generic, 101-item instrument that assesses function in 10 domains, with emphasis on musculoskeletal function: self-care, emotional status, recreation, household work, employment, sleep and rest, relationships, thinking, activities using arms and legs, and activities using hands. It is responsive, reliable, and validated, and the MFA has been published with reference values to population norms. The MFA requires approximately 15 to 20 minutes to complete and can be either self- or interviewer-administered. The MFA provides a means by which the effectiveness of treatment and functional impact of musculoskeletal disease may be analyzed. The MFA is thought to avoid the ceiling effect evident in other generic instruments.[53]

The MFA may be more detailed and more demanding on office staff than is appropriate for routine use or for outcome studies. The SMFA was developed for this reason. Investigators selected questions from the longer MFA based on universality, applicability, uniqueness, reliability, and validity. The SMFA is a 46-question, self-administered instrument that can be completed in approximately 10 to 15 minutes, thereby facilitating data collection in a busy office setting. This instrument is divided into two parts. Part 1 has four categories: daily activities, emotional status, arm/hand function, and mobility, with an accompanying five-point scale for patients to estimate their function; part 1 questions are then totaled to create the "dysfunction index." Part 2 contains 12 questions that assess the degree to which patients are bothered in recreation and leisure, sleep and rest, work, and family, also with an accompanying five-point scale; responses from part 2 are combined to create the "bother index." The SMFA has been field tested in academic and community offices with excellent compliance and utility.[1] The SMFA is particularly useful to clinicians who routinely and quantitatively monitor patient progress over time as well as against patients from other settings. The SMFA has recently been translated into Spanish, making it even more practical. Both the MFA and the SMFA are somewhat resistant to the floor and ceiling effects that can be problematic for SF-36 data.

The above examples are commonly used general health status instruments that allow for comparison of the functional impact of various diseases. Disease- or condition-specific instruments offer increased sensitivity and limit the floor and ceiling effects. Table 24-1 lists the general health status instruments individually with their attributes and identifies sources for the reader.

Disease-Specific Instruments

Functional outcomes instruments for specific diseases have been developed for a wide range of ailments, ranging from cardiovascular disease to colorectal cancer to closed head injuries. The most commonly used disease-specific outcome instrument in orthopaedics is the Western Ontario and McMaster University Osteoarthritis Index (WOMAC), which is worth mentioning because it was designed to assess osteoarthritis of the upper and lower extremities. The WOMAC is a self-administered, 24-question, scaled-response instrument divided into the dimensions of pain, stiffness, and physical function. Importantly, the WOMAC has been validated in patient populations with hip and knee osteoarthritis; it has been used widely in both clinical and interventional studies.

The Toronto Extremity Salvage Score is a 30-question instrument used to measure physical function after tumor resection, specifically in those who have undergone musculoskeletal oncology limb salvage surgery. This instrument has been shown to be valid and responsive in this patient population. Toronto Extremity Salvage Score results are widely reported in clinical musculoskeletal oncological research.

The Roland-Morris Low Back Pain and Disability Questionnaire is a derivation of the SIP but specifically designed to assess low back pain. It is a short (24 questions), scaled-response instrument and can be self-administered. These features facilitate its use in clinical settings, and therefore it is widely used in studies regarding low back pain.

Region-Specific Instruments

Valiant attempts have been made to expand the repertoire of musculoskeletal-specific generic and region-specific instruments. In 1993, the American Academy of Orthopaedic Surgeons (AAOS) and members of the Council of Musculoskeletal Specialty Societies pooled resources to develop general health and region-specific questionnaires that could be used for patients with musculoskeletal injuries and diseases.[69] The goal was to create questionnaires that would be usable in an office setting. Patient-derived outcome data were collected on the local, regional, and national levels via a central database, the Musculoskeletal

Outcomes Data Collection and Management System (MODEMS). The database incorporated the demographic and co-morbidity information and SF-36 and questionnaires for the upper extremity, lower extremity, and pediatric and spine patients. This combined instrument was validated and takes 10 to 30 minutes to complete. The AAOS conducted a preliminary trial to post national data and collected data from more than 30,000 patients in 3 months.[69] The AAOS sponsored a national database for MODEMS collection, but it was discontinued in 2000 because of physician concerns regarding a central data registry. However, MODEMS questionnaires are still available for use at www.aaos.org. These questionnaires provide HRQOL data via the SF-36 as well as area/disease specific information, so they are a good choice for comprehensive evaluation (Table 24-2).

The Upper Extremity Function Scale is an eight-item, self-administered questionnaire. It was designed to measure the impact of upper extremity dysfunction on overall patient function. This instrument has been validated and has shown few floor effects.

The Disabilities of the Arm, Shoulder, and Hand (DASH) is a popular instrument in orthopaedic literature; it has been translated into at 17 languages. DASH is a 30-question, self-administered evaluation of physical activity, pain, symptom severity, and impact of upper extremity disease on everyday activities. Answers are weighted and compiled to produce a single score for intra- and inter-patient comparison.

Joint-Specific Instruments

Perhaps one of the most famous functional instruments in orthopaedics is the Harris Hip Score, commonly used to compare the preoperative versus postoperative status of patients who have undergone total hip arthroplasty. The Harris Hip Score includes questions regarding pain assessment, walking distances, physical function, and range of motion, and creates a single score. Although widely used in the orthopaedic literature, it has yet to be validated (see Table 24-1).

Table 24-2	
Useful Web Sites	
Organization	**Address**
Orthopaedic Trauma Association	http://www.ota.org
American Academy of Orthopaedic Surgeons	http://www.aaos.org/research
Agency for Healthcare Research and Quality (AHRQ)	http://www.ahcpr.gov
SF-36 Questionnaire	http://www.sf-36.com/general
MODEMS Questionnaires	http://www.aaos.org/outcomes/outcomes.asp
MFA/SMFA	http://www.ortho.umn.edu/research/clinicaloutcomes.htm
Cochrane Collaboration	http://Hiru.mcmaster.ca/cochrane/

Multiple instruments exist to evaluate knee function. The Iowa Knee Score instrument was developed for the evaluation of patients with tibia fractures, along with the Iowa Ankle Score. The Iowa Knee Score is based on a 100-point scale incorporating patient-based assessment of pain and physical function as well as objective clinical data—range of motion, gait, and deformity. The Knee Society Knee Score and International Knee Documentation Committee Ligament Evaluation Form are other examples of instruments that were created to evaluate knee pain and function. Again, although widely used in the literature, not all of these instruments have been validated.

The Iowa Ankle Score, the Foot and Ankle Score, and the Foot Function Index are commonly encountered instruments in the foot and ankle literature. The Iowa Ankle Score is also a 100-point scale combining patient-based data as well as objective clinical data. The Foot and Ankle Score and Foot Function Index are each self-administered forms that were scientifically developed, and both have been validated (see Table 24-1).

Shoulder instruments abound in the orthopaedic literature. The Simple Shoulder Test evaluates patients' ability to perform extremes of motion. These clinical data are combined with 12 patient-based endorsed-statement questions. The Simple Shoulder Test is most commonly used in studies of shoulder degenerative joint disease as well as rotator cuff tears. In addition, the American Shoulder and Elbow Surgeons Shoulder Evaluation, UCLA Shoulder Rating Scale, Constant Score, and Western Ontario Shoulder Index are all commonly used instruments in the shoulder literature, although again, not all have been validated. See Table 24-1 for details.

Patient-Specific Instruments

Patient-specific instruments are outcome questionnaires that use item-response theory in a computer-adaptive testing mode.[2,24,29,33] This is also known as "dynamic assessment." With sophisticated software, computerized testing alters future questions based on answers to previous questions. This process can significantly decrease the number of questions a patient is required to answer in outcome assessment. This, in theory, decreases the "patient burden" of outcome assessment.[12] Several available instruments are the patient-specific functional scale, the measure-yourself medical outcome profile, and the "adaptive" SF-36.[36,59,60,71,81] These instruments are reproducible and reliable at the individual level but may not be adequate for assessment of outcome of groups of patients with a specific injury or illness. Individual scores are applicable to a particular individual but are not easily generalized.

RECOMMENDATIONS FOR CLINICAL OUTCOMES RESEARCH AND OUTCOMES ASSESSMENT

Outcome assessment involves the routine collection of HRQOL data to evaluate the effectiveness of patient care. Patient-satisfaction and HRQOL data are routinely collected in the clinician's office from a specific segment of patients at predetermined intervals, both before and after treatment. These results provide the basis for outcome assessment, including data of interest to health care payers. Cost-benefit analysis of orthopaedic surgery interventions benefits both orthopaedists and their patients and justifies orthopaedic surgical care as payers and government agencies evaluate the effect of treatment given limited resources.[19,58] Often this research begins by collecting data on all patients within a practice, resulting in time-consuming data accumulations. Nonselective data collection can be frustrating for office staff responsible for administration and collection of questionnaires. However, patient cooperation and support of these projects is rarely problematic— patients tend to be most receptive to completing these types of questionnaires and believe that this process, as well as satisfaction surveys, represents an effort on behalf of the practice to meet their needs.

Outcome assessment should begin by selection of a target musculoskeletal condition or injury that is frequently treated in the practice. Institutional Review Board approval should be obtained if the practice is affiliated with a medical center, or from an outside agency, to ensure compliance with standard ethics and Health Insurance Portability and Accountability Act requirements of consent and follow-up. Prior to data collection, investigators should decide which clinical data are necessary to properly analyze HRQOL data. Data points, including clinical, demographic, or radiographic assessments, should be collected before treatment and at predetermined intervals. Patients should be approached before treatment and asked to complete an HRQOL questionnaire, and then notified that they will be contacted at predetermined intervals to complete the same survey. The intervals of data collection are not standardized, and the appropriate time intervals may vary for different musculoskeletal injuries and conditions. A patient with an isolated ankle fracture will return to normal function more quickly than a patient with a tibial plafond fracture, for which more frequent data collections may be required. A driving unmet need exists for studies that better characterize the rate of functional recovery of musculoskeletal injuries in order to answer patient questions and accurately address work-related and legal issues. Regarding the number of conditions studied, a minimalist approach is most beneficial when starting outcome assessment in clinical practice. Identification of an injury or disease common to the practice, and subsequent data collection on patients with this condition, will lead to useful data for evaluating current practice protocols.

Data collection must be done as simply and cost-efficiently as possible to ensure long-term success. In the past, language has prevented patient-based outcome assessment for a large percentage of the U.S. population. However, many outcome instruments are being or have been validated in different languages. Technology will also provide significant changes in the ability to provide outcome instruments to patients. The development of scanned forms, touch screens, and wireless Web-based real-time entry will improve the quality and efficiency of data collection. The quality of orthopaedic studies improves with increased awareness of study design, statistical impact, and adequate follow-up of clinical and functional outcomes.[4,11,15,34,44,47,48] A single surgeon (expert) study design may provide an estimate of optimal outcome that can be obtained from a specific intervention[54] but may not be generalizable to the general community for realistic surgeon and patient expectations. A multicenter multiple surgeon design will provide results more akin to what should be expected from an orthopaedic intervention.[54] Information derived from pooled orthopaedic practice data will be instrumental in improving the quality of musculoskeletal care, allowing rapid patient enrollment and encouraging timely analysis of clinical uncertainties.[39]

Randomized controlled trials have become the "gold standard" of outcome studies, but other study designs may be valid as well. Prospective cohort designs can also provide quality data if a defined injury/condition is studied with inclusion/exclusion criteria, standardized interventions, and follow-up parameters. This study design does not seem to bias data and can produce results similar to a randomized trial.[6,21,46,52]

Patient-based outcome measurement has increased significantly in the past 10 years and is likely to continue. Future clinical research studies will define the sensitivity to change over time of various functional outcome instruments. Outcome data facilitate comparison of individual patients' scores to normal general population scores, allowing physicians to predict and determine when patients reach maximal improvement. Patient-based outcome measurements may improve identification of the patients who score better on classic outcome measurements, such as range of motion, strength, and radiographic union, on the basis of their ability to adapt to their injury. Orthopaedic research needs to identify factors outside the control of the orthopaedist that may have a great effect on outcomes. For instance, education level, income, family support, employment, addiction status, personality type, emotional status, and genetics have significant impacts on long-term outcomes and may be more important than the severity or treatment of injury. Intervention in these areas by the health care team may be as important as standard medical and surgical care.

REFERENCES

1. Agel, J.; Obremsky, W.; Kregor, P.; et al. Administration of the Short Musculoskeletal Function Assessment: Impact on office routine and physician-patient interaction. Orthopaedics 26:783–788, 2003.
2. Andres, P.L.; Black-Schaffer, R.M.; Ni, P.; et al. Computer adaptive testing: A strategy for monitoring stroke rehabilitation across settings. Top Stroke Rehabil 11(2):33–39, 2004.
3. Atlas, S.J.; Deyo, R.A.; Keller, R.B.; et al. The Maine Lumbar Spine Study. II. One-year outcomes of surgical and nonsurgical management of sciatica. Spine 1:1777–1786, 1996.
4. Aune, A.K.; Ekeland, A.; Odegaard, B.; et al. Gamma nail vs. compression screw for trochanteric femoral fractures: Fifteen reoperations in a prospective, randomized study of 378 patients. Acta Orthop Scand 65:127–130, 1994.
5. Beaton, D.E.; Schemitsch, E. Measures of health-related quality of life and physical function. Clin Orthop Relat Res 413:90–105, 2003.
6. Benson, K.; Hartz, A.J. A comparison of observational studies and randomized, controlled trials. N Engl J Med 342:1878–1886, 2000.
7. Bergner, M.; Bobbitt, R.A.; Carter, W.B.; et al. The Sickness Impact Profile: Development and final revision of a health status measure. Med Care 19:787–805, 1981.
8. Bergner, M.; Bobbitt, R.A.; Kressel, S.; et al. The Sickness Impact Profile: Conceptual formulation and methodology for the development of a health status measure. Int J Health Serv 6(3):393–415, 1976.
9. Bergner, M.; Bobbitt, R.A.; Pollard, W.E.; et al. The Sickness Impact Profile: Validation of a health status measure. Med Care 14:57–67, 1976.
10. Bijur, P.E.; Silver, W.; Gallagher, E.J. Reliability of the visual analog scale for measurement of acute pain. Acad Emerg Med 8:1153–1157, 2001.
11. Blachut, P.A.; O'Brien, P.J.; Meek, R.N.; et al. Interlocking intramedullary nailing with and without reaming for the treatment of closed fractures of the tibial shaft: A prospective, randomized study. J Bone Joint Surg Am 79:640–646, 1997.
12. Bode, R.K.; Lai, J.S.; Dineen, K.; et al. Expansion of a physical function item bank and development of an abbreviated form for clinical research. J Appl Meas 7:1–15, 2006.
13. Bone, L.B.; Johnson, K.D.; Weigelt, J.; et al. Early versus delayed stabilization of femoral fractures: A prospective randomized study. J Bone Joint Surg Am 71:336–340, 1989.
14. Bone, L.B.; McNamara, K.; Shine, B.; et al. Mortality in multiple trauma patients with fractures. J Trauma 37:262–264, 1994.
15. Bracken, M.B.; Shepard, M.J.; Collins, W.F.; et al. A randomized, controlled trial of methylprednisolone or naloxone in the treatment of acute spinal-cord injury: Results of the Second National Acute Spinal Cord Injury Study. N Engl J Med 322:1405–1411, 1990.
16. Chapman, C.R.; Syrjala, K.L. Measurement of pain. In Loeser, J.D.; Butler, S.H.; Chapman, C.R.; et al., eds. Bonica's Management of Pain. Philadelphia, Lippincott Williams & Wilkins, 2001, pp. 310–328.
17. Codman, E.A. The product of a hospital, 1914. Arch Pathol Lab Med 114:1106–1111, 1990.
18. Codman, E.A. The Shoulder. Malaber, Florida, Krieger, 1934, pp. 1–29.
19. Committee on Medical Aspects of Automotive Safety. Rating the severity of tissue damage. JAMA 215:277–286, 1971.
20. Committee on Quality of Health Care in America, Institute of Medicine. Crossing the Quality Chasm: A New Health System for the 21st Century. Washington, D.C., National Academy Press, 2001.
21. Concato, J.; Shah, N.; Horwitz, R.I. Randomized, controlled trials, observational studies, and the hierarchy of research designs. N Engl J Med 342:1887–1892, 2000.

22. Coughlin, M.J.; Freund, E.; Roger, A. Mann Award: The reliability of angular measurements in hallux valgus deformities. Foot Ankle Int 22:369–379, 2001.

23. Deyo, R.A.; Inui, T.S.; Leininger, J.D.; et al. Measuring functional outcomes in chronic disease: A comparison of traditional scales and a self-administered health status questionnaire in patients with rheumatoid arthritis. Med Care 21:180–192, 1983.

24. Downing, S.M. Item response theory: Applications of modern test theory in medical education. Med Educ 37:739–745, 2003.

25. Engelberg, R.; Martin, D.P.; Agel, J.; et al. Musculoskeletal Function Assessment instrument: Criterion and construct validity. J Orthop Res 14:182–192, 1996.

26. Fakhry, S.M.; Rutledge, R.; Dahners, L.E.; et al. Incidence, management, and outcome of femoral shaft fracture: A statewide population-based analysis of 2805 adult patients in a rural state. J Trauma 37:255–260, 1994.

27. Gartland, J.J. Orthopaedic clinical research: Deficiencies in experimental design and determinations of outcome. J Bone Joint Surg Am 70:1357–1364, 1988.

28. Geisler, F.H.; Dorsey, F.C.; Coleman, W.P. Recovery of motor function after spinal-cord injury: A randomized, placebo-controlled trial with GM-1 ganglioside. N Engl J Med 324:1829–1838, 1991.

29. Gershon, R.C. Computer adaptive testing. J Appl Meas 6:109–127, 2005.

30. Gross, M. A critique of the methodologies used in clinical studies of hip-joint arthroplasty published in the English-language orthopaedic literature. J Bone Joint Surg Am 70:1364–1371, 1988.

31. Guyatt, G.H.; Feeny, D.H.; Patrick, D.L. Measuring health-related quality of life. Ann Intern Med 118:622–629, 1993.

32. Hardy, D.C.; Descamps, P.Y.; Krallis, P.; et al. Use of an intramedullary hip screw compared with a compression hip screw with a plate for intertrochanteric femoral fractures. J Bone Joint Surg Am 80:618–630, 1998.

33. Hays, R.D.; Morales, L.S.; Reise, S.P. Item response theory and health outcomes measurement in the 21st century. Med Care 38(9):II28–II42, 2000.

34. Horne, G.; Iceton, J.; Twist, J.; et al. Disability following fractures of the tibial shaft. Orthopaedics 13:423–426, 1990.

35. Johnson, K.D.; Cadambi, A.; Seibert, G.B. Incidence of adult respiratory distress syndrome in patients with multiple musculoskeletal injuries: Effect of early operative stabilization of fractures. J Trauma 25(5):375–384, 1985.

36. Jolles, B.M.; Buchbinder, R.; Beaton, D.E. A study compared nine patient-specific indices for musculoskeletal disorders. J Clin Epidemiol 58:791–801, 2005.

37. Kane, R.L.; Bershadsky, B.; Rockwood, T.; et al. Visual Analog Scale pain reporting was standardized. J Clin Epidemiol 58:618–623, 2005.

38. Keller, R.B. Outcomes research in orthopaedics. J Am Acad Orthop Surg 1:122–129, 1993.

39. Keller, R.B.; Atlas, S.J.; Singer, D.E.; et al. The Maine Lumbar Spine Study. I. Background and concepts. Spine 21:1769–1776, 1996.

40. Keller, R.B.; Rudicel, S.A.; Liang, M.H. Outcomes research in orthopaedics. J Bone Joint Surg Am 75:1562–1574, 1993.

41. Keller, R.B.; Soule, D.N.; Wennberg, J.E.; et al. Dealing with geographic variations in the use of hospitals: The experience of the Maine Medical Assessment Foundation Orthopaedic Study Group. J Bone Joint Surg Am 72:1286–1293, 1990.

42. Keller, R.B.; Wennberg, D.E.; Soule, D.N. Changing physician behavior: The Maine Medical Assessment Foundation. Qual Manag Health Care 5:1–11, 1997.

43. Kristianson, T.K.; Ryaby, J.P.; McCabe, J.; et al. Accelerated healing of distal radius fractures with the use of specific, low-intensity ultrasound: A multicenter, prospective, randomized, double-blind, placebo controlled study. J Bone Joint Surg Am 79:961–973, 1997.

44. L'Abbe, K.A.; Detsky, A.S.; O'Rourke, K. Meta-analysis in clinical research. Ann Intern Med 107:224–233, 1987.

45. Labelle, H.; Guibert, R.; Joncas, J.; et al. Lack of scientific evidence for the treatment of lateral epicondylitis of the elbow: An attempted meta-analysis. J Bone Joint Surg Br 74:646–651, 1992.

46. Loannidis, J.P.A.; Haidich, A.B.; Pappa, M.; et al. Comparison of evidence of treatment effects in randomized and nonrandomized studies. JAMA 286:821–830, 2001.

47. Loucks, C.; Buckley, R. Bohler's angle: Correlation with outcome in displaced intra-articular calcaneal fractures. J Orthop Trauma 13:554–558, 1999.

48. Lowe, D.K.; Gately, H.L.; Goss, J.R.; et al. Patterns of death, complication, and error in the management of motor vehicle accident victims: Implications for a regional system of trauma care. J Trauma 23:503–509, 1983.

49. Lu-Yao, G.L.; Keller, R.B.; Littenberg, B.; et al. Outcomes after displaced fractures of the femoral neck: A meta-analysis of one hundred and six published reports. J Bone Joint Surg Am 76:15–25, 1994.

50. MacKenzie, E.J.; Burgess, A.R.; McAndrew, M. P.; et al. Patient-oriented functional outcome after unilateral lower extremity fracture. J Orthop Trauma 7:393–401, 1993.

51. MacKenzie, E.J.; Cushing, B.M.; Jurkovich, G. J.; et al. Physical impairment and functional outcomes six months after severe lower extremity fractures. J Trauma 34:528–538, 1993.

52. MacLehose, R.R.; Reeves, B.C.; Harvey, I.M.; et al. A systemic review of comparisons of effect sizes derived from randomised and non-randomised studies. Health Technol Assess 4(34):1–154, 2000.

53. Martin, D.P.; Engelberg, R.; Agel, J.; et al. Development of a musculoskeletal extremity health status

instrument: The Musculoskeletal Function Assessment instrument. J Orthop Res 14:173–181, 1996.

54. Matta, J.M. Operative treatment of acetabular fractures through the ilioinguinal approach: A 10-year perspective. J Orthop Trauma 20(1):S20–S29, 2006.

55. Mattox, K.L.; Bickell, W.H.; Pepe, P.E.; et al. Prospective randomized evaluation of antishock MAST in post-traumatic hypotension. J Trauma 26:779–786, 1986.

56. Meek, R.N.; Vivoda, E.E.; Pirani, S. Comparison of mortality of patients with multiple injuries according to type of fracture treatment: A retrospective age- and injury-matched series. Injury 17:2–4, 1986.

57. Obremskey, W.T.; Brown, O.; Driver, R.; et al. Comparison of SF-36 and Short Musculoskeletal Functional Assessment in recovery from fixation of unstable ankle fractures. Orthopaedics 30:145–151, 2007.

58. Parker, M.J.; Myles, J.W.; Anand, J.K.; et al. Cost-benefit analysis of hip fracture treatment. J Bone Joint Surg Br 74:261–264, 1992.

59. Paterson, C.; Britten, N. In pursuit of patient-centred outcomes: A qualitative evaluation of the "Measure Yourself Medical Outcome Profile." J Health Serv Res Policy 5:27–36, 2000.

60. Paterson, C.; Langan, C.E.; McKaig, G.A.; et al. Assessing patient outcomes in acute exacerbations of chronic bronchitis: The measure your medical outcome profile (MYMOP), medical outcomes study 6-item general health survey (MOS-6A), and EuroQoL (EQ-5D). Qual Life Res 9:521–527, 2000.

61. Patrick, D.L.; Bergner, M. Measurement of health status in the 1990s. Annu Rev Public Health 11:65–83, 1990.

62. Pynsent, P.B. Choosing an outcome measure. J Bone Joint Surg Br 83:792–794, 2006.

63. Resnick, D.K.; Choudhri, T.F.; Dailey, A.T.; et al. Guidelines for the performance of fusion procedures for degenerative disease of the lumbar spine. 5. Correlation between radiographic and functional outcome. J Neurosurg Spine 2:658–661, 2005.

64. Schroder, S.A. Outcome assessment 70 years later: Are we ready? N Engl J Med 316:160–162, 1987.

65. Seibel, R.; LaDuca, J.; Hassett, J.M.; et al. Blunt multiple trauma (ISS 36), femur traction, and the pulmonary failure-septic state. Ann Surg 202:283–295, 1985.

66. Sjoden, G.O.; Movin, T.; Guntner, P.; et al. Poor reproducibility of classification of proximal humeral fractures: Additional CT of minor value. Acta Orthop Scand 68:239–242, 1997.

67. Smith, S.W.; Meyer, R.A.; Connor, P.M.; et al. Interobserver reliability and intraobserver reproducibility of the modified Ficat classification system of osteonecrosis of the femoral head. J Bone Joint Surg Am 78:1702–1706, 1996.

68. Stewart, A.L.; Ware, J.E.; Brook, R.H.; et al. Conceptualization and Measurement of Health for Adults in the Health Insurance Study. Vol. II: Physical Health in Terms of Functioning. Santa Monica, California, The Rand Corporation, 1978.

69. Swiontkowski, M.F.; Chapman, J.R. Cost and effectiveness issues in care of injured patients. Clin Orthop Relat Res (318):17–24, 1995.

70. Tarlov, A.R.; Ware, J.E., Jr.; Greenfield, S.; et al. The Medical Outcomes Study: An application of methods for monitoring the results of medical care. JAMA 262:925–930, 1989.

71. Tonidandel, S.; Quinones, M.A.; Adams, A.A. Computer-adaptive testing: The impact of test characteristics on perceived performance and test takers' reactions. J Appl Psychol 87:320–332, 2002.

72. Turner, J.A.; Ersek, M.; Herron, L.; et al. Surgery for lumbar spinal stenosis: Attempted meta-analysis of the literature. Spine 17:1–8, 1992.

73. Vrbos, L.A.; Lorenz, M.A.; Peabody, E.H.; et al. Clinical methodologies and incidence of appropriate statistical testing in orthopaedic spine literature: Are statistics misleading? Spine 18:1021–1029, 1993.

74. Ware, J.E. SF-36 Health Survey: Manual and Interpretation Guide. Boston, Massachusetts, The Health Institute, New England Medical Center Hospitals, 1996.

75. Ware, J.E.; Johnston, S.A.; Davies-Avery, A.; et al. Conceptualization and Measurement of Health for Adults in the Health Insurance Study. Vol. III. Mental Health. Santa Monica, California, The Rand Corporation, 1979.

76. Ware, J.E., Jr.; Sherbourne, C.D. The MOS 36-item short-form health survey (SF-36). I. Conceptual framework and item selection. Med Care 30:473–483, 1992.

77. Ware, J.E.; Sherbourne, C.D.; Davies, A.R. Developing and testing the MOS 20-item short-form health survey: A general population application. In Stewart, A.L.; Ware, J.E., eds. Measuring Function and Well-Being: The Medical Outcomes Study Approach. Durham, North Carolina, Duke University Press, 1992, pp. 277–290.

78. Wennberg, J.; Gittelsohn, A. Small area variations in health care delivery. Science 182(117):1102–1108, 1973.

79. Wennberg, J.E.; Roos, N.; Sola, L.; et al. Use of claims data systems to evaluate health care outcomes: Mortality and reoperation following prostatectomy. JAMA 257:933–936, 1987.

80. Williams, A. Setting priorities in health care: An economist's view. J Bone Joint Surg Br 73:365–367, 1991.

81. Wright, J.G.; Young, N.L.; Waddell, J.P. The reliability and validity of the self-reported patient-specific index for total hip arthroplasty. J Bone Joint Surg Am 82:829–837, 2000.

82. Xuan, J.; Kirchdoerfer, L.J.; Boyer, J.G.; et al. Effects of comorbidity on health-related quality-of-life scores: An analysis of clinical trial data. Clin Ther 21:383–403, 1999.

SECTION 2

Spine

Section Editor: Alan M. Levine, M.D.

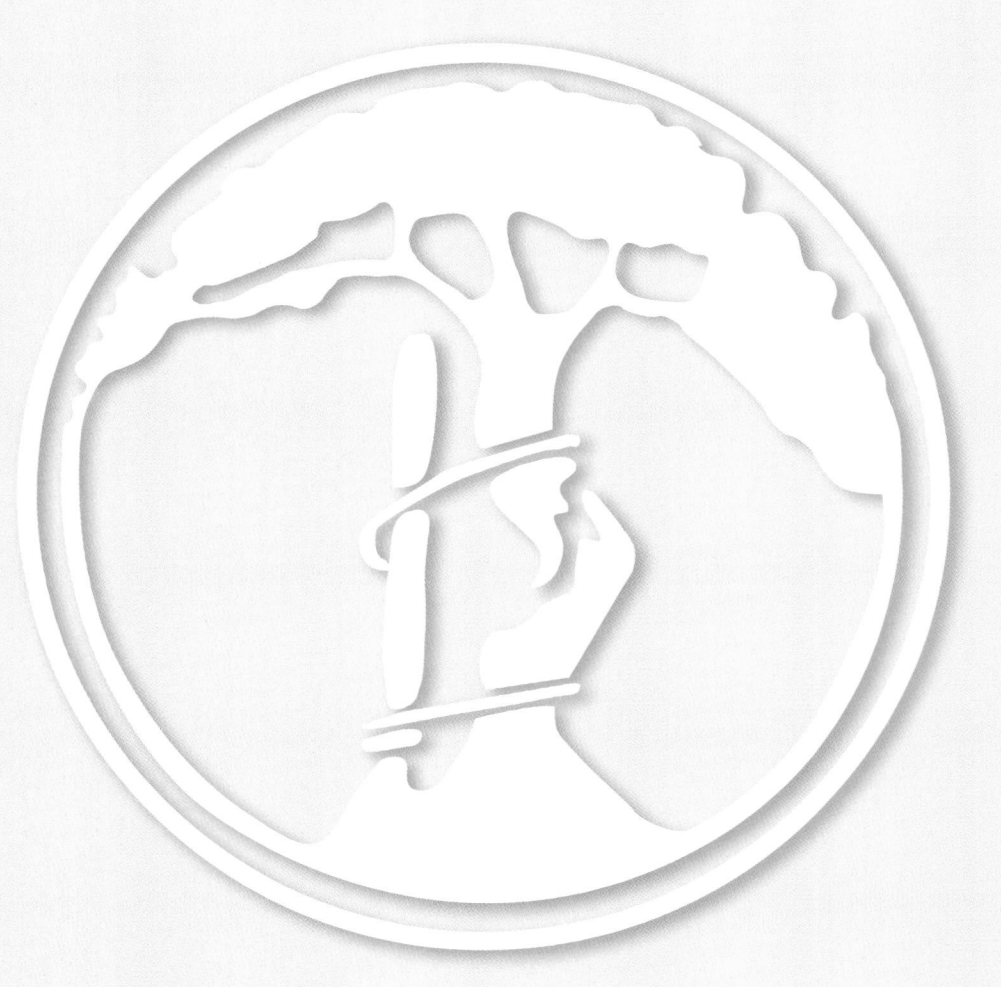

727

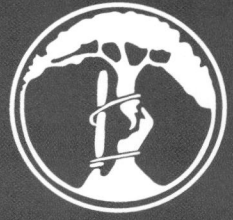

CHAPTER 25

Initial Evaluation and Emergency Treatment of the Spine-Injured Patient

....

Munish C. Gupta, M.D., Daniel R. Benson, M.D., and Timothy L. Keenen, M.D.

BASIC CONSIDERATIONS

Incidence, Etiology, and Demographics

Injury to the spinal column can be devastating. Some degree of neurologic deficit occurs in 10 to 25 percent of patients at all levels of injury,[10,89] in 40 percent at cervical spine levels,[10,12,89] and in 15 to 20 percent at thoracolumbar levels.[10,27] Even with the development of specialized spinal injury centers, the cost to society per patient remains staggering.[28] The ultimate solution rests in prevention of the original injury, but in the meantime, those managing a spine injury can minimize the risk of further damage by using accepted techniques of initial transportation and treatment. A thorough understanding of the demographics, anatomy, and pathophysiology of spinal cord injury, use of logical algorithms for initial evaluation and treatment, and knowledge of the potential complications seen with specific patient populations are critical for optimal patient treatment.

The magnitude of the problem and the difficulties with past studies on the incidence rates of spinal injuries prompted the U.S. Centers for Disease Control and Prevention to establish spinal cord injury surveillance systems.[22] The most recent estimates of incidence are generally unchanged from the previous estimates[36,111] of approximately 4.0 to 5.3 per 100,000 population.[114] This incidence corresponds to 12,000 new spinal cord injuries every year for which treatment is sought and an additional 4800 patients who sustain spinal cord injuries but die before arrival at the hospital.[111]

The causes of spinal column and spinal cord injury are illustrated in Figure 25-1.[10,12,13,27,89,111] The most significant cause of spinal column injury is motor vehicle accidents (45%), followed by falls (20%), sports-related accidents (15%), acts of violence (15%), and miscellaneous causes (5%). At the extremes of age, the role of falls increases from 9 percent in the 0- to 15-year-old group to 60 percent in those older than 75 years.[111] The male-to-female ratio is 4:1. When a neurologic deficit is associated with spinal column injury, the overall survival rate

for all levels of injury is 86 percent at 10 years.[112] The survival rate drops off for patients injured after age 29 to about 50 percent at 10 years. In patients older than 55 years, in nonwhites, and in quadriplegics, the leading cause of death is pneumonia. Accidents and suicides are most common in those younger than 55 years of age, in nonwhites, and in paraplegics.[112]

Although improvements in prevention and treatment have been slow in developing, they are clearly represented in the national statistics. The National Spinal Cord Injury Data Base reported fewer complete injuries and a higher percentage of incomplete spinal cord injuries in 1985 than in 1973,[111] an improvement that can be attributed to better initial management. These changes evolved from severe deficiencies in the emergency medical services, which were described in a classic report released by the National Academy of Sciences National Research Council Committee on Shock and the Committee on Trauma in 1966.[24,49] Progress in prevention was seen in a 14-year report from the National Football Head and Neck Injury Registry,[115] which noted a decrease in the number of football-related cases of permanent quadriplegia and cervical fractures between 1976 (34 and 110 cases, respectively) and 1984 (5 and 42 cases, respectively). This decrease was attributed to tackling rules instituted in 1975 in which deliberate "spearing" and the use of the top of the helmet as the initial point of contact were banned.

The establishment of spinal cord injury centers and the improvement in prehospital management of spinal cord injuries have been of significant benefit in the overall outcome for such patients. The concept of a spinal cord injury center as a separate unit began at the Ministry of Pensions Hospital, Stoke Mandeville, England, under the supervision of Sir Ludwig Guttman in 1943. Founding of this unit was followed by the establishment in 1945 of a unit in Toronto, Canada, and later by the creation of eight units in Veterans Affairs hospitals in the United States. When compared with the outcomes in other centers, such specialized facilities in the United States are credited with a shorter length of

729

FIGURE 25-1 *Causes of spinal column and spinal cord injury. MVA, motor vehicle accidents.*

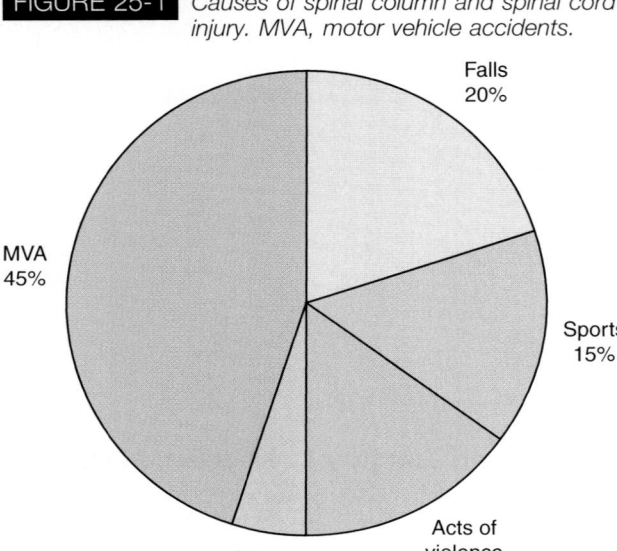

Falls
20%

MVA
45%

Sports
15%

Acts of
violence
15%

Other
5%

hospitalization, a lower rate of complications (e.g., urinary tract infection, pulmonary complications, decubitus ulcers), and therefore an overall lower cost of patient care. In addition, these centers have greatly lowered the percentage of complete versus incomplete injuries, with a decrease of 65 to 46 percent in one study[113] and 20 to 9 percent in another.[79]

Anatomy and Pathophysiology

Understanding the conclusions drawn from the initial physical examination of a spine-injured patient requires a basic knowledge of the osseous and neurologic structures of the spinal column. Details of osseous structures and fracture patterns are presented in Chapters 28 through 31. Knowledge of fracture patterns allows the examining physician to assess the relative stability of the injury, the risk of an associated neurologic deficit, and the indications for treatment.

SPINAL CORD ANATOMY

The spinal cord fills about 35 percent of the canal at the level of the atlas and then about 50 percent in the cervical and thoracolumbar segments. The remainder of the canal is filled with cerebrospinal fluid, epidural fat, and dura mater. The diameter of the cord varies, with swellings in the cervical and lumbar regions for the exiting nerve roots of the plexuses. The myelomere, or segment of cord from which a nerve root arises, lies one level above the same-numbered vertebral body in the cervical and high thoracic levels. For example, the T7 myelomere lies at the level of the T6 vertebral body. The lumbar and sacral myelomeres are concentrated between the T11 and L1 vertebral bodies. The end of the spinal cord (i.e., the conus medullaris) is most commonly located at the level of the L1-L2 intervertebral disk. The conus medullaris consists of the myelomeres of the five sacral nerve roots.

The spatial relationships of the gray and white matter structures remain consistent throughout the length of the cord, but their proportions change according to the level.

Because the white matter carries the long tract fibers from the sacral, lumbar, thoracic, and cervical levels, it constitutes more of the cervical than the sacral cross-sectional area. The gray matter, with its concentration of lower motor neurons, is predominant in the cervical and lumbar swellings, where the axons exit to the upper and lower extremities. Accurate examination of a patient with a spinal cord injury depends on understanding the reflex arc and the organization of motor and sensory elements.

Figure 25-2 presents a cross-sectional view of the spinal cord in the cervical region. The upper motor neuron, which originates in the cerebral cortex, crosses to the opposite side in the midbrain and then descends in the lateral corticospinal tract to synapse with its respective lower motor neuron in the anterior horn of the gray matter. The sacral fibers of the corticospinal tract are the most peripheral and the cervical fibers the most central (see Fig. 25-2). The lower motor neurons in the gray matter are organized with the extensor neurons anterior to the flexor neurons. Upper motor neurons not crossing in the midbrain descend in the smaller ventral corticospinal tract. The ascending sensory input originates in an axon from a cell body located in the dorsal root ganglion within the vertebral foramen. Sensory input enters the posterior horn of the gray matter and travels beyond, depending on the type of sensation. Pain and temperature sensations cross immediately to the opposite level of the cord and ascend in the lateral spinothalamic tract. Touch sensation also crosses immediately and ascends diffusely but is carried primarily in the ventral spinothalamic tract. Proprioceptive position and vibratory sensation fibers ascend in the posterior column (funiculus cuneatus, funiculus gracilis) and cross higher in the brainstem. The posterior column is structured with the sacral elements more peripheral and posterior relative to the lumbar, thoracic, and cervical levels. The reflex arc (Fig. 25-3; e.g., bulbocavernosus) is a simple sensory motor pathway that can function without using ascending or descending white matter long tract axons. If the level of the reflex arc is both physiologically and anatomically intact, the reflex can function despite disruption of the spinal cord at a higher level.

Below the level of the conus medullaris (L1-L2 interspace), the spinal canal is filled with the cauda equina, with the motor and sensory roots yet to exit their respective intervertebral foramina distally. These roots are less likely to be injured because they have more room within the canal and are not tethered to the same degree as is the spinal cord. Furthermore, the motor nerve root is the lower motor neuron axon (peripheral nerve), which is known to be more resilient to trauma than central nervous tissue.

PATHOPHYSIOLOGY OF SPINAL CORD INJURY

The pathophysiology of spinal cord injury can be divided into two parts: primary and secondary. Primary injury occurs at the moment of impact to the spine. When the energy transmitted to the spinal column musculature, ligaments, and osseous structures exceeds the flexibility of the spinal column, the spinal column and cord become injured. Primary injury to the spinal cord can develop in two ways: (1) direct injury by means of excessive flexion, extension, or rotation of the spinal cord and (2) indirect

Transverse view of the spinal cord in the cervical region. Note that the sacral structures (S) are most peripheral in the posterior columns and the lateral corticospinal tracts. The extensors are also more lateral than the flexors in the gray matter. C, cervical structures; L, lumbar structures; T, thoracic structures.

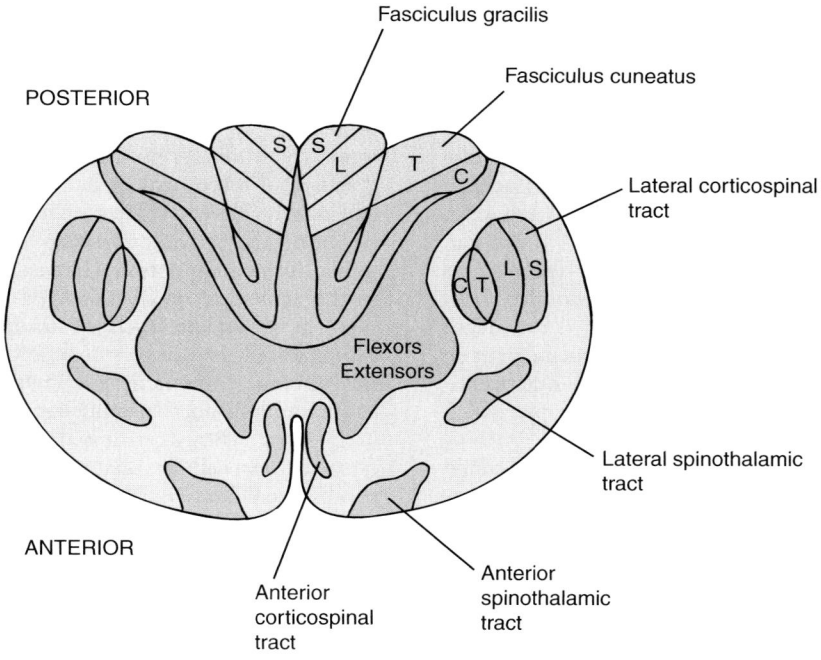

The bulbocavernosus, a reflex arc that is a simple sensorimotor pathway, can function without using ascending or descending white matter long tract axons.

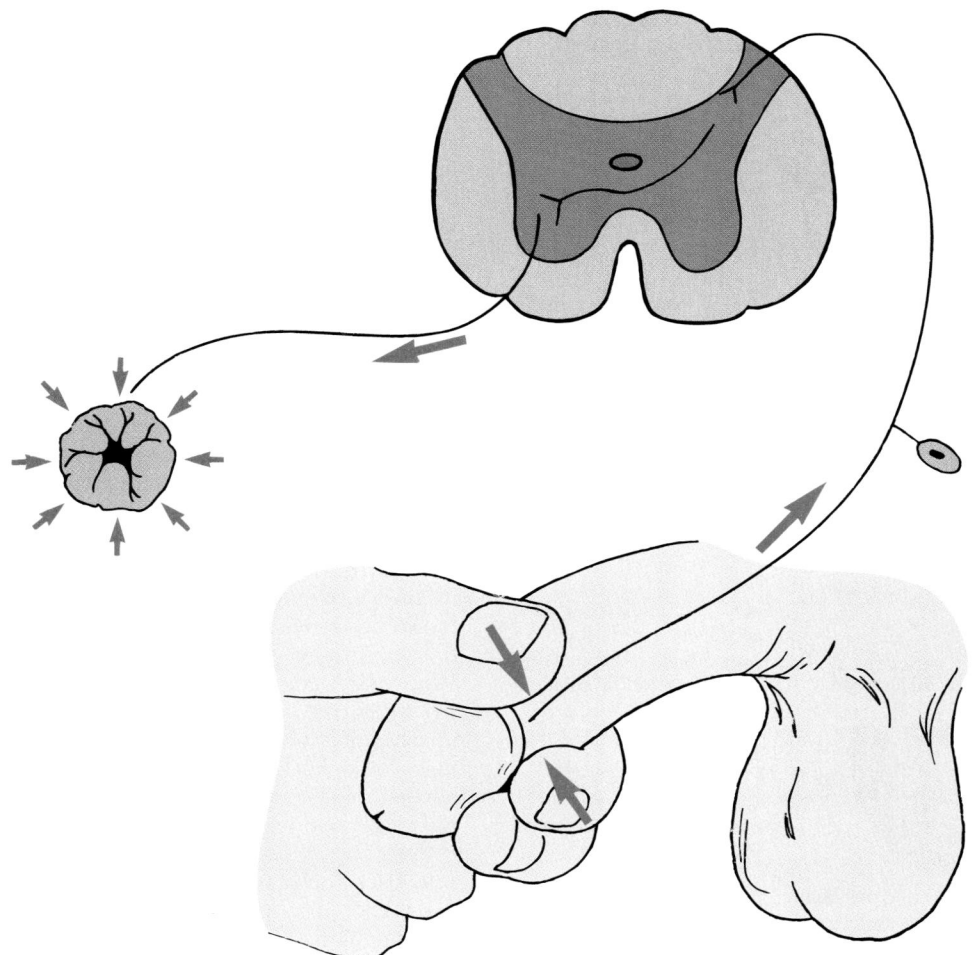

injury by impaction of displaced bone or disk material. Injury secondary to contusion and compression is most common and causes physiologic interruption rather than physical transection of the spinal cord.

Secondary injury to the spinal cord occurs after the initial direct injury to neural tissue. The complicated events that take place on a chemical, cellular, and tissue level are not completely understood, however (Fig. 25-4). The cascade is interrelated and eventually leads to cavitation, largely because of cell death (Fig. 25-5). Cell death can occur as a result of necrosis or apoptosis. Necrosis is brought on by cellular swelling and mitochondrial and membrane damage. Apoptosis is programmed cell death that occurs normally but is evident to a greater extent in spinal cord injury. Chromatin aggregation and intact cellular organelles can be seen by electron microscopy, which can differentiate between apoptosis and necrosis.[72]

Secondary injury is produced by various interrated pathophysiological mechanisms, which include inflammatory injury, excitotoxicity, apoptosis, free radical damage, and oxidative stress.[64a] The inflammatory response is initiated by neutrophils, which infiltrate the injury site and recruit other inflammatory cells. They produce cytokine such as Tumor Necrosis Factor (TNF) that can cause further tissue damage.[62a] As cells die they release

FIGURE 25-4 *An illustrated sequence of the progression from acute primary to late secondary injury. (From Lu, J.; Ashwell, K.W.; Waite, P. Advances in secondary spinal cord injury: Role of apoptosis. Spine 25:1859–1866, 2000.)*

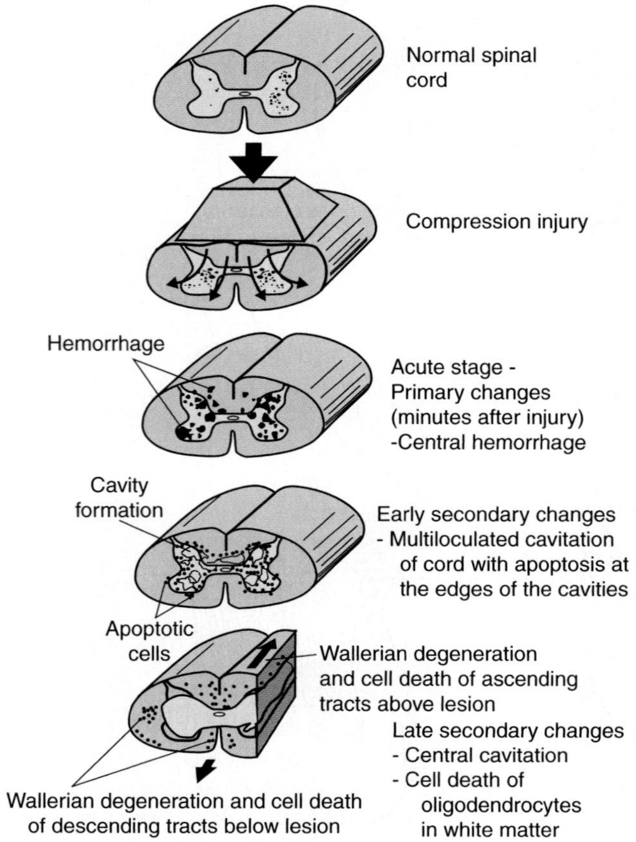

molecules that trigger cellular receptors that stimulate the generation of pro-inflammatory sources. This can lead to an elevation in the levels of excitatory amino acids, especially glutamate, which initiates a cascade called excitotoxicity. The excessive amount of glutamate causes an over-activation of N methyl D asparatate (NMDA) receptors, which results in too many calcium ions entering through the receptors ion channel.[71a] The excessive amount of calcium ions stimulates many other processes to occur including the activation of calpin, which has been shown to play a role in apoptosis. The excessive calcium also leads to the activation of several other intracellular messengers such as guanylate cyclase, arachidonic acid, increased expression of the proto-oncogene C-fos, and an increase in the number of free radicals,[23a] which disrupts normal processes and kills neurons and oligodendrocylotes. The action of the free radicals can initiate a progressive oxidation of fatty acids in cellular membranes such that the oxidation process generates more free radicals than can be moved across the cell membrane. The result of the oxidative stress is the disruption of organelle and nuclear proteins, which can lead to cell death and further injury.[64a]

Inflammatory mediators such as prostaglandins and cytotoxins are produced by inflammatory cells that enter the area of spinal cord damage through a break in the blood-brain barrier. Cytokines such as tumor necrosis factor-α can lead to damage to oligodendrocytes. Arachidonic acids break down to prostaglandins, and eicosanoids can lead to an increase in free radicals, vascular permeability, change in blood flow, and cell swelling.

The anatomic and morphologic changes in the spinal cord after injury have been well defined.[3,30,31] Within 30 minutes of injury, multiple petechial hemorrhages are seen within the central cord gray matter. Direct disruption of the myelin sheath and axoplasm is also seen. Over the course of 1 hour, these changes extend progressively to the posterior of the cord. Several hours after injury, the hemorrhages tend to coalesce, and progressive longitudinal necrosis is seen. Histologic and ultrastructural changes characteristic of edema are seen within 6 hours and are most severe 2 to 3 days after trauma. At 1 week after injury, cystic degeneration of the previously necrotic areas of the cord develops.

Clinically, progressive neurologic deterioration after the initial spinal cord injury is uncommon.[106] It is difficult to define a point in the anatomic injury cascade at which secondary injury factors become important, but the recent success of some pharmacologic agents directed at the agents of secondary injury implies that intervention is possible to some degree.

The initial mechanical injury disrupts neuronal activity in several ways. Microvascular endothelial damage and thrombus formation decrease local blood flow dramatically in the central gray matter without reperfusion. This effect is in contrast to the reperfusion that is frequently seen in the peripheral white matter at about 15 minutes after injury and that is probably induced by vasospasm. Primary injury also leads to altered systemic vascular tone and hypotension, thus worsening this probably reversible white matter hypoperfusion.

Relative cord ischemia can play a major role in the secondary metabolic derangements of nervous tissue. A decrease in membrane-bound sodium, potassium adenosine triphosphatase (N^+,K^+-ATPase) causes severe alterations

FIGURE 25-5 *Pathways involved in cell death after spinal cord injury. (From Lu, J.; Ashwell, K.W.; Waite, P. Advances in secondary spinal cord injury: Role of apoptosis. Spine 25:1859–1866, 2000.)*

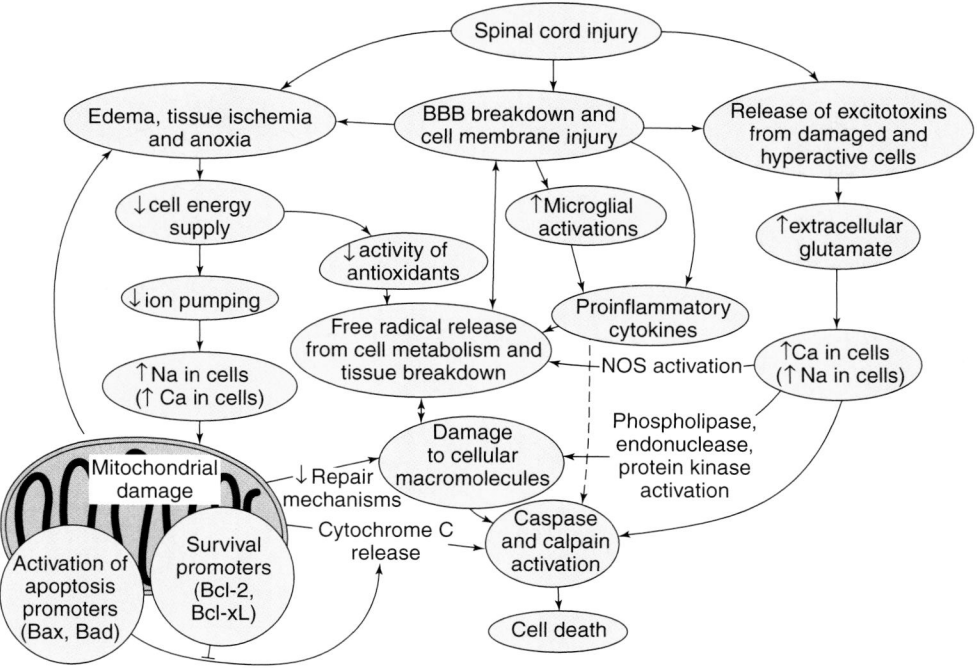

in the product of high-energy phosphorylation and the subsequent lactic acidosis. Abnormalities in electrolyte concentration are believed to be associated with abnormal axonal conduction. Membrane damage and direct damage to intracellular organelles cause severe derangements in calcium homeostasis. Large intracellular shifts of calcium (Ca^{2+}) induce further mitochondrial dysfunction with decreased energy production and eventual cell death. Uncontrolled influx of Ca^{2+} leads to the activation of phospholipases A_2 and C, thereby resulting in accelerated breakdown of cellular membranes and the production of arachidonic acid and free radicals.[59] Many recent advances in the treatment of acute spinal cord injuries have attacked this secondary injury cascade at various levels, with varying degrees of success.

SPINAL CORD REGENERATION

The promotion of regeneration of spinal cord axons after injury so that the cord again becomes functional is a monumental challenge that has been approached in many ways. The use of neurotrophic factors such as nerve growth factor, brain-derived neurotrophic factor, neurotrophic factor 3, and ciliary neurotrophic factor has been shown to be helpful in vitro in regenerating axons. Delivery of these factors by cells programmed to secrete them has helped in long-term release directly inside the central nervous system (CNS) so that they do not also have to cross the blood-brain barrier. Growth-inhibiting factors have been identified that may inhibit axonal regeneration in the CNS. Antibodies to these factors increase the regeneration of axons.[97] Electrical stimulation has also been shown to effect axonal growth, but the exact mechanism is unclear.

Peripheral nerve and Schwann cell transplants have shown the ability to lead to regeneration of motor pathways.[23,51] Fetal spinal cord tissue has been successfully

transplanted in neonates. Considerable functional recovery along with growth and regeneration of the cells has been observed.[21,116] Similar success has not occurred with transplantation in adults. Transplantation of olfactory glial cells, which appear to continue to divide in adulthood, has been reported to regenerate corticospinal tracts in an adult rat.[70]

Classification of Neurologic Injury

An initial responsibility of the examining physician in evaluating a patient with a spinal cord injury is to determine the extent of neurologic deficit. A patient with an incomplete neurologic deficit has a good prognosis for at least some functional motor recovery, whereas functional motor recovery is seen in only 3 percent of those with complete injuries in the first 24 hours after injury and never after 24 to 48 hours.[12,108] According to the Standards for Neurological Classification published by the American Spinal Injury Association (ASIA), a complete injury is one in which no "motor and/or sensory function exists more than three segments below the neurological level of injury."[5] Likewise, an incomplete injury is one in which some neurologic function exists more than three segments below the level of injury. Critical to this determination is the definition of level of injury. The ASIA defines it as the most caudal segment that tests intact for motor and sensory functions on both sides of the body. A muscle is considered intact if it has at least antigravity power (grade 3 out of 5) and if the next most cephalic level is graded 4 or 5.[5] These definitions can make determination of completeness of an injury somewhat difficult. At least one study has found the simple presence or absence of sacral nerve root function to be a more stable and reliable indicator of the completeness of an injury.[118]

The concept of sacral sparing in an incomplete spinal cord injury is important because it represents at least partial

FIGURE 25-6 | *Sacral sparing may include perianal sensation, rectal tone, and great toe flexion.*

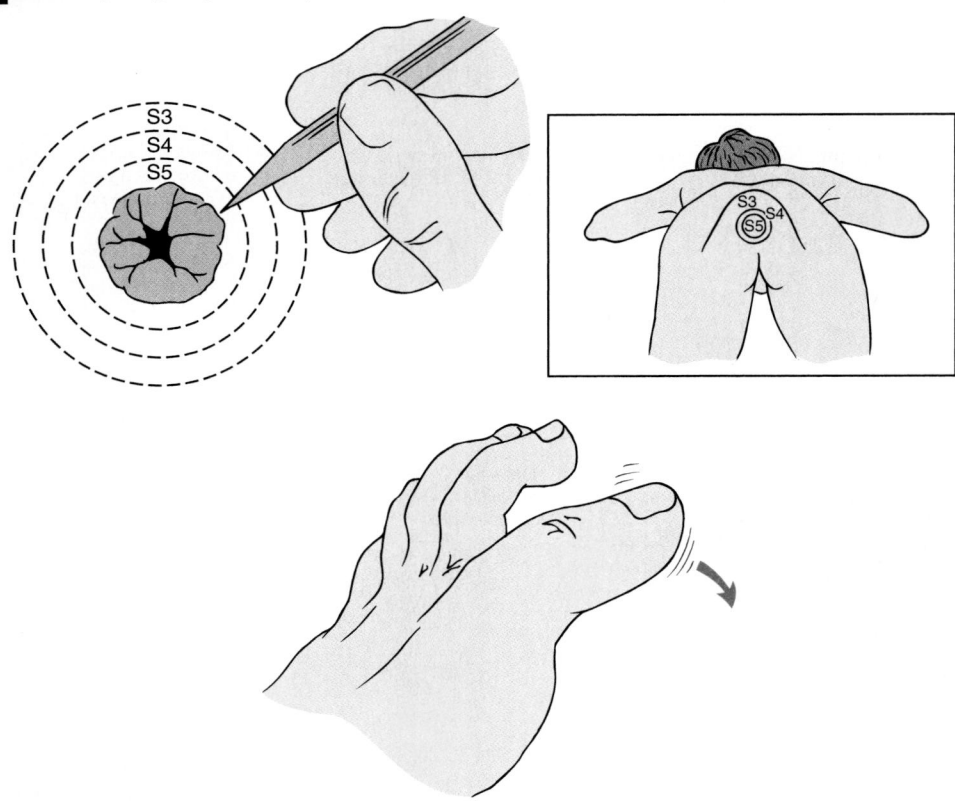

structural continuity of the white matter long tracts (i.e., corticospinal and spinothalamic tracts). Sacral sparing is demonstrated by perianal sensation, rectal motor function, and great toe flexor activity (Fig. 25-6). Electrical detection of sacral sparing by dermatomal somatosensory potentials has been reported but is not in common use.[99] Comparison of the normal anatomy in Figure 25-2 with that of the injury depicted in Figure 25-7A reveals how preservation of only the sacral white matter is possible. Sacral sparing is defined as continued function of the sacral lower motor neurons in the conus medullaris and their connections through the spinal cord to the cerebral cortex. The presence of sacral sparing therefore indicates an incomplete cord injury and the potential for more function after the resolution of spinal shock. At the time of physical examination in the emergency department, sacral sparing may be the only sign that a lesion is incomplete; documentation of its presence or absence is essential. Waters and coauthors[118] found that the presence of external anal sphincter or toe flexor muscle power or the presence of perineal sensation accurately predicted the completeness of injury in 97 percent of 445 consecutive patients. In addition, for prognostic purposes, no patients with initial sacral sparing were found to have had complete injuries.

After a severe spinal cord injury, a state of complete spinal areflexia can develop and last for a varying length of time. This state, conventionally termed *spinal shock,* is classically evaluated by testing the bulbocavernosus reflex, a spinal reflex mediated by the S3-S4 region of the conus medullaris (see Fig. 25-3). This reflex is frequently absent for the first 4 to 6 hours after injury but usually returns within 24 hours. If no evidence of spinal cord function is noted below the level of the injury, including sacral

sparing, and the bulbocavernosus reflex has not returned, no determination can be made regarding the completeness of the lesion. After 24 hours, 99 percent of patients emerge from spinal shock, as heralded by the return of sacral reflexes.[107] If no sacral function exists at this point, the injury is termed *complete,* and 99 percent of patients with complete injuries will have no functional recovery.[107] One exception to this dictum is an injury to the distal end of the spinal cord itself. A direct injury to the conus medullaris can disrupt the bulbocavernosus reflex arc and thus make its absence an unreliable indicator of spinal shock.

CLASSIFICATION SYSTEMS

After a determination of its completeness, an injury can be further classified according to the severity of the remaining paralysis. Classification systems are useful because they allow patient outcomes to be compared within and between clinical studies. The most commonly used classification system is that of Frankel and colleagues,[39] which divides spinal cord injuries into five groups (Table 25-1). The ASIA has put forth the Motor Index Score, which uses a standard six-grade scale to measure the manual muscle strength of 10 key muscles or functions in the upper and lower extremities (Fig. 25-8). All the individual muscle groups, both right and left, are measured, with a possible maximal score of 100. The disadvantage of the Frankel score is that an infinite continuum of injury severity is divided into five discrete groups. However, because recovery and repair of injured neural tissue must occur through the injury site for an injury to move to a higher grade, improvement by one Frankel grade, especially

FIGURE 25-7 **A,** *This illustration of a central cord syndrome can be compared with Figure 25-2 to appreciate the spinal cord abnormality. An incomplete spinal injury can affect the more central but not the peripheral fibers, thereby preserving the sacral white fibers.* **B,** *Anterior cord syndrome. The dorsal columns are spared, so that the patient retains some deep pressure sensation and proprioception over the sacral area and lower extremities.* **C,** *Posterior cord syndrome, a very rare traumatic lesion with clinical features similar to those of tabes dorsalis.* **D,** *Brown-Séquard syndrome, also known as hemisection syndrome. Patients have motor paralysis on the ipsilateral side distal to the lesion and sensory hypoesthesia on the contralateral side distal to the level of the lesion. C, cervical structures; L, lumbar structures; S, sacral structures; T, thoracic structures.*

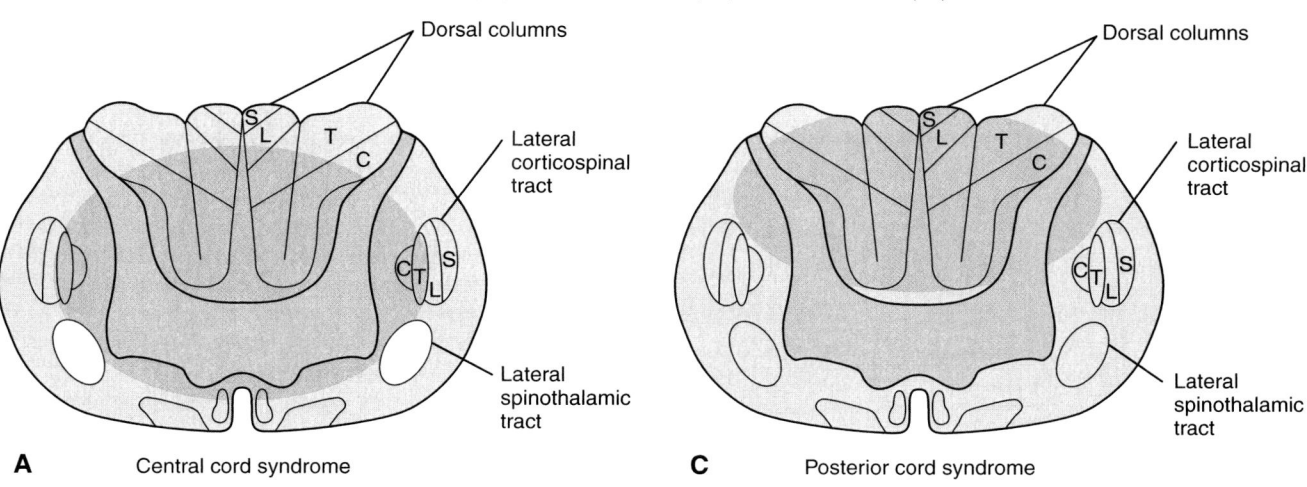

A   Central cord syndrome   **C**   Posterior cord syndrome

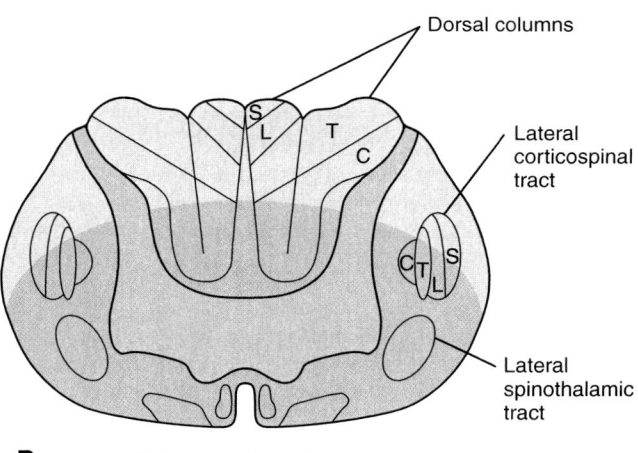

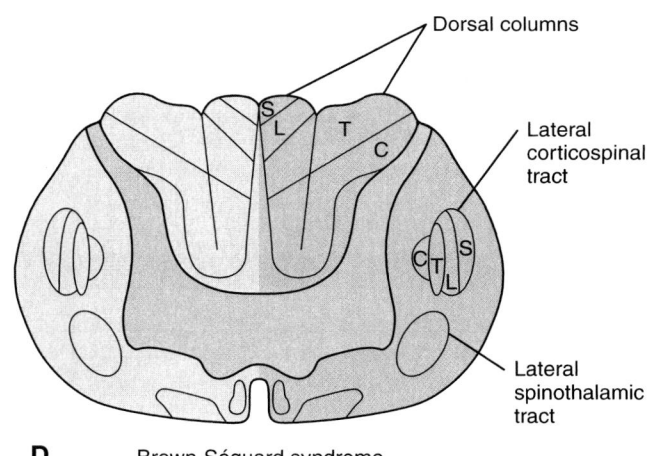

B   Anterior cord syndrome   **D**   Brown-Séquard syndrome

Table 25-1		
Frankel Classification of Neurologic Deficit		
Type	**Characteristics**	
A	Absent motor and sensory function	
B	Sensation present, motor function absent	
C	Sensation present, motor function active but not useful (grades 2/5 to 3/5)	
D	Sensation present, motor function active and useful (grade 4/5)	
E	Normal motor and sensory function	

improvement by two grades, is functionally quite significant. On the other hand, the ASIA Motor Index Score represents injuries along a continuum, but an improvement does not necessarily represent recovery in the injured spinal segment. Instead, the improved score may represent recovery in the most caudal level of function in a complete injury or a generalized recovery of motor strength in previously weak but functioning muscles.

INCOMPLETE SPINAL CORD INJURY SYNDROMES

If an incomplete spinal cord injury is diagnosed by the protocols discussed, it can usually be described by one of several syndromes (Table 25-2). As a general rule, the greater the function distal to the injury, the faster the recovery and the better the prognosis.[73]

FIGURE 25-8 | *The worksheet for the American Spinal Injury Association (ASIA) Motor Index Score. The motor strengths for the 10 muscles on the left side of the worksheet are graded on a scale of 0 to 5. All scores are added, for a total maximal score of 100. (Copyright, American Spinal Injury Association, from International Standards for Neurological and Functional Classification, Revised 1996.)*

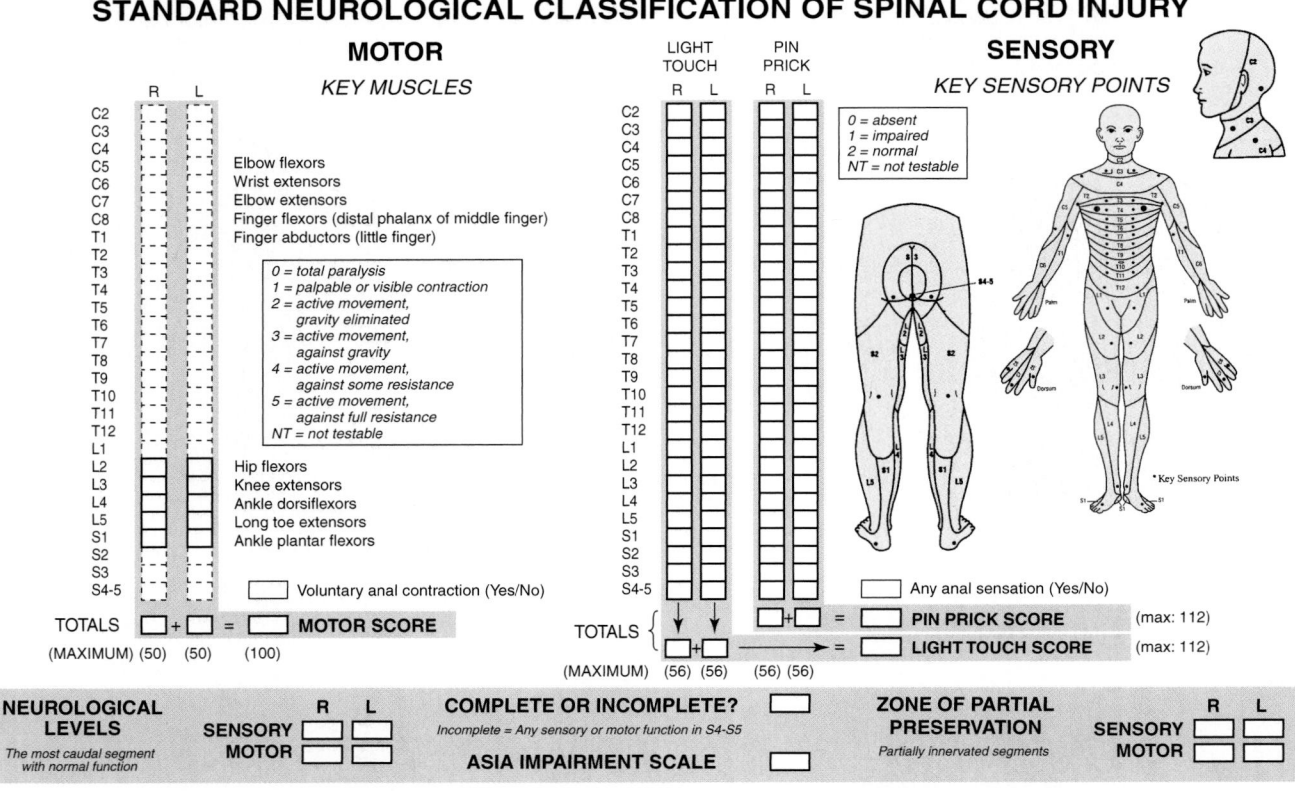

STANDARD NEUROLOGICAL CLASSIFICATION OF SPINAL CORD INJURY

Table 25-2
Incomplete Cord Syndromes

Syndrome	Frequency	Description	Functional Recovery (%)
Central	Most common	Usually quadriplegic, with sacral sparing; upper extremities affected more than lower	75
Anterior	Common	Complete motor deficit; trunk and lower extremity deep pressure and proprioception preserved	10
Posterior	Rare	Loss of deep pressure, deep pain, and proprioception	
Brown-Séquard	Uncommon	Ipsilateral motor deficit; contralateral pain and temperature deficit	>90
Root	Common	Motor and sensory deficit in dermatomal distribution	30–100

CENTRAL CORD SYNDROME Central cord syndrome, the most common pattern of injury, represents central gray matter destruction with preservation of only the peripheral spinal cord structures, the sacral spinothalamic and corticospinal tracts (see Fig. 25-7A). The patient usually presents as a quadriplegic with perianal sensation and has an early return of bowel and bladder control. Any return of motor function usually begins with the sacral elements (toe flexors, then the extensors), followed by the lumbar elements of the ankle, knee, and hip. Upper extremity functional return is generally minimal and is limited by the degree of central gray matter destruction. The chance of some functional motor recovery has been reported to be about 75 percent.[109]

ANTERIOR CORD SYNDROME A patient with anterior cord syndrome has complete motor and sensory loss, with the exception of retained trunk and lower extremity deep pressure sensation and proprioception.[98] This syndrome carries the worst prognosis for return of function, and only a 10 percent chance of functional motor recovery has been reported (see Fig. 25-7B).[108]

POSTERIOR CORD SYNDROME Posterior cord syndrome is a rare syndrome consisting of loss of the sensations of deep pressure and deep pain and proprioception, with otherwise normal cord function. The patient ambulates with a foot-slapping gait similar to that of someone afflicted with tabes dorsalis (see Fig. 25-7C).

BROWN–SÉQUARD SYNDROME Brown–Séquard syndrome is anatomically a unilateral cord injury, such as a missile injury (see Fig. 25-7D). It is clinically characterized by a motor deficit ipsilateral to the spinal cord injury in combination with contralateral pain and temperature hypoesthesia. Almost all these patients show partial recovery, and most regain bowel and bladder function and the ability to ambulate.[109]

ROOT INJURY The spinal nerve root can be injured along with the spinal cord at that level, or an isolated neurologic deficit of the nerve root can occur. The prognosis for motor recovery is favorable, with approximately 75 percent of patients with complete spinal cord injuries showing no root deficit at the level of injury or experiencing return of function.[108] Those with higher cervical injuries have a 30 percent chance of recovery of one nerve root level, those with midcervical injuries have a 60 percent chance, and almost all patients with low cervical fractures have recovery of at least one nerve root level.[109]

MANAGEMENT

Accident Scene Management

The initial evaluation of any trauma patient begins at the scene of the accident with the time-honored ABCs of resuscitation, such as the advanced trauma life support (ATLS) method described by the American College of Surgeons.[1] The ABC (airway, breathing, and circulation) method can be described more accurately as A (airway), B (breathing), and C (circulation and cervical spine). All patients with potential spine injuries arriving at the emergency department should be on a backboard with the cervical spine immobilized. A spinal column injury should be considered in all polytrauma patients, especially those who are unconscious or intoxicated and those who have head and neck injuries. Suspicion of a spine injury must begin at the accident scene so that an organized extrication and transport plan can be developed to minimize further injury to neural tissue.

Regardless of the position in which found, the patient should be placed in a neutral spine position with respect to the long axis of the body. This position is achieved by carefully placing one hand behind the neck and the other under the jaw and applying only gentle stabilizing traction.[49] An emergency two-piece cervical collar is then applied before extrication from the accident scene. Any patient wearing a helmet at the time of injury should arrive at the emergency department with it still in place unless a face shield that cannot be removed separately from the helmet is obstructing ventilation, a loose-fitting helmet is preventing adequate cervical spine immobilization, or the paramedic has been trained in helmet removal.[4] A scoop-style stretcher is now recommended for transfer; previously recommended maneuvers such as the four-man lift and the log roll have been shown to cause an excessive amount of motion at thoracolumbar fracture sites.[77] The victim on a scoop stretcher is then placed immediately onto a rigid full-length backboard and secured with sandbags on either side of the head and neck and the forehead taped to the backboard.[86] The method of transportation and initial destination are determined by a multitude of factors, including but not limited to the medical stability of the patient, distance to emergency centers, weather conditions, and the availability of resources. Vale and colleagues[117] have shown that keeping the mean blood pressure above 85 mm Hg results in a better neurologic outcome.

Resuscitation

Patients with spinal injuries are frequently the victims of major trauma and as such are at high risk for multiple injuries. Experience with such patients has documented a clear relationship between head and facial trauma and cervical spine injuries and between specific intrathoracic and abdominal injuries and thoracolumbar fractures. The evaluation and management of hypotension in these multiply injured patients have been the subject of much discussion. Although hemorrhage and hypovolemia are significant causes of hypotension, one must be aware of the syndrome of neurogenic shock in patients with cervical and high thoracic spinal cord injuries. Neurogenic shock is defined as vascular hypotension plus bradycardia occurring as a result of spinal injury. In the first few minutes after spinal cord injury, a systemic pressor response occurs through activation of the adrenal medulla. This state of hypertension, widened pulse pressure, and tachycardia subsequently gives way to a drop in pressure and pulse. Neurogenic shock is attributed to the traumatic disruption of sympathetic outflow (T1-L2) and to unopposed vagal tone, with resultant hypotension and bradycardia.[50,85]

Hypotension with associated tachycardia is not caused by neurogenic shock, so another cause must be sought. A review of 228 patients with cervical spine injury revealed that 40 (69%) of 58 patients with systolic blood pressure lower than 100 mm Hg had neurogenic shock.[103] The remaining 18 patients had hypotension caused by other associated major injuries. Another study demonstrated that victims of blunt trauma with associated cervical spinal cord injury rarely sustain significant intra-abdominal injuries (2.6%).[2] Nonetheless, hemodynamic instability strongly suggested occult intra-abdominal injuries. The degree of hypotension and bradycardia and the incidence of cardiac arrest are directly related to the Frankel grade. For example, in a study of 45 patients with acute cervical spinal cord injury, 87 percent of Frankel A patients had a daily average pulse rate lower than 55 beats per minute, 21 percent had a cardiac arrest, and 39 percent required the administration of atropine or a vasopressor. Among the Frankel B patients, 62 percent had average pulses lower than 55 beats per minute, and none had cardiac arrest or needed vasopressors.[85]

A more recent study demonstrated that spinal cord injury secondary to penetrating trauma is distinctly different from that caused by blunt trauma with respect to the origin of hypotension.[119] Penetrating injuries rarely result in neurogenic shock. Of 75 patients with a penetrating spinal cord injury, only 5 (7%) showed classic signs of neurogenic shock, and of the patients in whom hypotension developed, only 22 percent were found to have a neurogenic origin of their shock. As in all patients with major trauma, hypotension should be assumed to be caused by an injury involving major blood loss, especially in those with penetrating trauma.[119]

Whatever the cause of the hypotension, support of blood pressure is critical in the early hours after spinal cord injury. As described previously, localized spinal cord ischemia is an important cause of late neurologic disability. As the injured spinal cord loses its ability to autoregulate local blood flow, it is critically dependent on systemic arterial pressure.[32] Hypotension needs to be aggressively treated by blood and volume replacement and, if indicated, by emergency surgery for life-threatening hemorrhage and appropriate management of neurogenic shock. The initial treatment of neurogenic shock is volume replacement, followed by vasopressors if hypotension without tachycardia persists despite volume expansion. The patient's legs should be elevated to counteract venous pooling in the extremities. Fatal pulmonary edema can result from overinfusion of a hypotensive patient with a spinal cord injury.[50] Endotracheal suctioning is a cause of severe bradycardia and can induce cardiac arrest, which is attributed to vagal stimulation. Repeated doses of atropine may be necessary to maintain the heart rate, and vasopressors may be necessary to maintain blood pressure. Use of a gentle sympathomimetic agent (e.g., phenylephrine) may also be helpful.

Assessment

After the patient arrives at the emergency department, rapid assessment of life-threatening conditions and emergency treatment are begun in a logical, sequential manner as dictated by the ATLS protocols.[1] The primary survey includes assessment of airway, breathing, circulation, disability (neurologic status), and exposure (undress the patient) (ABCDE). As resuscitation (described earlier) is initiated, a secondary survey is begun that includes evaluation of spinal column and spinal cord function. The evaluation usually starts with a physical examination, with a more detailed history elicited later. The only part of the initial assessment that absolutely pertains to the spine is the emergency need for a lateral cervical spine radiograph (from the occiput to the superior end plate of T1) to establish the safest means of maintaining an airway. A patient thought to have a spine injury should, before intubation, have the airway maintained with a jaw thrust maneuver rather than a head tilt method.

An unconscious or intoxicated patient is difficult to assess in terms of pain and motor sensory function. Careful observation of spontaneous extremity motion may be the only information that can be obtained about spinal cord function, and a detailed examination may have to be delayed until the patient can cooperate. An unconscious patient's response to noxious stimuli and the patient's reflexes and rectal tone can provide some information on the status of the cord. Similarly, spontaneous respirations with elevation and separation of the costal margins on inspiration indicate normal thoracic innervation and intercostal function. Unconscious patients should be rolled onto their side with the cervical spine immobilized while on a full-length backboard, and the entire length of the spine should be inspected for deformity, abrasions, and ecchymosis. The spine should be palpated for a stepoff or interspinous widening.

The locations of lacerations and abrasions on the skull are critical for determination of cervical injuries. Occipital lacerations suggest flexion injuries, whereas frontal or superior injuries suggest extension or axial compression, respectively. The presence of a single spinal injury does not preclude inspection of the rest of the spine.

Any associated head and neck trauma should increase the suspicion of cervical spine injury, and any thoracic or abdominal trauma (e.g., shoulder or lap seat belt markings) should raise suspicion of a thoracolumbar spine injury. Clear patterns of associated injuries should be recognized. For example, in addition to the relationship between head trauma and cervical spine injury, the presence of multiple fractured ribs and chest trauma can suggest thoracic spine injury. Massive pelvic injuries are frequently associated with flexion–distraction injuries of the lumbar spine. Finally, falls from heights resulting in calcaneal or tibial plafond fractures are frequently associated with injuries to the lumbar spine.

A responsive patient who is hemodynamically stable can be examined in greater detail. Inspection and palpation of the entire spine should be performed as described for an unconscious patient. The patient should be asked to report the location of any pain and to move the upper and lower extremities to help localize any gross neurologic deficit. If possible, the patient should be questioned about the mechanism of injury, any transient neurologic symptoms or signs, and any preexisting neurologic signs or symptoms. The upper (Fig. 25-9) and lower (Fig. 25-10) extremities are examined for motor function by nerve root level. The motor examination includes a digital rectal examination for voluntary or reflex (bulbocavernosus) anal sphincter contraction.

The sensory examination includes testing of the dermatomal pattern of the proprioceptive and pain temperature pathways, as described previously (Fig. 25-11). The sharp-dull sensation of a pin tip is considered to reflect a pain pathway (lateral spinothalamic tract), and this sensation should also be tested in the perianal region. The presence of pin-prick sensation around the anus or perineal region may be the only evidence of an incomplete lesion. Proprioception (posterior columns) can be tested easily by having the patient report the position of the toes as up, down, or neutral as the examiner moves them. Temperature sensation (lateral spinothalamic tract) is difficult to establish in the often loud and busy emergency department setting, and testing for this function is usually deferred until a later time. The areas of sensory deficit should be accurately recorded, dated, and timed on the medical record progress note or a spinal injury flow sheet. It is also recommended that the sensory level be marked, dated, and timed in ink on the patient's skin at the affected level. The practice of marking the sensory level on the skin can avoid much uncertainty when a number of examiners are involved.

Figure 25-12 reviews the locations of the upper and lower extremity stretch reflexes and their nerve roots of origin. If spinal shock is present, all reflexes may be absent for up to 24 hours, only to be replaced by hyper-reflexia, muscle spasticity, and clonus. If a spine injury patient with a neurologic deficit has a concomitant head injury, it is important to distinguish between the cranial upper motor neuron lesion and a spinal cord lower motor neuron injury. The presence of extremity stretch reflexes in a patient without spontaneous motion of the extremities or a

FIGURE 25-9 *An examination of the upper extremities must include, at a minimum, the muscle groups that are designated by their respective nerve root innervation. These are C5, elbow flexion; C6, wrist extension; C7, finger extension; C8, finger flexion; and T1, finger abduction. The strength (0 to 5) should be listed on the time-oriented flow sheet.*

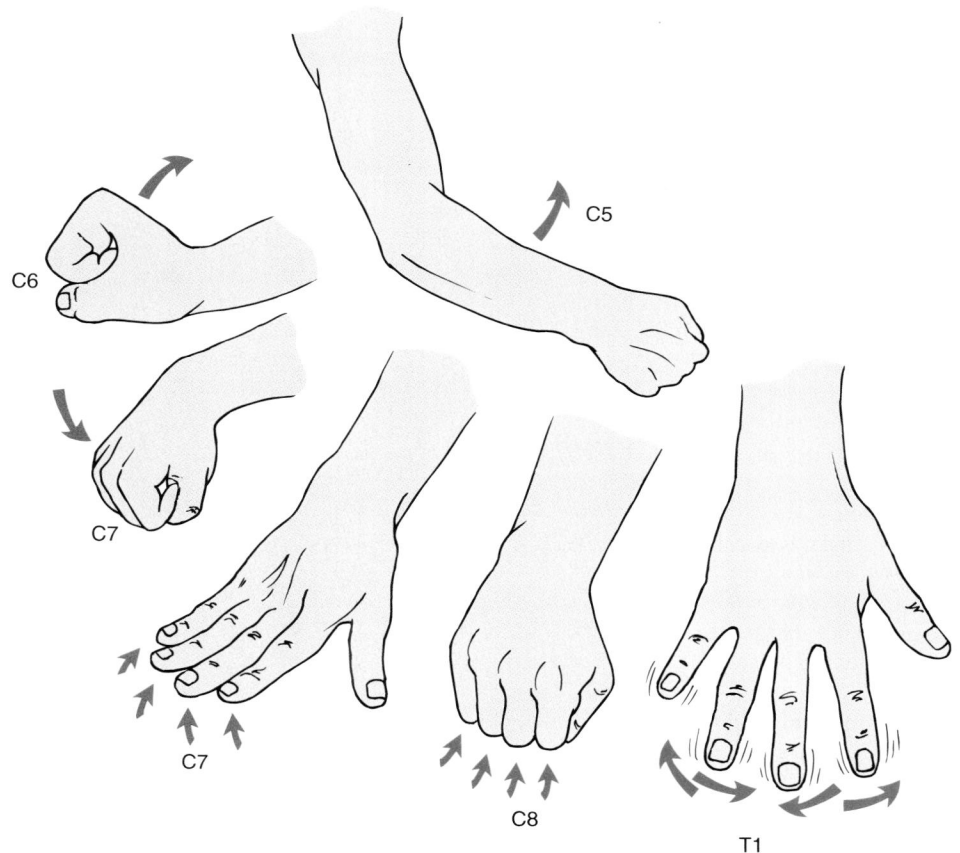

response to noxious stimuli implies an upper motor neuron lesion. The absence of these reflexes in the same setting implies lower motor neuron injury of the spinal cord.

The plantar reflex in the lower extremity is elicited by stroking the plantar aspect of the foot firmly with a pointed object and watching the direction of motion of the toes. A normal plantar reflex is plantar flexion of the toes. An abnormal plantar reflex (Babinski's sign), in which the great toe extends and the toes splay out, represents an upper motor neuron lesion. Similar information can be obtained by running a finger firmly down the tibial crest; abnormal great toe extension with splaying of the toes (Oppenheim's sign) constitutes evidence of an upper motor neuron lesion.

Other significant reflexes include the cremasteric, the anal wink, and the bulbocavernosus reflexes. The cremasteric reflex (T12-L1) in the male is elicited by stroking the proximal aspect of the inner part of the thigh with a pointed instrument and observing the scrotal sac. A normal reflex involves contraction of the cremasteric muscle and an upward motion of the scrotal sac, whereas an abnormal reflex involves no motion of the sac. The anal wink (S2, S3, S4) is elicited by stroking the skin around the anal sphincter and watching it contract normally; an

abnormal reflex involves no contraction. The bulbocavernosus (S3, S4) reflex (see Fig. 25-3) is obtained by squeezing the glans penis (in a male) or applying pressure to the clitoris (in a female) and feeling the anal sphincter contract around a gloved finger. This response can usually be elicited more easily by gently pulling the Foley catheter balloon against the bladder wall and feeling the anal sphincter contract. The bulbocavernosus reflex examination in a catheterized female can be misleading; the Foley balloon can be pulled up against the bladder wall and thus be felt by a fingertip that is past the anal sphincter, with this response being misinterpreted as contraction of the anal sphincter.

Not uncommonly, a more detailed history is delayed until the patient is hemodynamically stable and the overall neurologic status can be determined. In addition to a routine review of systems, the patient should be specifically questioned regarding previous spine injury, previous neurologic deficit, and details of the mechanism of injury. If the patient cannot respond, an attempt should be made to interview family members in person or by telephone.

At some time during the physical examination, the initial lateral cervical spine radiograph should be available

FIGURE 25-10   *An examination of the lower extremities needs to include at least these muscle groups, designated by their respective nerve root innervation: L1-L2, hip abductors; L3-L4, knee extension; L5-S1, knee flexion; L5, great toe extension; and S1, great toe flexion.*

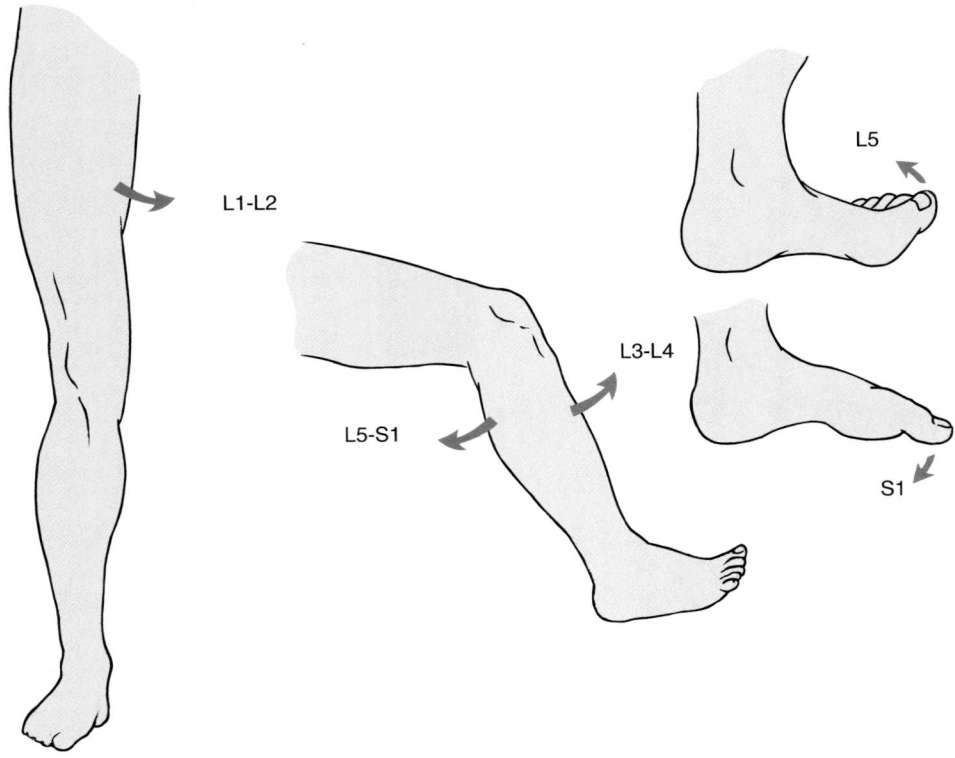

for review. It should first be examined to ensure that the interval from the occiput to the superior end plate of T1 can be seen clearly. If the radiographic appearance is normal, the remainder of the cervical spine series is obtained. Interpretation of the film is discussed in Chapter 26. Under no circumstances should spine precautions be removed until the cervical spine and any suspicious areas of the thoracolumbar spine have been cleared radiographically. In the assessment of a polytraumatized patient, the association between thoracolumbar fractures and other high-energy internal injuries (i.e., aortic and hollow viscus injuries) must be kept in mind. Because these patients' thoracolumbar spines cannot be cleared of injury on clinical grounds, anteroposterior and lateral thoracic and lumbar spine films should be obtained on a routine basis. In addition, the 10 percent incidence of noncontiguous fractures must be kept in mind in a patient with multiple injuries.[61] For example, the presence of a thoracolumbar burst fracture requires review of a complete plain radiographic series of the cervical, thoracic, and lumbar spine in any patient who is unable to fully cooperate or accurately report pain during the physical examination.

Special Studies

After the initial cross-table lateral cervical spine radiograph, a complete cervical spine series should be obtained. Several studies have reported that a technically adequate radiographic series consisting of a cross-table lateral view, an anteroposterior view, and an open-mouth odontoid view is almost 100 percent sensitive for detecting cervical injuries.[29] In the trauma situation, it can be difficult to see the atlantoaxial articulation and the cervicothoracic junction, so additional studies may be needed. A limited computed tomographic (CT) scan through the C7 to T1 levels can rule out significant cervicothoracic junction injuries; however, most studies have shown such imaging to have very low yield. In addition, CT may be required to clear the C1-C2 levels if plain radiographs are equivocal.[94] In an awake, conversant patient, the physical examination can be used to guide further imaging studies. Numerous studies have demonstrated the occurrence of concomitant spinal fractures.[61] Therefore, if a cervical fracture is identified, especially in a patient with a spinal cord lesion, radiographs of the entire thoracic and lumbar spine are indicated.

Magnetic resonance imaging (MRI) has found an increasing role in the evaluation of patients with spine injuries. In a patient who has a clinical spinal cord injury and minimal or no bony or ligamentous injury on other imaging studies, MRI is useful for the identification of soft tissue (ligamentous or disk) injuries, as well as abnormalities of the spinal cord itself. Findings on MRI have been shown to have some prognostic significance with respect to the severity of spinal cord injury and neurologic recovery.[55,83] In children, the syndrome of spinal cord injury without radiographic abnormality (SCIWORA) has been

FIGURE 25-11 *Sensory dermatome chart. Note that C4 includes the upper chest just superior to T2.*

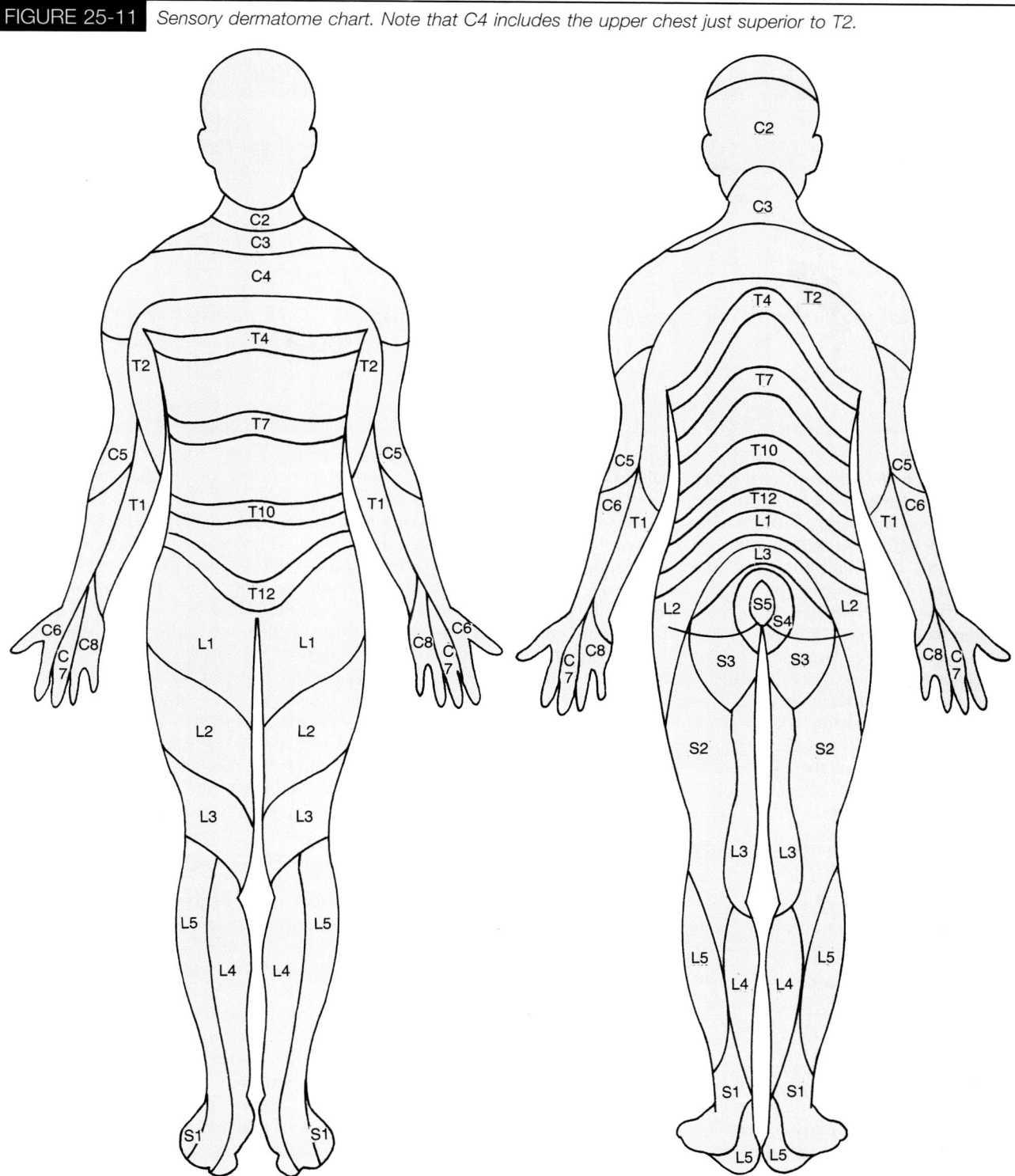

described,[8,56] and more recently, the use of MRI to better define these injuries has proved useful.[48] MRI has found an important role in the evaluation of intervertebral disks in cervical dislocations[35,91] (see later discussion and ligamentous description[66]).

Transportation of a cervical spine injury patient in skull traction can be done safely with the patient in a hospital bed, on a gurney, or in a Stryker frame, as long as a traction pulley unit is used. The use of a Stryker frame has been associated with loss of reduction after turning and with worsening of neurologic deficits, especially in those with lumbar spine injuries.[75,102] Traction can be compromised while the patient lies on the radiographic table and the rope hangs over the table edge without the use

FIGURE 25-12 *Stretch reflexes and nerve roots of origin.*

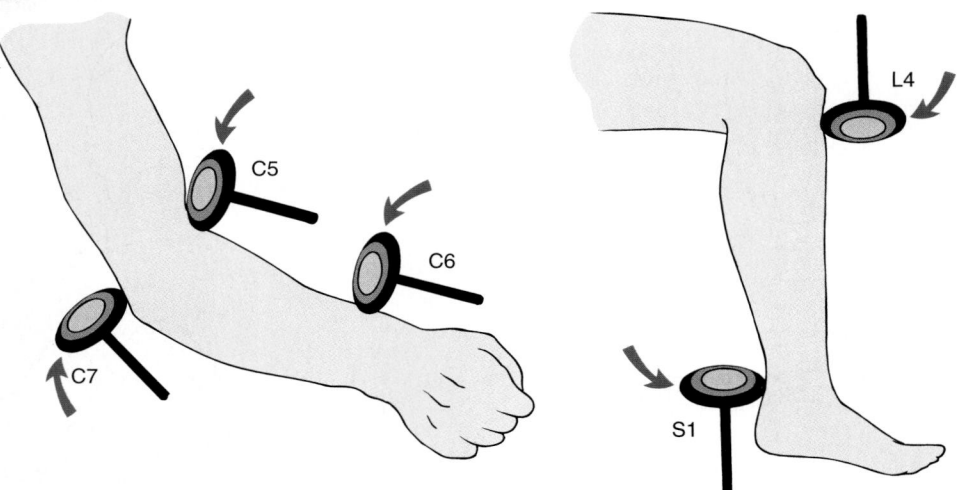

of a pulley. Disturbance of the magnetic field of MRI by the ferrous elements of traction equipment presents a problem, but solutions are being sought. A traction system has been described in which nonferrous zinc pulleys are bolted to an aluminum ladder with water traction bags attached to the halo ring by nylon traction rope.[76] A patient with a high cervical spine injury and dependence on a ventilator who needs MRI studies must be ventilated by hand or with a nonferrous ventilator.[80] A patient with a thoracolumbar spine injury is easier to manage because plastic construction backboards can now be used during conventional radiographic and MRI studies. Experimental in-board traction sets can allow transport of cervical cord injury patients without the danger of free weights.

Intervention

Once a spine-injured patient is resuscitated adequately, the mainstay of treatment is prevention of further injury to an already compromised cord and protection of uninjured cord tissue. Realignment and immobilization of the spinal column remain critical to this end. Other life-threatening issues in a multiply injured trauma patient may take precedence over time-consuming interventions related to the spine. Perhaps the most rapidly evolving interventions toward limiting the degree of neurologic injury have been pharmacologic.

PHARMACOLOGIC INTERVENTION

Pharmacologic intervention in an effort to improve the outcomes in spinal cord injury patients has been increasingly utilized over the last 20 years. In fact the efficacy of glucocorticoids for this purpose has been studied since the mid-1960s. In animal studies, high doses of methyl prednisolone (MPS) given intravenously after spinal cord injury has been shown to lessen the degree of post-traumatic lipid peroxidation and ischemia, prevent neuronal degradation, and allow improved neurologic recovery.[52,53] The initial National Acute Spinal Cord Injury Study (NASCIS I) attempted to work out an appropriate dosage for MPS but failed to show a difference in outcome between patients who received a 100 mg bolus per day for 10 days and those who received 1000 mg/day for 10 days. In fact, the

high dose regimen was associated with an increased risk of complications.[16]

A second multicenter randomized trial compared MPS, naloxone, and placebo. The results of NASCIS II completed in 1990 showed that patients who were treated with MPS within 8 hours of injury had improved neurologic recovery at one year, regardless of whether their injury was complete or incomplete.[18,19] Naloxone treatment was no better than placebo. When MPS was given sometime after 8 hours postinjury, patients recovered less function than did placebo patients and this paradoxical result caused some to question the overall results of the study. A predictable trend toward increased complications was seen in the steroid group including a twofold higher incidence of wound infection (7.1%); these differences, however, were not statistically significant in this study. Critics of this study question the significance of the improvement in treated patients because the neurologic grading system used did not report a true level of patient function.[34] Nonetheless the results of this study made treatment with MPS a standard of care for patients with spinal cord injury in North America. The NASCIS II trial established the dosage schedule as an initial bolus of 30 mg/kg followed by a continuous infusion of 5.4 mg/kg/hr for 23 hours.

The third multicenter randomized trial NASCIS III was completed in 1997.[20] One treatment arm in this study was the standard MPS bolus and 23-hour infusion; a second arm extended the infusion another 24 hours and the third arm consisted of the initial MPS bolus followed by a 10 mg/kg/day dose of tirilazad for 48 hours. Tirilazad mesylate is a 21-aminosteroid compound, a group of MPS analogues that lack the hydroxyl function necessary for glucocorticoid receptor binding. Theoretically these drugs possess no glucocorticoid activity but are potent inhibitors of lipid peroxidation. The negative systemic effects seen with prolonged use of high-dose MPS should be significantly reduced.[15] The study showed that high-dose steroid regimen was effective only when given within 8 hours after injury. They recommended that if the steroid bolus were given within 1 to 3 hours, the drip should continue for 24 hours. If the bolus was given between 3 and 8 hours, the drip should continue for 48 rather than 24 hours.

While it was recognized that the increase in steroid dose duration would increase complications, it was the opinion of the authors that it might improve neurologic outcome. However, reanalysis of the data from NASCIS II and NASCIS III has not demonstrated a statistically beneficial effect, which has resulted in some heated debate in the literature.[82,101]

In addition subsequent studies evaluating complications between MPS treated patients and non-MPS patients have shown a statistically significant increase in respiratory infections, total infections, and hyperglycemia.[112a] Since these studies have also failed to show differences in neurologic outcome the role of MPS has been called into question.[112a] However, even with that information, the usage of MPS was continued in the United States for mainly medical legal reasons. In a recent study from Canada the practice patterns for the use of MPS administration were re-evaluated. In a survey of both Orthopaedic and Neurosurgical spine surgeons 76 percent were no longer prescribing MPS for spinal cord injury whereas 5 years prior 76 percent utilized it. Of the 24 percent who still used it, one third did so because of fear of litigation.[57a] Studies in humans evaluating the extent of spinal edema on MRI postinjury with and without MPS have failed to show any differences.[69a] Newer animal model information has shown that while MPS administration in rat models has a protective effect on oligodendrocytes it has failed to show any rescue of neurons.[66a]

Gangliosides are complex acidic glycolipids present in high concentration in the membranes of CNS cells. Experimental evidence has shown that these compounds augment regeneration and sprouting of neurons in vitro and restore neural function after injury in vivo.[45] A prospective, randomized, placebo-controlled trial of GM_1 ganglioside in patients with spinal cord injury showed that GM_1 enhanced motor recovery when compared with placebo controls.[45] However, only 16 patients received GM_1 once a day for 18 to 32 days, with the first dose given within 72 hours. All patients received initial treatment with steroids at a dose much less than the current standard dose. Analysis of the results showed that improved motor scores in both the Frankel and ASIA grading systems were attributable to restoration of power in initially paralyzed muscles rather than improvement in strength in previously weak muscles. The authors postulated that GM_1 allows for enhanced recovery of effectiveness in initiating the motor response of the circumferential white matter. Current trials exploring combination therapy with GM_1 and MPS are under way. The combination of the early antioxidant effects of high-dose bolus MPS and the late neuronal recovery effects of GM_1 may produce greater than additive benefits.[44]

Opiate receptor blockade has been an attractive target for pharmacologic manipulation of the injury process. Theoretically, release of endogenous opiates can cause systemic hypotension and a decrease in spinal cord blood flow. Naloxone and thyrotropin-releasing hormone (TRH) have been studied extensively in animal models and have shown variable success in improving neurologic recovery.[24,54,78,106] The results of the NASCIS do not support the use of naloxone in humans because it performed no better than controls. Clinical trials of a more stable analogue of TRH (longer half-life) are under way.

Various other agents have shown variable promise in the laboratory but remain unproven in clinical trials. The antioxidant effects of vitamin E have be shown to be useful but the need to administer the drug before injury limits its application.[6] Calcium channel blockers have been used in an attempt to minimize the calcium-modulated elements of the secondary injury cascade, but published reports have been variable and clinical use is controversial.[100] An endothelial receptor antagonist has been shown to prevent and delay the degeneration of axons after spinal cord injury in rats. Osmoitic diuretics used to reduce edema in head trauma (mannitol, low molecular weight dextran) failed to provide evidence of clinical effectiveness with regard to spinal cord injury[59,87] Table 25-3 summarizes the most frequently studied drugs used for the treatment of spinal cord injury in humans. Finally to date, while numerous other agents have been tried, no pharmacologic agent has been shown to be definitively effective in modulating secondary damage.[53a] However, many new approaches are being investigated including sodium channel blocker riluzole, the tetracycline derivative minocycline, fusogen copolymer polyethylene glycol, the Rho pathway anatagonist, Cethrin (Biaone Therapeutic Inc.), and erythropoetin.[8a,8b,64a]

PHYSICAL INTERVENTION

After administration of any indicated pharmacologic agents, an assessment of the overall alignment of the spinal column (and therefore the cord) should be made. Any malalignment or dislocation causing the neural elements to be under a severe degree of tension should be noted. Although treatment of the spinal injury cannot alter the initial trauma, experimental evidence has shown that immediate immobilization protects the spinal cord.[33] In addition, it has been demonstrated experimentally that continued compression causes additive detrimental effects that result in ischemia and electrophysiologic changes in the injured spinal cord.[47] A highly unstable situation may allow an already severely injured cord to undergo repeated injury with the slightest movement. Examination of the dorsal skin may reveal an impending breakdown over a kyphotic deformity, in which case urgent reduction is imperative. If the neurologic injury can be determined to be a complete injury (i.e., the bulbocavernosus reflex is intact), realignment may proceed at a less urgent pace. An exception may be in the cervical spine, where urgent reduction may improve the rate of "root-sparing" recovery.

Table 25-3	
Pharmacologic Agents for Spinal Cord Injury	
Agent	**Mechanism of Action**
Methylprednisolone (MPS)	Membrane stabilization by decrease in lipid peroxidation, prevention of inflammatory cascade
Tirilazad mesylate	Same as MPS, lacks glucocorticoid activity
GM_1 ganglioside	Augmentation of neuron regeneration
Naloxone	Blocks effects of endogenous opiates that cause local and systemic hypotension and spinal cord ischemia
Thyrotropin-releasing hormone	Same as naloxone

In an incomplete lesion, reduction and stabilization should be performed as quickly as possible to minimize continued neurologic injury. In the cervical spine, such management frequently involves the application of skull traction. In the thoracolumbar spine, traction is less successful, so if positioning does not restore anatomic alignment, emergency surgical reduction is required.

The role of pretraction MRI became a focus of debate after Eismont and colleagues,[35] among others,[74,93] reported neurologic deterioration in patients with cervical dislocations after they underwent traction and reduction. The high incidence of disk herniations with facet dislocations[91] prompted these authors to advocate that an MRI study be obtained before closed reduction of the cervical spine is attempted. Several large studies have refuted this contention by showing no worsening of neurologic levels with closed traction and reduction in awake, cooperative patients.[25,65,105] Nonetheless, expediency is of the utmost importance in the reduction of incomplete injuries. If it can be obtained quickly without putting an unstable patient at risk during transportation, pretraction MRI is reasonable. In many centers, such studies are difficult to obtain within several hours. MRI is required if the patient is otherwise uncooperative, closed reduction fails, or the injury requires reduction under anesthesia for any reason. If MRI demonstrates disk herniation, anterior discectomy plus fusion is performed before other surgery is attempted. If operative reduction of a thoracolumbar dislocation is planned, MRI should be obtained and operative plans modified based on the results.

After adequate alignment and stabilization, further diagnostic studies, such as CT (or MRI, if not obtained previously), can be performed on a less urgent basis. Frequent neurologic examinations, preferably by the same physician, should be documented and recorded, especially when the patient is returned after diagnostic tests. If worsening of a neurologic deficit is documented, emergency surgical decompression is indicated. In a patient with a stable or improving spinal cord injury, the timing of surgical stabilization, if needed, is controversial. In the case of a polytrauma victim, early stabilization, whether in a halo vest or by surgery, has been shown to improve overall outcome and shorten the hospital stay.[37]

An overview of a suggested algorithmic approach to a spine-injured patient is shown in Figure 25-13. Although such an algorithm tends to oversimplify a complicated decision-making process, adherence to a dedicated protocol provides a basic framework from which to treat these often multiply injured, complicated patients.

In patients with isolated injuries, as well as those with complicated multiple injuries, a simple, reliable method of cervical and thoracolumbar immobilization is necessary to safely perform a complete evaluation. The most effective method of initial cervical immobilization is the use of bilateral sandbags and taping of the patient across the forehead to a spine board, along with the use of a Philadelphia collar (which serves to limit extension).[86] In the cervical spine, a soft collar, extrication collar, hard collar, or Philadelphia collar alone is probably not sufficient for immobilization.[60,86] A poster brace (e.g., four-poster brace) or cervicothoracic brace (SOMI brace) is not practical in the emergency setting. A standard long spine board is adequate for immobilization and turning of the thoracolumbar spine.[77] Immobilization gear is removed only after radiographs have been interpreted as normal.

An unstable or malaligned cervical spine requires either more stable immobilization or axial traction to achieve reduction. Specific indications for skull traction are discussed in Chapters 28 and 29. The concept of skull traction was introduced by Crutchfield in 1933,[26] but the Crutchfield skull tongs for traction have been replaced by the Gardner-Wells[40] and halo immobilization devices. Gardner-Wells tongs are a simple, effective means of applying axial traction for reduction, but they do not significantly limit voluntary rotation, flexion, or extension in an uncooperative patient. Gardner-Wells tongs can be applied with minimal skin preparation and without assistance. The halo ring allows axial traction for reduction and provides rather stable immobilization with the application of a vest, but in a busy polytrauma setting, its application requires an assistant, and it takes longer to apply than Gardner-Wells tongs.

Gardner-Wells Tongs

The halo should be applied for initial stabilization of cervical spine injuries only if prolonged halo vest or cast immobilization is planned. If short-term traction followed by surgical stabilization and nonhalo external immobilization is planned, the use of Gardner-Wells tongs is preferred. Gardner-Wells tongs are easily applied by one person and without anterior pin sites.

Gardner-Wells tongs (Fig. 25-14) are fast and easy to apply, with no assistance required. Directions for use are generally located on the tongs (Fig. 25-15). The pins should be positioned below the temporal ridges at a point 2 cm above the external auditory canal and above the temporalis muscle (Fig. 25-16). After shaving, the skin is infiltrated with local anesthetic after the application of an antiseptic. The screws must be tightened symmetrically. The tongs are secure when the metal pressure pin protrudes 1 mm (Fig. 25-17). Protrusion of the pressure indicator pin by 1 mm has been demonstrated in cadavers to provide a pull-off strength of 137 ± 34 lb.[64] Pressure indicator pin protrusion of as little as 0.25 mm can support up to 60 lb.[64] It is recommended that the pin be tightened to 1 mm on the next day, but not again thereafter.

Traction should be initiated at 10 lb and increased by 5- to 10-lb increments. Reduction should be performed in awake patients with administration of intravenous midazolam if needed. Fluoroscopy or serial radiographs and serial neurologic examinations should be performed to avoid injury. In patients with neurologic symptoms or signs or 1-cm distraction of a disk space, closed reduction should be stopped and further images taken.

Gardner-Wells tongs have been reported to undergo pin and spring wear with repeated use. The pins and the tongs should be inspected and replaced if necessary or the indicator given a lower pin pressure to prevent pull-out.[67] Blumberg and associates[11] have reported that the MRI-compatible titanium alloy Gardner-Well tongs are more predisposed to plastic deformation and slippage than stainless steel Gardner-Wells tongs. They warned against using MRI-compatible tongs for reduction, especially with weights greater than 50 lb. Tongs may be switched after reduction to a lower weight if MRI is needed. A halo ring compatible with MRI would be another option if MRI is needed.

FIGURE 25-13 | *An algorithmic approach to the spine injury patient. Abbreviations: ATLS, advanced trauma life support; CT, computed tomography; MPS, methylprednisolone; MRI, magnetic resonance imaging; R/O, rule out.*

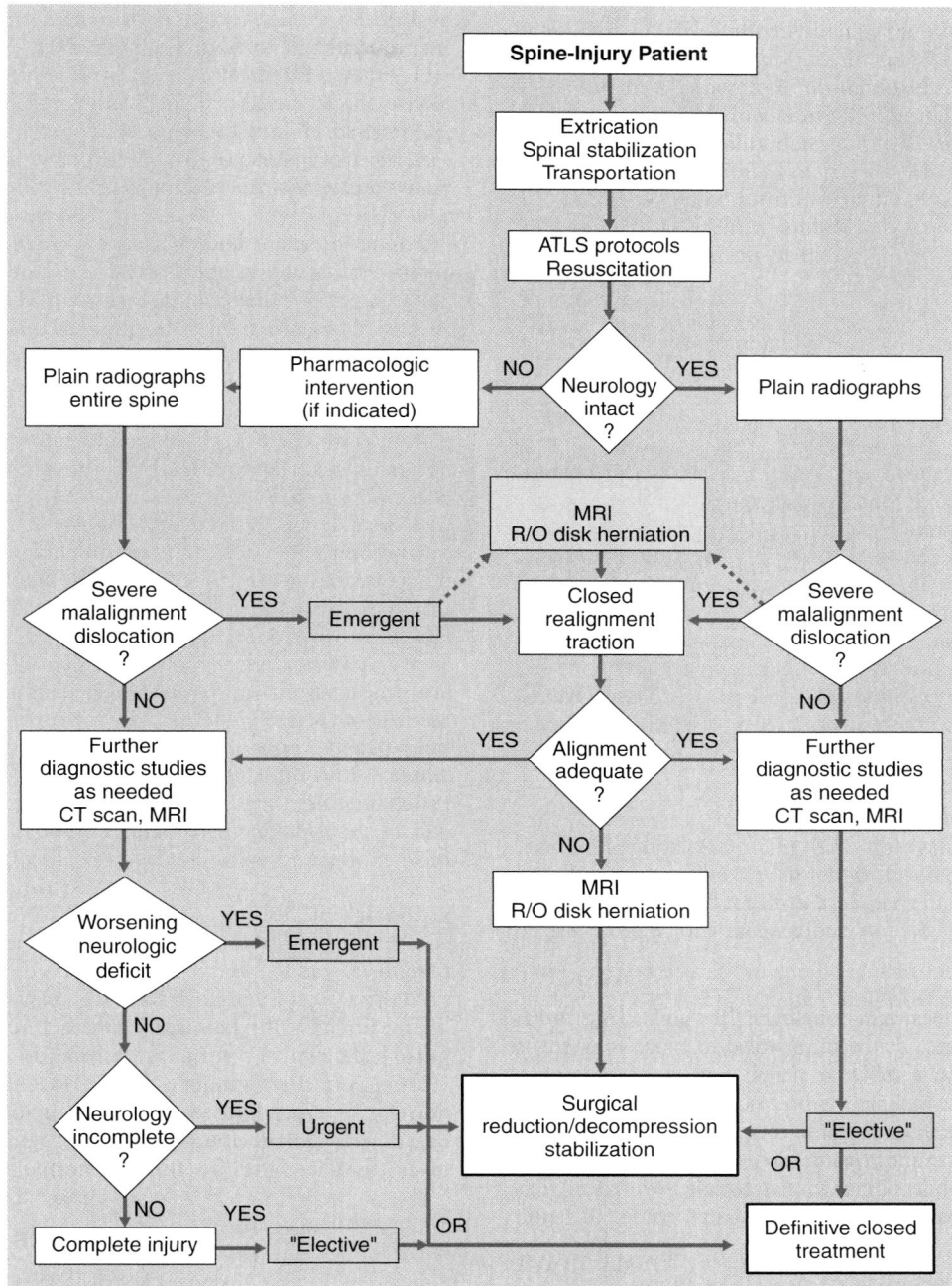

Halo Ring Application

A halo ring can be applied in the emergency department when definitive treatment is anticipated to be in a halo or in cases in which distraction should not be applied through Gardner-Wells tongs. Placing a halo vest underneath the patient during transfer to the bed can help attach the ring to the vest while the patient is in traction after reduction. Open halo rings offer the advantage over previous whole rings of being able to put the ring on without putting the patient's head on a head holder off the stretcher. The correct ring size is selected according to head circumference. The ring is placed around the head, the pin holes in the ring are used to identify the posterolateral pin sites, and the hair is shaved in these areas. The ring can be held in place temporarily with three plastic pod attachments. The skin is prepared, and local anesthetic is infiltrated through the ring holes.

Placement of the halo pins too high on the convexity of the skull can result in slippage of the ring, especially with traction. Placement of the anterior pin, as determined by skull osteology[41] and by supraorbital nerve anatomy, is best at a point in the middle to lateral third of the forehead,

FIGURE 25-14 *MRI-compatible graphite Gardner-Wells tongs.*

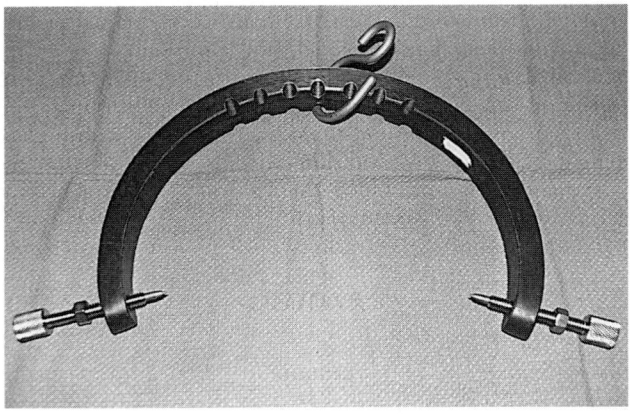

just above the eyebrow (Fig. 25-18). Although not supported by osteologic studies, placement of the anterior pin more laterally and just into the hairline for cosmetic reasons has been reported to give good clinical results.[46] This more lateral pin placement has been used by one of the authors (Benson), with similarly good clinical results. If the more lateral position is to be used, care must be taken to palpate and avoid penetration of the temporal muscle and temporal artery on each side. The posterior pin is placed in the posterolateral position on the halo ring, with care taken to avoid skin contact with the ring because pressure ulceration can result.

All pins are first secured to finger tightness. As the pins are tightened, the patient should be encouraged to keep both eyes tightly closed to avoid stretching the skin, which limits the patient's ability to close the eyes. Once the pins are finger tight, the ring is inspected carefully to ensure a symmetrical fit. The pins are then tightened sequentially in a diagonally opposite manner (i.e., right front with left rear and left front with right rear) to 2 inch-lb, then 4 inch-lb, and finally 8 inch-lb in an adult or 4 to 6 inch-lb in a child younger than 5 years. The pins should be retightened within 24 hours (and thereafter) only if they are loose and resistant to tightening. A loose pin without resistance to tightening should be moved to another position on the skull. Traction can then be applied with the traction bar attachment. If a vest is to be applied, the size should be equal to the chest diameter measured in inches at the level of the xiphoid process. MRI-compatible halo vests with graphite rings are used routinely, as shown in Figure 25-19.

Fleming and co-workers[38] devised instrumented halo vest orthoses with gauges that can measure pin force and showed an 83 percent decrease in compressive force during approximately a 3-month typical halo vest wear period. All patients had some symptoms caused by the degradation in pin force, which signified some loosening. The high stress on the bone may cause resorption and is thus one of the postulated causes of loosening. This potential complication highlights the importance of clinical vigilance during treatment of patients with halo vests. Attention to detail such as pin site care is essential, as well as alertness to symptoms of loosening or other complications during treatment.

Reports of complications with use of the halo ring and vest[42,46] have indicated significant rates of pin loosening (36%), pin site infection (20%), pressure sores under the vest or cast (11%), nerve injury (2%), dural penetration (1%), cosmetically disfiguring scars (9%), and severe pin

FIGURE 25-15 *Directions for use of the Gardner-Wells tongs are usually attached to the traction hook.*

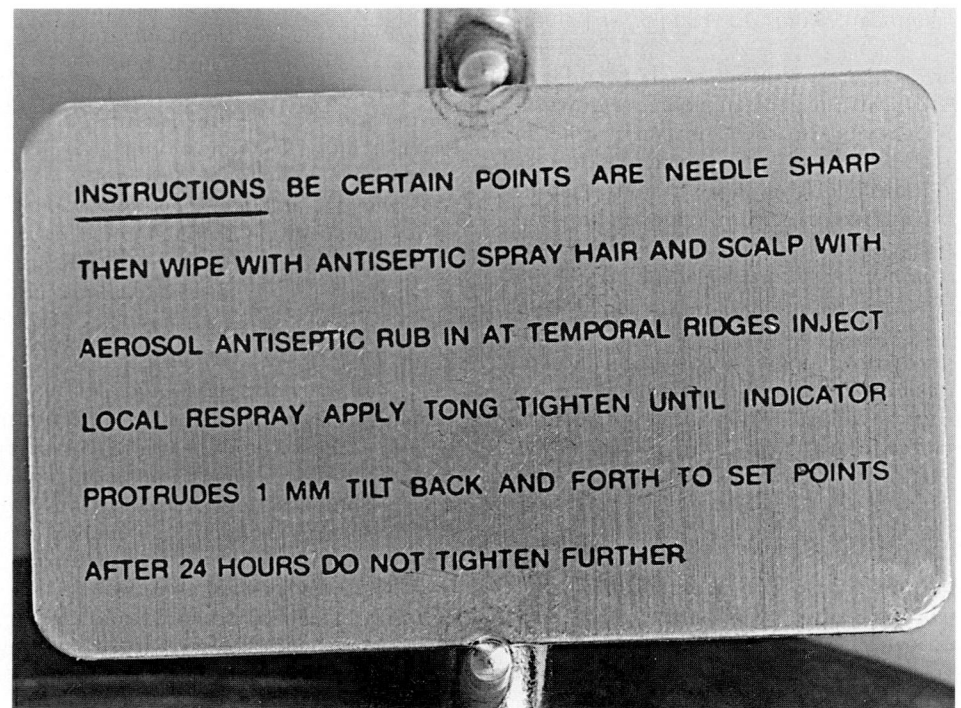

FIGURE 25-16 *Correct position for the Gardner-Wells tongs is 1 to 2 cm above the external auditory canal and below the temporal ridge.*

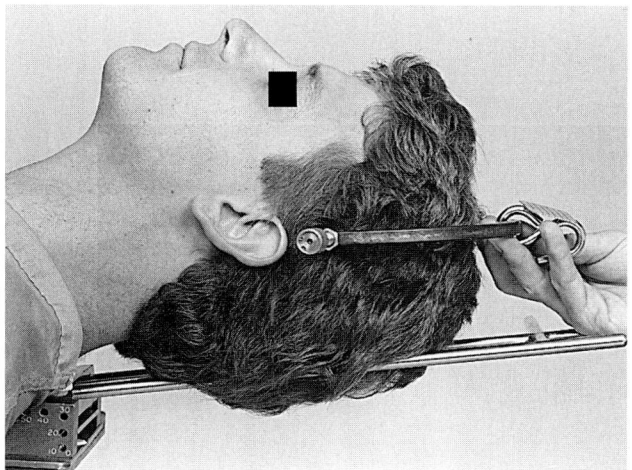

FIGURE 25-17 *Pressure indication pins of the Gardner-Wells tongs should protrude 1.0 mm.*

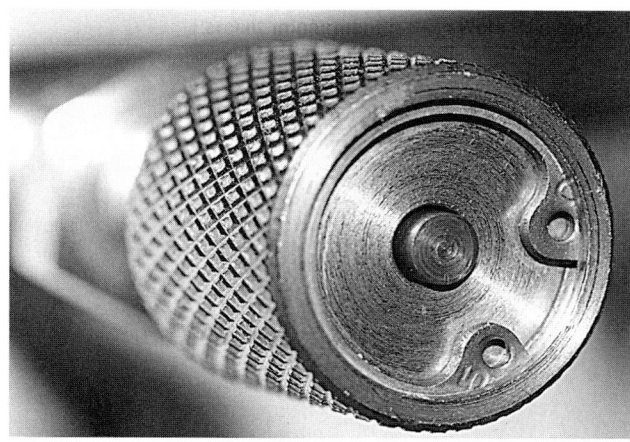

discomfort (18%). Skull osteomyelitis and subdural abscess have also been described. A lower rate of pin loosening and infection has been reported with an initial torque of 8 inch-lb rather than 6 inch-lb in adults.[14] A prospective randomized study has, however, shown that 6- or 8-lb torque does not lead to any significant difference in pin loosening.[92]

The use of a halo ring in children requires special consideration[43,63,81] because of a higher complication rate in this population.[9] The calvaria develops in three significant phases: by age 1 to 2 years, when interdigitation of the cranial sutures ends; by age 2 to 5 years, a period of rapid growth in diameter; and by age 5 to 12 years, when skull growth ceases.[43] Overall, the calvaria is thinner in a child

12 years or younger than in an adult, and the middle layer of cancellous bone may well be absent. CT studies have demonstrated that the standard adult anterolateral and posterolateral pin positions correspond to the thickest bone in a child, and they are recommended as the site of halo pin placement.[41,43] In children younger than 3 years, a multiple-pin, low-torque technique is recommended.[81] In this age group, custom fabrication of the halo ring and vest may be required. Ten to 12 standard halo pins can be used. The pins are inserted to a torque tightness of 2 inch-lb circumferentially around the temporal and frontal sinus regions. Halo placement in children younger than 2 years is complicated because of incomplete cranial suture interdigitation and open fontanels.[81]

FIGURE 25-18 *The anterior pin should be placed above the eyebrow in the medial to lateral third, avoiding the supraorbital nerve.*

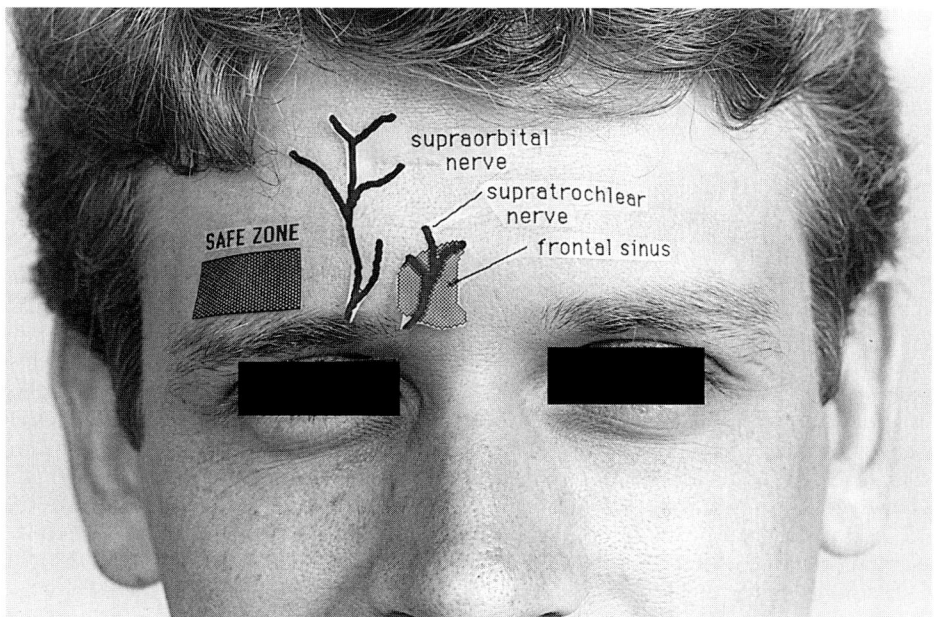

FIGURE 25-19   *MRI-compatible halo vests.*

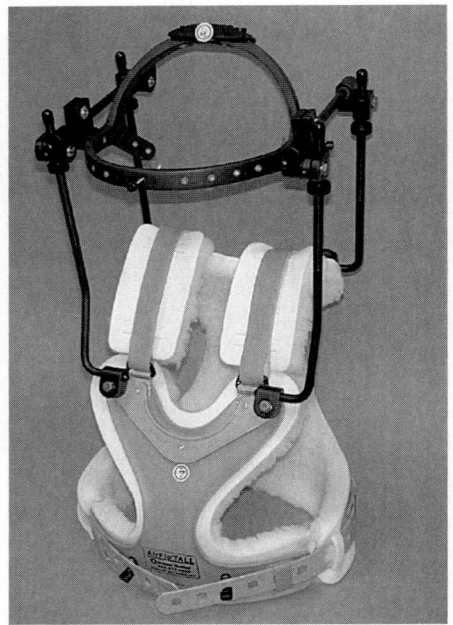 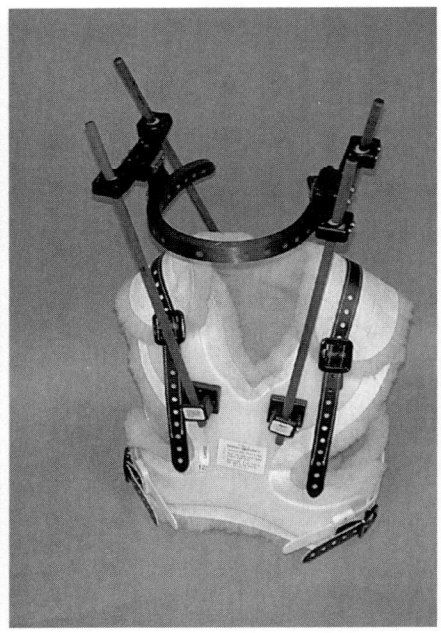

SPECIAL CONSIDERATIONS

Pediatric Patients

The spine is thought to behave biomechanically as an adult spine by about the age of 8 to 10 years.[8,56,57] Until then, spinal column injury is uncommon, usually involves soft tissues, and therefore is not seen on plain radiographs in the emergency department. In patients younger than 10 years, the most common injury occurs in the occiput to C3 region.[57,110] The entire spectrum of neurologic involvement is associated with these injuries, including cranial nerve lesions and vertebral basilar signs such as vomiting and vertigo. SCIWORA is most common in children younger than 10 years. Flexion, extension, and distraction cervical spine views and MRI scans can be helpful in identifying the level, but they should be used with extreme care to avoid further injury. After the age of 10 years, the pattern of injury is similar to that of adults, except for flexion-distraction injuries in the lumbar spine. As a result of seat belt injuries, pediatric patients can have a lumbar fracture with a more proximal thoracic level of paraplegia.

Initial immobilization of a pediatric patient requires an understanding of the supine kyphosis anterior translation (SKAT) phenomenon.[56] A young child lying supine on a standard backboard can have the head forced into kyphosis because of the normally disproportionate relationship of the larger head and smaller trunk in a child. Cases of forced kyphosis causing anterior translation of an unstable pediatric spine have been reported.[56] In normal development of a child, head diameter grows at a logarithmic rate, with 50 percent of adult size achieved by the age of 18 months, and chest diameter grows at an arithmetic rate, with 50 percent of adult size achieved by the age of 8 years. The problem can be avoided by elevating the thorax of a child on a spine board with a folded sheet to bring the shoulders to the level of the external auditory meatus or by the use of a pediatric backboard with a cutout to compensate for the prominent occiput of a young child.

Elderly Patients

Spinal trauma and spinal cord injury have traditionally been thought of as conditions of youth, but as many as 20 percent of all spinal cord injuries occur in patients older than 65 years.[17] Some particular characteristics and injury patterns are specific to elderly patients. For example, elderly patients with spinal cord injuries are more likely to be female. Whereas spinal injury is commonly associated with high-energy trauma in young adults, simple falls are the most common mechanism in patients older than 65 years.[71,95,104] Cervical spine injury predominates in the elderly population and accounts for 80 percent or more of traumatic spinal injuries. Injury to the C1-C2 complex is significantly more common in elderly people and accounts for a higher percentage of the total number of spinal injuries, with odontoid fractures being the single most common spinal column injury in these patients.[96,104]

Elderly patients are more likely to have an incomplete injury.[95,104] The frequent incidence of spondylosis in this population predisposes this patient group to central cord syndromes. Most importantly, the overall mortality rate for the initial hospitalization period has been reported to be 60 times higher in patients older than 65 years than in those younger than 40 years.[104] The causes of death are more commonly related to the stress of the treatment (immobilization, recumbency) than to the injury itself.

Treatment of this patient population is problematic. The overall priority in treatment should be early mobilization of the patient to avoid respiratory and other complications. Although previous reports have suggested that halo vests are poorly tolerated by the elderly population,[84] these patients are frequently poor surgical candidates. A high index of suspicion must be maintained when evaluating an elderly patient with neck pain, even after relatively trivial trauma.

Multiply Injured Patients

Several important issues should be raised regarding multiply injured patients with spinal trauma. Delay in diagnosis of a spine injury is a significant problem that can affect a trauma patient's care. The rate of delay in diagnosis in spinal trauma is 23 to 33 percent in the cervical spine[12,88] and about 5 percent in the thoracolumbar spine. As many as 22 percent of all delays in diagnosis in one series occurred after arrival at a tertiary referral center.[88] The main cause is a low level of suspicion, as represented by the following: (1) failure to obtain a radiograph, (2) missing the fracture on radiography, or less commonly, (3) failure of the patient to seek medical attention. A secondary neurologic deficit developed in 10 percent of patients with a delayed diagnosis as compared with 1.5 percent of those in whom spinal injury was diagnosed on initial evaluation,[88] but no progression of an already recognized deficit was observed. Other factors associated with a delay in diagnosis include intoxication, polytrauma, decreased level of consciousness, and noncontiguous spine fractures. Knowledge of the relationships between specific injury patterns and spinal injuries should decrease the incidence of serious missed spinal injuries. Patients with severe head injuries, as evidenced by a decreased level of consciousness or complex scalp lacerations, have a high incidence of cervical spine injuries, which may be difficult to diagnose clinically.[12,58] The incidence of noncontiguous spine fractures is about 4 to 5 percent of all spine fractures[10,61,62] but is higher in the upper cervical spine.[68] Therefore, diagnosis of a spinal fracture should in itself be an indication for aggressive investigation to rule out other, noncontiguous spinal injuries.

Conversely, the presence of a spinal fracture should heighten the awareness of the possibility of a serious, occult visceral injury. Thoracic fractures resulting in paraplegia have a high incidence of associated multiple rib fractures and pulmonary contusions. Translational shear injuries at these levels have significant associations with aortic injuries.[69] A delay in the diagnosis of a visceral injury can occur in up to 50 percent of patients with spinal injuries.[90] The relationship between the use of lap-style seat belts and Chance-type flexion-distraction injuries of the thoracolumbar spine is now well appreciated.[7] Almost two thirds of patients with flexion-distraction injuries from lap belts have an associated injury to a hollow viscus. Overall, approximately 50 to 60 percent of spine-injured patients have an associated nonspinal injury, ranging from a simple closed extremity fracture to a life-threatening thoracic or abdominal injury.[10,62]

REFERENCES

1. Advanced Trauma Life Support Student Manual. Chicago, American College of Surgeons, 1989.
2. Albuquerque, F.; Wolf, A.; Dunham, C.M.; et al. Frequency of intraabdominal injury in cases of blunt trauma to the cervical spinal cord. J Spinal Disord 5:476–480, 1992.
3. Allen, A.R. Remarks on the histopathological changes in the spinal cord due to impact: An experimental study. J Nerv Ment Dis 41:141–147, 1914.
4. American Academy for Orthopedic Surgeons. Emergency Care and Transportation of the Sick and Injured, 4th ed. Menasha, WI, George Banta, 1987.
5. American Spinal Injury Association. Standards for Neurological Classification of Spinal Injury. Chicago, American Spinal Injury Association, 1990.
6. Anderson, D.K.; Waters, T.R.; Means, E.D. Pretreatment with alpha tocopherol enhances neurologic recovery after experimental spinal cord injury. J Neurotrauma 5:61–67, 1988.
7. Anderson, P.A.; Rivara, F.P.; Maier, R.V.; et al. The epidemiology of seatbelt-associated injuries. J Trauma 31:60–67, 1991.
8. Apple, J.S.; Kirks, D.R.; Merten, D.F.; et al. Cervical spine fracture and dislocations in children. Pediatr Radiol 17:45–49, 1987.
8a. Baptiste, D.C.; Fehlings, M.G. Emerging drugs for spinal cord injury. Expert Opin Emerg Drugs 13:63–80, 2008.
8b. Baptiste, D.C.; Fehlings, M.G. Pharmacological approaches to repair the injured spinal cord. J Neurotrauma 23:318–334, 2006.
9. Baum, J.A.; Hanley, E.N.; Pullekines, I. Comparison of halo complications in adults and children. Spine 14:251–252, 1989.
10. Benson, D.R.; Keenen, T.L.; Antony, J. Unsuspected associated findings in spinal fractures. J Orthop Trauma 3:160, 1989.
11. Blumberg, K.D.; Catalano, J.B.; Cotler, J.M.; et al. The pullout strength of titanium alloy MRI-compatible and stainless steel MRI-incompatible Gardner-Wells tongs. Spine 18:1895–1896, 1993.
12. Bohlman, H.H. Acute fractures and dislocations of the cervical spine. J Bone Joint Surg [Am] 61:1119–1142, 1979.
13. Bosch, A.; Stauffer, E.S.; Nickel, V.L. Incomplete traumatic quadriplegia: A ten year review. JAMA 216:473–478, 1971.
14. Botte, M.J.; Byrne, T.P.; Garfin, S.R. Application of the halo device for immobilization of the cervical spine utilizing an increased torque pressure. J Bone Joint Surg [Am] 69:750–752, 1987.
15. Bracken, M.B. Pharmacological treatment of acute spinal cord injury: Current status and future projects. J Emerg Med 11:43–48, 1993.
16. Bracken, M.B.; Collins, W.F.; Freeman, D.; et al. Efficacy of methylprednisolone in acute spinal cord injury. JAMA 251:45–52, 1984.
17. Bracken, M.B.; Freeman, D.H.; Hellenbrand, L. The incidence of acute traumatic spinal cord injury in the U.S., 1970–1977. Am J Epidemiol 113:615–622, 1980.
18. Bracken, M.B.; Shepard, M.J.; Collins, W.F.; et al. A randomized controlled trial of methylprednisolone or naloxone in the treatment of acute spinal cord injury: The results of the National Acute Spinal Cord Injury Study. N Engl J Med 322:1405–1411, 1990.
19. Bracken, M.B.; Shepard, M.J.; Collins, W.F.; et al. Methylprednisolone or naloxone treatment after acute spinal cord injury: 1 year follow-up data. Results of the second National Acute Spinal Cord Injury Study. J Neurosurg 76:23–31, 1992.

20. Bracken, M.B.; Shepard, M.J.; Holford, T.R.; et al. Administration of methylprednisolone for 24 and 48 hours or tirilazad mesylate for 48 hours in the treatment of acute spinal cord injury: Results of the third National Acute Spinal Cord Injury Randomized Controlled Trial. JAMA 277:1597–1604, 1997.

21. Bregman, B.S.; Kunkel-Bagden, E.; Reier, P.J.; et al. Recovery of function after spinal cord injury: Mechanisms underlying transplant-mediated recovery of function differ after cord injury in newborn and adult rats. Exp Neurol 11:49–63, 1991.

22. Centers for Disease Control. Acute traumatic spinal cord injury surveillance—U.S.: 1987. MMWR CDC Surveill Summ 37:285–286, 1987.

23. Cheng, H.; Cao, Y.; Olson, L. Spinal cord repair in adult paraplegic rats: Partial restoration of hind limb function. Science 273:510–513, 1996.

23a. Coderre, T.J.; Katz, J.; Vaccarino, A.L.; et al. Contribution of central neuroplasticity to pathological pain: review of clinical and experimental evidence. Pain 52:259–285.

24. Committee on Trauma of the American College of Surgeons. Hospital and prehospital resources for optimal care of the injured patient. Bull Am Coll Surg 71:4–23, 1986.

25. Cotler, J.M.; Herbison, G.J.; Nasuti, J.F.; et al. Closed reduction of traumatic cervical spine dislocations using traction weights up to 140 pounds. Spine 18:386–390, 1993.

26. Crutchfield, W.G. Skeletal traction for dislocation of the cervical spine: Report of a case. South Surg 2:156–159, 1933.

27. Denis, F. The three-column spine and its significance in the classification of acute thoracolumbar spinal injuries. Spine 8:817–831, 1983.

28. Devivo, M.J.; Kartus, P.L.; Stover, S.L.; et al. Benefits of early admission to an organised spinal cord injury care system. Paraplegia 28:545–555, 1990.

29. Dilberti, T.; Lindsey, R.W. Evaluation of the cervical spine in the emergency setting: Who does not need an x-ray? Orthopedics 15:179–180, 1992.

30. Dohrmann, G.J.; Wick, K.M.; Bucy, P.C. Transitory traumatic paraplegia: Electron microscopy of early alterations in myelinated nerve fibers. J Neurosurg 36:425–429, 1972.

31. Ducker, T.B.; Kindt, G.W.; Kempe, L.G. Pathological findings in acute experimental spinal cord trauma. J Neurosurg 35:700–708, 1971.

32. Ducker, T.B.; Saleman, M.; Perot, P.L.; et al. Experimental spinal cord trauma, I: Correlation of blood flow, tissue oxygen and neurologic status in the dog. Surg Neurol 10:60–63, 1978.

33. Ducker, T.B.; Solomon, M.; Daniel, H.B. Experimental spinal cord trauma, III: Therapeutic effect of immobilization and pharmacologic agents. Surg Neurol 10:71–76, 1978.

34. Ducker, T.B.; Zeidman, S.M. Spinal cord injury: Role of steroid therapy. Spine 19:2281–2287, 1994.

35. Eismont, F.G.; Arena, M.J.; Green, B.A. Extrusion of intervertebral disc associated with traumatic subluxation or dislocation of cervical facets. J Bone Joint Surg [Am] 73:1555–1559, 1991.

36. Ergas, A. Spinal cord injury in the United States: A statistical update. Cent Nerv Sys Trauma 2:19–32, 1985.

37. Fellrath, R.F.; Hanley, E.N. Multitrauma and thoracolumbar fractures. Semin Spine Surg 7:103–108, 1995.

38. Fleming, B.C.; Krag, M.H.; Huston, D.R.; et al. Pin loosening in a halo-vest orthosis: A biomechanical study. Spine 25:1325–1331, 2000.

39. Frankel, H.; Hancock, D.O.; Hyslop, G.; et al. The value of postural reduction in the initial management of closed injuries to the spine with paraplegia and tetraplegia. Paraplegia 7:179–192, 1969.

40. Gardner, W. The principle of spring-loaded points for cervical traction. J Neurosurg 39:543–544, 1973.

41. Garfin, S.R.; Botte, M.J.; Centeno, R.S.; et al. Osteology of the skull as it affects halo pin placement. Spine 10:696–698, 1985.

42. Garfin, S.R.; Botte, M.J.; Waters, R.L.; et al. Complications in the use of the halo fixation device. J Bone Joint Surg [Am] 68:320–325, 1986.

43. Garfin, S.R.; Roux, R.; Botte, M.S.; et al. Skull osteology as it affects halo pin placement in children. J Pediatr Orthop 6:434–436, 1986.

44. Geisler, F.H. GM₁ ganglioside and motor recovery following human spinal cord injury. J Emerg Med 11:49–55, 1993.

45. Geisler, F.H.; Dorsey, F.C.; Coleman, W.P. Recovery of motor function after spinal cord injury: A randomized, placebo-controlled trial with GM₁ ganglioside. N Engl J Med 324:1829–1838, 1991.

46. Glaser, J.A.; Whitehill, R.; Stamp, W.G.; et al. Complications associated with the halo vest. J Neurosurg 65:762–769, 1986.

47. Gooding, M.R.; Wilson, C.B.; Hoff, J.T. Experimental cervical myelopathy: Effects of ischemia and compression of the canine spinal cord. J Neurosurg 43:9–17, 1975.

48. Grabb, P.A.; Pang, D. Magnetic resonance imaging in the evaluation of spinal cord imaging without radiographic abnormality in children. Neurosurgery 35:406–414, 1994.

49. Green, B.A.; Eismont, F.J.; O'Heir, J.T. Prehospital management of spinal cord injuries. Paraplegia 25:229–238, 1987.

50. Grundy, D.; Swain, A.; Russell, J. ABC of spinal cord injury: Early management and complications, I. BMJ 292:44–47, 1986.

51. Guest, J.D.; Rao, A.; Olson, L.; et al. The ability of human Schwann cell grafts to promote regeneration in the transected nude rat spinal cord. Exp Neurol 148:502–522, 1997.

52. Hall, E.D. The neuroprotective pharmacology of methyl prednisolone. J Neurosurg 76:13–22, 1992.

53. Hall, E.D.; Braughler, J.M. Nonsurgical management of spinal cord injuries: A review of studies with the glucocorticoid steroid methylprednisolone. Acta Anaesthesiol Belg 38:405–409, 1987.

53a. Hall, E.D.; Springer, J.E. Neuroprotection and acute spinal cord injury: a reappraisal. Neuro RX 1:80–100, 2004.

54. Hamilton, A.J.; McBlack, P.; Carr, D. Contrasting actions of naloxone in experimental spinal cord trauma and cerebral ischemia: A review. Neurosurgery 17:845–849, 1985.

55. Hayashi, K.; Yone, K.; Ito, H.; et al. MRI findings in patients with a cervical spinal cord injury who do not show radiographic evidence of a fracture or dislocation. Paraplegia 33:212–215, 1995.

56. Herzenberg, J.E.; Hensinger, R.N.; Dedrick, D.K.; et al. Emergency transport and positioning of young children who have injury of the cervical spine: The standard backboard may be hazardous. J Bone Joint Surg [Am] 71:15–22, 1989.

57. Hill, S.A.; Miller, C.A.; Kosimils, E.J.; et al. Pediatric neck injuries. J Neurosurg 60:700–706, 1984.

57a. Hurlbert, R.J.; Hamilton, M.G. Methyl prednisolone for acute spinal cord injury: 5-year practice reversal. Can J Neurol Sci 35:41–45, 2008.

58. Irving, M.K.; Irving, P.M. Associated injuries in head trauma patients. J Trauma 7:500–504, 1967.

59. Janssen, C.; Hansebout, R.R. Pathogenesis of spinal cord injury and newer treatments. Spine 14:23–32, 1989.

60. Johnson, R.M.; Hart, D.L.; Simmons, E.F.; et al. Cervical orthoses. J Bone Joint Surg [Am] 59:332–339, 1977.

61. Keenen, T.L.; Anthony, J.; Benson, D.R. Noncontiguous spinal fractures. J Trauma 30:489–501, 1990.

62. Kewalramani, L.S.; Taylor, R.G. Multiple noncontiguous injuries to the spine. Acta Orthop Scand 47:52–58, 1976.

62a. Klusman, I.; Schwab, M.E. Effects of pro-inflammatory cytokines in experimental spinal cord injury. Brain Res 762:173–184, 1997.

63. Kopits, S.E.; Steingass, M.H. Experience with the halo cast in small children. Surg Clin North Am 50:934–935, 1970.

64. Krag, M.H.; Byrt, W.; Pope, M. Pulloff strength of Gardner-Wells tongs from cadaveric crania. Spine 14:247–250, 1989.

64a. Kwon, B.K.; Tetzialaff, W.; Grauer, J.N.; et al. Pathophysiology and pharmacological treatment of acute spinal cord injury. Spine J 4:451–461, 2004.

65. Lee, A.S.; MacLean, J.C.B.; Newton, D.A. Rapid traction for reduction of cervical spine dislocations. J Bone Joint Surg [Br] 76:352–356, 1994.

66. Lee, H.M.; Kim, H.S.; Kim, D.J.; et al. Reliability of magnetic resonance imaging in detecting posterior ligament complex injury in thoracolumbar spinal fractures. Spine 25:2079–2084, 2000.

66a. Lee, J.M.; Yan, P.; Xiao, Q.; et al. Methylprenisolone protects oligodendrocytes but not neurons after spinal cord injury. J Neurosci 28:3141–3149, 2008.

67. Lerman, J.A.; Haynes, R.J.; Koeneman, E.J.; et al. A biomechanical comparison of Gardner-Wells tongs and halo device used for cervical spine traction. Spine 19:2403–2406, 1994.

68. Levine, A.M.; Edwards, C.C. Treatment of injuries in the C1-C2 complex. Orthop Clin North Am 17:31–44, 1986.

69. Levine, A.M.; McAfee, P.C.; Anderson, P.A. Evaluation and treatment of patients with thoracolumbar trauma. Instr Course Lect 44:33–45, 1995.

69a. Leypold, B.G.; Flanders, A.E.; Schwartz, E.D.; et al. The impact of methylprednisolone on lesion severity following spinal cord injury. Spine 32:373–378, 2007.

70. Li, Y.; Field, P.M.; Raisman, G. Repair of adult rat corticospinal tract by transplants of olfactory ensheathing cells. Science 237:642–645, 1987.

71. Lieberman, I.H.; Webb, J.K. Cervical spine injuries in the elderly. J Bone Joint Surg [Br] 76:877–881, 1994.

71a. Lipton, S.; Failures and successes of NMDA receptor antagonists: Molecular basis for the use of open-channel blockers like memantine in the treatment of acute and chronic neurologic insults. NeuroRX 1(1):101–110, 2004.

72. Lu, J.; Ashwell, K.W.S.; Waite, P. Advances in secondary spinal cord injury: Role of apoptosis. Spine 25:1859–1866, 2000.

73. Lucas, J.T.; Ducker, T.B. Motor classification of spinal cord injuries with mobility, morbidity and recovery indices. Am Surg 45:151–158, 1979.

74. Mahale, Y.J.; Silver, J.R.; Henderson, N.J. Neurological complications of the reduction of cervical spine dislocations. J Bone Joint Surg [Br] 75:403–409, 1993.

75. Marshall, L.F.; Knowlton, S.; Garfin, S.R.; et al. Deterioration following spinal cord injury. J Neurosurg 66:400–404, 1987.

76. McArdle, C.B.; Wright, J.W.; Prevost, W.J. MR imaging of the acutely injured patient with cervical traction radiology. Radiology 159:273–274, 1986.

77. McGuire, R.A.; Neville, S.; Green, B.A.; et al. Spinal instability and the log-rolling maneuver. J Trauma 27:525–531, 1987.

78. McIntosh, T.K.; Faden, A.I. Opiate antagonists in traumatic shock. Ann Emerg Med 15:1462–1465, 1986.

79. Midwestern Regional Spinal Cord Injury Care System. Northwestern University and Rehabilitation Institute of Chicago Progress Report No. 9. Chicago, Northwestern University, 1980.

80. Mirvis, S.E.; Borg, U.; Belzberg, H. MR imaging of ventilator-dependent patients: Preliminary experience. Am J Radiol 149:845–846, 1987.

81. Mubarak, S.J.; Camp, J.F.; Vuletich, W.; et al. Halo application in the infant. J Pediatr Orthop 9:612–614, 1989.

82. Nesathurai, S. Steroids and spinal cord injury: Revisiting the NASCIS 2 and NASCIS 3 trials. J Trauma 45:1088–1093, 1998.

83. O'Beirne, J.; Cassidy, N.; Raza, K.; et al. Role of magnetic resonance imaging in the assessment of spinal injuries. Injury 24:149–154, 1993.

84. Pepin, J.W.; Bourne, R.B.; Hawkins, R.J. Odontoid fracture, with special reference to the elderly patient. Clin Orthop 193:178–183, 1985.

85. Piepmeier, J.M.; Lehmann, K.B.; Lane, J.G. Cardiovascular instability following acute cervical spinal cord trauma. Cent Nerv Sys Trauma 2:153–160, 1985.

86. Podolsky, S.; Baraff, L.J.; Simon, R.R. Efficacy of cervical spine immobilization methods. J Trauma 23:461–465, 1983.

87. Reed, J.E.; Allen, W.E.; Dohrmann, G.J. Effect of mannitol on the traumatized spinal cord. Spine 4:391–397, 1979.

88. Reid, D.C.; Henderson, R.; Saboe, L.; et al. Etiology and clinical course of missed spine fractures. J Trauma 27:980–986, 1987.

89. Riggins, R.S.; Kraus, J.F. The risk of neurologic damage with fractures of the vertebrae. J Trauma 7:126–133, 1977.

90. Ritchie, W.P.; Ersek, R.A.; Bunch, W.L.; et al. Combined visceral and vertebral injuries from lap style seat belts. Surg Gynecol Obstet 131:431–435, 1970.

91. Rizzolo, S.J.; Piazza, M.R.; Cotler, J.M.; et al. Intervertebral disc injury complicating cervical spine trauma. Spine 16(Suppl):187–189, 1991.

92. Rizzolo, S.J.; Piazza, M.R.; Cotler, J.M.; et al. The effect of torque pressure on halo pin complication rates. Spine 18:2163–2166, 1993.

93. Robertson, P.A.; Ryan, M.D. Neurological deterioration after reduction of cervical subluxation: Mechanical compression by disc tissue. J Bone Joint Surg [Br] 74:224–227, 1992.

94. Ross, S.E.; Schwab, C.W.; David, E.T.; et al. Clearing the cervical spine: Initial radiographic evaluation. J Trauma 27:1055–1060, 1987.

95. Roth, E.J.; Lovell, L.; Heinemann, A.W.; et al. The older adult with a spinal cord injury. Paraplegia 30:520–526, 1992.

96. Ryan, M.D.; Henderson, J.J. The epidemiology of fractures and fracture dislocations of the cervical spine. Injury 23:38–40, 1992.

97. Schell, L.; Schwab, M.E. Sprouting and regeneration of lesioned corticospinal tract fibres in the adult rat spinal cord. Eur J Neurosci 5:1156–1171, 1993.

98. Schneider, R.C. The syndrome of acute anterior cervical spinal cord injury. J Neurosurg 12:95–122, 1955.

99. Schrader, S.C.; Sloan, T.B.; Toleikis, R. Detection of sacral sparing in acute spinal cord injury. Spine 12:533–535, 1987.

100. Shi, R.Y.; Lucas, J.H.; Wolf, A.; et al. Calcium antagonists fail to protect mammalian spinal neurons after physical injury. J Neurotrauma 6:261–278, 1989.

101. Short, D.J.; Masry, W.S.; Jones, P.W. High dose methylprednisolone in the management of acute spinal cord injury—a systematic review from a clinical perspective. Spinal Cord 38:273–286, 2000.

102. Slabaugh, P.B.; Nickel, V.L. Complications with the use of the Stryker frame. J Bone Joint Surg [Am] 60:111–112, 1978.

103. Soderstrom, C.A.; McArdle, D.Q.; Ducker, T.B.; et al. The diagnosis of intraabdominal injury in patients with cervical cord trauma. J Trauma 23:1061–1065, 1983.

104. Spivak, J.M.; Weiss, M.A.; Cotler, J.M.; et al. Cervical spine injuries in patients 65 and older. Spine 19:2302–2306, 1994.

105. Star, A.M.; Jones, A.A.; Cotler, J.M.; et al. Immediate closed reduction of cervical spine dislocation using traction. Spine 15:1068–1072, 1990.

106. Starr, J.K. The pathophysiology and pharmacological management of acute spinal cord injury. Semin Spine Surg 7:91–97, 1995.

107. Stauffer, E.S. Diagnosis and prognosis of the acute cervical spinal cord injury. Clin Orthop 112:9–15, 1975.

108. Stauffer, E.S. Neurologic recovery following injuries to the cervical spinal cord and nerve roots. Spine 9:532–534, 1984.

109. Stauffer, E.S. A quantitative evaluation of neurologic recovery following cervical spinal cord injuries. Presented at the Third Annual Meeting of the Federation of Spine Associates, Paper 39. Atlanta, Georgia, February 1988.

110. Steel, H.H. Anatomical and mechanical consideration of the atlantoaxial articulation. J Bone Joint Surg [Am] 50:1481–1482, 1968.

111. Stover, S.L.; Fine, P.R. Spinal Cord Injury: The Facts and Figures. Birmingham, AL, The University of Alabama, 1986.

112. Stover, S.L.; Fine, P.R. The epidemiology and economics of spinal cord injury. Paraplegia 25:225–228, 1987.

112a. Suberviola, B.; Gonzales-Castro, A.; Liorca, J.; et al. Early complications of high-dose methylprednisolone in acute spinal cord injury patients. Injury 39:748–752, 2008.

113. Tator, C.H.; Duncan, E.G.; Edmonds, V.E.; et al. Demographic analysis of 552 patients with acute spinal cord injury in Ontario, Canada, 1947–1981. Paraplegia 26:112–113, 1988.

114. Thurman, D.J.; Burnett, C.C.; Jeppson, L.; et al. Surveillance of spinal cord injuries in Utah, USA. Paraplegia 32:665–669, 1994.

115. Torg, J.S.; Vegso, J.; Sennett, B.; et al. The National Football Head and Neck Injury Registry. JAMA 254:3439–3443, 1985.

116. Uesugi, M.; Kasuya, Y.; Hayashi, K.; et al. SB20967, a potent endothelin receptor antagonist, prevents or delays axonal degeneration after spinal cord injury. Brain Res 786:235–239, 1998.

117. Vale, F.L.; Burns, J.; Jackson, A.B.; et al. Combined medical and surgical treatment after spinal cord injury: Result of a prospective pilot study to assess the merits of aggressive medical resuscitation and blood pressure management. J Neurosurg 87:129–146, 1997.

118. Waters, R.L.; Adkins, R.H.; Yakura, J.S. Definition of complete spinal cord injury. Paraplegia 29:573–581, 1991.

119. Zipnick, R.I.; Scalea, T.M.; Trooskin, S.Z.; et al. Hemodynamic responses to penetrating spinal cord injuries. J Trauma 35:578–583, 1993.

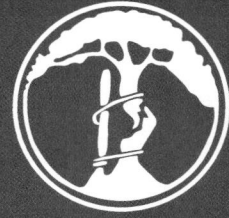

CHAPTER 26

Spinal Imaging

Stuart E. Mirvis, M.D., F.A.C.R.

INTRODUCTION

Spinal imaging must be considered in the context of the clinical presentation of the entire patient, which dictates management priorities as well as the type and sequence of diagnostic imaging evaluations. Acutely injured patients with back or neck pain or clinical signs of spine or spinal cord injury and all noncommunicative patients in whom the account of the mechanism of injury is consistent with spine or spinal cord injury should have an imaging assessment of the spine. While traditionally the initial radiographic imaging of the spine has been with radiographs, typically using the anteroposterior (AP) and lateral views, increasingly computed tomography (CT) is being employed as the initial and definitive screening examination of the spine. This is due to both its frequent general use in polytrauma patients and its substantially greater diagnostic accuracy than radiographs. If the potentially injured spine cannot be "cleared" (i.e., declared negative for injury) by initial clinical or imaging assessment or if the patient's condition requires immediate surgical intervention or more complex imaging procedures for other organ systems (i.e., interventional angiography), the spine *must remain immobilized* to protect the cord until the patient has been stabilized sufficiently to complete *definitive clinical and imaging examinations* of the spine.

Spinal imaging refers to evaluation of the spine by any of the various imaging modalities and techniques, or by any combination of such techniques, generally included in radiology. Diagnostic imaging of the spine is the definitive method for determining the presence, location, extent, and nature of injury to the spinal column (including the spinal soft tissues using magnetic resonance imaging [MRI]). Diagnostic imaging is essential to the accurate identification, characterization, and planning management of spinal injury. The efficient and economic application of diagnostic imaging of spinal trauma requires a thorough knowledge of the indications for and limitations of the various imaging techniques available and the sequence in which they should be applied.

In this chapter the diagnostic imaging of each region of the spine is considered separately because of differences in anatomy and injury patterns. The first section of the chapter considers currently available imaging modalities for evaluating acute spinal injury, highlighting their relative strengths and weaknesses. Illustrations of normal imaging

anatomy and examples of common injuries, as they relate to the imaging concepts discussed, are shown. The next section describes the types and sequence of recommended imaging techniques, as dictated by the patient's clinical condition, that culminate in a definitive diagnosis as rapidly as possible. The final brief section discusses imaging the traumatized spine of patients with special circumstances such as preexisting conditions that affect the spine, which may significantly alter its normal appearance, penetrating spinal trauma, and spinal trauma in the patient with immediately life-threatening conditions. The diagnostic approach presented reflects experience in the imaging evaluation of acute spinal injuries within the environment of a Level I trauma center, but it is applicable to spinal injuries seen in any setting (Fig. 26-1).

DIAGNOSTIC IMAGING OF THE SPINE: AN OVERVIEW OF IMAGING MODALITIES— ADVANTAGES AND DISADVANTAGES

The diagnostic imaging modalities useful in the evaluation of spinal trauma include plain film radiography, computed tomography including two- and three-dimensional data re-formation, CT myelography (CTM), MRI, and occasionally nuclear scintigraphy. Cervical vascular injury, with the potential for devastating neurologic consequences, is not uncommonly associated with cervical spine trauma and may require use of catheter angiography in selected cases. Vascular injuries may be initially recognized using CT angiography (CTA) with intravenous contrast or with MRI or magnetic resonance angiography (MRA), and Doppler sonography in areas where an acoustic window is available. The development and increasing availability of ultrafast multidetector CT (MDCT) has led to its use as a screening technique for cervical vascular injury for patients with and without cervical spine injury, as discussed in detail below.

Plain Radiography

CERVICAL SPINE

Imaging examination of patients with potential spinal trauma often begins with plain radiographic studies. Plain

754 SECTION 2 • *Spine*

FIGURE 26-1 *Algorithm for imaging diagnosis of cervical spine injury.* Abbreviations: *AP, anteroposterior; CT, computed tomography; MRI, magnetic resonance imaging; OMO, open-mouth odontoid.*

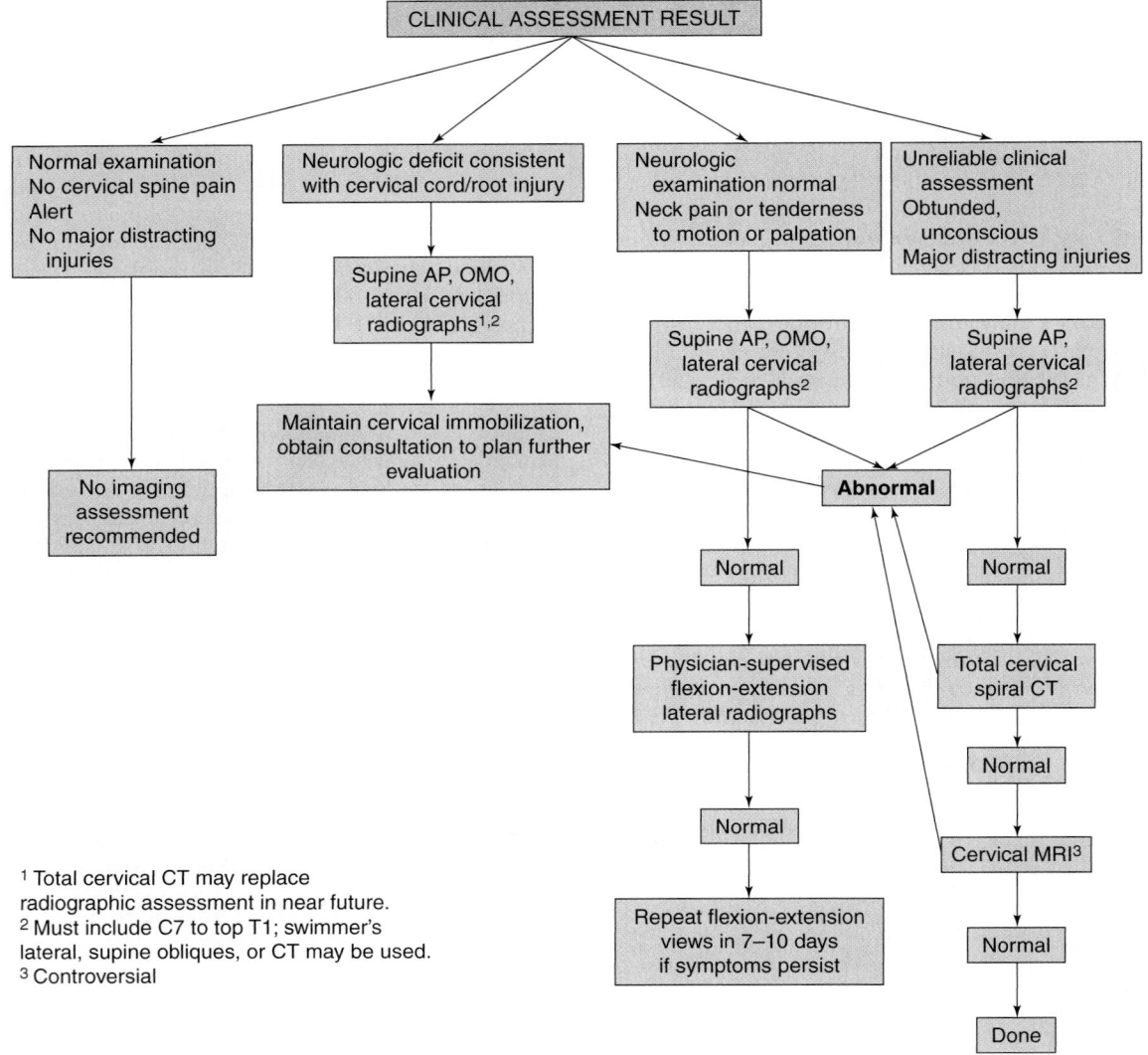

¹ Total cervical CT may replace radiographic assessment in near future.
² Must include C7 to top T1; swimmer's lateral, supine obliques, or CT may be used.
³ Controversial

film radiography is readily available in all emergency centers and is a reliable and quick method for evaluation of patients that can be performed with portable or fixed equipment. Radiography usually provides an excellent overview of the extent and magnitude of injury and makes a definitive and specific diagnosis possible in certain spinal injuries. The flexibility of the x-ray tube film geometry provides the positioning latitude necessary for obtaining a comprehensive examination without special positioning of the patient, which is essential for patients in whom a spinal injury is suspected.

The quality of the plain radiographic study is of paramount importance to the identification of cervical spine injury. A properly exposed radiograph must display both the skeleton and the soft tissues and must be free of motion or artifacts that could obscure or mimic fractures. The prevention of artifact is of primary importance in detecting subtle, minimally displaced osseous injuries. A properly collimated plain film study limits patient

radiation exposure and is relatively inexpensive. Most unstable cervical spine injuries can be diagnosed by adequately experienced interpreters using technically adequate cervical spine radiographs.

LATERAL VIEW The lateral cervical spine projection offers the most informative view of the cervical spine for injury detection.[13] An adequate study must include the cervicothoracic junction at least to include the top of T1. The patient should be positioned without rotation of the head. Every reasonable effort must be made to visualize the cervicothoracic junction on the initial plain radiographic examination. If the C7–T1 level is not adequately visualized on the lateral radiograph, the cervical spine cannot be cleared (i.e., declared negative), and other plain film studies (see later discussion) or CT must be performed.

The cross-table lateral radiograph ranges from 74 to 93 percent sensitive for detection of cervical spine injuries, but this sensitivity depends to a large extent on the expertise and experience of the examiner.[54,71] However, studies comparing cervical spine radiographs to CT interpretation indicate that at least 40 percent of cervical fractures are missed on radiographs, although the majority of these injuries are mechanically stable.[33] Missed injuries may result from (1) overlapping of bone, particularly involving the cervicocranial junction, the articular masses, and the laminae; (2) nondisplaced or minimally displaced fractures, particularly involving the atlas and axis; and (3) ligament injuries that may not be manifested when the radiograph is taken with the patient in a supine position with the neck in slight extension and stabilized by a cervical collar (i.e., no stress applied). Some cervical spine subluxations or dislocations can reduce spontaneously or be reduced with placement in a cervical collar before imaging evaluation, making their detection more difficult. Obviously, poor imaging technique related to positioning, exposure, or motion can significantly impair diagnostic accuracy.

Review of the lateral cervical radiograph involves assessment of anatomic lines, including the anterior and posterior vertebral margins, alignment of the articular masses, and alignment of the spinolaminar junctions (Fig. 26-2).

FIGURE 26-2 *Normal lateral cervical spine radiograph. Proper alignment of the cervical spine is seen as smooth continuity of the anterior vertebral margins* (open black arrows), *posterior vertebral margins* (open white arrows), *and spinolaminar junction lines* (solid black arrows). *The anterior atlantodental space* (curved white arrow) *should measure 2.5 to 3 mm or less.*

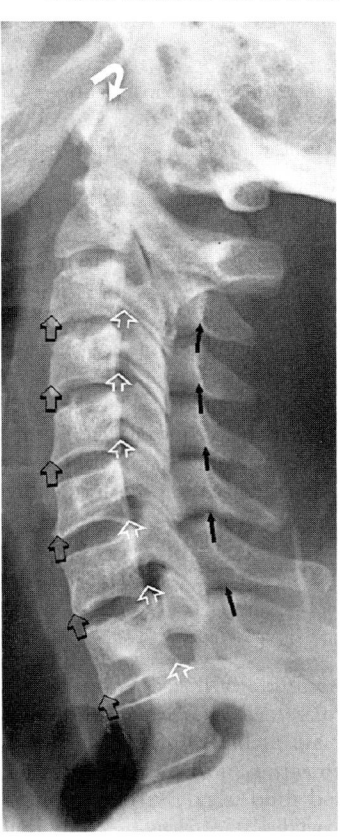

FIGURE 26-3 *Physiologic subluxation. Lateral cervical radiograph in flexion (**A**) shows slight anterolisthesis at several levels* (arrows). *Relative lack of articular process overlap at C5–C6 is also physiologic. Extension (**B**) view shows physiologic retrolisthesis at C2–C3 and C3–C4* (arrows).

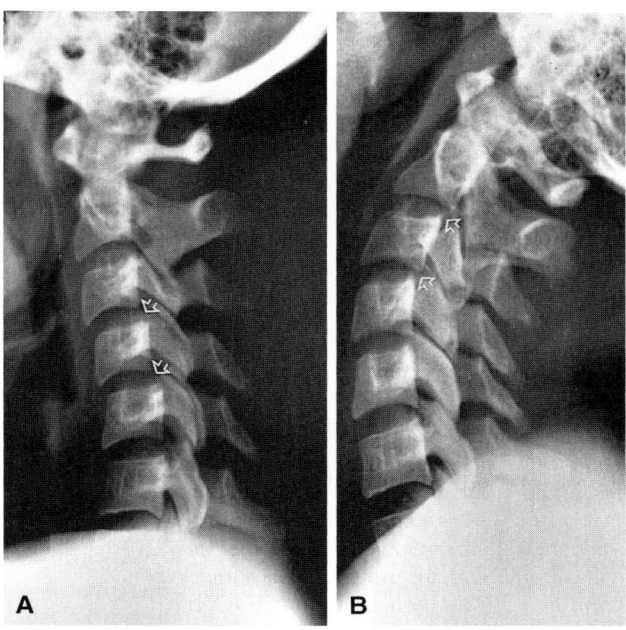

It is important to recognize minimal degrees of anterior and posterior intervertebral subluxation that occur normally with physiologic motion with cervical flexion and extension (Fig. 26-3) and involve multiple levels. Such physiologic displacement typically occurs at multiple contiguous levels and usually does not exceed 2 mm.[77] Spacing between laminae, articular facets, and spinous processes should be similar at contiguous levels (see Fig. 26-2). The intervertebral disk spaces should appear nearly uniform in height across the disk space. The orientation of each vertebra should be assessed for rotational abnormalities. On a true lateral radiograph, the articular pillars should be superimposed (see Fig. 26-2). An *abrupt offset* of the pillars indicates a rotational injury such as a unilateral interfacet dislocation (UID). Similarly, an abrupt change in the distance from the posterior margin of the articular pillar to the spinolaminar line (the laminar space) indicates a rotational injury[88] (Fig. 26-4).

Focal prevertebral or retropharyngeal soft tissue edema or hematoma can sometimes indicate an otherwise radiographically occult injury. However, absolute measurements of the prevertebral soft tissues are not particularly useful indicators of injury and can vary with head position, body habitus, time from imaging, and phase of inspiration, among other factors. Herr and colleagues[42] evaluated prevertebral soft tissue measurements at the C3 level in 212 patients with blunt trauma using a 4-mm upper limit of normal. They found that a measurement greater than 4 mm was only 64 percent sensitive for detecting cervical spine fractures involving the anterior, posterior, upper, or

FIGURE 26-4 *Unilateral facet dislocation. Lateral cervical radiograph shows anterior subluxation of C5 on C6. There is offset of the articular masses at C5 (single-headed arrows) and superimposition of these at C6, indicating rotation of the articular masses. There is an abrupt alteration in the distance from the back of the articular mass to the spinolaminar line (laminar space), also indicating rotation of the C5 vertebral body relative to C6 (double-headed arrows).*

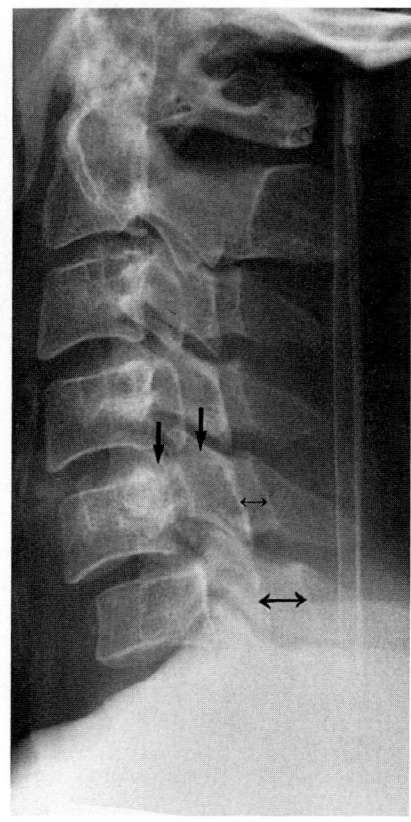

lower cervical spine. Precervical soft tissue prominence from the skull base to the axis is particularly important to recognize, since injuries at the craniocervical junction are often not apparent on the lateral radiograph. Harris[36] has shown that the analysis of the contour of the cervicocranial prevertebral soft tissues can be particularly useful in detecting subtle upper cervical spine injuries (Fig. 26-5).

Assessment of the axis in the lateral view is aided by identification of the Harris ring,[37] a composite shadow of cortical bone along the margins of the neurocentral synchondrosis (Fig. 26-6). In a true lateral projection, the Harris rings from both sides of C2 are superimposed, whereas two parallel Harris rings result from an oblique (off-lateral) projection. The Harris ring of cortical bone is normally incomplete in its posteroinferior aspect owing to the foramen transversarium. The Harris ring is particularly helpful in detecting atypical cases of traumatic spondylolisthesis[37] (Hangman's fracture) and the classical type III or low odontoid fracture (Fig. 26-7; see also Fig. 26-6).[1]

Radiologic identification of subluxation at the atlanto-occipital articulation can be difficult. Alignment at this articulation can be assessed by reference to three anatomic landmarks with the neck in the neutral position. First, the occipital condyle should lie within the condylar fossae of the atlas ring, with no gap between them in the adult patient. Second, a line drawn along the posterior surface of the clivus should intercept the superior aspect of the odontoid process. Third, a line drawn along the C1 spinolaminar line should intercept the posterior margin of the foramen magnum (opisthion) (Fig. 26-8).

A more precise assessment of this anatomic relationship can be determined by a direct measurement, regardless of the degree of cervical flexion and extension. The tip of the odontoid process should lie within 12 mm of the basion (inferior tip of the clivus), and a vertical line drawn along the posterior cortex of C2 (posterior axial line) should lie within 12 mm of the basion[38,39] (Fig. 26-9). Cranial distraction and anterior displacement are indicated by measurements greater than 12 mm. The atlantodental space at the C1–C2 articulation should be evaluated; it normally measures less than 3 mm in the adult.[21] A larger atlantodental space associated with a cervicocranial hematoma indicates acute transverse atlantal ligament injury and instability of the articulation (Fig. 26-10).

ANTEROPOSTERIOR VIEW The AP radiograph of the cervical spine supplements information provided on the lateral cervical radiograph and can identify additional injuries.[71] On the normal AP view, the spinous processes are vertically aligned, the lateral masses form smoothly undulating margins without abrupt interruption, the disk spaces are uniform in height, and the alignment of the vertebral bodies in the transverse (horizontal) plane is easily assessed (Fig. 26-11). Typically, the craniocervical junction region and the odontoid process are not well seen, being obscured by the face, mandible, and occipital skull. Lateral flexion injuries compressing an articular pillar or lateral portion of a vertebral body are seen to advantage. Rotational injuries are indicated by an abrupt offset of spinous process alignment, as occurs with unilateral facet dislocation.

Fractures of the vertebral body in the sagittal plane are also often evident on the AP view. Facet and articular mass fractures can sometimes be visualized as well. Laminopedicular separation (fracture separation of the articular mass), which may occur with hyperflexion-rotation injuries[78] or rarely hyperextension[40] mechanisms, can produce a horizontal orientation of the articular mass, leading to an open-appearing facet joint (Fig. 26-12). Normally, these joints are not seen in tangent on the AP view because of their 35° inclination from the horizontal plane. Some studies suggest that the AP view provides no significant diagnostic information in addition to that available from the lateral and open-mouth projection.[44] West and co-workers[86] have shown that a single lateral cervical spine radiograph is as sensitive for injury diagnosis as the standard three-view series for experienced interpreters.

OPEN-MOUTH ODONTOID VIEW The open-mouth odontoid (OMO) or atlantoaxial view requires patient cooperation for optimal studies. Ideally, the skull base (occiput), atlas, and axis are well displayed without overlap from the mandible or dentition (Fig. 26-13). The normal OMO

FIGURE 26-5 *Subtle soft tissue abnormality indicating fracture.* **A,** *Coned-down lateral view of the craniocervical junction shows normal prevertebral soft tissue configuration with a slight soft tissue fullness (convex bulge) at the level of the C1 anterior arch and a slight concavity below* (arrows). **B,** *Coned-down lateral view from another patient with cervical pain shows loss of these contours with uniform prevertebral soft tissue fullness above, at, and below the C1 anterior tubercle. A subtle odontoid fracture* (arrows) *is present. The fracture interrupts the Harris composite ring shadow.* **C,** *Lateral cervical radiograph from another patient shows prevertebral soft tissue prominence at the cervicocranial junction with loss of normal contours around the C1 anterior tubercle* (arrowheads), *indicating prevertebral hematoma and edema. The spinolaminar line of C2 is also posteriorly displaced* (solid arrows *and* black line). *There is a subtle traumatic spondylolisthesis* (open arrow). *(B, From Mirvis, S.E.; Young, J.W.R. In Mirvis, S.E.; Young, J.W.R., eds. Imaging in Trauma and Critical Care. Baltimore, Williams & Wilkins, 1992, p. 343.)*

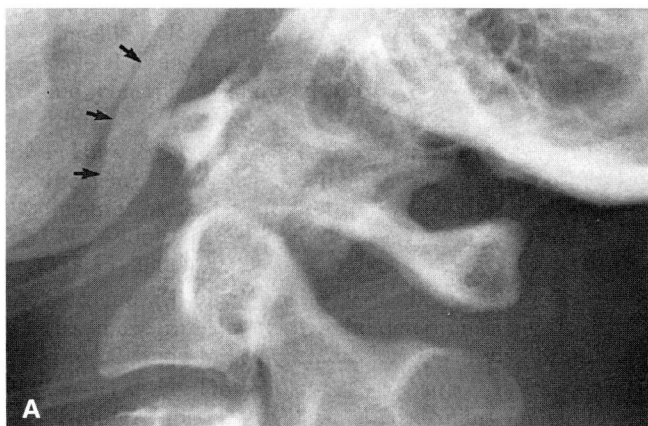
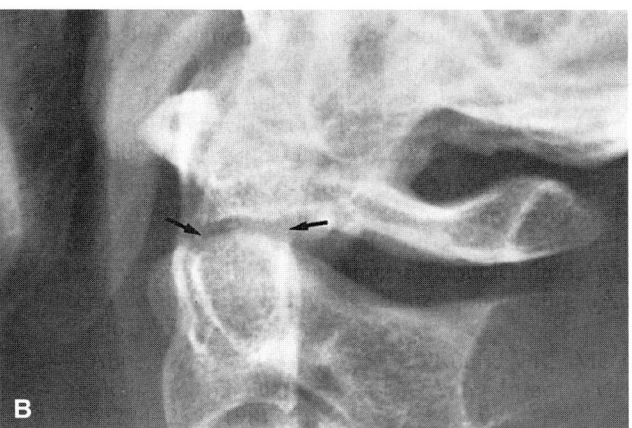
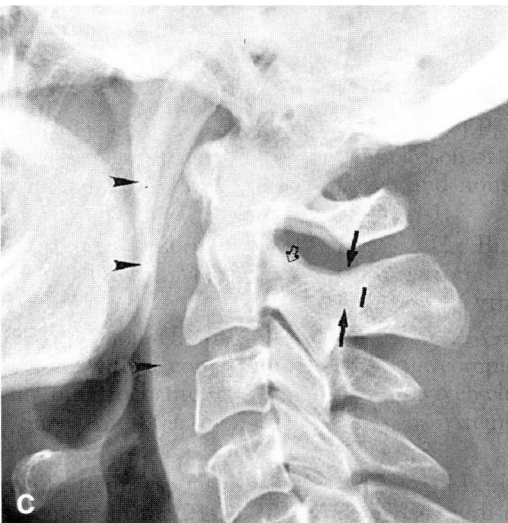

view demonstrates the lateral margins of the C1 ring aligned within 1 or 2 mm of the articular pillars of the axis. The articular masses of C2 should appear symmetrical, as should the joint spaces between C1 and C2 as long as there is no head rotation. The measured distance between the odontoid and the C1 medial border (i.e., the lateral atlantodental space) should be equal, but a discrepancy of 3 mm or greater is often seen in patients without pathology.[48] Finally, a vertical line bisecting the odontoid process should form a 90° angle with a line placed horizontally across the superior aspect of the C2 articular masses[83] (Fig. 26-14).

Voluntary rotation, head tilting, or torticollis can be difficult to distinguish from atlantoaxial rotatory subluxation on the basis of radiography alone.[62] Dynamic CT studies can be useful in differentiating a locked atlantoaxial

dislocation from subluxation without locking (Fig. 26-15).[62] Injuries that are best seen on the OMO view include the C1 burst fracture (Jefferson fracture) (Fig. 26-16), odontoid fracture (see Fig. 26-14), and lateral flexion fracture of the axis. Lateral spreading of the C1 lateral masses of greater than 6 to 7 mm in the Jefferson burst fracture suggests coexisting disruption of the transverse portion of the cruciate ligament, producing an unstable "atypical" Jefferson fracture (Fig. 26-17).[25] This pattern usually creates two fractures on one side of the C1 ring and probably results from asymmetrical axial loading or bending forces.

SUPINE OR TRAUMA OBLIQUE VIEW The supine oblique, or "trauma" oblique, projection is obtained with the patient maintained in collar stabilization in the supine

FIGURE 26-6 *C2 composite ring shadow. In the lateral projection, portions of the C2 cortex form a composite shadow of bone density (arrows). A small circle of the foramen transversarium interrupts the ring in its posterior inferior margin (arrowhead). Discontinuity or irregularity of the ring shadow indicates probable type III odontoid fracture or atypical traumatic spondylolisthesis.*

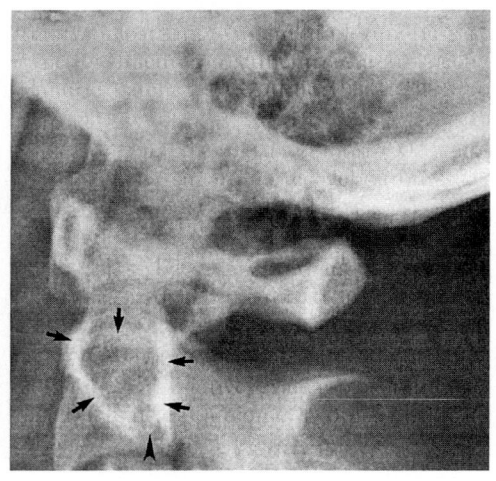

FIGURE 26-7 *Type III odontoid fracture. Coned-down lateral view shows complete disruption of the Harris composite ring shadow, indicating odontoid fractures (arrows). The atlas is anteriorly displaced relative to the axis, as indicated by respective spinolaminar lines (arrowheads). (From Mirvis, S.E.; Shanmuganathan, K. Trauma radiology. 5. Imaging of acute cervical spine trauma. J Intensive Care Med 10:15, 1995.)*

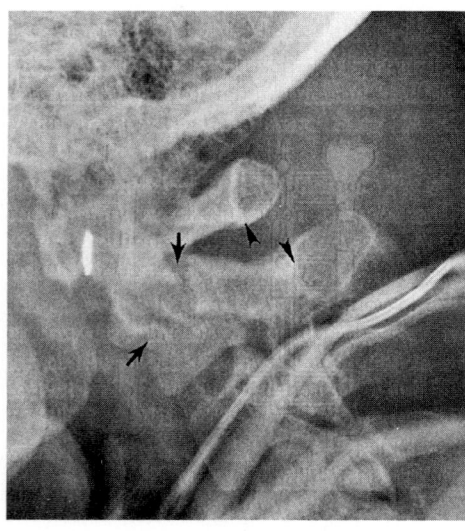

FIGURE 26-8 *Normal atlanto-occipital anatomic relationships. In a coned-down lateral view from a normal patient, the spinolaminar line of C1 aligns with the posterior foramen magnum (double-headed black arrow), and the occipital condyle sits within the fossae of the C1 ring without a gap (black arrowheads). The distance between the basion (tip of clivus, asterisk) and the top of the odontoid process (plus sign) is less than 12 mm. The posterior axial line (white arrows) drawn along the posterior margin of the C2 body lies within 12 mm of the basion.*

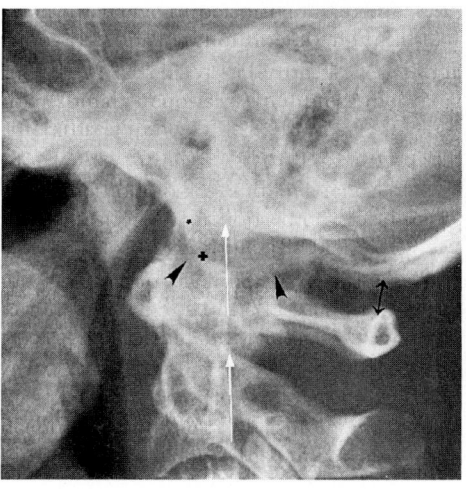

FIGURE 26-9 *Atlanto-occipital subluxation. Lateral view of the upper cervical spine shows anterior displacement of the posterior margin of the foramen magnum relative to the C1 spinolaminar line (short arrows). The occipital condyles are displaced from the condylar fossae of the atlas (arrowheads), and a line drawn along the clival posterior margin intercepts the odontoid process along its anterior surface (long arrow). Finally, the distance between the tip of the odontoid (plus sign) and the basion (asterisk) exceeds 12 mm, as does the distance from the posterior axial line (interrupted line) to the basion.*

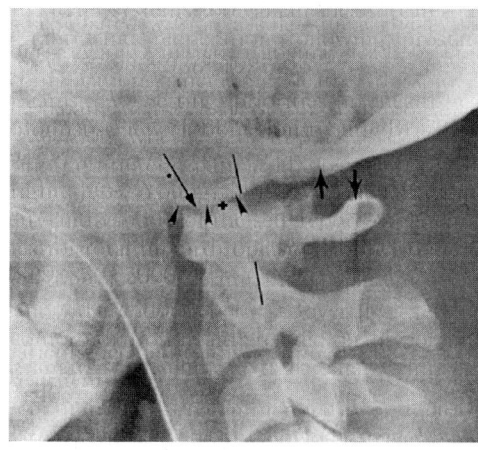

FIGURE 26-10 *Atlantoaxial dislocation. Lateral coned-down cervical view shows marked widening of the atlantodental space, indicating disruption of the transverse atlantal ligament. Note the anterior displacement of the C1 spinolaminar junction line relative to that of C2. (From Mirvis, S.E.; Shanmuganathan, K. Trauma radiology. 5. Imaging of acute cervical spine trauma. J Intensive Care Med 10:15, 1995.)*

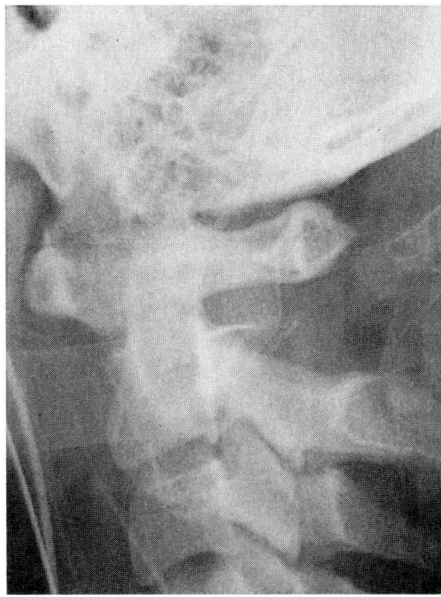

FIGURE 26-11 *Normal anteroposterior (AP) cervical radiograph. In the normal AP view, a smoothly undulating lateral border is created by the lateral masses, the spinous processes are vertically aligned, and the spacing of the intervertebral disks and uncovertebral joints (arrows) is uniform. The facet joints cannot be visualized because they are inclined about 35° to the horizontal. Enlarged C7 transverse processes (cervical ribs) are seen as a variant. In general, C2 and C1 are poorly seen in this projection. (From Mirvis, S.E.; Young, J.W.R. In Mirvis, S.E.; Young, J.W.R., eds. Imaging in Trauma and Critical Care. Baltimore, Williams & Wilkins, 1992, p. 298.)*

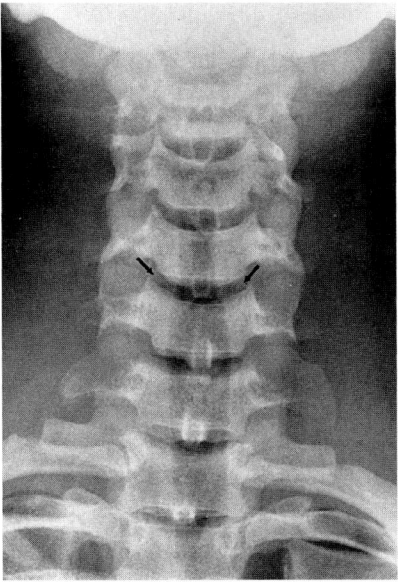

and neutral position. The film or computed radiography cassette is placed alongside the patient's neck, and the x-ray tube is angled 45° from the vertical. Normal supine oblique views show the neural foramina on one side and the pedicles of the contralateral side. The laminae are normally aligned like shingles on a roof (Fig. 26-18).

This projection can be used to improve visualization of the cervicothoracic junction when the lateral view is insufficient.[51] Subluxation or dislocation of the articular masses and laminae that may not be seen on other standard views may be well demonstrated in this projection. If the cervicothoracic junction cannot be adequately visualized on the neutral lateral view, most institutions obtain a swimmer's lateral radiograph (89%) as opposed to a bilateral supine oblique (11%) as the next imaging study.[50] The supine oblique views are cost-effective compared with CT scanning for *selectively clearing the cervicothoracic junction.*[51]

SWIMMER'S LATERAL VIEW This view is often acquired to visualize the cervicothoracic junction when it is obscured by the density of shadows produced by the shoulders in the true lateral projection. Optimal positioning requires that one of the patient's arms be abducted by 180° and extended above the head, which may be difficult or impossible for patients with arm and shoulder injuries, while the opposite shoulder is extended posteriorly to decrease overlapping of skeletal structures. This projection requires the patient to be rotated slightly off true lateral.

Positional changes required to obtain the swimmer's view are contraindicated for patients who are unconscious or who have cervical cord injuries.

The swimmer's view results in a somewhat distorted oblique projection of the cervicocranial junction, with the vertebrae obscured by portions of the shoulder girdle or the ribs, or both. Even with its limitations, however, this view is generally suitable to assess alignment and detect gross injuries.

PILLAR VIEW The pillar view (Fig. 26-19) is designed to visualize the cervical articular masses directly in the frontal projection. It is generally agreed, however, that this view should be reserved for neurologically intact patients in whom articular mass fractures are suspected on the basis of radiography, and it is now rarely used.

To obtain the view, the patient must be able to voluntarily rotate the head, and the presence of an upper cervical injury must have been previously excluded in the initial plain radiographic evaluation. Because articular pillar and pedicle fractures often occur with rotational injuries, further rotation is contraindicated when assessing these injuries. If injuries to the lateral cervical pillars are suspected on the basis of the initial radiographs, they are best further assessed by CT.

FIGURE 26-12 *Isolation of articular pillar. This anteroposterior view shows direct visualization of the facet articulations of C4–C5 and C5–C6 on the left caused by rotation of the articular mass (arrow). This finding requires combined fractures of the C5 right lamina and ipsilateral pedicle.*

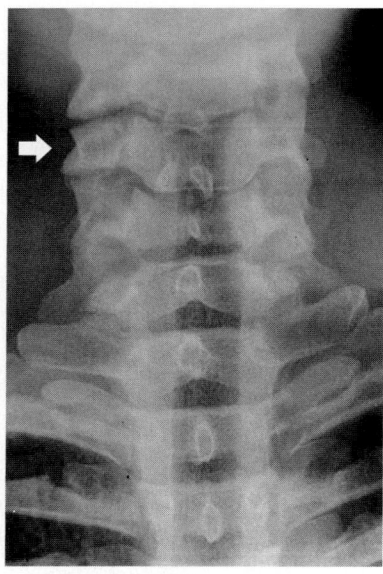

FLEXION-EXTENSION STRESS VIEWS

Demonstration of ligament injury may require placing stress on the cervical ligaments. It is imperative that cervical flexion and extension views be obtained only for *alert, cooperative, and neurologically intact patients* who can describe pain or

FIGURE 26-13 *Normal open-mouth odontoid (OMO) view. The lateral borders of the lateral masses of the atlas are aligned with the lateral borders of the axis. Without rotation of the head, the lateral atlantodental spaces are equivalent. A thin radiolucent Mach line at the base of the odontoid is created by the overlapping inferior surface of the posterior atlas ring (arrow).*

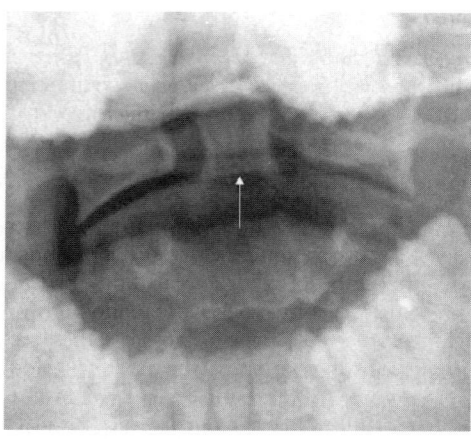

FIGURE 26-14 *Odontoid fracture with tilt. The open-mouth odontoid view shows a fracture across the base of the odontoid (arrows) and lateral tilting of the odontoid process.*

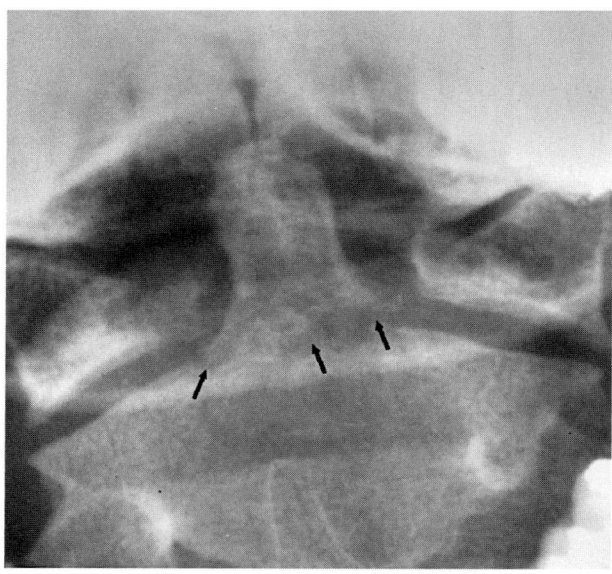

initial onset of any subjective neurologic symptoms. During the evaluation of acute injuries, active flexion-extension radiographs should be supervised by a physician. The use of fluoroscopically guided passive flexion-extension cervical spine assessment is discussed in detail in the following section on imaging approaches. Although for most patients evidence of cervical instability is apparent on the neutral radiographs, some injuries can be effectively reduced to an anatomic position with the patient in a cervical collar and may be completely invisible in the stabilized neutral position (Figs. 26-20 to 26-22).

Normally, flexion and extension produce minimal physiologic motion of adjacent vertebrae and anterior or posterior sliding movement across the articular facets. An abrupt change in facet coverage at one level indicates injury to the ligament support. Finally, degenerative disease (cervical spondylosis) of the facet articulations with loss of the interarticular fibrocartilage may allow excessive anterior translation at one or more levels that can mimic pathologic movement related to acute injury (Fig. 26-23). In degenerative antero- or retrolisthesis, the shape of the articular facet and width of the facet joint spaces may be normal; however, in most cases the articular facet has become "ground down," the facet joints narrowed, and the articular processes thinned. In traumatic subluxation, the articular facets are either normally shaped or fractured and the joint spaces are widened.

In a national survey of 165 trauma centers, Grossman and associates[35] found that flexion-extension views were more likely to be obtained as part of cervical spine imaging evaluation in Level I as opposed to Level II or lower level centers. Brady and colleagues[12] evaluated use of dynamic flexion-extension views in 451 patients with blunt trauma who manifested neck pain, midline tenderness, or an abnormal spinal contour on static cervical radiographs.

FIGURE 26-15 *3-D computed tomography (CT) scan (volume rendering) of atlantoaxial rotatory subluxation. **A,** Volume-rendered inferior view of the cervical spine from 16-slice multidetector CT shows patient's head turned to the left with marked anterior subluxation of the right C1 articular mass (arrow) with uncovering of about 80 percent of the facet surface. **B,** Another volume-rendered view from the inferior perspective with patient's head rotated to the right shows a lesser degree of anterior subluxation of the left C1 lateral mass (arrow). The fact that the patient can rotate the head in both directions excludes locked facets.*

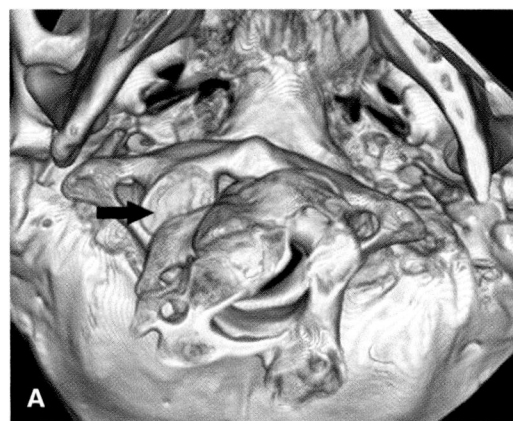 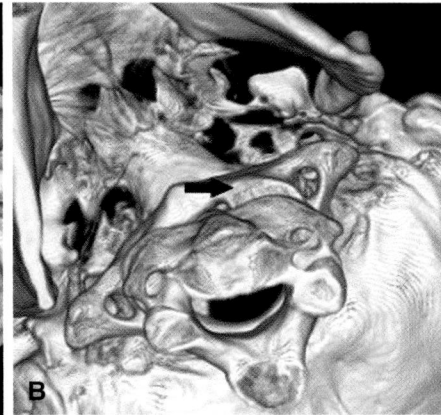

Patients with abnormal static cervical radiographs were statistically more likely to have abnormal active flexion-extension studies than those with normal static studies and therefore more likely to require definitive stabilization.

Lateral flexion-extension cervical radiographs are often unsuccessful owing to the inability of the patient to attain an adequate degree of flexion and extension stress or to the inability to visualize the lower cervical spine or cervicothoracic junction. In addition, they have not been shown to be cost-effective and tend to add little useful information to the workup.[2,49,66] Verifying that the patient can indeed flex and extend the cervical spine without limitation of pain or neurologic symptoms prior to attempting radiographic assessment is advised. Assessment of the patient for potential ligament injury or spine instability may require MRI in the acute setting, or flexion-extension views may be reattempted after a period of cervical immobilization if symptoms persist.

FIGURE 26-16 *Jefferson burst fracture. The open-mouth odontoid view shows lateral displacement of the C1 articular masses relative to those of C2 (double-headed arrows), indicating a C1 burst fracture.*

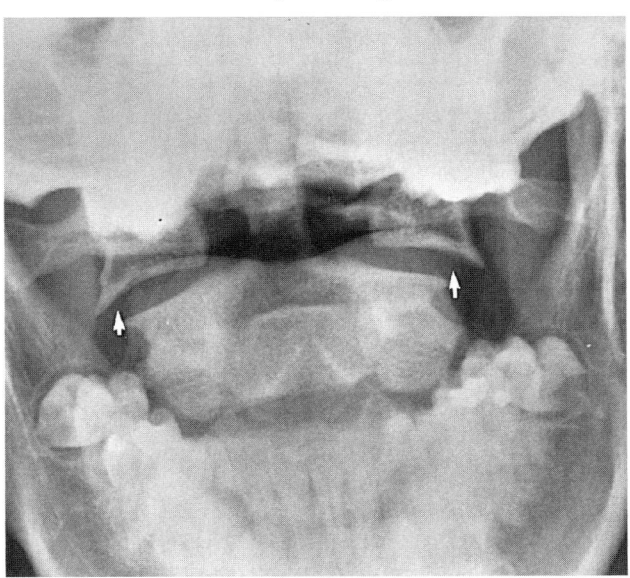

FIGURE 26-17 *Unstable Jefferson fracture. Axial CT scan through the atlas shows wide displacement of parts of the ring (double-headed arrows), indicating probable disruption or avulsion of the transverse atlantal ligament, creating both mechanical and neurologic instability.*

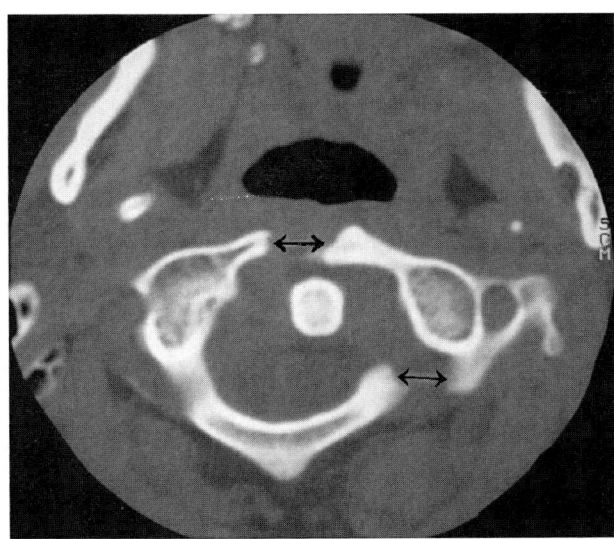

FIGURE 26-18 | *Normal "shingles-on-the-roof" orientation of laminae seen in an oblique projection of the cervical spine.*

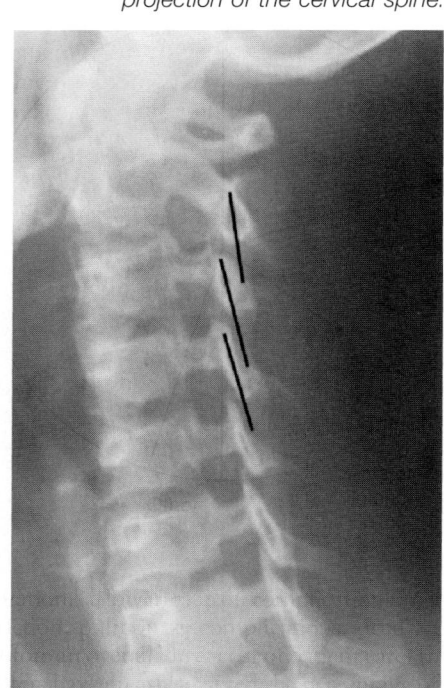

FIGURE 26-19 | *Pillar view of the right articular masses of the cervical spine.*

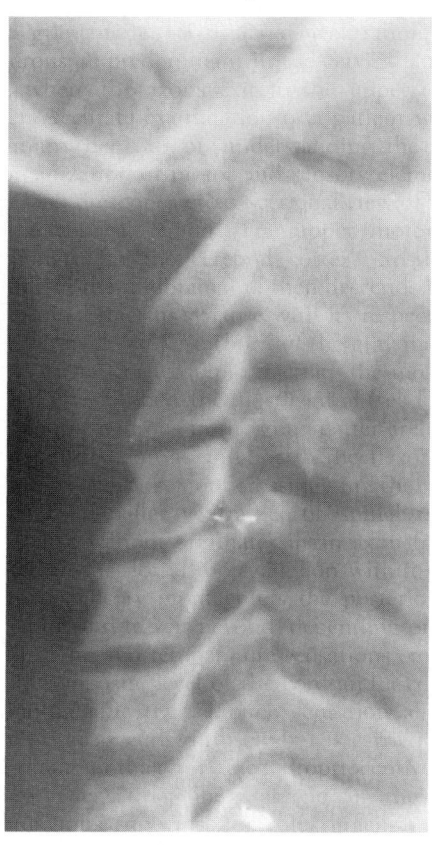

FIGURE 26-20 | *Subtle hyperflexion injury. **A,** Hyperflexion sprain not visible on neutral lateral cervical radiograph. **B,** Sagittal CT re-formation in slight flexion shows a narrowed disk space at C5–C6 (arrow) and widened interspinous space (white line) indicating flexion sprain. Stability cannot be determined even from CT appearance.*

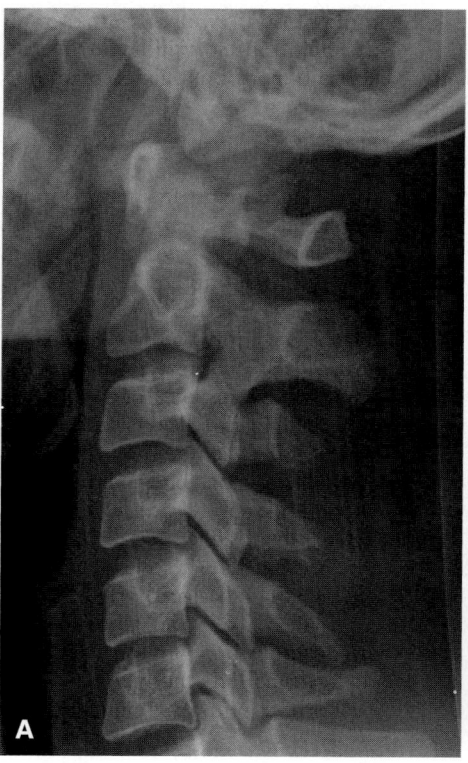
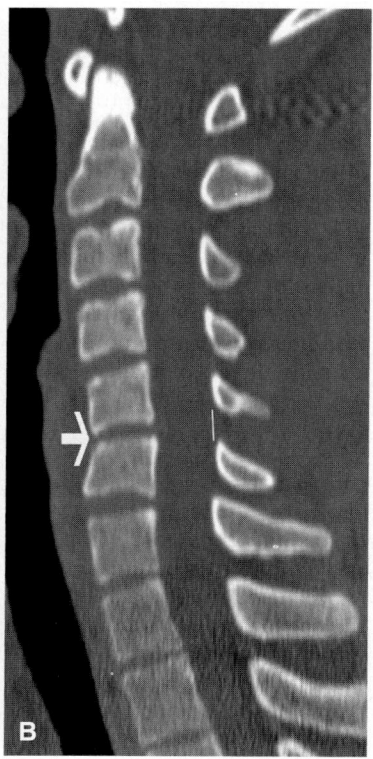

FIGURE 26-21 *Hyperflexion ligament injury not apparent on neutral position lateral view radiograph. **A,** Lateral cervical radiograph in a trauma patient with cervical spine pain is unremarkable. **B,** Flexion lateral view (physician supervised) shows hyperflexion subluxation at C5–C6 (white arrow) and unilateral facet dislocation at C4–C5 (black arrow). (From Mirvis, S.E.; Shanmuganathan, K. Trauma radiology. 5. Imaging of acute cervical spine trauma. J Intensive Care Med 10:15, 1995.)*

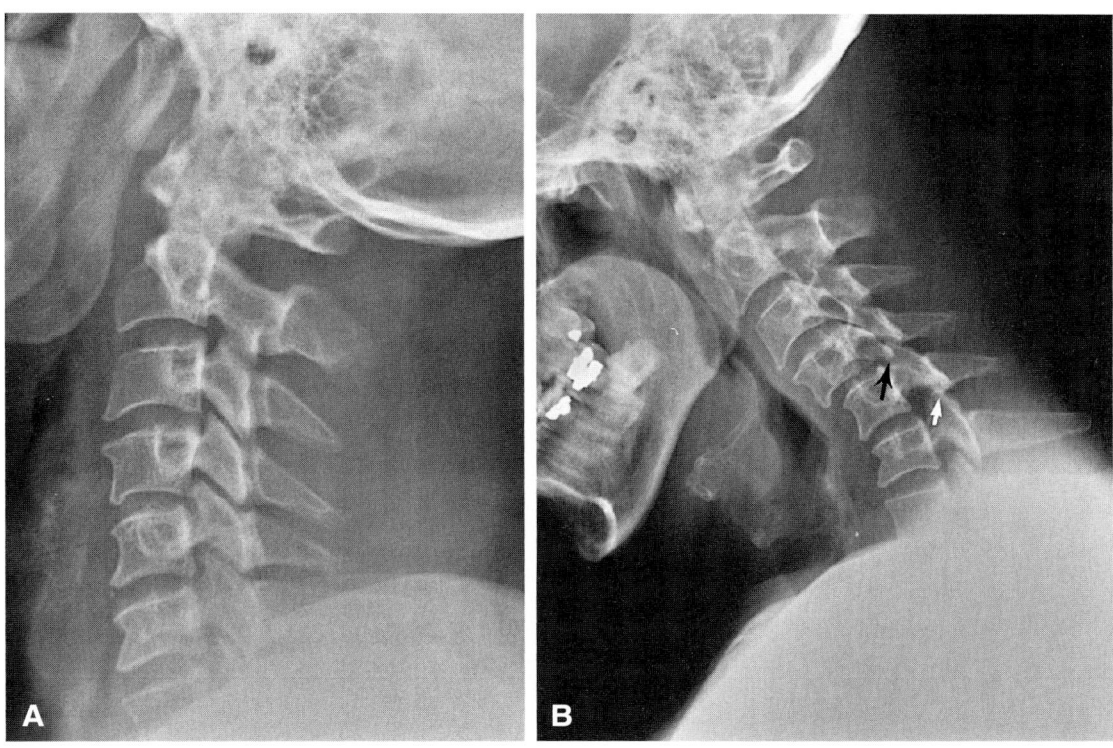

FIGURE 26-22 *Hyperflexion ligament injury not apparent on neutral lateral cervical radiograph. **A,** Neutral position lateral radiograph of a trauma patient with cervical spine tenderness is unremarkable. **B,** Repeated view with flexion limited by pain shows hyperflexion sprain at C4–C5 (arrowhead) with mild flaring of the spinous processes (open arrow).*

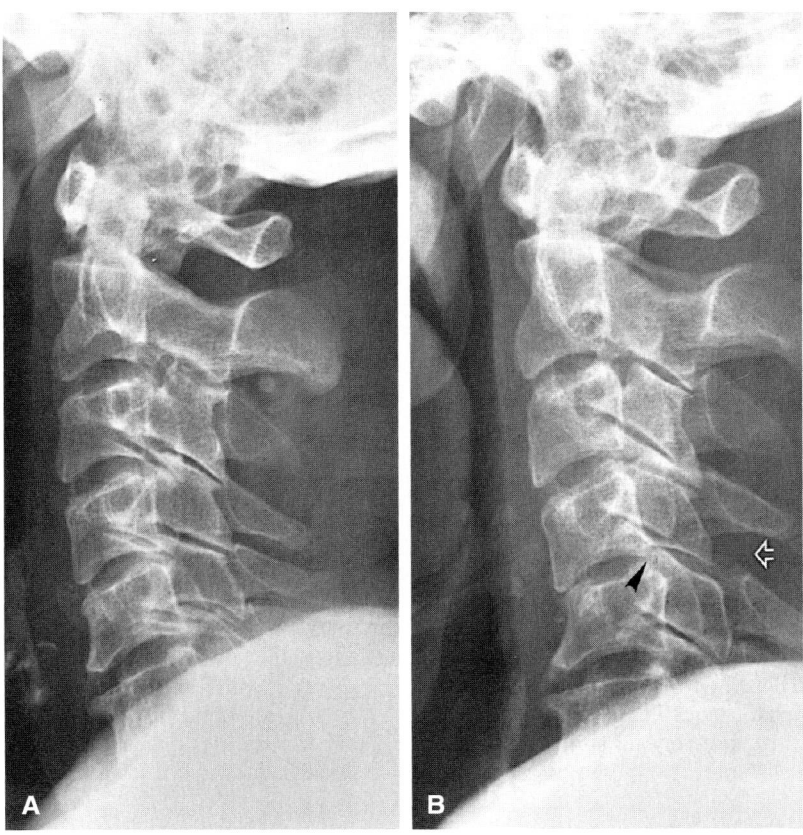

FIGURE 26-23 *Degenerative subluxation. Lateral cervical radiograph shows slight anterolisthesis of C4 on C5 (arrow). There is diffuse degenerative change. Note narrowing of the facet joints and sclerosis of the facet surfaces (arrowheads).*

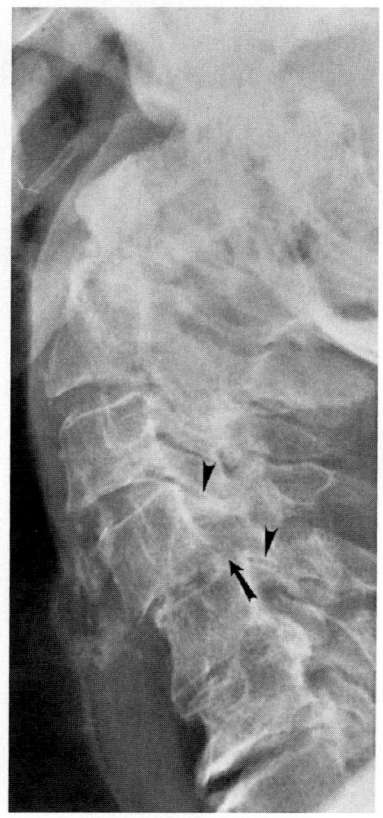

THORACIC SPINE

Imaging of the thoracic spine is a less complex procedure than that of the cervical spine. The influence of the patient's overall condition on the type and sequence of imaging procedures used to evaluate the thoracic and lumbar areas is identical to that discussed for the cervical spine. Routine AP and lateral plain radiographs often constitute the initial evaluation of the thoracic spine, with the exception of the upper thoracic vertebrae (discussed separately later in this chapter). Unilateral or bilateral focal bulging of the thoracic paraspinous soft tissue shadows (the mediastinal stripe or paraspinal line) due to hematoma is an important marker of thoracic fractures (Fig. 26-24). Alteration of the contour of the paraspinous shadow is not specific for hematoma unless there is an appropriate history and corresponding findings on physical examination. Paraspinous fat, abscess, or neoplasm can produce a soft tissue density similar to that caused by a localized traumatic hematoma.

The great majority of acute thoracic spine injuries are recognizable on the initial plain film examination, and it is not so frequently necessary to use CT to establish the primary diagnosis as it is for the cervical spine. The only segment of the thoracic spine that requires special attention with plain radiography is the cervicothoracic junction. It is essential to be aware that the upper four or five thoracic vertebrae are not routinely visible on lateral radiographs of the thoracic spine because of the density of the superimposed shoulders. It is therefore incumbent on the attending physician *to indicate specifically* to the radiologist when the upper thoracic spine is the area of suspected injury so that additional views can be obtained.

The AP view of both the thoracic and the lumbar spine is also quite helpful in plain film evaluation. Vertebral alignment is assessed using the position of the pedicles, the presence or absence of scoliosis, and alignment of the spinous processes. The architecture of the pedicles at the affected level is important, as the relationship between the spinous processes can be helpful in demonstrating ligament disruption. A sudden increase in distance between two adjacent spinous processes, as determined from the AP view, is frequently associated with disruption of the intraspinous and supraspinous ligaments and of the facet capsules (Fig. 26-25). Widening of the distance between the pedicles at one level compared to adjacent levels is associated with burst fractures with lateral spreading of the vertebral body (Fig. 26-26). Lateral translation on the AP view, combined with anterior translation on the lateral view, suggests a grossly unstable shearing injury. Supine oblique views, which can be invaluable in the evaluation of the lower cervical region, are of little use in the upper thoracic spine because of superimposition of the ribs and the complexity of the costovertebral articulations.

LUMBAR SPINE

Radiographic evaluation of the acutely injured lumbar spine, like that of other segments of the spinal column, often begins with AP and lateral plain radiographs. When it is clinically inappropriate to place the patient in the true lateral position, the lateral examination should be carried out using a horizontal beam with the patient recumbent. For patients with a history of acute trauma, the lateral "spot" radiograph of the lumbosacral junction is neither indicated nor necessary.

On initial evaluation, the overall alignment of the thoracolumbar junction and lumbar spine is most clearly assessed with a lateral radiograph taken in the supine position. Many fractures demonstrate not only comminution of the vertebral body but also a local area of kyphosis. The complete loss of lumbar lordosis in the absence of obvious pathology may still be suggestive of injury. As in the cervical spine, subtle rotational injuries are often evident on the lateral projection. In burst fractures of the lumbar spine, the degree of canal compromise can frequently be estimated by observing the posterosuperior corner of the injured vertebral body (see Fig. 26-26).

The AP view provides the same information as described previously for the thoracic spine. Oblique projections of the lumbar spine should be obtained only when the AP and lateral radiographs are grossly negative and inconsistent with the clinical evaluation. Also, the patient's condition must allow rotation into the oblique position. The oblique projection provides another perspective of the lumbar vertebral body and excellent visualization of the pars interarticularis and the facet joints.

FIGURE 26-24 *Paraspinal hematomas indicating thoracic spine fracture.* **A,** *The anteroposterior coned-down view of the lower thoracic spine shows bulging of the paraspinal stripes* (arrowheads) *accompanied by a widened disk space at T11–T12* (open arrow). **B,** *The coned-down lateral projection shows hyperextension injury with partial inferior end-plate avulsion from T11* (arrow).

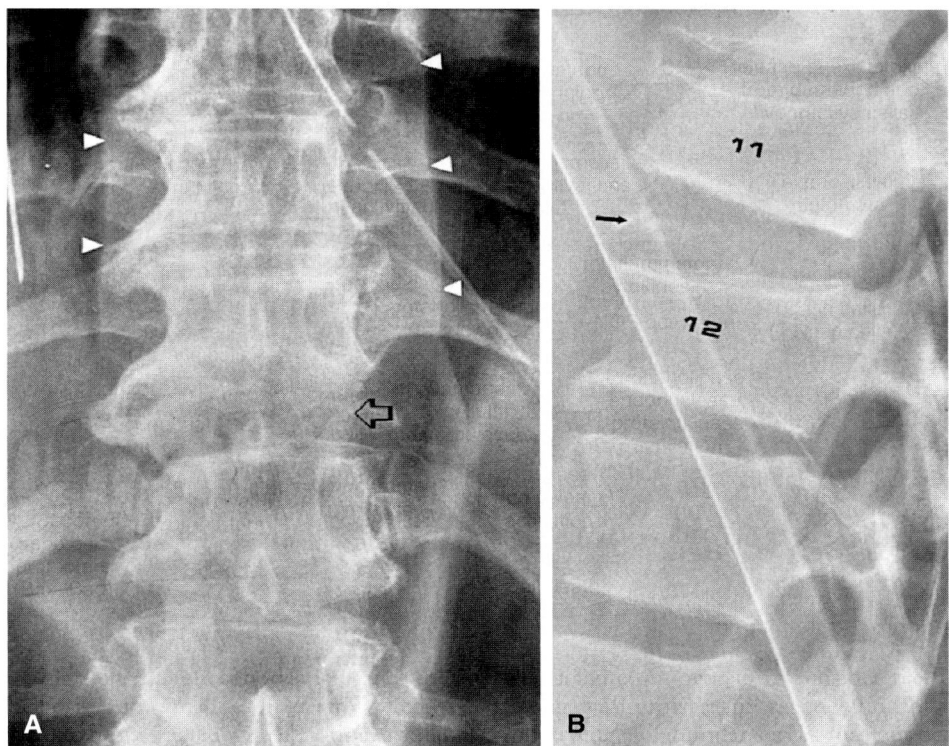

FIGURE 26-25 *Hyperflexion lumbar fracture.* **A,** *Anteroposterior view of lumber spine shows widening between the spinous processes of T12–L1 indicating hyperflexion injury* (black arrows). *There is a fracture of the left L1 transverse process* (white arrow). **B,** *Lateral view demonstrates interspinous flaring* (white arrow) *and anterior L1 vertebral compression* (black arrow).

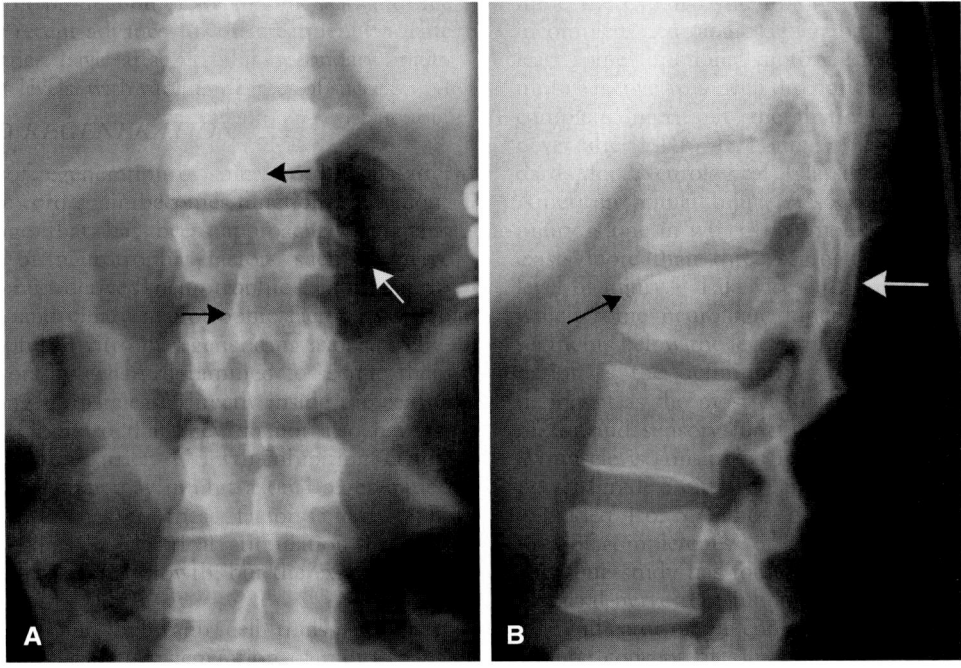

FIGURE 26-26 | *Lumbar burst fracture.* **A,** *Anteroposterior radiograph shows loss of height of L2 and widening of the pedicles are forced laterally* (double-headed arrow) *with body compression.* **B,** *Lateral view shows significant loss of height of L2 and marked posterior retropulsion of the posterior cortical bone nearly occluding the spinal canal.*

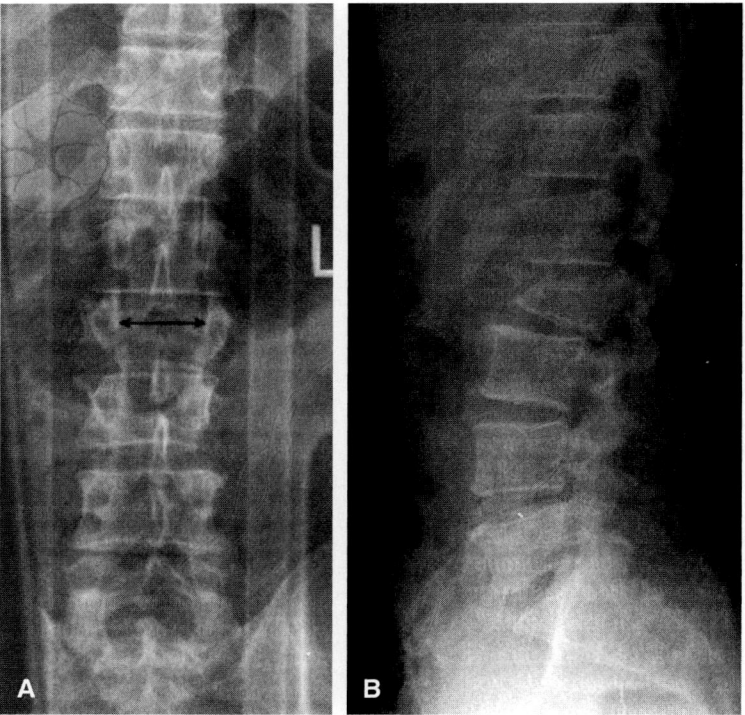

SACRUM AND COCCYX

Acute injuries involving the sacrum are commonly associated with pelvic ring disruption. However, isolated injuries of the lower sacral segments and coccyx do occur and require special imaging techniques. The sacral and coccygeal concavity makes adequate visualization of all these segments on a single AP projection impossible. Consequently, in addition to the straight AP radiograph, standard plain radiographic examination of the sacrum and coccyx must include rostrally and caudally angulated AP views as well as a true lateral projection. Superimposition of intestinal artifacts, pelvic calcifications, and soft tissue structures can obscure minimally displaced fractures of the sacral and coccygeal segments in the AP projection. In such a case, the fracture is usually evident on the lateral radiograph. In all areas of the thoracic-lumbar-sacral spine, CT may be needed to detect subtle injuries not evident by radiography. Sacrococcygeal dislocation, even when grossly displaced, is difficult to diagnose radiographically because of the range of normal variation at this level and the effects of pelvic delivery in women. Clinical correlation is particularly important for these patients.

Computed Tomography of the Spine

CT allows images to be obtained in any plane determined by the radiologist to demonstrate the pathology in question to maximal advantage. Multiplanar computed tomography is CT with routinely obtained sagittal and coronal reformatted images. The role of multiplanar CT in the evaluation of injuries of the axial skeleton has been well established. Simply put, multiplanar CT (including three-dimensional CT) is currently the imaging technique of choice for spinal injury.

The principal value of CT is in the axial image, which demonstrates the neural canal and the relationship of fracture fragments to the canal. Axial data obtained in the supine patient are converted electronically to images displayed in the sagittal and coronal planes, without requiring movement of the injured patient. The development of multidetector CT technology with 0.4-second or less gantry rotation time allows up to 128 axial images to be acquired per second and is expected to continue to expand to more images per second in the near future. The speed of data acquisition decreases the effects of patient motion and permits thinner image slices to be routinely obtained than with single-slice spiral CT. These factors contribute to a major improvement in the quality of reformatted two-dimensional (2-D) and three-dimensional (3-D) images. The volume elements obtained (voxels) with multidetector spiral scanning can be made equivalent in size in all three orthogonal axes (isotropic), permitting image quality equivalent to that of axial images in any orientation. Addition of detector arrays leads to increases in the speed of image acquisition and improvements in image quality. Cervical CT studies, particularly using state-of-the-art equipment, are far more rapidly obtained than bedside cervical spine radiographs.[14]

Spinal CT imaging is performed without intrathecal contrast to (1) evaluate uncertain radiologic findings,

(2) provide details of osseous injury as an aid to surgical planning, (3) assess focal or diffuse spine pain when no radiologic abnormalities are demonstrated, (4) clear the lower cervicothoracic region in symptomatic patients in whom cervical radiography provides inadequate visualization, (5) assess the adequacy of internal fixation and detect postoperative complications, and (6) localize foreign bodies and bone fragments in relation to neural elements.

CT imaging is not indicated for some spinal injuries identified radiographically. These include simple wedge compression, clay-shoveler's fracture, anterior subluxation of the cervical spine, hyperextension teardrop fracture, typical hangman's fractures, and typical odontoid fractures. In the thoracic, lumbar, and sacrococcygeal spine, CT is used primarily to assess the relationship of bone fragments to the neural canal, localize penetrating foreign bodies, record the details of complex fracture patterns, and exclude osseous injury with greater accuracy when plain radiographs are negative in symptomatic patients. Ballock and colleagues[4] have shown that CT is more accurate than plain radiography in distinguishing wedge compression fractures from burst fractures in the thoracolumbar spine. Hauser et al. and Sheridan et al. have shown that screening of the thoracolumbar spine as part of a thoracic-abdominal-pelvic CT survey excludes the need for radiography in blunt trauma patients.[41,79]

CT often shows additional injuries not suspected on review of plain radiographic views (see below). CT is particularly useful in identifying fractures of the occipital condyles (Fig. 26-27), articular mass, and laminae, which may occur in association with hyperflexion facet dislocations[78] (Fig. 26-28), hyperextension fracture-dislocations, hyperflexion teardrop fractures (Fig. 26-29), axial loading fractures of C1 (Jefferson fracture) (Fig. 26-30), odontoid process fractures,[1] and vertebral body burst fractures (Fig. 26-31).

Assessment of subluxation and dislocation is aided by 2-D multiplanar as well as surface contour 3-D image re-formation (Figs. 26-32 and 26-33). The quality of both 2-D re-formations and 3-D surface contour images is improved by the use of thinner axial CT slices and by

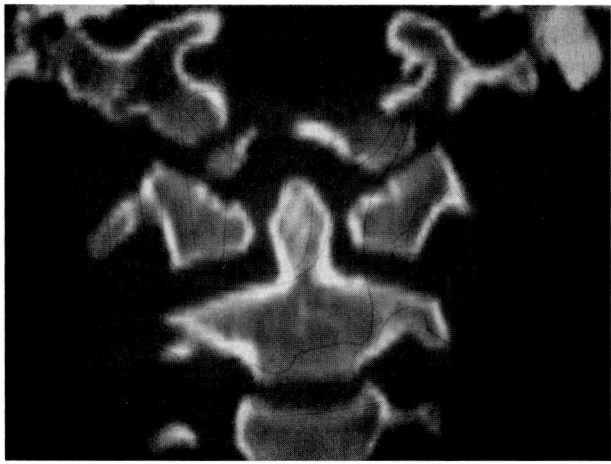

FIGURE 26-27 CT scan of type III occipital condyle fracture. Coronal reformatted image at craniocervical junction shows bilateral avulsions of the occipital condyles due to distraction forces. There is also widening of the C1–C2 joint spaces below, reflecting distraction force at this level as well.

overlapping axial CT images. Axial CT slice thickness should be no greater than 3 mm in the cervical spine and 5 mm in the thoracic and lumbar spine and can be routinely made thinner by means of MDCT scanners. Spiral CT scanners allow reconstruction of images at any slice thickness down to 0.5 mm and therefore generally provide higher quality reformatted images. Use of such thin-section scans and slice overlap assists in detection of fractures that are oriented in the plane of scanning (axial) such as the type II or low odontoid fracture as well as any minimally displaced fracture (Fig. 26-34).

Potential limitations of axial CT include volume averaging (accentuated by use of thick and nonoverlapping

FIGURE 26-28 Unilateral facet dislocation. **A,** Sagittal CT re-formation reveals anterolisthesis of C3 on C4 by about 20 percent with slight flexion at this level. **B,** Axial CT image shows a fracture through the articular pillar of C3 with the superior articular processes of the left C4 pillar embedded between fragments. **C,** A volume-rendered view of the same injury showing posterior displacement of the posterior aspect of the C3 articular mass and mild anterolisthesis of C3 on C4.

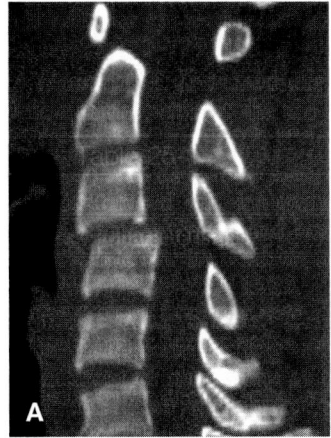 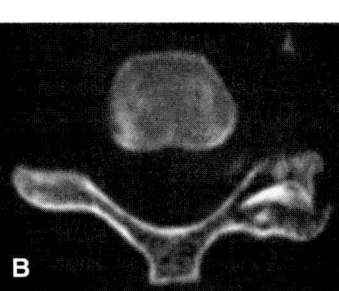 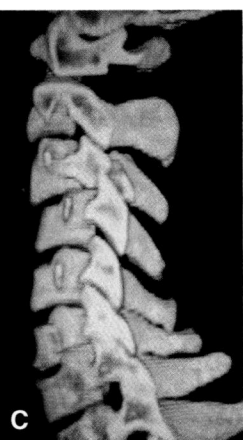

FIGURE 26-29 *CT scan of hyperflexion teardrop fracture. **A,** Lateral cervical radiograph shows a triangular, anteriorly displaced fragment at C5 with retrolisthesis of the C5 body. Posterior elements appear intact. **B,** Axial CT image reveals that the fracture has three-column involvement, with two fractures in the laminae. A vertical splitting fracture of C5 is observed in addition to anterior compressions, and there is diastasis of the right facet articulation. In certain complex fracture patterns, CT is far more useful than plain radiography to elucidate the spectrum of injuries. **C,** A sagittal inversion recovery MR image shows marked C6 on C7 posterior displacement (arrow), bright signal adjacent cord contusion, bright signal contusion of the C6 and C7 vertebral bodies, and generous pre-cervical high signal edema. The lower cervical spinous processes are flared due to hyperflexion stress.*

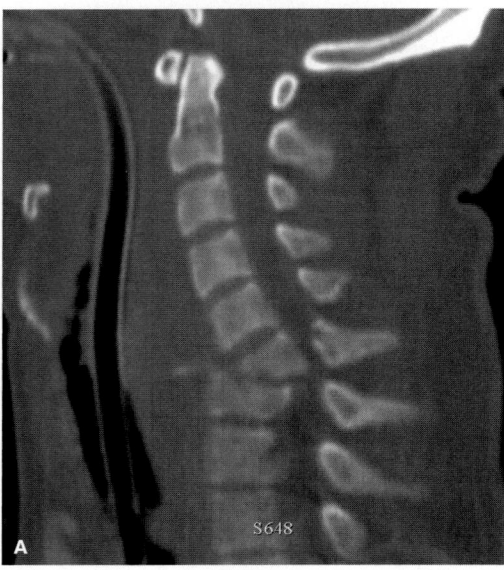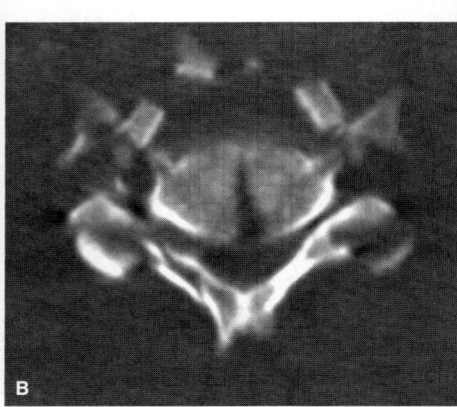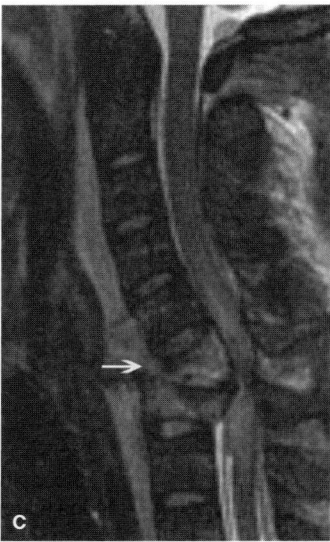

images that may simulate or obscure a fracture, particularly those oriented along the axial imaging plane), radiation exposure, and time constraints. Minimally displaced fractures may be difficult to identify on reformatted sagittal and coronal images because of degradation in spatial resolution inherent in these images. CT quality is also adversely affected by patient motion. As described earlier, multidetector spiral CT with 0.5-second tube rotation *significantly diminishes problems with volume averaging and patient motion artifacts and is extremely rapid to acquire.*

FIGURE 26-30 *CT scan of a Jefferson burst fracture. Axial image through the C1 level shows a five-part fracture of the C1 ring. Fractures are minimally displaced, making plain radiographic diagnosis more difficult.*

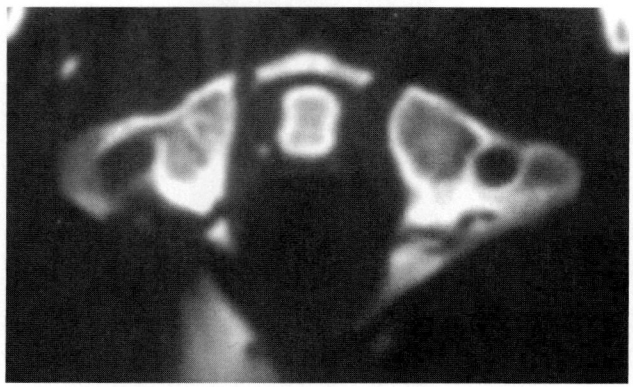

COMPUTED TOMOGRAPHY WITH INTRATHECAL CONTRAST

CTM is multiplanar CT performed after the intrathecal introduction of nonionic water-soluble contrast medium. Depending on the patient's condition and the level of suspected cord involvement, the contrast medium can be introduced in the usual myelographic fashion or, more often, laterally at the C1–C2 level with the patient supine. Because it is nonviscid, nonionic contrast medium can be introduced through a 22-gauge needle, which can then be removed, and absorbed through the meninges and subarachnoid villi. The water-soluble contrast medium diffuses through the cerebrospinal fluid; as a result, less movement of the patient is required to visualize the clinically indicated areas of the spine. Typically, the area of interest is examined fluoroscopically with spot and overhead radiography. If desired, CTM can be performed immediately after introduction of nonionic contrast medium, since current CT scanners can easily produce good-quality images despite the high density of the contrast material.

CTM provides direct visualization of the spinal cord, cauda equina, and nerve roots, thereby permitting distinction between extramedullary and intramedullary cord or root injury, and between localization of cord compression by fracture fragments or herniated disk, and it can identify root avulsion (Fig. 26-35), partial or complete block of cerebrospinal fluid, dural tear, or post-traumatic syringomyelia. The presence of contrast medium in the cord itself indicates a penetrating injury, such as might be caused by a fracture fragment displaced into the canal.

Many applications of CTM for the evaluation of spinal cord injury have been replaced by MRI. In institutions

FIGURE 26-31 | *Imaging of vertebral burst fracture.* **A,** *Lateral cervical radiograph shows loss of height of the C7 body, indicating compression of the anterior and posterior cortices.* **B,** *The extent of the injury is better seen by CT, which shows a significant retropulsed fragment.*

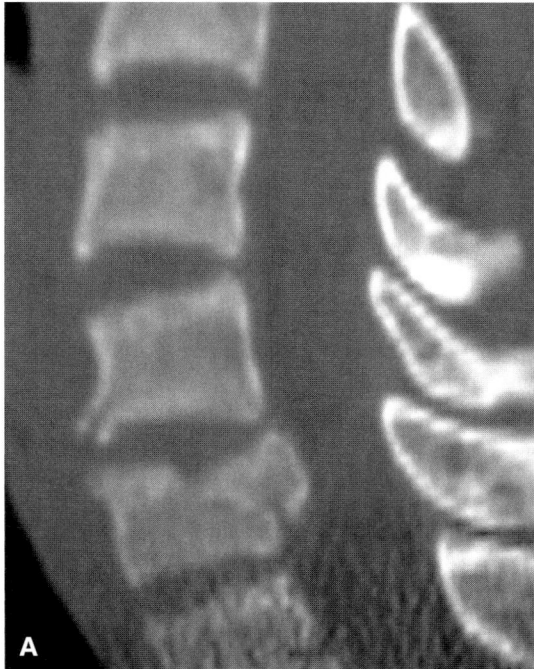

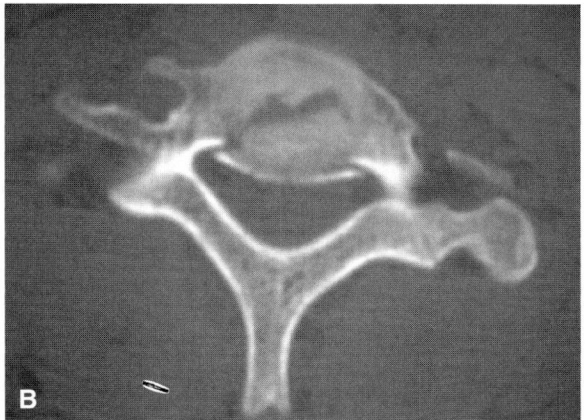

in which magnetic field–compatible immobilization, support, and monitoring systems are available, MRI of the spinal cord should be performed as soon as clinically feasible in all patients with myelopathy. If MRI is not available,

the traditional indications for CTM remain valid. CTM, however, remains the imaging technique of choice for demonstrating the presence and extent of dural tears, nerve root herniation, and root avulsion (see Fig. 26-35).

FIGURE 26-32 | *3-D volume-rendered Chance fracture of the thoracic spine. Note horizontal split through the posterior elements and antero-superior compression fracture.*

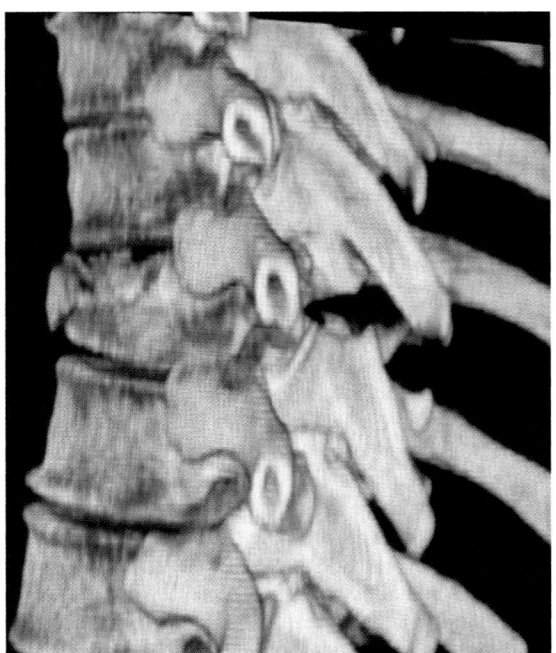

FIGURE 26-33 | *3-D volume-rendered facet dislocation of the C4–C5 level.*

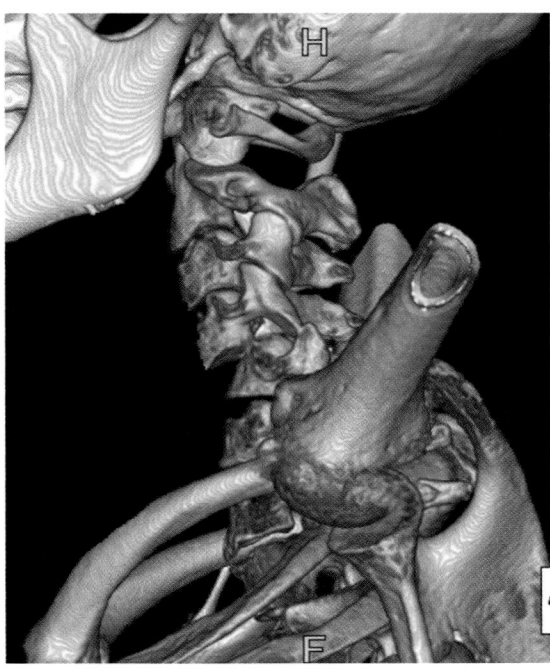

FIGURE 26-34 *Subtle type II odontoid fracture.* ***A,*** *Coned-down lateral cervical radiograph shows mild soft tissue swelling anterior to C2. There is a subtle step-off in the anterior cortex (arrow) and posterior cortex at the dens–C2 body junction.* ***B,*** *A sagittal CT re-formation nicely depicts the horizontal fracture plane at the base of the odontoid process.*

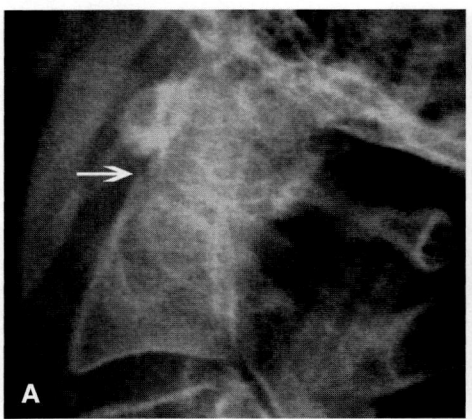
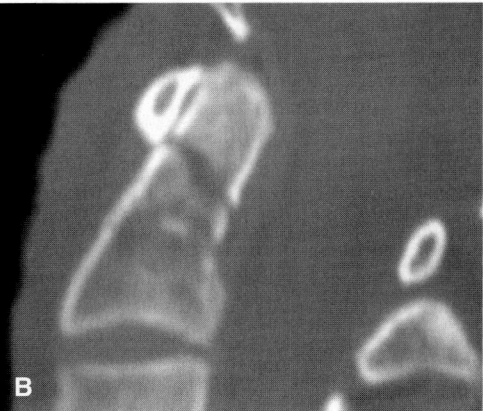

COMPUTED TOMOGRAPHY WITH TWO-DIMENSIONAL MULTIPLANAR AND VOLUME-RENDERED IMAGES

3-D CT is the logical extension of the concept of sagittal and coronal re-formation of axial image data sets. In essence, 3-D CT software programs transform axial CT data into a 3-D optical illusion of the portion of the spinal skeleton being examined. The 3-D images are derived from the data of the axial CT scan.[84] Consequently, 3-D re-formation increases neither examination time nor radiation dose to the patient.

In contemporary CT systems (MDCT), CT data are transferred immediately upon acquisition to independent work stations dedicated to manipulation of large-image data sets. Some work stations can be programmed to present "instant" preselected 3-D renderings of the spine with or without adding surrounding soft tissues. Tissues of different density are assigned different colors and degrees of transparency to enhance distinction. The 3-D volume images can then be manipulated in real-time to find the preferred angle of viewing or perspective to enhance appreciation of pathology. The spine can be electronically cut along any axis to view the neural canal from within or to delete anatomic structures that might obscure the skeletal pathology. The surface contour–rendered 3-D image clearly defines and reduces or eliminates ambiguity of complex fractures and fracture-dislocations (see Figs. 26-15, 26-32, and 26-33).

While in many institutions the radiologic evaluation typically begins with plain radiographs, increasingly CT, particularly multidetector MDCT, is completely replacing

FIGURE 26-35 *Myelography and CT myelography for evaluation of cervical nerve root avulsion.* ***A,*** *Anteroposterior view from the cervical myelogram reveals post-traumatic pseudomeningoceles arising from the torn nerve roots at the C7 and T1 levels (arrows).* ***B,*** *Axial CT scan through the C7 level after injection of contrast medium shows a small left pseudomeningocele (arrow).*

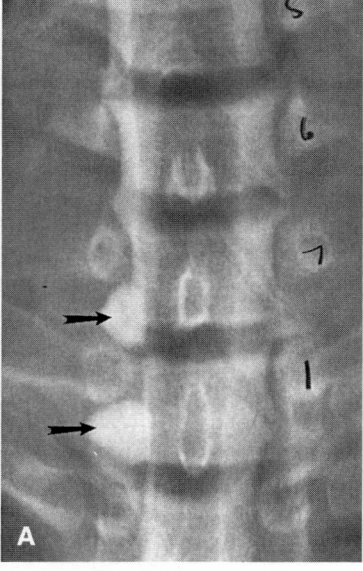
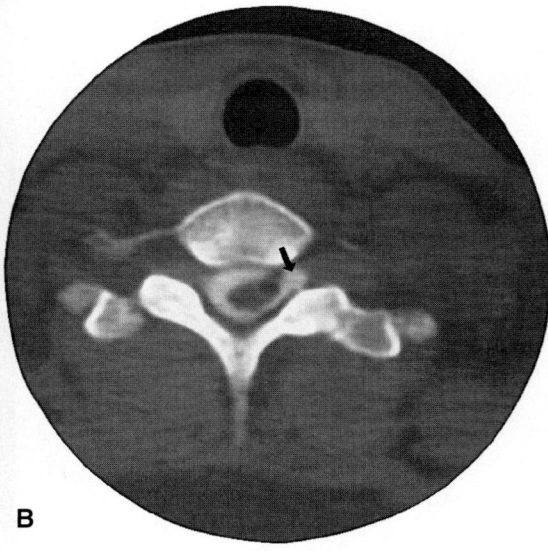

radiography or routinely supplementing admission cervical radiographs for many trauma patients. Comparison of cervical spine CT, particularly MDCT, has shown significant improved diagnostic accuracy over plain radiographic assessment. Although many of the additional injuries diagnosed by CT are trivial, perhaps one-third will lead to changes in management. CT acquires very thin axial sections (1 mm or less) that can be used to reconstruct images in any other plane with spatial resolution equivalent to the original axial acquisition (termed isotopic voxels, i.e., having the same dimensions on all sides). Moreover, with much faster image processing, these nonaxial images can be prepared rapidly, even concurrently, with the axial image reconstruction, for quick post-scan access. MDCT with 4, 8, 16, 40, 64, or more rows of detectors can image the cervical spine in a few seconds with decreased motion artifacts as compared with conventional or single-detector helical CT. The spinal anatomy can be displayed in a variety of 3-D volume-rendered orientations (see Figs. 26-32 and 26-33) to enhance understanding of pathologic anatomy. The spine can be quickly imaged as part of a global (total body) CT examination in polytrauma cases with minimal increase in irradiation and little or no increase in study time. Finally, the cervical spine examination can be performed with intravenous contrast to assess the entire neck including the cervical vessels (Figs. 26-36 and 26-37). The same intravenous contrast dose can be used to scan the entire chest and abdomen in a single scan.

FIGURE 26-36 *3-D volume-rendered CT scan with intravenous contrast shows a dissection of the left internal carotid artery with about 30 percent luminal narrowing. CT data acquired on a 40-slice multidetector system.*

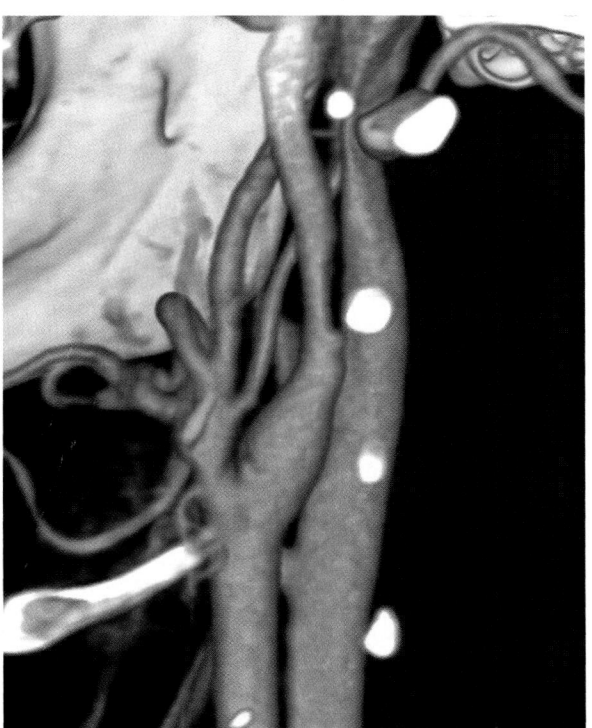

FIGURE 26-37 *3-D volume-rendered CT scan with intravenous contrast demonstrates a diffuse dissection of the internal carotid artery with a small pseudoaneurysm (arrow). All soft tissues around the carotid arteries and jugular vein have been electronically subtracted based on CT density. CT data acquired on a 40-slice multidetector system.*

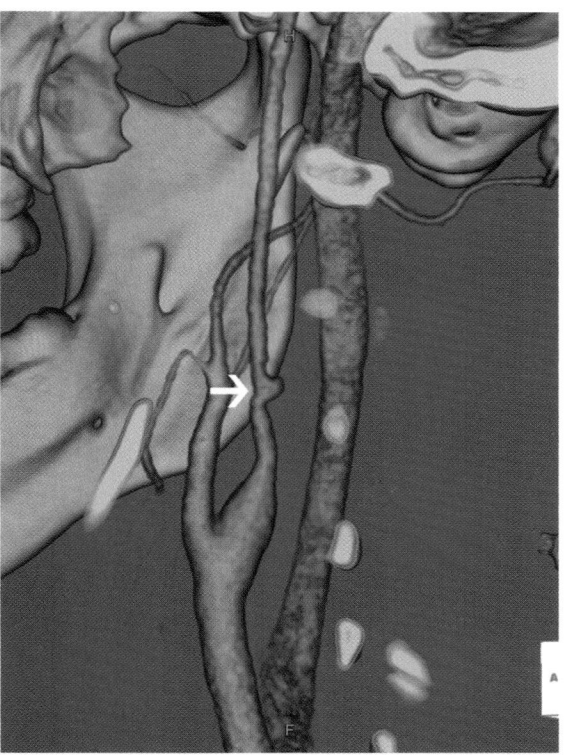

CERVICAL CT ANGIOGRAPHY

CT angiography is a technique in which fast, thin-section CT imaging is used to visualize the major cranial arteries in their cervical and intracranial course. This technique has been fostered by the availability of MDCT systems, particularly those with 16 or more rows of x-ray detectors. The large number of detectors, fast gantry rotation (0.5 sec per rotation or less), thin detector thickness, and very rapid data collection have made routine CT angiography practicable. These factors allow for high spatial resolution acquisition in all imaging planes and a marked decrease in artifacts from patient motion.

In the author's experience, CTA can be used both to assess trauma patients with risk factors for blunt cerebrovascular injury and to screen for injury in those without. The capabilities of MDCT-16 and above are so robust in this regard that blunt trauma patients can be easily screened as part of a total body survey using contrast-enhanced CT.

The carotid and vertebral arteries are assessed based on axial images, multiplanar re-formations, color-coded volume rendered images, and virtual endovascular views (Fig. 26-38; see also Figs. 26-36 and 26-37). Vascular injuries can include wall contusion, dissection with or without significant flow compromise, pseudoaneurysm, occlusion, and active

FIGURE 26-38 *Multiplanar reformatted image from CT angiogram shows abrupt occlusion of the left vertebral artery (arrow) with a pseudoaneurysm (P) arising from the termination of the injured artery. The right vertebral artery is intact.*

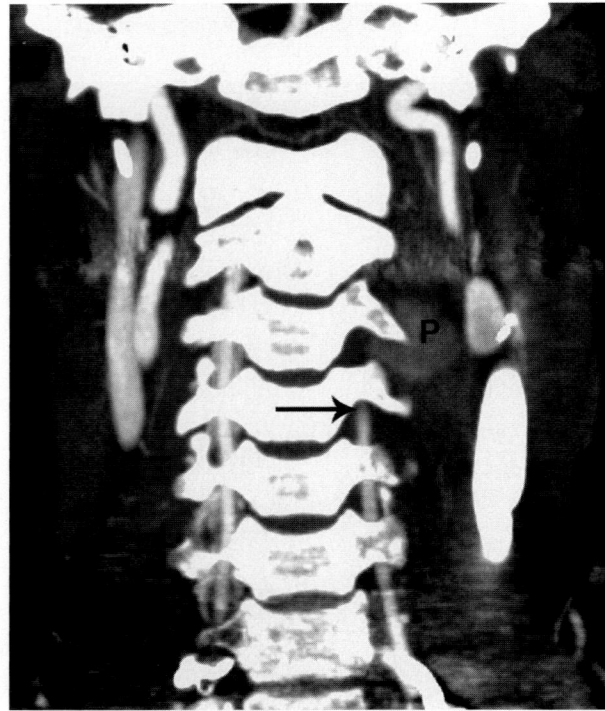

hydrogen protons with the external magnetic field. A map is created of the location and energy intensity at each point in a slice that reflects the magnetic properties of the particular tissues within the slice. MR images are also influenced by the number of protons within a tissue relative to other tissues, the bulk and microscopic movement of protons, and the chemical state of some tissues such as hemoglobin. Contrast agents such as gadolinium chelates can be used to manipulate tissue relaxation properties and increase or decrease signal and therefore intensity.

The intrinsic advantages of MRI have made it the imaging technique of choice for the central nervous system, including the spinal cord, its meninges, and its roots. These advantages include the following:

1. Direct imaging of the spine in any orientation
2. Superior contrast resolution, when compared with other techniques, in the detection of soft tissue injury, including ligaments, with greater sensitivity
3. Creation of myelography-equivalent images to assess the epidural space for evidence of hematoma, bone fragments, herniated disk material, and osteophytes without the use of instilled intrathecal contrast medium
4. Direct imaging of the spinal cord to detect evidence of contusion, hematoma, or laceration
5. Provision of prognostic information regarding the potential for recovery of function based on the MRI appearance of cord injuries
6. Visualization of flowing blood—which appears dark or bright, depending on the imaging sequence used—for assessment of major blood vessels, such as the vertebral arteries, without the necessity for intravascular contrast enhancement
7. No requirement for intravenous contrast material or ionizing radiation

Several imaging sequences are routinely performed to emphasize various aspects of normal and pathologic anatomy. In general, most centers employ the following sequences:

1. Sagittal T1-weighted spin-echo to define basic anatomy (Fig. 26-39)
2. Sagittal proton and fast T2-weighted spin-echo sequence to emphasize pathologic processes and ligamentous structures (Fig. 26-40)
3. Sagittal gradient-echo sequence to optimize detection of hemorrhage and distinguish osteophytes from disk material (Fig. 26-41)
4. Axial T1-weighted spin-echo to assess the epidural space, spinal cord, and neural foramen through areas of interest seen on sagittal sequences (Fig. 26-42)
5. Axial gradient-echo sequences to visualize gray-white matter delineation and exiting nerve roots and neural foramen (Fig. 26-43)
6. Optional MRA sequence to assess cervical arteries, depending on the type of spinal injury (Fig. 26-44)

A variety of other sequences are now available that may improve detection of certain types of spinal pathology. The use of a particular sequence (short tau inversion recovery [STIR]) can improve detection of subtle spinal cord contusions compared with other standard imaging sequences (Fig. 26-45).

bleeding (see Figs. 26-36 to 26-38). Injuries must be carefully sought in all vessels in patients with or without risk factors for cervical artery injury. The type of injury diagnosed will directly influence the type of treatment possible including anticoagulants, antiplatelet agents, endovascular stents, and surgery. CTA can also be used to follow injuries for signs of healing or progression.

It is estimated that the use of screening cervical CTA detects at least eight-fold more cervical arterial injuries than does selective arteriographic evaluation. This is an area of active research, and more information defining the use of CTA to assess the cervical vessels will clarify its role.[8] It must be appreciated that particular cervical spine injures including major subluxations and dislocations, and cervical spine fractures that cross the foramen transversarium, significantly increase risk for injury to the cervical parts of the cranial vessels.[8]

Magnetic Resonance Imaging

Simplistically, MRI scans are derived from the energy released by the hydrogen protons of the body. When placed in a magnetic field, these protons change their orientation and energy state because of an additional radio-frequency signal introduced into the static uniform external magnetic field. Only tissues within a specific slice within the body have protons precessing at the correct frequency to absorb the radio-frequency energy. Release of this excess applied radio-frequency energy (relaxation) accompanies reorientation of

FIGURE 26-39 *MRI of normal sagittal T1-weighted sequence. On T1 weighting, the cerebrospinal fluid (CSF) appears dark and the cord intermediate in signal. The anterior anulus and anterior longitudinal ligament appear as a low-signal band (arrowheads)* outlined by brighter signals from the disk material (open arrow) *and prevertebral fat. The ligamentum flavum appears as a dark signal outlined by brighter signal fat on the posterior aspect (closed arrows). The low-signal posterior anulus fibrosus and posterior longitudinal ligament are poorly seen because of the dark CSF. (From Mirvis, S.E.; Ness-Aiver, M. In Harris, J.H., Jr.; Mirvis, S.E., eds. Radiology of Acute Cervical Spine Trauma. Baltimore, Williams & Wilkins, 1995, p. 140.)*

FIGURE 26-40 *MRI of normal sagittal T2-weighted sequence. The sagittal T2-weighted spin-echo image shows the cerebrospinal fluid (CSF) as bright, surrounding an intermediate-signal cord. The vertebral bodies are less dark than on gradient-echo sequences and show less contrast with disk material. The posterior longitudinal ligament–anulus fibrosus complex (closed arrows) is dark between the disk and the CSF. The ligamentum flavum (arrowheads) appears dark, outlined anteriorly by bright CSF. The open arrow shows an artifact. (From Mirvis, S.E.; Ness-Aiver, M. In Harris, J. H., Jr.; Mirvis, S.E., eds. Radiology of Acute Cervical Spine Trauma. Baltimore, Williams & Wilkins, 1995, p. 143.)*

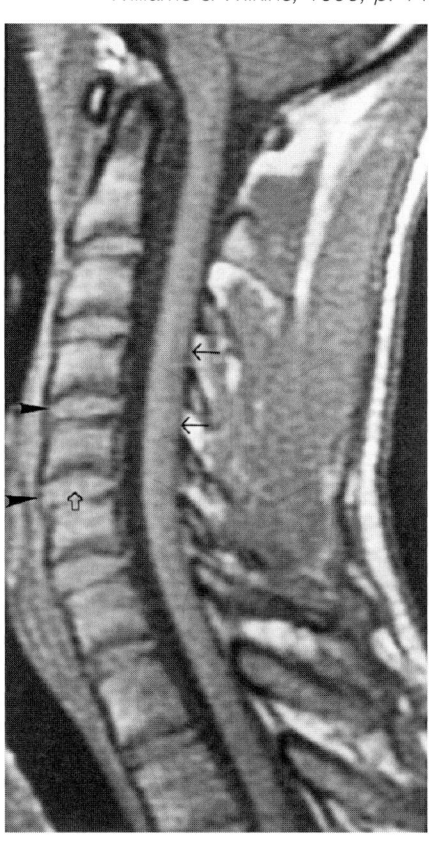

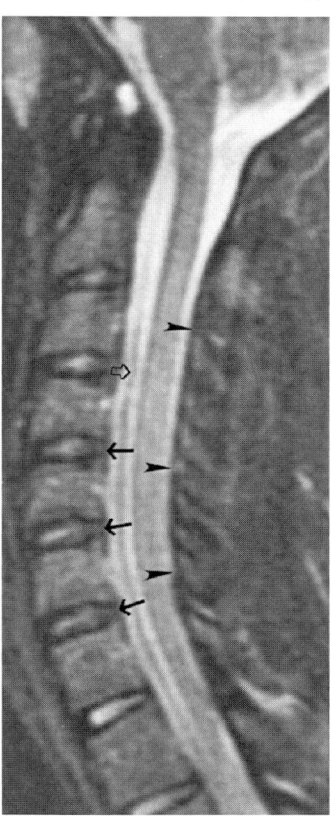

The limitations of MRI are few but should be mentioned. Because cortical bone contains essentially no hydrogen atoms, it is not well visualized by MRI. Bone is identified by the proton signal of blood and fat in its medullary portion. Consequently, only major osseous injuries are reliably shown by MRI, and MRI cannot be depended on for the diagnosis of subtle bone injury, particularly that involving the posterior spinal elements. Comprehensive MRI examinations of the spine require more time than comparable CT studies because of the longer data acquisition. New image acquisition sequences and MRI hardware changes (parallel processing) can potentially make MRI as fast as or faster than CT scanning.[47]

Hemodynamically *unstable* patients should not be studied by MRI, because acute cardiopulmonary resuscitation is not easily or safely performed in the MRI environment. The need for sophisticated physiologic monitoring and support requires MRI-compatible systems that can function reliably with the fringe magnetic field around the MRI machine and that do not create radio-frequency noise in the image acquisition process. The development of such systems has made the application of MRI to patients with acute spinal injury possible. However, patients with ferromagnetic intracranial aneurysm clips and pacemakers are excluded from the MRI environment. Some aneurysm clips undergo torque when moved through the external

FIGURE 26-41   *MRI of normal sagittal gradient-echo sequence. The sagittal gradient-echo sequence normally shows the vertebral bodies as relatively low in signal (because fat signal decreases). The intervertebral disks and cerebrospinal fluid (CSF) remain bright, allowing demonstration of the combined low signal of the anulus fibrosus and longitudinal ligaments. The intermediate signal intensity of the cord is easily seen, surrounded by bright CSF.*

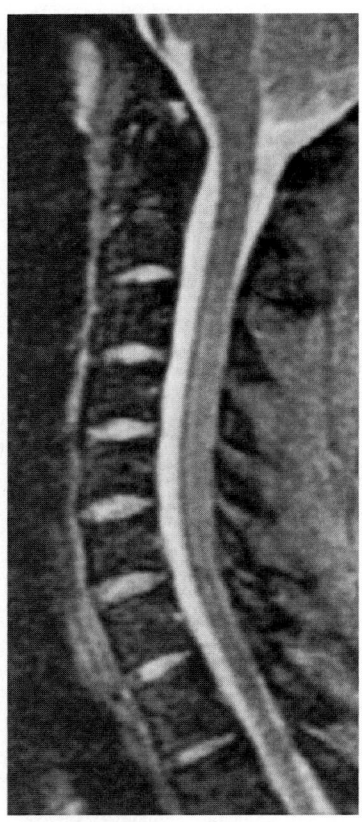

FIGURE 26-42   *MRI of normal axial T1-weighted sequence. The axial T1-weighted image shows an intermediate signal cord surrounded by dark cerebrospinal fluid. The nerve roots are seen traversing the subarachnoid space (open white arrows) and exiting the neural foramen (arrowheads). The cortical bone is dark, with brighter signal marrow. The vertebral arteries (open black arrows) are dark in this sequence (flow void). No internal anatomy in the cord is discerned. (From Mirvis, S.E.; Ness-Aiver, M. In Harris, J.H., Jr.; Mirvis, S.E., eds. Radiology of Acute Cervical Spine Trauma. Baltimore, Williams & Wilkins, 1995, p. 144.)*

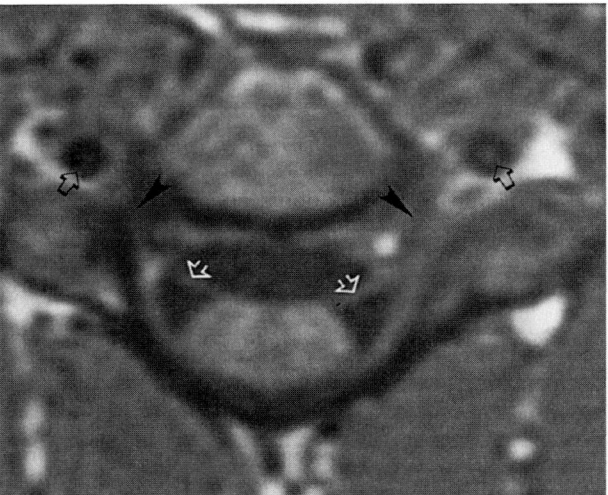

magnetic field, and pacemakers can malfunction. Also, patients with metal in close proximity to vital soft tissue structures such as the spinal cord, nerve roots, or orbit are at increased risk for further tissue injury when positioned in the magnet, particularly when metal foreign body penetration is acute. Patients for whom a history regarding possible exposure to metal fragments cannot be obtained (e.g., welders who are unconscious) must be screened radiographically for the presence of metal foreign bodies. Finally, approximately 3 percent of patients are sufficiently claustrophobic to preclude their being placed inside the magnet bore.[52]

MRI is uniquely suited to directly demonstrate injuries to the soft tissues of the spine and paraspinal region. While spatial resolution for MRI is less than that provided by CT, it has far better contrast sensitivity allowing greater discrimination among various soft tissues including muscle, fat, cerebrospinal fluid, ligaments, intervertebral disk material, fluid, and hematoma. The diminished spatial resolution of

MRI makes *it relatively insensitive* for detection of spinal fractures, particularly when nondisplaced or involving the relatively small posterior portions of the vertebral bodies. On the other hand, soft tissue injuries are directly visualized, and knowledge of these injuries is vital in determining overall extent of injury and potential for mechanical instability (Fig. 26-46; see also Fig. 26-45). In general, MRI is indicated to examine patients with neurologic deficits, particularly those that are partial or fluctuating. MRI is also occasionally used for patients with persistent neck pain, without CT evidence of fracture, to exclude major ligament disruption. The use of MRI for any patient who cannot provide an adequate clinical examination is also commonly practiced to facilitate early removal of the cervical collar, but is a subject of debate (see below). MRA can be performed with or without gadolinium contrast enhancement to assess the craniocerebral vessels (Figs. 26-47 and Fig. 26-48), but few studies have described its use and accuracy in the acute trauma setting.[58]

Most MR examinations include a variety of image acquisition sequences that accentuate different tissues and pathologies (as described above). Spin-echo T1-weighted images provide the best overall image quality and anatomic delineation (see Fig. 26-39), proton-weighted sequences distinguish the cervical ligaments (dark signal due to lack of

FIGURE 26-43   *MRI of normal axial gradient-echo sequence.* **A** *and* **B,** *Gradient-echo images produce very dark bone and bright cerebrospinal fluid (CSF). The dura is outlined by CSF (arrows in* **A***). Internal architecture of the cord, with brighter central gray and darker white matter tracts, can be observed (* **A***). Vertebral arteries appear bright on this sequence (open arrows in* **B***). Nerve roots can be seen within the neural foramen surrounded by high-signal CSF (white arrows in* **B***). Facet articular spaces contain high-signal fluid (arrowheads in* **B***). (From Mirvis, S.E.; Ness-Aiver, M. In Harris, J.H., Jr.; Mirvis, S.E., eds. Radiology of Acute Cervical Spine Trauma. Baltimore, Williams & Wilkins, 1995, p. 145.)*

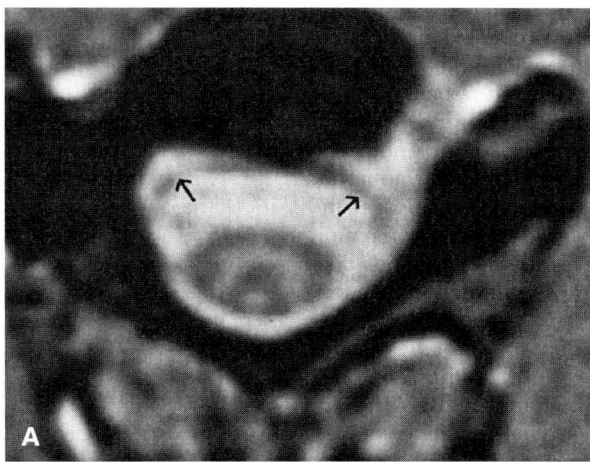
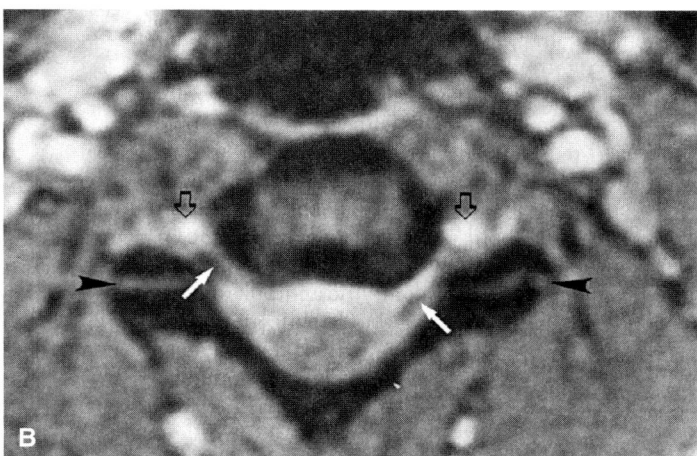

mobile hydrogen atoms) from adjacent higher signal tissues (see Fig. 26-46), and T2-weighted fast spin-echo sequences show edema with high sensitivity and accentuate injured sites (Fig. 26-49; see also Fig. 26-40). STIR images offer somewhat higher sensitivity for edema in the bone marrow and spinal cord owing to improved contrast sensitivity and suppression of fat signal (see Fig. 26-45), but these are also generally "noisier" images.[19] Gradient-echo sequences (2-D) usually performed in the axial plane are particularly sensitive to the signal strength lowering influence of hemorrhage in some chemical forms within the spinal cord (Fig. 26-50; see also Fig. 26-43).[19]

FIGURE 26-44   *Magnetic resonance angiography (MRA) study of normal time-of-flight cervical vessels demonstrating anteroposterior (***A***) and oblique (***B***) views of the cervical vasculature. All vessels appear bright on the gradient-echo sequence used to acquire images. The venous flow signal is selectively negated. Note the bright signal from moving cerebrospinal fluid in the AP projection. (From Mirvis, S.E.; Ness-Aiver, M. In Harris, J.H., Jr.; Mirvis, S.E., eds. Radiology of Acute Cervical Spine Trauma. Baltimore, Williams & Wilkins, 1995, p. 146.)*

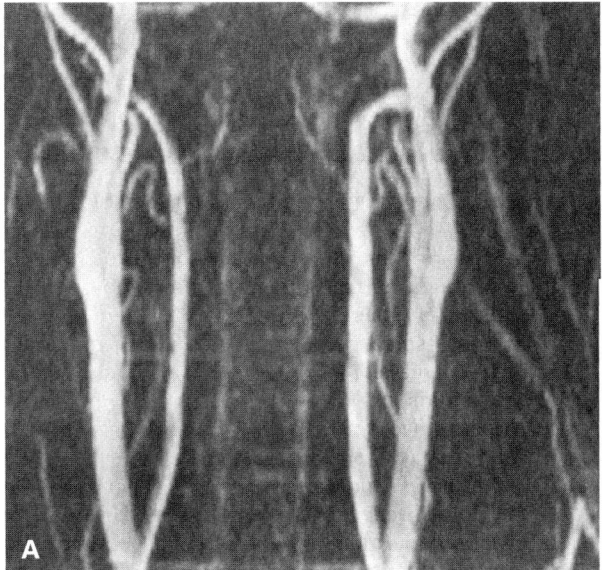
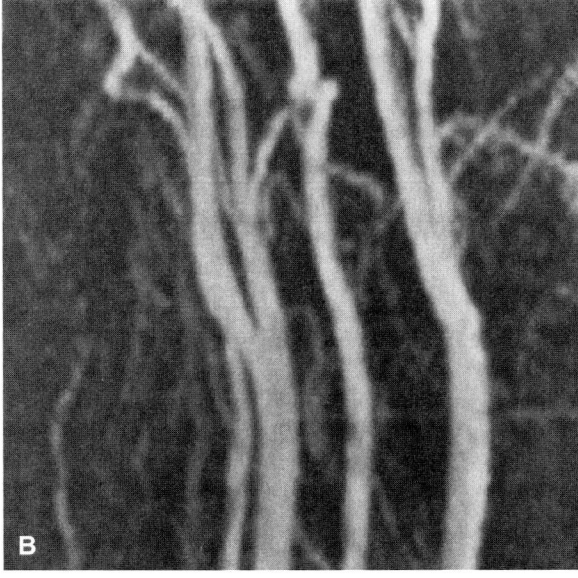

FIGURE 26-45 *Increased sensitivity for cord edema with inversion recovery sequence (STIR). Inversion recovery provides a higher level of contrast in MR images and often accentuates edema compared with other sequences such as T2-weighted spin echo. This image shows a C4–C5 hyperflexion injury with tearing of the anterior and posterior longitudinal ligaments and ligamentum flavum. A cord contusion is seen at C4 and C5 as higher signal intensity (between arrows) than spinal cord with a low signal focus at the C4–C5 disk space from hemorrhage. Disk material herniates through the torn ligaments and annulus fibers. The signal of fat is relatively suppressed by inversion recovery excitation sequences.*

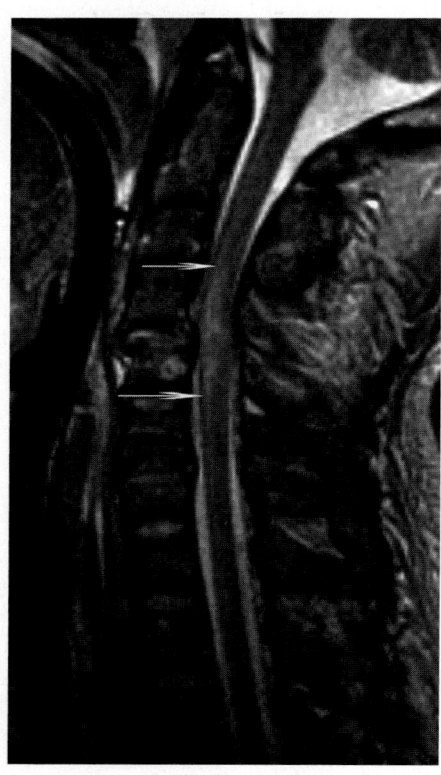

MRI is indicated in the evaluation of all patients with incomplete or progressive neurologic deficits after cervical spinal injury if permitted by the patient's overall clinical status. Patients with complete deficits should also undergo MRI assessment to demonstrate any cord-compressing lesions, e.g., herniated disk material (Fig. 26-51; see also Figs. 26-46 and 26-49), epidural hematoma, or bone fragments, the removal of which may allow some neurologic improvement. Other patients for whom spinal MRI is indicated include those with myelopathy or radiculopathy after spinal trauma but with radiographic or CT studies that are negative or fail to account for the deficit. Another strong indication is that the level of the deficit does not correlate with the injury location depicted by radiography or CT.

FIGURE 26-46 *MRI showing ligament injury. This mid-sagittal MR image of the cervical spine obtained with proton-density weighting (optimizing ligament visualization) reveals a hyperflexion sprain at C5–C6. The anterior and posterior (white arrow) longitudinal low signal lines are disrupted. The disk is herniated posterior to C5, and the dark signal line of the ligamentum flavum (black arrow) is interrupted from posterior distraction. The anterior disk space is narrowed and the posterior aspect widened from the hyperflexion force.*

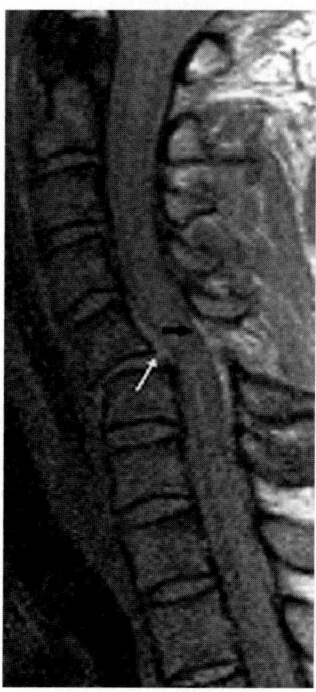

MRI can demonstrate the level and extent of ligament disruption and intervertebral disk herniation. This information helps determine the need for and the type of internal fixation required to restore a patent spinal canal and ensure mechanical stability. MRI is useful in defining the extent of posterior ligament injury in thoracolumbar spine injuries, which increases instability when associated with anterior column fractures. MRI is particularly helpful in determining the extent of ligament injury and instability that typically accompany injuries occurring in the fused spine, such as ankylosing spondylitis and diffuse idiopathic skeletal hyperostosis.

MAGNETIC RESONANCE IMAGING OF SPECIFIC SPINE AND SPINAL CORD PATHOLOGY

PARENCHYMAL LESIONS MRI is unique in its ability to detect acute injury to the spinal cord, including edema, hemorrhage, and laceration. Cord edema appears isointense or slightly hypointense in relation to the normal cord on T1-weighted spin-echo images but becomes brighter in signal than the normal cord on T2-weighted

FIGURE 26-47 | MR angiography using time-of-flight sequence shows absence of the right vertebral artery signal in a patient with blunt cervical spine trauma. The normal left vertebral artery is marked (arrows).

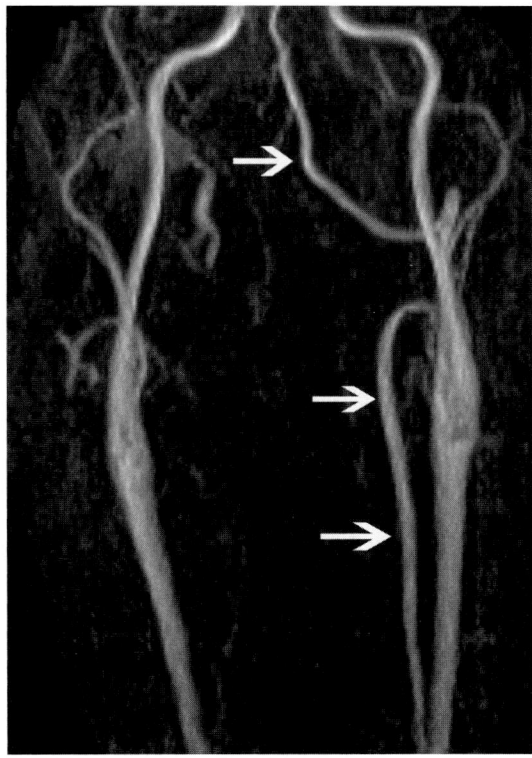

FIGURE 26-48 | Axial T2-weighted MR image shows a normal signal void for the left vertebral artery. There is increased signal in the thrombosed right vertebral artery due to clotted blood (arrow) obstructing flow in the vessel.

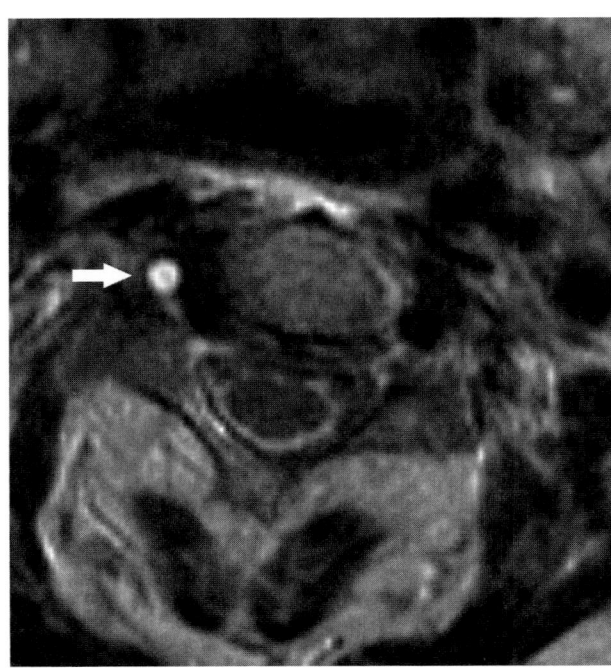

FIGURE 26-49 | Burst fracture of L1 with marked retropulsion creating cord contusion. The sagittal T2-weighted image shows herniation of the L1–L2 disk material and posterior cortical bone into the region of the conus. High signal edema is present in the cord (arrow) above the level of injury.

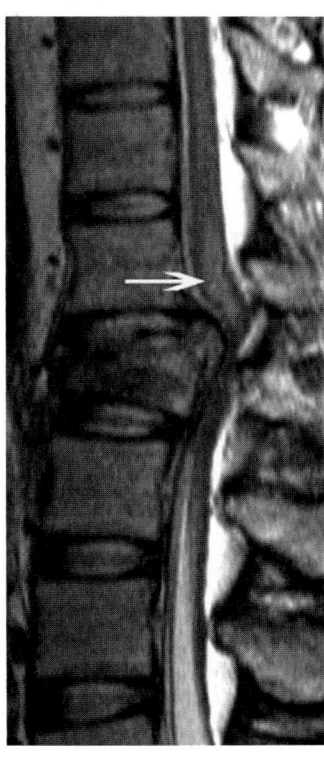

FIGURE 26-50 | Axial gradient-echo image sequence shows a lower signal area in the cord (arrow) representing blood products (usually subacute 7–14 days). The patient has a flexion teardrop fracture that often caused cord contusion. Note that the vertebral arteries appear bright on this sequence.

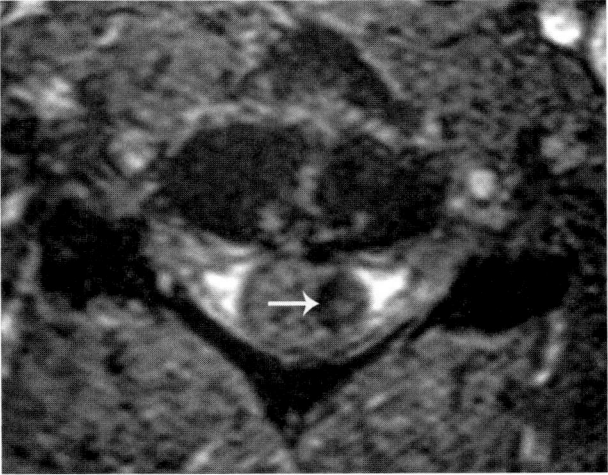

FIGURE 26-51 *Sagittal proton-density MR sequence demonstrates a C4–C5 disk herniation anteriorly and posteriorly associated with intervertebral disk space narrowing and interruption of the annulus fibers, longitudinal ligaments, and ligamentum flavum at the injury level (arrow). The anterior and posterior longitudinal ligaments are stretched but appear intact.*

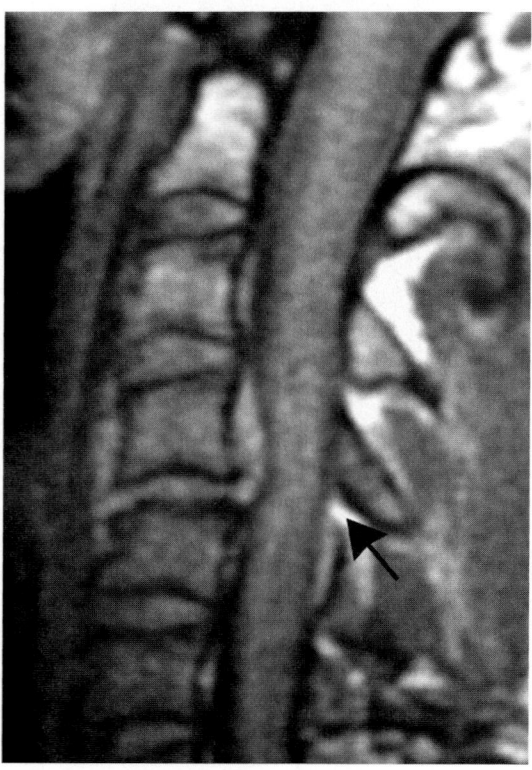

FIGURE 26-52 *MRI of spinal cord contusion. Mid-sagittal T2-weighted sequence indicates a hyperflexion injury at C5–C6 with posterior herniation of disk material. Areas of bright signal in the cord represent edema (contusion), and there is complete interruption of the ligamentum flavum.*

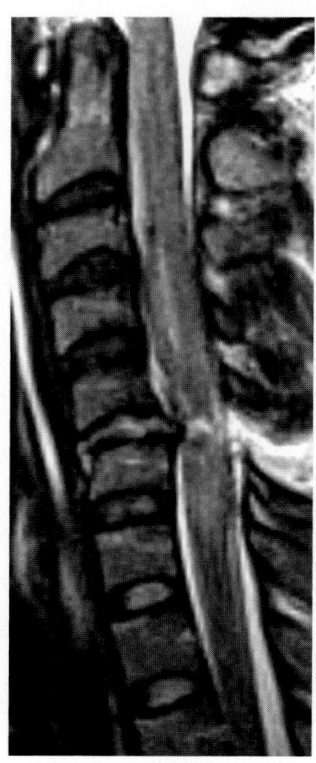

image sequences (Fig. 26-52; see also Fig. 26-49). When hemorrhage is present within the cord, its MRI appearance depends on a complex relationship between the chemical state of the blood, the field strength of the magnet, and the imaging sequence used.[12] In the acute to subacute period after injury (1 to 7 days), blood generally appears dark (low-intensity signal) on T2-weighted sequences, whereas edema has a bright signal. After about 7 days, as red cells are lysed, blood acquires a high-intensity signal in both T1- and T2-weighted studies.

Kulkarni and colleagues[53] were the first to describe a relationship between the characteristics of the MRI cord signal and the patient's outcome, suggesting that MRI cord signal characteristics reflect the type of cord histopathology. The prognostic information provided by MRI regarding potential recovery of function has been verified by several other studies.[24,56,74] The ability of the MRI signals to identify the histopathology of acute cord injury has been confirmed by direct comparison of the MRI signal with histologic findings in experimentally induced spinal cord injuries.[69]

LIGAMENT INJURY Ligament injury sustained in acute spinal trauma is inferred from the mechanism of injury, the fracture pattern, and the alignment of the spine

after injury. However, even significant ligament injury leading to spinal mechanical instability, particularly hyperflexion and hyperextension sprains without concurrent fractures, may not be apparent when the spine is studied radiographically in a neutral position. Furthermore, the spinal alignment demonstrated by plain radiographs may serve to reveal the site of major or principal mechanical instability but may not demonstrate all major ligament injuries and other potential sites of immediate or delayed instability.

MRI depicts normal ligaments as regions of low signal intensity because of lack of mobile hydrogen. Disruption of the ligament is seen on MRI scans as an abrupt interruption of the low signal, ligament attenuation or stretching of the ligament, or association of a torn ligament with an attached avulsed bone fragment (see Figs. 26-46, 26-51, and 26-52). Determination of the status of the major support ligaments of the spine as revealed by MRI has a definite bearing on management approaches. MRI can demonstrate unsuspected ligament injury or injury that is greater than anticipated from the results of other available imaging modalities.

INTERVERTEBRAL DISK HERNIATION Acute intervertebral disk herniation may accompany fractures or dislocations or may occur as an isolated lesion. If the disk impinges on the spinal cord or roots, a neurologic injury may result. MRI demonstration of a single-level acute intervertebral disk herniation that impinges on the spinal cord is crucial in surgical management of spinal trauma to optimize neurologic recovery. MRI clearly depicts disk material herniation with essentially all imaging sequences (Fig. 26-53; see also Figs. 26-46 and 26-51) but best separates disk material from posterior osteophyte with the gradient-echo sequence, on which relatively bright disk material is visualized against a dark background of bone.

The advantage of MRI over CTM in detecting acute traumatic disk herniation was shown clearly by Flanders and associates.[24] In their study, 40 percent of acute disk herniations producing neurologic deficits were demonstrated by MRI but not by CTM. Rizzolo and colleagues[71] found a 42 percent incidence of herniated nucleus pulposus in 53 patients studied by MRI at 1.5 T within 72 hours of injury. The highest incidence occurred among patients with bilateral facet dislocations (80%) and anterior cord syndromes (100%). Doran and co-workers[22] described a high incidence of traumatic disk herniation among patients with both unilateral and bilateral facet dislocations. Patients with traumatically herniated intervertebral disks may sustain a neurologic deterioration when the cervical spine is reduced, as

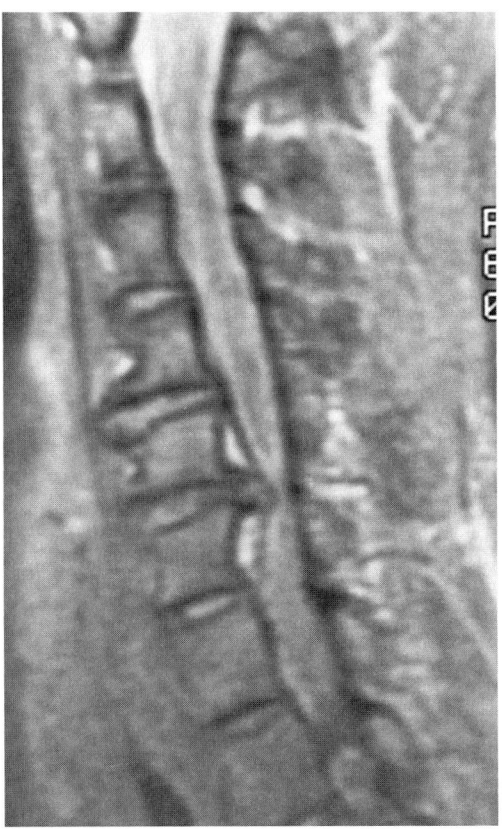

FIGURE 26-53 *MRI of disk herniation. Off-midline sagittal proton density scan shows chronic disk herniation at the C6–C7 level indenting the spinal cord. The presence of low-signal osteophytes around the disk suggests chronicity, possibly with acute exacerbation after trauma.*

the disk may then compress neural tissue.[22,31,67] However, this point is controversial, since others have found no evidence of neurologic deterioration when closed reduction is performed for patients with disk herniation or disruption.[31]

EPIDURAL HEMATOMA Epidural hematomas (EDHs) are an uncommon sequela of spinal trauma and occur in 1 to 2 percent of cervical spine injuries.[28] The cervical spine is the most common location of EDHs of traumatic origin.[28] EDH most commonly occurs in the dorsal epidural space as a result of close adherence of the ventral dura to the posterior longitudinal ligament.[28] Bleeding most likely arises from sudden increases in pressure in the rich epidural venous plexus, which comprises valveless veins.[28] EDHs may develop acutely after trauma, in a delayed fashion, or after open or closed spinal column reduction. Up to 50 percent of post-traumatic EDHs may occur among patients without overt cervical spine injuries.[28] For this reason, the presence of myelopathy without an injury demonstrated by radiography or CT without intrathecal contrast should suggest an EDH. Garza-Mercado[28] described an increased likelihood of cervical spine EDH in younger trauma victims owing to increased elasticity of the vertebral column and among patients with fused cervical spines, including those with ankylosing spondylitis and diffuse idiopathic skeletal hyperostosis. The development of progressive, unexplained neurologic deterioration among patients sustaining spinal trauma may herald the onset of cord compression by an expanding EDH.

Again, the MRI appearance of EDH depends on the age of the blood, magnetic field strength, and imaging sequence used. In the acute phase of trauma (1 to 3 days after injury), blood appears isointense (bright) relative to the spinal cord on the T1-weighted sequence (Fig. 26-54) and hypointense (dark) relative to the spinal cord on T2-weighted sequences. At 3 to 7 days after injury, the central portion of the hematoma, which contains intact red blood cells, has low signal intensity on T2-weighted sequences, whereas the periphery, composed of lysed red blood cells, shows increased signal strength on both T1- and T2-weighted sequences (Fig. 26-55).[11]

CONGENITAL OR ACQUIRED SPINAL STENOSIS Spinal cord injury may be caused by impaction of posteriorly projecting osteophytes or hypertrophied, calcified, or ossified ligaments on the anterior surface of the cord during traumatic deformation of the cervical spine. Posterior spinal cord injury can result from buckling of hypertrophied ligamentum flavum during hyperextension. Patients with congenital spinal stenosis or spinal stenosis acquired from degenerative changes (spondylosis) have an increased likelihood of injury from cervical spine trauma or even physiologic cervical spine motion. The occurrence of post-traumatic myelopathy without radiologic evidence of acute injury among older patients with posterior spinal osteophytes, ossification of the posterior longitudinal ligament, or congenital spine stenosis suggests that these conditions are etiologic. Cervical spinal cord impaction by posterior cervical osteophytes typically produces a central cord syndrome.

MRI in the sagittal and axial orientation depicts spinal canal compromise produced by degenerative processes. Comparison of T2-weighted spin-echo and T2-weighted gradient-echo sequences can be helpful in differentiating

FIGURE 26-54   *MRI of epidural hematoma (acute). Lateral **(A)** and axial **(B)** T1-weighted MRI scans of a patient with cervical flexion injury show an epidural hematoma (arrowheads) isointense with the spinal cord, displacing the cord posteriorly. There is C5 on C6 anterior subluxation. (From Mirvis, S.E.; Ness-Aiver, M. In Harris, J.H., Jr.; Mirvis, S.E., eds. Radiology of Acute Cervical Spine Trauma. Baltimore, Williams & Wilkins, 1995, p. 160.)*

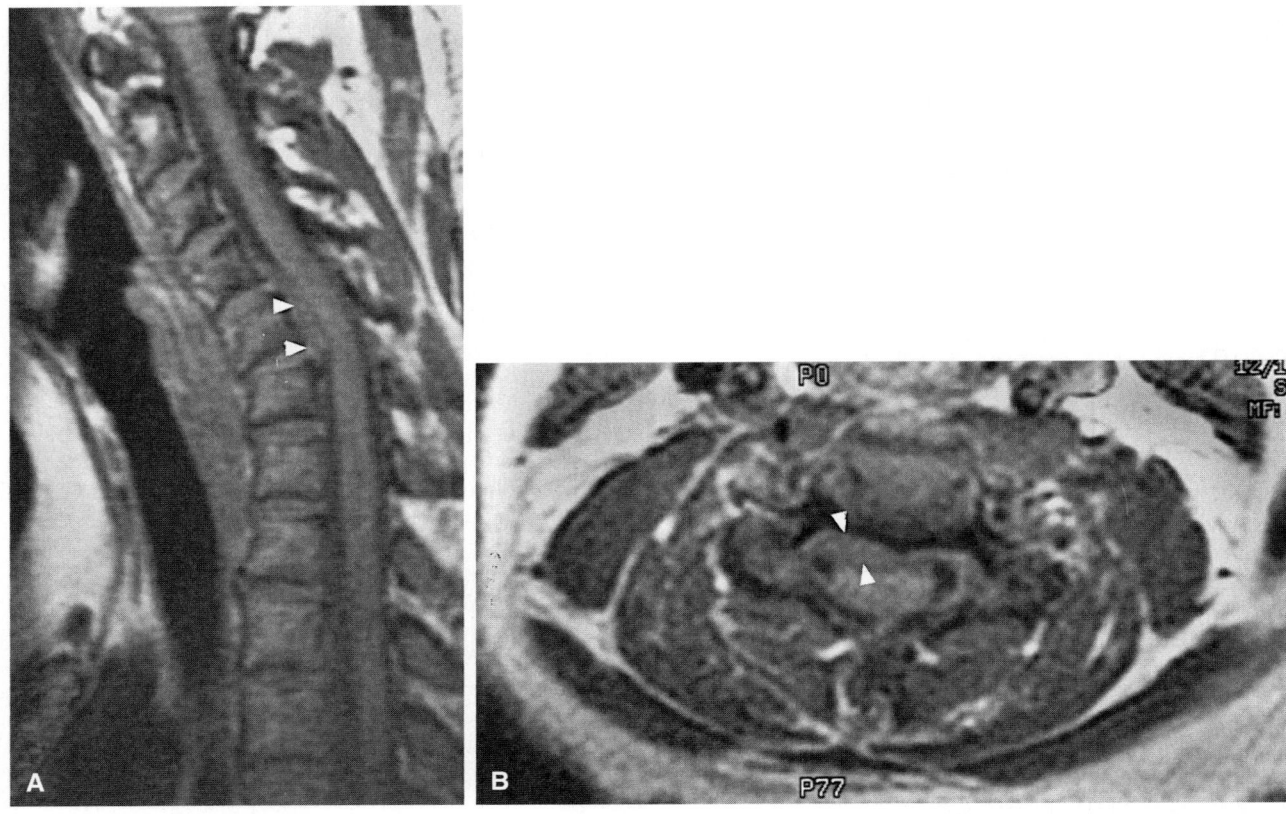

acutely herniated soft disk material from osteophytes surrounding chronic disk herniations. Both sequences produce a myelographic appearance that demonstrates the relationship of osteophytes and intervertebral disks to the spinal cord. However, gradient-echo sequences produce very dark-appearing osteophytes and increased contrast with brighter signal disk material compared with these features on T2-weighted spin-echo sequences. MRI is crucial in planning the extent of posterior surgical decompression by showing the points at which the thecal sac and direct spinal cord compression occur. It should be noted that the gradient-echo pulse sequence tends to make bone appear larger than in actuality ("blooming"), and this may accentuate the apparent degree of spinal canal encroachment.

MAGNETIC RESONANCE IMAGING OF CHRONIC AND POSTOPERATIVE SPINE INJURIES

It has been well documented that MRI is superior to myelography, CT, and CTM in the evaluation of chronic injuries of the spinal cord, particularly for the differentiation of myelomalacia and post-traumatic spinal cord cyst.[65] Myelomalacia typically appears as a focal low-signal area on T1-weighted sequences and as a high-signal area on T2-weighted sequences in a cord of normal or decreased caliber (Fig. 26-56). Syringomyelia has a similar

appearance but is more sharply delineated and typically occurs in an expanded cord. Flow-sensitive imaging sequences may help demonstrate a syrinx by showing movement of cerebrospinal fluid within the cavity. Postoperative MRI studies of patients with internal fixation devices are improved when titanium fixation devices are used.[60] These produce far less magnetic susceptibility artifact than stainless steel fixation devices and permit visualization of the cord and surrounding epidural space without artifact.[60]

MAGNETIC RESONANCE ANGIOGRAPHY

MRA is used as a screening assessment of the vertebral arteries. The exact incidence of vertebral artery injury occurring after cervical spine fracture-dislocation is unknown, but the injury is being reported with increasing frequency especially since the increased use of CT angiography of the spine.[58,82] Vertebral artery injuries from cervical spine trauma generally involve the second portion of the artery extending from C6 to C2. Fixation of the artery within the confines of the transverse foramina predisposes this vessel to injury from cervical dislocations. Although a variety of cervical spine injuries have been associated with vertebral artery injury, unilateral and bilateral dislocations are most commonly implicated.[64] Vertebral artery injury

FIGURE 26-55 *Thoracolumbar epidural hematoma. A mixed signal intensity collection displaces the spinal cord anteriorly, producing some posterior compression on this T1-weighted spin-echo sagittal study. The brighter peripheral areas represent effects of extracellular hematoma (T1 shortening or paramagnetic). Hemoglobin in still intact red cells centrally does not show this effect and is darker in signal on this imaging sequence.*

FIGURE 26-56 *MRI of titanium implant internal fixation. Sagittal T2-weighted MR image shows a titanium fixation plate at C4–C6 used to fix a hyperflexion teardrop fracture at C5, producing local magnetic field inhomogeneity and signal dropout. However, the spinal canal and cord are still well seen, with a focal area of post-traumatic cyst formation or myelomalacia visible at the C5 level (white arrow). There is minimal retrolisthesis of C5.*

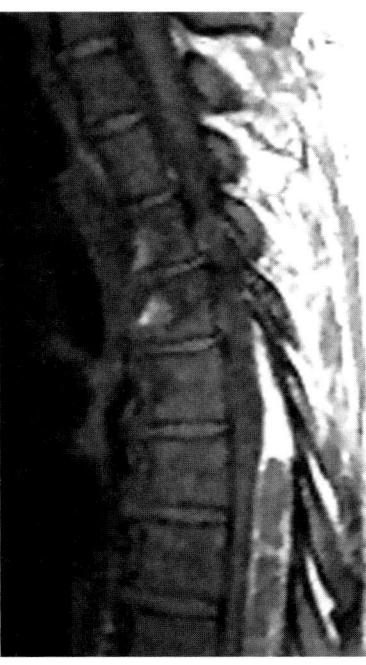

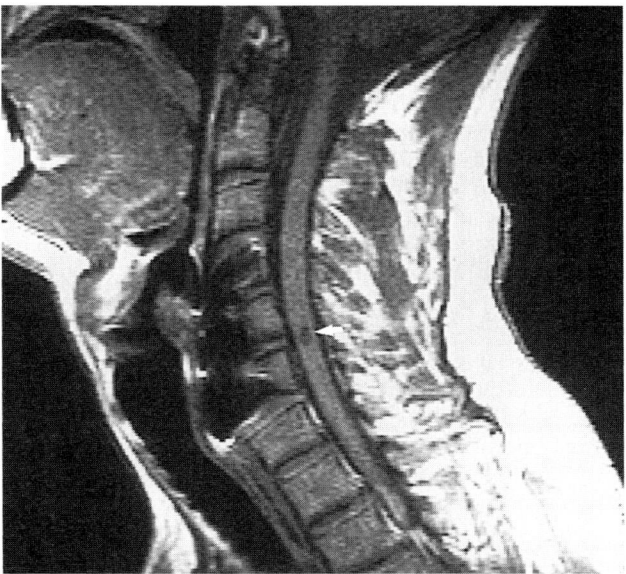

can occur from fractures extending across the foramen transversarium and has been reported with lateral cervical dislocations.[64,82]

MRA screening of the vertebral arteries should be considered for all patients with blunt cervical spine trauma with significant degrees (>1 cm) of dislocation or subluxation or fracture of the foramen transversarium or with neurologic deficits consistent with vertebral vessel insufficiency.[29] Routine assessment of the cervical spine by MRI should include axial T1-weighted images. On these sequences, flowing blood creates a signal void (dark image) and non-flowing blood has an increased signal (see Fig. 26-48). Conversely, on gradient-echo sequences, flowing blood creates a bright image. Inspection of the major cervical arteries for the anticipated signal characteristics should be performed as part of overall assessment of the MRI study. Absence or irregularity of the expected flow signal should raise a question of vascular injury. Injuries identifiable by MRA include intimal flaps, intramural dissection or hematoma, pseudoaneurysm, and thrombosis. Care must be taken to distinguish injury from vessel hypoplasia or atherosclerotic disease. Positive MRA findings of vessel injury are confirmed and better characterized by direct contrast angiography, which offers spatial resolution greater than that possible with MRA. MRA can be performed with or without gadolinium contrast enhancement to assess the craniocerebral vessels, but few studies have described its use and accuracy in the acute trauma setting.[58]

RADIONUCLIDE BONE IMAGING

Radionuclide bone imaging (RNBI) has been used in the assessment of trauma to the spine primarily to determine whether a radiographic abnormality represents an acute process that is potentially responsible for the patient's pain or to exclude an osseous abnormality as a source of spine pain when radiographs are normal. In the cervical spine, image resolution is improved by placing the patient's neck directly on the collimator surface, decreasing distance from the nuclide activity. Slightly posterior oblique images of the cervical spine can also assist diagnostically.

Reports[57,81] and anecdotal experience indicate that an acute, nondisplaced cervical fracture cannot be entirely excluded even when the initial RNBI scan is normal. RNBI was assessed in patients with whiplash, and no correlation was found between symptoms and signs of injury and scintigraphic findings.[5] However, one retrospective study of 35 cases[5] found that a negative bone scan excluded a skeletal injury, and in another prospective study of 20 patients[43] with whiplash injuries, no patients had bone scan findings suggestive of fracture and none had a subsequent diagnosis of fracture. Increased activity within the cervical spine on delayed bone imaging includes a differential diagnosis of nonspecific stress response, degenerative arthritis, and healing fracture. Use of single photon emission computed tomography may increase diagnostic accuracy in bone imaging of acute spine trauma.

RNBI in the thoracic and lumbar spine is technically easier than in the cervical spine. Acute fractures can be detected on both blood pool and delayed images (Fig. 26-57). Increased linear activity at the superior end plate is characteristic of traumatic fracture. RNBI may be particularly helpful in detecting acute compression fractures in patients with severe osteoporosis that may be quite subtle radiographically. Increased lateral activity on the concave side of a scoliotic spine that is not sharply marginated most likely represents stress-related or degenerative change. In patients with nonlocalized lower back pain after trauma and normal lumbar radiographs, large-field-of-view RNBI can screen for small laminar, transverse process or articular process fractures that might otherwise require multilevel CT scanning to detect.

CATHETER ANGIOGRAPHY

Conventional angiography is used to detect or confirm vertebral artery injury resulting from cervical spine trauma (Fig. 26-58). Although associated with higher procedure-related morbidity than MRA or CT angiography, the technique offers greater spatial resolution for detection and characterization of vascular injuries. Conventional angiography is the current study of choice for assessment of potential vertebral artery injury resulting from penetrating injury to the cervical spine. In addition, angiography can provide the potential for intravascular thrombolysis and endovascular stent treatment of selected vertebral injuries[68] (Fig. 26-59).

IMAGING APPROACH TO THE POTENTIALLY INJURED CERVICAL SPINE

The evaluation of cervical spinal injury must begin with clinical examination of the patient by an experienced physician. The spine must remain immobilized to protect it and the cord during any imaging examination until the spine has been declared negative or mechanically stable. The type, extent, and order of the cervical spine and overall imaging evaluation are governed by the patient's clinical condition, particularly hemodynamic status, and neurologic status, as well as the evolution of the patient's status in the early post-admission period. In recent years, as noted above, fast CT has become more tightly integrated into cervical spine screening, as well as clearing areas not well delineated radiographically. CT has become the study of choice in many clinical post-trauma settings for general assessment of the patient's injuries and has, by choice and default, become more commonly used to initially screen the cervical and entire spine. The high sensitivity of CT for fracture detection and its ability to provide advanced analysis of complex osseous injuries have fostered this trend.

FIGURE 26-57 *Nuclear scintigraphy of a lumbar compression fracture.* **A,** *Lateral lumbar spine radiograph in a trauma patient with mild back pain shows possible L3 compression fracture (X) versus Schmorl's node deforming the superior end-plate.* **B,** *Static images from bone scintigraphy show end-plate increased tracer activity, indicating acute fracture.*

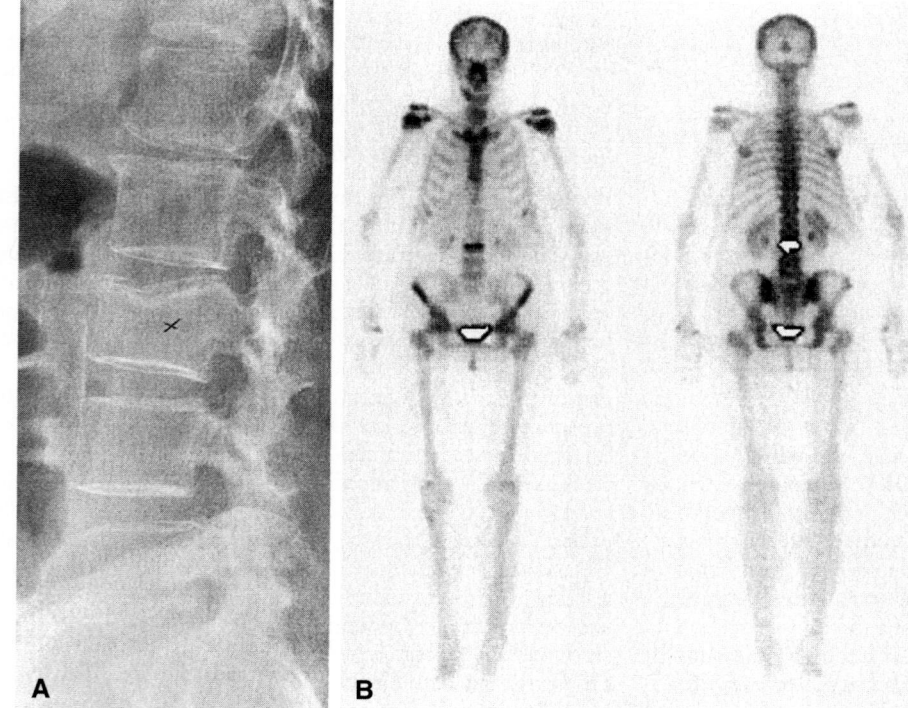
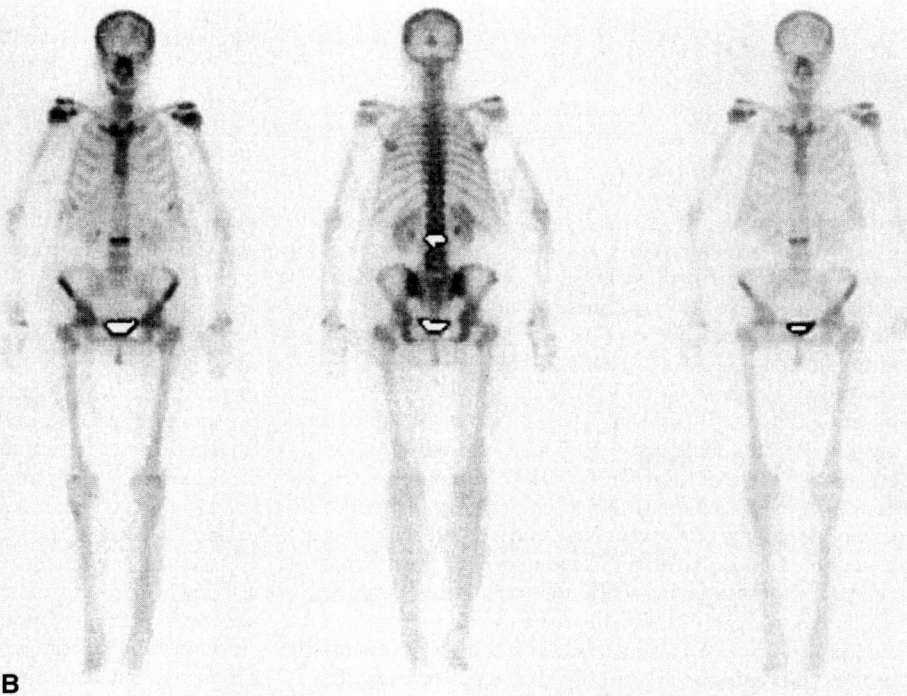

A   **B**

FIGURE 26-58   *Acute vertebral artery injury. **A,** Axial CT image with intravenous contrast shows absence of left vertebral artery density. **B,** Catheter angiogram shows multiple areas of thrombus along the course of the left vertebral artery.*

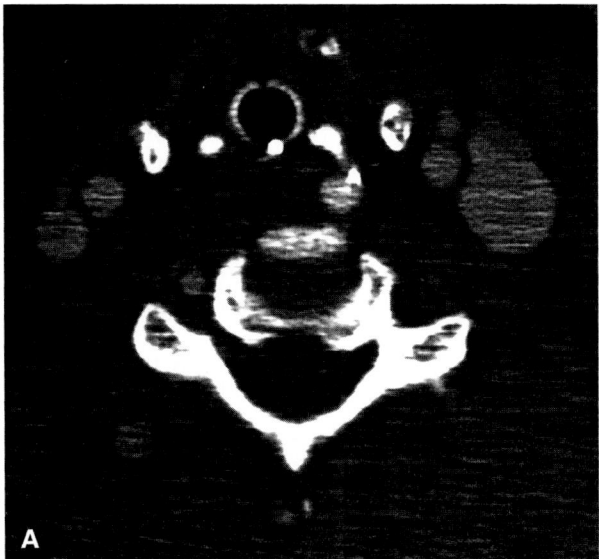
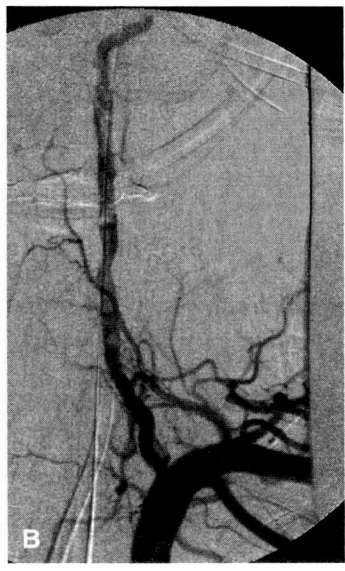

FIGURE 26-59   *CT angiography of cervical vascular injury. CT angiogram acquired on 40-slice multidetector CT with automatic contrast bolus timing demonstrates occlusion of the right external carotid artery (long black arrow), a pseudoaneurysm of the right internal carotid artery below the skull base (short black arrow), and an intravascular stent treating a dissection of the left internal carotid artery (white arrow).*

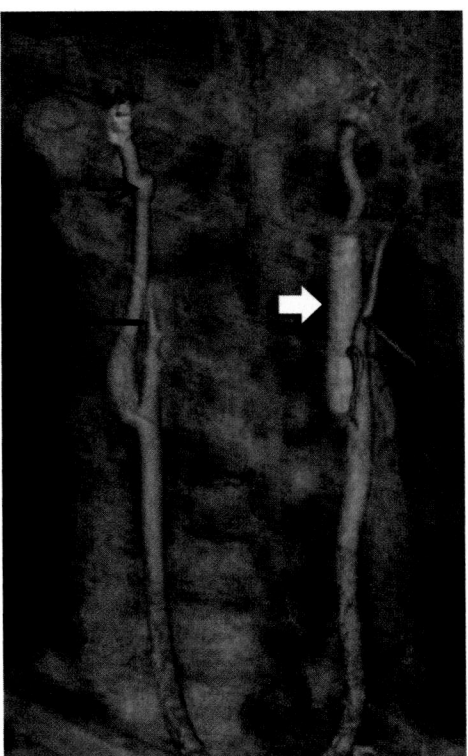

In many medical centers, the imaging workup of the cervical spine will be strongly influenced by the particular imaging equipment available, its location relative to the patient resuscitation area, and the image interpretation expertise available. Although certain imaging guidelines are suggested herein, based on the clinical circumstances of the patient, it must be acknowledged that these recommendations are best supported in a major trauma center environment and must be tailored to fit other emergency care settings.

Imaging Approach for Potential Cervical Spine Based Injury on Clinical Presentation

TRAUMA PATIENT WITH A NEUROLOGIC DEFICIT REFERABLE TO THE CERVICAL SPINAL CORD

Trauma patients *with spinal injury and signs of cord damage* may undergo lateral or three-view radiography in the admissions area to obtain a general appreciation of the nature of the injury (see Fig. 26-1). Some centers will also use the lateral cervical spine view to ascertain previous endotracheal tube positioning, to assess the upper airway, and to plan the intubation method in the presence of cervical spine injury. For some injuries, such as an isolated odontoid fracture or Jefferson fracture, the diagnostic information may not be significantly improved by performing CT, although additional injuries, not suspected from plain radiographs, may be detected by CT. The cervical spine CT study must include at least sagittal and coronal re-formations and, in the case of complex injuries, should be supplemented by volume-rendered images from various perspectives to enhance anatomic understanding of the injury. When there are clinical indications of potential cervical vascular injury, such as significant displaced fractures (unilateral or bilateral facet dislocations, flexion tear-drop fracture-dislocations, or extension fracture-dislocation) or fractures crossing the foramen transversarium, thin-section (2 mm or less) CT should be performed with intravenous contrast (CTA). Reconstruction of the axial images with overlapping will improve the quality of 2-D and 3-D re-formations. Some centers will proceed *directly to CT* in these cases without performing cervical radiographs.

Usually, MRI is subsequently performed to evaluate for soft tissue injuries including the intervertebral disks and ligaments and to assess the spinal canal for narrowing. The presence of a herniated disk or hematoma compressing the cord might have significant therapeutic indications for patients with incomplete or fluctuating neurologic deficits. Knowing the precise location and extent of ligament damage can help determine the most appropriate method and levels for spinal fixation. Finally, the cord can be assessed for the presence of edema or hemorrhage, which provide prognostic information. Trauma patients with definite myelopathy but negative plain radiographs and CT are best served by MRI or, if MRI is unavailable, myelography and CT myelography as the next study.

ALERT TRAUMA PATIENT WITH CERVICAL PAIN AND POSITIVE PHYSICAL FINDINGS

The attending physician must always initially approach a traumatized patient with a high index of suspicion regarding the presence of spinal injury, since failure to recognize and treat an unstable injury can lead to devastating, irreparable cord damage.[3] A history of trauma that could produce spinal injury or the presence of objective physical signs consistent with spinal injury is of particular importance in determining which patients should undergo imaging evaluation. However, radiographic or other imaging of the spine is clearly not indicated for every patient who complains of minimal symptoms after minor trauma. The NEXUS (National X-ray Utilization Study) project indicated that the absence of certain combined criteria could virtually exclude cervical injury and not require imaging assessment.[45,61] Other studies assessing risk of cervical spine injury under various clinical scenarios can also be used to triage patients regarding the need to proceed to an imaging assessment.[10,45]

The appropriate radiologic evaluation of the cervical spine is controversial, particularly with regard to the number of views that constitute an adequate radiologic assessment. As noted above, thin-section CT provides much greater sensitivity for diagnosis of cervical spine fractures and is gradually becoming the imaging test of choice to assess patients with post-traumatic neck pain or findings indicating possible injury on physical examination. This development is based on the recognized improved accuracy of CT over radiography for osseous pathology, the increased use of CT in general for assessing stable patients with blunt trauma in multiple body regions, the increased speed of image acquisition and processing, and its general cost-efficacy.[9,34] Although plain radiographs can be used to assess neurologically intact patients with positive physical findings on cervical spine examination, the potential for missing some fractures or ligament injuries should be kept in mind despite apparently negative radiography.[27,32]

If all cervical radiographs are normal and of adequate technical quality, including the C7–T1 region, the possibility of a significant missed skeletal cervical spine injury is relatively low, but ligamentous injuries, including potentially neurologically unstable injuries such as reduced bifacet dislocations or reduced hyperflexion or hyperextension subluxations, may still be present (Fig. 26-60).[32] If CT of the cervical spine is normal, osseous injury is virtually excluded. Several plans of action are then open. The patient with persistent pain may be placed in a cervical collar and followed clinically. MRI can be performed to look for ligament and other soft tissue injury. Active (patient-controlled) flexion-extension views can be performed if the patient is able to perform these maneuvers without limiting pain or neurologic symptoms.

The use of routine flexion and extension stress lateral cervical radiographs is by no means universal and should not be considered standard of practice.[51] The procedure should be *carefully supervised by a physician, and the patient should be alert and cooperative.* A radiography technologist should never perform the study alone. At least one third of these studies are inadequate for interpretation, mainly owing to limited cervical spine excursions and inability to visualize the entire cervical spine.[2] The patient should flex and extend the neck to the limit of pain tolerance or onset of subjective neurologic symptoms. Obviously, any suggestion of an onset of neurologic impairment mandates return to the neutral position and reapplication of cervical immobilization. If adequate flexion and extension views are acquired with visualization of the spine through C7–T1, the vast majority of potentially unstable injuries are excluded. Flexion and extension lateral cervical views should not be obtained in uncooperative patients or those with decreased mental acuity and should not be obtained with passive movement of the patient's cervical spine by a physician.[17,18,33,80]

The accuracy of spiral CT in detecting all potentially unstable ligament injuries is not known, although some of these injuries would be suggested by soft tissue swelling or subtle abnormalities of alignment. For this reason, active flexion-extension views are still needed in some circumstances to ensure cervical spine ligament integrity. When cervical flexion-extension views cannot be performed or when clinical follow-up may be in doubt, some clinicians would opt for cervical MRI to definitively clear the cervical spine.

PATIENT WITH UNRELIABLE PHYSICAL EXAMINATION OR ABILITY TO ASSESS CERVICAL PAIN

Trauma patients without evidence of myelopathy but whose physical examination cannot be considered reliable or who are distracted by significant pain of noncervical spine origin should be regarded as potentially having unstable spinal injuries until proved otherwise. The radiographic assessment of such patients should include at least lateral and AP cervical spine views. Open-mouth views are often difficult to obtain and technically suboptimal in this population. In addition, supine oblique views of the cervicothoracic junction region can be obtained if needed. Often, CT is used to assess the cervicocranial junction if not well demonstrated by radiography, depending on its

FIGURE 26-60 *Subtle hyperflexion injury on CT.* **A,** *Mid-sagittal CT re-formation in a blunt trauma patient with neck pain reveals a slight anterolisthesis at C4–C5 (arrow) associated with slight widening of the spinous processes.* **B,** *A parasagittal re-formation through a facet joint shows subluxation of articular facets (arrow), indicating significant ligament injury.* **C,** *Subsequently, in a collar the patient had further subluxation involving about 40 percent of the AP diameter of the vertebral bodies indicating an underlying unstable injury at C4–C5.* **D,** *A sagittal T2-weighted MR image shows marked narrowing of the spinal canal at the level of the subluxation. Increased linear signal present in the adjacent spinal cord indicates contusion.*

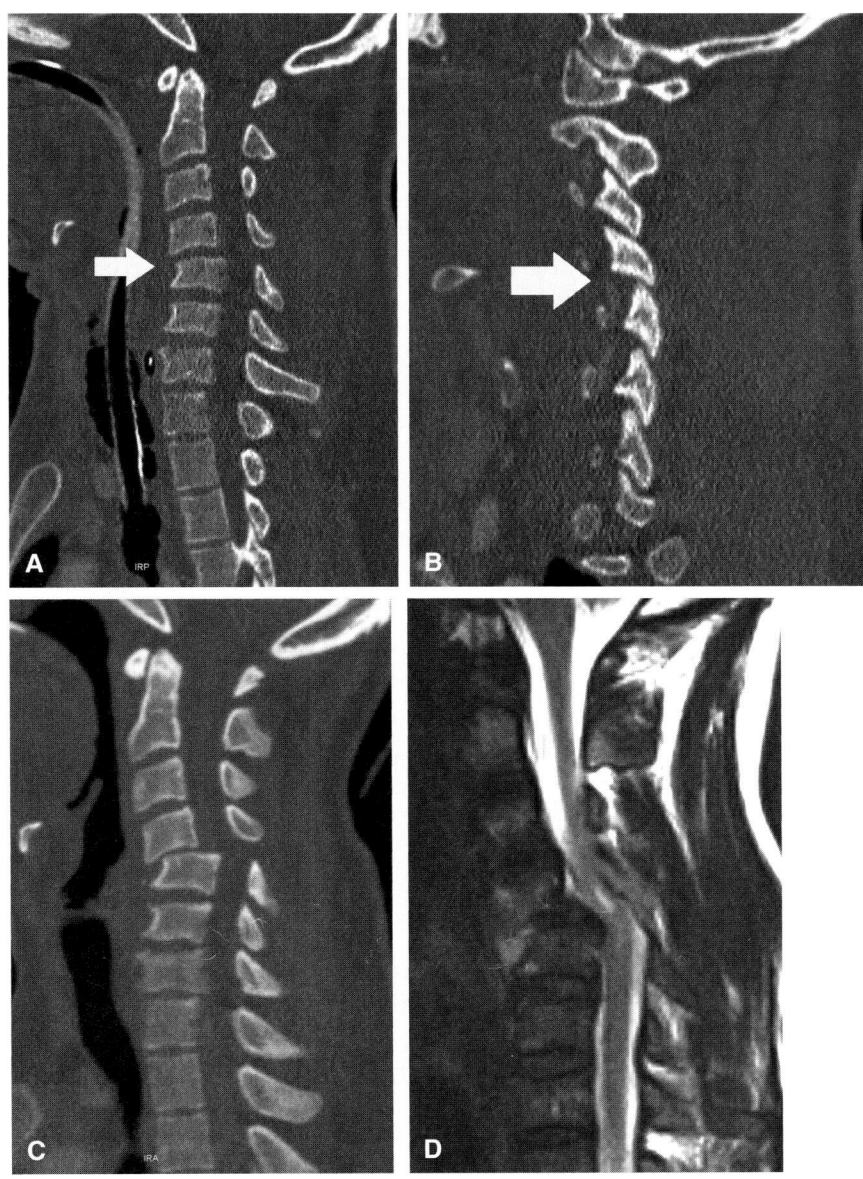

availability and indication for CT of other body regions. If injuries are identified, spine immobilization is maintained and further imaging workup performed when clinically feasible. Again, CT, especially MDCT, has assumed an increasing role in the initial screening of the *entire* cervical spine, particularly for patients with this clinical scenario.[87]

If all radiographic evaluations of the spine are negative, the vast majority of unstable injuries are excluded, but again, some potential for a neurologically unstable injury persists and some cervical fractures will not be diagnosed. The use of MRI in this setting involves some controversy when both cervical radiographs and complete cervical spine CT are normal.

D'Alise and colleagues[16] performed limited cervical spine MRI within 48 hours of trauma in 121 patients who had no obvious injury shown by plain radiography. There were 31 patients (25.6%) who had significant injury to paravertebral ligamentous structures, the intervertebral disk, or bone. Eight of these patients required surgical fixation of the injury. Hogan and associates studied 366 obtunded trauma patients using both 16-slice MDCT and 1.5 T MRI. All MDCT studies were interpreted as negative in this population. Follow-up cervical MRI studies were negative for any acute cervical spine injury in 354 (96.7% of patients) and negative specifically for ligament injury in 362 (99%). Among the four patients with ligament injury, all had only one-column involvement and were mechanically stable. In this study, MDCT had a 99 percent negative predictive value for ligament injury and 100 percent negative predictive value for a mechanically unstable cervical spine.[46] Another study by Schuster et al. also indicated that MRI added no useful information in 93 patients who had a normal admission motor examination and negative cervical spine CT with sagittal re-formation, but with persistent cervical spine pain.[75] However, the subject of supplemental MRI screening remains controversial, as Diaz et al. found that *single-slice helical* CT had only a 78 percent negative predictive for ligament injury and concluded that while helical CT was the most sensitive, specific, and cost-effective modality for screening the cervical spine for bony injuries, it was not an effective modality for screening for cervical ligament injury.[20] Clearly, further studies are needed using state-of-the-art MDCT to evaluate this issue.

If MRI is not available, an alternative approach is to obtain an erect AP and lateral cervical radiograph with the patient in collar stabilization to allow limited physiologic stress on the cervical spine. If these films are normal, erect AP and lateral views are repeated out of collar with the cervical spine slightly extended and the head supported by a pillow. If these views are normal, the cervical collar is permanently removed. Although these approaches are considered prudent to avoid missing a cervical spine injury, they are by no means universally followed. In some sites the cervical collar is removed on the basis of negative AP and lateral supine radiography alone, suggesting the rarity with which neurologically unstable cervical spine injuries occur with normal-appearing cervical radiographs interpreted by appropriately trained physicians.

Some authors have suggested the use of passive flexion and extension imaging under fluoroscopic guidance for patients who do not have a reliable physical examination.[18,73,76] The limited data available do not provide sufficient evidence to support routine use of this technique. A number of cervical spine injuries are not detected by this method, including herniated intervertebral disks and epidural hematomas. These lesions may cause spinal cord compression that creates or worsens a neurologic deficit without evidence of overt subluxation on fluoroscopy. More recent studies have demonstrated that this approach can induce a neurologic deficit, is limited in visualization of the lower cervical spine, is not cost effective, and has low sensitivity for ligament injury detection.[17,26,33,80]

Cervical disk herniation is a more common cause of central cord syndrome than previously suspected.[15] Benzel and co-workers[7] found 27 acute cervical disk herniations among 174 trauma patients with negative cervical radiographs having cervical MRI. Rizzolo and colleagues[70] observed acute cervical disk herniation in 42 percent of 55 patients with blunt cervical trauma with cervical fractures or neurologic deficits. In addition, either congenital or acquired spinal stenosis can produce spinal cord lesions in association with blunt trauma when there is no radiographic evidence of injury. Flexion and extension in this population could worsen cord compression and ischemia. To date, only MRI has proven diagnostic accuracy for direct diagnosis of ligament injury from blunt spinal trauma.[6,16]

ALERT PATIENT WITH NORMAL CERVICAL SPINE EXAMINATION

The need to perform imaging in alert, appropriately oriented trauma victims without evidence of cervical pain, tenderness to palpation of the cervical spine, or major distracting injuries has been highly controversial. Most patients admitted to emergency centers from the scene of a major blunt force trauma are placed in cervical immobilization and are presumed to have a cervical injury until proved otherwise. This scenario places a great deal of pressure on the admitting physician to exclude an injury with an extremely high degree of certainty. There are case reports describing so-called painless cervical spine fractures. A close review of many such articles typically reveals that the patient either had symptoms or was not truly alert.[21,55,72]

Many large series published to date indicate that alert trauma patients without major distracting injuries and without subjective complaints of neck pain or positive physical findings invariably have normal imaging evaluations.[21,44,89] A prospective series of alert trauma patients without symptoms who underwent cervical spine CT to clear the cervicothoracic junction revealed one nondisplaced C7 transverse process fracture in 146 patients at a cost of more than $58,000.[59] Diliberti and Lindsey[21] recommended omission of radiologic assessment of the cervical spine in any trauma patient with class 1 level of consciousness (i.e., able to follow complex commands, responds immediately) and without evidence of intoxication, neurologic deficit, cervical spine pain, or pain elicited on palpation. Gonzales and associates[30] found that clinical assessment was more sensitive than radiography in detecting cervical spine injury even in intoxicated patients. As noted above the NEXUS study indicates that significant cervical spine injury could be virtually excluded in patients without midline cervical tenderness or focal neurologic deficit, normal level of alertness, no intoxication, and no painful distracting injuries.[44] Other similar decision rules have been developed to help confidently exclude cervical spine injury in the vast majority of certain patient populations.[10]

Imaging in Spinal Trauma: Special Situations

CONCOMITANT CERVICAL SPINE AND LIFE-THREATENING INJURIES

As stated throughout this chapter, the imaging evaluation of the spine must be performed in the total context of the trauma patient's management. The radiographic examination of patients with concomitant acute spinal injury and life-threatening injuries should consist only of AP and horizontal beam lateral projections obtained in the emergency center during the clinical evaluation. If a radiologic diagnosis can be made from this limited study (e.g., traumatic spondylolisthesis, bilateral facet dislocation, burst fracture), management of the injury consistent with the patient's clinical condition can be initiated. If results of the initial limited examination are equivocal or if the spinal injury is one that requires additional evaluation by CT or MRI, the spine must be appropriately immobilized until the life-threatening injury has been stabilized and the radiologic evaluation can be continued.

PENETRATING CERVICAL SPINE TRAUMA

CERVICAL SPINE INJURY Instability of the cervical spine as a result of penetrating trauma is most unusual. When patients sustaining penetrating neck trauma are fully conscious and have no neurologic deficits, spine immobilization is not required, although one case report does describe cervical instability in a patient without spinal cord injury. In most cases, assessment of cervical soft tissue injuries including the vessels and aerodigestive tract will be required either by imaging or exploration, or both, in select cases. CT can document the extent of bony injury and localize retained foreign bodies. When a neurologic deficit is present after any penetrating spine injury, MRI can determine the level of injury, the presence of residual cord compression, and direct signs of cord damage (Fig. 26-61). Neurologic deficits can occur from gunshot injury without direct trauma to the cord from dispersion of the ballistic object's kinetic injury around the tract.

VERTEBRAL ARTERY INJURY Penetrating injury accounts for the majority of cervical vertebral injuries resulting from trauma.[29] The presence of retained metal fragments from ballistic injury precludes vascular MRA assessment because of artifacts created by the close proximity of metal. In addition, because MRA is less sensitive for detection of subtle intimal injuries or mural hematoma, conventional arteriography is generally recommended for evaluation of suspected vertebral artery injury caused by penetrating force. Although the incidence of vertebral artery injury from blunt trauma to the cervical spine appears to be higher than previously suspected, the injury usually results in complete thrombosis without producing neurologic deterioration.[85] It also appears that thrombosed

vessels remain occluded on long-term follow-up without the need to perform endovascular occlusion. Most acutely occluded vertebral arteries remain clinically silent, but vessels that are injured but patent can lead to formation of clot with extension or embolization resulting in posterior circulation infarction (Fig. 26-62). These injuries, when identified, require treatment to prevent or minimize the chance of embolization using antiplatelet or anticoagulant therapy as permitted by the patient's condition or open surgical or endovascular treatment.

PREEXISTING PATHOLOGIC CONDITIONS

Trauma patients with various conditions that lead to fusion of the spine are at increased risk for spinal injury compared with patients with normal spine mobility. Patients with ankylosing spondylitis can sustain spinal injury from minimal amounts of blunt force impact. Because the spine has undergone bony ankylosis, it is fragile and fractures equally easily across the bone or disk spaces (Fig. 26-63). Usually, these injuries completely traverse all supporting ossified spinal ligaments, creating marked instability. In my experience, these injuries are typically evident in extension or extension-dislocation patterns. It has been noted that spinal fractures in patients with underlying ankylosing spondylitis are not uncommonly occult radiographically.[23] Fractures and dislocations most typically occur in the lower cervical followed by the thoracic spine. This finding may be due to spontaneous reduction of the fracture, generalized osteoporosis that often occurs in patients with advanced disease, and failure to appreciate noncontiguous injuries.[23]

Although patients with ankylosing spondylitis may present with well-established neurologic deficits and obvious imaging abnormalities, about one third have delayed

---

FIGURE 26-61 *Gunshot wound of the cervical spine. **A,** Lateral cervical radiograph of victim of gunshot wound with quadriplegia shows bullet track though the C1–C2 level with comminution of the C2 body and bone fragments on the spinal canal. **B,** Sagittal MRI, T2-weighted fast spin-echo shows the tract through the cord at the C2 level with increased signal (contusion) extending from the medulla to the C6 level (arrows). Bright signal edema is seen in the prevertebral soft tissues.*

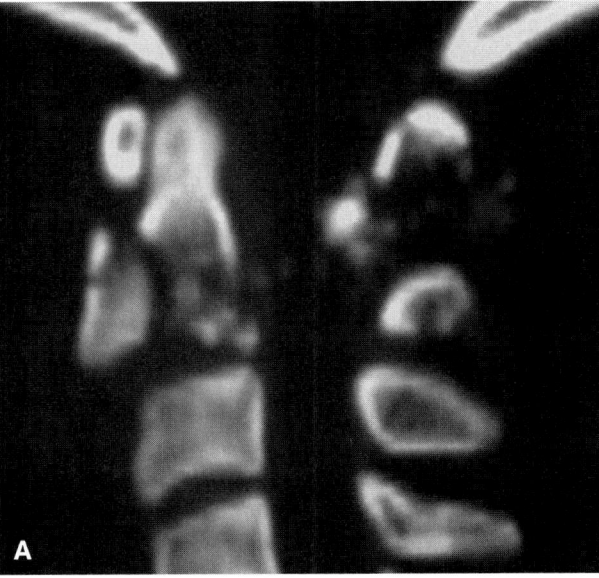
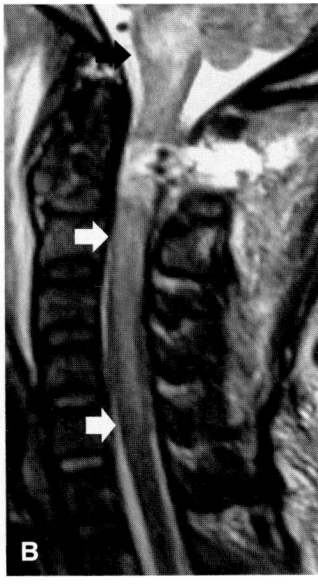

FIGURE 26-62   *Cervical vertebral injury from blunt trauma leading to cerebral infarct. **A,** Axial CT image shows a low attenuation area in the midbrain (arrows), of concern for contusion of infarct in this blunt trauma patient. **B,** CT image of the C1 body after intravenous contrast enhancement shows a nondisplaced linear fracture of the right anterior ring. Note the absence of the expected opacified right vertebral artery (arrow). **C,** Volume-rendered image from a cerebral CT angiogram shows complete occlusion of brainstem circulation, presumably from progression of thrombosis or emboli from the injured right vertebral artery.*

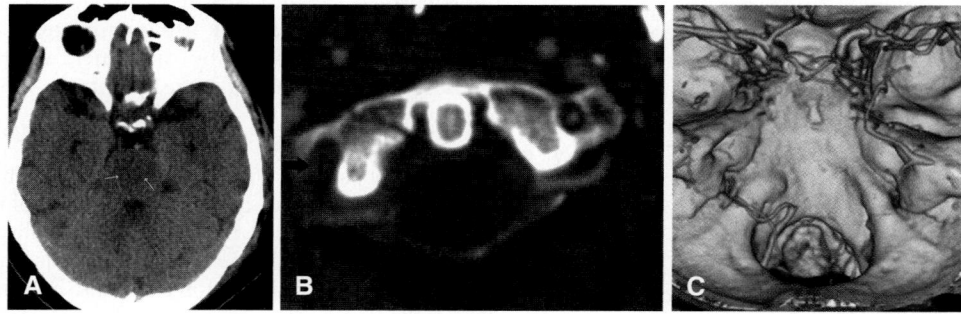

onset of neurologic deficits as a result of failure to diagnose or properly immobilize the very unstable spine. In general, patients with blunt trauma who have ankylosing spondylitis should be regarded as having unstable injuries until definitely proved otherwise. If radiographs appear normal, further evaluation by thin-section CT is recommended to detect subtle fractures. CT may also assist in differentiating acute fractures from pseudarthrosis related to previous injury. If the patient has cervical pain, further assessment by MRI to detect subtle soft tissue edema or bone marrow edema is also indicated to avoid misdiagnosing a highly unstable injury.

Other preexisting conditions that may be associated with an increased risk of spinal fracture with lower energy blunt trauma include diffuse idiopathic skeletal hyperostosis (DISH) or Forestier disease (also called ankylosing hyperostosis), spinal spondylosis, and osteoporosis. DISH is similar to ankylosing spondylitis in the sense that the spine contains a segment of bone fusion. DISH may be differentiated from ankylosing spondylitis by the absence of squared vertebral body corners; the larger, coarser, and predominantly anterior syndesmophytes of DISH; and lack of sacroiliac and apophyseal changes that occur in ankylosing spondylitis. Fractures in DISH may occur through the mid-portion of a fused segment or at the top or bottom through a disk space or odontoid process.[63] The long lever arm created by the fused segment focuses all the energy of the applied force onto a single disk space,

FIGURE 26-63   *Spinal injury with underlying ankylosing spondylitis. **A,** Lateral thoracic spine study in paraplegic trauma patient shows marked dislocation at the T9–T10 level with posterior displacement of the superior spine indicating extension injury. **B,** Sagittal CT re-formation confirms a complete fracture-dislocation. Note the disruption of the bony ankylosis spanning the anterior vertebral bodies. **C,** Corresponding coronal re-formation showing widened disk space at injury level and lateral translation of the spine.*

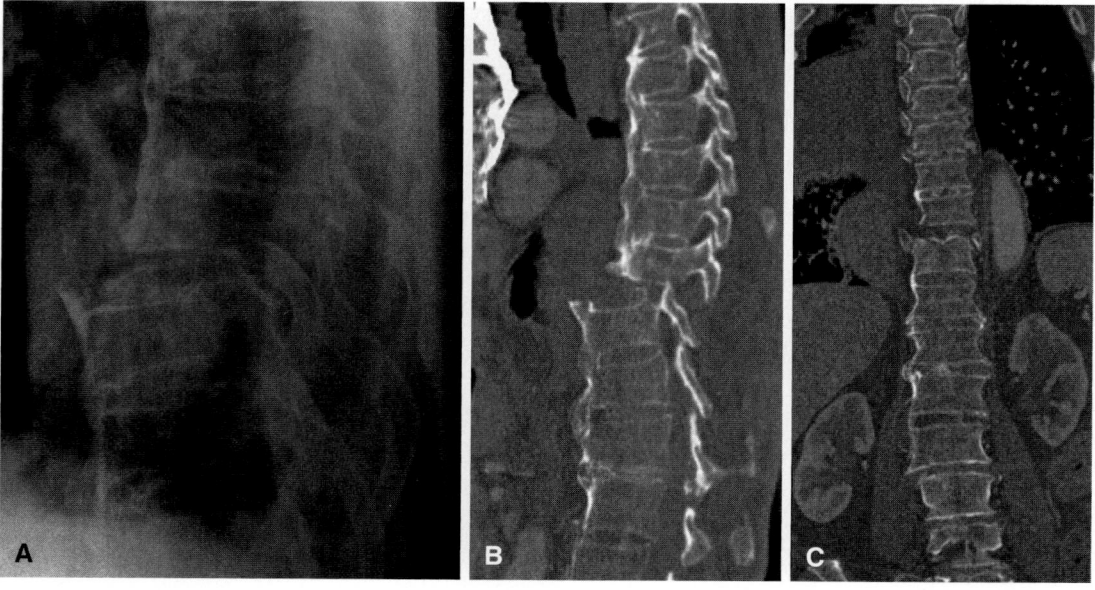

increasing the risk of injury. Similarly, spines that are fused because of multiple contiguous levels of degenerative spondylosis are also at increased risk for injury because of inability to distribute straining forces across multiple spinal levels.

Patients with severe osteoporosis are at increased risk for fracture resulting from minor injury or activities of daily living. In the spine, such injuries may appear as minor loss of height of a vertebral body. The age of the injury may not be apparent, and it may be assumed in some cases to be a remote lesion. Compression fractures in patients with structural bone weakness can progress to significant compression with physiologic loading and produce acute or delayed onset of radicular or complete neurologic deficits. The diminished density of demineralized bone associated with suboptimal film technique renders radiographic interpretation of the spine difficult and insensitive to detection of subtle fractures.

If the patient has persistent spinal pain, examination by thin-section CT is recommended initially, as it often demonstrates subtle end-plate fractures and paraspinal hematoma not detected by radiography. If clinical symptoms remain unexplained or CT is not definitive, MRI is suggested. MRI shows paraspinal edema, hematoma, and bone edema with high sensitivity, improving the level of confidence in injury detection or exclusion. Nuclear bone scintigraphy can also play a role in diagnosing fractures in this setting. However, acute fractures may not have abnormal bone turnover activity in the acute phase, particularly in elderly people. Also, foci of increased nuclide deposition in the spine may be due to chronic abnormalities such as seen with spondylosis or subacute injuries as well as acute pathology, making this examination less useful. In general, careful attention to imaging for these subsets of patients combined with a low threshold for performing additional diagnostic studies in symptomatic patients is warranted.

SUMMARY

Advances in diagnostic imaging in recent years have significantly changed the approach to imaging acute spinal trauma. Whereas spinal radiography was considered routine for essentially all major trauma patients, with the advent of MDCT this study is no longer mandated. Many emergency or trauma physicians will opt for CT screening of the entire body including the entire spine in one CT sweep. The information provided by CT is considerably more accurate than that based on plain radiographic interpretation alone. The advent of faster computer processing and more accessible user interfaces has made the creation of high-resolution 2-D and 3-D spine images straightforward and available for use in a timely fashion for making patient management decisions. Additionally, MRI has continued to improve in speed of data acquisition and image quality. Newer sequences that provide information about spinal cord ischemia (diffusion weighting) and the integrity of axonal tracks (diffusion tensor imaging) will continue to expand the types of anatomic and physiologic information that MRI can provide. It is vital that the sequence of imaging studies performed relate to the specific clinical presentation of the patient and be altered as required by changes in the patient's condition. Maintenance of spinal immobilization before, during, and after imaging evaluation is critical until potentially unstable spinal injury has been excluded.

REFERENCES

1. Anderson, L.D.; D'Alonzo, T.R. Fractures of the odontoid process of the axis. J Bone Joint Surg Am 56:1663, 1974.
2. Anglen, J.; Metzler, M.; Bunn, P.; et al. Flexion and extension views are not cost-effective in a cervical spine clearance protocol for obtunded trauma patients. J Trauma 52:54, 2002.
3. Bachulis, B.L.; Long, W.B.; Hynes, G.D.; et al. Clinical indications for cervical spine radiographs in the traumatized patient. Am J Surg 153:473, 1987.
4. Ballock, R.T.; MacKersie, R.; Abitbol, J.; et al. Can burst fractures be predicted from plain radiographs? J Bone Joint Surg Br 74:147, 1992.
5. Barton, D.; Allen, M.; Findlay, D.; et al. Evaluation of whiplash injuries by technetium 99m isotope scanning. Arch Emerg Med 10:197, 1993.
6. Benzel, E.C.; Hart, B.L.; Ball, P.A.; et al. Fractures of the C2 vertebral body. J Neurosurg 81:206, 1994.
7. Benzel, E.C.; Hart, B.L.; Ball, P.A.; et al. Magnetic resonance imaging for the evaluation of patients with occult cervical spine injury. J Neurosurg 85:824, 1996.
8. Biffl, W.L.; Moore, E.E.; Elliott, J.P.; et al. The devastating potential of blunt vertebral arterial injuries. Ann Surg 23:672, 2000.
9. Blackmore, C.C.; Mann, F.A.; Wilson, A.J. Helical CT in the primary trauma evaluation of the cervical spine: An evidence-based approach. Skeletal Radiol 29:632, 2000.
10. Blackmore, C.C.; Ramsey, S.D.; Mann, F.A.; et al. Cervical spine screening with CT in trauma patients: A cost-effectiveness analysis. Radiology 212:117, 1999.
11. Bradley, W.G. MR appearance of hemorrhage in the brain. Radiology 189:15, 1993.
12. Brady, W.J.; Moghtader, J.; Cutcher, D.; et al. ED use of flexion-extension cervical spine radiography in the evaluation of blunt trauma. Am J Emerg Med 17:504, 1999.
13. Christensen, P.C. The radiologic study of the normal spine. Radiol Clin North Am 15:133, 1977.
14. Daffner, R.H. Helical CT of the cervical spine for trauma patients: A time study. AJR Am J Roentgenol 177:677, 2001.
15. Dai, L.; Jia, L. Central cord injury complicating acute cervical disc herniation in trauma. Spine 25:331, 2000.
16. D'Alise, M.D.; Benzel, E.C.; Hart, B.L. Magnetic resonance imaging evaluation of the cervical spine in the comatose or obtunded patient. J Neurosurg 91:54, 1999.

17. Davis, J.W.; Kaups, K.L.; Cunningham, M.A.; et al. Routine evaluation of the cervical spine in head-injured patients with dynamic fluoroscopy: A reappraisal. J Trauma 50:1044, 2001.

18. Davis, J.W.; Parks, S.N.; Detlefs, C.L.; et al. Clearing the cervical spine in obtunded patients: The use of dynamic fluoroscopy. J Trauma 39:435, 1995.

19. Demaerel, P.; Sunaert, S.; Wilms, G. Sequences and techniques in spinal MR imaging. JBR-BTR 86:221, 2003.

20. Diaz, J.J., Jr.; Aulino, J.M.; Collier, B.; et al. The early work-up for isolated ligamentous injury of the cervical spine: Does computed tomography scan have a role? J Trauma 59:897, 2005.

21. Diliberti, T.; Lindsey, R.W. Evaluation of the cervical spine in the emergency setting: Who does not need an x-ray? Orthopedics 15:170, 1992.

22. Doran, S.E.; Papadopoulos, M.; Ducker, T.; et al. Magnetic resonance imaging documentation of coexistent traumatic locked facets of the cervical spine and disc herniation. J Neurosurg 79:341, 1993.

23. Finkelstein, J.A.; Chapman, J.R.; Mirza, S. Occult vertebral fractures in ankylosing spondylitis. Spinal Cord 37:444, 1999.

24. Flanders, A.E.; Schaeffer, D.M.; Doan, H.T.; et al. Acute cervical spine trauma: Correlation of MR imaging findings with degree of neurologic deficit. Radiology 177:25, 1990.

25. Flee, C.; Woodring, J.H. Unstable Jefferson variant atlas fracture: An unrecognized cervical injury. AJNR Am J Neuroradiol 12:1105, 1992.

26. Freedman, I.; van Gelderen, D.; Cooper, D.J.; et al. Cervical spine assessment in the unconscious trauma patient: A major trauma service's experience with passive flexion-extension radiography. J Trauma 58:1183, 2005.

27. Gale, S.C.; Gracias, V.H.; Reilly, P.M.; et al. The inefficiency of plain radiography to evaluate the cervical spine after blunt trauma. J Trauma 59:1121, 2005.

28. Garza-Mercado, R. Traumatic extradural hematoma of the cervical spine. Neurosurgery 24:410, 1989.

29. Giacobetti, F.B.; Vaccaro, A.R.; Bos-Giacobetti, M.A.; et al. Vertebral artery occlusion associated with cervical spine trauma: A prospective analysis. Spine 22:188, 1997.

30. Gonzales, R.P.; Fried, P.O.; Bukhalo, M.; et al. Role of clinical examination in screening for blunt cervical spine injury. J Am Coll Surg 189:152, 1999.

31. Grant, G.A.; Mirza, S.K.; Chapman, J.R.; et al. Risk of early closed reduction in cervical spine subluxation injuries. J Neurosurg 90:13, 1999.

32. Griffen, M.M.; Frykberg, E.R.; Kerwin, H.A.; et al. Radiographic clearance of blunt cervical spine injury: Plain radiography or computed tomography scan? J Trauma 55:222, 2003.

33. Griffiths, H.J.; Wagner, J.; Anglen, J.; et al. The use of forced flexion/extension views in the obtunded trauma patient. Skeletal Radiol 31:587, 2002.

34. Grogan, E.L.; Morris, J.A., Jr.; Dittus, R.S.; et al. Cervical spine evaluation in urban trauma centers: Lowering institutional costs and complications through helical CT scan. J Am Coll Surg 200:160, 2005.

35. Grossman, M.D.; Reilly, P.M.; Gillet, T.; et al. National survey of the incidence of cervical spine injury and approach to cervical spine clearance in U.S. trauma centers. J Trauma 47:684, 1999.

36. Harris, J.H., Jr. Abnormal cervicocranial retropharyngeal soft-tissue contour in the detection of subtle acute cervicocranial injuries. Emerg Radiol 1:15, 1994.

37. Harris, J.H., Jr.; Burke, J.T.; Ray, R.D.; et al. Low (type III) odontoid fracture: A new radiologic sign. Radiology 153:353, 1984.

38. Harris, J.H., Jr.; Carson, G.C.; Wagner, L.K. Radiologic diagnosis of traumatic occipitovertebral dissociation. 1. Normal occipitovertebral relationships on lateral radiographs of supine subjects. AJR Am J Roentgenol 162:881, 1994.

39. Harris, J.H., Jr.; Carson, G.C.; Wagner, L.K.; et al. Radiologic diagnosis of traumatic occipitovertebral dissociation. 2. Comparison of three methods of detecting occipitovertebral relationships on lateral radiographs of supine subjects. AJR Am J Roentgenol 162:887, 1994.

40. Harris, J.H. The radiographic examination. In Harris, J.H.; Mirvis, S.E., eds. Radiology of Acute Cervical Spine Trauma, 3rd ed. Baltimore, Williams & Wilkins, 1995, p. 180.

41. Hauser, C.J.; Visvikis, G.; Hinrichs, C.; et al. Prospective validation of computed tomography screening of the thoracolumbar spine in trauma. J Trauma 55:228, 2003.

42. Herr, C.H.; Ball, P.A.; Sargent, S.K.; et al. Sensitivity of prevertebral soft tissue measurement of C3 for detection of cervical spine fractures and dislocations. Am J Emerg Med 16:346, 1998.

43. Hildingsson, C.; Hietala, S.O.; Toolanen, G. Scintigraphic findings in acute whiplash injury of the cervical spine. Injury 20:265, 1989.

44. Hoffman, J.R.; Mower, W.R.; Wolfson, A.B.; et al. Validity of a set of clinical criteria to rule out injury to the cervical spine in patients with blunt trauma. National Emergency X-Radiography Utilization Study Group. N Engl J Med 343:94, 2000. Erratum in N Engl J Med 344:464, 2001.

45. Hoffman, J.R.; Schriger, D.L.; Mower, W.; et al. Low-risk criteria for cervical-spine radiography in blunt trauma: A prospective study. Ann Emerg Med 21:1454, 1992.

46. Hogan, G.J.; Mirvis, S.E.; Shanmuganathan, K.; et al. Exclusion of unstable cervical spine injury in obtunded patients with blunt trauma: Is MR imaging needed when multi-detector row CT findings are normal? Radiology 237:106, 2005.

47. Hyslop, W.B.; Balci, N.C.; Semelka, R.C. Future horizons in MR imaging. Magn Reson Imaging Clin N Am 3:211, 2005.

48. Iannacone, W.M.; DeLong, W.G.; Born, C.T.; et al. Dynamic computerized tomography of the occiput-atlas-axis complex in trauma patients with odontoid lateral mass asymmetry. J Trauma 3:1501, 1990.
49. Insko, E.K.; Gracias, V.H.; Gupta, R.; et al. Utility of flexion and extension radiographs of the cervical spine in the acute evaluation of blunt trauma. J Trauma 53:426, 2002.
50. Jenkins, M.G.; Curran, P.; Rocke, L.G. Where do we go after the three standard cervical spine views in the conscious trauma patient? A survey. Eur J Emerg Med 6:215, 1999.
51. Kaneriya, P.P.; Schweitzer, M.E.; Spettell, C.; et al. The cost-effectiveness of oblique radiography in the exclusion of C7–T1 injury in trauma patients. Skeletal Radiol 28:271, 1999.
52. Katz, R.C.; Wilson, L.; Fraser, N. Anxiety and its determinants in patients undergoing magnetic resonance imaging. J Behav Ther Exp Psychiatry 25:131, 1994.
53. Kulkarni, M.V.; McArdle, C.B.; Kopanicky, D.; et al. Acute spinal cord injury: MR imaging at 1.5 T. Radiology 164:837, 1987.
54. MacDonald, R.L.; Schwartz, M.L.; Mirich, D.; et al. Diagnosis of cervical spine injury in motor vehicle crash victims: How many x-rays are enough? J Trauma 30:392, 1990.
55. Mace, S.E. Unstable occult cervical spine fracture. Ann Emerg Med 20:1373, 1992.
56. Mascalchi, M.; Pozzo, G.D.; Dini, C.; et al. Acute spinal trauma: Prognostic value of MRI appearances at 0.5T. Clin Radiol 48:100, 1993.
57. Matin, P. The appearance of bone scans following fractures, including immediate and long-term studies. J Nucl Med 20:1227, 1979.
58. Miller, P.R.; Fabian, T.C.; Croce, M.A. Prospective screening for blunt cerebrovascular injuries: Analysis of diagnostic modalities and outcomes. Ann Surg 236:386, 2002.
59. Mirvis, S.E.; Diaconis, J.N.; Chirico, P.A.; et al. Protocol driven radiologic evaluation of suspected cervical spine injury: Efficacy study. Radiology 170:831, 1989.
60. Mirvis, S.E.; Geisler, F.H.; Joslyn, J.N.; et al. Use of titanium wire in cervical spine fixation as a means to reduce MR artifacts. AJNR Am J Neuroradiol 9:1229, 1988.
61. Mower, W.R.; Hoffman, J.R.; Pollack, C.V., Jr.; et al. Use of plain radiography to screen for cervical spine injuries. Ann Emerg Med 38:1, 2001.
62. Murray, J.B.; Ziervogel, M. The value of computed tomography in the diagnosis of atlanto-axial rotatory fixation. Br J Radiol 63:894, 1990.
63. Paley, D.; Schwartz, M.; Cooper, P.; et al. Fractures of the spine in diffuse skeletal hyperostosis. Clin Orthop 267:22, 1991.
64. Parent, A.D.; Harkey, H.L.; Touchstone, D.A.; et al. Lateral cervical spine dislocation and vertebral artery injury. Neurosurgery 31:501, 1992.
65. Pathria, M.N.; Petersilge, C.A. Spinal trauma. Radiol Clin North Am 29:847, 1991.
66. Pollack, C.V., Jr.; Hendey, G.W.; Martin, D.R.; NEXUS Group. Use of flexion-extension radiographs of the cervical spine in blunt trauma. Ann Emerg Med 38:8, 2001.
67. Pratt, E.S.; Green, D.A.; Spengler, D.M. Herniated intervertebral discs associated with unstable spine injuries. Spine 15:662, 1990.
68. Price, R.F.; Sellar, R.M.; Leung, C.; et al. Traumatic vertebral arterial dissection and vertebrobasilar arterial thrombosis successfully treated with endovascular thrombolysis and stenting. AJNR Am J Neuroradiol 19:1677, 1998.
69. Quencer, R.M.; Bunge, R.P.; Egnor, M.; et al. Acute traumatic central cord syndrome: MRI-pathologic correlation. Neuroradiology 34:85, 1992.
70. Rizzolo, S.J.; Piazza, M.R.; Cotler, J.M.; et al. Intervertebral disc injury complicating cervical spine trauma. Spine 16:187, 1991.
71. Rizzolo, S.J.; Vaccaro, A.R.; Cotler, J.M. Cervical spine trauma. Spine 19:2288, 1994.
72. Roth, B.J.; Martin, R.R.; Foley, K.; et al. Roentgenographic evaluation of the cervical spine: A selective approach. Arch Surg 129:643, 1994.
73. Scarrow, A.M.; Levy, E.L.; Resnick, D.K.; et al. Cervical spine evaluation in obtunded or comatose pediatric trauma patients: A pilot study. Pediatr Neurosurg 30:169, 1999.
74. Schaeffer, D.M.; Flanders, A.E.; Osterholm, J.L.; et al. Prognostic significance of magnetic resonance imaging in the acute phase of cervical spine injury. J Neurosurg 76:218, 1992.
75. Schuster, R.; Waxman, K.; Sanchez, B.; et al. Magnetic resonance imaging is not needed to clear cervical spines in blunt trauma patients with normal computed tomographic results and no motor deficits. Arch Surg 140:762, 2005.
76. Sees, D.W.; Rodriguez Cruz, L.R.; Flaherty, S.F.; et al. The use of bedside fluoroscopy to evaluate the cervical spine in obtunded trauma patients, J Trauma 45:768, 1998.
77. Seybold, E.A.; Dunn, E.J.; Jenis, L.G.; et al. Variation on the posterior vertebral contour line at the level of C-2 on lateral cervical roentgenograms: A method for odontoid fracture detection. Am J Orthop 28:696, 1999.
78. Shanmuganathan, K.; Mirvis, S.E.; Levine, A.M. Isolated articular pillar fractures of the cervical spine: Imaging observations in 20 patients. AJR Am J Roentgenol 166:897, 1996.
79. Sheridan, R.; Peralta, R.; Rhea, J.; et al. Reformatted visceral protocol helical computed tomographic scanning allows conventional radiographs of the thoracic and lumbar spine to be eliminated in the evaluation of blunt trauma patients. J Trauma 55:665, 2003.
80. Sliker, C.W.; Mirvis, S.E.; Shanmuganathan, K. Assessing cervical spine stability in obtunded blunt trauma patients: Review of medical literature. Radiology 234:733, 2005.

81. Spitz, J.; Laer, I.; Tillet, K.; et al. Scintimetric evaluation of remodeling after fractures in man. J Nucl Med 34:1403, 1993.

82. Taneichi, H.; Duda, K.; Kalino, T.; et al. Traumatically induced vertebral artery occlusion associated with cervical spine injuries: Prospective study using magnetic resonance angiography. Spine 30:1955, 2005.

83. Thomeir, W.C.; Brown, D.C.; Mirvis, S.E. The "tilted" odontoid: A sign of subtle odontoid fracture. AJNR Am J Neuroradiol 11:605, 1990.

84. Vannier, W.; Marsh, J.L.; Warren, J.O. Three-dimensional CT construction images for craniofacial surgical planning and evaluation. Radiology 150:179, 1984.

85. Weller, S.J.; Rossitch, E., Jr.; Malek, A.M. Detection of vertebral artery injury after cervical spine trauma using magnetic resonance angiography. J Trauma 46:660, 1999.

86. West, O.C.; Anbari, M.M.; Pilgram, T.K.; et al. Acute cervical spine trauma: Diagnostic performance of single-view versus three-view radiographic screening. Radiology 204:819, 1997.

87. Widder, S.; Doig, C.; Burrowes, P.; et al. Prospective evaluation of computed tomographic scanning for the spinal clearance of obtunded trauma patients: Preliminary results. J Trauma 56:1179, 2004.

88. Young, J.W.R.; Resnick, C.S.; DeCandido, P.; et al. The laminar space in the diagnosis of rotational flexion injuries of the cervical spine. AJR Am J Roentgenol 152:103, 1989.

89. Zabel, D.D.; Tinkoff, G.; Wittenborn, W.; et al. Adequacy and efficacy of lateral cervical radiography in alert, high-risk blunt trauma patient. J Trauma 43:952, 1997.

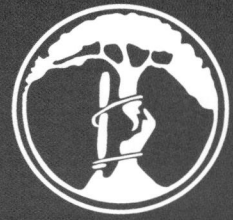

CHAPTER 27

Spinal Orthoses

Theodore J. Fisher, M.D., M.S., Susan L. Williams, M.D., and Alan M. Levine, M.D.

Spinal orthoses are used for external immobilization of the spine in order to treat a number of spinal disorders or simply protect the spine or spinal cord. Indications for use include immobilization to allow for fracture healing, diminish nerve root irritation, decrease pain or weakness, and prevent deformity. The basic concepts of spinal orthoses have changed little throughout history. Spinal injury and deformities were described in ancient Egyptian writings and in ancient Hindu mythologic epics.[34] The earliest evidence of external spine manipulation was documented in the Hindu epic Srimad Bhagwat Mahapuranam sometime between 3500 and 1800 B.C.E.[20] Two of the earliest mechanical devices for spinal manipulation were described by the Greek philosopher Hippocrates of Cos (c. 460–370 B.C.E.).[24] Thoracic binders and jackets for the treatment of spinal disorders were first described by the Greek physician Galen of Pergamum circa 158 C.E.[27] Currently, many types of orthoses are available that share some similarities and many variations. They are grossly divided into broad categories defined by the part of the spine they effectively immobilize. These include cervical orthoses (COs), high and low cervicothoracic orthoses (CTOs), thoracolumbar orthoses (TLOs), lumbar corsets, and thoracolumbosacral orthoses (TLSOs). Most orthoses work in a similar fashion by indirectly applying force to the spine by pressing on the head, neck, chest, abdomen, or pelvis.

To better understand the magnitude of the problem of immobilization, it is necessary to consider the normal range of motion and the normal biomechanics of the various regions of the spine. Many factors make immobilizing the spine challenging—some unique to the region of the spine to be immobilized. Biomechanically the range of motion of the spine can be described as having six degrees of freedom, but each area has a unique pattern defined by the shape, size, and orientation of the facet joints; the characteristics of the intervertebral disks; the extrinsic stabilizing structures (e.g., ribs and muscles); and the orientation of the individual vertebral segments in space. For the cervical spine the motions are broken down into flexion-extension, rotation, and lateral bending. The normal passive motion from the occiput to C7 allows for 156 degrees (±19) of flexion-extension, 97 degrees (±14) of lateral bending, and 179 degrees (±22) of axial rotation.[7] Each vertebral segment can move independently. This makes it difficult to stabilize

the spine using a brace. When attempting to control motion in the cervical spine it is important to understand that even different regions of the cervical spine may have different predominant motion characteristics. For example the C1-C2 complex accounts for 50 percent of rotation in the cervical spine, and therefore any orthosis that does not securely control the head will not effectively reduce control rotation in the cervical spine. On the other hand C5-C6 has the most flexion and extension (each level averages about 13 degrees), and C2-C4 the most lateral bending.

The thoracic spine has far less motion that the cervical or lumbar vertebrae, but the junction levels (cervicothoracic and thoracolumbar) are subjected to higher bending forces because of the relatively immobile thoracic segment. The thoracic spine has more flexion than extension. The upper thoracic spine (T1-T6) has less total flexion-extension, with only four degrees per level, than the lower thoracic spine (T7-T12), which gradually increases from 5 to 12 degrees with distal migration.[41] The thoracic spine also has much less lateral bending than either the cervical or lumbar portions as a result of the stabilization afforded by the rib cage. Axial rotation is the most mobile range in the thoracic spine, averaging about eight degrees per level except at the lower end; this is the result of the coronal plane orientation of the facet joints in the thoracic spine.

Motion in the lumbar spine is greatest in flexion-extension, again related to the orientation of the facet joints, averaging 15 degrees per level (range 12–20 degrees).[41] In the lumbar spine lateral bending averages only six degrees while axial rotation is on average only two degrees. In addition the lordotic orientation of the lumbar spine makes immobilization in flexion and extension even more difficult, as the lordosis must be decreased to allow adequate purchase in this region.

Other anatomic factors in the thoracic and lumbar spines present significant challenges to orthotic immobilization. The spine is much more difficult to immobilize than the extremities. The large amount of soft tissue between the surface and the bony structure of the spine makes it difficult to gain points of contact to effectively prevent motion. This problem is accentuated in obese patients. Anterior bony structures for point of contact include the sternum, the symphysis pubis, and the anterior superior iliac spine (ASIS). Posterior points are the spinous processes of the thoracic and lumbar spine and the posterior aspect of the sacrum. In females, breast tissue is often an obstacle to the anterior pads of the brace. In obese patients, a pendulous panniculus obstructs the bony contact points of the pubis and ASIS. In addition, the volumes of the thorax and abdomen fluctuate with everyday physiologic functions. Inhalation and exhalation, as well as forceful motion during coughing and sneezing, constantly move the rib cage in the thoracic spine. In the lumbar region, the abdomen is a soft structure that fluctuates in girth with breathing and feeding. For example, a trauma patient may have an ileus that produces a temporarily protuberant abdomen. After the ileus resolves, a brace that was fitted during the ileus no longer fits well. The soft tissues also change dimensions in different positions such as sitting, standing, or supination. For instance, in the seated position the flexed thighs can impinge on the anterior distal part of the brace, pushing it upward and changing its fit. Spine orthoses rely on indirect stabilization, such as hydrostatic pressure and ligamentaxis, and the surrounding tissues, such as joint capsules, intervertebral disks, ligaments, and muscles, to limit intervertebral motion.

GENERAL CONCEPTS

A number of critical design features are very important in the effective application of spinal orthoses. The first is the *material* out of which the orthosis is made. This influences the *weight* of the orthosis, and, clearly, lighter yet stronger devices are more desirable and accepted by the patient than heavier ones. The material should be relatively *durable* so that the orthosis retains its shape and effectiveness over the period of treatment, which ranges from 3 to 6 months, and does not have to be replaced during treatment. The material should be reasonably *priced*. It should be *adjustable* for *comfort* as well as accommodating various shapes and sizes of patients. It should be *cosmetically* acceptable so it can be used with normal clothing and not destroy clothing during use. It should be relatively easy to take on and off and should provide acceptable access to surgical sites for wound care as well as tracheotomies and gastrostomies, for instance. It should not be overly warm and should avoid trapping moisture to prevent maceration of the skin beneath it. It should fit snugly to minimize chaffing or abrasion of the skin.

Wearing any orthosis for 3 months or more can have a number of drawbacks and even complications, including local pain and irritation or even skin breakdown. Localized pressure from an orthosis can cause ingrown hairs on the face or chest. Local nerve compression can result from the edge of the brace directly weighing on the nerve (lateral femoral cutaneous) or continuous pressure when sleeping or sitting (brachial plexus). Muscle atrophy of the abdominal or erector spinae is common in both the lumbar and cervical spine. Decreased pulmonary capacity occurs with braces in the thoracic region and early satiety from those immobilizing the lumbar region. Orthoses can case significant difficulty with activities of daily living such as sitting (lumbosacral orthosis) and transfers (thoracolumbar orthosis). Inappropriate application of an orthosis can increase motion in the segment that needs to be immobilized, such as using a thoracolumbar orthosis without a leg extension when attempting to immobilize L5-S1.

CERVICAL TRACTION

Cervical traction is frequently indicated for the treatment of cervical spine injury to achieve (1) reduction of cervical spine deformity, (2) indirect decompression of traumatized neural elements, and (3) cervical spine stability. Familiarity with the use of cervical traction is essential in the treatment of cervical spine trauma because of its ease of application and low morbidity when applied properly.

Cervical traction can be applied with a head halter, tongs, or a halo ring. Head halter traction consists of straps that attach to the head at the chin and the occiput, but only small amounts of weight (5–10 lb) can be applied safely. In addition to limited traction weight, the disadvantages of head halter traction include poor attachment to the head and an ability to control only axial compression through distraction. Excessive weight over an extended period can cause pressure ulcerations at the chin or occiput. Currently, halter traction is rarely indicated for spine trauma.

Tongs Traction

When applying traction with tongs, in contrast to head halters, fixation into the skull is achieved through the use of special pins with a pointed tip that abruptly flares out. This design allows for pin insertion through the outer cortex of the skull without penetration of the inner cortex. The flared nature of the pin design distributes pin pressure over its entire width on insertion while engaging the outer table.

Several types of tongs presently exist, including the Gardner-Wells or Trippi-Wells models. Tongs, similar to head halters, essentially control motion in a single plane through the application of longitudinal traction. Gardner-Wells tongs (Fig. 27-1) have achieved the widest acceptance because of their ability to withstand high loads and

FIGURE 27-1 *Gardner-Wells tongs have angulated pins designed to better counteract traction forces. The tongs can be made from magnetic resonance imaging-compatible materials (carbon fiber, titanium), which obviates the need for removal of the tongs and facilitates head and cervical spine imaging.*

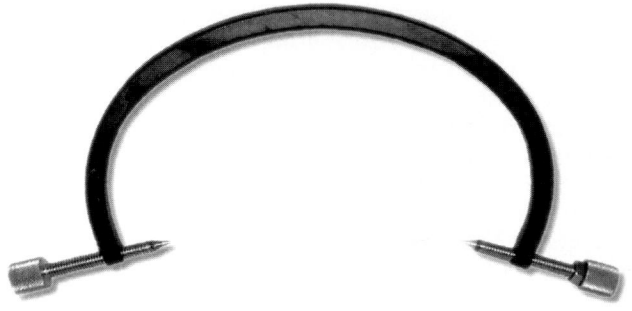

their ease of application. Gardner-Wells tongs can be applied quickly by a single physician. Trippi-Wells tongs use the same pins as Gardner-Wells tongs, but they are used in a multipin fashion. Because of the ability of tongs to resist motion in only one plane, they are associated with a high incidence of loosening. Tongs are typically indicated when longitudinal traction is to be temporarily applied or the patient is to remain bedridden.

APPLICATION OF TONGS

In preparation for the application of tongs, the patient is positioned supine with the head resting on the tabletop and no pillow support. The physician stands at the top (head) of the table above the patient for easy access to either side of the head. Pins should be placed just below the greatest diameter (equator) of the skull in a manner that avoids the temporalis muscle and superficial temporal artery and vein (Fig. 27-2). The standard site for pin insertion is approximately 1 cm posterior to the external auditory meatus and 1 cm superior to the pinna of the ear. Asymmetrical pin placement, either slightly posterior to affect flexion or slightly anterior to affect extension, can either facilitate or inhibit fracture reduction.

The use of Gardner-Wells tongs does not require shaving of the pin site. The skin and hair are prepared with an iodine solution, and the pin can be inserted directly into the skin without an incision. Before pin placement, local anesthetic is injected into the skin with care taken to infiltrate the periosteum down to the galea. The pins, which must be sterile and handled accordingly, are positioned orthogonally on either side of the skull before tightening. Tightening the pins by alternating from side to side will maintain pin symmetry. Gardner-Wells tongs are spring-loaded and thereby prevent perforation of the inner table of the skull. The force of pin insertion is gauged by the spring-loaded force indicator contained in

one of the pins, and optimal insertion torque is typically 6 to 8 in-lb. After the tongs are in place, the pins should be cleaned once a day with hydrogen peroxide at the skin-pin interface. After the first 24 hours of tongs application, the spring-loaded pins must be retightened; additional tightening should not be done thereafter to avoid the risk of perforating the inner table.

Halo Ring Traction

Cervical traction can be applied more efficiently through a halo ring. The multipin attachment of the halo to the skull reduces the distribution of the pin load, thereby allowing for greater traction loads to be applied for an extended period. Experimentally, the measured pull-out strength for a halo ring is almost twice that of Gardner-Wells tongs (440 vs. 233 lb).[22] Furthermore, the circumferential pin fixation to the skull better resists multiplane spine motion and allows for traction in flexion, extension, or simultaneous bivector traction techniques.[33] Finally, a major advantage of halo ring traction is that it can be rapidly converted to a halo vest orthosis once spinal reduction has been achieved.

The design of the halo ring has dramatically improved since its advent as a device for stabilization of facial fractures.[4] Currently available halo rings are made of light and radiolucent materials (titanium, carbon composites) that permit computed tomography (CT) and magnetic resonance imaging (MRI). Open-ring and crown-type halo designs that encircle only a part of the head have also been developed. These devices are open posteriorly to avoid the need to pass the head through a ring and thus ease application and improve safety. With some crown designs, the posterior ends of the incomplete ring must be angled inferiorly to ensure posterior pin placement below the equator of the skull. Halo rings are available in a variety of sizes to fit virtually any patient, including young children. A properly fitted halo ring provides 1 to 2 cm of clearance around every aspect of the patient's skull. The appropriate ring size can usually be determined by measuring the circumference of the skull 1 cm above the ears and eyebrows and then referring to the manufacturer's chart for preferred ring sizes.

HALO RING APPLICATION

A halo ring is routinely applied under local anesthesia; occasionally, light pharmacologic sedation may be necessary. The patient is positioned supine, and, to permit application of a full-ring halo, the patient's occiput is elevated with a folded towel or the head is gently positioned beyond the edge of the bed. Open-back halo rings can be applied without these maneuvers and are therefore preferred. Before application of a halo ring, all patients, including those who will undergo conversion of traction tongs to halo immobilization, should be in a hard collar. The halo ring is temporary positioned equidistant from the patient's head, 1 cm above the eyebrows and 1 cm above the tip of the ears. It is extremely important that the ring be positioned just below the greatest circumference of the patient's skull to prevent the halo ring from becoming displaced upward and out of position. The halo ring is provisionally stabilized with three blunt positioning

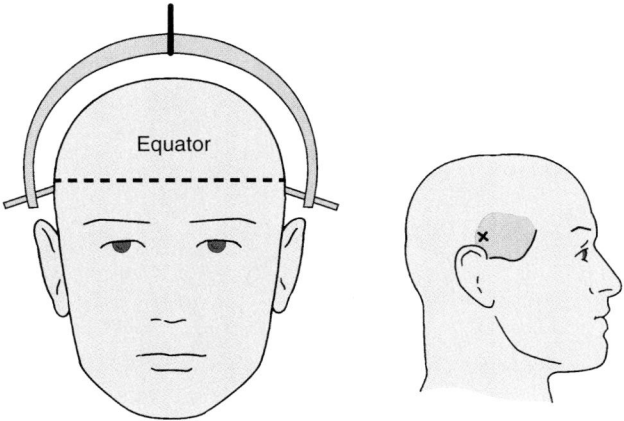

FIGURE 27-2 *Pins for traction tongs are placed below the cranial brim or the widest diameter of the skull (equator), anterior and superior to the earlobe. Care must be taken to position the pins posterior to the temporalis muscle. Precalibrated indicator pins are set to protrude at 8 lb of pressure.*

*The halo ring is held in a temporary position equidistant from the patient's head, 1 cm above the eyebrows and 1 cm above the tip of the ears, with the use of blunt positioning pins (**A**). With the halo ring held in place, sharp halo pins are then placed just below the skull equator. Spring-loaded pins are placed in front and a blank pin on the back (**B**). The pins are inserted and tightened in a diagonal fashion.*

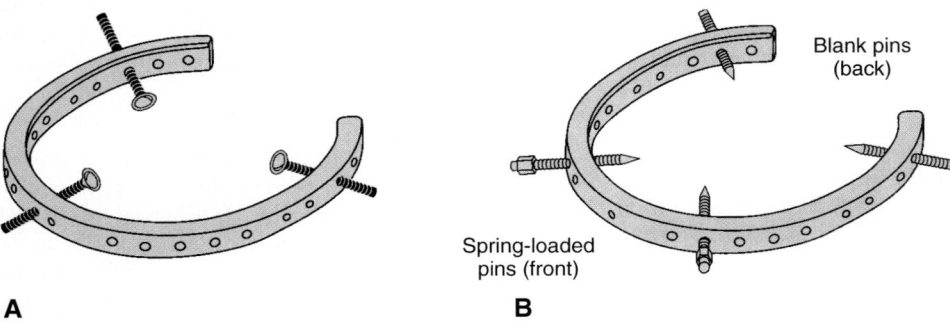

A   **B**

pins, and locations for the sharp head pins are then determined (Fig. 27-3). The optimal location for the anterior pins is 1 cm superior and two-thirds lateral to the orbital rim, just below the greatest circumference of the skull (Fig. 27-4A), and is considered the safe zone. This avoids injury to the supraorbital nerve and supratrochlear nerves and penetration of the frontal sinus (Fig. 27-5). Some authors advocate hiding the pin sight behind the hairline over the ear. Placement of pins in the temporalis region behind the hairline confers a cosmetic advantage but is, however, anatomically and biomechanically inferior.[6,15] Insertion sites for the posterior pins are less critical because neuromuscular structures are lacking and the skull is thicker and more uniform in that area. The posterior sites should be inferior to the widest portion of the skull, yet superior enough to prevent impingement of the ring or crown on the upper helix of the ear (see Fig. 27-4B). These pins are placed 180° opposite the anterior pins below the widest equator of the skull.

While the halo is held in position, the skin is shaved and prepared with an iodine solution. Local anesthetic, typically a 1 percent lidocaine solution, is injected with the needle passed through the holes for the sharp pins until the periosteum is elevated. Small stab incisions are made and the pins inserted in a diagonal fashion to maintain equal distance between the halo ring and skull. Pins should be inserted perpendicular to the skull because angulated pin insertion has been reported to be biomechanically inferior.[38] The pins are tightened with a torque screwdriver, and during this maneuver the patient is asked to close the eyes and relax the forehead to prevent eyebrow tenting or tethering. When all sharp pins are in place, the blunt pins are removed and the sharp pins tightened in a diagonal fashion up to a torque of 6 to 8 in-lb.[5] Pin torque should never exceed 10 in-lb because of the risk of penetration of the outer cortex.[5] Breakaway wrenches can be used to prevent the pins from being tightened past the maximal torque; however, torque limits are more

*The safe zone for the anterior pins is located 1 cm superior and two-thirds lateral to the orbital rim, just below the greatest circumference of the skull. On the medial aspect of the safe zone are the supraorbital (SO) and supratrochlear (ST) nerves (**A**). The zone for the posterior pins is inferior to the widest portion of the skull, yet superior enough to prevent ring or crown impingement on the upper helix of the ear (**B**).*

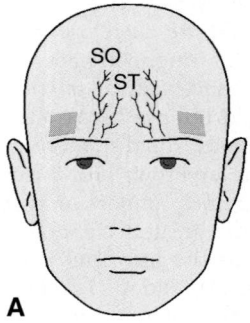 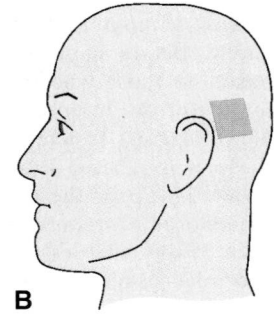

A   **B**

Anterior halo pins should be placed within the safe zone.

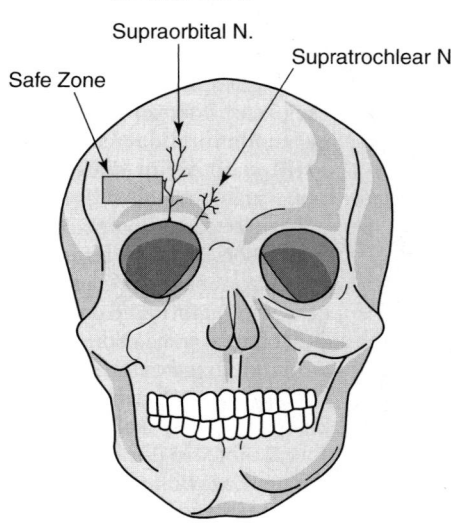

Supraorbital N.

Supratrochlear N.

Safe Zone

reliably measured with a calibrated torque screwdriver. Locknuts are then placed on each pin and gently tightened to secure the pin to the ring. Once the halo application is complete, a traction bow can be mounted. The traction weight protocol for halo rings can be much more aggressive than that for tongs, and weights can exceed 100 lb when indicated.

Cervical Traction Weight

After tongs or a halo ring has been applied, cervical traction can begin at approximately 10 to 15 lb, with immediate evaluation by lateral radiographs to avoid overdistraction (Fig. 27-6). Traction weight can be increased by 5- to 10-lb increments, depending on the size and weight of the patient. Serial lateral radiographs should be obtained approximately 10 to 15 minutes after each application of weight to allow for soft tissue creep. Fluoroscopy can be used instead of plain radiographs to facilitate this process. The patient must be completely relaxed, and analgesics or muscle relaxants can often assist in minimizing muscle spasm or tension. At higher weights (greater than 40 lb), 30 to 60 minutes should elapse before further load increase. The head of the bed should be slightly elevated to provide body weight resistance to traction.

The maximal amount of weight that can safely be applied for closed traction reduction of the cervical spine remains controversial. It has been suggested that a slow, gradual increase in traction weight effects spinal reduction at a lower total traction load.[26] Some physicians support a more rapid incremental increase in weight and have applied weights up to 150 lb without any adverse effects.[21] Typically, the maximal weight tolerated is limited by the skeletal fixation used, and for cranial tongs, the limit is up to 100 lb.

Cervical traction is used to achieve the maximal effect from the weight being applied. The maximal traction weight should be considered to be a function of the patient's size, body weight, or body habitus (or any combination of these attributes) rather than an absolute number (100-lb cervical traction may be well tolerated by a burly 300-lb male weightlifter, but not appropriate for a 115-lb female). The greater the associated ligamentous disruption, the less the appropriate total weight. The maximal weight should also correspond to the level of the cervical injury; specifically, upper cervical injuries require less weight than do injuries at the cervicothoracic junction. When these parameters are respected and sufficient time is permitted between incremental increases in traction weight, the maximal weight can usually be limited to 70 lb or less for lower cervical injury in an average-sized adult. Regardless of whether spinal reduction has been achieved, it is imperative that the maximal traction weight be decreased to 10 to 15 lb once the monitored reduction process has been terminated.

FIGURE 27-6 *A, Admission lateral radiograph showed no abnormal distraction. **B,** Cervical traction initiated at 20 lb resulted in marked overdistraction. Traction should always be initiated at 10 lb.*

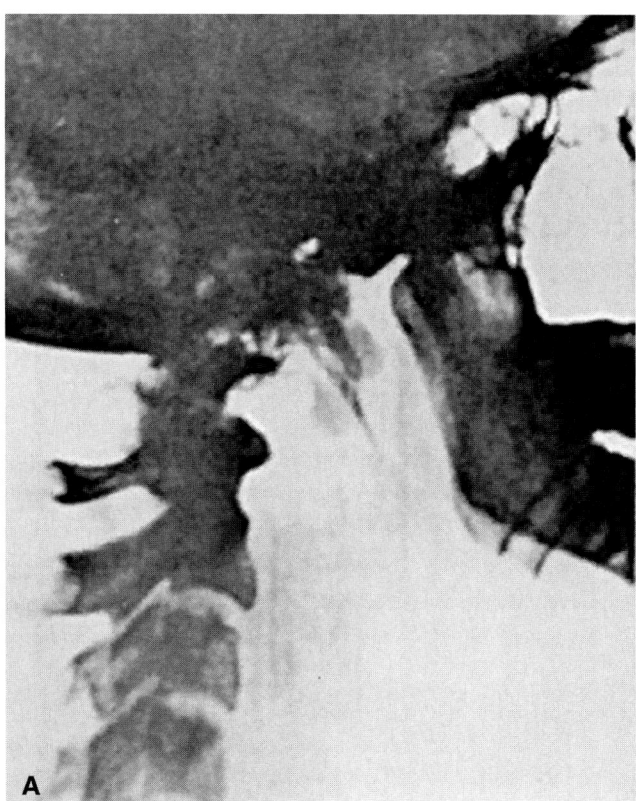

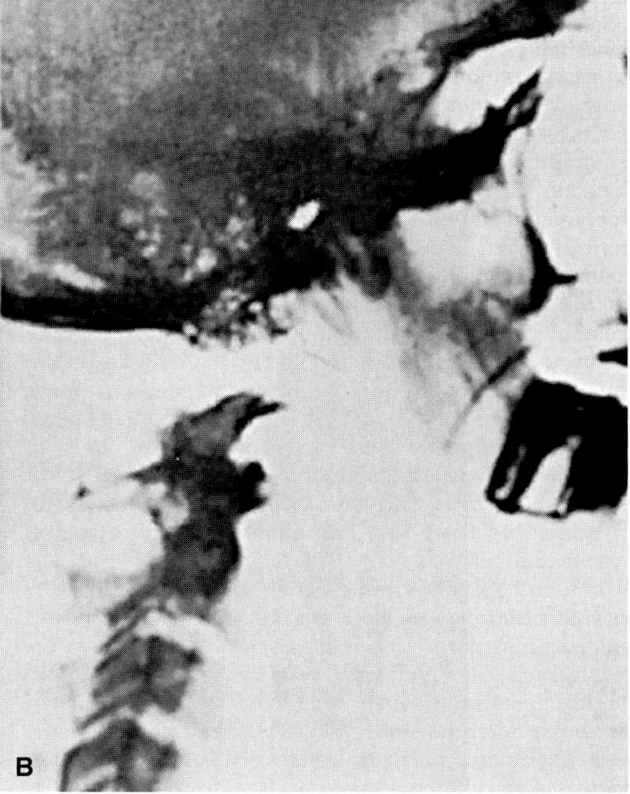

A

B

Most cervical spine injuries can be reduced with only longitudinal traction, but small changes in the vector of traction (i.e., slightly more flexion or more extension) can be helpful in some cases. Spinal manipulation can be hazardous and is therefore controversial.[23] Lee and associates compared cervical traction and manipulation under anesthesia and determined that traction alone was preferable.[21] Cotler and co-workers suggested that gentle manipulation in combination with traction could be of benefit in awake patients.[11] Manual manipulation as a means of achieving cervical spine reduction should never be performed in a patient under general anesthesia or in an unconscious patient. Light sedation in an otherwise alert patient allows the physician to detect neurologic alterations. In general, the authors do not support manual manipulation and prefer that patients who do not respond to traction be treated surgically.

The Halo Vest

Modern halo vest orthoses are widely considered the most stable fixation for the cervical spine.[31] Halos are essentially a hybrid between a brace and an external fixator. They firmly attach to the skull with sharp pins and a lightweight, radiolucent, nonferromagnetic ring. In some designs the posterior portion of the ring is removed to limit the shearing forces and flexion moment on supine patients. In a standard construct, the neck is generally spanned by four rigid posts to a thoracic jacket much like the four-post low CTO braces. The halo is more invasive than TLSOs and carries the additional risk of pin infections, skull penetration, and abscess formation.[16] Much like TLSOs its ability to stabilize is limited by the fit of the thoracic jacket. Another drawback of the halo vest is that it bypasses fixation to the neck itself and can allow paradoxical "snaking" of vertebral segments. This is where the gross flexion and extension angle of the spine remains constant, but intersegmental motion allows different vertebrae to flex and extend simultaneously.

Standard application protocols for cervical spine immobilization with halo vests have developed over the past 50 years since their first use in patients with polio undergoing cervical fusion.[29] Four skull fixation pins are generally used in adults, although using more has been described. The pins are placed perpendicular to the skull below its widest equator in order to prevent pin loosening and slippage.[2,38] The pins are retightened to 8 ft-lb once at 48 hours. Additionally, all the bolts on the halo vest should also be checked for tightness at the same time since mobilization of the patient could cause loosening of the uprights. It has been shown that mean compression force of the pins decreases by 6.4 percent in the first 18 hours and by 35 percent at 6 weeks.[14] Additional tightening is performed cautiously. If no resistance is met, the pin should be replaced by another one at an adjacent site to avoid skull penetration. Pin loosening is often an indicator of pin tract infections. Infected pins should be treated for local wound care and with systemic antibiotics. If the infection persists, the pin should be replaced by a new one at an adjacent site. Pediatric patients have thinner skulls. Additional pins at a lesser torque are often used to spread the forces along more points of fixation.

There is an inherent difficulty in performing in vivo studies of intravertebral motion with halo fixation. Cadaveric studies have shown that halo vests are superior to rigid cervical collars in minimizing upper cervical C1-C2 and C2-C3 segmental motion in both the intact and unstable cervical spine.[25,31] Other studies have shown halo vests to be superior to rigid collars such as the NecLoc, Philadelphia, or Stifneck collars in their ability to stabilize cadaveric specimens that were surgically destabilized at C4-C5 when a flexion moment was applied.

CERVICAL ORTHOSES

The simplest cervical orthoses are soft collars that are foam cylinders that minimally restrict motion but act as proprioceptive reminders that can prevent extreme or sudden movements (Fig. 27-7). Studies have shown that soft collars restrict less than 20 percent of normal motion in flexion-extension, lateral bending, or rotation.[31,35] Collars are available from various sources in a variety of heights and circumferences for a more customized fit. They are most appropriate for cervical sprain and are inexpensive.

FIGURE 27-7   *Appropriate application of a soft cervical collar requires that the both the circumference and the height of the front of the collar are correct. The anterior height should allow it to fit comfortably under the mandible, placing the neck in slight extension without impinging on the ears or causing the chin to fall inside of the collar. For obese patients a Velcro extension can be added to any collar height.*

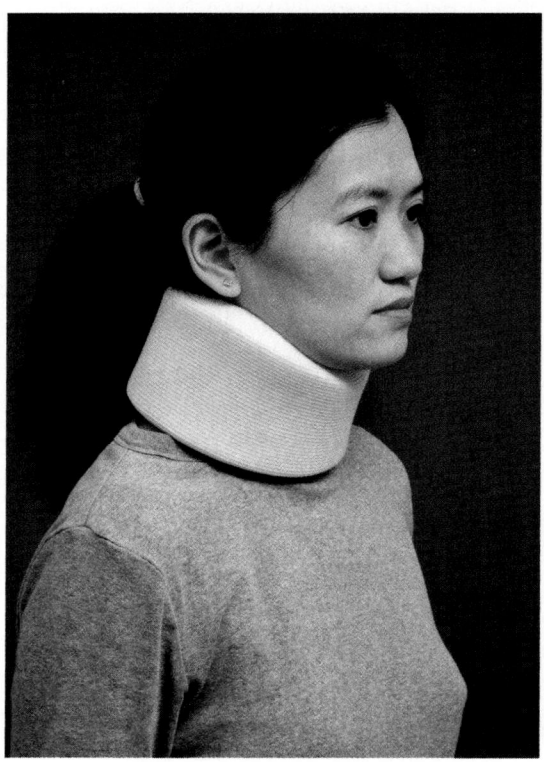

HIGH CERVICOTHORACIC ORTHOSES

High cervicothoracic orthoses (CTOs) have molded occipital and mandibular supports that span the cervical spine and extend to the upper part of the thorax (Fig. 27-8A, B). Many varieties of high CTOs are currently on the market. They vary in design, comfort, rigidity, materials, and sizes. Commonly used CTOs include the Miami J (Jerome Medical, Moorestown, NJ), Philadelphia (Philadelphia Collar Co., Thorofare, NJ), NecLoc (Jerome Medical, Moorestown, NJ), Aspen (also called the Newport), Stifneck (Laerdal Medical, Wappinger Falls, NY), PMT cervical collar (PMT Corp., Chanhassen, MN), Malibu, and Nebraska orthoses.

The Philadelphia collar (Fig. 27-9) and the Malibu collar consist of a semirigid, two-piece, closed-cell Plastazote foam collar with the addition of two outer plastic shell supports. The Miami J collar, Newport/Aspen collar, PMT cervical collar, and the NecLoc collar consist of a two-piece rigid polyethylene shell with soft open-cell foam liners. All are available in multiple styles and are adjustable at the chin, occiput, and sternum for a more customized fit.[40] All are available with access holes for tracheotomies.

Other collars such as the Stifneck collar are designed for their ease of use in emergency situations such as extrications or transport. The Stifneck collar consists of a one-piece polyethylene rigid collar that can quickly and easily be applied to the neck with the patient seated or supine. It is generally used for temporary immobilization and replaced with more comfortable braces if needed for long-term use.

Many biomechanical studies have compared the efficacy of high CTOs in stabilizing the cervical spine. One such study compared the Miami J and Aspen high CTOs using optoelectronic motion measurement systems and video fluoroscopy to evaluate cervical spine motion in 20 healthy volunteers. This study found that both the Miami J and Aspen collars significantly reduced gross neck motion. In addition there was no difference between the Miami J and Aspen collars in reducing gross movement of the neck. This remained true when evaluating intervertebral sagittal motion, except at C6-C7, where neither collar significantly reduced motion, and at C5-C6, where the Aspen collar was found to be more restrictive in flexion than the Miami J collar.[17]

Other studies have used radiographs and goniometer measurements to compare high CTOs such as the Philadelphia collar, Aspen, Stifneck, Miami J, and NecLoc in resisting occiput-to-C7 motion in flexion, extension, lateral tilt, and rotation. The NecLoc cervical orthosis demonstrated statistically superior restriction of cervical motion in flexion, extension, rotation, and lateral tilt compared with the other four orthoses. The Miami J cervical orthosis was found to be the next most restrictive.[1]

FIGURE 27-8 **A, B,** *This figure shows the front and back views of a Miami J collar, with a mandibular as well as occipital mold. It more rigidly maintains the position of the head relative to the shoulders and can even be fitted with an opening for tracheotomy care.*

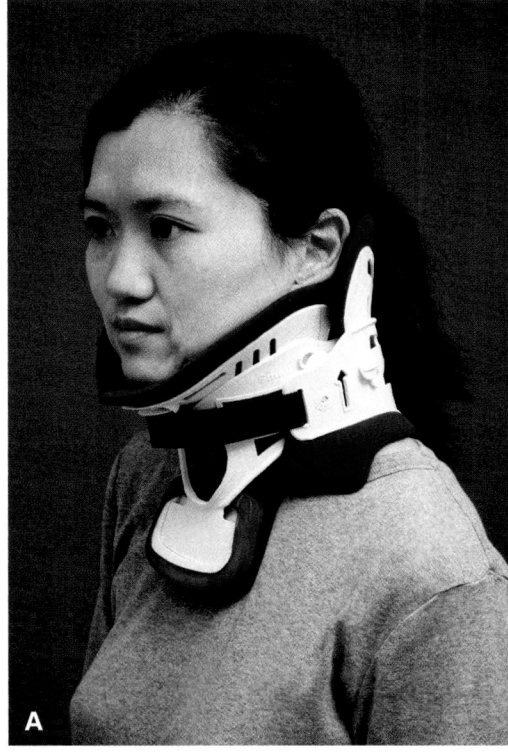
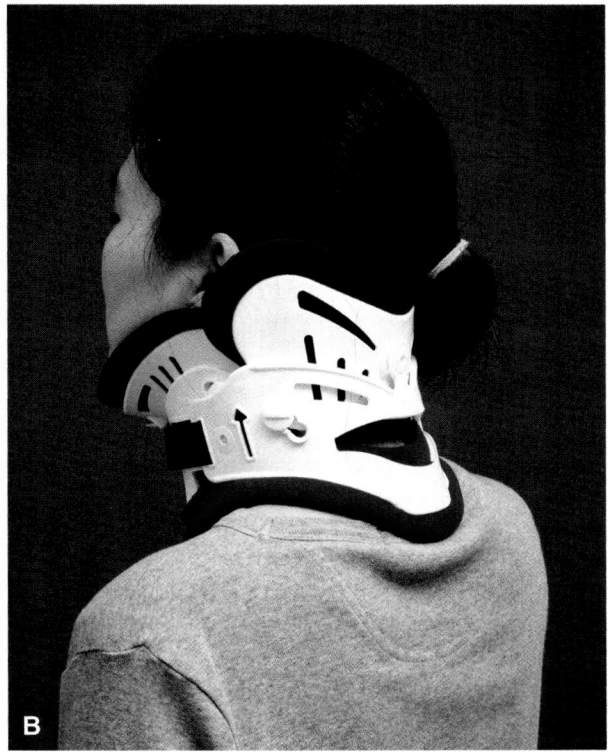

FIGURE 27-9   *A, B, The Philadelphia collar is commonly used for in-field and initial trauma immobilization before ruling out a spinal injury. It is a common postoperative form of immobilization since it is reasonably well tolerated. Sizing can be difficult because appropriate front height may result in impingement on the ear.*

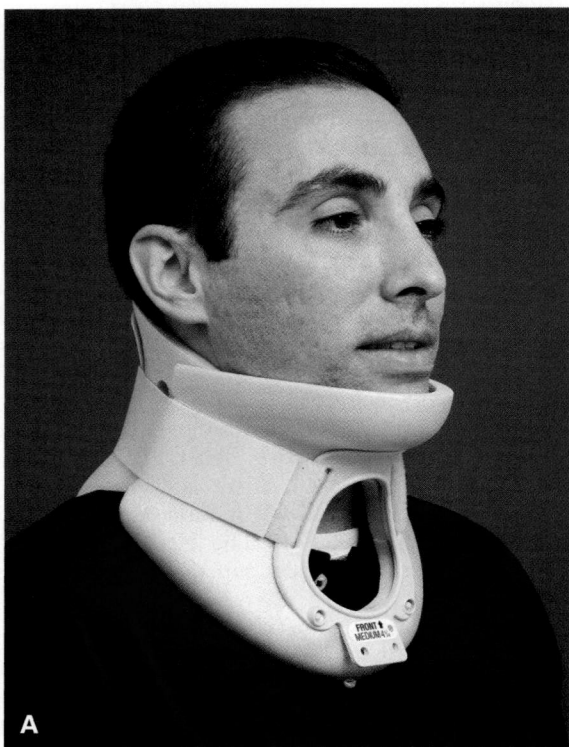

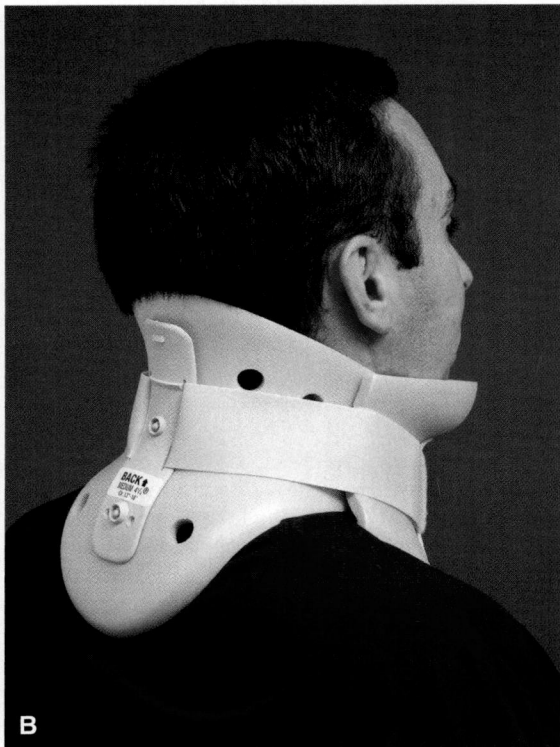

Three-dimensional digital tracking sensors have also been used to compare gross head and cervical spine motion in the sagittal, coronal, and axial planes. One such study of 45 healthy volunteers wearing the Miami J, Aspen, PMT, and Philadelphia collars found that all of the orthoses significantly resisted gross vertebral motion in all planes compared with controls wearing no brace (Fig. 27-10). Intervertebral segmental motion was also evaluated using fluoroscopic techniques. The tested orthoses were found to be variably effective at different vertebral levels[36] (Fig. 27-11).

FIGURE 27-10   *Graph comparing subjects wearing no brace with subjects wearing each of the seven braces. This graph shows the mean sagittal plane rotation of the head from maximum flexion (F) to maximum extension (E), the mean axial head rotation from maximum left (L) to maximum right (R) turn, and mean coronal plane tilt of the head from maximum left to maximum right tilt of the head toward the shoulders. The error bars show one standard deviation. deg indicates degrees. (Reprinted, with permission, from Schneider, A.M.; Hipp, J.A.; Nguyen, L.; et al. Reduction in head and intervertebral motion provided by seven contemporary cervical orthoses in 45 individuals. Spine 32:E1–E6, 2007.)*

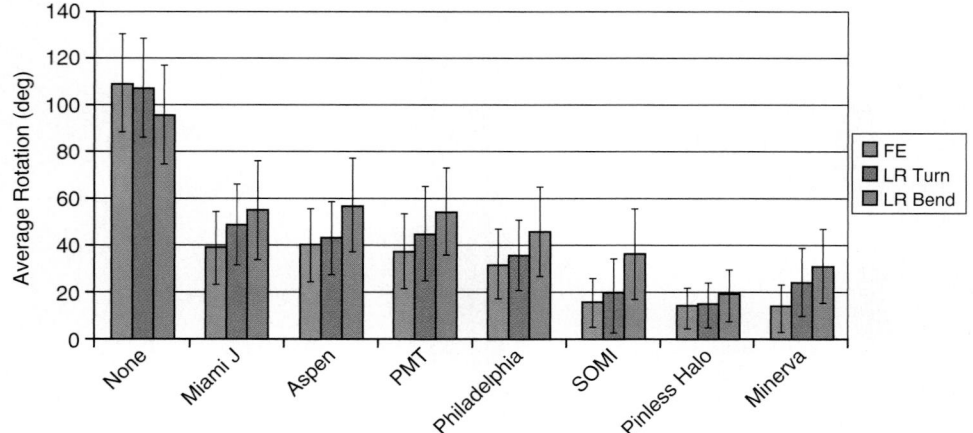

FIGURE 27-11 | *Sagittal plane intervertebral rotation by level and brace. The error bars show one standard deviation. deg indicates degrees. (Reprinted, with permission, from Schneider, A.M.; Hipp, J.A.; Nguyen, L.; et al. Reduction in head and intervertebral motion provided by seven contemporary cervical orthoses in 45 individuals. Spine 32:E1–E6, 2007.)*

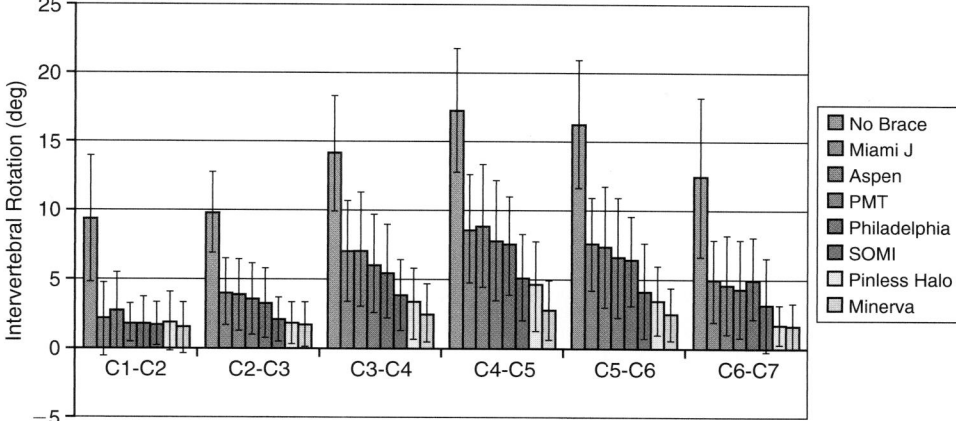

LOW CERVICAL THORACIC ORTHOSES

Low CTOs are similar to high CTOs except that they extend down to encompass more of the thorax. This provides a firmer base to stabilize the cervical spine and allows increased control of lower C-spine and upper T-spine vertebrae. Commonly used low CTOs include the sternal-occipital-mandibular immobilizer (SOMI) (Seattle Systems, Seattle, WA), Yale, and Aspen two-post and four-post. The Aspen two- and four-post collars consist of two padded rigid breast and back plates connected to a high thoracic Aspen CTO by either two or four rigid posts (Fig. 27-12A–C). The SOMI brace has a similar thoracic

FIGURE 27-12 | *A–C, The Aspen two- and four-post collars consist of two padded rigid breast and back plates connected to a high thoracic Aspen CTO by either two or four rigid posts.*

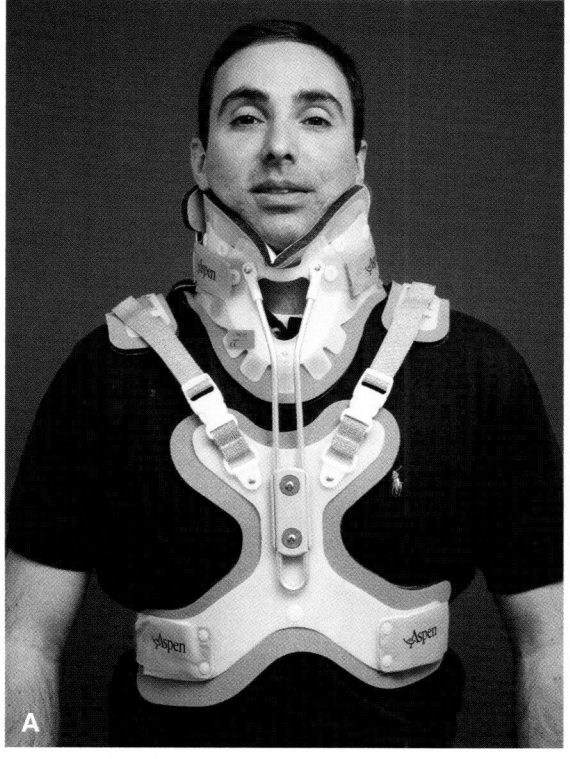

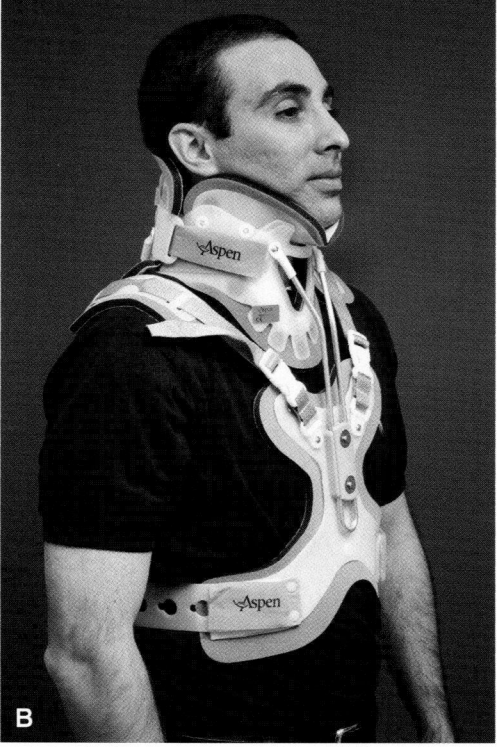

(Continued)

FIGURE 27-12 *(Continued)*

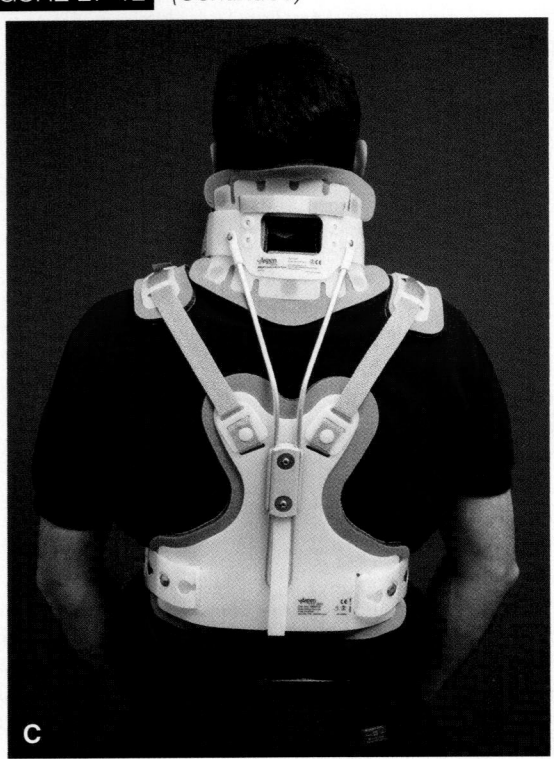

C

back and breast plate connected to an occipital plate by two rigid bars (Fig. 27-13A, B). In addition the SOMI brace has a chin rest that can be removed for mastication when eating. The Yale CTO brace is a two-piece rigid foam and plastic clamshell low CTO that is similar to the Philadelphia collar but encompasses the entire thorax. It is held in place with a strap around the neck and the lower chest.

Biomechanical studies have shown that CTOs provided significantly more restriction of gross and intervertebral flexion and extension motion than simpler COs.[17,31,35,36] The Aspen two-post and four-post CTO performed similarly in flexion, but the Aspen four-post provided significantly more restriction of extension motion.[17] It is important to monitor cervical collars for possible complications. Cervical collars help restrict cervical spine motion, but do not eliminate it. After the application of a cervical orthosis, additional spinal cord injuries have been found in 3 to 25 percent of patients with cervical spine trauma. In addition, it has been shown that up to 55 percent of patients who have had a hard cervical collar on for more than 5 days may develop full-thickness skin ulcers.[3,40] This is especially true in elderly patients or those who by trauma or surgery have an injury to the greater occipital nerve. All of these classes of patients are at increased risk for an occipital decubitus within days of application of the collar. Marginal mandibular nerve palsy has been reported from pressure points on the mandible.[32] Patients with cervical orthoses are at increased aspiration risk secondary to limitations in swallowing, coughing, breathing, and vomiting. It also has been shown that cervical collars can delay

FIGURE 27-13 *A, B, The chin plate on the SOMI brace can be removed for eating, and doing so may reduce the motion in the cervical spine caused by the jaw striking the front piece of the brace during the chewing motion.*

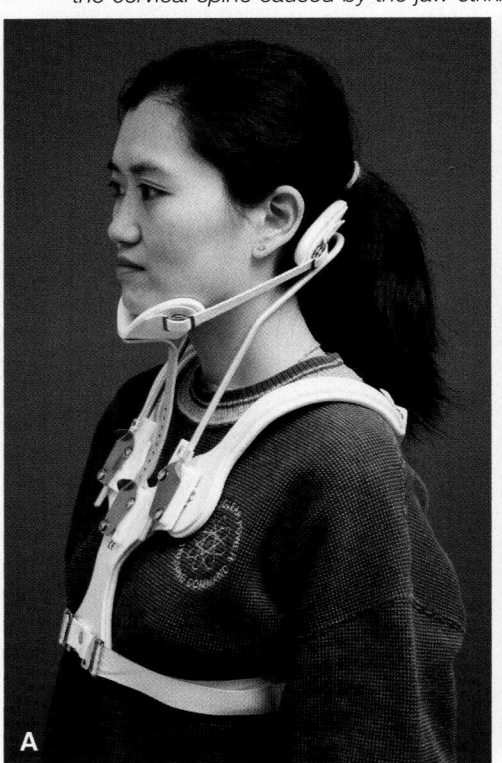

A

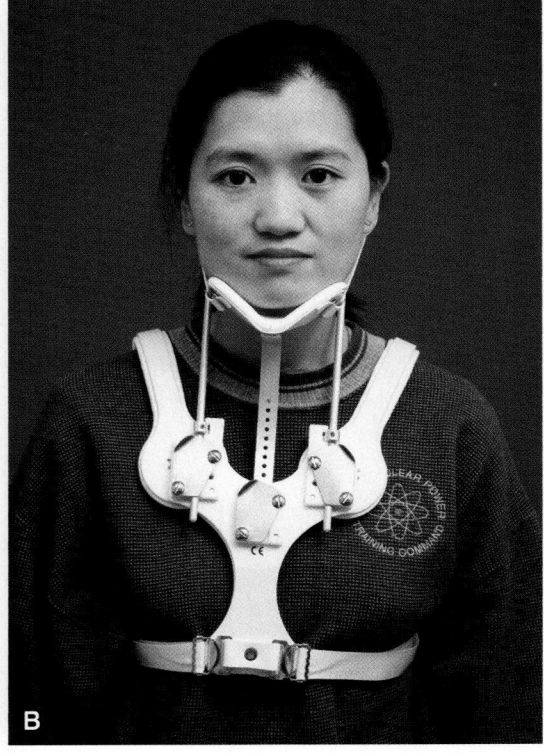

B

weaning from a ventilator.[40] Studies have shown that a rigid collar significantly increases intracranial pressure by theoretically causing a venous outflow obstruction.[12,18] Activities of daily living such as mastication can cause significant upper cervical spine segmental motion particularly at occiput-C1 and C1-C2. It has been proposed that wearing a soft collar backward or removing the chin plate on SOMI braces during eating decreases this segmental motion.[8]

THORACIC AND LUMBAR SPINE ORTHOSES

An array of spinal orthoses on the market range in their rigidity and comfort. Rigidity and comfort are typically inversely related, although there are some exceptions. A balance must be attained. If a brace is too uncomfortable, patients are less likely to comply with its use. On the other hand, if the brace is not rigid enough to protect the spine, then wearing it is futile. With an understanding of the biomechanics of the injury and an understanding of the different brace designs an appropriate orthosis can be chosen to maximize stability and comfort. Thoracic and lumbar orthoses typically are able to partially immobilize T7-L2. With a thigh extender, L4-S1 can be included. Luckily the inherent stability afforded by the rib cage prevents as well as protects injuries in the T1-T10 region. Because T11 and T12 are floating ribs, they do not share in the same protective effect. Injuries and thus the need for immobilization typically occur at the thoracolumbar region between T11 and L2.

A spinal orthosis should provide a force vector opposite to the force of the injury. The concept of a three-point molding to create such a force vector applies in the spine as it does in the extremities. For example, a properly molded extension thoracolumbar cast can effectively oppose the progression of a kyphotic deformity following a flexion distraction injury. It is applied with the patient lying prone between two operating room tables causing the spine to go into extension. The three-point mold is applied on the sternum and iliac crests anteriorly opposing the third point in the posterior region centered over the level of injury. The drawbacks of the extension thoracolumbar cast are the difficulty of application and its permanence. The only way to remove the cast is to cut it off. This presents issues for periodic skin checks for breakdown and access to the abdomen for serial exams by the general surgeons.

Lumbar Corset

The least rigid brace is the lumbar corset. The corset is made of canvas or a similar type of flexible fabric combined with elastic bands running through a series of eyelets allowing for cinching of the brace under tension. Some designs include removable steel bars that can be placed within the brace (Fig. 27-14). Lumbar corsets increase intra-abdominal pressure, contributing some indirect stability to the spine; however, they do not really limit spinal motion. They serve more as a proprioceptive reminder to the patient to voluntarily limit movement. Some patients also feel psychologically more secure with the brace, so it can be used to encourage early immobilization. Even though it is not terribly rigid, it still

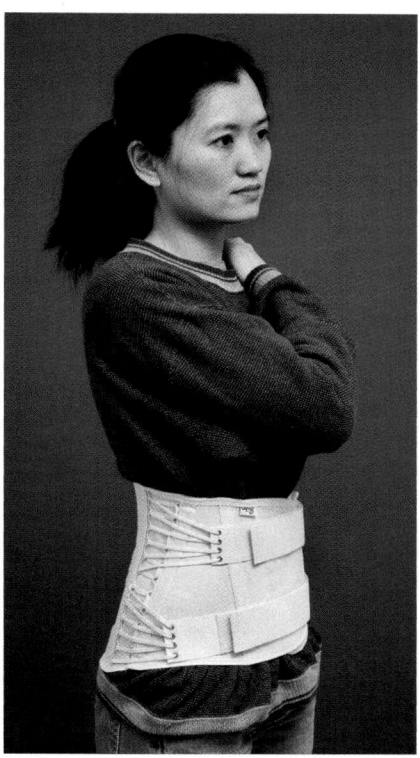

FIGURE 27-14 *The least rigid lumbar orthosis, the corset, is made of canvas or a similar type of flexible fabric combined with elastic bands running through a series of eyelets allowing for cinching of the brace under tension. Some designs include removable steel bars that can be placed within the brace.*

alters breathing patterns. Puckree and associates found that after a canvas thoracolumbar corset was worn for 1 hour, tidal volumes decreased by 24 percent.[30] In five of eight patients, a compensatory increase in breathing frequency to maintain minute ventilation occurred. It is important to keep this in mind, especially in treating traumatically injured and postoperative patients who are at risk of atelectasis and pneumonia.

TLSO Body Jacket

The thoracolumbosacral orthosis body jacket is the most rigid brace (Fig. 27-15A-C). It is custom-molded by an orthotist and is fabricated from polypropylene or ethylene plastic. The brace is circumferentially rigid around the trunk but allows for full motion of the upper and lower extremities. It is often referred to as a clamshell brace with overlapping anterior and posterior pieces held together by multiple Velcro straps that are tightened to create a snug fit. The brace works by both contact with bony prominences as well as circumferential closure increasing intra-abdominal pressure. The pressure of the brace is distributed throughout the entire torso. It can be made either by making a mold from a cast of the patient or by taking measurements and adapting a prefabricated mold to the unique dimensions of the patient. Measurements are taken vertically between the sternum, xiphoid,

FIGURE 27-15   ***A–C,*** *The thoracolumbar orthosis, or body jacket, is the most rigid brace and is effective from T7 through L4. It is custom-molded by an orthotist and is fabricated from polypropylene or ethylene plastic. It can be made as a two-piece clamshell, which is less rigid than the one-piece, which opens in the front and has overlapping edges.*

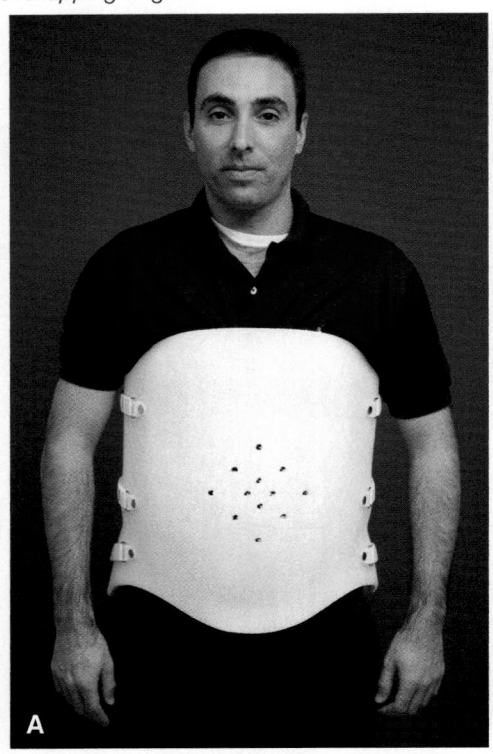
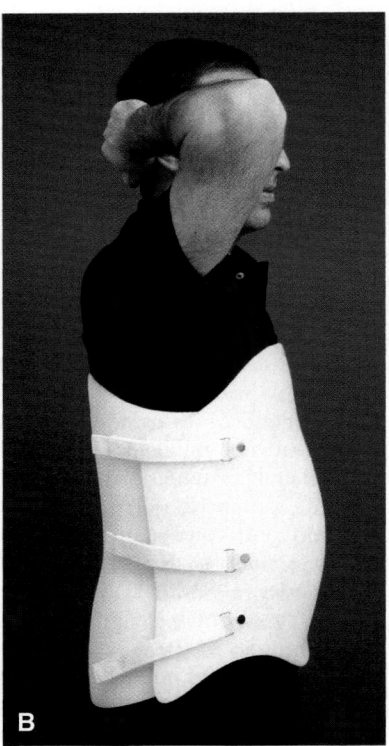
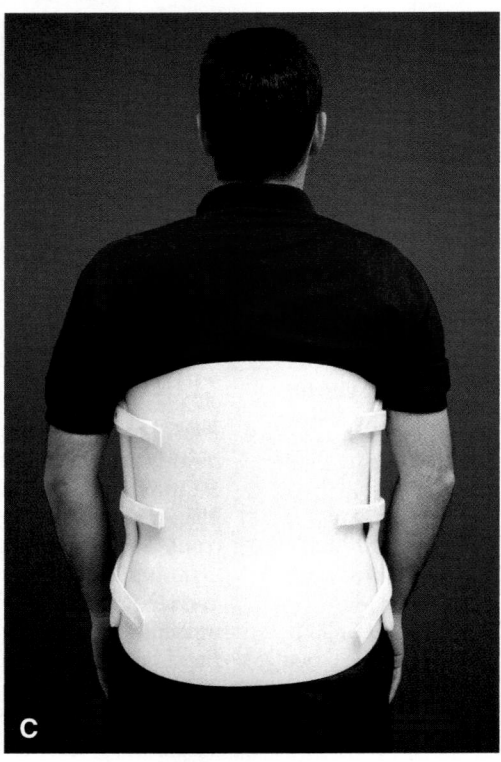

umbilicus, and pubic symphysis. Horizontal measurements are taken of the distance between the anterior ribs and the anterior superior iliac spines. Circumferential measurements are taken at the level of the axilla, xiphoid process, small of the waist, and greater trochanters. Additional lordosis can be added to the molding process if a hyperextension force is needed. A thigh extension or hip spica can be added at any specified angle. The thigh extender is usually placed with a degree of flexion to allow the patient to sit, but not so much that ambulation would be difficult.

TLSOs can contribute to immobilization of the T7-L4 levels.[37] The addition of a thigh extender allows for effective immobilization of L4-S1. Vander Kooi and colleagues used video fluoroscopy to study the effective motion restriction of the lower lumbar spine by a TLSO.[39] They found that the TLSO reduced intervertebral motion by 40 percent at L3-L4 and L4-L5 At L3, total rotation with respect to the horizontal was 70 degrees without a brace, 50 degrees with a TLSO, and 10 degrees with a TLSO with thigh extender. This is an 85 percent reduction of total rotation. Both positions of the thigh extender tested (0 degrees or 15 degrees flexion) were equally effective in reducing motion. Cholewicki and co-workers used strain-gauge devices to measure spinal motion and showed a 45 percent restriction in motion in the thoracic spine and 39 percent restriction in the lumbar spine.[10] In postoperative lumbar fusion patients, Krag and associates found a 20 percent restriction of motion when performing activities of daily living such as sitting up, standing up, lifting a 2-lb box, and putting on a lightweight jacket.[19] Electromyography (EMG) has been used to study the spine unloading effect of a lumbosacral orthosis on trunk muscle contractions. Cholewicki found a 4.9 percent decrease of maximum voluntary activation (MVA) on EMG of isometric trunk extension. Lesser decreases in MVA were seen in flexion, axial rotation, and lateral bending. The spine compression force decreased on average by 26.6 percent.[9]

The custom-molded body jacket has several advantages and disadvantages. One advantage is the distribution of force over a large surface area instead of concentrating on areas on the brace pads. If superficial bruising occurs at the level of injury the posterior pad of the Jewett brace can be quite uncomfortable, whereas the custom-molded orthosis can distribute the pressure more evenly. The body jacket also fits better, at least initially, because it is molded to each person's unique dimensions. It is quite straightforward to don because it has only two pieces that fit together perfectly, rather than the many buckles and parts present in other orthoses. The main drawback is that the orthosis is custom-fitted to the patient at one point in time, and gross changes can occur shortly after fitting, especially in trauma and postoperative patients. Decreased swelling, resolution of an ileus, weight loss, and muscle atrophy can result in significant changes that affect brace fit. The Velcro straps can only be tightened or loosened to a limited extent due to the rigidity of the brace. It is like two pieces of a puzzle with specific contours that must fit in a certain way. Another drawback is the fact that it needs to be custom-fitted, which entails either taking measurements or creating a mold with casting material. First, this can delay obtaining the orthosis. Turnaround time between fitting and fashioning the orthosis can vary from

a few hours to days. Second, the process of measuring or molding can be very difficult because of pain and stability issues in an acute injury or a new postoperative patient. Efforts have been made to try to use measurements or special computer programs based on CT or MRI. These have been found to have comparable volumetric accuracy but less circumferential accuracy especially in the distal axial plane.[13] Also, since measurements are generally taken in the supine position, the orthosis does not fit properly in the standing or sitting positions. Problems with sweating also arise because such a large surface area is completely covered by plastic. A cotton T-shirt can help absorb the sweat and prevent skin maceration. Overall the body jacket's greatest asset is its total contact rigidity, which also contributes to its weaknesses.

Aspen Orthosis

The makers of the Aspen cervical collar also make a TLSO and LSO (Fig. 27-16A, B). These orthoses have inner soft pads and an outer layer of plastic with buckles, straps, and bars connecting them together. The four bars, two anterior and two posterior, act as vertical struts. The buckles and straps allow for adjustments at several crucial connections to form a personal fit. The Aspen TLSO has shoulder straps to connect the sternal portion and the upper lumbar portion to help control more of the thoracic spine. The LSO is a simpler design without the shoulder straps if control of the thorax is not necessary. A thigh extender can also be added to either orthosis. Two studies comparing the Aspen and the custom-molded Boston brace showed equivalent motion restriction as measured by strain gauge devices, however, unequal subjective comfort.[10,19] In one of the studies, the Aspen was rated 2/10 for comfort by the visual analogue scale (VAS) and the Boston brace was rated 4/10.[19] Interestingly even though the Aspen was more comfortable, the subjects did not report a difference in the perceived restriction of spine motion.[10] Because the adjustments are made with buckles and straps, fitting can be completed at one visit. The drawback is that the material is not as rigid and durable. Also since there are so many adjustable parts, some settings may come undone and the patient may not be able to restore them to the correct fit. On the other hand, with changes in body contour or with different supine, standing, or sitting positions, the brace can be adjusted for maximal fit at all times. This is ideal with a knowledgeable and compliant patient. In a noncompliant or neurologically or cognitively impaired patient, this modularity may be undesirable. The Aspen orthosis is similar in cost to the clamshell custom-molded body jacket.

Several other companies make their own version of a rigid TLSO; however, all braces are not created equal. One study compared the Aspen, Boston, and CAMP TLSO. The CAMP is similar to the Aspen in that it is an off-the-shelf brace and not custom-molded. By using strain gauge devices, they found all the braces were equivalent in motion restriction; however, the Aspen was rated significantly more comfortable by the patients.[10] Another study looked at motion restriction in the Aspen, Boston, and Cybertech TLSOs. The patients were studied 3 months after surgery for lumbar fusions; all had been braced for those 3 months in a Boston brace. At the 3-month visit,

FIGURE 27-16 | *A, B,* The Aspen lumbosacral orthosis has inner soft pads and an outer layer of plastic with buckles, straps, and bars that connect them together. The four bars, two anterior and two posterior, act as vertical struts. The buckles and straps allow for adjustments at several crucial connections to form a personal fit.

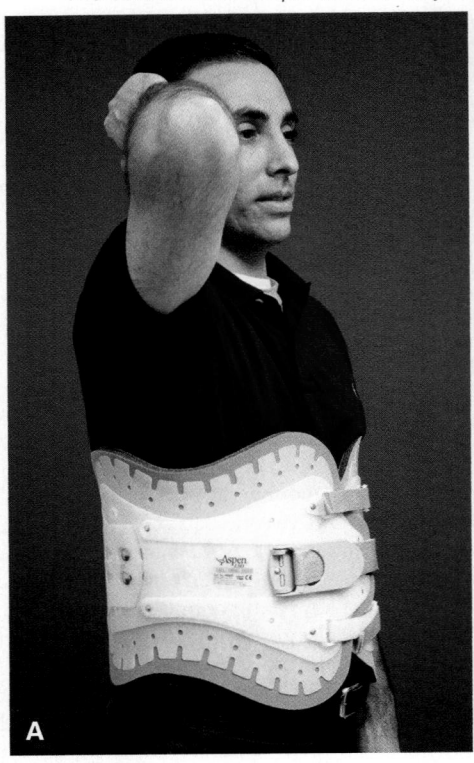
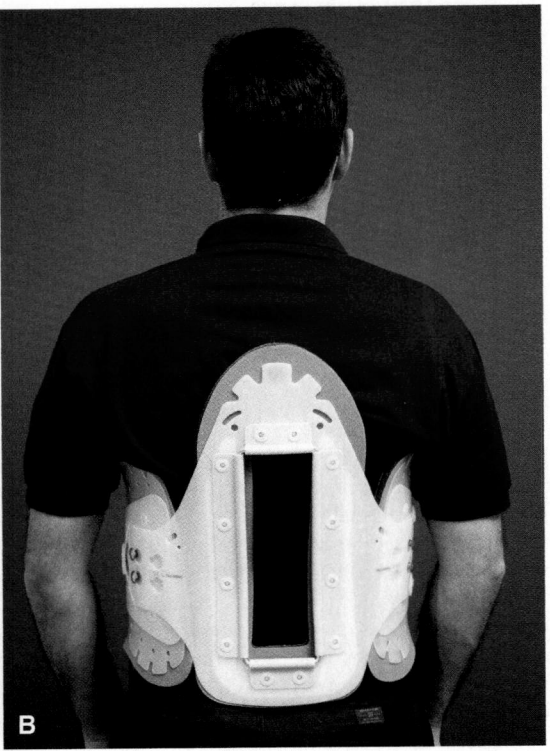

the patients tried each of the braces while performing activities of daily living tasks such as sitting up, standing up, lifting a 2-lb box, and putting on a lightweight jacket. They found that the Aspen and Boston braces restricted approximated 20 percent of motion compared with a no brace condition, but the Cybertech orthosis restricted only 3 percent.[19] One problem with the study is that the patients were likely stiff even in the no brace condition because they had been previously in a brace full time for 3 months after surgery. Even so, the Cybertech is still not as effective at restricting motion as the Aspen and Boston braces. In both studies, the Aspen was rated more comfortable than the others.

Jewett Hyperextension Brace

The Jewett hyperextension brace is designed as a three-point pressure system with two anterior pads over the sternum and pubic symphysis opposed by a posterior pad in the midthoracic region to hold the spine in an extended position (Fig. 27-17A-C). The pads are easily adjustable where they are connected to metal sidebars that run in the midaxillary line. The Jewett brace is effective for one- and two-column injuries of the thoracolumbar region T10-L2. Biomechanical studies using finite-element analysis showed that the Jewett brace restored stiffness to normal values in one- and two-column injuries, but was ineffective in treating three-column injuries.[28] It is effective over a relatively short span of the spine but ineffective for most of the lumbar spine. The major disadvantage occurs in the elderly or very thin. Because control is

achieved through the placement of three small pads, the increased relative contact pressures on the skin areas covered by the pads heighten the potential for discomfort or skin breakdown. The Jewett brace has better air circulation and less moisture retention than a TCO. However, the Jewett provides no support over the abdomen, does not restrict lateral bending, and concentrates pressure on the small surface areas of the pads. Advantages include lighter weight, fitting in one sitting, and less expensive than the custom-molded body jacket and Aspen brace.

Cruciform Anterior Spinal Hyperextension Brace

The cruciform anterior spinal hyperextension (CASH) brace is similar to the Jewett in that it has two anterior pads over the sternum and pubis, opposed by a pad in the thoracolumbar region. The pads are connected to bars that cross anteriorly and can be bent to provide varying degrees of hyperextension. The brace is easy to put on and take off but more difficult to adjust than the Jewett. The Korsain brace is a Jewett brace with added abdominal support at a price similar to that for the Jewett.

Knight–Taylor Brace

The Knight-Taylor brace is a corset-type brace (Fig. 27-18A-C). It has posterior and lateral rigid aluminum or polyvinylchloride slats and shoulder straps. The anterior portion of the brace is made of canvas with several eyelets that can be laced and tightened. This brace is a hybrid

FIGURE 27-17 *A–C,* The Jewett is designed as a three-point pressure system with two anterior pads over the sternum and pubic symphysis opposed by a posterior pad in the midthoracic region to hold the spine in an extended position.

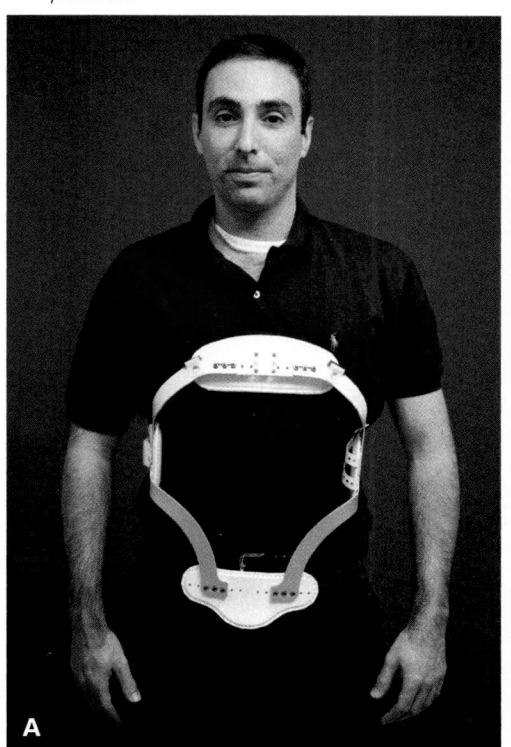
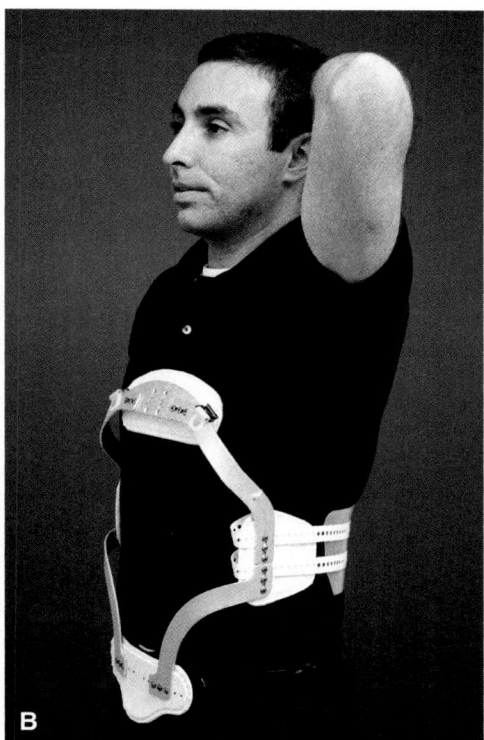
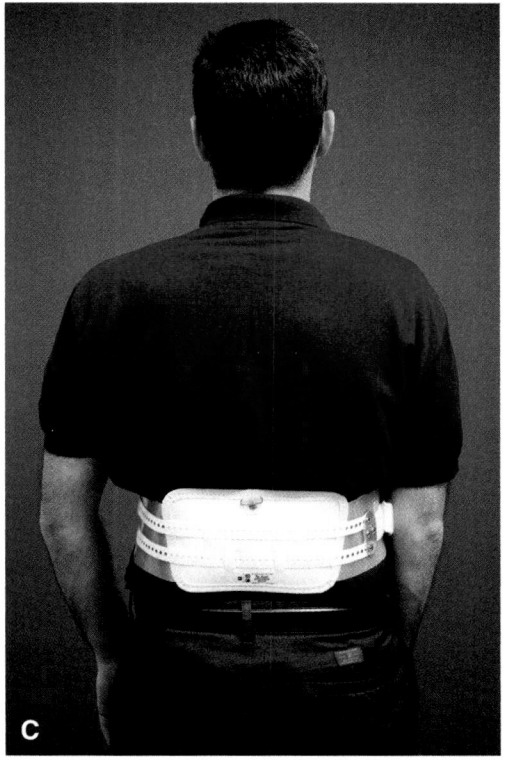

of the corset and TLSO. Although orthopaedists previously suggested that the Knight-Taylor brace was effective in immobilizing regions of the thoracic spine, it has proved inadequate and has little practical use today except in the elderly patient requiring only a very mild degree of support. The shoulder straps may cause discomfort in some patients. It has very poor rotational control but limits to a mild degree flexion, extension, and lateral bending.

FIGURE 27-18 | **A–C,** *This brace, built of a corset bottom with uprights secured to the torso by shoulder straps, is supposed to give some control to the thoracic spine. The brace is used often in the elderly in whom more rigid braces are not well tolerated. Control is minimal, however, and the shoulder straps can cause skin irritation in the axilla.*

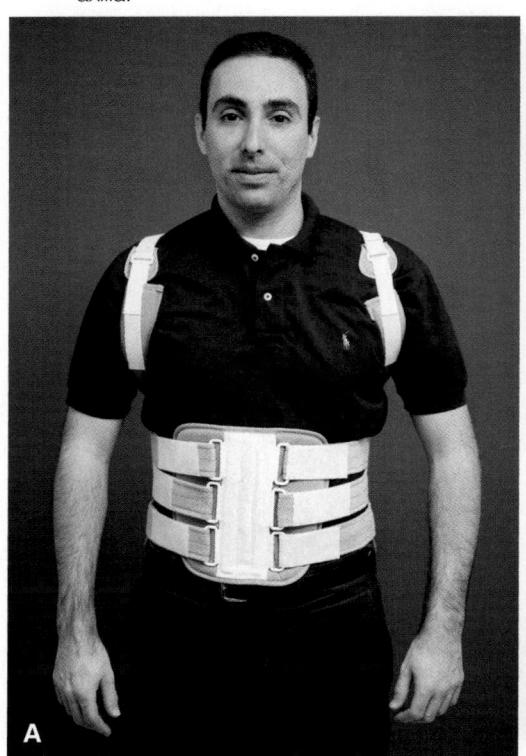
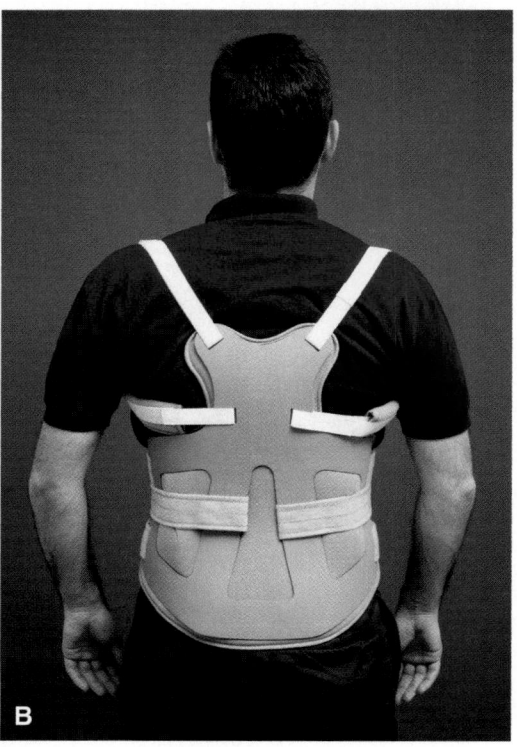
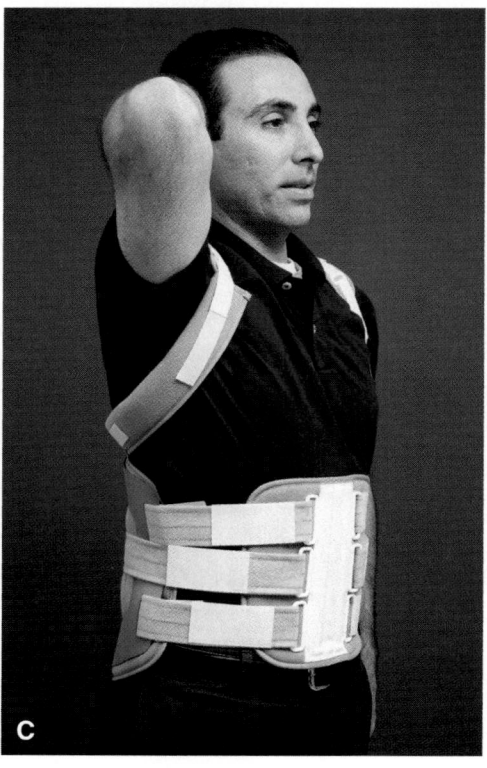

Chairback Brace

The chairback brace is also a hybrid brace with a rigid posterior piece attached to a corset-like anterior (Fig. 27-19 A-C). Its like strapping the back of a chair to the torso with a corset. The posterior piece can be a single solid piece or a rectangle with a thoracic band just below the inferior angle of the scapula, a pelvic band at the midtrochanteric line, and two vertical uprights along the

FIGURE 27-19   ***A–C,*** *The chairback brace is also a hybrid brace with a rigid posterior piece attached to a corset-like anterior. This brace provides some flexion-extension motion restriction in the L1–L4 region, minimal control of rotation, and about 45 percent lateral bending at the thoracolumbar junction.*

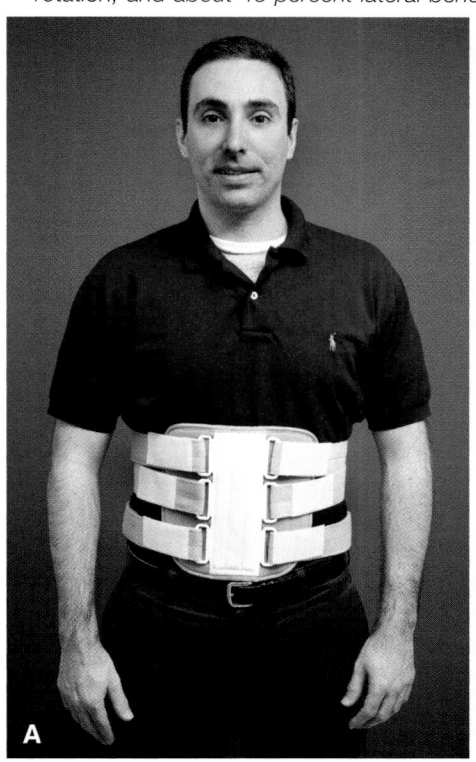
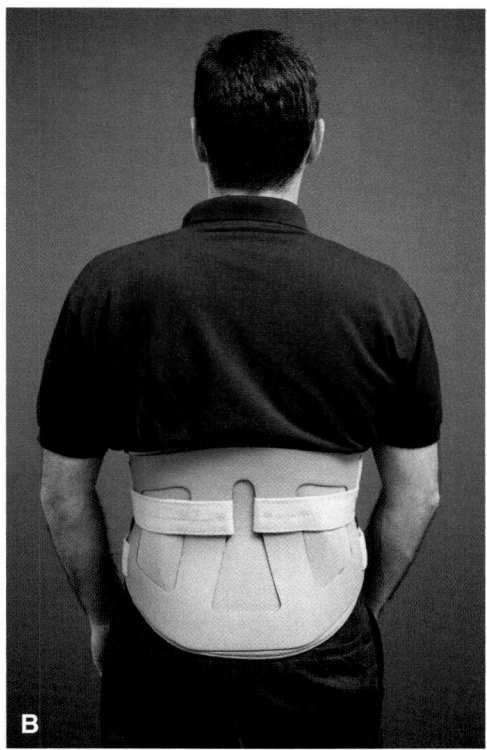
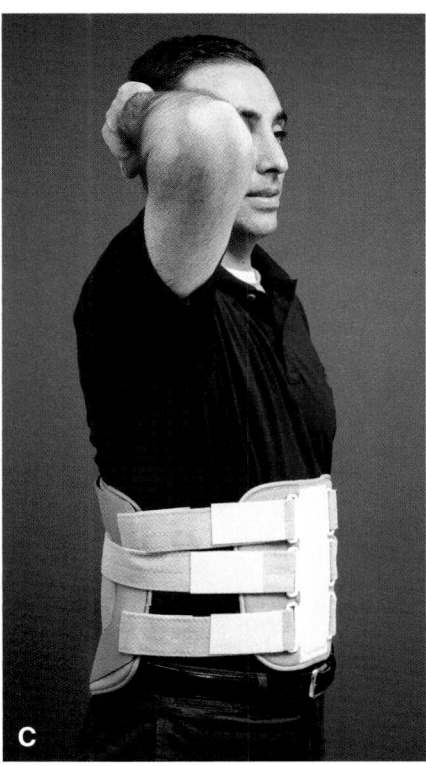

paraspinal muscles. This brace achieves moderate motion restriction, with some flexion-extension in the L1-L4 region, minimal control of rotation, and about 45 percent of lateral bending at the thoracolumbar junction. This brace is infrequently used in trauma care today except in the elderly patient.

Williams Brace

The Williams brace is designed to limit extension while allowing flexion. It is used for treating spondylolysis and spondylolisthesis. The brace has a rigid posterior portion with horizontal thoracic and pelvic bands connected to lateral uprights with reinforcing oblique struts. The rigid posterior portion is attached to an elastic abdominal apron allowing forward flexion. It limits some extension and side bending at the terminal ends only.

CONCLUSIONS

Successful nonoperative treatment of many types of traumatic injuries of the spine requires effective use of an orthosis. Matching the type and degree of instability with the appropriate orthosis is critical in restricting motion for the involved segment of the spine in that particular range of motion. It is also vital to understand that no brace effectively applies axial traction or even adequately counteracts axial compression. Even the halo vest has been shown to allow axial compression to be applied to the cervical spine under certain conditions. Effective use of an orthosis should provide the patient pain relief, a sense of stability of the fracture, and a kinesthetic reminder to avoid certain motions that may be either painful or detrimental to fracture healing.

REFERENCES

1. Askins, V.; Eismont, F.J. Efficacy of five cervical orthoses in restricting cervical motion. A comparison study. Spine 22:1193–1198, 1997.
2. Ballock, R.T.; Lee, T.Q.; Triggs, K.J.; et al. The effect of pin location on the rigidity of the halo pin-bone interface. Neurosurgery 26:238–241, 1990.
3. Blaylock B. Solving the problem of pressure ulcers resulting from cervical collars. Ostomy Wound Manage 42:26–33, 1996.
4. Botte, M.J.; Byrne, T.P.; Abrams, R.A.; et al. Halo skeletal fixation: Techniques of application and prevention of complications. J Am Acad Orthop Surg 4:44–53, 1996.
5. Botte, M.J.; Byrne, T.P.; Garfin, S.R. Application of the halo device for immobilization of the cervical spine utilizing an increased torque pressure. J Bone Joint Surg [Am] 69:750–752, 1987.
6. Botte, M.J.; Garfin, S.R.; Byrne, T.P.; et al. The halo skeletal fixator. Principles of application and maintenance. Clin Orthop Relat Res 239:12–18, 1989.
7. Castro, W.H.; Sautmann, A.; Schilgen, M.; et al. Non-invasive three-dimensional analysis of cervical spine motion in normal subjects in relation to age and sex. An experimental examination. Spine 25:443–449, 2000.
8. Chin, K.R.; Auerbach, J.D.; Adams, S.B., Jr.; et al. Mastication causing segmental spinal motion in common cervical orthoses. Spine 31:430–434, 2006.
9. Cholewicki, J. The effects of lumbosacral orthoses on spine stability: What changes in EMG can be expected? J Orthop Res 22:1150–1155, 2004.
10. Cholewicki, J.; Alvi, K.; Silfies, S.P.; et al. Comparison of motion restriction and trunk stiffness provided by three thoracolumbosacral orthoses (TLSOs). J Spinal Disord Tech 16:461–468, 2003.
11. Cotler, H.B.; Miller, L.S.; DeLucia, F.A.; et al. Closed reduction of cervical spine dislocations. Clin Orthop Relat Res 214:185–199, 1987.
12. Davies, G.; Deakin, C.; Wilson, A. The effect of a rigid collar on intracranial pressure. Injury 27:647–649, 1996.
13. Eldeeb, H.; Boubekri, N.; Asfour, S.; et al. Design of thoracolumbosacral orthosis (TLSO) braces using CT/MR. J Comput Assist Tomogr 25:963–970, 2001.
14. Fleming, B.C.; Krag, M.H.; Huston, D.R.; et al. Pin loosening in a halo–vest orthosis: A biomechanical study. Spine 25:1325–1331, 2000.
15. Garfin, S.R.; Botte, M.J.; Centeno, R.S.; et al. Osteology of the skull as it affects halo pin placement. Spine 10:696–698, 1985.
16. Garfin, S.R.; Botte, M.J.; Waters, R.L.; et al. Complications in the use of the halo fixation device. J Bone Joint Surg [Am] 68:320–325, 1986.
17. Gavin, T.M.; Carandang, G.; Havey, R.; et al. Biomechanical analysis of cervical orthoses in flexion and extension: A comparison of cervical collars and cervical thoracic orthoses. J Rehabil Res Dev 40:527–537, 2003.
18. Kolb, J.C.; Summers, R.L.; Galli, R.L. Cervical collar-induced changes in intracranial pressure. Am J Emerg Med 17:135–137, 1999.
19. Krag, M.H.; Fox, M.J.; Haugh, L.D. Comparison of three lumbar orthoses using motion assessment during task performance. Spine 28:2359–2367, 2003.
20. Kumar, K. Spinal deformity and axial traction. Spine 21:653–655, 1996.
21. Lee, A.S.; MacLean, J.C.; Newton, D.A. Rapid traction for reduction of cervical spine dislocations. J Bone Joint Surg [Br] 76:352–356, 1994.
22. Lerman, J.A.; Haynes, R.J.; Koeneman, E.J.; et al. A biomechanical comparison of Gardner–Wells tongs and halo device used for cervical spine traction. Spine 19:2403–2406, 1994.
23. Mahale, Y.J.; Silver, J.R.; Henderson, N.J. Neurological complications of the reduction of cervical spine dislocations. J Bone Joint Surg [Br] 75:403–409, 1993.
24. Marketos, S.G.; Skiadas, P. Hippocrates. The father of spine surgery. Spine 24:1381–1387, 1999.
25. McGuire, R.A.; Degnan, G.; Amundson, G.M. Evaluation of current extrication orthoses in immobilization

of the unstable cervical spine. Spine 15:1064–1067, 1990.

26. Miller, L.S.; Cotler, H.B.; De Lucia, F.A.; et al. Biomechanical analysis of cervical distraction. Spine 12:831–837, 1987.

27. Moen, K.Y.; Nachemson, A.L. Treatment of scoliosis. An historical perspective. Spine 24:2570–2575, 1999.

28. Patwardhan, A.G.; Li, S.P.; Gavin, T.; et al. Orthotic stabilization of thoracolumbar injuries. A biomechanical analysis of the Jewett hyperextension orthosis. Spine 15:654–661, 1990.

29. Perry, J.; Nickel, V.L. Total cervical spine fusion for neck paralysis. J Bone Joint Surg [Am] 41-A:37–60, 1959.

30. Puckree, T.; Lauten, V.A.; Moodley, S.; et al. Thoracolumbar corsets alter breathing pattern in normal individuals. Int J Rehabil Res 28:81–85, 2005.

31. Richter, D.; Latta, L.L.; Milne, E.L.; et al. The stabilizing effects of different orthoses in the intact and unstable upper cervical spine: A cadaver study. J Trauma 50:848–854, 2001.

32. Rodgers, J.A.; Rodgers, W.B. Marginal mandibular nerve palsy due to compression by a cervical hard collar. J Orthop Trauma 9:177–179, 1995.

33. Rushton, S.A.; Vaccaro, A.R.; Levine, M.J.; et al. Bivector traction for unstable cervical spine fractures: A description of its application and preliminary results. J Spinal Disord 10:436–440, 1997.

34. Sanan, A.; Rengachary, S.S. The history of spinal biomechanics. Neurosurgery 39:657–668, 1996.

35. Sandler, A.J.; Dvorak, J.; Humke, T.; et al. The effectiveness of various cervical orthoses. An in vivo comparison of the mechanical stability provided by several widely used models. Spine 21:1624–1629, 1996.

36. Schneider, A.M.; Hipp, J.A.; Nguyen, L.; et al. Reduction in head and intervertebral motion provided by 7 contemporary cervical orthoses in 45 individuals. Spine 32:E1–E6, 2007.

37. Spivak, J.M.; Vaccaro, A.R.; Cotler, J.M. Thoracolumbar spine trauma: II. Principles of management. J Am Acad Orthop Surg 3:353–360, 1995.

38. Triggs, K.J.; Ballock, R.T.; Lee, T.Q.; et al. The effect of angled insertion on halo pin fixation. Spine 14:781–783, 1989.

39. Vander, K.D.; Abad, G.; Basford, J.R.; et al. Lumbar spine stabilization with a thoracolumbosacral orthosis: Evaluation with video fluoroscopy. Spine 29:100–104, 2004.

40. Webber-Jones, J.E.; Thomas, C.A.; Bordeaux, R.E., Jr. The management and prevention of rigid cervical collar complications. Orthop Nurs 21:19–25, 2002.

41. White, A.A., III; Panjabi, M.M. The basic kinematics of the human spine. A review of past and current knowledge. Spine 3:12–20, 1978.

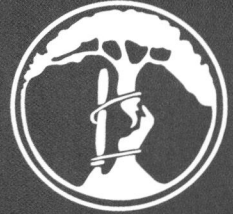

CHAPTER 28

Injuries of the Cervicocranium

John C. France, M.D. and Ryan T. Gocke, M.D.

The upper cervical spine encompasses a highly specialized anatomic arrangement that functionally allows increased mobility for the head. This mobility is necessary in humans to compensate for a limited ocular motion and to increase the field of vision. As with the more caudal portions of the spine, the cervicocranium also functions to protect the spinal cord. Injuries to the cervicocranium have the potential for acute catastrophic neurologic compromise as well as chronic disability. Although relatively rare in younger patients in clinical practice, these injuries are more common among elderly osteoporotic patients. The spectrum of injuries in the cervicocranium includes occipital condyle fractures, occipitoatlantal dislocations, dislocations and subluxations of the atlantoaxial joint, fractures of the ring of the atlas, odontoid fractures, fractures of the arch of the axis, and lateral mass fractures of the axis. Although similar in their mechanism of injury patterns, each specific injury requires a unique treatment algorithm to optimize outcomes. Many of the injuries may be treated conservatively; others, however, require a more aggressive surgical approach.

These injuries are often missed or not reported, so the true incidence is difficult to estimate. Most craniocervical injuries are the result of automobile accidents or falls.[5,28,39,62,156,187] The predominant mechanism of injury is usually forced flexion or extension secondary to unrestrained deceleration forces, resulting in either anterior or posterior displacement of the occiput and the upper two cervical segments in relation to the more caudal segments. A less common mechanism is axial load that causes compression injury to the condyles, lateral mass, or splaying of the atlas as in a true Jefferson's fracture.

Alker and colleagues[5] noted the devastating nature of these injuries in their analysis of 312 victims of fatal traffic accidents, with 24.4 percent showing evidence of injury to the cervical spine, mostly involving the cervicocranium. Bohlman[28] in his analysis of 300 patients who sustained acute cervical spine injuries noted that the correct diagnosis was missed in one third of patients. Of these injuries, 30 percent involved the cervicocranium. The presence of a head injury, decreased level of consciousness, alcohol intoxication, multiple injuries, and inadequate radiographs were the extenuating factors that led to delay in diagnosis.

ANATOMY

Traumatic injuries with fracture displacement in the upper cervical spine tend to occur with fewer neurologic deficits than occur in lower cervical spine fractures due to a relatively greater space available for the cord at this level of the spine.[334] Proper treatment of these traumatic injuries requires an essential knowledge of the intricate regional anatomy and the kinematic relationships of the occipitoatlantoaxial complex (Figs. 28-1 through 28-3). The skull and atlas are bound together by the paired occipitoatlantal joints laterally. The atlanto-occipital joint is a shallow ball-in-socket joint. Two condyle surfaces are convex in the caudal direction, whereas the C1 articular surfaces are reciprocally concave. The joint is shallower in the sagittal plane than in the coronal plane, which may explain the predisposition to anteroposterior displacement or dislocations. Two groups of ligaments stabilize this structure: (1) those that connect the atlas to occiput, and (2) those that connect the axis to occiput. The first group comprises the anterior and posterior atlanto-occipital membranes; the second group includes the tectorial membrane, two alar ligaments, and the apical ligament. The articular capsular ligaments are very thin and provide very little stability. The anterior occipitoatlantal membrane is a structural extension of the anterior longitudinal ligament, and the tectorial membrane is a continuation of the posterior longitudinal ligament (PLL). It extends from the dorsal surface of the odontoid process to the ventral surface of the foramen magnum. It is thought to be the prime ligament responsible for stability of the occipitoatlantal articulation.[329] A posterior occipitoatlantal membrane also connects the posterior rim of the foramen magnum to the posterior C1 arch (similar to the ligamentum flavum in the lower cervical spine). In biomechanical cadaveric testing, the ligamentous upper cervical spine was shown to be significantly stronger in extension than flexion.[227] This may help to explain the pattern of injuries that is seen with upper cervical spine trauma.

The atlas is essentially a bony ring with two lateral masses. Mechanically, the superior and inferior articular facets lie anterior to the posterior facets of the subaxial spine. The superior articular surfaces face upward and

FIGURE 28-1 *Sagittal anatomy of the cervicocranium.*

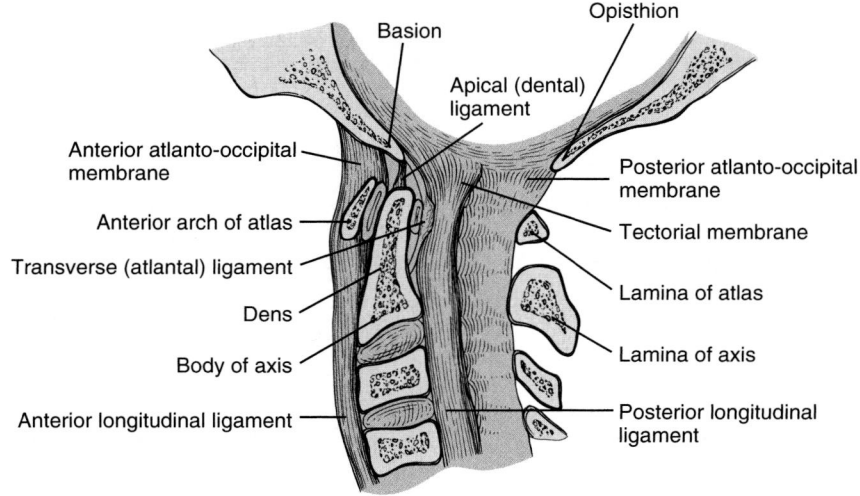

FIGURE 28-2 *Coronal anatomy of the cervicocranium.*

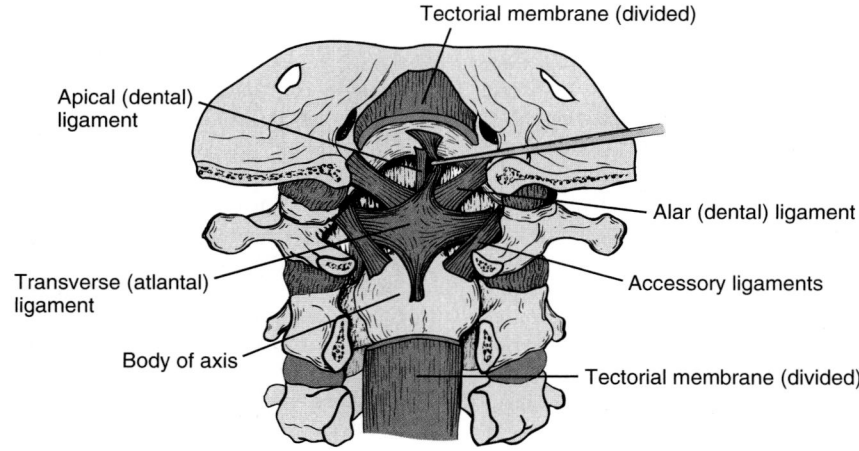

FIGURE 28-3 *Anatomy of the atlantoaxial articulation.*

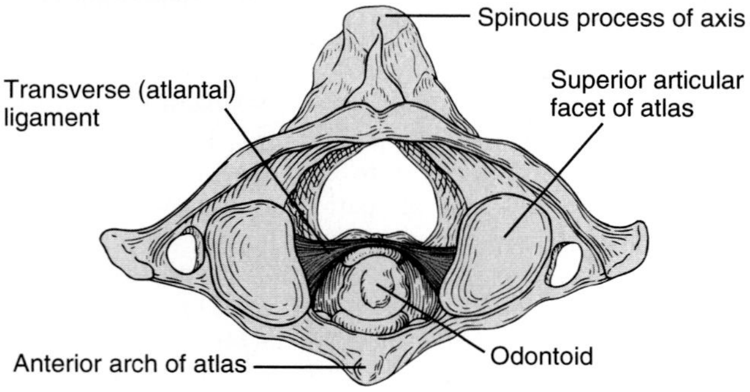

medially to receive the occipital condyles of the skull, which face laterally. The inferior articulating surfaces face downward and slightly medially and rotate on the corresponding anteriorly placed superior facets of the axis. The posterior arch consists of a modified lamina with a posterior tubercle that gives rise to the suboccipital muscles. The anterior arch connects the lateral masses and has a tubercle on which the longus colli muscles insert.

Range of motion between the occiput and atlas is 25° of flexion-extension, 5° of lateral bending, and 5° of rotation. Between the atlas and axis is 20° of flexion-extension, 5° of lateral bending, and 40° of rotation.[334] The atlantoaxial articulation comprises three joints: the paired lateral atlantoaxial facet joints and the central atlantoaxial joint. The lateral atlantoaxial facet joints are covered by thin, loose capsular ligaments that accommodate the large amount of rotation at this level. The central atlantoaxial joint, making up the atlantodens interval, is the articulation of the odontoid process with the posterior aspect of the C1 anterior arch. The crucial stabilizing structure is the transverse atlantal ligament (cruciform ligament), which essentially serves to harness the atlas to the dens of the axis. This ligament originates from two internal tubercles on the posterior aspect of the anterior arch of C1 (see Fig. 28-3) and functions to stabilize the dens against the anterior arch of the atlas during rotation and translation. The paired alar ligaments are expansions of the transverse ligament that attach to tubercles on the lateral rim of the foramen magnum and provide additional stability to the occipito-atlantal articulation. The apical dental ligament runs from the tip of the odontoid process to the ventral surface of the foramen magnum and is only a minor stabilizer of the craniocervical junction.[85,114]

The axis provides a bearing surface on which the atlas rotates. The vertically projecting odontoid (dens) process mechanically abuts the posterior aspect of the C1 arch, acting as a pivot point for rotations of the C1 ring and preventing posterior C1 translation. The angulation of the dens in the sagittal plane varies, ranging from 2° anterior to 42° posterior. There is no correlation between the height of the dens and the space available for the cord.[68] The superior articulating surfaces of the axis are convex and directed slightly laterally to articulate with the medially oriented C1 inferior facets. It is important to remember that the articular surfaces of the axis represent a transition point from the anteriorly located occiput–C1-C2 joints to the posteriorly located facet joints of the subaxial spine. Thus, the inferior articulating surfaces are typical of those of the more caudal cervical vertebrae. The pedicles of the axis project 20° superiorly and 33° medially.[348] The pedicles' dimensions average 7 to 8 mm in height and width, with slight variations between males and females.[348]

The vertebral artery exits out of the C1 foramen transversarium and lies directly on the posterior C1 arch within a groove while traveling medially and superiorly into the foramen magnum. Its course through the C2 foramen can vary significantly and be at risk during screw insertions, and, thus, should be studied for each individual patient. The carotid artery courses along the anterolateral aspect of the C1 lateral mass. Vital neurologic structures occur within close proximity to the atlanto-occipital joint. Within the base of the occipital condyle lies the hypoglossal canal through which the hypoglossal nerve (CN XII) passes. Just lateral to the occipital condyle and posterior to the carotid canal is the jugular foramen that contains cranial nerves IX–XI.[196] The jugular foramen lies in close proximity to the hypoglossal canal within 3 mm on the extracranial side and 7 mm on the intracranial side[183] (Fig. 28-4).

OCCIPITAL CONDYLE FRACTURES

Fractures of the occipital condyle are rarely reported; they usually occur in conjunction with other cervical spine injuries and are associated with high mortality rates. In patients who manage to survive these injuries, the incidence of these fractures remains unknown because such fractures often go undiagnosed and may present only with vague complaints of neck pain. With the increased use of

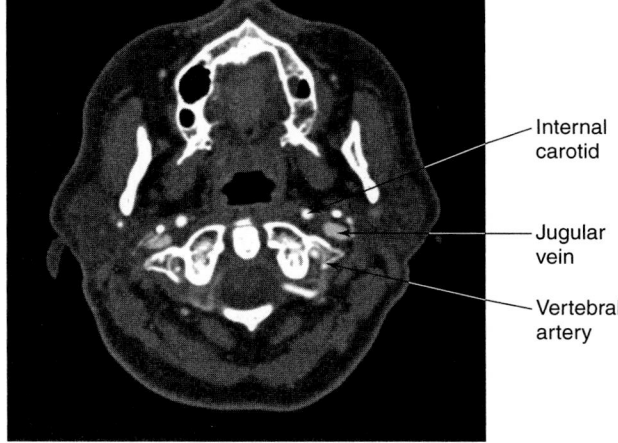

FIGURE 28-4 *An axial CT image at the level of the C1 lateral masses showing the structures at risk from a screw that penetrates the anterior cortex. This will be soft tissue anatomy around upper cervical spine.*

Internal carotid

Jugular vein

Vertebral artery

helical computed tomography (CT), a greater number of stable occipital condyle fractures are being identified. The injury may be difficult to detect with plain radiographs. Anterior soft tissue swelling may be the best parameter for predicting occipitocervical injury on plain radiographs. One study found that maximum soft tissue thickness of 7 mm, or approximately 30 percent of the width of the adjacent vertebral body at C1 through C4, should prompt suspicion of injury.[250] A review of literature by Hadley calculated plain films to be 3.2 percent sensitive. The clinical criteria he considered important to consider included altered consciousness (Glasgow Coma Scale, GCS), impaired craniocervical motion, occipital pain or tenderness, lower cranial nerve paresis, and retropharyngeal soft tissue swelling as seen on plain films.[135] Evaluation of the craniovertebral junction by CT has enabled more subtle detection. Bloom and colleagues reported a significant discrepancy between occipital condyle fractures diagnosed with CT versus with nondiagnostic plain cervical radiographs.[24] Important physical findings to consider are prevertebral swelling, impaired skull mobility, torticollis, and acute or delayed cranial nerve symptoms (CN IX–XII).[32,45,49,64,183,188,215,313] In their review of the reported cases, Alcelik and associates noted that the twelfth cranial nerve is the most commonly affected due to the close relationship of the hypoglossal canal to the occipital condyles, with palsy also having occurred in the third, fourth, fifth, seventh, eighth, ninth, tenth, and eleventh nerves in 1, 1, 9, 10, 3, 19, 22, and 16 cases, respectively.[4]

Occipital condyle fractures can be divided into three injury patterns, depending on whether the injury was produced by axial compression, a direct blow, or shear or lateral bending (or both). The Anderson and Montesano classification of occipital condyle fractures is based on the mechanism of injury.[9] Type I injuries are impact fractures of the condyle secondary to an axial load. Type II injuries are basilar skull fractures that extend through the condyle and communicate with the foramen magnum. These

FIGURE 28-5 *Axial computed tomography (CT) of a Tuli type IIB unstable occipital condyle fracture.*

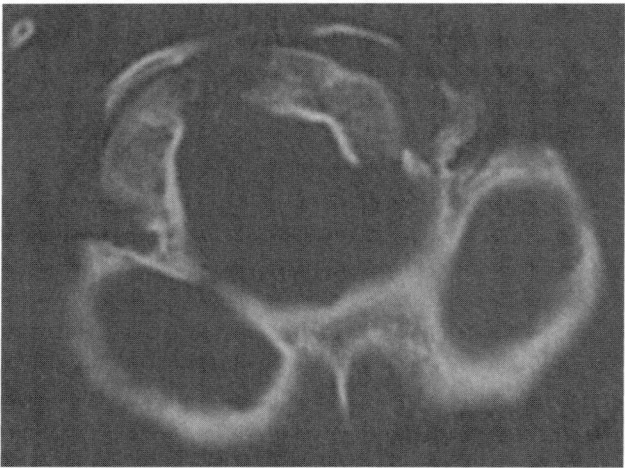

injuries are due to a direct blow to the occipital region. Type III injuries are avulsion fractures of the condyle caused by tension placed on the alar ligaments secondary to shear, lateral bending, rotational forces, or a combination of these mechanisms.

Tuli and colleagues proposed a more recent classification because of difficulty in predicting stability of the injury simply by judging displacement of the fracture. A type I fracture is nondisplaced and stable, and a type IIA is displaced but stable at the occiput–C1-C2 level. Type IIB fractures are unstable at the occiput–C1-C2 level.[312] Higher rates of mortality are associated with type IIB (57.1%) versus 11.6 percent for the other patients[15] (Fig. 28-5).

CT is the study of choice for identifying the bony injury and is used for the purpose of classification (Fig. 28-6A,B). Magnetic resonance imaging (MRI) may play a limited role in determining craniocervical instability and is useful for diagnosing cord injury. However, it is difficult to visualize the individual craniocervical ligaments with MRI, and joint effusions seen on MRI are common in asymptomatic individuals.[242] Furthermore, Hanson and co-workers in their study (retrospective review of 107 cases) noted that no patient with completely normal lateral radiographs, including normal prevertebral soft tissue shadows, had an unstable occipital condyle fracture. They also propose that instability should be defined as a "bilateral occipito-atlantoaxial joint complex injury" (defined as either bilateral occipital condyle fractures or unilateral occipital condyle fracture with contralateral widening of the occipitoatlantal joint greater than 2 mm or atlantoaxial joint greater than 3 mm as seen on CT). They note the importance of considering the occipital condyle fracture as a component of a more extensive injury to the craniocervical junction.[140]

Treatment of these injuries is essentially based on the degree of associated occipitoatlantal instability. Any evidence of displacement in the anteroposterior (AP) plane, diastasis, or joint incongruity implies instability of the injury and may necessitate occiput–C2 fusion.[8] Type I and type II fractures (in the Anderson-Montesano classification) are stable injuries and are therefore best treated with a rigid cervical orthosis or halo vest for 3 months. A recent case report of a patient developing delayed onset of Collet-Sicard syndrome (CN IX, X, XI, XII dysfunction without associated Horner's syndrome) was noted. In this case report, the authors note that the fracture was initially nondisplaced and that because the patient was not immobilized, progressive subluxation of the occipital condyle fragments occurred. The authors believe that the type I fracture in this particular patient actually represented an unstable subtype of the type I fracture. They believe that comminuted "type I" fractures should be treated with halo immobilization.[252]

Surgical indications for type III injuries are not well defined. In his review of literature, Hadley noted that 12 out of 23 patients who sustained type III injuries developed delayed neurologic deficits without treatment, and thus he states that the literature suggests patients with type III injuries should at least be treated with external immobilization.[135] Regardless of fracture type, flexion-extension views should be obtained after treatment to assess residual instability. Strong indications for surgery are few and include brainstem compression, vertebral artery injury, and concomitant suboccipital injury.[17,24] Any findings of

FIGURE 28-6 *Axial (A) and coronal (B) computed tomography (CT) image of an occipital condyle fracture.*

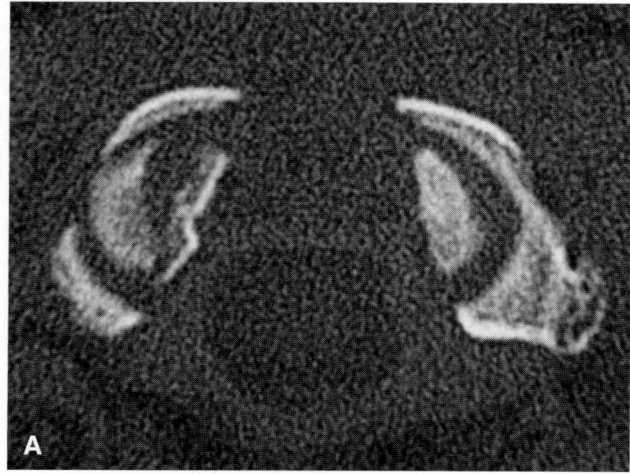

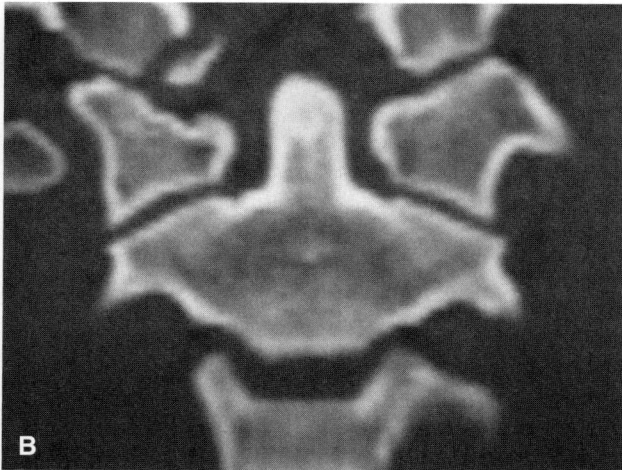

FIGURE 28-7 *Lateral radiograph demonstrating posteriorly placed screws across the atlanto-occipital joint for an occipital cervical fusion isolated to occipital–C1 level.[127]*

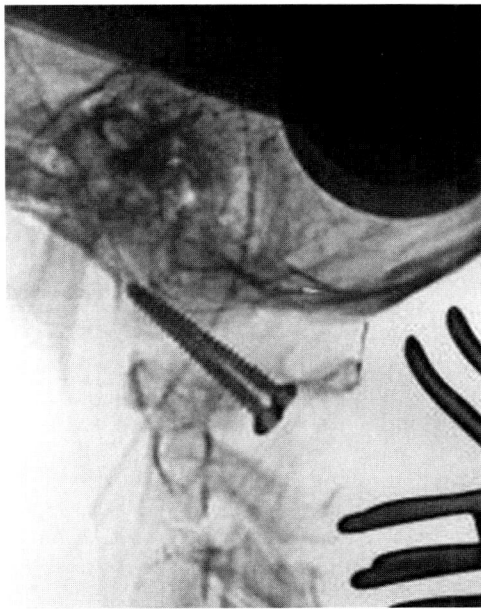

instability of the occipitoatlantal joint should prompt the surgeon to pursue surgical options. Transarticular atlantocondylar screws[6,116,126] (Fig. 28-7) as well as posterior occiput to C1 fusion[208] have recently been used in the context of preserved atlantoaxial stability, depending on the integrity of the majority of the occipital condyle. However, Vishteh and colleagues performed a cadaveric study in which they showed that unilateral resection of an occipital condyle results in statistically significant hypermobility at the occiput-C1 joint as well as at the atlantoaxial junction.[322] This increased mobility at the C1-C2 junction may have important clinical implications, and the traditional surgical treatment would be a posterior occiput-C2 fusion.

OCCIPITOATLANTAL DISLOCATIONS

Occipitoatlantal dislocations are rarely seen in patients fortunate enough to survive an injury that may disrupt the remarkably strong supporting ligament seen at the occiput-C1 junction.[81,105] Like many other injuries of the upper cervical spine, the true incidence is unknown due to the fatal nature of these injuries.[22] The dislocations occur in 0.67 to 1.0 percent of all acute cervical spine injuries and are present in 8 percent of victims of fatal motor vehicle accidents.[28,36,245] These injuries are frequently associated with submental lacerations, mandibular fractures, and posterior pharyngeal wall lacerations.[36,51,71,85,105,114,233,345]

Craniocervical dislocations have been classified according to the direction of the dislocation.[18,79,171] Anterior dislocations are most common, although posterior and vertical dislocations can occur as well.[113,245] However, classification

based on the direction of displacement is faulty in that these injuries are so highly unstable that the direction of displacement on any static film depends on the head position at that time. This injury is thought to be roughly twice as common in children as in adults,[36,85] possibly due to smaller occipital condyles and a more horizontal occipito-atlantal joint line seen in the immature skeleton.[36,51,81,85]

The injury was first described anatomically in post-mortem specimens by Kissinger[175] and Malgaigne.[201] Anatomic studies were first done by Werne and showed that flexion is limited by abutment of the basion against the dens and extension was limited by both the tectorial membrane and bony contact between the occiput and the posterior arch of C1. Lateral tilting is controlled by the alar ligaments. Most importantly, Werne was able to produce anterior dislocations cadaverically by sectioning the tectorial membrane and the alar ligaments.[329]

Although frequently overlooked, radiographic diagnosis of the injury can sometimes be made from lateral cervical spine radiographs and can incidentally be made from flexion-extension views done to diagnose other pathology. However, if an occipitocervical injury is suspected, then flexion-extension views would be contraindicated. Soft tissue swelling in this region is often present and should not be overlooked (Fig. 28-8). The soft tissue swelling results from hemorrhage into the retropharyngeal space. Interestingly, cervicocranial CT performed in the setting of abnormal prevertebral soft tissue contours has yielded a 16 percent positive injury rate. Other important radiographic diagnostic parameters include the Powers ratio, the "rule of twelve," and the dens-basion relationship. The Powers ratio[245] assesses the ratio of two distances measured between four points: the distance between the basion and the posterior arch of C1 is measured in relation to the

FIGURE 28-8 *Soft tissue swelling associated with occipital cervical injury indicated by the arrow.*

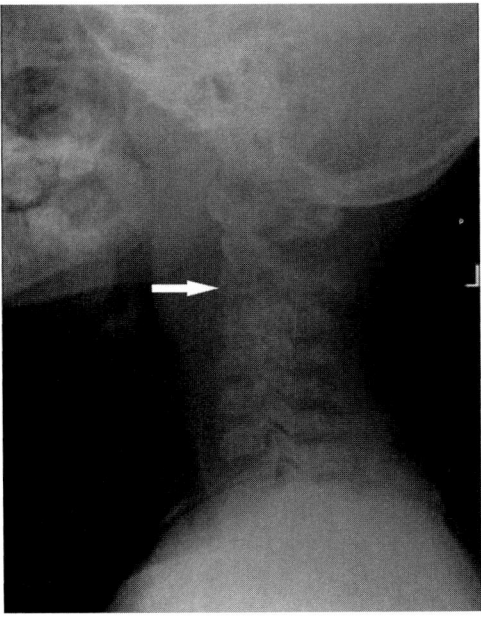

distance between the opisthion and the anterior arch of C1. A ratio greater than 1 is significant for an anterior atlanto-occipital dislocation (Fig. 28-9A, B). Ratios less than 1 are normal except in posterior occipitoatlantal dislocations, associated fractures of the odontoid process of the ring of C1, and congenital abnormalities of the foramen magnum.[51,245] The Powers ratio is helpful because the measurements do not depend on the position of head flexion or extension. Furthermore, if the clinician finds plain films to be difficult to interpret, the ratio can be calculated with sagittal CT reconstructed images. The "rule of twelve," or Harris' lines, can also be used to detect occipital cervical dissociation and is superior to the Powers ratio. The measurement uses three landmarks: the basion, the rostral tip of the odontoid, and the posterior axial line (cephalad extension of the posterior cortical margin of the axis). Two distances are measured; basion-atlanto interval (BAI) and the basion-dens interval (BDI). The authors state that both distances should be less than 12 mm in normal individuals older than 13 years of age[143] (Fig. 28-10). A more simplistic approach involves simply looking at the dens-basion relationship. In a normal cervical spine with the head in neutral, the tip of the odontoid should be in vertical alignment with the basion at a distance of 4 to 5 mm.[10,31,119,280,299,337,338] Furthermore, on flexion-extension films, the treating physician should be looking for no more than 1 mm of horizontal translation of the odontoid tip in relation to the basion.[279,329,338] Wackenheim's line runs along the posterior aspect of the clivus and should pass the tip of the odontoid and abut the posterior edge of the tip.[48] On CT, the occipital condyle should be perfectly congruent with the C1 superior articular surface, and any incongruity should raise

suspicion for this injury pattern (Fig. 28-11). Also, recent evidence suggests that MRI can be used to visualize the alar ligaments,[341] important stabilizing structures for the occipitocervical junction. Soft tissue swelling anteriorly is also a hallmark of MRIs for these injuries.

Associated injuries are noted frequently in survivors. The most susceptible areas of neurologic injury are the 10 caudal pairs of cranial nerves (with the abducens nerve being most frequently injured), the brainstem, the proximal portion of the spinal cord, and the upper three cervical nerves.[71,85,105,114,233,245] Fatalities are usually caused by transection of the medulla oblongata or the spinomedullary junction and are due to respiratory compromise secondary to compression or injury to the respiratory centers in the lower brainstem. The clinical manifestations may vary from mild to catastrophic, depending on the nature and degree of injury. Peripheral motor defects are relatively common and may often demonstrate improvement. Neurologic lesions secondary to central cranial nerve lesions are frequent as well, and most appear to be permanent.[114] In addition, injuries to the vertebral artery are occasionally seen.[97,108,345] Lesions include vasospasm, intimal tears, thrombosis, dissection, and pseudoaneurysmal dilatation. Vertebral artery injuries can result in a neurologic deficit that is acute or delayed from minutes to days. They can appear even with normal-appearing radiographs. Carotid artery injuries have also been reported secondary to compression by the malrotated lateral mass of C1. Typical clinical features of a vertebral artery injury include altered consciousness, nystagmus, ataxia, diplopia, and dysarthria. The diagnosis is made by magnetic resonance angiograms, CT angiography, or conventional arteriography.[65]

FIGURE 28-9 **A, B,** *Powers ratio. If BC/OA is greater than 1, an anterior occipitoatlantal dislocation exists. Ratios less than 1 are normal except in posterior dislocations, associated fractures of the odontoid process or ring of the atlas, and congenital anomalies of the foramen magnum. Abbreviations: B, basion; C, posterior arch of C1; O, opisthion; A, anterior arch of C1.*

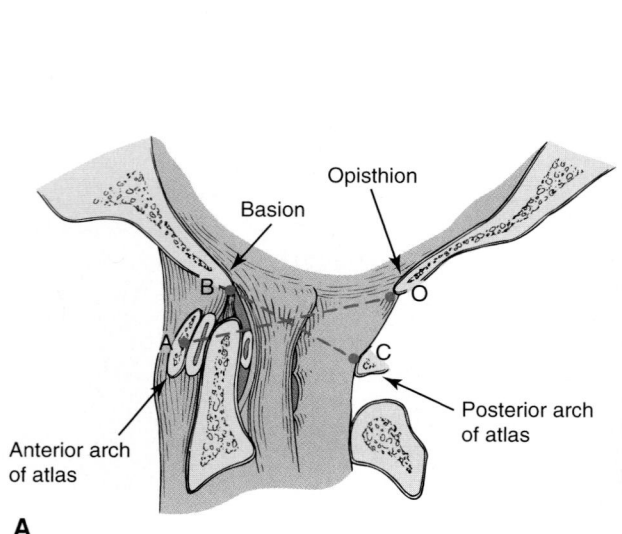

A

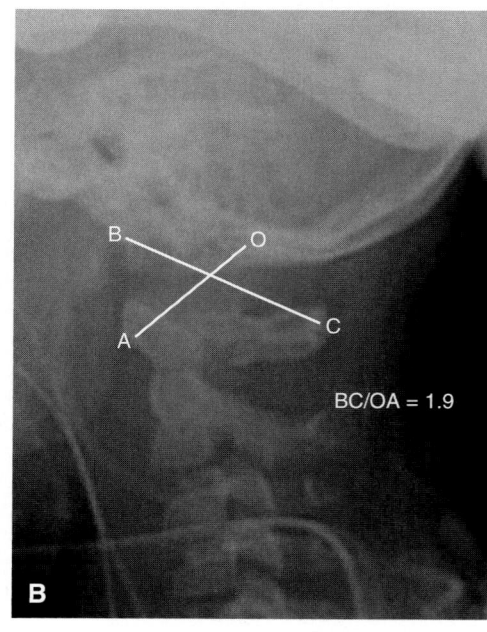

B

FIGURE 28-10 *A, Wackenheim's line drawn along the clivus should abut the posterior aspect of the tip of the dens as shown in this normal individual. Harris's line should both be less than 12 mm in adults and include the basion-dens interval (BDI) **(B)** (line **B** from basion to tip of odontoid) and the basion-atlanto interval (BAI) **(C)** (line **A** from basion to a line parallel to the posterior wall of the odontoid).*

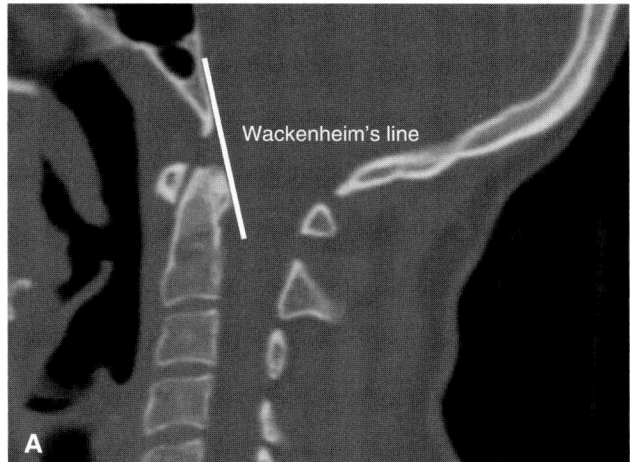
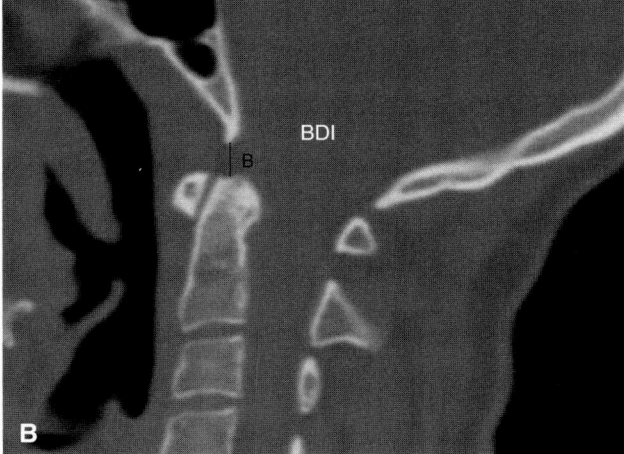
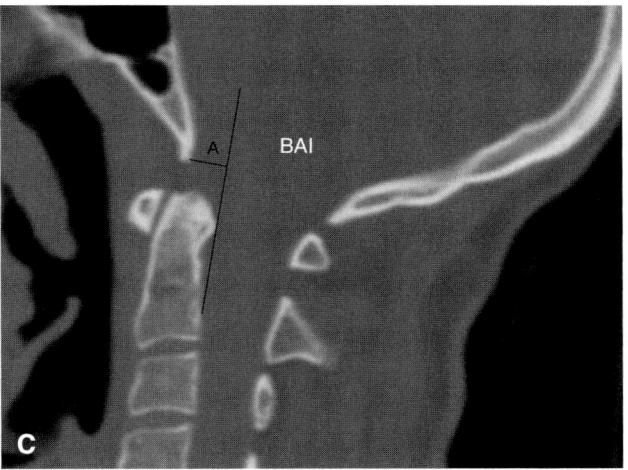

FIGURE 28-11 *Any incongruity of the occipital–C1 joint, like that shown here, is considered abnormal and indicative of instability.*

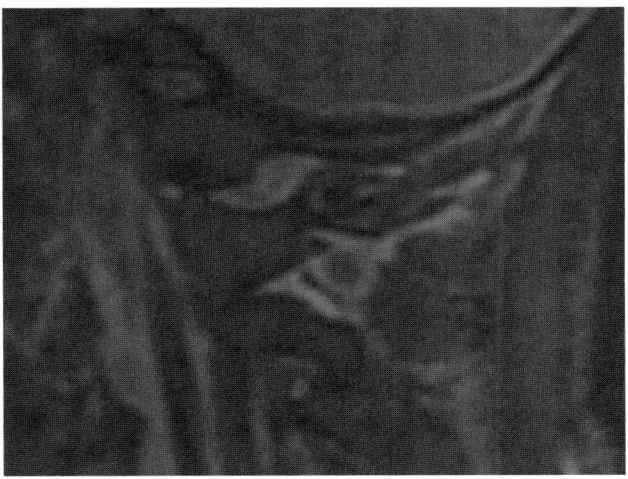

Respiratory support and immediate stabilization of the injury are the mainstays of initial treatment to avoid further neurologic injury. It is critical to observe the occipitoatlantal interval during closed reduction of other injuries while using traction. Traction should be avoided if this injury has been identified. Any radiographic evidence of occipitoatlantal widening should alert the physician to the possibility of occipitoatlantal instability as a concomitant injury. For vertical displacement, reduction can be performed via downward pressure or elevation of the bed.[8] Surgical stabilization[85,108,114,233,245,345] is usually preferred to prolonged immobilization.[245,345] Occipitocervical fusion is the preferred method of internal stabilization, given the potential for catastrophic neurologic deterioration. Furthermore, because it is a ligamentous injury, the likelihood of healing with external immobilization is significantly reduced.[321] As with most ligamentous injuries in the cervical spine, nonoperative treatment rarely results in stability. When determining the type of fixation, it is important to keep in mind the presence of other injuries in the cervical spine, which may or may not play a role in presurgical planning. Posterior arch fractures, for example, may preclude the possibility of wiring to the C1 lamina.

ATLAS FRACTURES

As with other upper cervical spine injuries, atlas fractures are usually the result of falls or automobile accidents.[54,138,276] Isolated fractures of the ring of the atlas are rarely associated with neurologic deficit.[83] This is mainly because of the wide space available for the cord at the C1 level, as well as the tendency of atlas fractures to expand and create more space. They account for 2 to 13 percent of all cervical spine fractures and approximately 1.3 percent of all spine fractures.[83,132,281] Although neurologic deficit from cord compression is rare, associated injuries can occur. Neuropraxia of the suboccipital and greater occipital nerves as they course around the posterior arch of C1 result in suboccipital scalp dysaethsias. Cranial nerve palsies of the lower six pairs of cranial nerves, and injuries to the vertebral artery or vein as they cross the posterior atlantal arch, can also occur.[111,112,152,154,164,180] Vertigo, dizziness, blurred vision, and nystagmus are all suggestive of injury to the vertebral artery.

Jefferson, whose name is usually associated with the bursting type of atlas fracture, described an anatomic classification system[164] that included posterior arch fractures, anterior arch fractures, and lateral mass and transverse process fractures (Fig. 28-12). With the introduction of CT, Segal and associates in 1987 expanded Jefferson's original fracture classification to include six subtypes,[164] followed by a seventh subtype added by Levine and Edwards:[188]

1. Burst fractures (33%), as seen in other areas of the spine, are usually the result of an axial loading force. The force is transmitted through the occipital condyles to the medially oriented superior articulations of C1, which are forced apart, and either three- or four-part fractures are produced.[243,264] Although most common, they are the least likely to cause neurologic injury (Fig. 28-13). The degree of displacement dictates treatment, as will be discussed shortly.

2. Posterior arch fractures (28%), resulting from cervical hyperextension, are important to recognize because they are often (greater than 50% chance) associated with odontoid fractures, traumatic spondylolisthesis of the axis, or occipital condyle fractures.[83,187,194,276] The presence of additional injuries alters the treatment plan and outcomes, although when posterior arch fractures occur in isolation, nonoperative treatment is recommended with rigid collar immobilization.

3. Comminuted fractures (22%) are defined anatomically by combined unilateral transverse ligament avulsion with an ipsilateral anterior or posterior arch fracture. They result from combined forces: axial compression and lateral flexion. They generally include an avulsion fracture of the transverse ligament with ipsilateral anterior and posterior arch fractures. More aggressive treatment is warranted with these injuries because they are the most likely to result in nonunion and a poor functional outcome (Fig. 28-14).

4. Anterior arch fractures occur with failure of the anterior arch while abutting the dens during hyperextension.[180,294] Associated disruption of the PLL (tectorial membrane) can lead to instability with this variant.[181] In the absence of associated atlantooccipital instability, the treatment is rigid collar immobilization.

5. Lateral mass fractures are generally the result of combined axial loading and lateral compression. If severe enough, the occipital condyle can settle onto the lateral mass of C2, creating a "cock-robin" deformity.

FIGURE 28-12   *Classification of fractures of the atlas.*

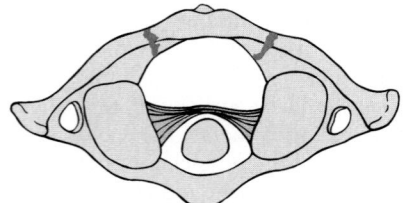

Posterior arch fracture

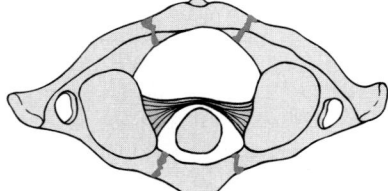

Burst fracture

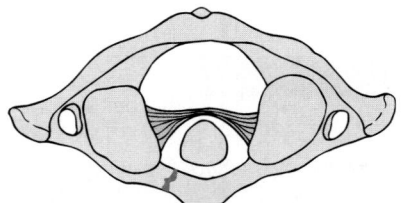

Anterior arch fracture

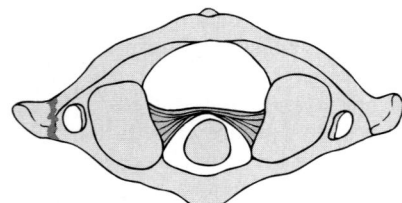

Transverse process fracture

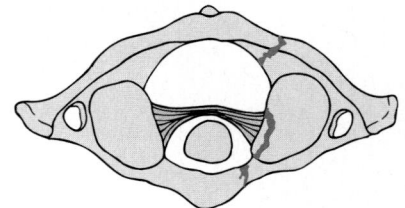

Comminuted, or lateral mass, fracture

FIGURE 28-13   *Burst type, true Jefferson's fracture.* **A,** *An anteroposterior tomogram demonstrates splaying of the lateral mass of C1.* **B,** *Computed tomographic scan in the plane of C1 demonstrates the four fractures of the ring: two anterior and two posterior (arrows). (From Levine, A.M.; Edwards, C.C. Treatment of injuries in the C1-C2 complex. Orthop Clin North Am 17:31–44, 1986.)*

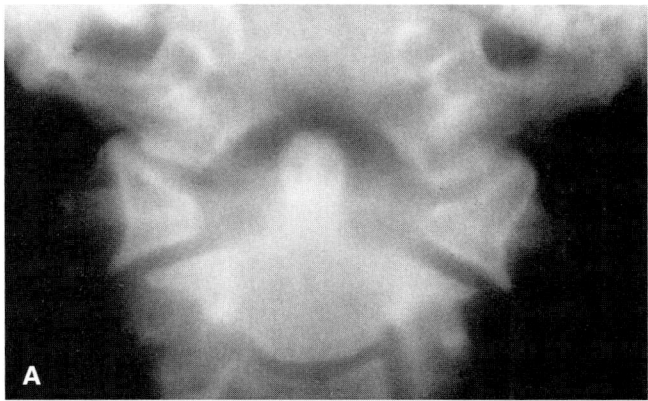
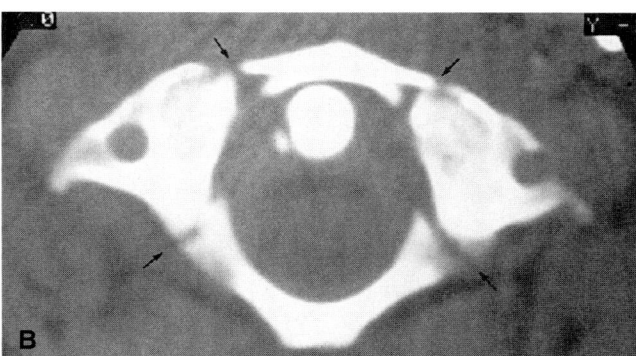

6. Transverse process fractures may be unilateral or bilateral, resulting from an avulsion with lateral bending. These are usually considered benign injuries when in isolation.

7. Inferior tubercle avulsion fractures are thought to be avulsion injuries of the longus colli muscle caused by hyperextension of the neck. Nonoperative treatment is recommended.

These fractures tend to decompress the spinal canal, and thus rarely produce neurologic symptoms. Most isolated injuries heal with conservative nonoperative treatment.[205] As is true for other spine fractures, it is important to assess atlas fracture stability when deciding treatment. Bursting atlantal fractures have been subdivided by Spence and colleagues into stable and unstable types based on the integrity of the transverse ligament as determined radiographically.[294] In their classic study, the atlantoaxial offset was measured in experimentally produced burst fractures.

Burst fractures in which the transverse ligament remained intact produced an atlantoaxial offset of less than 5.7 mm, whereas those associated with rupture of the transverse ligament produced an atlantoaxial offset greater than 6.9 mm (Fig. 28-15 A, B). When looking at plain films, however, it should be appreciated that simple rotation and lateral bending of the normal cervical spine may produce up to 4 mm of lateral offset on the open-mouth odontoid view at the C1-C2 articulation.[138,281] Congenital anomalies including clefts and aplasias should also be considered because they may produce a falsely positive lateral offset.[112] The "odontoid–lateral mass interspace" was evaluated by Sutherland and co-workers, who noted that asymmetry can occur in the neutral position and that the interspace tended to increase with ipsilateral rotation of the head.[302] Stability can also be assessed with evaluation of the atlantodens interval (ADI) in lateral flexion and extension radiographs. In normal individuals, the maximum ADI should be less than 3 mm in adults and less than 5 mm

FIGURE 28-14   **A,** *An axial and* **B,** *coronal CT image of a comminuted C1 ring fracture with transverse ligament unilateral avulsion.*

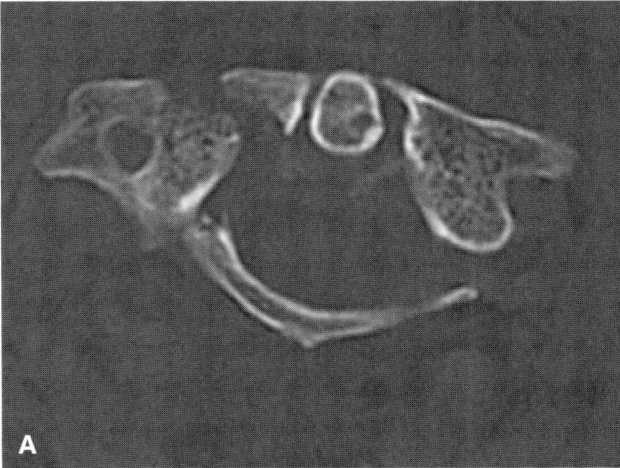
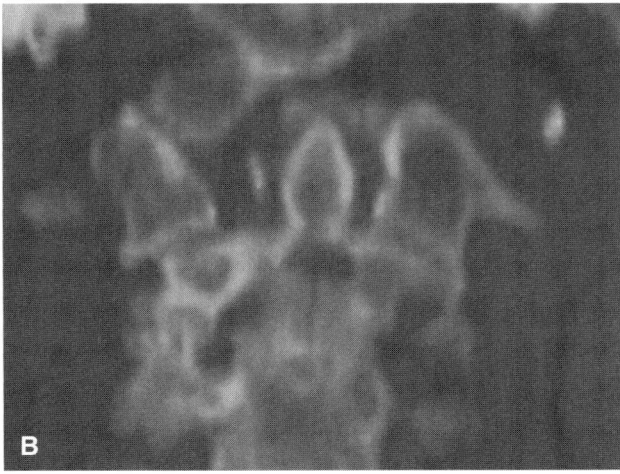

A, Atlantoaxial offset. If X + Y is greater than 6.9 mm, transverse atlantal ligament rupture is implied. (Redrawn from White, A.A., 3rd; Johnson, R.M.; Panjabi, M.M.; et al. Biomechanical analysis of clinical stability in the cervical spine. Clin Orthop Relat Res 109:85, 1975.) B, Admission open-mouth plain film view demonstrating the method for determining total lateral translation. 6, 6 mm offset; 7, 7 mm offset. (From Levine, A.M.; Edwards, C.C. Treatment of injuries in the C1-C2 complex. Orthop Clin North Am 17:31–44, 1986.)

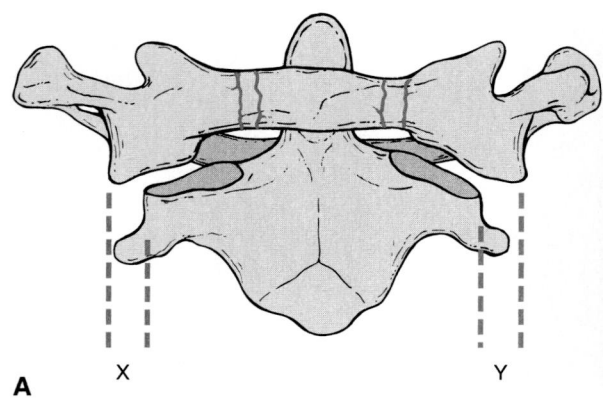

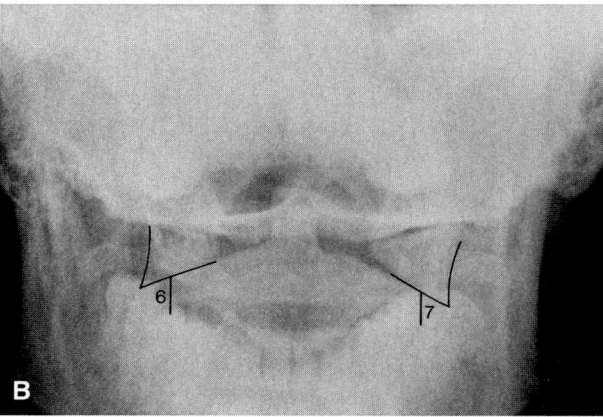

in children[90,132,296] (Fig. 28-16). In the case of a unilateral lateral mass or comminuted fracture, there may be significant lateral offset on one side only; this can allow the occipital condyle to displace vertically and create late pain and deformity. When this is recognized, operative treatment should be considered.

As mentioned previously, inferior tubercle (see item 7 of the preceding list) avulsion fractures typically involve a transverse fracture of the inferior pole or midportion that usually results from a distraction mechanism with neck hyperextension. This occurs at the attachment site of the longus colli muscle and is thought to be mechanically stable.[253] Simple, uncomplicated arch fractures, minimally displaced burst and lateral mass fractures (combined

atlantoaxial offset by <5.7 mm), and transverse process fractures can be reliably managed with halo or semirigid collar immobilization until union occurs.[182,187]

Levine and Edwards have devised a treatment algorithm for atlas fractures depending on the atlantoaxial offset.[189] For atlas fractures that show 2 to 7 mm of combined lateral mass, halo vest immobilization for 3 months is appropriate. However, for fractures with an offset greater than 7 mm, they recommend an initial period of axial traction for 4 to 6 weeks followed by 1 to 2 months of halo vest wear. In either case, after 3 months of immobilization, the stability of the atlantoaxial articulation should be verified with lateral flexion-extension films. Any significant instability (atlantodental interval >5 mm

A, An extension lateral radiograph with normal antlantodens interval (ADI) followed by a widened ADI on flexion as indicated by the arrow (B).

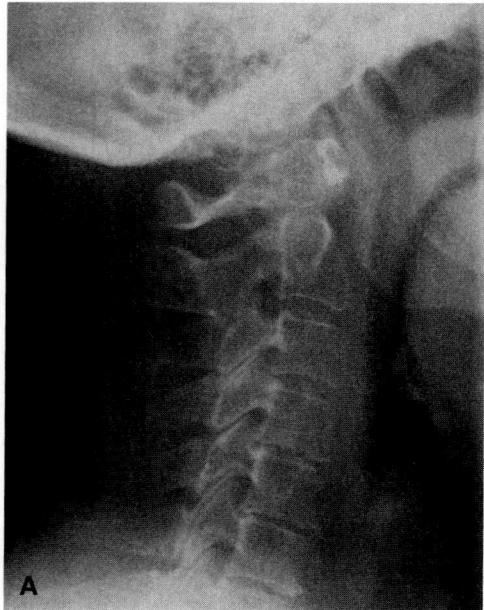

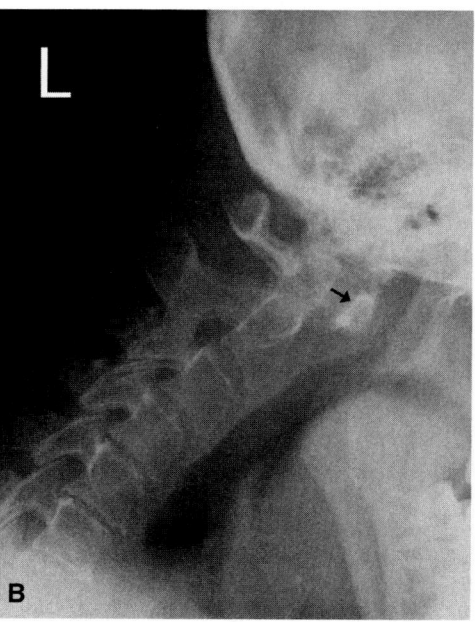

in adults, >4 mm in children) at that point warrants posterior C1-C2 fusion. In addition to Levine and Edwards, other authors have reported a very low incidence of residual instability with the use of this algorithm.[180,187,229,276,284,294,321] As shown by Fielding and co-workers, the atlantodental interval increases to approximately 5 mm when the transverse ligament is transected alone and the alar ligaments, the apical ligament, and facet capsules are left intact.[90] This may explain the low incidence of residual instability that presumably results from intact secondary stabilizers.[187,229] Thus, the axial compression-type injury described here is not nearly as unstable as a hyperflexion-type atlantoaxial dissociation (to be discussed later). The latter type injury results in tearing of the accessory ligaments, including the alar and apical ligaments and facet capsule, along with the transverse ligament, which is the reason for its instability.

With modern surgical techniques, prolonged traction followed by halo immobilization is seldom used. Surgical treatment options of massively unstable atlas fractures include traction to realign the C1 lateral masses with the C2 facets followed by posterior fixation-fusion of C1-C2 with transarticular screw (Fig. 28-17) fixation[128,163,213] or occipitocervical fusion to span the injury.[258,333] Alternatively, the fracture can be repaired more directly with lateral mass screws in C1 and a rod to reconnect them to each other avoiding fusion across motion segments, but this technique does not have a long track record (Fig. 28-18). Many patients with fractures of the atlas have long-term clinical complaints of scalp dysaesthesias, neck pain, and decreased range of motion.[189,276] The incidence of these long-term complications increases with involvement of the lateral masses, as well as with other injuries to the occiput or C1-C2 articulation.[286] Other reported complications include nonunion.[276] A recent retrospective long-term analysis noted significantly lower of quality of life in those patients with Jefferson's fractures greater than 7 mm displacement as well as in those individuals with associated injuries.[74] This could suggest that more aggressive surgical management of these injuries may result in better long-term outcomes; however, no current literature exists on this topic. Recently, a new method involving transoral reduction and osteosynthesis for unstable Jefferson's fractures was reported by Ruf and co-workers. The authors cite excellent outcomes in six patients with maintenance of rotatory movement at C1-C2 and congruent occipital-atlantoaxial joints. No patients in their group had postoperative instability.[263]

ATLANTOAXIAL INSTABILITY

Traumatic rupture of the transverse ligament leading to atlantoaxial instability is a relatively rare injury.[41,53,63] These injuries are commonly fatal, and, if the patient survives, there is almost always some degree of spinal cord injury.[85,149,150,339] These injuries are more frequently seen in older patients with post-traumatic instability developing in the fifth decade of life and beyond.[160,188] These are high-energy injuries typically resulting from hyperflexion of the neck.[63,160,188]

The stability of these areas depends not only on the transverse ligament, but also on the alar ligaments, the apical ligaments, and facet capsules, as well as the accessory atlantoaxial ligaments (see Fig. 28-2). The alar ligaments become more important in anterior stability with an insufficient transverse ligament. As revealed by Fielding and associates, if the alar and apical ligaments remain intact, the maximum amount of translation from a resected transverse ligament is 5 mm.[90] However, the secondary stabilizers are unable to withstand significant forces, as seen in high-energy automobile accidents or falls. Posterior stability depends directly on the bony odontoid providing direct mechanical abutment to the posterior aspect of the anterior atlantal arch.

Survivors from this usually fatal injury may have a clinical picture ranging from a dense, mixed neurologic deficit to only severe upper neck pain.[72,115,160,188] Radiographic analysis can be misleading to physicians not familiar with injuries in this area and due to the normal hypermobility of the C1-C2 segment.[63] Although cervical spine radiographs can typically be part of most trauma patient evaluations, recent evidence suggests that helical CT can be used alone to detect osseous abnormalities.[211] If a purely ligamentous injury such as this is suspected, supervised flexion-extension radiographs with constant neurologic monitoring are indicated to assess the atlantodental interval. It should be kept in mind that a lack of apparent instability may be caused by protective paraspinous muscle spasm. Furthermore, flexion-extension radiographs in a patient with a swollen spinal cord and neurologic deficit are contraindicated. When reading flexion-extension films, 3 mm of anterior displacement of C1 on C2, as measured by the atlantodental interval, implies that the transverse ligament is intact. A displacement of 3 to 5 mm is indicative of transverse ligament rupture, and a displacement greater than 5 mm implies probable rupture and functional incompetence of the transverse and accessory ligaments[90,132,153,187,206,296,323] (Fig. 28-19). MRI with fine, properly oriented cuts in the coronal and axial planes can also aid the documenting upper cervical ligamentous injury such as transverse ligament disruption. Children, patients with Down syndrome, and those with rheumatoid arthritis may all exhibit chronic instability with a widened atlantodens interval.

Vertical instability can be seen with traumatic ligamentous C1-C2 injuries, and a high index of suspicion should be maintained when attempting manual reduction. When examining the C1-C2 facet space and vertical translation, Gonzalez and colleagues noted that 95 percent of healthy individuals have a C1-C2 lateral mass interval (LMI) of between 0.7 and 2.6 mm. The authors concluded that an LMI greater than 2.6 mm should alert the physician to the possibility of a distraction injury.[117] A recent case report discussed a patient with traumatic anterior atlantoaxial dislocation in whom atlantoaxial vertical dissociation developed after Gardner-halo skull traction with 4.02 lb (1.5 kg). In addition to monitoring the C1-C2 LMI, the occiput to C1 interval should be observed during traction reduction. Furthermore, the closed-reduction attempt should be done only in a patient who is alert and oriented enough to cooperate with sequential neurologic exams. Some authors report, however, that longitudinal instability usually occurs with atlantoaxial dissociation and that longitudinal traction should be avoided.[248,351]

FIGURE 28-17 **A,** *An open-mouth odontoid view of a C1 ring fracture with significant spread of the lateral masses.* **B,** *The corresponding axial CT image.* **C,** *A closed reduction of the lateral masses of C1 onto the lateral masses of C2 in traction then stabilization using C1-C2 transarticular screws* **(D, E)**. *(Courtesy Robert McGuire, M.D., Mississippi University.)*

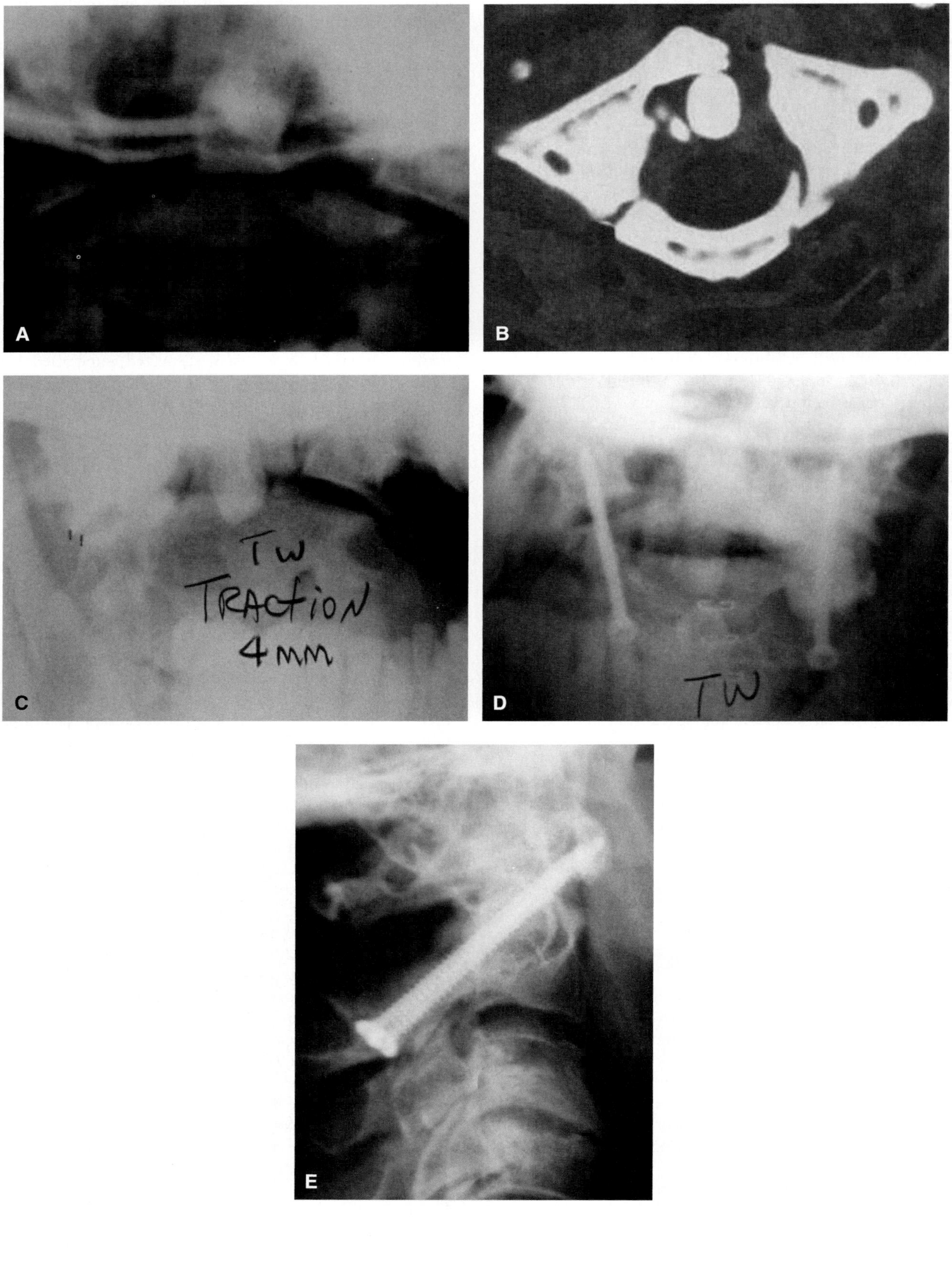

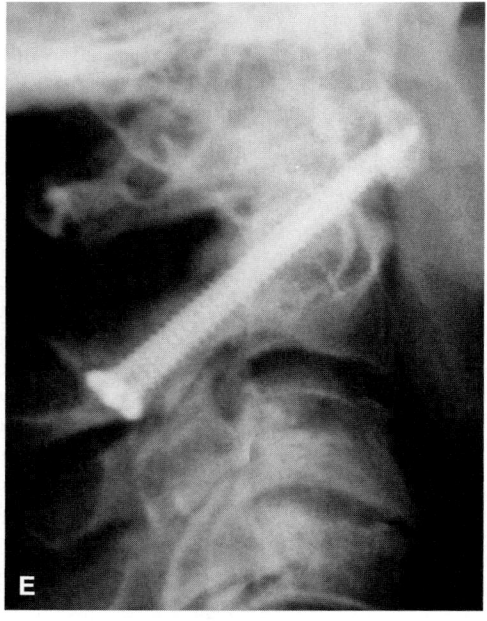

FIGURE 28-18 | *A saw bones demonstration of utilizing C1 lateral mass screws and transverse connecting rod to reduce a classic Jefferson's fracture, thus achieving direct fracture healing and avoiding a fusion. (Courtesy Jens Chapman, M.D., University of Washington.)*

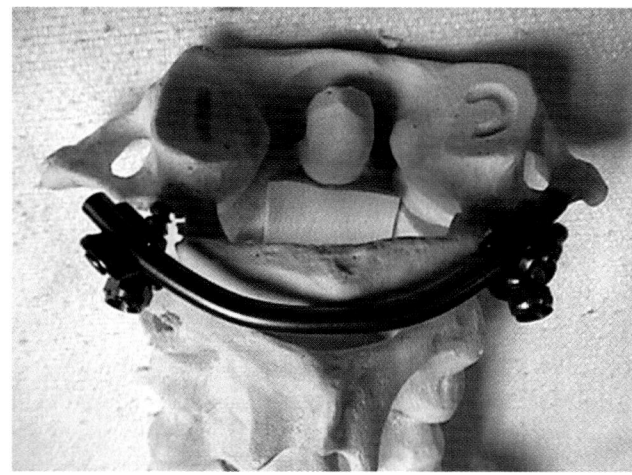

Treatment of atlantoaxial instability depends to some degree on whether the transverse ligament injury is a midsubstance tear or an avulsion of the ligament from the C1 lateral mass. One study showed that midsubstance tears have a higher likelihood of not healing and usually require arthrodesis, but that 74 percent of avulsion-type injuries heal with immobilization.[66] However, most authors agree that nonoperative management is not indicated and that reduction followed by posterior fusion is the treatment of choice.[63,90,93,160,188] The time at which surgery should be performed to optimize outcome is unclear. Because axial rotation is the major motion that occurs at the C1-C2 articulation, it would seem that a fusion that resists this type of motion is most appropriate. Biomechanical studies have compared axial rotation stiffness in the Brooks-type fusion[34] with that of Gallie wiring, Halifax clamps, Magerl's transarticular screw technique, and Harm's technique with C1 lateral mass/C2 pedicle screws.[127,141,255] One study found that rotational stability was least with the Gallie wiring technique and was greatest with the transarticular screw and Brooks' fusion techniques. The strongest overall fixation was seen with C1-C2 transarticular screws.[127] However, other authors advocate the importance of reestablishing anterior stability and claim that

FIGURE 28-19 | ***A,*** *Atlantodental interval (ADI). If the ADI is greater than 3 mm on flexion and extension radiographs, rupture of the transverse ligament is implied. If the ADI is larger than 5 mm, the accessory ligaments are also functionally incompetent.* ***B,*** *Lateral flexion radiograph showing an atlantodental interval of 12 mm, which is diagnostic of complete rupture of the transverse ligament and the alar and apical ligaments as well as disruption of some fibers of the C1-C2 joint capsule. (From Levine, A.M; Edwards, C.C. Traumatic lesions of the occipitoatlantoaxial complex. Clin Orthop Relat Res 239:53–68, 1989.)*

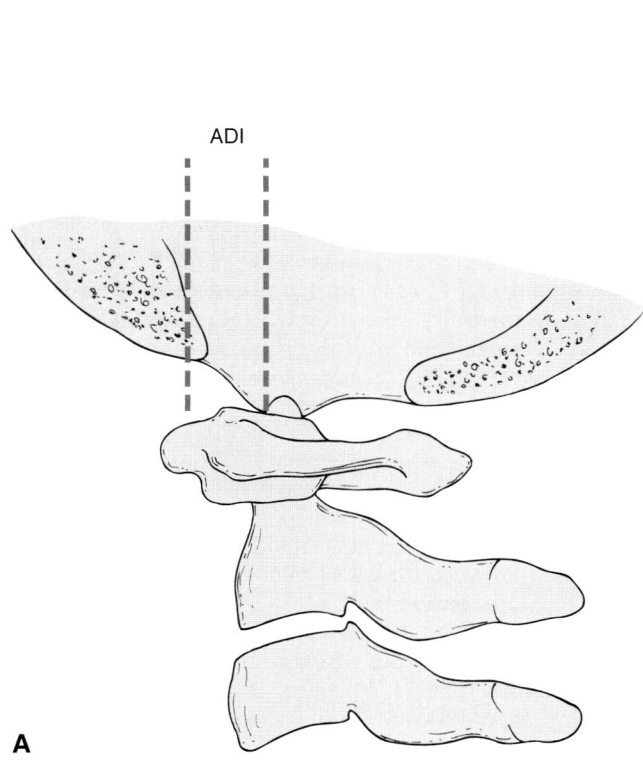

ADI

A

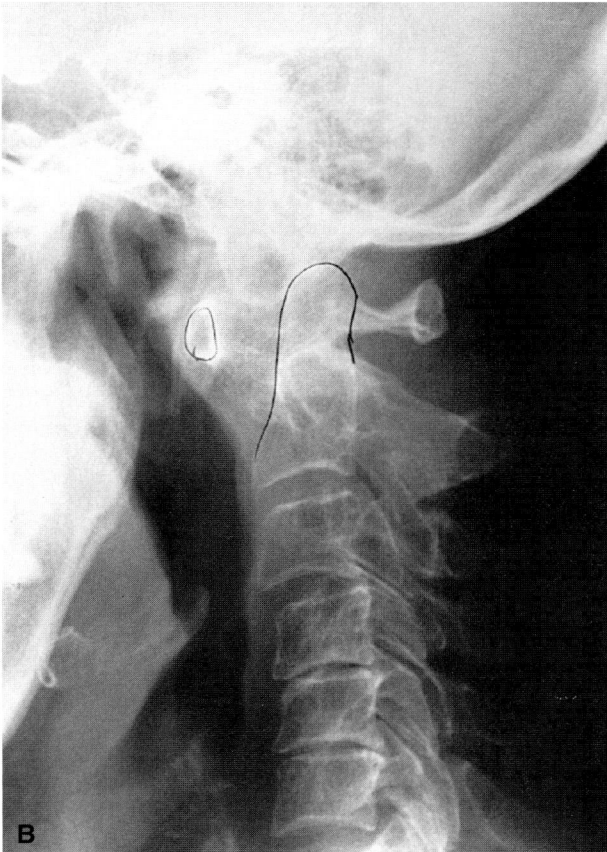

B

transarticular screws or a Gallie wiring technique should be considered for the reason that anterior translation is best prevented with these two techniques.[109,127,141,160,186] Any concurrent injury may be treated with immobilization until it heals, followed by posterior C1-C2 fusion to address the atlantoaxial instability. However, in that situation, anterior C1-C2 stability should be reassessed with flexion-extension radiographs prior to proceeding with posterior fusion. An alternative treatment plan with concomitant injuries would be the transarticular screw technique, which would allow for immediate surgical stabilization. Recently, C1-C3 lateral mass/sublaminar axial cable fixation was performed in 10 patients with atlantoaxial instability. All patients had vertebral artery anomalies that precluded C1-C2 transarticular screws. The authors concluded that it is a safe and effective way to treat patients needing C1-C2 fusion but who have unfavorable anatomy.[157] This may be a suitable alternative in patients with concomitant injuries that preclude the use of more traditional surgical techniques. Modern techniques for C1-C2 posterior fusions that involve screws in the C1 lateral mass, C2 pedicles, short C2 pars screws, and C2 laminar screws have become more popular.[67,142]

ATLANTOAXIAL ROTATORY SUBLUXATIONS AND DISLOCATIONS

Rotatory injuries of the atlantoaxial joint were first described by Corner in 1907.[56] Rotatory injuries, which usually result from flexion and rotation, can occur with or without a concomitant transverse ligament tear. At approximately 65° of atlantoaxial rotation, ensuing narrowing of the neural canal and subsequent potential damage to the spinal cord usually occur when the transverse ligament is intact.[58] Alternatively, with a deficient transverse ligament, complete unilateral facet dislocation can occur at approximately 45° of rotation with similar consequences. In addition to spinal cord impingement, the vertebral arteries can be compromised by excessive rotation with resultant brainstem or cerebellar infarction and death.[274,329] As pointed out by Levine and Edwards, rotatory dislocations at the C1-C2 articulation rarely occur in adults and are significantly different from those in children.[92,95,188] Subluxations in children rarely involve severe neurologic manifestations, are related to a viral illness or minor trauma, are almost always self-limited, and generally resolve with conservative treatment. Additionally, the adult form is frequently associated with fracture of a portion of one or both lateral masses.

The diagnosis of atlantoaxial rotatory subluxation can be difficult. Physical findings may vary, with minimal amounts of subluxation resulting in only neck pain and more severe involvement leading to neurologic injury. Torticollis may be noted, and the patient may present with the typical "cock-robin" posture with the head tilted toward one side and rotated toward the other and in slight flexion. The anterior arch of the atlas and the step-off at C1-C2 may be palpable orally. Plagiocephaly is commonly seen in younger patients as a late symptom.[95] Although rare, catastrophic neurologic deterioration as a result of

compromise of the neural canal at the medullocervical junction[95,187] mandates a high index of suspicion in trauma patients with neck injuries.

Using CT, Pang and Li were able to define normal rotatory C1-C2 movement in children. They found that with 0° to 23° of turning, C1 moves alone, with C2 remaining in a fixed position. From 24° to 65° of rotation, both C1 and C2 move together, but C1 rotates at a faster rate. After 65° of rotation, C1 and C2 remain at a relatively fixed angle, measuring 43° from each other, and further head rotation is carried out exclusively by the subaxial segments.[235] Adler Jacobson in 1956 and Fiorani-Gallotta and Luzzatti in 1957 were the first to describe the radiologic manifestations of these injuries, which were also seen in cases of torticollis.[2,98] Wortzman and Dewar suggested a dynamic method of differentiating rotatory fixation from torticollis by using plain radiographs, and Fielding and co-workers suggested cineradiography and CT as additional tools for evaluating these injuries.[92,95,346] On an open-mouth odontoid radiograph with the atlantoaxial joint in neutral rotation, the articular masses of the atlas and axis are symmetrically located with the odontoid midway between the lateral masses of the atlas (Fig. 28-20). With rotation to the right, the left lateral mass of C1 travels forward and to the right with an apparent approximation of the left atlantal articular mass to the odontoid process. Associated with forward movement of the left articular mass and posterior movement of the right articular mass, the leftward lateral mass increases in width because of a larger radiographic shadow, whereas the right lateral mass demonstrates a diminished width because of a narrower radiographic shadow. The facet joint on the left appears widened, and the right facet joint appears narrowed because of the corresponding slope of these joints. This abnormality produces the so-called wink sign[187] (Fig. 28-21). When plain cervical spine radiographs demonstrate evidence of a rotational anomaly at the atlantoaxial joint, additional radiographic investigation is indicated and should consist of open-mouth odontoid views with the patient's head rotated 15° to each side to determine whether true atlantoaxial fixation is present. Persistent asymmetry of the odontoid and its relationship to the articular masses of the atlas, with the asymmetry not being correctable by rotation, forms the basic radiologic criteria for the diagnosis of atlantoaxial rotatory fixation.[346] Additionally, cineradiography in the lateral projection may be considered if it is available. Alternatively, a CT scan through the C1-C2 articulation with the patient's head rotated to the right and to the left approximately 15° confirms or disproves the presence or absence of rotatory fixation at the atlantoaxial joint. Most commonly, acute or chronic traumatic injuries are in a fixed position. Currently, CT with two- or three-dimensional reconstruction gives the most accurate delineation of the injury. Flexion-extension lateral radiographs are also essential to inspect the integrity of the transverse atlantal ligament.

Rotatory fixation is a more appropriate term to describe the injury because rotatory subluxation of the atlas on the axis may be indicative of injury or may represent normal atlantoaxial rotation.[91,95] The radiographic classification system (types I–IV) by Fielding and associates[167] (Fig. 28-22)

FIGURE 28-20 | *The atlantoaxial joint in neutral position **(A)** and on rotation to the right **(B)**. With rotation, the anteroposterior view demonstrates (1) an apparent approximation of the left atlantal articular mass to the odontoid, (2) an increase in width of the left atlantal articular mass with decreased width of the right atlantal articular mass, and (3) a widened left and a narrowed right atlantoaxial joint because of the slope of these joints, as is evident on a lateral view. (Redrawn from Wortzman, G.; Dewar, F.P. Rotary fixation of the atlantoaxial joint: Rotational atlantoaxial subluxation. Radiology 90:479–487, 1960.)*

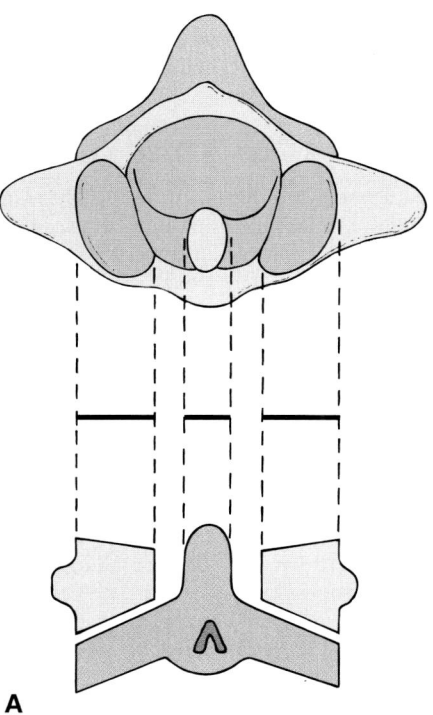

A

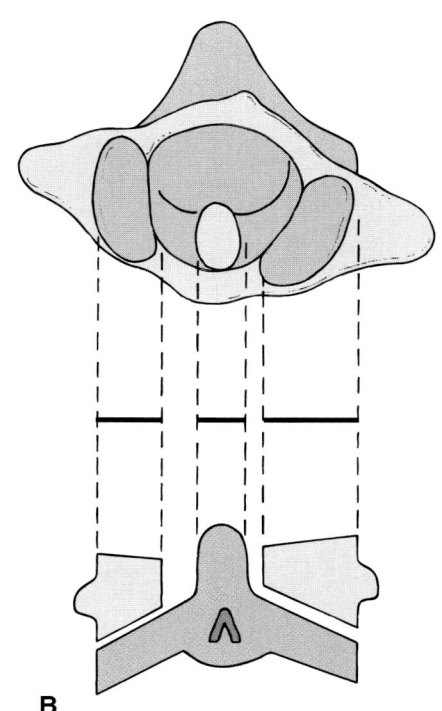

B

takes into account the integrity of the transverse ligament and the position of the facet joints. It was expanded on by Levine and Edwards to include frank rotatory dislocation (type V).[187]

Type I rotatory fixation, the most common, was seen in 47 percent of Fielding and associates' series and occurs within the normal range of motion.[167] The transverse ligament is intact and acts as the pivot point with anterior subluxation of one facet and posterior subluxation of the contralateral facet.

Type II rotatory fixation occurred with an associated deficiency of the transverse ligament and 3 to 5 mm anterior displacement of the atlas. It was the second most common injury (30%) and occurs with unilateral anterior displacement of one lateral mass of the atlas when the opposite intact joint acted as a pivot.

Type III rotatory fixation was seen with greater than 5 mm anterior displacement of the atlas on the axis and occurs with both transverse ligament and secondary stabilizer (alar ligaments, apical ligament, facet capsules) insufficiency. Both lateral masses of the atlas were subluxated anteriorly, one more than the other, thus producing the rotated position.

Type IV rotatory fixation, the most uncommon, was observed when there was posterior displacement of the atlas on the axis due to a deficient dens.

Type V, frank rotatory dislocation, may also be seen, although it is extremely uncommon.[167,187] The cause of this injury in adults is almost universally associated with trauma involving a flexion-rotation mechanism of injury. The atraumatic form in adults is very rare. Many different theories have been proposed, including effusion of the synovial joint producing attenuation of the ligaments,[343] facet synovial fringes from inflammation blocking atlantoaxial reduction,[58] rupture of one or both of the alar ligaments and transverse ligament,[98] or hyperemic decalcification with loosening of the ligaments.[326] Muscle spasms in addition to a combination of any one of the aforementioned possibilities may also play a role.[124,151] More recently, Fielding and colleagues noted that this injury is occasionally associated with lateral mass articular fractures and that muscle spasms occur secondarily as a result of inflammation.[92] They postulated that ligament and capsular contractures result in a fixed deformity.

Because of the rarity of the injury in adults, treatment recommendations in the literature are sparse. Although atlantoaxial rotatory instability in children usually responds to either immobilization or combined traction and immobilization,[300] this has yet to be proven in adults. In children, the most important factor in determining the efficacy of nonoperative management is the duration of rotatory subluxation. However, a recent adult case report

FIGURE 28-21 *Open-mouth radiograph showing a wink sign in which the lateral mass of C1 overlaps the lateral mass of C2 on the affected side (arrow). (From Levine, A. M.; Edwards, C.C. Traumatic lesions of the occipitoatlantoaxial complex. Clin Orthop Relat Res 239:53–68, 1989.)*

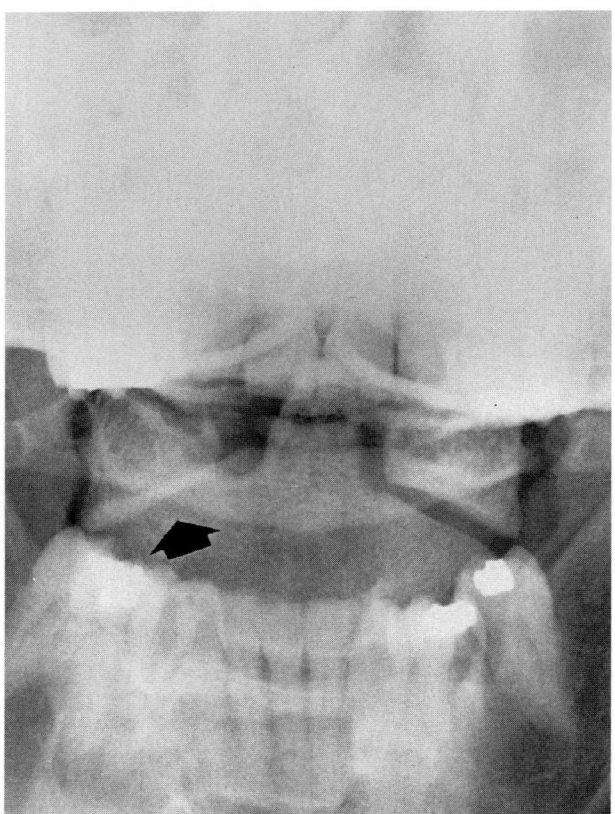

noted a rugby player presenting with a 4-week history of torticollis who was treated with halo traction for 10 days followed by gentle manipulation. The transverse ligament at that time was noted to be intact and the patient was treated in a Minerva jacket for 6 weeks, after which no rotatory instability was noted with dynamic CT studies.[46]

Levine and Edwards advocate manipulation for acute cases due to trauma. Traction should be applied to the patient while he or she is awake, and because the reduction can usually be heard and palpated transorally, topical anesthetic should be applied to the posterior pharynx. A halo should be applied if the injury is stable. C1-C2 arthrodesis is performed in the unstable injury. Arthrodesis can be done in situ and should be reserved for those cases that involve instability, neurologic involvement, or failure to maintain reduction.[187]

ODONTOID FRACTURES

As a result of their significant potential for neurologic injury and nonunion, no other injury of the upper cervical spine has generated as much controversy as fractures of the odontoid process. In the early 1900s, odontoid fractures were thought to be almost uniformly fatal. Later evaluations dropped the estimated mortality rate to approximately 50 percent, and more recent figures indicate that the mortality rate is approximately 4 to 11 percent.[7,12,16,94,125] These figures may be misleading in that some patients with this injury may never reach the hospital because of rapidly fatal brainstem or spinal cord injury. This scenario is probably more a possibility than a reality inasmuch as Bohler in an autopsy series reported only one case of fatal quadriplegia from an odontoid fracture.[26] The overall incidence of odontoid fractures ranges from 7 to 14 percent of all cervical fractures,[16,26,61,223,266] and as with most other injuries to the upper cervical spine, they are usually the result of falls or motor vehicle accidents.[12,16,50,125,217,292]

An understanding of the ligamentous anatomy of this region allows the physician to understand the problems associated with fractures of the dens such as instability and incorrect healing. The dens is connected to the occiput and the atlas by a number of small structures, the importance of which has been recently unveiled (see Fig. 28-2). From the cephalic aspect of the dens, the single apical ligament extends vertically to attach to the anterior rim of the foramen magnum. Furthermore, the paired alar ligaments fan out in a rostral direction and have multiple fibers or bands with different attachment sites. The occipital portion, or band, attaches to the anterior lip of the foramen magnum and occipital condyles on either side. An atlantal portion, or band, is also present in some people that attaches to the

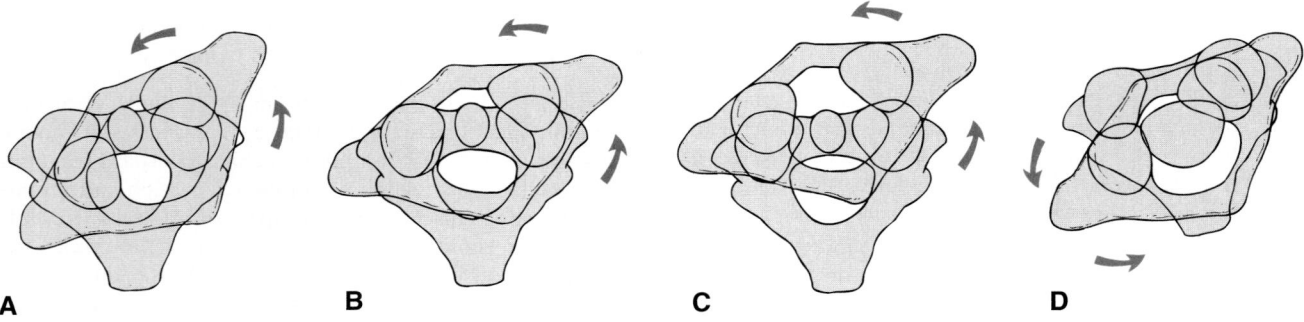

FIGURE 28-22 *Drawings showing the four types of rotatory fixation.* **A,** *Type I: rotatory fixation with no anterior displacement and the odontoid acting as the pivot.* **B,** *Type II: rotatory fixation with anterior displacement of 3 to 5 mm and one lateral articular process acting as the pivot.* **C,** *Type III: rotatory fixation with anterior displacement of more than 5 mm.* **D,** *Type IV: rotatory fixation with posterior displacement.*

A   **B**   **C**   **D**

lateral aspect of the anterior arch of C1.[75] The transverse ligament arises from the anteromedial aspect of the lateral masses of the atlas, curves posteriorly around the dens, and is separated from the dens by a small synovial joint (see Fig. 28-3). Furthermore, accessory ligaments arise in conjunction with the transverse ligament along the C1 lateral masses and insert near the base of the dens.

The odontoid is the main stabilizer to posterior displacement of the atlas on the axis (see Fig. 28-2). It functions to mechanically abut the posterior aspect of the anterior atlantal arch. It also serves as the point at which the transverse ligament is attached so as to prevent anterior translation. The facet joints of the atlantoaxial complex provide minimal stability, and the secondary stabilizers (e.g., the cruciform ligament and the atlantal portion of the alar ligament) become disrupted with odontoid fractures. Therefore, depending on the level at which the dens is fractured, anterior-posterior stability may be lost.[271] The exact mechanism of injury is unknown but probably involves a combination of forces.[5,36,217,287]

The vascular anatomy is important to consider given the problems with healing. The paired right and left posterior and anterior ascending arteries, arising from the vertebral arteries, form the principal blood supply to the dens. Although they do not provide direct branches to the dens, the paired carotid arteries have perforating branches that anastomose with the anterior ascending arteries. The ascending arteries penetrate the axis at the base of the dens and also continue outside the dens in a cephalad direction to form the apical arcade over the tip of the dens. Thus, although regarded as tenuous, the blood supply to the dens is provided from both a cephalad and caudal entrance point, and the concept of end-vessel supply does not exist as is seen with the scaphoid in the wrist. Certainly, fractures of the base of the dens may cause damage to the vessels in this area and create problems with healing[272] (Fig. 28-23). However, Govender and

associates showed that blood supply to the odontoid fragment is not compromised with odontoid fractures. In their study, they did selective vertebral angiography on 18 patients, 10 with acute fractures and 8 with nonunion, and found no differences between the two groups.[119] Therefore, the high nonunion rates of many odontoid fractures may result from other factors such as the degree of displacement, motion, the presence of synovial fluid, and soft tissue interposition.[292] Furthermore, autopsy retrieval studies of odontoid nonunion have not shown evidence of osteonecrosis, so this notion has for the most part been discarded, and many authors espouse the view that the odontoid actually has a rich blood supply.[7]

As alluded to previously, the dens is essentially an intra-articular structure that is bathed in synovial fluid that creates an unfavorable internal milieu around the fracture.[36] Also, with all the soft tissue stabilizers attaching to the dens, it is plausible that distraction of the fractured ends from each other allows soft tissue interposition to occur as shown by Crockard and co-workers. They reported several cases in which the transverse ligament was caught between the fracture fragment of the odontoid process and the body of C2.[60] Another factor was brought into question by Govender and associates when they showed that the difference in surface area between type II and type III fractures was statistically significant;[119] this may account for the discrepancy in healing rates between the two fracture types.

As with other injuries to the craniocervical junction, most of these injuries result from motor vehicle accidents or falls, and a high percentage of patients have distracting injuries, which may make diagnosis difficult.[36,282] Other factors such as head trauma, drug and alcohol abuse, fractures in the elderly with dementia, and the occurrence of concomitant cervical spine fractures may cause these injuries to be overlooked on initial evaluation.[125,204,292] Neurologic deficit, which is seen in only 25 percent of patients, may range from high tetraplegia with respiratory

FIGURE 28-23 *Vascular anatomy of the odontoid process.*

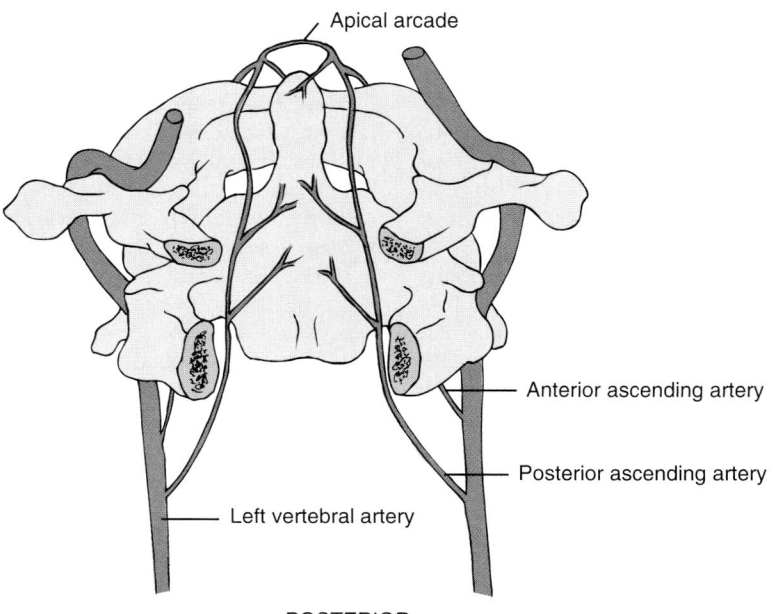

POSTERIOR

center involvement to minimal motor and sensory weakness.[7,292] In addition, some of these injuries are not evident initially, but patients may present much later in life with neck pain or spasms, myelopathic symptoms, or accident-induced neurologic deficit secondary to nonunion.[37,236]

Because of the variations in dens fracture presentation and natural history, it is important to appropriately image and rule out associated cervical spine injuries by appropriate plain radiographs and CT.[78] This is particularly true in the elderly, as they may sustain an odontoid facture with very low energy injury such as a fall from standing height and then only present with neck pain. Widening of the prevertebral soft tissue space, as is occasionally found in lower cervical spine injuries, is relatively less frequent with injuries to C1 and C2.[222] However, an increase in the prevertebral soft tissue shadow greater than 10 mm anterior to the ring of C1 suggests an anterior fracture. In looking at the use of standard CT with minimally displaced fractures, Rubinstein and colleagues noted that 1-mm cuts should be used, and that the absence of a fracture line on reformatted images (coronal and sagittal) does not rule out the diagnosis.[262] Because standard CT images are gathered as axial slices, the odontoid fracture that lies in the same plane as the axial slice can go undetected. Even the reformatted coronal and sagittal images would not detect it since they are reconstructed from the axials. With the advent of helical CT scanning this shortcoming has been overcome, since the images are gathered in a spiral fashion. Multislice CT was recently been able to diagnose odontoid fractures more precisely, better visualizing the extent of comminution.[177] This might play a role in fracture classification and treatment.

Anderson and D'Alonzo classified these injuries into three anatomic types based on the location of the fracture line[7] (Fig. 28-24). Type I fractures are the least common and represent avulsion fractures via the alar ligament attachment and are more likely as part of an occipitocervical dissociation. Type II fractures, which account for approximately 60 percent in most series, occur at the junction of the vertebral body with the base of the odontoid. Management of these injuries is most controversial because of the significant potential for nonunion.[70,93,125,222,282] Type III fractures involve the body of the axis and account for approximately 30 percent of odontoid fractures. Not included in the Anderson and D'Alonzo classification is a vertical fracture extending from the odontoid process continuing inferiorly through the body of C2.[21] It may represent a variant of a C2 traumatic spondylolisthesis to be discussed later.

Recently a study was performed to look at the reliability and reproducibility of diagnosis using plain films and CT. In this study, the authors look specifically at the distinction between type II and type III fractures using the Anderson and D'Alonzo classification. They found that inter- and intraobserver reliability was increased by the use of CT; however, there was still a wide range of interobserver reliability with the use of CT, albeit better than the range of reliability that was noted using plain films. Thus the authors question the validity of fracture classification data even with the use of CT and point out that previous studies based on the Anderson and D'Alonzo system may be affected by data reliability and

FIGURE 28-24	*Three types of odontoid fractures as seen in the anteroposterior (left) and lateral (right) planes. Type I is an oblique fracture through the upper part of the odontoid process itself. Type II is a fracture at the junction of the odontoid process and the vertebral body of the second cervical vertebra. Type III is really a fracture through the body of the atlas. (Redrawn from Anderson, L.D.; D'Alonzo, R.T. Fractures of the odontoid process of the axis. J Bone Joint Surg [Am] 56:1663–1674, 1974.)*

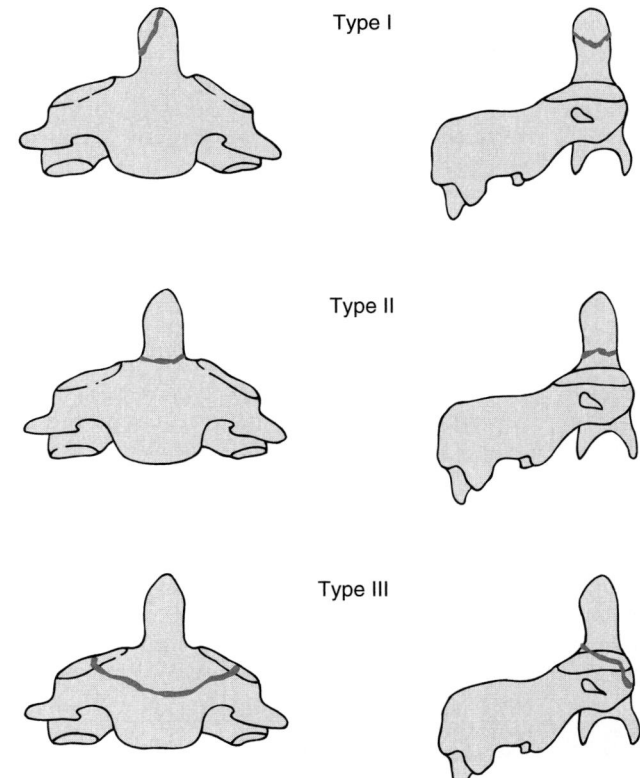

Type I

Type II

Type III

reproducibility.[19] A more recent classification method proposed by Grauer and co-workers focuses on a treatment-oriented classification system. Type II fractures are located below the inferior aspect of the C1 ring and do not involve superior articular facets of C2. Type II fractures are broken down into subtypes: IIA—no comminution and displacement less than 1 mm; IIB—fractures that pass obliquely anterior–superior to posterior-inferior or greater than 1 mm displacement; and IIC—anterior–inferior to posterior–superior with comminution.[120]

Treatment for odontoid fractures depends on the type of fracture as well as patient factors. Type I fractures represent an avulsion fracture of the alar or apical ligaments and are typically treated nonoperatively. These injuries do not compromise the integrity of the atlanto-dens articulation, but they may be of more clinical significance than once thought. Some authors have noted that type I odontoid fracture requires disruption of the occipital portion of at least one of the alar ligaments as well as disruption of part of tectorial membrane.[310] Furthermore, avulsion of the alar ligament off the odontoid process may, in fact, radiographically point to occipital-cervical instability.[275] As such, one must at least consider injury to the occipitoatlantal region with flexion-extension lateral radiographs or MRI. As an isolated fracture, these injuries tend to heal quite well with a brief period of simple collar immobilization.[7]

Surgical versus nonsurgical treatment for type II and III fractures has been reported. Attaining union with type II fractures is the most problematic and will be discussed in depth shortly. Problems associated with obtaining union with type III fractures are relatively less common.[292] Nondisplaced and minimally displaced type III fractures can be managed with external immobilization. Whether the immobilization method employs a halo vest or other lesser device such as a Minerva jacket or simple hard collar depends on various factors such as energy of the injury, comorbidities, and patient age. Some type III injuries can be more problematic to treat than previously thought.[50] Cervical orthoses are probably not adequate to manage significantly displaced or angulated type III injuries. These fractures should be reduced in halo traction and held in rigid external immobilization until union is achieved.[2] Alternatively, "shallow" type III (type II by the Grauer classification) fractures have been found to heal well with screw osteosynthesis.[47,82,84,88] Bear in mind that malunion of odontoid fractures can ultimately lead to cervical myelopathy[60] and post-traumatic C1-C2 arthrosis. Furthermore, vertically unstable type III odontoid fractures with distraction of atlantoaxial facet joints, cranial nerve palsy, or craniocervical subarachnoid hemorrhage have been reported.[162,248] With type III odontoid fractures and vertical instability, some recommend 5 mm of vertical displacement as the cut-off point for surgical stabilization with C1-C2 posterior arthrodesis.[174] These injuries can be associated with circumferential disruption of anterior atlantoaxial ligament, tectorial membrane, and facet joint capsules.[1]

Type II odontoid fractures are by far the most problematic to treat, and a great deal of controversy surrounds how best to do so based on the likelihood of achieving union and how to avoid creating additional complications. Patients with type II odontoid fractures fall into two groups: the young patient who suffers a high-energy injury and the elderly who usually suffer a low-energy impact via a fall from a standing height. In the next section we devote more time to discussing the elderly subgroup, since they generate the most controversy. Three modes of treatment are available: a simple hard collar, a halo vest, and surgery (surgery can be via an anterior odontoid screw or posterior C1-C2 fusion). Many studies of odontoid fractures include type III fractures, and the following sections will discuss type III as well as type II patterns.

Information in the literature regarding successful healing of type II odontoid fractures varies to a great extent, with the reported incidence of nonunion ranging from 10 to 60 percent.[271,304] As is the case with fractures elsewhere in the body, odontoid fracture healing in large part depends on a good reduction and subsequent stabilization. Factors associated with nonunion include displacement greater than 4 to 5 mm[12,50,119,139] and angulation greater than 10°.[50] Nonunion rates of up to 40 percent can be seen with significant displacement regardless of the treatment method. When angulation is greater than 10°, the nonunion rate approximates 22 percent.[50] In addition, posterior displacement and delays in beginning treatment negatively affect union rates.[178] Successful healing of type II odontoid fractures varies to a great extent depending on the type of treatment.

Some recent evidence suggests that even nonrigid immobilization with hard collars for odontoid fractures may be suitable. Muller and colleagues retrospectively reviewed 26 patients with acute type II and III fractures of the odontoid with an average follow-up of 25.4 months. The study variables included a fracture gap of less than 2 mm, initial anteroposterior displacement of less than 5 mm, angulation of less than 11°, less than 2 mm of displacement on lateral flexion-extension views, and no neurologic deficits. Only two patients eventually had internal stabilization due to persistent instability defined as more than 2 mm of motion of the dens in flexion–extension views.[218]

Union rates with halo immobilization for type II and type III fractures have been reported to be 66 percent and 93 percent, respectively.[12,50] A meta-analysis to determine the outcome of immobilization in a halo vest revealed an 85 percent union rate with type II fractures, and a 96 percent union rate for type III odontoid fractures.[321] A recent case-control study by Lennarson and co-workers defined cases as those with nonunion after halo immobilization and controls as those with successful bony union attained with halo immobilization. The groups were similar with respect to concomitant medical conditions, gender ratios, amount of fracture displacement, direction of fracture displacement, length of hospital stay, and length of follow-up. The authors found age to be a significant factor in outcomes, with the odds ratio indicating that the risk of failure of halo immobilization is 21 times higher in patients 50 years or older.[185] Koivikko and associates retrospectively identified factors contributing to nonunion in patients treated with halo vest immobilization. Factors that were identified included (1) fracture gap greater than 1 mm, (2) posterior displacement greater than 5 mm, (3) delayed start of treatment (>4 days), and (4) posterior redisplacement greater than 2 mm. Interestingly, the authors did not identify the variables associated with decision to perform primary surgical stabilization.[178]

Surgical treatment can be via anterior screws or posterior C1-C2 fusion. Screw fixation union rates range from 92 to 100 percent,[47,84,88,269] and stabilization rates associated with posterior spinal fusion have been reported to be on the order of 96 to 100 percent.[12,50,130,163,288] In looking at factors affecting screw fixation, Fountas and colleagues performed a retrospective analysis on 50 consecutive patients with reducible type II or rostral type III odontoid fractures treated with anterior screw fixation. Age, gender, and number of screws implanted had no effect on fusion rates or clinical outcomes.[101] Borm and co-workers, however, specifically looked at the effect of age on screw fixation outcomes. They demonstrated in a case-control study that fusion rates were similar between a group of patients younger than 70 and a group older than 70.[29] Greene and associates suggested that MRI can be used to detect concomitant transverse ligament injury with odontoid fractures and suggested that nonoperative treatment in such a situation should be avoided because of the possibility of late instability.[122] Anterior screw fixation is also relatively contraindicated in such situations due to the potential risk of rotation instability. Posterior wiring or C1-C2 transarticular screws and fusion produce good results in stabilization of C1-C2[134,170] in such circumstances. Posterior fusion is also preferred for nonunions, in reverse oblique fractures such as a IIC fracture according to Grauer, and in cases of an osteoporotic C2 vertebral body. In some atypical fractures, the usual bony fixation points are not available and techniques to span the fractured vertebrae may be necessary (Fig. 28-25).

In addition to considering factors that contribute to nonunion, the possibility of acute or late-presenting neurologic deficits must be considered when determining treatment. Przybylski and colleagues noted a 55 percent prevalence of subarachnoid hemorrhage at the C2 level and a 15 percent rate of dural laceration or brainstem injury in odontoid fractures

with atlantoaxial dislocation.[246] A retrospective analysis looked at the direction of displacement and respiratory compromise. The study showed that 13 of 32 patients with posteriorly displaced type II fractures experienced respiratory problems during reduction, whereas only 1 of 21 patients with anterior displacement had problems during reduction. The authors felt that closed reduction using a flexed position in patients with posterior displacement should undergo elective intubation prior to performing reduction, although this is not commonly done.[247] Also worth considering is the posterior atlanto-dens interval (PADI). In looking at the PADI in rheumatoid patients (without odontoid fractures) Boden and co-workers noted that less than 14 mm of PADI was the critical value below which neurologic compromise became more frequent.[25] Hart and associates retrospectively looked at nonoperative management of dens nonunions that were classified as chronic, unstable injuries. All patients had a minimum PADI of 14 mm at initial presentation and none of

---

FIGURE 28-25 *A C2 lateral mass fracture shown on axial **(A)**, coronal **(B)**, and sagittal **(C)** CT study with an associated base of the dens fracture. This complicates the surgical treatment options because the lateral mass at C2 is not available as a fixation point. **D**, A posterior fusion spanning C1 to C3 was used in this patient.*

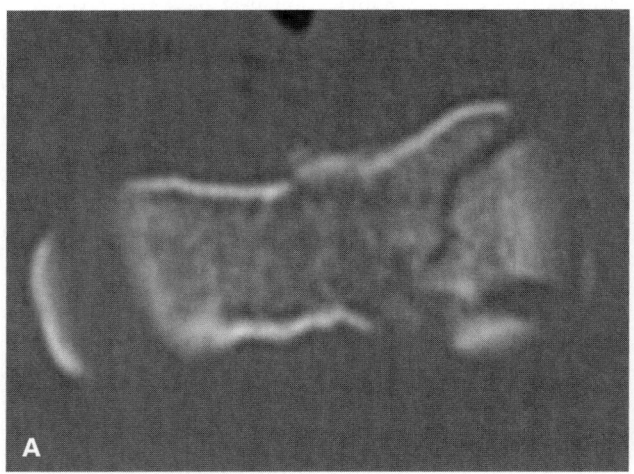

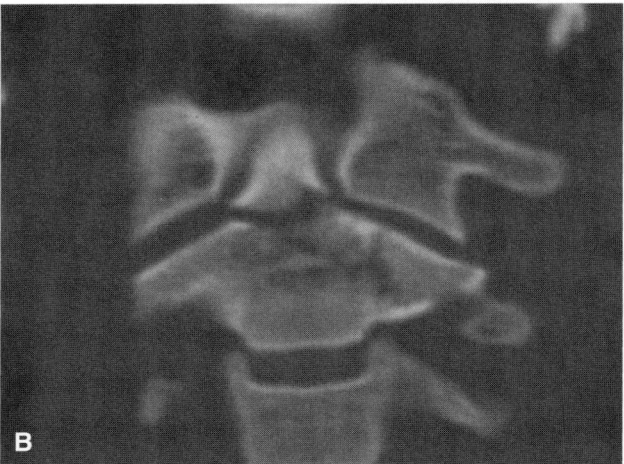

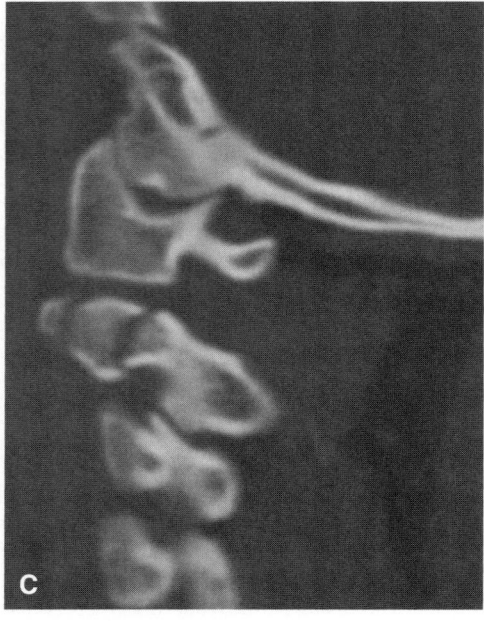

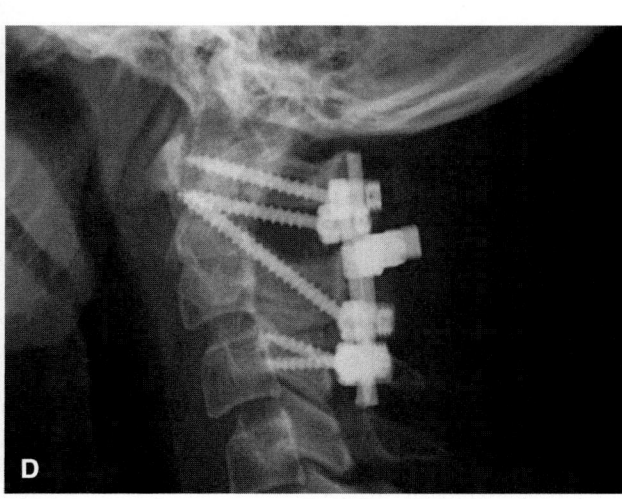

the patients developed neurologic symptoms or significant radiographic changes.[144] The existence of late neurologic problems has been reported and studied by Kirankumar and colleagues, who looked at 19 patients with myelopathy and remote, isolated type II odontoid fractures (defined as presenting at more than 6 months after injury) with atlantoaxial dislocation. Patients were excluded if they had any signs or symptoms of myelopathy prior to initial date of injury, and the majority of patients presented with spasticity and limb weakness. The authors divided the patients into two groups based on dynamic radiographic findings (reducible and irreducible). Reducible lesions were treated by realignment and posterior fusion, whereas irreducible fractures were treated with transoral decompression and posterior fusion. All but three patients in the study showed improvement in their neurologic status with a mean follow-up of 15 months, and no patients showed deterioration.[173]

The correct decision to proceed with surgical fixation versus nonoperative management has not been borne out in randomized clinical studies. An evidence-based analysis of odontoid fracture management reviewed 95 articles based on the American Medical Association data classification schema. No class I or class II papers could be identified, and thus the observations made were based on class III data. The authors noted that the evidence reviewed is insufficient to accurately determine optimal treatment guidelines.[168]

Nonetheless, despite the confusion and inconsistency in the literature, some generally accepted guidelines can be noted. It is reasonable initially to manage nondisplaced or minimally displaced type II injuries by attempting closed reduction and halo immobilization for 12 weeks, particularly in younger patients. Although C1-C2 fusion is a reasonable alternative with good results shown in the literature, 50 percent of normal cervical rotation is also sacrificed. The attractiveness of odontoid screw fixation lies in preservation of atlantoaxial motion, as well as negation of the need for halo immobilization or posterior fusion.[147] As such, patients with type II injuries that demonstrate inadequate reduction or redisplacement and those initially seen more than 2 weeks after injury[266] should be considered candidates for surgical stabilization. It is important to note that one study revealed type II fractures fixed within first 6 months of injury with direct screw fixation had a fusion rate of 88 percent, whereas those fractures treated after 18 months had only a 25 percent fusion rate.[11] Thus, if the fracture does not heal with external fixation within 6 months, then surgical intervention should be considered, keeping in mind that anterior odontoid screw fixation may still have reasonable success.[11,47,88]

FRACTURES IN OLDER PATIENTS

Upper cervical spine fractures in older patients are important to recognize and treat appropriately due to mortality rates approaching 25 to 30 percent.[26,328] These injuries are relatively more frequent in the elderly and can occur via lower energy mechanisms. They account for up to 23 percent of all cervical fractures.[187] The incidence of C1-C2 fractures progressively rises with age because of the higher incidence of odontoid fractures in this patient group,[265] although there is a high incidence of combination

C1 and C2 fractures.[136,328] The effect of aging was studied by Lakshmanan and co-workers, who proposed that the atlanto-odontoid joint is significantly affected by osteoarthritis, whereas the atlantoaxial facet joints are relatively unaffected. The odontoid becomes fixed to the anterior arch of the atlas, but the atlantoaxial facet joints still maintain their mobility. This, combined with limitation of movement and stiffness of osteoarthritic facet joints more caudally, results in biomechanical vulnerability of the odontoid in the elderly.[179]

Management of cervical spine fractures in older patients is made difficult by preexisting medical conditions, poor ability to tolerate halo immobilization, and poor healing potential. The decision to treat with immobilization or surgery remains controversial. As previously mentioned, most studies provide only level III evidence with limited numbers, so definite conclusions cannot be drawn[26,166,192,193,231,239,291,306,328] although certain trends can be identified. Olerud and colleagues retrospectively noted that cervical spine fractures carried an increased risk of death in patients older than 65 years. In addition to age, they found that severe comorbidity (ASA physical status classification >2), neurologic injury (Frankel grades A to C), and ankylosing spondylitis were also significant risk factors for death.[231] Likewise, Finelli and colleagues found that for a given level of injury severity, trauma in the elderly population results in increased mortality in comparison with younger persons.[96]

Many investigators have noted that halos can be tolerated by patients in this subset.[26,166,328] The purported advantages are no surgical risks and rapid mobilization. However, several studies also maintain that halos are fraught with a high complication[278] and nonunion rate.[185] Lennarson and co-workers found that an age older than 50 years was found to be a highly significant risk factor for nonunion of odontoid fractures in patients treated with halo immobilization. In their case-control study, these investigators found that the risk of nonunion with halo immobilization is 21 times higher in patients 50 years or older. They thus advocate surgical intervention in this patient cohort who have a type II dens fracture, if the procedure can be performed with acceptable risks of morbidity and death.[185] Taitsman et al. recently examined the rate of complications associated with halo immobilization in patients older than 65[306] and found a relatively high complication rate, including pin problems (29%), aspiration pneumonia (23%), and significant respiratory compromise or arrest necessitating intubation or tracheostomy and intensive care management (17%). In looking at short-term morbidity and mortality rates with halo vest versus without halo vest immobilization (HVI) in patients older than 65, a recent study showed statistically greater and clinically significant complications rates in the HVI group than in the non-HVI group. The authors report no baseline difference between the two groups in injury severity or medical conditions.[307] Another recent study examined different types of treatment in the young versus the old, including HVI, collar, and surgery. Patients with any type of cervical spine fracture were divided retrospectively into two groups: those older than 65 and those between the ages of 18 and 65. Older patients had much higher mortality rates than younger ones among those treated with HVI, and there was no baseline difference between young and old in injury severity score (ISS), Glasgow Coma Score (GCS), or emergency department systolic blood pressure. Older patients treated with HVI also had much higher mortality rates than other elderly patients treated with surgery or collar, with no statistical difference evident in age, ISS, GCS, or comorbidities between the two groups.[200]

Seybold and Bayley evaluated the functional outcome of surgically (posterior fusion) and conservatively managed dens fractures with regard to age and fracture type.[278] They found that the long-term functional outcome of halo immobilization is not significantly worse than that for surgical patients. However, patients older than age 60 had significantly higher complication rates (increased pin loosening rates, shoulder discomfort, dysphagia) and decreased cervical range of motion when treated with HVI. Furthermore, although not statistically significant, some trends toward improved outcome scores were seen in the elderly treated operatively.

Screw osteosynthesis versus posterior spinal fusion in the elderly has also been studied retrospectively. In their retrospective analysis, Andersson and colleagues note that anterior screw fixation is associated with an unacceptably high rate of problems in the elderly population. This may be due to osteoporotic bone or difficulty with optimal patient positioning intraoperatively to obtain correct screw trajectory. They also cite pitfalls with nonoperative treatment and advocate posterior C1-C2 fusion.[10,23] To the contrary, a long-term fusion rate of 87 percent has been reported for anterior screw fixation, which is comparable to other large, but short-term clinical studies. Time to fusion can average 11.2 months,[100] although in some other studies it ranges from 14.1 weeks to 8 months.[3,147] An alternative safe option that avoids anterior screw fixation and HVI is posterior C1-C2 fusion.[43] Keep in mind, however, the long-term morbidity due to neck pain and pain associated with autogenous bone graft harvesting in posterior spinal fusions.[89]

The most recent literature seems to suggest that, although more uniformly successful in younger patients, halo treatment of odontoid fractures in the elderly remains an option but should be exercised with caution given the much higher complication and failure rates. Furthermore, fusion for those patients who can tolerate surgery, and especially those with significant angulation and displacement, results in more predictable outcomes. The surgeon who favors aggressive treatment should bear in mind that odontoid fracture nonunion can ultimately lead to acceptable clinical results. Nonoperative treatment with a simple collar can be considered in this group of patients, particularly if dementia is present or the patient has low functional demands.[198,244]

TRAUMATIC SPONDYLOLISTHESIS OF THE AXIS

Due to the radiographic similarities, the term *hangman's fracture*, also known as traumatic spondylolisthesis of the axis, has been used extensively in the literature to describe both the injury produced by judicial hanging as well as similar fractures from other mechanisms.[33,35,57]

The historic nature of these injuries has been described,[146,319,344] but Schneider and co-workers in 1965 actually coined the phrase hangman's fracture because of the radiographic similarity they detected to the injuries produced by judicial hanging.[273] The judicial hanging uniformly results in hyperextension and distraction with complete disruption of the C2-C3 disk space and associated ligaments between them.[283,319,344] The bilateral fractures through the C2 pars interarticularis observed with hanging can also occur via falls and motor vehicle accidents from various combinations of extension, axial compression, and flexion and consequent varying degrees of disk disruption.[57,110,132,273,308,342] In fatal motor vehicle accidents, only occipitoatlantal dislocations are more common.[35] Traumatic spondylolisthesis of the axis is also noted to be approximately half as common (a reported incidence of 27%) as odontoid fractures in patients who have sustained cervical trauma in motor vehicle accidents.[137] The anatomic nomenclature must be kept in mind when describing these injuries. Although the pars interarticularis of the axis and the pedicle of the axis are, strictly speaking, two distinct anatomic structures, the two terms have been used interchangeably in the literature. The C2 pedicle is the area between the vertebral body and the articular column, whereas the pars interarticularis is the thin, bony bridge between the superior and inferior axis facets.

The axis is mechanically vulnerable due to its anatomy and corresponding function. The articulating surfaces of the axis serve as a transition point between the more anterior occiput–dens–atlas articulation and the posterior facet articulations of the subaxial spine. The pars interarticularis functions as a bridge between the two points and essentially acts as a fulcrum in flexion and extension between the cervicocranium (skull, atlas, dens, and body of the axis) and the relatively fixed lower cervical spine, to which the neural arch of the axis is anchored by its inferior articular facets, stout bifid spinous process, and strong nuchal muscles.[33,342]

As with most injuries of the upper cervical spine, traumatic spondylolisthesis tends to produce acute decompression of the neural canal, and neurologic involvement is relatively uncommon in survivors (seen in 6–10%).[33,35,57,102,103,273] However, reports of atypical hangman's fractures that involve the posterior C2 vertebral body have shown the potential for spinal canal compromise[295] with displacement of the vertebral body fragment into the canal (Fig. 28-26). Some case reports of these injuries describe treatment in a closed fashion with subsequent neurologic deterioration due to development of a large epidural hematoma.[38] Craniofacial trauma is very common with these injuries,[103,240] and vertebral artery and cranial nerve injuries have also been reported.[238] Associated cervical spine injuries with C2 traumatic spondylolisthesis almost always involve the upper three cervical vertebrae.[102,103]

Stability of this injury has been shown to be related to the integrity of the ligaments and disk between the C2-C3 bodies[35] and can be determined radiographically.[77] The most recent and most useful classification is that proposed by Levine and Edwards, which is essentially a modification of Effendi and associates' radiographic

FIGURE 28-26 | *The typical hangman's fracture **(B)** displaces the vertebral body anteriorly and its corresponding posterior element posteriorly, thus creating increased space for the spinal cord. Whereas, the atypical hangman's fracture line **(A)** leaves the canal circumferentially intact and puts the spinal cord at risk if displaced.*

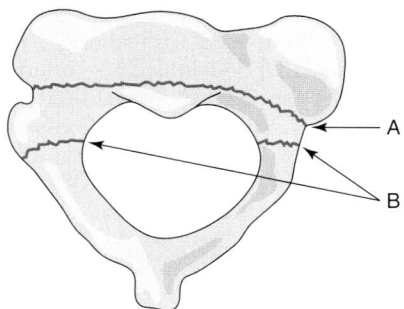

system.[77,186] The classification system takes into account both angulation of the dens and displacement of the C2 body in relation to the C3 body. The integrity of the C2-C3 discoligamentous complex (disk proper, anterior longitudinal ligament, and posterior longitudinal ligament) is considered based on the radiographic findings:

Type I fractures are nondisplaced and show no angulation and less than 3 mm of displacement (Fig. 28-27A). They usually result from a hyperextension and axial loading force that fractures the neural arch through the pars, and there is minimal disruption to the C2-C3 disk.

Type II fractures have significant translation and some angulation (Fig. 28-27B). They usually result from a hyperextension and axial load (as seen with type I injuries) followed by flexion and compression. The combined forces result in disruption of the posterior longitudinal ligament and disk in a posterior-to-anterior direction and, frequently, a compression fracture of the C3 anterior-superior end plate.

FIGURE 28-27 | *Classification of traumatic spondylolisthesis of the axis. **A,** Type I injuries have a fracture through the neural arch with no angulation and as much as 3 mm of displacement. **B,** Type II fractures have both significant angulation and displacement. **C,** Type IIA fractures show minimal displacement, but severe angulation is present. **D,** Type III axial fractures combine bilateral facet dislocation between C2 and C3 with a fracture of the neural arch of the axis. (**A-C,** From Levine, A.M.; Edwards, C.C. The management of traumatic spondylolisthesis of the axis. J Bone Joint Surg [Am] 67:217–226, 1985. **D,** From Levine, A.M.; Edwards, C.C. Treatment of injuries in the C1-C2 complex. Orthop Clin North Am 17:42, 1986.)*

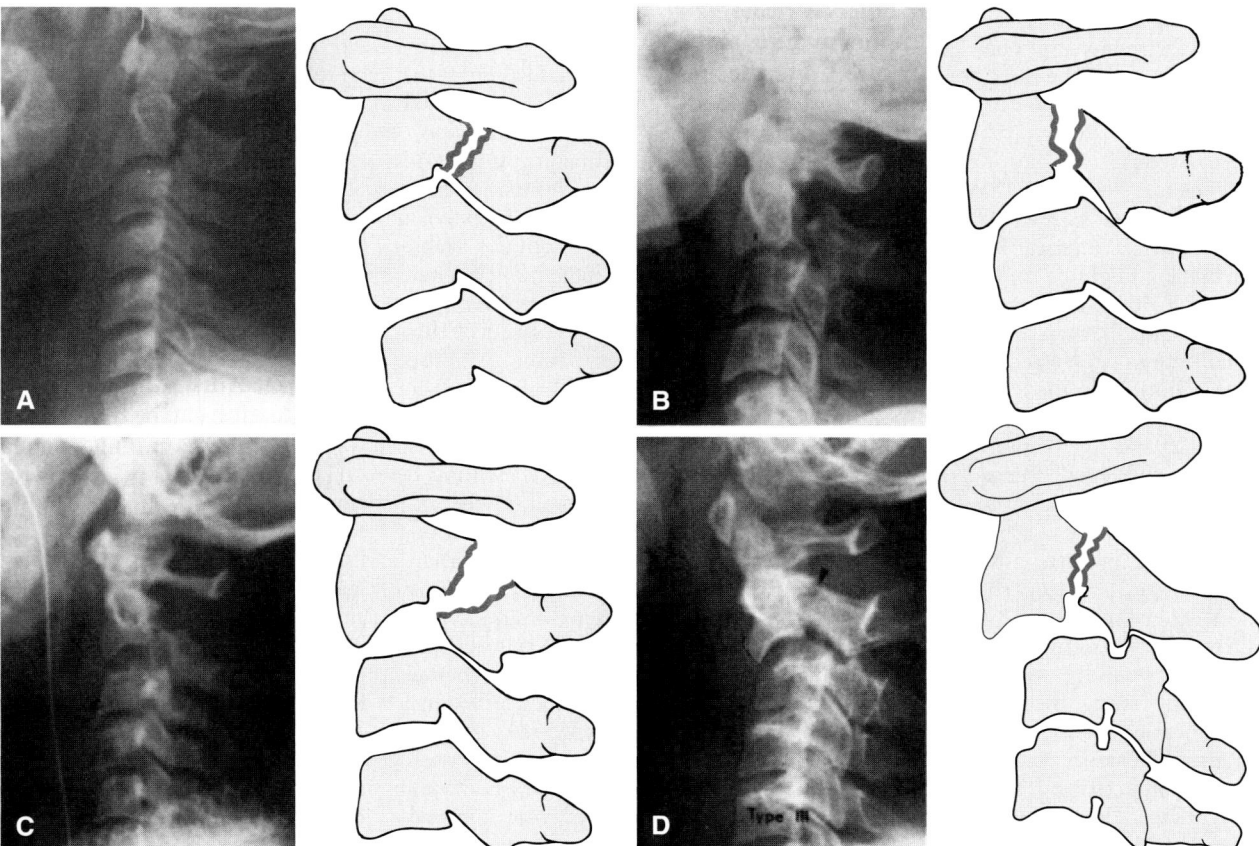

Type IIA fractures show slight or no translation but severe angulation of the fracture fragments (Fig. 28-27C). This fracture pattern is seen with flexion and distraction and results in a vertical tear of the posterior longitudinal ligament and the disk.

Type III fractures have severe angulation and severe displacement, as well as concomitant unilateral or bilateral facet dislocations at the level of C2 and C3 (Fig. 28-27D). This pattern is thought to result from flexion and compression resulting in complete disruption of the discoligamentous complex.

Generally speaking, type I fractures are thought to be stable due to an intact C2-C3 discoligamentous complex; types II, IIA, and III are somewhat unstable because of some degree of disruption at the C2-C3 interspace. Type II fractures are the most common and are seen in 55.8 percent of patients, followed by type I injuries, type IIA, and type III, which account for 28.8 percent, 5.8 percent, and 9.6 percent of patients, respectively.

Although relatively benign, management of hangman's fractures is somewhat controversial.[33,203,273] The vast majority of these injuries do well with conservative treatment,[33,77,103,133,186,203,240,277,308] and the nonunion rate with external immobilization is approximately 5 percent.[33,102,331] However, because of problems associated with external immobilization, persistent neck pain, instability, and variations in functional outcomes, some authors have continued to advocate primary surgical treatment.[30,57,203,259,308,342] Given the relatively good prognosis, a nonoperative approach is reasonable in most cases. Gross and Benzel reviewed a large number of nonoperatively managed hangman's fractures of any type that were available for follow-up. They noted a 98.5 percent union rate and found that the cases of nonunion were complicated by complex additional cervical injuries and completely disrupted C2-C3 intervertebral discs.[123,133] The ability to achieve osseous union despite incomplete or nonanatomic closed fracture reduction is well recognized;[55] thus, operative management is reserved for compressive type injuries (type II and III injuries) and for situations in which external bracing might be contraindicated.

As with other injuries involving the spine, the treatment depends largely on associated instability. Marton and colleagues suggested that instability of hangman's fractures be determined by the integrity of the C2-C3 disk–ligament entity, and that angulation of the dens between 20 and 35° or more would suggest that the posterior longitudinal ligament and posterior disk must be disrupted.[207] Coric and co-workers defined instability with static and dynamic plain films, suggesting that instability occurs with more than 6 mm of anterior displacement and greater than 2 mm of movement on flexion-extension radiographs. All patients in their study had stability as defined by their criteria and all were treated successfully with nonrigid immobilization.[55] A cadaveric study by Arand and associates looked at the implication of an insufficient posterior longitudinal ligament. The authors showed that stability in flexion was most affected by an intact PLL and that direct osteosynthesis alone in such situations does not provide adequate stability. They recommend that anterior plating should be performed in the presence of damage to the posterior discoligamentous structures.[13] Muller and colleagues used Effendi's classification to correlate with stability. The authors state that with "type II flexion injuries" (IIA as proposed by Levine and Edwards) the axis body hinges on the intact anterior longitudinal ligament (ALL), and they recommend treatment with rigid external fixation. With "type II extension injuries" the axis body hinges around an intact PLL with the ALL and disk both being disrupted. These injuries, however, are stable and can be treated with nonrigid immobilization. The "type II spondylolisthesis injuries," which include rupture of the C2-C3 disk as well as the ALL and PLL, are highly unstable and have greater potential for neurologic compromise.[219] The relationship between asymmetry and instability has also been evaluated. Many authors have alluded to the idea that asymmetry (fracture through the pars interarticularis on one side, and through pedicle/anterior articular column on the other) in hangman's fractures may result in instability and consequent nonunion. Asymmetry may be due to a rotational component of the mechanism of injury. The authors in one study noted 60 percent of patients with hangman's fractures had asymmetry, compared with 18 percent noted in previous studies.[40] More importantly, they found no relationship between asymmetry of the fracture (determined with CT) and instability as defined by greater than 3 mm of anterior translation and kyphosis greater than 15° or lordosis of more than 5°.[267]

According to Levine and Edwards, the stability of type I fractures should be assessed by physician-supervised flexion-extension radiographs.[186] Although varying degrees of reduction are noted with extension, these injuries are stable, and treatment with the Philadelphia collar or a halo until healing of the fracture is satisfactory. Type II and IIA fractures are noted to be unstable on physician-supervised flexion-extension radiographs, making such dynamic imaging unnecessary in these grades of injury. Treatment of these injuries is usually conservative, with halo or tongs traction in extension for a variable period of time depending on the stability of the reduction. Specific fracture reduction parameters that result in consistently good clinical outcomes have not been identified. However, less than 4 to 5 mm of displacement or less than 10 to 15° of angulation would be acceptable reduction parameters by most physicians for nonoperative management.

Although clear-cut indications for nonoperative management have not been established, some pertinent points deserve mention here. Watanabe and co-workers reviewed a small number of patients who were treated nonoperatively for an average of 62 months after injury and found that average angulation and translation were greater in patients who had residual neck pain. They also noted that the presence of an intra-articular fracture involving the inferior facet of the axis was present in patients with cervical pain.[325] Furthermore, it should be realized that longitudinal traction without an extension force causes further displacement of type IIA injuries and should be avoided.[161] Recently, Vaccaro and associates[316] retrospectively reviewed the effects of fracture angulation and displacement on outcomes with halo immobilization. In their study, type IIA fractures were reduced, and reduction was maintained after halo application. However, type II fractures that had initial angulation greater than 11.5° were less likely to maintain reduction after traction was removed. The authors also noted that the degree of initial versus "postreduction" fracture translation and angulation did not affect fracture healing or maintenance of reduction.

In their review of literature, Li and colleagues looked at healing rates (determined radiographically) of conservatively treated injuries with regard to fracture type. Rates decreased sequentially from type I to type III fractures. They reported healing rates of type IIa and III below 50 percent.[191] Alternatives to conservative treatment of type II and IIA fractures include the use of C2 direct osteosynthesis with screws, posterior C1-C2 fusion, or anterior C2-C3 cervical plate. The fracture must first be reduced either intraoperatively or with extended halo traction, and then fixation can be achieved with lag screws through the pars interarticularis (transpedicular technique) (Fig. 28-28) as described by Roy-Camille and co-workers.[176,260,261] However, it should be noted that in their reported series of 104 cases the results showed that screw fixation only (of the pars fractures) would be inadequate in patients with instability of the C2-C3 mobile segment because the construct did not prevent loss of disk height and kyphosis.

Anterior cervical plating for unstable, inadequately reduced Effendi type II fractures has also been reported with good results with no complications.[311] Advantages with anterior plating are the reconstitution of two columns of vertebral stability, the ability to address the disruption to the C2-C3 discoligamentous complex when it exists, as well as allowing for decompression in the presence of a herniated disk. Citing the results from other studies, Vichard and associates noted the value of anterior arthrodesis for C2 pedicle fractures and stated that posterior arthrodesis should be reserved for those injuries with concomitant odontoid fractures or other complex patterns (Fig. 28-29).[320] Verheggen and Jansen advocate surgical treatment for types II and III due to anatomic reduction, which better preserves atlantoaxial mobility, and recommend anterior C2-C3 discectomy and fusion in cases with traumatic disk herniation.[318]

Type III fractures (with unilateral or bilateral C2-C3 facet dislocations) almost always require surgery because of the difficulty in attaining reduction or persistent instability. In addition to the need for surgical stabilization, type III injuries are important to recognize because of higher mortality rates (33% vs. 5%), a higher incidence of permanent neurologic injury (11% vs. 1%), and a higher incidence of cerebral concussion (55% vs. 21%).[73] In dealing with these injuries, the treating physician must remember that the C2-C3 facet dislocation(s) is irreducible by closed means if the ipsilateral pars interarticularis is disrupted. Furthermore, if a facet fracture-dislocation occurs, or if an ipsilateral C2 laminar fracture occurs, then surgical stabilization by bilateral oblique wiring or lateral mass plating is necessary after reduction of the dislocation because the reduced facet dislocation is usually unstable. An alternative technique, when appropriate, would be transpedicular screws (through the pars interarticularis) in C2 and lateral mass screws in C3 along with the application of lateral mass plates (Fig. 28-30). Advantages and

disadvantages of the different techniques will be discussed in the next section. Keep in mind that HVI of the pars component is a reasonable option after open reduction internal fixation of the C2-C3 facets, assuming the fracture pattern is stable (i.e., the C2 fracture is anterior to the C2-C3 facet dislocation).

MISCELLANEOUS C2 FRACTURES

Lateral mass fractures of the C2 vertebra are rarely reported injuries and have a mechanism of injury similar to those causing lateral mass fractures of the atlas. Axial compression and lateral bending forces combine to compress the C1-C2 articulation and result in a depressed fracture of the articular surface of C2 (see Fig. 28-25). Patients generally have a history of pain without neurologic deficit. Plain radiographs may be unremarkable, although anteroposterior and open-mouth views sometimes demonstrate lateral tilting of the arch of C1 and asymmetry of the height of the C2 lateral mass. If lateral mass fracture is suspected, CT of the area is helpful to more clearly delineate the injury. A search for additional fractures in the cervical spine should also be made because these injuries are frequently combined with other C1-C2 fractures.[188,285]

Treatment is based on the degree of articular involvement. In patients in whom depression of the articular surface is slight and incongruity is minimal, simple collar immobilization is sufficient. More extensive involvement of the lateral mass may require cervical traction to realign the lateral mass, followed by HVI until healing has occurred. In those in whom articular incongruity remains, degenerative changes may occur after injury and necessitate C1-C2 or C1-C3 stabilization at a later date.

Teardrop fractures involving the axis are unusual but stable injuries associated with an extension-type mechanism and are not associated with neurologic injury. It should be recognized that they are very different from lower cervical spine teardrop injuries resulting from flexion, which are unstable and associated with neurologic injury 75 percent of the time. A distinguishable radiographic feature of extension-type (C2) teardrop fracture is rotation of the fragment 35° anteriorly. Conversely, a flexion-type teardrop fracture remains aligned with the anterior margin of the spine. A C2 extension-type teardrop fracture can be associated with traumatic spondylolisthesis of C2 and, if a stable concomitant spondylolisthesis exists, can be treated conservatively.

SURGICAL TECHNIQUES

Skeletal traction with either tongs or a halo is frequently indicated in the initial stabilization and ultimate management of upper cervical spine injuries. If traction is temporary for reduction and is to be followed by definitive surgical stabilization, then Gardner-Wells tongs would be used; but if traction reduction is to be followed by HVI, then traction can be applied with the halo. Considerations should include the nature of the injury, the presence or absence of other injuries such as skull fractures, and the estimated duration of treatment. Indications for the use of skeletal traction, as well as HVI, were discussed earlier in this chapter.

FIGURE 28-28 *Technique for screw fixation of a type II hangman's fracture. Fluoroscopy should be used, preferably biplanar, to visualize reduction of the fracture, as well as screw trajectory. **A,** The medial wall of the C2 pedicle should be visualized. Dissection performed in a posterior-to-anterior direction usually exposes the fracture of the pedicle. **B,** The trajectory of the screws should be along the line of the pedicle just lateral to the medial wall of the pedicle and slightly convergent. **C,** The screw should be oriented to capture the distal fragment with the screw threads. A lag screw can be used. The C1-C2 facet joint should be avoided. **D,** The final axial view. **E,** The patient has a markedly displaced type II traumatic spondylolisthesis of the axis, which can be totally reduced with traction **(F)**. **G,** Rather than prolonged traction, the patient elected operative treatment with lag screw fixation. (From Levine, A.M.; Eismont, F.J.; Garfin, S.R.; et al., eds. Spine Trauma. Philadelphia. W.B. Saunders, 1998, p. 293.)*

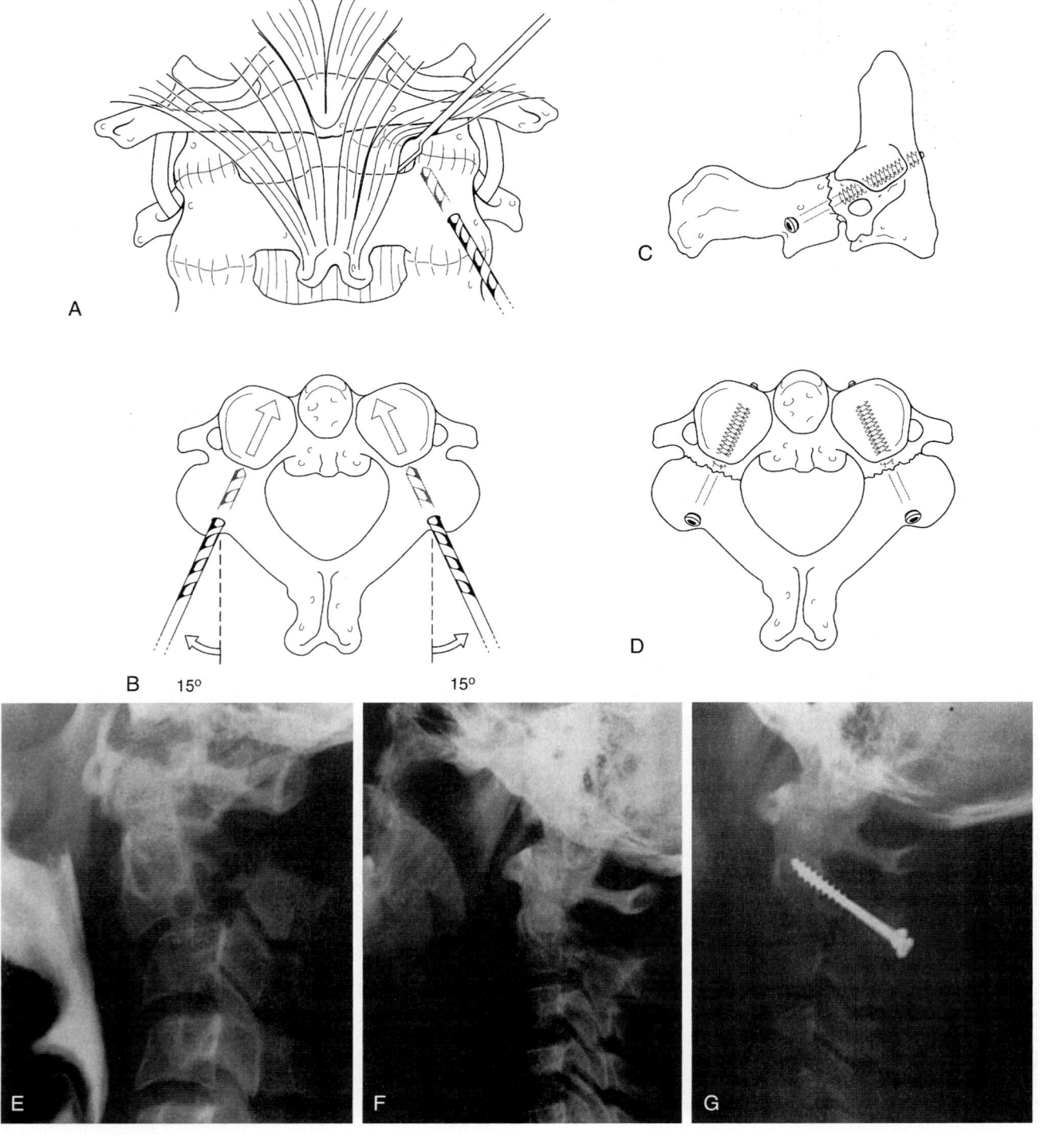

FIGURE 28-29   *A complex hangman's fracture with an associated odontoid fracture treated by posterior open reduction and C1-C3 instrumentation and fusion.* **A,** *Lateral x-ray with a displaced hangman's fracture and associated odontoid fracture.* **B,** *Sagittal CT scan demonstrating the odontoid component.* **C,** *The pars fracture.* **D,** *A lateral radiograph of the C1–C3 posterior fusion.*

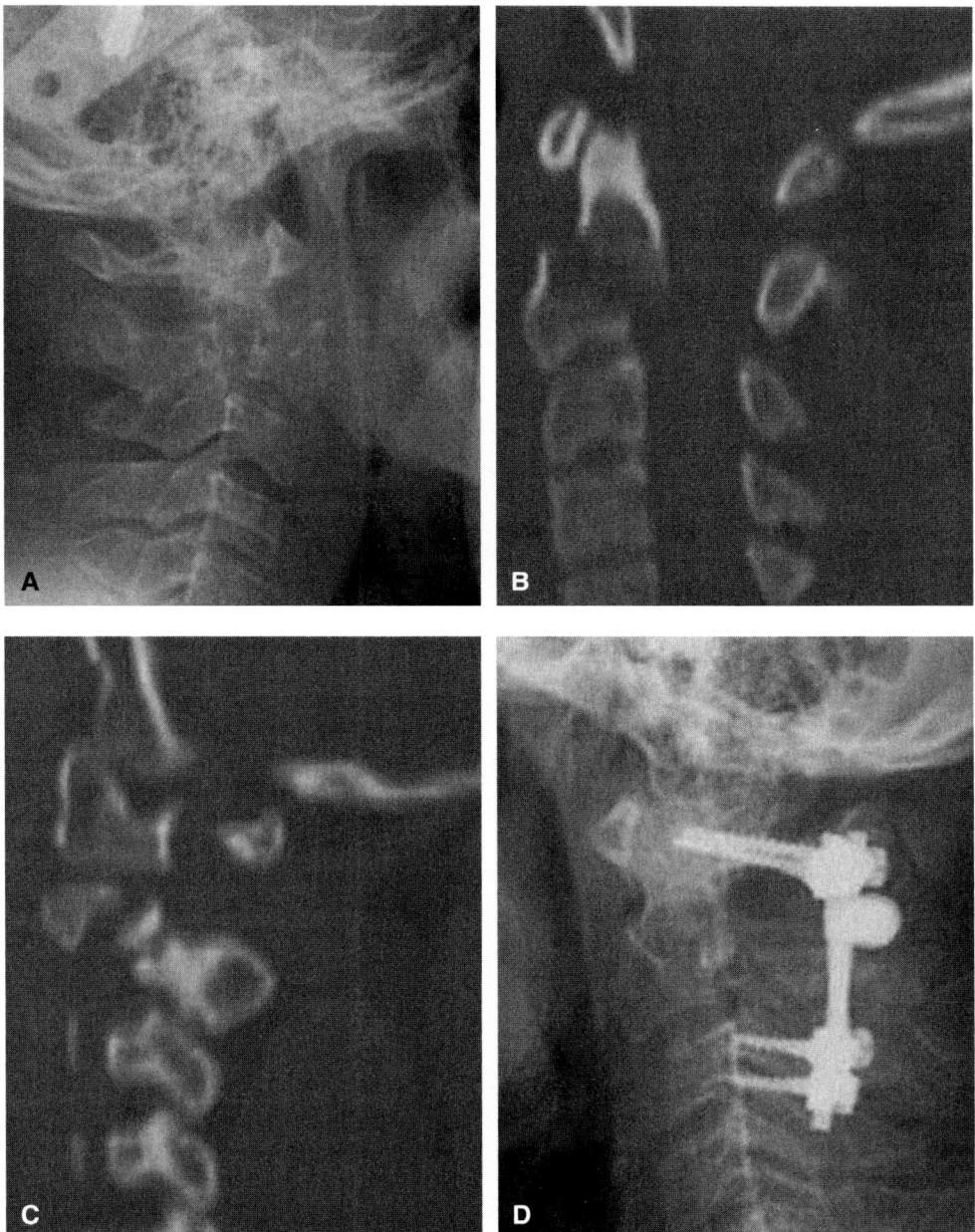

Many different design constructs have recently been described to stabilize upper cervical spine injuries. These include occipital screws, C1 lateral mass screws, C2 pedicle–isthmus screws, and C2 laminar screws, as well as C1-C2 transarticular screws. Prior to further discussion, the following general points (including entry points and trajectories) will better familiarize you with the different techniques.[118,315]

1. *C1 (atlas) lateral mass screws:* The lateral mass screw has become popular as a means of fixation for the C1 level. The insertion site is the midpoint of the lateral mass in the medial-to-lateral direction. Two

approaches are possible in the cephalad-caudal direction: the first begins just below the posterior arch and the second begins directly on the posterior arch. Each has benefits and risks, and the anatomy of an individual patient may be more conducive to one or the other. If the first is chosen, care must be taken in retracting the C2 root caudally, and the surgeon must be particularly careful of the venous plexus in that location. Usually the venous plexus can be dealt with effectively using bipolar electrocautery and packing temporarily with hemostatic gelatin (Gelfoam) and patties while working side to side. If the posterior arch approach is chosen, the surgeon

FIGURE 28-30   *A, A type III hangman's fracture with the pars fracture (white arrow) and facet dislocation (black arrow) treated with an open reduction of the facet dislocation, direct osteosynthesis of the pars fracture, and posterior C2-C3 fusion (B).*

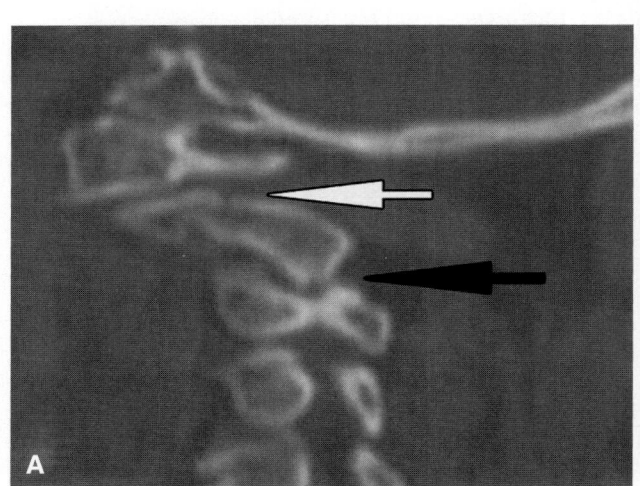

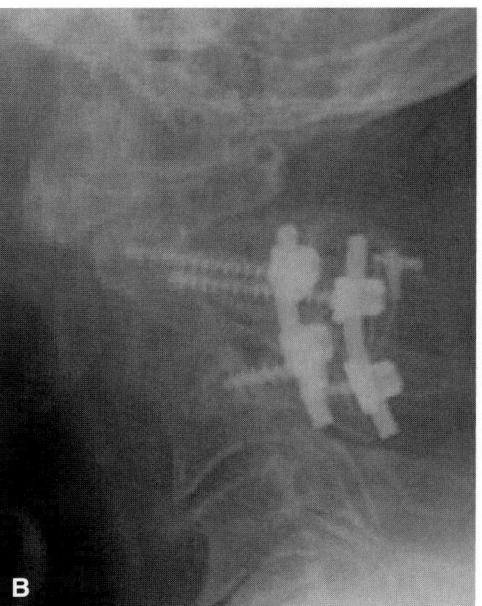

must be sure it is wide enough but is not a ponticulus posticus,[350] which can put the vertebral artery at risk. The mean angle of medialization from the midline in one study was noted to be approximately 16.7° to avoid the transverse foramen, and the mean superior angulation was 21.7° but is easily judged using lateral fluoroscopy[155] (Fig. 28-31).

2. *C2 (axis) pedicle screw:* This screw has also become more popular with the advent of polyaxial screws.

The starting point is roughly the upper outer quadrant of the C2 lateral mass, and the screw should be directed medially approximately 30° and cephalad 20° to avoid the vertebral artery. The preoperative CT should be analyzed to ensure that the artery does not have an aberrant tract.[349] The medial rim of the pars/pedicle area can be directly visualized to aid drill trajectory[158,232] (Fig. 28-32).

FIGURE 28-31   *Screw positions for C1 lateral fixation as shown on a lateral view (A), axial view (B), and posterior view (C). The two alternative starting points are noted.*

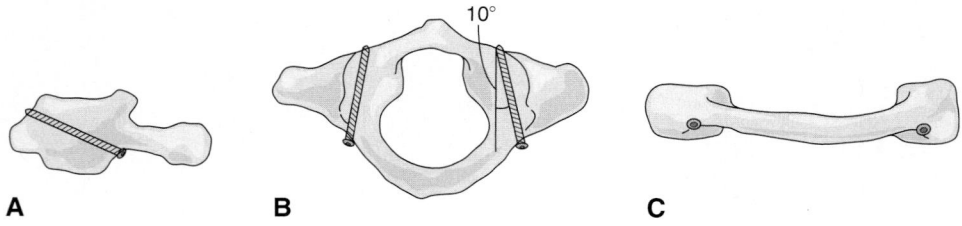

FIGURE 28-32   *Screw positions for C2 pedicle screws on a lateral (A), axial (B), and posterior (C) view.*

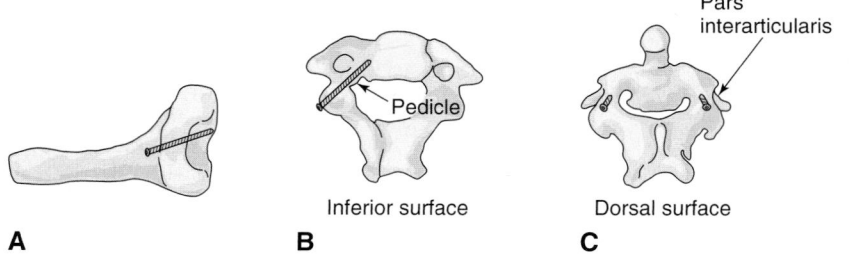

3. *C2 (axis) pars screw and C1-C2 transarticular screw:* These two screws have the same insertion point, which is approximately 2 to 3 mm lateral to the junction between the C2 lamina and the inferior facet, and 2 to 3 mm cephalad to the C2-C3 facet joint. A small divot or flat spot often occurs in the bone at that junction. Both screws are aimed about 5° medially (it is better to err in the medial rather than the lateral direction because the medial aspect affords more room before the cord is encountered as opposed to the position of the vertebral artery laterally), and the medial border of the pars can be directly visualized to aid trajectory. The cephalad direction is judged from the lateral fluoroscopy. For the pars screw, it is more like 30 to 40° upward, which can usually be accomplished through the wound used to expose the C1-C2 posterior elements. The screw is stopped short of the vertebral foramen. For a transarticular screw the angle is more like 60 to 65°, again judged by the lateral fluoroscopy, and is extended across the C1-C2 articulation aiming at the cephalad end of the anterior arch of C1. Preoperative CT is essential in determining that there is adequate room within the pars for the screw to pass safely above the vertebral artery (Fig. 28-33).

4. *C2 laminar screw:* This screw avoids the vertebral artery altogether and has good bony purchase.[347] The entry point is at the junction between the lamina and spinous process, midway between the cranial and caudal aspects. The endpoint of the screw should lie caudal to the junction between the pars interarticularis and the C2 lateral mass to ensure optimal screw length. The spinolaminar angle in one study was found to be 48.47°[324] (Fig. 28-34).

If in the course of drilling, tapping, or screw insertion a vertebral artery injury is recognized, then the other screw should not be inserted to avoid a potentially deadly bilateral vertebral artery injury. The screw on the side of the injury can still be inserted and may help control bleeding. Consideration should be made for a postoperative angiogram to rule out psuedoaneurysm formation that could lead to embolization.

Before discussing the different techniques, the nomenclature deserves mentioning here. There is a very important distinction between a "C2 pedicle screw" and a "C2 isthmus screw," also known as a "C2 pars screw." As mentioned previously, the C2 pedicle lies anterior to the superior articular process of C2, whereas the pars interarticularis is the bony bridge connecting the C2 superior and inferior articular facets. The two separate screw techniques have very different starting sites (albeit both in the same vicinity), trajectories, and screw tip endpoints. However, the term *pedicle screw* has been used most consistently in the literature and was described earlier. It is worth mentioning that a recent study by Dmitriev and colleagues looked at three different C2 fixation techniques comparing C2 pars, pedicle, and laminar screws biomechanically at the bone-screw interface. The C2 pedicle screws were found to have the highest peak pull-out force followed by intralaminar screws and pars screws.[67]

Occipitocervical Athrodesis

Many different techniques have been described for occipitocervical arthrodesis, especially recently with newer technology. The purpose of this section is to describe some of the more popular techniques, to discuss the advantages and disadvantages and most recent literature concerning more traditional methods, and to briefly mention some of the newer techniques. The reader is referred to separate texts that deal primarily with surgical techniques for more in-depth discussion of surgical methods and materials. Some general points about occipitocervical fusion can be made. As with any other surgery, proper patient positioning is crucial to optimize the likelihood of success for a surgical technique and to avoid undue harm to the patient. No accepted method ensures proper alignment; this is generally done by careful inspection of the head–neck–body relationship once positioned. This should be done clinically and radiographically. No specific radiographic lines or measurements have consistently proved reliable. One method is to place patients in a halo preoperatively, giving them the opportunity to assess their position themselves; then the fusion can be done with them in the halo vest to maintain that position. Malposition can create difficulty with line of site and dysphagia. After standard skin preparation and draping, a longitudinal midline skin incision is fashioned from the inion to the midcervical spine. The simplest method for obtaining fusion involves careful decortication of the posterior elements of C1, C2, and the suboccipital area, the application of bone graft, followed by HVI. Because early fixation is not obtained and the risk of nonunion is considerable,[80,221] occipital and cervical wires have been used in conjunction with structural grafts. Either iliac corticocancellous grafts or rib grafts are obtained to span the occiput to the upper cervical spine.[52,195,254,257,340] Autologous rib is excellent for the young pediatric patient (Fig. 28-35).

The technique of Robinson and Southwick, which involves the use of iliac crest grafts, was most popular in the past and is summarized here.[254] After exposure of the base of the occiput and upper cervical spine, two 1-cm bur holes are created in the occiput. In their technique, Robinson and Southwick place the bur holes for wire passage 0.5 cm from the midline and 0.5 mm from edge of the foramen magnum. To safely pass the wires, the underlying dura and periosteum adherent to the posterior arches of C1, C2, and the occiput are then carefully separated from the bone with small, angled curettes and a dural dissector. Two 24-gauge twisted wires are then passed so as to lie just anterior to the occiput and the posterior arches of C1 and C2. The wires are then looped through or around a previously harvested iliac crest graft and gently secured in place by gradually twisting the wires tight. The patient is then immobilized in a halo until healing has occurred.

More involved methods of performing occipitocervical arthrodesis incorporate different types of metal fixation devices, such as plates and screws, and are intended to add immediate stability to the fusion construct[44,128,129,209,241,251,335,336] (Fig. 28-36). Studies have reported fusion rates varying from 94 percent to 100 percent when posterior occipitocervical plates were used[128,129,270,288]

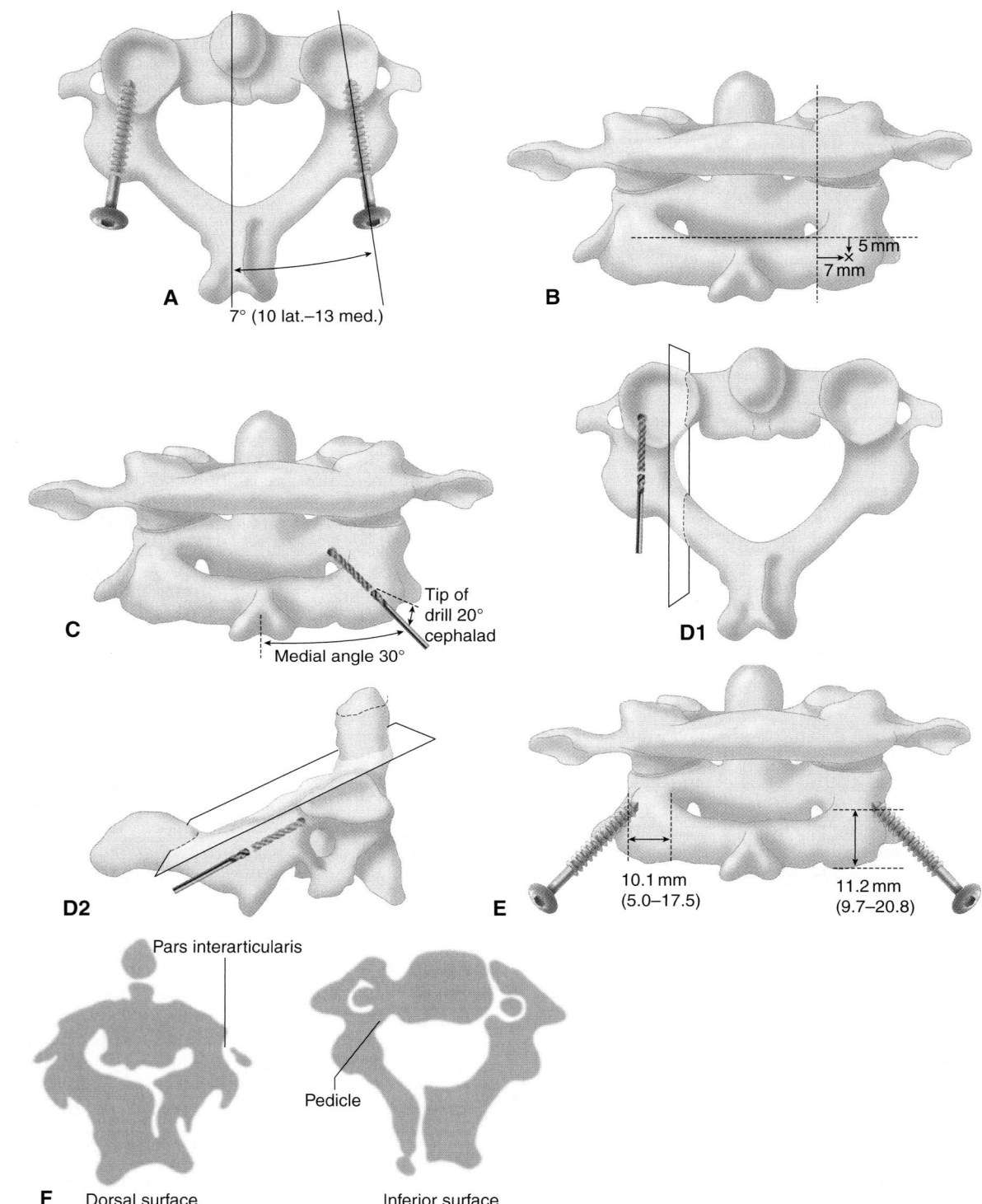

FIGURE 28-33 *Screw positions for C1-C2 transarticular screws in lateral **(A)**, axial **(B)**, and posterior **(C)** views. A short pars screw can be used to C2 fixation and is similarly placed to the transarticular screw but stops short of risking vertebral foramen penetration **(D)**.*

A

7° (10 lat.–13 med.)

B

5 mm
7 mm

C

Tip of drill 20° cephalad
Medial angle 30°

D1

D2

E

10.1 mm (5.0–17.5)

11.2 mm (9.7–20.8)

Pars interarticularis

Pedicle

F   Dorsal surface   Inferior surface

FIGURE 28-33 *(Continued)*

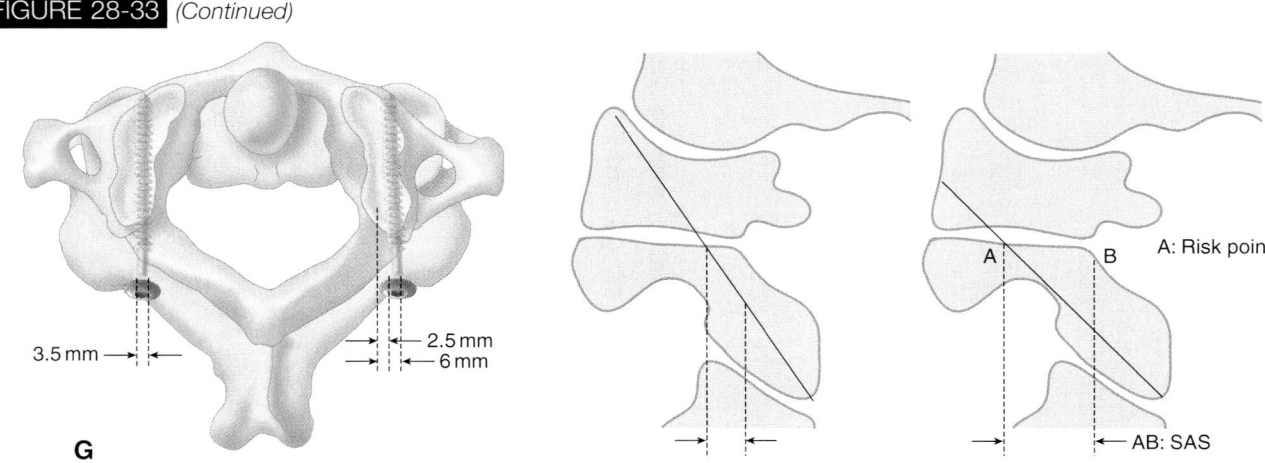

G   3.5 mm   2.5 mm   6 mm

A: Risk point   AB: SAS

without the use of HVI. Furthermore, no significant complications occurred with the use of posterior occipitocervical plates.[129]

Application of posterior occipitocervical plates requires the same surgical dissection as described previously. Ebraheim and co-workers[76] suggested that 8-mm screws can be safely placed at multiple points so as to avoid the dural sinuses: 2 cm lateral to the midline at the level of the inion, 1 cm below the inion and 1 cm lateral to the midline, or 2 cm below and 0.5 cm lateral to midline. The thickest bone is in the midline, and longer screws can be used there.[220,224] Care must also be taken to stay below the transverse venous sinus[224] (Fig. 28-37). One advantage of this type of fixation is that screws involving C1 and

C2 can be placed to attain stronger fixation than wiring techniques allow. Different options include C1 lateral mass screws, C2 pedicle screws, or C1-C2 transarticular screws. Variable types of plates can be used (e.g., dual plating or Y plates) and should be contoured to restore the normal curvature of the occipital cervical region (105°). Corticocancellous and cancellous bone grafts can then be placed into the area between the plates.[128,131,261]

Oda and colleagues found that the addition of C2 transpedicular or C1-C2 transarticular screws significantly

FIGURE 28-34 *Screw positions for C2 laminar screws in an axial (A) and posterior (B) view.*

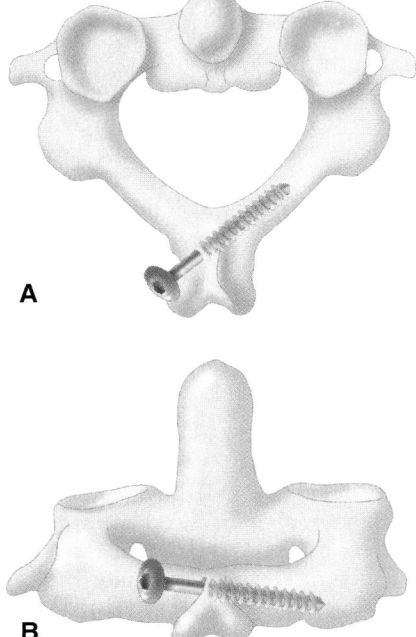

A

B

FIGURE 28-35 *A pediatric posterior occipital-cervical fusion done with cables and autologous rib graft. This technique is particularly valuable in very young patients because the ribs have a good natural contour, excellent healing potential, low morbidity, low profile, and good structural support.*

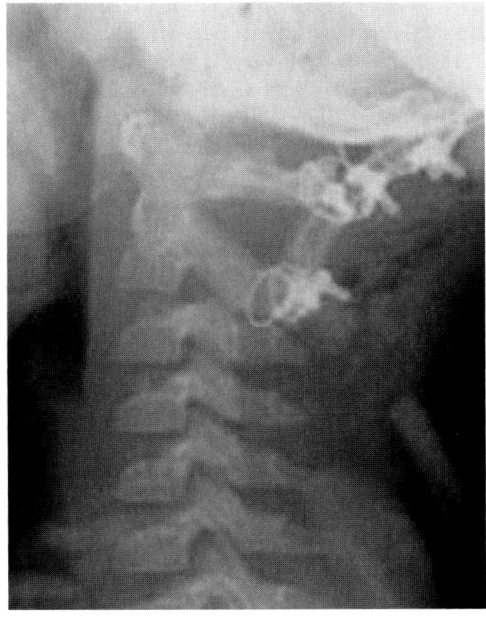

FIGURE 28-36 *Method of posterior occipitocervical plating and fusion. This type of rigid internal fixation allows for postoperative cervical immobilization with a soft collar. (Redrawn from Frymoyer, J.W., ed. The Adult Spine: Principles and Practice, 2nd ed. Philadelphia, Lippincott-Raven, 1997, p. 1428.)*

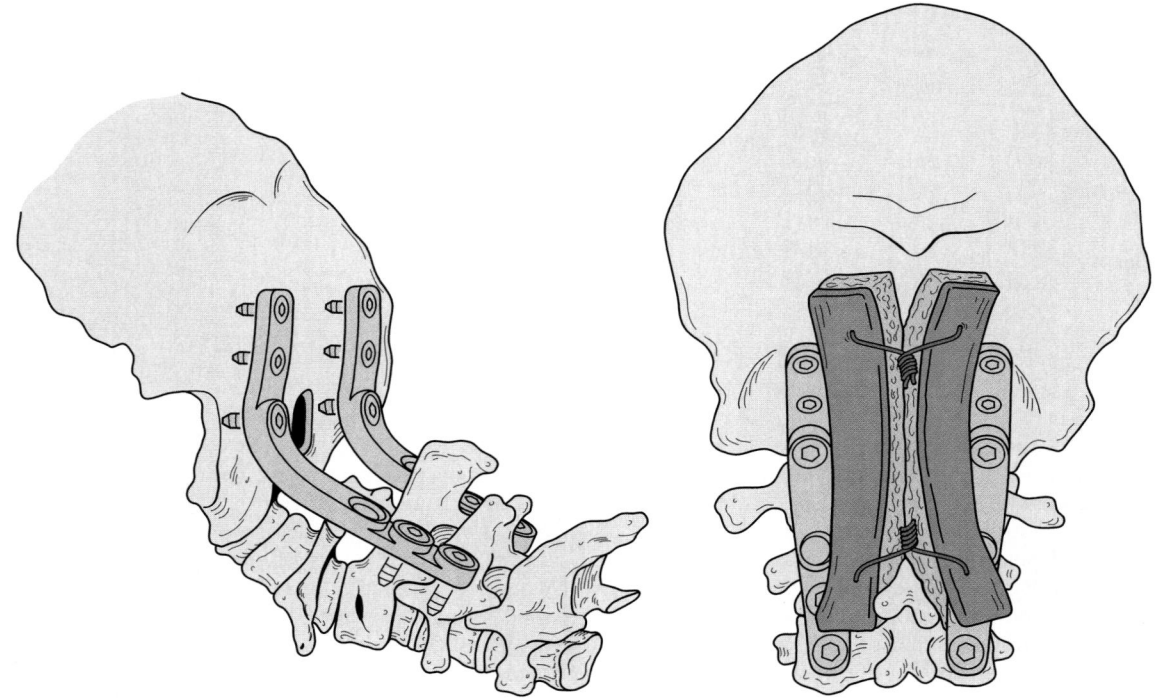

increased the stabilizing effect that was achieved with sublaminar wiring and laminar hooks.[230] A recent cadaveric study was performed looking at a polyaxial rod-screw construct (C1 lateral mass screws with C2 pedicle screws connected to a rod and transoccipital plating) versus a C1-C2 transarticular screw–plate construct (C1-C2 transarticular screws with occipital plating). All specimens were destabilized via odontoidectomy, and measurements were performed in axial rotation and lateral bending. The authors cite several advantages to the polyaxial rod-screw construct, including relative technical simplicity, easier application for various deformities, and the ability to contour the rods and reduce varying cervical segments independently.[249] The disadvantages with the C1-C2 transarticular screw–plate construct include the technically demanding nature of the procedure along with significant risk to the vertebral arteries, and the difficulty in attaining the proper entry point in severely kyphotic individuals. Furthermore, the latter technique necessitates the surgeon precontouring the plate, which limits screw placement and precludes the possibility of additional compression or distraction after the hardware is secured to bone.

Several other techniques that allow rigid fixation of the occipitocervical spine use rod-wire constructs such as contoured Wisconsin or Luque rods with occipital wires or cables.[59] These techniques have likewise been highly successful, with fusion rates ranging from 89 to 93 percent.[216] The "inside-outside" occipital bolt fixation technique is achieved with a flathead bolt that is placed into the epidural space with the threads facing outward engaging a cervical plate or longitudinal rod.[234] The primary advantages are safe lateral placement of fixation within the occiput,

more resistance to torsion than midline occipital screws,[303] greater pull-out strength,[42] and satisfactory clinical results.[268] With more advanced stabilization techniques, halo immobilization has not been necessary with these methods.

Atlantoaxial Arthrodesis

Gallie in 1939 first popularized a technique for atlantoaxial arthrodesis involving midline posterior wiring with bone grafting and facet joint arthrodesis.[109] Because of reported failure rates with this technique ranging from 60 to 80 percent,[104,212] other techniques were designed that include a posterior bone block and wiring between the posterior C1 and C2 arches to create a "wedge compression arthrodesis." These techniques include the modified Gallie fusion as described separately by Fielding and co-workers (Fig. 28-38) and by McGraw and Rusch, as well as the Brooks or modified Brooks technique.[34,93,125] The techniques are associated with clinically better fusion rates ranging from 92 to 100 percent.[34,256,327,332]

The Brooks technique creates the greatest stability of the wiring techniques and is discussed here (Fig. 28-39). Once a satisfactory level of general anesthesia has been obtained and reduction radiographically confirmed, a standard posterior exposure of the upper cervical spine is carried out. A number 2 Mersilene suture is passed on either side of the midline in a cranial-to-caudal direction under the arch of the atlas and then the axis. Two doubled 20-gauge stainless steel wires or titanium cables[59] are then passed into place by using the previously placed suture as a guide, or they can be passed directly with the use of the

FIGURE 28-37 *A diagram of the location of the transverse venous sinus, which must be avoided when using occipital screws.*

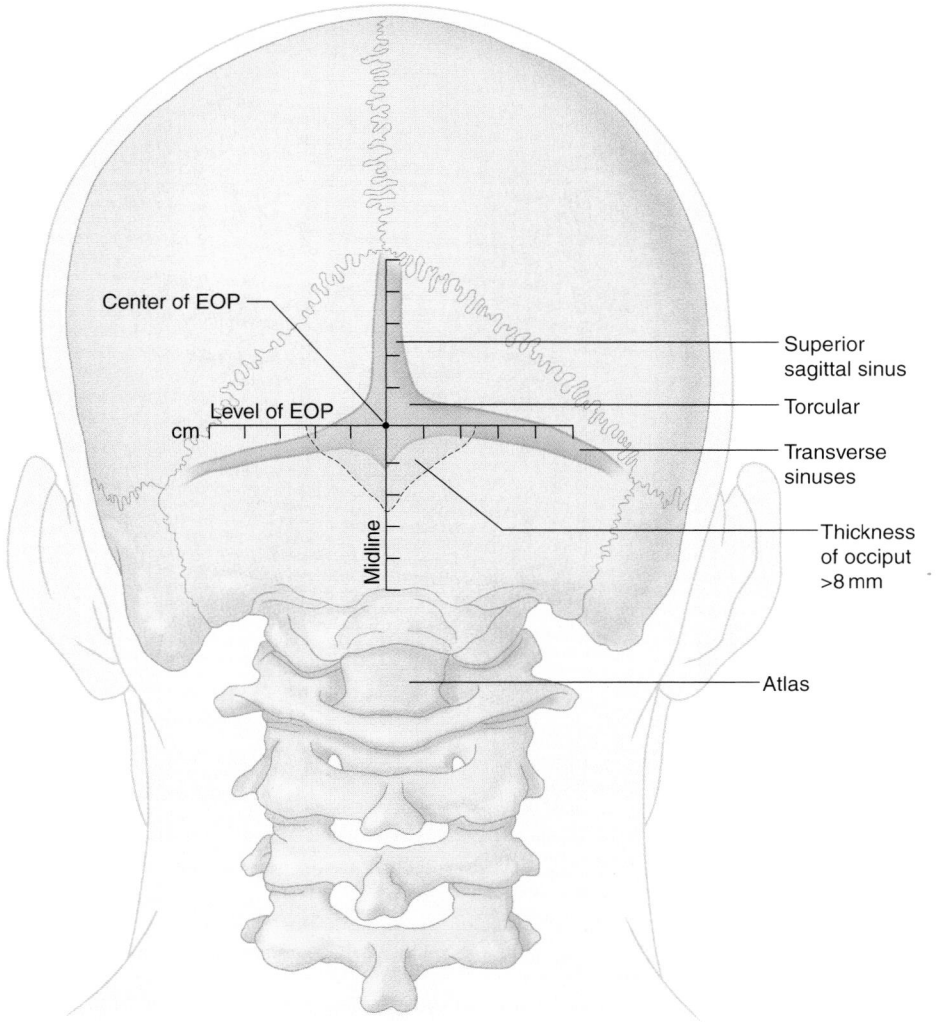

soft lead wire on the current cables. Two full-thickness bone grafts measuring 1.25 × 3.5 cm are then harvested from the posterior iliac crest. These grafts are beveled to fit between the posterior arches of the atlas and the axis on either side of the midline, and the wires are tightened while held in place to maintain the width of the interlaminar space. If the atlantoaxial membrane has been left intact, it helps prevent displacement of the grafts into the neural canal. Postoperatively, the patient can then be mobilized in a sternal-occipital-mandibular immobilizer (SOMI) or four-poster brace until the arthrodesis is solidly united. Griswold and colleagues described a modification of the original Brooks technique that incorporates the use of four doubled 24-gauge wires to hold trapezoidal grafts measuring 1.55 × 1.2 to 1.5 × 1.0 cm in place.[126]

More recent biomechanical testing has found the C1-C2 transarticular screw technique (TAS) to be superior to Gallie wiring, Brooks–Jenkins wiring, and Halifax clamp fixation.[127] A recent case-control study (level II) was performed comparing C1-C2 TAS to posterior wiring techniques. Twenty-seven patients were followed for a mean of 31 months, and union was assessed radiographically. Cases were defined as nonunions, and controls as unions. Patients with fusion were 21 times more likely to have undergone TAS rather than posterior wiring.[305] The procedure, however, is technically more demanding.[163] As such, CT must be done preoperatively to evaluate the bone morphology for such measures as isthmus diameter and to avoid damaging neurovascular structures, such as the vertebral artery and hypoglossal nerve.[87,106,169,199,202,225,237,309,348] One interesting CT study was performed by Solanki and Crockard, who showed that the vertical depth of the C2 transverse foramen is inversely related to the internal height of the C2 lateral mass as well as the length and width of the C2 pedicle.[289] Anatomic contraindications to TAS placement include pathologic destruction or collapse of C2, an aberrant vertebral artery anatomy or a large vertebral artery groove with a secondarily narrow C2 isthmus (20% of cases), or cranial assimilation of C1. A recent cadaveric

FIGURE 28-38   *Surgical technique.* **A,** *Exposure, with the wire loop being passed under the arch of the atlas. Note the proximity of the vertebral vessels.* **B,** *Wire passed below the spine of the axis. Note the decortication of the atlas and axis.* **C,** *The graft configuration.* **D,** *The graft and wire in place, with the wire being tightened over the graft.*

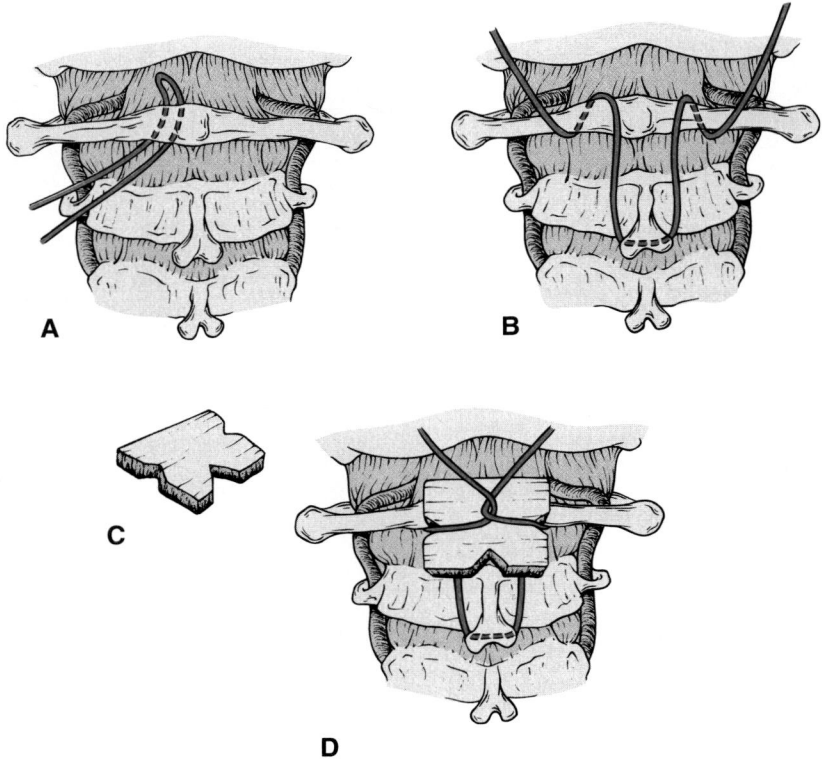

study of the axis showed that the isthmus size and width were not symmetrical in 41 percent of the specimens, and, as demonstrated in other studies, 20 percent of the specimens revealed a C2 isthmus diameter that was smaller than that of the 3.5-mm screw.[159] Because some patients have unilateral anomalies that prevent bilateral TAS placement, one study looked at the outcomes with the use of a unilateral TAS.[290] The authors in this study report successful treatment in 18 out of 19 patients (solid fusion achieved), with 1 patient presenting with a broken screw. Their mean follow-up was 31 months.

Correct screw placement and trajectory are technically demanding (Fig. 28-40). Visualization of the C2 pars or isthmus allows the surgeon to aim just lateral to the pars medial wall to avoid penetration of the spinal canal. If the screw trajectory is too far lateral, the vertebral artery is threatened. Furthermore, the screws must be angled sufficiently cephalad through the facet joint to achieve purchase on the C1 articular mass. If screw placement is too caudal, then fixation is achieved in only the anterior-inferior lip of the C1 lateral mass and could easily fail in extension.[130] Other factors that may influence screw trajectory include the patient's size and the amount of thoracic kyphosis present. After positioning and prior to draping, a Steinmann pin can be laid alongside the patient's head and neck and then imaged with lateral fluoroscopy to verify that a proper trajectory can be achieved. Although controversial, Jeanneret and Magerl[163] did not recommend postoperative immobilization when the

technique is augmented with sublaminar wiring. In the event that wiring is not used in addition to screw placement and posterior fusion, immobilization with a semirigid collar brace has been recommended.[297]

Other constructs that involve C1 pedicle and lateral mass screws as well as C2 laminar screws have been described. Ma and colleagues recently performed a combined cadaveric and clinical study. The authors note that 3.5-mm screws can be safely used for C1 pedicle screw fixation, and they use the center of the C2 lateral mass as the landmark for screw entry in the transverse plane. Rostrocaudal height of the posterior arch under the vertebral artery groove was measured in 50 cadaveric specimens and noted to be 3.88 mm medially and 4.25 mm laterally. By ensuring a larger rostrocaudal height to avoid damage to the vertebral artery, the center C2 lateral mass line, when used as a reference point, safely accommodated C2 pedicle screw placement under the vertebral artery groove of C1.[197] The authors report 100 percent fusion rates.

Alternatively, the use of C1 lateral mass and C2 pedicle screws for a posterior screw-rod construct has recently been described by Harms and co-workers and has gained widespread popularity.[142] The purported advantages include the ability to achieve stable internal fixation without anatomic reduction and the ability to avoid a high riding vertebral artery groove in C2. A cadaveric study comparing polyaxial screw-rod technique versus combined Gallie-Magerl technique on 10 cadaveric specimens after odontoidectomy was performed. No significant differences

FIGURE 28-39 *A, The occipital nerves emerge through the interlaminar space between the atlas and the axis; the vertebral arteries are more lateral. With a midline approach, the arteries and nerves are fairly well protected by the neck muscles. B, On the left, a suture is passed under the posterior arch of the atlas. On the right, the suture is used to guide the wire under the arch of the atlas and the lamina of the axis. C, The wires are now in place and lie anterior to the anterior portion of the atlantoaxial membrane, which was not removed during exposure of the posterior elements of the atlas and axis. On the right, the graft, with edges beveled to fit in the interval between the atlas and the axis, is being held with a towel clip. When wired in place, the beveled edges are in contact with the arch of the atlas and the lamina of the axis. D, The grafts are secured, and stability is maintained by the wires.*

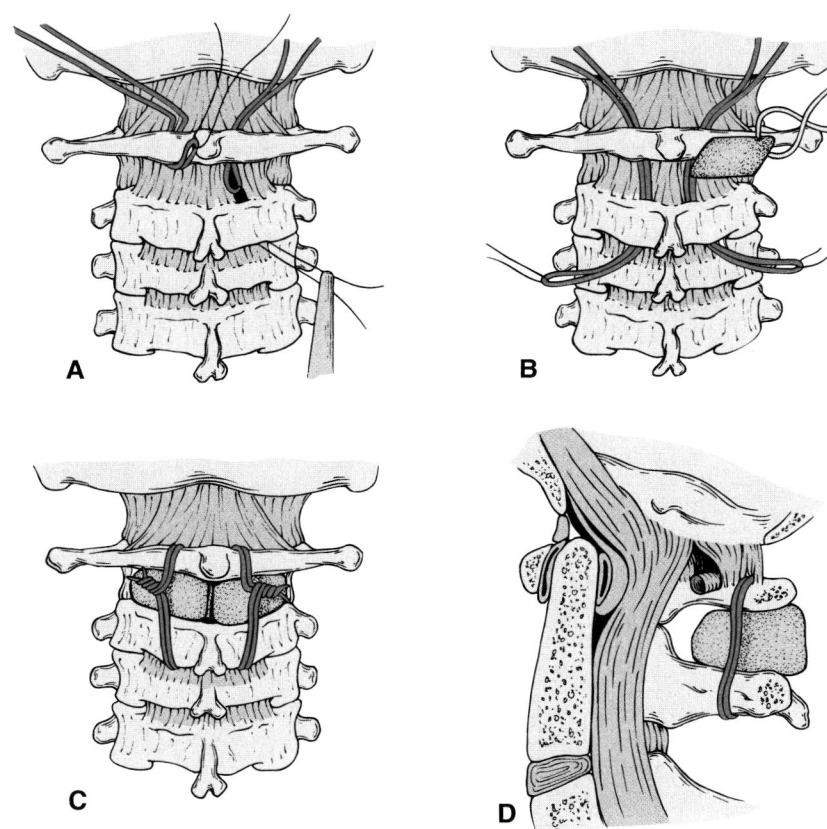

arose between techniques in mechanical testing in axial rotation and lateral bending, and the authors concluded the techniques were biomechanically equivalent.[214] Fiore and associates cite anatomic factors, such as an aberrant vertebral artery, significant cervical thoracic kyphosis, irreducible odontoid fractures, or poor bone quality, that often preclude the use of transarticular C1-C2 screw techniques. They report the use of 14 C1 lateral mass screws in eight patients for multiple pathologies. At 7.4 month average follow-up, rigid fixation was obtained in all patients, and there were no complications related to screws.[99] Other authors[298] have looked at C1 lateral mass screws with C2 pedicle screws for atlantoaxial fusions, noting that it is technically less demanding than C1-C2 TAS, and that the technique can be used when posterior elements are disrupted.

More recently, the use of C2 translaminar screws has been described. In one study, the authors report successful follow-up in 20 patients with bilateral, crossing translaminar axis screws. They note that C2 translaminar screw fixation is technically less demanding, is not affected by variations in anatomy, and does not place the vertebral artery at risk. They reported a 100 percent fusion rate with

no vascular or neurologic complications.[347] To better determine the stability of the construct, a cadaveric study compared C2 pedicle screw fixation versus C2 laminar screw fixation. All specimens were destabilized via odontoidectomy, and no statistically significant difference was noted between the two constructs.[118] However, Lehman and colleagues recently suggested that C2 pedicle screws may have some biomechanical advantage over C2 intralaminar and pars screws for atlantoaxial fixation.[184]

Anterior stabilizing techniques for atlantoaxial stability, such as anterior cervical plating or anterior C1-C2 TAS placement, may also be used.[14,27] For anterior TAS, Vaccaro and colleagues [314] described the use of a cannulated screw set with starting points being at the midpoint of the C2 body in the transverse plane and the respective medial thirds of the C1-C2 facets in the sagittal planes. The screws should be angulated laterally in the coronal plane approximately 30 to 35° to allow for perpendicular screw placement across facet joints. There are many advantages to using the anterior techniques. When cord compression occurs anteriorly, such as with irreducible atlantoaxial dislocations or a nonunited or malunited

FIGURE 28-40   *Magerl method of fixation with transarticular C1-C2 screws. The patient is placed prone and the head immobilized with Mayfield skull tongs. The position of the neck needed for reduction of the deformity influences the exposure. **A1,** If the head can be flexed forward, the transarticular screws can be placed through the same posterior incision; however, if extension is needed to maintain the reduction of C1 **(A2)**, a shorter incision is needed for exposure of the posterior elements of C1-C2, and the drill bit and instrumentation are passed into the wound through percutaneous incisions. **B,** The medial wall of the C2 pedicle should be exposed to aid in orienting the direction of the drill. The starting point for drilling is just medial to the edge of the facet joint and the inferior margin of the lamina of C2. Progress of the drill bit across the C1-C2 facet should be monitored using lateral image intensification for cephalad–caudal trajectory and direct visualization of the pars to assess medial-lateral trajectory. (From Levine, A.M., Eismont, F.J.; Garfin, S.R.; et al., eds. Spine Trauma. Philadelphia, W.B. Saunders, 1998, pp. 274, 275.)*

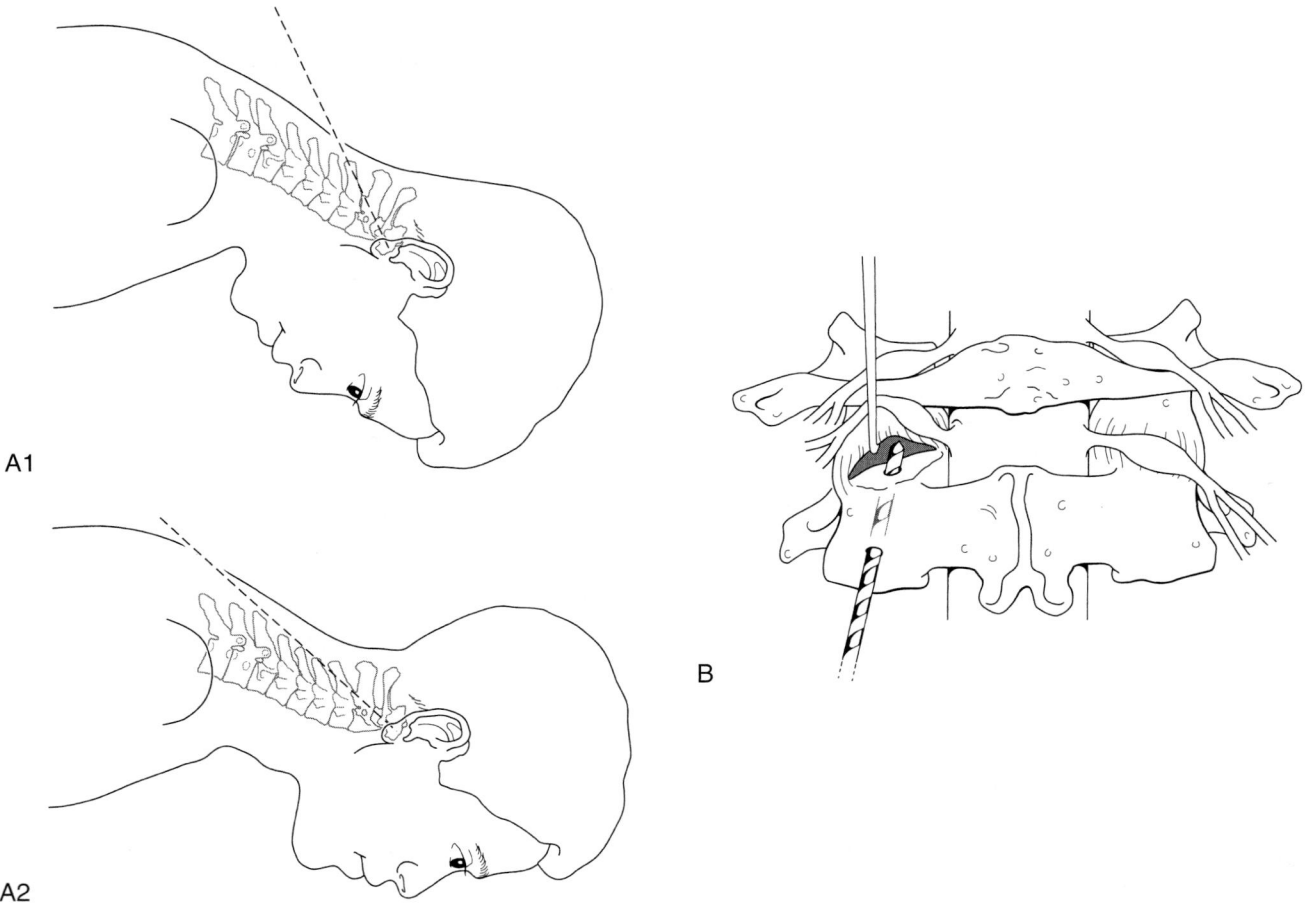

A1

A2

B

dens,[301] it may be difficult to perform a reduction from a posterior approach. Furthermore, flexion of the neck is sometimes necessary for certain posterior techniques, but may result in fatal cord damage. In the presence of a failed posterior stabilizing technique, anterior techniques may be the surgeon's only option. Last, an anterior approach allows acute decompression of the spinal canal when needed. The literature on optimal biomechanical properties in both anterior and posterior stabilizing techniques for cervicocranial injuries is sparse. However, a recent cadaveric study looked a biomechanical stability of different fusion methods including anterior cervical plating, anterior TAS, posterior rod-screw construct, and posterior TAS. The posterior rod-screw construct was found to have the highest biomechanical stiffness, followed by posterior TAS, then anterior TAS, and lastly anterior cervical plating.[172]

Anterior Stabilization of the Dens

First introduced in 1980 by Nakanishi,[226] screw osteosynthesis of the dens has the advantages of preserving atlantoaxial motion and minimizing the need for postoperative immobilization.[27,107,226] It can be used for type II and some type III fractures, and union rates of 92 to 100 percent have been achieved.[27,47,80,82,88,107] The procedure is technically difficult with the potential for catastrophic neurologic complications, as well as injury to the adjacent segment (C2-C3).[317] Short-necked patients, patients with stiff cervical spines or extreme thoracic kyphosis, a barrel-chested habitus, and fracture configurations that can be held reduced only while in flexion create difficulty with drill and screw trajectory and may make the surgeon opt for another treatment method.[84]

Similar to C1-C2 posterior TAS, positioning is critical, and after positioning but prior to draping a Steinmann pin can be laid alongside the patient's head and neck and then imaged with lateral fluoroscopy to verify that a proper trajectory can be achieved. It is essential to use two simultaneous C-arms because the open-mouth odontoid view requires a great deal of adjustment to achieve the proper view, and once it is achieved the C-arm should not be moved. After gaining access through a standard C5-C6 anterior approach, the anterior longitudinal ligament is split longitudinally over the body of the axis. Using fluoroscopy, drill holes are made starting at the anteroinferior aspect of C2 toward the cranial tip of the dens. Care must be taken to start within the C2-C3 disk to get into the inferior aspect of the C2 body and avoid starting on the anterior portion of the body, which can lead to screw cut out. Drill trajectory should be checked in multiple planes, and after gauging depth and tapping the hole, a small-fragment (3.5 mm) lag screw is inserted (Fig. 28-41). It is important that a lag screw effect is achieved by overdrilling the proximal cortex or using a partially threaded screw (in this case one must be certain that the threads do not span the fracture site). If the obliquity of the fracture is from posterior-cephalad to anterior-caudal (opposite the usual obliquity), then this technique is relatively contraindicated because the fracture will displace anteriorly and inferiorly as the screw is tightened. Recently, endoscopically assisted anterior screw fixation has also been used, with some authors citing a 17.4 percent major complication rate (minor rate of 13%) with the open technique[84] to justify use of the endoscopic

technique. In this technique, the authors use a 10-mL polyethylene syringe as a tubular retractor and a much smaller 2-cm skin incision.[145] Furthermore, the recent introduction of computer navigation prompted a cadaveric comparison of standard fluoroscopy with fluoroscopy-based computer navigation. The study showed no difference in accuracy of screw placement or procedural time. However, the study was limited by an intact odontoid model rather than a fracture model. Also worth noting was that the radiation exposure was less with virtual fluoroscopy.[20]

Some debate exists over the use of one or two interfragmentary screws for fixation.[82,88,121] It was shown recently, in looking at adult odontoid morphology, that the average transverse outer diameter was 10.4 mm (ranging from 8.2 to 13.2 mm) and that the average transverse inner diameter was 7.2 mm (ranging from 4.4 to 11.0 mm). The authors conclude that variations in adult odontoid anatomyinvolve thick irregular cortices and cite that in the coronal plane the critical diameter for two 3.5-mm cortical screws with tapping is 9.0 mm.[228] Some biomechanical studies suggest that no significant biomechanical difference occurs between the use of one or two screws.[69,121,269] Although clinically similar success rates have been observed with one- and two-screw fixation,[165] a recent cadaveric study showed different biomechanical results. Twelve cadavers were treated (six in each group) with either one 4.5-mm cannulated Herbert screw or two 3.5-mm AO cannulated screws. Torsional stiffness was found to be greater with the Herbert screw, sheer stiffness showed no statistical difference.[210] As far as

---

FIGURE 28-41 *Patient positioning for anterior odontoid screw fixation (A). Screw positions show in anteroposterior (B) and lateral (C) views.*

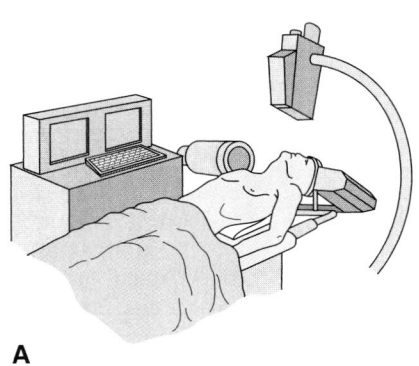

A

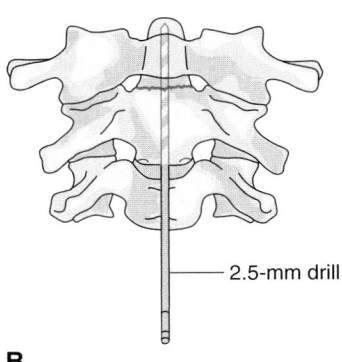

2.5-mm drill

B

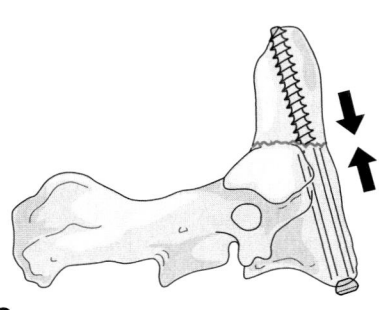

C

different screw designs are concerned, some surgeons use double-threaded compression screws, and most surgeons prefer a single midline screw.[47,176] Postoperatively, rigid collar immobilization is recommended until union is solid.

SURGICAL APPROACHES TO THE CERVICOCRANIUM

Four separate approaches are possible to the upper cervical spine. The indications, advantages, and disadvantages will be discussed along with a brief anatomic-surgical description. The different approaches include the posterior approach, the transoral approach (also known as transmucosal approach), the lateral retropharyngeal approach, and the anterior retropharyngeal approach.

Posterior Approach

The main advantage to the posterior approach is the relative ease of dissection, familiarity, a lower incidence of complications, and a high success rate for fusions. After standard skin preparation and draping, a longitudinal midline skin incision is made over the area of pathology. With meticulous hemostasis, the upper cervical spine is exposed, paying close attention to the midline raphe. This technique helps prevent excessive hemorrhage, as deviation off midline into more vascular muscle tissue may bleed more. Care should be taken to expose only the number of levels in the planned fusion to minimize damage to adjacent levels and avoid the risk of autofusion in the pediatric population. It is crucial to appreciate that the vertebral vessels lie on the superior aspect of the posterior arch of C1 approximately 1.5 to 2.0 cm lateral to the midline. Furthermore, defects in the posterior arch can be seen in approximately 1.4 percent of atlases, especially in those with congenital occipitoatlantal fusion.[330]

Transoral Approach to C1-C2

The direct transoral approach to the upper cervical spine, first described by Southwick and Robinson and later popularized by Fang and Ong, is optimal when anterior decompression is needed.[86,293] To gain access with the transoral approach, the surgeon only encounters the pharyngeal mucosa, the constrictor muscles, the buccopharyngeal fascia, and the prevertebral muscle. Wound infection rates, initially reported to occur in 33 to 50 percent of cases,[86,336] have dropped tremendously more recently.[14,190] In addition, initial studies reported a 25 percent perioperative death rate, whereas more recent series have not found perioperative mortality to be a problem.[14,190] The surgeon must be wary of excessive lateral soft tissue dissection or distraction so as to avoid inadvertent damage to the vertebral vessels. Furthermore, the potential for bone graft dislodgement exists due to the difficulty in obtaining stable bony anchorage. This may lead to irritation of the pharyngeal soft tissue or further increase the likelihood of infection.[314]

Reconstructive procedures can be difficult through this approach due to the depth of the field, the stereotactic restriction due to the mandible, and limited visibility. The approach is most commonly reserved for biopsies, aspirations, odontoid resection in rheumatoid arthritis, and drainage of infection. In the trauma setting, however, the primary indication for this approach is the need for anterior decompression of the atlantoaxial region because of fracture displacement, nonunion, or malunion.[14,301]

After establishing the endotracheal airway, the skin and hypopharynx are prepared and draped. A self-retaining oral retractor is inserted. This retractor depresses the tongue as well as the soft palate. A separate arm of the retractor holds the endotracheal and nasogastric tubes to the side. After infiltrating the posterior pharyngeal wall with a dilute epinephrine solution, a longitudinal midline incision measuring approximately 5 to 6 cm is made at the center of the anterior tubercle of the atlas. The anterior arch of the atlas and the body of the axis, as well as the atlantoaxial joints on either side, are then exposed. After the conclusion of the procedure, wound cultures are obtained in the event that the patient shows any signs of infection postoperatively. The wound is closed in layers, and antibiotic use is discontinued at 72 hours.

Retropharyngeal Approaches to the Upper Cervical Spine (Lateral and Anterior)

The lateral and anterior retropharyngeal approaches, which are very similar, are advantageous for several reasons. First, both approaches preclude the possibility of bone graft contamination from the nasopharyngeal bacterial flora. Both approaches allow dissection caudally and utilize the interval that is anterior to the sternocleidomastoid muscle and posterior to the cervical strap muscles. The complications from these approaches are numerous. Problems with swallowing or breathing can occur due to retropharyngeal edema or hematoma formation. Nerve dysesthesias involving the greater auricular, hypoglossal, facial, recurrent laryngeal, and spinal accessory nerves can all occur[148,332,335] (Fig. 28-42). The two approaches are quite similar with one difference. The anterior approach involves dissection anterior to the carotid sheath, whereas the lateral approach involves retracting the sheath and its contents anteriorly. Because of this, the anterior approach involves extensive dissection of the external carotid artery, its branches, and the superior laryngeal nerve.[314,335] In the absence of contraindications, the neck is extended and rotated to the opposite side. After induction of anesthesia and sterile preparation, a "hockey stick" incision is begun transversely across the tip of the mastoid process and carried distally along the anterior border of the sternocleidomastoid muscle. The greater auricular nerve is identified and retracted cephalad; if it is in the way, it may be resected with a negligible sensory deficit. In most cases, the sternocleidomastoid muscle is detached from the mastoid process. The spinal accessory nerve is then identified at its entrance into the sternocleidomastoid muscle approximately 3 cm from the mastoid tip. If only the C1-C2 area needs to be approached, it is retracted anteriorly. If a more extensive approach is necessary, the nerve is dissected from the jugular vein up to an area near the jugular foramen and retracted laterally with the sternocleidomastoid muscle (Fig. 28-43).

FIGURE 28-42 **A, B,** *Lateral retropharyngeal approach to the upper cervical spine. (Redrawn from Whitesides, T.E.; Kelly, R.P. Lateral approach to the upper cervical spine for anterior fusion. South Med J 59:879–883, 1966.)*

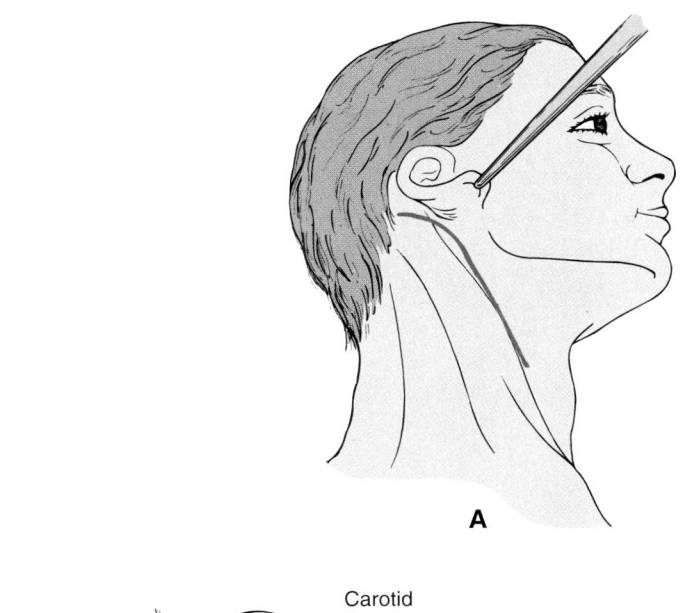

A

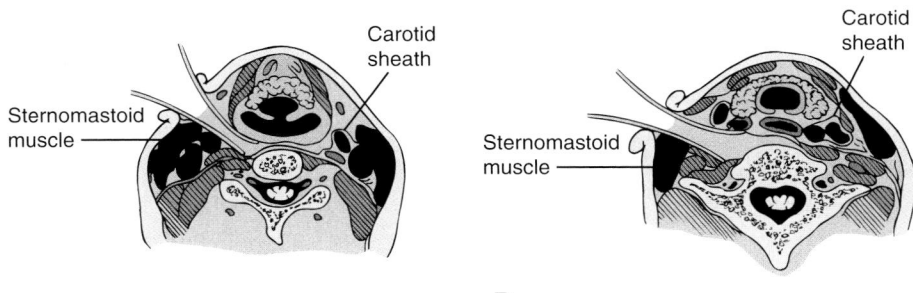

B

FIGURE 28-43 *Diagrammatic illustration of neurovascular structures uniquely at risk during a high anterior cervical approach.*

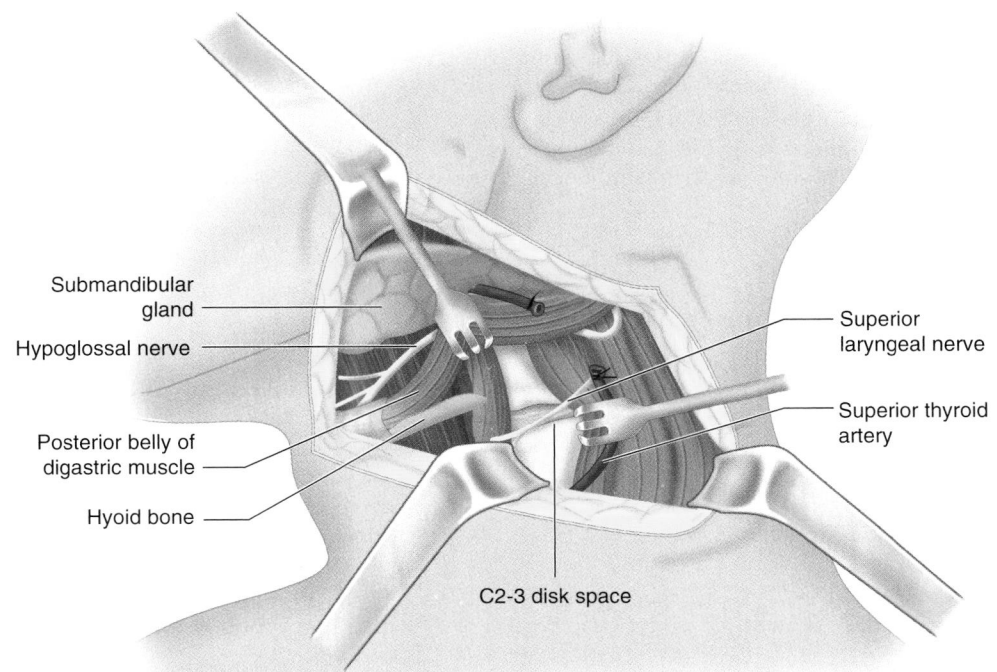

After eversion of the sternocleidomastoid muscle, the transverse processes of the cervical vertebrae are easily palpable. The transverse process of C1 extends more laterally than the rest and is thus especially prominent. With the anterior approach, the surgeon must dissect the branches of the external carotid artery and laryngeal nerves, retracting the carotid sheath posteriorly. The lateral approach avoids these structures, dissecting posterior to the carotid sheath and retracting it anteriorly. With further medial dissection, Sharpey's fibers can be divided and the retropharyngeal space entered.

Exposure of the appropriate vertebral bodies is then possible with subperiosteal stripping and, if necessary, removal of the anterior cervical muscles down to the upper thoracic region. Localization is easy because of the prominent, transversely oriented anterior arch of C1 and the prominent vertical midline ridge of the base of the odontoid and body of C2. At the conclusion of the procedure, the sternocleidomastoid is sewn back into place over suction drains. The platysma and skin are closed in layers. Because of the potential for significant retropharyngeal edema, postoperative intubation or prophylactic tracheostomy should be considered.

REFERENCES

1. Adams, V.I. Neck injuries: II. Atlantoaxial dislocation—A pathologic study of 14 traffic fatalities. J Forensic Sci 37:565–573, 1992.
2. Adler, D.C.; Jacobson, G. Examination of the atlanto-axial joint following injury with particular emphasis on rotational subluxation. Am J Roentgenol Radium Ther Nucl Med 76:1081–1094, 1956.
3. Aebi, M.; Etter, C.; Coscia, M. Fractures of the odontoid process. Treatment with anterior screw fixation. Spine 14:1065–1070, 1989.
4. Alcelik, I.; Manik, K.S.; Sian, P.S.; et al. Occipital condylar fractures. Review of the literature and case report. J Bone Joint Surg [Br] 88:665–669, 2006.
5. Alker, G.J., Jr.; Oh, Y.S.; Leslie, E.V. High cervical spine and craniocervical junction injuries in fatal traffic accidents: A radiological study. Orthop Clin North Am 9:1003–1010, 1978.
6. Anderson, A.J.; Towns, G.M.; Chiverton, N. Traumatic occipitocervical disruption: A new technique for stabilisation. Case report and literature review. J Bone Joint Surg [Br] 88:1464–1468, 2006.
7. Anderson, L.D.; D'Alonzo, R.T. Fractures of the odontoid process of the axis. J Bone Joint Surg [Am] 56:1663–1674, 1974.
8. Anderson, P.A.; Mizra, S.K.; Chapman, J.R. Injuries to the atlantooccipital articulation. In Clark, C.R.; Dvorak, J.; Ducker, T.B.; et al., eds. The Cervical Spine. Philadelphia, Lippincott-Raven, 1998, pp. 387–399.
9. Anderson, P.A.; Montesano, P.X. Morphology and treatment of occipital condyle fractures. Spine 13:731–736, 1988.
10. Andersson, S.; Rodrigues, M.; Olerud, C. Odontoid fractures: High complication rate associated with anterior screw fixation in the elderly. Eur Spine J 9:56–59, 2000.
11. Apfelbaum, R.I.; Lonser, R.R.; Veres, R.; et al. Direct anterior screw fixation for recent and remote odontoid fractures. J Neurosurg 93(2 Suppl):227–236, 2000.
12. Apuzzo, M.L.; Heiden, J.S.; Weiss, M.H.; et al. Acute fractures of the odontoid process. An analysis of 45 cases. J Neurosurg 48:85–91, 1978.
13. Arand, M.; Neller, S.; Kinzl, L.; et al. The traumatic spondylolisthesis of the axis. A biomechanical in vitro evaluation of an instability model and clinical relevant constructs for stabilization. Clin Biomech (Bristol, Avon) 17:432–438, 2002.
14. Ashraf, J.; Crockard, H.A. Transoral fusion for high cervical fractures. J Bone Joint Surg [Br] 72:76–79, 1990.
15. Aulino, J.M.; Tutt, L.K.; Kaye, J.J.; et al. Occipital condyle fractures: Clinical presentation and imaging findings in 76 patients. Emerg Radiol 11:342–347, 2005.
16. Aymes, E.W.; Anderson, E.M. Fracture of the odontoid process: Report of sixty-three cases. Arch Surg 72:377–393, 1956.
17. Bailey, D.K. The normal cervical spine in infants and children. Radiology 59:712–719, 1952.
18. Banna, M.; Stevenson, G.W.; Tumiel, A. Unilateral atlanto-occipital dislocation complicating an anomaly of the atlas. A case report. J Bone Joint Surg [Am] 65:685–687, 1983.
19. Barker, L.; Anderson, J.; Chesnut, R.; et al. Reliability and reproducibility of dens fracture classification with use of plain radiography and reformatted computer-aided tomography. J Bone Joint Surg [Am] 88:106–112, 2006.
20. Battaglia, T.C.; Tannoury, T.; Crowl, A.C.; et al. A cadaveric study comparing standard fluoroscopy with fluoroscopy-based computer navigation for screw fixation of the odontoid. J Surg Orthop Adv 14:175–180, 2005.
21. Bergenheim, A.T.; Forssell, A. Vertical odontoid fracture. Case report. J Neurosurg 74:665–667, 1991.
22. Blackwood, N.J. Atlantooccipital dislocations. Ann Surg 47:654–658, 1908.
23. Blauth, M.; Lange, U.F.; Knop, C.; et al. [Spinal fractures in the elderly and their treatment]. Orthopade 29:302–317, 2000.
24. Bloom, A.I.; Neeman, Z.; Slasky, B.S.; et al. Fracture of the occipital condyles and associated craniocervical ligament injury: Incidence, CT imaging and implications. Clin Radiol 52:198–202, 1997.
25. Boden, S.D.; Dodge, L.D.; Bohlman, H.H.; et al. Rheumatoid arthritis of the cervical spine. A long-term analysis with predictors of paralysis and recovery. J Bone Joint Surg [Am] 75:1282–1297, 1993.
26. Bohler, J. Fractures of the odontoid process. J Trauma 5:386–390, 1965.

27. Bohler, J. Anterior stabilization for acute fractures and non-unions of the dens. J Bone Joint Surg [Am] 64:18–27, 1982.

28. Bohlman, H.H. Acute fractures and dislocations of the cervical spine. An analysis of three hundred hospitalized patients and review of the literature. J Bone Joint Surg [Am] 61:1119–1142, 1979.

29. Borm, W.; Kast, E.; Richter, H.P.; et al. Anterior screw fixation in type II odontoid fractures: Is there a difference in outcome between age groups? Neurosurgery 52:1089–1992; discussion 1092–1094, 2003.

30. Borne, G.M.; Bedou, G.L.; Pinaudeau, M. Treatment of pedicular fractures of the axis. A clinical study and screw fixation technique. J Neurosurg 60:88–93, 1984.

31. Botelho, R.V.; de Souza Palma, A.M.; Abgussen, C.M.; et al. Traumatic vertical atlantoaxial instability: The risk associated with skull traction. Case report and literature review. Eur Spine J 9:430–433, 2000.

32. Bozboga, M.; Unal, F.; Hepgul, K.; et al. Fracture of the occipital condyle. Case report. Spine 17:1119–1121, 1992.

33. Brashear, R., Jr.; Venters, G.; Preston, E.T. Fractures of the neural arch of the axis. A report of twenty-nine cases. J Bone Joint Surg [Am] 57:879–887, 1975.

34. Brooks, A.L.; Jenkins, E.B. Atlanto-axial arthrodesis by the wedge compression method. J Bone Joint Surg [Am] 60:279–284, 1978.

35. Bucholz, R.W. Unstable hangman's fractures. Clin Orthop Relat Res 154:119–124, 1981.

36. Bucholz, R.W.; Burkhead, W.Z. The pathological anatomy of fatal atlanto-occipital dislocations. J Bone Joint Surg [Am] 61:248–250, 1979.

37. Buchowski, J.M.; Kebaish, K.M.; Ahn, N.U.; et al. Odontoid fracture in a 50-year-old patient presenting 40 years after cervical spine trauma. Orthopedics 26:1061–1063, 2003.

38. Buchowski, J.M.; Riley, L.H., 3rd. Epidural hematoma after immobilization of a "hangman's" fracture: Case report and review of the literature. Spine J 5:332–335, 2005.

39. Bundens, D.A.; Rechtines, G.R.; Bohlman, H.H. Upper cervical spine injuries. Orthop Rev 13:556–563, 1984.

40. Burke, J.T.; Harris, J.H., Jr. Acute injuries of the axis vertebra. Skeletal Radiol 18:335–346, 1989.

41. Cabot, A.; Becker, A. The cervical spine in rheumatoid arthritis. Clin Orthop Relat Res 131:130–140, 1978.

42. Caglar, Y.S.; Torun, F.; Pait, T.G.; et al. Biomechanical comparison of inside-outside screws, cables, and regular screws, using a sawbone model. Neurosurg Rev 28:53–58, 2005.

43. Campanelli, M.; Kattner, K.A.; Stroink, A.; et al. Posterior C1-C2 transarticular screw fixation in the treatment of displaced type II odontoid fractures in the geriatric population—Review of seven cases. Surg Neurol 51:596–600; discussion 600–601, 1999.

44. Cantore, G.; Ciappetta, P.; Delfini, R. New steel device for occipitocervical fixation. Technical note. J Neurosurg 60:1104–1106, 1984.

45. Cartmill, M.; Khazim, R.; Firth, J.L. Occipital condyle fracture with peripheral neurological deficit. Br J Neurosurg 13:611–613, 1999.

46. Castel, E.; Benazet, J.P.; Samaha, C.; et al. Delayed closed reduction of rotatory atlantoaxial dislocation in an adult. Eur Spine J 10:449–453, 2001.

47. Chang, K.W.; Liu, Y.W.; Cheng, P.G.; et al. One Herbert double-threaded compression screw fixation of displaced type II odontoid fractures. J Spinal Disord 7:62–69, 1994.

48. Chirossel, J.P.; Passagia, J.G.; Gay, E.; et al. Management of craniocervical junction dislocation. Childs Nerv Syst 16:697–701, 2000.

49. Cirak, B.; Akpinar, G.; Palaoglu, S. Traumatic occipital condyle fractures. Neurosurg Rev 23:161–164, 2000.

50. Clark, C.R.; White, A.A., 3rd. Fractures of the dens. A multicenter study. J Bone Joint Surg [Am] 67:1340–1348, 1985.

51. Collalto, P.M.; DeMuth, W.W.; Schwentker, E.P.; et al. Traumatic atlanto-occipital dislocation. Case report. J Bone Joint Surg [Am] 68:1106–1109, 1986.

52. Cone, W.T.; Turner, W.G. The treatment of the fracture-dislocation of the cervical vertebrae by skeletal traction and fusion. J Bone Joint Surg [Am] 19:584–602, 1937.

53. Conlon, P.W.; Isdale, I.C.; Rose, B.S. Rheumatoid arthritis of the cervical spine. An analysis of 333 cases. Ann Rheum Dis 25:120–126, 1966.

54. Cooper, A.A. Treatise on Dislocations and Fractures of the Joints. In: Cooper B.B. ed. London, Longman, Hurst Rees, Orme Browne, E. Cox & Son, 1823.

55. Coric, D.; Wilson, J.A.; Kelly, D.L., Jr. Treatment of traumatic spondylolisthesis of the axis with nonrigid immobilization: A review of 64 cases. J Neurosurg 85:550–554, 1996.

56. Corner, E.S. Rotary dislocations of the atlas. Ann Surg 45:9–26, 1907.

57. Cornish, B.L. Traumatic spondylolisthesis of the axis. J Bone Joint Surg [Br] 50:31–43, 1968.

58. Coutts, M.B. Rotary dislocations of the atlas. Ann Surg 29:297–311, 1934.

59. Crockard, A. Evaluation of spinal laminar fixation by a new, flexible stainless steel cable (Sofwire): Early results. Neurosurgery 35:892–898; discussion 898, 1994.

60. Crockard, H.A.; Heilman, A.E.; Stevens, J.M. Progressive myelopathy secondary to odontoid fractures: Clinical, radiological, and surgical features. J Neurosurg 78:579–586, 1993.

61. Crooks, F.B.; Birkett, A.N. Fractures and dislocations of the cervical spine. Br J Surg 31:252–265, 1944.

62. Davis, D.; Bohlman, H.; Walker, A.E.; et al. The pathological findings in fatal craniospinal injuries. J Neurosurg 34:603–613, 1971.

63. De Beer, J.D.; Thomas, T.M.; Walter, J.; Anderson, P. Traumatic atlantoaxial subluxation. J Bone Joint Surg [Am] 70:652–655, 1988.

64. Devi, B.I.; Dubey, S.; Shetty, S.; et al. Fracture occipital condyle with isolated 12th nerve paresis. Neurol India 48:93–94, 2000.

65. Dickman, C.A.; Papadopoulos, S.M.; Sonntag, V.K.; et al. Traumatic occipitoatlantal dislocations. J Spinal Disord 6:300–313, 1993.

66. Dickman, C.A.; Sonntag, V.K. Injuries involving the transverse atlantal ligament: Classification and treatment guidelines based upon experience with 39 injuries. Neurosurgery 40:886–887, 1997.

67. Dimtriev, A.E.; Lehman, R.A.; Helgeson, M.D.; Riew, K.D.; et al. Acute and Long Term Fatigue Stability Three Axial Fixation Methods: A Biomechanical Comparison of Pars, Pedicle, and Intralaminar Screws. In Cervical Spine Research Society [abstract]. Presented, Palm Springs, Florida, 2006.

68. Doherty, B.J.; Heggeness, M.H. Quantitative anatomy of the second cervical vertebra. Spine 20:513–517, 1995.

69. Doherty, B.J.; Heggeness, M.H.; Esses, S.I. A biomechanical study of odontoid fractures and fracture fixation. Spine 18:178–184, 1993.

70. Donovan, M.M. Efficacy of rigid fixation of fractures of the odontoid process. Retrospective analysis of fifty-four cases. Orthop Trans 4:46, 1980.

71. Dublin, A.B.; Marks, W.M.; Weinstock, D.; et al. Traumatic dislocation of the atlanto-occipital articulation (AOA) with short-term survival. With a radiographic method of measuring the AOA. J Neurosurg 52:541–546, 1980.

72. Dunbar, H.S.; Ray, B.S. Chronic atlanto-axial dislocations with late neurologic manifestations. Surg Gynecol Obstet 113:757–762, 1961.

73. Dussault, R.G.; Effendi, B.; Roy, D.; et al. Locked facets with fracture of the neural arch of the axis. Spine 8:365–367, 1983.

74. Dvorak, M.F.; Johnson, M.G.; Boyd, M.; et al. Long-term health-related quality of life outcomes following Jefferson-type burst fractures of the atlas. J Neurosurg Spine 2:411–417, 2005.

75. Dvorak, J.; Panjabi, M.M. Functional anatomy of the alar ligaments. Spine 12:183–189, 1987.

76. Ebraheim, N.A.; Lu, J.; Biyani, A.; et al. An anatomic study of the thickness of the occipital bone. Implications for occipitocervical instrumentation. Spine 21:1725–1729; discussion 1729–1730, 1996.

77. Effendi, B.; Roy, D.; Cornish, B.; et al. Fractures of the ring of the axis. A classification based on the analysis of 131 cases. J Bone Joint Surg [Br] 63-B:319–327, 1981.

78. Ehara, S.; el-Khoury, G.Y.; Clark, C.R. Radiologic evaluation of dens fracture. Role of plain radiography and tomography. Spine 17:475–479, 1992.

79. Eismont, F.J.; Bohlman, H.H. Posterior atlanto-occipital dislocation with fractures of the atlas and odontoid process. J Bone Joint Surg [Am] 60:397–399, 1978.

80. Elia, M.; Mazzara, J.T.; Fielding, J.W. Onlay technique for occipitocervical fusion. Clin Orthop Relat Res 280:170–174, 1992.

81. Englander, O. Nontraumatic occipitoatlantoaxial dislocation. A contribution to the radiology of the atlas. Br J Radiol 15:341–345, 1942.

82. Esses, S.I.; Bednar, D.A. Screw fixation of odontoid fractures and nonunions. Spine 16(10 Suppl):S483–S485, 1991.

83. Esses, S.; Langer, F.; Gross, A. Fracture of the atlas associated with fracture of the odontoid process. Injury 12:310–312, 1981.

84. Etter, C.; Coscia, M.; Jaberg, H.; et al. Direct anterior fixation of dens fractures with a cannulated screw system. Spine 16(3 Suppl):S25–S32, 1991.

85. Evarts, C.M. Traumatic occipito-atlantal dislocation. J Bone Joint Surg [Am] 52:1653–1660, 1970.

86. Fang, H.S.Y.; Ong, G.B. Direct anterior approach to the upper cervical spine. J Bone Joint Surg [Am] 44:1588–1604, 1962.

87. Farey, I.D.; Nadkarni, S.; Smith, N. Modified Gallie technique versus transarticular screw fixation in C1-C2 fusion. Clin Orthop Relat Res 359:126–135, 1999.

88. Fehlings, M.G.; Errico, T.; Cooper, P.; et al. Occipitocervical fusion with a five-millimeter malleable rod and segmental fixation. Neurosurgery 32:198–207; discussion 207–208, 1993.

89. Fernyhough, J.C.; Schimandle, J.J.; Weigel, M.C.; et al. Chronic donor site pain complicating bone graft harvesting from the posterior iliac crest for spinal fusion. Spine 17:1474–1480, 1992.

90. Fielding, J.W.; Cochran, G.B.; Lawsing, J.F., 3rd; et al. Tears of the transverse ligament of the atlas. A clinical and biomechanical study. J Bone Joint Surg [Am] 56:1683–1691, 1974.

91. Fielding, J.W.; Hawkins, R.J. Atlanto-axial rotatory fixation. (Fixed rotatory subluxation of the atlanto-axial joint). J Bone Joint Surg [Am] 59:37–44, 1977.

92. Fielding, J.W.; Hawkins, R.J.; Hensinger, R.N.; et al. Atlantoaxial rotary deformities. Orthop Clin North Am 9:955–967, 1978.

93. Fielding, J.W.; Hawkins, R.J.; Ratzan, S.A. Spine fusion for atlanto-axial instability. J Bone Joint Surg [Am] 58:400–407, 1976.

94. Fielding, J.W.; Hensinger, R.N.; Hawkins, R.J. Os odontoideum. J Bone Joint Surg [Am] 62:376–383, 1980.

95. Fielding, J.W.; Stillwell, W.T.; Chynn, K.Y.; et al. Use of computed tomography for the diagnosis of atlanto-axial rotatory fixation. A case report. J Bone Joint Surg [Am] 60:1102–1104, 1978.

96. Finelli, F.C.; Jonsson, J.; Champion, H.R.; et al. A case control study for major trauma in geriatric patients. J Trauma 29:541–548, 1989.

97. Finney, H.L.; Roberts, T.S. Atlantooccipital instability. Case report. J Neurosurg 48:636–638, 1978.

98. Fiorani-Gallotta, G.; Luzzatti, G. [Lateral subluxation & rotatory subluxation of the atlas.]. Arch Orthop 70:467–484, 1957.

99. Fiore, A.J.; Haid, R.W.; Rodts, G.E.; et al. Atlantal lateral mass screws for posterior spinal reconstruction: Technical note and case series. Neurosurg Focus 12:E5, 2002.

100. Fountas, K.N.; Kapsalaki, E.Z.; Karempelas, I.; et al. Results of long-term follow-up in patients undergoing anterior screw fixation for type II and rostral type III odontoid fractures. Spine 30:661–669, 2005.

101. Fountas, K.N.; Machinis, T.G.; Kapsalaki, E.Z.; et al. Surgical treatment of acute type II and rostral type III odontoid fractures managed by anterior screw fixation. South Med J 98:896–901, 2005.

102. Francis, W.R.; Fielding, J.W. Traumatic spondylolisthesis of the axis. Orthop Clin North Am 9:1011–1027, 1978.

103. Francis, W.R.; Fielding, J.W.; Hawkins, R.J.; et al. Traumatic spondylolisthesis of the axis. J Bone Joint Surg [Br] 63-B:313–318, 1981.

104. Fried, L.C. Atlanto-axial fracture-dislocations. Failure of posterior C.1 to C.2 fusion. J Bone Joint Surg [Br] 55:490–496, 1973.

105. Fruin, A.H.; Pirotte, T.P. Traumatic atlantooccipital dislocation. Case report. J Neurosurg 46:663–666, 1977.

106. Fuji, T.; Oda, T.; Kato, Y.; et al. Accuracy of atlantoaxial transarticular screw insertion. Spine 25:1760–1764, 2000.

107. Fujii, E.; Kobayashi, K.; Hirabayashi, K. Treatment in fractures of the odontoid process. Spine 13:604–609, 1988.

108. Gabrielsen, T.O.; Maxwell, J.A. Traumatic atlantooccipital dislocation; with case report of a patient who survived. Am J Roentgenol Radium Ther Nucl Med 97:624–629, 1966.

109. Gallie, W.E. Fractures and dislocations of the cervical spine. Am J Surg 46:495–499, 1939.

110. Garber, J.N. Abnormalities of the atlas and axis vertebrae—Congenital and traumatic. J Bone Joint Surg [Am] 46:1782–1791, 1964.

111. Gaudagni, A.P. Fracture of the first cervical vertebra, complicated by a cervical rib. JAMA 130: 276–277, 1946.

112. Gehweiler, J.A., Jr.; Daffner, R.H.; Roberts, L., Jr. Malformations of the atlas vertebra simulating the Jefferson fracture. AJR Am J Roentgenol 140:1083–1086, 1983.

113. Gehweiler, J.O.; Osborn, R.L., Jr.; Becker, R.F, eds. The Radiology of Vertebral Trauma. Philadelphia, W.B. Saunders, 1980.

114. Georgopoulos, G.; Pizzutillo, P.D.; Lee, M.S. Occipito-atlantal instability in children. A report of five cases and review of the literature. J Bone Joint Surg [Am] 69:429–436, 1987.

115. Goel, A.; Muzumdar, D.; Dindorkar, K.; et al. Atlantoaxial dislocation associated with stenosis of canal at atlas. J Postgrad Med 43:75–77, 1997.

116. Gonzalez, L.F.; Crawford, N.R.; Chamberlain, R.H.; et al. Craniovertebral junction fixation with transarticular screws: Biomechanical analysis of a novel technique. J Neurosurg 98(2 Suppl):202–209, 2003.

117. Gonzalez, L.F.; Fiorella, D.; Crawford, N.R.; et al. Vertical atlantoaxial distraction injuries: Radiological criteria and clinical implications. J Neurosurg Spine 1:273–280, 2004.

118. Gorek, J.; Acaroglu, E.; Berven, S.; et al. Constructs incorporating intralaminar C2 screws provide rigid stability for atlantoaxial fixation. Spine 30:1513–1518, 2005.

119. Govender, S.; Maharaj, J.F.; Haffajee, M.R. Fractures of the odontoid process. J Bone Joint Surg [Br] 82:1143–1147, 2000.

120. Grauer, J.N.; Shafi, B.; Hilibrand, A.S.; et al. Proposal of a modified, treatment-oriented classification of odontoid fractures. Spine J 5:123–129, 2005.

121. Graziano, G.J.; Jaggers, C.; Lee, M.; et al. A comparative study of fixation techniques for type II fractures of the odontoid process. Spine 18: 2383–2387, 1993.

122. Greene, K.A.; Dickman, C.A.; Marciano, F.F.; et al. Transverse atlantal ligament disruption associated with odontoid fractures. Spine 19:2307–2314, 1994.

123. Greene, K.A.; Dickman, C.A.; Marciano, F.F.; et al. Acute axis fractures. Analysis of management and outcome in 340 consecutive cases. Spine 22:1843–1852, 1997.

124. Grisel, P. Enucleation de l'atlas et torticollis nasopharyngien. Presse Med 38:50–53, 1930.

125. Griswold, D.M.; Albright, J.A.; Schiffman, E.; et al. Atlanto-axial fusion for instability. J Bone Joint Surg [Am] 60:285–292, 1978.

126. Grob, D. Transarticular screw fixation for atlanto-occipital dislocation. Spine 26:703–707, 2001.

127. Grob, D.; Crisco, J.J., 3rd; Panjabi, M.M.; et al. Biomechanical evaluation of four different posterior atlantoaxial fixation techniques. Spine 17:480–490, 1992.

128. Grob, D.; Dvorak, J.; Panjabi, M.; et al. Posterior occipitocervical fusion. A preliminary report of a new technique. Spine 16(3 Suppl):S17–24, 1991.

129. Grob, D.; Dvorak, J.; Panjabi, M.M.; et al. The role of plate and screw fixation in occipitocervical fusion in rheumatoid arthritis. Spine 19:2545–2551, 1994.

130. Grob, D.; Jeanneret, B.; Aebi, M.; et al. Atlantoaxial fusion with transarticular screw fixation. J Bone Joint Surg [Br] 73:972–976, 1991.

131. Grob, D; An, H.S. Posterior occiput and C-1/C-2 instrumentation. In An, H.S.; Colter, J.M., eds. Spinal Instrumentation, 2nd ed. Philadelphia, Lippincott, Williams & Wilkins, 2000, pp. 191–201.

132. Grogano, B.J.S. Injury of the atlas and axis. J Bone Joint Surg [Br] 33:397–410, 1954.

133. Gross, J.D.; Benzel, E.C. Non-operative treatment of hangman's fracture. In Zdeblick, T.A.; Anderson, P.A.; Stillerman, C.B., eds. Controversies in Spine Surgery. St. Louis, Quality Medical Publishing, 1999, pp. 51–71.

134. Hacker, R.J. Screw fixation for odontoid fracture; a comparison of the anterior and posterior technique. Nebr Med J 81:275–278, 1996.

135. Hadley, M.N. Occipital condyle fractures. Neurosurgery 50:S114–S119, 2002.

136. Hadley, M.N.; Dickman, C.A.; Browner, C.M.; et al. Acute traumatic atlas fractures: Management and long term outcome. Neurosurgery 23:31–35, 1988.

137. Hadley, M.N.; Sonntag, V.K.; Grahm, T.W.; et al. Axis fractures resulting from motor vehicle accidents. The need for occupant restraints. Spine 11:861–864, 1986.

138. Han, S.Y.; Witten, D.M.; Mussleman, J.P. Jefferson fracture of the atlas. Report of six cases. J Neurosurg 44:368–371, 1976.

139. Hanigan, W.C.; Powell, F.C.; Elwood, P.W.; et al. Odontoid fractures in elderly patients. J Neurosurg 78:32–35, 1993.

140. Hanson, J.A.; Deliganis, A.V.; Baxter, A.B.; et al. Radiologic and clinical spectrum of occipital condyle fractures: Retrospective review of 107 consecutive fractures in 95 patients. AJR Am J Roentgenol 178:1261–1268, 2002.

141. Hanson, P.B.; Montesano, P.X.; Sharkey, N.A.; et al. Anatomic and biomechanical assessment of transarticular screw fixation for atlantoaxial instability. Spine 16:1141–1145, 1991.

142. Harms, J.; Melcher, R.P. Posterior C1-C2 fusion with polyaxial screw and rod fixation. Spine 26:2467–2471, 2001.

143. Harris, J.H., Jr.; Carson, G.C.; Wagner, L.K.; et al. Radiologic diagnosis of traumatic occipitovertebral dissociation: 2. Comparison of three methods of detecting occipitovertebral relationships on lateral radiographs of supine subjects. AJR Am J Roentgenol 162:887–892, 1994.

144. Hart, R.; Saterbak, A.; Rapp, T.; et al. Nonoperative management of dens fracture nonunion in elderly patients without myelopathy. Spine 25:1339–1343, 2000.

145. Hashizume, H.; Kawakami, M.; Kawai, M.; et al. A clinical case of endoscopically assisted anterior screw fixation for the type II odontoid fracture. Spine 28:E102–105, 2003.

146. Haughton, S. On hanging, considered from a mechanical and physiological point of view. Lond Edinb Dublin Philos Mag J Sci 32:23–34, 1886.

147. Henry, A.D.; Bohly, J.; Grosse, A. Fixation of odontoid fractures by an anterior screw. J Bone Joint Surg [Br] 81:472–477, 1999.

148. Henry, A.K. Extensile Exposure. Edited, Baltimore, Williams & Wilkins, 1957.

149. Hensinger, R.N.; MacEwen, G.D. Congenital anomalies of the spine. In Rothman, R.H.; Simeone, F.A., eds. The Spine, Philadelphia, W.B. Saunders, 1982, pp. 194–201.

150. Hentzer, L.; Schalimtzek, M. Fractures and subluxations of the atlas and axis. A follow-up study of 20 patients. Acta Orthop Scand 42:251–258, 1971.

151. Hess, J.H.; Bronstein, I.P.; Abelson, S.M: Atlantoaxial dislocations unassociated with trauma and secodary to inflammatory foci in the neck. Am J Dis Child 49:1137–1147, 1935.

152. Hinchey, J.J.; Bickel, W.H. Fracture of the atlas, review and presentation of data on eight cases. Ann Surg 121:826–832, 1945.

153. Hinck, V.C.; Hopkins, C.E.; Savara, B.S. Sagittal diameter of the cervical spinal canal in children. Radiology 79:97–108, 1962.

154. Hohl, M.; Baker, H.R. The atlanto-axial joint. Roentgenographic and anatomical study of normal and abnormal motion. J Bone Joint Surg [Am] 46:1739–1752, 1964.

155. Hong, X.; Dong, Y.; Yunbing, C.; et al. Posterior screw placement on the lateral mass of atlas: An anatomic study. Spine 29:500–503, 2004.

156. Horlyck, E.; Rahbek, M. Cervical spine injuries. Acta Orthop Scand 45:845–853, 1974.

157. Horn, E.M.; Hott, J.S.; Porter, R.W.; et al. Atlantoaxial stabilization with the use of C1-3 lateral mass screw fixation. Technical note. J Neurosurg Spine 5:172–177, 2006.

158. Howington, J.U.; Kruse, J.J.; Awasthi, D. Surgical anatomy of the C-2 pedicle. J Neurosurg 95 (1 Suppl):88–92, 2001.

159. Igarashi, T.; Kikuchi, S.; Sato, K.; et al. Anatomic study of the axis for surgical planning of transarticular screw fixation. Clin Orthop Relat Res 408:162–166, 2003.

160. Jackson, H. The diagnosis of minimal atlanto-axial subluxation. Br J Radiol 23:672–674, 1950.

161. Jackson, R.S.; Banit, D.M.; Rhyne, A.L., 3rd; et al. Upper cervical spine injuries. J Am Acad Orthop Surg 10:271–280, 2002.

162. Jea, A.; Tatsui, C.; Farhat, H.; et al. Vertically unstable type III odontoid fractures: Case report. Neurosurgery 58:E797; discussion E797, 2006.

163. Jeanneret, B.; Magerl, F. Primary posterior fusion C1/2 in odontoid fractures: Indications, technique, and results of transarticular screw fixation. J Spinal Disord 5:464–475, 1992.

164. Jefferson, G. Fracture of the atlas vertebra. Report of four cases and a review of those previously recorded. Br J Surg 7:407–422, 1920.

165. Jenkins, J.D.; Coric, D.; Branch, C.L., Jr. A clinical comparison of one- and two-screw odontoid fixation. J Neurosurg 89:366–370, 1998.

166. Johnston, R.A. Management of old people with neck trauma. BMJ 299:633–634, 1989.

167. Jones, R.N. Rotatory dislocation of both atlantoaxial joints. J Bone Joint Surg [Br] 66:6–7, 1984.

168. Julien, T.D.; Frankel, B.; Traynelis, V.C.; et al. Evidence-based analysis of odontoid fracture management. Neurosurg Focus 8:e1, 2000.

169. Jun, B.Y. Anatomic study for ideal and safe posterior C1-C2 transarticular screw fixation. Spine 23:1703–1707, 1998.

170. Jun, B.Y. Complete reduction of retro-odontoid soft tissue mass in os odontoideum following the posterior C1-C2 transarticular screw fixation. Spine 24:1961–1964, 1999.

171. Kaufman, R.A.; Dunbar, J.S.; Botsford, J.A.; et al. Traumatic longitudinal atlanto-occipital distraction injuries in children. AJNR Am J Neuroradiol 3:415–419, 1982.

172. Kim, S.M.; Lim, T.J.; Paterno, J.; et al. Biomechanical comparison of anterior and posterior stabilization methods in atlantoaxial instability. J Neurosurg 100 (3 Suppl Spine):277–283, 2004.

173. Kirankumar, M.V.; Behari, S.; Salunke, P.; et al. Surgical management of remote, isolated type II odontoid fractures with atlantoaxial dislocation causing cervical compressive myelopathy. Neurosurgery 56:1004–1012; discussion 1004–1012, 2005.

174. Kirkpatrick, J.S.; Sheils, T.; Theiss, S.M. Type-III dens fracture with distraction: An unstable injury. A report of three cases. J Bone Joint Surg [Am] 86-A:2514–2518, 2004.

175. Kissinger, O. Lexations Fraktur im Atlantooccipitagelenke. Zentralbl Chir 27:933–934, 1900.

176. Knoringer, P. Osteosynthesis of injuries and rheumatic or congenital instabilities of the upper cervical spine using double-threaded screws. Neurosurg Rev 15:275–283, 1992.

177. Koivikko, M.P.; Kiuru, M.J.; Koskinen, S.K. Occurrence of comminution (type IIA) in type II odontoid process fractures: A multi-slice CT study. Emerg Radiol 10:84–86, 2003.

178. Koivikko, M.P.; Kiuru, M.J.; Koskinen, S.K.; et al. Factors associated with nonunion in conservatively-treated type-II fractures of the odontoid process. J Bone Joint Surg [Br] 86:1146–1151, 2004.

179. Lakshmanan, P.; Jones, A.; Howes, J.; et al. CT evaluation of the pattern of odontoid fractures in the elderly—relationship to upper cervical spine osteoarthritis. Eur Spine J 14:78–83, 2005.

180. Landells, C.D.; Van Peteghem, P.K. Fractures of the atlas: Classification, treatment, and morbidity. Spine 13:450–452, 1988.

181. Lee, C.; Woodring, J.H. Unstable Jefferson variant atlas fractures: An unrecognized cervical injury. AJNR Am J Neuroradiol 12:1105–1110, 1991.

182. Lee, T.T.; Green, B.A.; Petrin, D.R. Treatment of stable burst fracture of the atlas (Jefferson fracture) with rigid cervical collar. Spine 23:1963–1967, 1998.

183. Legros, B.; Fournier, P.; Chiaroni, P.; et al. Basal fracture of the skull and lower (IX, X, XI, XII) cranial nerves palsy: Four case reports including two fractures of the occipital condyle—a literature review. J Trauma 48:342–348, 2000.

184. Lehman, R.A., Jr.; Dmitriev, A.E.; Helgeson, M.D.; et al. Salvage of C2 Pedicle and Pars Screws Using the Intralaminar Technique: A Biomechanical Analysis. In Cervical Spine Research Society. Edited, Palm Springs, Florida, 2006.

185. Lennarson, P.J.; Mostafavi, H.; Traynelis, V.C.; et al. Management of type II dens fractures: A case-control study. Spine 25:1234–1237, 2000.

186. Levine, A.M.; Edwards, C.C. The management of traumatic spondylolisthesis of the axis. J Bone Joint Surg [Am] 67:217–226, 1985.

187. Levine, A.M.; Edwards, C.C. Treatment of injuries in the C1-C2 complex. Orthop Clin North Am 17:31–44, 1986.

188. Levine, A.M.; Edwards, C.C. Traumatic lesions of the occipitoatlantoaxial complex. Clin Orthop Relat Res 239:53–68, 1989.

189. Levine, A.M.; Edwards, C.C. Fractures of the atlas. J Bone Joint Surg [Am] 73:680–691, 1991.

190. Levine, A.M. Lutz, B. Extension teardrop injuries of the cervical spine. In Annual Meeting of the Cervical Spine Research Society. Edited, New York, 1993.

191. Li, X.F.; Dai, L.Y.; Lu, H.; et al. A systematic review of the management of hangman's fractures. Eur Spine J 15:257–269, 2006.

192. Lind, B.; Bake, B.; Lundqvist, C.; et al. Influence of halo vest treatment on vital capacity. Spine 12:449–452, 1987.

193. Lind, B.; Nordwall, A.; Sihlbom, H. Odontoid fractures treated with halo-vest. Spine 12:173–177, 1987.

194. Lipson, S.J. Fractures of the atlas associated with fractures of the odontoid process and transverse ligament ruptures. J Bone Joint Surg [Am] 59:940–943, 1977.

195. Louis, R. Anterior surgery of the upper cervical spine. Chir Organi Mov 77:75–80, 1992.

196. Lustrin, E.S.; Robertson, R.L.; Tilak, S. Normal anatomy of the skull base. Neuroimaging Clin N Am 4:465–478, 1994.

197. Ma, X.Y.; Yin, Q.S.; Wu, Z.H.; et al. Anatomic considerations for the pedicle screw placement in the first cervical vertebra. Spine 30:1519–1523, 2005.

198. Maak, T.G.; Grauer, J.N. The contemporary treatment of odontoid injuries. Spine 31(11 Suppl): S53–60; discussion S61, 2006.

199. Madawi, A.A.; Casey, A.T.; Solanki, G.A.; et al. Radiological and anatomical evaluation of the atlantoaxial transarticular screw fixation technique. J Neurosurg 86:961–968, 1997.

200. Majercik, S.; Tashjian, R.Z.; Biffl, W.L.; et al. Halo vest immobilization in the elderly: A death sentence? J Trauma 59:350–356; discussion 356–358, 2005.

201. Malagaigne, J. Traite des Fractures et des Luxations. Edited, Paris, J.B. Bailliere, 1847.

202. Mandel, I.M.; Kambach, B.J.; Petersilge, C.A.; et al. Morphologic considerations of C2 isthmus dimensions for the placement of transarticular screws. Spine 25:1542–1547, 2000.

203. Marar, B.C. Fracture of the axis arch. "Hangman's fracture" of the cervical spine. Clin Orthop Relat Res 106:155–165, 1975.

204. Marar, B.C.; Tay, C.K. Fracture of the odontoid process. Aust N Z J Surg 46:231–236, 1976.

205. Marlin, A.E.; Williams, G.R.; Lee, J.F. Jefferson fractures in children. Case report. J Neurosurg 58:277–279, 1983.

206. Martel, W. The occipitoatlantoaxial joints in rheumatoid arthritis and ankylosing spondylitis. AJR Am J Roentgenol 86:223–240, 1960.

207. Marton, E.; Billeci, D.; Carteri, A. Therapeutic indications in upper cervical spine instability. Considerations on 58 cases. J Neurosurg Sci 44:192–202, 2000.

208. Maughan, P.H.; Horn, E.M.; Theodore, N.; et al. Avulsion fracture of the foramen magnum treated with occiput-to-C1 fusion: Technical case report. Neurosurgery 57:E600; discussion E600, 2005.

209. McAfee, P.C.; Cassidy, J.R.; Davis, R.F.; et al. Fusion of the occiput to the upper cervical spine. A review of 37 cases. Spine 16(10 Suppl):S490–494, 1991.

210. McBride, A.D.; Mukherjee, D.P.; Kruse, R.N.; et al. Anterior screw fixation of type II odontoid fractures. A biomechanical study. Spine 20:1855–1859; discussion 1859–1860, 1995.

211. McCulloch, P.T.; France, J.; Jones, D.L.; et al. Helical computed tomography alone compared with plain radiographs with adjunct computed tomography to evaluate the cervical spine after high-energy trauma. J Bone Joint Surg [Am] 87:2388–2394, 2005.

212. McGraw, R.W.; Rusch, R.M. Atlanto-axial arthrodesis. J Bone Joint Surg [Br] 55:482–489, 1973.

213. McGuire, R.A., Jr.; Harkey, H.L. Trauma update: Unstable Jefferson's fracture treated with transarticular screws. Orthopedics 18:207–209, 1995.

214. Melcher, R.P.; Puttlitz, C.M.; Kleinstueck, F.S.; et al. Biomechanical testing of posterior atlantoaxial fixation techniques. Spine 27:2435–2440, 2002.

215. Miyazaki, C.; Katsume, M.; Yamazaki, T.; et al. Unusual occipital condyle fracture with multiple nerve palsies and Wallenberg syndrome. Clin Neurol Neurosurg 102:255–258, 2000.

216. Montesano, P.X.; Anderson, P.A.; Schlehr, F.; et al. Odontoid fractures treated by anterior odontoid screw fixation. Spine 16(3 Suppl): S33–37, 1991.

217. Mouradian, W.H.; Fietti, V.G., Jr.; Cochran, G.V.; et al. Fractures of the odontoid: A laboratory and clinical study of mechanisms. Orthop Clin North Am 9:985–1001, 1978.

218. Muller, E.J.; Schwinnen, I.; Fischer, K.; et al. Nonrigid immobilisation of odontoid fractures. Eur Spine J 12:522–525, 2003.

219. Muller, E.J.; Wick, M.; Muhr, G. Traumatic spondylolisthesis of the axis: Treatment rationale based on the stability of the different fracture types. Eur Spine J 9:123–128, 2000.

220. Mullett, J.H.; McCarthy, P.; O'Keefe, D.; et al. Occipital fixation: Effect of inner occipital protuberance alignment on screw position. J Spinal Disord 14:504–506, 2001.

221. Murphy, M.J.; Southwick, W.O. Posterior approaches and fusions. In Clark, C.R.; Dvorak, J.; Ducker, T.B.; et al., eds. The Cervical Spine. Philadelphia, Lippincott-Raven, 1998, pp. 775–791.

222. Murphy, M.J.; Wu, J.C.; Southwick, W.O. Complications of halo fixation. Orthop Trans 3:126, 1979.

223. Nachemson, A. Fracture of the odontoid process of the axis: A clinical study based on 26 cases. Acta Orthop Scand 29:185–217, 1959.

224. Naderi, S.; Usal, C.; Tural, A.N.; et al. Morphologic and radiologic anatomy of the occipital bone. J Spinal Disord 14:500–503, 2001.

225. Nadim, Y.; Sabry, F.; Xu, R.; et al. Computed tomography in the determination of transarticular C1-C2 screw length. Orthopedics 23:373–375, 2000.

226. Nakanishi, T. Internal fixation of odontoid fracture. Orthop Traumat Surg 23:399–406, 1980.

227. Nightingale, R.W.; Winkelstein, B.A.; Knaub, K.E.; et al. Comparative strengths and structural properties of the upper and lower cervical spine in flexion and extension. J Biomech 35:725–732, 2002.

228. Nucci, R.C.; Seigal, S.; Merola, A.A.; et al. Computed tomographic evaluation of the normal adult odontoid. Implications for internal fixation. Spine 20:264–270, 1995.

229. O'Brien, J.J.; Butterfield, W.L.; Gossling, H.R. Jefferson fracture with disruption of the transverse ligament. A case report. Clin Orthop Relat Res 126:135–138, 1977.

230. Oda, I.; Abumi, K.; Sell, L.C.; et al. Biomechanical evaluation of five different occipito-atlanto-axial fixation techniques. Spine 24:2377–2382, 1999.

231. Olerud, C.; Andersson, S.; Svensson, B.; et al. Cervical spine fractures in the elderly: Factors influencing survival in 65 cases. Acta Orthop Scand 70:509–513, 1999.

232. Ondra, S.L.; Marzouk, S.; Ganju, A.; et al. Safety and efficacy of C2 pedicle screws placed with anatomic and lateral C-arm guidance. Spine 31: E263–267, 2006.

233. Page, C.P.; Story, J.L.; Wissinger, J.P.; et al. Traumatic atlantooccipital dislocation. Case report. J Neurosurg 39:394–397, 1973.

234. Pait, T.G.; Al-Mefty, O.; Boop, F.A.; et al. Inside-outside technique for posterior occipitocervical spine instrumentation and stabilization: Preliminary results. J Neurosurg 90(1 Suppl):1–7, 1999.

235. Pang, D.; Li, V. Atlantoaxial rotatory fixation: Part 1—Biomechanics of normal rotation at the atlantoaxial joint in children. Neurosurgery 55:614–625; discussion 625–626, 2004.

236. Paradis, G.R.; Janes, J.M. Posttraumatic atlantoaxial instability: The fate of the odontoid process fracture in 46 cases. J Trauma 13:359–367, 1973.

237. Paramore, C.G.; Dickman, C.A.; Sonntag, V.K. The anatomical suitability of the C1-2 complex for transarticular screw fixation. J Neurosurg 85:221–224, 1996.

238. Pelker, R.R.; Dorfman, G.S. Fracture of the axis associated with vertebral artery injury. A case report. Spine 11:621–623, 1986.

239. Pepin, J.W.; Bourne, R.B.; Hawkins, R.J. Odontoid fractures, with special reference to the elderly patient. Clin Orthop Relat Res 193:178–183, 1985.

240. Pepin, J.W.; Hawkins, R.J. Traumatic spondylolisthesis of the axis: Hangman's fracture. Clin Orthop Relat Res 157:133–138, 1981.

241. Perry, J.; Nickel, V.L. Total cervical spine fusion for neck paralysis. J Bone Joint Surg [Am] 41-A:37–60, 1959.

242. Pfirrmann, C.W.; Binkert, C.A.; Zanetti, M.; et al. MR morphology of alar ligaments and occipitoatlantoaxial joints: Study in 50 asymptomatic subjects. Radiology 218:133–137, 2001.

243. Pierce, D.S.; Ojemann, R.G. Injuries of the spine, neurologic considerations. Fractures and dislocations. In Cave, E.F.; Burke, J.F.; Boyd, R.J., eds., Trauma Management. Chicago, YearBook Medical Publishers, 1974, pp. 343–397.

244. Polin, R.S.; Szabo, T.; Bogaev, C.A.; et al. Nonoperative management of Types II and III odontoid fractures: The Philadelphia collar versus the halo vest. Neurosurgery 38:450–456; discussion 456–467, 1996.

245. Powers, B.; Miller, M.D.; Kramer, R.S.; et al. Traumatic anterior atlanto-occipital dislocation. Neurosurgery 4:12–27, 1979.

246. Przybylski, G.J.; Clyde, B.L.; Fitz, C.R. Craniocervical junction subarachnoid hemorrhage associated with atlanto-occipital dislocation. Spine 21:1761–1768, 1996.

247. Przybylski, G.J.; Harrop, J.S.; Vaccaro, A.R. Closed management of displaced Type II odontoid fractures: More frequent respiratory compromise with posteriorly displaced fractures. Neurosurg Focus 8:e5, 2000.

248. Przybylski, G.J.; Welch, W.C. Longitudinal atlantoaxial dislocation with type III odontoid fracture. Case report and review of the literature. J Neurosurg 84:666–670, 1996.

249. Puttlitz, C.M.; Melcher, R.P.; Kleinstueck, F.S.; et al. Stability analysis of craniovertebral junction fixation techniques. J Bone Joint Surg [Am] 86-A:561–568, 2004.

250. Raby, N.; Berman, L.; de Lacey, G. Accident and Emergency Radiology. Philadelphia, Saunders, 2005.

251. Ransford, A.O.; Crockard, H.A.; Pozo, J.L.; et al. Craniocervical instability treated by contoured loop fixation. J Bone Joint Surg [Br] 68:173–177, 1986.

252. Rao, R.D.; Singhal, P. Delayed development of neurological deficit from an occipital fracture. A case report. J Bone Joint Surg [Am] 86-A:1047–1050, 2004.

253. Rao, S.K.; Wasyliw, C.; Nunez, D.B., Jr. Spectrum of imaging findings in hyperextension injuries of the neck. Radiographics 25:1239–1254, 2005.

254. Robinson, R.A.; Southwick, W.O. Surgical approaches to the cervical spine. Instr Course Lect 17:299–330, 1960.

255. Rocha R.; Baek, S.; Safavi-Abbasi, S.; et al. Biomechanical study of atlantoaxial rotary subluxation and related surgical fusion methods. In Cervical Spine Research Society. Presentation, Palm Beach, Florida, 2006.

256. Rodrigues, F.A.; Hodgson, B.F.; Craig, J.B. Posterior atlantoaxial arthrodesis. A simplified method. Spine 16:878–880, 1991.

257. Rogers, W.A. Treatment of fracture-dislocation of the cervical spine. J Bone Joint Surg [Am] 24:245–258, 1942.

258. Rogers, W.A. Fractures and dislocations of the cervical spine; an end-result study. J Bone Joint Surg [Am] 39-A:341–376, 1957.

259. Roy-Camille, R. Recent Advances in Orthopaedics. In Apley, A.G.; McKibbin, B. eds. Edinburgh, Churchill-Livingstone, 1979.

260. Roy-Camille, R. Fractures des pedicules de l'axis. Journees d'orthopedie a la Pitie. Edited, Paris, Masson, 1984.

261. Roy-Camille, R.; Saillant, G.; Mazel, C. Internal fixation of the unstable cerivcal spine by a posterior osteosynthesis with plates and screws. In Sherk, H.H.; Dunn, H.J.; Eismont, J.J.; et al. The Cervical Spine, Philadelphia, J.B. Lippincott, 1989, pp. 390–403.

262. Rubinstein, D.; Escott, E.J.; Mestek, M.F. Computed tomographic scans of minimally displaced type II odontoid fractures. J Trauma 40:204–210, 1996.

263. Ruf, M.; Melcher, R.; Harms, J. Transoral reduction and osteosynthesis C1 as a function-preserving option in the treatment of unstable Jefferson fractures. Spine 29:823–827, 2004.

264. Ruge, D.; Wiltse, L.L. Spinal Disorders: Diagnosis and Treatment. Philadelphia, Lea & Febiger, 1977.

265. Ryan, M.D.; Henderson, J.J. The epidemiology of fractures and fracture-dislocations of the cervical spine. Injury 23:38–40, 1992.

266. Ryan, M.D.; Taylor, T.K. Odontoid fractures. A rational approach to treatment. J Bone Joint Surg [Br] 64:416–421, 1982.

267. Samaha, C.; Lazennec, J.Y.; Laporte, C.; et al. Hangman's fracture: The relationship between asymmetry and instability. J Bone Joint Surg [Br] 82:1046–1052, 2000.

268. Sandhu, F.A.; Pait, T.G.; Benzel, E.; et al. Occipitocervical fusion for rheumatoid arthritis using the inside-outside stabilization technique. Spine 28:414–419, 2003.

269. Sasso, R.; Doherty, B.J.; Crawford, M.J.; et al. Biomechanics of odontoid fracture fixation. Comparison of the one- and two-screw technique. Spine 18:1950–1953, 1993.

270. Sasso, R.C.; Jeanneret, B.; Fischer, K.; et al. Occipitocervical fusion with posterior plate and screw instrumentation. A long-term follow-up study. Spine 19:2364–2368, 1994.

271. Schatzker, J.; Rorabeck, C.H.; Waddell, J.P. Fractures of the dens (odontoid process). An analysis of thirty-seven cases. J Bone Joint Surg [Br] 53:392–405, 1971.

272. Schiff, D.C.; Parke, W.W. The arterial supply of the odontoid process. J Bone Joint Surg [Am] 55:1450–1456, 1973.

273. Schneider, R.C.; Livingston, K.E.; Cave, A.J.; et al. "Hangman's fracture" of the cervical spine. J Neurosurg 22:141–154, 1965.

274. Schneider, R.C.; Schemm, G.W. Vertebral artery insufficiency in acute and chronic spinal trauma, with special reference to the syndrome of acute central cervical spinal cord injury. J Neurosurg 18:348–360, 1961.

275. Scott, E.W.; Haid, R.W., Jr.; Peace, D. Type I fractures of the odontoid process: Implications for atlanto-occipital instability. Case report. J Neurosurg 72:488–492, 1990.

276. Segal, L.S.; Grimm, J.O.; Stauffer, E.S. Non-union of fractures of the atlas. J Bone Joint Surg [Am] 69:1423–1434, 1987.

277. Seljeskog, E.L. Non-operative management of acute upper cervical injuries. Acta Neurochir (Wien) 41:87–100, 1978.

278. Seybold, E.A.; Bayley, J.C. Functional outcome of surgically and conservatively managed dens fractures. Spine 23:1837–1845; discussion 1845–1846, 1998.

279. Shapiro, R.; Youngberg, A.S.; Rothman, S.L. The differential diagnosis of traumatic lesions of the occipito-atlanto-axial segment. Radiol Clin North Am 11:505–526, 1973.

280. Sharma, B.S.; Mahajan, R.K.; Bhatia, S.; et al. Collet-Sicard syndrome after closed head injury. Clin Neurol Neurosurg 96:197–198, 1994.

281. Sherk, H.H. Lesions of the atlas and axis. Clin Orthop Relat Res 109:33–41, 1975.

282. Sherk, H.H. Fractures of the atlas and odontoid process. Orthop Clin North Am 9:973–984, 1978.

283. Sherk, H.H.; Howard, T. Clinical and pathologic correlations in traumatic spondylolisthesis of the axis. Clin Orthop Relat Res 174:122–126, 1983.

284. Shilke, L.H.; Callahan, R.A. A rational approach to burst fractures of the atlas. Clin Orthop Relat Res 154:18–21, 1981.

285. Signoret, F.; Feron, J.M.; Bonfait, H.; et al. Fractured odontoid with fractured superior articular process of the axis. Report of three cases. J Bone Joint Surg [Br] 68:182–184, 1986.

286. Silveri, C.P.; Nelson, M.C.; Vaccaro, A.; et al. Traumatic injuries of the adult upper cervical spine. In Cotler, J.M.; Simpson, J.M.; An, H.S.; et al., eds. Surgery of Spinal Trauma, pp. 179–217. Philadelphia, Lippincott Williams & Wilkins, 2000.

287. Skold, G. Fractures of the neural arch and odontoid process of the axis: A study of their causation. Z Rechtsmed 82:89–103, 1978.

288. Smith, M.D.; Anderson, P.; Grady, M.S. Occipitocervical arthrodesis using contoured plate fixation. An early report on a versatile fixation technique. Spine 18:1984–1990, 1993.

289. Solanki, G.A.; Crockard, H.A. Preoperative determination of safe superior transarticular screw trajectory through the lateral mass. Spine 24:1477–1482, 1999.

290. Song, G.S.; Theodore, N.; Dickman, C.A.; et al. Unilateral posterior atlantoaxial transarticular screw fixation. J Neurosurg 87:851–855, 1997.

291. Sonntag, V.K.; Hadley, M.N. Nonoperative management of cervical spine injuries. Clin Neurosurg 34:630–649, 1988.

292. Southwick, W.O. Management of fractures of the dens (odontoid process). J Bone Joint Surg [Am] 62:482–486, 1980.

293. Southwick, W.O.; Robinson, R.A. Surgical approaches to the vertebral bodies in the cervical and lumbar regions. J Bone Joint Surg [Am] 39-A:631–644, 1957.

294. Spence, K.F., Jr.; Decker, S.; Sell, K.W. Bursting atlantal fracture associated with rupture of the transverse ligament. J Bone Joint Surg [Am] 52:543–549, 1970.

295. Starr, J.K.; Eismont, F.J. Atypical hangman's fractures. Spine 18:1954–1957, 1993.

296. Steel, H.H. Anatomical and mechanical considerations of the atlantoaxial articulations. Proceedings of the American Orthopedic Association. J Bone Joint Surg [Am] 50:543–549, 1968.

297. Stillerman, C.B.; Wilson, J.A. Atlanto-axial stabilization with posterior transarticular screw fixation: Technical description and report of 22 cases. Neurosurgery 32:948–954; discussion 954–955, 1993.

298. Stokes, J.K.; Villavicencio, A.T.; Liu, P.C.; et al. Posterior atlantoaxial stabilization: New alternative to C1-2 transarticular screws. Neurosurg Focus 12:E6, 2002.

299. Stoney, J.; O'Brien, J.; Wilde, P. Treatment of type-two odontoid fractures in halothoracic vests. J Bone Joint Surg [Br] 80:452–455, 1998.

300. Subach, B.R.; McLaughlin, M.R.; Albright, A.L.; et al. Current management of pediatric atlantoaxial rotatory subluxation. Spine 23:2174–2179, 1998.

301. Subin, B.; Liu, J.F.; Marshall, G.J.; et al. Transoral anterior decompression and fusion of chronic irreducible atlantoaxial dislocation with spinal cord compression. Spine 20:1233–1240, 1995.

302. Sutherland, J.P., Jr.; Yaszemski, M.J.; White, A.A., 3rd. Radiographic appearance of the odontoid lateral mass interspace in the occipitoatlantoaxial complex. Spine 20:2221–2225, 1995.

303. Sutterlin, C.E., 3rd; Bianchi, J.R.; Kunz, D.N.; et al. Biomechanical evaluation of occipitocervical fixation devices. J Spinal Disord 14:185–192, 2001.

304. Sweigel, J.G. Halothoracic brace in the management of odontoid fractures. Orthop Trans 3:126, 1979.

305. Taggard, D.A.; Kraut, M.A.; Clark, C.R.; et al. Case-control study comparing the efficacy of surgical techniques for C1-C2 arthrodesis. J Spinal Disord Tech 17:189–194, 2004.

306. Taitsman, L.; Hecht, A.C.; Pedlow, F.X. Complications of halo treatment in elderly patients with cervical spine fractures.

307. Tashjian, R.Z.; Majercik, S.; Biffl, W.L.; et al. Halo-vest immobilization increases early morbidity and mortality in elderly odontoid fractures. J Trauma 60:199–203, 2006.

308. Termansen, N.B. Hangman's fracture. Acta Orthop Scand 45:529–539, 1974.

309. Tominaga, T.; Dickman, C.A.; Sonntag, V.K.; et al. Comparative anatomy of the baboon and the human cervical spine. Spine 20:131–137, 1995.

310. Traynelis, V.C.; Marano, G.D.; Dunker, R.O.; et al. Traumatic atlanto-occipital dislocation. Case report. J Neurosurg 65:863–870, 1986.

311. Tuite, G.F.; Papadopoulos, S.M.; Sonntag, V.K. Caspar plate fixation for the treatment of complex hangman's fractures. Neurosurgery 30:761–764; discussion 764–765, 1992.

312. Tuli, S.; Tator, C.H.; Fehlings, M.G.; et al. Occipital condyle fractures. Neurosurgery 41:368–376; discussion 376–377, 1997.

313. Urculo, E.; Arrazola, M.; Arrazola, M., Jr.; et al. Delayed glossopharyngeal and vagus nerve paralysis following occipital condyle fracture. Case report. J Neurosurg 84:522–525, 1996.

314. Vaccaro, A.R.; Lehman, A.P.; Ahlgren, B.D.; et al. Anterior C1-C2 screw fixation and bony fusion through an anterior retropharyngeal approach. Orthopedics 22:1165–1170, 1999.

315. Vaccaro, A.R.; Lim, M.R.; Lee, J.Y. Indications for surgery and stabilization techniques of the occipito-cervical junction. Injury 36(Suppl 2):B44–53, 2005.

316. Vaccaro, A.R.; Madigan, L.; Bauerle, W.B.; et al. Early halo immobilization of displaced traumatic spondylolisthesis of the axis. Spine 27:2229–2233, 2002.

317. Verheggen, R.; Jansen, J. Fractures of the odontoid process: Analysis of the functional results after surgery. Eur Spine J 3:146–150, 1994.

318. Verheggen, R.; Jansen, J. Hangman's fracture: Arguments in favor of surgical therapy for type II and III according to Edwards and Levine. Surg Neurol 49:253–261; discussion 261–262, 1998.

319. Vermooten, V. A study of the fracture of the epistropheus due to hanging with a note of the possible causes of death. Anat Rec 20:305–311, 1921.

320. Vichard, P.; Mirbey, J.; Pinon, P. [Value of anterior arthrodesis in the treatment of fractures of the pedicles of the axis (author's transl)]. J Chir (Paris) 118:565–572, 1981.

321. Vieweg, U.; Schultheiss, R. A review of halo vest treatment of upper cervical spine injuries. Arch Orthop Trauma Surg 121:50–55, 2001.

322. Vishteh, A.G.; Crawford, N.R.; Melton, M.S.; et al. Stability of the craniovertebral junction after unilateral occipital condyle resection: A biomechanical study. J Neurosurg 90(1 Suppl):91–98, 1999.

323. von Torklus, D.; Gehle, W. The Upper Cervical Spine: Regional Anatomy, Pathology, and Traumatology; A Systematic Radiological Atlas and Textbook. New York, Grune and Stratton, 1972.

324. Wang, M.Y. C2 crossing laminar screws: Cadaveric morphometric analysis. Neurosurgery 59(1 Suppl 1):ONS84-88; discussion ONS84-88, 2006.

325. Watanabe, M.; Nomura, T.; Toh, E.; et al. Residual neck pain after traumatic spondylolisthesis of the axis. J Spinal Disord Tech 18:148–151, 2005.

326. Watson-Jones, R. Spontaneous hyperaemic dislocation of the atlas. Proc Soc Med 25:586–590, 1932.

327. Weiland, D.J.; McAfee, P.C. Posterior cervical fusion with triple-wire strut graft technique: One hundred consecutive patients. J Spinal Disord 4:15–21, 1991.

328. Weller, S.J.; Malek, A.M.; Rossitch, E., Jr. Cervical spine fractures in the elderly. Surg Neurol 47:274–280; discussion 280–281, 1997.

329. Werne, S. Studies in spontaneous atlas dislocation. Acta Orthop Scand Suppl 23:1–150, 1957.

330. Wheeler, T. Variability in the spinal column as regards defective neural arches (rudimentary spina bifida). Contrib Embryol 9:97–107, 1920.

331. White, A.A. Hangman's fractures with nonunion and late cord compression. A case report. J Bone Joint Surg [Am] 60:839–840, 1978.

332. White, A.A., 3rd; Panjabi, M.M. Biomechanics of the occipitoatlantoaxial complex. Orthop Clin North Am 9:867–883, 1966.

333. White, A.A., 3rd; Panjabi, M.M. Clinical Biomechanics of the Spine. Philadelphia, Lippincott, 1978.

334. White, A.A.; Panjabi, M.M. Clinical Biomechanics of the Spine. Philadelphia, Lippincott, 1990.

335. Whitesides, T.E., Jr.; and Kelly, R.P. Lateral approach to the upper cervical spine for anterior fusion. South Med J 59:879–883, 1966.

336. Whitesides, T.E., Jr.; McDonald, A.P. Lateral retropharyngeal approach to the upper cervical spine. Orthop Clin North Am 9:1115–1127, 1978.

337. Wholey, M.H.; Bruwer, A.J.; Baker, H.L., Jr. The lateral roentgenogram of the neck; with comments on the atlanto-odontoid-basion relationship. Radiology 71:350–356, 1958.

338. Wiesel, S.W.; Rothman, R.H. Occipitoatlantal hypermobility. Spine 4:187–191, 1979.

339. Wigren, A.; Sweden, U.; Amici, F., Jr. Traumatic atlanto-axial dislocation without neurological disorder. A case report. J Bone Joint Surg [Am] 55:642–644, 1973.

340. Willard, D.P.; Nicholson, J.T. Dislocation of the first cervical vertebra. Ann Surg 113:464–475, 1941.

341. Willauschus, W.G.; Kladny, B.; Beyer, W.F.; et al. Lesions of the alar ligaments. In vivo and in vitro studies with magnetic resonance imaging. Spine 20:2493–2498, 1995.

342. Williams, T.G. Hangman's fracture. J Bone Joint Surg [Br] 57:82–88, 1975.

343. Wittek, A. Ein Fall von distensionsluxation im Atlantoepistrophealgelenke. Muench Med Wochenschr 55:1836–1837, 1908.

344. Wood-Jones, F. The ideal lesion produced by judicial hanging. Lancet 1:53, 1913.

345. Woodring, J.H.; Selke, A.C., Jr.; Duff, D.E. Traumatic atlantooccipital dislocation with survival. AJR Am J Roentgenol 137:21–24, 1981.

346. Wortzman, G.; Dewar, F.P. Rotary fixation of the atlantoaxial joint: Rotational atlantoaxial subluxation. Radiology 90:479–487, 1968.

347. Wright, N.M. Translaminar rigid screw fixation of the axis: Technical note. J Neurosurg Spine 3:409–414, 2005.

348. Xu, R.; Nadaud, M.C.; Ebraheim, N.A.; et al. Morphology of the second cervical vertebra and the posterior projection of the C2 pedicle axis. Spine 20:259–263, 1995.

349. Yoshida, M.; Neo, M.; Fujibayashi, S.; et al. Comparison of the anatomical risk for vertebral artery injury associated with the C2-pedicle screw and atlantoaxial transarticular screw. Spine 31:E513–517, 2006.

350. Young, J.P.; Young, P.H.; Ackermann, M.J.; et al. The ponticulus posticus: Implications for screw insertion into the first cervical lateral mass. J Bone Joint Surg [Am] 87:2495–2498, 2005.

351. Zimmerman, E.; Grant, J.; Vise, W.M.; et al. Treatment of Jefferson fracture with a halo apparatus. Report of two cases. J Neurosurg 44:372–375, 1976.

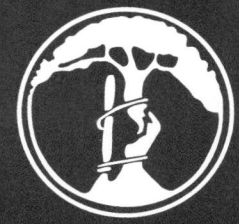

CHAPTER 29

Injuries of the Lower Cervical Spine

Brian K. Kwon, M.D., Ph.D., F.R.C.S.(C.) and Paul A. Anderson M.D.

•••

Injuries of the lower, "subaxial" cervical spine (C3 to C7 inclusive) occur along a wide spectrum of severity, from minor soft tissue "strains" to disastrous fracture dislocations with spinal cord injury. The incidence of cervical spine injuries in patients sustaining blunt trauma is relatively low. In a review of almost 34,000 blunt trauma patients, Lowery and colleagues identified only 818 patients with cervical injuries (approximately 2.4%).[56] Nonetheless, the associated risk of quadriplegia in the setting of unstable cervical spine injuries underscores the need to develop a sound and rational approach to their diagnosis and management. Few other injuries have the potential for such catastrophic morbidity when missed. Approximately two thirds of these cervical injuries occur within the lower cervical spine, with fractures occurring most often in C6 and C7 and dislocations most commonly occurring between C5-C6 and C6-C7.[36] Nearly one fifth of the injuries occur at C7-T1, making the visualization of the cervicothoracic junction critically important.

There are a number of pertinent considerations for the diagnosis and management of lower cervical spine injuries. The anatomy of the subaxial cervical spine is unique, and the widespread use of spinal instrumentation in the surgical treatment of subaxial injuries has placed substantial importance on this region of the cervical spine.

Understanding the principles of cervical biomechanics and the concepts of cervical stability is critical to deciding on the definitive treatment. Definitive treatment for some fracture patterns with external orthoses can be reviewed (see Chapter 27), but open surgical techniques employing anterior or posterior fixation are necessary for others.

ANATOMY OF THE SUBAXIAL CERVICAL SPINE

General Anatomy

OSSEOUS STRUCTURES

The osseous constituents of each vertebra and the structure of its articulations with adjacent vertebrae are relatively constant from C3 to C7 (Fig. 29-1). Each cervical vertebra consists of an anterior body, from which the pedicles extend posteriorly to meet the lateral masses and lamina, thus forming an osseous canal that envelopes the spinal cord. An important structure arising from the posterolateral corner of the vertebral body's superior surface is the uncinate process, which forms the uncovertebral joint of Luschka with a complementary convexity on the inferior surface of the suprajacent vertebral body. The uncinate process is an

---

FIGURE 29-1 | *Osseous constituents of the lower cervical spine. This illustrates the typical osseous anatomy of the vertebral bodies in the subaxial cervical spine, viewed from above (A) and from the left side (B). Note that the pedicle (6) is very short and extends at a sharp medial angle from the superior articular process (1). Note also how the lateral mass (consisting of the superior [1] and inferior [7] articular process) appears rhomboid in shape from the lateral view. The superior surface of the vertebral body (5) is raised at the posterolateral corners to form the uncovertebral joints (arrows). (From Mirza, S.K.; Anderson, P.A. Skeletal Trauma, 3rd ed., New York, W.B. Saunders, 2003.)*

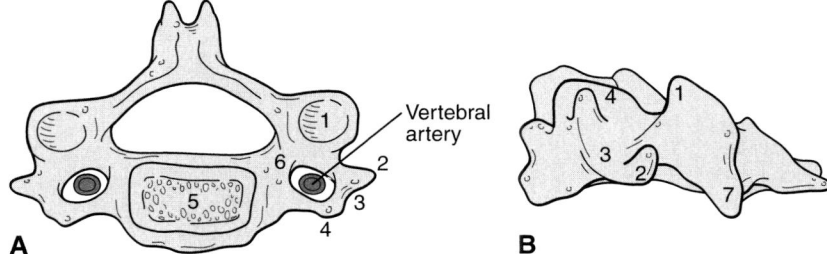

1 Superior articular process
2 Posterior tubercle ⎤
3 Costotransverse bar ⎥ of transverse process
4 Anterior tubercle ⎦
5 Body
6 Pedicle
7 Inferior articular process

Vertebral artery

A   B

important landmark for defining the lateral boundary of the vertebral body when performing an anterior diskectomy or corpectomy.

Extending laterally off the pedicle and anteriorly from the lateral mass are tubercles that form the transverse process, which cradles the nerve root exiting along its superior surface. Within the transverse process is a round defect called the foramen transversarium, through which the vertebral artery ascends, typically by skipping the foramen at C7 and entering at C6.

The lateral mass consists of the superior and inferior articular facets, which, when viewed from the side, give the lateral mass a rhomboid-shaped appearance (see Fig. 29-1). When viewed in cross section, the inferior articular facet lies posterior to the superior articular facet of the subjacent vertebrae. This "shingling" configuration can cause confusion when interpreting axial computed tomography (CT) scans (Fig. 29-2).

The laminae extend posteromedially from the lateral masses and converge on the midline to form the spinous process. At C3, C4, C5, and often at C6, the spinous process is bifid. The C7 spinous process is usually the most prominent dorsal structure in the lower cervical spine and, when palpable, represents a useful landmark for making the skin incision for posterior approaches.

NONOSSEOUS STRUCTURES

The most important nonosseous structure of the spinal column is the intervertebral disk. Like that of the lumbar

---

FIGURE 29-2   *Shingling of facets in lower cervical spine. The rhomboid-shaped facets overlap in a "shingling" pattern in the subaxial cervical spine. This is well visualized in the sagittal computed tomographic reconstructions of the right **(A)** and left **(B)** facets. Note the left-sided C5-C6 facet fracture dislocation **(B)**. On the axial cuts of the normal C3-C4 level **(C),** note that with the shingling pattern of the facets, the superior facet of C4 is anterior to the inferior facet of C3. At the level of the injury, note that the right-sided facets have maintained their alignment, with the superior facet of C6 being anterior to the inferior facet of C5. However, on the left, the C5 inferior facet is anterior to the C6 superior facet.*

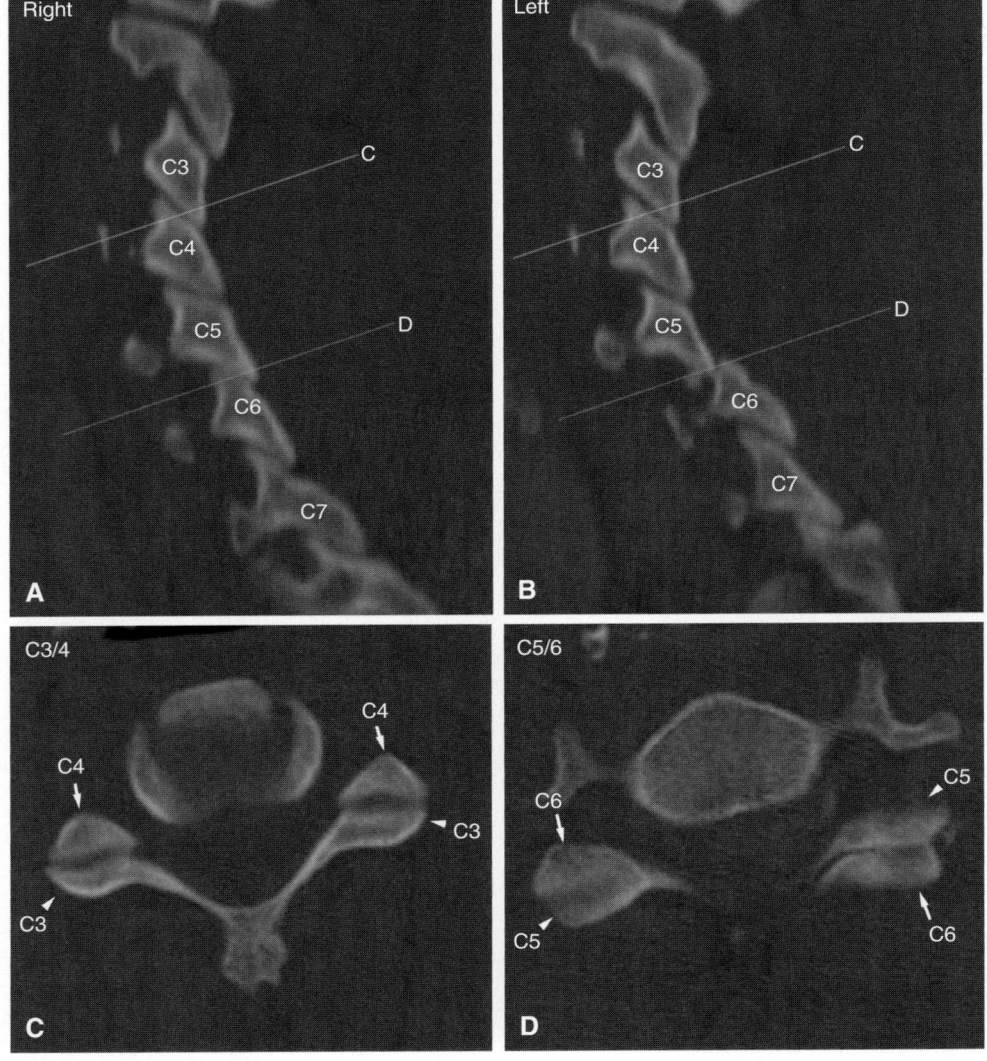

FIGURE 29-3 *Ligamentous restraints in the lower cervical spine. This illustrates the important ligamentous structures that support the vertebral bodies of the lower cervical spine, viewed from the side **(A)** and from above **(B)**. (From Mirza, S.K.; Anderson, P.A. Skeletal Trauma, 3rd ed., New York, W.B. Saunders, 2003; **A,** redrawn from Anderson, P.A. In: Hansen, S.T.; Swiontkiowski, M.F. Orthopaedic Trauma Protocols, New York, Raven, 1993. **B,** from White, A. A.; Panjabi, M.M. Clinical Biomechanics of the Spine, 2nd ed. Philadelphia, J.B. Lippincott, 1990.)*

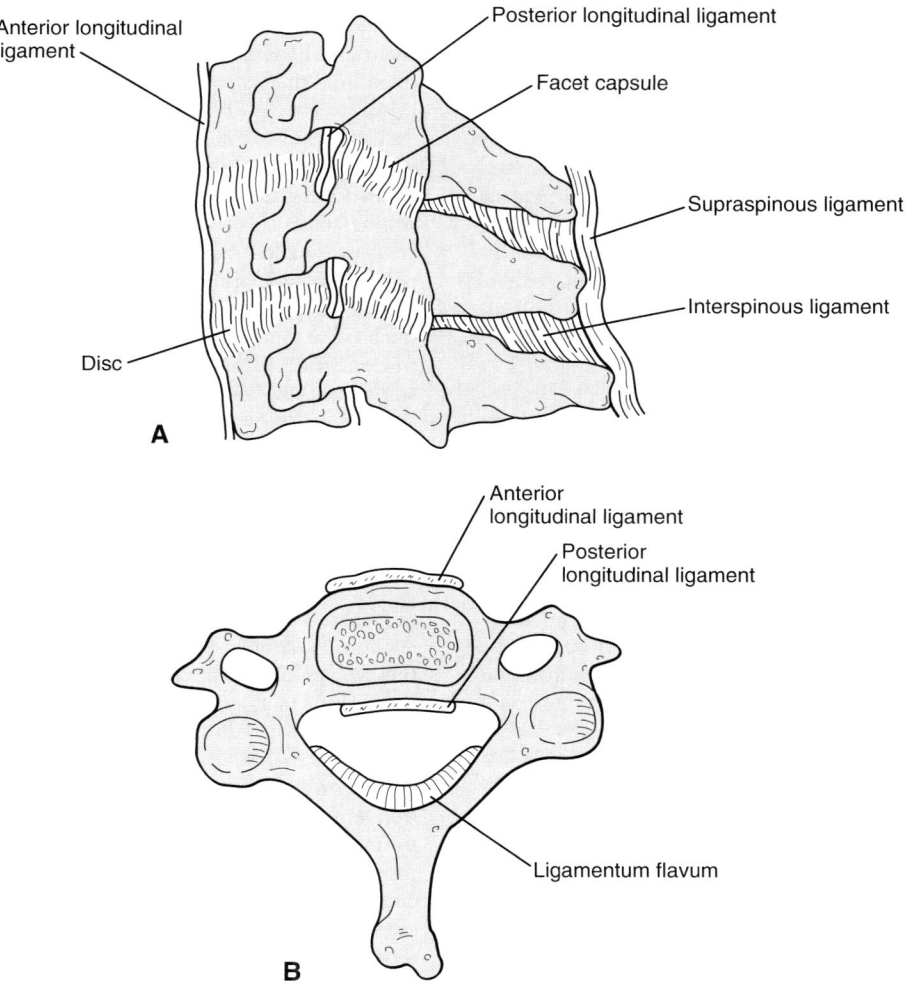

spine, the intervertebral disk consists of a central, gelatinous nucleus pulposus surrounded by the tough, fibrous annulus fibrosus. The disk is bordered superiorly and inferiorly by a cartilaginous end plate, and laterally by the uncovertebral joints. The disk represents an important stabilizing structure for the motion segment.

A number of important ligamentous structures exist within the subaxial cervical spine and also contribute to stability (Fig. 29-3). The anterior and posterior longitudinal ligaments run cephalocaudal along the anterior and posterior aspects of the vertebral body. The ligamentum flavum extends between the laminae. The interspinous and supraspinous ligaments run between the spinous processes and their tips, respectively. Although distinguished in most anatomic textbooks, the interspinous and supraspinous ligaments are essentially continuous and form a "nuchal ligament" complex with the ligamentum nuchae.

BIOMECHANICAL STABILITY OF THE CERVICAL SPINE

The cervical spine provides mobility and flexibility, and yet it normally does so without pain or injury to the neurovascular structures contained within. Unfortunately, this mobility makes the cervical spine susceptible to indirect injury when the head is subjected to a blow or rapid deceleration. The upper part of the cervical spine (C0-C1 and C1-C2) is responsible for most of the rotational and bending motion, but each level in the subaxial cervical spine contributes approximately 8° to 10° of flexion-extension and 3° to 5° of axial rotation.[72] Lateral bending is more evenly distributed among the entire cervical spine and, in fact, is highest at C2-C3, C3-C4, and C4-C5.

Understanding the concept of spinal instability is important when evaluating and treating spinal trauma. Clinical *spinal instability* has been defined by White and Panjabi as "the loss of the ability of the spine under physiologic loads to maintain its pattern of displacement so that there is no initial or additional neurological deficit, no major deformity, and no incapacitating pain."[113] In essence, the spine is *stable* when it is able to withstand the loads to which it is subjected during normal activity, without pain, neurologic injury, or deformity.

In general, the osseous anatomy of the subaxial cervical spine provides little intrinsic stability. This is well demonstrated in cases of severe bilateral facet dislocations, where the soft tissues from the intervertebral disk anteriorly to the capsuloligamentous structures posteriorly have been completely disrupted. Such cases are highly unstable, despite the absence of injury to the osseous structures of the cervical spine. Hence, the nonosseous structures of the subaxial cervical spine, such as the ligaments and intervertebral disks, are important stabilizing structures.

Anatomic Elements of the Subaxial Cervical Spine

The anterior elements include the anterior longitudinal ligament (ALL), intervertebral disk, vertebral body, intertransverse ligament, and posterior longitudinal ligament (PLL).[113] The ALL is a multilayered ligament that runs along the anterior aspect of the vertebral bodies and disks, covering the central half of the ventral surface of both. The superficial fibers of the ALL cross multiple levels, and the deeper fibers are associated with a single motion segment.[61] In this ventral position, the ALL and the anterior collagen fibers of the annulus fibrosus are important restraints to extension forces. It is important to recognize that the structure of the cervical intervertebral disk is substantially different from that of its lumbar counterpart. Mercer and Bogduk demonstrated that the cervical annulus fibrosus is thick anteriorly, thins as it approaches the uncinate processes, and is very thin posteriorly.[61] This gives it a crescent-shaped appearance when viewed axially, quite unlike the typical "jelly-donut" appearance of the lumbar disk. In contrast to the lamellar pattern of a lumbar disk, the anterior annular fibers of the cervical disk are vertically and obliquely oriented in an interwoven fashion, akin to an interosseous ligament between the two end plates.[61] This serves as an important restraint to hyperextension, in conjunction with the confluent ALL. Because the anterior annular fibers are shorter and deeper than the multilayered ALL, they fail in extension before the ALL,[106] thus explaining how disruption can occur through the anterior disk without apparent mechanical failure of the ALL.[99] In severe hyperextension injuries, however, the two structures fail together.[41]

Because the posterior annulus fibrosus is thin, it is unlikely to serve as much of a restraint to flexion forces. The PLL, however, covers the floor of the cervical canal and reinforces the posterior annulus. Like the ALL, the PLL is also a multilayered structure, with the deep layers adhering to adjacent vertebral bodies and the superficial layers crossing multiple levels. Throughout the subaxial cervical spine, the PLL is similar to the ALL in terms of its strength and biomechanical properties, and thus is likely to resist bending moments similarly.[82] At each level of the cervical spine, the PLL is slightly wider than the ALL.[83] However, neither the PLL nor the posterior annulus reinforces the region posterior and superior to the uncinate

process in the posterolateral corner—an anatomic feature that may predispose to disk protrusions through this area.[61]

Posterior Elements of the Subaxial Cervical Spine

The posterior elements lie posterior to the PLL.[113] These structures include the facets, laminae, and spinous processes, as well as the facet capsules, ligamentum flavum, and spinous processes. The ligamentum flavum runs from the anteroinferior surface of one lamina to the superoposterior surface of its subjacent lamina. At approximately 5 mm in thickness, the ligamentum flavum in the cervical spine is thinner than that of the thoracolumbar spine.[74] Its elastin content gives it both a yellowish appearance and elastic properties that promote extension and restrict flexion. How effectively the ligamentum flavum restrains motion likely changes as it degenerates with age and becomes thicker and stiffer, and it may itself contribute to dorsal spinal cord compression during cervical hyperextension.

The capsules of the facet joints are relatively thin and more patulous than those of the thoracolumbar spine.[74] The capsule bridges the osseous lateral mass on either side of the superior and inferior articular surfaces and is thinnest posteriorly and thickest along its anterolateral region.[107] In a cadaveric model, Onan and co-workers demonstrated that the subaxial cervical facets were highly mobile, and when the facets were isolated by disconnecting them from the surrounding lamina and vertebral body, the facet capsules by themselves did little to restrict joint motion due to their laxity.[68] In fact, capsular strain was not observed in flexion until the joint had almost dislocated anteriorly. This suggests that the facet capsules act as a posterior restraint to flexion only at the extremes of facet motion and are thus less frequently injured. Panjabi and colleagues supported this notion in simulations of frontal impact, during which the cervical spine rapidly flexes forward when the "torso" decelerates.[75] They found that the capsules (and PLL) rarely experienced significant strain during this injury model and thus are not prone to disruption during accidents involving frontal impact. Although these data may suggest that the capsules contribute little to the stability of the subaxial cervical spine, one should be careful not to disrupt the capsules at the nonfused levels when performing posterior approaches to the cervical spine, as this may lead to subluxation at the level above or below (Fig. 29-4).

The interspinous and supraspinous ligaments run between the spinous processes of each vertebra. They are poorly developed in the cervical spine compared with the thoracolumbar spine. These ligaments are confluent with the ligamentum nuchae, which is a triangular fibrous membrane that extends from the spinous processes to the skin between the external occipital protuberance and the C7 spinous process. The interspinous and supraspinous ligaments are farthest away from the anterior aspect of the spine, and thus they have the longest moment arm to resist bending forces, making them important restraints to flexion. In Panjabi and colleagues' aforementioned frontal impact simulations, the interspinous and supraspinous ligaments were stretched or disrupted most commonly, even at the lowest impact forces tested.[75] The role of the ligamentum nuchae is overlooked in such biomechanical

FIGURE 29-4 *Caudal subluxation after posterior fixation. It is important to leave the facet capsules intact at levels that will not be incorporated into the fixation construct. This patient presented with an incomplete spinal cord injury and a unilateral C4-C5 facet dislocation (**A**), which the MRI (**B**) demonstrated was associated with disk material behind the body of C4 (white arrowhead). A C4-C5 anterior diskectomy and fusion was therefore performed first, followed by posterior reduction and fixation of C3-C5. **C,** No injury was noted at the C5-C6 level on preoperative imaging, nor during the posterior fixation. Ten days postoperatively, severe kyphosis was noted at the C5-C6 level (**D**) that required extension of the fixation to C7. **E,** The C5-C6 facet capsules were found to be disrupted at her revision surgery.*

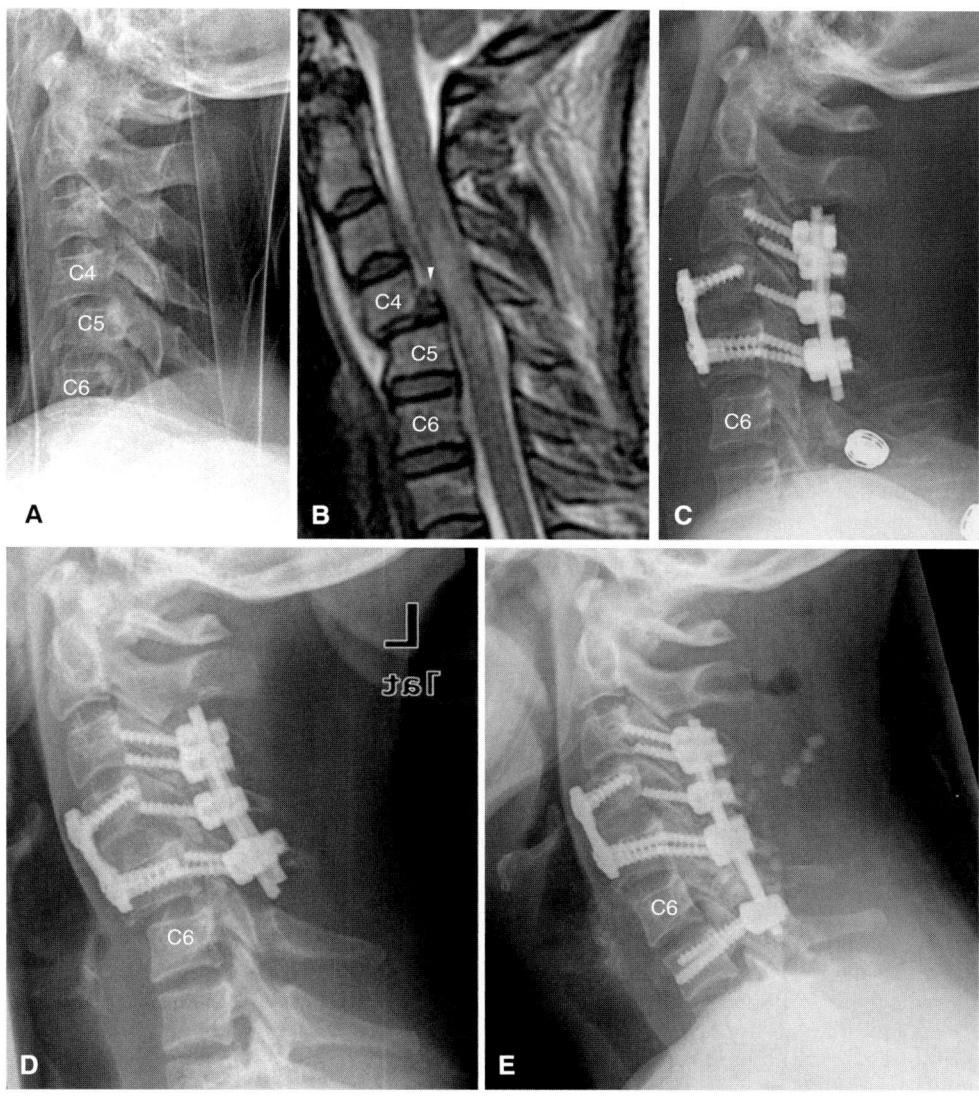

studies because it is typically removed from the cadaveric specimens prior to testing. Takeshita and associates demonstrated that the ligamentum nuchae indeed contributes as a posterior restraint to flexion, as one might expect from its posterior position.[105] Resection of the ligamentum nuchae alone increased the flexion range of the cervical spine by 28 percent. Further resection of the supraspinous, interspinous, and ligamentum flavum increased the flexion range by 52 percent.

Quantifying Instability

The extent of instability is a critical factor in deciding how to treat lower cervical spine injuries. Most importantly,

one should recognize that cervical instability is not a binary phenomenon (i.e., "stable" or "unstable") but, rather, exists along a spectrum of severity. The great challenge in managing cervical spine injuries is defining this spectrum of instability and deciding at what threshold external immobilization or surgical fixation is warranted.

THE WHITE AND PANJABI "CHECKLIST" FOR CERVICAL INSTABILITY

In 1975, Drs. Panjabi, White, Southwick, and Johnson published the results of an important biomechanical experiment in lower cervical trauma.[77,115] This experiment evaluated the role of the soft tissue stabilizers in a "functional spinal unit (FSU)," which consisted of two adjacent vertebrae and their connecting soft tissues. With a constant axial load of 25 percent body weight, the FSU was tested in simulated flexion and extension, and the relative motion of the upper vertebrae on the lower, fixed vertebra was measured. The relative motion was then assessed after sequentially cutting the soft tissue structures in either an anterior-to-posterior or posterior-to-anterior direction.

The authors observed that, in general, sectioning of the ligamentous structures led to only minor increases in relative motion (over the intact condition) prior to sudden and catastrophic disruption of the spinal unit. They reported that the spinal unit was unstable or on the "brink of instability" when all of the anterior elements or all of the posterior elements were destroyed, when more than 2.7 mm of relative vertebral body translation was observed, either in a resting position or on flexion-extension, and when the sagittal angulation between the two vertebral bodies was 11° more than that of the adjacent interspaces (to account for the normal lordosis of the cervical spine). With an assumed radiographic magnification of 30 percent on a standard lateral radiograph, they concluded that a 2.7 mm vertebral body translation would be seen on the lateral film as 3.5 mm. Such magnification is not relevant for CT technology, making the actual limit to vertebral body translation 2.7 mm.

Panjabi and colleagues also developed an axial stretch test to "dynamically" evaluate cervical instability.[94,114] It was theorized that controlled axial distraction would be less likely to cause a neurologic injury than flexion and extension. In this test, the patient is lying supine, and a lateral radiograph is taken at the standard 72 inches from the film. Traction is then applied to the head in 10-lb increments until one third of the body weight is applied, with a radiograph repeated at each increment. A positive stretch test is denoted by any neurologic alteration, a 1.7-mm increase in interspace distance, or a greater than 7.5° change in sagittal angulation.

From this biomechanical work, White and Panjabi developed a checklist to calculate the biomechanical severity of injury. In this checklist, the patient is assigned 2 points for each of the following: destruction of the anterior elements, destruction of the posterior elements, a positive stretch test, sagittal plane displacement of greater than 3.5 mm, or sagittal plane angulation of greater than 11° on a resting radiograph. Additional points in this checklist were added for other factors considered to be important in determining instability. The presence of a spinal cord injury was given 2 points. One point was given for the presence of each of the following: abnormal disk narrowing, a developmentally narrow spinal canal, the presence of a nerve root injury, and the anticipation of dangerous loading by the patient. White and Panjabi proposed that a score of 5 or more points on this checklist represented an "unstable" lower cervical spine injury.[113]

The White and Panjabi checklist provided, for the first time, a rational guideline for clinicians to look at a lateral C-spine radiograph and provide an estimation of cervical instability. Although based on sound biomechanical experiments, this checklist has never been tested for reliability or validity in the clinical setting. Furthermore, it does have significant limitations in the contemporary evaluation of in vivo cervical trauma. The experiments on which the checklist is based only considered ligamentous, not osseous, injuries. Biomechanical testing was limited to flexion and extension and involved only a single motion segment, not the entire cervical spine. The application of the checklist was based on a single lateral radiograph and did not utilize current technology, such as helical CT scanning and magnetic resonance imaging (MRI), which was unavailable at the time. The stretch test described by Panjabi and colleagues and even dynamic flexion-extension radiography are rarely, if ever, performed in the setting of acute cervical injury. The role of some of the secondary parts of the checklist such as "abnormal disk narrowing" and "dangerous loading anticipated" is arbitrary and subject to interpretation, and the relevance of a developmentally narrowed spinal canal is uncertain. Furthermore, the radiographic measurements of sagittal angulation or translation can be very misleading. Although the checklist suggests that the spine is not unstable unless the sagittal plane displacement and angulation exceed thresholds of 3.5 mm and 11°, respectively, it is possible that a patient with no sagittal angulation or translation can have quite an unstable lower cervical spine injury. In fact, many patients with obvious anterior column or posterior column injuries present with less than 3.5 mm of translation. The checklist produces a binary result of "stable" or "unstable" and does not recognize the potential ranges of instability that might exist. Finally, the checklist does not provide any definitive guidance on how to treat these injuries.

Others have also attempted to quantify mechanical instability after cervical injury. Louis proposed that the cervical spine was similar to a tripod with three columns: the anterior column and two lateral pillars (lateral columns).[55] The injury to each column was given a score of 0.25, 0.5, or 1.0 point, depending on its severity, and the value for each column was totaled. Cervical injuries with a sum of 2 points or more were deemed "unstable." Similar to the checklist system of White and Panjabi, this system has never been tested for reliability.

Allen and Ferguson proposed a mechanistic classification system to stratify the severity of injury for those that shared similar mechanisms.[6] Describing cervical spine injuries and their severity according to this classification has been done extensively in biomechanical research and clinical studies. However, it too has never been tested for its reliability.

Anderson and co-workers[11] and Moore and associates[63] have recently developed the Cervical Spine Injury Severity Score, a quantitative system to evaluate instability. The score is based on the integrity of four spinal columns: the anterior and posterior columns, and the right and left lateral masses. The anterior column is similar to that described by White and Panjabi.[113] Each lateral column includes the lateral masses, pedicles, and facet articulations with their joint capsules. The posterior column includes the laminae, spinous processes, ligamentum flavum, and nuchal ligaments. Each column is scored independently from 0 to 5 using a visual analogue scale, similar to that used to document pain. Increasing scores are assigned for increased degrees of displacement or disruption. For example, a nondisplaced fracture is given a score of 1, and the worst or most displaced injury that could occur is given a maximal score of 5. If the column is uninjured it is given a score of 0. Fractional values can be used. The analogue scale and representative displacements are shown in Fig. 29-5. The Cervical Spine Injury Severity Score is the sum of the scores from each of the four columns and, therefore, can range from 0 to 20 (Fig. 29-6).

FIGURE 29-5 *The Cervical Spine Injury Severity Score. This newly developed algorithm can be used to quantify the mechanical instability of the injury with the intention of guiding treatment decisions. The cervical spine is divided into four columns (anterior, posterior, and two lateral columns), and the severity of injury to each column is assessed using whatever imaging modalities are available (e.g., plain film radiography, CT, MRI). The severity of the bony or ligamentous injury to each column is then assigned a number according to the analogue scale shown below the films, with 0 being uninjured, and 5 being the most severely injured. The sum of the scores for each of the four columns then represents the Cervical Spine Injury Severity Score.*

Anterior Column Injury

Lateral Column Injury (Right)

Lateral Column Injury (Left)

Anterior Column

Lateral Column

Lateral Column

Posterior Column

Posterior Column Injury

Cervical Spine Injury Severity Scale

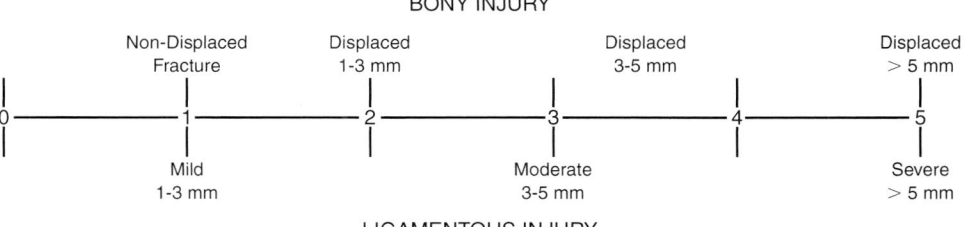

BONY INJURY

Non-Displaced Fracture	Displaced 1-3 mm	Displaced 3-5 mm	Displaced > 5 mm

0 — 1 — 2 — 3 — 4 — 5

| Mild 1-3 mm | Moderate 3-5 mm | Severe > 5 mm |

LIGAMENTOUS INJURY

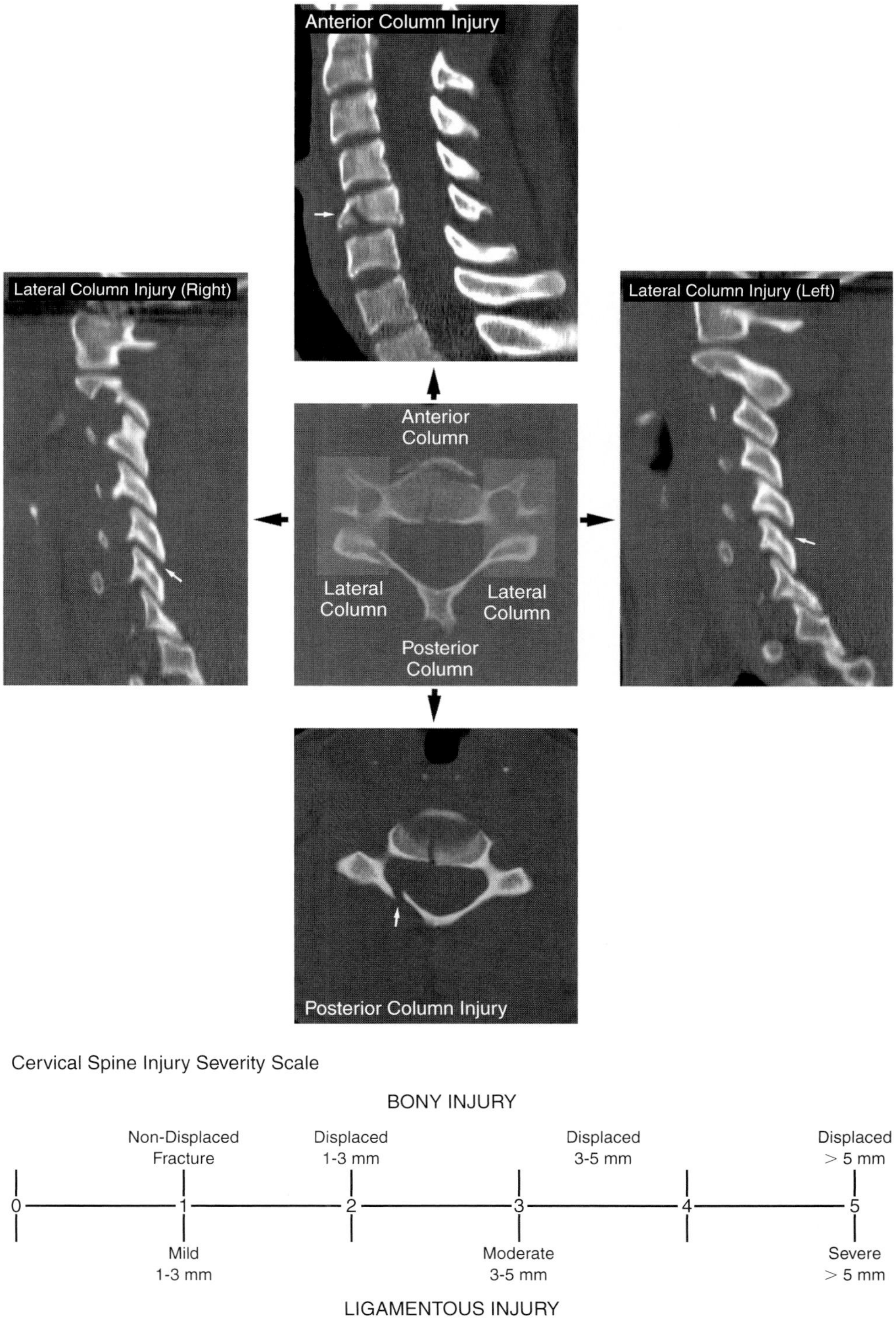

FIGURE 29-6 | *Application of the Cervical Spine Injury Severity Score. This patient presents with a compressive flexion injury. The midsagittal CT reformat **(A)** shows a fracture of the anterior body of C6, retrolisthesis of the C6 body into the spinal canal, and wide separation of the C5 and C6 spinous processes. Based on this, the anterior column injury was graded a "4," and the posterior column injury graded a "5." The left sagittal reformat **(B)** with axial cut (inset) shows the C5-C6 facet dislocation, giving the left lateral pillar a score of "4.5." The inset axial CT shows dislocation of left C5-C6 facet. The right sagittal reformat **(C)** shows diastasis of the C6-C7 facet, giving the right lateral pillar a score of "2.5." The sum of these four pillars is the Cervical Spine Injury Severity Score; in this case, 16. Scores greater than 7 indicate sufficient instability to warrant surgical stabilization.*

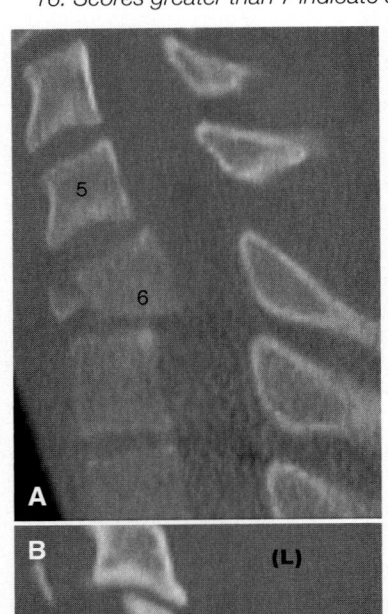

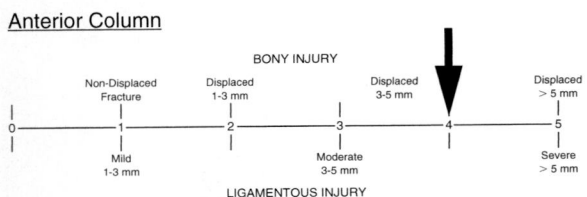

Anterior Column

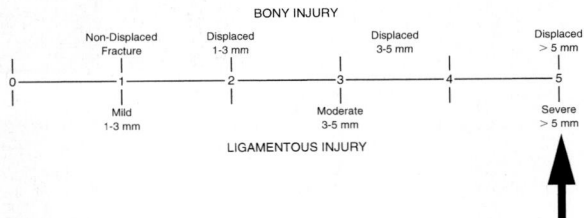

Posterior Column

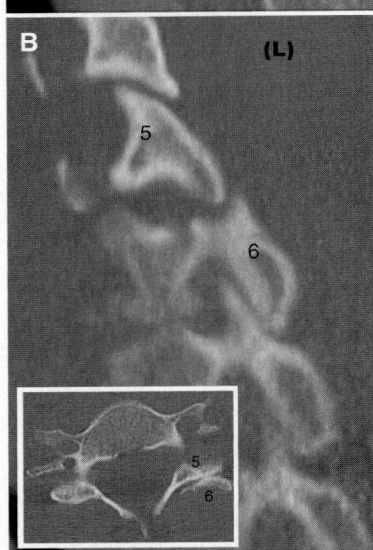

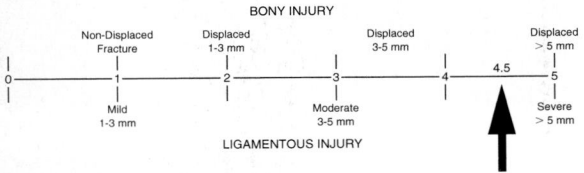

Left Lateral Pillar

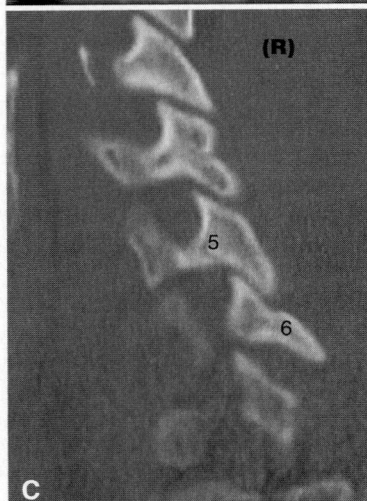

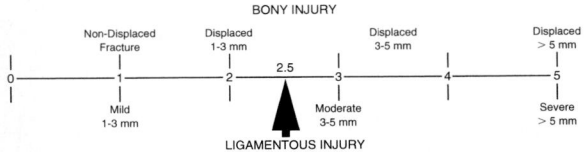

Right Lateral Pillar

Cervical Spine Injury Severity Score=
$4 + 5 + 4.5 + 2.5 = \underline{16}$

Unique to the Cervical Spine Injury Severity Score is that it has been tested for observer reliability and for validity in predicting injury severity (and thus, management). Fifteen examiners evaluated 40 cases based on plain radiographs and CT. The intraobserver reliability was excellent, with a mean intraclass correlation coefficient (ICC) of 0.98. Similarly, the interobserver reliability was excellent, with a mean ICC of 0.88.[63] No correlation to examiners' experience or which column was observed. The system appeared to be valid at predicting injury severity, as all cases with scores greater than 7 were treated surgically. Neurologic injury was seen in 65 percent of patient with scores greater than 7, with only 15 percent below.[11]

INJURY MECHANISMS AND CLASSIFICATION

A significant challenge for clinicians is to reconstruct how the injury occurred based on the history of the accident. With an understanding of the injury mechanism, one is theoretically able to infer what stabilizing structures were disrupted and then utilize this in the treatment decision. Unfortunately, it is often difficult, if not impossible, to know exactly what forces were applied to the cervical spine at the moment the trauma occurred. In the majority of cases, the spine injury occurs indirectly, by impact to the head (e.g., diving into a shallow pool headfirst), or acceleration-deceleration of the thorax (e.g., getting rear-ended at high speed). How these forces are transferred to the cervical spine depends on many factors, such as the magnitude and direction of impact, the position of the cervical spine at the time of impact, and the biomechanical characteristics of the cervical spine (e.g., the stiff, spondylotic spine of an elderly individual versus the supple spine of a young individual). Piecing all of these factors together into a unified description of "injury mechanism" is fraught with difficulty.

In biomechanical studies, even when the conditions are well controlled and the injury mechanism is fairly well understood, the resultant injuries are often unpredictable. Interestingly, how the head moves at the time of impact may not explain the given injury. Nightengale and colleagues dropped 11 cadaveric specimens with a simulated torso weight from a height of approximately 60 cm directly onto the head, with the neck held in a neutral lordotic position.[66] Surprisingly, the authors found that the direction of head motion on impact did not correspond to the types of injuries that occurred. The head flexed on impact in 6 of 11 specimens, but only 1 vertical compression and 4 *extension*-type injuries were induced. Remarkably, no flexion-type injuries were observed in these six specimens. The head extended on impact in the other five specimens, resulting in three vertical compression, nine extension, and two flexion-type injuries. The explanation for these unexpected and paradoxical results was that the entire cervical spine did not behave as one single entity on impact, but rather, the cervical spine "buckled" after impact, such that some parts of the spine were forced into extension, and others were forced into flexion (Fig. 29-7). A limitation of this in vitro experiment was that only simple forces were created (i.e., that of dropping straight down onto the top of the neutrally positioned head).

FIGURE 29-7 *Multiple injury mechanisms may occur in a single trauma. Even if a clear history of how the patient was injured allows one to estimate the mechanism of cervical injury, the resultant injury may not be so simply explained. This 67-year-old farmer was injured when a 500-lb bale of hay fell directly onto his head. This sagittal CT demonstrates widening of the C3-C4 disk space with retrolisthesis and compressive fracturing of the posterior elements (top arrow)—an injury characteristic of severe hyperextension. However, he also has anterolisthesis of C6 on C7 with bilateral facet dislocations and a spinous process fracture—an injury characteristic of severe hyperflexion (bottom arrow). The complex "buckling" of his cervical spine due to the severe axial loading (as described by Nightengale and colleagues) may explain these seemingly contradictory injury patterns.*

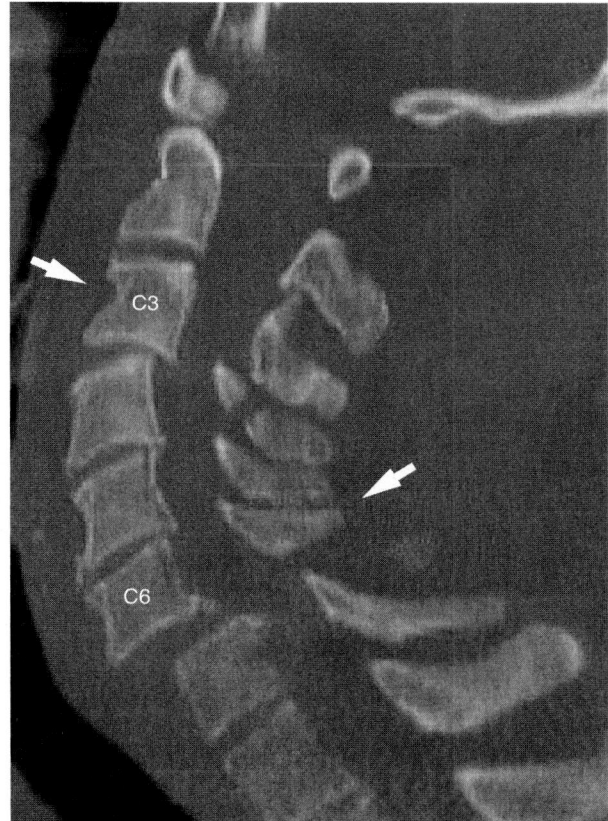

An important factor to consider when using the radiographic findings to infer biomechanical mechanism is that radiographs often underestimate the extent of bony retropulsion and collapse that occurs at the time of injury. At the time of initial evaluation, the displacement visualized on the static imaging—be it kyphotic angulation, distraction, or compression with canal compromise—is likely much less than what occurred during the injury. In an axial loading injury model, Chang and co-workers measured that the amount of residual spinal canal compression after injury was significantly less than the sudden and rapid bony retropulsion that occurred during injury.[18] Also, the amount of axial vertebral height loss that was seen after the injury was significantly less than what occurred at the time of injury. Hence, interpretation of the extent of displacement, angulation, or canal occlusion if using these parameters in treatment decisions must be done cautiously. Also unstable fractures may be in a relatively reduced state and therefore underappreciated on plain films.

Thus, our ability to reconstruct the mechanism of injury for lower cervical trauma is limited. Nonetheless, the most universally accepted classification scheme for lower cervical injuries is based on injury mechanism. This is the classification system of Allen and Ferguson, and we discuss it here as the framework for the description of specific lower cervical injuries.

The Allen and Ferguson Classification of Lower Cervical Injuries

In 1982, Allen and co-workers proposed a cervical spine injury classification scheme based on injury mechanism.[6] These authors retrospectively analyzed 165 subaxial cervical injuries and attempted to document "an unequivocal history" of a specific injury mechanism, noting the posture of the head and neck at the time of injury, the location and direction of the force being applied, and the exact circumstances of the trauma. They then divided the injuries into six "phylogenies" according to the "initial, dominant mode of failure," based on the presumed injury mechanism and the radiographic appearance. The basic phylogenies included (1) compressive flexion (CF), (2) vertical compression (VC), (3) distractive flexion (DF), (4) compressive extension (CE), (5) distractive extension (DE), and (6) lateral flexion (LF). Distractive flexion injuries were the most common (61 cases, 37%), followed by compressive extension (40 cases, 24%), compressive flexion (36 cases, 22%), and vertical compression (14 cases, 8%). Distractive extension (9 cases, 5%) and lateral flexion injuries (5 cases, 3%) were comparatively rare. Within each phylogeny a number of "stages" of severity were defined to distinguish different degrees of instability.

The mechanistic Allen and Ferguson classification scheme has several very important limitations. It was based on plain radiographs and does not include more sophisticated imaging such as CT and MRI. The postulated mechanism of injury was reconstructed retrospectively from the available accident details, and the authors hypothesized that the injury was the result of a single primary mechanism (although they did recognize that minor injury vectors likely also were relevant). The Allen and Ferguson classification has never been tested for reliability, and thus its utility is quite limited. Nonetheless, the different phylogenies of the Allen and Ferguson classification system serve as a useful framework for the subsequent discussion on the various injuries to the lower cervical spine.

PATIENT ASSESSMENT

The principles of patient evaluation, including history, physical examination, and imaging, are discussed in Chapter 25, Initial Evaluation and Emergency Treatment of the Spine-Injured Patient.

GENERAL MANAGEMENT CONSIDERATIONS

The goals of treatment are to prevent further neurologic injury, to reduce fractures and dislocations, and to provide a stable painless spine. The assessment process is aimed at identifying spine injuries and then placing the injury into a specific injury category. For each injury category, an individualized and rational approach is required that takes into account three major considerations.

First, the extent of *mechanical instability* inherent to the injury must be considered. In general, the greater the instability, the more likely the need for surgical fixation. The converse is also true for injuries that are less mechanically unstable—external immobilization may be all that is required.

Second, the possibility of *neurologic compromise* requiring decompression should be investigated. For example, the presence of ongoing spinal cord compression in a lower cervical injury plays a role in determining treatment. Decompression may be performed directly by surgically removing compressive lesions, or it may be achieved indirectly by reducing or realigning the spine.

Third, one should consider any unique circumstances relevant to the individual patient that might influence treatment. Such *patient factors* include the presence of noncontiguous spinal injuries or severe multisystem injuries, smoking history, medical comorbidities, and social considerations. For example, a patient's obesity or body habitus may negate any realistic chance of treating an otherwise mechanically stable injury with external immobilization.

Patients with severe spinal cord injuries often have many other injuries and are at risk for respiratory complication requiring lengthy stays in an intensive care setting. Generally speaking, multitraumatized patients are best treated with rigid internal fixation of the spinal injuries. This approach facilitates mobilization and makes both the patient and the clinical treatment team less dependent on a bulky, cumbersome external orthosis.

Considering these three issues—mechanical instability, neurologic compromise, and patient factors—allows for a rational decision about how to treat any given injury to the lower cervical spine. The Cervical Spine Injury Severity Score developed by Anderson and colleagues provides a simple algorithm for reproducibly quantifying mechanical instability of the injury and also provides guidance for treatment decisions.

Principles of Nonoperative Management

If the decision is made to manage the cervical injury nonoperatively, a wide variety of cervical immobilization devices are commercially available from which to choose the most appropriate orthosis. Conceptually these may be divided into those that secure the head to a thoracic vest (a cervicothoracic orthosis) and those that encircle the neck alone (a cervical collar). Cervicothoracic braces hold the head either rigidly with pins (i.e., the halo ring and vest) or nonrigidly with straps (e.g., Minerva and SOMI braces). Cervical collars are either *hard*, such as the Philadelphia, Aspen, and Miami J collars, or *soft*, such as a simple foam collar. Chapter 27 is devoted to such devices; the reader is directed there for a more comprehensive discussion.

In general, the rigidity of a cervical orthosis is theoretically improved by extension to a thoracic vest, which envelops the chest with pads and straps. The halo vest provides the greatest extent of immobilization of all the cervical orthoses, but correct pin placement, pin care, and a cooperative patient are essential to its safe and effective use and for the avoidance of pin tract complications. Furthermore, the halo vest does not provide rigid spinal fixation, and hence one must be very cautious in interpreting the extent of mechanical instability before deeming it suitable for such immobilization.

In an in vivo radiographic study, Anderson and associates demonstrated in patients treated with halo vests that significant fracture motion can still occur merely by changing from a supine to a seated position.[9] During this simple maneuver, they observed over 3° of angulation and 1 mm of translation in more than 75 percent of the injured levels. These findings have been corroborated in clinical experience by comparisons between halo vest and surgical stabilization for flexion-compression injuries.[35,50] In these studies, the clinical results of halo immobilization were clearly inferior to that achieved with surgery, both with respect to late nonunion and deformity. Although these observations do not negate the role of the halo vest in managing cervical injuries, they should inform the determination of whether the amount of immobilization it provides is sufficient for the degree of mechanical instability that exists. For hard cervical collars, the ability to restrict motion is greater in the midcervical spine and less so in the lower cervical spine, where larger bending moments cannot be resisted. Soft collars provide little intersegmental instability and should not be relied on as immobilization devices for unstable injuries. They may be used for minor soft tissue injuries such as whiplash.

After placement of the orthosis, patients should have upright radiographs to confirm the maintenance of satisfactory cervical alignment before discharge. Again, the importance of this radiographic reassessment is highlighted by Anderson and associates' demonstration of the significant motion that can occur when moving to an upright position, even with a halo vest.[9] This simple test occasionally identifies patients with significantly unstable injuries. If the alignment is satisfactory, follow-up radiographs within the first 1 to 2 weeks can be helpful for ensuring that the alignment is being maintained, that the orthosis is fitting properly, and that the patient is tolerating the brace without pin site infections or skin breakdown. Regular follow-up every 4 to 6 weeks is then important, with flexion and extension films being obtained after 8 to 12 weeks to confirm adequate healing.

Principles of Operative Management

The use of internal fixation for the management of subaxial cervical trauma has become increasingly more widespread as intervention has improved instability and ease of application. Surgical stabilization provides many of the same advantages to the cervical spine as internal fixation does over casting or traction for appendicular trauma. The stabilization conferred by internal fixation is superior to any external orthosis, providing more reliable healing in better cervical alignment.

Surgical management has a particularly important role in patients with cervical spinal cord injuries. Direct removal of impinging bone or disk may be the only means by which to effectively decompress the spinal cord. Even if decompression is not needed, the injury itself is likely to be more mechanically unstable than a radiographically similar injury without neurologic deficit, and so operative stabilization may still be warranted on the basis of mechanical instability. It also allows earlier mobilization of the patient without neurologic injury. Furthermore, it is generally believed that persistent motion is detrimental to the acutely injured spinal cord. The superior stabilization provided by spinal instrumentation may therefore be advantageous over external immobilization in this setting, even if it were felt that the latter could provide sufficient stability to heal the osseoligamentous injury.

Specific Anatomy Relevant to Surgical Stabilization

Understanding the basic anatomic groundwork relevant to screw placement within the lower cervical spine is essential to avoiding significant iatrogenic complications. However, although the available morphometric data provide useful guidelines for such things as screw length and trajectory, variation among individuals makes it critical for the surgeon to scrutinize preoperative imaging to plan the fixation placement for each patient.

THE LATERAL MASS

The lateral mass serves as a useful fixation point for screws in the subaxial cervical spine, as it represents the lateral osseous "pillar" of the spinal column. It is bordered superiorly and inferiorly by articular surfaces that slope upward, giving the lateral mass a rhomboid appearance when viewed from the side. The slope of the articular surfaces increases and becomes more vertical in the most caudal aspects of the lower cervical spine. For example, the facet joints are angled at approximately 35° in the upper part of the subaxial cervical spine, and closer to 65° in the lower cervical spine.[62] Accordingly, as the articular facets become more vertically sloped, the thickness of the lateral mass decreases, such that the C7 lateral mass is often too thin to serve as a fixation point for screws (Fig. 29-8). This limitation of the C7 lateral mass has popularized the use of the C7 pedicle for segmental fixation at this level.

The relationships of the lateral mass to the surrounding nonosseous structures are critical. The nerve root, which emerges directly in front of the lateral mass within the transverse process, is vulnerable to screw perforation. Ebraheim and colleagues reported in a cadaveric study that the distance between the ventral cortex of the lateral mass and the nerve root was, on average, as little as 1.2 mm at C7 and as much as 2.3 mm at C5, although distances as low as 0.3 mm were also measured in some specimens.[28] Ventral to the nerve root is the vertebral artery. The vertebral artery ascends within the foramen transversarium, which can be found approximately 15 mm directly anterior to the medial aspect of the lateral mass (Fig. 29-9).[70]

LATERAL MASS SCREW FIXATION Given the close anatomic relationships among the nerve root, vertebral

FIGURE 29-8 *Changing anatomy of the lateral mass in the lower cervical spine. This 39-year-old patient with a Hangman's fracture of C2 demonstrates the progressive sloping of the facet joints as one descends through the subaxial cervical spine. Note that at C6 and at C7, the lateral masses are very thin in the anteroposterior plane as compared with C3, C4, and C5, making it difficult to obtain stable screw fixation.*

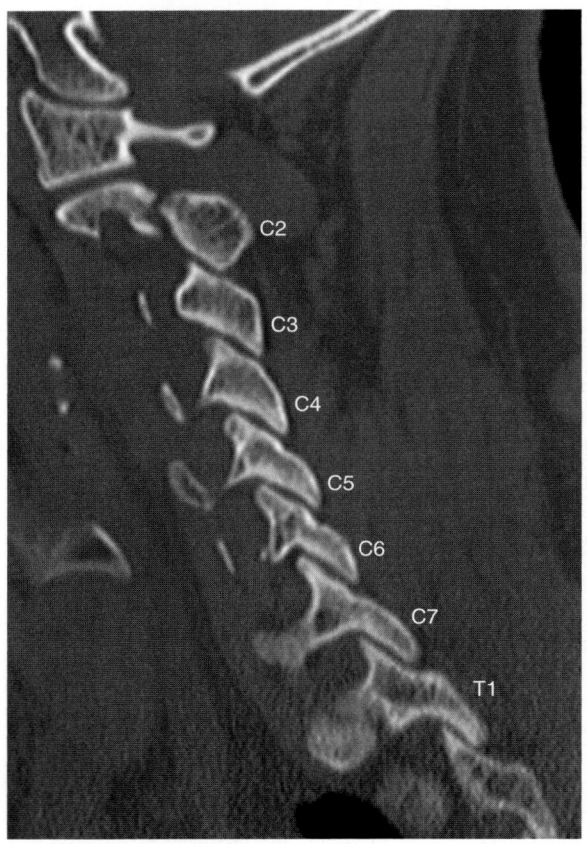

FIGURE 29-9 *Relationship between the foramen transversarium and the lateral mass. From the posterior approach, the surgeon is able to see and feel the posterior surface of the lateral mass (arrowheads). In the placement of lateral mass screws, it is important to remember that the foramen transversarium (arrows) through which the vertebral artery traverses is directly anterior to the medial half of the lateral mass. Hence, directing the screw outward lessens the risk of injuring the vertebral artery.*

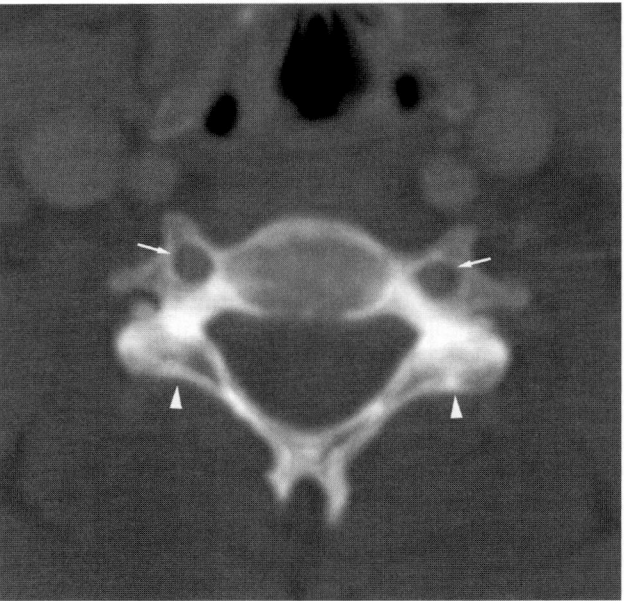

The Roy-Camille technique advocates starting to drill within the midpoint of the lateral mass, then drilling out laterally 10° in the transverse plane and straight ahead in the rostrocaudal plane.[92] Because the drill is not aimed upward, the tip of the screw can inadvertently end up in the inferior, nonfused facet joint. The Magerl, Anderson, and An trajectories all direct the screw upward in the rostrocaudal plane to be more parallel with the articular facet joints.[8,10,46] These techniques advocate starting slightly medial to the midline, then aiming superiorly in the sagittal plane and out laterally in the transverse plane 15 to 25°. To guide this drill trajectory, the drill guide can be laid down along the spinous processes (Fig. 29-12). If one were to divide the lateral mass into quadrants, these techniques aim to leave the tip of the screw in the upper and outer quadrant. Aiming the screw laterally reduces the risk of injuring the vertebral artery. Aiming it superiorly reduces the risk of drilling into the inferior facet. Additionally, an oblique trajectory is longer than the straight-ahead trajectory of the Roy-Camille technique, thus allowing for the placement of a slightly longer screw. Always consider that failure to angle the screw outward increases the risk of injuring the vertebral artery (Fig. 29-13).[20]

Although there are theoretical advantages to placing as long a screw as possible and achieving bicortical purchase,

artery, and spinal cord, errors in the placement of lateral mass screws can result in undesirable complications.[44] Lateral mass screw fixation requires identification of the borders of the lateral mass. The medial border is at the "valley" where the lamina and lateral mass meet (Fig. 29-10). The lateral border is the lateral edge as the lateral mass drops down into soft tissue. The cranial and caudal borders are the respective facet joints. In an effort to balance ease of placement, safety, and biomechanical strength, several techniques have been described that guide the starting point and trajectory of lateral mass screws.[8,10,46,92] It is important to remember that when viewing the posterior cortex of the lateral mass, the lateral mass forms a parallelogram-shaped osseous box with walls that slope superiorly along the articular surfaces of the surrounding facet joints. With this concept in mind, the various techniques for screw trajectory merely attempt to remain safely within this box so as to minimize the chance that the screw tip might exit and cause neurovascular injury (Fig. 29-11).

FIGURE 29-10 *Lateral mass anatomy. Appreciation for the borders of the lateral mass is critical for the selection of an appropriate starting point for screw insertion. The lateral mass is shaped like a rectangle when viewed posteriorly* ***(A)***. *The medial border of the lateral mass is drawn on this model, and is appreciated on the inferior view* ***(B)*** *as the "valley" where the lateral mass and lamina meet (arrows). The superior and inferior borders are defined by the facet joint surfaces, and the lateral border is where the lateral mass ends. A proposed starting point for screw insertion is depicted as black dots.*

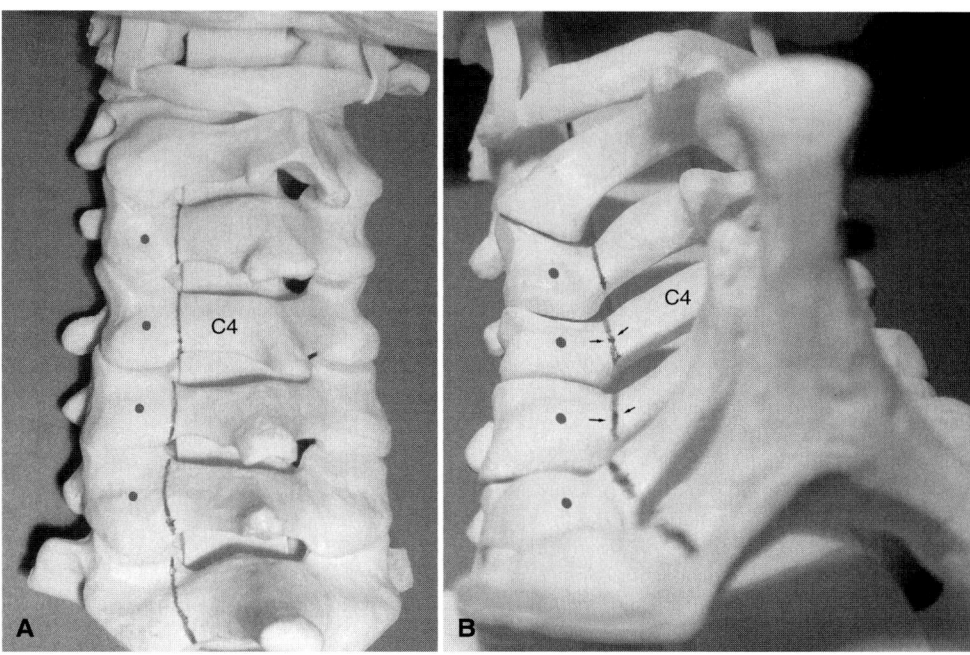

in vitro biomechanical testing has revealed little advantage in screw purchase between bicortical and unicortical screws.[97] An advantage to bicortical purchase may have been realized in screw-plate systems in which the screws did not lock rigidly to the plate. However, this is of less relevance with contemporary screw-rod instrumentation systems. Therefore, except in unusual conditions, the authors recommend unicortical purchase to avoid the risk of endangering surrounding neurovascular structures.

When employing an "upward-and-outward" technique for lateral mass screw placement, a few technical aspects should be considered. First, to get the appropriate upward trajectory, the hand should be lowered in a caudal direction. In placing screws at C3 or C4, this is not a problem. However, more caudally, the soft tissues of the wound impede the ability to drop the drill down far enough; hence, the skin and fascial incision may need to be extended caudally to achieve the appropriate trajectory. Second, when drilling upward into the lateral mass, it is important to keep a downward force on the drill guide, so that the drill does not fracture off the dorsal cortex of the lateral mass. It is not uncommon, particularly in osteoporotic bone, for the dorsal cortex to fracture when drilling at a steep angle, and also when tapping the outer cortex. Finally, if the starting point is too lateral, drilling in an upward and outward direction may fracture off the lateral aspect of the lateral mass. To salvage this situation, a more medial starting point can be chosen and the

Roy-Camille technique of drilling employed in a more straight-ahead trajectory. However, screws no longer than 8 to 10 mm should be used to avoid vertebral artery injury (see Figs. 29-9 and 29-13).

CERVICAL PEDICLES

Cervical pedicle screw fixation has been advocated as a method for improving construct stability, but it also significantly increases the risk of neurovascular injury. With the exception of C7, pedicle screw placement is technically very challenging and not recommended by the authors except in exceptional circumstances. Anatomically, the cervical pedicles diverge posteriorly from the vertebral body at an angle of approximately 40 to 45° away from the midsagittal plane (Fig. 29-14). The pedicles are typically taller than they are wide, with outer diameters of approximately 7.0 mm in height and between 4.5 and 6.0 mm in width.[12,58,85] The actual inner cancellous diameters are smaller due to the thickness of the cortical bone, with a mean width reported by Rezcallah and co-workers to be approximately half of the outer diameter (between 2.3 and 3.0 mm).[85] Occasionally the pedicle is solid cortical bone.[48] The cortical bone is thinnest along the lateral aspect of the pedicle, adjacent to which runs the vertebral artery.[76]

The vertebral artery ascends just lateral to the pedicle. The placement of screws at C7 is safer than in the rest of

FIGURE 29-11 *Lateral mass anatomy and techniques for placing lateral mass screws. A variety of techniques have been described to guide the safe placement of lateral mass screws. In general, these techniques represent subtle modifications of the starting point and angulation. In the Magerl technique **(A),** the starting point is 1 to 2 mm medial and cephalad to the center of the lateral mass and angled 25° outward and 30° upward, parallel to the facet joint. In the Roy-Camille technique **(B),** the starting point is the center of the lateral mass, and the screws are directed straight forward and 10° outward. In the Anderson technique **(C),** the starting point is 1 to 2 mm medial to the center of the lateral mass and angled 15 to 20° outward, and 20 to 30° upward. (From Mirza, S.K.; Anderson, P.A. Skeletal Trauma, 3rd ed., New York, W.B. Saunders, 2003. Originally redrawn from Abdu, W.A.; Bohlman, H.H. Techniques of subaxial posterior cervical spine fusions: An overview. Orthopedics, 15:293, 1992.)*

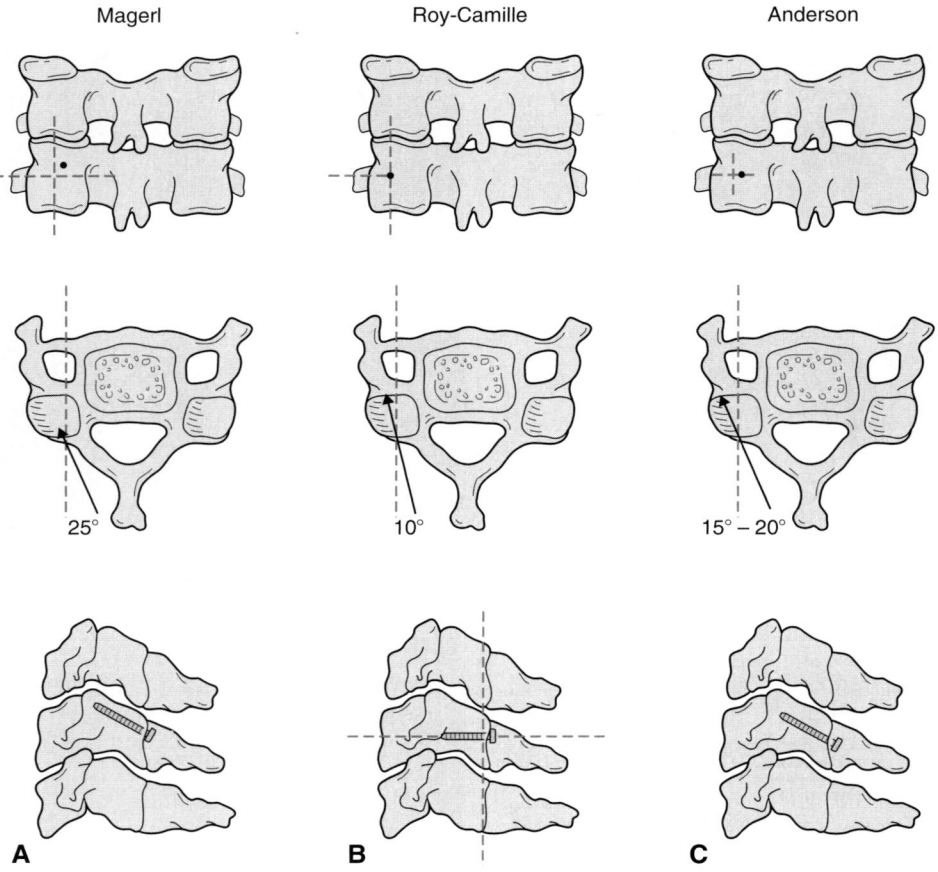

the subaxial cervical spine as the artery is extraosseous. The dural sac runs directly along the medial aspect of the pedicle. Unlike in the lumbar spine where the exiting nerve root curves under the pedicle, the exiting nerve root in the cervical spine lies on the superior border of the pedicle. Ugur and associates revealed in a cadaveric study that there is direct approximation of these structures to the pedicle, such that no space exists between the medial and superior surface of the pedicle and the dural sac and exiting nerve root, respectively.[108] Approximately 1.0 to 2.5 mm separates the inferior border of the pedicle and the subjacent nerve root.

Females have generally smaller cervical pedicles than males. The same can be said for Asians, who have smaller cervical pedicles than non-Asians (making Asian females likely the worst candidates for pedicle screw fixation).[117] Arthropathies such as rheumatoid arthritis can significantly alter the pedicular anatomy. Careful scrutinization of the pedicular anatomy by CT is essential before attempting to place cervical pedicle screws.

CERVICAL PEDICLE SCREW FIXATION With the exception of C7, pedicle screw placement is technically challenging. Although pedicle screws may have a biomechanical advantage over lateral mass screws in terms of bicolumnar purchase,[51,78,87] this needs to be weighed against the potential neurovascular hazards of placing such screws compared with the relative ease and safety of lateral mass screws. The greatest hazard in placing pedicle screws from C3 to C6 is injury to the vertebral artery by deviating laterally, which is more likely due to small pedicle size and weakness of the lateral cortical bone, making transgression into the foramen transversarium more likely. The steep medial angulation of the pedicle (40–45°) also makes it more likely to exit laterally and into the foramen. Ludwig and colleagues demonstrated that inserting cervical pedicle screws using anatomic guidelines resulted in a cortical perforation rate of 87.5 percent, with a neurovascular structure (usually the vertebral artery) being encroached on in two thirds of these cases.[58] The accuracy

FIGURE 29-12 *Technique for lateral mass screw insertion. To aid in directing the screw out laterally, one can rest the drill guide against the spinous processes **(A)**. The upward direction of drilling places the screws parallel to the facet joints **(B)**. To promote fusion, the facet joints should be burred and bone graft placed **(C)**. (Modified from Mirza, S.K.; Anderson, P.A. Skeletal Trauma, 3rd ed., New York, W.B. Saunders, 2003.)*

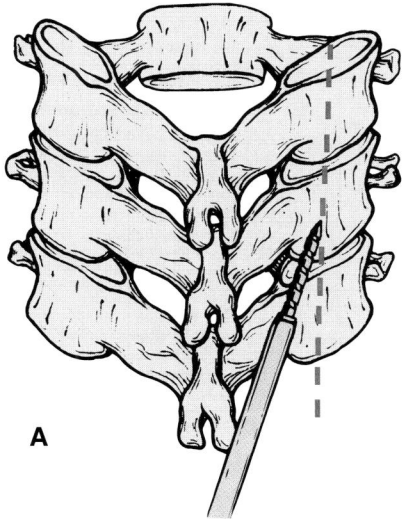

A

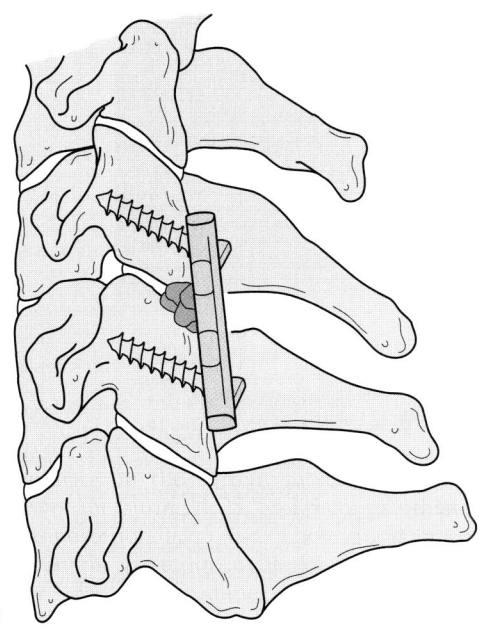

B

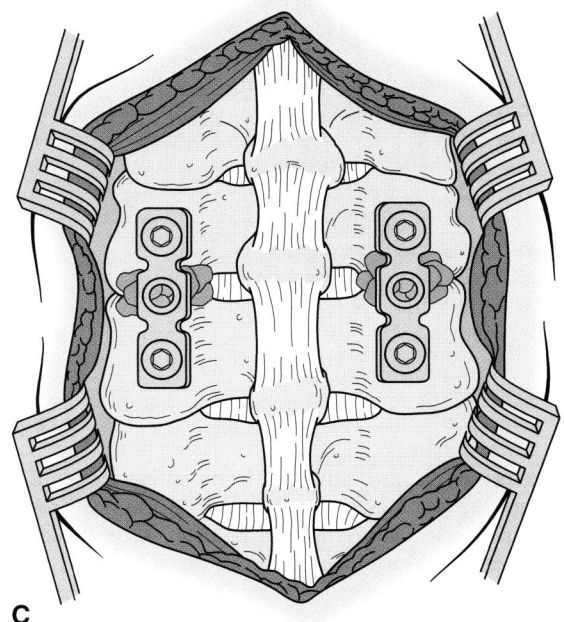

C

was improved by performing a laminoforaminotomy to palpate and visualize the pedicle, but even with this technique, cortical perforation occurred in 55 percent. At C3 to C6, 25 percent of the screws impinged on a neurovascular structure, suggesting that even when palpating the pedicle at these levels, and within the controlled lab environment with a cadaveric cervical spine specimen devoid of blood and posterior musculature, the risk of a "critical breach" was still high.

Abumi and colleagues championed the application of pedicle screw fixation in the subaxial cervical spine.[1] In their technique, a bur is used to decorticate the lateral mass until the cancellous bone of the pedicle is identified. A 2-mm probe is tapped down the pedicle, using lateral fluoroscopy to guide the rostrocaudal trajectory. The mediolateral trajectory is guided by preoperative CT. Abumi has reported a 6.7 percent pedicle violation rate, with 1 patient in 180 suffering a vertebral artery injury (controlled with bone wax), and 2 patients sustaining radiculopathies.[2] Other experience has been less favorable; Neo and co-workers reported a 29 percent pedicle breach rate, with 15 percent deviating the vertebral artery more than 2 mm.[65] Kast and associates reported from a review of 26 patients a correct pedicle screw placement rate of only

FIGURE 29-13 | *Vertebral artery injury secondary to misplaced lateral mass screw. This case report by Cho and colleagues demonstrates a 41-year-old male who underwent posterior fixation for a C5-C6 facet dislocation (**A** and **B**). The patient suffered a vertebral artery injury as seen on angiography (**D**) and a posterior cerebellar infarction (**E**). Axial computed tomography (**C**) and anteroposterior radiograph (**A**) demonstrate that the screws were not directly outward, and the starting point on the left was too medial. This case demonstrates the importance of appreciating the surgical anatomy and directing the screws laterally. (Reprinted from Cho, K.H.; Shin, Y.S.; Yoon, S.H.; et al. Poor surgical technique in cervical plating leading to vertebral artery injury and brain stem infarction—case report. Surg Neurol 64:222–223, 2005. Reprinted with permission from Elsevier.)*

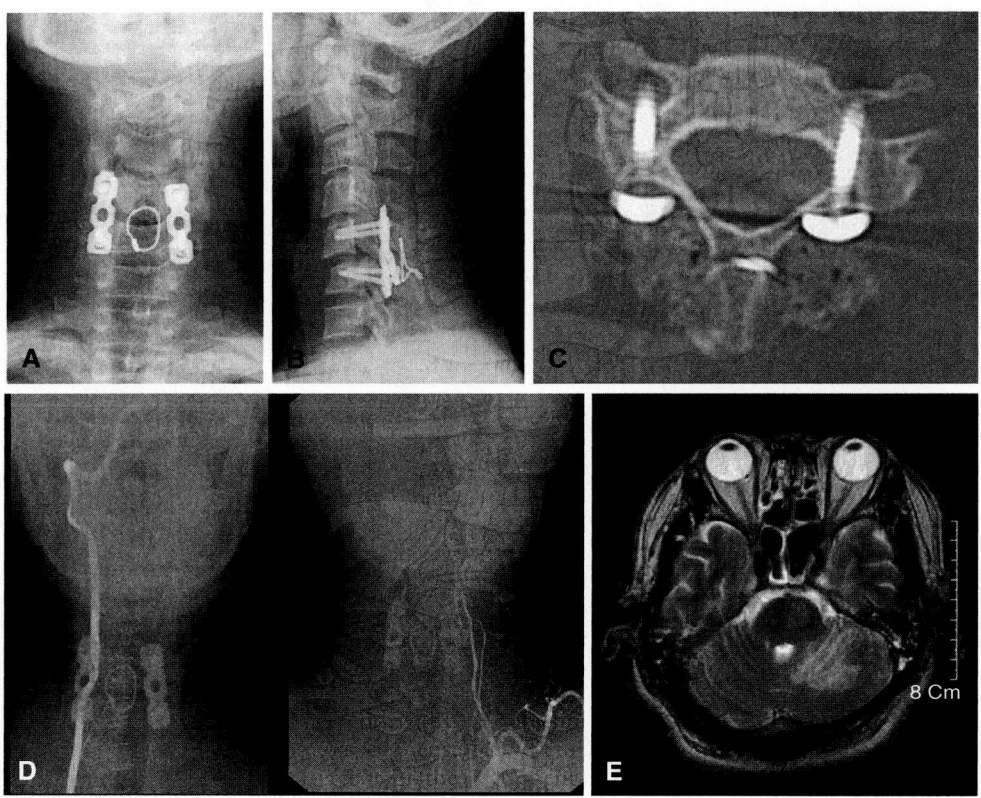

70 percent; 21 percent of the screws breached in a "minor" fashion, and 9 percent of the screws were considered to be "critically" misplaced, causing neurologic symptoms in 2 patients.[49] Image-guided technology may help in the future to make screw placement from C3 to C6 safer, but until then, we recommend it only in rare instances and for surgeons with substantial cervical spine experience.

Conversely, pedicle screw cannulation can be safely performed at C7. Because the C7 lateral mass is thin, and the vertebral artery does not enter the transverse foramen until C6, the C7 pedicle is an attractive fixation point for screws. Enough variation exists in the anatomy of the C7 pedicle that performing a small laminoforaminotomy is useful for palpating the medial, superior, and inferior borders of the

FIGURE 29-14 | *Pedicular and vertebral body anatomy in the subaxial cervical spine. This figure depicts the vertebral bodies and pedicles for each level of the subaxial cervical spine in a healthy 42-year-old male. Note particularly the steep medial angulation of the pedicle from the lateral mass (approximately 40–45°) and the close proximity of the vertebral artery (arrow) within the foramen transversarium along the anterior border of the pedicle from C3 to C6. At C7, the vertebral artery (arrowhead) is not intimately related to the pedicle, making screw placement at this level much safer. Note also that the vertebral bodies widen toward the caudal end of the subaxial cervical spine.*

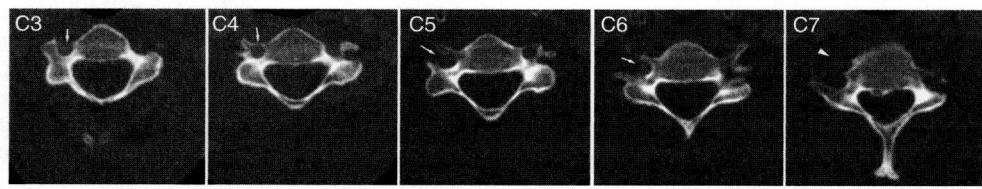

C7 pedicle.[5] This provides direct visualization of the pedicle location and establishes the starting point on the lateral mass for drilling. In Ludwig and colleagues' cadaveric study, no C7 screws encroached on a neurovascular structure when placed with the guidance of a laminoforaminotomy.[58] Remember that the exiting nerve root is along the superior border of the pedicle, and as such, the superior and medial border of the pedicle should be most carefully appreciated prior to drilling. A common mistake with the placement of the pedicle screw at C7 is the failure to medially direct the drill and thus exit laterally.

VERTEBRAL BODY

Approaching the cervical spine anteriorly, the longus colli muscles lie in a rostrocaudal direction and are important landmarks for determining the midline. Retracting the longus colli muscles reveals the rectangular aspect of the anterior vertebral bodies. The anteroinferior corner of the superior vertebral body often hangs over the disk space, which can often be exposed more easily if this anterior "lip" is resected. The vertebral bodies are wider in the transverse than in the sagittal plane. On average, the vertebral bodies are approximately 22 to 28 mm wide in males, and 21 to 27 mm in females and increase in size from C3 to C7.[54,57,71] At the superior end plate, the lateral borders of the vertebral body are outlined by the uncinate processes (Fig. 29-15). Together, the position of the longus colli muscles, the location of the uncinate processes, and the knowledge of vertebral body width are all important factors to keep in mind when performing a vertebrectomy, so as to remain midline and to avoid straying too far laterally and into the transverse foramen. These considerations are particularly important in the case of anterior column injuries, in which the native anatomy and alignment of the cervical spine may be altered.

VERTEBRAL BODY SCREW FIXATION AND INTERBODY RECONSTRUCTION Familiarity with the sagittal, or anteroposterior, depth of the vertebral body is important when inserting screws for anterior cervical plates. Measured at midbody, the average sagittal depth is approximately 17 to 18 mm in males and 15 to 16 mm in females. In a morphometric CT study of the cervical spine, Kwon and co-workers reported that out of 50 males, none had a midsagittal depth of 12 mm or less, but 8 were 14 mm or less.[54] In females, 8 of 50 had a midsagittal depth of 12 mm or less, and 35 were 14 mm or less. However, there is enough individual variation amongst individuals to necessitate careful evaluation using radiographic imaging and direct intraoperative intradiskal measurements to determine screw lengths.

The anatomy of the end plate is often underappreciated, but is important to consider for placement of interbody or vertebrectomy grafts, particularly in osteoporotic patients. The uncinate processes are critical landmarks for the superior end plate, as they define the lateral boundaries and help to keep one from straying into the vertebral artery during diskectomies or vertebrectomies (see Fig. 29-15). The superior end plate, which is generally thicker than the inferior end plate, is thickest posteriorly and thinnest anteriorly; conversely, the inferior end plate is thinnest posteriorly and thickest anteriorly.[71,95] The peripheral aspects of the end plates are also thicker than the central aspect. An interbody or vertebrectomy graft that is sized appropriately to rest on the thicker parts of the end plate is less likely to subside, which may indeed be very important in osteoporotic bone.

VERTEBRAL ARTERY

The vertebral artery is discussed here due to its relevance in both anterior and posterior stabilization surgery for the subaxial cervical spine. The vertebral artery arises off the subclavian artery, courses between the scaleneus anterior and longus colli muscles, passes anterior to the transverse process of C7, and enters the foramen transversarium at C6 (see Fig. 29-15). The artery is approximately 3 to 4 mm in width and is often larger on the left than on the right.[16] The foramen transversarium moves posteriorly as one ascends from C6 to C3. As it traverses within the foramen transversarium, the vertebral artery is vulnerable to injury in cervical fractures and dislocations (Fig. 29-16). The vertebral arteries pierce the dura at the foramen magnum, course medially along the ventral medulla and inferior pons, then coalesce to form a single basilar artery. As the basilar artery ascends it gives off bilateral posterior cerebellar arteries, internal acoustic arteries, and superior cerebellar arteries, which supply the cerebellum, pons, and middle ear structures. At the superior pons it divides into the left and right posterior cerebral arteries, which contribute to the arterial circle of Willis, and then continues to supply the occipital lobes of the cerebral cortex. This anatomy explains some of the neurologic manifestations of a vertebral artery injury, which include visual deficits, dizziness, nausea and vomiting, vertigo, tinnitus, dysphagia, hoarseness, and ataxia. It also explains how unilateral injuries are typically compensated for by collateral circulation and are thus often asymptomatic.

The position of the vertebral artery directly anterior to the medial aspect of the lateral mass and along the lateral aspect of the pedicle was discussed earlier (see Fig. 29-9, 29-13, and 29-14). During anterior cervical diskectomy or vertebrectomy, the vertebral artery is potentially vulnerable along the lateral aspect of the vertebral body. An iatrogenic injury to the vertebral artery can cause catastrophic bleeding with possibly devastating neurologic consequences.[101] Keeping a constant perspective on location of the anatomic midline is critical to avoiding injury to the vertebral artery. Injury can occur with a high-speed bur when widening a vertebrectomy trough, or with a Kerrison rongeur when doing an aggressive uncinate process resection. Within the disk space, the uncinate processes are the reliable landmarks, and having good exposure of them bilaterally is important for not only demonstrating the lateral border of the vertebral body, but also calculating where midline is. In a detailed cadaveric study, Pait and colleagues reported that the vertebral artery is located, on average, 0.8 to 1.6 mm lateral to the lateral tip of the uncinate process.[69] The close proximity of the vertebral artery to the uncinate process strongly suggests that one avoid passing surgical instruments lateral to this anterior landmark. Heary and co-workers reported the distance between the medial borders of the foramen transversarium to decrease as the vertebral artery ascends through the subaxial spine, with an average of 32 mm at C6 to 25 mm at C3.[43] In general, a corpectomy trough of 15

Anterior anatomy of the subaxial cervical spine. When viewed from the anterior approach **(A),** *the uncinate processes at the posterolateral corners of the superior end plates are important landmarks for defining the lateral borders of the disk space. On the coronal computed tomographic reconstruction* **(B),** *the uncinate processes (arrows) form the uncovertebral joint with the convex undersurface of the suprajacent vertebral body. (Modified from Mirza, S.K.; Anderson, P.A. Skeletal Trauma, 3rd ed., New York, W.B. Saunders, 2003.)*

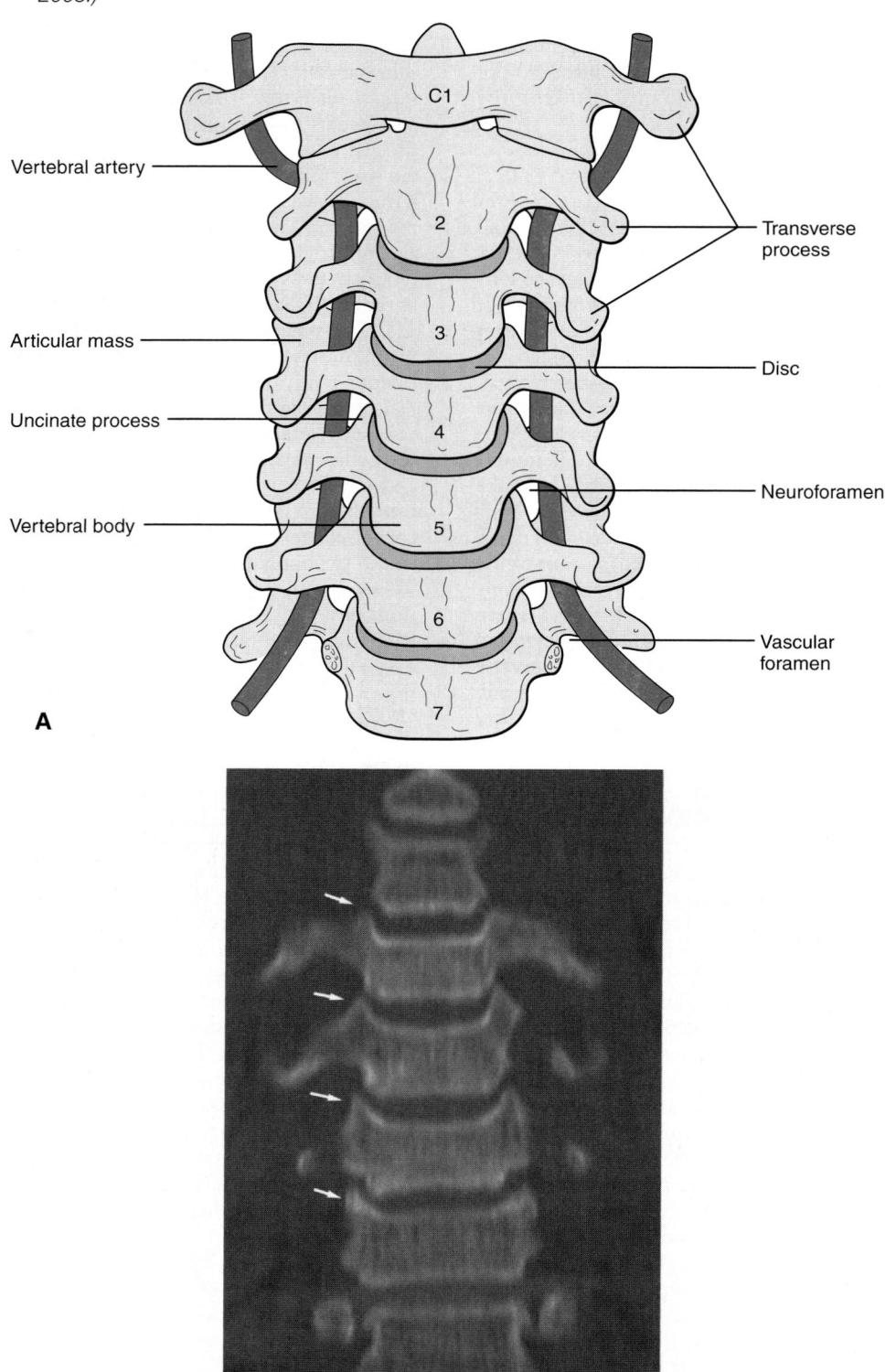

FIGURE 29-16 *Vertebral artery injury in blunt cervical trauma. **A,** This 35-year-old male sustained a C7 compressive flexion injury (burst fracture). **B,** Although he was not symptomatic, the fracture of his right C6 transverse process (*) prompted a computed tomography (CT) angiogram, which demonstrated occlusion of the right vertebral artery. The CT angiogram is a rapid and relatively noninvasive method for identifying such vascular injuries. Note the filling of the left foramen transversarium (arrow) on the axial **(B)** and coronal **(C)** reconstructions. In contrast to the vast majority of vertebral artery injuries, like this patient's, most cases are asymptomatic.*

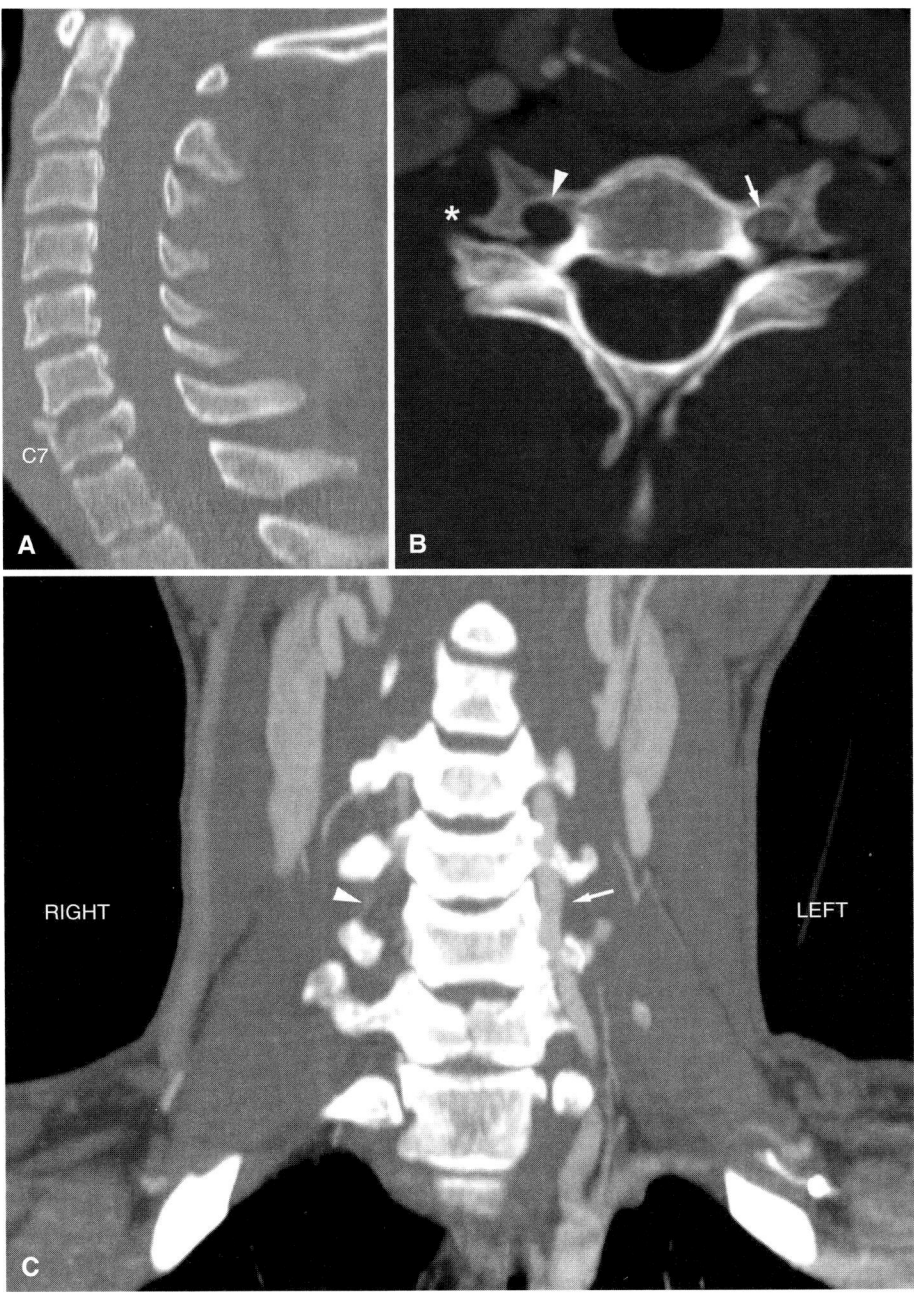

to 16 mm in width would therefore leave a few millimeters of bone on either side, provided that the trough was centered along the midline. Given that the uncinate process is typically 5 to 6 mm in width,[57] using the medial aspects of the uncinate processes to define the lateral boundaries of the bony resection provides a 5-mm margin for error from the medial border of the foramen transversarium. One should also be prepared for the fact

that, particularly when treating a burst fracture anteriorly, the uncinate processes may not be visualized all that well due to bony comminution and bleeding.

Knowledge of surgical anatomy does not substitute for careful review of preoperative imaging. This is especially true of the vertebral artery, which can have many anomalous courses such as having a tortuous course that migrates medially in the vertebral body (Fig. 29-17). This occurs in

FIGURE 29-17 *Tortuous vertebral artery with medial encroachment within the vertebral body. These two cases at C3 in a 39-year-old female (A) and at C5 in a 48-year-old male (B) illustrate the need to carefully assess the position of the vertebral artery when planning a cervical diskectomy or corpectomy. The right lateral border of the vertebral body is marked with a line, and the corresponding position on the left is marked with an arrow to demonstrate how far medial the vertebral artery has deviated. Recognizing this before embarking on a diskectomy or vertebrectomy can help prevent iatrogenic injury and major blood loss.*

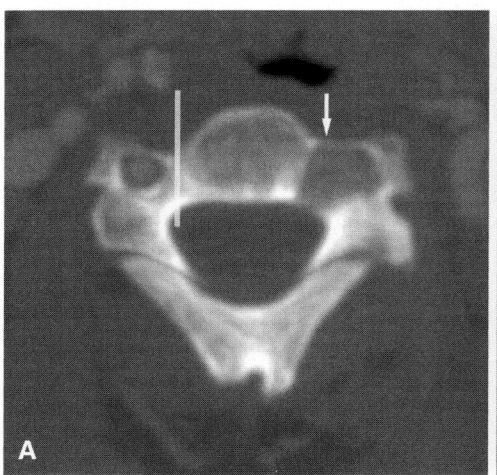 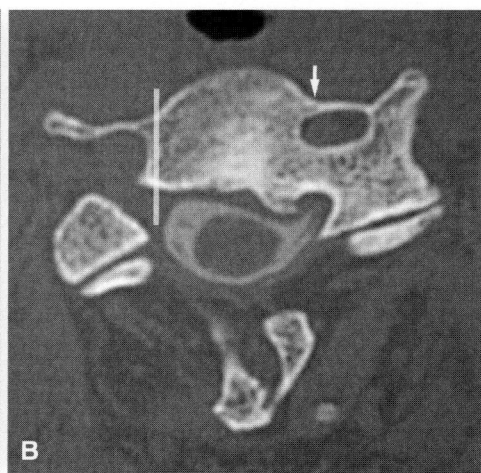

up to 2.7 percent of patients.[23] Typically, the artery is in its expected position at the level of the disk space, being held laterally by the end plate and uncinate processes. However, at the midbody level, the artery has the potential to migrate medially. In such a case, the typical anatomic landmarks described earlier may not be reliable for preventing an iatrogenic injury to the vessel during a vertebrectomy or by screw placement within the body. There is, however, no recourse for the more medially deviated vertebral artery other than recognizing its presence preoperatively and planning for its avoidance intraoperatively.

Management of such iatrogenic vertebral artery injuries should be considered before one occurs. Smith and associates reported on 10 patients who suffered iatrogenic vertebral artery injuries during anterior cervical decompressions.[101] Hemostasis was fortunately achieved in three patients with local tamponade, using various hemostatic agents. In five patients, the artery was directly exposed and either electrocoagulated or ligated, and in two the artery was blindly ligated. Three patients suffered neurologic deficits related to the vertebral artery injury. Options other than local tamponade and direct ligation include direct arterial repair[80] and endovascular techniques, such as coil occlusion or stenting.[32] In general, an intraoperative injury to the vertebral artery during an anterior cervical procedure should prompt several responses. The anesthesiology team should prepare for rapid and catastrophic blood loss—hemostatic agents and extra suction should be made available to gain visualization and local control. A vascular surgeon should be contacted for assistance in either ligating or repairing the vessel, and the interventional radiology suite should be alerted to the possibility of requiring an emergent endovascular procedure. Obviously, avoiding such an emergency with careful preoperative planning and operative technique is preferable.

SURGICAL TECHNIQUES

Anterior Stabilization

The primary advantages of an anterior approach to the cervical spine are the ability to directly decompress the spinal cord from ventral compression secondary to displaced bone or disk and the ability to reconstruct the anterior weight-bearing column.

Anterior stabilization is performed through a standard Smith-Robinson anteromedial approach to the cervical spine. In severe fractures and dislocations, the anterior longitudinal ligament may be disrupted and the longus colli muscles injured, making it more difficult to assess true midline. One should be cautious in such situations where the anatomy is obscured to use the uncovertebral joints within the disk space to define the lateral boundaries of safe dissection. Straying off to one side or the other may result in an incomplete decompression or vertebral artery injury. Decompression is performed by diskectomy or corpectomy, making sure to remove sufficient bone from both right and left sides because the tendency is to remove less bone on the side of the surgical approach (Fig. 29-18). Bleeding may be greater in patients with acute fractures and should be anticipated.

Following decompression, numerous choices exist for the interbody or vertebral body reconstruction. These include tricortical iliac crest bone graft, allograft, or interbody cage devices. In the last instance, local autogenous bone can be used to fill the cage. After the decompression, lordosis may be restored by either extending the patient's neck or using a distractor to allow placement of a slightly longer cage. In addition to restoring a more physiologic alignment, lowering the head into extension can help to lock the facets into a fully reduced position and provide some degree of posterior resistance to shear forces. Restoring lordosis by distracting and forcing in a large graft may result in overdistraction,

FIGURE 29-18 *Technique of anterior vertebrectomy. In this illustration of a burst fracture with posterior ligamentous disruption (A) the extent of kyphosis is exaggerated (normally, one would realign such an injury with traction or gentle extension of the head). The diskectomies are carried out first (B), then bone is removed from the injured vertebral body (C). This bone should be saved for use within a reconstruction cage or allograft fibula if tricortical iliac crest autogenous bone graft is not to be used. The decompression is carried out all the way back to the posterior lateral ligament (D), which in such injuries may be disrupted as well. The reconstruction is then completed (E) with bone or alternative reconstruction devices (F). (From Mirza, S.K.; Anderson, P.A. Skeletal Trauma, 3rd ed., New York, W.B. Saunders, 2003.)*

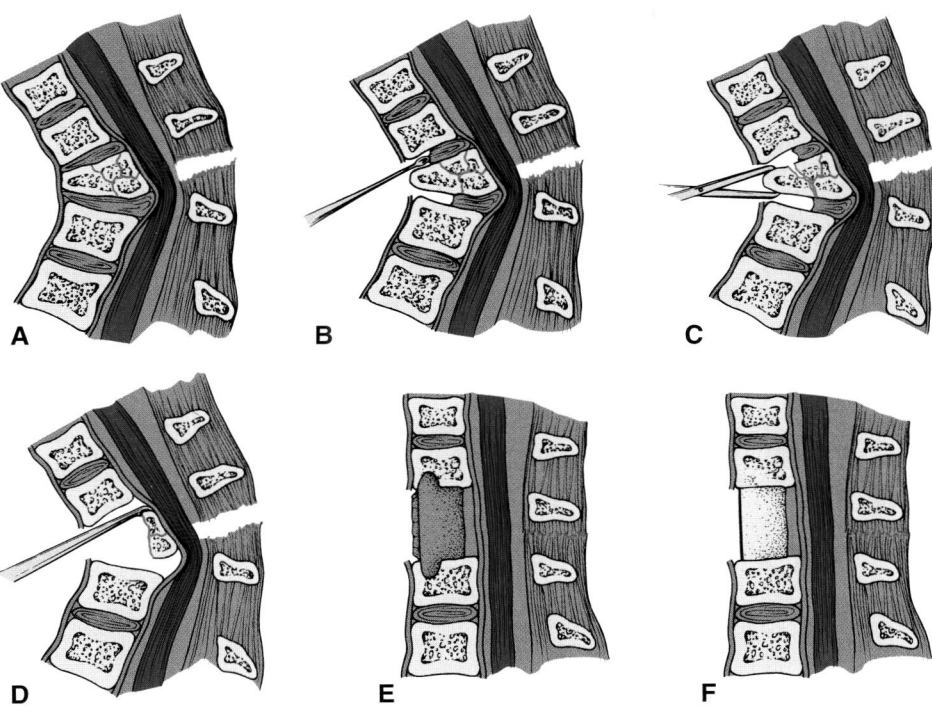

because the disrupted posterior elements may not provide any resistance to excessive lengthening.

Finally, anterior cervical plate fixation is used to stabilize the injured segments (Fig. 29-19). Static plating systems in which the screws lock rigidly to the plate or dynamic systems that allow for relative motion between the screw and plate are both in common use. Whether there is an advantage to dynamic plating systems in the setting of trauma is unclear. The screws should be started as close to the end plates as possible, so as to use as short of a plate as possible and reduce the risk that the edge of the plate will encroach on the adjacent disk space.

Posterior Stabilization

Posterior stabilization is performed through a posterior midline incision. The primary advantages of the posterior approach are the superior biomechanical characteristics of posterior lateral mass fixation, as compared with anterior fixation, and the ability to easily decompress the spinal cord over multiple levels. The exposure is straightforward, but in cases of severe posterior ligamentous and bony disruption, the typical landmarks may be obscured. Normally, once incising the fascia, one can descend midline to the

posterior elements and dissect them in a bloodless manner. This is often difficult with severe posterior ligamentous and bony injury. When laminar and spinous process fractures are present, care should be taken during exposure to avoid neurologic injury. When exposing laterally, it is important to spare the facet capsules at the levels above and below the injured segments.

Lateral mass fixation is the most common form of posterior stabilization. The method by which lateral mass screws are inserted has already been described. At C6-C7, it can be difficult to fit a lateral mass screw in C6 and a pedicle screw at C7, because the heads of their screws can abut one another. In general, the C7 pedicle is placed first, because there is less flexibility in the placement of this screw. The C6 lateral mass is then drilled, the angulation of which can be modified by starting slightly more superiorly than normal. The C6 lateral mass screw is then inserted first, followed by the C7 screw.

The decompression is achieved by laminectomy (Fig. 29-20). Often, the cord needs to be decompressed over a long distance, making the posterior approach ideal. Laminoplasty may also be performed to decompress the cord, although it should be reserved for cases of central cord syndrome in which there is no associated mechanical instability.

FIGURE 29-19 | *Technique of anterior cervical plating. Contemporary plating systems **(A)** prevent the screws from backing out from the plate. Either the screw locks rigidly to the plate, or the system allows for limited rotational or translational motion between the screw and plate for "dynamization" of the graft. Contemporary plating systems do not require bicortical screw fixation, and the screws are typically drilled to a predetermined distance **(B)**. In this system, a locking screw **(D)** prevents the screws from backing out. (From Mirza, S.K.; Anderson, P.A. Skeletal Trauma, 3rd ed., New York, W.B. Saunders, 2003.)*

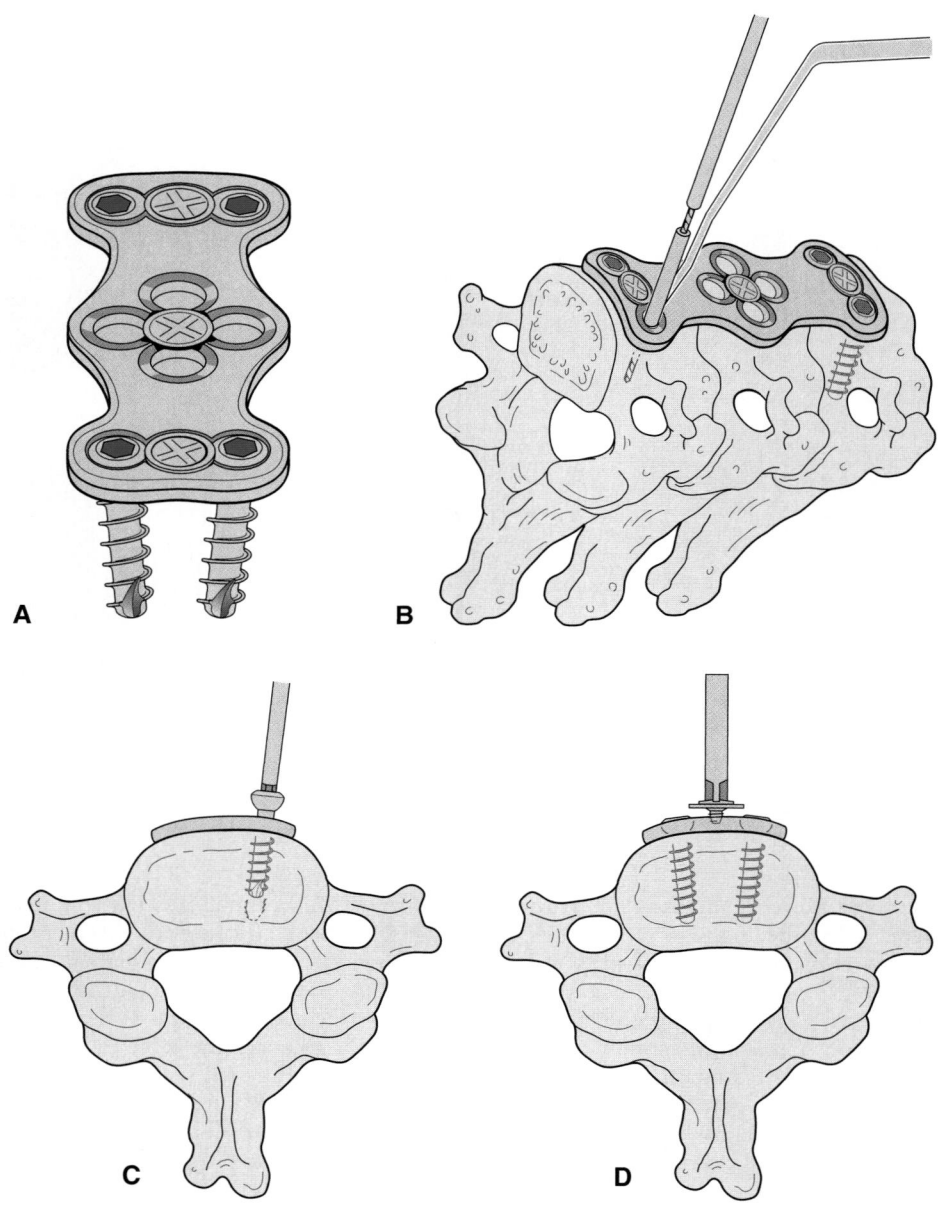

Anterior Versus Posterior Stabilization of the Cervical Spine

Many factors should be considered when choosing between an anterior and posterior surgical approach. In general, if cord decompression is required, the surgical approach that provides direct access to the compressive pathology should be chosen. In anticipation of inserting internal fixation, one should determine where the osseous elements are least compromised and thus able to accept screws or reconstruction devices. For example, a C5-C6 facet fracture-dislocation with a C6 end plate fracture might be best treated posteriorly with lateral mass fixation because of the inability of the C6 end plate to support an interbody graft.[47] Alternatively, a C5-C6 facet fracture-dislocation with a comminuted C6 lateral mass might be better treated anteriorly with a diskectomy and fusion because of the inability to achieve secure fixation in the lateral mass posteriorly.

Advantages of the anterior approach include direct decompression of ventral compressive pathologies, reconstruction of the anterior weight-bearing column, lower

FIGURE 29-20 *Technique of posterior laminectomy-decompression.* ***D,*** *illustrates the basic technique for performing a decompressive laminectomy, although in the setting of trauma with any spinal instability, it must be combined with lateral mass stabilization. In the setting of multilevel stenosis* ***(A),*** *a posterior laminectomy is a far easier method of achieving spinal cord decompression than an anterior procedure. If the spine is lordotic or is brought back into lordosis after the decompression is complete, the spinal cord will drift posteriorly, away from the ventral compressive pathology* ***(B)****. The laminectomy is performed by burring troughs along the lateral borders of the lamina* ***(C)****, and lifting the lamina/ligamentum flavum off en bloc* ***(D)****. (From Mirza, S.K.; Anderson, P.A. Skeletal Trauma, 3rd ed., New York, W.B. Saunders, 2003.* ***A*** *and* ***B*** *redrawn from Epstein, J.A.; Epstein, M.E. Surgical Management of Cervical Spine Stenosis, Spondylosis and Myeloradiculopathy by Means of Posterior Approach. In: The Cervical Spine Research Society Staff, eds. The Cervical Spine, 2nd ed. Philadelphia, J.B. Lippincott, 1989; from Epstein, J.A., Contemp Neurosurg 7:3, 1985.* ***C*** *and* ***D*** *redrawn from Dante, S.J.; Heary, R; Kramer, D. Cervical laminectomy for myelopathy. Oper Tech Orthop 6:30–37, 1996.)*

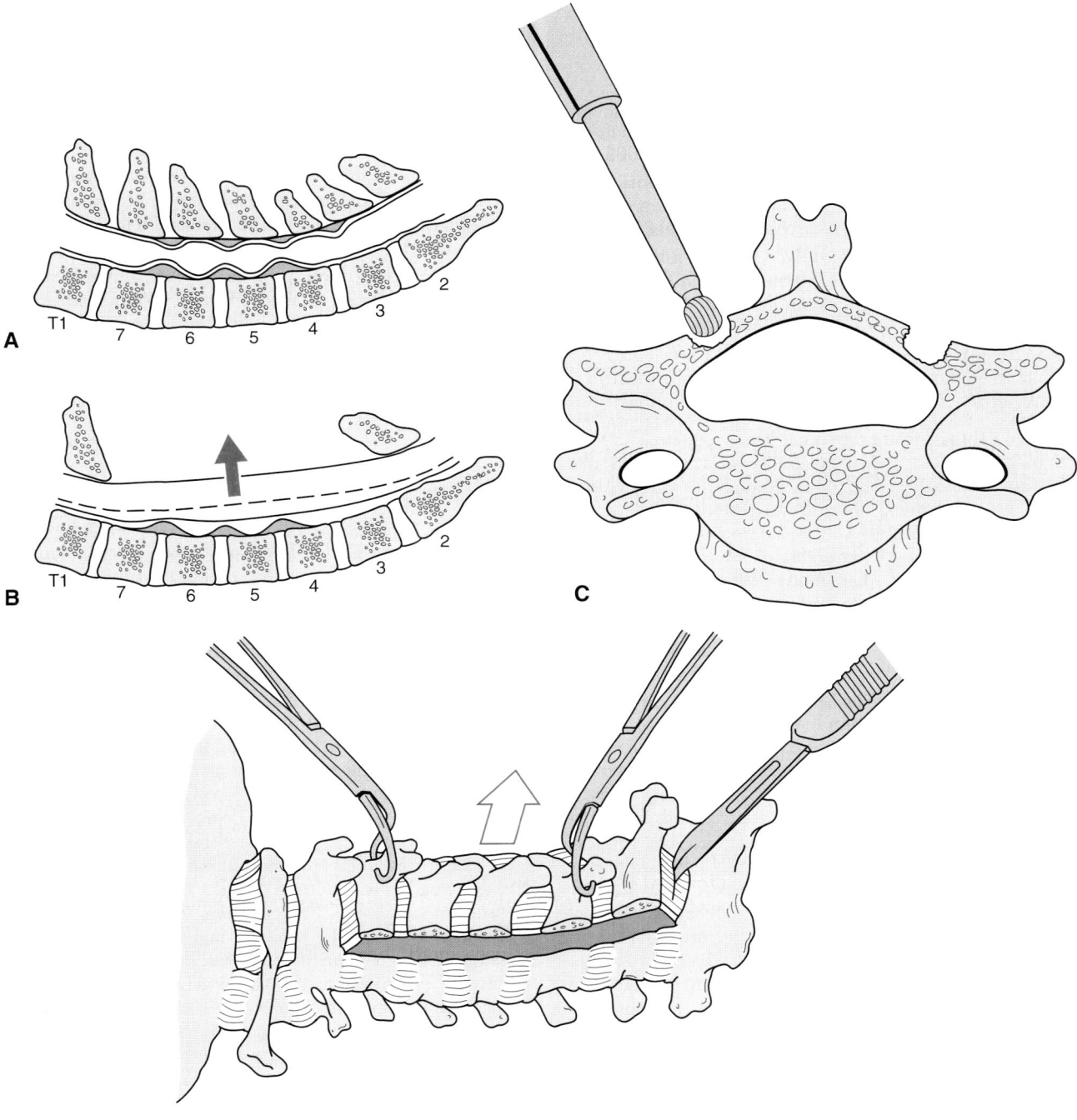

infection rate, and minimal muscle trauma. One avoids turning the patient prone, which can be dangerous in patients with unstable spinal injuries, hemodynamic instability, pulmonary injuries, or obesity. Disadvantages of the anterior approach include the reduced biomechanical rigidity of anterior compared with posterior fixation, which potentially predisposes to a higher pseudarthrosis rate, and greater difficulty in correcting kyphosis or translation. The approach itself can inflict further damage in patients with significant laryngeal or tracheal injury, and in large patients the sternum may obstruct distal access to the cervicothoracic junction.

The anterior approach is technically simple and is well tolerated. However, in the elderly or in those with cervical spinal cord injuries, postoperative swallowing and airway problems associated with an anterior approach to the cervical spine can lead to pneumonia and severe respiratory sepsis. Even if such alterations are minor, in the elderly patient who may already have subtle, subclinical abnormalities in swallowing mechanics, they can precipitate a major aspiration risk. Postoperative delirium and diminished levels of consciousness after a general anesthetic also contribute to this risk in elderly individuals. In the quadriplegic patient, pulmonary function is already compromised due to the loss of intercostal muscle function and inability to clear secretions.

The posterior approach has a number of advantages as well. From a mechanical perspective, lateral mass fixation reestablishes the posterior tension band of the cervical spine and thus resists further kyphotic forces. Also, its position more laterally than a centrally placed anterior cervical plate allows lateral mass fixation to better resist rotational and lateral bending forces. In general, most in vitro studies that have simulated various types of cervical injuries have demonstrated a biomechanical advantage to posterior over anterior fixation, which potentially improves fusion rates. In a randomized comparison between anterior and posterior fixation for 52 unstable cervical spine injuries, Brodke and colleagues reported that the fusion rate was slightly higher in the posteriorly treated patients (100 vs. 90%), although this difference was not statistically significant.[13] Further published comparisons between anterior and posterior approaches are lacking.

Other advantages of the posterior approach include its extensile nature, which allows for easier exposure of the entire cervical spine and, if necessary, the upper thoracic spine as well. When multiple vertebral bodies are fractured anteriorly, achieving a solid reconstruction anteriorly may be impractical, and a long posterior fixation construct through this extensile approach may suffice. Decompression over multiple segments can also be achieved more easily from the posterior side. With respect to deformity correction, it is technically easier to reduce translational malalignment, such as that seen in fracture-dislocations or facet dislocations, from a posterior approach. Also, compression of posterior segmental instrumentation such as lateral mass screws or pedicle screws helps to restore cervical lordosis. The airway problems associated with an anterior approach are obviated by approaching posteriorly. The posterior exposure does, however, require dissection and denervation of the dorsal musculature and iatrogenic injury to adjacent ligaments, with the possibility of exacerbating instability of the adjacent segment.

CIRCUMFERENTIAL FUSION

Circumferential anteroposterior fixation provides the most biomechanically rigid and stable construct.[4] When severe comminution of the anterior weight-bearing column and gross posterior ligamentous disruption occur, the mechanical instability makes it rational to proceed with immediate combined anterior and posterior fixation, rather than doing one side only and endeavoring to "follow it closely" radiographically for postoperative failure. Unfortunately, insufficient literature is available to establish which cases warrant this approach. In cases in which circumferential stabilization is planned, doing the anterior aspect first so as to decompress and "provisionally" stabilize the motion segments makes the subsequent turn into the prone position safer.

MANAGEMENT OF SPECIFIC INJURIES

For descriptive purposes, we divide the discussion of specific injuries of the lower cervical spine according to the phylogeny of Allen and Ferguson, recognizing the limitations of this classification system. Commonly used nomenclature for specific injuries is also included. The spectrum of severity within each phylogeny is discussed, and specific surgical and nonsurgical recommendations are offered for guidance.

Compressive Flexion Injuries

Compressive flexion injuries, or flexion teardrop fractures, occur most commonly at C5 and are frequently the result of diving injuries, football spearing injuries, and motor vehicle accidents. These injuries were postulated to occur with a compressive force being applied "obliquely downward and posterior in the sagittal plane, with the stress concentration at the anterior-superior margin of the vertebral body."[6] In essence, these are axial loading injuries in which the motion segment is flexed, thus concentrating the compressive forces on the anterior aspect of the vertebral body and imposing varying degrees of distraction on the posterior elements (Fig. 29-21). Although the primary mechanical insult is compression, the stability of these injuries is influenced by the extent to which the posterior elements are disrupted by the resultant distraction applied posterior to the center of rotation.

Within the compressive flexion (CF) phylogeny are five stages, representing increasing degrees of anterior and posterior element injury. The first two stages (CFS1 and CFS2) involve injury to the anterior lip of the vertebral body, creating a blunting (CFS1) of the anterosuperior corner or beaking (CFS2) of the anterior vertebral body. The latter stages (CFS3, CFS4, and CFS5) are characterized by a coronally oriented fracture that extends obliquely from the anterior cortex of the vertebral body to the inferior end plate. This fracture line separates a triangular anterior "teardrop" fragment from the posterior vertebral body. In CFS4 and CFS5, retrolisthesis of the posterior vertebral body into the spinal canal is present. This extent of posterior vertebral body retrolisthesis and posterior element injury distinguishes these two stages, with CFS5 injuries representing >3 mm of retrolisthesis and complete

FIGURE 29-21 *Compressive flexion mechanism of injury. The increasing stages of compressive flexion injuries represent increasing forces being applied to the spine, with eventual tensile failure of the posterior ligamentous structures. In the lower stages of injury* **(A)**, *the flexion and compression cause only a blunting of the anterior lip of the vertebral body. Because the posterior ligamentous complex is intact, these are considered to be relatively stable. With higher energy injuries, the flexion and compression cause a shear, compressive fracturing of the vertebral body, and tensile failure of the posterior ligamentous complex* **(B)**. *(From Mirza, S.K.; Anderson, P.A. Skeletal Trauma, 3rd ed., New York, W.B. Saunders, 2003.* **A** *redrawn from Holdsworth F.; J Bone Joint Surg 45: 6–20, 1963.* **B** *redrawn from White, A.A.; Panjabi, M.M. Practical Biomechanics of Spine Trauma. In: White, A.A.; Panjabi, M.M., eds. Clinical Biomechanics of the Spine, 2nd ed. Philadelphia, J.B. Lippincott.)*

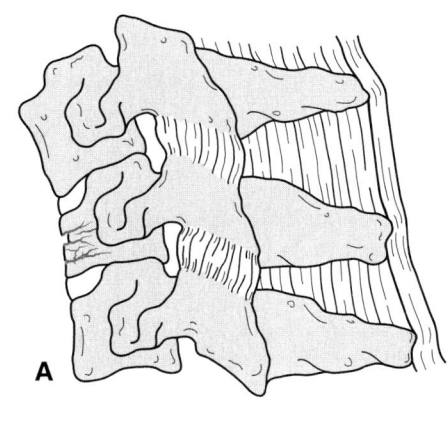

A

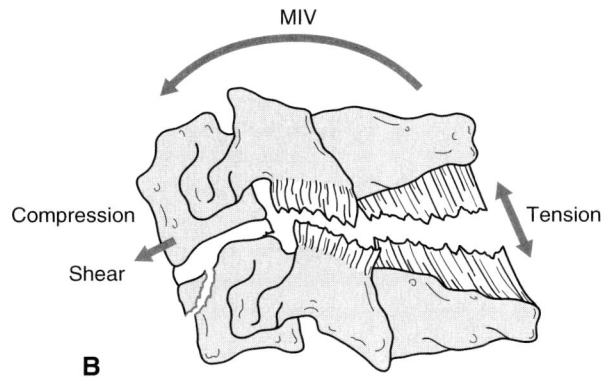

MIV

Compression

Shear

Tension

B

failure of the posterior ligamentous complex. Associated osseous injuries observed with these higher stages of injury include sagittal fractures through the vertebral body and fractures of the lamina or spinous processes. Favero and van Peteghem in 1989 described a variant of the CFS5 injury that they called the "quadrangular fragment fracture."[33] They hypothesized that this injury pattern was caused by a greater degree of axial loading than in other CFS5 lesions, which produced a large "quadrangular" shaped anterior vertebral body fragment instead of the triangular "teardrop" fragment (Fig. 29-22). The purpose of distinguishing this quadrangular fragment fracture was to highlight the poor clinical and radiographic results that the authors achieved with nonoperative management and to make recommendations regarding its surgical management.

More important than memorization of specific stages is understanding how the compressive flexion forces create this spectrum of injuries. These injuries begin with anterior vertebral body failure secondary to the anterior compressive forces, either by blunting-beaking of the anterior body or fracturing off the teardrop fragment. With increased energy, the spine continues to flex forward, and the injury is propagated posteriorly through the intervertebral disk, and then through the posterior longitudinal ligament, the facets and their capsules, and finally the interspinous and supraspinous ligaments. This divides the cervical spine into a "caudal" segment consisting of the anterior teardrop fragment and the subjacent vertebral body, and a "cranial" segment consisting of the posterior vertebral body and posterior elements with the suprajacent vertebral body (Fig. 29-23).

The extent to which the posterior vertebral body fragment is translated into the spinal canal as the spine continues to flex forward determines whether the spinal cord is injured and the severity of the resultant neurologic deficit. In Allen and colleagues' description of these compressive flexion injuries, the higher stages of injury had an increased incidence of spinal cord injury, as a result of the retrolisthesis of the posterior vertebral body. In general this type of injury has the highest rate of neurologic injury of all cervical injuries including burst fractures. The site of maximal cord injury is adjacent to the posterior inferior corner of the vertebral body.

It is quite likely that immediately after the posterior vertebral body displaces back into the spinal canal in a severe compressive flexion injury, it is reduced forward to some degree (possibly even completely). This produces a radiograph that underestimates the extent of retrolisthesis and possibly also the degree of posterior ligamentous disruption. To illustrate this point, it is noted that a quarter of the patients with stage 3 lesions (anterior teardrop fracture with no retrolisthesis) had spinal cord injuries in the Allen and Ferguson series. Clearly, the static radiographs in these patients did not fully represent the severity of their osteoligamentous injury and displacement. This serves as a reminder that one must be extremely cautious in interpreting the static supine radiographs and should utilize advanced imaging studies such as CT and MRI to develop a more complete understanding of the extent of the injury.

DEFINITIVE TREATMENT

As mentioned in the preceding section, the decision-making process should take into account the mechanical stability of the injury, the presence or absence of a neurologic deficit, and other patient factors that might be relevant to the particular individual.

FIGURE 29-22 *Severe compression-flexion injury (quadrangular pattern). This patient presented with a severe C5 compression-flexion injury and complete quadriplegia. Notice on the sagittal (A) and axial (B) cuts the large anterior fragment of the C5 vertebral body (arrow), consistent with a quadrangular fracture (rather than a teardrop fracture). There is a sagittal split in the C5 vertebral body, bilaminar fractures, and facet disruption (arrowheads), as seen on sagittal computed tomography (C) and confirmed on the T2-weighted magnetic resonance imaging (D). Due to the severe instability, a circumferential stabilization was performed (E). The autogenous bone from the C5 vertebrectomy was used to fill a titanium reconstruction cage, followed by anterior plating and posterior lateral mass fixation from C4 to C6.*

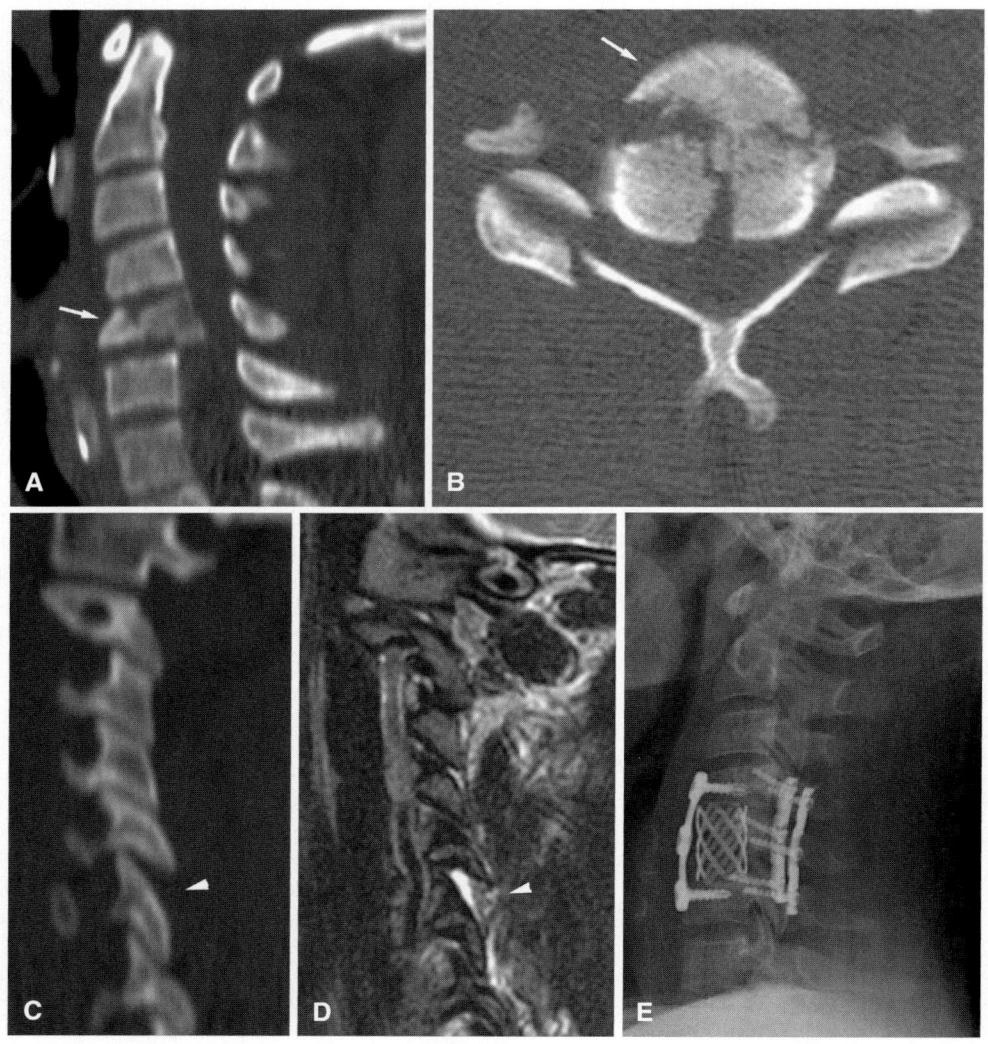

COMPRESSIVE FLEXION INJURIES WITH NEUROLOGIC DEFICIT If a neurologic deficit exists, one needs to decide if the spinal cord remains compressed due to retropulsed bone or malalignment, and thus is in need of direct or indirect decompression. If compression exists, an initial reduction with Gardner-Wells traction should be attempted. Definitive surgical treatment in the presence of residual compression from retropulsed bone should include a direct decompression by anterior corpectomy, followed by strut graft reconstruction and anterior cervical plate stabilization.

Biomechanical studies using nonlocking anterior cervical plates reported poor stabilization of the cervical spine with this approach.[21,104] Do Koh and co-workers compared fixation techniques in a cervical corpectomy model and demonstrated that posterior fixation with lateral mass plates and screws was significantly better than contemporary anterior plate fixation in reducing motion in extension, lateral bending, and axial rotation.[25] Anterior reconstruction and plate fixation was slightly better at reducing motion in flexion testing, as one might expect from a restoration and stabilization of the anterior weight-bearing column. However, Adams and associates reported more recently in an in vitro model of severely unstable compressive flexion injuries that contemporary locking plates provide significant stability for such fracture patterns.[4] These data correlated with clinical experience in the management of such injuries.[13,50]

FIGURE 29-23 | *Resolution of forces in a compression-flexion injury. Computed tomography **(A)** and magnetic resonance imaging **(B)** demonstrate how the spine is ultimately divided in compression-flexion injuries. As the compressive and flexion forces are applied, the anterior column fractures, often producing the triangular teardrop fragment (arrowhead). The forces then propagate posteriorly through the disk and posterior ligamentous structures. This divides the spine into a caudal segment consisting of the teardrop fragment (arrowhead) attached to C5 and the segments below, and the cranial segment consisting of the C4 posterior vertebral body (arrow) attached to C3 and the segments above. Similar to the injury in Fig. 29-21, significant retropulsion of the posterior vertebral body fragment is apparent, with spinal cord injury.*

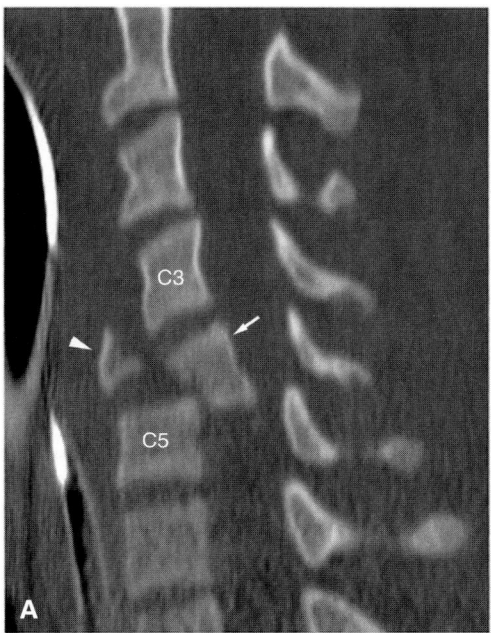
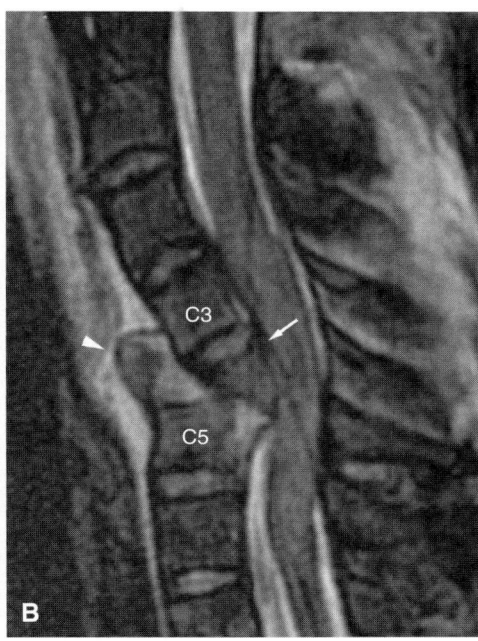

Alternatively, in patients without residual ventral cord compression following traction, the need for a direct anterior decompression is obviated. Realignment of the cervical spine can be achieved with extension, and stabilization can be achieved with posterior stabilization with lateral mass fixation.

COMPRESSIVE FLEXION INJURIES WITHOUT NEUROLOGIC DEFICIT

In the absence of a neurologic deficit, the treatment decision is based primarily on mechanical instability. The stability of the injury is heavily influenced by the integrity of each lateral mass and the strength of the posterior column, because the ability of the cervical spine to resist further kyphosis is highly dependent on these posterior and lateral structures. The Cervical Spine Injury Severity Score is useful for defining the extent of this injury and for guiding treatment. As a reminder, it is established by scoring the displacement-disruption of each column (anterior, posterior, and lateral columns) on a scale of 0 to 5, and then totaling them. In general, when the score exceeds 7, the extent of mechanical instability warrants surgical stabilization.

The less severe stages of compressive flexion injuries (CFS1 and CFS2) are relatively stable and can be treated nonoperatively with an external orthosis (Fig. 29-24) unless additional patient circumstances make effectively immobilizing the neck impossible. The higher stage injuries (CFS4 and CFS5) are unstable mechanically and associated with a significant chance of neurologic injury (see Figs. 29-21 and 29-22). An associated spinal cord injury mandates operative intervention, but even without such a neurologic deficit, the degree of mechanical instability in such injuries (CFS4, CFS5) warrants surgical stabilization. The management of such injuries with halo immobilization alone has been associated with late instability, deformity, and neurologic deterioration.[14,35,50,90] The choices include anterior vertebrectomy and fusion, posterior stabilization and fusion, or a combined circumferential fusion. Each has its advantages, and unfortunately, there is little objective clinical literature to delineate which is best.

The midlevel CFS3 injury compromises the anterior weight-bearing column of the cervical spine, but there is no vertebral body retrolisthesis. The integrity of the posterior ligamentous structures is the key factor to consider in these injuries. If the posterior ligaments are truly intact, then external immobilization may lead to a good clinical and radiographic outcome. Besides avoiding the risks of surgical intervention, achieving healing with an external orthosis may maintain some mobility at the two motion segments that would be otherwise fused. Because of the importance of posterior ligamentous integrity on the success of nonoperative treatment, radiographs and CT scans should be scrutinized for evidence of interspinous or facet widening, and an MRI scan should be obtained to assess

Flexion-compression injury without severe posterior element disruption. This 54-year-old male was struck by a falling log and presented with neck pain but no neurologic deficit. His radiograph (A) and sagittal computed tomographic (CT) reconstruction (B) demonstrate a compression fracture of the anterior aspect of C7 (arrow). Note that the overall sagittal alignment is well maintained. The left parasagittal CT reconstruction (C) demonstrates that the C6-C7 facet is well aligned. The axial cuts, however, (D and E) demonstrate an undisplaced fracture through the left superior facet of C7 (arrowhead), which is oriented in the sagittal plane (and hence not visualized on the sagittal reconstruction). Due to the relatively minor anterior column fracture, the lack of displacement of the facet fracture, and the lack of any kyphotic deformity suggestive of more severe ligamentous disruption, this injury was considered stable and treated with an external orthosis (Philadelphia collar). His lateral radiograph at 3 months after injury (F) shows that C6 has subluxed forward approximately 1 mm, but the injury has healed in acceptable alignment with a good clinical result.

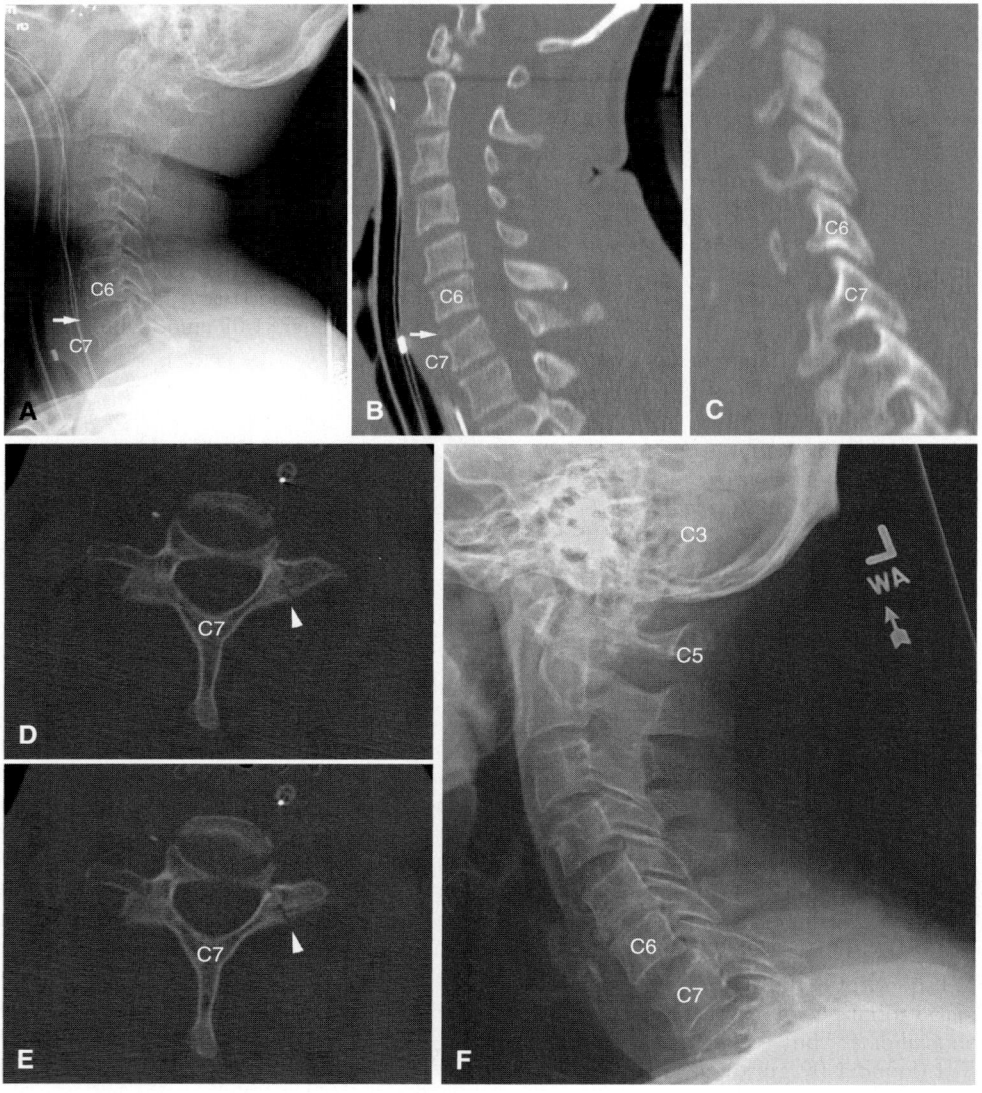

the status of the interspinous ligament, facet capsules, and ligamentum flavum.

For CFS3 injuries with disruption of the posterior ligamentous complex, surgery is likely warranted. With disruption of the posterior ligamentous structures, a stage 3 injury differs from a stage 4 or 5 injury only by the lack of retrolisthesis, which may in fact be grossly underestimated on the static radiograph. Hence, a strong rationale exists for surgically stabilizing such injuries.

Several studies have compared the results of anterior vertebrectomy and plate fusion against nonoperative management of compressive flexion injuries (flexion teardrop injuries). Fisher and co-workers compared 22 patients treated with halo immobilization with 17 treated with anterior fusion.[35] The radiographic and clinical outcomes were inferior in the patients treated with halo immobilization. The average residual kyphosis was 11.4° in the halo immobilization group, and 4 of 22 eventually required surgery, 2 for kyphotic collapse and neurologic deterioration. For the anterior vertebrectomy and fusion group, the average residual kyphosis was 3.5°, and all successfully healed with no major early or late local complications. Because a quarter of the nonoperative and almost two thirds of the operative patients were motor-complete quadriplegics, we can infer that many of the patients in this study had high-stage compressive flexion injuries. Thus, the primary message from this study is that for the mechanical instability inherent to high-stage compressive flexion injuries, surgical fixation is warranted.

Koivikko and associates also performed a comparison between surgical and nonsurgical management, although the patients included in this study had both "cervical burst fractures" and "flexion teardrop fractures."[50] Again, the surgically treated patients had an improved radiographic outcome. The authors described a mean kyphosis of 12.6° in the 34 patients treated conservatively, and a mean lordosis of 2.2° in the 35 treated with anterior vertebrectomy, iliac crest reconstruction, and Caspar plate fixation. Similar to the study by Fisher and co-workers,[35] many had cervical spinal cord injuries, suggesting a high level of mechanical instability.

Vertical Compression Injuries (Burst Fractures)

Vertical compression injuries are postulated to occur by compressive forces being applied directly vertically instead of obliquely, as they are with the compressive flexion injuries. This fracture pattern is commonly referred to as "cervical burst fracture," in which vertical compression causes a "bursting" of the vertebral body with potential retropulsion into the spinal cord, but without tensile failure of the posterior elements. Pure vertical compression forces, technically speaking, cause compressive failure of the anterior column and leave the posterior ligaments intact. This injury leads to a symmetrical loss of vertebral body height and little kyphosis or translational malalignment.

Three stages of these injuries were proposed, based on the severity of vertebral body fracturing. Stage 1 (VCS1) is characterized by a "cupping" failure of the center of either the superior or inferior end plate, stage 2 (VCS2) has involvement of both end plates with or without an undisplaced fracture through the vertebral body, and stage 3 (VCS3) involves comminution of the vertebral body with displacement in "multiple directions," including posteriorly into the spinal canal. All of the patients who sustained VCS1 or VCS2 injuries in the Allen and Ferguson series were neurologically intact, whereas of five patients who sustained a stage 3 injury had complete spinal cord injuries. Allen and colleagues postulated that in the highest stage injury (VCS3), after the characteristic vertical compressive failure of the vertebral body, the spinal unit might be subjected to either late flexion or extension forces that could injure the posterior elements.[6] Late extension could cause severe comminution of the posterior vertebral arch, which they observed in two of the five patients. Alternatively, late flexion could cause posterior ligamentous disruption, which would make the injury similar in nature to severe compressive flexion injuries, with disruption of both the anterior weight-bearing column and the posterior tensile restraints. The combination of the bony retropulsion into the canal and disruption of the posterior elements resulted in a high incidence (80%) of complete spinal cord injury in the patients with VCS3 injuries.

It is important to recognize, however, that these vertical compression injuries represented only a small proportion of the total in the original Allen and Ferguson series. This is likely explained by the fact that it is difficult to apply pure axial compression without additional bending forces on the cervical spine. Even with compressive force applied directly onto the top of the head, as in Nightingale and co-workers' previously mentioned biomechanical study, the cervical spine buckles, causing extension of some regions and flexion in others.[66] Panjabi and colleagues also reported in cadaveric studies of cervical spine trauma that it is difficult to apply pure vertical compression to a single spinal unit.[73,103]

TREATMENT RECOMMENDATIONS

Vertical compressive injuries are assessed and treated similarly to flexion compressive injuries. Retropulsion of the anterior column into the spinal canal is best addressed directly with an anterior vertebrectomy and fusion (Fig. 29-25). Associated injury to the posterior ligamentous structures from flexion forces confers a high degree of mechanical instability. Comminuted fracturing of the posterior vertebral arch from extension also influences the mechanical stability.

Also similar to compressive flexion injuries is the fact that the static radiographs often underestimate the extent of bony retropulsion and collapse that occurs at the time of the vertical compression injury. This important concept was elegantly demonstrated by Chang and colleagues in an in vitro study of vertical compression injuries.[18] These authors observed that following an axial loading injury, the amount of residual spinal canal compression present after the injury was significantly less than the sudden and rapid bony retropulsion that occurred at the time of injury. In most cases the maximal area of cord compression is near the posterior superior corner of the body. Also, the amount of axial vertebral height loss seen after the injury was significantly less than that which occurred at the time of injury. Hence, one must be cautious in interpreting the extent of vertebral body height loss and canal occlusion secondary to bony retropulsion if using these parameters in treatment decisions.

Distractive Flexion Injuries

Distractive flexion was the most common mechanism of injury in Allen and colleagues' series,[6] characterized primarily by the tensile or shear failure of the posterior elements, resulting in facet fracture or dislocation and anterior displacement of the vertebral body. The original Allen and Ferguson description of these distractive flexion injuries acknowledged that a compressive "minor injury vector" was also frequently present, manifested as a compressive fracturing of the subjacent end plate. The common feature of distractive flexion injuries is that they all involve injury to the facet joints. The flexion mechanism may result from a blow or fall onto the occiput, or from a deceleration mechanism associated with motor vehicle collisions. The center of rotation of this flexion moment is thought to occur anterior to the vertebral body, resulting in progressive tensile failure of the posterior elements.

FIGURE 29-25   *Vertical compression injury with no posterior element injury. This 32-year-old cyclist suffered an isolated C7 vertical compression injury when hit by a car. On plain film **(A)** and sagittal computed tomographic (CT) reconstruction **(B)**, the C7 injury has the classic "burst fracture" appearance, with superior end plate rupture and retropulsion of the posterior vertebral body into the spinal canal. The overall sagittal alignment of the cervical spine is well maintained. No interspinous widening occurred, and the facet joints **(C)** appear intact. The axial CT **(D)** demonstrates the retropulsed posterior body of C7 (arrows), which narrow the canal. Fortunately, there was no neurologic injury. The patient underwent a C7 vertebrectomy, with titanium cage reconstruction and anterior cervical plating, and went on to heal uneventfully **(E)**.*

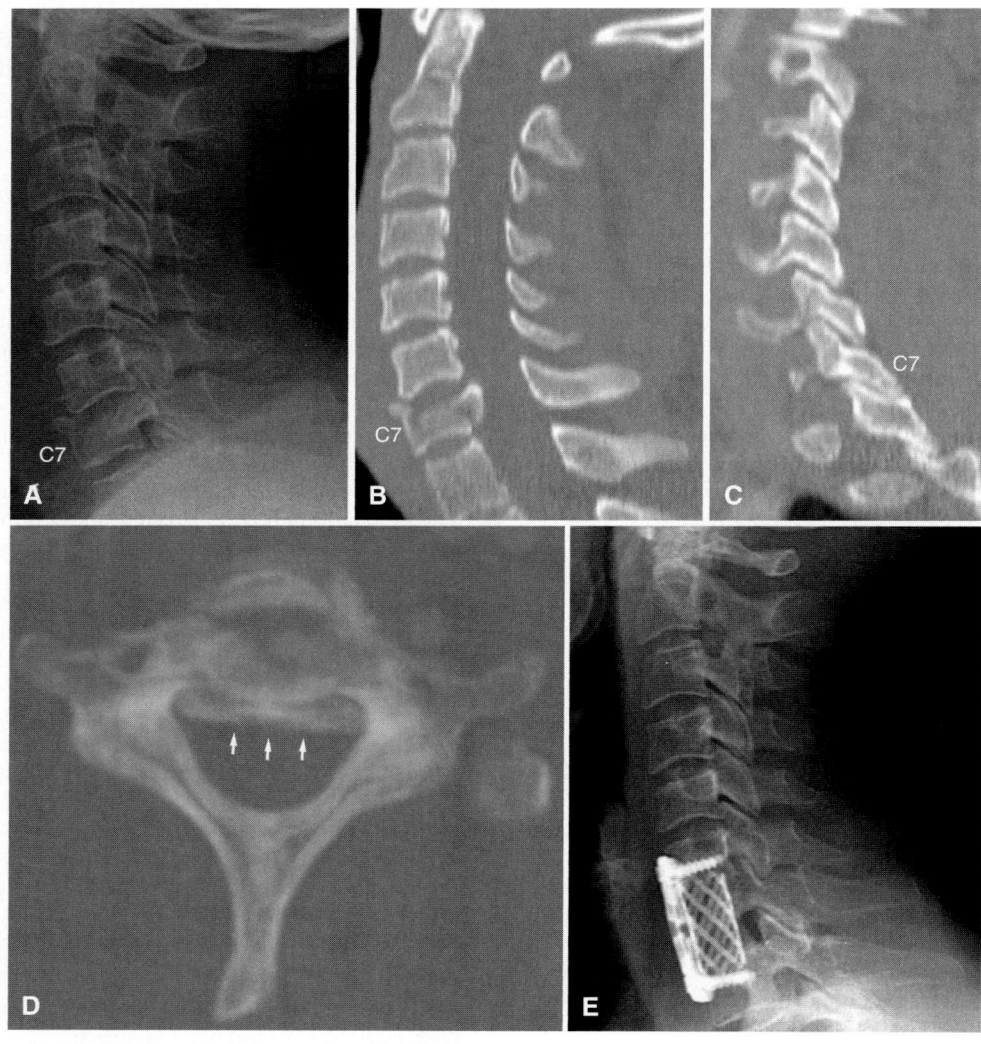

Four stages, representing an increasing extent of posterior and anterior soft tissue disruption, were described within the distractive flexion phylogeny. Similar to the other phylogenies, the Allen and Ferguson staging refers to the static position of the injury on radiographic evaluation, which may underrepresent the extent of displacement that occurred at the time of the accident. For example, both facets may dislocate at the time of injury but then reduce completely, leaving behind only subtle radiographic features of a highly unstable injury (see Figs. 28-5 and 28-6, Chapter 25—Initial Evaluation and Emergency Treatment of the Spine-Injured Patient).

Stage 1 (DFS1) injuries, also known as facet sprains, occur when facet capsule disruption results in slight widening of the facet joints and interspinous distance, causing mild focal kyphosis (less than 10°). Plain radiographs may show subtle facet joint widening, which can be more apparent on oblique views, as well as interspinous widening on anteroposterior and lateral radiographs. CT demonstrates facet widening, which may be more obvious on sagittal reformations. Facet widening or ligamentum flavum disruption with increased T2 signal intensity is the typical finding on MRI (Fig. 29-26).

Stage 2 (DFS2) injuries are unilateral facet dislocations and fracture-dislocations, with the etiologic difference between the two being the amount of flexion. Their defining characteristic is a rotational deformity in the axial plane, and to a lesser extent in the coronal plane, the latter being more difficult to identify radiographically. The mechanism of injury is believed to involve a flexion injury

FIGURE 29-26 *Distractive flexion injury to the cervical spine with minor ligamentous disruption. This 46-year-old male was under the influence of alcohol when he crashed his all-terrain vehicle. He had a brief episode of bilateral upper and lower extremity weakness at the time of injury. On presentation he had regained full strength and his only complaint was mild paresthesias in both arms. His radiograph **(A)** demonstrates straightening of his cervical lordosis and significant anterior soft tissue swelling (outlined by arrows). The T2-weighted magnetic resonance image (MRI) **(B)** and fat-suppression MRI **(C)** demonstrate the significant anterior edema (arrows), diffuse posterior bright signal, and a discrete disruption of his ligamentum flavum (arrowhead). There were no fractures, the facets were intact, and the disks all appeared normal. It was therefore felt that this was a relatively stable injury and could be managed in a cervical orthosis. He went on to heal uneventfully with full neurologic recovery.*

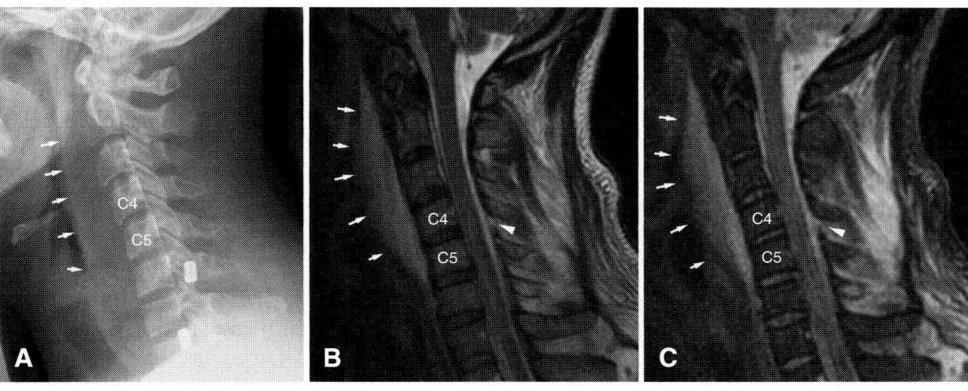

with resulting distraction of the posterior elements, coupled with a rotational force. This rotational force is not considered to be a key mechanistic component of the subsequent distractive flexion stages, and so in this regard the Allen and Ferguson staging of this phylogeny does not represent a continuum of the same injury vector. The magnitude of the rotational force required to produce this injury in vivo is unclear, since a cadaveric biomechanical study has shown that a purely distractive force applied unilaterally results in coupled rotation sufficient to produce a unilateral facet dislocation.[100] Although less severe than their bilateral equivalent, unilateral facet dislocations are usually high-energy injuries that result in complete disruption of the involved facet capsule, as well as disruption or severe attenuation of the interspinous ligament, annulus fibrosus, and uncovertebral joints.[111] The annular disruption and thus the potential for extrusion of nucleus pulposus into the spinal canal may have important implications in the management of unilateral facet injuries, as discussed later in greater detail.

Several radiographic features are characteristic of unilateral facet dislocations in which significant asymmetrical rotational displacement has occurred. Assuming that the caudal part of the cervical spine is viewed perfectly laterally on the lateral radiograph, the rotational deformity is manifested as displacement of the right and left facet joints relative to each other at and above the level of injury (the "bow-tie" sign) (Fig. 29-27), non-superimposition of the cortical lines representing the posterolateral edges of the vertebral body above the injured level, and by lack of end plate parallelism above the level of injury (although this is more commonly due to parallax). Anterolisthesis of the dislocated vertebral body usually does not exceed 25 percent of the anteroposterior diameter of the vertebral body. The rotated vertebral bodies may also appear longer in their anteroposterior diameter than the normally aligned

vertebral bodies below. On the anteroposterior radiograph, the spinous processes are malaligned and the lamina is tilted (see Fig. 29-27). These are all important hallmarks of the rotational deformity; visualizing the actual facet dislocation on the lateral radiograph may be difficult because of superimposition of the uninjured facet. Axial CT demonstrates the rotational deformity and the typical appearance of the facet joints due to the reversal of the relative position of the superior and inferior facets with respect to one another (see Fig. 29-2). The juxtaposition of the two articular processes is not seen in unilateral facet fractures. The facet alignment is best appreciated on the sagittal CT reformats.

Stage 3 and 4 (DFS3 and 4) injuries were described by Allen and Ferguson as bilateral facet dislocations and fracture-dislocations. With the increased forward flexion force permitting complete dislocation of the facet joint (Fig. 29-28), there is 50 percent anterior translation of the dislocated body (DFS3) or more (DFS4). When fully dislocated or perched, bilateral facet injuries are obviously recognizable on radiographic imaging, although it is still important to visualize the entire cervical spine (Fig. 29-29). One should be wary, however, of bilateral facet subluxations with only mild displacement, as these may have been completely displaced at the time of injury and then came to rest in a near-reduced position.

The distractive flexion mechanism, combined with some degree of compression or axial rotation, can produce a wide spectrum of injuries (Fig. 29-30).[98] In pure distraction, the facet joints are likely to be subluxed or dislocated with disruption of the soft tissues alone; however, shear forces applied by added rotation, compression, or forward translation can cause the facets to fracture. This is particularly seen in unilateral facet injuries, where it is common for the superior facet to be fractured off and displaced forward into the foramen by the inferior facet of the

FIGURE 29-27 | *Rotational deformity of a facet dislocation. This 23-year-old male was under the influence of alcohol when he was involved in a rollover motor vehicle accident. He complained of neck pain and left arm numbness and was taken to a local hospital where the lateral and anteroposterior (AP) plain films (**A** and **B**) were taken. Note the inability to visualize the C7 and T1 levels on his lateral radiograph (**A**). On this lateral film, one can appreciate the "bow-tie" appearance of his facets (outlined with an arrow at C4). The AP radiograph (which is often neglected) provided the most obvious sign of a rotational injury, with the sudden change in the spinous process alignment (arrow and arrowheads). These clues were missed, and the patient was discharged home from the emergency department. Six days later, he returned, and computed tomography (**C** and **D**) demonstrated the severe facet injury at C6-C7. The axial view (**C**) demonstrates the rotational deformity of C6 on C7, and the fractured superior facet of C7 (double arrow). This fragment gets dragged forward into the foramen (**D**) where it contributes to the nerve root compression and radiculopathy.*

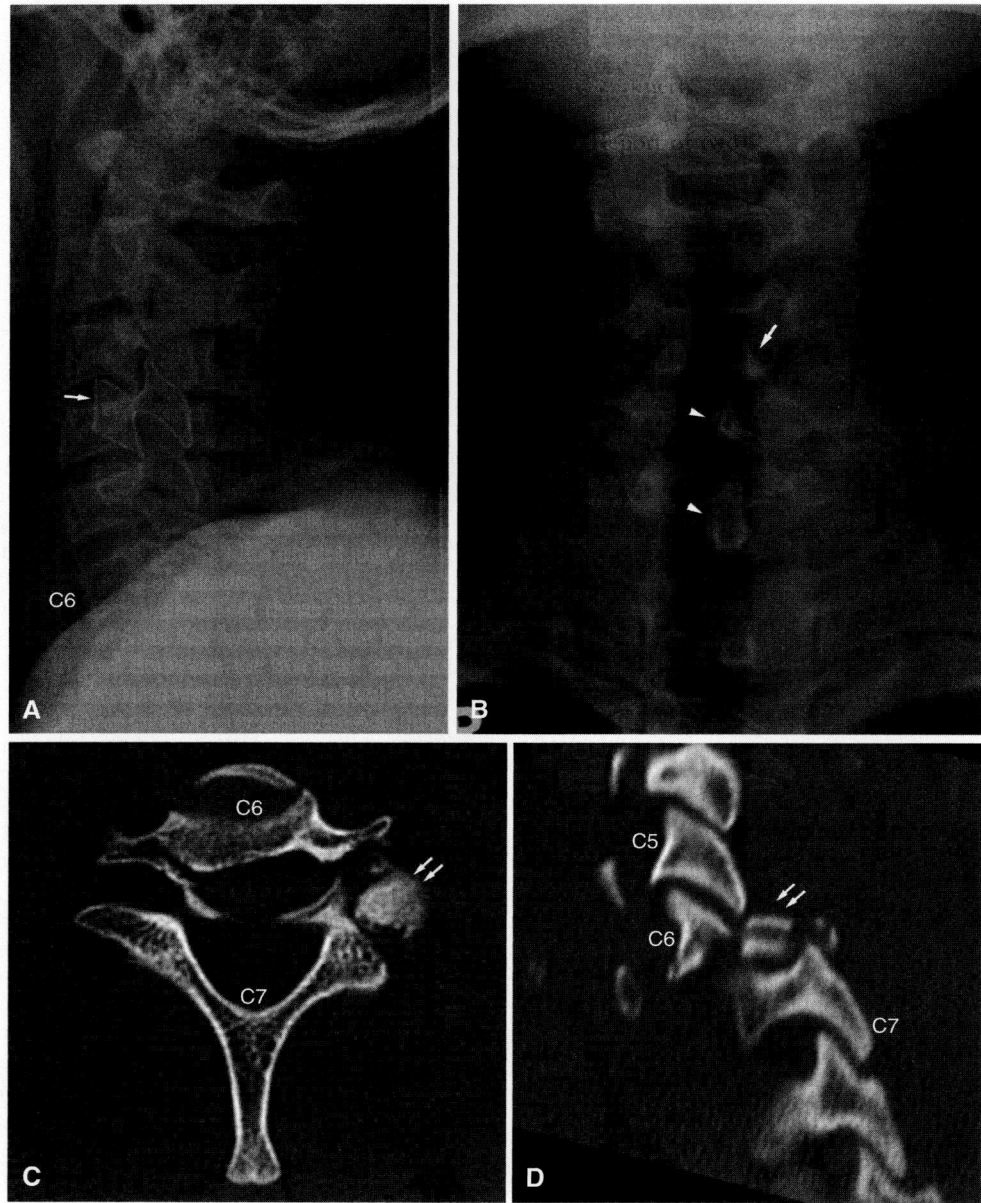

suprajacent vertebrae. For example, a C5-C6 facet fracture-dislocation in which the superior facet of C6 is fractured and displaced anteriorly will embarrass the C6 nerve root, leading to a radicular pattern of pain. The lamina and spinous process may also be fractured in these injuries (the former often being an extension of the facet fracture).

MRI has been helpful in defining the soft tissues that are disrupted in flexion-distraction injuries. Vaccaro and colleagues performed MRIs on 48 patients with unilateral

FIGURE 29-28 *Bilateral facet dislocation mechanism. With sufficient forward flexion with distraction **(A)**, both facets can be dislocated **(B)**. Illustrated is a purely ligamentous bilateral facet injury that occurs with the combination of flexion and distraction. With less distraction and more forward translation, the facets can be fractured. In the dislocated position, one may need to bur down some of the superior facet (hashed) to facilitate reduction. **C,** Lateral radiograph showing bilateral facet dislocation. (Modified From Mirza, S.K.; Anderson, P.A. Skeletal Trauma, 3rd ed., New York, W.B. Saunders, 2003.)*

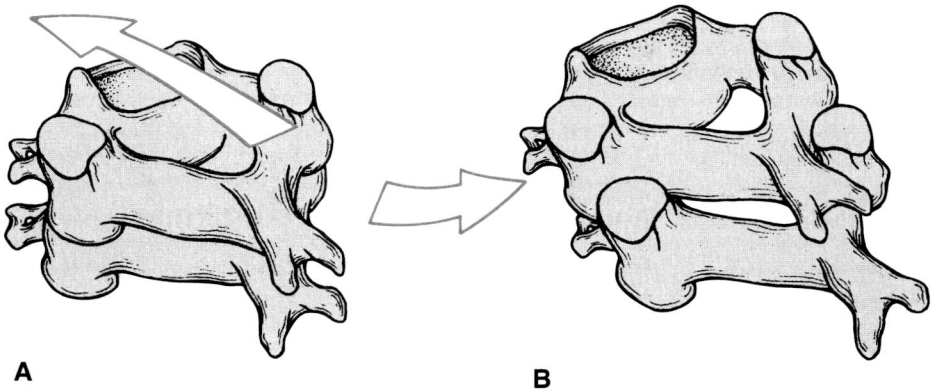

A   B

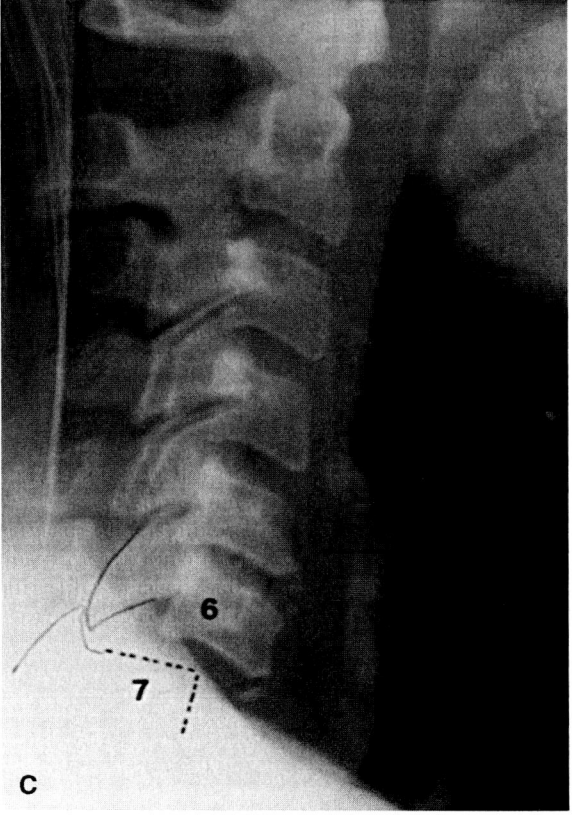

C

or bilateral facet dislocations.[111] As expected, the patients with both unilateral and bilateral facet dislocations had a high rate of disruption through the posterior ligamentous complex (posterior muscles, interspinous and supraspinous ligaments, ligamentum flavum, and facet capsules). Injuries to the disk were also very common, with disk herniations observed in 56 percent of unilateral and 82.5 percent of bilateral facet dislocations. A more recent study of bilateral facet injuries from the same institution reported that MRI evidence of anterior and posterior longitudinal ligament disruption was found in only 27 percent and 40 percent of cases, respectively, suggesting that the PLL (a posterior stabilizing element) is not necessarily torn in these highly unstable distractive flexion injuries.[17] Disk herniation or disruption, however, was observed in 90 percent of these bilateral facet injuries.

FIGURE 29-29 *Bilateral facet dislocation. This 54-year-old male was involved in a high-speed motor vehicle accident and presented with complete quadriplegia. He sustained a bilateral C7-T1 facet dislocation. With the injury being so low, even the lateral swimmer's view radiograph **(A)** needs close scrutiny to see the injury, serving as a reminder that the entire cervical spine and cervicothoracic junction must be visualized. The anterior borders of the C7 and T1 vertebral body are outlined. The midsagittal reconstruction **(B)** demonstrates the characteristic 50 percent anterior displacement of the vertebral body. In this case, there is a compression fracture of T1 and bilateral laminar fractures, which in the very lucky few prevent serious spinal cord injury Parasagittal computed tomography **(C)** shows the facet dislocation. Magnetic resonance imaging **(D)** demonstrates the disruption of all soft tissue restraints, from the anterior longitudinal ligament through the disk, posterior longitudinal ligament, and posterior bony arch. Note the collection of blood (high signal) behind the body of C7. No disk fragment is seen behind C7 or T1.*

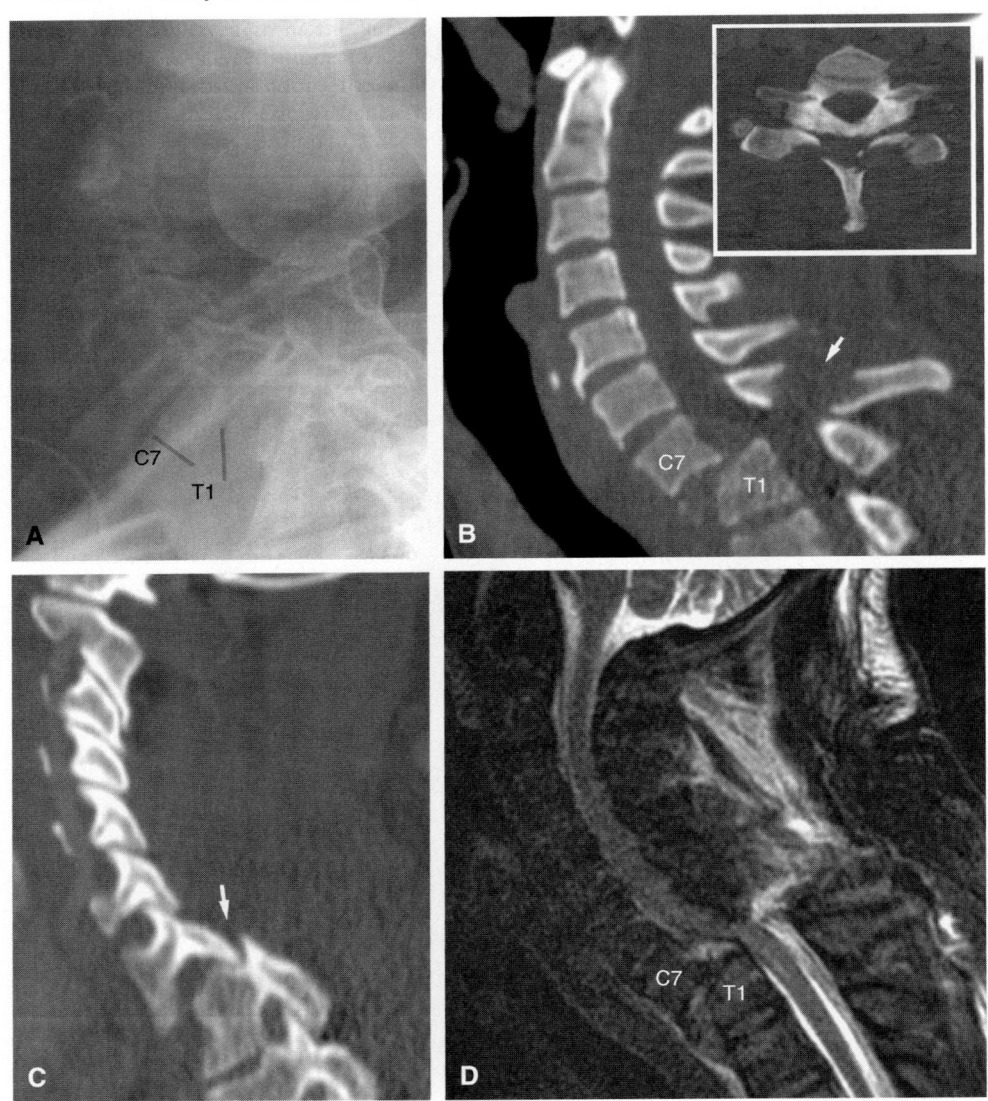

TREATMENT RECOMMENDATIONS

The issue of disk herniations is particularly relevant in the treatment of unilateral and bilateral facet dislocations because of the potential risk of displacing a herniated fragment of disk back into the spinal cord when realigning such injuries (Fig. 29-31). Widespread recognition of this catastrophic complication is best attributed to a case report by Eismont and colleagues in 1991.[30] In this report, the authors described a 33-year-old woman who sustained a C6-C7 bilateral facet dislocation after a fall. Her clinical presentation was that of neck pain, left arm paresthesias, bilateral triceps weakness (grade 4 of 5), and a "positive Lhermitte's sign involving both upper and lower extremities." A closed reduction was attempted unsuccessfully, and she was then taken to the operating room for a posterior open reduction, wiring, and arthrodesis under anesthesia. *She awoke quadriplegic.* An urgent CT-myelogram revealed anterior thecal compression, and a subsequent anterior diskectomy removed a large extruded disk fragment from behind the body of C6. It was felt that this disk fragment had been pushed into the spinal cord on

ac

FIGURE 29-30 *Different facet injuries that result from various combinations of flexion, compression, rotation. Many different configurations of facet injuries can occur, depending on the extent and timing of the various forces that the spine may be subjected to during the injury. The top row (A–E) demonstrates a spectrum of purely ligamentous injuries, starting from the normally aligned facet (A). The facet capsule may be disrupted with subtle widening (B), and greater soft tissue disruption leads to facet subluxation (C), perching (D), and frank dislocation (E). The bottom row (F–J) demonstrates a number of different fracture patterns. Most commonly, the superior facet is fractured and pushed forward into the foramen (F). Superior facet fracturing can be associated with facet subluxation or dislocation as well (G). Less commonly, the inferior facet is fractured— a pattern that may be associated with extension injuries (H). This fracture significantly compromises the ability to achieve stable screw fixation in this lateral mass. Both the inferior and superior facets may be fractured (I). Finally, significant comminution of the facet (J) may preclude stable screw fixation.*

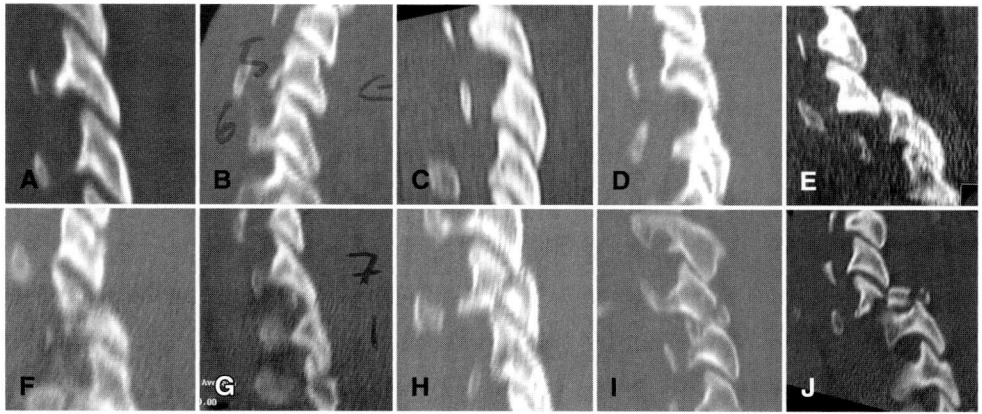

realignment of her dislocation. Despite a rapid ventral decompression, she remained completely paralyzed. One of the most critical factors is the differentiation between disk disruption (which must occur in the majority of facet injuries) and disk herniation in which a fragment occurs posterior to the annulus.

DISK HERNIATIONS AND THE REDUCTION OF FACET DISLOCATIONS The potential to cause a neurologic injury in a patient with a facet dislocation during a closed or open reduction has prompted much debate on the role of disk herniations with these injuries.[3,26,37,40,42,60,67,89,112] The initial reports (including

FIGURE 29-31 *Disk herniation causing cord compression after facet reduction. One of the great fears in reducing a bilateral facet dislocation (A) (or unilateral facet dislocation for that matter) is the potential for a herniated fragment of disk to be pushed back into the spinal cord. In this illustration, the disk fragment has flipped behind the dislocated vertebral body and is pushed into the spinal cord on realignment (B). Descriptions of this causing catastrophic paralysis have come from patients who are not examinable during the closed reduction.*

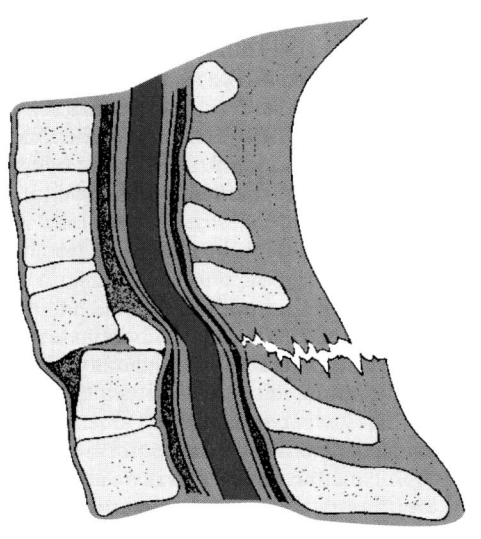
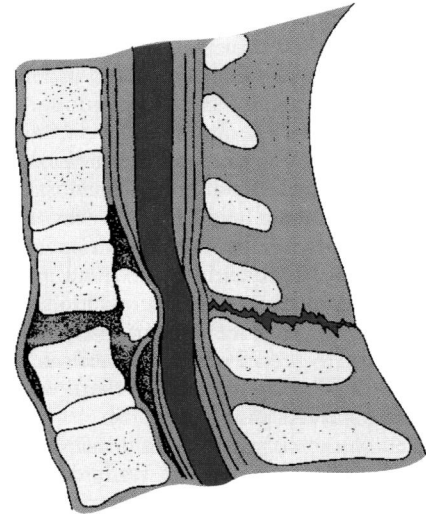

A   **B**

that of Eismont and colleagues[30]) of catastrophic worsening of neurologic function after the reduction of cervical facet injuries occurred in patients who were *not* examinable during the reduction process. Such patients are clearly different from the awake, alert, and examinable patient, and hence a single approach to the closed reduction of facet dislocations cannot be applicable to both. Nevertheless, this topic continues to engender much debate, with a number of pertinent questions arising from its discussion. How often does an associated disk herniation occur? Whom is it safe to perform a closed reduction on? Is there a safe technique for performing a closed reduction?

The prevalence of a concomitant disk disruption or herniation with either a unilateral or bilateral facet injury has been variably reported in the literature, most likely because of differing imaging technology used to identify the injury (e.g., MRI, CT, myelography) and varying criteria for what constitutes a "herniation." Vaccaro and co-workers, for example, defined a disk herniation on MRI studies to be present when material with signal intensity consistent with nucleus pulposus protruded posteriorly to the posterior cortex of the subjacent vertebral body.[109] In a series of 11 patients, disk herniations were found in 2 (18%): 1 unilateral and 1 bilateral facet injury. Others have defined disk herniations as the presence of any thecal sac or nerve root deformation on MRI and have reported rates of 19 percent[37] and 50 percent.[3] Rizzolo and associates reported, in a consecutive series of 55 patients, a rate of herniated nucleus pulposus in 46 percent of patients with unilateral facet injuries and 62 percent in those with bilateral facet injuries.[88] A neurologic deficit on presentation correlates strongly with the presence of a disk herniation,[37,88] and for this reason, the possibility of a disk herniation should be considered (as evidenced by the experience of Eismont and colleagues[30]) (Fig. 29-32). Narrowing of the disk space may also be suggestive of prolapsed disk material,[3,30,89] although the reliability of this radiographic feature is inconsistent.[109]

Although disk disruption can be significant, how its management should be influenced by this risk is less definitive. Vaccaro and co-workers performed prereduction MRIs on 11 patients with unilateral and bilateral facet injuries, documenting 2 patients with disk herniations.[109] They then went ahead and performed closed reductions of these awake and alert patients using a standard protocol for applying traction and monitoring the neurologic status. Following successful reduction, a postreduction MRI revealed three additional disk herniations, in addition to the worsening (enlargement) of one of the two preexisting disk herniations. None of these patients, however, sustained any neurologic injury. This raises an important problem for the strategy of obtaining MRIs in every patient with a cervical facet dislocation prior to performing a closed reduction—that is, what constitutes a sufficient degree of disk protrusion to preclude a safe closed reduction? The experience of Vaccaro and co-workers would indicate that the mere presence of a disk herniation is not necessarily a neurologic risk.[109] Without being able to rationally establish criteria for what constitutes a "dangerous" disk herniation versus one that would not pose a risk to the spinal cord, it is likely—given the reported incidence of disk herniations with facet dislocations—that

many patients will have their closed reduction delayed unnecessarily in favor of an open procedure.

This experience in 11 patients does not discount the risk of reducing facet dislocations, as has been borne out in the experience of other authors.[26,30,60] However, we suggest that in the awake, alert, and cooperative patient whose neurologic status can be monitored, a carefully performed closed reduction with skull traction can be safely performed. *The obvious corollary to this principle is that a closed reduction should not be attempted in an obtunded patient or in one for whom a reliable neurologic examination cannot be performed.* Wimberely and colleagues subsequently published a case report of an awake and alert individual with a C5-C6 bilateral facet dislocation who did have a neurologic deficit after a closed reduction.[116] This patient had ossification of the posterior longitudinal ligament, and it would appear that a detached segment of this ossified ligament caused the spinal cord compression following reduction. Because the patient was alert and his neurologic function was monitored throughout the reduction, the neurologic deficit was rapidly detected, imaging studies were performed to delineate the pathology, and urgent operative decompression was achieved with a good recovery of neurologic function. Although this experience might urge more clinicians to acquire MRI for all such injuries prior to a closed reduction, the basic principle remains the same: the undertaking of a closed reduction should be done only in an awake, alert, examinable patient, with judicious monitoring of the neurologic function throughout.

Darsaut and associates performed closed reduction on 17 awake patients monitored with MRI.[24] With progressive increasing traction weight, a gradual reduction of malalignment was observed. Reduction of the disk herniation was observed in all four cases in which it was present. No cases had disk displacement into the canal during reduction, including the 11 patients in whom a description was present. No neurologic deterioration occurred. The authors concluded that closed reduction "appears to be safe and is useful in achieving spinal cord decompression."

The technique for achieving such a closed reduction is therefore worth discussing. The first thing to consider (apart from the disk herniation risk) is whether any factors preclude a successful closed reduction. For example, if the patient is large and radiographic visualization of the dislocation in the lower cervical spine is impossible, there is little sense in initiating a closed reduction. Such a patient needs an MRI to rule out a disk herniation and then an open reduction. Patients with distraction injuries in whom the disk space and facets are already vertebrally separated are poor candidates for traction. One should be certain that no other noncontiguous cervical injuries are present, particularly in the upper cervical spine, that may be displaced during traction. Injuries in which the facets are fractured may be impossible to reduce, as the ability to apply traction on the fractured fragment may be impaired.[39,102] In the setting of an ankylosed cervical spine, traction may not be recommended, and the recent report by Wimberley and colleagues[116] of the awake and alert patient with ossification of the PLL who deteriorated during a closed reduction also suggests that one carefully consider whether proceeding in this patient population is justified.

FIGURE 29-32 *The evaluation of disk herniations in facet dislocations. These three patients presented with unilateral facet dislocations and associated spinal cord injuries. **A–D**, A 45-year-old male mountain-biker with C3-C4 dislocation and incomplete quadriplegia. Magnetic resonance image (MRI, **B**) shows a peeling off of his posterior longitudinal ligament (PLL, arrowhead), but no disk herniation behind C3 or C4. He deteriorated neurologically in the MRI suite, and an urgent closed reduction was performed, with assurance that there was no disk herniation. The postreduction MRI **(C)** confirms this and demonstrates the reapproximation of the PLL to the vertebral bodies. He underwent posterior lateral mass fixation **(D)**. **E–G**, A 25-year-old male in motor vehicle accident with C5-C6 dislocation and complete quadriplegia. MRI **(F)** shows a dark mass with the signal consistent with disk material (arrowhead) behind the body of C5 and even behind the body of C6. An anterior diskectomy was performed prior to open reduction, then interbody fusion **(G)**. **H–J**, A 60-year-old male after a fall from a balcony shows a C6-C7 dislocation and incomplete quadriplegia. MRI **(I)** shows flattening of the C6-C7 disk space and a large dark mass behind the body of C6 (arrowhead). He underwent anterior diskectomy, open reduction, and fusion, followed by posterior stabilization due to posterior element fractures.*

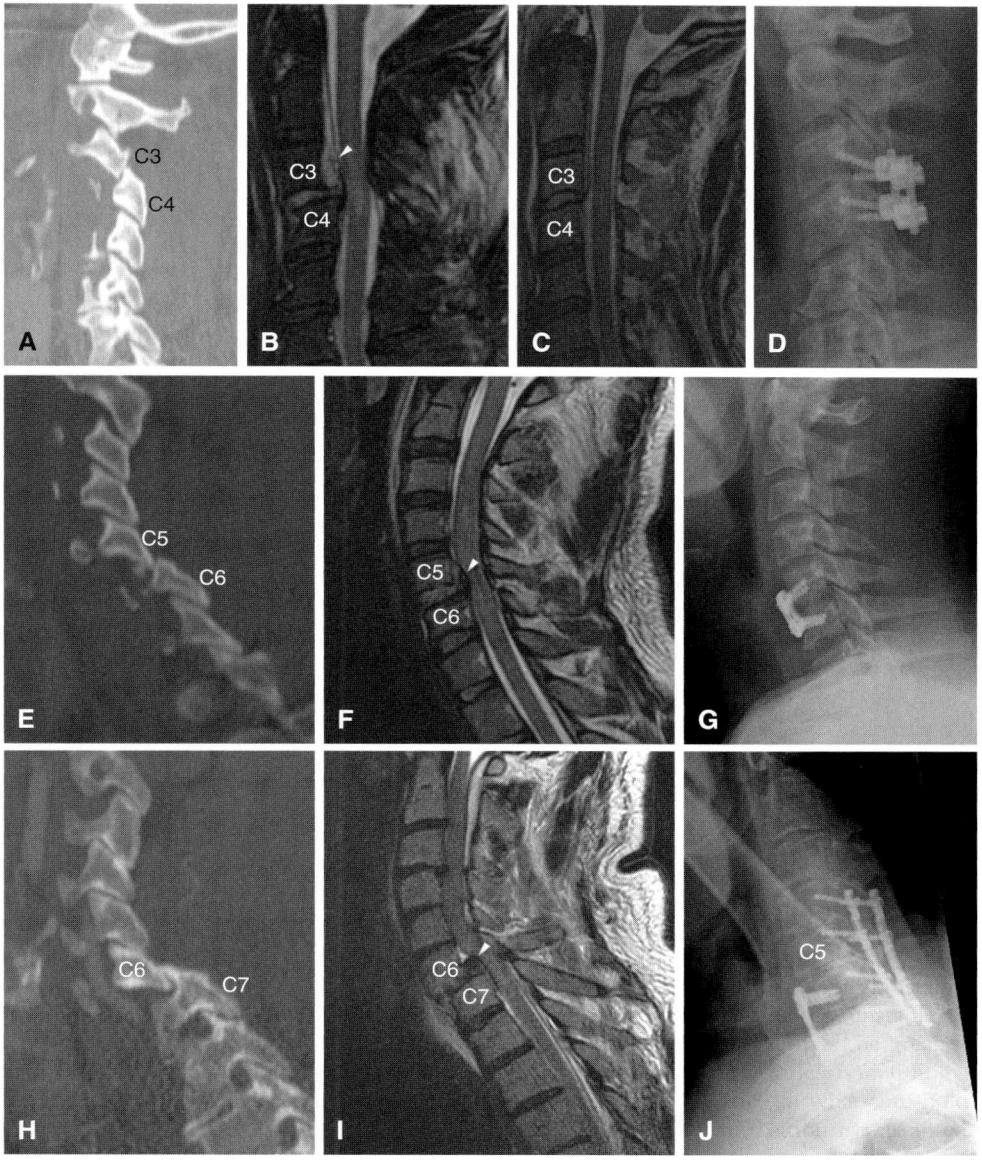

The setting is the next thing to consider. The patient certainly requires systemic analgesia and sedation; the procedure should, therefore, take place in an area where support, including airway control, is either present or readily available (remembering also that these patients have an unstable cervical spine that may preclude a standard intubation). These procedures are most commonly performed in the emergency department, which is acceptable if the necessary medical staff and radiologic support are available. A fluoroscopy unit is very helpful for obtaining real-time imaging of the cervical spine as the traction is applied. The operating room is also an excellent setting, especially with the anesthesiology support on standby, the ability to bring in a fluoroscopy unit to radiographically assess the cervical spine, and, if need be, the ability to rapidly intervene surgically if necessary.

The patient is supine on a bed or stretcher that can be tipped into reverse Trendelenburg's position to provide some countertraction. A roll can be placed between the scapulae, and the shoulders can be pulled and taped distally to improve radiographic visualization of the lower cervical region and provide countertraction. The authors recommend the use of stainless steel Gardner-Wells tongs for the initial reduction, as deformation of the MRI-compatible materials at weights above 80 lb may result in disengagement from the skull. After local anesthetic is injected into the skin, stainless steel pins are inserted 1 cm above the pinna in line with the external auditory meatus. Shaving is typically not necessary, although preparing the area with chlorhexidine or covering the pin tip with an antibacterial ointment prior to insertion may prevent infection. The pins are tightened until the spring strain gauge extends outward approximately 1 mm (flush with the knob of the pin). The side locking nuts are then tightened (Fig. 29-33 and Fig. 29-34).

Traction pulleys are arranged in a manner that allows for some flexion of the neck during the initial phase of reduction to facilitate disengagement of the dislocated facet. Initial traction weights of 5 and then 10 lb should be followed by scrutiny of the craniocervical junction to evaluate for previously undetected injuries that may distract with minimal weight. As with the addition of all subsequent weight, the injured level and all other intervertebral levels should be evaluated for unacceptable distraction, normally defined as disk space widening of greater than 1.5 times that of adjacent uninjured levels. A thorough sensorimotor evaluation must be performed after the addition of each weight, and the patient should be questioned regarding the development or evolution of any neurologic symptoms. Weight is generally added in 5- to 10-lb increments until the dislocated facet appears to have "cleared" its more caudal counterpart. A more longitudinal traction vector may then facilitate the final phase of reduction and can be achieved by lowering the height of the traction pulley or placing an interscapular bump beneath the patient (Fig. 29-35). This maneuver helps the dislocated facet ride back to its native position posterior to the more caudal adjacent facet. Although generally discouraged, in the case of unilateral facet dislocations a

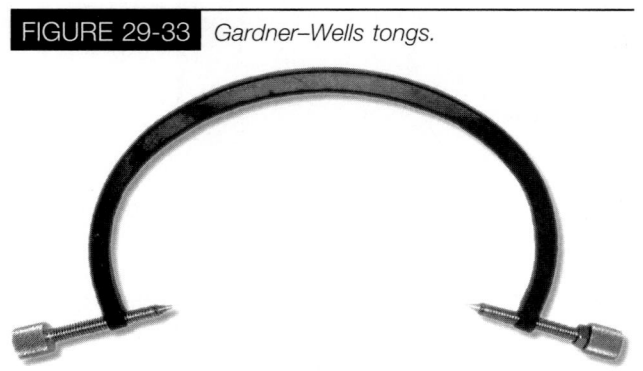

FIGURE 29-33 *Gardner–Wells tongs.*

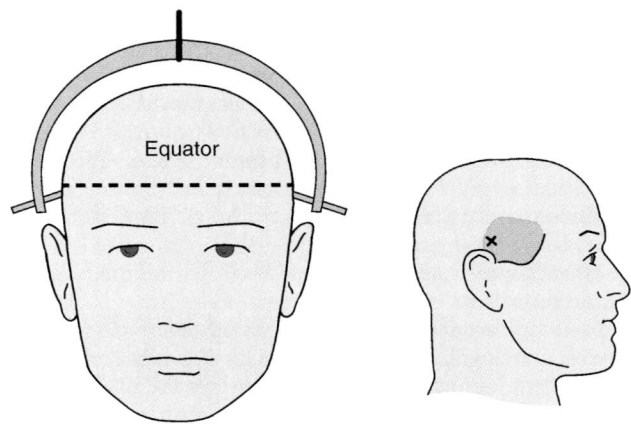

FIGURE 29-34 *The pins are located above the pinna in line with the external auditory meatus.*

derotation reduction maneuver may be required and should be performed by an individual experienced in the treatment of these injuries. Once reduction has been achieved, traction weight is incrementally reduced under fluoroscopic evaluation to between 15 and 25 lb depending on which level is involved. Higher weights may be required if radiographs during the reduction of weight suggest gradual recurrence of subluxation. Following completion of the reduction maneuver, MRI-compatible tongs are substituted for the stainless steel Gardner-Wells tongs while manual axial traction stabilizes the cervical spine. To evaluate the spinal cord and establish the presence of any compressive lesions an MRI of the cervical spine is obtained at the earliest possibility, regardless of whether one was obtained prior to reduction.

Opinions vary widely regarding the maximal weight that should be applied before abandoning attempts at closed reduction. Many factors must be taken into account when making this decision other than simply adhering to empirically accepted and unvalidated dogma. One should anticipate that dislocations become harder to reduce the lower down in the cervical spine they occur, and hence more weight will likely be needed to reduce a C7-T1 dislocation than a C3-C4 dislocation. The presence of a facet fracture might preclude a successful reduction, and hence it may be irrational to keep adding more weight to such an injury. The foremost considerations are the patient's neurologic status and the radiographic observation of the cervical spine (i.e., overdistraction of the disk spaces). Cotler and co-workers reported safe closed reductions of facet dislocations with weights as high as 140 lb.[22] As long as the patient remains neurologically stable and shows no sign of excessive distraction on sequential radiographs, the authors have no absolute, preconceived limit on the amount of traction that can be applied, and the decision regarding when to abandon closed reduction is made on an individualized basis.

If neurologic deterioration does occur during or after the closed reduction, one should consider the possible causes, which are not limited solely to a disk herniation. The development of a posterior epidural hematoma has been reported to cause neurologic worsening after the closed reduction of a bilateral facet injury.[59] Rhee and

FIGURE 29-35 *Traction is applied in line with the spine (A). As weight is applied the facets are almost reduced but still locked (B). Slight flexion unlocks facets and allows reduction (C). Manual reduction can be utilized by laterally bending each side, unlocking facet (D). E, Reduction has been achieved.*

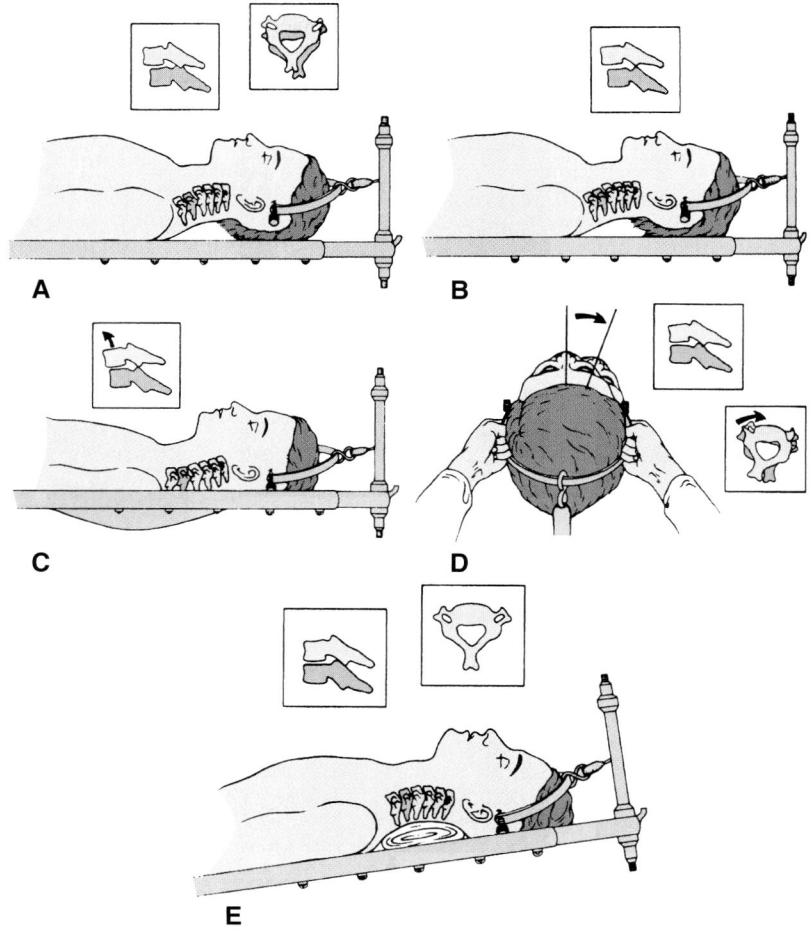

associates recently reported on two patients whose condition deteriorated due to infolding of the ligamentum flavum from the caudal lamina after reduction.[86] Further injury to the spinal cord can occur due to the movement of the spinal column with the traction and manipulation, particularly if the canal is already stenotic.[60] The onset of neurologic worsening should prompt the physician to cease further attempts to reduce the injury, reverse any reduction maneuvers (if applicable), and call for an immediate MRI. Warning the operating room immediately in anticipation of an urgent decompression may save valuable time.

In summary, this collective experience would suggest the following approach to the closed reduction of facet injuries. If the patient is neurologically intact and is awake, alert, and cooperative, the literature to date indicates that it is reasonable to proceed with a closed reduction, as described earlier. Given that there is not a great urgency to the matter, it would also be reasonable in such a patient to obtain an MRI first to evaluate the status of the disk herniation. If taking this route, one should recognize that if a disk herniation *is* seen on MRI, it may not be possible to determine whether it would actually cause a neurologic injury if a closed reduction were carried out. This almost predisposes the patient to having an anterior diskectomy.

If the patient has a complete spinal cord injury, then relieving the pressure on the spinal cord should take precedence and provides the rationale for proceeding with an urgent closed reduction without MRI.

It is the patient with an incomplete spinal cord injury who presents the greatest challenge, as he or she likely has the most to gain from an urgent decompression of the cord, and yet such a patient may also have a great deal of function to lose. As discussed earlier, the presence of a neurologic deficit is itself correlated to the presence of a disk herniation,[37,88] and so one needs to carefully consider this in the patient with incomplete quadriplegia (see Fig. 29-31). Balanced against the risk of pushing a disk fragment back into the spinal cord is the possibility that an urgent realignment of the spinal column might alternatively be of neurologic benefit. How to best proceed in this situation is, unfortunately, ill-defined, and decisions must be made on an individual basis. If the neurologic deficit is improving (which often occurs in incomplete cord injuries) or is mild to begin with, then taking the time to do an expeditious MRI would be reasonable before undertaking a closed reduction. If the patient's incomplete neurologic injury is severe or is deteriorating, then one may be compelled to urgently realign the spine without further imaging.

DEFINITIVE TREATMENT

The options for the definitive management of distractive flexion injuries include external immobilization and cervical fixation performed anteriorly, posteriorly, or circumferentially. DFS1 injuries, which include facet sprains, generally require external immobilization in a rigid orthosis for 6 to 12 weeks. They need to be followed radiographically in the early stages to ensure that what appeared radiographically as a DFS1 injury was not something more unstable that had reduced spontaneously prior to presentation.

Isolated nondisplaced unilateral facet fractures (DFS2 injuries) can similarly be treated with external immobilization due to the propensity of the bony surfaces to eventually unite (see Fig. 29-24). Close radiographic follow-up is again required to ensure that significant fracture displacement and kyphosis are not occurring. Nondisplaced or minimally displaced facet fractures in association with anterior column injuries or other posterior osseous or ligamentous injuries should prompt serious consideration for operative stabilization (Fig. 29-36). As stated earlier, the Cervical Spine Injury Severity Score is helpful in quantifying the mechanical instability of such fractures and guiding an individualized treatment for each injury. Unilateral facet dislocations and displaced fracture-dislocations generally require operative stabilization as definitive treatment. The treatment of such injuries with external orthoses or halo immobilization has been associated with a high rate of radiographic failure.[15,39,91,96] This failure likely relates to the inability of halo immobilization to adequately stabilize such injuries. Anderson and associates performed a radiographic study of patients with cervical spine fractures treated with halo braces, and demonstrated that patients with facet fracture dislocations had 1.6 mm of translational motion and 3.3° of angular motion at the injured segment when moving from a supine to upright position.[9]

The surgical stabilization of displaced unilateral facet injuries can be achieved either anteriorly with an anterior cervical diskectomy and fusion, or posteriorly with lateral mass fixation. A recent biomechanical comparison of anterior cervical nonlocking plates versus posterior lateral mass plates reported that lateral mass plating provided superior biomechanical immobilization of the injured segment.[27]

FIGURE 29-36 *Failure of cervical orthoses to immobilize a distractive flexion injury. This 48-year-old woman was involved in a rollover motor vehicle accident. She complained of neck pain, but was neurologically normal. Her radiograph (**A**) demonstrates a compression fracture of C7 with very mild C6 subluxation on C7. Computed tomography (CT, **B**) shows undisplaced fractures through a number of posterior osseous elements, including the right C6 pedicle (arrowhead), left C6 lamina and facet, and left C7 facet (arrows). Her overall alignment was considered acceptable (**A**) and she was treated in a Philadelphia collar. Seven days later, her upright plain film (**C**) demonstrates widening of the C5-C6 and C6-C7 interspace (arrows) and progressive collapse of the C6-C7 disk space with further C6 subluxation. CT (**D**) shows displacement of all the fractures, including the right C6 pedicle, left lamina, and left C7 facet. Interestingly, magnetic resonance imaging (MRI, **E**) shows a ligamentous disruption at C5-C6 (arrow). The disk herniation at this level was considered to be chronic. She underwent posterior open reduction and fixation (**F**).*

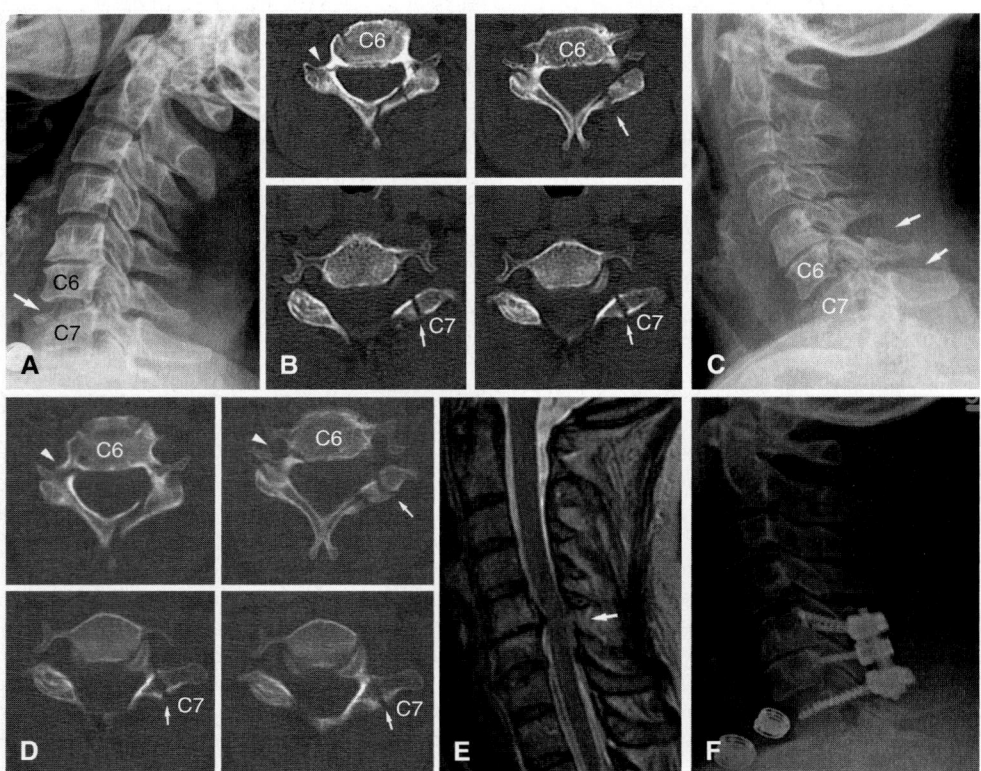

Despite this, in a prospective randomized comparison between anterior cervical locking plates versus posterior lateral mass plating or wiring for unilateral facet injuries, Kwon and co-workers reported a 100 percent fusion rate in patients randomized to anterior fixation.[53] This high fusion rate was corroborated by Henriques and colleagues, who also reported a 100 percent fusion rate for single-level unilateral facet injuries treated with anterior fixation.[45] These results suggest that for these unilateral facet injuries, sufficient stability can be achieved with either anterior or posterior fixation.

Bilateral facet injuries (DFS3 and DSF4) require operative stabilization as the definitive treatment. Numerous cadaveric biomechanical studies that have simulated bilateral facet injuries with complete ligamentous disruption report superior stabilization with lateral mass fixation posteriorly compared with anterior cervical plate fixation.[21,25,81] As such, posterior stabilization is appropriate for these injuries, provided that a disk herniation requiring ventral decompression does not exist.[13,34] Severe fracturing of the facets may preclude obtaining secure fixation with lateral mass screws, warranting extension of the fixation construct above or below the injury (or both).

In addition to the biomechanical advantage of lateral mass fixation, the posterior approach is favored for performing an open reduction of facet dislocations if irreducible by closed means. The ability to directly visualize and control the posterior elements makes this technically easier than reducing from the anterior approach. Accomplishing the open reduction often requires placing a narrow curved instrument between the dislocated facets to lever them into a reduced position. Towel clamps can be placed on the spinous processes of the dislocated segment to provide some distraction and control of the proximal and distal vertebrae. Removal of the superior part of the more caudal facet may help the dislocated facet to clear the caudal facet and slip back posteriorly into its native position. If the head has been held rigidly in a head clamp system (e.g., a Mayfield head clamp), having someone loosen the attachments of the head clamp to the operating table so that the head (and dislocated segment) can be moved obviously facilitates the reduction.

Although biomechanically inferior in this setting, anterior cervical diskectomy and fusion (ACDF) for the stabilization of bilateral facet injuries has also been reported with clinical success. For example, Razack and co-workers reported a 100 percent fusion rate with anterior plating alone in a series of 22 patients with bilateral facet fracture dislocations.[84] This would suggest that ACDF can provide sufficient immobilization for these highly unstable injuries. Others, however, have not had the same experience. Henriques and colleagues found that 7 of their 13 patients with bilateral facet injuries suffered redisplacement or loss of alignment with anterior plating alone.[45] A major consideration for anterior fixation in the setting of bilateral facet injuries is the recognition that the severe flexion-distraction forces are often accompanied by compressive failure of the anterior column. This can result in an end plate fracture, compression fracture, or even burstlike fractures of the anterior vertebral body in association with bilateral ligamentous disruption and facet dislocation posteriorly. One should be aware of such anterior injuries in

the planning of anterior column reconstruction and fixation (Fig. 29-37). In an analysis of 87 patients with distractive flexion injuries (most of whom had bilateral facet injuries), Johnson and associates found that the presence of an end plate fracture was strongly associated with radiographic failure of anterior fixation when used alone.[47] It was postulated that even with minor fracturing of the end plate, the subsequent resorptive biologic phenomenon compromised the stability of the interbody graft and possibly also the screw fixation for the locking plate. The presence of facet fractures (vs. dislocations) also was associated with radiographic failure of anterior fixation, perhaps due to the loss of the posterior "buttressing" effect that an intact facet joint might have once reduced.

As a technical note, care should be taken to avoid overdistraction when performing anterior fusion for flexion-distraction injuries. Due to the disruption of the posterior complex and possibly also the PLL, distraction of the disk space may be unrestrained and can potentially cause a neurologic deficit. Following the anterior diskectomy, the head can be carefully lowered to increase the lordosis of the injured segment and "lock" the reduced facets into place if they are not fractured. Accepting a looser interbody graft and performing a secondary posterior stabilization procedure is preferable to aggressively overdistracting the disk space to fit in a large interbody graft.

The primary indication for anterior diskectomy and fusion in a bilateral facet injury may be to decompress the spinal cord in the presence of a large disk herniation detected on MRI either before or after reduction. However, the criteria for determining when a disk herniation requires removal prior to reduction are unknown. Nonetheless, if anterior decompression is to be done prior to reduction, one should be prepared for the possibility that a partial corpectomy of the suprajacent vertebral body may be needed to gain access to the herniated disk. Particularly if the facets are perched, the segment will be quite kyphotic, and access to the disk may be limited without resecting some of the inferior aspect of the vertebral body. Once the diskectomy is complete, an open reduction can be performed by various means, including the standard sequential application of weight under lateral fluoroscopy as previously discussed, or direct manipulation of the vertebral bodies with a lamina spreader or Caspar pins.[52] The need for caution in the application of traction is emphasized again here, because once the diskectomy is complete, the dislocated segment will be circumferentially devoid of any soft tissue restraints to distraction across the disk space.

If an open reduction cannot be achieved after performing the anterior diskectomy, the patient should be turned for a posterior open reduction and fixation, and then returned to place an anterior interbody graft and plate. To obviate the need for this last step of returning to the anterior exposure after the posterior open reduction and fixation, Allred and Sledge described a technique in four patients of placing an interbody graft and a buttress anterior cervical plate fixed to only the suprajacent vertebral body.[7] The anterior plate helps to hold the interbody graft in place when the reduction is accomplished posteriorly, and in their experience of four patients, the combination of posterior fixation with the anterior interbody graft was sufficiently stable to promote union.

FIGURE 29-37 | *Failure of anterior fixation in distractive flexion injury. This 55-year-old woman sustained a C5-C6 bilateral facet dislocation in a motor vehicle accident. Note on the midsagittal magnetic resonance image **(A)** and computed tomograph (CT, **B**) the subluxation of C5 on C6, the interspinous widening (arrow), and the subtle superior end plate fracture of C6 (arrowhead). The parasagittal CT **(C)** shows the facet dislocation (arrow). She underwent a C6 anterior vertebrectomy, followed by an open reduction, cage reconstruction, and plating **(D)**. Five days postoperatively, her upright plain film **(E)** and sagittal CT **(F)** suggest subsidence of the cage anteriorly into C6 with resubluxation and interspinous widening (arrow). Conservative management was chosen. Fourteen days postoperatively, kyphosis has increased **(G),** and the repeat CT **(H)** shows complete dislocation of the facets again. She underwent posterior lateral mass fixation **(I)**. This case illustrates the dangers of depending solely on anterior reconstruction in distractive flexion injuries, particularly in the setting of an end plate fracture, a point made by Johnson and co-workers in their radiographic review of such injuries.*

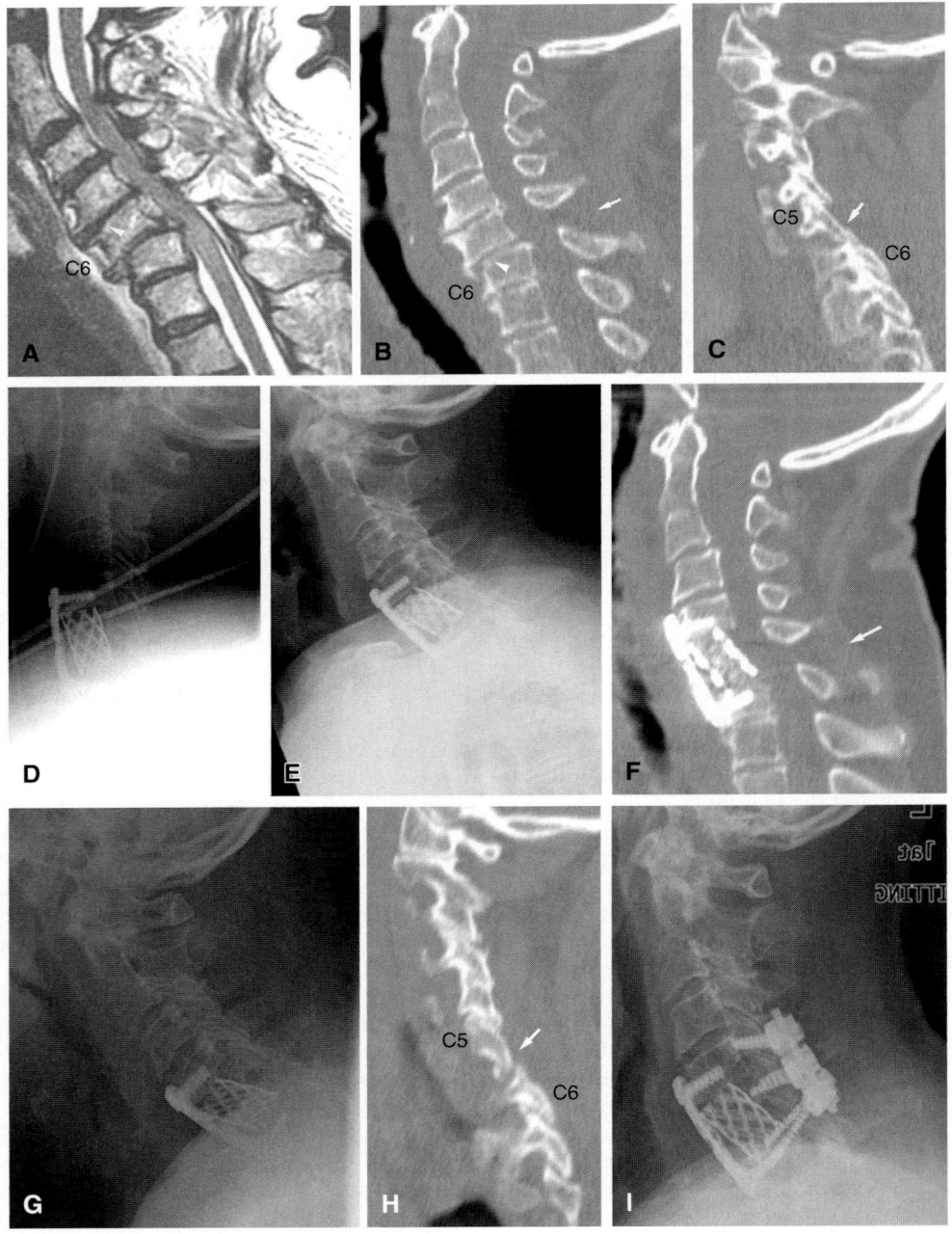

It is unclear which injuries require both anterior and posterior stabilization. Clearly, good clinical results have been achieved with posterior fixation alone and anterior fixation alone. The experiences of Johnson and associates[47] and Henriques and colleagues[45] suggest that anterior fixation alone may not suffice when the bony anterior column is compromised, due to end plate or vertebral body fracture, or to osteoporosis (see Fig. 29-37). Poor neuromuscular control in patients with cord injuries may also contribute to fixation failure of isolated anterior constructs. In the setting of severe anterior column injury in association with the posterior ligamentous disruption characteristic of distractive flexion injuries, circumferential fixation is likely warranted.

Compressive Extension Injuries

The compressive extension phylogeny comprised nearly a quarter of the Allen and Ferguson series and consisted of injuries at two ends of the severity spectrum. Stage 1 (CES1) injuries are unilateral arch fractures and comprised the vast majority of these injuries (32 of 40). Included in CES1 injuries was the pattern of ipsilateral pedicle and laminar fractures, which produce what is commonly referred to as a "floating lateral mass" injury. These injuries are currently viewed as a variant of unilateral facet injuries (DFS2 injuries), but involve both the rostral and caudal facet joints. Stage 2 (CES2) injuries are bilaminar fractures without vertebral body displacement. At the other end of the spectrum, stage 5 (CES5) injuries (of which there were only three in the Allen and Ferguson series) were characterized by bilateral pedicle fractures with full vertebral body width displacement anteriorly (traumatic spondylolisthesis). Interestingly, none of the three patients with the severe CES5 injuries suffered a cord injury. It is unclear whether these injuries were in fact severe distractive flexion injuries in which the patients were fortunate enough to have "laminectomized" themselves with the fractured vertebral arch. Stages 3 and 4 were deemed "hypothetical" in the Allen and Ferguson classification but were described as representing increasing degrees of vertebral body displacement from stage 2 injuries.

TREATMENT RECOMMENDATIONS

Compressive extension injuries are similar in nature to distractive extension injuries, and as such their treatment will be discussed in more detail in the following section. In general, isolated minimally displaced laminar fractures can be treated with external immobilization alone. The CES1 injuries that involve ipsilateral pedicle and laminar fractures warrant some discussion here, though, as they behave more like unilateral facet injuries (DFS2).

An ipsilateral pedicle and laminar fracture in which the lateral mass is disconnected from the vertebral body and the lamina can potentially lead to rotational instability at both the facet above and facet below. If nondisplaced, treatment with external immobilization may be considered. However, if displaced even minimally, external immobilization may fail to provide sufficient stability,

given that the "floating" C5 lateral mass provides support to neither the rostral C4-C5 nor the caudal C5-C6 facet joints. Fixation of these generally requires stabilization across both motion segments (Fig. 29-38).

Distractive Extension Injuries

Distractive extension injuries represent a small but extremely important subset of subaxial cervical injuries because of their prevalence in individuals with spondylotic or ankylosed cervical spines (patients with ankylosing spondylitis and diffuse idiopathic skeletal hyperostosis, or DISH). Allen and Ferguson identified only nine patients in their series, five of whom sustained their injuries after a minor fall. Stage 1 (DES1) injuries consisted of ALL rupture with abnormal widening of the disk space but no posterior displacement (Fig. 29-39). Stage 2 (DES2) injuries share the same features as DES1 injuries but include some retrolisthesis of the suprajacent vertebral body. In such injuries, neurologic deficits occur with high frequency. Extension injuries usually result from a blow to the face or forehead. The sequence of injury to the spinal column begins from the ALL and progresses posteriorly. The extension forces may tear the ALL, anterior annulus, or even cause a transverse fracture of the vertebral body. Tensile forces through the ALL may cause an avulsion fracture of the anterior body (an extension "teardrop" fracture) or fracture off an osteophyte or syndesmophyte overlying the disk space. Depending on how far posterior the axis of rotation exists, tensile failure of the anterior column may be accompanied by compressive fracturing of the posterior neural arch, lateral masses, and pedicles or, alternatively, by progressive disruption of the posterior ligamentous complex.

Extension injuries are observed in younger patients after high-energy trauma and in older patients with spondylotic or ankylosed spine after seemingly trivial injuries. In elderly individuals with spinal canals already narrowed by diffuse spondylotic changes, the sudden extension mechanism can induce a pincer-like compression on the spinal cord (Fig. 29-40), causing severe neurologic injuries even in the absence of anterior column failure. This is the most common cause of the so-called central cord pattern of incomplete quadriplegia, with a disproportionate upper extremity deficit.

DISH represent a unique subset of these injuries. In patients with ankylosis of the cervical spine, spinal fractures behave more like long-bone fractures and are unstable, even in the absence of displacement. The long lever arms applied to even the undisplaced fracture can lead to progressive displacement and kyphosis, with potentially catastrophic neurologic consequences. The most significant pitfalls in the management of these injuries are in the failure to recognize the ankylosing condition and in the failure to visualize the injury. Many patients with ankylosing spondylitis or particularly those with DISH are reported as having "advanced degenerative changes," and hence the presence of neck pain does not raise the alarms that it should. *Any patient with ankylosing spondylitis or DISH who presents with neck pain after even trivial*

FIGURE 29-38 *"Floating lateral mass" injury treated conservatively with progressive subluxation. This 26-year-old male was involved in a motorcycle accident and presented with neck pain but no neurologic deficits. His radiograph (A) and midsagittal computed tomographic (CT) reconstruction (B) show the mild subluxation and kyphosis at C3-C4. Axial CTs (C and D) show an ipsilateral C4 pedicle and laminar fracture (arrows) on the right, which disconnects the C4 lateral mass from the body anteriorly and lamina posteriorly—hence the "floating lateral mass." On the axial cut (D) kyphosis of the lateral mass is evident by the diastasis of the facet joint and the posterior migration of the posteroinferior corner of the lateral mass (arrowhead). This is viewed more easily on the parasagittal CT reconstruction (E). The fat suppression magnetic resonance image (F) does not show distinct disruption of the facet capsules at C3-C4 or C4-C5. He was placed in a firm cervical orthosis. Two weeks later, his upright plain film (G) shows progressive C3-C4 subluxation and kyphosis, and further kyphosis of the C4 lateral mass is evident, which is now almost horizontally oriented (arrowhead points to the posteroinferior corner of the lateral mass). The patient underwent posterior fixation to stabilize both the C3-C4 and C4-C5 levels (H).*

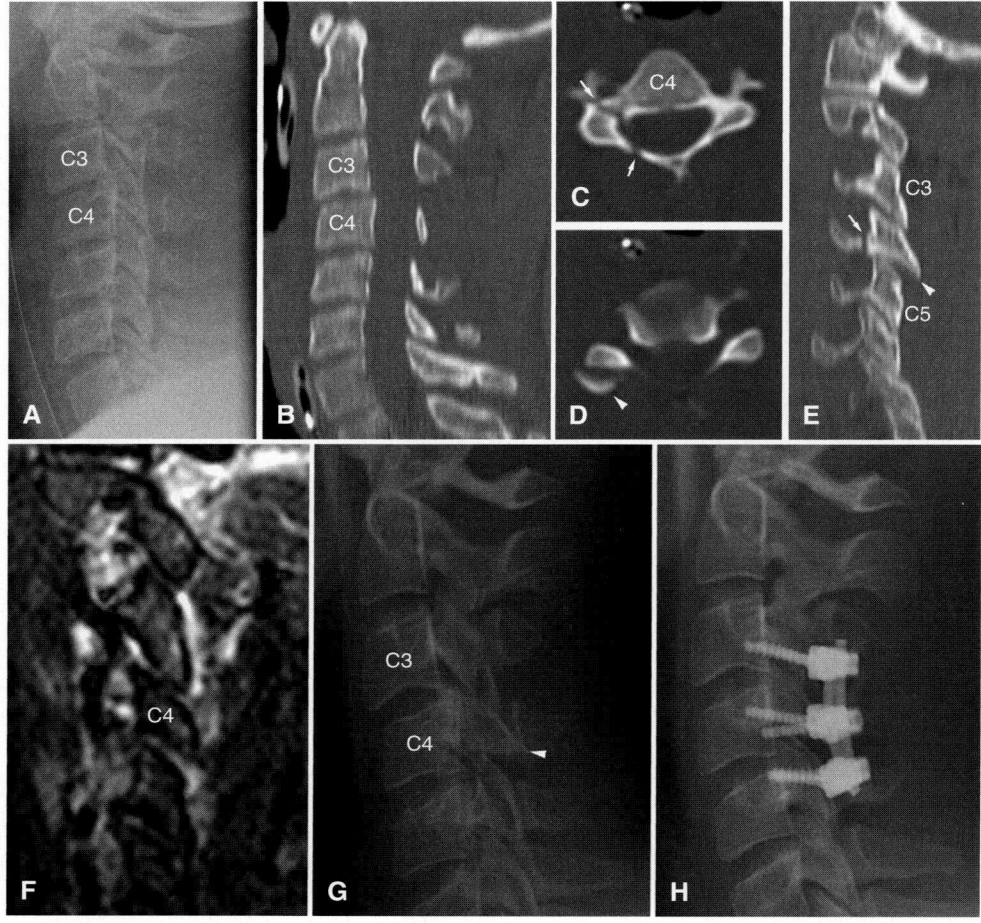

trauma has an unstable cervical fracture until proven otherwise with advanced imaging studies. Alternatively, the fractures themselves may be missed because of their lack of displacement, or because visualization of the lower cervical spine is obscured on plain radiographs due to the cervicothoracic kyphosis characteristic of ankylosing spondylitis or in the elderly (in whom DISH is most prevalent). CT imaging with sagittal and coronal reconstruction is crucial for the identification of such injuries. MRI is also useful for identifying acute bony or soft tissue edema in subtle injuries. The identification of a cervical spine fracture in a patient with ankylosing spondylitis or DISH should prompt a repeat CT or MRI through the rest of the thoracolumbar spine to look for additional noncontiguous injuries (Fig. 29-41).[93]

TREATMENT RECOMMENDATIONS FOR THE NONANKYLOSED SPINE

Patients who present with hyperextension injuries but without significant anterior column injury can be treated nonoperatively with an external orthosis for comfort. The most common scenario for this is the patient who suffers a hyperextension injury and presents with a central cord pattern of incomplete quadriplegia due to the pincer-like compression of his or her spinal cord. If the cervical spinal

FIGURE 29-39 *Extension distraction injuries with disk space disruption. This figure depicts a spectrum of anterior column disruption that can be observed with an extension mechanism of injury in the nonankylosed spine. **A–C**, This 29-year-old mountain-biker went over his handlebars at high speed and struck his helmeted chin on a log, sustaining a mild, incomplete spinal cord injury (ASIA D). Midsagittal computed tomographic (CT) reconstruction **(A)** shows very subtle widening of the C4-C5 disk space and an avulsion fracture (arrow). Magnetic resonance imaging (MRI, **B**) shows disruption of the anterior longitudinal ligament and the very anterior aspect of his C4-C5 disk (arrow). He demonstrates severe anterior soft tissue swelling characteristic of a hyperextension injury (outlined by arrowheads). He has signal change within his spinal cord, consistent with his neurologic deficit. Despite the neurologic deficit, there was no need for surgical decompression, and his spine was considered to be relatively stable, as his injury was confined to the anterior column. He was treated in a Philadelphia collar, and his upright plain film **(C)** shows good alignment of his spine, with the severe anterior soft tissue swelling (arrowheads). **D–F,** This 62-year-old male was involved in a head-on motor vehicle accident. He was neurologically intact. CT shows obvious disruption of the C5-C6 disk (arrow) **(D)** with compressive fractures of the facets posteriorly at C5 and C6 (arrow) **(E)**. He underwent an anterior diskectomy and fusion, followed by posterior stabilization **(F)**. Turning the patient prone for his posterior fixation is made much safer by performing the anterior fixation first.*

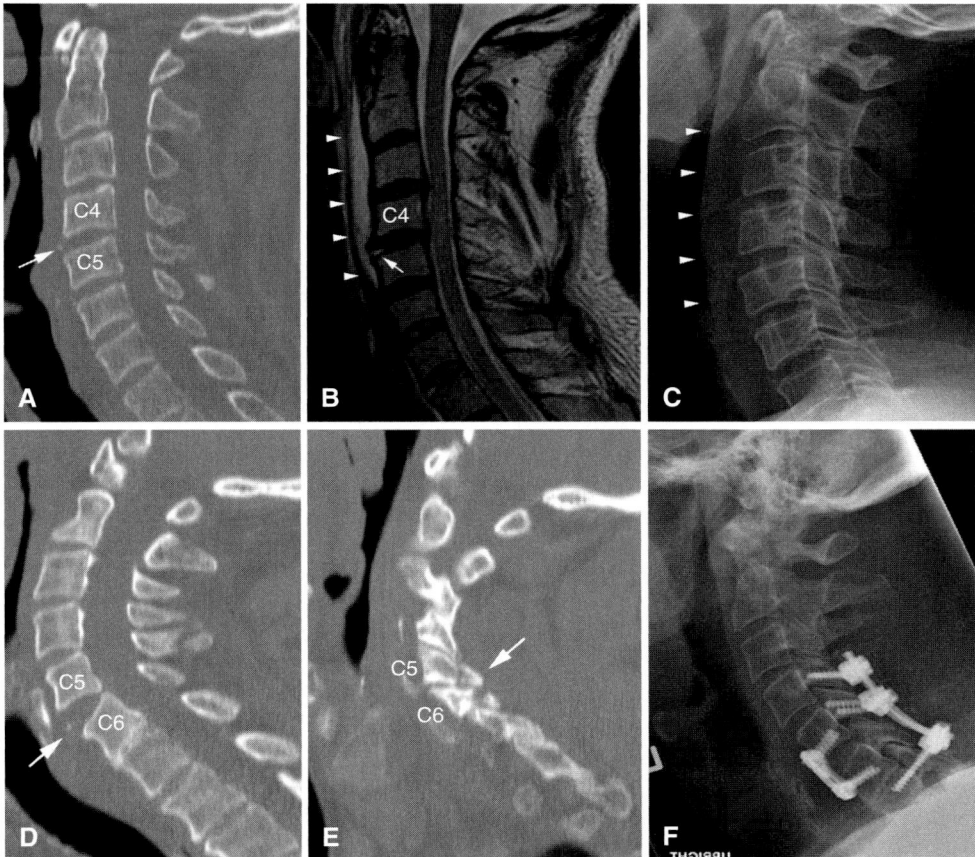

column is deemed to be stable after CT and MRI, there is no reason to operate to provide stability. However, for the issue of optimizing neurologic recovery, there is an ongoing debate about whether these patients should undergo acute operative decompression or wait and reconsider surgery after their neurologic improvement plateaus over the first 6 to 12 weeks. A prospective randomized evaluation to address this important question has not yet been performed, but the retrospective literature to this date has failed to demonstrate a long-term neurologic benefit to early decompression in these patients with central cord injuries secondary to low-energy hyperextension injuries in a spondylotic spine.[19,38]

For stage 1 (DES1) injuries, in which tensile failure of the anterior column has occurred without vertebral body retrolisthesis, nonoperative management with a firm cervical orthosis or halo-vest immobilization is reasonable. To some extent, the management strategy for these injuries depends on how significant the anterior column injury is. For example, if it appears that the extension forces have merely torn the ALL and disrupted only the anterior annulus, then it seems reasonable, given the intact PLL and posterior osseous and ligamentous structures, to treat this condition with a firm cervical orthosis. However, if the extension forces have disrupted everything from the ALL back to the PLL, such an injury may be quite

FIGURE 29-40   *Extension-distraction injury causing "pincer-like" compression of spinal cord. Extension injuries frequently cause spinal cord injuries in elderly individuals who have narrowing of the spinal canal secondary to cervical spondylosis. The forced hyperextension causes a pinching of the spinal cord between bulging disk–osteophyte complexes anteriorly and the infolding ligamentum flavum posteriorly. (From Mirza, S.K.; Anderson, P.A. Skeletal Trauma, 3rd ed., New York, W. B. Saunders, 2003.)*

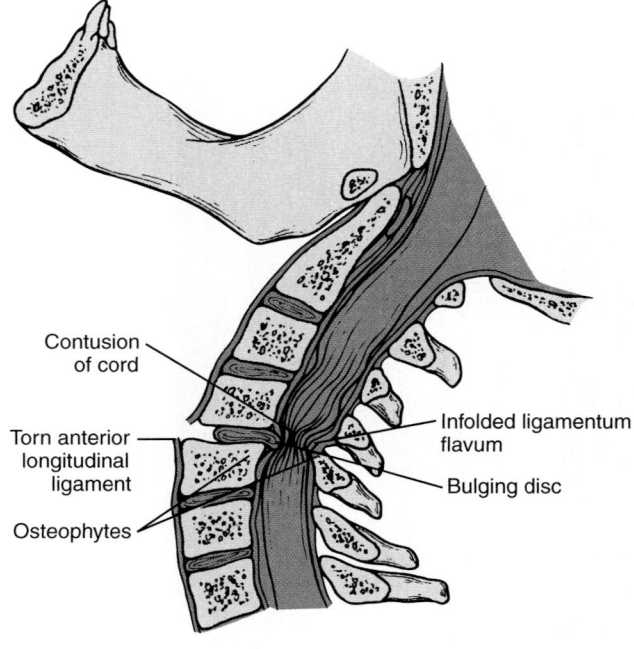

Contusion of cord

Torn anterior longitudinal ligament

Osteophytes

Infolded ligamentum flavum

Bulging disc

unstable even in the absence of retrolisthesis, and even a halo vest may not provide sufficient immobilization. In Vaccaro and colleagues' review of 24 patients with distractive extension injuries (8 of whom had stage 1 injuries), successful union was achieved with halo-vest immobilization of most bony DES1 injuries, but persistent displacement and progressive kyphosis were recognized limitations of this nonoperative approach.[110] They reported good clinical and radiographic success in DES1 injuries treated operatively with anterior cervical diskectomy and fusion.

For stage 2 (DES2) injuries, anterior cervical diskectomy and fusion is the recommended treatment. The presence of significant translational malalignment or fractures of the posterior elements provides some rationale for secondary posterior fixation as well. An important technical point was raised by Vaccaro and colleagues in the performance of anterior fixation for these patients.[110] They experienced deteriorations in the intraoperative spinal cord monitoring waveforms during the insertion of the interbody grafts in two patients, a problem they attributed to overdistraction of the disk space. The authors emphasized

that "overstuffing" the interspace with a large graft in such extension-distraction injuries must be avoided.

TREATMENT RECOMMENDATIONS FOR THE ANKYLOSED SPINE

Immobilization in the patient who presents with acute ankylosing spondylitis or DISH and a cervical fracture must be evaluated with extreme caution. Particularly for patients with ankylosing spondylitis who have significant cervicothoracic kyphosis, an attempt at immobilization using a standard cervical collar may only worsen the neck extension. One should endeavor to immobilize the neck in its native, kyphotic position, which may involve placing many layers of padding underneath the head.[64] If traction is used, it should be done with great caution, minimal weight, and biplanar traction pulleys to provide force vectors both anteriorly and posteriorly. Alternatively, the patient may be fitted with a halo vest while awaiting definitive operative stabilization. In all cases, with or without neurologic deficit, these patients represent a high risk for developing airway problems, and an early anesthesiology consultation is warranted.

The long lever arms make these fractures highly unstable, and as such, operative stabilization is recommended. Although anterior diskectomy and fusion may, in theory, restore the anterior tension band of an extension-distraction injury, posterior fixation may also be warranted due to the forces across the injury site (Fig. 29-42). Furthermore, in patients with ankylosing spondylitis, the opened disk space may be almost vertical to the ground due to the severe cervicothoracic kyphosis. In such cases, posterior instrumentation over multiple levels is advisable (Fig. 29-43). Anterior reconstruction and fixation can help to restore the anterior tension band. Numerous authors have recently advocated a circumferential stabilization approach for the surgical management of these injuries.[29,31,79]

Other factors to consider in patients with ankylosing spondylitis include exposure, positioning, and bleeding. Due to the cervicothoracic kyphosis, it may be difficult, if not impossible, to obtain sufficient access to the anterior cervical spine to place a graft and plate. For the same reasons, posterior positioning can also be quite challenging, because standard bed frames may not allow the head to fall far enough forward (the head is forward due to the kyphosis across the cervicothoracic spine). In such cases, the patient may need to be kept in a seated position for the posterior exposure, as is done for realignment osteotomies. Because sparing motion segments is not an issue and stability is needed, multilevel segmental constructs should be used. Finally, bleeding can be quite excessive in patients with ankylosing spondylitis and should be planned for.

Lateral Flexion Injuries

Lateral flexion injuries are unusual, and this phylogeny comprised only 5 injuries of the 165 studied by Allen and Ferguson. Two injury types were described. Stage 1 (LFS1) injuries were identified as unilateral arch fractures with lateral compression of the vertebral body, and stage 2 (LFS2) injuries were described as having associated contralateral posterior ligament injury manifested primarily as facet widening. Although spinal cord injury is unusual,

FIGURE 29-41 *Segmental spine injury in ankylosing spondylitis. This 58-year-old male was found down on his bathroom floor and presented with a Brown-Séquard pattern of incomplete quadriplegia. Two years prior to his injury he had a cervical radiograph taken **(A)**, which shows fusion of his facets (arrowheads) characteristic of ankylosing spondylitis. Midsagittal computed tomographic (CT) reconstruction **(B)** demonstrates an obvious extension injury (arrow) of his cervical spine with gross widening of the C3-C4 disk space and retrolisthesis of C3 on C4. The parasagittal CT reconstructions demonstrate the posterior injury through the facets **(C,** arrow) and how the spine behaves like a long bone, with displacement of the posterior elements of the "distal fragment" into the spinal canal **(D,** arrowhead). His right-sided weakness was well explained by the right-sided cord compression **(D,** inset). Prior to his operation, he underwent magnetic resonance imaging screening of his entire spine, which revealed an extension injury of his thoracic spine at T8-T9 (arrow) **(E)**. The subsequent CT **(F)** demonstrates the propagation of the fracture from the anterior column through the pedicle and out the back (arrow). He underwent an anterior diskectomy and fusion, which was made quite challenging by his cervicothoracic kyphosis. This was supplemented by a long posterior cervical instrumentation **(G** and **H)**.*

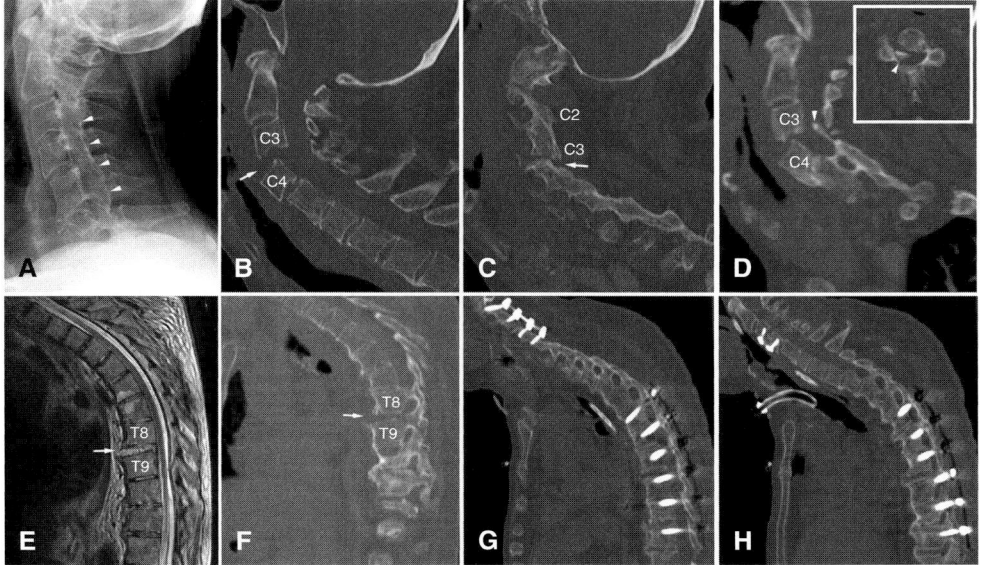

FIGURE 29-42 *Extension-distraction injury in diffuse idiopathic skeletal hyperostosis (DISH). This 62-year-old male fell off a ladder while doing yard work and presented with incomplete quadriplegia. The radiograph **(A)** demonstrates gross disruption of the C3-C4 disk space with severe distraction, focal lordosis, and retrolisthesis of C3 on C4. Note the "flowing" osteophytes bridging the anterior aspects of the vertebral bodies, and what appears to be a fractured anterior osteophyte at C4 (arrow). Sagittal magnetic resonance imaging **(B)** shows the distinct appearance of the C2-C3 and C3-C4 disks compared with the disks within the fused subaxial cervical spine. This suggests that C3-C4 may have been his most caudal mobile segment, and thus the most likely to fail in extension. He was treated **(C)** with an diskectomy and fusion first, then long posterior fixation with a multisegment decompression. Notice that during the anterior procedure the spine was brought back into a relatively kyphotic position to reduce the "pinching" effect of the posterior ligamentum flavum, and that a short interbody graft was inserted to prevent overdistraction.*

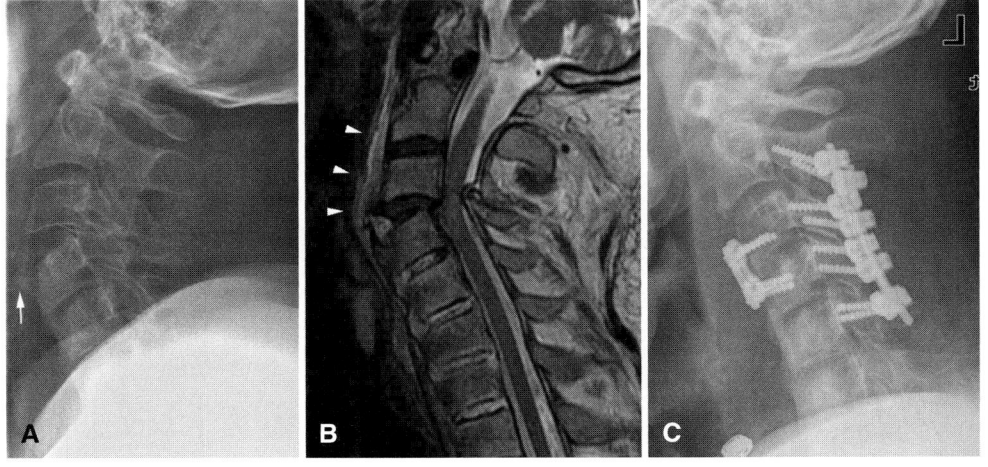

FIGURE 29-43 *Failure of fixation in ankylosing spondylitis. This 52-year-old male with known ankylosing spondylitis tripped and fell in a parking lot. He presented to his local emergency department with neck pain and facial injuries. Radiographs were taken, and he was discharged home. Despite repeated films and clinical follow-up for his persistent neck pain, no advanced imaging was performed until he began having myelopathic symptoms, 4 weeks later. At that stage, he was found to have a displaced C5-C6 fracture dislocation (A) that was most certainly undisplaced at the time of his injury. The sagittal computed tomographic (CT) reconstruction clearly demonstrates the posterior element injury (B, arrow). He underwent an anterior C5-C6 diskectomy and fusion with autogenous bone graft, followed by posterior C5-C6 lateral mass fixation (C). Notice on the upright plain film (C), his cervicothoracic kyphosis makes the screws in the short anterior and posterior fixation construct almost horizontal, a clearly suboptimal biomechanical result. Repeat imaging 14 months later due to persistent pain revealed failure to unite either anteriorly (D) or posteriorly along the right (E) or left (F) facets. He underwent a revision posterior procedure with long proximal and distal extension of the instrumentation and a T1 pedicle subtraction osteotomy to correct the overall sagittal alignment (G). CT 9 months postrevision reveals osseous union both anteriorly (H) and posteriorly (I). This case illustrates the ease at which such fractures can be missed in patients with ankylosing spondylitis and serves as a reminder that such patients must have advanced imaging to rule out fracture, no matter how trivial the trauma. Furthermore, this case illustrates the biomechanical challenges of fusing the ankylosed spine when such large lever arms are present. Posterior fixation over multiple segments would have been preferable at his index surgery.*

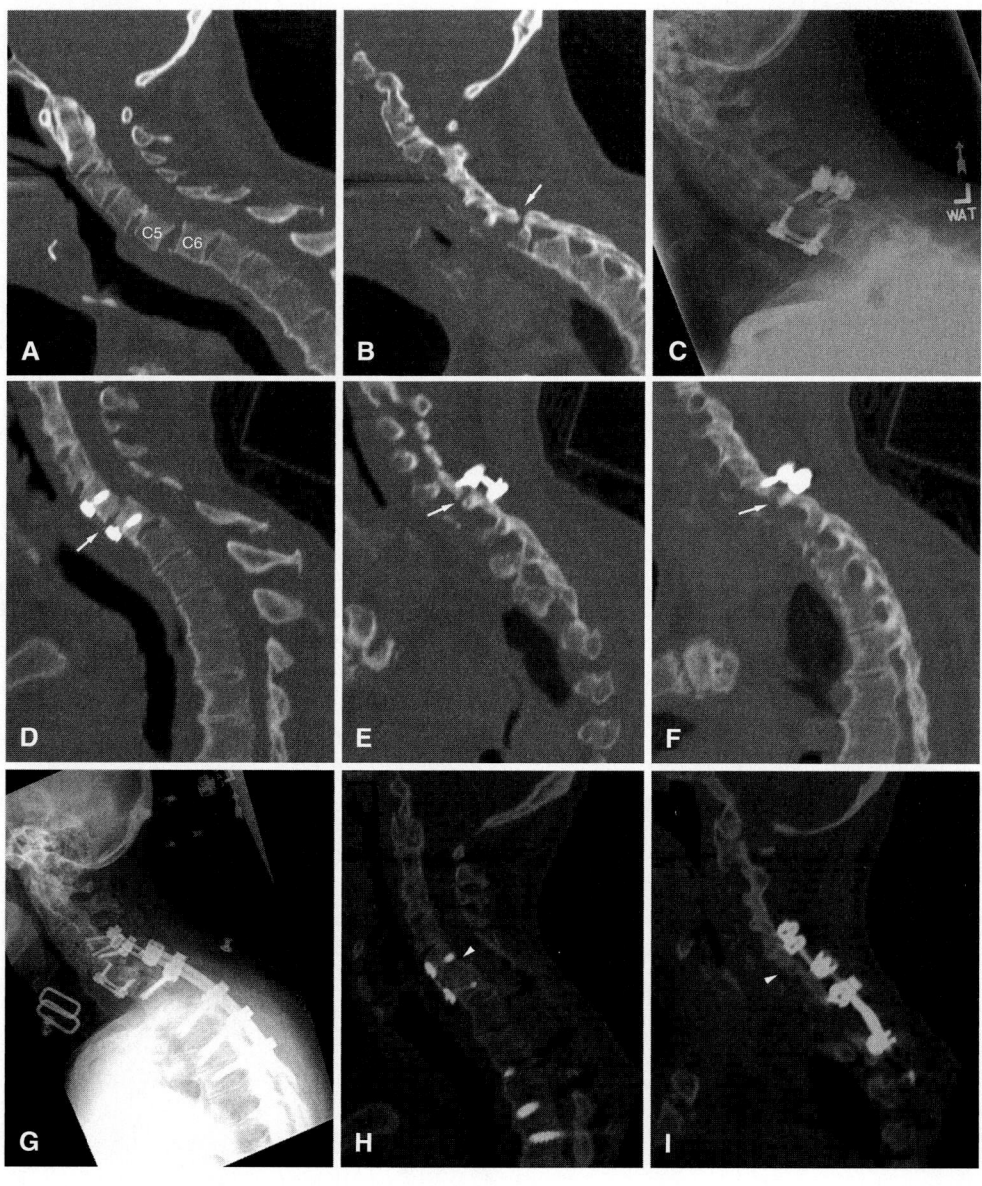

since the mechanism is thought to involve violent lateral flexion of the neck, nerve root injuries, including root avulsions and brachial plexus injuries, may occur.

TREATMENT RECOMMENDATIONS

The majority of patients with LFS1 injuries can be successfully treated with 6 to 12 weeks of collar immobilization. LFS2 injuries, because of their greater coronal plane deformities and associated posterior ligamentous injuries, warrant reduction with cranial tong traction followed by posterior stabilization. Secondary anterior intervention can be performed if warranted due to neurologic deficits with anterior neural compression.

SUMMARY

Injuries to the subaxial cervical spine encompass a wide spectrum of osseous and ligamentous pathologies, in addition to being frequently associated with neurologic injury. Adhering to the basic principles of assessing stability, neurology, and relevant patient factors can help guide rational decisions regarding definitive treatment. A recent algorithm, outlined in this chapter, will help the clinician in assessing the stability of the injury. Considering the injury mechanism and understanding the pathoanatomy are important for deciding the surgical or nonoperative treatment.

REFERENCES

1. Abumi, K.; Itoh, H.; Taneichi, H.; et al. Transpedicular screw fixation for traumatic lesions of the middle and lower cervical spine: Description of the techniques and preliminary report. J Spinal Disord 7:19–28, 1994.
2. Abumi, K.; Shono, Y.; Ito, M.; et al. Complications of pedicle screw fixation in reconstructive surgery of the cervical spine. Spine 25:962–969, 2000.
3. Abumi, K.; Shono, Y.; Kotani, Y.; et al. Indirect posterior reduction and fusion of the traumatic herniated disc by using a cervical pedicle screw system. J Neurosurg 92:30–37, 2000.
4. Adams, M.S.; Crawford, N.R.; Chamberlain, R.H.; et al. Biomechanical comparison of anterior cervical plating and combined anterior/lateral mass plating. Spine J 1:166–170, 2001.
5. Albert, T.J.; Klein, G.R.; Joffe, D.; et al. Use of cervicothoracic junction pedicle screws for reconstruction of complex cervical spine pathology. Spine 23:1596–1599, 1998.
6. Allen, B.L., Jr.; Ferguson, R.L.; Lehmann, T.R.; et al. A mechanistic classification of closed, indirect fractures and dislocations of the lower cervical spine. Spine 7:1–27, 1982.
7. Allred, C.D.; Sledge, J.B. Irreducible dislocations of the cervical spine with a prolapsed disc: Preliminary results from a treatment technique. Spine 26:1927–1930, 2001.
8. An, H.S.; Gordin, R.; Renner, K. Anatomic considerations for plate-screw fixation of the cervical spine. Spine 16:S548–S551, 1991.
9. Anderson, P.A.; Budorick, T.E.; Easton, K.B.; et al. Failure of halo vest to prevent in vivo motion in patients with injured cervical spines. Spine 16:S501–S505, 1991.
10. Anderson, P.A.; Henley, M.B.; Grady, M.S.; et al. Posterior cervical arthrodesis with AO reconstruction plates and bone graft. Spine 16:S72–S79, 1991.
11. Anderson, P.A.; Moore, T.A.; Davis, K.W.; et al. The Cervical Spine Injury Severity Score: Assessment of reliability. J Bone Joint Surg [Am] 89:1057–1065, 2007.
12. Bozbug, M.; Ozturk, A.; Ari, Z.; et al. Morphometric evaluation of subaxial cervical vertebrae for surgical application of transpedicular screw fixation. Spine 29:1876–1880, 2004.
13. Brodke, D.S.; Anderson, P.A.; Newell, D.W.; et al. Comparison of anterior and posterior approaches in cervical spinal cord injuries. J Spinal Disord Tech 16:229–235, 2003.
14. Bucci, M.N.; Dauser, R.C.; Maynard, F.A.; et al. Management of post-traumatic cervical spine instability: Operative fusion versus halo vest immobilization. Analysis of 49 cases. J Trauma 28:1001–1006, 1988.
15. Bucholz, R.D.; Cheung, K.C. Halo vest versus spinal fusion for cervical injury: Evidence from an outcome study. J Neurosurg 70:884–892, 1989.
16. Cagnie, B.; Petrovic, M.; Voet, D.; et al. Vertebral artery dominance and hand preference: Is there a correlation? Man Ther 11:153–156, 2006.
17. Carrino, J.A.; Manton, G.L.; Morrison, W.B.; et al. Posterior longitudinal ligament status in cervical spine bilateral facet dislocations. Skeletal Radiol 35:510–514, 2006.
18. Chang, D.G.; Tencer, A.F.; Ching, R.P.; et al. Geometric changes in the cervical spinal canal during impact. Spine 19:973–980, 1994.
19. Chen, T.Y.; Dickman, C.A.; Eleraky, M.; et al. The role of decompression for acute incomplete cervical spinal cord injury in cervical spondylosis. Spine 23:2398–2403, 1998.
20. Cho, K.H.; Shin, Y.S.; Yoon, S.H.; et al. Poor surgical technique in cervical plating leading to vertebral artery injury and brain stem infarction—Case report. Surg Neurol 64:221–225, 2005.
21. Coe, J.D.; Warden, K.E.; Sutterlin, C.E., III; et al. Biomechanical evaluation of cervical spinal stabilization methods in a human cadaveric model. Spine 14:1122–1131, 1989.
22. Cotler, J.M.; Herbison, G.J.; Nasuti, J.F.; et al. Closed reduction of traumatic cervical spine dislocation using traction weights up to 140 pounds. Spine 18:386–390, 1993.
23. Curylo, L.J.; Mason, H.C.; Bohlman, H.H.; et al. Tortuous course of the vertebral artery and anterior cervical decompression: A cadaveric and clinical case study. Spine 25:2860–2864, 2000.

24. Darsaut, T.E.; Ashforth, R.; Bhargava, R.; et al. A pilot study of magnetic resonance imaging-guided closed reduction of cervical spine fractures. Spine 31:2085–2090, 2006.

25. Do Koh, Y.; Lim, T.H.; Won, Y.J.; et al. A biomechanical comparison of modern anterior and posterior plate fixation of the cervical spine. Spine 26:15–21, 2001.

26. Doran, S.E.; Papadopoulos, S.M.; Ducker, T.B.; et al. Magnetic resonance imaging documentation of coexistent traumatic locked facets of the cervical spine and disc herniation. J Neurosurg 79:341–345, 1993.

27. Duggal, N.; Chamberlain, R.H.; Park, S.C.; et al. Unilateral cervical facet dislocation: Biomechanics of fixation. Spine 30:E164–E168, 2005.

28. Ebraheim, N.A.; Klausner, T.; Xu, R.; et al. Safe lateral-mass screw lengths in the Roy-Camille and Magerl techniques. An anatomic study. Spine 23:1739–1742, 1998.

29. Einsiedel, T.; Schmelz, A.; Arand, M.; et al. Injuries of the cervical spine in patients with ankylosing spondylitis: Experience at two trauma centers. J Neurosurg Spine 5:33–45, 2006.

30. Eismont, F.J.; Arena, M.J.; Green, B.A. Extrusion of an intervertebral disc associated with traumatic subluxation or dislocation of cervical facets. Case report. J Bone Joint Surg [Am]. 73:1555–1560, 1991.

31. El Masry, M.A.; Badawy, W.S.; Chan, D. Combined anterior and posterior stabilisation for treating an unstable cervical spine fracture in a patient with long standing ankylosing spondylitis. Injury 35:1064–1067, 2004.

32. Epstein, N.E. From the neurointerventional lab… intraoperative cervical vertebral artery injury treated by tamponade and endovascular coiling. Spine J 3:404–405, 2003.

33. Favero, K.J.; Van Peteghem, P.K. The quadrangular fragment fracture. Roentgenographic features and treatment protocol. Clin Orthop Relat Res 239:40–46, 1989.

34. Fehlings, M.G.; Cooper, P.R.; Errico, T.J. Posterior plates in the management of cervical instability: Long-term results in 44 patients. J Neurosurg 81:341–349, 1994.

35. Fisher, C.G.; Dvorak, M.F.; Leith, J.; et al. Comparison of outcomes for unstable lower cervical flexion teardrop fractures managed with halo thoracic vest versus anterior corpectomy and plating. Spine 27:160–166, 2002.

36. Goldberg, W.; Mueller, C.; Panacek, E.; et al. Distribution and patterns of blunt traumatic cervical spine injury. Ann Emerg Med 38:17–21, 2001.

37. Grant, G.A.; Mirza, S.K.; Chapman, J.R.; et al. Risk of early closed reduction in cervical spine subluxation injuries. J Neurosurg 90:13–18, 1999.

38. Guest, J.; Eleraky, M.A.; Apostolides, P.J.; et al. Traumatic central cord syndrome: Results of surgical management. J Neurosurg 97:25–32, 2002.

39. Hadley, M.N.; Fitzpatrick, B.C.; Sonntag, V.K.; et al. Facet fracture–dislocation injuries of the cervical spine. Neurosurgery 30:661–666, 1992.

40. Harrington, J.F.; Likavec, M.J.; Smith, A.S. Disc herniation in cervical fracture subluxation. Neurosurgery 29:374–379, 1991.

41. Harris, J.H.; Yeakley, J.W. Hyperextension–dislocation of the cervical spine. Ligament injuries demonstrated by magnetic resonance imaging. J Bone Joint Surg [Br] 74:567–570, 1992.

42. Hart, R.A. Cervical facet dislocation: When is magnetic resonance imaging indicated? Spine 27:116–117, 2002.

43. Heary, R.F.; Albert, T.J.; Ludwig, S.C.; et al. Surgical anatomy of the vertebral arteries. Spine 21:2074–2080, 1996.

44. Heller, J.G.; Silcox, D.H., III; Sutterlin, C.E., III. Complications of posterior cervical plating. Spine 20:2442–2448, 1995.

45. Henriques, T.; Olerud, C.; Bergman, A.; et al. Distractive flexion injuries of the subaxial cervical spine treated with anterior plate alone. J Spinal Disord Tech 17:1–7, 2004.

46. Jeanneret, B.; Magerl, F.; Ward, E.H.; et al. Posterior stabilization of the cervical spine with hook plates. Spine 16:S56–S63, 1991.

47. Johnson, M.G.; Fisher, C.G.; Boyd, M.; et al. The radiographic failure of single segment anterior cervical plate fixation in traumatic cervical flexion distraction injuries. Spine 29:2815–2820, 2004.

48. Karaikovic, E.E.; Daubs, M.D.; Madsen, R.W.; et al. Morphologic characteristics of human cervical pedicles. Spine 22:493–500, 1997.

49. Kast, E.; Mohr, K.; Richter, H.P.; et al. Complications of transpedicular screw fixation in the cervical spine. Eur Spine J 15:327–334, 2006.

50. Koivikko, M.P.; Myllynen, P.; Karjalainen, M.; et al. Conservative and operative treatment in cervical burst fractures. Arch Orthop Trauma Surg 120:448–451, 2000.

51. Kothe, R.; Ruther, W.; Schneider, E.; et al. Biomechanical analysis of transpedicular screw fixation in the subaxial cervical spine. Spine 29:1869–1875, 2004.

52. Kwon, B.K.; Beiner, J.; Grauer, J.N.; et al. Anterior/posterior operative reduction of cervical spine dislocations: Techniques and literature review. Curr Opin Orthop 14:193–199, 2003.

53. Kwon, B.K.; Dvorak, M.F.; Fisher, C.G.; et al. A Prospective Randomized Comparison of Anterior Versus Posterior Stabilization for Unilateral Facet Injuries. Banff, Alberta, 2005.

54. Kwon, B.K.; Song, F.; Morrison, W.B.; et al. Morphologic evaluation of cervical spine anatomy with computed tomography: Anterior cervical plate fixation considerations. J Spinal Disord Tech 17:102–107, 2004.

55. Louis, R. Spinal stability as defined by the three-column spine concept. Anat Clin 7:33–42, 1985.

56. Lowery, D.W.; Wald, M.M.; Browne, B.J.; et al. Epidemiology of cervical spine injury victims. Ann Emerg Med 38:12–16, 2001.

57. Lu, J.; Ebraheim, N.A.; Yang, H.; et al. Anatomic bases for anterior spinal surgery: Surgical anatomy of the cervical vertebral body and disc space. Surg Radiol Anat 21:235–239, 1999.

58. Ludwig, S.C.; Kramer, D.L.; Balderston, R.A.; et al. Placement of pedicle screws in the human cadaveric cervical spine: Comparative accuracy of three techniques. Spine 25:1655–1667, 2000.

59. Ludwig, S.C.; Vaccaro, A.R.; Balderston, R.A.; et al. Immediate quadriparesis after manipulation for bilateral cervical facet subluxation. A case report. J Bone Joint Surg [Am] 79:587–590, 1997.

60. Mahale, Y.J.; Silver, J.R.; Henderson, N.J. Neurological complications of the reduction of cervical spine dislocations. J Bone Joint Surg [Br] 75:403–409, 1993.

61. Mercer, S.; Bogduk, N. The ligaments and annulus fibrosus of human adult cervical intervertebral discs. Spine 24:619–626, 1999.

62. Middleditch, A.; Oliver, J. Functional Anatomy of the Spine. Oxford, Butterworth Heinemann, 1991.

63. Moore, T.A.; Vaccaro, A.R.; Anderson, P.A. Classification of lower cervical spine injuries. Spine 31: S37–S43, 2006.

64. Mountney, J.; Murphy, A.J.; Fowler, J.L. Lessons learned from cervical pseudoarthrosis in ankylosing spondylitis. Eur Spine J 14:689–693, 2005.

65. Neo, M.; Sakamoto, T.; Fujibayashi, S.; et al. The clinical risk of vertebral artery injury from cervical pedicle screws inserted in degenerative vertebrae. Spine 30:2800–2805, 2005.

66. Nightingale, R.W.; McElhaney, J.H.; Richardson, W.J.; et al. Experimental impact injury to the cervical spine: Relating motion of the head and the mechanism of injury. J Bone Joint Surg [Am] 78:412–421, 1996.

67. Olerud, C.; Jonsson, H., Jr. Compression of the cervical spine cord after reduction of fracture dislocations. Report of 2 cases. Acta Orthop Scand 62:599–601, 1991.

68. Onan, O.A.; Heggeness, M.H.; Hipp, J.A. A motion analysis of the cervical facet joint. Spine 23:430–439, 1998.

69. Pait, T.G.; Killefer, J.A.; Arnautovic, K.I. Surgical anatomy of the anterior cervical spine: The disc space, vertebral artery, and associated bony structures. Neurosurgery 39:769–776, 1996.

70. Pait, T.G.; McAllister, P.V.; Kaufman, H.H. Quadrant anatomy of the articular pillars (lateral cervical mass) of the cervical spine. J Neurosurg 82:1011–1014, 1995.

71. Panjabi, M.M.; Chen, N.C.; Shin, E.K.; et al. The cortical shell architecture of human cervical vertebral bodies. Spine 26:2478–2484, 2001.

72. Panjabi, M.M.; Crisco, J.J.; Vasavada, A.; et al. Mechanical properties of the human cervical spine as shown by three-dimensional load-displacement curves. Spine 26:2692–2700, 2001.

73. Panjabi, M.M.; Duranceau, J.S.; Oxland, T.R.; et al. Multidirectional instabilities of traumatic cervical spine injuries in a porcine model. Spine 14:1111–1115, 1989.

74. Panjabi, M.M.; Oxland, T.R.; Parks, E.H. Quantitative anatomy of cervical spine ligaments. Part II. Middle and lower cervical spine. J Spinal Disord 4:277–285, 1991.

75. Panjabi, M.M.; Pearson, A.M.; Ito, S.; et al. Cervical spine ligament injury during simulated frontal impact. Spine 29:2395–2403, 2004.

76. Panjabi, M.M.; Shin, E.K.; Chen, N.C.; et al. Internal morphology of human cervical pedicles. Spine 25:1197–1205, 2000.

77. Panjabi, M.M.; White, A.A., III; Johnson, R.M. Cervical spine mechanics as a function of transection of components. J Biomech 8:327–336, 1975.

78. Papagelopoulos, P.J.; Currier, B.L.; Neale, P.G.; et al. Biomechanical evaluation of posterior screw fixation in cadaveric cervical spines. Clin Orthop Relat Res 411:13–24, 2003.

79. Payer, M. Surgical management of cervical fractures in ankylosing spondylitis using a combined posterior–anterior approach. J Clin Neurosci 13:73–77, 2006.

80. Pfeifer, B.A.; Freidberg, S.R.; Jewell, E.R. Repair of injured vertebral artery in anterior cervical procedures. Spine 19:1471–1474, 1994.

81. Pitzen, T.; Lane, C.; Goertzen, D.; et al. Anterior cervical plate fixation: Biomechanical effectiveness as a function of posterior element injury. J Neurosurg 99:84–90, 2003.

82. Przybylski, G.J.; Carlin, G.J.; Patel, P.R.; et al. Human anterior and posterior cervical longitudinal ligaments possess similar tensile properties. J Orthop Res 14:1005–1008, 1996.

83. Przybylski, G.J.; Patel, P.R.; Carlin, G.J.; et al. Quantitative anthropometry of the subatlantal cervical longitudinal ligaments. Spine 23:893–898, 1998.

84. Razack, N.; Green, B.A.; Levi, A.D. The management of traumatic cervical bilateral facet fracture–dislocations with unicortical anterior plates. J Spinal Disord 13:374–381, 2000.

85. Rezcallah, A.T.; Xu, R.; Ebraheim, N.A.; et al. Axial computed tomography of the pedicle in the lower cervical spine. Am J Orthop 30:59–61, 2001.

86. Rhee, J.M.; Kimmerly, W.S.; Smucker, J.D. Infolding of the ligamentum flavum: A cause of spinal cord compression after reduction of cervical facet injuries. J Spinal Disord Tech 19:208–212, 2006.

87. Rhee, J.M.; Kraiwattanapong, C.; Hutton, W.C. A comparison of pedicle and lateral mass screw construct stiffnesses at the cervicothoracic junction: A biomechanical study. Spine 30:E636–E640, 2005.

88. Rizzolo, S.J.; Piazza, M.R.; Cotler, J.M.; et al. Intervertebral disc injury complicating cervical spine trauma. Spine 16:S187–S189, 1991.

89. Robertson, P.A.; Ryan, M.D. Neurological deterioration after reduction of cervical subluxation. Mechanical compression by disc tissue. J Bone Joint Surg [Br] 74:224–227, 1992.

90. Rockswold, G.L.; Bergman, T.A.; Ford, S.E. Halo immobilization and surgical fusion: Relative indications and effectiveness in the treatment of 140 cervical spine injuries. J Trauma 30:893–898, 1990.

91. Rorabeck, C.H.; Rock, M.G.; Hawkins, R.J.; et al. Unilateral facet dislocation of the cervical spine. An analysis of the results of treatment in 26 patients. Spine 12:23–27, 1987.

92. Roy-Camille, R.R.; Sailant, G.; Mazel, C. Internal fixation of the unstable cervical spine by posterior osteosynthesis with plate and screws. In Cervical Spine Research Society, ed. The Cervical Spine, 2nd ed. Philadelphia, Lippincott, pp. 390–404, 1989.

93. Samartzis, D.; Anderson, D.G.; Shen, F.H. Multiple and simultaneous spine fractures in ankylosing spondylitis: Case report. Spine 30:E711–E715, 2005.

94. Schlicke, L.H.; White, A.A., III; Panjabi, M.M.; et al. A quantitative study of vertebral displacement and angulation in the normal cervical spine under axial load. Clin Orthop Relat Res 140:47–49, 1979.

95. Schmitz, B.; Pitzen, T.; Beuter, T.; et al. Regional variations in the thickness of cervical spine endplates as measured by computed tomography. Acta Radiol 45:53–58, 2004.

96. Sears, W.; Fazl, M. Prediction of stability of cervical spine fracture managed in the halo vest and indications for surgical intervention. J Neurosurg 72:426–432, 1990.

97. Seybold, E.A.; Baker, J.A.; Criscitiello, A.A.; et al. Characteristics of unicortical and bicortical lateral mass screws in the cervical spine. Spine 24:2397–2403, 1992.

98. Shanmuganathan, K.; Mirvis, S.E.; Levine, A.M. Rotational injury of cervical facets: CT analysis of fracture patterns with implications for management and neurologic outcome. AJR Am J Roentgenol 163:1165–1169, 1994.

99. Shea, M.; Wittenberg, R.H.; Edwards, W.T.; et al. In vitro hyperextension injuries in the human cadaveric cervical spine. J Orthop Res 10:911–916, 1992.

100. Sim, E.; Vaccaro, A.R.; Berzlanovich, A.; et al. In vitro genesis of subaxial cervical unilateral facet dislocations through sequential soft tissue ablation. Spine 26:1317–1323, 2001.

101. Smith, M.D.; Emery, S.E.; Dudley, A.; et al. Vertebral artery injury during anterior decompression of the cervical spine. A retrospective review of ten patients. J Bone Joint Surg [Br] 75:410–415, 1993.

102. Sonntag, V.K. Management of bilateral locked facets of the cervical spine. Neurosurgery 8:150–152, 1981.

103. Southern, E.P.; Oxland, T.R.; Panjabi, M.M.; et al. Cervical spine injury patterns in three modes of high-speed trauma: A biomechanical porcine model. J Spinal Disord 3:316–328, 1990.

104. Sutterlin, C.E., III; McAfee, P.C.; Warden, K.E.; et al. A biomechanical evaluation of cervical spinal stabilization methods in a bovine model. Static and cyclical loading. Spine 13:795–802, 1988.

105. Takeshita, K.; Peterson, E.T.; Bylski-Austrow, D.; et al. The nuchal ligament restrains cervical spine flexion. Spine 29:E388–E393, 2004.

106. Taylor, J.R.; Twomey, L.T. Acute injuries to cervical joints. An autopsy study of neck sprain. Spine 18:1115–1122, 1993.

107. Tonetti, J.; Peoc'h, M.; Merloz, P.; et al. Elastic reinforcement and thickness of the joint capsules of the lower cervical spine. Surg Radiol Anat 21:35–39, 1999.

108. Ugur, H.C.; Attar, A.; Uz, A.; et al. Surgical anatomic evaluation of the cervical pedicle and adjacent neural structures. Neurosurgery 47:1162–1168, 2000.

109. Vaccaro, A.R.; Falatyn, S.P.; Flanders, A.E.; et al. Magnetic resonance evaluation of the intervertebral disc, spinal ligaments, and spinal cord before and after closed traction reduction of cervical spine dislocations. Spine 24:1210–1217, 1999.

110. Vaccaro, A.R.; Klein, G.R.; Thaller, J.B.; et al. Distraction extension injuries of the cervical spine. J Spinal Disord 14:193–200, 2001.

111. Vaccaro, A.R.; Madigan, L.; Schweitzer, M.E.; et al. Magnetic resonance imaging analysis of soft tissue disruption after flexion–distraction injuries of the subaxial cervical spine. Spine 26:1866–1872, 2001.

112. Vaccaro, A.R.; Nachwalter, R.S. Is magnetic resonance imaging indicated before reduction of a unilateral cervical facet dislocation? Spine 27:117–118, 2002.

113. White, A.A.; Panjabi, M.M. Clinical Biomechanics of the Spine, 2nd ed. Philadelphia, Lippincott, 1990.

114. White, A.A.; Panjabi, M.M.; Saha, S.; et al. Biomechanics of the axially loaded cervical spine: Development of a safe clinical test for ruptured cervical ligaments. J Bone Joint Surg [Am] 57:582, 1975.

115. White, A.A., III; Johnson, R.M.; Panjabi, M.M.; et al. Biomechanical analysis of clinical stability in the cervical spine. Clin Orthop Relat Res 109:85–96, 1975.

116. Wimberley, D.W.; Vaccaro, A.R.; Goyal, N.; et al. Acute quadriplegia following closed traction reduction of a cervical facet dislocation in the setting of ossification of the posterior longitudinal ligament: Case report. Spine 30:E433–E438, 2005.

117. Yusof, M.I.; Ming, L.K.; Abdullah, M.S.; et al. Computerized tomographic measurement of the cervical pedicles diameter in a Malaysian population and the feasibility for transpedicular fixation. Spine 31:E221–E224, 2006.

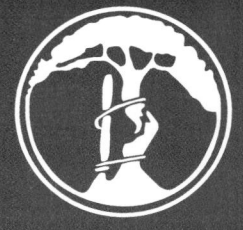

CHAPTER 30

Thoracic and Upper Lumbar Spine Injuries

**Yu-Po Lee, M.D., Cary Templin, M.D.,
Frank Eismont, M.D., and Steven R. Garfin, M.D.**

The primary goals in caring for patients who have sustained thoracolumbar spinal trauma include preservation of life, protection of neurologic function, and the restoration and maintenance of spinal stability and alignment. Accomplishing these goals while managing thoracolumbar fractures can be challenging as these patients often have other injuries that also must be concurrently addressed. Furthermore, patients with neurologic compromise or spinal instability must have their injuries taken care of in a timely fashion, which adds to the complexity of caring for them. The chances of a successful outcome can be optimized, however, when the treating physician understands the anatomy of the spinal column, appreciates the biomechanics of the injury, and is aware of the expanding treatment options available for the care of a spine-injured patient.

HISTORICAL BACKGROUND

The earliest written record of spinal cord injury is found in the Edwin Smith Papyrus (3000 BCE).[26] Later, Egyptian physicians noted that patients with vertebral trauma often had paralysis of the arms and legs and urinary incontinence, thus suggesting an association among vertebral injuries, spinal cord damage, and loss of function.

Celsus made the next important contribution of spinal cord trauma when he distinguished cervical from thoracolumbar spinal cord injuries. He reported that fractures of the cervical spine produced respiratory embarrassment and vomiting, whereas trauma to the lower portion of the spinal column produced paralysis of the lower extremities and urinary incontinence. He also expanded on Hippocrates' concept of manual extension for reduction of spinal deformities.[26]

In the 16th century, Ambroise Paré readdressed the problem of spinal injury.[19] He accurately described the symptoms of cord compression as follows:

"Amongst the symptoms are the stupidity, or numbness or palsy of the arms, legs, fundament and bladder, which take away their sense and motion, so that their urine and excrements come from them against their wills and knowledge, or else are wholly suppressed. Which when they happen saith Hippocrates, you may foretell that death is

at hand, by reason that the spinal marrow is hurt. . . . Having made such a prognostication, you may make an incision so to take forth the splinters of the broken vertebrae, which driven in press the spinal marrow in the nerves thereof."

Modern management of vertebral column trauma arrived with the development of anesthesia and radiography. In the 1920s, based heavily on principles advocated by Guttman, treatment of vertebral trauma emphasized closed reduction of fractures.[68] Davis proposed a method of reduction in which the patient was anesthetized and placed in a prone position.[33] An overhead pulley suspension raised the lower limbs and produced marked hyperextension. The physician then made a manual thrust over the fractured vertebra in an attempt to realign the fracture. When reduction was achieved, the patient was immobilized in a plaster jacket. In 1931, Watson-Jones modified this technique by using tables of different heights to hyperextend the spine and obtain reduction.[168]

Internal fixation of thoracic and lumbar spinal fractures began after World War II with the development of spinous process plating for unstable fractures. Later, Dickson and colleagues revolutionized spinal care and rehabilitation with the introduction of his posterior spinal instrumentation devices.[40] Since then surgical techniques and instruments have proliferated and have continued to improve the ability to anatomically reduce and internally stabilize the injured spinal column. Neurologic recovery, however, has remained unchanged or only slightly improved over the results obtained with postural reduction and nonoperative care.[158,162,178] At this time, the major predictable benefits of internal fixation of spinal fractures are decreased hospital stay, early rehabilitation, and prevention of deformity.[158,162,178]

ANATOMY

The thoracolumbar spine is characterized by a dynamic and complex interaction between the bony vertebral elements, disks, and interconnecting ligaments. A solid understanding of this anatomy is helpful in making sound diagnostic and therapeutic decisions.

The human spine has 12 thoracic and 5 lumbar vertebrae with interspaced intervertebral disks. Stagnara and associates studied spinal alignment in healthy persons age 20 to 29 years without back complaints.[153] Wide variation was noted in this healthy population, the range of thoracic kyphosis being 7 to 63°, with 91 percent between 18 and 51° (Fig. 30-1 A). In the thoracic spine, this configuration is maintained by the wedge-shaped vertebral bodies and disks, which are larger posteriorly than anteriorly. Across the thoracolumbar junction (T10-L2), where most injuries occur,

the normal range his reported to be 0 to 10° kyphosis. In the lumbar spine, the average lordosis in this same group of normal people was 50°, with a range of 32 to 84°; 92 percent of these individuals had between 42 and 74° of lordosis (Fig. 30-1, B). In the lumbar spine, the disks have an increased height anteriorly, which helps create lordosis.

White and Panjabi investigated the types of motion present throughout the spine (Fig. 30-2).[171,172] The thoracic spine has significantly less flexion–extension motion than the cervical or lumbar spines. In the cervical spine

---

FIGURE 30-1 | **A,** *The distribution of thoracic kyphosis in 100 French people (43 women and 57 men). The distribution of lumbar lordosis in the same group of 100 French people. (**A, B,** Data from Stagnara, P.; De Mauroy, J.C.; Dran, G.; et al. Reciprocal angulation of vertebral bodies in a sagittal plane: Approach to references for the evaluation of kyphosis and lordosis. Spine 7:335–342, 1982.)*

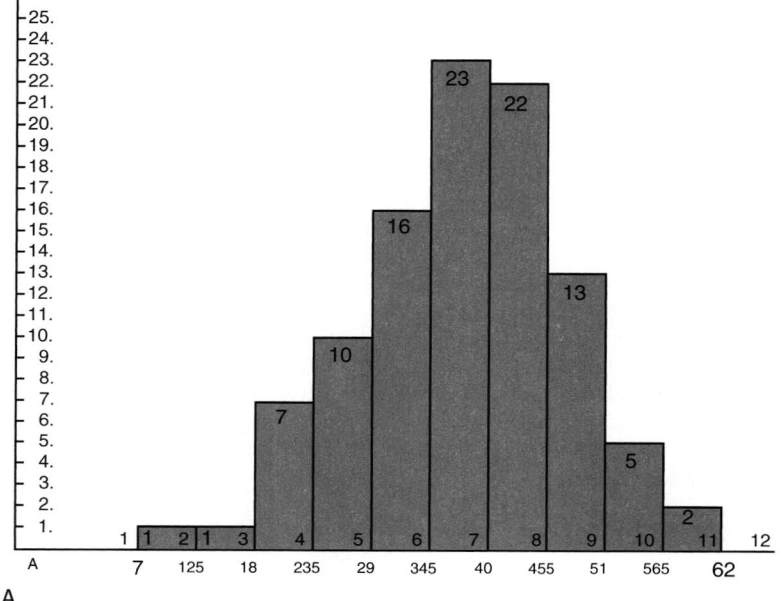

A

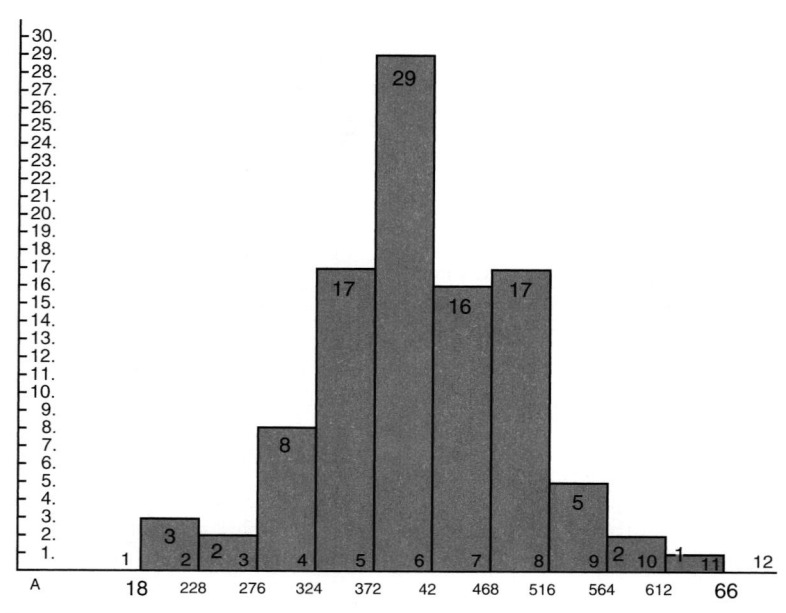

B

FIGURE 30-2 *The motion present at each level of the spine. (Data from multiple reviews and from the experimental work of White, A.A.; Panjabi, M.M. The basic kinematics of the human spine: A review of past and current knowledge. Spine 3:12–20, 1978.)*

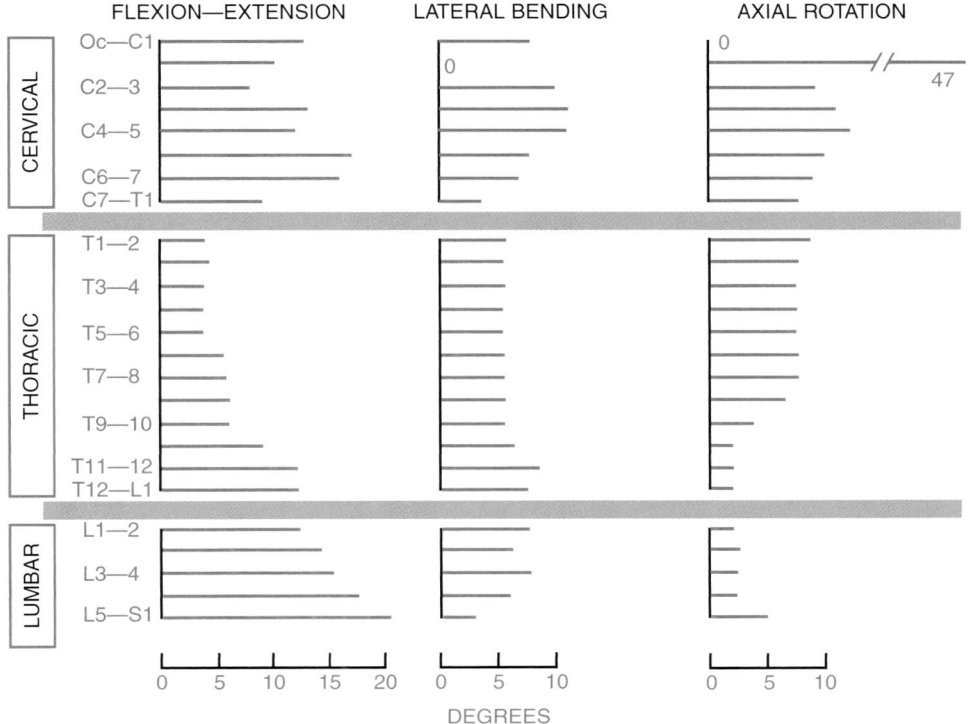

from the occiput to C7, the average motion between flexion and extension is 13° per level, with a range of 8 to 17°. At C7-T1 this motion decreases to 9°, and in the thoracic spine from T1 to T6, each level has only 4° of total flexion–extension motion. From the T6-T7 to the T12-L1 levels, flexion–extension motion gradually increases from 5 to 12°, in contrast to the average 15° flexion–extension motion at each lumbar level (range of 12–20°).

The thoracic spine is less capable of bending laterally than the cervical spine. Lateral bending in the cervical spine from occiput to C7 average 8° per level, whereas it is only about 6° per level from T1 to T10. At the area of the T10-L1 thoracolumbar junction, lateral bending increases to an average of 8° per level. In the lumbar spine, this motion decreases to about 6° per level. Much of the thoracic-level rigidity is related to the presence of the rib cage and the costovertebral articulations.[123,154,167]

Axial rotation in the thoracic spine averages 8° from T1 to T8 but decreases to approximately 2° per level below T10. Axial rotation is greater in the thoracic spine than in the lumbar spine because the facets are aligned in the coronal plane, as opposed to the more sagittal alignment that occurs in the lumbar spine (Fig. 30-3).[33,171] The transition region for facet orientation is the area from T10 to T12. Because of this alteration in facet orientation, the motion characteristics of the lower thoracic spine more closely resemble those of the lumbar spine. In the lumbar spine, the facet joints gradually attain an almost true sagittal orientation at the L4-L5 level. Such alignment provides significant restriction to rotation and side bending.

The thoracolumbar junction is more susceptible to injury than any other adjacent portions of the spine. Approximately 50 percent of all vertebral body fractures and 40 percent of all spinal cord injuries occur from T11 to L2. This greater susceptibility to injury can be explained by the decease in rib restraint, changes in stiffness for flexion–extension and rotation, and changes in disk size and shape, which occur relatively acutely in the transitional area between the upper thoracic and the midlumbar spine.

The conus medullaris usually begins at T11 and, in most males, ends at the L1-L2 disk space. The conus in females frequently stops slightly more proximally. The conus medullaris can occasionally extend much lower into the lumbar spine and is often associated with a hypertrophic filum terminale. The neural elements of the lumbar spine below the L1-L2 disk are usually purely spinal nerve rootlets (cauda equine). In addition, an extensive collateral circulation is located distal to the nerve roots and proximal to the spinal cord, thus making this region less prone to vascular compromise and more likely to recover from a spinal cord injury.[127] The thoracic spinal cord has relatively poor vascularity and limited collateral circulation compared with the cervical spinal cord and conus medullaris.[41,42] Adamkiewicz in 1882 described the blood supply of the spinal cord, including a relatively constant medullary artery known as the great medullary artery or the artery of Adamkiewicz. This artery may be injured as a result of trauma to or thoracic disk herniation of one of the lateral or posterolateral extracavitary approaches. Injury to this artery may cause serious ischemic insult to the cord and

FIGURE 30-3 *The rotation in the midthoracic spine and at the thoracolumbar junction. **A,** The rotation at T5-T6 is represented by the arrow between the spinous processes. The inset shows how the lamina of T5 glides over the posterior elements of T6 with no resistance to rotation. **B,** Following facetectomy, the motion present between T5 and T6 (arrow) is unchanged from A. **C,** The rotation present between T12 and L1 is represented by the arrow between the spinous processes. Because of the sagittal orientation of the facets (inset), rotation is markedly restricted. **D,** Following a bilateral facetectomy, the motion between T12 and L1 (arrow) is markedly increased. The restriction from the sagittally oriented facets has been eliminated.*

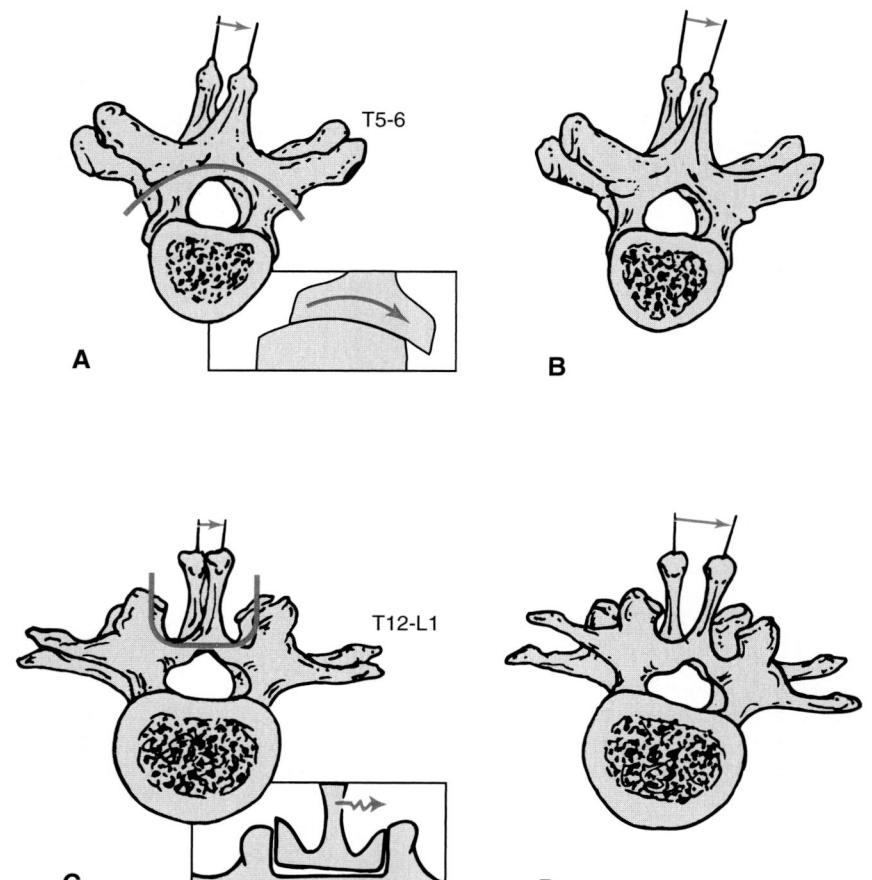

lead to paralysis. In most people, the artery of Adamkiewicz originates from the intercostal, artery on the left side between T10 and T12, where it joins the nerve root sleeve and becomes intradural. The artery then crosses one to three disk spaces, at which point it anastomoses with the anterior spinal artery. Knowledge of this artery and its course is important during certain approaches and may explain certain neurologic deficits that may not recover despite adequate anterior decompression.[107]

The spinal canal in the midthoracic region is considerably narrower than in the cervical or lumbar region.[46,136] At the T6 level, the spinal canal has a circular configuration with a 16-mm diameter. In the middle to lower cervical spine, the canal is 23 × 14 mm, and in the lumbosacral region, it is 26 × 17 mm. The small size of the thoracic spinal canal must be appreciated for two reasons. First, because less space is available, even minor spinal column displacement may produce significant spinal cord compression.

As Dommisse and others have shown, in the thoracic spine the free space between the spinal cord and the borders of the spinal canal is relatively small.[41,42] Although the thoracic cord tends to be smaller than the cervical and lumbar

enlargements, the free space also narrows. In addition, the blood supply in the middle and lower thoracic spine is less abundant than elsewhere in the spinal cord. Adding to the variability is the location of the conus medullaris, with terminations in the general population following almost a bell-shaped curve from the T12 to the L3 level.[41,42]

The cord is usually wider in the lateral plane than in the anterior-to-posterior direction. Elliott demonstrated that the largest diameter of the cervical enlargement, which is at approximately C5-C6, was 13.2 mm in the lateral plane and 7.7 mm from anterior to posterior.[46] In the thoracic region, the smallest measurements were 8 mm laterally and 6.5 mm from anterior to posterior, and the lumbosacral enlargement was 9.6 and 8.0 mm, respectively.[46] The dimensions can be correlated with the space available within the spinal canal. Aebi and Thalgott demonstrated that the largest area (i.e., the space available in the cervical canal) was 24.5 mm laterally and 14.7 mm from anterior to posterior in the thoracic region, thus correlating with the small size of the spinal cord at this location.[3] The largest space available was 17.2 mm in the lateral plane and 16.8 mm anterior to posterior. At the level of the lumbar enlargement, it was 23.4 mm laterally and 17.4 mm from anterior to posterior. In general, the cord occupies approximately half the space available in each direction. In the thoracic spine, according to Dommisse, the anterior-to-posterior diameter of the spinal canal changes minimally; it averages approximately 13 mm throughout but increases to 15 mm in the lower thoracic spine.[42] His measurements of interpedicular distance (lateral measurement) averaged about 15 mm at the smallest point (approximately T6) and increased to 17 mm at T10-T11.

The morphometry of the pedicles of the thoracic and lumbar spines varies considerably from level to level, as well as from patient to patient.[17,98] Zindrick and colleagues, in an evaluation of 2900 pedicles, determined pedicle isthmus widths and pedicle angles in the sagittal and transverse planes.[182] In general, pedicle isthmus widths were significantly smaller in the thoracic spine than in the lumbar spine (Fig. 30-4, A, B). The pedicle angles in the transverse plane varied from 27° medial inclination (in a posterior-to-anterior direction) in the proximal thoracic spine to approximately 1° at T11 and −4° at T12. At L1, the angle again inclines medially at 11° and gradually increases to approximately 30° at L5 (Fig. 30-4, C). In an anatomic study investigating the internal architecture of thoracic pedicles,

Kothe and associates showed that the medial wall is two to three times thicker than the lateral wall.[95] This difference in thickness could explain the fact that most pedicle fractures related to pedicle screw insertion occur laterally. An understanding of these dimensions and angles is important when considering the use of pedicle screw fixation systems to stabilize thoracic and thoracolumbar spinal injuries.

The flexion axis of the normal thoracic spine and the thoracolumbar junction occurs at the middle to posterior third junction of the vertebral body.[135,174] This location of the axis results in an anterior compressive force moment that is approximately one fourth the length of the posterior tensile force.[150] Brown and colleagues in 1957 demonstrated that posterior elements fail under tension at approximately 400 lb.[27] This amount of posterior force corresponds to a resultant anterior compressive force of approximately 1200 to 1600 lb. Comprehension of this biomechanical principle is essential to gain an understanding of spinal stability (described later). In the thoracic spine, the human body's center of gravity is anterior to the spine. As a result, the resting condition in the thoracic spine and at the thoracolumbar junction is one of vertebral body compression and posterior ligamentous complex tension. In the thoracic spine, the ribs anterior to the spinal

FIGURE 30-4 *An analysis of the morphometric characteristics of the thoracic and lumbar pedicles.* **A,** *The transverse width of the pedicle at each level of the thoracic and lumbar spine is shown. The average pedicle width of the lumbar spine ranges from 9 to 18 mm. In the thoracic spine, all pedicles are smaller than 9 mm.* **B,** *The longitudinal pedicle width of each level in the thoracic and lumbar spine is represented. This peaks at 17 mm at the T11 vertebra, decreasing to 10 mm at T1 and to 14 mm at L5.* **C,** *The transverse angle of the pedicles for each level of the thoracic and lumbar spine is shown. The angle is −4° at the T12 vertebra and increases to 30° at L5 and to 27° at T1. (Redrawn from Zindrick, M.R.; Wiltse, L.L.; Doornik, A.; et al. Analysis of the morphometric characteristics of the thoracic and lumbar pedicles. Spine 12:160–166, 1987.)*

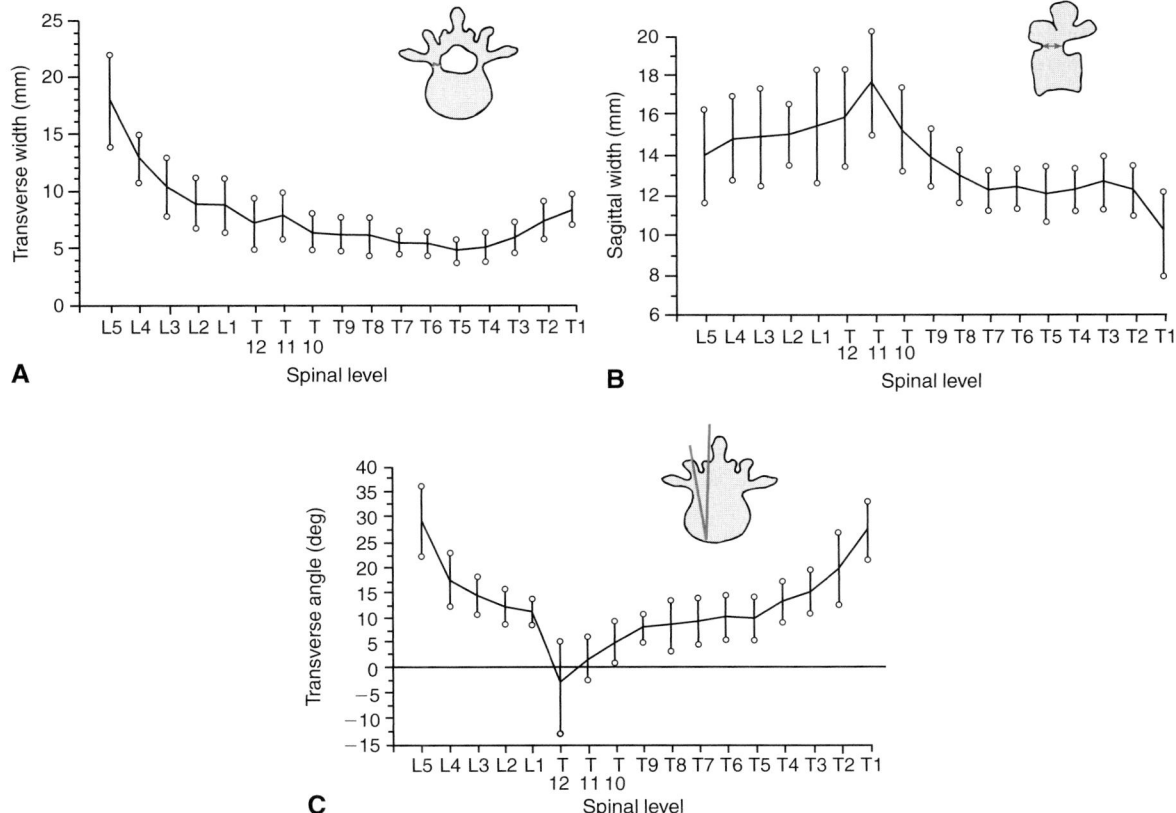

column and the thick ligaments posteriorly, acting in tension, restrict any further forward flexion in the normal situation.[123,154,167] In the lumbar spine, particularly in the more lordotic lower lumbar region, the center of gravity is located more posteriorly, and the posterior elements provide approximately 30% of the weight-bearing support. These considerations are important for realignment or for maintenance of alignment after spinal injury.

One of the important components of the thoracolumbar spinal anatomy is the soft tissue that interconnects the bony elements. The complex interaction of ligaments, disks, and musculature allows for both controlled motion and stability of the spine. Trauma to the soft tissues of the thoracolumbar spine can have profound effects on function and stability.

The anterior longitudinal ligament is a strong, broad-based ligament that runs on the anterior aspect of the vertebral body from the atlas to the sacrum. It is firmly attached to both the ventral aspect of the disk and periosteum of the vertebral body. It is a major contributor to spinal stability and limits hyperextension of the vertebral column. The posterior longitudinal ligament also runs the length of the spinal column, but it is narrower and weaker than its anterior counterpart. Its primary function is to limit hyperflexion. The intervertebral disk is composed of the annulus fibrosus and the nucleus pulposus. The annulus is formed by concentric bands of fibrocartilage that run obliquely from one vertebral body to another. This arrangement allows for some motion, yet is one of the strongest connections between vertebral segments. The nucleus, which is encased in the annulus, acts as a shock absorber for axial forces. Of importance in thoracolumbar trauma is that the disk is essentially an avascular structure that relies on passive diffusion through the end plates and peripheral aspect of the annulus for nutrition. When this structure is disrupted, the potential for healing is limited.

Posteriorly, the lamina are joined by the ligamentum flavum, a broad band of elastic fiber. The spinous processes are joined by a weak interspinous ligament and a strong supraspinous ligament. The intrinsic muscles of the back include the erector spinae group of muscles (spinalis, longissimus, iliocostalis) and the transversospinalis group (rotators, multifidus, and semispinalis). The intrinsic muscles maintain posture and provide movement of the vertebral column. Any deformity resulting from trauma can alter the function of these muscles. In addition, it is important to have an understanding of these muscle groups when considering the various anatomic approaches to the spine described later in this chapter.

MECHANISMS OF INJURY

Frequently, many complex forces occur at the time of injury, each of which has the potential to produce structural damage to the spine. Most often, however, one or two forces account for most of the bone or ligamentous injuries encountered. The forces most commonly associated with thoracic, thoracolumbar, and lumbar spine injuries are axial compression, flexion, lateral compression, flexion–rotation, shear, flexion–distraction, and extension. Each is discussed from a mechanical viewpoint, and their effect on the bone–disk–ligament complex of the spine is described.

Axial Compression

Because of the normal thoracic kyphosis, axial loading in this area usually results in an anterior flexion load on the vertebral body. The resultant spine injuries are discussed under the following section on Flexion.

An axial load in the straight thoracolumbar region (Fig. 30-5) often results in pure compressive loading of the vertebral body.[90] As described by Roaf, this mechanism produces end plate failure, followed by vertebral body compression.[135] With sufficient force, vertical fractures develop through the vertebral body and produce a burst fracture (Fig. 30-6).[39,91] Frederickson and co-workers observed that

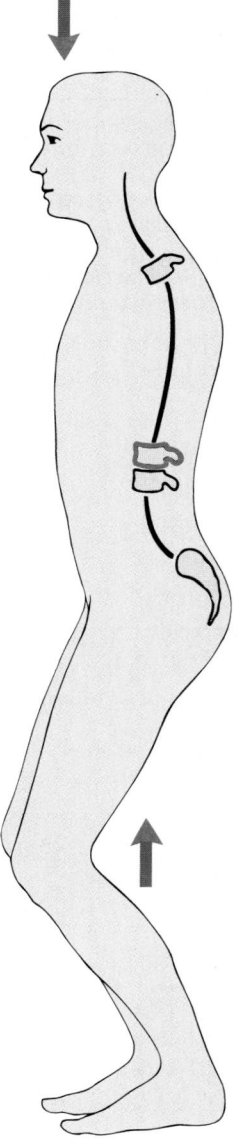

FIGURE 30-5 *Axial compression across the straight thoracolumbar regions results in pure compressive loading of the vertebral body, most often resulting in a thoracolumbar burst fracture.*

FIGURE 30-6 *This burst injury is a result of a fall from height. The patient sustained an incomplete spinal cord injury.* **A,** *An anteroposterior radiograph demonstrates loss of height and interpedicular widening at L2.* **B,** *A lateral radiograph confirms multicolumn involvement, with collapse of the anterior and posterior vertebral walls.* **C,** *Computed tomography reveals a large retropulsed fragment causing considerable compromise of the canal.* **D,** *This patient was treated with anterior decompression and humeral allograft strut and anterior instrumentation augmented with posterior pedicle screws.*

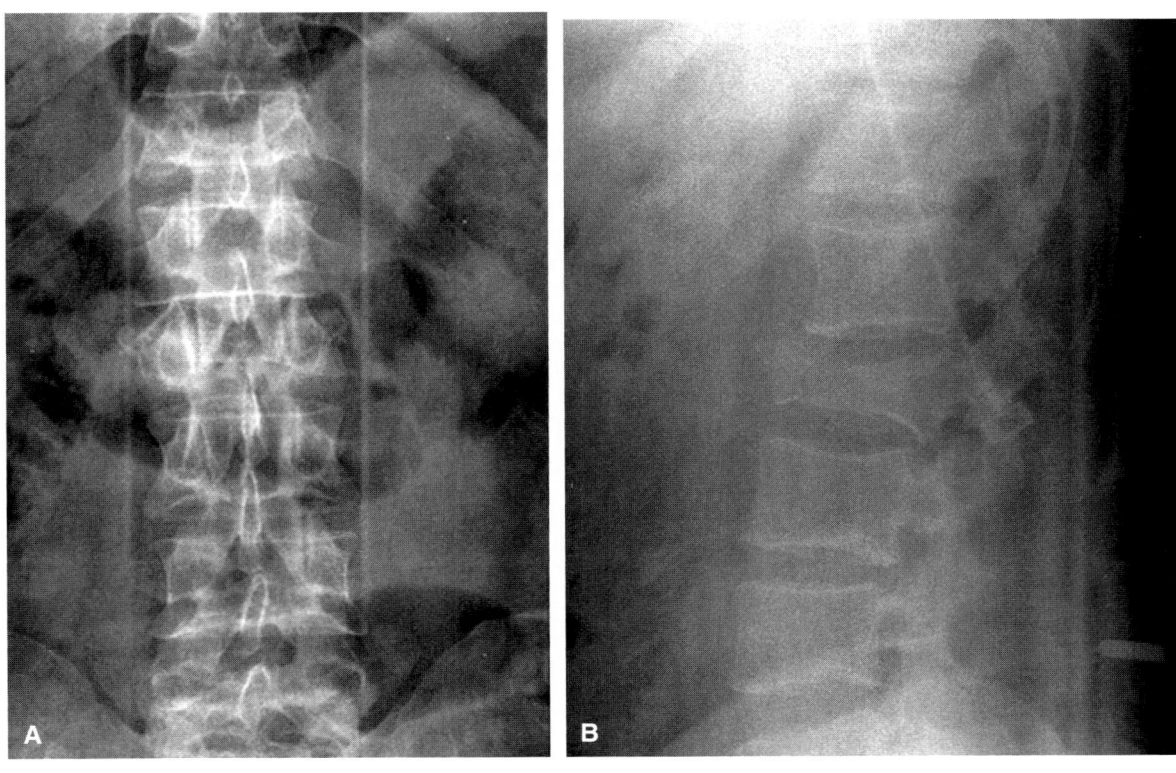

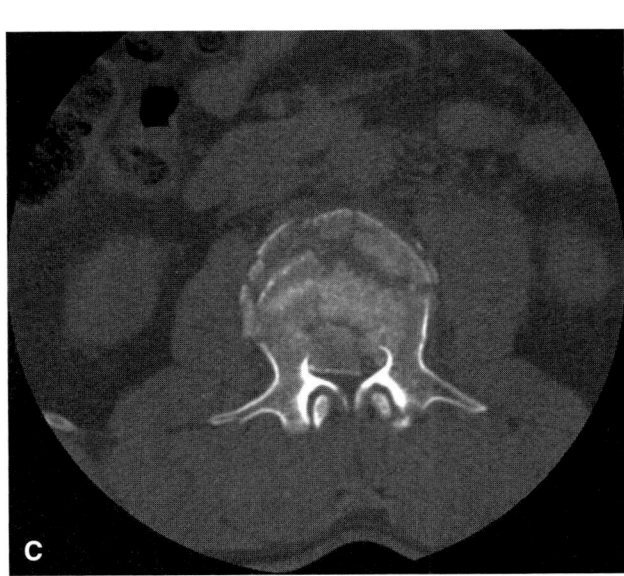

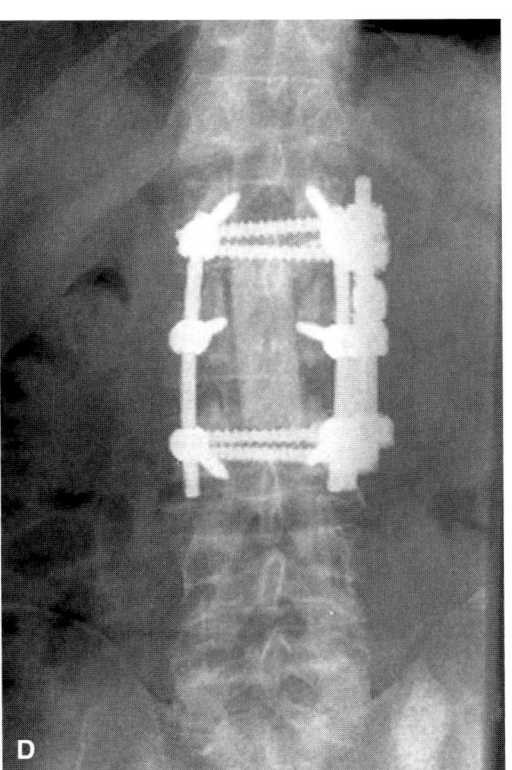

(Continued)

FIGURE 30-6 *(Continued)* **E,** *A lateral radiograph shows reestablishment of the vertebral height and restoration of lordosis.*

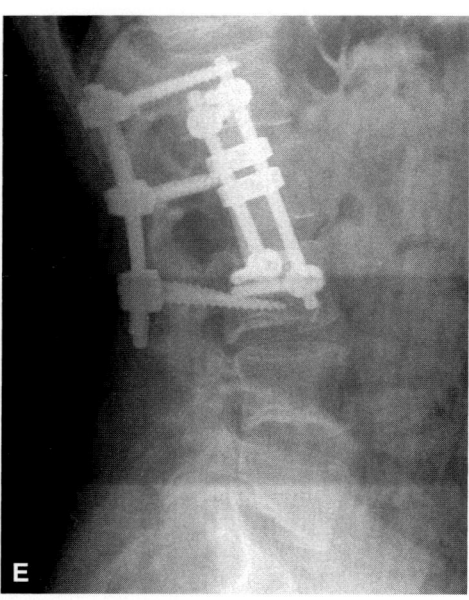

this fracture then propagates through the midportion of the posterior cortex of the vertebral body through vascular foramina.[55,56] With further loading, centripetal displacement of the bone occurs, frequently with disk fragmentation and posterior disruption. This centripetal force can produce fractures at the pedicle–body junction and result in widening of the interpedicular distance and, particularly if a flexion component is present, a greenstick fracture of the lamina. With severe compression, significant disruption of the posterior elements may occur.

Heggeness and Doherty studied the trabecular anatomy of the thoracolumbar vertebrae and documented a trabecular framework that originates from the medial corner of the base of the pedicle and extends in a radial fashion throughout the vertebral body, with thinning of the vertebral cortex near the base of the pedicle at the origin of this trabecular array.[74] Such anatomy may produce a site of stress concentration and may explain the trapezoidal shape of the bony fragments that are frequently retropulsed into the spinal canal in burst-type fractures caused by an axial load (Fig. 30-7).

Flexion

Flexion forces (Fig. 30-8) cause compression anteriorly along the vertebral bodies and disks, with tensile forces

FIGURE 30-7 **A,** *Line drawing of a coronal and sagittal section from a vertebral body illustrating the trabecular array.* **B,** *Computed tomographic image of a burst injury with a typical trapezoidal-shaped fragment taking origin from the point in the posterior cortex where it thins abruptly. Also note that the trapezoidal shape of the fragment roughly parallels the direction of the trabecular arrays. (Line drawing from Heggeness, M.H.; Doherty, B.J. The trabecular anatomy of thoracolumbar vertebrae: Implications for burst fractures. J Anat 191(Pt 2):309–312, 1997.)*

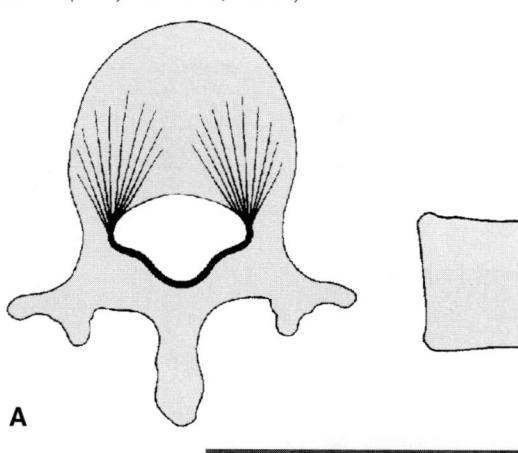
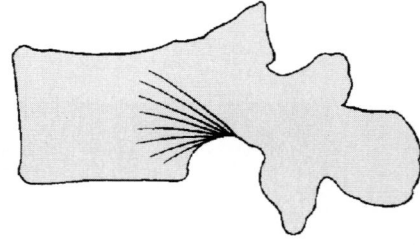

A

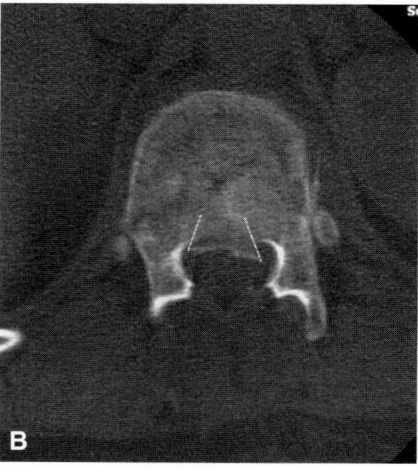

B

FIGURE 30-8 *Flexion forces cause anterior compression of the vertebral bodies and disks and tension in the posterior elements. This usually results in a stable compression fracture of the vertebral bodies anteriorly, but as the force continues, posterior ligamentous disruption may occur.*

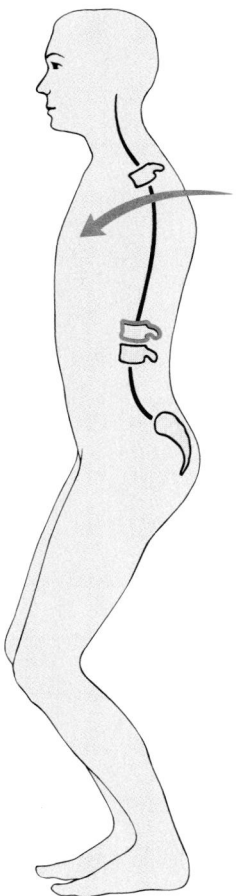

developed posteriorly. The posterior ligaments may not tear, particularly with rapid loading rates, but posterior avulsion fractures may develop.[135] Anteriorly, as the bone fractures and angulation increase, the force is dissipated. With intact posterior ligaments, a stable fracture pattern most often results. Frequently, the middle column remains intact with no subluxation or retropulsion of bone or disk fragments (Fig. 30-9). However, with disrupted posterior ligaments and facet capsules, instability may occur.[171-173] If the anterior wedging exceeds 40 to 50 percent, posterior ligamentous and facet joint failure can be assumed, and late instability with progressive deformity may occur.[174] Flexion–compression injuries with concomitant middle element failure have a higher potential for causing mechanical instability, progressive deformity, and neurologic deficit.[85]

Lateral Compression

Lateral compression forces produce an injury similar to the anterior wedge compression injuries previously described, except that the force is applied laterally (Fig. 30-10). Lesions may be limited to vertebral body fractures, or associated posterior ligamentous injury may occur (Fig. 30-11).[49,50] The former are usually stable injuries, whereas the latter may be chronically unstable and lead to progressive pain and deformity.

Flexion–Rotation

A flexion–rotation injury pattern includes a combination of flexion and rotation forces (Fig. 30-12). As described previously for pure flexion, the predominant injury pattern may be anterior bone disruption. However, as rotational forces increase, the ligaments and facet capsules tend to fail, with subsequent disruption of both the anterior and posterior columns.[76-78,135] A highly unstable injury pattern frequently develops, with the posterior ligaments and joint capsules ruptured and the anterior disk and

FIGURE 30-9 *Radiographs and computed tomography (CT) of a compression fracture in a 48-year-old woman who was involved in a motor vehicle accident. **A,** An anteroposterior radiograph of the thoracolumbar junction shows a slight irregularity of the superior end plate of the body of L1 with minimal interspinous widening between T12 and L1. **B,** A lateral radiograph shows loss of height anteriorly and preservation posteriorly at L1. **C,** CT through the body of L1 shows disruption of the cortex anteriorly with an intact posterior cortex.*

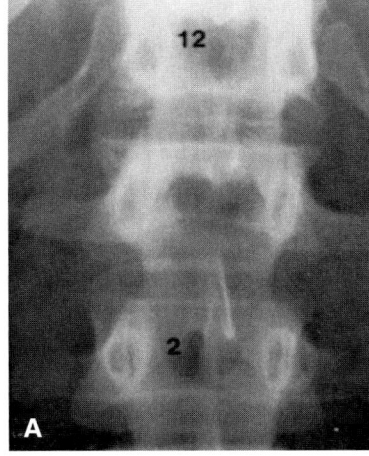
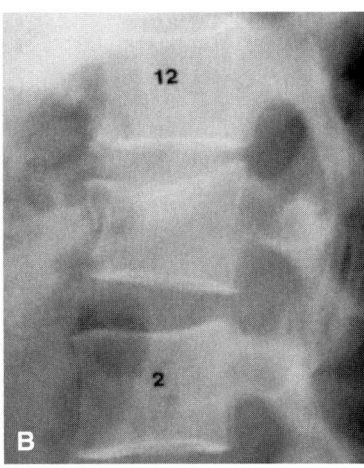
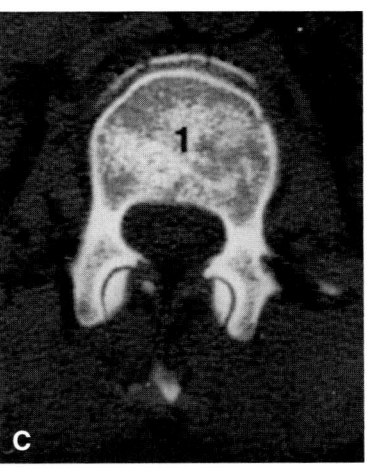

FIGURE 30-10   *Lateral compression forces may produce stable lateral wedge compression injuries. These are most often not associated with posterior ligamentous injury.*

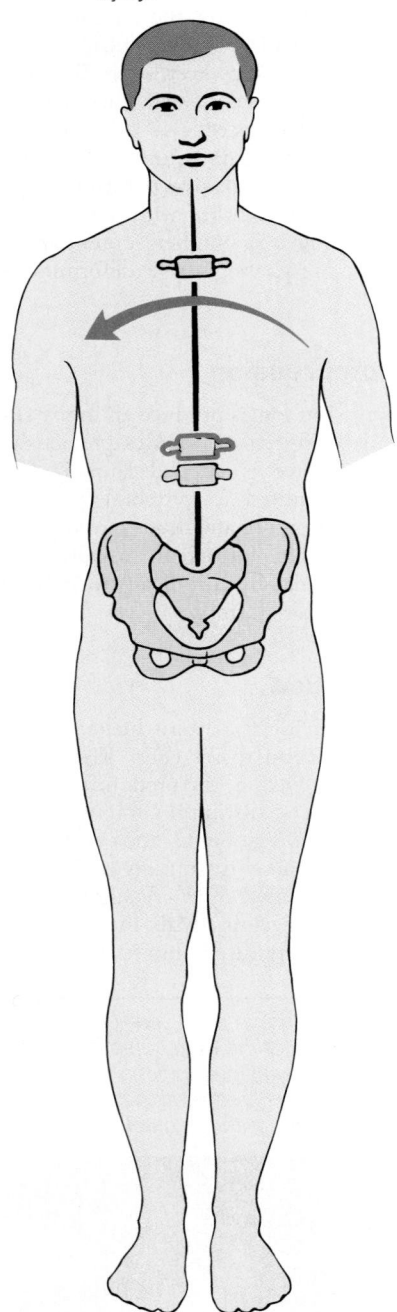

FIGURE 30-11   *An example of a lateral compression fracture.* ***A,*** *An anteroposterior radiograph demonstrates lateral compression with an asymmetrical loss of height. There is no interspinous process widening.* ***B,*** *A lateral radiograph confirms a wedge compression injury with maintenance of height of the posterior portion of the vertebral body.* ***C,*** *Computed tomography through the injured vertebra shows that the injury is limited to the right anterolateral aspect (arrows), with the remaining cortex intact.*

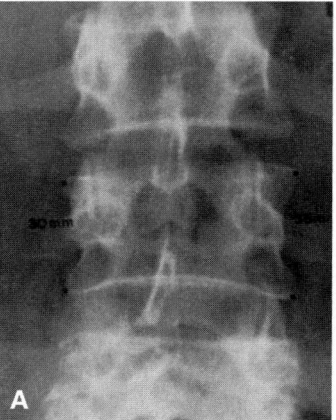

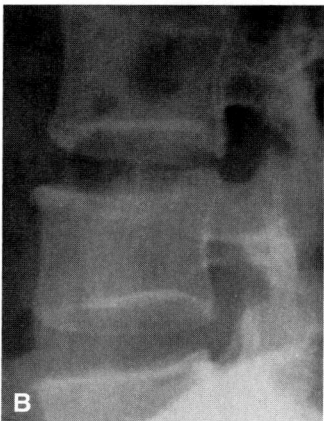

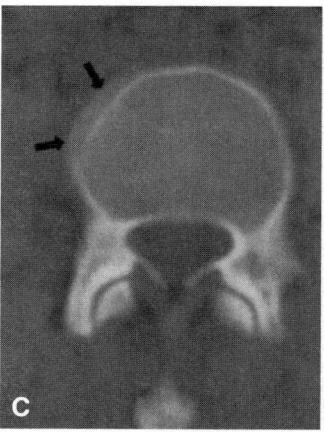

vertebral body disrupted obliquely. This mechanism can result in the classic slice fracture originally described by Holdsworth.[76-78]

In contrast to the cervical spine, pure dislocations are uncommon in the thoracic or lumbar spine because of the size and orientation of the facets, which require

FIGURE 30-12 *Flexion–rotation forces are much more liable to produce serious spinal injuries than flexion alone. The combination frequently disrupts the posterior ligaments and joint capsules and obliquely disrupts the anterior disk and vertebral body.*

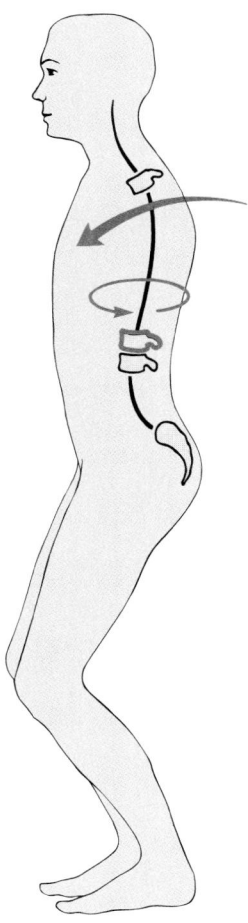

distraction in addition to flexion and rotation for dislocation to occur.[61,105] With a flexion–rotation mechanism of injury, fracture of the facets or other posterior elements will occur more commonly and allow the spine to dislocate (Fig. 30-13).[106]

Flexion–Distraction

Flexion–distraction lesions were first demonstrated radiographically by Chance in 1948,[31] but the mechanism of this so-called seat belt injury was not fully elucidated until later.[81,137] In this injury pattern (Fig. 30-14), the axis of flexion is moved anteriorly (usually toward the anterior abdominal wall), and the entire vertebral column is subjected to large tensile forces. The posterior elements, disks, and ligaments are torn or avulsed, not crushed as typically occurs in most spinal injuries. These forces can produce a pure osseous lesion, a mixed osteoligamentous lesion, or a pure soft tissue (ligamentous or disk) injury. The pure

osseous lesion, described by Chance, involves a horizontal fracture beginning in the spinous process, progressing through the lamina, transverse processes, and pedicles, and extending into the vertebral body (Fig. 30-15). This pure osseous lesion usually occurs in the region of L1-L3. Even though it is acutely unstable, it has excellent potential for healing with good long-term stability if alignment can be obtained. Combined osteoligamentous or pure soft tissue injuries most commonly occur from T12 to L2 and should be considered unstable with low spontaneous healing potential (Fig. 30-16).

Flexion–distraction can cause a bilateral facet dislocation in the thoracic or thoracolumbar spine (Fig. 30-17).[61,105] The ligaments, capsules, and disks are disrupted, but the anterior longitudinal ligament usually remains intact; however, it is sometimes stripped off the anterior aspect of the caudal vertebra. If the axis of flexion is far enough anterior and the energy is sufficient, rupture of the anterior longitudinal ligament may occur and result in a severely unstable injury.[87,150] Generally, this injury is a pure distraction rather than a flexion–distraction injury. If the axis of rotation is at the anterior border of the vertebral bodies, compression may occur. This locus of the axis of rotation changes the nature of the injury.

Shear

A pure shear force (Fig. 30-18) was found by Roaf to produce severe ligamentous disruption, similar to the combination of flexion and rotation described previously.[135] This force can result in anterior, posterior, or lateral spondylolisthesis of the superior vertebral segments on those inferior. Traumatic anterior spondylolisthesis is most common and usually results in a complete spinal cord injury. Occasionally, concomitant fractures through the pars interarticularis may occur and result in an autolaminectomy with neural sparing.[71,141] Shear is frequently combined with other mechanisms to cause complex injuries.

Extension

Extension forces (Fig. 30-19) are created when the head or upper part of the trunk is thrust posteriorly; these forces produce an injury pattern that is the reverse of that seen with pure flexion. Tension is applied anteriorly to the strong anterior longitudinal ligaments and the anterior portion of the annulus fibrosus, whereas compression forces are transmitted to the posterior elements (Fig. 30-20). This mechanism may result in facet, lamina, and spinous process fractures. Avulsion fractures of the anteroinferior portion of the vertebral bodies may occur, but they are not pathognomonic of extension injuries, as previously thought. Most of these injuries are stable unless significant retrolisthesis of the upper vertebral body on the lower vertebral body has occurred or they are combined with shear forces.[28,34] Denis and Burkus reported on a hyperextension injury pattern that they termed a *lumberjack fracture–dislocation*.[38] The mechanism of this injury is a falling mass, often timber, striking the midportion of the patient's back. The injury involves complete disruption of the anterior ligaments and is an extremely unstable injury pattern.

FIGURE 30-13 *This patient sustained a bilateral facet dislocation at T12-L1 as a result of a flexion–distraction/rotation mechanism.* **A,** *A lateral radiograph shows the significant translation of T12 over L1 with maintenance of the integrity (height) of the posterior wall of L1 but with some slight comminution of the anterosuperior portion of the body.* **B,** *This relationship is well demonstrated on the midsagittal reconstruction of the computed tomography (CT) scan.* **C,** *The characteristic findings on the axial images of the CT scan are the double body image and the empty facet sign (arrows).*

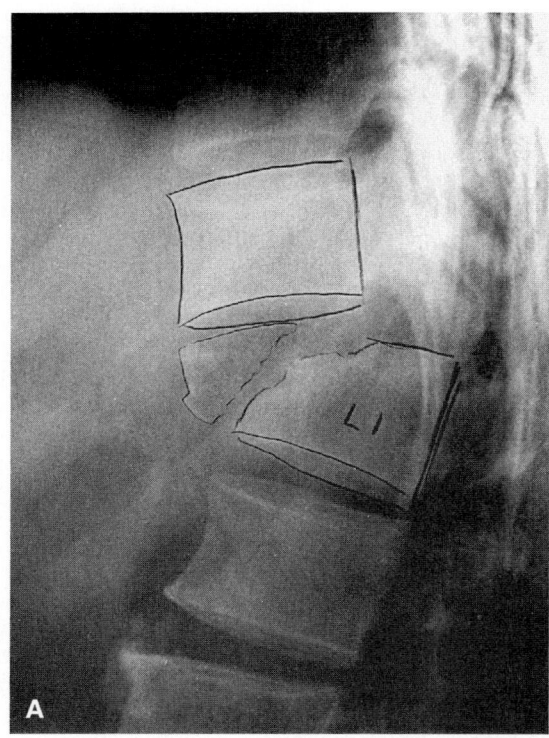
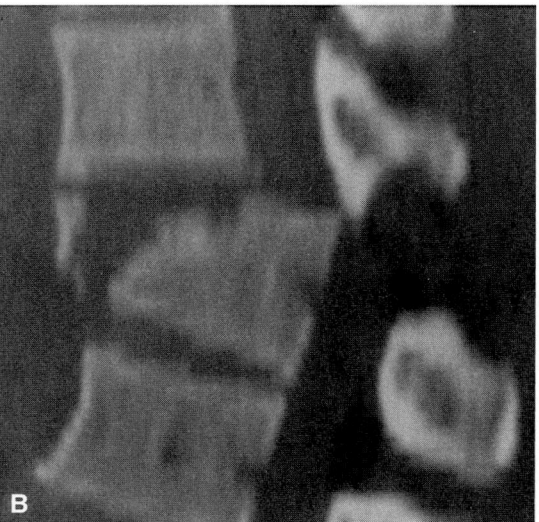
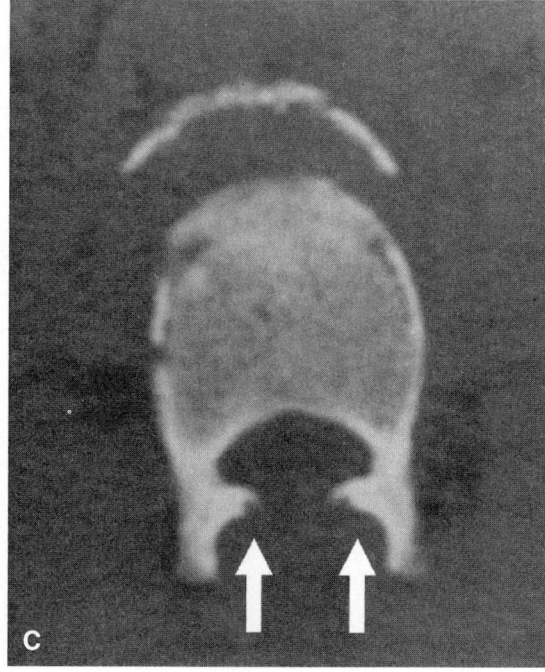

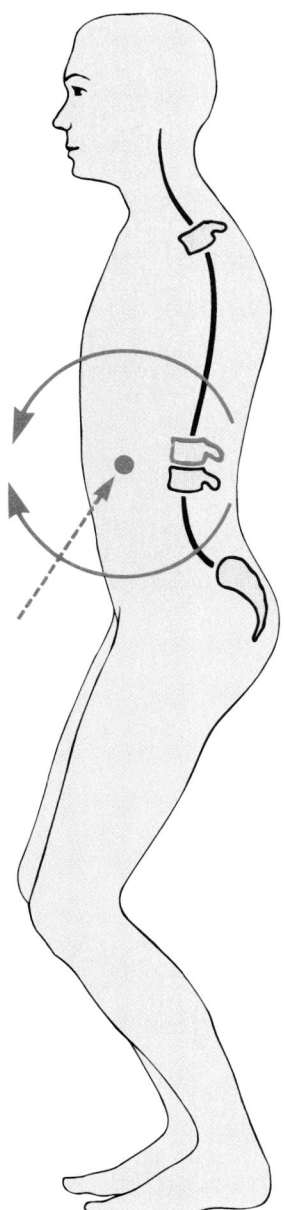

FIGURE 30-14 *Flexion–distraction forces across the thoracolumbar spine frequently produce the typical seat belt injury. The axis of rotation is anterior to the spine with all of the elements of the spine in tension. If this axis of rotation is moved posteriorly into the vertebral body, it is possible to have compressive forces across the anterior vertebral body and distraction forces across the posterior elements and middle column of the spine.*

SPINAL STABILITY

The concept of thoracic, thoracolumbar, and lumbar stability after trauma continues to evolve. Work by Nicoll[122] and Holdsworth[76-78] suggested that the posterior ligamentous complex was the major determinant of spinal stability. They considered fracture–dislocations and severe shear injuries with complete disruption of the posterior ligamentous complex to be highly unstable injuries and most other injuries to be stable. Roaf biomechanically confirmed that gross instability was produced by flexion–rotation forces and shear stress.[135]

Bedbrook disagreed with the importance given to the posterior ligamentous complex and believed that the anterior disk and vertebral body were the prime determinants of stability.[15,16] He cited the lack of instability after laminectomy as an example of the relative importance of the anterior spinal elements, as opposed to the posterior structures, in providing stability.

These two concepts gradually merged into a two-column concept of spinal stability: an anterior weight-bearing column of vertebral bodies and disks and a posterior column of neural arches and ligaments resisting tension.[88,174] It was believed that destruction of either of these columns was enough to produce stability. This model helped explain the chronic instability often seen after spinal injuries, especially those that result in a kyphotic deformity. However, it was unable to fully explain all cases of acute instability. Experiments had shown that complete section of the posterior elements alone does not result in acute instability with flexion, extension, rotation, or shear.[126] It was necessary to also section the posterior portion of the anterior column to produce acute instability, at least in flexion.

Further progress was made when Denis proposed his three-column model of the spine (Fig. 30-21) to better reconcile these clinical and biomechanical observations.[36] In his classification system, the posterior column is composed of the posterior body arch (including the spinous process, the lamina, the facets, and the pedicles) and the interconnecting posterior ligamentous structures (including the supraspinous ligament, interspinous ligament, ligamentum flavum, and facet joint capsules). The middle column is composed of the posterior aspects of the vertebral body, the posterior portion of the annulus fibrosus, and the posterior longitudinal ligament. The anterior column includes the anterior longitudinal ligament, the anterior portion of the annulus fibrosus, and the anterior vertebral body. Though useful in helping define vertebral column instability, this basic anatomic description of the support columns of the spine does not include the spinal cord and spinal nerves. The neural elements, although they do not directly contribute to spinal stability, cannot be forgotten or ignored in stability and treatment considerations.

Denis reviewed his fracture classification system and proposed four categories based on the presence and type of instability.[36] These categories were stable injuries, mechanical instability, neurologic instability, and mechanical and neurologic instability.

Stable injuries include minimal and moderate compression fractures with an intact posterior column, which prevents abnormal forward flexion. By definition, the middle column is intact; it prevents any extrusion of bone or disk into the spinal canal and protects against significant subluxation. A compression fracture without posterior column involvement is an example of a stable injury.

Mechanical instability includes injuries in which two of the three columns are injured, thereby allowing abnormal motion. An example is a severe compression fracture with disruption of the anterior and posterior columns, which allows abnormal flexion across an intact middle column.

FIGURE 30-15 *An example of a flexion–distraction injury with disruption through bone.* ***A,*** *An anteroposterior (AP) radiograph shows a fracture line through the body of the L2 vertebral body (arrow).* ***B,*** *A lateral radiograph confirms the pure osseous lesion, with a compression fracture of the vertebral body anteriorly and a fracture line coursing posteriorly through the upper portion of the lamina anteriorly into the vertebral body (arrow).* ***C,*** *This patient was treated nonoperatively in a thoracolumbrosacral orthosis (TLSO) brace. AP radiograph showing healing at 6 months (arrow).* ***D,*** *Lateral radiograph at 6 months.*

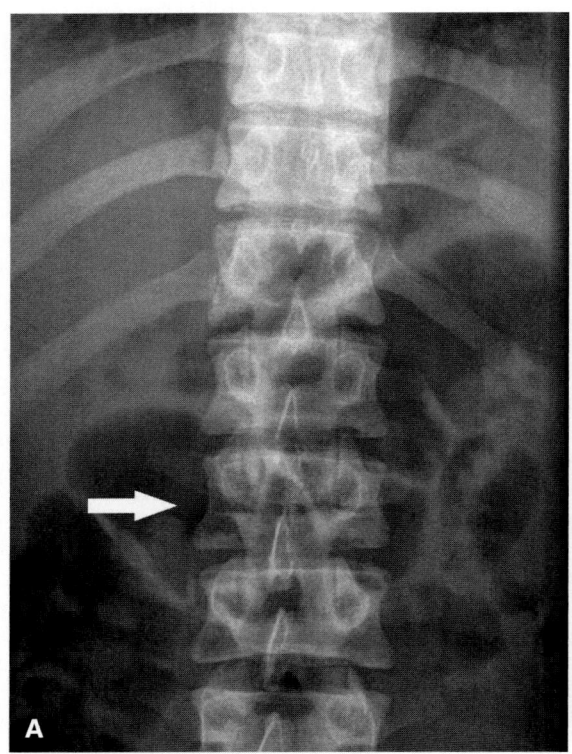
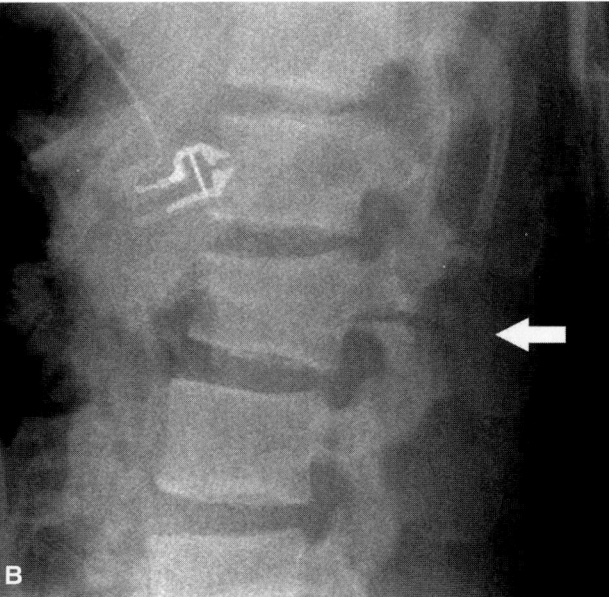
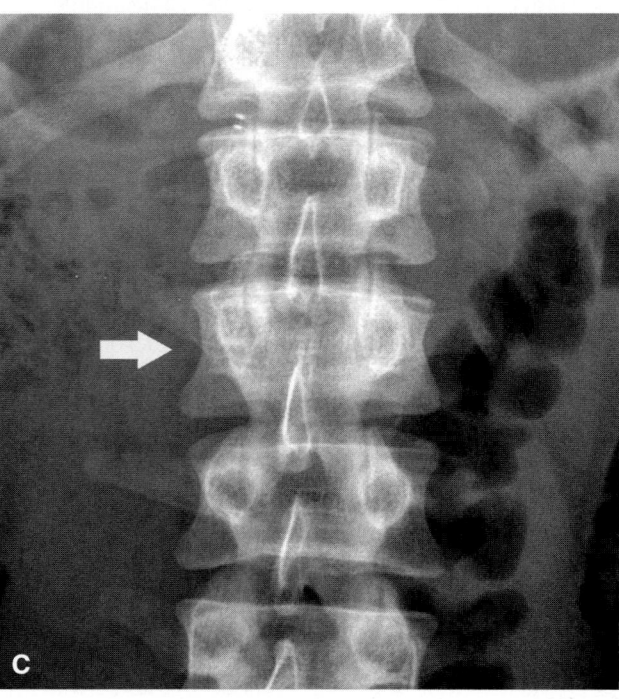
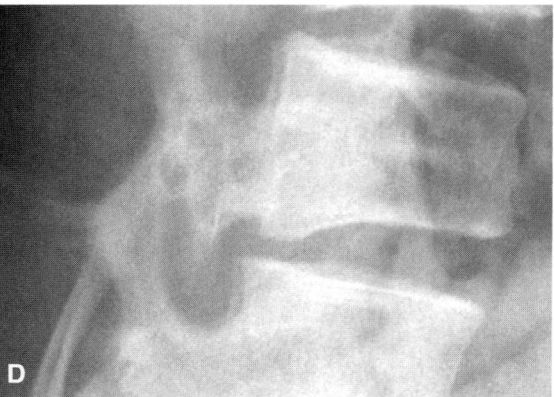

FIGURE 30-16 *An example of a combined osteoligamentous flexion–distraction injury at L1.* **A,** *Lateral radiograph demonstrates a compression injury in the vertebral body and widening of the spinous processes posteriorly, indicating that the posterior ligamentous structures have been injured.* **B,** *T2 sagittal magnetic resonance imaging (MRI) shows that the posterior wall of the L1 body is intact.* **C,** *An MRI short tau inversion recovery (STIR) image shows that the fracture extends into the pedicle* (white arrow).

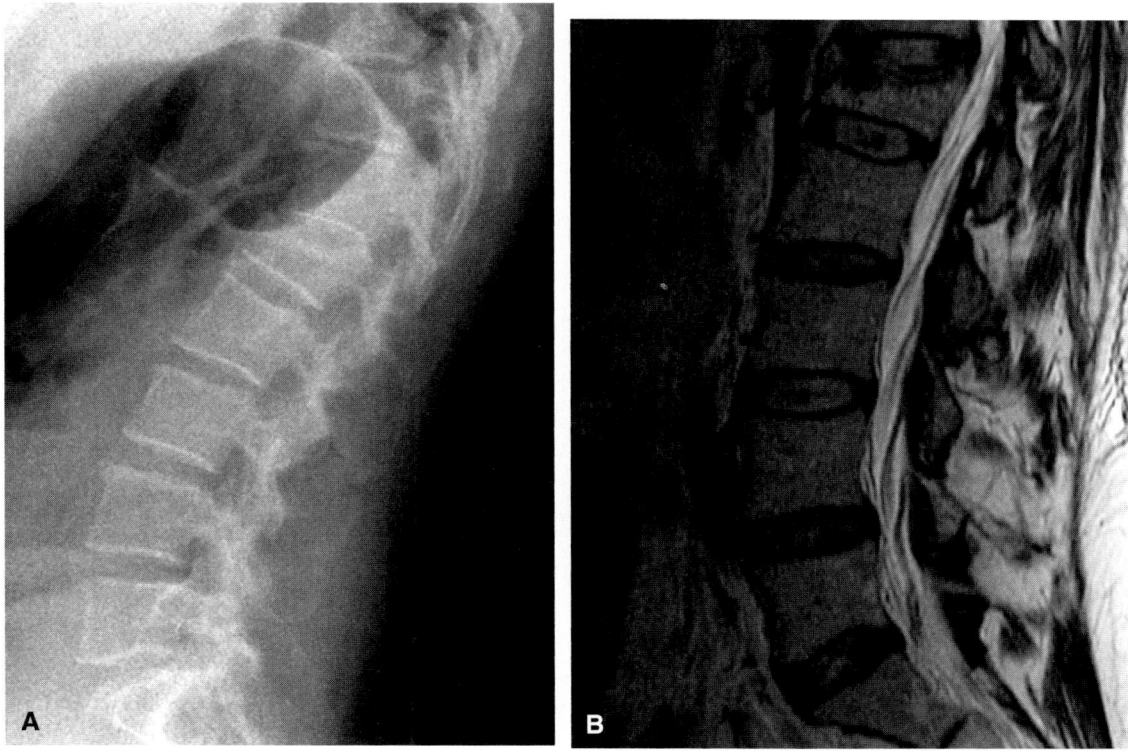

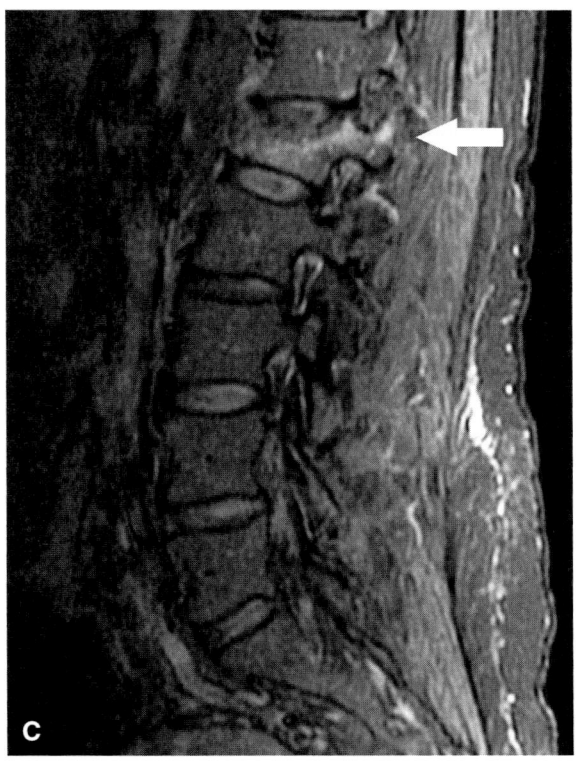

(Continued)

FIGURE 30-16 *(Continued)* ***D, E,*** *This injury was treated with a posterior pedicle-screw-and-rod construct with reduction of the fracture and realignment of the spine. Anteroposterior and lateral views.*

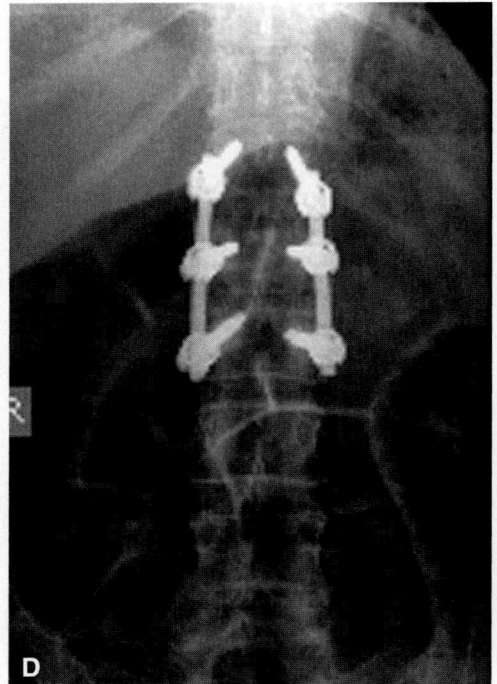
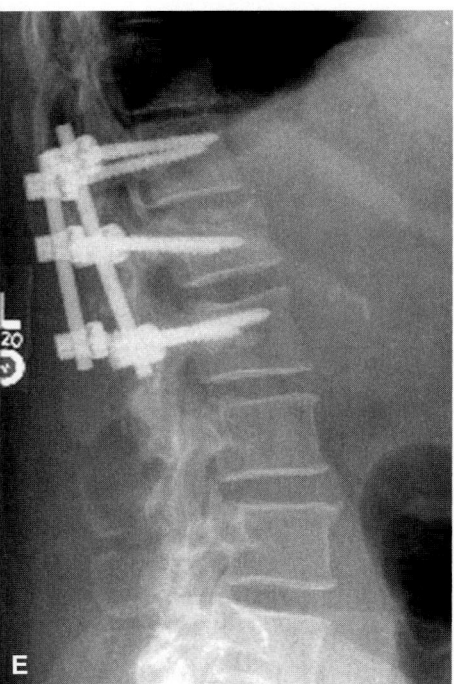

This instability is often associated with pain, but not necessarily with a neurologic deficit. It is important to closely determine the status of the posterior elements when evaluating this type of injury. The position of these elements in relation to one another in the horizontal and vertical planes can give clues regarding flexion and rotatory deformity and possible instability. A second example is a flexion–distracting injury with disruption of the posterior and middle columns; this mechanism causes abnormal flexion with a fulcrum at the intact anterior column, which functions as a hinge. Chronic instability and pain may result, but again, the injury does not necessarily jeopardize neurologic function. Panjabi and colleagues performed a biomechanical study on a high-speed trauma model and measured multidirectional flexibility.[126] The results of this study supported the three-column theory of Denis and also showed that the middle column appears to be the primary determinant of mechanical stability in the thoracolumbar spine.

Neurologic instability refers specifically to a burst fracture. Denis believed that most of these lesions heal and that they often become mechanically stable. However, he found that a neurologic deficit developed in 20 percent of his patients with a burst fracture after mobilization as a result of middle column failure and protrusion of bone into the spinal canal. Neurologic compromise is a strong indication for surgical stabilization and decompression. The decompression may be accomplished either directly or indirectly by reduction of deformity and rigid internal immobilization of the segment. It is generally assumed that injuries severe enough to cause neurologic deficits are unstable. The index of suspicion should remain high when evaluating these patients.

The typical example of *mechanical and neurologic instability* is a fracture–dislocation with disruption of all three columns and either a neurologic deficit or "impending neurologic deterioration" with the neural elements either being compressed or "threatened."

As with the use of any classification system, treatment failure may result from rigid adherence to definitions without individualizing treatment for each patient. To keep the use of these definitions in proper perspective, White and Panjabi defined generic clinical instability as "the loss of the ability of the spine under physiologic conditions to maintain relationships between vertebrae in such a way that there is neither damage nor subsequent irritation to the spinal cord or nerve root and, in addition, there is no development of incapacitating deformity or pain from structural changes."[171]

White and Panjabi defined physiologic loads as loads incurred during normal activity, *incapacitating deformity* as gross deformity unacceptable to the patient, and *incapacitating pain* as discomfort uncontrolled by non-narcotic analgesics.[171] This definition addresses both the acute and the late stages of vertebral column trauma. It also draws attention to the neural elements as a major structure of the spinal column and requires the physician to consider these structures, in addition to bones, ligaments, disks, and other soft tissues, as determinants of stability. Though less specific than Denis' classification, it requires a basic understanding of spinal anatomy, the mechanism of injury, and modes of failure when undertaking treatment.

The preceding discussion should be supplemented with a reminder that instability does not always require surgical treatment. In some cases, prolonged bedrest may be able

FIGURE 30-17 *An example of a flexion–distraction injury at T12-L1, predominantly disrupting ligamentous structures.* **A,** *An anteroposterior (AP) radiograph shows disruption between T12 and L1.* **B,** *A lateral radiograph shows complete dislocation of the T12 and L1 vertebral bodies. This 18-year-old female was involved in a motor vehicle collision while wearing a lap belt.* **C, D,** *AP and lateral radiographs after posterior reduction and instrumented fusion with pedicle screws and rods.*

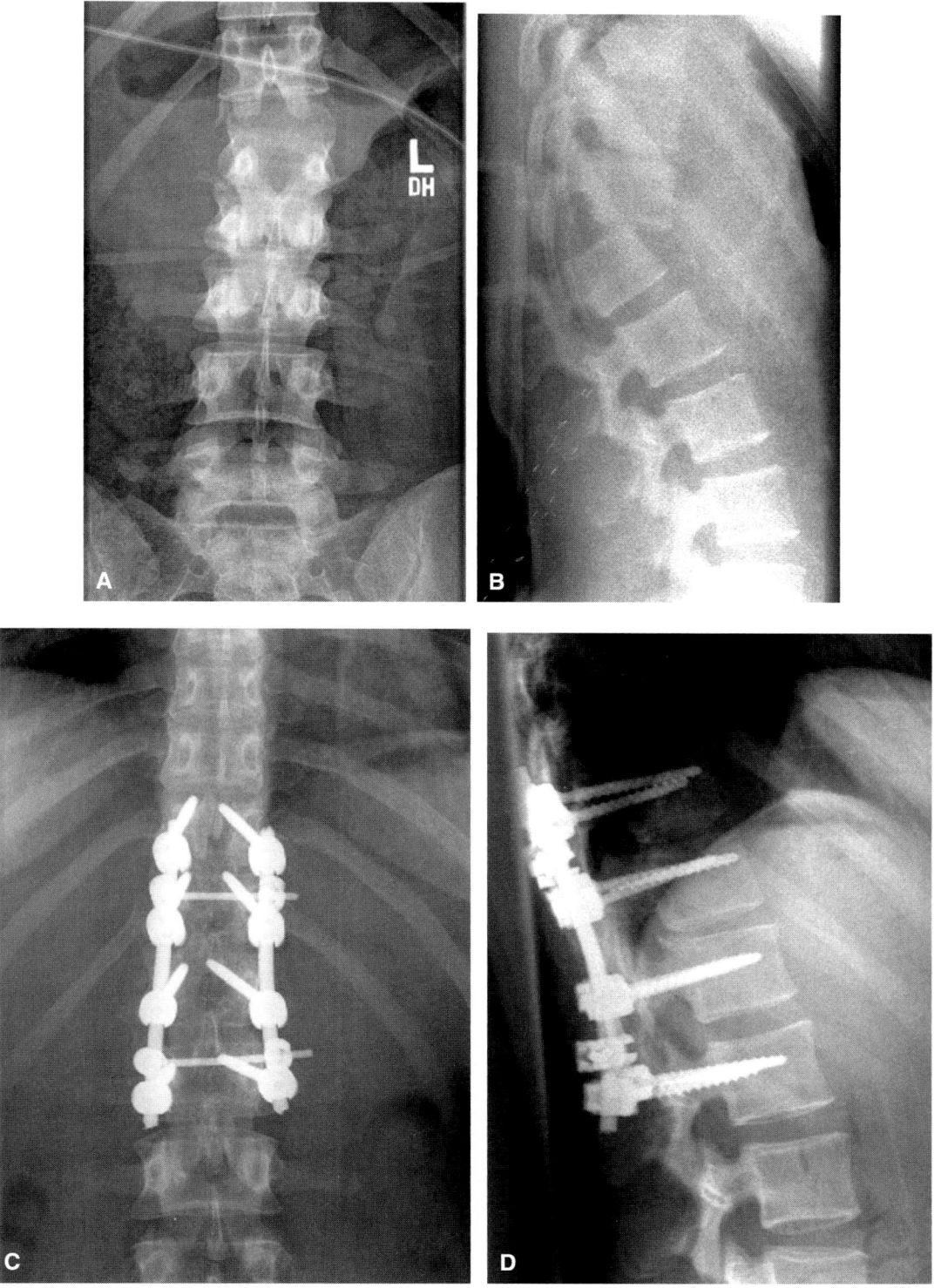

FIGURE 30-18 | *Shearing requires forces from opposing directions to pass through the spine at slightly different levels. This tends to produce extremely unstable injuries with disruption of all columns of the spine and may produce severe spondylolisthesis with the cephalic spine positioned anteriorly, posteriorly, or laterally in relation to the caudal portion of the spine.*

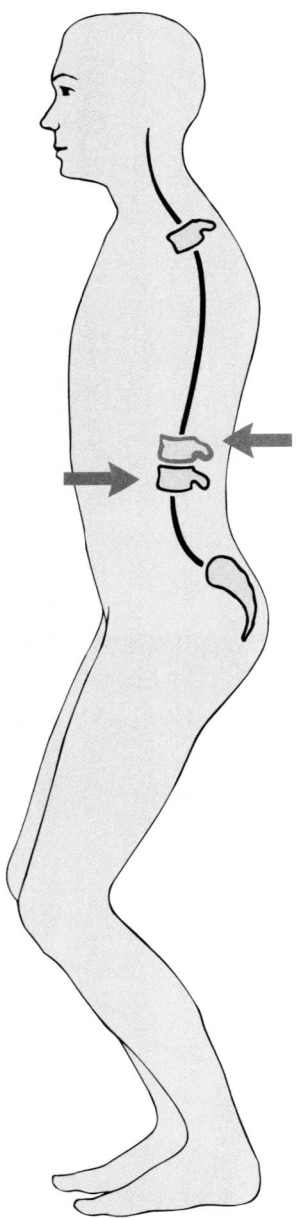

FIGURE 30-19 | *Extension forces occur when the upper trunk is thrust posteriorly, and this applies anterior tension and posterior compression. Most of these injuries are stable unless there is retrolisthesis of the upper on the lower vertebral body.*

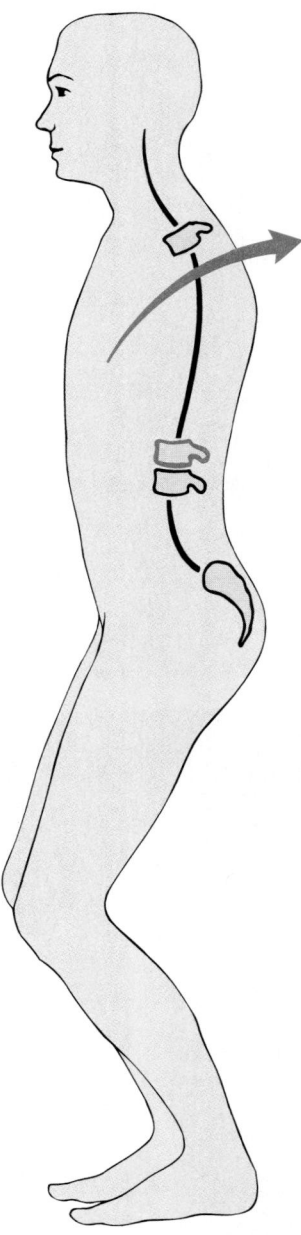

to achieve the same long-term degree of spinal stability as surgery, and it may be appropriate for the particular circumstances of an individual patient.

CLASSIFICATION

There is no universally accepted classification system for fractures of the thoracic and thoracolumbar region. It is difficult to group these injuries because of the broad variability of symptoms with which patients may present. Proposed systems have focused on fracture pattern and mechanism of injury and fracture biomechanics. It is important, however, in treating these fractures to also consider the patient's degree of neurologic injury when attempting classification.

The ideal classification system would allow for high inter- and intrarater reliability. The classification system should also offer prognostic information and provide a guideline for treatment. Historic classification systems have failed to consider factors such as neurologic injury and thus were not ideal for dictating treatment plans.

FIGURE 30-20 | *This 26-year-old man was involved in a motor vehicle accident, sustaining an extension injury to the lower spine. **A,** An anteroposterior radiograph shows a fracture line coursing through the lamina of L4 (arrows). Arrowheads point to transverse process fractures. **B,** A lateral radiograph was unremarkable. **C,** Computed tomography through the injured body of L4 with multiple fracture lines noted in the posterior column (arrowheads).*

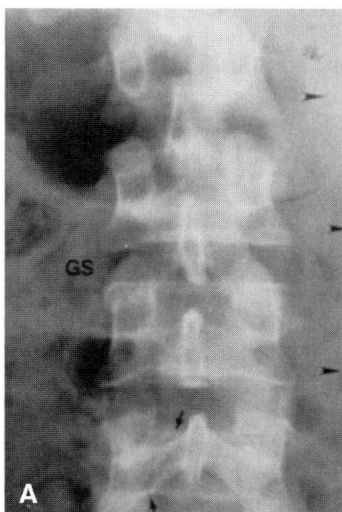
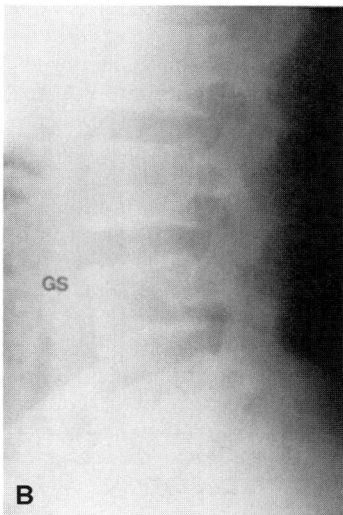
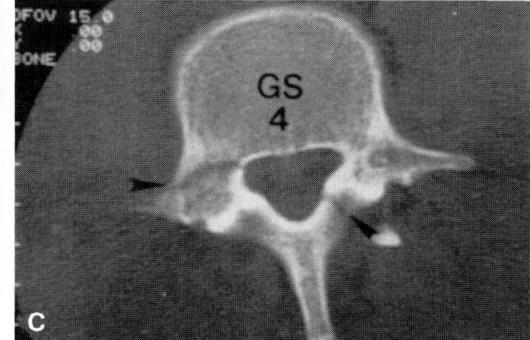

The initial standard classification which was offered by Holdsworth consisted of a two-column system: an anterior column that resists compressive loads, and a posterior osteoligamentous complex that resists tensile forces.[76] This system was later replaced by Denis' classification, which incorporated the middle column.[36] (The proposed importance of the middle column was its propensity for retropulsion into the spinal canal.) This system was based on computed tomography (CT) findings, which could reliably visualize bony fragments that had retropulsed. The Denis classification continues to be commonly referred to today, likely due to its relative ease of use. The basic classifications serve as the basis for more recent systems and therefore, it is covered in depth.

FIGURE 30-21 | *Denis' three-column model of the spine. The middle column is made up of the posterior longitudinal ligament, the posterior annulus fibrosis, and the posterior aspects of the vertebral body and disk.*

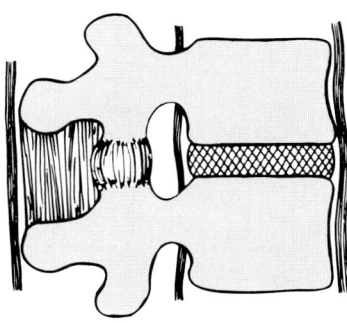

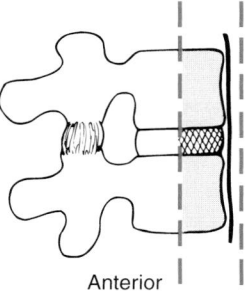
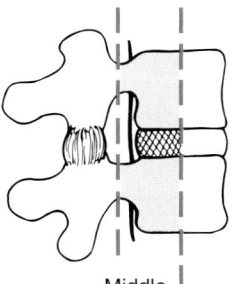
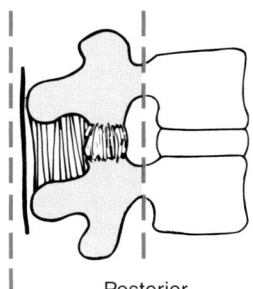

Anterior   Middle   Posterior

Denis' Classification of Spinal Injuries

Many classification systems have been designed to describe thoracic and thoracolumbar injuries. They may be based on the mechanism of injury, radiologic/descriptive characteristics, or stability. Denis' three-column concept is frequently used because it includes each of the injury patterns most commonly seen and relates them to a specific mechanism of injury.[36] Denis developed his classification system after a review of 412 patients with thoracic and lumbar spinal injuries. He divided them into minor and major injuries. Minor injuries included isolated articular process fractures (0.7%), transverse process fractures (13.6%), spinous process fractures (1.7%), and pars interarticularis fractures (1.0%). The four major injury types were compression fractures (47.8%), burst fractures (14.3%), flexion–distraction (seat belt) injuries (4.6%), and fracture-dislocations (16.3%). Each of these major injuries was further subdivided, depending on the specific radiographic findings.

COMPRESSION FRACTURES

By definition, compression fracture injuries are associated with fracture of the anterior portion of the vertebral body, but the middle column of the spine is intact (see Fig. 30-21). In some cases, the posterior column may be disrupted in tension as the upper segments hinge forward on the intact middle column. The mechanism of the injury is either anterior or lateral flexion.

Compression fractures may be anterior or lateral, with the former accounting for 89 percent of this group. Fractures may involve both end plates (type A, 16%), the superior end plate only (type B, 63%), the inferior end plate only (type C, 6%), or a buckling of the anterior cortex but with both end plates intact (type D, 15%) (Fig. 30-22).

None of the 197 patients with compression fractures reported by Denis had a neurologic deficit related to the spinal fracture. Compression fractures with less than 40 to 50 percent compression and without posterior ligamentous disruption tend to be stable, low-energy injuries.

FIGURE 30-22   *Denis' classification of compression fractures. These fractures may involve both end plates (**A,** type A), the superior end plate only (**B,** type B), the inferior end plate only (**C,** type C), or a buckling of the anterior cortex with both end plates intact (**D,** type D).*

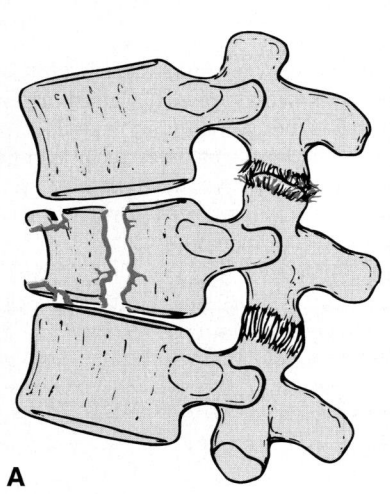

A

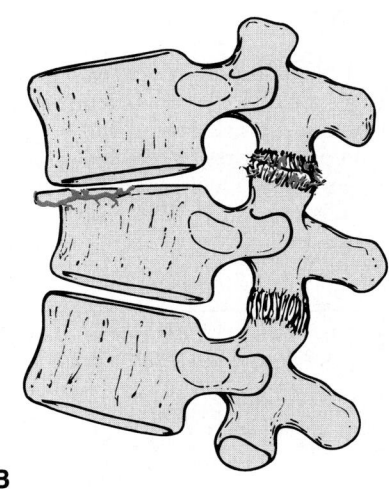

B

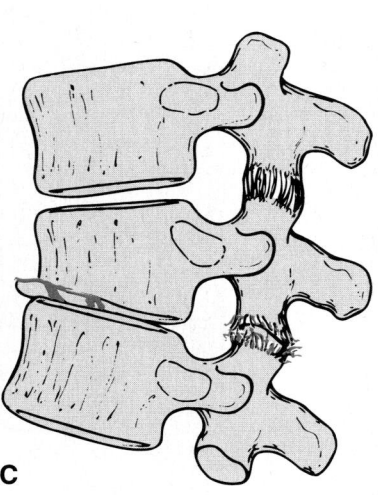

C

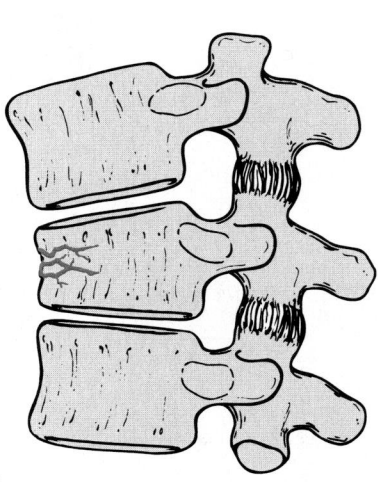

D

However, it is still important to assess the patient for noncontiguous spinal fractures.[6] A 40 to 50 percent anterior body compression fracture with the posterior body intact in a physiologically young individual (with no osteoporosis) strongly suggests that the posterior ligaments were disrupted.

BURST FRACTURES

Burst fractures are characterized by disruption of the posterior wall of the vertebral body (middle column of the spine), which differentiates them from compression fractures (Figs. 30-23, 30-24, and 30-6). Spreading of the posterior elements may occur and can be seen as a widening of the interpedicular distance on a plain anteroposterior (AP) radiograph of the spine.

Lamina fractures may also occur. Cammisa and associates found that lamina fractures were present on CT in 50 percent of patients with severe burst fractures, especially in the lower lumbar spine.[29] In this surgical series, 11 of 30 patients with burst fractures and lamina fractures also had posterior dural tears located at the site of the posterior lamina fracture (Fig. 30-25). The incidence was almost 70 percent in those with burst fractures, retropulsed bone in the canal, and neurologic injury. The possibility of a dural tear should be taken into consideration if posterior decompression and stabilization procedures are planned. It should not, however, mandate treatment to routinely repair the dural laceration. Some burst fractures are accompanied by horizontal fractures of the posterior column. In a retrospective study by Abe and colleagues, nine patients with a thoracolumbar burst fracture and an associated horizontal fracture of the posterior column were studied.[1] They found that this type of fracture pattern is not rare; it represented 21 percent of the burst fractures treated by them over an 8-year period. It is best visualized on plain radiographs because it is not easily seen on CT axial cuts. This type of burst fracture differs from flexion–distraction injuries combined with a burst fracture, which are accompanied by horizontal fractures not only in the posterior but also in the middle column. This fracture pattern seems to be more unstable than burst fractures with no horizontal splitting and may require surgical stabilization to prevent progression of kyphosis.

The mechanism of injury for burst fractures is primarily axial loading. Axial loading is combined with other forces such as flexion (either anterior or lateral) or rotation to account for the different fracture patterns seen.

Denis noted that burst injuries can be divided into five frequently observed subgroups (Fig. 30-26). One involves fractures of both end plates (type A, 24%) and is usually seen in the lower lumbar spine. Another involves fracture of only the superior end plate (type B, 49%) and usually occurs at the thoracolumbar junction. Fracture of only the inferior end plate is much less common (type C, 7%). A fourth pattern is diagnosed by the presence of a burst fracture of the middle column in combination with a rotational injury leading to some degree of lateral subluxation or tilt (type D, 15%); this pattern is best seen on a plain AP radiograph. The final subgroup is a burst fracture of the middle column associated with asymmetrical compression of the anterior column, as seen in a lateral compression fracture (type E, 5%).

Willen and co-workers verified these injury types anatomically in autopsy specimens.[177] Neurologic deficits were seen in 47 percent of the 59 patients studied with burst fractures. There did not appear to be a simple, direct relationship between the extent of spinal canal compromise and the severity of neurologic deficit. Willen and co-workers found increased neurologic damage with type D fractures, whereas Gertzbein[62] found only a weak correlation between canal compromise and neurologic deficit in a study of more than 1000 patients with thoracolumbar spine injuries. Gertzbein thought that most trauma to the neural elements probably occurred at the instant of injury. A relationship was, however, found between the location of injury and subsequent neurologic deficit, with the incidence of complete neurologic injury being significantly lower below the thoracolumbar junction (T12-L1).

Burst fractures may be unstable because they represent at least a minimum of a two-column injury, but additionally, they may also be accompanied by extensive disk injury at the levels directly adjacent to the fracture. This possibility has to be considered when deciding on treatment options.

FLEXION–DISTRACTION INJURIES

The flexion and distraction mechanism of injury, which most commonly occurs in a motor vehicle accident when the passenger is using a lap seat belt with no shoulder harness, results in failure of the posterior and middle columns in tension, with the anterior column serving as the fulcrum (see Figs. 30-15 to 30-17).

Denis divided these injuries into one-level and two-level lesions (Fig. 30-27). A one-level lesion can occur through bone, as described by Chance (type A, 47%), or it may be primarily ligamentous (type B, 11%). Two-level injuries involve the middle column by disruption through bone (type C, 26%) or through the ligaments and disk with no middle column fractures (type D, 16%).

One weakness of this classification system is that it does not include a category for patients who have distraction failure of the posterior column with axial load failure of the middle and anterior columns resulting in a compression or burst fracture. This shortcoming has been noted by several authors, who have added additional categories for seat belt injury.[64,65]

None of the 19 patients with a seat belt injury in Denis' series developed a neurologic deficit related to the spinal fracture. In other series, the incidence is also low, usually less than 10%.[62] Injuries with ligamentous involvement should be considered acutely and chronically unstable, whereas those with significant bone involvement are acutely unstable but may heal well.

FRACTURE–DISLOCATIONS (SHEAR)

Fracture–dislocations are caused by failure of all three columns of the spine as a result of compression, tension, rotation, or shear forces (see Figs. 30-17, 30-28, and 30-29).

FIGURE 30-23 *A 43-year-old man sustained a T12 burst fracture when a mobile home roof fell on him during a storm. The patient was neurologically intact. **A,** A preoperative anteroposterior (AP) radiograph shows approximately 50 percent loss of height at T12 and L1. **B,** A preoperative lateral view shows local kyphosis measuring 27°. **C,** Axial computed tomography shows a minimal burst component at L1. **D,** This injury was stabilized with posterior pedicle screws and rods. A pedicle screw was placed in the burst-fractured vertebra of T12 (the pedicles were intact) to act as a fulcrum in the reduction of his kyphosis. **E,** Postoperative AP radiograph showing two cross-connectors used for additional stability.*

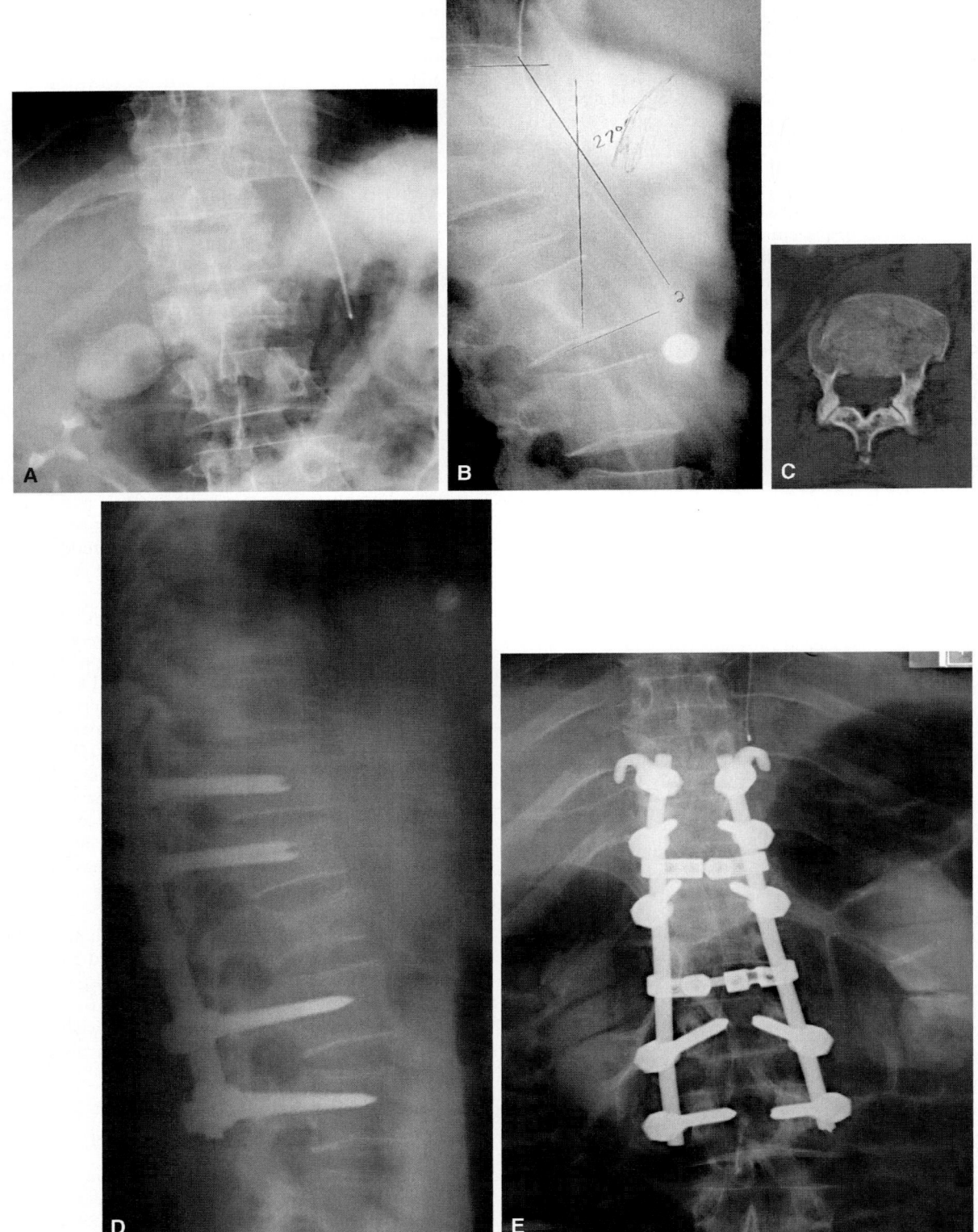

*An example of a stable burst fracture (Denis' type B) in a 52-year-old man who was neurologically intact. The fracture was treated nonoperatively. **A,** An anteroposterior radiograph demonstrates loss of height of the body of T12, with minimal interpedicular widening and no interspinous separation noted. **B,** A lateral radiograph confirms involvement of the anterior and middle columns with loss of height at both sites. **C,** Computed tomography through T12 demonstrates disruption of the posterior vertebral cortex (arrow) but only minimal displacement of the fragment. The posterior ring remains intact.*

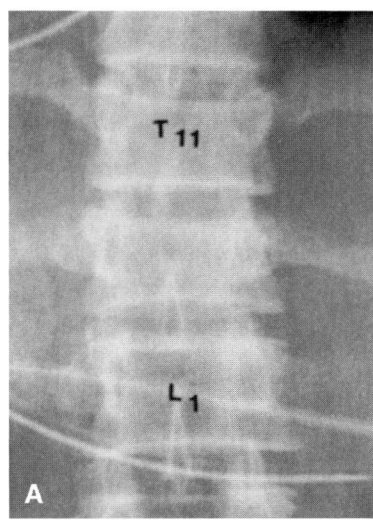
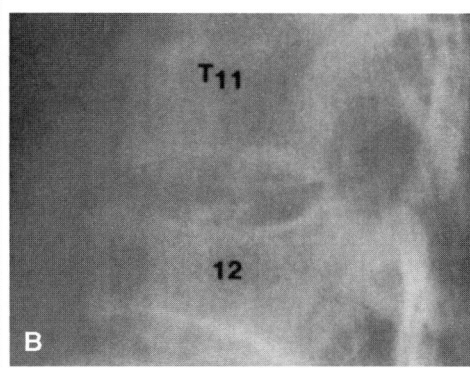
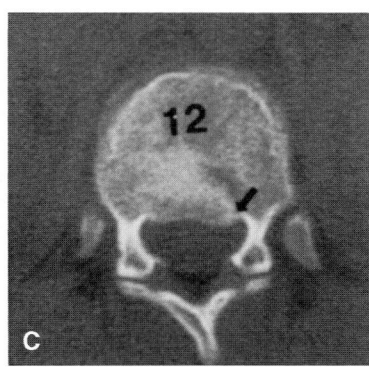

*Illustration of the proposed mechanism of injury in patients with burst fractures with associated lamina fractures and posterior dural tears. **A,** With axial loading and spreading of the pedicles, the lamina fracture is produced, and bone is retropulsed from the vertebral body into the spinal canal. This may result in protrusion of the dura between the lamina fracture fragments. **B,** As the axial load is dissipated, the lamina fracture fragments recoil and may entrap the dura and nerve rootlets. **C,** If approached posteriorly, the lamina fracture is difficult to visualize, and if not carefully sought, dura and nerve rootlets may be further injured. (Redrawn from Camissa, F.P., Jr.; Eismont, F.L.; Green, B.A. Dural laceration occurring with burst fractures and associated laminar fractures. J Bone Joint Surg [Am] 71:1044–1052, 1989.)*

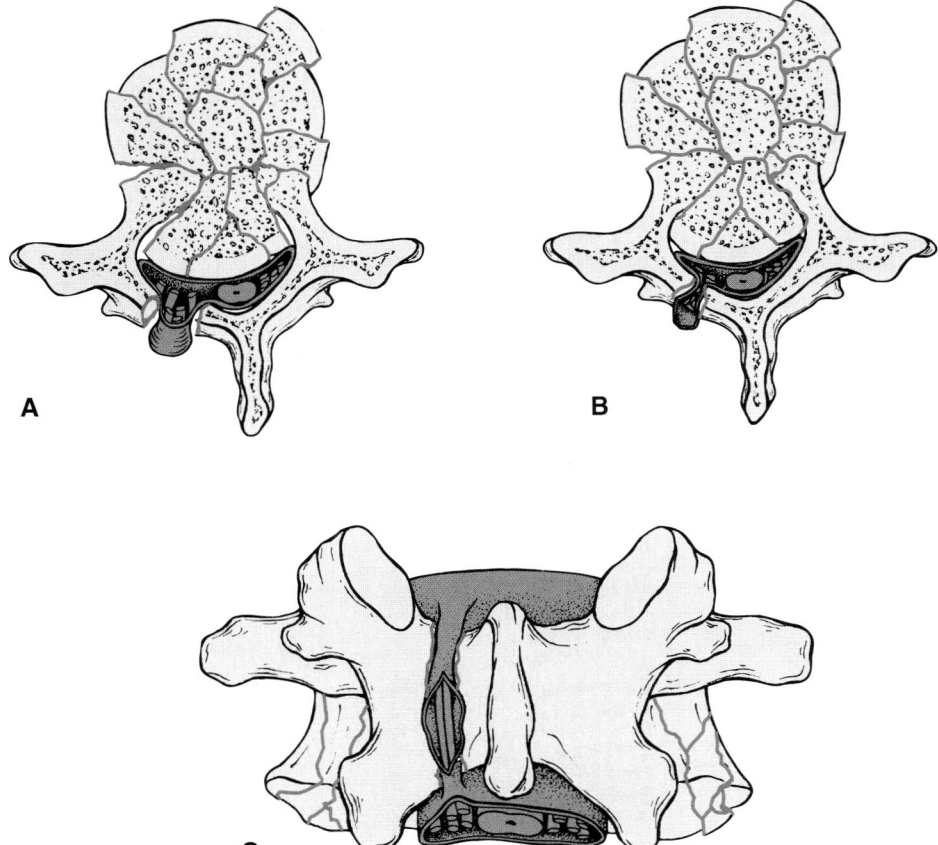

Three different mechanisms (i.e., three types of fracture–dislocation) can occur (Fig. 30-30). One pattern (type A) is a flexion–rotation injury, which was originally described by Holdsworth in victims of mining accidents.[76,78] This type may also occur after ejection from a motor vehicle or a fall from a height (Fig. 30-30, A). A shear fracture–dislocation (type B) can be caused by a violent force directed across the long axis of the trunk. One such example, as described by Denis and Burkus, occurs when a lumberjack is struck across the midportion of his back by a falling tree (see Fig. 30-30, B).[38] Denis' third type (type C) is a bilateral facet dislocation (see Fig. 30-30, C) caused by a flexion–distraction injury. It resembles the seat belt injury previously described, but with failure of the anterior column. This injury most commonly occurs with failure of either the anterior intervertebral disk or the anterior vertebral body. The anterior longitudinal ligament is usually stripped off the inferior vertebral body, thereby allowing significant subluxation to occur.

Denis described 67 patients with fracture–dislocations. Of these patients, 56 had flexion–rotation injuries, 7 had shear injuries, and 4 had bilateral facet dislocations resulting from flexion–distraction injuries. All these injuries involve significant destruction of each of the three columns. This group of injuries was associated with the highest incidence of neurologic deficit. Of the patients with flexion–rotation injuries, only 25 percent were neurologically normal, and 39 percent had complete spinal cord injuries. All seven patients with shear injuries had complete neurologic deficits. Of the four patients with flexion–distraction injuries, three had incomplete neurologic deficits, and one was neurologically normal. Other investigators have also reported a significantly higher incidence of neurologic deficit in patients with fracture–dislocations than in those with other injury patterns.[62] These injuries are acutely highly unstable.

FIGURE 30-26 *Denis' classification of burst fractures. **A–C,** Types A, B, and C represent fractures of both end plates, the superior end plate, and the inferior end plate, respectively. **D,** Type D is a combination of a type A burst fracture with rotation, which is best appreciated on an anteroposterior (AP) radiograph. **E,** Type E burst fracture is due to a laterally directed force and hence appears asymmetrical on an AP radiograph. The superior or inferior end plate, or both, may be involved with this fracture.*

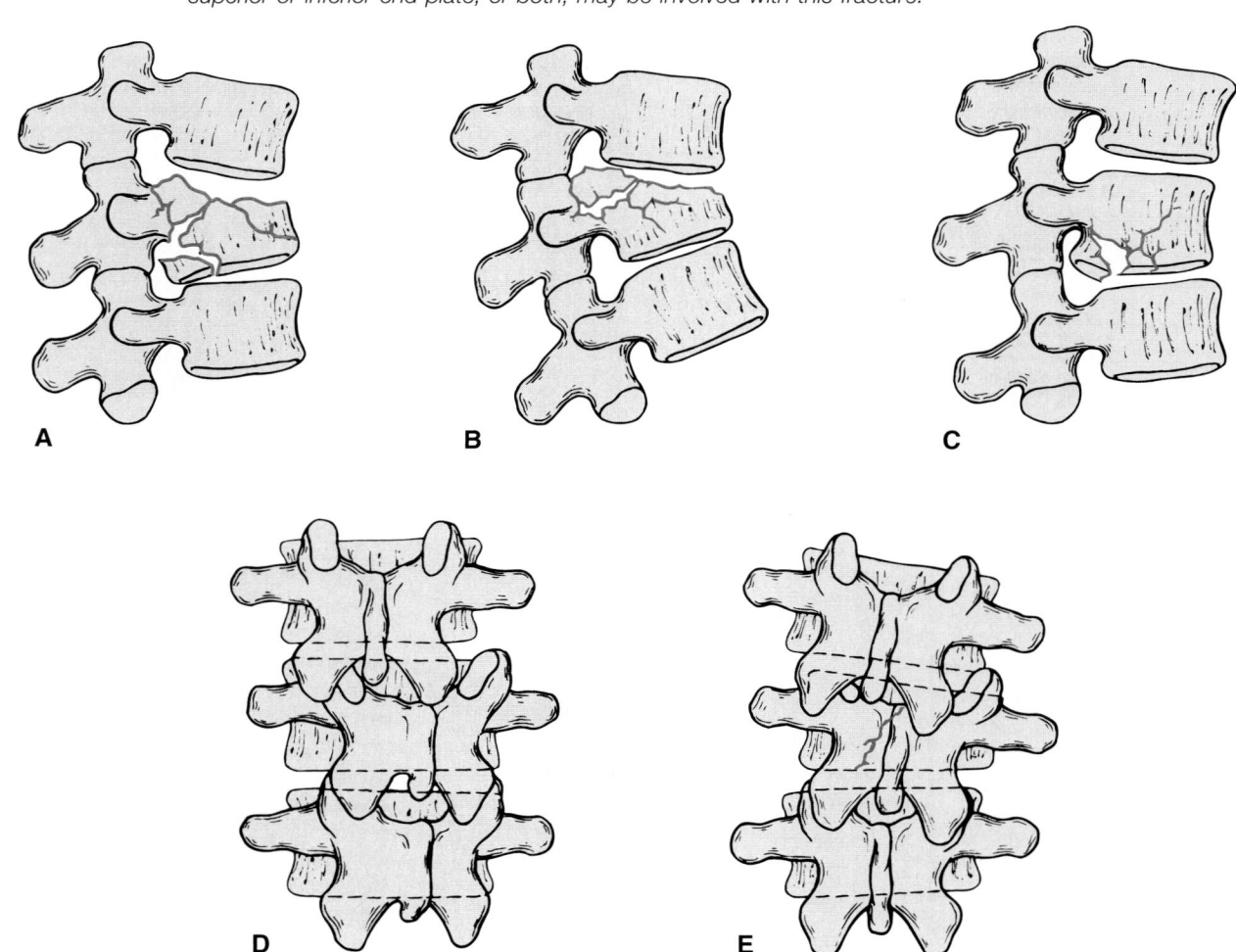

FIGURE 30-27 *Denis' classification of flexion–distraction injuries. These may occur at one level through bone **A,** at one level through the ligaments and disk **B,** at two levels, with the middle column injured through bone **C,** or at two levels with the middle column injured through ligament and disk **D**.*

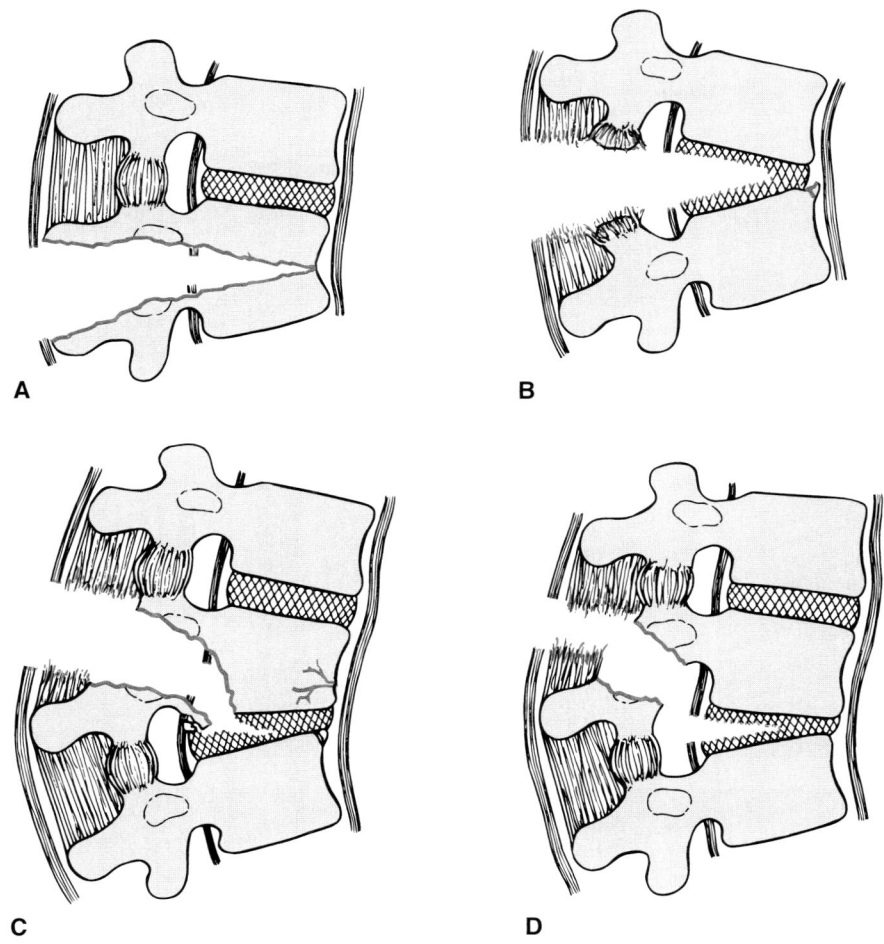

A B

C D

FIGURE 30-28 *This 24-year-old man was a victim of a fall from a height, which resulted in a fracture–dislocation at L1-L2 and a complete spinal cord injury. **A,** An anteroposterior radiograph highlights the malalignment at L1-L2 with a significant rotatory component and lateral slip at this level. **B,** A lateral radiograph confirms the displacement with forward subluxation and overlap at L1-L2. **C,** A computed tomographic scan through L1-L2 highlights the displacement and malalignment, resulting in significant canal compromise and spinal cord injury.*

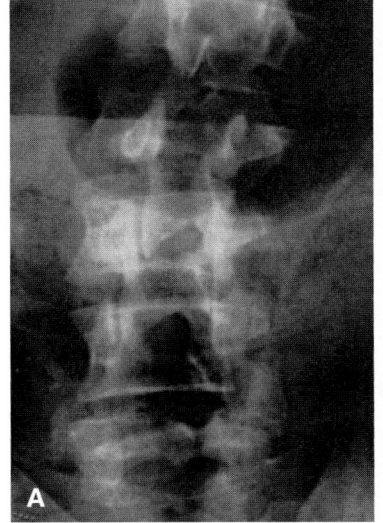

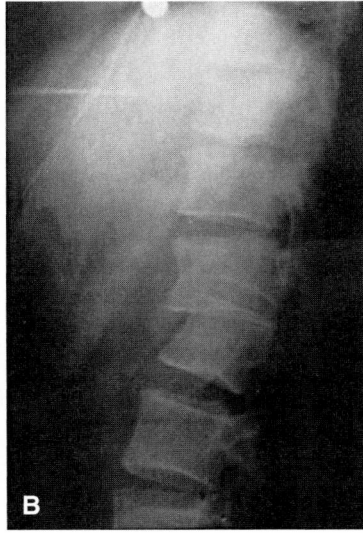

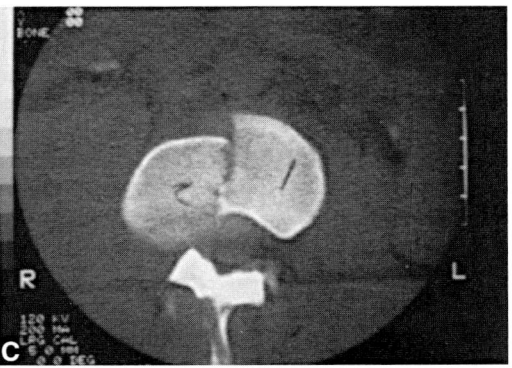

FIGURE 30-29 | *This 20-year-old female was involved in a motor vehicle accident that resulted in a fracture–dislocation of the thoracolumbar spine and a complete spinal cord injury.* **A,** *An anteroposterior (AP) radiograph demonstrates a loss of height at L1 with a rotatory component.* **B,** *A lateral radiograph confirms a fracture through the body of L1 and dislocation of T12 on L1.* **C,** *Sagittal computed tomography shows a fracture–dislocation injury.* AP **(D)** *and lateral* **(E)** *radiographs showing reduction of the fracture–dislocation and stabilization with posterior pedicle screws and rods.*

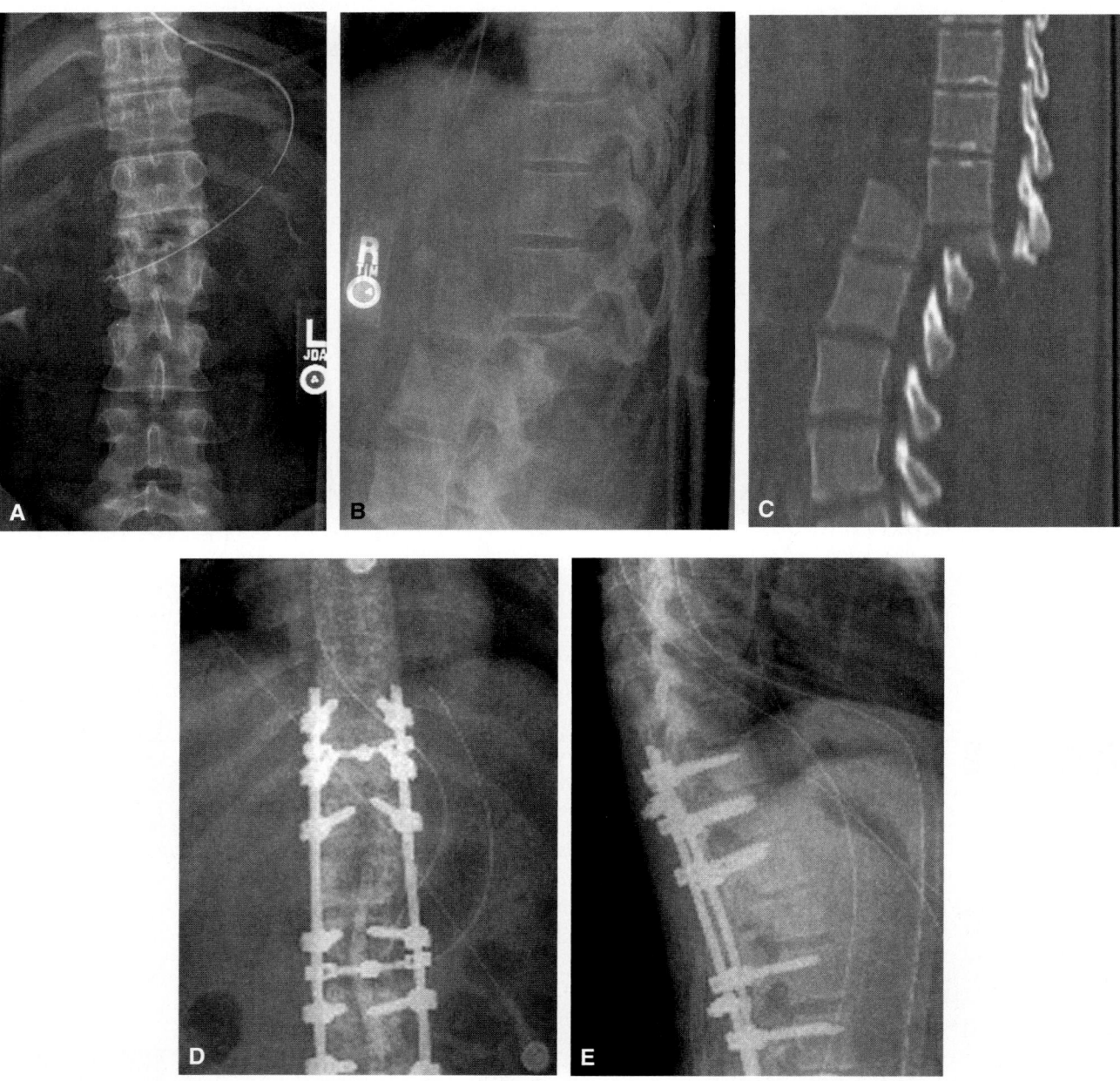

AO "Comprehensive" Classification

Various attempts have been made to develop a universal classification of spinal injuries. The Arbeitsgemeinschaft für Osteosynthesefragen (AO) classification system, commonly referred to as the Magerl or Gertzbein system was intended to allow specific classification of fractures based on fracture mechanics with modifiers that further delineate the specific fracture pattern.[63] To be effective, such a classification must include structural injury to both bone and soft tissue, as well as consideration of the patient's neurologic status. Gertzbein and colleagues formulated a classification system dealing with the structural components of spinal injury, similar to the AO fracture classification used for the extremities. The lesions are differentiated on the basis of not only the mechanism and radiographic appearance of the injury

FIGURE 30-30   *Denis' classification of fracture–dislocation of the spine.* ***A,*** *Type A is a flexion–rotation injury, occurring either through bone or through the disk. There is a complete disruption of all three columns of the spine, usually with the anterior longitudinal ligament remaining the only intact structure. Commonly, this is stripped off the anterior portion of the vertebral body below. These injuries are usually associated with fractures of the superior facet of the more caudal vertebra.* ***B,*** *Type B is a shear injury. The type that produces anterior spondylolisthesis of the more cephalad vertebra usually fractures a facet, but the type that causes a posterior listhiasis of the more cephalad vertebra normally does not cause a fracture of the facet joint.* ***C,*** *Type C is a bilateral facet dislocation. This is a flexion–distraction injury but with disruption of the anterior column in addition to the posterior and middle columns. This disruption through the anterior column may occur through either the anterior intervertebral disk or the anterior vertebral body.*

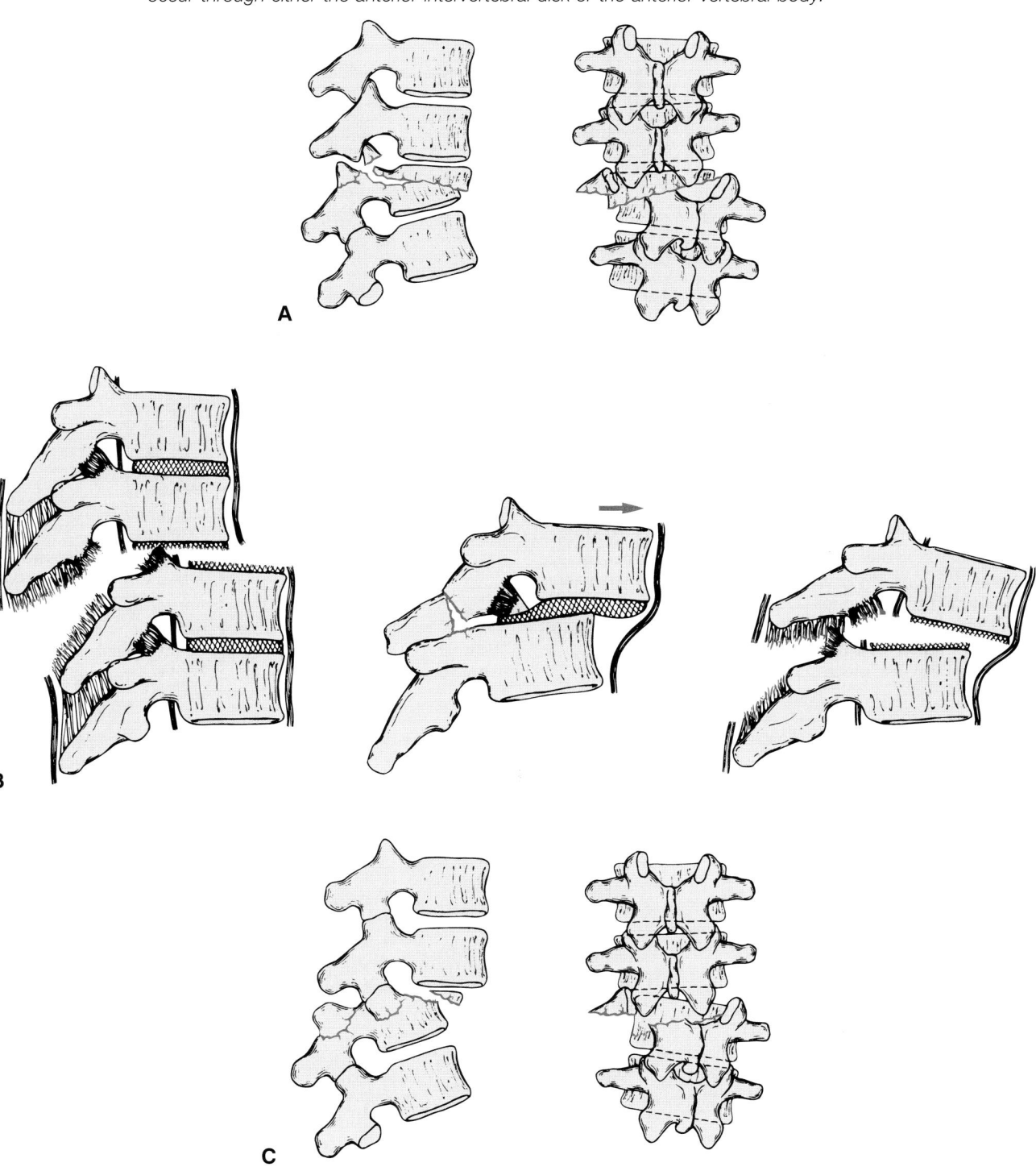

FIGURE 30-31   *Comprehensive classification of spine injuries.* **A,** *Type A vertebral body compression.* **B,** *Type B anterior and posterior element injury with distraction.* **C,** *Type C anterior and posterior element injury with rotation. (Redrawn by permission from Gertzbein, S.D. Classification of thoracic and lumbar fractures. In: Gertzbein, S.D., ed. Fractures of the Thoracic and Lumbar Spine. Baltimore, Williams and Wilkins, 1992.)*

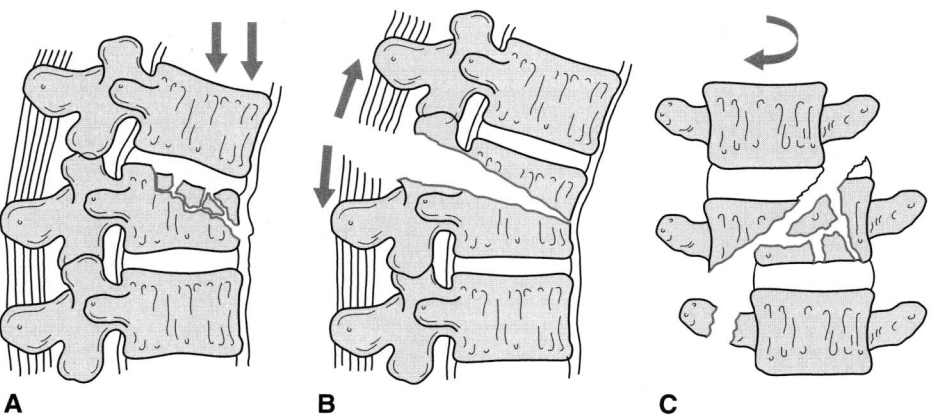

but also the associated soft tissue disruption. The classification consists of well-defined categories based on common morphologic characteristics, as well as common primary forces producing the particular injury pattern (Fig. 30-31).

Three main injury types are recognized. Type A injuries are vertebral body compression fractures (Fig. 30-32). They are caused by axial loading with or without additional flexion forces and are associated with loss of vertebral height. Type B injuries involve both the anterior and the posterior elements and are caused by distraction forces (Fig. 30-33). The hallmark of these injuries is elongation of the distance between portions of the adjacent vertebrae. In type C injuries, anterior and posterior disruption is present along with associated evidence of rotational instability, such as offset vertebral bodies, unilateral facet fracture–dislocations, or fractured transverse processes (Fig. 30-34).

The three major patterns and their associated subtypes represent a continuum of injury severity, from type A lesions, which are axially unstable, to type B lesions, which have additional sagittal plane instability, to type C, with instability in all three planes. Because the classification progresses according to the severity of bony and soft tissue disruption, as well as stability, it may be used as a guide for treatment, with injuries more advanced on the classification being more likely to benefit from surgical treatment. However, it has not been validated as a reproducible classification and is unlikely to be validated because of its extreme complexity.

Because of the complexity of the AO system and simplicity of the Denis classification schemes, an effort has been made to formulate a comprehensive system that more reliably offers treatment recommendations to the surgeon. Wood and co-workers found that both systems produce only moderate reliability and reproducibility when

FIGURE 30-32   *Comprehensive classification of spine injuries—type A injuries. The three categories of type A fractures include impaction injuries* **(A1),** *of which wedge fractures are most commonly seen; split fractures* **(A2),** *of which the pincer fracture is the typical injury; and the burst fracture* **(A3)**. *(Redrawn by permission from Gertzbein, S.D. Classification of thoracic and lumbar fractures. In: Gertzbein, S.D., ed. Fractures of the Thoracic and Lumbar Spine. Baltimore, Williams and Wilkins, 1992.)*

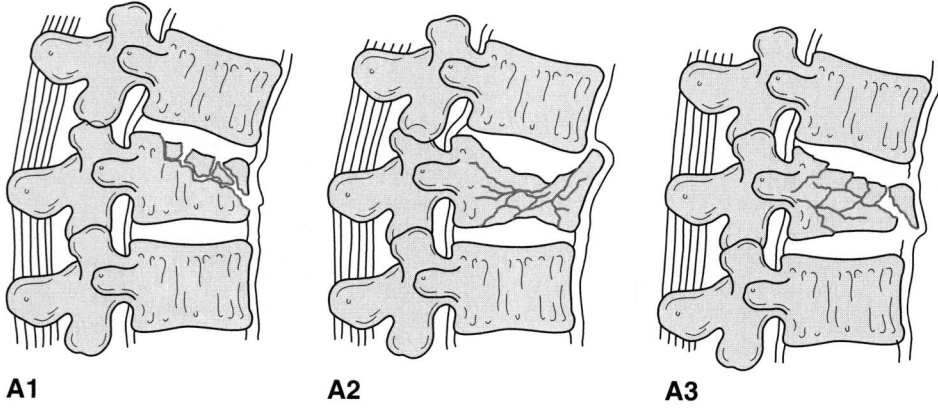

FIGURE 30-33 | *Comprehensive classification of spine injuries—type B injuries. Flexion–distraction injuries can result in disruption of soft tissues posteriorly through the capsule of the facet joints **(B1)** or through the body arch **(B2)**. If distraction and extension occur, anterior disruption through the disk often may be seen **(B3)**, with or without associated fractures or soft tissue injuries of the posterior elements. (Redrawn by permission from Gertzbein, S.D. Classification of thoracic and lumbar fractures. In: Gertzbein, S.D., ed. Fractures of the Thoracic and Lumbar Spine. Baltimore, Williams and Wilkins, 1992.)*

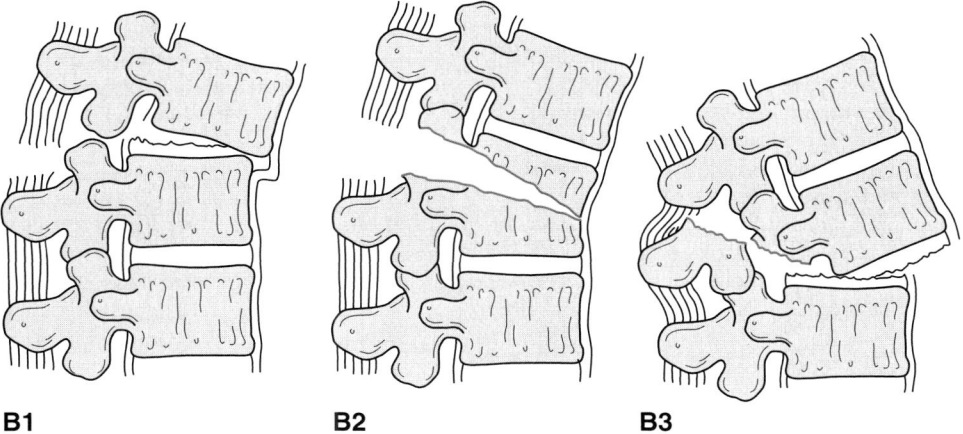

B1   **B2**   **B3**

classified by fellowship-trained spine surgeons.[178] Although the initial fracture types had 82 and 79 percent intra-rater agreement for the AO and Denis systems, respectively, those numbers decreased to 67 and 56 percent, respectively, for the subgroup classifications.

Thoracolumbar Injury Severity Score

Because of the lack of understanding of the natural history of various subtypes of thoracolumbar fractures and the absence of a universally accepted classification system, the Spine Trauma Study Group developed the Thoracolumbar Injury Severity Score system for these fractures.[160,161] This system bases its scoring on three major variables: the mechanism of injury, neurologic status, and integrity of the posterior ligamentous complex. The goal of the system is to determine which fractures are at risk for clinical instability and to address those fractures surgically to ensure mechanical and neurologic stability. The combined score in these categories assists the surgeon in choosing a treatment course, either operative or nonoperative. By reviewing a selection of cases, retrospectively, which involved the three major injury patterns, including compression, translational–rotational, and distraction injuries, they were able to determine the validity of the scoring system.

The initial step in this classification is to determine the mechanism of injury or fracture morphology. The worst level of fracture is scored when there are multiple fractures, and combined mechanisms are additive. Compression

FIGURE 30-34 | *Comprehensive classification of spine injuries—type C injuries. The common feature of these injuries is rotation, associated with compression **(C1)**, distraction **(C2)**, or rotational shear **(C3)**. (Redrawn by permission from Gertzbein, S.D. Classification of thoracic and lumbar fractures. In: Gertzbein, S.D., ed. Fractures of the Thoracic and Lumbar Spine. Baltimore, Williams and Wilkins, 1992.)*

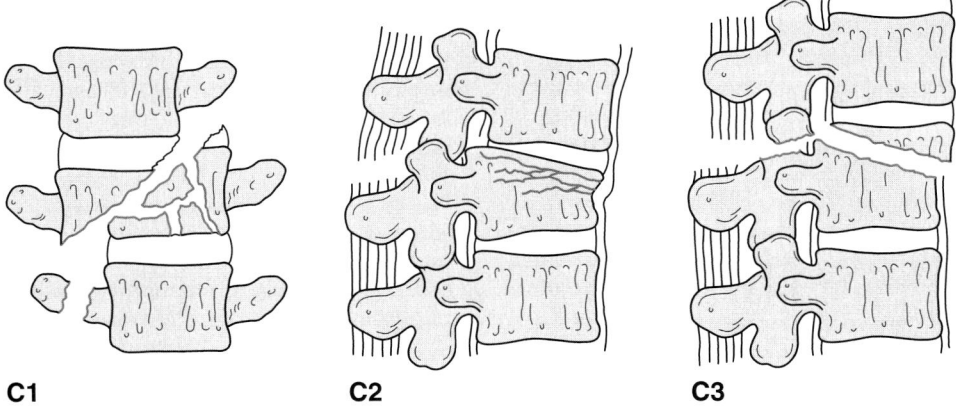

C1   **C2**   **C3**

injuries involving only the anterior aspect of the vertebral body are scored with 1 point, and burst fractures involving the posterior vertebral body cortex are scored as 2 points. Coronal plane deformity >15° adds an additional point. Translational–rotational injuries, which represent a more significant shear or torsional injury, are scored with 3 points, and distraction injuries, which result from tensile forces, are assigned 4 points. These fractures are inherently unstable due to circumferential disruption of the spinal elements, either osseous or ligamentous.

Secondly, the patient's neurologic status is determined. Scoring is divided into four subcategories based on the severity of the deficit and the potential for recovery. Intact patients are scored 0 points, and nerve root injury is scored 2 points. Complete spinal cord injury is scored 2 points, whereas patients with incomplete injuries or cauda equine are scored 3 points, given the potential benefits of decompression of the neural elements.

The third component of the system is to determine the integrity of the posterior ligamentous complex, based on exam, radiographic, CT, or magnetic resonance imaging (MRI) findings. When no injury is present, 0 points are assigned. If the studies and exam are indeterminate, then 2 points are assigned, and definite disruption is assigned 3 points.

Treatment is based on the total score. Patients with 3 points are treated nonoperatively. Patients with 5 points are treated with surgery. Those patients who score 4 points may be treated surgically or nonoperatively, and the surgeon must weigh clinical qualifiers such as age, concomitant injury, and comorbidities (Table 30-1).

Although this classification system has shown acceptable reliability,[160,161,170] a more definitive description

of posterior ligamentous complex integrity and fracture morphology and mechanism of injury may improve its reproducibility, and the idea of considering fracture morphology rather than mechanism of injury has been raised. A recent study has suggested that mechanism of injury may be a more valuable parameter to consider than fracture morphology for classification and treatment of thoracolumbar fractures.[170] Treatment recommendations, however, agree in the vast majority of cases between surgeons, achieving greater than 90 percent agreement. This classification is currently progressing into the clinical validation phase through prospective study.

Other useful classification systems are described by Ferguson and Allen[49] and by McAfee and co-workers.[112,113] These classification systems focus primarily on the mechanical forces involved and describe the type of bone or ligamentous injuries associated with these forces. The American Spinal Injury Association (ASIA) classification system for neurologic injury is the most commonly used system to describe spinal cord injury.

In order to provide clinical guidelines for diagnosing and treating specific injuries, we have chosen to employ the Thoracolumbar Injury Severity Score used in conjunction with the Denis classification for describing the injuries. For purposes of consistency, a nomenclature and classification system consisting of a combination of mechanistic and descriptive features is used; it is the same for thoracic, thoracolumbar, and lumbar injuries. The first group of injuries consists of minor injuries, such as avulsion and minor fractures. The second group includes compression fractures or injuries generated by a combination of flexion and bending that can be either stable or unstable, depending on the degree of anterior compression and ligamentous disruption. The third major group represents burst fractures caused by a combination of flexion and axial loading in varying proportion, and they are easily subdivided by Denis' classification. The fourth group is flexion–distraction injuries, which are subdivided according to the injured tissues: the pure bony form is a Chance fracture, the purely ligamentous form is a bilateral facet dislocation, and the combination form is either an anterior bony injury with posterior ligamentous disruption or a posterior bony injury with anterior disk disruption. The fifth group of injuries results from an extension force. The final type is caused by shear. No comprehensive or universal system exists because the optimal classification system would have to combine the fracture pattern with instability and neural status.

TREATMENT OPTIONS

Nonoperative treatment of thoracic and thoracolumbar spine injuries can be extremely effective. The data presented by Frankel and associates in 1969 remain the standard against which most treatments and final outcomes are measured.[54] Similar excellent results were published by Davies and colleagues.[32] If surgery is to be considered for these patients, the outcomes of surgery must be superior to nonoperative treatment in order to justify the increased risks of surgery.

Table 30-1

TLISS System

Injury mechanism: worst level is used and injury is additive (e.g., a distraction injury with a burst component without lateral angulation would receive 1 [simple compression] + 1 [burst] + 4 [distraction] = 6)

	Qualifier	Points
1. Description		
a. Compression	Simple compression	1
	Lateral angulation >15°	1
	Burst	1
b. Translational/ rotational		3
c. Distraction		4
2. PLC disrupted in tension, rotation, or translation		
a. Intact		0
b. Suspected/indeterminate		2
c. Injured		3
3. Neurologic status		
Nerve root involvement		2
Cord, conus medullaris involvement	Incomplete	3
	Complete	2
Cauda equina involvement		3

The score is the total of three components: injury mechanism, neurologic status, and PLC disruption. A score of ≤3 suggests nonoperative treatment, 4, operative or nonoperative treatment, and ≥5 suggests operative treatment.
From Vaccaro, A.R.; et al. Spine 31:11(Suppl) 562–569, 2006.

A comparison of the results of surgical and nonsurgical treatment in the literature is difficult because of the variations in injury type and differences in severity in the two groups, with surgically treated groups often containing patients with more severe injuries.[63] There is little or no level I evidence comparing outcomes for similar degrees of bony and neurologic injury. Some series show a slight trend toward better neurologic improvement with surgical treatment, but the statistical significance is not high.[92] Most investigators describing better neurologic improvement with surgery have directed their attention at neural decompression through either an anterior or posterior approach.[3,62,80,180] Edwards and Levine described better neurologic recovery than would be expected with nonoperative treatment by using the Edwards instrumentation system posteriorly while depending on indirect decompression based on improved fracture reduction.[43] Gertzbein, in a study of 1019 spine fractures, found no significant improvement in neurologic function with operative treatment.[62] In addition, Bravo and co-workers did not find a significant difference in neurologic improvement in patients treated with surgery versus those treated by postural reduction and immobilization.[25]

Neurologic deterioration can occur during nonoperative treatment and was documented in 6 of 33 patients with burst fractures of the thoracic or thoracolumbar spine.[37] In that study Denis and co-workers concluded that surgical treatment was a safer treatment option for this specific injury. However, Frankel and associates, in their review of 371 patients with thoracic or thoracolumbar fractures, found that only 0.5 percent had neurologic deterioration when treated by postural reduction and recumbency.[54] Mumford and co-workers reported a 2.4 percent incidence of neurologic deterioration in patients with burst fractures treated nonoperatively.[121] If patients experience neurologic deterioration during nonoperative treatment, surgical treatment, including decompression by an anterior approach, can be performed. Finally, whether surgical treatment or nonoperative treatment is safer depends to some degree on the experience and preference of the treating physician and the medical team.[62]

Deformity can be corrected with surgery, but it is unclear whether it is clinically relevant.[158,162,178] Nicoll[122] noted no correlation between deformity and symptoms, whereas Soreff and colleagues[151] found a significant correlation. McAfee and associates,[111] in their review of later anterior decompression and fusion for thoracolumbar and lumbar injuries, found that residual kyphosis did not inhibit neural improvement. Gertzbein, however, reported that kyphosis of more than 30° was associated with a significantly increased amount of back pain at 2-year follow-up.[62] Edwards and Levine's data also suggest that anatomic restoration is important in obtaining good long-term results.[44]

Some authors believe that chronic back pain is diminished in operatively treated patients compared with those treated nonoperatively.[62] This improvement in relief of pain may be a result of better correction and maintenance of alignment with operative treatment. In addition, operative treatment includes fusion of motion segments with significantly damaged soft tissue elements. These injured tissues often have poor healing potential, and the patient is left with an abnormal motion segment even after adequate healing of bone.

Most authors agree that hospitalization time can be shortened by surgical stabilization in patients with paralysis.[40,53,82,134] Mobilization and rehabilitation can be facilitated by rigid surgical stabilization, which decreases the associated morbidity of prolonged immobilization. However, Gertzbein, in a multicenter spinal fracture study, found the complication rate in surgical patients to be more than 25 percent, whereas patients treated nonoperatively had a complication rate of only 1 percent.[62] The patients treated surgically tended to have more severe injuries and a higher incidence of neurologic deficit, both of which increase the likelihood of complications regardless of treatment type. Place and colleagues compared operative and nonoperative treatment of patients who sustained spinal fractures with resultant complete spinal cord injuries.[130] The length of inpatient hospital and rehabilitation stay was 19% less for the surgically treated group, even though their rate of complications was almost twice as high as that in the nonoperative group. At this time, early mobilization remains the primary predictable advantage of instrumentation.

In rare instances in which surgery poses an extremely high risk, patients with unstable fractures may be treated with extended bedrest and spinal precautions. The benefits of this treatment, however, must be weighed against the potential complications of decubitus ulcers and pulmonary compromise. The use of rotating beds may help decrease the incidence of decubitus ulcers. The formation of deep venous thrombosis is also a risk in these patients. The use of chemical thromboprophylaxis is recommended in these patients to offset this risk.[148] It is recommended that anticoagulation be delayed 72 hours from the time of injury to avoid the formation of epidural hematomas.

TREATMENT OF SPECIFIC INJURIES

Minor Fractures

Fractures of the transverse processes usually occur either from direct trauma or as a result of violent muscular contraction (avulsion injuries) in response to injury. Isolated fractures of the spinous processes may result from a direct blow over the posterior aspect of the spine. Similarly, a fracture of the articular process may occur as a result of direct trauma. In each of these cases, even though the injury may appear trivial, further evaluation is necessary to be certain that no other associated spinal injuries are present. Such evaluation is most easily accomplished by obtaining a thin-cut CT scan through the index vertebra and the adjacent vertebrae. If the CT scan is negative (no other injuries detected), lateral flexion and extension radiographs should be considered if dynamic instability is a concern. Once other major injuries to the spine have been excluded, these patients can be mobilized without brace or activity restrictions, except as needed for relief of pain. Because transverse process fractures are associated with underlying soft tissue injury, they can be painful and an orthotic may be helpful. The primary exception to this is an L5 transverse process fracture. This may be associated with a sacral fracture and a neurogenic bladder. A CT extending into the sacrum should routinely be performed.

Another minor injury is an isolated fracture of the pars interarticularis at one level, either unilaterally or bilaterally. In Denis' series, four individuals had this type of fracture, with all four being the result of a sports injury.[36] If the patient has this injury along with a negative previous history of local spine pain (particularly in a young adult or teenager), it can be assumed that this fracture is an acute injury that is best treated with immobilization. In the thoracolumbar and upper lumbar regions of the spine, a total-contact thoracolumbosacral orthosis (TLSO) is appropriate. At the L5 level of the spine, it may be necessary to include one thigh to provide adequate immobilization (see Chapter 27).

Compression Fractures

Compression fractures involve disruption of the anterior column with an intact middle column and differentiation from a minimally displaced burst fracture (with associated middle column involvement) may be difficult on plain radiograph. McGrory and colleagues described the use of the posterior vertebral body angle (PVBA) measured on a lateral plain radiograph.[116] The PVBA is the angle formed by either the superior or the inferior end plate and the posterior vertebral body wall. An angle greater than 100° for either the superior or the inferior PVBA is considered diagnostic of a burst fracture. A slight decrease in height of the posterior wall relative to the vertebra above and below and loss of the biconcave contour may also suggest the presence of a burst rather than a compression fracture. Even with careful scrutiny, 20 percent or more of subtle burst fractures can be misdiagnosed on plain radiographs. Therefore, the routine use of CT for patients with probable compression fractures is a better method for evaluating the middle column.[14] Treatment of these injuries depends on the status of the posterior elements, which may or may not be disrupted. If the anterior column is compressed 40 percent or more or if the kyphosis exceeds 25 to 30°, it can be inferred that the ligaments of the posterior column have been attenuated to the point that they can no longer function normally. MRI has been shown to be a useful adjunct for identifying the presence of posterior ligamentous injury.[89] In addition, MRI may be helpful in differentiating benign from pathologic compression fractures.[8]

Nonoperative treatment is adequate in most compression fractures with less than 40 percent anterior compression and less than 25 to 30° kyphosis. These patients can usually be treated with an orthosis, such as a total-contact TLSO orthosis or, occasionally a Jewett or Boston brace for young patients with fractures of the thoracolumbar junction. They can be allowed to participate in most of their normal activities while wearing the brace. They should be discouraged from lying supine on a soft mattress with multiple pillows because this position can accentuate the deformity. Hazel and associates reviewed the long-term outcome of neurologically intact patients with compression fractures treated nonoperatively.[73] Of the 25 patients monitored, 8 had no symptoms, 11 had occasional back pain, 5 needed treatment or modification of activity because of frequent pain, and only 1 had chronic disabling back pain.

The brace should be worn for at least 3 months with standing lateral flexion and extension radiographs out of the brace obtained at the end of that time. If no abnormal motion is seen through the fractured vertebra or disk above and if the deformity has not progressed, use of the orthosis can be discontinued. Muscle weakness may be marked, and gradual cessation of bracing over a few weeks may be beneficial, along with a muscle-strengthening program to help support the spine. In those patients with abnormal motion at the level of injury, continued pain, or unacceptable progression of deformity, surgery may be indicated. Some authors believe that stable fractures in the upper and middle thoracic spine do not require brace treatment at all because of the inherent stability of the rib cage. Most authors, however, tend to be more cautious and recommend external immobilization at the thoracolumbar junction or in the lumbar spine. Schlickewei and associates compared a group of patients with stable thoracolumbar injuries treated by early mobilization with or without a brace.[142] After an average of 2.5 years' follow-up, they found good or excellent results in both groups, without clinically significant differences in progression of deformity between groups.

Initial surgical treatment should be considered if the anterior column is compressed more than 40 percent, if the kyphosis exceeds 25 to 30°, or if the posterior ligamentous structures are disrupted. MRI can be helpful in borderline cases for determining if the posterior ligaments are injured.

If surgery is indicated, a posterior surgical approach using pedicle screw and rod fixation is preferred. Although hooks and rods have been used in the past with good results, the use of pedicle screws provides purchase in all three columns and has been shown to be biomechanically superior to hooks and rods.[18,75] The goal of surgery is to restore coronal and sagittal alignment and to provide rigid fixation until a solid fusion is achieved. The use of neuromonitoring can be helpful if any correction is being performed.

Anterior surgery for neural decompression is not required for patients with these fractures because the middle column remains intact and thus any canal compromise is typically not clinically relevant. However, supplemental anterior surgery may occasionally be necessary for patients with marked anterior destruction to restore bone stock. This situation is usually seen in patients with severe osteopenia who are involved in high-energy injuries. In these patients, however, kyphoplasty or vertebroplasty may be a better alternative if there is not any posterior ligamentous injury.[58,60,155]

Burst Fractures

By definition, all burst fractures include disruption of the anterior and middle columns, with or without disruption of the posterior column. The type of treatment depends on the severity of the injury. The three most important factors to be considered are the percentage of spinal canal compromise, the degree of angulation present at the site of injury, and the presence or absence of a neurologic deficit.

No strong clinical basis has been established for a consensus on the best treatment of patients with burst fractures. James and co-workers, using a cadaver L1 burst fracture model, showed that the condition of the posterior column was the most important factor in determining the acute stability of a burst fracture and, therefore, the suitability for nonoperative treatment.[83] They went on to review a series of patients with intact posterior columns, but varying degrees of anterior and middle column disruption, and noted that they healed without further deformity. Willen and colleagues reported on 54 patients with thoracolumbar burst fractures treated nonoperatively, including patients with neurologic deficit.[176] Most of the deformity occurred on initial mobilization, with little progression of deformity noted at follow-up. Patients with more than 50 percent loss of height or more than 50 percent canal compromise were found to have significantly increased complaints of pain at follow-up. Cantor and co-workers also recommended operative treatment for patients with evidence of posterior column disruption.[30] Treatment of burst fractures can be directed by the goals of surgery. Three parameters determine these goals: neurologic status, instability, and deformity. In patients with neurologic compromise accompanied by instability, cord compression, marked deformity, or any combination of these conditions, surgical intervention is the most appropriate treatment. It should be emphasized that a neurologic deficit includes not only lower extremity motor and sensory dysfunction but also perineal sensory loss and bowel or bladder dysfunction. Nonoperative treatment of a patient with a neural deficit can be considered in the rare instance of a stable burst fracture without deformity or residual cord compression. If the patient is neurologically intact and has less than 50 percent canal compromise and less than 30° kyphosis, nonoperative treatment is indicated. Patients with minimal angulation and a two-column or stable burst pattern should be placed in a total-contact orthosis with early ambulation as tolerated. Surgery is the preferred treatment in patients with more than 50 percent canal compromise or more than 30° kyphosis at the level of injury, even if they do not have any neurologic deficit. It is believed that patients who have more than 50 percent canal compromise or more than 30° kyphosis have disrupted the posterior ligaments.[36] Surgery is also recommended if disruption of the posterior ligaments is seen on MRI. Surgical intervention is recommended in these patients to prevent progressive deformity and chronic pain.

Controversies in the nonoperative treatment of burst fractures include the appropriateness of bedrest and the duration and types of orthosis. The duration of using a total-contact orthosis should be at least 3 months. During that time, once ambulation is initiated and no change in alignment is observed on standing lateral radiographs, an increase in activities can be allowed. Some progressive loss of height across the involved disk space is to be expected; however, if posterior spinous process widening is noted or angulation increases to more than 30°, surgical treatment is recommended.[83] Mumford and co-workers studied 41 patients with thoracolumbar fractures and no neurologic deficit who were treated nonoperatively.[121]

The average collapse at follow-up was only 8 percent, with significant resorption of protruding bone and diminution in canal compromise (22%). Almost 90 percent of patients had satisfactory work status at last follow-up. The authors were unable to correlate residual deformity with symptoms. Cantor and associates reported their results on 18 neurologically intact patients with burst fractures treated nonoperatively.[30] They found no prolonged hospital stay, no significantly increased kyphosis, and little or no restriction of function at follow-up.

If nonoperative treatment is used, prolonged riding in automobiles and participation in impact activities should be discouraged for 3 to 6 months. The patient should also be instructed to avoid marked flexion at the level of injury while lying in bed and to avoid lying supine with multiple pillows because this position could increase the deformity. If they are unable to understand or follow these instructions, either a cast or surgery should be considered. Patients should be instructed to notify the physician immediately if any paresthesias, cramping in their lower extremities, weakness in their legs, or a change in bowel or bladder control develops. Patients should be evaluated frequently (1 week, 1 month, 2 months, and 3 months after injury) with standing lateral radiographs to be certain that the angulation at the level of injury has not increased. After healing appears to be adequate, flexion–extension radiographs are taken with the patient out of the brace to ensure that no excessive motion has occurred at the fracture level. If nonoperative treatment fails and either progressive deformity or a neurologic deficit develops, surgical intervention should be considered. The type of surgery depends on the method of failure of nonoperative treatment. If a neurologic deficit develops, anterior decompression should be considered because posterior instrumentation performed more than 2 to 3 weeks after injury will not adequately indirectly reduce the canal compromise. Similarly, posterolateral decompression may be difficult as the fragment begins to heal into position. However, if nonoperative treatment because of persistent pain or increasing deformity, posterior surgery is usually adequate. If the deformity is partially corrected on flexion–extension views, satisfactory reduction of kyphosis may be achieved with posterior instrumentation and fusion. However, the longer the time from injury, the less successful, and higher the risk with posterior correction and instrumented fusion.

Burst fractures that require operative treatment should be reviewed on a case by case basis because these fractures can be treated anteriorly, posteriorly, or combined anteriorly and posteriorly depending on the amount of canal compromise and posterior ligamentous disruption.

Zou and colleagues studied the use of various posterior fixation devices for the treatment of burst fractures in a cadaver model.[183] They noted that devices capable of providing distraction and restoration of sagittal alignment resulted in significantly better canal decompression than did systems that used only distraction. Mann and associates compared the Syracuse I Plate (applied anteriorly) with the AO Fixateur Interne pedicle screw system for the treatment of burst fractures.[110] They found that both systems provided adequate stability in patients without posterior column disruption. In the presence of posterior disruption, posterior instrumentation provided significantly increased stability. Gurwitz and colleagues compared the use of the Kaneda device for anterior fixation with pedicle screws and a variable spinal plate (VSP) posteriorly for fixation of a corpectomy model used to simulate a burst fracture.[67] They found that short-segment posterior instrumentation did not adequately restore spinal stability. Farcy and co-workers reported that posterior fixation does not adequately prevent collapse if significant anterior destruction with concomitant kyphosis has occurred.[48] They recommended the addition of an anterior strut graft for mechanical reasons, in addition to posterior instrumentation. Surgeons who perform posterior stabilization procedures should be aware that patients who have burst fractures with concomitant lamina fractures and a neurologic deficit have a 50 to 70 percent chance that a posterior dural laceration secondary to the injury is also present.[29] Should this complication be encountered, the surgical team should be prepared to make appropriate repairs. It is not, however, an indication to perform posterior surgery to treat the dural tear.

Anterior decompression and fusion (with instrumentation) may be performed to treat burst injuries. This procedure is best for patients with significant neural compression and neurologic deficit, particularly those with minimal kyphotic deformity. Anterior decompression and fusion should be routinely considered if the injury occurred 3 or more weeks previously. The use of this approach best ensures complete neural decompression, and although more residual deformity may remain than with most posterior instrumentation systems, it is tolerated by the patient if the anterior fusion is solid. With the use of anterior instrumentation it is possible to obtain adequate correction of deformity, as well as decompression and rigid stabilization in the thoracolumbar, midlumbar, and low lumbar spine. In a study by McDonough and co-workers, 35 patients with thoracolumbar fractures treated with anterior corpectomy and instrumented fusion without supplemental posterior instrumentation were evaluated.[114] Indications for anterior corpectomy were neurologic injury, segmental kyphosis, and severe vertebral body comminution. They noted that all 16 patients who presented with a neurologic injury improved at least one Frankel grade, whereas 69 percent improved completely. Sagittal alignment also improved from 18° kyphosis at presentation to 6° kyphosis at the end of 2 years. In another study by Sasso and associates, 40 patients who had a thoracolumbar fracture treated by anterior corpectomy and fusion without posterior instrumentation were compared with 13 patients treated by short-segment posterior instrumentation and fusion.[140] They noted that although both groups had good initial correction, the posteriorly treated patients lost 8.1° of correction at final follow-up but the anteriorly treated patients lost only 1.8° of correction. Although patients in both groups did well, it is difficult to project what long-term consequences the lost correction will have. Thus, anterior decompression and fusion should be considered in patients who have neurologic compromise or who have severe vertebral body comminution. Posterior instrumentation and fusion may be considered in patients with posterior element disruption but no neurologic compromise and little vertebral body comminution. Combined anterior and posterior fusions should be considered in patients with severe vertebral body comminution and posterior element disruption. If there is also neurologic compromise, the anterior corpectomy will decompress the nerves. Bear in mind, however, that these are general guidelines for evaluating patients with thoracolumbar burst fractures in whom surgery is being considered. They are not absolute rules, and there may be exceptions to these guidelines.

Laminectomy *by itself* is not indicated for the treatment of burst fractures. It cannot relieve the anterior neural compression, further destabilizes the spine, and is often associated with an increase in neurologic deficit.[20,21]

Flexion–Distraction Injuries

Flexion–distraction injuries are characterized by disruption of the posterior and middle columns of the spine in tension, whereas the anterior column usually remains intact and acts as a hinge. The decision to perform nonoperative rather than operative treatment depends primarily on whether this injury is through bone, as originally described by Chance (Denis' type A), or it also involves significant ligamentous injuries, as seen in atypical Chance fractures (Denis' types B, C, and D).[31] A Chance fracture extending only through bone has an excellent prognosis for healing, although it may be unstable early and difficult to hold in anatomic reduction without surgery. Injuries with significant ligamentous disruption tend to heal in a less predictable fashion and should be considered unstable both acutely and chronically.

Nonoperative care of a patient with a seat belt injury through bone may consist of bedrest for 2 weeks or longer, followed by mobilization in a total-contact TLSO molded in hyperextension. This orthosis is best molded with the patient in the prone position or supine on an extension frame. The patient should be instructed to wear the TLSO and participate in activities as tolerated while wearing the brace. Frequent evaluation with radiographs taken in the standing position should be made to ensure that the deformity has not progressed. After 3 to 4 months, the level of injury should be assessed for excess motion with flexion–extension radiographs obtained out of the brace. If nonoperative treatment has failed to produce a stable spine with minimal deformity, surgical treatment consisting of posterior fusion with a compression system is indicated. Even if treatment is performed late after injury, the chance of obtaining successful fusion and satisfactory alignment of the spine is good. Alternatively, early posterior fixation with instrumentation and fusion can be considered if fracture–ligament stability or patient compliance is a concern or if body habitus precludes application of a well-fitting brace.

If a seat belt injury is to be treated operatively, posterior pedicle screws and rods are generally used. Positioning the patient in the prone position with support under the chest and pelvis can often anatomically reduce the fracture. Anterior decompression is not usually appropriate or necessary (unless a large disk herniation is present at the level).

Fracture–Dislocations

In fracture–dislocations, all three columns of the spine are disrupted. These injuries have the highest incidence of neurologic deficit. Most patients with this injury pattern should be treated surgically. If a fracture–dislocation is present and the patient is neurologically normal, surgery is performed to stabilize the spine and prevent the occurrence of a neurologic deficit while allowing the patient to be mobilized. If a fracture–dislocation is present and the patient has an incomplete neurologic deficit, surgery should be performed to stabilize the spine and decompress the neural elements. If a fracture–dislocation is present and the patient has a complete neurologic deficit, surgery should be performed to stabilize the spine, shorten the hospital stay, minimize the need for rigid external immobilization, and maximize the patient's potential for rehabilitation.

The surgical management of fracture–dislocations varies according to the type of injury. If the patient is neurologically normal or has an incomplete neurologic deficit, it is best to intubate and turn the patient to the prone position while still awake. The patient's muscle tone helps stabilize the spine during turning, and the patient can be quickly monitored after turning to make certain that neurologic function is unchanged. Most patients do not find this maneuver particularly distressful, provided that they are informed of it in advance. It makes the turning and positioning maneuvers safer than logrolling an anesthetized patient with a spinal column injury who has no inherent ability to protect the cord. After positioning has been completed and neurologic assessment has been performed, the patient may be anesthetized. An alternative method is to perform an awake intubation with the patient supine on an Orthopedic Systems, Inc. (OSI) table. Once the patient is intubated, the anterior portion can be secured to the patient and table and the patient is then rotated 180° to the prone position and the posterior portion is removed.

In both flexion–rotation and flexion–distraction injuries, the anterior longitudinal ligament most often remains intact. These injuries can be adequately treated with a pedicle screw and rod system.

Primary acute anterior decompression rarely has a role in fracture–dislocations because the main problem in these injuries is usually stability and malalignment. Realignment by itself frequently decompresses the compromised neural elements. Anterior decompression may be used in conjunction with posterior instrumentation if adequate decompression cannot be achieved from a posterior procedure alone. This option is particularly important in a patient with a partial neurologic deficit.

Soft Tissue Injuries

Soft tissue injuries (grades 1 and 2 sprains) involving the thoracic and lumbar spine without complete ligamentous disruption are diagnosed by exclusion after obtaining a detailed history, performing a thorough physical examination, and ordering appropriate tests. Treatment is symptomatic, as for soft tissue injuries that occur elsewhere in the body. Standard physical therapy measures coupled with short-term bedrest may prove helpful, if necessary, to relieve symptoms. Provided that structural integrity is present, gradual mobilization of the patient should be encouraged. The administration of analgesics, including nonsteroidal anti-inflammatory drugs, may shorten the course of disability and decrease symptoms. Two treatment options to be avoided are prolonged rigid immobilization and chronic use of narcotic analgesics.

If symptoms of the soft tissue injury persist, the patient should be reevaluated with the use of plain radiographs with flexion–extension lateral views. If results are negative, a bone scan or MRI may be performed to rule out an occult spinal fracture or ligamentous injury. If any area is abnormal in the bone scan, a thin-section CT scan with reconstructions should be obtained. Additionally, if the symptoms warrant, MRI can be performed to rule out disk herniation or other soft tissue injury.

Disk Injuries

High-energy injuries of the intervertebral disks in the thoracic and thoracolumbar spine are uncommon, but they can be a significant source or morbidity and cause pain or even paralysis. Disk herniations down to the T12-L1 and sometimes the L1-L2 interspaces can involve spinal cord compression, whereas in disk herniations below these levels, compression is limited to the cauda equina. As stated previously, the spinal cord is more susceptible to injury and less likely to recover once injured. This discussion is limited to disk herniations in the thoracic and thoracolumbar regions.

The classification of disk herniations in the thoracic spine is the same as for herniations in the low lumbar spine. Disk abnormalities are defined as bulging, protruded, extruded, or sequestered. A *bulging,* or *protruded,* disk is defined as an injury in which the nucleus pulposus migrates posteriorly but remains confined within the annulus fibrosis. With an *extruded* disk, the nucleus pulposus ruptures through the annulus fibrosis but is still confined anterior to the posterior longitudinal ligament. When a disk is *sequestered,* the nucleus pulposus has ruptured through the annulus fibrosis, as well as the posterior longitudinal ligament, and lies within the spinal canal, separated from the disk space. The thoracic and thoracolumbar regions of the spine are less tolerant than the lumbar spine of any of these disk abnormalities. Even a protruded intervertebral disk may be symptomatic because the spinal canal is narrower than in the cervical and low lumbar regions and the thoracic cord is more susceptible to pressure because of the limited vascular supply and small space.

Though significantly less common, limbus fractures of the lumbar spine must be considered in the differential diagnosis of any adolescent or young adult thought to have a traumatic herniated nucleus pulposus. Fracture of the lumbar vertebral limbus consists of a fracture of the peripheral apophyseal ring from either the posterosuperior or the posteroinferior aspect of the vertebra, and the symptoms are similar to those seen with a herniated nucleus pulposus. Although they were originally thought to occur exclusively in the pediatric population, a number of studies have shown the existence of fragmented, unfused apophyseal rings in adults. Epstein and Epstein reported on

27 patients who sustained limbus vertebral fractures at an average age of 32 years and range extending to 44 years of age.[47] Treatment of these lesions is by surgical excision.

Symptoms of thoracic and thoracolumbar disk herniation include pain, paresthesias, and neurologic deficits. The pain may be local and axial at the level of injury, or it may be radicular in nature, with radiation to the flank, along a rib, or down toward the groin if the disk herniation is at the thoracolumbar junction. Less commonly, pain may involve all areas distal to the spinal cord compression. When this type of dysesthetic pain occurs, significant neural compression and weakness are usually present.

Neurologic findings can include a wide-based, ataxic gait. Sensation may be decreased either in a radicular distribution or in a distribution involving all regions distal to the level of spinal cord compression. Weakness may be present and may follow any of the patterns of spinal cord syndromes. Complete paralysis may also be associated with thoracic or thoracolumbar disk herniation. In addition, abnormal findings related to rectal tone, perineal sensation, and bladder function may be observed. Subtle changes may be detected with cystometric evaluation. The reflexes may range from normal in patients with minimal spinal cord compression to marked hyper-reflexia with a positive Babinski sign in patients with significant spinal cord compression.

Thoracic disk herniation can be detected by MRI, myelography, or myelography followed by CT (which has the added advantage over just myelography of demonstrating spinal cord deformity at the level of the disk herniation). CT alone is not usually adequate to demonstrate thoracic disk herniation or accurately assess the extent of spinal cord compression. Plain radiographs are seldom diagnostic. Plain films can, however, be helpful if the patient has Scheuermann's disease because thoracic disk herniation is more likely to develop in these patients.

Appropriate treatment of thoracic and thoracolumbar disk herniation is surgical, provided that the herniation is associated with incapacitating pain or abnormal neurologic findings. Surgical approaches to treatment of disk herniation in this region include anterior transthoracic diskectomy with or without fusion, posterolateral decompression from a transpedicular approach, and a costotransversectomy approach. Standard laminectomy should not be used to remove a thoracic or thoracolumbar herniated disk. Because spinal cord manipulation is required to remove a disk through a standard posterior laminectomy, worsening of the neurologic condition can occur and has been reported in up to 45 percent of patients treated with this approach. The results reported for the anterior transthoracic, costotransversectomy, and posterolateral transpedicle approaches all show that 80 to 90 percent of patients improve after surgery, with the remainder being without change or deterioration.[22,109] Because the condition is traumatically induced, internal fixation and fusion should be considered, concurrent with the diskectomy.

Bohlman and Zdeblick reviewed 19 patients treated surgically for thoracic disk herniations; 8 were treated with a transthoracic approach, and the remaining 11 were treated with a costotransversectomy approach.[22] They concluded that the transthoracic approach was preferable because it greatly improved visualization of the pertinent anatomic structures, including the disk and the neural elements. All seven patients with paralysis improved after anterior transthoracic decompression.

Thorascopy can be successfully used in complex surgical procedures, including thoracic diskectomy. The potential benefits of video-assisted thorascopic surgery include reduced postoperative pain, improved early shoulder girdle function, and a shorter hospital stay.[103] Regan and associates reported on video-assisted thorascopic surgery performed on 12 thoracic spinal patients, including 5 diskectomies.[132] Postoperative CT showed adequate spinal cord decompression. Pain was relieved in all patients.

OPERATIVE TREATMENT

Selection of the instrumentation and type of construct is not random, nor should it be based entirely on the preference of the surgeon. All systems have relative strengths and weaknesses that can be used to advantage. The optimal system and construct for a given fracture should counteract the deforming forces and maximally diminish the degree of instability.

Pedicle screw fixation has been shown to be more resistant to pull-out than cables or claw hooks.[75] For the treatment of adult spinal deformity, thoracic pedicle screw instrumentation offers superior results for deformity correction and fusion rate.[18] An and co-workers found superior stability with pedicle screw fixation compared with hook–rod constructs in an in vitro burst fracture model.[9] In a study comparing pedicle screws to hook–rod constructs at the caudal end of a construct, pedicle screws were associated with improved anterior height restoration and maintenance of spinal canal clearance.[94]

Advances in pedicle screw systems have improved the ease of transpedicular instrumentation in both the thoracic and lumbar spine. This coupled with increasing use of pedicle screw instrumentation by spine surgeons has resulted in widespread application of pedicle screw-based constructs to the treatment of thoracic and thoracolumbar trauma. Bransford and associates demonstrated that fluoroscopy can facilitate safe thoracic screw placement in trauma patients.[23] Of 1533 screws in 245 patients, only 0.26% of screws required revision placement, with no major complications related to screw placement. Fisher and colleagues found a 98.5 percent rate of acceptable screw placement in a similar review.[52] In a cadaveric study, Hart and co-workers found that the use of fluoroscopic assistance may increase confidence in thoracic pedicle screw placement, but emphasized that surgeons should exercise caution when instrumenting the T4-T7 levels (the most narrow pedicles anatomically), as pedicle diameter inversely corresponded to the rate of pedicle breach.[72]

Siebenga and associates showed in a prospective study that patients with AO type A thoracolumbar fractures have superior results with posterior short-segment fixation than with nonoperative management.[146] Patients in this study had no neurologic deficit. At an average follow-up of 4.3 years with 94 percent of patients reporting, patients were found to have improved local and regional sagittal alignment after surgical intervention. Operative patients also showed improved scores in functional outcome as well as improvement in ability to return to work. Wang and associates further evaluated the results of burst fracture treatment with posterior short-segment fixation.[166] In their study, patients were randomly assigned to instrumentation and fusion versus instrumentation alone. These investigators found superior maintenance of correction in the nonfusion group with decreases in operative time and blood loss. Patients also experienced similar functional outcome at 41-month average follow-up. Sanderson and colleagues reported similar satisfactory results; however, they reported a 14 percent instrumentation failure rate, which was comparable with results of patients treated with fusion.[139]

The question of short-segment (one level above and below the fractured vertebra) versus long-segment instrumentation and fusion (more than one level above or below the fractured vertebra) has been debated. The goal of short-segment fixation is to preserve motion segments in the mobile thoracolumbar and lumbar spine. Kramer and associates reported on the results of 11 patients treated with short-segment constructs and found 36 percent failure of the caudad screws with increasing kyphotic deformity postoperatively.[99] McClain and co-workers reported their prospective results with segmental instrumentation.[118] They reported a high failure rate (6/11) for short-segment fixation in burst fractures without anterior reconstruction. This subset of patients had fair to poor outcomes and a higher rate of instrumentation complications compared with other patients treated with segmental instrumentation. Alvine and colleagues recommended instrumentation of at least three to four motion segments rather than two based on their experience with short-segment fixation.[7] Terezen and Kuru reported a failure rate of 55 percent with short-segment pedicle fixation in thoracolumbar burst fractures, although long-segment fixation required prolonged operative time and increased blood loss.[156] There was no difference between groups in regards to the Low Back Outcome Score. They did suggest that anterior column support would obviate the need for long-segment fixation. McLain's recent literature review recommends against short-segment instrumentation without supplemental anterior column support.[117]

Using the load-sharing classification to grade anterior column support, Parker and associates achieved 100 percent success with short-segment transpedicular fixation.[128] There were no failures of instrumentation. Patients were treated with a postoperative spinal orthosis for 3 to 4 months and were followed for an average of 66 months. Scholl and co-workers found acceptable results in extending the cephalad fixation to two levels and felt that this achieved the goal of limiting loss of lumbar motion while improving survival of the construct.[143] Razak and colleagues reported an average loss of 2° of correction at 24-month follow-up with the use of short-segment instrumentation in 26 patients.[131]

Anekstein and associates showed biomechanically that insertion of an intermediate pedicle screw into the pedicle of the fractured vertebra can increase the stiffness of a short-segment construct.[12] This added stiffness and extra point of fixation may reduce the load imparted to the caudal screw and may serve to improve construct survival and thus maintain alignment.

The addition of anterior and middle column support by transpedicular grafting has been performed in an attempt to improve the outcome of short-segment constructs. Knop and co-workers reported on late outcomes using transpedicular bone grafting and found no improvement in loss of correction with the technique.[93] Alanay and colleagues found similar results in their prospective, randomized study comparing patients receiving grafts with those not receiving grafts.[5] Of the patients in the grafted group, 50 percent lost at least 10° of their correction, whereas in the ungrafted group, only 40 percent did. Toyone and associates, however, reported on their results with hydroxyapatite grafting of the anterior column in combination with posterior instrumentation, without fusion, in 15 patients.[159] Instruments were removed at 1 year and patients were followed until at least 2 years. They experienced no loss of fixation, minimal loss of sagittal alignment, and excellent spinal canal clearance.

Recently, there have been reports of balloon-assisted reduction of the vertebral end plate and injection of transpedicular anterior column support (calcium phosphate or polymethylmethacrylate in conjunction with posterior short-segment instrumentation).[2,125,163] Although long-term results have not been reported, this technique has been shown to allow reduction of the fractured end plate with maintenance of vertebral height. Although cement leakage was reported, there were no significant clinical implications.[163] Long-term results of this technique will further clarify its utility in selected fractures.

Sasso and colleagues compared posterior short-segment instrumentation with anterior alone instrumentation for unstable burst fractures.[140] Although both methods achieved significant postoperative improvement in sagittal alignment, the posterior group lost 8.1° on average compared with only 1.8° in the anterior group. However, at the thoracolumbar junction the morbidity associated with the anterior approach is greater than for the posterior approach.

In the thoracic spine, the preservation of motion segments is less a concern than in the thoracolumbar and lumbar spine due to the rigidity of the thoracic structures. In these situations, posterior pedicle screw instrumentation at least two levels above and below the fractured level is recommended. Transpedicular instrumentation in the thoracic spine permits three-column control of the vertebral segment and fixation in the absence of intact posterior structures. It also eliminates the need for intracanal dissection or instrumentation. Yue and associates studied 32 patients treated with transpedicular instrumentation in the thoracic spine from T2-L1. They found there to be no complications with 222 screw placements from T2-L1.[181] Patients had improvements in vertebral body height and sagittal alignment. Fusion was achieved at an average of 4.8 months' follow-up with no failures of instrumentation, loss of reduction, or painful hardware.

Verlaan and co-workers systematically reviewed the literature on the treatment of thoracic and lumbar trauma.[164] The evidence that they found was largely based on retrospective studies regarding surgical approaches (anterior, posterior, and combined) and encompassed 5748 patients treated surgically. They found that patients with worse injuries (higher Cobb's angle, polytrauma, and neurologic deficit) tended to be treated anteriorly, and those with less severe injuries were treated with short-segment posterior instrumentation. Complications were relatively infrequent in all groups, and differences between groups were small. All groups, including anterior, posterior short- and long-segment, and combined, achieved excellent correction of preoperative deformity immediately after surgery. Follow-up showed loss of correction in all groups with an average loss of 7.6° in the posterior short-segment group compared with 3.1° in the anterior group. Postoperative pain scores at follow-up were comparable between groups, with greater than 80 percent satisfaction for each group. Return to work was similar for anterior and posterior short-segment groups as well, with 84 and 83 percent returning to work, respectively. Implant failures were less common after anterior procedures or combined procedures, 5 percent, compared with posterior alone procedures, 10 percent. Overall, patient outcomes were better than expected, but no surgical method was able to maintain corrected kyphosis to physiologic levels.

SURGICAL TECHNIQUE

Because many different pedicle screw fixation devices are currently available and more are in the process of development, this surgical description is general, with emphasis on proper positioning of the pedicle screws. As stated in the previous section, fixation of one pedicle above and one pedicle below the level of injury may be adequate, provided that the anterior fragmentation is minimal. If the anterior comminution is more significant, the alternatives are to extend the instrumentation to two levels above and two levels below the injury or plan to perform anterior corpectomy and fusion of the fractured vertebra to provide anterior support.

The patient is placed in the prone position, and a midline incision is made to expose the spinous processes, laminae, facet joints, and transverse processes of each level to be instrumented. The orientation of the pedicles is approximately −4° from sagittal at T12 and 11° from sagittal at L1, slowly increasing to 30° from sagittal at the L5 level. Pedicle diameter similarly varies and is approximately 8 mm at T12, L1, L2, and L3. It increases to approximately 1 cm at L4 and almost 1.3 cm at L5. A helpful way to assess angulation from the sagittal plane is to measure it on the patient's CT scan. Pedicle diameter can also be determined from the CT scan.

The central portion of the pedicle in a cranial-to-caudal direction can be approximated by passing a line through the center of the transverse processes of the vertebral body bilaterally. This line bisects the midpoint of the pedicles. The midportion crosses the transverse process line in a medial-to-lateral direction at a point defined by a line drawn through the facet joints (Fig. 30-35, A). In the lumbar spine, the mammillary process, just lateral to the facets, is useful for guiding entry into the pedicle.

Once the soft tissues have been completely removed and the bone in the area exposed, a high-speed bur can be used to remove the outer cortex over the chosen entry point. An awl or pedicle finder is next used to create a channel through the central portion of the pedicle into the vertebral body while maintaining the appropriate inclination in the sagittal plane. Craniocaudal tilt is best discerned from a lateral scout radiograph. The awl or pedicle finder should be guided down along the path of least resistance. The softer cancellous bone in the central portion of the pedicle should give way easier than the harder cortical bone in the walls of the pedicle. If resistance is met, the awl or pedicle finder should be redirected so that it passes easily down. Intraoperative radiography

FIGURE 30-35 *Proper positioning of pedicle screw instrumentation. **A,** The central portion of the pedicle can be identified by the intersection of two lines. The transverse line bisects the transverse process of each level, and the longitudinal line runs cephalad to caudal, bisecting the facet joints. **B,** After application of the pedicle screws, the screws are connected with a plate or rod construct. (Redrawn from Leona Allison.)*

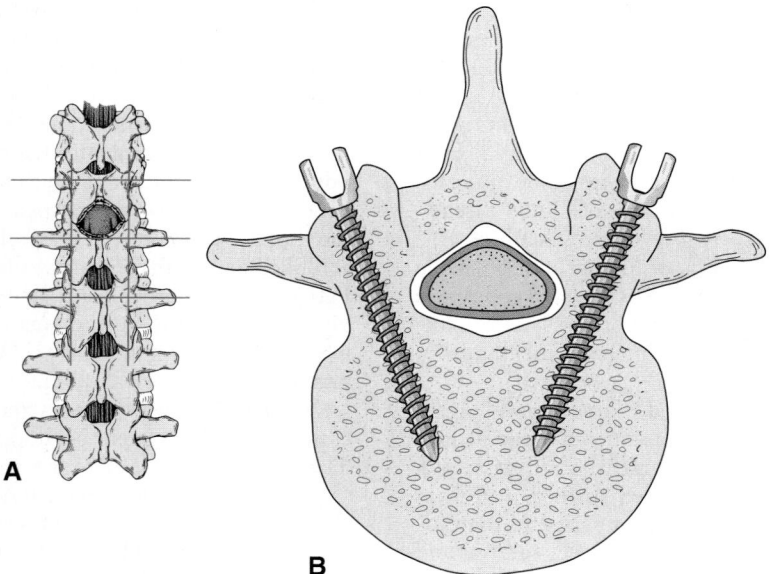

or fluoroscopy with drill bits placed in the hole can be used to assess the position if the path created is in question. If insertion of these screws is based only on anatomic landmarks and the experience of the spinal surgeon, the chance of having a screw outside the desired boundaries of the pedicle may be as high as 30 percent.[169] The use of intraoperative radiographs and fluoroscopy helps decrease this risk. Each hole can be probed with a pedicle probe, in all four quadrants to see if the cortex has been violated. The hole may be tapped. This is recommended in younger patients with strong bone. The pedicle screws are then inserted.

Regardless of the type of instrumentation, care should be taken to insert the screws down to an appropriate depth. Fixed-angle screws are better for achieving reduction. Polyaxial screws should only rarely be used, and overinsertion of the screw will hinder the mobility of the head of the screw if the pedicle screw is polyaxial. Because of the high risk of vascular and visceral injury, the anterior cortex of the vertebra should not be violated from the midthoracic region to L5. This problem can be avoided by selecting the appropriate screw length. This can be facilitated by preoperatively measuring the screw lengths on CT or MRI.

Another consideration during placement of these screws is whether the pedicle screw or rod will violate an adjacent normal joint. The potential for this complication is determined by the basic design of the pedicle screw fixation device and cannot usually be altered by the surgeon, so it must be considered when initially selecting the pedicle screw instrumentation system.

Achievement of reduction and normal sagittal alignment is one of the primary goals of surgical treatment. Both lordosis forces and distracting forces can be applied through short-segment pedicle screw constructs to achieve these desired outcomes (Fig. 30-36). Radiographs in both the AP and the lateral planes should be obtained with the final instrumentation system in place to be certain that the fracture is adequately reduced, sagittal spinal alignment is satisfactory, and each of the pedicle screws is in the desired position (see Fig. 30-35 A, B).

There are a number of different methods for decreasing kyphosis (in the thoracic spine and at the thoracolumbar junction) or actually restoring lordosis (in the lumbar spine). Whichever method is used, care should be taken that fixation with the bone is solid so that reduction does not pull out the screws. Also, reduction should be done using both rods simultaneously to prevent overstressing fixation on one side. In most cases, fixed-angle screws facilitate reduction, especially in short constructs. In slightly longer constructs (two above and two below) one screw of each pair can be fixed and one polyaxial to improve ease of assembly. The rod should be contoured to the desired degree of correction and fixed in the proper orientation in the proximal screw or screws (see Fig. 30-36). The distal screw or two screws can be inserted and the reduction achieved by gradually tightening the caps (see Fig. 30-36) or by placing a rod pusher on the distal end of each rod and reducing it into the screw slots before placing the caps (see Fig. 30-36). Slight distraction can be applied to complete the reduction.

A useful method for re-creating lordosis is placement of a screw at the level of injury. When used in conjunction with contouring of the rod, excellent three-point fixation may be achieved. Another method of restoring lordosis is to leave the caudal aspect of the rod angled at approximately 15° up from the caudal screw (best performed with screw heads that allow angulation), with the cephalad aspect fixed to the screw. The rods are then forced down to engage the caudal screws at the same time with the use of persuaders. This technique provides distraction and lordosis of the proximal segments.

As with all other instrumentation systems, solid fusion is one of the primary goals of surgery. Adequate care should be taken to decorticate the transverse processes and the lateral aspects of the superior facets to increase the chance of achieving fusion. Inserting the bone graft prior to placing the rod or plate to the pedicle screws may facilitate placement of the bone graft. Finally, a number of newer instrumentation systems are made of titanium, which allows for better postoperative imaging, particularly MRI.

Posterolateral Decompression

Surgical reduction of the fracture often results in indirect surgical decompression of thoracolumbar spine injuries. If complete reduction can be achieved, a formal decompression is often not necessary. Edwards and Levine[43] and Edwards and colleagues[44] showed that surgical reduction performed within 2 days of injury restores the spinal canal area by an additional 32 percent, whereas surgery performed between 3 and 14 days after injury restores 23 percent. They also found that little or no improvement occurs when posterior instrumentation is delayed for more than 2 weeks.

The adequacy of reduction cannot be easily assessed by plain radiography. A postoperative myelo-CT scan, or MRI, are effective ways of assessing for residual neural compression if there are any concerns.[24] If a significant abnormality is found, anterior decompression can be performed at a later date.

In addition, if anatomic realignment has been achieved, some resorption of bone from within the spinal canal will occur over the course of the next year, thereby lessening the extent of neural compression. Krompinger and colleagues reviewed 29 patients with injuries of the thoracic or lumbar spine treated nonoperatively; 14 had canal compromise greater than 25 percent on initial evaluation.[101] Bone remodeling of the compromised canal was noted in 11 of these 14 patients, and canal compromise of less than 25 percent resolved completely in four of eight cases. Similar results during nonoperative treatment of burst fractures have been reported by others.[30] Sjöström and colleagues noted resorption of intracanal fragments after the application of pedicle screw constructs and fusion.[149] Willen and co-workers, however, reported that patients with more than 50 percent canal compromise rarely had significant resorption.[176] With these factors kept in mind, some patients in whom significant neural compression remains and is not improved by posterior instrumentation and reduction may still benefit from late operative treatment of fractures of the thoracic or thoracolumbar spine. Posterolateral decompression has also been used at the time of instrumentation.

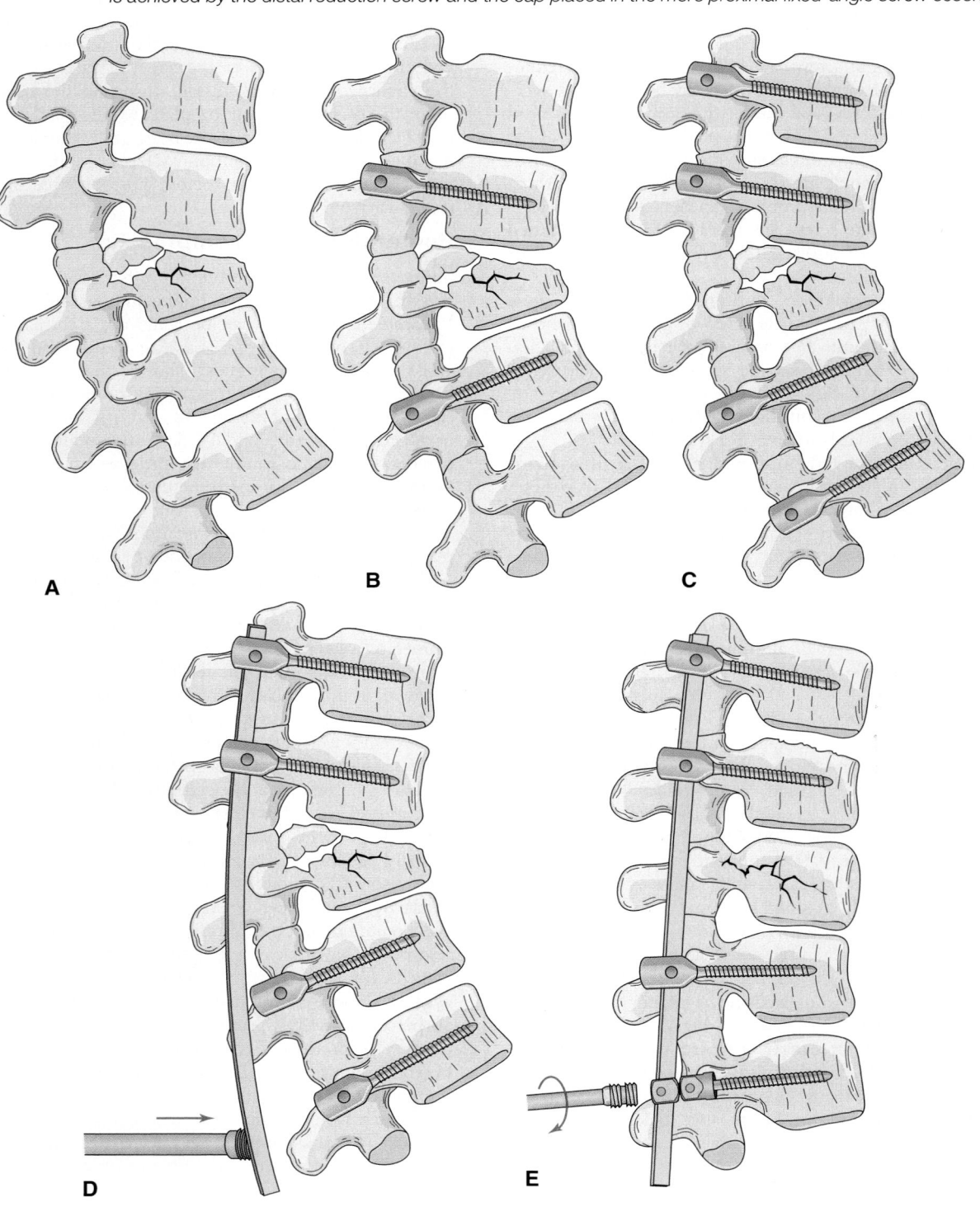

FIGURE 30-36 **A,** There are several different instrumentation constructs and methods of reduction that can be used for posterior reduction and stabilization of a burst fracture. **B,** Generally a short construct with only two screws above and two below should not be used as it is more likely to fail. Four screws above and four below will allow sufficient fixation for achieving and maintaining a reduction. In certain circumstances four screws above and two below may be adequate. **C,** Screw placement is critical and each screw should be aligned parallel to the superior endplate of the vertebra, which can be difficult when the patient is unreduced and kyphotic. Several different combinations of screw types can be used which allow different reduction maneuvers. In all constructions however it is recommended that the upper four screws all be fixed angle to allow the best capture of the segments above the fracture for subsequent reduction of the kyphotic component of the fracture. If four fixed-angle screws are also used below, reduction is achieved by placing rod pushers on the ends of both rods simultaneously **(D)** followed by cap placement. Alternatively rod reduction devices can be placed on the distal screw and the reduction achieved more gradually. The rod should be bent to the final desired alignment and distraction (restoration of height) should never be done until kyphosis is fully reduced. Alternatively a combination of a fixed-angle and a reduction screw can be used **(E)** if the kyphosis is not severe and the reduction is achieved by the distal reduction screw and the cap placed in the more proximal fixed-angle screw second.

FIGURE 30-36 *(Continued) The final method of reduction is with four reduction screws **(F)** reducing the rod just far enough to engage the proximal reduction screw and placing the cap **(G)**. **H,** The distal cap can often then be engaged without any further use of rod pushers or sometimes both can be engaged simultaneously. **I,** In all cases the reduction of kyphosis should be complete before use of distraction to achieve final reduction.*

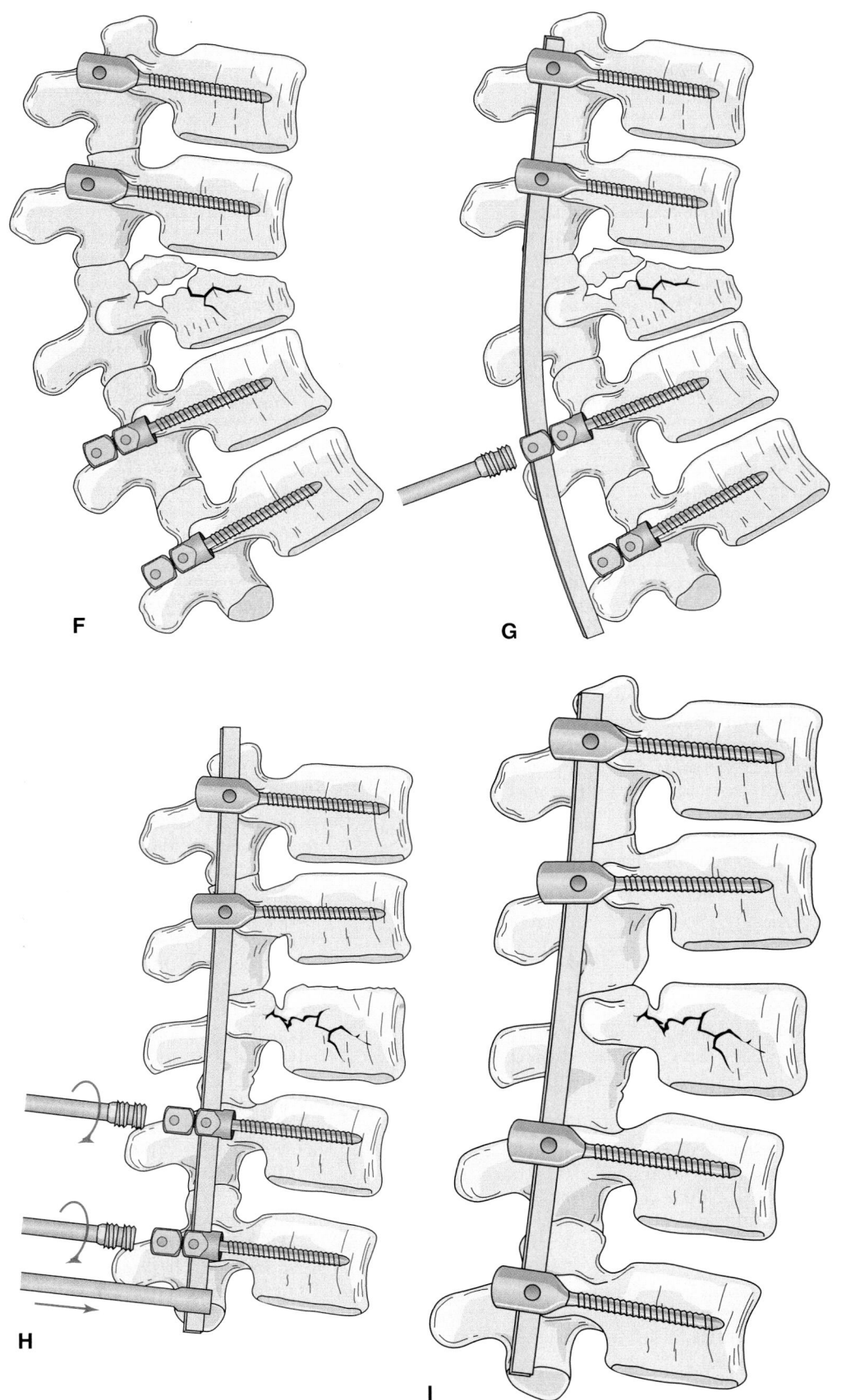

F

G

H

I

The advantage of the posterolateral technique is that it allows stabilization of severe spine injuries, including fracture–dislocations, and at the same time allows some degree of neural decompression without requiring a second surgical procedure. One disadvantage of this technique is that it necessarily requires removal of posterior and posterolateral bone and may thus further jeopardize spinal stability and eventual fusion. The second major disadvantage is that it is a relatively blind procedure because the dural and neural elements lie between the surgeon and the anterior compressive tissue.

The posterolateral technique has been evaluated by Garfin and colleagues.[59] In that series, nine patients with burst fractures of the thoracic or lumbar spine were treated by posterolateral decompression and evaluated with postoperative CT. Postoperative CT showed only one patient with bone remaining in the canal. Hardaker and co-workers reported the use of bilateral transpedicular decompression with instrumentation and fusion for severe burst fractures with an average canal compromise of more than 65 percent.[69] Although anterior decompression would normally be required for such extreme amounts of canal compromise, only one patient in the study underwent an additional anterior procedure. Seventy-seven percent of the patients with neurologic deficit had significant improvement, and significant kyphotic deformity had not developed in any patient at follow-up. Hu and associates compared anterior decompression with transpedicular decompression in patients with incomplete neurologic deficits and found no additional benefit for anterior vertebrectomy over transpedicular decompression.[80] Both treatments resulted in significant neurologic improvement compared with a similar group of patients treated by indirect reduction maneuvers alone. Others have reported comparable results with the use of transpedicular decompression. In contrast, Lemons and colleagues compared direct decompression by a posterolateral route with indirect reduction and found no significant differences in improvement in canal clearance or neurologic function.[104] They concluded that the posterolateral transpedicular approach is of questionable value for the treatment of burst fractures.

SURGICAL TECHNIQUE

Posterolateral decompression is performed as part of a posterior stabilizing operation in patients with thoracic, thoracolumbar, or lumbar spine injuries. Before the instrumentation system is applied and before any posterolateral decompression, the CT transverse sections at the level of the injury should be studied to determine which side of the spinal canal has the more severe neural compression. The instrumentation should be inserted first on the side with the smaller amount of neural compression and corrective forces then applied to reduce the spine injury. In most cases, these forces include a combination of distraction and lordosis with three- or four-point fixation and the force vector directed anteriorly at the level of injury.

Attention is then directed to the side of the spine that is free of instrumentation (Fig. 30-37, A). A laminotomy is performed at the level of maximal neural compression, which is most commonly the area of the pedicles of the fractured vertebra. At this level, the adjacent spinous processes are each trimmed and the intervening ligamentum flavum is excised. Adjacent bone is removed, including portions of the cephalic and caudal laminae, as well as the medial portion of the facet joint at that level.

The posterior edge of the fracture (anterior to the dura) can be palpated with an angled dural elevator to assess the degree of residual canal compromise. The laminotomy should be extended distally at least to the inferior edge of the pedicle. Once the medial border of the pedicle is identified, a power bur is used to drill into the central portion of the pedicle with all cortices left intact (Fig. 30-37, B). A thin rongeur or curette is then used to remove the medial cortex of the pedicle, with care taken to preserve the nerve root exiting below it (Fig. 30-37, C). A trough is cut 1 cm into the vertebral body anterior to the medial portion of the pedicle that has been thinned. Reverse-angle curettes can be inserted through this opening, and any bone fragments compressing the anterior neural elements can be impacted into the vertebral body or brought out through the lateral trough previously made (Fig. 30-37, D). Mimatsu and co-workers have designed a variety of impactors specifically for use in the transpedicular approach.[120] It is possible to extend this decompression slightly past midline through this unilateral exposure (Figs. 30-37, E and 30-38).

If the decompression is adequate on both sides of the canal, no further decompression is needed. If further decompression is needed on the side that has already been instrumented, a second rod is inserted on the side already decompressed, the instrumentation is removed, transpedicular decompression is performed on the first side, and the instrumentation is reinserted.

Anterior Transthoracic Decompression and Fusion

Anterior transthoracic decompression and fusion may be used for the treatment of thoracic and thoracolumbar spine fractures (T2 to L1), either as a single operative procedure or in conjunction with a posterior stabilization procedure. It is most indicated in patients with maximal anterior neural compression, patients with an incomplete spinal cord injury, and those with minimal instability, as well as for the delayed treatment of injuries, including late post-traumatic deformities.

This transthoracic approach for trauma was first described by Paul and colleagues,[129] and detailed techniques along with long-term results of this treatment have been published by Bohlman and associates.[21] In a review of acute injuries of the upper thoracic spine with paralysis, eight patients were treated by anterior decompression and fusion for residual neural compression. All had reached a plateau in terms of neurologic recovery at the time of anterior decompression. Postoperatively, five patients were able to walk without aid, two recovered partially and were able to walk with crutches and braces, and one patient improved but remained unable to ambulate. No patient lost neurologic function as a result of this procedure, and solid fusion developed in all patients, even though three had previously undergone laminectomy. None was

FIGURE 30-37 *Technique of posterolateral decompression of the spinal canal. **A,** A posterior view of the spine shows the region of exposure and the amount of pedicle resection required to achieve posterolateral decompression. Care should be taken to not cut inferolaterally across the pars interarticularis. **B,** The ligamentum flavum has been resected at the level of injury, and the dura has been exposed. Bone is resected laterally up to the medial extent of the pedicle and caudally to the inferior extent of the pedicle. A bur is used to make a hole in the central portion of the pedicle, with the hole proceeding anteriorly toward the vertebral body. A circumferential rim of cortical bone is left in place. The nerve root is shown medial to the pedicle and exiting below the pedicle. Care should be taken to not injure this nerve root. **C,** The medial wall of the pedicle is removed with a rongeur, such as a pituitary rongeur. **D,** A transverse section shows the hole bured down through the pedicle and into the vertebral body. A reverse-angle curet is used to tap bone out of the spinal canal and into the trough that has been drilled out of the vertebral body. Large bone fragments may also be pulled out through this lateral trough. Care must be taken not to hook the anterior aspect of the dura. **E,** A transverse section shows the final result after decompression. Unilateral posterolateral transpedicular decompression usually enables adequate decompression slightly past the midline.*

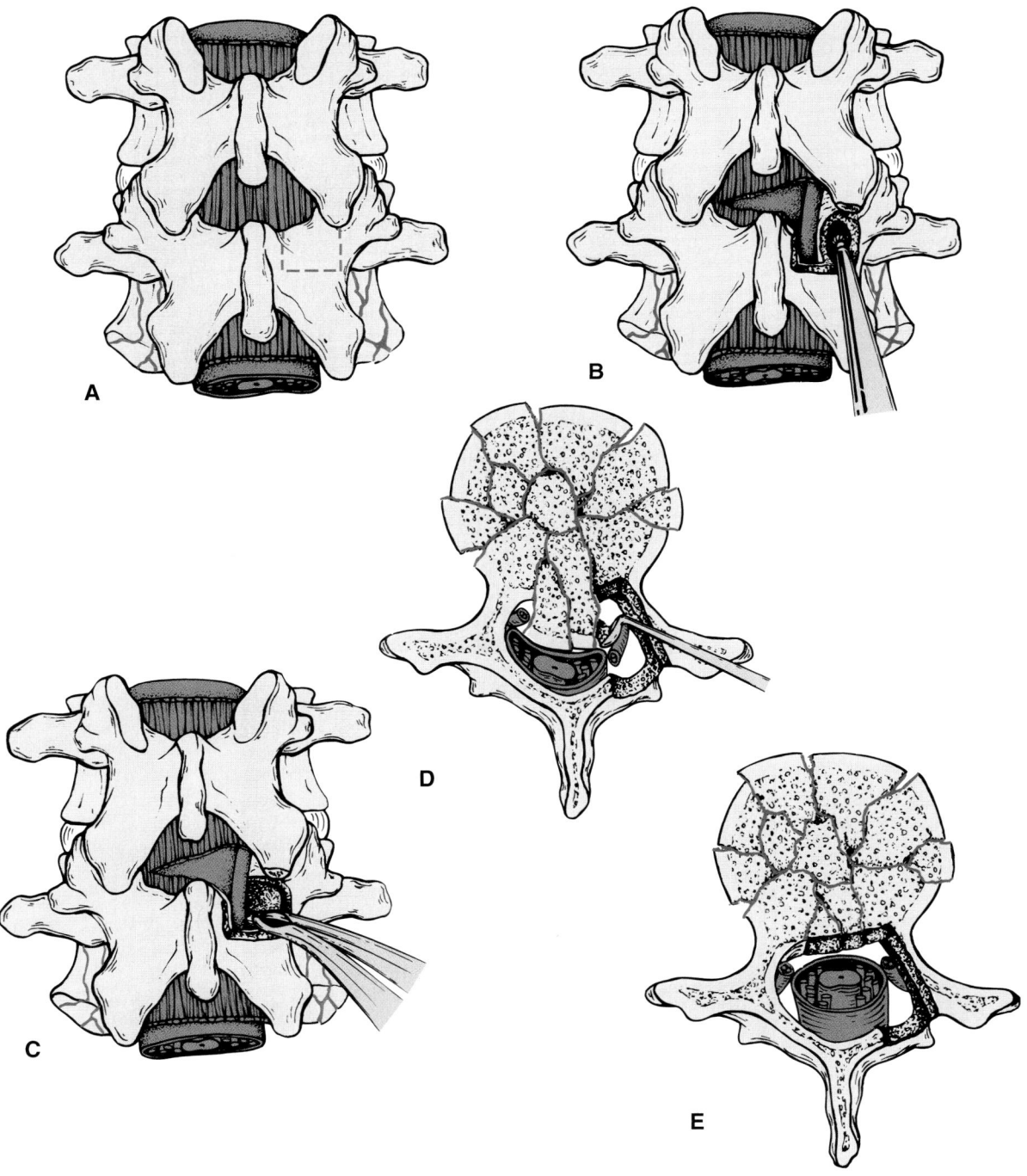

augmented with any type of instrumentation either anteriorly or posteriorly. No data were given concerning residual angulation at the site of injury.

Most published series of transthoracic decompression for treatment of spinal trauma review either patients with minimal to moderate levels of instability or those who are no longer in the acute stage after their injury. In the latter group, some healing with partial stabilization may already have occurred. Gurr and colleagues showed in an animal corpectomy model that the strength of the spine is markedly reduced after corpectomy in comparison with the strength of an intact spine.[66] This reduction in strength is true for axial loading, flexion loading, and rotation testing. The addition of an iliac graft still allows three times the displacement with axial compression, as well as displacement with flexion testing, and torsional stiffness

FIGURE 30-38 *This is a 42-year-old female who fell from approximately 20 feet.* ***A,*** *Lateral radiograph showing L1 burst fracture.* ***B,*** *Sagittal computed tomography (CT) showing retropulsion of posterior bony fragment into canal.* ***C,*** *Axial CT showing retropulsion of posterior bony fragment.*

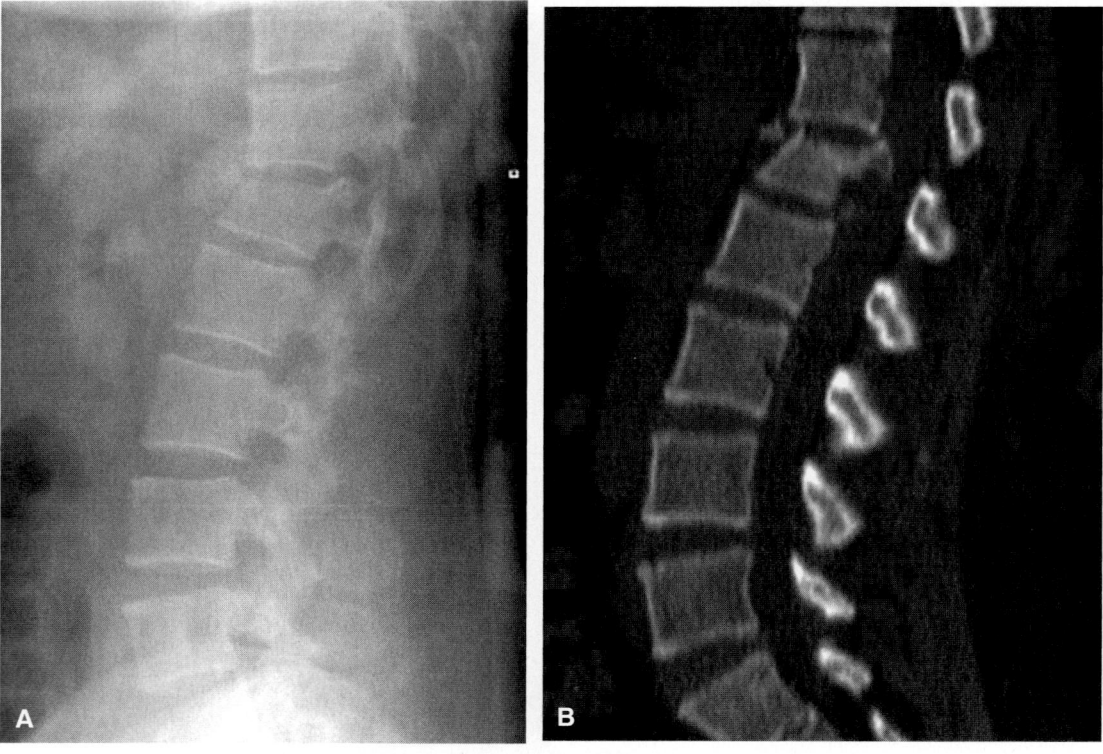

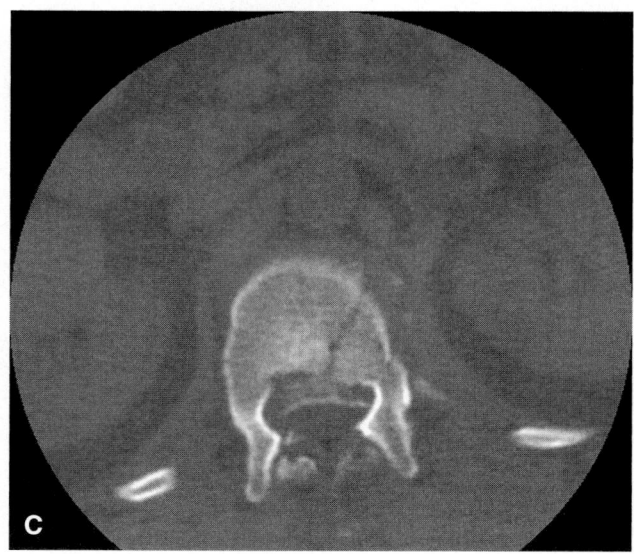

FIGURE 30-38 *(Continued)* **D, E,** *This patient was treated with posterolateral decompression with posterior instrumented fusion with pedicle screws and rods.* **F,** *Postoperative sagittal CT showing realignment of spine with reduction of the retropulsed fragment.* **G,** *Postoperative axial CT showing reduction of retropulsed fragment.*

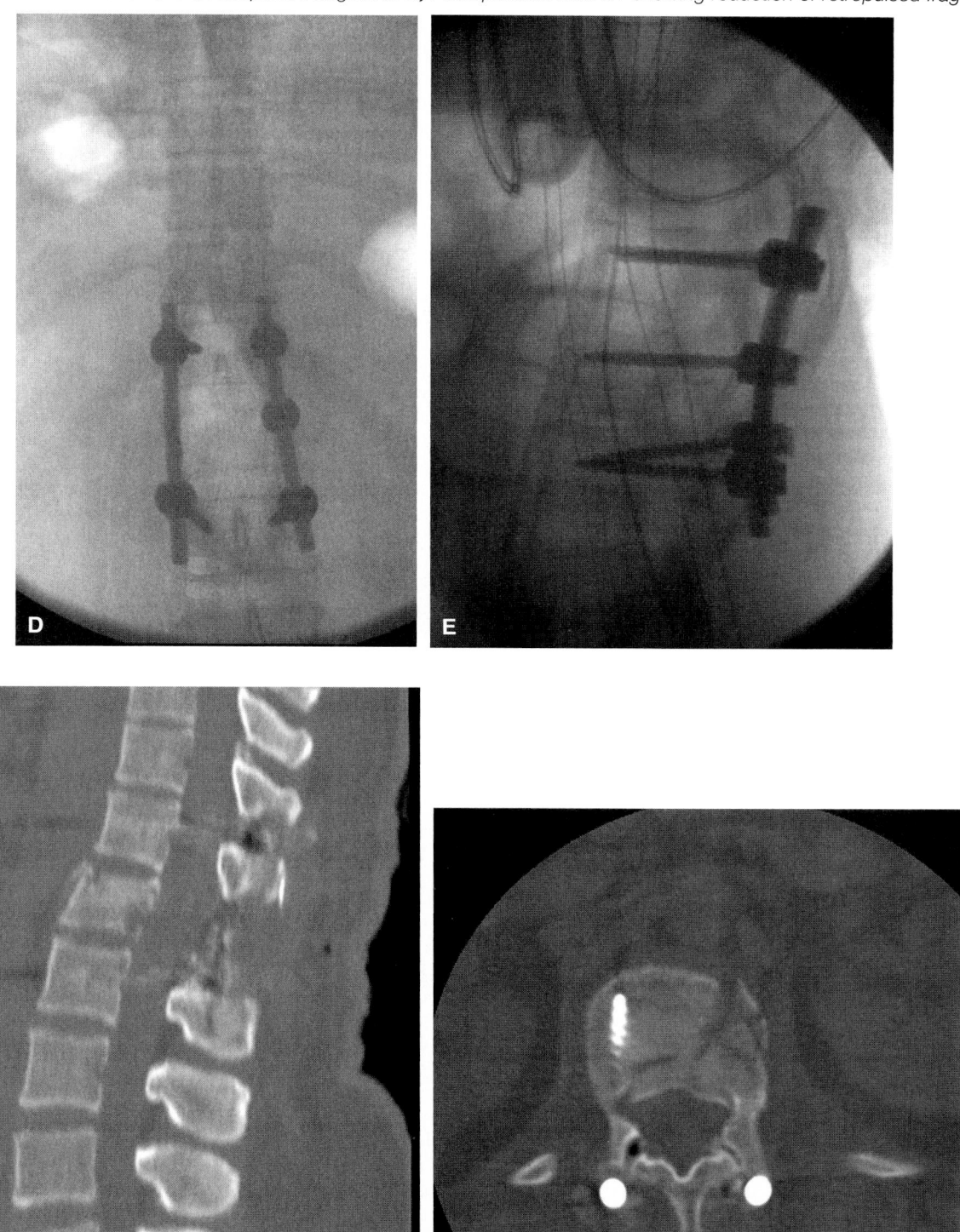

is less than one-third that of an intact spine. In trauma patients with significant posterior disruption and an anterior corpectomy, additional instability is probably present. For this reason, uninstrumented anterior transthoracic decompression plus fusion is rarely indicated and should be reserved for patients with significant neural compression and minimal instability. As the degree of instability increases, it becomes necessary to supplement the anterior decompression and fusion with either anterior instrumentation or posterior stabilization. In severe injuries associated with three-column disruption, some authors recommend supplementation of anterior instrumentation with posterior instrumentation and spinal fusion.[144,175] Almost all patients should have postoperative immobilization in a TLSO, except perhaps for those stabilized with rigid posterior segmental fixation devices.

Beginning in the late 1980s, the development of more sophisticated anterior plate systems improved the quality of anterior fixation in the thoracic and thoracolumbar spine.[114,180] However, anterior plate fixation to L4, L5, and S1 remains problematic. Most of the current systems are based on the principle of two screws per level, with one screw placed posteriorly, parallel to the posterior cortical wall of the vertebral body, and the second angled obliquely from anterior in the body to posterior. This triangular arrangement improves pull-out strength. In addition, in most systems an element of compression or distraction can be applied between the upper and lower segments of fixation before fixing the bolt or screw to the plate. This technique may improve incorporation of the graft anteriorly, as well as the stability of the construct.

Kaneda and associates reported their results in treating 150 consecutive patients with thoracolumbar burst fractures by anterior decompression and stabilization with the Kaneda device.[86] After a mean follow-up of 8 years, radiographs showed a successful fusion rate of 93 percent. Ten patients with a pseudoarthrosis were successfully managed by posterior spinal instrumentation and fusion. They believed that all their pseudoarthroses occurred in patients who had poor placement of the anterior strut graft. Kaneda thought that the success of his device relied directly on load transmission through a strong tricortical iliac crest graft, with placement of the tricortical portion beyond the contralateral pedicle. The mean percent canal obstruction preoperatively was 47 percent and, postoperatively, 2 percent. Neurologic function improved by at least one grade in 95 percent of patients. Breakage of the implant occurred in nine patients. There were no iatrogenically induced neurologic deficits. Of the patients who were employed before the injury, 96 percent returned to work. The average kyphosis was 19° preoperatively, 7° immediately postoperatively, and 8° at follow-up. In a separate report, Kaneda and co-workers used the Kaneda device after anterior decompression in patients with neurologic deficits caused by post-traumatic kyphosis. They reported excellent results in all patients.[85] Gardner and associates used the contoured anterior spinal plate (CASP) system for a variety of conditions, including acute burst fractures, and had a fusion rate of 100 percent.[57] McGuire reported 14 unstable three-column injuries treated by anterior decompression and stabilization with the University Plate (Acromed Corp.).[115] Radiographically, vertebral

height was maintained, and no measurable graft subsidence or kyphosis developed. He reported no implant failures. One nonunion was treated successfully with a posterior compression construct. Okuyama and associates reviewed 45 patients with unstable burst fractures treated by anterior decompression and stabilization.[124] They reported 84 percent with no or minimal pain, a 74 percent return-to-work rate, and minimal loss of the kyphotic angle until fusion. Other more recently published studies have shown similar results with anterior decompression and stabilization for thoracolumbar burst fractures.[114,140]

Most studies reporting the results of anterior decompression and stabilization have used rib or iliac crest bone grafts (or both) for their fusions. Finkelstein and associates reported the results of a prospective cohort study to evaluate the use of cortical allograft bone for anterior spine reconstruction in thoracolumbar fractures.[51] They packed the medullary canal of tibial allografts with autogenous bone from the corpectomy. Twenty-two patients underwent anterior surgery alone, and 14 patients had both anterior and posterior surgery. In the latter group, posterior instrumentation was combined with autogenous bone grafting. They reported an overall fusion rate of 81 percent, with a trend suggesting that patients undergoing anterior surgery alone had a higher rate of nonunion (5 of 22) than did those undergoing anterior and posterior instrumentation (2 of 14). In addition, of 8 patients who had loss of correction or loss of stability after anterior fixation alone, 3 required revision surgery with the addition of posterior instrumentation.

Other authors have noted high complication rates with anterior fixation (30%), as well as significant loss of the initial deformity correction over time (50%).[66] Yuan and co-workers, reporting on their results with the Syracuse I Plate, cautioned that osteoporosis and significant posterior column disruption are relative contraindications to anterior fixation.[180]

SURGICAL TECHNIQUE

The patient should be intubated with a double-lumen tube for approaches above T10 so that the left and right mainstem bronchi may be ventilated separately; this tube allows for later collapse of one lung to provide adequate exposure of the spine. From T10 distally, a single-lumen tube is adequate. For exposure of T10 and above, the patient is usually turned to the left lateral decubitus position. The right side of the chest is chosen as the side for surgery, assuming that the patient does not have any contraindications or exposure-related considerations. This position avoids any encroachment on the heart and great vessels, as would be encountered in a left-sided approach, especially in the middle and upper thoracic spine regions. A left-sided approach can be chosen if necessary, but prominent internal fixation has increased risk of vascular (aortic) injury over time due to palpitations against the metal.

Special care should be taken to place a pad just distal to the patient's downside axilla to prevent a stretch palsy of the brachial plexus. Also, an arm support should be used to hold the upper part of the arm in a neutral position: 90° forward flexion at the shoulder, neutral abduction–adduction, and almost straight at the elbow. Both arms should be adequately protected and padded, especially in the region of the radial nerve in the posterior aspect of the upper part of the arm and near the ulnar nerve at the elbow. Forward flexion of more than 90° at the shoulder should be avoided to minimize the risk of brachial plexus palsy. Tape can be securely placed across the patient, both at the level of the greater trochanter and across the shoulder, and then affixed to the table. A beanbag placed under the patient is also useful to help maintain this position.

The patient's entire right flank, anterior part of the chest, and posterior portion of the torso should be prepared from just inferior to the level of the axilla to inferior to the lateral aspect of the iliac crest. Care should be taken to prepare the skin to the midline anteriorly and beyond the midline posteriorly. Such preparation minimizes the chance of disorientation during the operation and also makes it possible to perform anterior transthoracic decompression and fusion and posterior instrumentation and fusion simultaneously, if necessary.

From T6 through T10, the incision should be made directly over the rib of the same number as the fractured vertebra (Fig. 30-39, A) or one level proximal to it. It is technically easier to work distally than proximally. Removal of a rib one to two levels higher works well, especially if the corpectomy involves more than one level. For fractures above T6, the skin incision should extend over the T6 rib anteriorly and laterally. Posteriorly, it should extend to the inferior tip of the scapula and then curve gently more cephalad, halfway between the medial border of the scapula and the midline spinous processes (Fig. 30-39, B). For exposure of T11, T12, or L1, the incision should be made over the T10 rib to simplify wound closure.

The incision should be made through skin and subcutaneous tissue down to the deep fascia. From T6 through T10, the deep fascia and underlying muscles are incised in line with the skin incision down to the rib, which is stripped subperiosteally on both its outer and inner

surfaces. The surgeon should be cautious in the use of electrocautery near the neurovascular bundle. A rib cutter is used to cut the rib at the costovertebral angle posteriorly and at the costochondral junction anteriorly. The remaining inner periosteum is then incised over the length of the rib bed. For T2 through T5, it is important to note that the long thoracic nerve courses in the midaxillary line from the region of the axilla to its innervation of the serratus anterior muscle. Rather than cut this nerve and lose innervation to the more caudal portion of the muscle, it is preferable to detach the serratus anterior muscle from the anterior chest wall and reflect it cephalad. This technique can be performed to provide exposure up to the T3 rib, with additional exposure achieved by mobilization of the scapula. Division of the dorsal scapular muscles, rhomboids, and trapezius allows the scapula to be elevated and displaced laterally from the midline. This maneuver offers a simple method of gaining a more extensive thoracotomy through the bed of the third rib.

After the chest has been opened, the surgeon should place a hand in the chest in the midlateral line and count the cephalad and caudal ribs because this is more accurate than counting the ribs outside the chest wall. The surgeon should make certain that the rib removed is the rib that was planned for removal. It should also be verified that the total number of ribs corresponds to that seen on a good-quality AP radiograph of the thoracic spine.

A self-retaining thoracotomy retractor is then inserted over moistened sponges in such a manner that the neurovascular bundle of the cephalad rib and the neurovascular bundle from the removed rib are not compressed by the retractor. The chest retractor is opened slowly to minimize the chance of fracture of adjacent ribs. At this point, the lung can be deflated on the ipsilateral side to provide adequate exposure to the spine.

The spine can be seen and palpated within the chest cavity. It is covered by the relatively thin and translucent

(Text continues on p. 966)

FIGURE 30-39 *Technique of anterior transthoracic corpectomy and fusion.* **A,** *The patient is placed in a straight decubitus position with the shoulders extended forward 90°, neutral in terms of abduction and adduction, and with the elbows straight. Care is taken to protect the downside brachial plexus by using a pad just distal to the axilla. The* dotted line *over the rib represents the incision one level above that of the spinal fracture.*

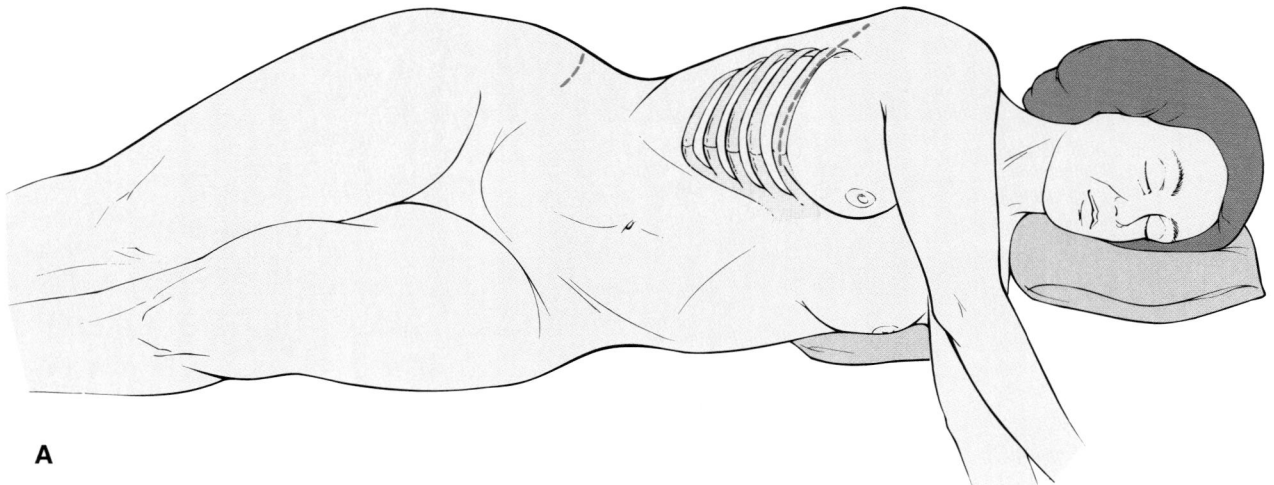

A

(Continued)

FIGURE 30-39 *(Continued)* **B,** *If the incision is used to expose above the T6 rib, the posterior limb of the incision is extended cephalad halfway between the medial border of the scapula and the spinous processes. All of the intervening muscles down to the chest wall are divided and tagged for later repair.* **C,** *After the thoracic cavity has been entered, the self-retaining chest retractor is inserted. The parietal pleura is incised halfway between the anterior great vessels and the posterior neural foramina, and the segmental vessels are ligated at this same level. The vertebra to be excised as well as one vertebra above and one vertebra below are exposed. Extraperiosteal dissection provides the best plane. A malleable retractor is placed on the opposite side of the spine and connected to the self-retaining chest retractor with a clamp. This malleable retractor serves to protect the great vessels during the vertebral corpectomy.*

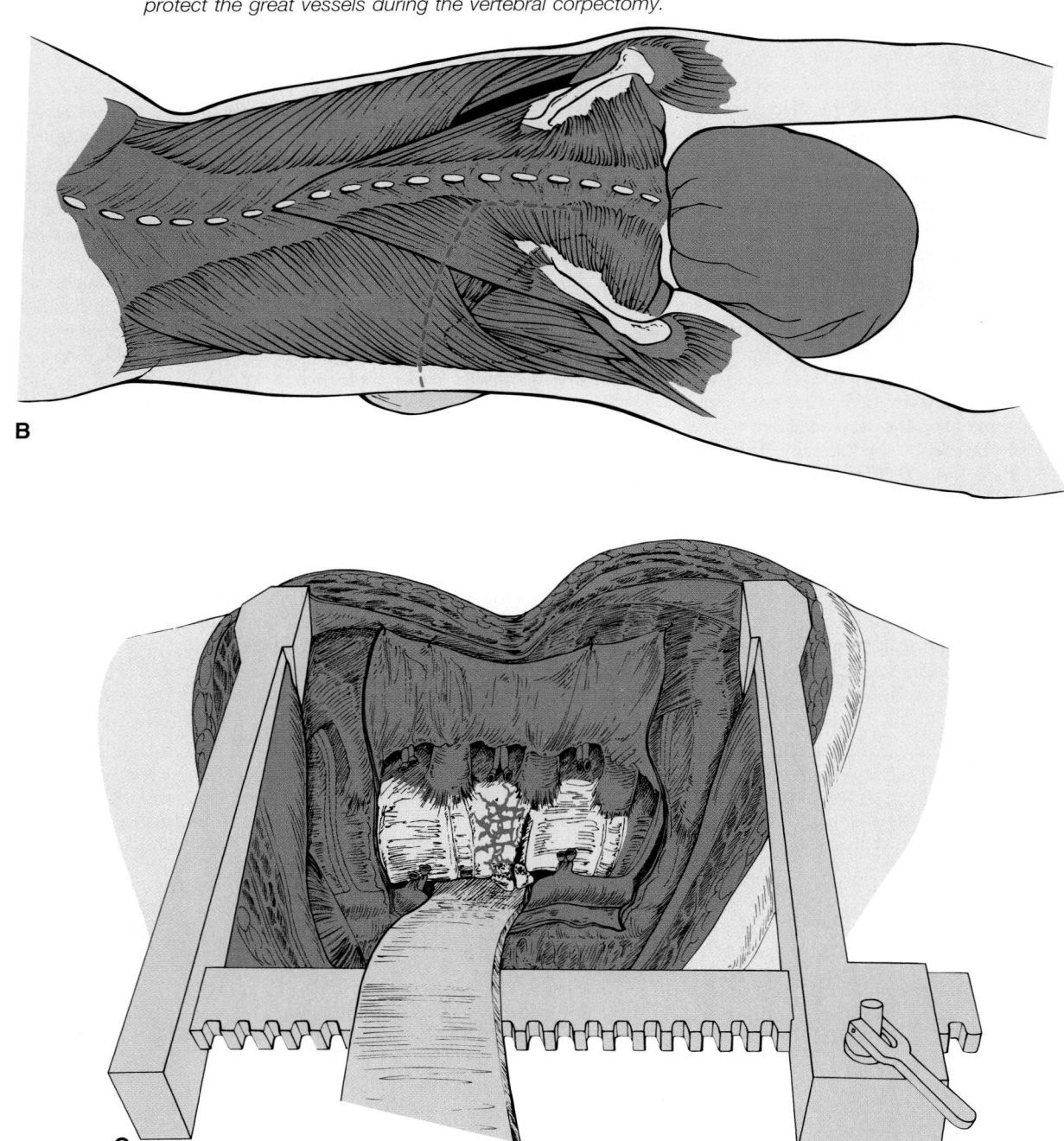

B

C

FIGURE 30-39 *(Continued)* ***D,*** *Scalpel and rongeur are used to remove the disks above and below the level of the vertebral fracture.* ***E,*** *Osteotome, chisel, or gouge is utilized to excise the vertebral body back to its posterior cortex. Special care is taken to originally position the patient exactly in the straight decubitus position. During the vertebral body resection, using these instruments, each of the cuts is made perpendicular to the floor. These instruments can be used as long as red cancellous bone is encountered. As soon as white cortical bone is encountered, these instruments should no longer be used.* ***F,*** *A high-speed bur can be used to perforate the posterior vertebral body cortex into the spinal canal. When the neural compression is significant, a diamond-tipped bur can be used to minimize the chances of dural or neural injury.*

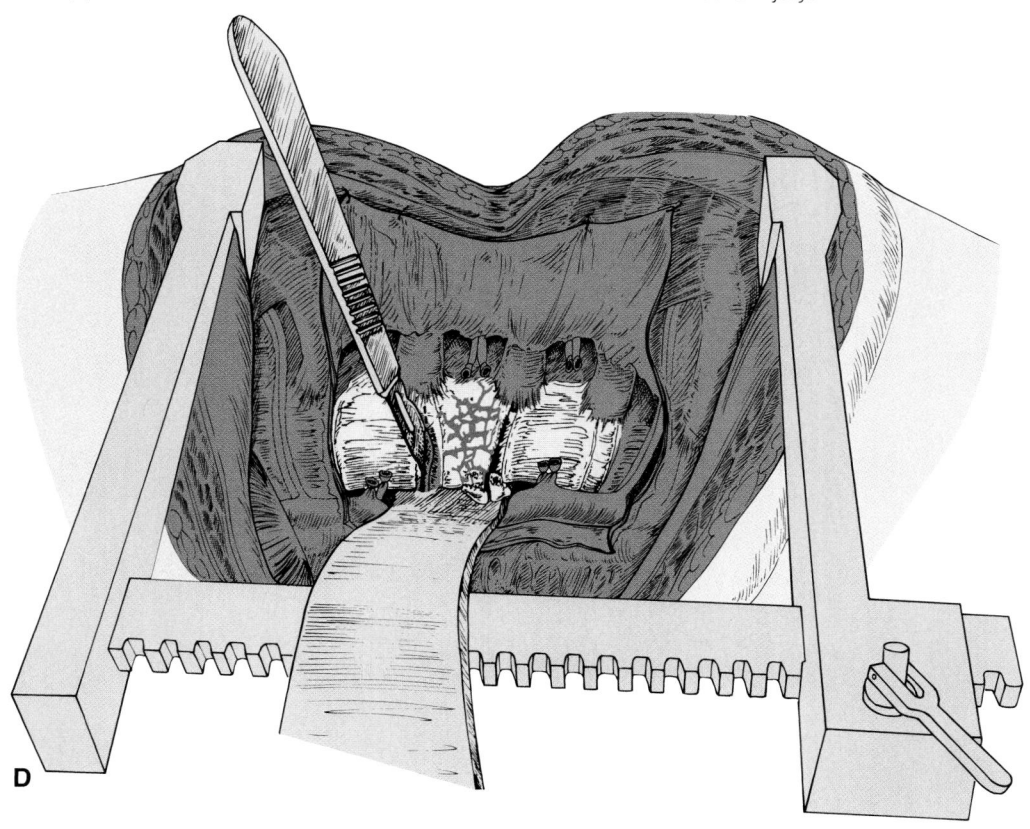

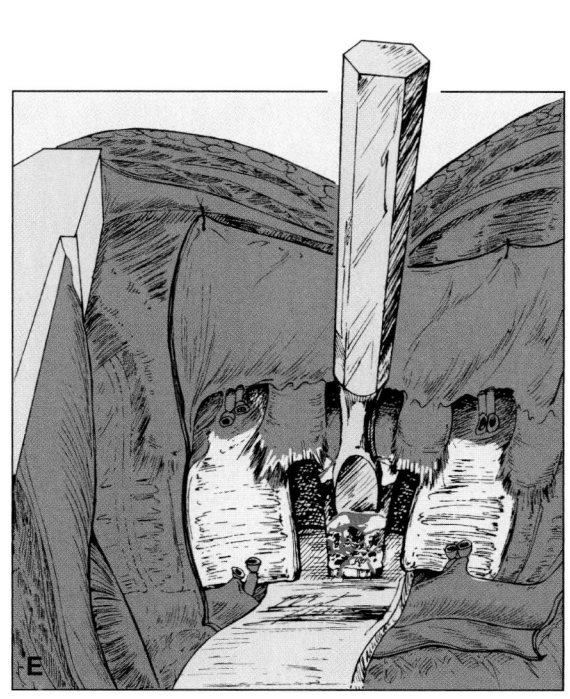

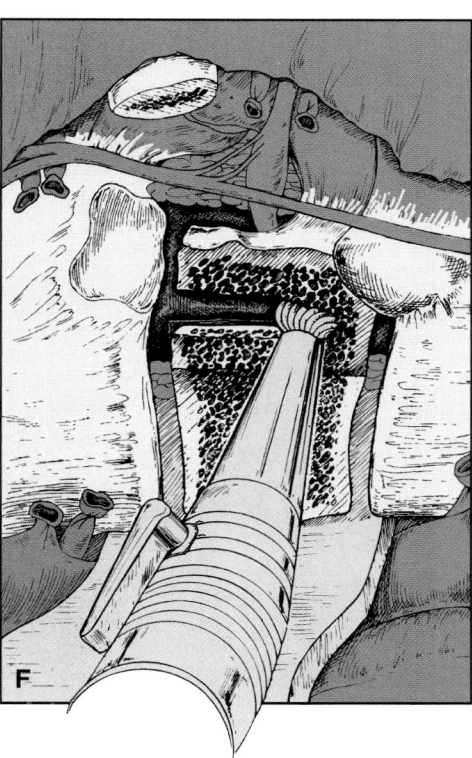

(Continued)

FIGURE 30-39 *(Continued)* **G,** Down-biting 90° Kerrison rongeurs are used to remove the bone on the most superficial portion of the vertebral body. **H,** Reverse-angle curets are utilized to carefully impact the bone from the spinal canal on the far side of the vertebral body. **I,** The bone resection at the end of the decompression should extend from the pedicle on one side to the pedicle on the opposite side. It is easy to underestimate the extent of bone removal necessary to achieve this. At the end of the neural decompression, the dura should bulge anteriorly in a uniform fashion from the end plate of the vertebra above to the end plate of the vertebra below and from pedicle to pedicle. If the dura does not bulge out concentrically, the surgeon should check for residual neural compression. **J,** After the corpectomy as well as resection of the disk above and below the corpectomy. If there is any degree of osteoporosis present, the trough should be cut through the cancellous bone up to the next intact end plate at the superior end of the cephalad vertebra and the inferior aspect of the caudal vertebra. A ridge of bone should be preserved at the posterior aspect of these adjacent vertebrae to prevent migration of the bone graft into the spinal canal.

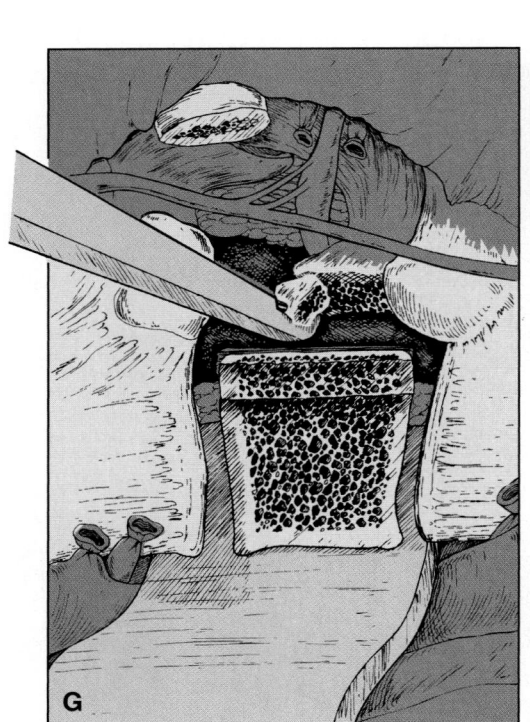

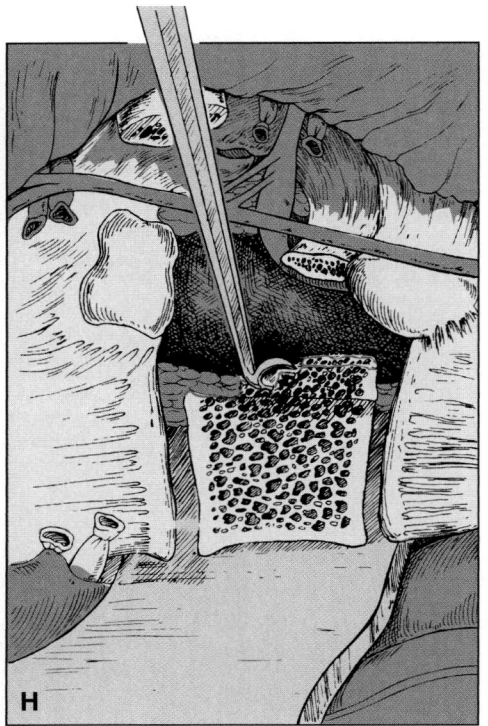

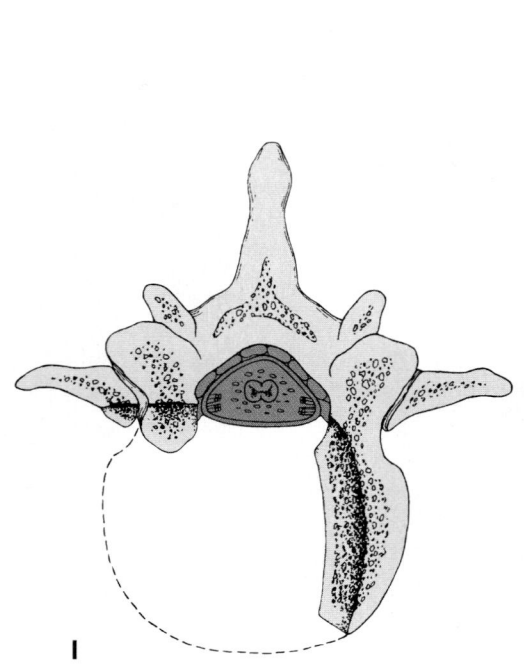

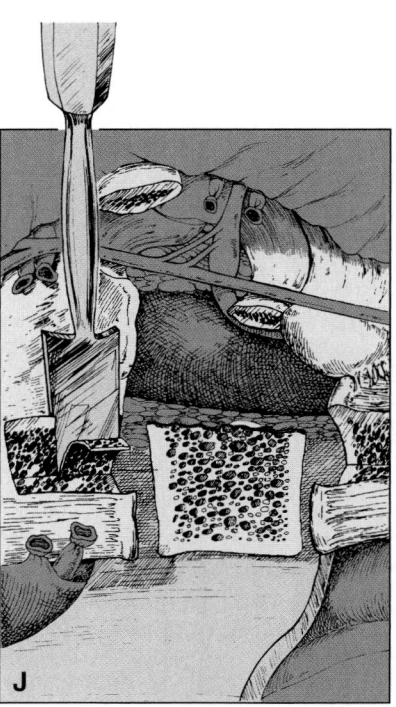

FIGURE 30-39 *(Continued) **K,** At the end of the neural decompression and fusion, there should be adequate space between the bone graft and the dura and neural elements to minimize the chance of producing any iatrogenic neural compression. This illustration shows three strips of rib being used as bone graft, but a single large piece of iliac crest can also be used and may actually provide a stronger anterior strut. A transverse section at the vertebrae above **(L)** and below **(M)** the level of the corpectomy should reveal an adequate posterior rim of cortical bone to prevent migration of the bone graft into the spinal canal and an anterior cortical and cancellous rim of bone to prevent dislodgement of the bone graft.*

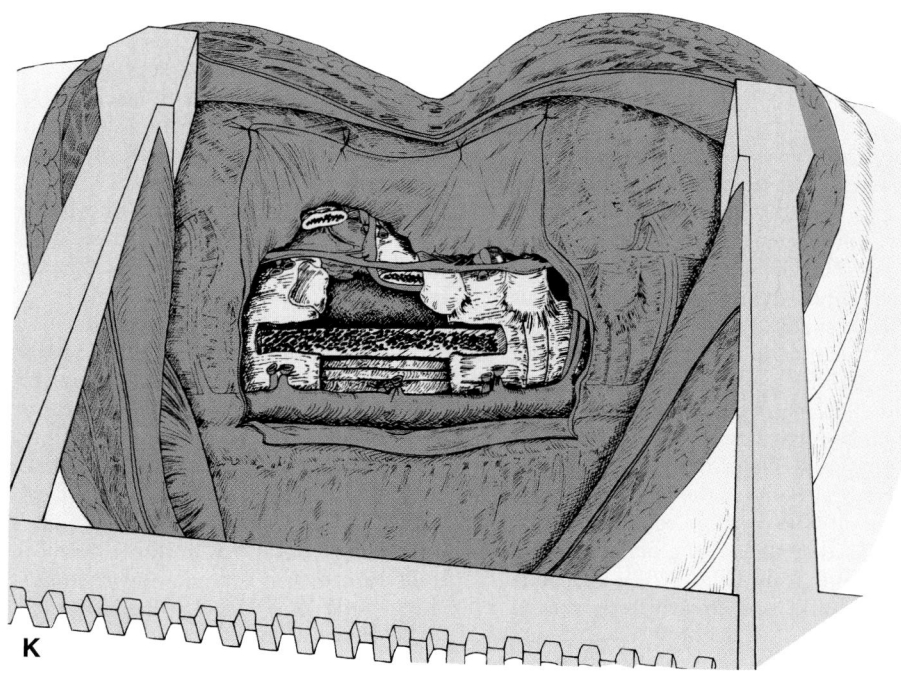

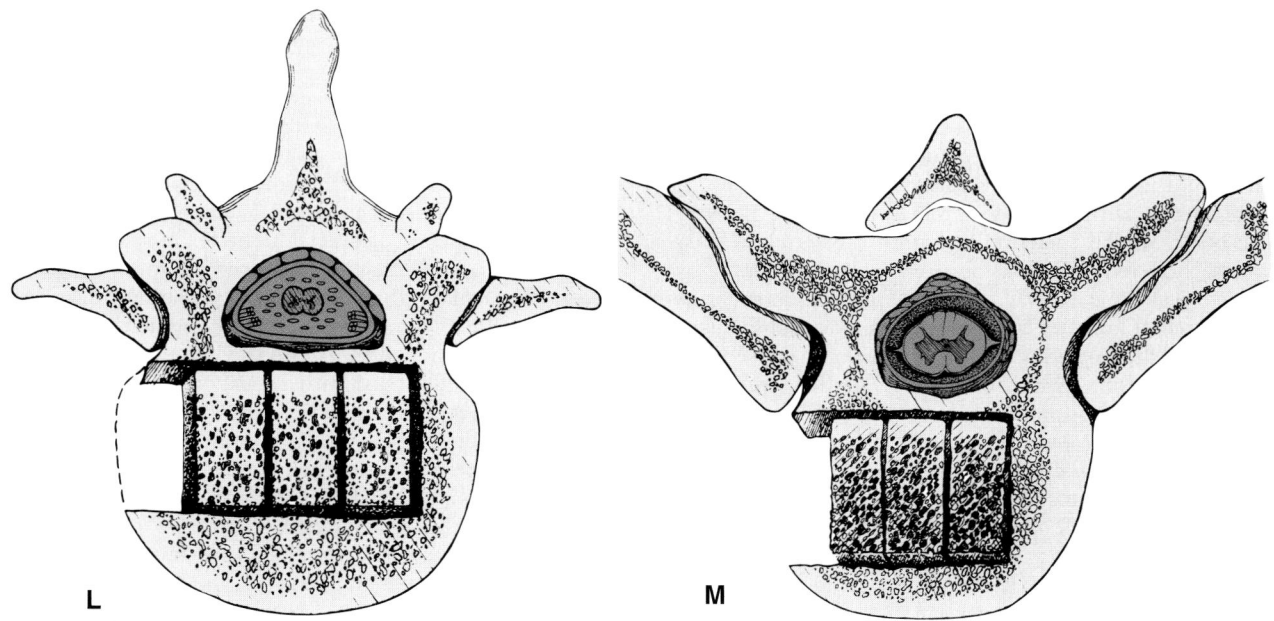

parietal pleura. The rib base of the previously resected rib is traced down to its costovertebral junction, and with the knowledge that each rib inserts at the cephalic quarter of its own vertebra, the levels of each of the vertebral bodies and disks can be determined. At this point, a spinal needle should be placed in a disk and a radiograph obtained to definitively identify the levels.

The parietal pleura is incised halfway between the vertebral neural foramina posteriorly and the anteriorly located azygos vein and inferior vena cava. After division of the parietal pleura one level above and one level below the vertebral body of interest, the segmental vessels are identified in the midportion of the vertebral body at each of these three levels. These segmental vessels should be isolated and either tied or ligated with vascular clips. The vessels should be cut over the anterior third of the vertebral bodies so that they do not interfere with any collateral flow to the spinal cord, which enters the segmental vessels near the neuroforamen. With a small sponge on a clamp or a periosteal elevator, the segmental vessels and parietal pleura can be swept anteriorly and posteriorly to expose the vertebral bodies and disks in an extraperiosteal fashion. Blunt dissection can then be carried out in this same plane, with a sponge on the surgeon's finger used to expose the opposite side of the vertebral body at the site of primary interest. At this time, a malleable or cobra retractor can be inserted between the exposed spine and the parietal pleura that have been dissected anteriorly (Fig. 30-39, C). The retractor protects the esophagus and great vessels during excision of the vertebral body.

Because the rib extends anteriorly over the lateral aspect of the vertebral body, it is necessary to cut it just anterior to the neural foramina. The disks above and below the vertebra to be resected can be removed with a scalpel and rongeurs (Fig. 30-39, D). The vertebral body may then be removed with a rongeur, as well as gouges, osteotomes, and power burs (Fig. 30-39, E). Loupe magnification and a headlamp should be used for this procedure. In the case of an acute fracture with many loose pieces of bone, a large curette can be used to remove the bulk of the vertebral body. As the posterior margin of the vertebral body is approached, red cancellous bone begins to be replaced by white cortical bone, which represents the posterior cortex of the vertebral body. A high-speed bur may then be used to perforate the posterior cortex at the point of minimal neural compression (Fig. 30-39, F). Another technique to gain access to the spinal canal is to use a small Kerrison rongeur to enter through the adjacent disk space. Alternatively, one can begin by removing the pedicle and following the nerve root to the spinal cord. Once a point of entry into the spinal canal has been made, the remainder of the posterior cortex of the vertebral body can be removed with appropriately shaped rongeurs and curettes (Fig. 30-39, G, H). Removal is often facilitated with the use of fine-angle curettes to allow the surgeon to push or pull the posterior cortex away from the spinal canal. This decompression should be performed from pedicle to pedicle to ensure that no spinal cord compression remains (Fig. 30-39, I). If the bone has been removed and the posterior longitudinal ligament does not bulge anteriorly, the ligament should be removed while at the same time looking for other disk or bone fragments that may be causing continued compression of the dura. At the end of the decompression, the ligament or dura, or both, should be bulging anteriorly.

A trough can be cut into the vertebral bodies through the end plates above and below the area of decompression (Fig. 30-39, J), but creation of a trough can weaken stabilization with the graft and is not routinely recommended. Alternatively, all the cartilage can be removed from the end plates, but care must be taken to maintain cortical integrity of the end plates. Appropriate bone graft is then obtained for insertion across this level of decompression. The patient's own iliac crest may be harvested; a tricortical bone graft provides maximal support. Another option, particularly if the injury is associated with minimal instability and the patient's rib is of adequate strength, is to impact three tiers of rib graft into this trough while an assistant pushes on the patient's gibbus to minimize the deformity (Fig. 30-39, J). Alternatively, fresh frozen corticocancellous allograft (iliac crest or distal end of the femur) can be used with good fusion success anteriorly; the use of metal or composite cages filled with autograft, from the corpectomy, is also another good option. At the end of the decompression and bone grafting, adequate space should be left between the neural elements and the bone graft (see Fig. 30-39, K), and a posterior ridge should be present on the vertebra both cephalad and caudal to the decompression to prevent migration of the bone graft toward the neural elements (Fig. 30-39, L, M).

After the corpectomy is completed, an appropriately sized plate is selected to center the two screws at the level above and below the corpectomy as closely as possible on the adjacent bodies. A template (if supplied) is used to place the drill holes parallel to the posterior cortex of the vertebral body so that they accept screws or bolts in that location; the screws or bolts are commonly used to provide compression or distraction. Care must be taken to precisely understand the orientation of the patient on the operating table and the resulting direction of drilling. A bicortical hole is drilled. It is then depth-gauged to determine the proper length screw or bolt. The bolts are screwed tightly into position and may then be used to apply distraction to the interspace, thereby achieving restoration of body height at the injured level. An appropriately sized bone graft can be fashioned to fit into the interspace. Placement of the graft should be slightly biased anteriorly in the corpectomy defect. The distraction can then be released and a plate of proper size selected so that it does not impinge on the open spaces above and below the stabilized levels. The plate (or rods) are placed over the bolts and nuts provisionally placed on the bolts. Slight compressive force is applied across the reconstructed level, and the nuts are tightened down to maintain position. Finally, the two anterior screw holes are drilled and the screws placed into position to complete the construct.

Retractors are removed and hemostasis is obtained before closure. The parietal pleura is reapproximated with the use of absorbable suture material. One or two large chest tubes are inserted. The thoracotomy is closed with sutures placed above the cephalic rib and below the caudal rib, with care taken to avoid the neurovascular bundle immediately beneath the caudal rib. A rib approximator is used to close the chest wall defect, and the pericostal sutures are tied. The muscles are sutured back to their original positions, including the serratus anterior if it was detached from the chest wall.

If the spine injury was relatively stable and is at a level of the spine that can be adequately braced with an orthosis, the patient may be mobilized while wearing the brace. The brace is worn until solid union is demonstrated radiographically. If the spinal fracture was judged to be moderately or severely unstable, the anterior procedure should be combined with posterior instrumentation (usually in compression) and fusion to allow early mobilization. As an alternative, anterior instrumentation can be used to supplement the anterior decompression and fusion, provided that the instability is only moderate (Figs. 30-40 and 30-41).

COMPLICATIONS

With the correct application of currently available spinal instrumentation, it is possible to stabilize and anatomically correct most disrupted spinal columns. However, these procedures are not risk-free and may be associated with major complications. This section does not address all complications related to spinal surgery but focuses on those associated with the treatments described in this chapter. Certain complications such as death, deep vein thrombosis, and pulmonary embolism, though intimately related to surgery, are not peculiar to spine surgery and are therefore not discussed here. Other complications such as iliac crest bone graft donor site morbidity are common to all spinal surgeries.[13,102,152] It cannot be emphasized strongly enough that many potential intraoperative complications may be avoided, or their severity reduced, by careful preoperative planning. Accurate identification of the mechanism of injury and selection of the appropriate instrumentation and levels constitute the first critical step. However, despite detailed planning, surgical complications may still occur.

Neurologic Deterioration

Neurologic deterioration can occur before initiation of definitive treatment. Gertzbein reported a 3.4 percent incidence of new or increased neurologic deficit after patients were admitted to trauma centers.[62] He noted, however, that this group of patients had a significantly increased return of neurologic function after initiation of treatment compared with those who initially had a neurologic deficit. For patients whose neurologic function deteriorates after the initial evaluation, surgical treatment is recommended. In addition, progressive deformity with associated late neurologic deterioration may develop in fractures managed nonoperatively, even if initially stable. Neurologic deficit occurring during or after treatment is one of the most serious complications associated with the surgical treatment of spinal injuries. The reported incidence is approximately 1 percent.[105] Neurologic deterioration may be associated with direct injury resulting from the introduction of instrumentation into the spinal canal or loss of position or reduction.

During instrumentation, if evoked potentials deteriorate or if an intraoperative wake-up test is not fully

achieved successfully, the instrumentation system should be altered, if possible.

Neurologic deterioration observed in the postoperative period may be related to disk herniation, loss of reduction, spinal cord edema, hematoma, or some combination of these complications. Immediate study with myelography, CT, or MRI should be considered, and the patient should be returned to the operating room as necessary to relieve any neural compression.

INJURY RESULTING FROM INSERTION OF PEDICLE SCREWS

The spinal nerves are particularly susceptible to injury if the pedicle is violated medially or inferiorly. In addition, a screw that is too long can transgress the anterior cortex of the vertebral body and injure a major vascular structure.

The risk of neural damage can be minimized if the surgeon is aware of the spinal anatomy and familiar with the process of localization and entering the pedicle. Careful identification of the pedicle and proper screw placement under radiographic control help minimize potential injuries. In earlier studies, some authors reported a 10 to 20 percent rate of inaccurate pedicle screw placement, even in well-controlled environments. This rate reportedly increased to as high as 41 percent in the thoracic spine.[147] It may also be increased with deformity and instability. Fortunately, not all errant screw placements lead to clinical consequences.

Neural damage can result from direct contact by a screw or by a drill, curette, or tap. Late screw cut-out through the pedicle may also result in nerve damage. If a postoperative radiculopathy is noted, CT evaluation of the screw and bone should be performed, with consideration of screw removal if the results are positive. However, stability issues must also be considered when making these decisions. Rose and associates described a technique involving persistently electrified pedicle stimulation instruments, which can be used to detect whether the pedicle screws have fractured or broached the cortical bone during placement.[138] This technique may help confirm intraosseous placement of pedicle screws and prevent neurologic injury.

Kothe and colleagues simulated pedicle fractures in an in vitro model to determine the effect on multidirectional stability when pedicle instrumentation is used.[96] After simulation of an intraoperative pedicle fracture, the results of three-dimensional flexibility testing showed a significant decrease in axial rotation and lateral bending stability provided by the instrumentation.

If screw loosening occurs, loss of correction may develop before the fusion heals. Loss of fixation can result from errant placement of a screw, fracture of the pedicle, inadequate purchase of the screw into bone, poor bone quality, or inadequate screw size. Pedicle fracture may occur if too large a screw is placed into the pedicle or the screw is driven out of the pedicular cortex. Sjöström and associates used CT to study the pedicles of patients after removal of pedicle screw instrumentation following fusion for burst fractures.[149] They found that 65 percent of instrumented pedicles increased in width, as did 85 percent of those in which the screw diameter was greater than 65 percent of the diameter of the pedicle. This result, however, may not have clinical consequences. The authors

FIGURE 30-40 *Technique for anterior spinal instrumentation following corpectomy. **A,** After utilizing a depth gauge directed on the exposed vertebral body, appropriately sized screw lengths are selected in order to engage the opposite cortex of the vertebral body. The bolts are placed parallel to the adjacent end plate to avoid intrusion into the disk space above and below the corpectomy site. **B,** Distraction is applied against the bolts, allowing easy insertion of the strut graft into the corpectomy site. **C,** Determination of proper length of plate via a template is important to avoid impingement of the superior or inferior disk space. Locking nuts are applied and provisionally tightened. **D,** Compressive forces are applied and locking nuts are tightened firmly. **E,** Finally, two anterior screws are placed and the nuts are crimped down, preventing possible backing out or loosening. (Redrawn with permission from Zdeblick, T.A. Z-Plate-ATL Anterior Fixation System: Surgical Technique. Sofamor Danek Group, Inc. All rights reserved.)*

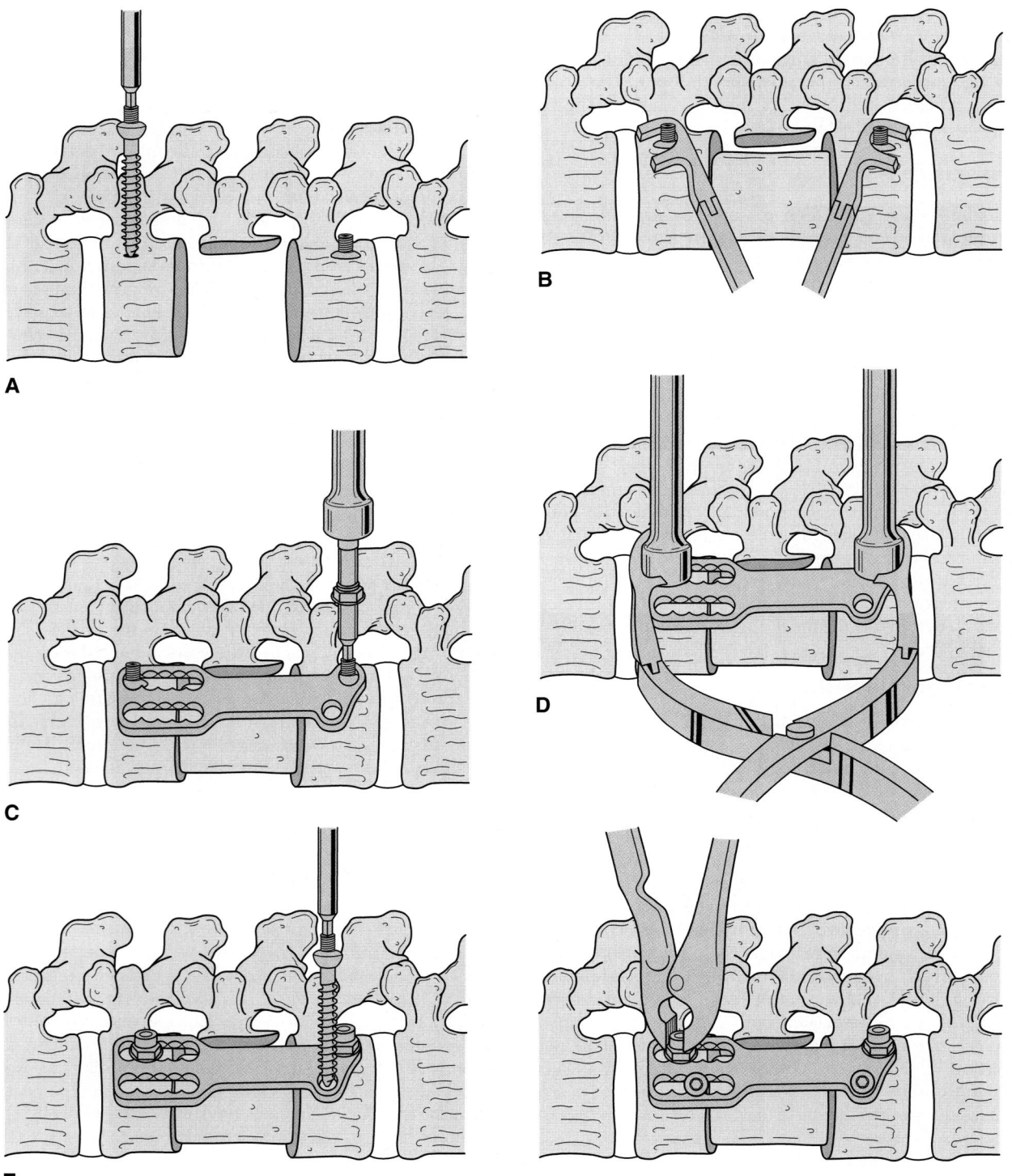

emphasized the importance of correct screw size to avoid injury to the pedicle and subsequent loosening of the implant.

Occasionally, with severe deformity or osteopenia, maximal bone–screw interface strength is required and necessitates placement of the screw deep within the vertebral body or through the anterior cortex. The need for anterior cortical fixation must be balanced against the risk of injury to the anterior vascular structures. This problem may be handled by adding screws at other levels or by augmenting the fixation with polymethylmethacrylate (rarely used in trauma). However, in fractures, alternatives are usually

FIGURE 30-41 *A 17-year-old female who sustained an L1 burst fracture in a motor vehicle accident.* **A,** *Lateral radiograph showing L1 burst fracture.* **B,** *Sagittal computed tomography (CT) showing burst fracture with retropulsion of posterior wall. Note that the relationship between the spinous processes is maintained without significant widening between the spinous processes of L1 and L2.* **C,** *Axial CT showing retropulsion of the posterior fragment with approximately 80% canal compromise.*

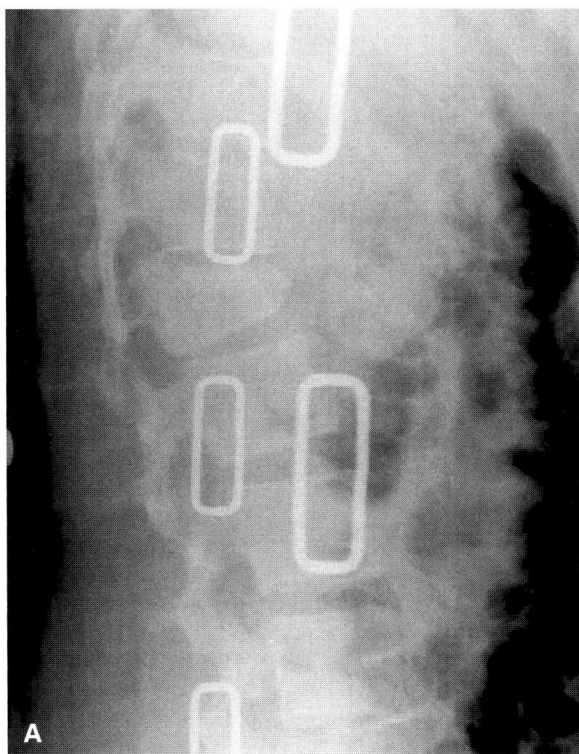
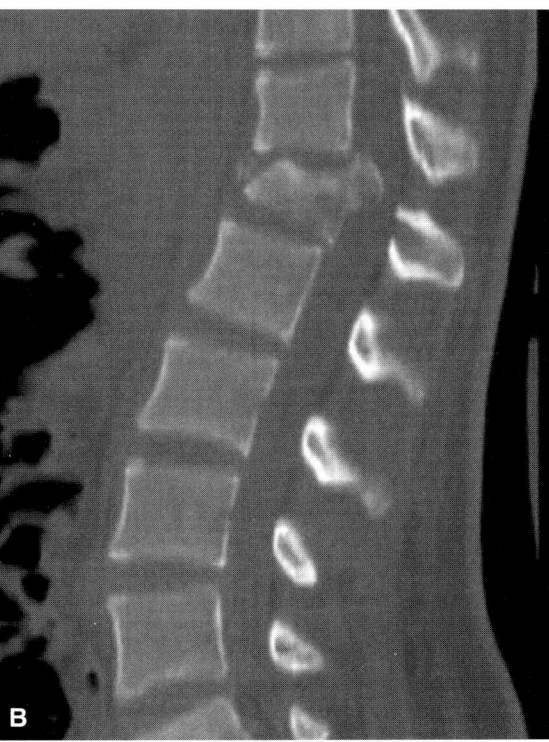
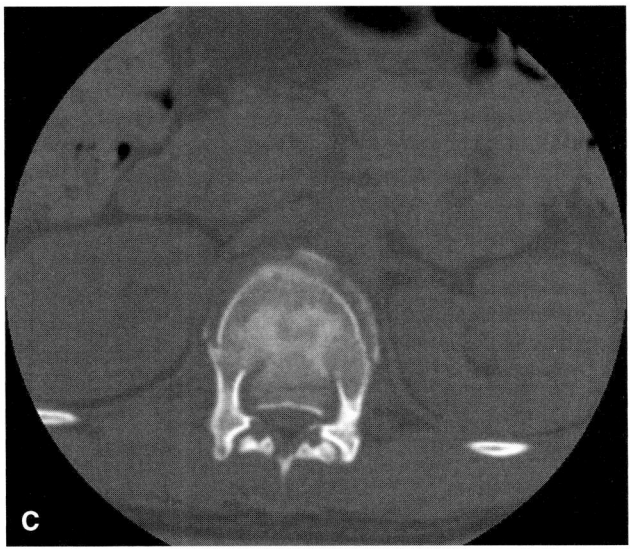

(Continued)

FIGURE 30-41 *(Continued)* ***D, E,*** *Based on the amount of canal compromise, it was decided that this patient would need an anterior decompression and fusion. As there was minimal posterior ligamentous disruption, and also because she was young and had good bone stock, the decision was made not to supplement the anterior fusion with posterior instrumentation. Bicortical purchase is recommended if the decision is made not to supplement with posterior instrumentation.*

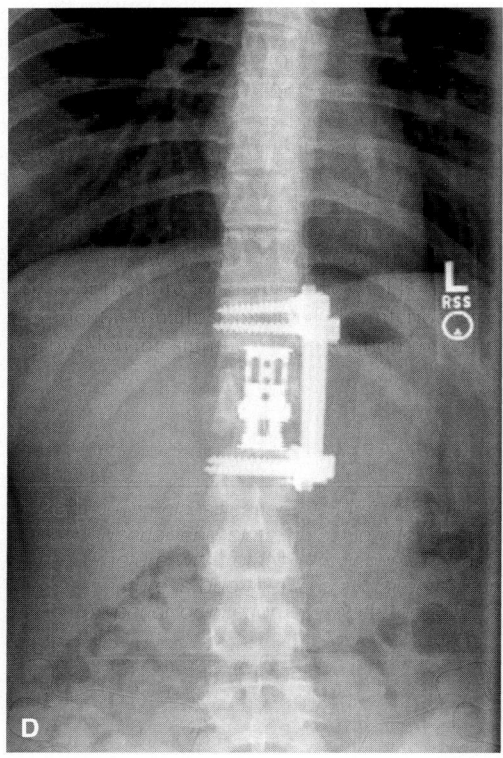
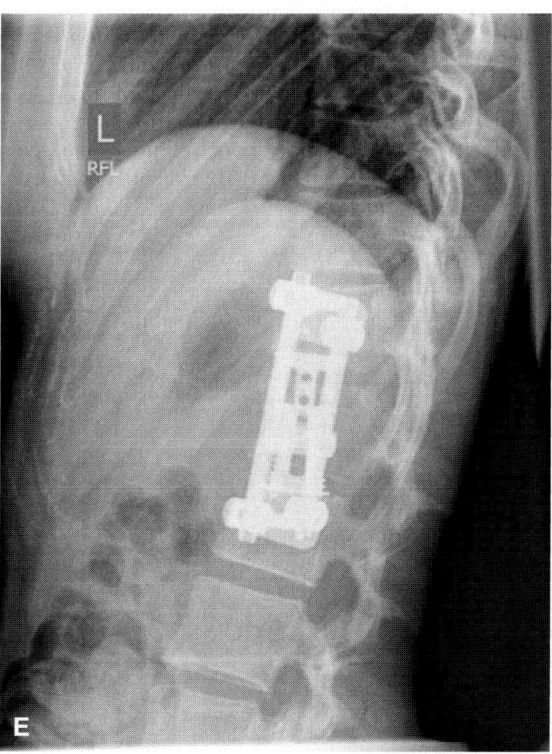

available, including noninstrumented fusion, bedrest, and alteration of the instrumentation to a system with laminar fixation.

Dural Tears

A dural laceration and concomitant leak of cerebrospinal fluid may result from the injury or from surgery. Intraoperatively, laceration can occur during exposure, instrumentation, or decortication. Regardless of the cause, the site of the injury, once identified, should be adequately visualized (with bone removed as necessary) and the dura repaired.[45] The repair may be augmented with a fibrin glue (e.g., Tisseal [Baxter Inc.]). If primary repair is not possible, muscle or fascia grafting should be performed to close the defect. In addition, if the seal is less than adequate, a lumbar transdural drain can be placed to reduce cerebrospinal fluid pressure and permit dural healing.

Infections

Infections can occur after spine surgery, but they are relatively less common than after instrumentation and fusion for degenerative conditions. Infections superficial to the fascia can be treated with early and aggressive débridement and either open packing of the wound or closure over a drainage tube.

Deep infections should be treated by aggressive irrigation and débridement as soon as the infection is noted.

If this complication occurs, we attempt to leave the bone graft and the metal instrumentation system in place. After thorough irrigation, drains are placed deep to the fascia and all layers are tightly closed. The drain is maintained for at least 4 days until cultures from the effluent are clear. Inflow–outflow systems may also be used. Because superinfections have been noted to occur 7 to 10 days after surgery, the tubes should be removed before this length of time, even if culture results are still positive. Vacuum-assisted closure (VAC) devices may also be used to help clean the wound and stimulate the formation of granulation tissue. Good results have been noted in a couple of studies where VAC devices were used in spine infections.[119,165] A delayed closure may be performed when the wound bed is clean. If the infection persists, the procedure can be repeated once, again trying to salvage the bone graft, the instrumentation, and the reduction. Occasionally, this treatment fails and it is necessary to remove the metal, the bone graft, or both to eradicate the infection. An alternative is to pack the wound open, deep to the fascia, and change the dressing at least daily.

Associated Medical Conditions

Improved medical management has reduced the complications associated with spinal cord injury and is responsible for a marked increase in life expectancy. However, head injury, musculoskeletal trauma, and visceral damage, which occur concomitantly in up to 60 percent of patients with spinal cord injury, often complicate treatment. If the patient is unconscious at initial evaluation, the diagnosis of spinal cord injury may be difficult to make. Screening radiographs of the spine and all long bones below the level of injury should be performed in all patients with head or spinal cord injury. Additionally, after blunt trauma, a significant number of spinal cord-injured patients have an associated abdominal injury and may be unable to feel or communicate the underlying problem. Reid and co-workers reported a 50 percent incidence of intra-abdominal injury associated with Chance fractures in children and adolescents.[133] Anderson and colleagues reported a 66 percent incidence of hollow viscus lesions associated with seat belt-type injuries, which climbed to 86 percent in a pediatric subset.[10] A perforated viscus with associated peritonitis may go undetected. Because this complication is responsible for significant morbidity and death, peritoneal lavage should be a routine part of the initial evaluation of all patients with spinal cord injury.

Renal failure is a frequent occurrence in patients with spinal cord injury. A gradual decline in the incidence of this problem, particularly as a cause of death, has occurred as a result of advances in bladder drainage techniques (e.g., intermittent catheterization). Once the fluid status (inflow and outflow) is normalized in the acute injury state, intermittent bladder catheterization should be considered for the management of a neurogenic bladder. After further urologic evaluation, individualized treatment may be instituted. Pulmonary complications, already increased in neurologically injured patients, are further worsened if the anterior transthoracic approach is used.[11]

Late complications in a spinal cord-injured patient can relate to painful nonunion of the spine, limited neurologic recovery of spinal cord or root function (particularly because limited recovery leads to persistent nerve compromise and pain), and medical complications associated with prolonged bedrest, many of which can be avoided by early, rigid immobilization, as discussed earlier in this chapter. In particular, disuse osteoporosis is a common problem in paraplegic patients immobilized for even short periods; it increases their susceptibility to recurrent injuries.[84]

Finally, individuals with spinal cord injuries may experience intractable spasticity. For this condition, studies have shown the efficacy of implantable intrathecal baclofen pumps, if oral medications are not effective.

CONCLUSION

The major objective of any treatment is to construct the most stable environment for the spinal cord, nerve roots, and spinal column to allow neurologic improvement. Although the emphasis in this chapter has been on rigid spinal stabilization, it should be stressed that such stabilization is only one means of achieving this goal. Its major advantage at this time, in addition to stabilizing and protecting the spinal cord, is that it allows the patient to rapidly initiate rehabilitation. Reversibility of spinal cord injury remains an unsolved medical and surgical problem. However, rehabilitation has greatly improved the quality of life of patients with spinal cord injuries.

Intensive rehabilitation should begin as early as possible, with the major objective being attainment of functional independence. The final functional level depends primarily on the level and severity of the neurologic deficit. Surgical instrumentation of the spine and effective use (and fit) of spinal orthoses permit earlier mobilization of the patient in the acute phase and may allow patients to reach their functional level sooner. The best selection of treatment depends on understanding the anatomy, the mechanics of the injury, the forces involved, and the options that are available to stabilize and protect the spinal column and cord.

Minimizing complications associated with the surgical treatment of spine injuries requires a thorough knowledge of the anatomy, an accurate diagnosis, and an understanding and experience with the implants chosen. Although complications can be minimized, they cannot be completely eliminated.

REFERENCES

1. Abe, E.; Sato, K.; Shimada, Y.; et al. Thoracolumbar burst fracture with horizontal fracture of the posterior column. Spine 22:83–87, 1997.
2. Acosta, F.L., Jr.; Aryan, H.E.; Taylor, W.R.; et al. Kyphoplasty-augmented short-segment pedicle screw fixation of traumatic lumbar burst fractures: Initial clinical experience and literature review. Neurosurg Focus 18: e9, 2005.
3. Aebi, M.; Thalgott, J.S. Fractures and dislocations of the thoracolumbar spine treated by the internal spinal skeletal fixation system. Proc North Am Spine Soc 68, 1987.
4. Agus, H.; Kayali, C.; Arslantas, M.; et al. Nonoperative treatment of burst-type thoracolumbar vertebrafractures: Clinical and radiological results of 29 patients. Eur Spine J 14:536–540, 2005.
5. Alanay, A.; Acaroglu, E.; Yazici, M.; et al. Short-segment pedicle instrumentation of thoracolumbar burst fractures: Does transpedicular intracorporeal grafting prevent early failure? Spine 26:213–217, 2001.
6. Albert, T.J.; Levine, M.J.; An, H.S.; et al. Concomitant noncontiguous thoracolumbar and sacral fractures. Spine 18:1285–1291, 1993.
7. Alvine, G.F.; Swain, J.M.; Asher, M.A.; et al. Treatment of thoracolumbar burst fractures with variable screw placement or Isola instrumentation and arthrodesis: Case series and literature review. J Spinal Disord Tech 17:251–264, 2004.
8. An, H.S.; Andreshak, T.G.; Nguyen, C.; et al. Can we distinguish between benign versus malignant compression fractures of the spine by magnetic resonance imaging? Spine 20:1776–1782, 1995.
9. An, H.S.; Singh, K.; Vaccaro, A.R.; et al. Biomechanical evaluation of contemporary posterior spinal internal fixation configurations in an unstable burst-fracture calf spine model: Special references of hook configurations and pedicle screws. Spine 29:257–262, 2004.

10. Anderson, P.A.; Rivara, F.P.; Maier, R.V.; et al. The epidemiology of seatbelt-associated injuries. J Trauma 31:60–67, 1991.

11. Anderson, T.M.; Mansour, K.A.; Miller, J.I., Jr. Thoracic approaches to anterior spinal operations: Anterior thoracic approaches. Ann Thorac Surg 55:1447–1451, 1993.

12. Anekstein, Y.; Brosh, T.; Mirovsky, Y. Intermediate screws in short segment pedicular fixation for thoracic and lumbar fractures: A biomechanical study. J Spinal Disord Tech 20:72–77, 2007.

13. Arrington, E.D.; Smith, W.J.; Chambers, H.G.; et al. Complications of iliac crest bone graft harvesting. Clin Orthop Relat Res 329:300–309, 1996.

14. Ballock, R.T.; Mackersie, R.; Abitbol, J.J.; et al. Can burst fractures be predicted from plain radiographs? J Bone Joint Surg [Br] 74:147–150, 1992.

15. Bedbrook, G.M. Treatment of thoracolumbar dislocation and fractures with paraplegia. Clin Orthop Relat Res 112:27–43, 1975.

16. Bedbrook, G.M. Spinal injuries with tetraplegia and paraplegia. J Bone Joint Surg [Br] 61:267–284, 1979.

17. Berry, J.L.; Moran, J.M.; Berg, W.S.; et al. A morphometric study of human lumbar and selected thoracic vertebrae. Spine 12:362–367, 1987.

18. Bess, R.S.; Lenke, L.G.; Bridwell, K.H.; et al. Comparison of thoracic pedicle screw to hook instrumentation for the treatment of adult spinal deformity. Spine 32:555–561, 2007.

19. Bishop, W.J. The Early History of Surgery. London, Robert Hale, 1960.

20. Bohlman, H.H. Treatment of fractures and dislocations of the thoracic and lumbar spine. J Bone Joint Surg [Am] 67:165–169, 1985.

21. Bohlman, H.H.; Freehafer, A.; Dejak, J. The results of treatment of acute injuries of the upper thoracic spine with paralysis. J Bone Joint Surg [Am] 67:360–369, 1985.

22. Bohlman, H.H.; Zdeblick, T.A. Anterior excision of herniated thoracic discs. J Bone Joint Surg [Am] 70:1038–1047, 1988.

23. Bransford, R.; Bellabarba, C.; Thompson, J.H.; et al. The safety of fluoroscopically-assisted thoracic pedicle screw instrumentation for spine trauma. J Trauma 60:1047–1052, 2006.

24. Brant-Zawadzki, M.; Jeffrey, R.B., Jr.; Minagi, H.; et al. High resolution CT of thoracolumbar fractures. AJR Am J Roentgenol 138:699–704, 1982.

25. Bravo, P.; Labarta, C.; Alcaraz, M.A.; et al. Outcome after vertebral fractures with neurological lesion treated either surgically or conservatively in Spain. Paraplegia 31:358–366, 1993.

26. Breasted, J.H. (ed). The Edwin Smith Papyrus. Chicago, University of Chicago Press, 1930.

27. Brown, T.; Hansen, R.J.; Yorra, A.J. Some mechanical tests on the lumbosacral spine with particular reference to the intervertebral discs: A preliminary report. J Bone Joint Surg [Am] 39:1135–1164, 1957.

28. Burke, D.C. Hyperextension injuries of the spine. J Bone Joint Surg [Br] 53:1–12, 1971.

29. Cammisa, F.P., Jr.; Eismont, F.J.; Green, B.A. Dural laceration occurring with burst fractures and associated laminar fractures. J Bone Joint Surg [Am] 71:1044–1052, 1989.

30. Cantor, J.B.; Lebwohl, N.H.; Garvey, T.; et al. Nonoperative management of stable thoracolumbar burst fractures with early ambulation and bracing. Spine 18:971–976, 1993.

31. Chance, C.Q. Note on a type of flexion fracture of the spine. Br J Radiol 21:452–453, 1948.

32. Davies, W.E.; Morris, J.H.; Hill, V. An analysis of conservative (non-surgical) management of thoracolumbar fractures and fracture–dislocations with neural damage. J Bone Joint Surg [Am] 62:1324–1328, 1980.

33. Davis, P.R. The medial inclination of the human thoracic intervertebral articular facets. J Anat 93:68–74, 1959.

34. De Oliveira, J.C. A new type of fracture–dislocation of the thoracolumbar spine. J Bone Joint Surg [Am] 60:481–488, 1978.

35. Denis, F. Updated classification of thoracolumbar fractures. Orthop Trans 6:8, 1982.

36. Denis, F. The three column spine and its significance in the classification of acute thoracolumbar spinal injuries. Spine 8:817–831, 1983.

37. Denis, F.; Armstrong, G.W.; Searls, K.; et al. Acute thoracolumbar burst fractures in the absence of neurologic deficit: A comparison between operative and nonoperative treatment. Clin Orthop Relat Res 189: 142–149, 1984.

38. Denis, F.; Burkus; J.K. Shear fracture–dislocations of the thoracic and lumbar spine associated with forceful hyperextension (lumberjack paraplegia). Spine 17: 156–161, 1992.

39. DeWald, R.L. Burst fractures of the thoracic and lumbar spine. Clin Orthop Relat Res 189:150–161, 1984.

40. Dickson, J.H.; Harrington, P.R.; Erwin, W.D. Results of reduction and stabilization of the severely fractured thoracic and lumbar spine. J Bone Joint Surg [Am] 60:799–805, 1978.

41. Dommisse, G.F. The blood supply of the spinal cord: A critical vascular zone in spinal surgery. J Bone Joint Surg [Br] 56:225–235, 1974.

42. Dommisse, G.F. The arteries, arterioles, and capillaries of the spinal cord: Surgical guidelines in the prevention of postoperative paraplegia. Ann R Coll Surg Engl 62:369–376, 1980.

43. Edwards, C.C.; Levine, A.M. Early rod-sleeve stabilization of the injured thoracic and lumbar spine. Orthop Clin North Am 17:121–145, 1986.

44. Edwards, C.C.; Rosenthal, M.S.; Gellard, F.; et al. The fate of retropulsed bone following vertebral body fractures. Orthop Trans 13:19, 1989.

45. Eismont, F.J.; Wiesel, S.W.; Rothman, R.H. Treatment of dural tears associated with spinal surgery. J Bone Joint Surg [Am] 63:1132–1136, 1981.

46. Elliott, H.C. Cross-sectional diameters and areas of the human spinal cord. Anat Rec 93:287–293, 1945.

47. Epstein, N.E.; Epstein, J.A. Limbus lumbar vertebral fractures in 27 adolescents and adults. Spine 16:962–966, 1991.

48. Farcy, J.P.; Weidenbaum, M.; Glassman, S.D. Sagittal index in management of thoracolumbar burst fractures. Spine 15:958–965, 1990.

49. Ferguson, R.L.; Allen, B.L., Jr. A mechanistic classification of thoracolumbar spine fractures. Clin Orthop Relat Res 189:77–88, 1984.

50. Ferguson, R.L.; Allen, B.L., Jr. An algorithm for the treatment of unstable thoracolumbar fractures. Orthop Clin North Am 17:105–112, 1986.

51. Finkelstein, J.A.; Chapman, J.R.; Mirza, S. Anterior cortical allograft in thoracolumbar fractures. J Spinal Disord 12:424–429, 1999.

52. Fisher, C.G.; Sahajpal, V.; Keynan, O.; et al. Accuracy and safety of pedicle screw fixation in thoracic spine trauma. J Neurosurg Spine 5:620–626, 2006.

53. Flesch, J.R.; Leider, L.L.; Erickson, D.L.; et al. Harrington instrumentation and spine fusion for unstable fractures and fracture–dislocations of the thoracic and lumbar spine. J Bone Joint Surg [Am] 59:143–153, 1977.

54. Frankel, H.L.; Hancock, D.O.; Hyslop, G.; et al. The value of postural reduction in the initial management of closed injuries of the spine with paraplegia and tetraplegia. I. Paraplegia 7:179–192, 1969.

55. Fredrickson, B.E.; Edwards, W.T.; Rauschning, W.; et al. Vertebral burst fractures: An experimental, morphologic, and radiographic study. Spine 17:1012–1021, 1992.

56. Fredrickson, B.E.; Mann, K.A.; Yuan, H.A.; et al. Reduction of the intracanal fragment in experimental burst fractures. Spine 13:267–271, 1988.

57. Gardner, V.O.; Thalgott, J.S.; White, J.I.; et al. The contoured anterior spinal plate system (CASP). Indications, techniques, and results. Spine 19:550–555, 1994.

58. Garfin, S.R. Buckley, R.A. Ledlie, J.; et al. Balloon kyphoplasty for symptomatic vertebral body compression fractures results in rapid, significant, and sustained improvements in back pain, function, and quality of life for elderly patients. Spine 31:2213–2220, 2006.

59. Garfin, S.R.; Mowery, C.A.; Guerra, J., Jr.; et al. Confirmation of the posterolateral technique to decompress and fuse thoracolumbar spine burst fractures. Spine 10:218–223, 1985.

60. Garfin, S.R.; Reilley, M.A. Minimally invasive treatment of osteoporotic vertebral body compression fractures. Spine J 1:76–80, 2002.

61. Gellad, F.E.; Levine, A.M.; Joslyn, J.N.; et al. Pure thoracolumbar facet dislocation: Clinical features and CT appearance. Radiology 161:505–508, 1986.

62. Gertzbein, S.D. Scoliosis Research Society. Multicenter spine fracture study. Spine 5:528–540, 1992.

63. Gertzbein, S.D. Classification of thoracic and lumbar fractures. In: Gertzbein S.D., ed. Fractures of the Thoracic and Lumbar Spine. Baltimore, Williams and Wilkins, 1992.

64. Gertzbein, S.D.; Court-Brown, C.M. Flexion–distraction injuries of the lumbar spine: Mechanisms of injury and classification. Clin Orthop Relat Res 227:52–60, 1988.

65. Gumley, G.; Taylor, T.K.; Ryan, M.D. Distraction fractures of the lumbar spine. J Bone Joint Surg [Br] 64:520–525, 1982.

66. Gurr, K.R.; McAfee, P.C.; Shih, C.M. Biomechanical analysis of anterior and posterior instrumentation systems after corpectomy: A calf-spine model. J Bone Joint Surg [Am] 70:1182–1191, 1988.

67. Gurwitz, G.S.; Dawson, J.M.; McNamara, M.J.; et al. Biomechanical analysis of three surgical approaches for lumbar burst fractures using short-segment instrumentation. Spine 18:977–982, 1993.

68. Guttman, L. Spinal Cord Injuries: Comprehensive Management and Research. Oxford, Blackwell, 1973.

69. Hardaker, W.T., Jr.; Cook, W.A., Jr.; Friedman, A.H.; et al. Bilateral transpedicular decompression and Harrington rod stabilization in the management of severe thoracolumbar burst fractures. Spine 17:162–171, 1992.

70. Harrop, J.S.; Vaccaro, A.R.; Hurlbert, R.J.; et al. Intrarater and interrater reliability and validity in the assessment of the mechanism of injury and integrity of the posterior ligamentous complex: A novel injury severity scoring system for thoracolumbar injuries. J Neurosurg Spine 4:118–122, 2006.

71. Harryman, D.T. Complete fracture–dislocation of the thoracic spine associated with spontaneous neurologic decompression: A case report. Clin Orthop Relat Res 207:64–69, 1986.

72. Hart, R.A.; Hansen, B.L.; Shea, M.; et al. Pedicle screw placement in the thoracic spine: A comparison of image-guided and manual techniques in cadavers. Spine 30:E326–E331, 2005.

73. Hazel, W.A., Jr.; Jones, R.A.; Morrey, B.F.; et al. Vertebral fractures without neurological deficit: A long-term follow-up study. J Bone Joint Surg [Am] 70:1319–1321, 1988.

74. Heggeness, M.H.; Doherty, B.J. The trabecular anatomy of thoracolumbar vertebrae: Implications for burst fractures. J Anat 191(Pt 2):309–312, 1997.

75. Hitchon, P.W.; Brenton, M.D.; Black, A.G.; et al. In vitro biomechanical comparison of pedicle screws, sublaminar hooks, and sublaminar cables. J Neurosurg 99(1 Suppl):104–109, 2003.

76. Holdsworth, F.W. Fractures, dislocations and fracture-dislocations of the spine. J Bone Joint Surg 45B:6, 1963.

77. Holdsworth, F.W. Fractures and dislocations of the lower thoracic and lumbar spines, with and without

neurological involvement. Curr Pract Orthop Surg 23:61–84, 1964.

78. Holdsworth, F.W. Fractures, dislocations and fracture–dislocations of the spine. J Bone Joint Surg [Am] 52:1534–1551, 1970.

79. Holdsworth, F.W.; Hardy, A. Early treatment of paraplegia from fractures of the thoracolumbar spine. J Bone Joint Surg [Am] 35:440–450, 1953.

80. Hu, S.S.; Capen, D.A.; Rimoldi, R.L.; et al. The effect of surgical decompression on neurologic outcome after lumbar fractures. Clin Orthop Relat Res 288:166–173, 1993.

81. Huelke, D.F.; Kaufer, H. Vertebral column injuries and seat belts. J Trauma 15:304–318, 1975.

82. Jacobs, R.R.; Asher, M.A.; Snider, R.K. Thoracolumbar spinal injuries: A comparative study of recumbent and operative treatment in 100 patients. Spine 5:463–477, 1980.

83. James, K.S.; Wenger, K.H.; Schlegel, J.D.; et al. Biomechanical evaluation of the stability of thoracolumbar burst fractures. Spine 19:1731–1740, 1994.

84. Jiang, S.D.; Dai, L.Y.; Jiang, L.S. Osteoporosis after spinal cord injury. Osteoporos Int 17:180–192, 2006.

85. Kaneda, K.; Asano, S.; Hashimoto, T.; et al. The treatment of osteoporotic-posttraumatic vertebral collapse using the Kaneda device and a bioactive ceramic vertebral prosthesis. Spine 17(8 Suppl): S295–303, 1992.

86. Kaneda, K.; Taneichi, H.; Abumi, K.; et al. Anterior decompression and stabilization with the Kaneda device for thoracolumbar burst fractures associated with neurological deficits. J Bone Joint Surg [Am] 79:69–83, 1997.

87. Kaufer, H.; Hayes, J.T. Lumbar fracture–dislocation: A study of twenty-one cases. J Bone Joint Surg [Am] 48:712–730, 1966.

88. Kelly, R.P.; Whitesides, T.E., Jr. Treatment of lumbodorsal fracture–dislocations. Ann Surg 167:705–717, 1968.

89. Kerslake, R.W.; Jaspan, T.; Worthington, B.S. Magnetic resonance imaging of spinal trauma. Br J Radiol 64:376–402, 1991.

90. King, A.G. Burst compression fractures of the thoracolumbar spine: Pathologic anatomy and surgical management. Orthopedics 10:1711–1719, 1987.

91. King, A.I.; Prasad, P.; Ewing, C.L. Mechanism of spinal injury due to caudocephalad acceleration. Orthop Clin North Am 6:19–31, 1975.

92. Klose, K.J.; Goldberg, M.L.; Smith, R.S.; et al. Neurologic change following spinal cord injury: An assessment technique and preliminary results: Model Sys Sci Digest 3:35–42, 1980.

93. Knop, C.; Fabian, H.F.; Bastian, L.; et al. Late results of thoracolumbar fractures after posterior instrumentation and transpedicular bone grafting. Spine 26:88–99, 2001.

94. Korovessis, P.; Baikousis, A.; Koureas, G.; et al. Correlative analysis of the results of surgical treatment of thoracolumbar injuries with long Texas Scottish rite hospital construct: Is the use of pedicle screws versus hooks advantageous in the lumbar spine? J Spinal Disord Tech 17:195–205, 2004.

95. Kothe, R.; O'Holleran, J.D.; Liu, W.; et al. Internal architecture of the thoracic pedicle: An anatomic study. Spine 21:264–270, 1996.

96. Kothe, R.; Panjabi, M.M.; Liu, W. Multidirectional instability of the thoracic spine due to iatrogenic pedicle injuries during transpedicular fixation: A biomechanical investigation. Spine 22:1836–1842, 1997.

97. Krag, M.H.; Beynnon, B.D.; Pope, M.H.; et al. Depth of insertion of transpedicular vertebral screws into human vertebrae: Effect upon screw-vertebra interface strength. J Spinal Disord 1:287–294, 1988.

98. Krag, M.H.; Weaver, D.L.; Beynnon, B.D.; et al. Morphometry of the thoracic and lumbar spine related to transpedicular screw placement for surgical spinal fixation. Spine 13:27–32, 1988.

99. Kramer, D.L.; Rodgers, W.B.; Mansfield, F.L. Transpedicular instrumentation and short-segment fusion of thoracolumbar fractures: A prospective study using a single instrumentation system. J Orthop Trauma 9:499–506, 1995.

100. Kriek, J.J.; Govender, S. AO-classification of thoracic and lumbar fractures: Reproducibility utilizing radiographs and clinical information. Eur Spine J 15:1239–1246, 2006.

101. Krompinger, W.J.; Fredrickson, B.E.; Mino, D.E.; et al. Conservative treatment of fractures of the thoracic and lumbar spine. Orthop Clin North Am 17:161–170, 1986.

102. Kurz, L.T.; Garfin, S.R.; Booth, R.E., Jr. Harvesting autogenous iliac bone grafts: A review of complications and techniques. Spine 14:1324–1331, 1989.

103. Landreneau, R.J.; Hazelrigg, S.R.; Mack, M.J.; et al. Postoperative pain-related morbidity: Video-assisted thoracic surgery versus thoracotomy. Ann Thorac Surg 56:1285–1289, 1993.

104. Lemons, V.R.; Wagner, F.C., Jr.; Montesano, P.X. Management of thoracolumbar fractures with accompanying neurological injury. Neurosurgery 30:667–671, 1992.

105. Levine, A.M.; Bosse, M.; Edwards, C.C. Bilateral facet dislocations in the thoracolumbar spine. Spine 13:630–640, 1988.

106. Lewis, J.; McKibbin, B. The treatment of unstable fracture–dislocations of the thoraco-lumbar spine accompanied by paraplegia. J Bone Joint Surg [Br] 56:603–612, 1974.

107. Lu, J.; Ebraheim, N.A.; Biyani, A.; et al. Vulnerability of great medullary artery. Spine 21:1852–1855, 1996.

108. Lukas, R.; Suchomel, P.; Sram, J.; et al. Classification-based surgical approach in surgical management of

thoracolumbar fractures of the spine. Rozhl Chir 85:365–372, 2006.

109. Maiman, D.J.; Larson, S.J.; Luck, E.; et al. Lateral extracavitary approach to the spine for thoracic disc herniation: Report of 23 cases. Neurosurgery 14: 178–182, 1984.

110. Mann, K.A.; McGowan, D.P.; Fredrickson, B.E.; et al. A biomechanical investigation of short segment spinal fixation for burst fractures with varying degrees of posterior disruption. Spine 15:470–478, 1990.

111. McAfee, P.C.; Bohlman, H.H.; Yuan, H.A. Anterior decompression of traumatic thoracolumbar fractures with incomplete neurological deficit using a retroperitoneal approach. J Bone Joint Surg [Am] 67:89–104, 1985.

112. McAfee, P.C.; Yuan, H.A.; Fredrickson, B.E.; et al. The value of computed tomography in thoracolumbar fractures: An analysis of one hundred consecutive cases and a new classification. J Bone Joint Surg [Am] 65:461–473, 1983.

113. McAfee, P.C.; Yuan, H.A.; Lasda, N.A. The unstable burst fracture. Spine 7:365–373, 1982.

114. McDonough, P.W.; Davis, R.; Tribus, C.; et al. The management of acute thoracolumbar burst fractures with anterior corpectomy and Z-plate fixation. Spine 29:1901–1908, 2004.

115. McGuire, R.A., Jr. The role of anterior surgery in the treatment of thoracolumbar fractures. Orthopedics 20:959–962, 1997.

116. McGrory, B.J.; VanderWilde, R.S.; Currier, B.L.; et al. Diagnosis of subtle thoracolumbar burst fractures: A new radiographic sign. Spine 18:2282–2285, 1993.

117. McLain, R.F. The biomechanics of long versus short fixation for thoracolumbar spine fractures. Spine 31(11 Suppl):S70–79, 2006.

118. McLain, R.F.; Burkus, J.K.; Benson, D.R. Segmental instrumentation for thoracic and thoracolumbar fractures: Prospective analysis of construct survival and five-year follow-up. Spine J 1:310–323, 2001.

119. Mehbod, A.A.; Ogilvie, J.W.; Pinto, M.R.; et al. Postoperative deep wound infections in adults after spinal fusion: Management with vacuum-assisted wound closure. J Spinal Disord Tech 18:14–17, 2005.

120. Mimatsu, K.; Katoh, F.; Kawakami, N. New vertebral body impactors for posterolateral decompression of burst fracture. Spine 18:1366–1368, 1993.

121. Mumford, J.; Weinstein, J.N.; Spratt, K.F.; et al. Thoracolumbar burst fractures: The clinical efficacy and outcome of nonoperative management. Spine 18:955–970, 1993.

122. Nicoll, E.A. Fractures of the dorso-lumbar spine. J Bone Joint Surg [Br] 31:376–394, 1949.

123. Oda, I.; Abumi, K.; Lu, D.; et al. Biomechanical role of the posterior elements, costovertebral joints, and rib cage in the stability of the thoracic spine. Spine 21:1423–1429, 1996.

124. Okuyama, K.; Abe, E.; Chiba, M.; et al. Outcome of anterior decompression and stabilization for thoracolumbar unstable burst fractures in the absence of neurologic deficits. Spine 21:620–625, 1996.

125. Oner, F.C.; Verlaan, J.J.; Verbout, A.J.; et al. Cement augmentation techniques in traumatic thoracolumbar spine fractures. Spine 31(11 Suppl):S89–95, 2006.

126. Panjabi, M.M.; Brand, R.A., Jr.; White, A.A., III. Three-dimensional flexibility and stiffness properties of the human thoracic spine. J Biomech 9:185–192, 1976.

127. Parke, W.W.; Gammell, K.; Rothman, R.H. Arterial vascularization of the cauda equina. J Bone Joint Surg [Am] 63:53–62, 1981.

128. Parker, J.W.; Lane, J.R.; Karaikovic, E.E.; et al. Successful short-segment instrumentation and fusion for thoracolumbar spine fractures: A consecutive 4 1/2-year series. Spine 25:1157–1170, 2000.

129. Paul, R.L.; Michael, R.H.; Dunn, J.E.; et al. Anterior transthoracic surgical decompression of acute spinal cord injuries. J Neurosurg 43:299-307, 1975.

130. Place, H.M.; Donaldson, D.H.; Brown, C.W.; et al. Stabilization of thoracic spine fractures resulting in complete paraplegia. A long-term retrospective analysis. Spine 19:1726–1730, 1994.

131. Razak, M.; Mahmud, M.M.; Hyzan, M.Y.; et al. Short segment posterior instrumentation, reduction and fusion of unstable thoracolumbar burst fractures—A review of 26 cases. Med J Malaysia 55(Suppl C):9–13, 2000.

132. Regan, J.J.; Mack, M.J.; Picetti, G.D., III. A technical report on video-assisted thoracoscopy in thoracic spinal surgery: Preliminary description. Spine 20:831–837, 1995.

133. Reid, A.B.; Letts, R.M.; Black, G.B. Pediatric Chance fractures: Association with intra-abdominal injuries and seatbelt use. J Trauma 30:384–391, 1990.

134. Rimoldi, R.L.; Zigler, J.E.; Capen, D.A.; et al. The effect of surgical intervention on rehabilitation time in patients with thoracolumbar and lumbar spinal cord injuries. Spine 17:1443–1449, 1992.

135. Roaf, R. A study of the mechanics of spinal injuries. J Bone Joint Surg [Br] 42:810, 1960.

136. Rockwell, H.; Evans, F.G.; Pheasant, J.C. The comparative morphology of the vertebral spinal column: Its form as related to function. J Morphol 63:87, 1938.

137. Rogers, L.F. The roentgenographic appearance of transverse or chance fractures of the spine: The seat belt fracture. Am J Roentgenol Radium Ther Nucl Med 111:844–849, 1971.

138. Rose, R.D.; Welch, W.C.; Balzer, J.R.; et al. Persistently electrified pedicle stimulation instruments in spinal instrumentation: Technique and protocol development. Spine 22:334–343, 1997.

139. Sanderson, P.L.; Fraser, R.D.; Hall, D.J.; et al. Short segment fixation of thoracolumbar burst fractures without fusion. Eur Spine J 8:495–500, 1999.

140. Sasso, R.C.; Renkens, K.; Hanson, D.; et al. Unstable thoracolumbar burst fractures: Anterior-only versus short-segment posterior fixation. J Spinal Disord Tech 19:242–248, 2006.

141. Sasson, A.; Mozes, G. Complete fracture–dislocation of the thoracic spine without neurologic deficit: A case report. Spine 12:67–70, 1987.

142. Schlickewei, W.; Schutzhoff, G.; Kuner, E.H. Early functional treatment of fractures of the lower thoracic and lumbar vertebrae with a 3-point brace. Unfallchirurg 94:40–44, 1991.

143. Scholl, B.M.; Theiss, S.M.; Kirkpatrick, J.S. Short segment fixation of thoracolumbar burst fractures. Orthopedics 29:703–708, 2006.

144. Schreiber, U.; Bence, T.; Grupp, T.; et al. Is a single anterolateral screw-plate fixation sufficient for the treatment of spinal fractures in the thoracolumbar junction? A biomechanical in vitro investigation. Eur Spine J 14:197–204, 2005.

145. Schweitzer, K.M., Jr.; Vaccaro, A.R.; Lee, J.Y.; et al. Confusion regarding mechanisms of injury in the setting of thoracolumbar spinal trauma: A survey of The Spine Trauma Study Group (STSG). J Spinal Disord Tech 19:528–530, 2006.

146. Siebenga, J.; Leferink, V.J.; Segers, M.J.; et al. Treatment of traumatic thoracolumbar spine fractures: A multicenter prospective randomized study of operative versus nonsurgical treatment. Spine 31:2881–2890, 2006.

147. Sim, E. Location of transpedicular screws for fixation of the lower thoracic and lumbar spine: Computed tomography of 45 fracture cases. Acta Orthop Scand 64:28–32, 1993.

148. Singh, K.; Vaccaro, A.R.; Eichenbaum, M.D.; et al. The surgical management of thoracolumbar injuries. J Spinal Cord Med 27:95–101. Review, 2004.

149. Sjöström, L.; Jacobsson, O.; Karlström, G.; et al. Spinal canal remodelling after stabilization of thoracolumbar burst fractures. Eur Spine J 3:312–317, 1994.

150. Smith, W.S.; Kaufer, H. Patterns and mechanisms of lumbar injuries associated with lap seat belts. J Bone Joint Surg [Am] 51:239–254, 1969.

151. Soreff, J.; Axdorph, G.; Bylund, P.; et al. Treatment of patients with unstable fractures of the thoracic and lumbar spine: A follow-up study of surgical and conservative treatment. Acta Orthop Scand 53:369–381, 1982.

152. St John, T.A.; Vaccaro, A.R.; Sah, A.P.; et al. Physical and monetary costs associated with autogenous bone graft harvesting. Am J Orthop 32:18–23, 2003.

153. Stagnara, P.; De Mauroy, J.C.; Dran, G.; et al. Reciprocal angulation of vertebral bodies in a sagittal plane: Approach to references for the evaluation of kyphosis and lordosis. Spine 7:335–342, 1982.

154. Takeuchi, T.; Abumi, K.; Shono, Y.; et al. Biomechanical role of the intervertebral disc and costovertebral joint in stability of the thoracic spine: A canine model study. Spine 24:1444–1420, 1999.

155. Taylor, R.S.; Fritzell, P.; Taylor, R.J. Balloon kyphoplasty in the management of vertebral compression fractures: An updated systematic review and meta-analysis. Eur Spine J 16:1085–1100, 2007.

156. Tezeren, G.; Kuru, I. Posterior fixation of thoracolumbar burst fracture: Short-segment pedicle fixation versus long-segment instrumentation. J Spinal Disord Tech 18:485–488, 2005.

157. Tezer, M.; Ozturk, C.; Aydogan, M.; et al. Surgical outcome of thoracolumbar burst fractures with flexion-distraction injury of the posterior elements. Int Orthop 29:347–350, 2005.

158. Thomas, K.C.; Bailey, C.S.; Dvorak, M.F.; et al. Comparison of operative and nonoperative treatment for thoracolumbar burst fractures in patients without neurological deficit: A systematic review. J Neurosurg Spine 4:351–358, 2006.

159. Toyone, T.; Tanaka, T.; Kato, D.; et al. The treatment of acute thoracolumbar burst fractures with transpedicular intracorporeal hydroxyapatite grafting following indirect reduction and pedicle screw fixation: A prospective study. Spine 31:E208–214, 2006.

160. Vaccaro, A.R.; Baron, E.M.; Sanfilippo, J.; et al. Reliability of a novel classification system for thoracolumbar injuries: The Thoracolumbar Injury Severity Score. Spine 31(11 Suppl):S62–69, 2006.

161. Vaccaro, A.R.; Zeiller, S.C.; Hulbert, R.J.; et al. The thoracolumbar injury severity score: A proposed treatment algorithm. J Spinal Disord Tech 18:209–215, 2005.

162. Van der Roer, N.; de Lange, E.S.; Bakker, F.C.; et al. Management of traumatic thoracolumbar fractures: A systematic review of the literature. Eur Spine J 14:527–534, 2005.

163. Verlaan, J.J.; Dhert, W.J.; Verbout, A.J.; et al. Balloon vertebroplasty in combination with pedicle screw instrumentation: A novel technique to treat thoracic and lumbar burst fractures. Spine 30:E73–79, 2005.

164. Verlaan, J.J.; Diekerhof, C.H.; Buskens, E.; et al. Surgical treatment of traumatic fractures of the thoracic and lumbar spine: A systematic review of the literature on techniques, complications, and outcome. Spine 29:803–814, 2004.

165. Vicario, C.; de Juan, J.; Esclarin, A.; et al. Treatment of deep wound infections after spinal fusion with a vacuum-assisted device in patients with spinal cord injury. Acta Orthop Belg 73:102–106, 2007.

166. Wang, S.T.; Ma, H.L.; Liu, C.L.; et al. Is fusion necessary for surgically treated burst fractures of the thoracolumbar and lumbar spine? A prospective, randomized study. Spine 31:2646–2652, 2006.

167. Watkins, R., IV.; Watkins, R., III.; Williams, L.; et al. Stability provided by the sternum and rib cage in the thoracic spine. Spine 30:1283–1286, 2005.

168. Watson-Jones, R. Fractures and Joint Injuries, 4th ed. Baltimore, Williams and Wilkins, 1960.

169. Weinstein, J.N.; Spratt, K.F.; Spengler, D.; et al. Spinal pedicle fixation: Reliability and validity of roentgenogram-based assessment and surgical factors on successful screw placement. Spine 13:1012–1018, 1988.

170. Whang, P.G.; Vaccaro, A.R.; Poelstra, K.A.; et al. The influence of fracture mechanism and morphology on the reliability and validity of two novel thoracolumbar injury classification systems. Spine 32: 791–795, 2007.

171. White, A.A.; Panjabi, M.M. Clinical Biomechanics of the Spine. Philadelphia, J.B. Lippincott, 1978.

172. White, A.A.; Panjabi, M.M. The basic kinematics of the human spine: A review of past and current knowledge. Spine 3:12–20, 1978.

173. White, A.A.; Panjabi, M.M. Clinical instability of the spine. In: Rothman, R.H.; Simeone, F.A., eds. The Spine vol. 4. Philadelphia, W.B. Saunders 1982, pp. 219–244.

174. Whitesides, T.E. Traumatic kyphosis of the thoracolumbar spine. Clin Orthop Relat Res 128:78–92, 1977.

175. Wilke, H.J.; Kemmerich, V.; Claes, L.E.; et al. Combined anteroposterior spinal fixation provides superior stabilisation to a single anterior or posterior procedure. J Bone Joint Surg [Br] 83:609–617, 2001.

176. Willen, J.; Anderson, J.; Toomoka, K.; et al. The natural history of burst fractures at the thoracolumbar junction. J Spinal Disord 3:39–46, 1990.

177. Willen, J.A.; Gaekwad, U.H.; Kakulas, B.A. Acute burst fractures: A comparative analysis of a modern fracture classification and pathologic findings. Clin Orthop Relat Res 276:169–175, 1992.

178. Wood, K.; Buttermann, G.; Mehbod, A.; et al. Operative compared with nonoperative treatment of a thoracolumbar burst fracture without neurological deficit: A prospective, randomized study. J Bone Joint Surg [Am] 85:773–781, 2003.

179. Wood, K.B.; Khanna, G.; Vaccaro, A.R.; et al. Assessment of two thoracolumbar fracture classification systems as used by multiple surgeons. J Bone Joint Surg [Am] 87:1423–1429, 2005.

180. Yuan, H.A.; Mann, K.A.; Found, E.M.; et al. Early clinical experience with the Syracuse I-Plate: An anterior spinal fixation device. Spine 13:278–285, 1988.

181. Yue, J.J.; Sossan, A.; Selgrath, C.; et al. The treatment of unstable thoracic spine fractures with transpedicular screw instrumentation: A 3-year consecutive series. Spine 27:2782–2787, 2002.

182. Zindrick, M.R.; Wiltse, L.L.; Doornik, A.; et al. Analysis of the morphometric characteristics of the thoracic and lumbar pedicles. Spine 12:160–166, 1987.

183. Zou, D.; Yoo, J.U.; Edwards, W.T.; et al. Mechanics of anatomic reduction of thoracolumbar burst fractures: Comparison of distraction versus distraction plus lordosis, in the anatomic reduction of the thoracolumbar burst fracture. Spine 18:195–203, 1993.

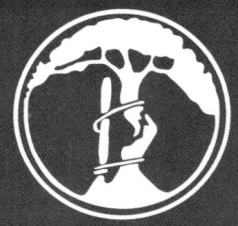

CHAPTER 31

Low Lumbar Fractures

Alan M. Levine, M.D.

Treatment of injuries to the low lumbar spine requires consideration of a number of additional factors beyond those relevant to injuries of the thoracic and thoracolumbar spine. These factors are related to the anatomic complexity of the lower lumbar spine, as well as the lordotic sagittal alignment and increased normal mobility of the lumbosacral junction. Prior to the advent of pedicle screw fixation, no satisfactory instrumentation or techniques were available for reduction and stabilization of injuries in the low lumbar spine. Fixation to the sacrum was problematic and stabilization with Harrington rods required decrease in lordosis and sufficient length of instrumentation to maintain tension, and Luque instrumentation did not maintain enough distraction to achieve any degree of reduction. Use of these techniques resulted in less than optimal results and led most authors to espouse nonoperative techniques as a better alternative.[21,42] Occasional reports, however, suggested that an operative approach yielded better anatomic results and perhaps even better functional outcomes.[71,104] Even with the more widely accepted use of pedicle screw fixation for the lumbar spine in the late 1980s and early 1990s combined with more effective methods of sacral fixation, some early, poorly conceptualized operative approaches to fractures in this region also led to early failure.[2,3,50,101] Although anterior approaches to these fractures have been advocated, rigid fixation to the sacrum from an anterior approach has been problematic and requires a combined approach if anterior decompression is used.[94] This problem caused some surgeons and their patients to accept chronic pain and the failure to return to preinjury occupation as the norm in this very young group. Additionally, the relatively high complication rate associated with operative treatment of low lumbar fractures[103] has caused some to advocate nonoperative over operative treatment for these patients. Since the neural canal is relatively large in the low lumbar area and the most common neurologic deficit is the result of root impingement, the need for operative stabilization to achieve an optimal functional result has been reexamined. A number of recent studies have suggested that nonoperative treatment yields satisfactory results in this group of patients, all of whom are relatively young at the time of injury (average age in most series, 27 years). Additionally the trend in the treatment of thoracolumbar spinal trauma in general has been toward nonoperative treatment in patients without neurologic deficit, as operative treatment

has demonstrated no conclusive advantage.[114,122,123] However, many problems still exist with regard to interpreting data on these fractures inasmuch as most series report short to intermediate follow-up (<4 years) in a group of predominantly young male patients (27 years old) more often than not employed in manual labor tasks.[17,40,86] Additionally, these conclusions are based on analysis of retrospective series with many discrepancies and inconsistencies, such as marked variation in the elements of "nonoperative care." In some series, recumbency for up to 6 weeks is included as part of treatment,[2,3,5,17,99,103,104] whereas in others, it is not used. The type and duration of immobilization have also varied. Finally, the severity of injury has likewise not been uniform in comparisons of types of treatment[2,3,103] in that patients with less structural instability and those without neurologic deficit are most commonly treated nonoperatively, whereas those with gross instability and neural deficit are treated with surgical decompression and stabilization. All these factors, in addition to studies suggesting comparable complication rates[99] for the two types of treatment, make selection of optimal therapy for an individual patient difficult.

In the lumbar spine, anatomic and motion considerations have made instrumentation more difficult than in other regions of the spine. Injuries to the lumbar spine and upper part of the sacrum disrupt the normal lordotic alignment of the spine, and restoration of that lordotic alignment is critical to overall vertebral mechanics and spinal alignment in the sagittal plane. Failure to maintain or restore normal sagittal alignment in the lower lumbar spine after either elective fusion or fracture has led to the occurrence of late symptoms and even degenerative changes in long-term follow-up. The lumbosacral junction in particular must resist a number of large forces, but it must also permit a significant amount of motion. It has therefore been difficult to achieve anatomic reduction and reconstruction of the lumbar spine and sacrum until the most recent advances in instrumentation. This difficulty has led many authors to suggest either limited procedures and goals or "benign neglect" as the method of treatment of low lumbar and sacral injuries. Fixation to the bone of the sacrum has been even more problematic. These numerous features and problems distinguish fractures of the lower lumbar spine from the more numerous and common fractures at the thoracolumbar junction.

More accurate diagnostic imaging studies, as well as advances in instrumentation techniques, should now allow us to treat injuries of the lumbar spine with the same degree of accuracy and competence as more proximal spinal injuries. To do so, however, we must have a clear understanding of the anatomic and functional differences that distinguish the lumbar spine from the remainder of the more proximal areas of the spine. As described in Chapter 30, a specific set of technical considerations and fixation methods is applicable to the treatment of spinal trauma in the thoracic region (T2–T10), and similarly, a set is applicable to the thoracolumbar junction (T10–L1). Fractures of the second lumbar vertebra form a transitional group, both functionally and technically, between those of the thoracolumbar junction (T10–L1) and those of the lumbar region (L3–S1). The major differences in anatomic considerations and techniques apply predominantly to L3–S1, whereas L2 should be considered the transitional level because treatment at this level involves borrowing techniques from above and below.

The treatment goals for spine trauma in general are (1) anatomic reduction of the injury, (2) rigid fixation of the fracture, and, when necessary, (3) decompression of the neural elements. For treatment of low lumbar fractures, we must add the considerations of (4) maintenance of sagittal alignment, (5) conservation of motion segments, and (6) prevention of frequent complications (e.g., recurrence of kyphosis, loss of sacral fixation, pseudarthrosis). As the characteristics of the lumbar spine are reviewed, it will become evident that techniques discussed previously for the treatment of cervical, thoracic, and thoracolumbar spine injuries are not applicable to the treatment of lumbar spine injuries.

ANATOMIC FEATURES

The first critical anatomic consideration is the sagittal alignment of the lumbar spine. Normal kyphosis of the thoracic spine falls within a range of 15 to 49°,[121] whereas normal lumbar lordosis is generally thought to be less than 60°. This curvature is in part determined by the slope of the sacral base, which averages approximately 45° from the horizontal. This angle is critical in determining the amount of shear force[109] to which the lumbosacral junction is subjected (Fig. 31-1). Anatomic differences in the structure of the lumbar vertebrae and sacrum influence therapeutic decisions and affect the attachment of fixation devices differently from those made at proximal levels in the thoracic and lumbar spine.

With caudal descent in the lumbar spine, the overall dimensions of the canal enlarge and the area occupied by the neural elements decreases. The cord in the thoracic region measures approximately 86.5 mm^2 and is housed within a canal that averages about 17.2 × 16.8 mm^2. Thus, in the thoracic region, the cord occupies about 50 percent of the canal area. In the thoracolumbar region, the conus broadens, as does the canal. The spinal cord usually terminates at approximately L1. In the lumbar region, the canal is typically large (23.4 × 17.4 mm^2).[36,98] Here, the roots of the cauda equina are the only contents. In the sacrum, however, the diameter of the canal again begins to narrow and flatten. In addition, with the normal, slightly kyphotic angle at the midpoint of the sacrum

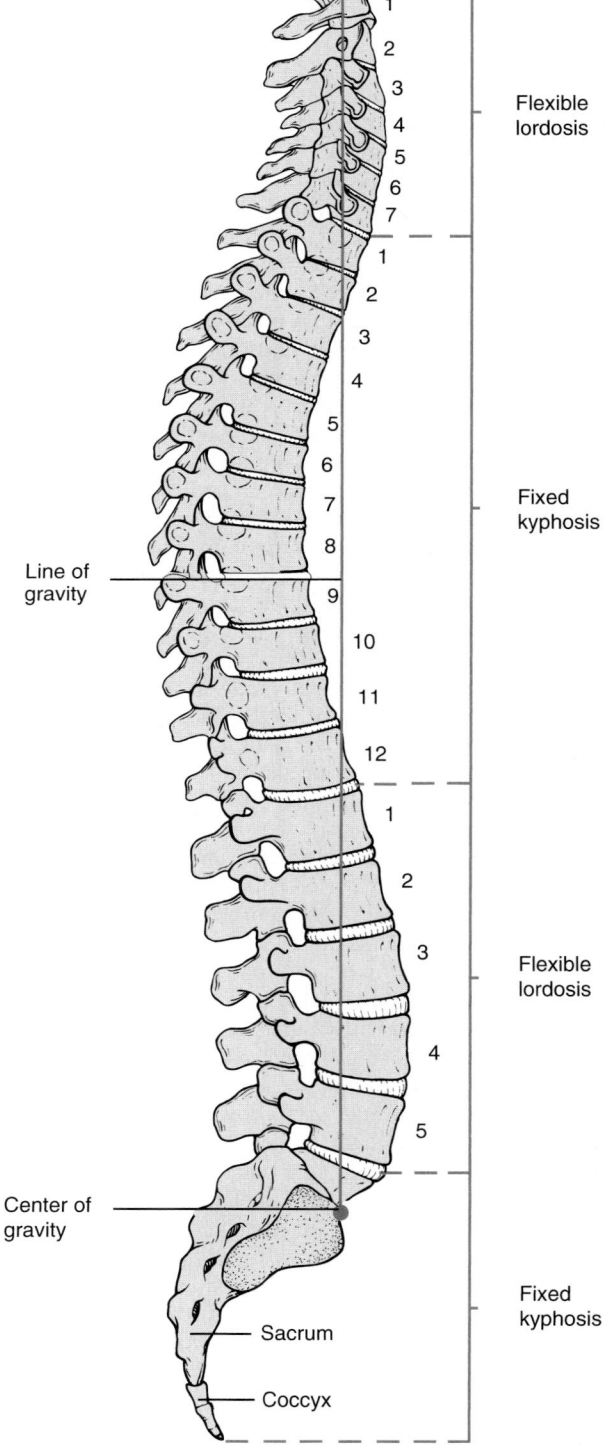

FIGURE 31-1   *The spine is divided into four segments: two with relatively fixed kyphosis (the sacral and thoracic spine) and two with relatively flexible lordosis (the cervical and lumbar spine). The weight-bearing axis is anterior to the thoracic spine and thoracolumbar junction. Because it falls posterior to the vertebral bodies of the lumbar spine, the pattern of fracture with axial loading injuries is significantly different in the lumbar spine from that in the thoracic and thoracolumbar spine.*

Flexible lordosis

Fixed kyphosis

Line of gravity

Flexible lordosis

Center of gravity

Fixed kyphosis

Sacrum

Coccyx

(S2-S3), the roots are tethered in a relatively fixed location. This anatomic arrangement allows less flexibility in placing fixation devices within the canal in the sacrum. In addition, the size and shape of the laminae change configuration at the various levels of the spine. The laminae in the thoracic and thoracolumbar region are rectangular, somewhat longer than wide. In the midlumbar spine, the width and length of the laminae equalize. At L5, the laminae are considerably wider than long (Fig. 31-2). The sacral laminae are extremely thin and might be absent in some areas. Similarly, it has been shown that in the lumbar spine, the minimal and maximal pedicle diameters increase to reach a mean minimal diameter of approximately 10 mm at L5 and 8.5 mm at L3.[102]

With the increasing emphasis on innovative methods of fixation for injuries in the low lumbar spine,[7,75,94] understanding the pertinent anatomic dimensions takes on new significance. Previously, with hook fixation or sublaminar wiring to the posterior elements, the only important consideration was posterior topographic anatomy. However, the dimensions, position, and orientation of the pedicles, as well as the shape of the vertebral body, are likewise critical. The initial anatomic description of pedicle morphology referable to pedicle screw fixation was made by Saillant[101] in 1976 and confirmed by two later studies from North America.[61,125] The critical features are sagittal and transverse width of the pedicles, pedicle length, pedicle angle, and chord length (depth to the anterior cortex along a fixed orientation). These dimensions vary widely within regions of the spine (thoracic versus lumbar), but they also vary within the lumbar spine, with progression from L1 to L5. The mean transverse diameter measured on either computed tomography (CT) or an anatomic specimen was approximately 9 mm at L1 and increased to as much as 18 mm at L5 (Fig. 31-3). The sagittal width in the lumbar spine is relatively constant, with a mean of between 14 and 15 mm at all levels (see Fig. 31-3B). The angle of the pedicle axis generally increases in the lumbar spine, with a mean of about 11° at L1, 15° at L3, and over 20° at L5 (see Fig. 31-3A). Finally, the angle of insertion of the screw is critically important inasmuch as the shape of the lumbar vertebrae changes dramatically from L1 to L5 (see Fig. 31-3C and D). Because the distance between the pedicles is greater at L5 and the anteroposterior (AP) diameter of the vertebral body is effectively less at that location, the chord length or distance from the posterior cortex to the anterior cortex can vary dramatically with the angle of insertion. If screws are inserted perpendicular to the posterior cortex along a 0° axis, as originally described by Roy-Camille, the mean depth at L1 is about 45 mm, whereas at L5 it is only 35 mm. Increasing the angle of insertion to 10 or 15° or to the angle of the axis of the pedicle can increase the cortex-to-cortex distance by as much as 5 mm at L1 (to 50 mm) and 15 mm at L5 (to about 50 mm).

For fractures of L5 or even very unstable shear injuries involving L4, fixation to the sacrum is a necessary component. Understanding the three-dimensional anatomy of the various sacral levels, as well as the position of the neurovascular structures applied to the anterior surface of the sacrum, is critical for the conceptualization of adequate and safe fixation to the sacrum. The anatomic structures

---

FIGURE 31-2 *A–D, The shape of the lumbar laminae and the relative size of the pedicles dramatically influence the ability to position hardware. From L2 to L5, the length of the laminae becomes less and the width becomes greater. Therefore, hook placement is easier proximally in the spine but may cause impingement when placed over the lamina of L5 because of its relatively short length. However, pedicle fixation is easier distally with the larger pedicle size.*

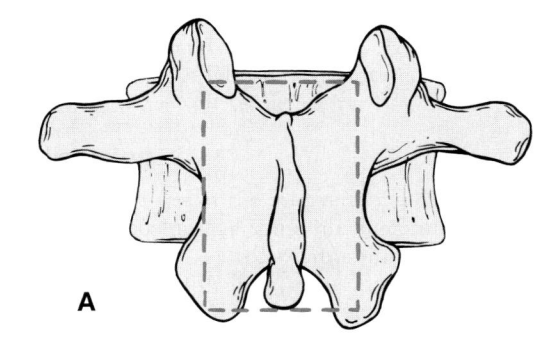

A   L2

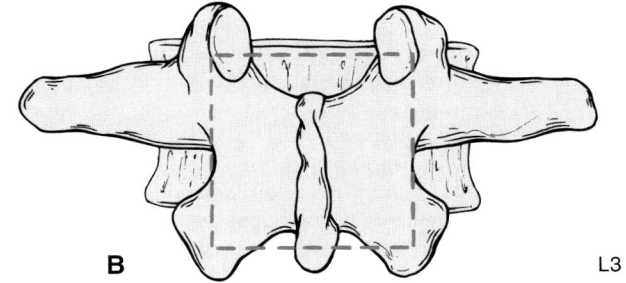

B   L3

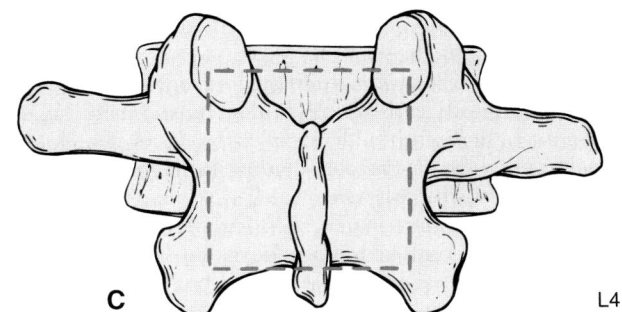

C   L4

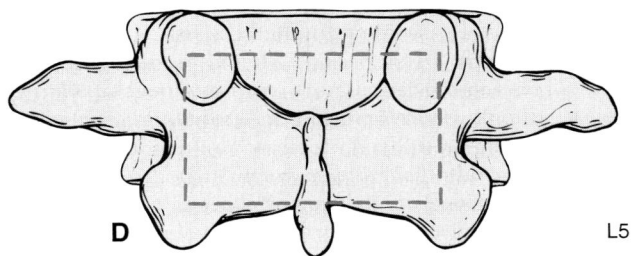

D   L5

FIGURE 31-3 **A,** *This axial view of a lumbar vertebral body shows the transverse pedicle width, which increases from L1 to L5. It also demonstrates the pedicle axis, which likewise increases from L1 to L5.* **B,** *A sagittal view of the vertebral body shows the sagittal pedicle width, which is relatively constant in the lumbar spine.* **C,** *This diagram shows an L1 axial view with the axis of the pedicle demonstrating the larger cortex-to-cortex distance.* **D,** *An axial view of L5 demonstrates how the anteroposterior length can increase with increasing angle.*

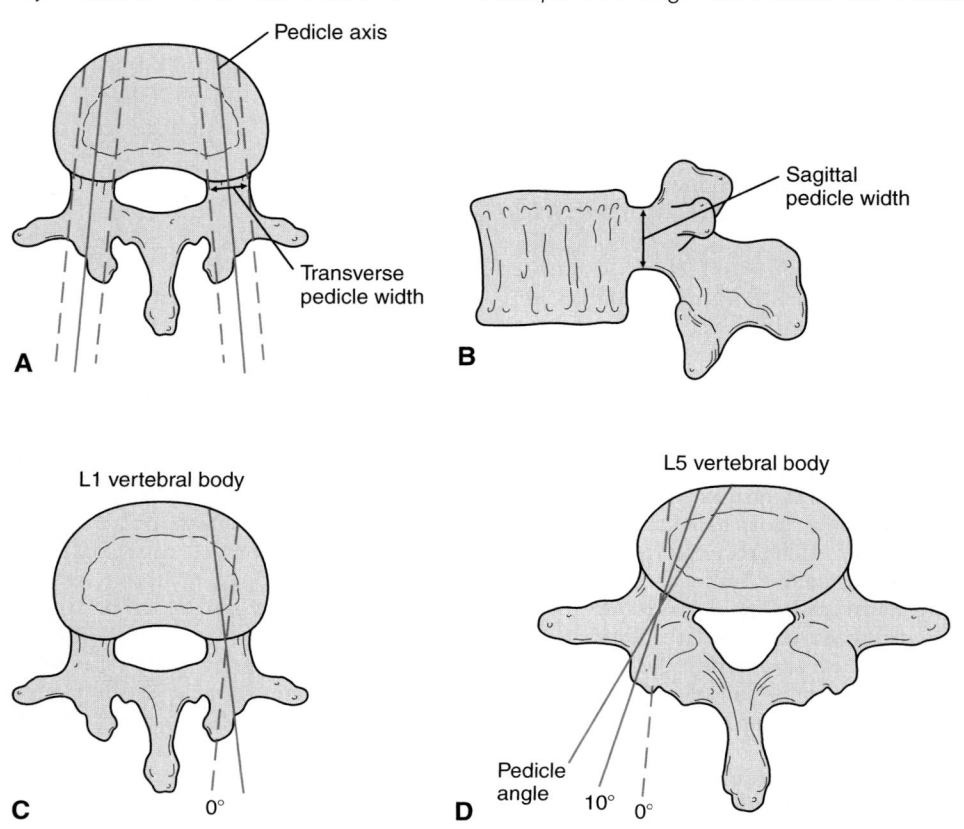

that may be encountered at the level of the S1 body are the internal iliac vein, the lumbosacral plexus, and the sacroiliac joint. A safe zone bordered by the sacral promontory medially and the iliac vein laterally can, however, be used for fixation; it is about 2 cm wide and is invariably entered by orientation of a screw along the S1 pedicle.[87] Screws placed laterally at either 30 or 45° are aimed at a smaller lateral safe zone. The more lateral orientation provides for a longer screw length of 44 mm.[87] At the S2 level, the only vulnerable structure is the sigmoid colon on the left side. Penetration through the cortex by more than 1 cm is usually necessary for injury. At the S2 level, the thickness of the sacral bone is significantly decreased from that of the S1 level, and thus, the holding power of the bone in an axis parallel to the placement of S1 would be significantly less. To compensate for these deficiencies, orientation of fixation devices both proximally and laterally significantly increases the length of screw purchase and thus pull-out strength. Variations in the amount of cancellous and cortical bone mass in different regions of the sacrum significantly affect fixation possibilities and the risk of fixation. Sacrum fixation is more secure in the sacral ala because of its increased bone mass or in the sacral vertebral bodies, as opposed to fixation in the very thin posterior laminar structures. Entry points for lateral and medial screw orientation at S1 are sufficiently separate to make

it technically feasible to obtain both medial and lateral fixation into S1, thus increasing stability and resistance to pull-out. As with sacral fractures (see Chapter 35), the alternative now exists to bypass the sometimes tenuous fixation into the sacral and achieve more stable fixation into the posterior ilium. Although this alternative is clearly attractive for certain types of severely comminuted sacral fractures in which the sacroiliac joints may be involved, it is less optimal for distal fixation for L5 burst fractures or fracture dislocations. In those patients the sacroiliac joints are generally uninjured and since the fixation will bypass the sacroiliac joints, subsequent motion causes either loosening of the screws or screw or rod fracture. No studies have been done to date evaluating the use of temporary fixation across the SI joints as distal fixation with later hardware removal.

The next significant anatomic feature is the extreme flexion-extension mobility of the lumbar spine in comparison with other areas. The thoracic spine is relatively stiff as a result of the orientation of the facet joints. Flexion-extension in the thoracic spine is limited, and in fact, rotation exceeds flexion-extension at each level. At the thoracolumbar junction, flexion-extension increases, whereas lateral bending and rotation decrease. The orientation of the facet joints in the lumbar spine becomes sagittal, and the facet joints become quite large.[117] Therefore, the degree of freedom of motion progressively increases in flexion-extension from L1 to L5 and decreases in rotation. Flexion-extension increases from approximately 12° at the L1-L2 level to 20° at the L5-S1 level, with lateral bending remaining similar at about 6°.[118] This extreme flexion-extension mobility needs to be taken into account when considering injuries to the lumbar spine and sacrum because the relative position and orientation of one vertebra to another can change according to the position of the victim at impact. The extreme lumbar lordosis and lumbosacral angle can be flattened dramatically by sitting and the spine oriented in a vertical rather than lordotic position. This change in angle and orientation contributes to differences in the relative incidence of specific types of injuries in the lumbar spine in comparison with those in more proximal regions.

LUMBAR SPINE INJURY PATTERNS

Most operatively treated fractures of the thoracic, thoracolumbar, and lumbar spine occur at the thoracolumbar junction. As a result of the anatomic differences previously discussed, the relative incidence of patterns of injuries is different in the lumbar spine than in the thoracic or thoracolumbar spine. The thoracic spine is additionally stabilized by the rib cage, whereas the thoracolumbar junction is a transitional zone at the end of a relatively stiffer segment. The lumbar spine is protected by only the abdominal and paraspinous musculature and is more subject to forces such as distraction and shear. In addition, factors extrinsic to the spine, such as the type of accident (motor vehicle accident vs. fall) and the use of restraints (e.g., lap belts vs. shoulder harnesses), also influence the number and types of injuries. For instance, the use of a lap belt alone by a passenger in a motor vehicle accident predisposes to flexion-distraction injuries of the lumbar spine.[4,90] Because the lower lumbar spine and lumbosacral junction are normally quite lordotic, severe flexion injuries are less common than in the thoracic or thoracolumbar spine. The extreme flexion-extension range of motion frequently tends to negate the flexion moment of an injury. Therefore, more low lumbar injuries are axial loading injuries as the spine is brought to a straight neutral position at the moment of impact and is then axially loaded. Some flexion-distraction injuries occur as the pelvis or low lumbar spine becomes fixed in a given position and the remainder of the body is flexed and distracted over it. A recent study of 54 patients[23] with low lumbar fractures had a relatively common distribution with 25 compression fractures, 21 burst fractures, 3 flexion-distraction injuries, and 5 fracture dislocations. Of those 3 had complete neurologic deficit, 17 had partial or root deficits, and 34 were neurologically intact.

A variety of different injury patterns can occur in the lumbar spine. The purpose of dividing them into subgroups and classifying the injuries is to be able to predict their natural history and behavior. Easy recognition of these subgroups is important for determining optimal treatment. In addition, such classification should help the treating physician understand the nature of the instability[11,30] and thus construct a treatment regimen based on

counteracting that instability. Although many classification systems exist, none has been totally successful in achieving those goals. Therefore, as in the other sections describing spinal injuries, these injuries are grouped and described by both radiologic criteria and their major deforming forces. The major forces contributing to the injuries are flexion, extension, compression, lateral bending, rotation, distraction, and shear. Most injuries are caused not by a single force but by a major force with minor components from other, different types of forces.

Soft Tissue Injuries, Avulsion Fractures, and Ligamentous Injuries

Although this group of injuries may conceptually appear to be quite simple to understand and treat, it may be the most challenging because the injuries encompass a large and highly variable group. Until the early 1990s, these injuries were very poorly imaged because we relied on plain radiographic and CT findings that were merely indirect evidence of the soft tissue and ligamentous injury. In some cases, these findings poorly reflect the force imparted to the spine or the subsequent severity of the injury. The use of magnetic resonance imaging (MRI) has allowed the physician to directly visualize the location of the injury; however, direct correlation between the visualized soft tissue or ligamentous injury and its effect on spinal stability has still not been clarified. The significant force needed to overcome the muscular and ligamentous restraints of the lumbar spine should be considered when evaluating these problems. For example, fractures of the transverse processes of the lumbar spine may represent several different injuries, depending on the mechanism. The significance of an L5 transverse process fracture associated with a vertical shearing injury to the pelvis is different from that of multiple transverse process fractures. A more severe injury would normally be expected from a direct blow, such as when a pedestrian is struck by a motor vehicle, and a less severe injury from indirect muscular tension. The significant force produced by the paraspinous musculature at the time of impact can result in an avulsion fracture of the transverse process (Fig. 31-4). More severe injuries can be accompanied by nerve root avulsion at the same level. Before any treatment and especially in combination with other significant bony injuries, avulsion fractures should be thoroughly investigated to ascertain that the nerve root exiting at the level of the transverse process is intact. Preoperative MRI or intraoperative exploration at the time of surgery for an associated injury can be used confirm the diagnosis (see Fig. 31-4).

End plate avulsion[85] is a recognized phenomenon in adolescent patients. Disk herniation can occur in an adult who sustains significant trauma, whereas in a child, the ligamentous attachments are somewhat stronger than the bony attachment of the end plate (Fig. 31-5). Therefore, end plate avulsion with displacement and neurologic findings might be present. This pattern of injury can be visualized by a combination of CT and MRI and should be treated by excision of the end plate fragment, which usually resolves the neurologic symptoms completely. End plate avulsion is most frequently seen in adolescents and young adults at the L4-L5 and L5-S1 levels.[37] In a

FIGURE 31-4 *Anteroposterior radiograph of the lumbar spine of a 24-year-old man involved in a motorcycle accident. The patient had a burst fracture of L1 and multiple avulsion fractures of the transverse processes at L1, L2, L3, and L4 (arrows).*

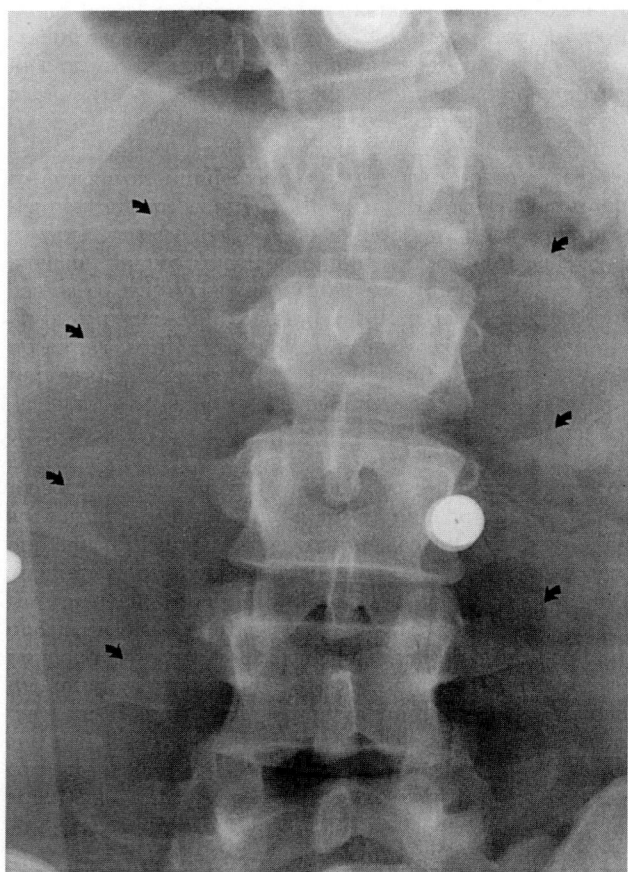

FIGURE 31-5 *Lateral radiograph of the lumbar spine of a 16-year-old girl demonstrating an end plate avulsion. She was involved in a motor vehicle accident and sustained complete paraplegia from the flexion-distraction injury several levels above the area of bone injury. Note the avulsion of the end plate of the vertebral body (arrows) with translation of the end plate anteriorly, in addition to the flexion and distraction of the posterior portion of the end plate.*

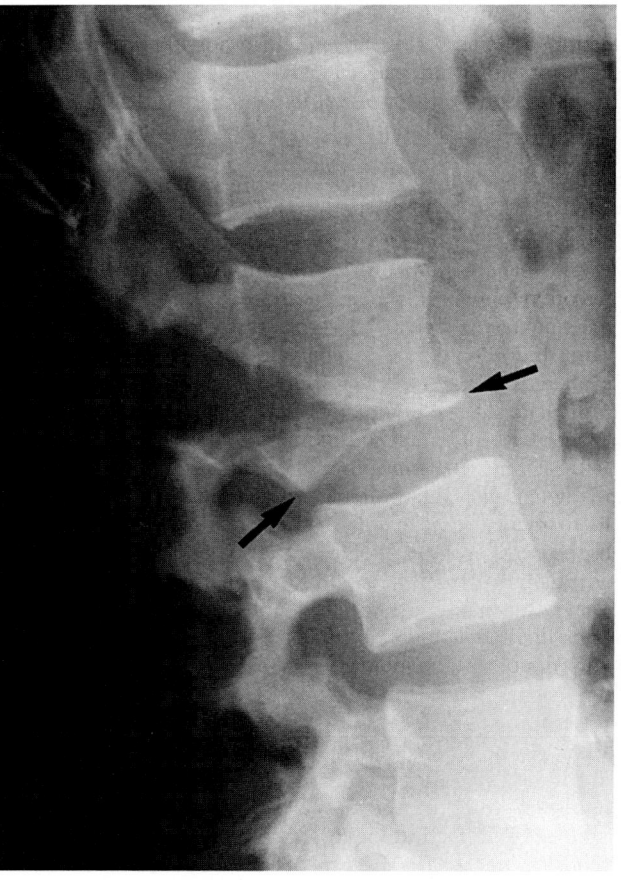

younger child, it might occur only with avulsion of the cartilaginous ring apophysis. In adolescents and young adults, an isolated portion of the limbus or the entire bony end plate can fracture off.[37] Neural impingement is the result of both the bony fragment and disk herniation.[37,49,113]

Disruption of the posterior ligamentous complex (i.e., supraspinous ligament, intraspinous ligament, facet capsules, ligamentum flavum, and annulus of the disk) constitutes a continuum of injuries usually occurring in concert with other bony flexion injuries.[45,46] If a significant ligamentous injury occurs alone or in combination with a very innocent-appearing bony injury, such as insignificant anterior compression of the vertebral body (Fig. 31-6), it may be easily overlooked initially. If the patient has considerable spasm from the soft tissue injury, the full significance of the ligamentous instability might be masked. CT does not help demonstrate the extent of the ligamentous injury. MRI can define the degree of ligamentous destruction, but not its effect on instability. Clinical correlation of these findings is yet to be proved. Most of these patients do not have any neurologic deficit.[108] If a lap belt has been used without a shoulder harness, the patient might have significant abdominal injuries. A high level of suspicion

for lumbar ligament disruption should be present in any patient with L3, L4, or L5 anterior compression who has sustained a high-impact injury. To achieve compression of the anterior portions of the low lumbar vertebrae, the entire lumbar lordosis needs to be overcome and the patient placed in significant flexion, which should lengthen the posterior ligamentous structures beyond their elastic limit. Supervised flexion-extension radiographs after resolution of the initial spasm can make the diagnosis evident. Indications for surgical intervention and techniques are discussed in Chapter 30.

Wedge Compression Fractures

Wedge compression fractures (less than 50% anterior compression) result from a predominantly flexion injury. They can vary from mild anterior compression with little or no instability to gross instability with significant posterior ligamentous disruption. In all cases, the middle column is

FIGURE 31-6 *A 44-year-old woman was involved in a motor vehicle accident and sustained bilateral tibial fractures in addition to a fracture of L4. **A,** Lateral admission radiograph demonstrating alignment of her low lumbar spine at the time of acute evaluation. She underwent anterior compression (arrow) with satisfactory alignment in the sagittal plane. **B,** The anteroposterior radiograph does not show any apparent disruption of the posterior elements. She was therefore placed in an orthosis. **C,** Five months after the injury, the patient had significant back pain after being out of the orthosis for 2 months. A lateral radiograph shows not only the anterior compression (arrow) but also disruption of the ligamentous restraints posteriorly with subluxation of the facets and apparent disruption of the interspinous ligament.*

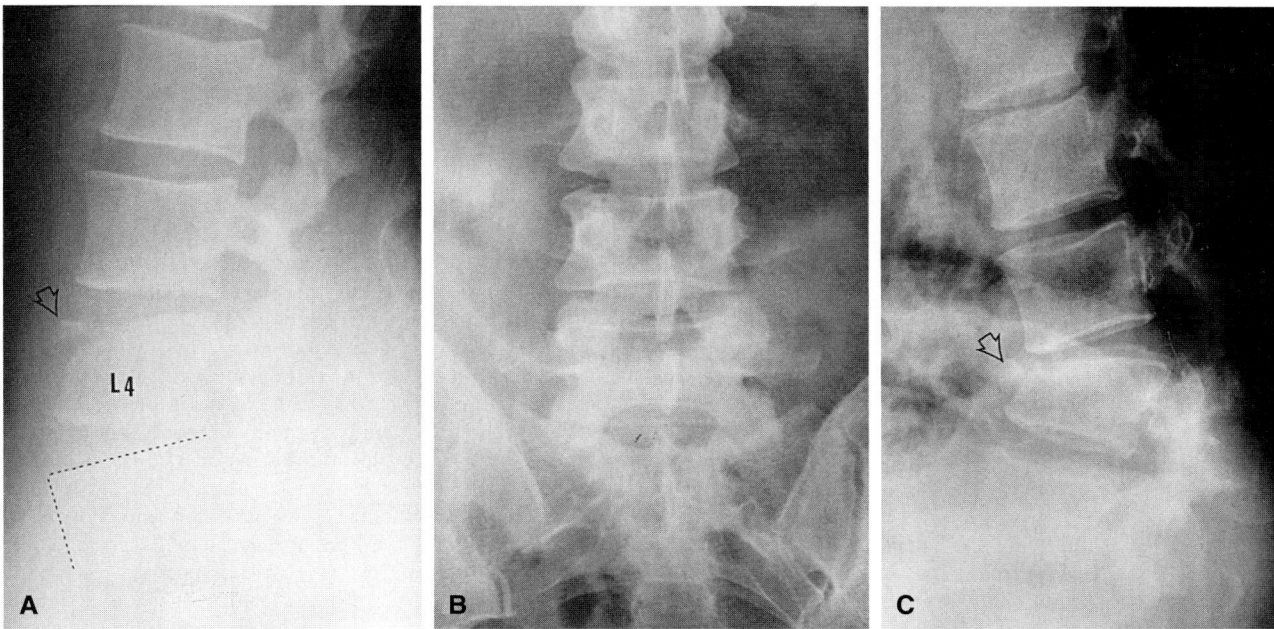

spared. By definition, the bony architecture of the posterior wall of the vertebral body must remain intact, and that is the critical defining difference between a compression fracture and a burst fracture. The degree of compression differs and results in the various fracture patterns. The flexion load applied to the spine causes it to rotate about its axis of rotation and produces a fracture of the superior subchondral plate of the vertebral body (Fig. 31-7). Such fractures can occur at multiple adjacent levels in the lumbar spine. Care must be taken to differentiate this injury from one with a distractive force; in the latter case, severe ligamentous disruption can occur and the patient has significant kyphosis and ligamentous instability.

Compression fractures of the lumbar spine are a frequent consequence of severe osteopenia in older men and women. Although fractures of the lumbar spine occur less frequently than fractures of the thoracic region, once a single fracture has occurred, the risk of another fracture in either location is increased.[91] Approximately 10 percent of white women older than 50 years have at least one fracture;[84] the proportion increases to almost 50 percent of women older than 80 years who have at least one fracture.[81] These fractures may be associated with trivial trauma or may have no apparent trauma associated with them. They differ from compression fractures observed with trauma in younger individuals in that they may have a progressive course. When initially diagnosed at the time of onset of pain, these fractures may exhibit as little as 10 percent anterior compression with preservation of the posterior wall. However,

over a period of 2 to 3 months, they can progress to almost 100 percent anterior compression with involvement of the posterior wall, canal compromise, and neurologic deficit. Intervention by vertebroplasty may be appropriate in patients with increasing compression and persistent pain.

Burst Fractures

The fractures of most patients who ultimately require operative treatment of injuries to the low lumbar spine fall into this category. The injury patterns can differ markedly, depending on the level of the injury, as well as the predominant forces responsible for causing the injury. All burst fractures are produced by a combination of forces that always include flexion and axial loading, with the pattern of the injury related to the relative proportions of the forces applied. These variations in pattern have been well described by Denis[29] (see Chapter 30). In the upper portion of the lumbar spine (L2 and L3), either a predominant axial loading injury (Denis type A) or a predominant flexion injury with some axial compression (Denis B) is possible. The former generally has little kyphosis but significant axial compression of the body with comminution of both the superior and inferior end plates. The body-pedicle junction is disrupted, and posterior element fractures also frequently occur. The latter consist of a fracture of the superior end plate and a portion of the body, with retropulsion of bone into the canal. The critical features on CT are that the lower portion of the pedicle remains intact and that it remains in continuity with the body.

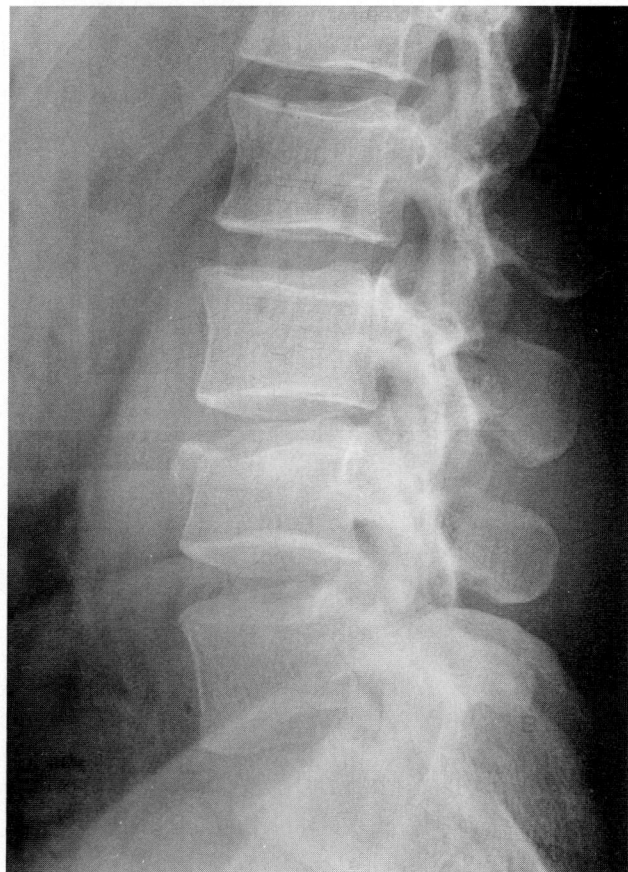

FIGURE 31-7 *Lateral radiograph of the lumbar spine demonstrating an L4 compression fracture sustained during a motor vehicle accident. Note the compression of the anterior portion of the vertebral body. However, the posterior wall of the L4 body importantly remains intact with its normal biconcave appearance. The interspinous distance is not widened, and overall alignment of the lumbar spine remains within physiologic norms.*

The retropulsed fragment is the posterosuperior portion of the vertebral body. These injuries usually involve significant anterior compression of the vertebral body, a variable amount of posterior ligament disruption, and sparing of the posterior elements (Fig. 31-8). A variant of this fracture type is the most common pattern that occurs in the low lumbar spine at the L4 and L5 levels. Fractures at L4 and L5 demonstrate little kyphosis but can nevertheless cause significant canal impingement.

Reports by Levine and Edwards[60,71,82,84] indicate that most of these injuries occur in younger patients, with slightly more than 50 percent younger than 20 years.[66,69,71] The fractures were equally divided between the L4 and the L5 levels and equally divided between patients with and without neurologic deficit. The mean canal compromise was only 47 percent, but in 5 of 22 patients, the retropulsed bone was so severe that it was in contact with the undersurface of the lamina. In 18 of 22 patients, the

vertebral comminution involved approximately the upper half of the vertebral body, and the inferior halves of the pedicles were not comminuted and remained connected to the lower portion of the body (Fig. 31-9). The inferior section of the vertebral body was split into two halves in the sagittal plane, as described by Lindahl and co-workers.[74] The mean loss of vertebral height was approximately 25 percent and was not as dramatic as in injuries to the thoracic and thoracolumbar spine. In addition, the measured kyphosis across the fracture level was only 8°. This figure is less than the average traumatic kyphosis of approximately 21° at the thoracolumbar junction, but it must be placed in context with the normal lordotic posture of the low lumbar spine. If a normal value of approximately 15° of lordosis is accepted for each level (L4-L5 and L5-S1), the total relative kyphosis is approximately 23° (although the absolute kyphosis is only 8°). These figures are compatible with the amount of deformity seen in comparable injuries at other levels.

A smaller number of patients with L4 and L5 fractures have a classic burst fracture pattern (Denis A) (Fig. 31-10). This pattern also occurs more commonly in the upper portion of the lumbar spine at L2 and L3 and is characterized by marked widening of the pedicles on the AP radiograph, along with comminution of the pedicles and disruption of the body-pedicle junction. A large retropulsed fragment of bone and severe comminution of the anterior portion of the body are frequently seen. This scenario represents one extreme of the spectrum of flexion-compression injuries, with the dominant force being axial loading. Such a force complex yields more impressive comminution of the vertebral body, with less kyphosis. If the force is applied asymmetrically or if the patient twists during impact, a rotational or lateral bending component of the injury can be involved and induce scoliosis or lateral wedging (Denis E) (Fig. 31-11).

More recent studies have emphasized an additional feature of these fractures that is clinically significant. A small proportion of patients have a longitudinal laminar fracture that seems to be associated with traumatic dural lacerations.[14,31,95] In patients with lumbar burst fractures, a sagittal split can occur in the spinous process. It can appear as an incomplete greenstick fracture. This split should be differentiated from a fracture or comminution of the lamina. An incomplete sagittal split of the spinous process is frequently recognized on CT. When combined with a burst fracture and neurologic deficit, a dural tear is usually indicated[67,95] (Fig. 31-12). Nerve roots can be outside the dural sac and might in fact be trapped in the split in the lamina. When evaluating these fractures, care should be taken to distinguish this feature so that appropriate surgical intervention can be undertaken.

Flexion-Distraction Injuries

Although most flexion-distraction fractures occur in the upper lumbar spine, less than 10 percent of all major fractures of the lumbar spine result from flexion-distraction forces. They are usually a result of the pelvis and lower part of the spine being anchored in a fixed position (e.g., by an automobile lap belt).[4] On impact, the upper portion of the spine accelerates and is thus distracted and flexed away from the fixed lower portion. Three major types of injuries

FIGURE 31-8 *A 19-year-old man sustained a flexion-compression variant of a burst fracture when thrown from a motorcycle. **A,** A lateral radiograph demonstrates kyphosis at the level of the fracture with compression of the anterior portion of the vertebral body. The posterior wall is likewise disrupted, but its height is diminished to a lesser extent. The posterosuperior corner of the vertebral body is retropulsed into the canal (arrow) and is causing significant compression of the dural sac. Some widening of the interspinous distance has occurred, along with disruption of the interspinous ligament from the extent of flexion. **B,** A computed tomography (CT) scan at the level of the injury demonstrates two important features. First, a large central fragment of bone has been retropulsed back into the canal and is causing high-grade neural compression. This fragment, at the level of the pedicles, is seen on the lateral view. Importantly, the pedicles are intact. No break is noted in the lateral wall of the pedicle, nor is the pedicle comminuted. The pedicle remains connected to the vertebral body, so any lordotic pressure applied to the pedicles will be translated to the vertebral body. The posterior neural arch is also intact, although it is not seen on this cut of the CT scan.*

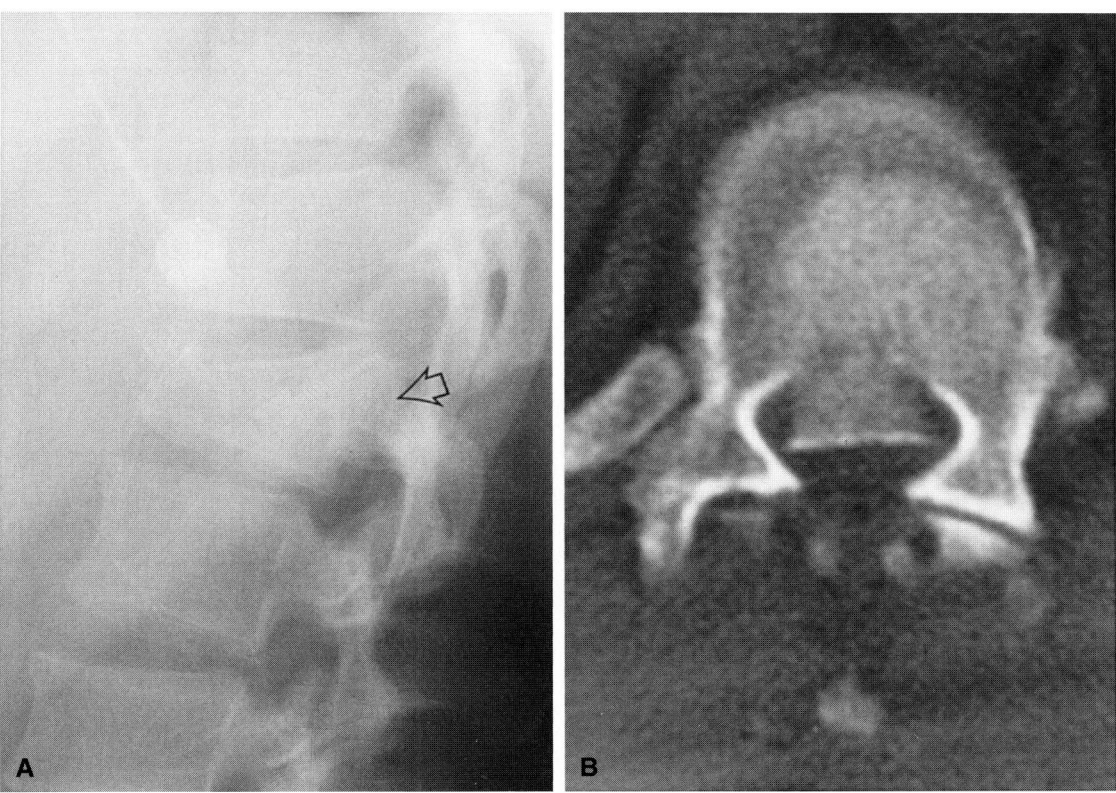

occur. The first is a completely bony injury (Chance fracture), the second is a completely ligamentous injury (facet dislocation), and the third is part ligamentous and part bony. The implications for stability and treatment differ tremendously.

The Chance fracture, described by Chance in 1948,[18] is a pure bony injury with a fracture line extending in a posterior-to-anterior direction through the spinous process, pedicles, and body. It is frequently associated with seat belt wear.[48] The injury generally hinges off the anterior longitudinal ligament. In its common form, it has no significant shear component nor is associated displacement present. It is infrequently associated with neurologic deficit. The diagnosis can be made from lateral and AP radiographs. The lateral radiograph demonstrates a split in the spinous process, whereas the AP radiograph demonstrates a coronal split through the pedicles on both sides (Fig. 31-13). Although a Chance fracture involves disruption of the posterior and anterior portions of the vertebral

body, it is considered to be a stable injury and does not tend to angulate further into kyphosis.

Two reviews of flexion-distraction injuries[45,46] showed that this injury occurred only between T12 and L4, and that approximately 50 percent of the injuries were at L2, L3, or L4. This injury has an extremely high incidence of associated intra-abdominal injuries (50%), including bowel rupture and liver or spleen lacerations. These injuries were originally classified by Gumley and associates,[46] but the classification system was modified by Gertzbein and Court-Brown, who added anterior body fractures.[45] Although the system is somewhat complex, the principle of differentiating the ligamentous from the bony component of the injury is critical. Injuries with a fracture line traversing the spinous process, pedicles, and body are likely to achieve satisfactory union and stability if acceptable sagittal alignment can be maintained (see Fig. 31-13). If the line of injury goes through the interspinous ligament and facets into the pedicle and body (Fig. 31-14), satisfactory

FIGURE 31-9 *The flexion-compression variant (Denis type B) of a burst fracture is the most commonly seen pattern in L4 and L5 fractures. An 18-year-old man involved in a motor vehicle accident has rather typical findings. **A,** A lateral radiograph of the metrizamide myelogram shows kyphosis of 8° across the L4 vertebral level. Minimal to moderate compression of the superior portion of the vertebral body can be noted. The degree of compression seen at this level is frequently less than that at more rostral levels. In spite of the minimal compression of the vertebra, a large retropulsed fragment can create significant compression on the dural sac (arrow); the dural sac compression may be asymmetrical, in which case it frequently traps a specific nerve root or roots and causes radicular symptoms. **B,** This patient had compression of his right-sided roots as a result of a retropulsed fragment (arrow) and a laminar fracture posteriorly on the same side with depression of the laminar fracture. The displaced posterior wall fragment and the depressed laminar fragment were in continuity on the right side and causing right-sided radicular symptoms. The pedicles remain intact in most patients with L4 and L5 burst fractures. The superior portion of the pedicle may be comminuted, but the lower portion remains attached to the vertebral body. **C,** In addition, the lower half of the vertebral body is most commonly split in half in the sagittal plane (arrows), with one pedicle remaining attached to each of the lower halves of the body.*

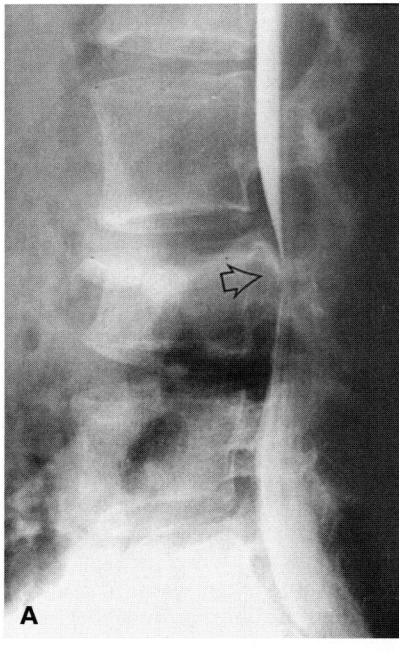
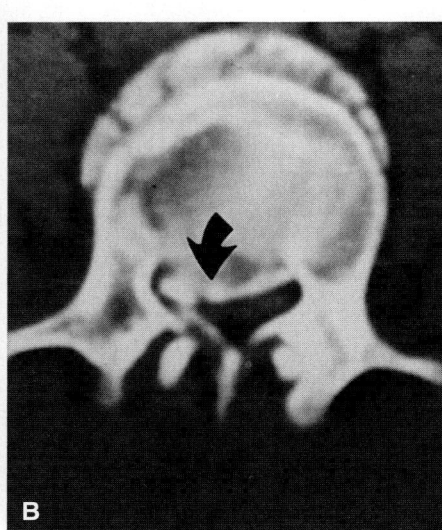
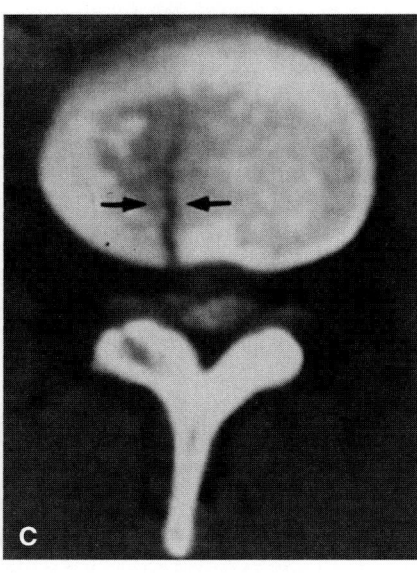

FIGURE 31-10 *A smaller number of patients with L4 and L5 burst fractures have a classic burst pattern with comminution of the vertebral body and the pedicles. This 46-year-old man represents a typical example after a fall. **A,** A lateral radiograph demonstrates complete destruction of the L4 body with comminution of the pedicles and vertebral body. Little kyphosis is present, but there is a moderate degree of loss of height. The overall sagittal configuration of the spine remains relatively normal. **B,** An anteroposterior (AP) radiograph demonstrates splaying of the pedicles (arrows). Loss of height at the vertebral body can be noted on the AP radiograph as well. **C,** Computed tomography demonstrates severe comminution of the vertebral body with marked retropulsion of bone into the neural canal. There is a disruption of the body at the pedicle junction and, in fact, comminution of the pedicles. This patient has a sagittal split of the spinous process at L4 as well.*

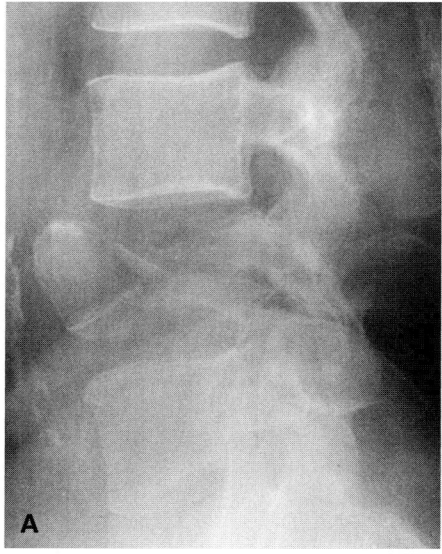
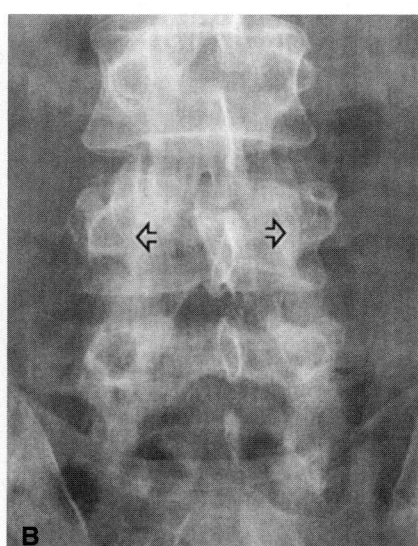
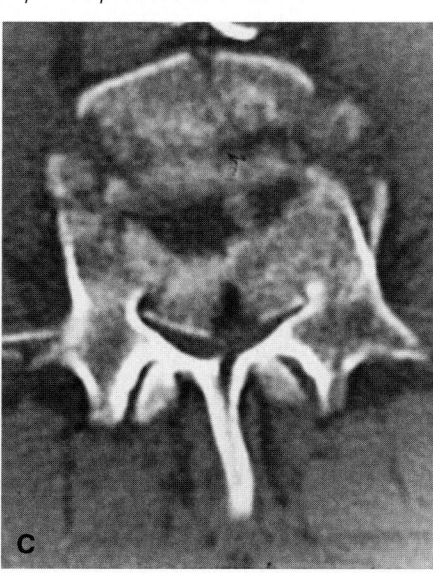

FIGURE 31-11 *A 17-year-old boy sustained a burst fracture of the L3 level with severe lateral compression. **A,** A lateral radiograph demonstrates loss of height of the disk space at L2-L3 and slight kyphosis between L2 and L3. Comminution of the posterior elements (the spinous processes) is also noted. **B,** An anteroposterior radiograph demonstrates the major deformity: severe lateral wedging to the left side with severe compression of the left lateral side of the vertebral body. In addition, the transverse process and lamina of L3 on the right side are split (arrow).*

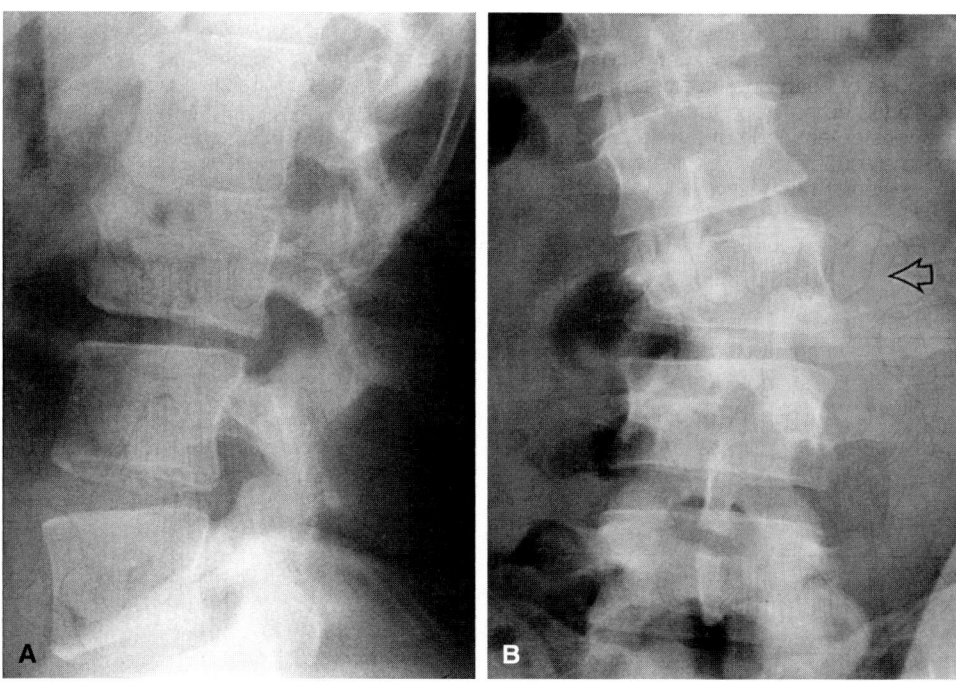

union of the body can occur, but residual instability can result from the posterior ligament disruption.

Facet injuries of the lumbar spine occur infrequently. Levine and colleagues noted that bilateral facet dislocations below L1-L2 represent only 10 percent of the total cases.[70] The important feature of this type of flexion-distraction injury is that it is mainly a soft tissue injury that results in complete disruption of the posterior ligamentous complex as well as the intravertebral disk. The bony architecture of the facets remains intact but totally dislocated. The minor compression of the anterior portion of the inferior body is merely a result of the severe ligamentous injury and does not contribute to the overall instability of the injury. The posterior walls of both vertebral bodies remain intact, and canal compromise results from the translation of one intact vertebral ring in reference to the adjacent ring. This injury must be differentiated from a facet fracture, which is mechanically a different injury with comminution of the facets and sometimes also the laminae, pars interarticularis, and vertebral body.

The severe translation seen in bilateral facet dislocations frequently results in significant neurologic injury (80%).[25,44,70] Then the injury occurs at the thoracolumbar junction, but complete neurologic injury does not usually occur with these injuries in the low lumbar spine. Although severe translation resulting from disruption of the posterior ligaments occurs in association with severe disk disruption, the canal area is large enough that the nerve roots may be at least partially spared. Denis[29] suggested that complete posterior disruption is insufficient to account for the degree of flexion instability seen in this injury. Only incompetence of the posterior longitudinal ligament, annulus fibrosus, and disk could produce such a degree of translational instability. The anterior longitudinal ligament is often stripped from the anterior portion of the inferior body but remains intact. A number of authors[54,73,83,119] have suggested that this injury is a flexion-distraction injury with the axis of rotation posterior to the anterior longitudinal ligament.

Radiographs of bilateral facet dislocations are usually diagnostic.[44,70,92] They demonstrate intact posterior walls of the vertebral bodies with significant translation (36%) and lesser degrees of anterior compression and loss of disk height (Fig. 31-15). AP radiographs of the lumbar spine often reveal the dislocation of the facets. CT confirms the pathology and demonstrates an empty facet sign,[92] as well as the severity of canal compromise on sagittal reconstructions.[44] The neurologic injury in patients with bilateral facet dislocations in the lumbar spine is less severe than in those with dislocations in the thoracic and thoracolumbar spine, 80 percent of whom are complete paraplegics. This decreased severity is clearly a result of the larger canal area and the resilience of the cauda equina. Unilateral and bilateral facet dislocations and fractures at the lumbosacral junction may be associated with sacral fractures and are therefore addressed in the chapter on fractures of the sacrum (Chapter 35).

FIGURE 31-12 | *A 62-year-old man sustained a severe burst fracture of L3 with an incomplete neurologic deficit from L3 distally. Computed tomography demonstrates a burst fracture of L3 with severe comminution of the vertebral body and pedicles. In addition, the spinous process of L3 is split in a sagittal plane within the spinous process (arrows). On dissection of the posterior of the spine, this sagittal split is not evident. However, the combination of a sagittal split with a burst fracture of the lower lumbar spine and neurologic deficit is pathognomonic of a posterior dural tear. On exploration, the patient was found to have a 3-cm laceration of the posterior aspect of the dural sac with herniation of nerve roots through the sac and entrapment of the roots within the sagittal split of the spinous process.*

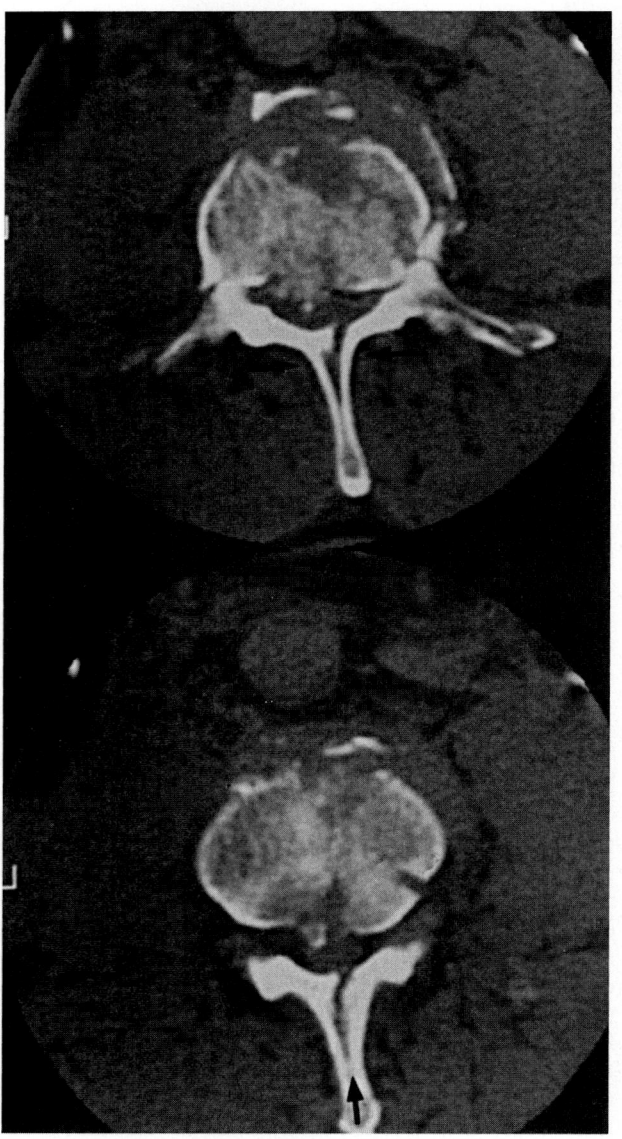

Shear Injuries and Mixed Instabilities

Only about 3 percent of all major lumbar spine injuries are complex combinations of deformities or significant shear injuries. The addition of a shear force in combination with any other injury type markedly complicates the instability and treatment (Fig. 31-16). For example, the combination of shear force with a bilateral facet fracture-dislocation or Chance fracture can cause complete rupture of the anterior longitudinal ligament and marked translation. "Stiff spines," especially those affected by diffuse idiopathic skeletal hyperostosis or ankylosing spondylitis, are extremely susceptible to shear-type injuries, and dramatic deformity is noted on admission (Fig. 31-17). Although not all shear injuries demonstrate tremendous deformity initially, a more subtle indicator of this extremely unstable injury is bidirectional translation (anterior as well as lateral) (Fig. 31-18) on initial radiography.

These injuries are most significant in that they are grossly unstable and compromise the surgeon's ability to achieve anatomically stable reduction. Recognition of disruption of the anterior longitudinal ligament and the circumferential nature of the injury is important. Most posterior fixation techniques rely in part for their stability on an intact anterior longitudinal ligament. Care must be taken to recognize this phenomenon and to be certain that the constructs used to reduce and stabilize the injury counteract the instability.

NEUROLOGIC DEFICIT

The anatomic relationship of the conus and cauda equina to the lumbar spine largely determines the pattern of neurologic deficit. At the upper end of the lumbar spine, the conus broadens and can occupy as much as 50 percent of the canal diameter.[98] In the distal portion of the canal, however, the cauda equina occupies less than a third of the cross-sectional area. Generally, spinal trauma from L2 down results in cauda equina (root-type) injuries, and thus recovery is different from that of injuries in the proximal portion of the canal. The relative position of the nerve roots within the dural sac is also important. The most posterior roots are usually those that exit more distally, because the more proximal roots are already anterior and lateral and somewhat more tethered by the bony foramen. This relationship is especially important for fractures of the lamina of L4 or L5, where roots may become entrapped after a traumatic dural laceration. These roots are generally the distal sacral roots, so injury to them may be evident only as changes in perineal sensation or subtle changes in bowel or bladder function.

Neurologic injuries related to lumbar spine injuries are usually of two types. The first is a complete cauda equina syndrome, which is often seen in severe burst fractures with canal retropulsion and large amounts of bone within the neural canal. The second type of injury is an isolated root injury or combinations of root injuries. These injuries may be nonrecoverable root avulsions and can occur in combination with avulsion of the transverse processes. Lesser degrees of root injury occur with canal impingement. Isolated root injury is common and is caused by a retropulsed fragment of bone catching the exiting root between it and the undersurface of the lamina. Root deficits are also frequent in patients with low lumbar fractures that have sagittal splits in the lamina associated with dural

An 11-year-old boy was a passenger restrained by only a seat belt (without a shoulder harness) in a motor vehicle accident. He sustained a flexion-distraction injury with paraplegia at the T12 level. **A,** A lateral radiograph demonstrates a Chance fracture with the fracture line proceeding through the pedicles and the vertebral body in a line between the arrows. **B,** An anteroposterior radiograph shows both the transverse processes and the pedicle to be split in a coronal plane as marked by the arrows. Because this injury is strictly a bony injury, adequate bone-to-bone contact can be maintained and healing achieved without ligamentous instability.

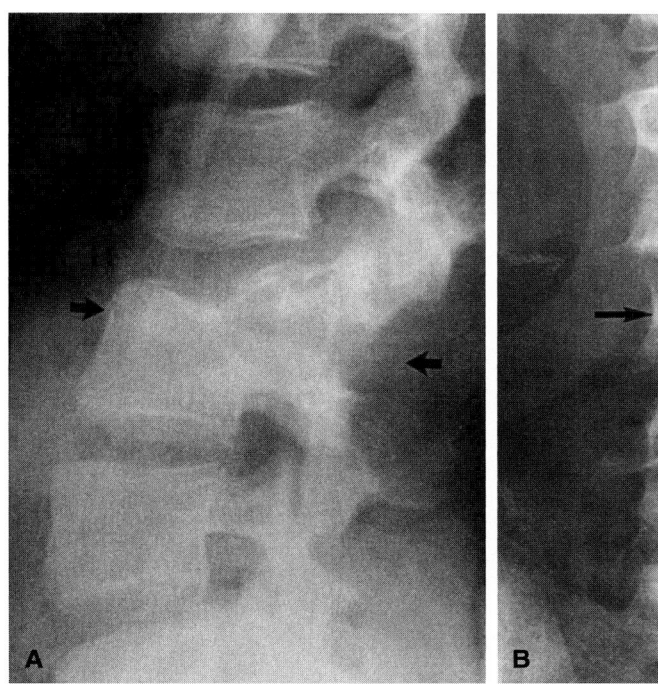

A 26-year-old man who had a car fall on him off a jack stand and cause severe flexion sustained a variant of a Chance fracture. **A,** On a lateral radiograph, kyphosis is centered at L1. The fracture line goes through the interspinous ligament and into the pedicle on one side and the pars on the other side and into the vertebral body. Both end plates are intact, and the fracture line is seen in the vertebral body (dotted line). Note the widening of the pedicles (arrows). **B,** Widening of the interspinous ligament is evident (arrows) on an anteroposterior radiograph, and the fracture line is seen obliquely traversing the pedicle on one side and the pars on the other (dotted line). Because the interspinous ligament is disrupted, residual posterior ligamentous instability occurs after healing of the bone injury.

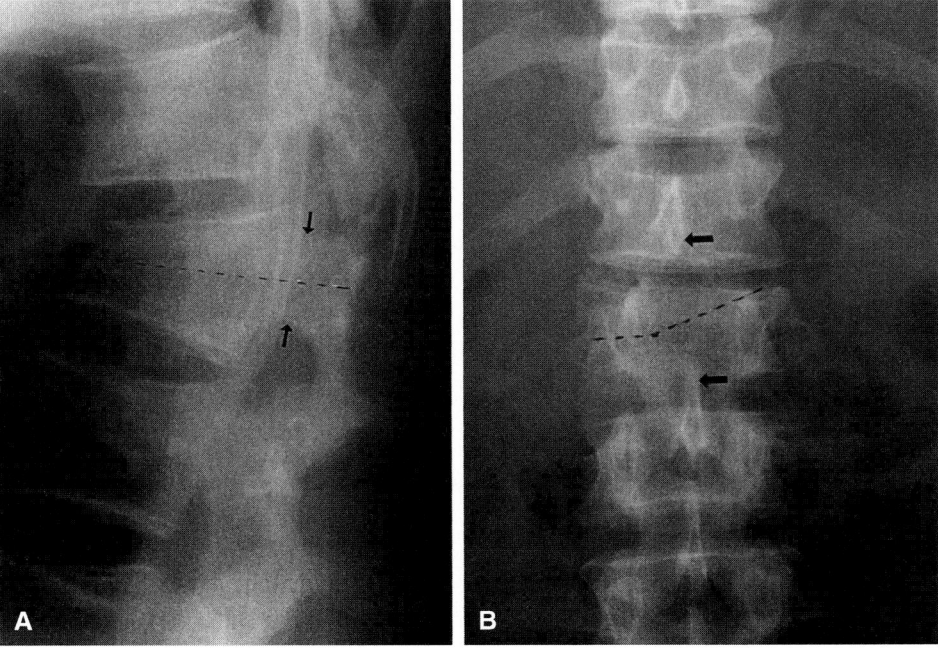

FIGURE 31-15   *A patient sustained a bilateral facet dislocation at L4-L5. **A,** He presented with severe back pain, diffuse weakness below L4, and severe kyphosis, as seen in this preoperative photograph. **B,** A lateral radiograph shows severe translation of L4 over L5 with maintenance of height of the vertebral bodies. No fractures of the posterior wall were evident, although slight comminution of the anterosuperior portion of L5 occurred. **C,** Computed tomography (CT) shows an empty facet sign. In addition, the translational and slight rotational deformities are apparent on this cut of the CT scan.*

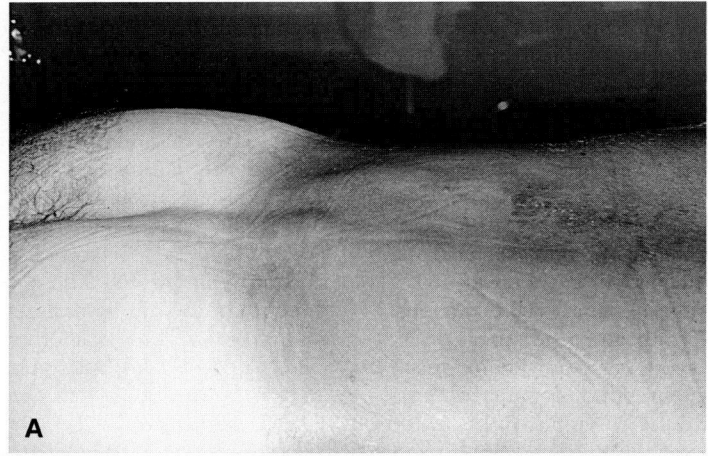

A

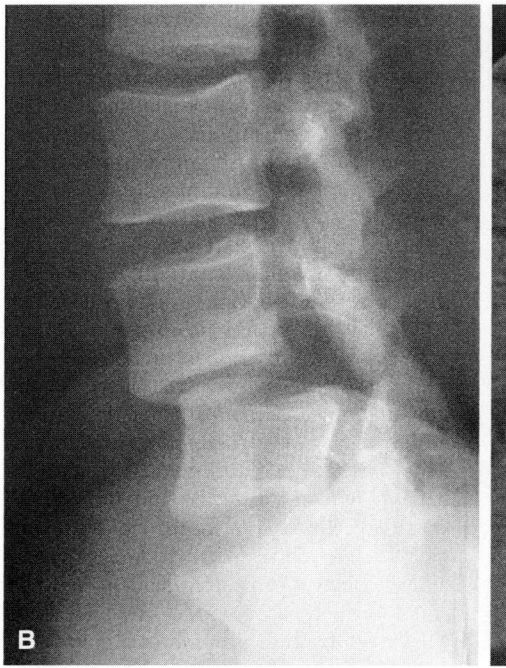

B

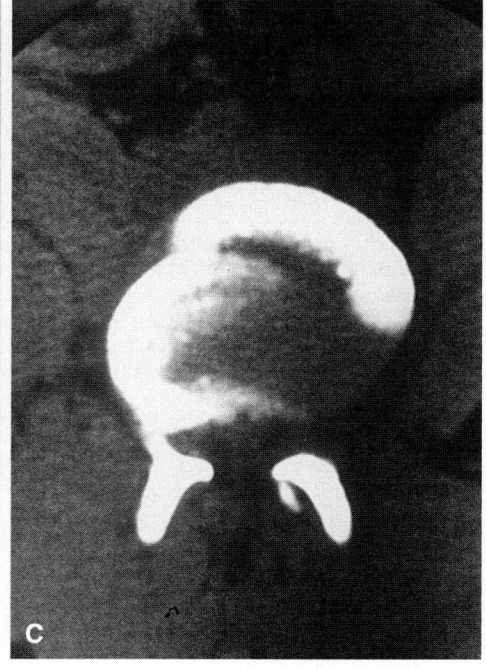

C

tears. Posterior dural tears allow herniation of the roots outside the dural sac or entrapment within the spinous process or laminar fracture.[14,31,67,95] Canal narrowing by translational deformity, such as in bilateral facet dislocation, is less likely to cause severe neurologic deficit in the low lumbar spine than at the thoracolumbar junction. Burst fractures of the lumbar spine are associated with neurologic deficit in about 50 percent of patients.

MANAGEMENT

Indications

Various systems have been devised in an attempt to classify spinal injuries according to both mechanism and degree of instability. In addition, a number of definitions have been proposed—for example, stable versus unstable. A generic definition of spinal stability includes fracture patterns that are not likely to change position with physiologic loads and will therefore not cause additional neurologic deficit or increasing deformity. Although many systems have been proposed that are applicable to lumbar spine injuries, no pragmatic system has been devised that clearly groups the injuries so that treatment approaches can be differentiated. Most classifications of thoracolumbar trauma have either an anatomic reference[8,53] or a mechanistic reference,[38] but all clearly fail to achieve the desired goal of classifying injuries according to subsequent treatment categories. Therefore, other criteria must be used to aid in

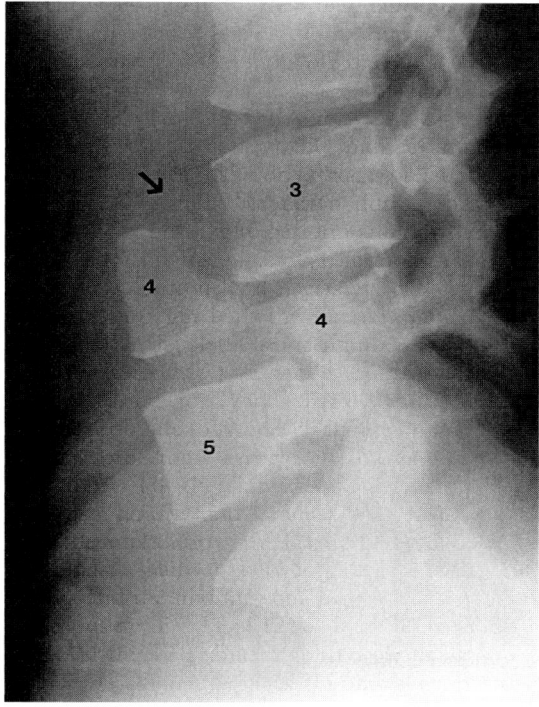

FIGURE 31-16 *This lateral lumbar radiograph demonstrates a severe shear injury in a 26-year-old man ejected from a motor vehicle. The spinal column is totally disrupted, and a fracture line (arrow) is traversing obliquely in an anterosuperior-to-posteroinferior direction through the body of L4.*

making decisions about the treatment of lumbar and sacral fractures.

In general terms, the indications for surgery in patients with lumbar and sacral injuries are the following: (1) the presence of detectable motion at the fracture site that cannot be controlled by nonoperative methods (instability), (2) neurologic deficit, and (3) severe disruption of axial or sagittal spinal alignment. In lumbar and sacral fractures, the presence of neurologic deficit can indicate gross instability. With a large canal–neural element ratio, significant translation or angulation must take place to have neural injury. This rule is not universal, however, because transverse process fractures and avulsions can have accompanying nerve root avulsions. Additionally, in children, neurologic injury can occur at a level above that of the actual bony injury because of the differential elasticity of the cord and spinal elements.

INSTABILITY

In lumbar fractures, certain patterns of injury can be defined as unstable, even in the absence of neurologic deficit. Patients with severe disruption of the posterior ligamentous complex from a flexion or flexion-distraction injury are considered to have unstable injuries. Treatment is clearly indicated, and there is little controversy regarding the appropriate treatment. Most authors believe that

nonoperative treatment of ligamentous injuries does not restore stability and prefer limited operative stabilization. Similarly, flexion-distraction injuries, such as bilateral facet dislocations with complete disruption of the posterior ligamentous complex and the disk, are considered to have gross ligamentous instability that will result in continued loss of sagittal alignment. In addition, shear injuries with circumferential disruption are known to be grossly unstable and in fact require operative stabilization. Burst fractures present a much more complex problem because they represent a spectrum of injuries. Patients who are neurologically intact with minimal deformity require less aggressive treatment than do those with more severe injuries. The majority of current studies show no significant differences in functional outcome or even radiographic outcome between operative and nonoperative treatment in those patients who have a burst fracture and are neurologically intact.[28,114,122,123] The real problem is predicting the future behavior of the injury based on static radiographic studies. Burst injuries that demonstrate greater than 50 percent canal compromise, disruption of the anterior and posterior portions of the vertebral body, and laminar fractures have been considered to be unstable and may require operative treatment to achieve a satisfactory long-term outcome. However, to this point there are very few well done randomized clinical trials, and even the meta-analyses do not give clear differentiation. Mixed instabilities with gross displacement and shear injuries demonstrate markedly unstable clinical behavior.

NEUROLOGIC DEFICIT

The second criterion that constitutes an indication for treatment is neurologic deficit. The benefits of operative treatment of spinal injury have stimulated considerable controversy with regard to neurologic recovery of cord-level injuries,[19,20,22,50,65,89,106] but it is generally agreed that surgery is needed in the lumbar spine for the reason that most injuries involve the nerve roots.[14,67] Because the canal–neural element ratio is very large, a small degree of canal compromise (30%) in the absence of severe deformity (kyphosis) tends to not be significant with regard to neural recovery. A larger degree of canal compromise (50%) accompanied by high-grade neurologic compromise (complete cauda equina syndrome) can often be treated successfully by direct neural decompression.[71,82] In addition, specific root involvement with localized compression of the root can be improved by direct exploration of the root and decompression. Finally, patients with sagittal spinous process fractures, neurologic deficit, and dural tears with roots outside the dural sac also benefit from direct decompression and dural repair.[14,31,67,95]

DISRUPTION OF AXIAL OR SAGITTAL SPINAL ALIGNMENT

The next indication for treatment is severe sagittal- or coronal-plane deformity. Most fractures of the lumbar spine result in kyphotic deformities and may be accompanied by translational and rotational deformities. Because normal lumbar sagittal alignment (i.e., lordosis) is critical to establishment of the normal weight-bearing axis of the body

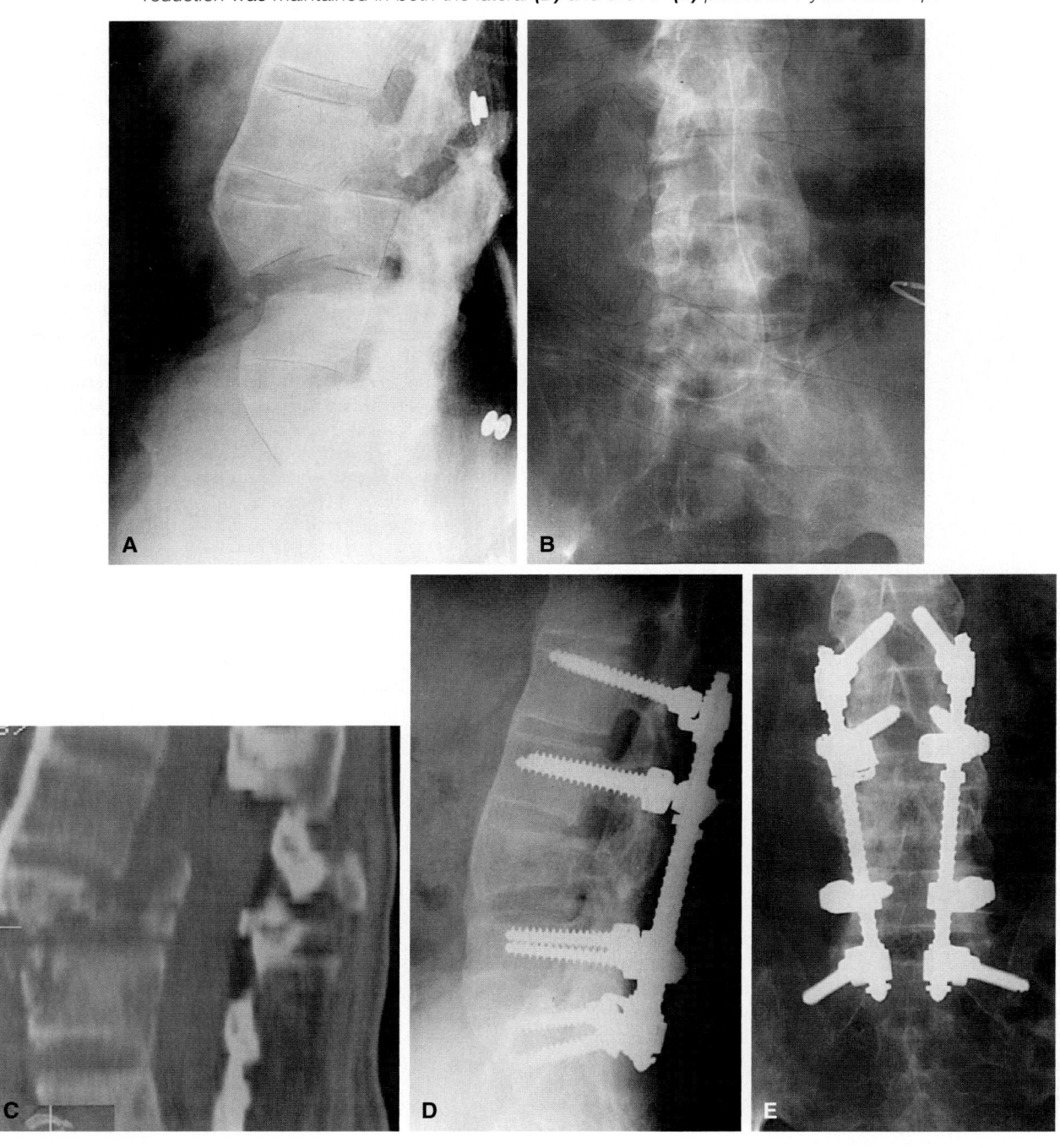

FIGURE 31-17 *A 31-year-old man with a known history of ankylosing spondylitis fell from a roof, landed on the upper part of his back, and sustained this shear injury. **A,** The lateral radiograph is the most dramatic, with the fracture line going through the ankylosed spine at the level of L4. There was 50 percent translation but relatively minimal angulation. **B,** The anteroposterior (AP) view shows little or no angulation or translation in this plane. **C,** Most likely as a result of the uniplanar translation and the significant comminution of the spinal canal without retropulsion seen on this computed tomographic reconstruction, the patient had minimal neural deficit. Anatomic reduction was achieved with multiple points of fixation on the two rigid segments, and reduction was maintained in both the lateral **(D)** and the AP **(E)** planes at 1-year follow-up.*

and to optimal function of the paraspinous musculature, restoration of sagittal alignment to normal is a critical element of treatment. It may be an important parameter in obtaining long-term, pain-free functional results. However, the validity of this statement has not been fully verified because most of these injuries occur in relatively young individuals and the follow-up in most operative and nonoperative series is still relatively short.[2,3,17,40,57,58,86,111] Clinically stable fractures that do not have significant associated kyphosis or scoliosis can

FIGURE 31-18 *A 44-year-old man was sitting in the bleachers as a spectator at a sporting event when a runaway van plowed into the stands. He sustained this L4-L5 shear injury with complete three-column disruption. **A,** The anteroposterior radiograph shows both angulation and translation, whereas the lateral film **(B)** shows predominantly translation (arrows). **C,** An axial cut of a computed tomographic scan through the disk space gives the best visualization of the severity of the injury, which consists of total disruption of the entire spinal column. **D,** Reduction and stabilization were achieved through the use of segmental fixation, including reapproximation of the fractured pedicles to the vertebral body with central screws.*

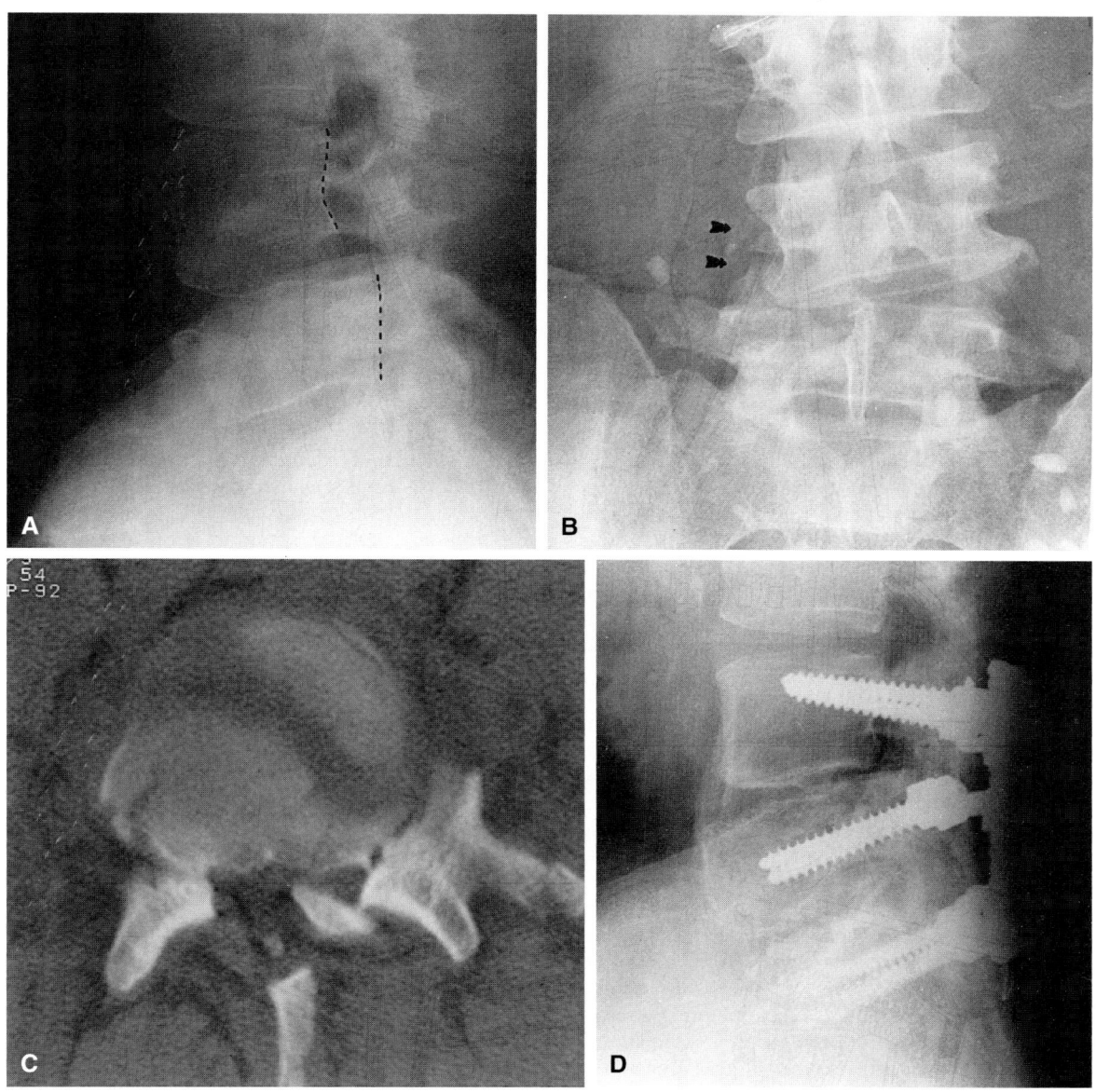

be optimally treated with external immobilization. However, fractures that have significant kyphosis or other deformities that cannot be reduced and maintained with external immobilization need operative intervention for reestablishment of normal spinal alignment. Less emphasis was previously given to operative intervention because of the lack of appropriate methods to restore spinal alignment in a predictable manner. In fact, the use of spinal instrumentation for fractures of the lumbar spine resulted not in restoration of spinal alignment but in iatrogenically induced flat back and other significant alignment deformities with secondary symptoms. If the aim of treatment is accurate restoration of alignment, the surgeon must be certain that the method selected can achieve that goal.

Treatment Options

A number of treatment measures can be used for the management of lumbar fractures and, in general, consist of nonoperative and operative treatment. Nonoperative treatment may include varying combinations of immobilization by cast or orthosis, postural reduction, recumbency, or immediate mobilization. For low lumbar injury, as with thoracolumbar injury, treatment regimens have not been very consistent from series to series. Operative intervention can involve various procedures, including (1) reduction, stabilization, and fusion of spinal fractures from a posterior approach; (2) indirect or direct decompression of neural elements from a posterior or posterolateral (transpedicular) approach; and (3) decompression or reduction, stabilization, fusion, and fixation from an anterior approach.

NONOPERATIVE TREATMENT

Nonoperative treatment can be used for both stable and unstable injuries in the lumbar region. It is most often indicated for minor fractures such as spinous process fractures, transverse process fractures, compression fractures with less than 50 percent anterior compression, and bony flexion-distraction injuries (Chance fractures). In addition, burst fractures[17,53] in patients without any neurologic deficit can in most cases be regarded as stable and therefore appropriate for nonoperative treatment. The trend in the last 5 to 10 years has been an overwhelming transition toward nonoperative treatment for burst fractures of the low lumbar spine.[12,23] This shift in approach has been the result of a number of factors, such as the relatively high complication rate with operative treatment of these fractures,[52] loss of correction after operative treatment, and finally, failure to demonstrate improved functional results in short- to intermediate-term follow-up with operative treatment.[28,114,122,123] However, there are few randomized studies and those that exist compare all thoracolumbar burst fractures and do not stratify those with low lumbar bursts. Currently, therefore, a major consideration in making the decision should be the degree of disruption of the posterior wall of the vertebral body and the extent of disruption in sagittal and axial alignment. Optimal nonoperative treatment of lumbar burst fractures should involve prolonged bed rest (3–6 weeks) before mobilization in an appropriate orthotic device. Failure to provide sufficient protection from axial loading forces by the use of bed rest can result in further deformity. At present, patients without neural deficit or with only isolated root deficit are optimal candidates for nonoperative treatment. Those with dense neural deficits or severe deformity are better treated operatively. Even advocates of postural reduction have indicated that certain fracture patterns, such as bilateral facet dislocations, are not amenable to postural reduction and must be treated surgically regardless of the patient's neurologic status.[53]

Optimal orthotic use for most fractures of the low lumbar spine requires immobilization of the pelvis by a single leg spica cast or a thoracolumbosacral orthosis to fix the relationship of the low lumbar spine. Immobilization by standard lumbar orthoses could actually accentuate motion at L4-L5 and L5-S1.[10,39,45,116] For upper lumbar fractures, a molded total-contact orthosis provides optimal immobilization. Care should be taken to not use an orthosis with a thoracolumbar extension (e.g., a Jewett brace) in the lumbar spine because it might increase motion at the index level by rigidly immobilizing more proximal levels. Thus, pain and deformity might increase in the low lumbar spine.

Some authors have advocated the use of nonoperative treatment for unstable injuries. Treatment consisted mainly of using bed rest to reduce gross malalignment and allow the fracture to begin to consolidate in the supine position before mobilization. Although such management was once an accepted method of treatment,[6,41] the current demands to reduce the length and cost of hospitalization, combined with the effectiveness of operative methods, render nonoperative treatment less desirable for unstable fractures.

OPERATIVE TREATMENT GOALS AND INSTRUMENTATION

Once the decision has been made to consider surgery for a patient with a spinal injury, the goals must be clearly defined to aid in selecting the appropriate procedure to achieve optimal results. With specific reference to the lumbar spine, the goals of operative treatment are reviewed here, and the various surgical methods by which those goals can be achieved are discussed. Details of the operative methods for specific injuries and their treatment plans are described subsequently.

The major goals in the treatment of lumbar spine injuries are anatomic reduction of the fracture, maintenance of correction, decompression of neural elements (when indicated), maintenance of sagittal alignment, minimization of fixation length, and minimization of the complication rate. The time from injury must also be considered because the efficacy of various methods changes with the time course.

The controversy concerning the relative benefits and risks of operative versus nonoperative treatment of fractures of the lumber spine continues to rage. Since the early 1990s, with the advent of patient satisfaction scales, measurement of the outcome of treatment has become more objective and is now considered to be as important as objective neurologic and radiologic criteria. A major problem still exists when attempting to decide on the optimal treatment for lumbar burst fractures. The average age of patients sustaining these injuries is around 27 years, and many are employed in manual labor at the time of injury. Although short-term studies have suggested that the fractures heal relatively reliably, the long-term outcome has not been clearly delineated. If we are technically able to restore anatomic alignment of the spine, do these patients do better with less pain and return to previous employment in both short- and long-term evaluation? Part of the problem in decision making is that some surgical techniques were used that either did not restore or did not maintain anatomic alignment.[3,111] Thus, the appropriate comparison is restoration of alignment with nonoperative treatment. With relatively short follow-up (<4 years), the trends in current studies suggest that patients with neurologic deficit appear to recover more quickly and more completely with surgical intervention.[55,86] Some authors believe that nonoperative treatment of low lumbar burst fractures will provide satisfactory short-term results, but when the data are critically analyzed, most patients have a significant degree of residual back pain and disability, even in the short term.[2,3,17,40] More accurate reduction and longer-term follow-up will yield different conclusions.

In a series of 30 patients with a range of follow-up of 5 to 11 years (mean, 8.2 years) and with anatomic restoration of alignment in most patients, the incidence of back pain was less than 20 percent and the norm was return to preinjury employment.[68] Thus, the current trend is non-operative treatment for patients who are neurologically intact and have minimal to moderate deformity. For those with significant deformity, neurologic deficit, or both, operative treatment should give better long-term results.

ANATOMIC REDUCTION OF THE FRACTURE The first goal of operative intervention is anatomic reduction of the fracture. A general principle of achieving anatomic reduction is that the deforming forces that caused the injury must be directly counteracted by the instrumentation system used to achieve the reduction. In addition, in the lumbar spine, the deforming influence of normal physiologic forces must also be counteracted, specifically, the shear force acting at the lumbosacral junction. For the lumbar spine, selection of an instrumentation system should be determined by the ability of that system to achieve reduction of the deformity and by the relative length of the instrumentation required. If a shorter construct can achieve the same degree of reduction and rigid fixation, it should be used preferentially to maintain as many mobile levels as possible in the lumbar spine. Flexion and axial loading contribute in varying degrees to most deformities in the lumbar spine, and counteracting these forces should be carefully considered. The fixation procedure should have an element of distraction and lordosis to restore normal alignment. Experimental data have demonstrated that devices offering variable and independent application of distraction and lordosis are more able to achieve anatomic reduction.[13,126]

Not all instrumentation systems can achieve optimal results in all portions of the spine. In the following sections, some general types of instrumentation and their feasibility for use with different types of injury in the lumbar spine are considered. Although in the past systems such as Harrington rods with or without rod sleeves[35] or contoured rod systems with segmental fixation by either wires or hooks (e.g., Moe rods, Harri-Luque, Cotrel-Dubousset, Synthes, TSRH [Texas Scottish Rite Hospital]) allowed some correction of deformity, they required long lengths of fixation and achieved little ultimate restoration of sagittal alignment. The advent of pedicle screw systems allowed fixation of lumbar injuries while immobilizing fewer levels with less hardware dislodgement. Whereas the early systems such as the Olerud device and the Fixateur Interne were bulky and complicated, more current systems have technical advantages over the early pedicle screw systems. However, little appreciable improvement in outcome was noted in the treatment of thoracolumbar fractures,[124] or in those in the low lumbar spine without neurologic deficit. In addition, most pedicle screw systems can achieve rigid fixation and maintenance of sagittal contours. Additionally, the length of instrumentation does not need to be increased when removing portions of the posterior elements for repair of dural lacerations or for direct root decompression.[95]

Pedicle screw systems are of two basic types: plate-based systems and rod-based systems. Most plate-based systems have no significant capability of achieving reduction other than by postural reduction on the operating table.[34,76,100,110] Rod-based pedicle fixation devices[32,60,77,78,93] allow progressive reduction of deformities after screw fixation, with maintenance of correction.

Anterior Procedures
Anterior procedures for decompression, reduction of deformity, and stabilization have been used in the acute setting. In the absence of instrumentation, the long-term results of anterior correction of deformity with the use of a strut graft have been poor in terms of maintenance of anatomic alignment.[82] A tricortical bone graft cannot provide progressive correction, but when augmented by the use of a plate, it may be a satisfactory alternative in certain L3 and L4 fractures. Wedge-shaped cages now allow more anatomic restoration of the body after corpectomy both for L3 and L4 as well as for L5. They are also better able to resist collapse from axial compression than most bone grafts, with the exception of femoral allograft, which can also be shaped appropriately to maintain lordosis. Fixation to the sacrum is difficult from an anterior approach although contoured anterior plates have been attempted, but fixation to L4 and L5 is hindered by the presence of the overlying iliac vessels. Lateral fixation to the sacrum is not possible but is more feasible at L4-L5. Cortical femoral allografts can be secured interiorly by lag screws into the sacrum and augmented with posterior fixation. The ability to slightly compress and distract is now built into the slotted holes and instrumentation of several different plate designs.[56] This addition is an improvement over previous plates that simply functioned as neutralization devices. These plate systems now allow decompression and reasonable stabilization to be accomplished from an anterior approach for upper lumbar spine fractures.

For the correction of deformity from spinal fractures that are more than 6 weeks old, the mechanics of correction are different because secondary changes have occurred that complicate the fracture deformity. Primary healing of the cancellous fractures has begun, along with scarring of the soft tissues. At this stage, an anterior procedure for release of tissues becomes important in achieving and maintaining correction as the complexity and stiffness of the deformity increase. When reduction is attempted with posterior instrumentation alone more than 6 weeks after injury, it is difficult to overcome the kyphosis resulting from the shortening of anterior structures and the formation of anterior bony bridges. Some preliminary evidence is now available that anatomic reduction can be achieved and maintained from a posterior approach with appropriate application of forces if no synostosis has formed anteriorly. Total reduction from an anterior approach alone can be difficult in these late cases because posterior scarring or healing of posterior element fractures may have occurred. In addition, most anterior spinal devices lack sufficient lever arms and rigidity of fixation points to be able to apply forces adequate for achieving total reduction.

MAINTENANCE OF CORRECTION The second goal of surgical treatment, maintenance of correction, is related to the rigidity of fixation and to the ability of the selected instrumentation to counteract both the deforming forces and the normal physiologic forces of the lumbar spine. In the lumbar spine, where construct length is important, shorter constructs impart more load bearing to the hardware and may therefore have a higher failure rate. The concept of load sharing either with intact posterior elements or with supplemental anterior graft should be considered. Experimental data on short constructs for the lumbar spine often lead to the conclusion that restoration of the anterior column with a strut graft is important,[34,47,59,79,107] although in practice, load sharing with the intact posterior elements, if properly applied, seems to be sufficient. In addition, in areas of the spine where stability of the construct is compromised by inadequate terminal fixation (e.g., the sacrum), maintenance of long-term anatomic restoration of alignment has been unsatisfactory. Posterior devices that achieve rigid fixation and counteract deforming forces should theoretically be able to produce satisfactory results with pedicle screw fixation. However, the majority of studies have shown that with burst fractures in the thoracolumbar and lumbar spine maintenance of reduction is suboptimal.[28,114,123] The use of anterior grafts as the sole stabilizer after anterior decompression and correction of deformity has had disappointing results. More rigid anterior devices have improved the outcome in maintaining satisfactory long-term results.[80] The combination of anterior surgery to restore stability of the anterior column plus posterior pedicle screw fixation can allow optimal stability, but it requires more extensive surgery with higher risk and is probably not indicated except when anterior decompression is necessary. Even when the anterior portion is performed thoracoscopically, the operative time and relative risks are still high.[94]

DECOMPRESSION OF NEURAL ELEMENTS The third goal, decompression of neural elements, is a less common goal for patients with low lumbar fractures, as the incidence of complete or even dense neurologic deficit is relatively low compared with other areas of the spine.[23] Although it was originally thought that a patient who was neurologically intact but had significant canal compromise might benefit from neural decompression, it has been shown that this assumption is false. Late spinal stenosis does not occur in either surgical or nonsurgical patients in whom reasonably normal anatomic reduction is achieved. It has been well demonstrated that resorption of residual bone within the canal predictably occurs both with and without surgery.[15,24,26,63,106,112] Thus, the sole indication for neural decompression is neural deficit. Neural decompression can be achieved in several different ways, both directly and indirectly, and the most favorable method depends on the specific clinical situation. Laminectomy alone rarely plays a role in decompression of retropulsed bone that has been retropulsed against the anterior portion of the dural sac. It is effective in removing pressure from a posterior fragment of lamina driven into the canal or in decompression of an isolated root. Significant experimental[42,51] and clinical evidence[22,33,72,105,116,120] has indicated that immediate indirect decompression by ligamentotaxis and complete correction of the deformity can provide adequate decompression of the neural elements although it is much more difficult to achieve in

the low lumbar spine than the thoracolumbar junction as a result of the normal lordotic sagittal alignment. This technique has been shown to be most effective in the first 48 hours after injury, however. Transpedicular decompression is a direct posterior technique,[50,115] but one with limited visibility of the anterior portion of the dural sac and with results that do not differ from those of indirect decompression. In the low lumbar spine and sacrum, however, indirect decompression is not as successful because the technique depends on distraction and tensioning of the posterior longitudinal ligament. It is therefore less effective in an area of extreme lordosis or kyphosis. Thus, at L4 and L5, direct decompression by laminectomy or laminotomy can be effective in revealing the area of compression and allowing decompression by removal of the bone fragments that are compressing the dural sac or nerve roots. This technique can be done because limited retraction of the dural sac to achieve exposure is possible at this level. It is recommended only for areas of the spine involving the cauda equina. Direct decompression is most easily performed when the compression is one-sided and bilateral exposure is not necessary. It is technically easier when carried out within the first 2 weeks after injury because the fragments are more mobile and more easily removed. In the upper lumbar spine, a transpedicular posterolateral approach to direct decompression might be indicated. In this case, removal of a portion of the lamina and the pedicle exposes the dural sac adequately on one side and allows direct decompression.

For patients who have had inadequate indirect decompression with posterior instrumentation or who are initially seen late (more than 2 weeks after injury) and require decompression of the dural sac, anterior corpectomy and direct decompression are the most effective procedures. Some authors have advocated direct anterior decompression and stabilization in the immediate acute setting for the treatment of lumbar trauma, but the increased morbidity and potential for decreased stabilization noted with the anterior approach make it a somewhat less attractive alternative. In addition, the use of pedicle fixation for the stabilization of especially low lumbar fractures allows laminectomy and posterior decompression along with a very short construct length, without compromising the quality of the reduction and stabilization.

MAINTENANCE OF SAGITTAL ALIGNMENT The next important goal in the treatment of low lumbar fractures is maintenance of sagittal alignment. Any treatment used for these fractures should be able to impart and maintain the lordosis of the lumbar spine and lumbosacral junction. When crossing the lumbosacral junction, as is the case with many low lumbar fractures, fixation to the pelvis needs to be accomplished to maintain lordosis. Although several systems have used rods driven into either the sacral ala or the ilium, they do not impart adequate stability and the latter has the disadvantage of crossing the sacroiliac joint. Direct screw fixation into the sacrum with the screws either directed medially into the body or laterally into the sacral ala generally give sufficient fixation to maintain sagittal plane alignment. Use of multiaxial screws makes attachment of the rod easier but compromises the ability to adjust alignment. Occasionally fixation to the posterior ilium in the region of S2 and S3 is necessary when the proximal sacrum is highly comminuted. Adequate and stable fixation is especially critical in maintaining the lumbosacral angle, lumbosacral lordosis, and overall sagittal alignment of the spine.

MINIMIZATION OF FIXATION LENGTH Minimizing fixation length to maintain the maximal number of mobile lumbar segments is the next important treatment goal and consideration in instrumentation of fractures of the lumbar spine. However, satisfactory balance must be maintained between the number of levels requiring instrumentation to achieve satisfactory reduction plus stabilization and preservation of important lumbar motion segments. Fixation rigidity should not be compromised to shorten levels. Relatively short constructs (one above and one below) have been shown to lack rigidity and result in loss of alignment in thoracolumbar fracture fixation. More comminuted fractures generally require two above and two below or short fixation with restoration of the anterior column to achieve maintenance of reduction. Parker and colleagues[97] attempted to quantify the degree of disruption of the anterior column to understand which fractures had sufficient residual integrity to allow short-segment posterior instrumentation. Although this concept is helpful, in reality, the most stable fracture patterns that would maintain alignment with short-segment fixation would also most probably maintain alignment with nonoperative treatment. Even anteriorly, attempts have been made to shorten the construct to only the injured segment.[88] Thus, when selecting a construct, the surgeon should keep in mind both the rigidity of fixation and the length of the construct to avoid compromising other treatment goals. Fractures of the low lumber spine are slightly different from those of the thoracolumbar spine in that the pedicles of the fractured level can often be used to achieve fixation. If the pedicles are not severely comminuted, the screw fixation at that level can capture the pedicle and then proceed into the body (see Fig. 31-18), allowing a much more stable construct than just one above and one below the fractured level.

MINIMIZATION OF THE COMPLICATION RATE The final treatment goal of lumbar and sacral fractures is to minimize the extremely high complication rate associated with instrumentation of these injuries. The major complications are pseudarthrosis, failure of sacral fixation, and iatrogenic flat back.[64] Care must be taken when achieving the other treatment goals so that the instrumentation system does not jeopardize the results with an unacceptably high complication rate.[52]

Standard Techniques for Specific Types of Injuries

MINOR BONY, DISKAL, AND LIGAMENTOUS INJURIES

Most minor bony injuries, such as avulsion fractures, spinous process fractures, and ligamentous strains, are satisfactorily treated by external immobilization for symptomatic relief. Patients with posterior ligamentous instability but no significant fracture might not be initially recognized, but once the spasm of the acute injury has subsided,

flexion-extension radiographs can usually demonstrate the instability. With a minor degree of disruption (sprain), external immobilization for 6 weeks to 2 months can allow sufficient healing to achieve symptomatic relief and stability. If the disruption is complete, with tearing of the ligamentum flavum and annulus and anterior wedging of the disk space on flexion-extension radiographs, arthrodesis may be necessary to restore sagittal alignment and control the ligamentous instability (Fig. 31-19). Avulsion fractures of the transverse processes can be treated symptomatically by external immobilization to support the severe muscular trauma associated with the more minor bony injury. Transverse process fractures associated with more severe bony injury can be secondarily treated by immobilization of the primary injury. End plate avulsions in children simulating disk herniation in the acute injury setting require surgical intervention for direct decompression after appropriate diagnostic studies.[35,37,113] A laminotomy, as used for diskectomy, is generally sufficient to allow excision of the protruding portion of the end plate. The remaining portion of the end plate generally heals without further intervention.

ANTERIOR WEDGE COMPRESSION FRACTURES
Compression fractures of the lumbar spine are relatively frequent as either single or multiple injuries. Their outcome is usually favorable, except in an osteopenic patient. The two most common diagnostic problems are failure to recognize accompanying severe ligamentous disruption and the incorrect identification of a burst fracture as merely a compression fracture. In evaluating these injuries, care must be taken to prove that the posterior wall of the vertebral body remains intact.

Another common pitfall in the treatment of these injuries is failure to recognize the extent of the injury. Although the degree of sagittal-plane deformity might not be severe, CT is indicated to confirm the integrity of the posterior wall of the vertebral body. Careful examination of centered AP and lateral plain radiographs will differentiate the two injuries in most cases. Often, the lateral radiograph shows displacement of the posterosuperior corner (Fig. 31-20). Comminution of the posterior wall converts the injury to the more significant burst pattern, which alters the prognosis and the treatment program. In addition, the surgeon must be certain that the compression fracture is not accompanied by ligament disruption (see Fig. 31-19).

For wedge compression fractures with loss of less than 50 percent of the height of the vertebral body, no ligamentous instability generally exists. The goal of treatment is to prevent further anterior compression and residual kyphosis.[62] Nonoperative treatment, even in hyperextension, cannot restore vertebral height, but affected patients are still best treated nonoperatively. Careful attention needs to be paid to the ability of the orthosis chosen to immobilize that segment of the spine. Compression fractures of L2-L4 are not hyperextended by a Jewett brace and might in fact be made worse. These fractures are best treated by use of a custom-molded total-contact orthosis made of one piece for increased rigidity (see Chapter 27). Compression fractures of L5 are not well immobilized by the standard lumbar orthoses, and, in fact, motion at the L5 level is accentuated by the use of a lumbar orthosis,

FIGURE 31-19 │ *A 44-year-old woman whose initial radiographs are shown in Figure 31-6 presented 5 months after injury with severe kyphosis and ligamentous instability.* **A,** *Unfortunately, her maximal hyperextension radiograph shows only minimal correction of kyphosis (arrows). The patient underwent posterior correction, stabilization, and fusion of her kyphosis.* **B,** *She eventually achieved solid arthrodesis and was pain-free with no evidence of instability.*

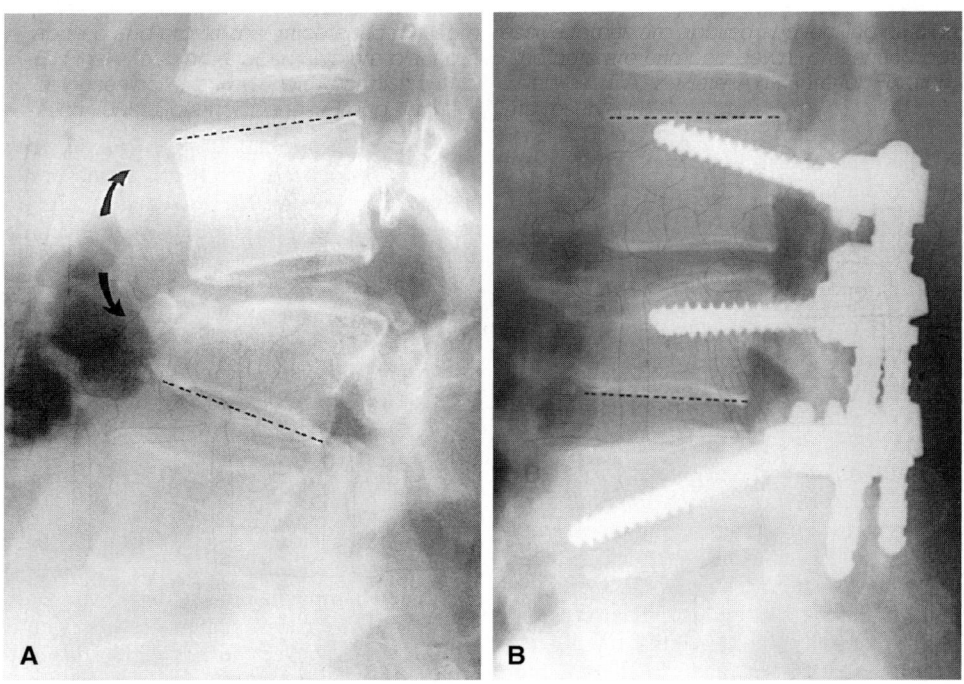

FIGURE 31-20 │ **A,** *An L4 burst fracture might be mistaken for a simple compression fracture of L4 on this lateral radiograph. The key to the diagnosis is the posterosuperior corner (arrow) of the affected vertebral body (L4).* **B,** *The posterosuperior corner is retropulsed into the canal as confirmed by computed tomography (CT). Although the comminution of the vertebral body and the loss of height are unimpressive, the degree of canal occlusion and the overall structural disruption of the vertebral body are not fully appreciated except on CT.*

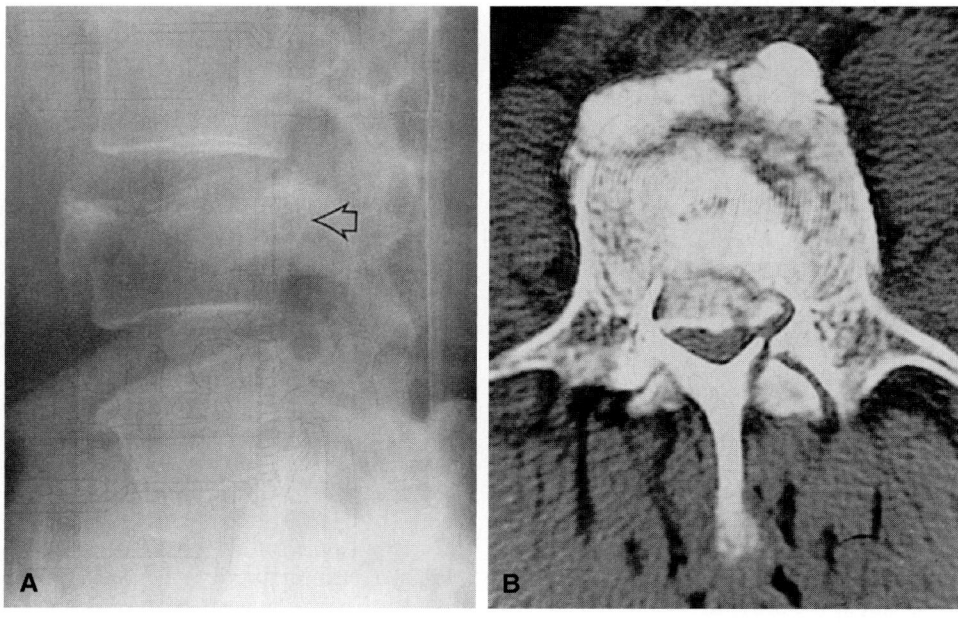

which blocks movement at the other levels.[10,39] Immobilization of L5 fractures requires a single leg included in the orthosis to immobilize the lumbosacral junction. Immobilization needs to be extended for a period of 3 months, until the vertebral body has consolidated. After immobilization, the patient should be checked with flexion-extension radiographs to determine whether any residual instability is present. Increasing compression during the course of treatment that interferes with the normal lordotic sagittal alignment of the spine might require a change in treatment, surgical restoration of alignment, and single-level arthrodesis.

Compression fractures secondary to osteoporosis require two critical elements in their treatment. First, compression fractures in the lumbar spine can result in a significant retroperitoneal hematoma, which in an elderly patient may result in an ileus. Additionally, establishment of a pain medication level that is tolerated by an elderly patient may be difficult. Therefore, it is recommended that the patient be admitted to the hospital for a period of 24 hours after the diagnosis is made to ascertain that an ileus that could potentially result in life-threatening dehydration does not develop. Second, the pain medication needs to be regulated so that the patient is functional but sufficiently comfortable. Next, if the patient is not already taking a bisphosphonate, a basic workup should be done to establish the level of osteopenia, and a treatment program should be initiated. Finally, immobilization should be applied to help relieve the pain. A semirigid corset is sufficient for lumbar fractures, and it is usually well tolerated and helps relieve pain. After discharge, follow-up should be scheduled in 1 week for repeat radiographs and to ascertain that the pain relief is acceptable. Follow-up should again be performed at 1 month for careful evaluation of healing of the fracture and for measurement to determine whether the vertebral body is continuing to collapse. If severe pain and continued collapse are still present at 4 weeks, consideration of vertebroplasty or kyphoplasty should be made at that time (see Chapter 18).

BURST FRACTURES OF THE LUMBAR SPINE

Most patients who sustain injuries to the lumbar spine that require operative stabilization have burst fractures. The key to selecting the most appropriate treatment for these patients is recognition of the components of the fracture pattern. As previously described, all burst injuries involve comminution of the anterior portion of the body and significant involvement of the posterior wall (middle column), along with retropulsion of bone into the canal. The types of burst fractures that occur most commonly in the lumbar spine are Denis A (comminution of the entire body and the body-pedicle junction with or without involvement of the posterior elements) and Denis B (comminution of only the upper end plate with an intact body-pedicle junction and usually sparing of the posterior elements). These two fracture types have reasonably equal distribution at L2 and L3, but the Denis B fracture predominates at L4 and L5. Lateral burst fractures (Denis E) are also occasionally seen. Review of the care of these injuries illustrates most of the techniques required for the surgical treatment of lumbar injuries. Differentiation between the types of treatment appropriate for fractures occurring in the upper and the lower lumbar spine is necessary for optimal results. However, with the adoption of pedicle screw fixation as the standard for the lumbar spine, constructs used in the upper and lower lumbar spine are not dissimilar, with the exception of length.

Flexion-compression (Denis B) injuries, a subset of burst fractures, are characterized by fracture of the posterior wall of the vertebral body with retropulsion of the postero-superior corner into the spinal canal causing compression. The critical feature on AP radiographs and CT is that the pedicles are not splayed. On CT, it is evident that they are still attached to the lateral sides of the vertebral body, although a large central fragment is present and can cause canal compression. This finding is usually accompanied by a significant degree of kyphosis. The instrumentation construct used for this area needs to be able to correct the kyphosis in the upper lumbar spine and restore lordosis in the lower lumbar spine. This ability is related to the length of fixation and thus the length of the lever arm applying the forces, as well as the rigidity of the system and the types of forces applied to the screws.[96]

Pedicle fixation constructs are now almost exclusively used for lumbar fixation and have replaced most of these other fixation systems and are likewise used as well for thoracolumbar and thoracic fractures. The application of these systems has been thoroughly discussed in Chapter 29. Before discussing the use of surgical techniques for lumbar fractures, it must be reemphasized that the role of surgical treatment of these injuries is still being defined. The most common current surgical indications are traumatic dural lacerations, neurologic deficit (other than isolated root deficit), and significant deformity (greater than 25° of relative kyphosis with or without deficit). Although most of the reports to date have relatively short (<5 years) follow-up,[2,3,86] data on intermediate-length (5–10 years) follow-up are now becoming available.[12,103]

Pedicle screw fixation for upper lumbar injuries can be used over more levels to achieve rigid fixation, especially for fractures with more disruption of the anterior column. Thus, for an L2 fracture, the type of construct applied can vary considerably. If it is a Denis B fracture, it may require only one screw above and below (L1 and L3) (Fig. 31-21A), or it may also accommodate a screw directed into the lower portion of the fractured body for a three-screw construct (two screws above and one below the fracture) to achieve greater reduction force (Figs. 31-21B and E and 31-22). For Denis A fractures (Fig. 31-23) with complete anterior disruption, the same two screws above (T12 and L1) and either one below (L2) or two below (L2 and L3) can be used (see Fig. 31-21B and C). Some authors advocate restoration of the anterior column with a cage or graft and an adjunctive one above and one below the posterior construct (see Fig. 31-21D). For fractures of the upper lumbar spine, the length of fixation is not as critical in terms of incorporating distal segments and maintaining motion. Stability and maintenance of correction are important. For the lower lumbar spine, the length of fixation becomes more critical. Pedicle fixation has the advantage of allowing fixation across short levels (three segments, two interspaces). For an L4 burst fracture, instrumentation extends from L3 to L5 (see Fig. 31-21E), and for an L5 burst fracture, instrumentation extends from L4 to S1. Various pedicle fixation systems that can achieve these goals are currently available.

A, The use of pedicle screw constructs or hybrid screw-hook constructs allows correction of both the flexion component and the compression component of a deformity. A number of options exist, and the length of the construct and the number of screws used depend on the stability of the fracture, as well as the level of the fracture. For relatively stable Denis B burst fractures, one screw above and below the fractured level is adequate at the L2 or L3 level. **B,** For Denis B fractures requiring a longer lever arm for reduction or those that are less stable (more disruption of the anterior column), two screws above and one below can be used. **C,** For Denis A fractures with severe comminution, two screws above and two below increase the stability of the construct and also increase the lever arms to achieve reduction. **D,** Alternatively, some authors suggest an anterior graft to restore the stability of the anterior column; however, this procedure increases the duration of surgery and risk and is harder to justify unless the patient requires anterior decompression to correct a neurologic deficit.

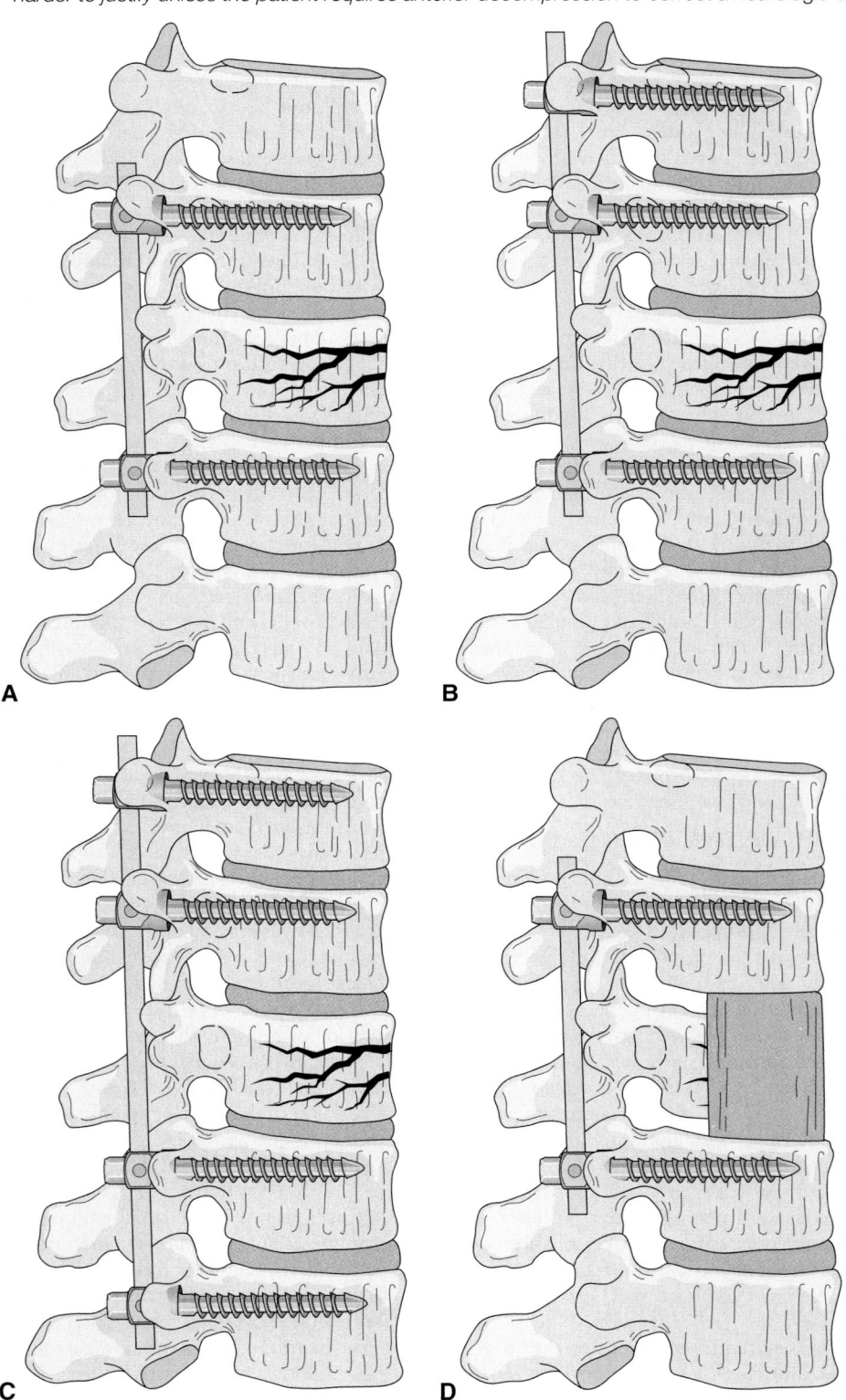

A

B

C

D

(Continued)

FIGURE 31-21 *(Continued)* **E,** *In certain fractures increased stability can be achieved by angling a screw into the noncomminuted portion of the fractured vertebral body.*

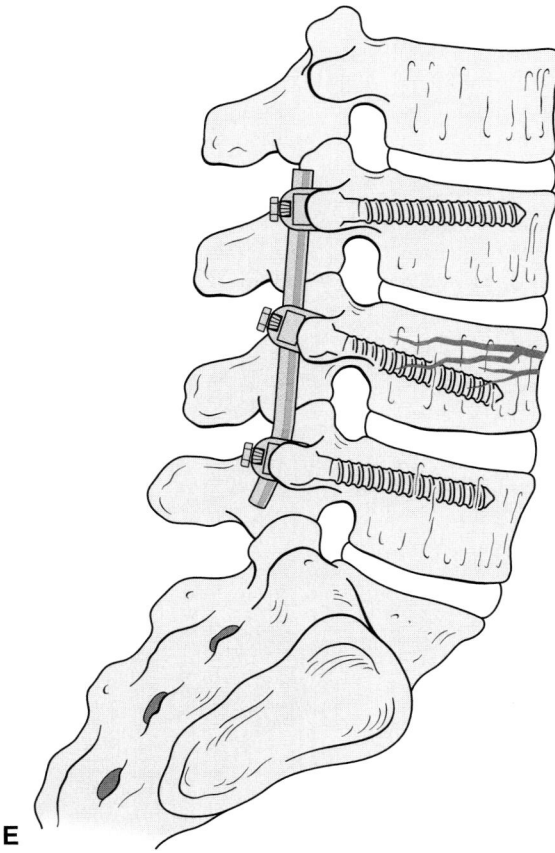

E

Technically, the existing fixation systems can use a variety of techniques to achieve reduction: these are based on the number of levels of fixation (two: one above/one below, or three: one above/one below/involved level) and the type of screw used (fixed or multiaxial). If only one level above and one below are used, reduction of kyphosis and restoration of lordosis can be more difficult. Although a precontoured rod can help, it is often necessary to use "joysticks" attached to the heads of fixed-angle screws to achieve the proper degree of lordosis before inserting the rod and caps for fixation (Fig. 31-24A–C). With three points of fixation, including the apical or fractured level (Fig. 31-24D,E), more options for reduction and restoration of lordosis exist depending on the screw configuration. Again the proximal and distal points of fixation should be fixed-angle screws, and the middle point may need in some instances to be a variable-angle screw so that both the pedicle and the body can be captured and the head still can align sufficiently to engage the rod. Reduction can then be achieved with a precontoured rod inserted into either the proximal or distal screw (depending on the level of fracture) and reduced into the other screws by use of a rod pusher, thus driving the middle screw anteriorly, reducing the kyphosis and recreating lordosis prior to inserting the caps. Alternatively a reduction screw can be used at one end or both ends that allows the caps to be put on the extended screw threads (Fig. 31-24E) and the lordosis recreated by gradually tightening down the screws prior to braking off the extended screw thread portion. The latter is a more progressive and gradual method of reduction. The direction of sacral fixation is down the pedicle of S1 into the body (see Fig. 31-24F) or laterally into the sacral ala (see Fig. 31-24G). Bidirectional or two-point fixation into the sacrum can be achieved with some systems to enhance the fixation of L5 fractures. The type of screw used in the sacrum (fixed or multiaxial) is determined by the position and the direction of the sacral screw, as certain positions require multiaxial screws to achieve rod capture, but use of the multiaxial screw makes active restoration of alignment more challenging.

The following description is a general discussion of pedicle screw application, fixation, and realignment illustrating the principles of this technique as applied to low lumbar fractures. Initial evaluation with appropriate AP and lateral plain radiographs and CT to determine pedicle and vertebral size and location is critical. Patients are positioned on a standard operating room table in a neutral position on longitudinal rolls, transverse rolls, or a radiolucent spinal frame depending on which technique can achieve the highest degree of passive reduction and sagittal realignment for the surgeon. A radiolucent operating table allows for easier radiographic control of screw placement. In either case, AP and lateral imaging or radiographic control for positioning of the pedicle screws is mandatory.

A midline posterior incision is used. Dissection is done carefully with a cautery to avoid excess motion of the injured spine. Frequently, spinous process and posterior element fractures are encountered when exposing L4 and L5 fractures. If there is a longitudinal fracture in the lamina or a greenstick fracture in the spinous process, care should be taken during the dissection to make certain that no nerve roots are trapped in the fracture. If a traumatic dural laceration is possible or extruded roots may be trapped in the laminar or spinous process fracture, they should be explored, replaced into the dural sac, and the laceration sutured before reduction is attempted. If reduction is done with the roots entrapped they may be further injured by complete closure of the fracture. The screws can be placed prior to exploration, but reduction should be done after exploration. If the spinous processes and the interspinous ligament are intact, the ligament should not be removed but instead preserved during the dissection. The integrity of the interspinous ligament should be maintained at the levels just proximal and distal to the construct to prevent hypermobility postoperatively. The ligament can also be used during closure to restore the integrity of the lumbodorsal fascia. Care is also taken while stripping soft tissue from the spine at the proximal level that the capsule of the adjacent facet joint that remains unfused not be disturbed when exposing the transverse process (Fig. 31-25A). Specifically, the L2-L3 facet joint (adjacent to the L3 transverse process) for an L4 burst fracture and the L3-L4 facet joint for an L5 burst fracture should remain unfused, and their capsules must be competent to resist the increased stress on adjacent instrumented levels. The pedicle screw can be placed inferior and lateral to that facet joint so that it does not impinge on the unfused facet and cause secondary changes. Exposure of the transverse

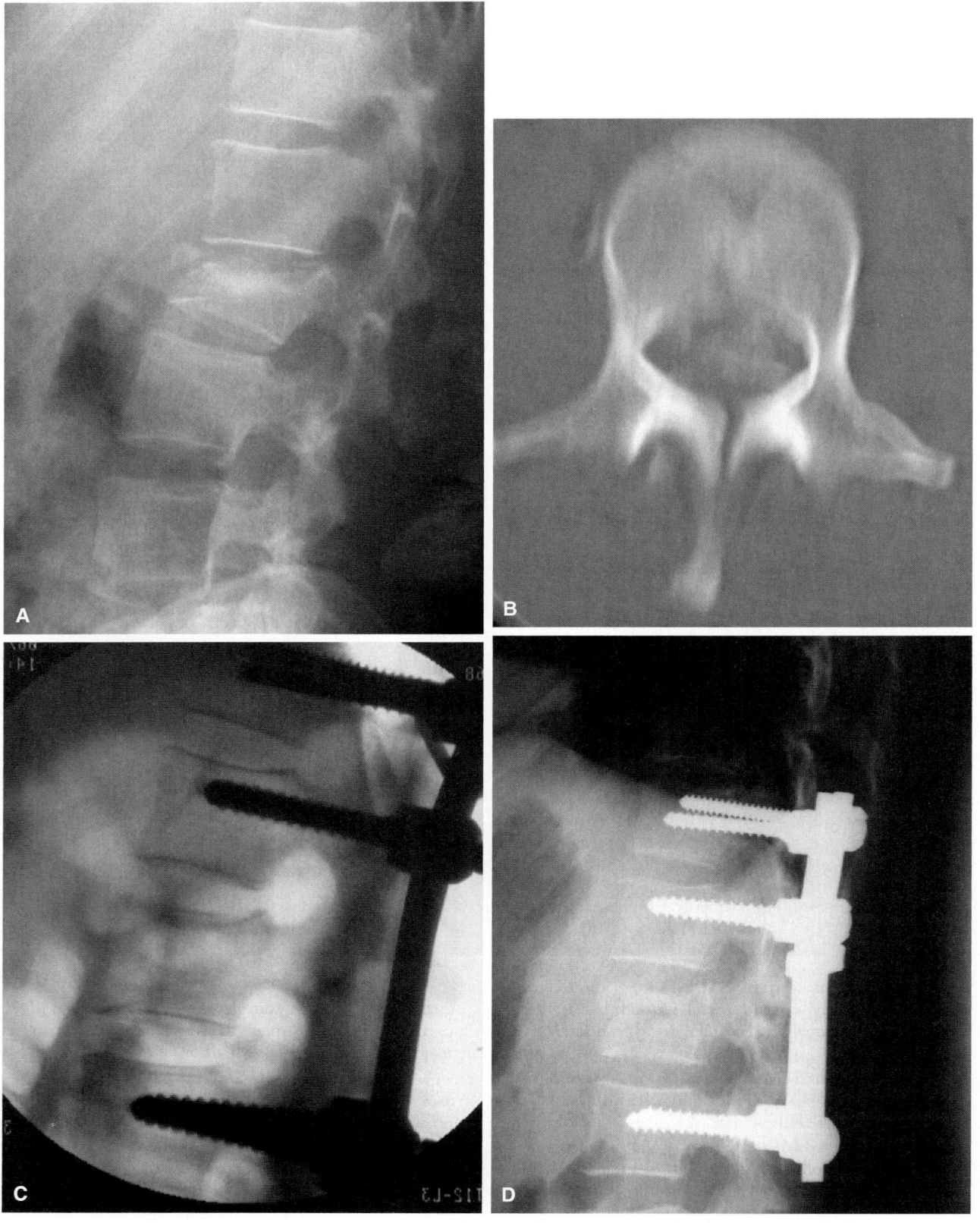

FIGURE 31-22 **A,** *A 44-year-old woman fell through the attic floor, landed on her buttocks, and sustained this burst fracture. It was an isolated injury; however, the patient had loss of movement and sensation in the lower extremities for approximately 10 minutes after the fall. By the time that she was seen at the trauma center, she had recovered all neurologic function. Computed tomography **(B)** showed greater than 50 percent canal compromise, and she had approximately 30° of kyphosis. After discussion of the alternatives, she underwent reduction and fixation with two screws above and one below. Intraoperative images **(C)** showed complete reduction of the deformity. Six months postoperatively, she had lost slight correction of height **(D)** but achieved solid painless arthrodesis.*

FIGURE 31-23 *A 63-year-old man sustained a burst fracture of L3.* **A,** *A lateral preoperative radiograph demonstrates severe destruction and axial compression of the L3 body. The fracture demonstrates slight posterior translation but little angulation.* **B,** *An anteroposterior radiograph demonstrates severe comminution of the vertebral body with spreading of the pedicles and posterior element fractures.* **C,** *Computed tomography of the affected level demonstrates the critical radiologic features. Complete comminution of the entire vertebral body is apparent, as well as significant retropulsion of bone into the canal with nearly complete occlusion of the canal and comminution of the pedicles. Pressure applied to these pedicles would only drive the pedicles into the severely comminuted body and would not cause resultant lordosis and ligamentotaxis.*

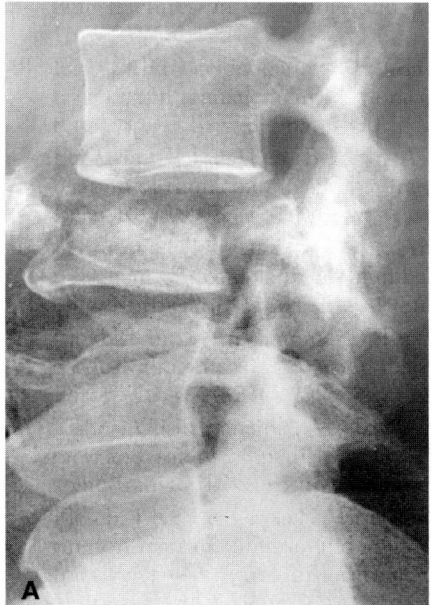

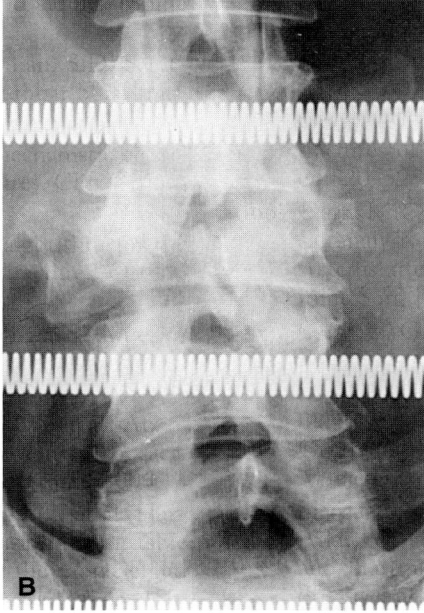

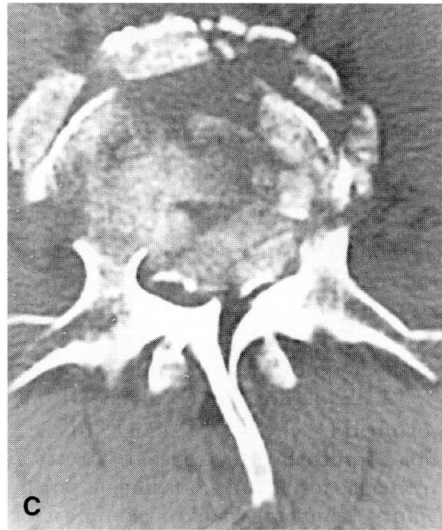

processes of the appropriate levels can reveal fractures and landmarks helpful in screw placement. The facet capsules are removed only at the two or more levels to be fused. When fusion is extended to the sacrum, the L5-S1 facet is cleared of all soft tissue and the sacrum is stripped back to the first dorsal foramen. Complete exposure of all landmarks is critical for accurate screw placement.

For positioning of screws in L3, L4, and L5, a line is drawn across the transverse processes and through the inferolateral edge of the facet, as suggested by Roy-Camille and associates[100] (Fig. 31-25B). Similarly, care must be taken to determine the proper angle of entry into the body. The orientation of the screws at each level is affected by several factors, including the positioning of the patient on the operating table, the amount of kyphotic deformity of the fracture, and the shape of the vertebra. In addition, distortion of the anatomy at the fractured apical level can make accurate placement difficult. Because laminectomy or laminotomy is frequently necessary, direct palpation of the pedicle might be possible and can be helpful in placement.

Beginning at the most proximal level, the facet joint is meticulously avoided and entry made through the posterior cortex with a 3-mm oval bur at the inferolateral corner of the pedicle. Such entry requires that the superior screw be angled approximately 15° superiorly toward the end plate and 10° medially to have it enter through the pedicle. Although most surgeons probe the pedicle when placing pedicle screws during elective fusions, that technique may require significant force in a young individual with hard bone and an unstable spine. The pedicle can also be drilled with a 2- or 3.2-mm bit until the surgeon has ascertained

that the pedicle has been entered. This technique is especially useful when attempting to place a screw in a fractured vertebra.

A 2.0-mm drill bit or Kirschner wire is then inserted, with care taken to not place it deeper than the depth of the pedicle. It should not be inserted into the body so that localizing radiographs or fluoroscopy can determine the site of entry accurately. Two drill bits at the same level can be reversed if AP and lateral radiographs are being used for localization, one with the point into the pedicle and one with the point out, so that the position of the two sides can be differentiated (see Fig. 31-25C). If image intensification is used, the image should be oriented parallel to the axis of each guide pin. The pin should appear in the inferolateral portion of the pedicle for the superior level and in the center of the pedicle for all other levels. The inferior level is at L5 for an L4 burst fracture and at S1 for an L5 burst fracture.

Screw placement at the L5 level is done in a fashion similar to that for the superior end of the construct, with several slight modifications. The position of the pedicle is determined in the same manner, although the starting hole for the screw is begun in the center of the pedicle with a high-speed bur to remove the inferior portion of the superior facet of L5. The angle of placement is inward approximately 10° and inferior approximately 15° (parallel to the superior L5 end plate as the patient is positioned on the table) (see Fig. 31-25D).

If the inferior screw is to be placed into the sacrum, two options are available. For placement of a screw into the sacral ala, visualization of several landmarks is necessary. The capsule is removed from the L5-S1 facet, and the inferior edge of the

FIGURE 31-24 *Multiple approaches to pedicle screw reduction and fixation of lumbar fractures may be used. The first variation is the number of points of fixation of the spine. **A,** When only one level above and below can be captured fixed-angle screws should be used at each level and the screw heads can be captured to allow restoration of lordosis prior to inserting the rods. **B,** If three points of fixation can be used the position of the central screw in the injured level can be used to achieve reduction of alignment and restoration of lordosis. The second variation is in the direction of sacral fixation. **C,** The fixation may be directed into the anterior portion of the S1 body, which is free of both vascular and neural structures. **D,** Alternatively, the fixation may be directed laterally out into the sacral alae and, if taken far enough, likewise lies in a zone free of both neural and vascular elements.*

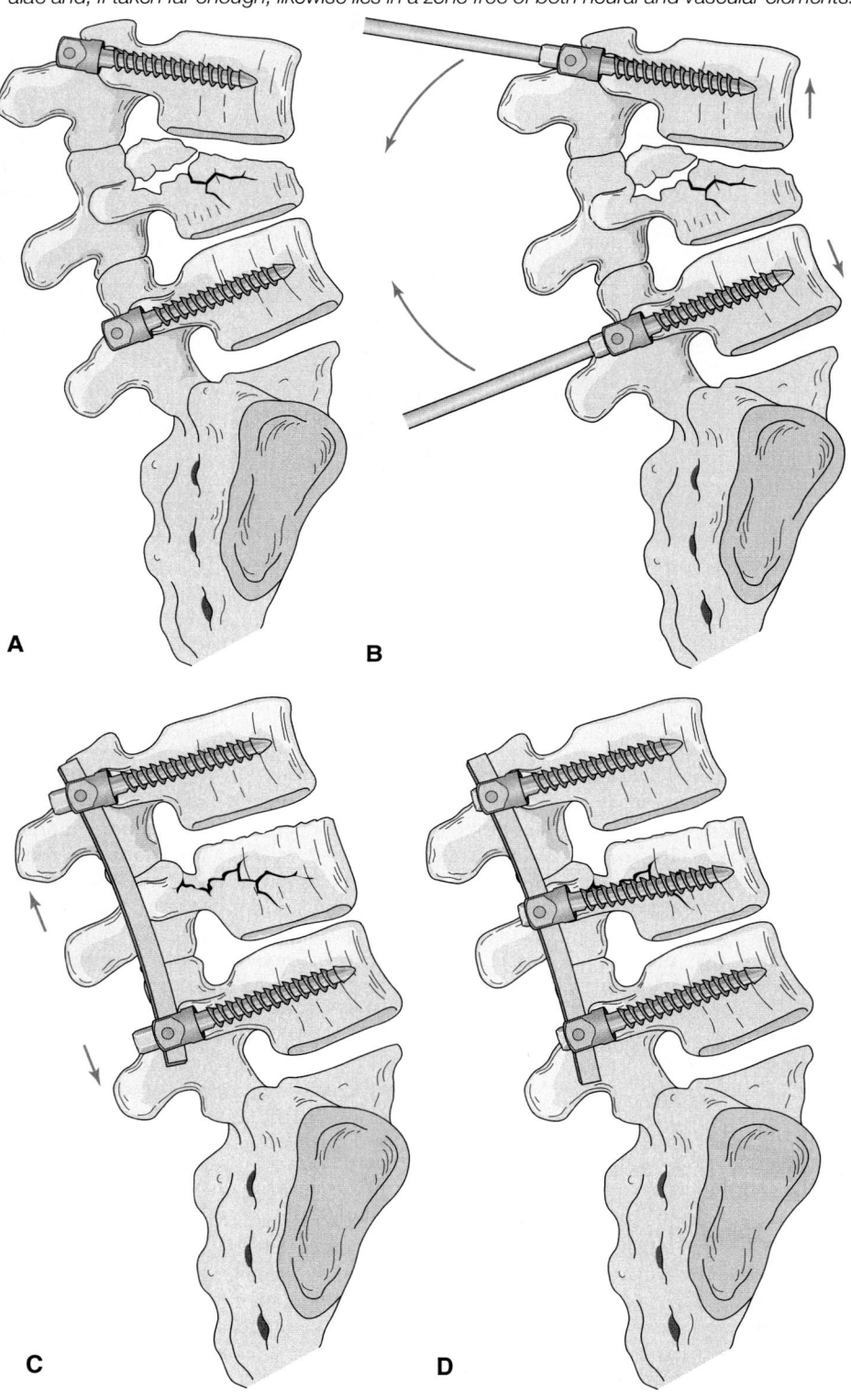

A

B

C

D

FIGURE 31-24	*(Continued)* **E,** *If the central screw can be used then an additional reduction alternative exists. Reduction screws can be used at one or both ends and by gradually tightening the caps into the screwheads over a contoured rod lordosis can be restored. The second variation is in the direction of sacral fixation.* **F,** *The fixation may be directed into the anterior portion of the SI body, which is free of both vascular and neural structures.* **G,** *Alternatively, the fixation may be directed laterally out into the sacral alae and, if taken for enough, likewise lies in a zone free of both neural and vascular elements.*

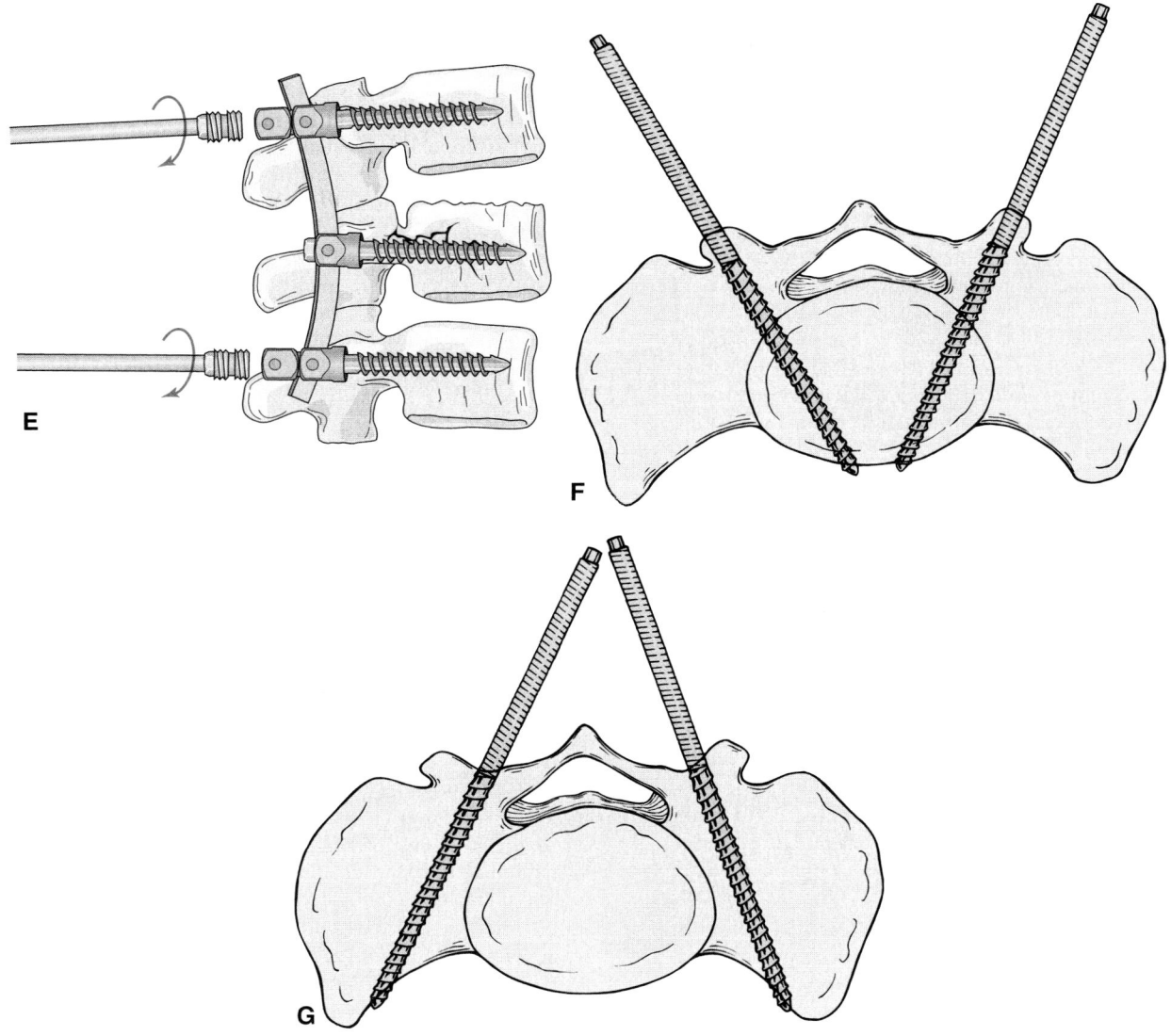

first dorsal foramen is exposed. At a point midway between the facet and the first dorsal foramen, a slight indentation, or "dimple," can be found and is the starting point for insertion of the screw. A 2.0-mm drill bit is placed into the indentation and aligned against the inferior edge of the L5 spinous process (if it exists). Such positioning should orient the drill with 35° of lateral tilt and 25° of inferior tilt (see Fig. 31-25E). The posterior cortex of the sacrum is then drilled in that orientation. The bit is advanced to the anterior cortex of the sacrum simply by pushing it through the soft cancellous bone until the anterior, dense cortical bone of the sacrum is encountered. The anterior cortex is not drilled at this point, but drill bits are placed as described previously, with one inverted, and their position is checked radiographically. On a true lateral view, the drill bit should be oriented parallel to or slightly

converging toward the superior end plate of the sacrum, approximately 1 cm inferior to it. After checking the position, the hole is overdrilled to a size appropriate for the screw.

When drilling the anterior cortex, a hand drill should be used and the drill steadied with both hands to prevent plunging. Once the anterior cortex is felt to be engaged by the drill bit, three quarters of an additional twist is necessary to penetrate the anterior cortex fully. A depth gauge is used to measure screw length, and care should be taken to medially orient the foot of the depth gauge so that the shortest possible length is used to engage the cortex (the ala slopes laterally, and therefore lateral measurements are always longer). If medial screw orientation into the vertebral body of S1 is necessary for the fixation device, the S1 pedicle must be located. An entrance hole

FIGURE 31-25 *The operative technique for pedicular fixation of low lumbar burst fractures has many similarities from one system to the next. The technique shown emphasizes the critical features. When exposing the spine, care must be taken to not disrupt the interspinous ligament or the facet capsules proximal to the level of instrumentation. In exposing the transverse process opposite the superior pedicle, it is critical that the facet capsule not be disrupted. In view of the location of the pedicle and its proximity to the capsule (A), great care should be taken in this dissection. Screw position can be determined by a number of different techniques. The technique of Roy-Camille (B) positions the entry point at the intersection of a line through the transverse processes and a line through the inferolateral edge of the facet joint. Entry into the pedicle can be facilitated by using a 3-mm oval bur to remove the cortical bone at the location of the suggested entry point. A small probe, sound, or curette can be used to easily traverse the cancellous bone of the pedicle. This technique prevents inadvertent perforation of the pedicle walls. Drill bits can be placed into pedicles so that the use of intraoperative image intensification or radiographs will allow identification of the position of the drill bits within the pedicles (C). The orientation of the drill bits within the vertebral bodies changes with the level. In view of the angle of the side wall of L5, the screws should be oriented approximately 10° medially and 15° caudally to accommodate the lordosis of L5 (D).*

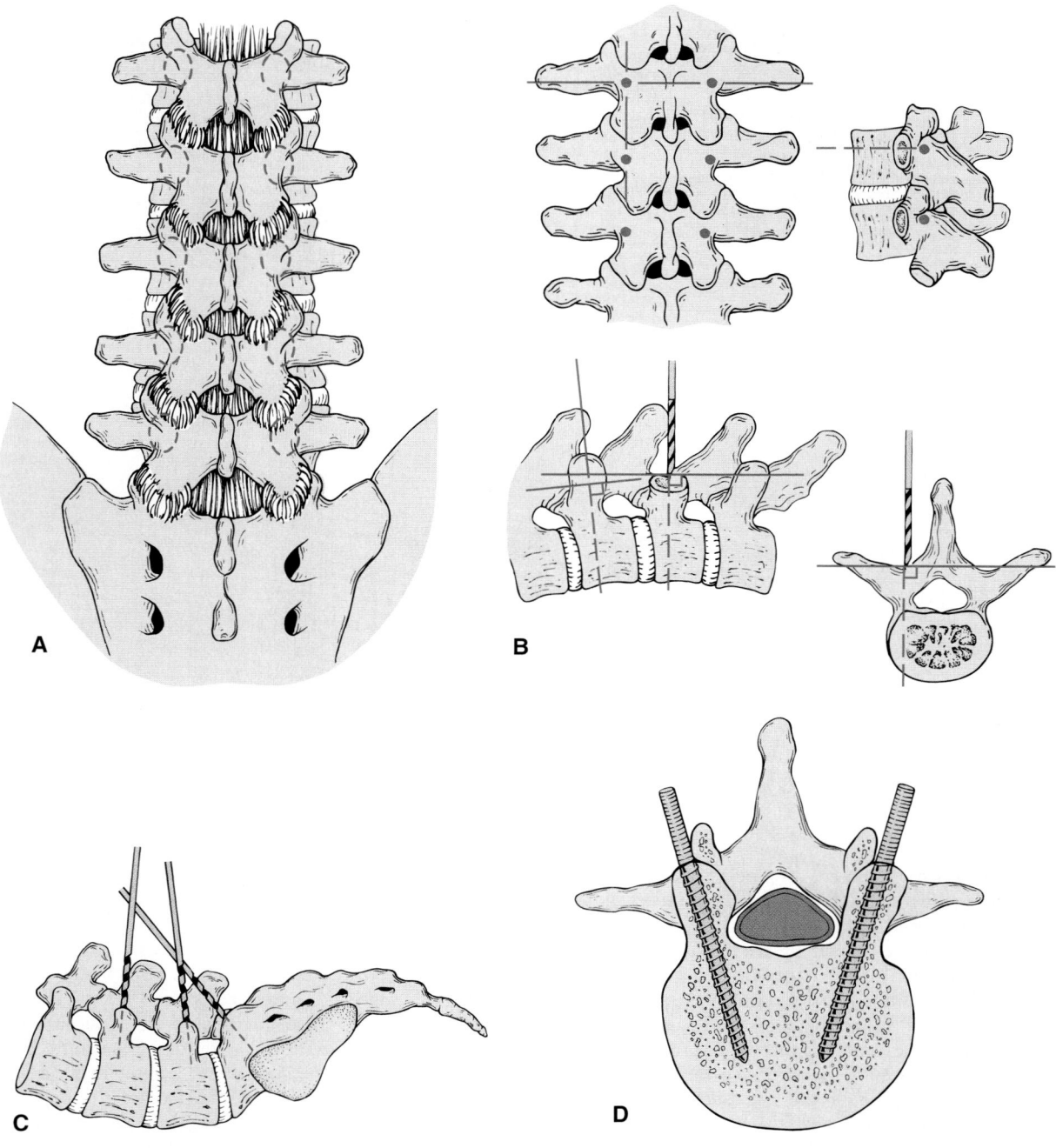

A

B

C

D

(Continued)

FIGURE 31-25 *(Continued) Orientation within the sacrum, as previously described, can be either medially into the body or laterally out into the sacral ala. Lateral orientation requires a 35° lateral tilt and a 25° inferior tilt (E). For a pedicle screw system requiring screw fixation into the apical fractured level, a number of specific considerations are necessary. The configuration of the fracture body must be clearly understood before attempting screw placement. If the body is split sagittally, the two halves may be oriented in different directions. Therefore (F), one side may require vertical placement of the screw, whereas the other side, because of orientation, may require slight angulation medially. In addition, the screw may traverse a fracture within the body. The surgeon should feel the fracture site as the screws are placed. A transverse connector is recommended to increase the rigidity of the construct.*

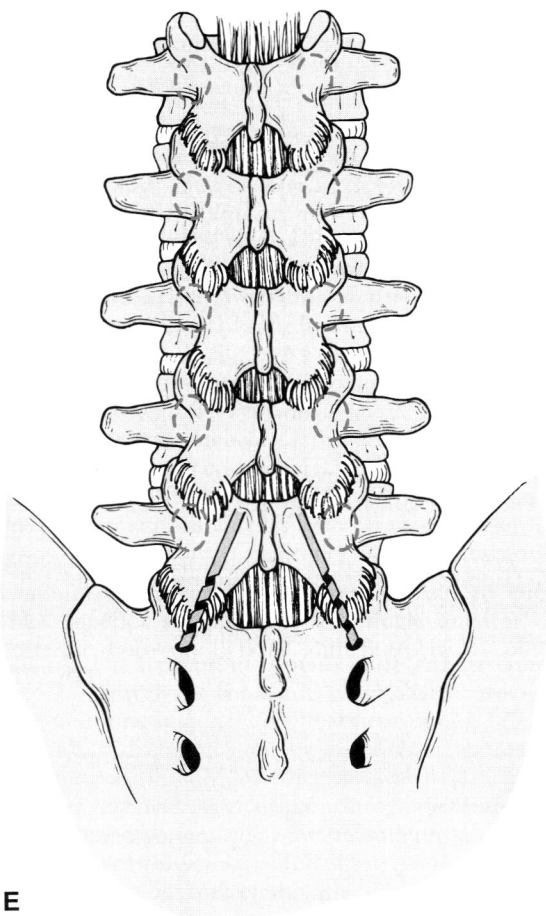

E

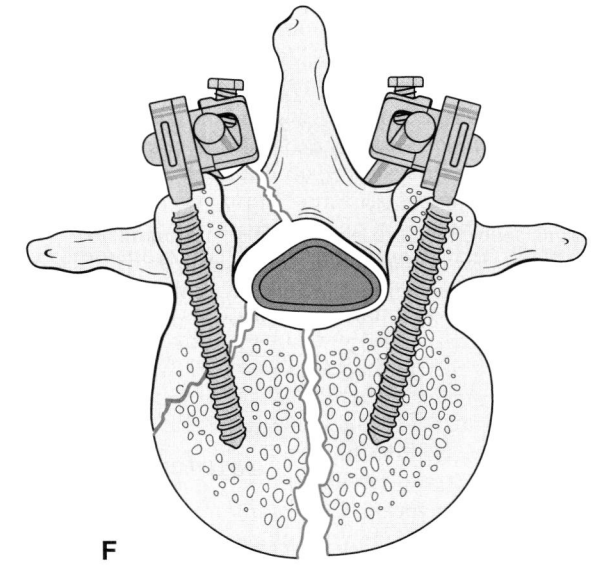

F

is made at the base of the superior facet of S1, and the pedicle is probed and located in standard fashion. Because of the severe medial slope of the sacrum, 20 to 30° of medial and 25° of inferior orientation of the screw are necessary to attain adequate fixation in the sacral body.

If the pedicle screw system being used can accommodate fixation or requires fixation in the apical or fractured level, certain other factors must be considered. First, the configuration of the fractured body must be clearly delineated on CT before attempting screw placement. The most common pattern for L4 and L5 burst fractures is that the superior portion of the body and the pedicle are comminuted but the inferior portion of the pedicle remains attached to the inferior portion of the vertebral body. This pattern can be accompanied by a sagittal split in the body so that the two halves of the vertebra are not attached. Most frequently, however, the area of best screw purchase is in the inferior portion of the body. Therefore, placement requires orientation of the drill bit in a much more inferiorly directed position than normal. In addition, if the two

halves are split, a more directly anterior position (rather than medial orientation) might also be necessary for good purchase[27] (see Fig. 31-25F).

A common variation is that one pedicle and the lateral cortex of the body on that side are displaced significantly. It might not be possible to reduce this injury or place the final screw in that pedicle until vertebral height has been restored.

Finally, when placing the screws, other cracks and fissures in the body might be palpable as the vertebral body is probed. The surgeon should always be aware of the exact dimensions of that vertebral body and the depth of insertion of any instrument so that the anterior cortex of the body is not penetrated through a fracture line. Screw placement at the fracture level is accomplished in a manner similar to that at other vertebral levels, by opening the posterior cortex over the center of the pedicle with a 3-mm bur. This technique usually requires removal of the inferior portion of the superior facet and probing with a 3-0 curette before placement of a 2.0-mm drill bit. With all three levels prepared for screw insertion, devices requiring three points of pedicle fixation can be applied. Consideration of preparation of the spine for fusion is also necessary before final insertion of the hardware.

Assembly of the construct varies with the system. However, certain principles should be observed independent of the type of system and the number of screws inserted. First, it is critical that the kyphosis be corrected before applying distraction. When the fractured level is not instrumented, a precontoured rod is inserted into the proximal screw or screws on both sides simultaneously. The rods are locked into the screw or screws in the correct orientation, and then by applying force to both rods either with a rod pusher or by using the reduction devices available with the system, the rods are reduced progressively down into the distal screw heads and preliminarily locked into position. If additional correction of kyphosis is necessary, the rods can be contoured with in situ bending irons. Once correction of the kyphosis has been achieved, the rod is loosened at one end and distraction applied until the interspinous ligament is appropriately tensioned, and then the quality of reduction is checked with image intensification. Additional distraction can be gradually applied while watching for restoration of body height of the fractured level.

If a screw is placed in the fractured vertebral level, as mentioned earlier a number of different methods of reduction can be utilized depending on surgeon preference and experience. If a fixed-angle screw is used or even a multi-axial screw in some cases, an anteriorly directed force can be applied through the middle screw to achieve reduction. In rod systems without the ability to gradually achieve reduction with the system in place, the rod can be precontoured to the appropriate lordosis and then, for smaller degrees of deformity, either rotated into position similar to correction of scoliosis or attached to the middle and distal screws and reduced into the proximal screw. The reduction process is done in this sequence because most deformity exists at the upper end of the fractured level and the disk space above. Correction of height is done by keeping the middle screw tight and first loosening the distal screw to allow distraction to be applied across the normal disk space so that it is comparable to the one below. That screw is tightened, and then the proximal screw is loosened and distraction applied across the injured level until it is restored to normal. The use of a reduction screw with added thread height that can later be removed is a very effective tool in applying gentle and controlled anterior force to the middle screw to achieve reduction (see Fig. 31-24E).

In most systems it is necessary to thoroughly decorticate the transverse processes and lateral sides of the facets before assembling the construct. Epinephrine-soaked sponges can be used to diminish bleeding. If laminectomy is required, usually only one side of the hardware is assembled—that on the side opposite the surgeon. Partial reduction of the deformity is preferable before laminectomy both to achieve some fracture stability and to attain some fracture reduction if repair of a traumatic dural laceration or removal of a bony fragment is thought necessary. After completing the decompression or repair of the dural laceration, the second side of the construct is placed. The

reduction is checked by either radiographic or image intensification; at least one cross lock should be placed, and the bone graft is harvested and placed in the decorticated lateral gutters.

Postoperatively, the patient is placed in a regular bed, and either a total-contact or a thoracolumbosacral orthosis, depending on the level of fracture, is applied on approximately the third postoperative day. If a thoracolumbosacral orthosis is used for an L5 fracture or for fixation extending to the sacrum, the leg extension is removed at 3 months and the patient is kept in the orthosis for an additional 3 months.

The three-screw technique is applicable to L4 and L5 burst fractures in which the body-pedicle junction is intact and to some L3 fractures. It relies on three-point fixation for applying slight distraction and lordosis to maintain sagittal alignment. This technique can also be used in patients with burst fractures and comminution of the pedicles at L3, as well as at L4 and L5. Difficulty might be encountered with severe comminution of the body or in obtaining solid screw fixation. By using the curette, the pedicle finder, and the 2.0-mm drill bit to feel through the pedicle and the body, however, it is possible to obtain reasonable fixation in most fractures. Small laminotomies at the apical level can aid in determining the orientation of the pedicle when fractured and in allowing solid fixation. Because the major force is a lordotic force at the apical level, satisfactory fixation in the pedicle and in some pieces of the body is all that is necessary to maintain three-point fixation, which achieves the reduction and rigid fixation. For most fractures at L2 and some at L3, fixation can be augmented by an additional level of purchase proximally or even, if necessary, an additional level distally with skipping of the fractured level.

ANTERIOR DECOMPRESSION AND FIXATION

Anterior surgical techniques are most beneficial for late direct decompression and stabilization of low lumbar fractures. Fractures in the lumbar spine from L2 to L5 can be visualized through a retroperitoneal approach, which is relatively straightforward. The technique allows excellent exposure to the vertebral bodies and the certainty of complete anterior decompression. In the acute trauma setting, the role of anterior surgery in the lumbar spine is somewhat less clear. The risks and complexity of direct anterior decompression and stabilization need to be balanced against the relative risks of the posterior surgery. In the lumbar spine, it has been demonstrated that the use of an anterior strut graft alone to reconstruct the spine is inadequate and results in anterior compression of the graft and kyphotic deformities. This complication can be avoided by applying posterior stabilization at the same sitting or by the use of some adjunctive anterior procedure. Use of anterior plating[1,43,56] for neutralization can augment the results and achieve more rigid fixation, and these measures are adequate for long-term stabilization. Care must be taken that the devices do not protrude against the aorta, or vascular complications can arise.[9] The technique of retroperitoneal dissection and direct anterior decompression was described in Chapter 30; it is essentially the same for the low lumbar spine. Dissection of L4 and especially L5 requires extreme care in handling the iliac vein.

FLEXION–DISTRACTION INJURIES

The two most common types of flexion-distraction injuries are Chance fractures (and related variants) and bilateral facet dislocation. As previously noted, the relative incidence of these two types of injury is reversed in the lumbar spine in comparison with the thoracolumbar junction. Flexion-distraction fractures, as classified by Gumley and associates[46] and by Gertzbein and Court-Brown,[45] are not generally amenable to any distraction techniques for stabilization. Fractures that traverse the spinous process, pedicle, and body can often be reduced in a hyperextension cast and heal predictably. Those that cannot be reduced, however, and that will result in significant residual lumbar kyphosis should undergo surgical reduction and stabilization. In addition, fractures that traverse the posterior ligamentous complex, pedicle, and body commonly result in ligamentous instability after fracture healing and should undergo stabilization and fusion initially for an optimal result. Both these injury types can be treated with a posterior compression/neutralization construct because of the absence of posterior wall comminution and disk involvement. Depending on the involvement of the posterior elements, the compression-neutralization instrumentation requires two levels (one interspace) or three levels (two interspaces) (Fig. 31-26) with a pedicle screw system. When the fracture line traverses the interspinous ligament and the posterior elements are left intact, the injury can be stabilized with a two-level (one interspace) construct. When pedicle fixation is considered, purchase in the fractured pedicle and body must be carefully assessed if two-level fixation is chosen (see Fig. 31-26). Severe comminution of the posterior elements of the involved level require use of a three-level (two interspace) compression-neutralization construct.

The most common flexion-distraction injury in the thoracolumbar spine is bilateral facet dislocation. This injury is distinctly rare in the lumbar spine but requires special consideration. Such injuries can result in severe posterior ligament and disk disruption. Patients with lumbar spine and lumbosacral dislocations tend to have incomplete neural injuries and thus increased potential for recovery. An L2-L3 bilateral facet dislocation should therefore be directly reduced, and a two-level (one interspace) neutralization construct with pedicle fixation used to limit the length of fixation. Because the disk disruption is so significant with this injury, care should be taken not to apply too much compression to the construct. Only enough compression should be used to keep the facets engaged but not enough to cause extrusion of disk material. If there is a question about the degree of disk disruption and potential herniation from the injury, after reduction the disk should be explored and extruded disk material removed. In patients in whom the lower vertebral body is fractured in combination with the bilateral facet dislocation, instrumentation may need to span two interspaces and three levels to achieve adequate reduction.

Bilateral facet dislocations in the upper lumbar spine can also be treated satisfactorily with a one- or two-level pedicle screw construct. This technique is extremely

FIGURE 31-26 *A 17-year-old girl sustained a Chance fracture of L4 and had flexion instability after nonoperative treatment. A posterior compression construct was able to reduce the kyphosis and eliminate the instability. One-level compression instrumentation can be used acutely in flexion-distraction injuries with posterior instability, but the purchase in the fractured body must be carefully assessed if a two-level/one-interspace construct is chosen.*

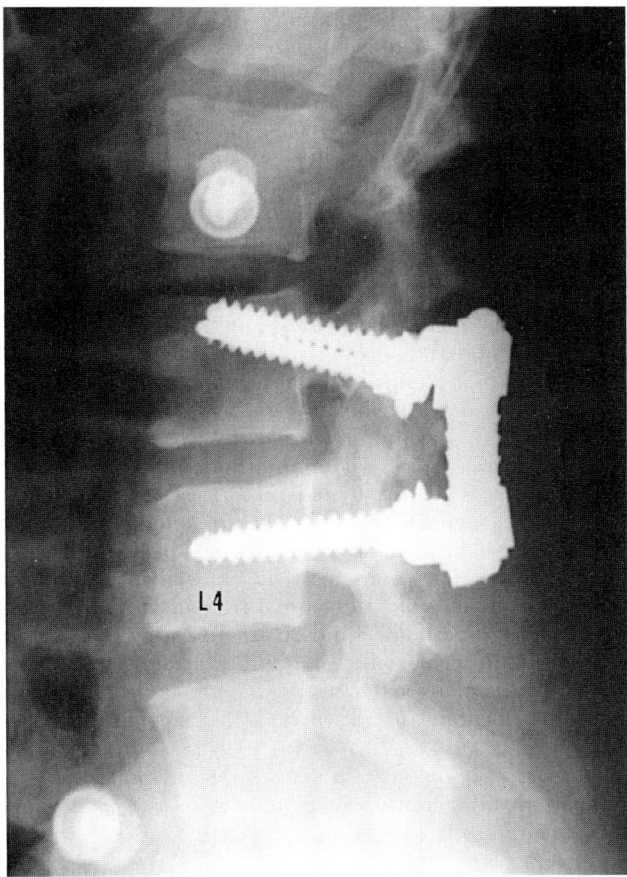

straightforward because the posterior elements and posterior wall of both vertebral bodies are intact. Once the facets have been reduced, screws are placed in the pedicles of the level above and below the dislocation (assuming that no body fractures are present) and connected by a straight rod. Lordosis is achieved first and then just enough distraction applied to place the vertebral levels in normal orientation and the disk at normal height. Compression should not be used. Care should be taken during reduction of the bilateral facet dislocation so that the facets are not damaged because they contribute significantly to the stability of the construct. Operative reduction of dislocated facets can be achieved with the following method: After complete delineation of the dislocated facets by meticulous dissection, the disrupted facet capsules and ligamentum flavum are resected. A laminar spreader is placed between the two spinous processes and gentle distraction applied until the tips of the facets are unlocked (Fig. 31-27A). The laminar spreader is twisted slightly to reduce the facet and then released to allow the facets to be reduced into normal position. An interspinous wire (18 gauge) is placed around the two spinous processes to complete the reduction (see Fig. 31-27B). The spine is now reduced and stabilized, and a pedicle screw construct can be applied to complete the construct. At the end of the procedure, the interspinous wire can be left in place or removed.

Other techniques that can maintain the reduction with a short fixation length and without the use of compression can also be effective. In the low lumbar spine, where conservation of levels is important and a one-level construct is considered, prophylactic diskectomy should be performed before a single-level compression construct. This procedure removes damaged disk material, prevents extrusion, and allows the use of a single-level compression construct. Specifically, an L4-L5 facet dislocation can be stabilized with a single-level L4-L5 compression construct and the proximal and distal levels left open.

FIGURE 31-27 *Reduction of a bilateral facet dislocation in the lumbar spine should be accomplished in a controlled fashion with preservation of the facets to allow reestablishment of stability. The soft tissues are dissected, and the facet dislocations are identified. The ruptured ligamentum flavum is removed, as are the disrupted facet capsules. Cartilage is removed from the superior facet of the lower level under direct vision. A laminar spreader is then placed between the two spinous processes and gently manipulated until the facets are distracted. When the tips of the facets are disengaged, the laminar spreader is tipped to push the inferior facet anteriorly and pull the superior facets posteriorly. The distraction on the laminar spreader is then released to allow the facets to engage in a normal position. **A,** An interspinous wire is placed across the involved level and tightened to complete the reduction and reestablish stability. If neither vertebral body is significantly fractured, then a two-level (one interspace) pedicle screw construct can be placed either before or after reduction. It is generally easier to place it after reduction when the spine is stable. If the lower vertebral body is fractured, then a three-level (two interspace) construct may be necessary to achieve adequate reduction. **B,** After complete reduction of the facet dislocation, screws are placed. Depending on the level of injury either a straight or precontoured rod is selected and placed into the screw heads. Caps are then placed on the screws; slight compression or neutralization is done to keep the facets engaged. The construct is locked in place, and alignment is checked on image intensification. The wire can be left in place or removed depending on whether the facets are fractured or intact.*

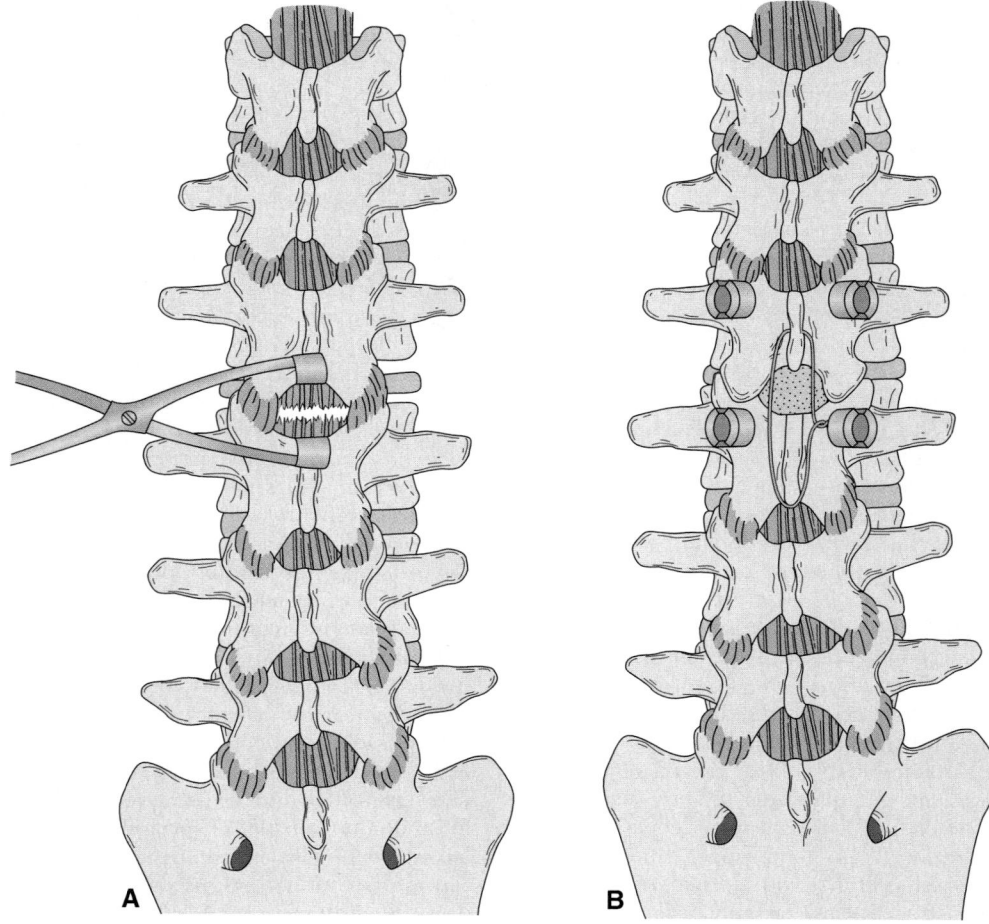

A   B

SHEAR INJURIES AND COMPLEX DEFORMITIES

The optimal stabilization construct for shear injuries and complex deformities generally involves posterior stabilization, which with an operative plan allows stabilization of the various deforming forces. Each one needs to be individualized for the particular situation. Segmental fixation is often necessary to control the abnormal forces, especially in patients with stiff spines (see Figs. 31-17 and 31-18). Other constructs[16] have been used with success; however, the more points of fixation, the greater the degree of stability that can be achieved with these injuries.

Complications of Surgical Treatment

Prevention of surgical complications is by far the best situation. Prevention requires a complete understanding of the injury mechanism and thorough preplanning of the surgical procedure.[52] However, in spite of adequate preoperative planning and imaging, a number of neurologic and mechanical complications can occur.

NEUROLOGIC DETERIORATION

Neurologic deterioration can occur intraoperatively and postoperatively. It has been demonstrated that a patient's lumbar spine is not well immobilized on a Stryker frame. As the patient rolls from a prone to a supine position, an unstable burst fracture can shift significantly, which could result in increased neurologic damage. Long-term immobilization on a logrolling frame can also cause shifting of fragments and potential neural damage. This situation is one indication for early surgical intervention. Intraoperative neurologic deterioration can be caused by applying distraction over a kyphotic segment of the lumbar spine, thus stretching the already tight neural elements over a prominent area. Reduction of kyphosis should be accomplished before any distraction maneuver. Postoperative neurologic complications can be caused by dislodgment of anterior grafts or by recurrence of deformity. Placement of pedicle screws may be associated with either root deficit or more severe deficits, depending on the degree of error in placement (Fig. 31-28).

NONUNION

Nonunion of lumbar spine fractures is a frequent complication that has been reported in as many as 40 percent of fractures at the lumbosacral junction. More rigid fixation techniques with segmental fixation, as well as meticulous fusion techniques, are required to prevent this complication. Care must be taken to extend bone graft proximally above the upper hook in a rod construct to the transverse process on that side to achieve solid arthrodesis. In addition, with bulky posterior hardware, care must be taken that the device does not obscure pertinent areas for bony fusion.

LOSS OF CORRECTION

Most reports on spinal injury have noted loss of correction, as well as residual kyphosis. This complication is related to the inability of the fixation system selected to achieve rigid fixation that does not change with the patient's position. Proper selection of hardware and meticulous application with concern for counteracting deforming forces can minimize loss of correction.

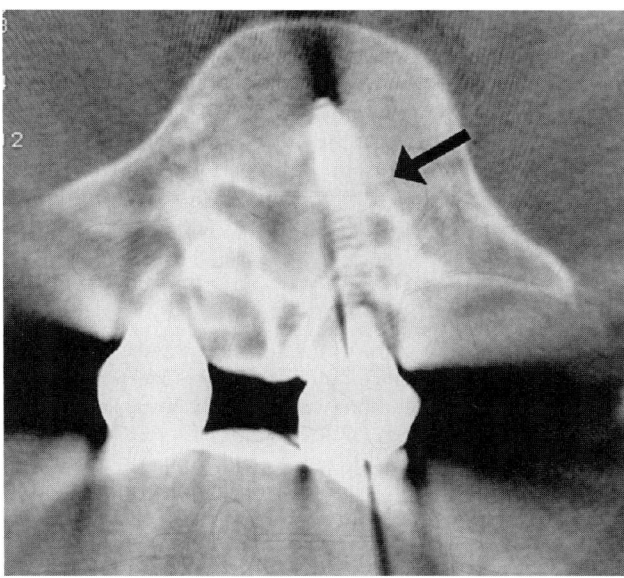

FIGURE 31-28 *Although segmental fixation with pedicle screws can shorten the construct and more rigidly fix the lumbar lordosis, the surgical technique is more exacting. Especially in a traumatized spine, where normal landmarks may be obscured, misplacement of screws (arrow) is a potential complication.*

SUMMARY

Treatment of lumbar fractures requires an understanding of the mechanics and normal functioning of the lumbar spine. Hardware selection depends on the goals to be achieved, the time to surgery, and the types of instabilities encountered. Appropriate consideration of the treatment goals for an individual patient and the injury is necessary for optimal results. The surgeon's selection of treatment should not be based on knowledge of a single technique, but rather on knowledge of the relative advantages and disadvantages of various nonoperative and operative procedures for the treatment of lumbar spine fractures.

REFERENCES

1. An, H.S.; Lim, T.H.; You, J.W.; et al. Biomechanical evaluation of anterior thoracolumbar spinal instrumentation. Spine 20:1979–1983, 1995.

2. An, H.S.; Simpson, J.M.; Ebraheim, N.A.; et al. Low lumbar burst fractures: Comparison between conservative and surgical treatments. Orthopedics 15:367–373, 1992.

3. An, H.S.; Vaccaro, A.; Cotler, J.M.; et al. Low lumbar burst fractures. Comparison among body cast, Harrington rod, Luque rod, and Steffee plate. Spine 16:S440–S444, 1991.

4. Anderson, P.A.; Rivara, F.P.; Maier, R.V.; et al. The epidemiology of seatbelt-associated injuries. J Trauma 31:60–67, 1991.

5. Andreychik, D.A.; Alander, D.H.; Senica, K.M.; et al. Burst fractures of the second through fifth lumbar vertebrae. Clinical and radiographic results. J Bone Joint Surg [Am] 78:1156–1166, 1996.

6. Bedbrook, G.M. Treatment of thoracolumbar dislocation and fractures with paraplegia. Clin Orthop Relat Res 112:27–43, 1975.

7. Benzel, E.C.; Ball, P.A. Management of low lumbar fractures by dorsal decompression, fusion, and lumbosacral laminar distraction fixation. J Neurosurg 92:142–148, 2000.

8. Boucher, M.; Bhandari, M.; Kwok, D. Health-related quality of life after short segment instrumentation of lumbar burst fractures. J Spinal Disord 14:417–426, 2001.

9. Brown, L.P.; Bridwell, K.H.; Holt, R.T.; et al. Aortic erosions and lacerations associated with the Dunn anterior spinal instrumentation. Orthop Trans 10:16, 1986.

10. Brown, T.; Nortron, P.L. The immobilizing efficiency of back braces; their effect on the posture and motion of the lumbosacral spine. J Bone Joint Surg [Am] 39:111–139, 1957.

11. Bucholz, R.W.; Gill, K. Classification of injuries to the thoracolumbar spine. Orthop Clin North Am 17:67–73, 1986.

12. Butler, J.S.; Fitzpatrick, P.; Ni Mhaolain, A.M.; et al. The management and functional outcome of isolated burst fractures of the fifth lumbar vertebra. Spine 32:443–447, 2007.

13. Cain, J.E., Jr.; DeJong, J.T.; Dinenberg, A.S.; et al. Pathomechanical analysis of thoracolumbar burst fracture reduction. A calf spine model. Spine 18:1647–1654, 1993.

14. Cammisa, F.P., Jr.; Eismont, F.J.; Green, B.A. Dural laceration occurring with burst fractures and associated laminar fractures. J Bone Joint Surg [Am] 71:1044–1052, 1989.

15. Chakera, T.M.; Bedbrook, G.; Bradley, C.M. Spontaneous resolution of spinal canal deformity after burst-dispersion fracture. AJNR Am J Neuroradiol 9:779–785, 1988.

16. Chaloupka, R. Complete rotational burst fracture of the third lumbar vertebra managed by posterior surgery. A case report. Spine 24:302–305, 1999.

17. Chan, D.P.; Seng, N.K.; Kaan, K.T. Nonoperative treatment in burst fractures of the lumbar spine (L2-L5) without neurologic deficits. Spine 18:320–325, 1993.

18. Chance, G.Q. Note on a type of flexion fracture of the spine. Br J Radiol 21:452–453, 1948.

19. Chapman, J.R.; Anderson, P.A. Thoracolumbar spine fractures with neurologic deficit. Orthop Clin North Am 25:595–612, 1994.

20. Clohisy, J.C.; Akbarnia, B.A.; Bucholz, R.D.; et al. Neurologic recovery associated with anterior decompression of spine fractures at the thoracolumbar junction (T12-L1). Spine 17:S325–S330, 1992.

21. Court-Brown, C.M.; Gertzbein, S.D. The management of burst fractures of the fifth lumbar vertebra. Spine 12:308–312, 1987.

22. Crutcher, J.P., Jr.; Anderson, P.A.; King, H.A.; et al. Indirect spinal canal decompression in patients with thoracolumbar burst fractures treated by posterior distraction rods. J Spinal Disord 4:39–48, 1991.

23. Dai, L.D. Low lumbar spinal fractures: Management options. Injury 33:579–582, 2002.

24. Dai, L.Y. Remodeling of the spinal canal after thoracolumbar burst fractures. Clin Orthop Relat Res 382:119–123, 2001.

25. Davis, A.A.; Carragee, E.J. Bilateral facet dislocation at the lumbosacral joint. A report of a case and review of literature. Spine 18:2540–2544, 1993.

26. de Klerk, L.W.; Fontijne, W.P.; Stijnen, T.; et al. Spontaneous remodeling of the spinal canal after conservative management of thoracolumbar burst fractures. Spine 23:1057–1060, 1998.

27. De, B.H.; Opdecam, P. Split coronal fractures of the lumbar spine. Treatment by posterior internal fixation and transpedicular bone grafting. Int Orthop 23:87–90, 1999.

28. Defino, H.L.; Canto, F.R. Low thoracic and lumbar burst fractures: Radiographic and functional outcomes. Eur Spine J 16:1934–1943, 2007.

29. Denis, F. The three column spine and its significance in the classification of acute thoracolumbar spinal injuries. Spine 8:817–831, 1983.

30. Denis, F. Spinal instability as defined by the three-column spine concept in acute spinal trauma. Clin Orthop Relat Res 189:65–76, 1984.

31. Denis, F.; Burkus, J.K. Diagnosis and treatment of cauda equina entrapment in the vertical lamina fracture of lumbar burst fractures. Spine 16:S433–S439, 1991.

32. Dick, W. The "fixateur interne" as a versatile implant for spine surgery. Spine 12:882–900, 1987.

33. Doerr, T.E.; Montesano, P.X.; Burkus, J.K.; et al. Spinal canal decompression in traumatic thoracolumbar burst fractures: Posterior distraction rods versus transpedicular screw fixation. J Orthop Trauma 5:403–411, 1991.

34. Ebelke, D.K.; Asher, M.A.; Neff, J.R.; et al. Survivorship analysis of VSP spine instrumentation in the treatment of thoracolumbar and lumbar burst fractures. Spine 16:S428–S432, 1991.

35. Edwards, C.C.; Levine, A.M. Early rod-sleeve stabilization of the injured thoracic and lumbar spine. Orthop Clin North Am 17:121–145, 1986.

36. Elliot, H.C. Cross sectional diameters and areas of human spinal cord. Anat Rec 93:287–293, 1945.

37. Epstein, N.E.; Epstein, J.A. Limbus lumbar vertebral fractures in 27 adolescents and adults. Spine 16:962–966, 1991.

38. Ferguson, R.L.; Allen, B.L., Jr. A mechanistic classification of thoracolumbar spine fractures. Clin Orthop Relat Res 189:77–88, 1984.

39. Fidler, M.W.; Plasmans, C.M. The effect of four types of support on the segmental mobility of the lumbosacral spine. J Bone Joint Surg [Am] 65:943–947, 1983.

40. Finn, C.A.; Stauffer, E.S. Burst fracture of the fifth lumbar vertebra. J Bone Joint Surg [Am] 74:398–403, 1992.

41. Frankel, H.L.; Hancock, D.O.; Hyslop, G.; et al. The value of postural reduction in the initial management of closed injuries of the spine with paraplegia and tetraplegia. I. Paraplegia 7:179–192, 1969.

42. Fredrickson, B.E.; Yuan, H.A.; Miller, H. Burst fractures of the fifth lumbar vertebra. A report of four cases. J Bone Joint Surg [Am] 64:1088–1094, 1982.

43. Gardner, V.O.; Thalgott, J.S.; White, J.I.; et al. The contoured anterior spinal plate system (CASP). Indications, techniques, and results. Spine 19:550–555, 1994.

44. Gellad, F.E.; Levine, A.M.; Joslyn, J.N.; et al. Pure thoracolumbar facet dislocation: Clinical features and CT appearance. Radiology 161:505–508, 1986.

45. Gertzbein, S.D.; Court-Brown, C.M. Flexion–distraction injuries of the lumbar spine. Mechanisms of injury and classification. Clin Orthop Relat Res 227:52–60, 1988.

46. Gumley, G.; Taylor, T.K.; Ryan, M.D. Distraction fractures of the lumbar spine. J Bone Joint Surg [Br] 64:520–525, 1982.

47. Gurwitz, G.S.; Dawson, J.M.; McNamara, M.J.; et al. Biomechanical analysis of three surgical approaches for lumbar burst fractures using short-segment instrumentation. Spine 18:977–982, 1993.

48. Haddad, G.H.; Zickel, R.E. Intestinal perforation and fracture of lumbar vertebra caused by lap-type seat belt. N Y State J Med 67:930–932, 1967.

49. Handel, S.F.; Twiford, T.W., Jr.; Reigel, D.H.; et al. Posterior lumbar apophyseal fractures. Radiology 130:629–633, 1979.

50. Hardaker, W.T., Jr.; Cook, W.A., Jr.; Friedman, A.H.; et al. Bilateral transpedicular decompression and Harrington rod stabilization in the management of severe thoracolumbar burst fractures. Spine 17:162–171, 1992.

51. Harrington, R.M.; Budorick, T.; Hoyt, J.; et al. Biomechanics of indirect reduction of bone retropulsed into the spinal canal in vertebral fracture. Spine 18:692–699, 1993.

52. Heary, R.F.; Salas, S.; Bono, C.M.; et al. Complication avoidance: Thoracolumbar and lumbar burst fractures. Neurosurg Clin N Am 17:377–388, viii, 2006.

53. Holdsworth, F.W. Fractures, dislocations and fracture–dislocations of the spine. J Bone Joint Surg [Br] 45:6–20, 1963.

54. Holdsworth, F.W.; Hardy, A. Early treatment of paraplegia from fractures of the thoraco-lumbar spine. J Bone Joint Surg [Br] 35:540–550, 1953.

55. Hu, S.S.; Capen, D.A.; Rimoldi, R.L.; et al. The effect of surgical decompression on neurologic outcome after lumbar fractures. Clin Orthop Relat Res 288:166–173, 1993.

56. Huang, T.J.; Chen, J.Y.; Shih, H.N.; et al. Surgical indications in low lumbar burst fractures: Experiences with Anterior Locking Plate System and the reduction–fixation system. J Trauma 39:910–914, 1995.

57. Jeanneret, B.; Ho, P.K.; Magerl, F. Burst–shear flexion–distraction injuries of the lumbar spine. J Spinal Disord 6:473–481, 1993.

58. Knight, R.Q.; Stornelli, D.P.; Chan, D.P.; et al. Comparison of operative versus nonoperative treatment of lumbar burst fractures. Clin Orthop Relat Res 293:112–121, 1993.

59. Kostuik, J.P.; Munting, E.; Valdevit, A. Biomechanical analysis of screw load sharing in pedicle fixation of the lumbar spine. J Spinal Disord 7:394–401, 1994.

60. Krag, M.H.; Beynnon, B.D.; Pope, M.H.; et al. An internal fixator for posterior application to short segments of the thoracic, lumbar, or lumbosacral spine. Design and testing. Clin Orthop Relat Res 203:75–98, 1986.

61. Krag, M.H.; Weaver, D.L.; Beynnon, B.D.; et al. Morphometry of the thoracic and lumbar spine related to transpedicular screw placement for surgical spinal fixation. Spine 13:27–32, 1988.

62. Kreitz, B.G.; Cote, P.; Cassidy, J.D. L5 vertebral compression fracture: A series of five cases. J Manipulative Physiol Ther 18:91–97, 1995.

63. Krompinger, W.J.; Fredrickson, B.E.; Mino, D.E.; et al. Conservative treatment of fractures of the thoracic and lumbar spine. Orthop Clin North Am 17:161–170, 1986.

64. Lagrone, M.O.; Bradford, D.S.; Moe, J.H.; et al. Treatment of symptomatic flatback after spinal fusion. J Bone Joint Surg [Am] 70:569–580, 1988.

65. Lemons, V.R.; Wagner, F.C., Jr.; Montesano, P.X. Management of thoracolumbar fractures with accompanying neurological injury. Neurosurgery 30:667–671, 1992.

66. Levine, A.M. The surgical treatment of low lumbar fractures. Semin Spine Surg 2:41–53, 1990.

67. Levine, A.M. Dural lacerations in low lumbar burst fractures. Presented at the AAOS Meeting, Washington, D.C., February 1992.

68. Levine, A.M. The long term follow-up of patients with L4 and L5 burst fractures treated with surgical stabilization. Submitted for publication.

69. Levine, A.M.; Edwards, C.C. In Camins, M., & O'Leary, P., eds. The Lumbar Spine. New York, Raven, 1987.

70. Levine, A.M.; Bosse, M.; Edwards, C.C. Bilateral facet dislocations in the thoracolumbar spine. Spine 13:630–640, 1988.

71. Levine, A.M.; Edwards, C.C. Low lumbar burst fractures. Reduction and stabilization using the modular spine fixation system. Orthopedics 11:1427–1432, 1988.

72. Levine, A.M.; Edwards, C.C.; Gellad, F.E. Indirect decompression of the spinal canal in the thoracolumbar spine. American Spinal Injury Association, Abstracts Digest March 20-22:16–18, 1987.

SECTION 2 • Spine

1016

SECTION 2 • Spine

73. Lewis, J.; McKibbin, B. The treatment of unstable fracture–dislocations of the thoraco-lumbar spine accompanied by paraplegia. J Bone Joint Surg [Br] 56:603–612, 1974.

74. Lindahl, S.; Willen, J.; Nordwall, A.; et al. The crush-cleavage fracture. A "new" thoracolumbar unstable fracture. Spine 8:559–569, 1983.

75. Louis, C.A.; Gauthier, V.Y.; Louis, R.P. Posterior approach with Louis plates for fractures of the thoraco-lumbar and lumbar spine with and without neurologic deficits. Spine 23:2030–2039, 1998.

76. Louis, R. Fusion of the lumbar and sacral spine by internal fixation with screw plates. Clin Orthop Relat Res 203:18–33, 1986.

77. Magerl, F.P. In Uhthoff, H.K. ed. Current Concepts of External Fixation of Fractures. New York, Springer-Verlag, pp. 353–366, 1982.

78. Magerl, F.P. Stabilization of the lower thoracic and lumbar spine with external skeletal fixation. Clin Orthop Relat Res 189:125–141, 1984.

79. Maiman, D.J.; Pintar, F.; Yoganandan, N.; et al. Effects of anterior vertebral grafting on the traumatized lumbar spine after pedicle screw–plate fixation. Spine 18:2423–2430, 1993.

80. Mann, K.A.; Found, E.M.; Yuan, H.A. Biomechanical evaluation of the effectiveness of anterior spinal fixation system. Orthop Trans 11:378, 1987.

81. Marshall, D.; Johnell, O.; Wedel, H. Meta-analysis of how well measures of bone mineral density predict occurrence of osteoporotic fractures. BMJ 312:1254–1259, 1996.

82. McAfee, P.C.; Bohlman, H.H.; Yuan, H.A. Anterior decompression of traumatic thoracolumbar fractures with incomplete neurological deficit using a retroperitoneal approach. J Bone Joint Surg [Am] 67:89–104, 1985.

83. McAfee, P.C.; Yuan, H.A.; Fredrickson, B.E.; et al. The value of computed tomography in thoracolumbar fractures. An analysis of one hundred consecutive cases and a new classification. J Bone Joint Surg [Am] 65:461–473, 1983.

84. Melton, L.J., III; Lane, A.W.; Cooper, C.; et al. Prevalence and incidence of vertebral deformities. Osteoporos Int 3:113–119, 1993.

85. Micheli, L.J. Low back pain in the adolescent: Differential diagnosis. Am J Sports Med 7:362–364, 1979.

86. Mick, C.A.; Carl, A.; Sachs, B.; et al. Burst fractures of the fifth lumbar vertebra. Spine 18:1878–1884, 1993.

87. Mirkovic, S.; Abitbol, J.J.; Steinman, J.; et al. Anatomic consideration for sacral screw placement. Spine 16:S289–S294, 1991.

88. Miyakoshi, N.; Abe, E.; Shimada, Y.; et al. Anterior decompression with single segmental spinal interbody fusion for lumbar burst fracture. Spine 24:67–73, 1999.

89. Mumford, J.; Weinstein, J.N.; Spratt, K.F.; et al. Thoracolumbar burst fractures. The clinical efficacy and outcome of nonoperative management. Spine 18:955–970, 1993.

90. Neumann, P.; Nordwall, A.; Osvalder, A.L. Traumatic instability of the lumbar spine. A dynamic in vitro study of flexion–distraction injury. Spine 20:1111–1121, 1995.

91. Nevitt, M.C.; Ross, P.D.; Palermo, L.; et al. Association of prevalent vertebral fractures, bone density, and alendronate treatment with incident vertebral fractures: Effect of number and spinal location of fractures. The Fracture Intervention Trial Research Group. Bone 25:613–619, 1999.

92. O'Callaghan, J.P.; Ullrich, C.G.; Yuan, H.A.; et al. CT of facet distraction in flexion injuries of the thoracolumbar spine: The "naked" facet. AJR Am J Roentgenol 134:563–568, 1980.

93. Olerud, S.; Karlstrom, G.; Sjostrom, L. Transpedicular fixation of thoracolumbar vertebral fractures. Clin Orthop Relat Res 227:44–51, 1988.

94. Olinger, A.; Hildebrandt, U.; Mutschler, W.; et al. First clinical experience with an endoscopic retroperitoneal approach for anterior fusion of lumbar spine fractures from levels T12 to L5. Surg Endosc 13:1215–1219, 1999.

95. Ozturk, C.; Ersozlu, S.; Aydinli, U. Importance of greenstick lamina fractures in low lumbar burst fractures. Int Orthop 30:295–298, 2006.

96. Panjabi, M.M.; Oda, T.; Wang, J.L. The effects of pedicle screw adjustments on neural spaces in burst fracture surgery. Spine 25:1637–1643, 2000.

97. Parker, J.W.; Lane, J.R.; Karaikovic, E.E.; et al. Successful short-segment instrumentation and fusion for thoracolumbar spine fractures: A consecutive 4½-year series. Spine 25:1157–1170, 2000.

98. Rauschning, W. In Post, J.D., ed. Computed Tomography of the Spine. Baltimore, Williams & Wilkins, pp. 20–67, 1984.

99. Rechtine, G.R.; Cahill, D.; Chrin, A.M. Treatment of thoracolumbar trauma: Comparison of complications of operative versus nonoperative treatment. J Spinal Disord 12:406–409, 1999.

100. Roy-Camille, R.; Saillant, G.; Mazel, C. Plating of thoracic, thoracolumbar, and lumbar injuries with pedicle screw plates. Orthop Clin North Am 17:147–159, 1986.

101. Saillant, G. Etude anatomique des pedicles, vertebraux, application chirurgicales. Rev Chir Orthop Rep Appar Mot 62:151–160, 1976.

102. Scoles, P.V.; Linton, A.E.; Latimer, B.; et al. Vertebral body and posterior element morphology: The normal spine in middle life. Spine 13:1082–1086, 1988.

103. Seybold, E.A.; Sweeney, C.A.; Fredrickson, B.E.; et al. Functional outcome of low lumbar burst fractures. A multicenter review of operative and nonoperative treatment of L3–L5. Spine 24:2154–2161, 1999.

104. Shen, W.J.; Liu, T.J.; Shen, Y.S. Nonoperative treatment versus posterior fixation for thoracolumbar junction burst fractures without neurologic deficit. Spine 26:1038–1045, 2001.

105. Shiba, K.; Katsuki, M.; Ueta, T.; et al. Transpedicular fixation with Zielke instrumentation in the treatment of thoracolumbar and lumbar injuries. Spine 19:1940–1949, 1994.

106. Sjostrom, L.; Jacobsson, O.; Karlstrom, G.; et al. Spinal canal remodelling after stabilization of thoracolumbar burst fractures. Eur Spine J 3:312–317, 1994.

107. Slosar, P.J., Jr.; Patwardhan, A.G.; Lorenz, M.; et al. Instability of the lumbar burst fracture and limitations of transpedicular instrumentation. Spine 20:1452–1461, 1995.

108. Smith, W.S.; Kaufer, H. Patterns and mechanisms of lumbar injuries associated with lap seat belts. J Bone Joint Surg [Am] 51:239–254, 1969.

109. Stagnara, P.; De Mauroy, J.C.; Dran, G.; et al. Reciprocal angulation of vertebral bodies in a sagittal plane: Approach to references for the evaluation of kyphosis and lordosis. Spine 7:335–342, 1982.

110. Steffee, A.D.; Biscup, R.S.; Sitkowski, D.J. Segmental spine plates with pedicle screw fixation. A new internal fixation device for disorders of the lumbar and thoracolumbar spine. Clin Orthop Relat Res 203:45–53, 1986.

111. Stephens, G.C.; Devito, D.P.; McNamara, M.J. Segmental fixation of lumbar burst fractures with Cotrel-Dubousset instrumentation. J Spinal Disord 5:344–348, 1992.

112. Stromsoe, K.; Hem, E.S.; Aunan, E. Unstable vertebral fractures in the lower third of the spine treated with closed reduction and transpedicular posterior fixation: A retrospective analysis of 82 fractures in 78 patients. Eur Spine J 6:239–244, 1997.

113. Takata, K.; Inoue, S.; Takahashi, K.; et al. Fracture of the posterior margin of a lumbar vertebral body. J Bone Joint Surg [Am] 70:589–594, 1988.

114. Thomas, K.C.; Bailey, C.S.; Dvorak, M.F.; et al. Comparison of operative and nonoperative treatment for thoracolumbar burst fractures in patients without neurological deficit: A systematic review. J Neurosurg Spine 4:351–358, 2006.

115. Viale, G.L.; Silvestro, C.; Francaviglia, N.; et al. Transpedicular decompression and stabilization of burst fractures of the lumbar spine. Surg Neurol 40:104–111, 1993.

116. Vornanen, M.J.; Bostman, O.M.; Myllynen, P.J. Reduction of bone retropulsed into the spinal canal in thoracolumbar vertebral body compression burst fractures. A prospective randomized comparative study between Harrington rods and two transpedicular devices. Spine 20:1699–1703, 1995.

117. White, A.A.; Panjabi, M.M. Clinical Biomechanics of the Spine. Philadelphia, Lippincott Williams & Wilkins, 1978.

118. White, A.A.; Panjabi, M.M. The basic kinematics of the human spine. A review of past and current knowledge. Spine 3:12–20, 1978.

119. Whitesides, T.E., Jr. Traumatic kyphosis of the thoracolumbar spine. Clin Orthop Relat Res 128:78–92, 1977.

120. Willen, J.; Lindahl, S.; Irstam, L.; et al. Unstable thoracolumbar fractures. A study by CT and conventional roentgenology of the reduction effect of Harrington instrumentation. Spine 9:214–219, 1984.

121. Winter, R.B. Congenital Deformities of the Spine. New York, Thieme-Stratton, 1983.

122. Wood, K.; Buttermann, G.; Mehbod, A.; et al. Operative compared with nonoperative treatment of a thoracolumbar burst fracture without neurological deficit. A prospective, randomized study. J Bone Joint Surg [Am] 85:773–781, 2003.

123. Yi, L.; Jingping, B.; Gele, J.; et al. Operative versus non-operative treatment for thoracolumbar burst fractures without neurological deficit. Cochrane Database Syst Rev CD005079, 2006.

124. Yuan, H.A.; Garfin, S.R.; Dickman, C.A.; et al. A historical cohort study of pedicle screw fixation in thoracic, lumbar, and sacral spinal fusions. Spine 19:2279S–2296S, 1994.

125. Zindrick, M.R.; Wiltse, L.L.; Doornik, A.; et al. Analysis of the morphometric characteristics of the thoracic and lumbar pedicles. Spine 12:160–166, 1987.

126. Zou, D.; Yoo, J.U.; Edwards, W.T.; et al. Mechanics of anatomic reduction of thoracolumbar burst fractures. Comparison of distraction versus distraction plus lordosis, in the anatomic reduction of the thoracolumbar burst fracture. Spine 18:195–203, 1993.

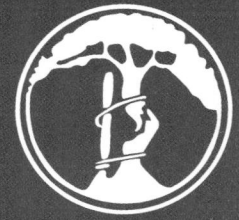

CHAPTER 32

Gunshot Wounds of the Spine

Frank Eismont, M.D. and Jonathan G. Roper, M.D.

DEMOGRAPHICS AND EPIDEMIOLOGY

Firearm injuries are a major cause of trauma worldwide, and in some cities they are the leading cause of death.[8] Legal owning of firearms, youth, and male gender have been reported risk factors for gunshot injuries.[75,77] Bahebeck looked at the incidence, case-fatality rate, and clinical pattern of firearm injuries in two large cities. In both cities firearms are forbidden, restricted to law enforcement officers and registered hunters. They found the incidence of firearm injuries to be 1.14 cases/100,000 per year, which is 5 to 50 times lower than in other cities the same size where firearms are legal, especially in western countries.[2]

Data from the Model Spinal Cord Injury Care Systems and published by the National Spinal Cord Injury Statistical Center are available from 1973 to 2006 and detail the demographics and long-term outcome of more than 24,000 patients with spinal cord injuries. The data list "violence" as the third most common cause of spinal cord injury (SCI) and admission to one of these centers (18.2% overall). The most common cause is motor vehicle accidents (43.4% overall). The second most common cause is falls (19.7% overall). Violence includes gunshot wounds (GSWs) and other activities such as knife injuries, but GSWs constitute the vast majority of the violence category. Over the period from 1973 to 2006, the percentage of patients admitted to these centers as the result of violence has risen and fallen. In the period from 1973 to 1979 the percentage of patients with SCI secondary to violence was 13.3 percent. It increased to 28.9 percent in the years between 1990 and 1994. It has subsequently decreased to 13.8 percent in the years 2000 to 2005. The percentage of patients with SCI secondary to violence from 1973 to 2005 is 18.2 percent. One center shows that violence is the most common cause of SCI at 48.5 percent over the 1973 to 2005 time period. Another center shows that violence is responsible for only 5.7 percent of admissions with SCI over the same period. Over this same period, 86.5 percent of SCIs due to violence were incurred by males. At these same centers, looking at age at admission, of those between birth and 15 years of age, 24 percent were due to violence; at age 16 to 30 years, 23 percent were due to violence; at age 31 to 45 years, 17 percent; at age 46 to 60 years, 8 percent; and at age 61 to 75, 3 percent. From data

published in 1982[84] only 9 percent of penetrating wounds of the spine were classified as job-related injuries, presumably affecting security guards, police officers, and workers shot during robberies. That same database showed that the incidence of SCI due to violence remained constant throughout the year and that 40 percent of SCI due to violence occurred on Saturday and Sunday.

For all SCIs, approximately 47 percent result in paraplegia and 53 percent in quadriplegia, with 60 percent of the thoracic and lumbar injuries being complete injuries and 48 percent of the cervical injuries being complete injuries. A significantly greater number of penetrating wounds of the spine result in complete injuries, with a much greater shift toward thoracic spine injuries, compared with those of the neck or lumbar spine (Fig. 32-1). The incidence of gunshot injuries to the spine is higher in urban areas.[84]

The number of patients with more minor gunshot injuries to the spine with no paralysis is more difficult to estimate because nationwide numbers are not available for this type of injury. Based on what is seen at our medical center and SCI unit, the incidence of GSWs with no paralysis would be very similar to the number of GSWs of the spine with associated paralysis. To broaden the perspective, in 1989 it was estimated that 48,700 people would be killed in motor vehicle accidents and that slightly more than 30,000 civilians would be killed with firearms in the United States.[41] Furthermore, five times as many people are wounded as are killed by gunshots.

WOUND BALLISTICS

The term *ballistics* is defined as "the modern science dealing with the motion and impact of projectiles, especially those discharged from firearms." In a medical sense, the term is described as "the study of effects on the body produced by penetrating projectiles."[13]

To understand the basic concepts of ballistics, it is important to define some other relevant terms:

Mass. The weight of the bullet is usually measured in grams; most range in weight from 2 to 10 g.

Velocity. Bullet velocity can be given in feet per second or in meters per second. A .45-caliber automatic handgun, for example, has a velocity of 869 ft/sec

FIGURE 32-1 | *The bar graphs on the left represent the distribution of the levels of injury for all incomplete and complete spinal cord injuries. The bar graph on the right shows the distribution for penetrating wounds of the spine. Penetrating wounds constitute a higher percentage of complete injuries and, as is evident, a proportionately higher number of thoracic injuries. (From Young, J.A.; Burns, P.E., McCutchen, R. Spinal Cord Injury Statistics: Experience of the Regional Spinal Cord Injury Systems. Phoenix, Good Samaritan Medical Center. pp. 1–152, 1982.)*

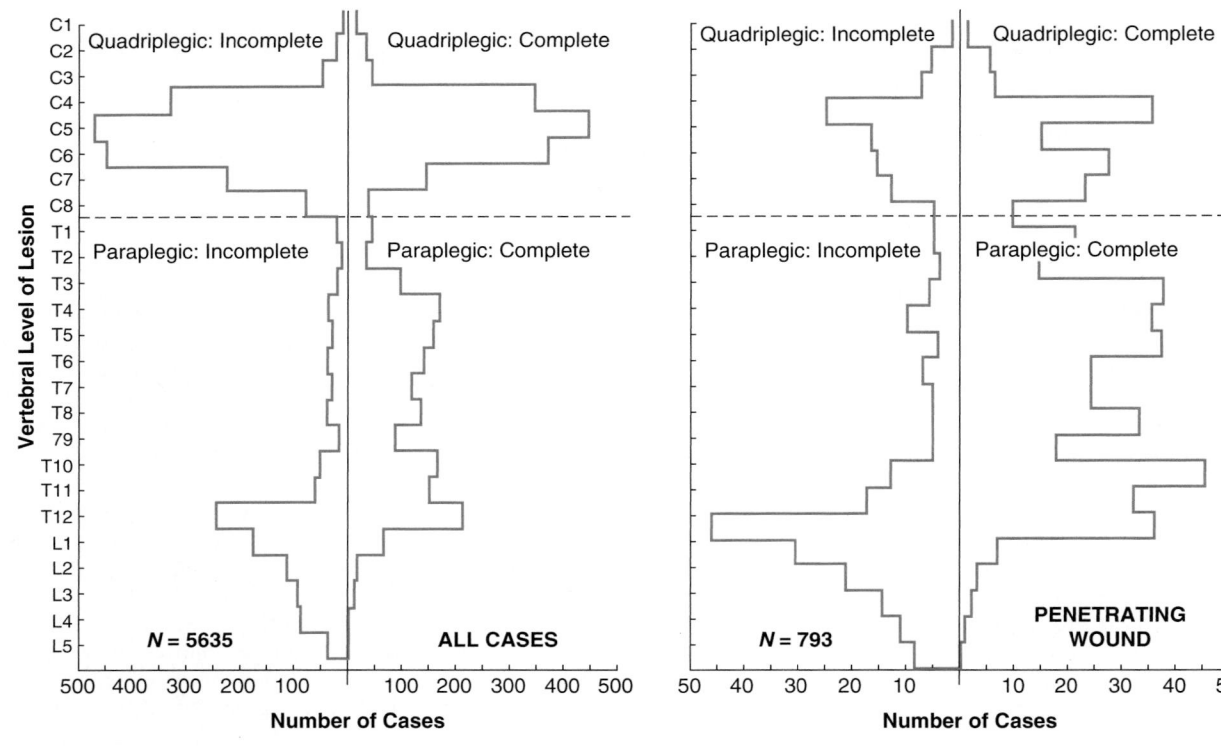

(265 m/sec), a 0.357-caliber Magnum has a velocity of 1393 ft/sec (425 m/sec), and an AK-47 has a velocity of 2340 ft/sec (713 m/sec).

Fragmentation. This describes the extent to which a bullet disintegrates into multiple pieces as it courses through tissue. This is often described by comparing the largest final bullet fragment to its original weight. This is one of the most important factors determining the extent of final tissue injury.

Permanent Cavity. This describes the permanent crushing of tissue resulting from the passage of the bullet.

Temporary Cavity. This describes the stretching of tissue as a result of the passage of the bullet. Elastic tissue, such as muscle, is relatively resistant to damage from this type of stretching, whereas more solid tissue is more significantly damaged under the same circumstances.

To better understand the mechanism of tissue injury with GSWs, it is helpful to study the courses of bullets in tissue or in gelatin tissue simulants.[14,15] Several such illustrations are shown (Figs. 32-2 through 32-4). It is most important to notice how the cross-sectional area of the permanent cavity

varies widely despite significant similarities in the velocities. The tissue effects of bullet fragmentation and yaw (the end-over-end rotation of the bullet) can be appreciated in these illustrations.

Fackler,[13] in an article on misconceptions about wound ballistics, makes the transition from the mechanical science of projectiles to the clinical art of patient care. Among the major misconceptions, he lists an overemphasis on bullet velocity and an exaggeration of tissue damage due to the effects of the temporary cavity. He also points out that many of the positive effects of the administration of systemic antibiotics have been incorrectly attributed to the surgical débridement of tissue. He points out that the incidence of clostridial myositis decreased from 5 percent in World War I to 0.08 percent in the Korean War, even though the débridement techniques remained relatively unchanged during that period. This improvement can be more appropriately attributed to the increasing use of antibiotics on the battlefield. Fackler emphasizes the importance of evaluating the patient both clinically, with a hands-on physical examination, and radiographically, with standard roentgenograms to look for bullet fragmentation, to arrive at the most appropriate treatment.

These figures represent the injury profile as seen after discharging weapons through a gelatin medium. Note that for the first 15 cm of travel through tissue, the injury patterns are extremely similar despite a significant difference in bullet velocity. It is not until the bullet yaws that the permanent cavity becomes significantly larger for a rifle injury as opposed to a handgun injury. (From Fackler, M.L.; Bellamy, R.F.; Malinowski, J.A. The wound profile: Illustration of the missile-tissue interaction. J Trauma 28 (Suppl):S21–S29, 1988.)

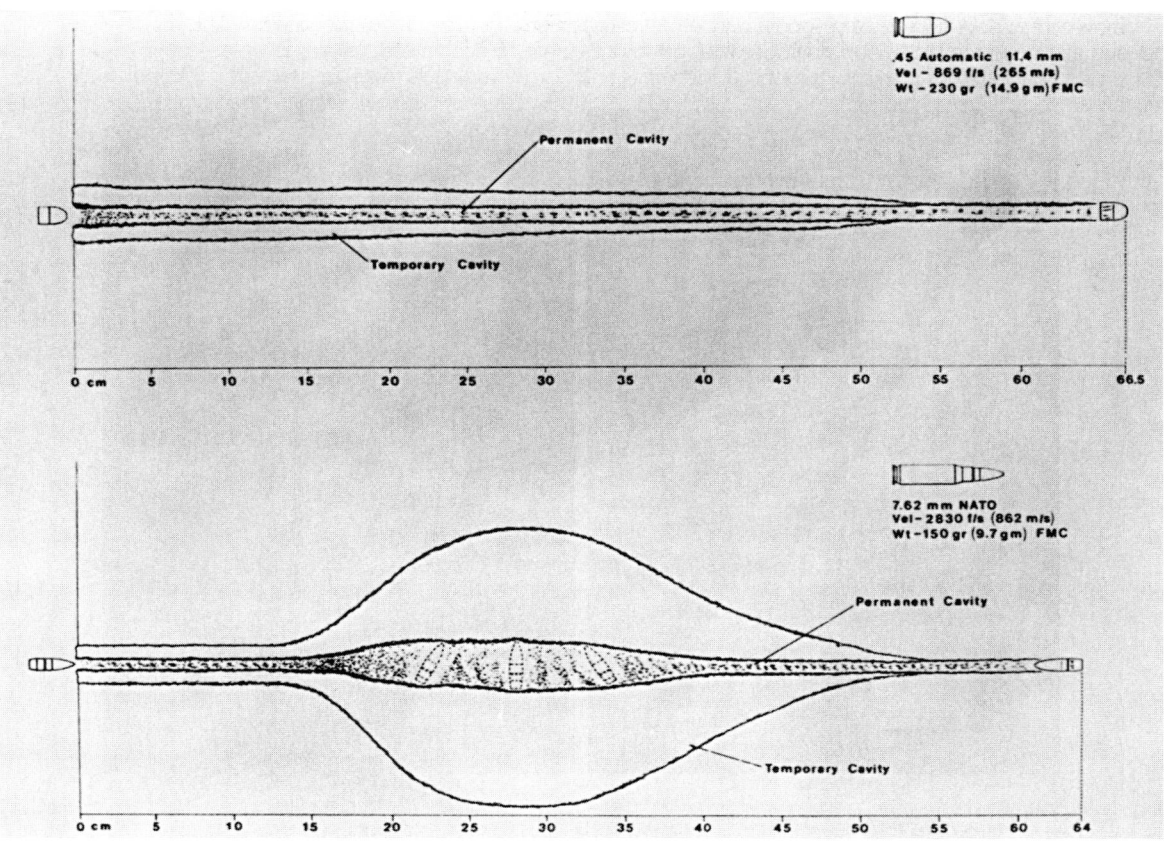

This wound profile is from the same rifle represented by the lower graph in Figure 32-2. The permanent cavity is significantly larger in this case, and this is entirely due to the use of a soft-point bullet, which leads to significant bullet fragmentation. (From Fackler, M.L.; Bellamy, R.F.; Malinowski, J.A. The wound profile: Illustration of the missile-tissue interaction. J Trauma 28 (Suppl):S21–S29, 1988.)

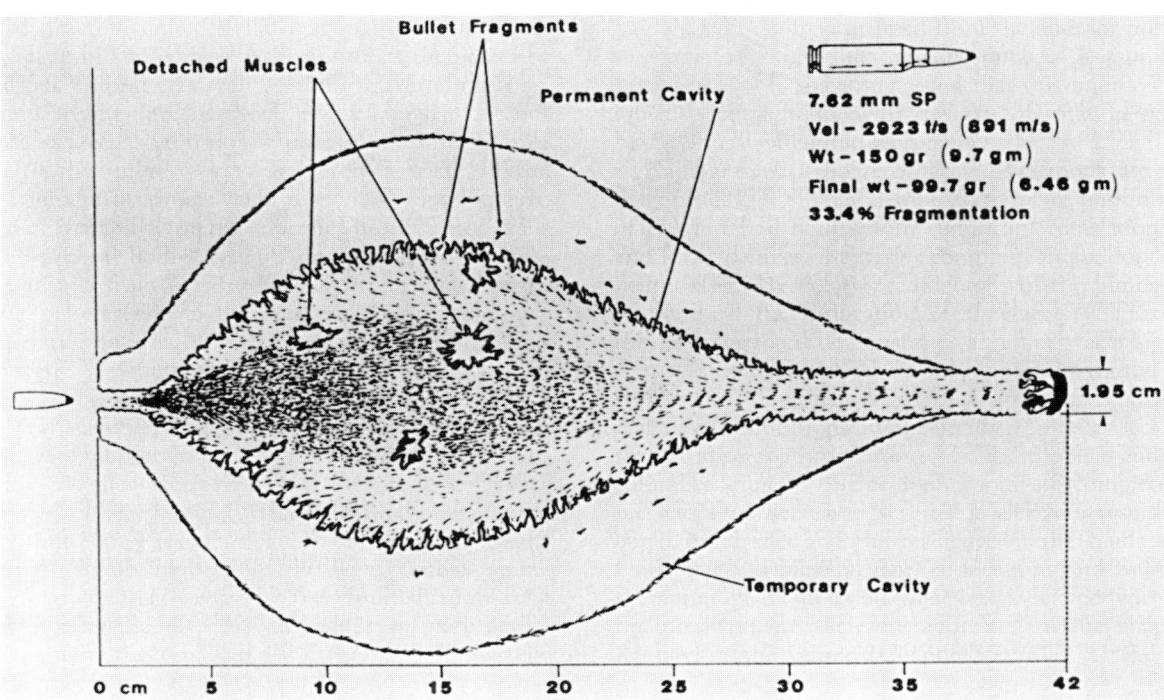

FIGURE 32-4   ***A, B,*** *These wound profiles were obtained using a small sphere at a high velocity to compare the injury with a large sphere at a slower velocity. The kinetic energy (E = mv^2) is the same in each of the two examples. However, the larger sphere penetrates 30 cm deeper and produces a permanent cavity more than 50 times the volume of that produced by the smaller sphere. (From Fackler, M.L. Wound ballistics: A review of common misconceptions. JAMA 259:2730–2736, 1988.)*

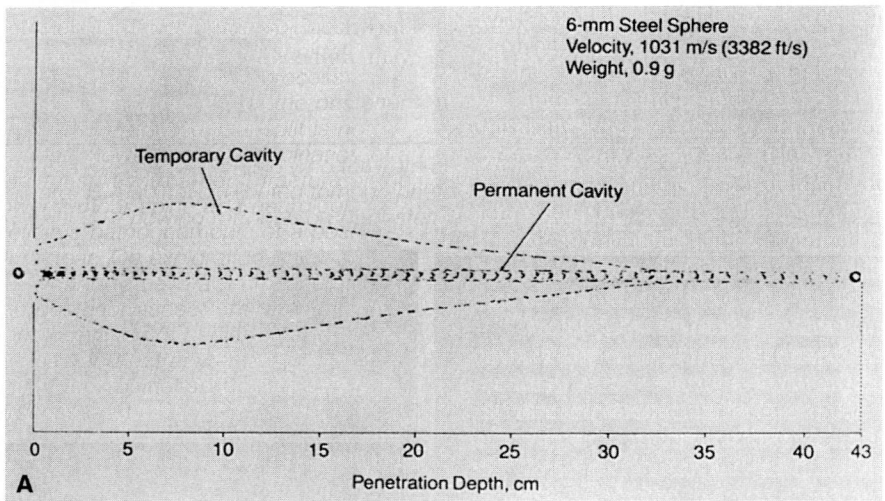

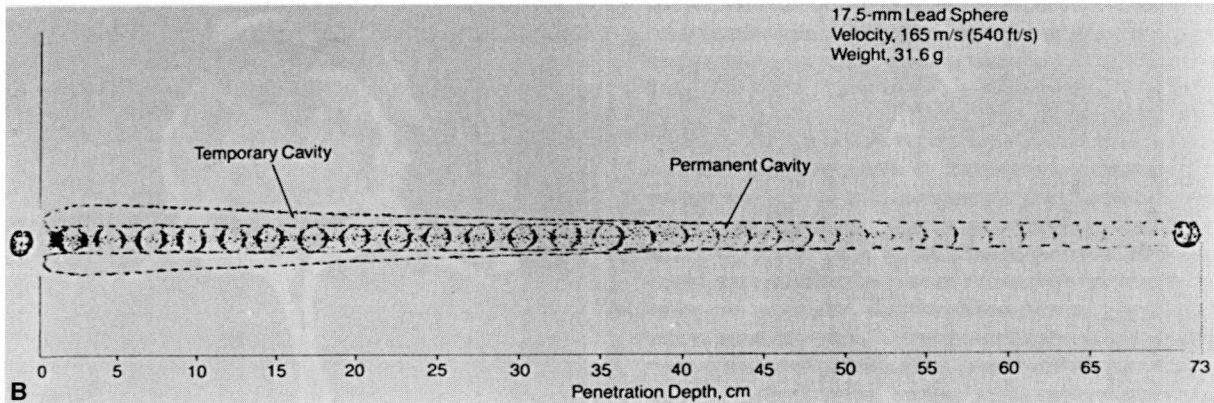

Composition of Bullets

The bullet projectile is most commonly composed of lead, but a portion of the bullet may occasionally consist of either copper or brass. It is known that a systemic toxic response may occur to the lead that leaches out of a bullet, and this has been well described when bullets are bathed in synovial joint fluid[38,72,79] or lodged in the intervertebral disk space.[20] The exact incidence of this problem with GSWs of the spine is unknown, but it is thought to be quite uncommon. If lead toxicity is suspected, serum lead levels are diagnostic; if lead levels are significantly elevated, a bone marrow aspiration may be required to assess hematopoietic toxicity. If lead toxicity can indeed be proved, then surgical excision of the bullet is indicated.

The toxicity of lead, copper, and brass at a more local level has been thoroughly investigated in brain tissue.[9,66,67] It has been found that copper, when evaluated in the monkey brain, causes a severe necrotic local reaction, which is minimally evident with lead and nickel-coated pellets. The necrotic reaction can be so severe as to allow significant migration of the copper-coated pellet through the brain, whereas the other metal pellets remain in place.[67] This is also seen when a copper powder is sprayed on monkey brain; again, a severe necrotizing foreign-body reaction is appreciated, which results in death of the animal.[9]

A study on the effects of bullet fragments on the spinal cord in a rabbit model has been published that shows a great variation depending on the intraspinal fragment location and the fragment metallic composition. Three types of fragments were tested, including aluminum ("silver-tipped" bullets), lead, and copper. If these were placed directly on the dura, none had any effect on the microscopic appearance of the spinal cord other than minor effects of a local spinal cord compression. If the fragments were placed intradurally and in contact with the spinal cord, there was a tremendous variation in local effect on the spinal cord. The aluminum fragment had minimal effect (Fig. 32-5), the lead produced moderate local myelin and axon destruction (Fig. 32-6), and the copper fragment produced severe local myelin and axon destruction (Fig. 32-7). The rabbits with implanted copper fragments were the only group with elevated serum levels of the metal.[74]

FIGURE 32-5 *Axial cross sections through a rabbit spinal cord with an implanted intradural aluminum fragment. **A,** Image showing some indentation of the spinal cord (arrowheads) (solochrome-cyanin, ×5). **B,** Image showing minimal-to-no gliosis of the underlying spinal cord tissue. The surrounding connective-tissue matrix remains well organized (solochrome-cyanin, ×20). (From Tindel, N.L.; Marcillo, A.E.; Tay, B.; et al. The effect of surgically implanted bullet fragments on the spinal cord in a rabbit model. J Bone Joint Surg [Am] 83:884–890, 2001.)*

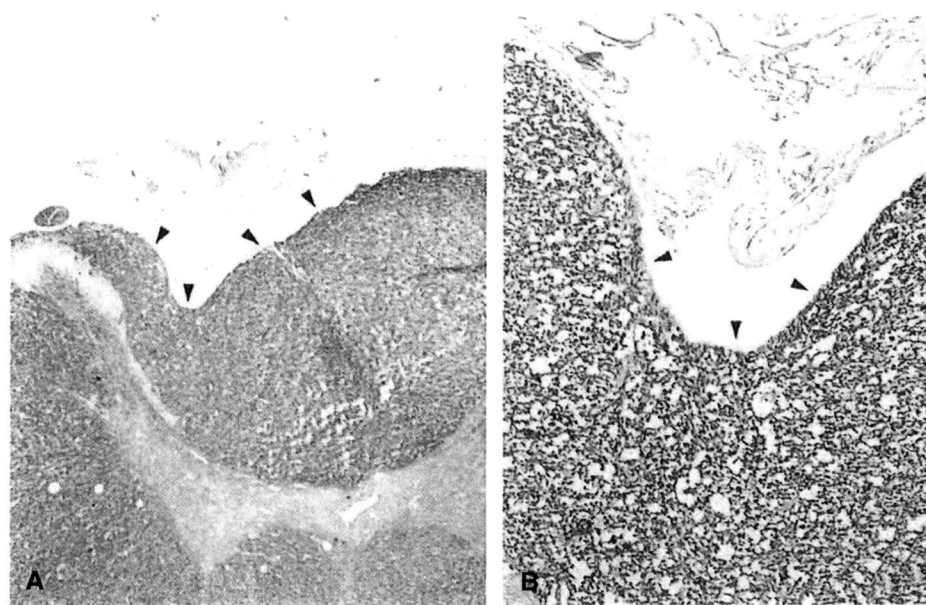

On the basis of this animal research, it is recommended that copper-jacketed bullets be removed from the spinal canal regardless of other considerations. Most often, however, it is not known if a bullet is copper-jacketed. The presence of wadding in the back of a shotgun cartridge must be appreciated for clinical reasons. Shotgun pellets are easily appreciated on plain radiographs, but the wadding of the shotgun is not apparent on plain radiograph, and it often acts as a significant foreign body unless it is removed. If a patient is shot with a shotgun at close range (≤6 m), the shotgun wadding should be sought within the wounds[4,61,42] (Fig. 32-8).

Pathology of Spinal Gunshot Wounds

Pathologic specimens have been collected and described following World War I. The War Office Collection contains 50 specimens, and these have been described in the

FIGURE 32-6 *Axial cross sections through a rabbit spinal cord with an implanted intradural lead fragment. **A,** Image showing indentation of the dorsal column with a small area of gliosis adjacent to the area of depression (arrow) (hematoxylin and eosin, ×20). **B,** Image showing areas of gliosis and breakdown of supporting matrix (arrows) (hematoxylin and eosin, ×40). **C,** Image demonstrating loss of axonal elements with disorganization of the surrounding connective tissue adjacent to the area of fragment implantation (arrows) (solochrome-cyanin, ×40). (From Tindel, N.L.; Marcillo, A.E.; Tay, B.; et al. The effect of surgically implanted bullet fragments on the spinal cord in a rabbit model. J Bone Joint Surg [Am] 83:884–890, 2001.)*

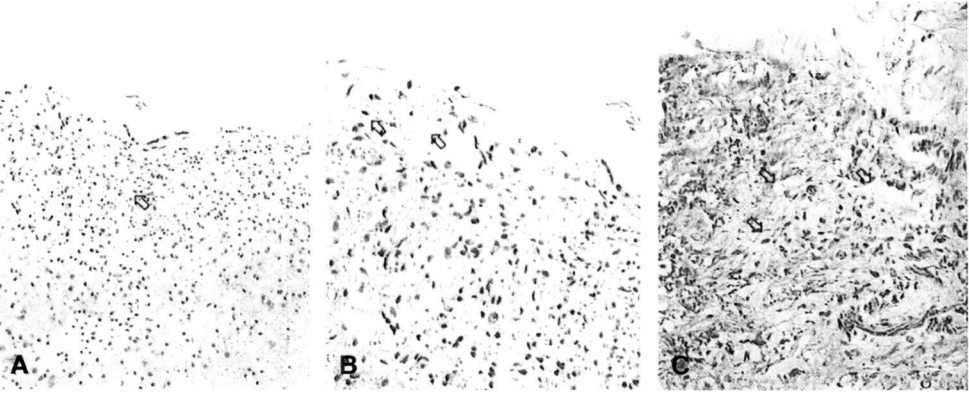

FIGURE 32-7   *Axial cross sections through the spinal cords of rabbits with an implanted copper bullet fragment. **A,** An extradurally placed fragment caused no deformation or injury to the underlying spinal cord (trichrome, ×5). **B,** Image showing indentation and injury to the underlying spinal cord tissue from an intradurally placed copper fragment (arrows) (×5). **C,** Image showing destruction of the spinal cord parenchyma (arrows). The damage is confined to the white matter (A); the gray matter (B) is preserved (hematoxylin and eosin, ×40). **D,** Image showing vacuolization of the adjacent spinal cord tissue (arrows) with damage localized to the white matter (A); there is no damage in the gray matter (B) (solochrome-cyanin, ×40). **E,** Image showing disruption of the connective-tissue matrix adjacent to the site of implantation of the bullet fragment (arrows) (trichrome, ×40). (From Tindel, N.L.; Marcillo, A.E.; Tay, B.; et al. The effect of surgically implanted bullet fragments on the spinal cord in a rabbit model. J Bone Joint Surg [Am] 83:884–890, 2001.)*

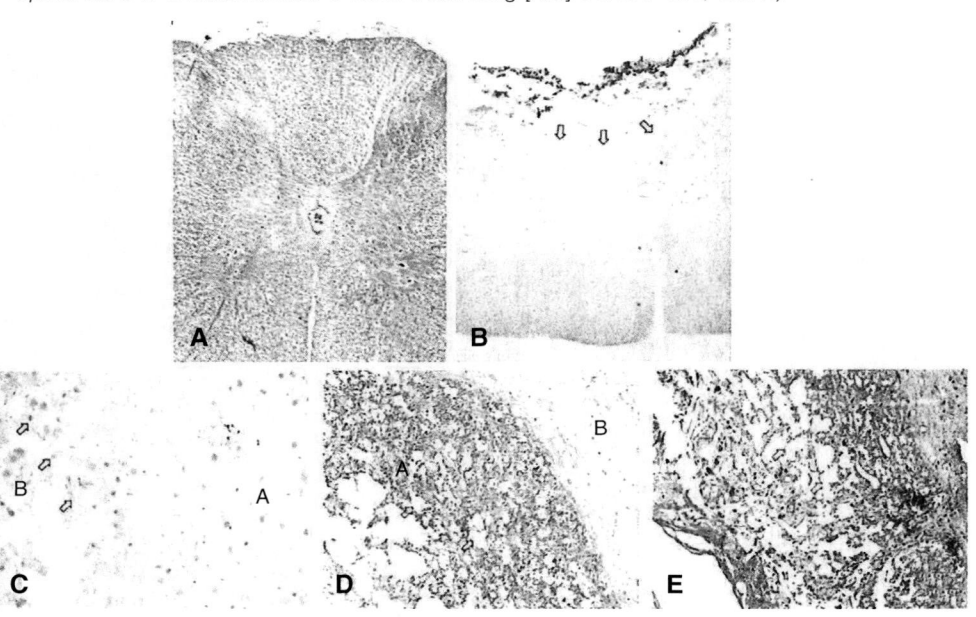

FIGURE 32-8   ***A, B,*** *This patient was shot in the back of the neck with a pellet shotgun. He sustained complete quadriplegia as a result of the injury. It is important to recognize that removal of the pellets is not indicated, but surgical débridement, and especially a removal of the shotgun wadding, is necessary to prevent infection as this was a close-range injury. (From Eismont, F.; Lattuga, S. Gunshot wounds of the spine. In: Browner, B.D.; Jupiter, J.B.; Levine, A.M.; et al. eds. Skeletal Trauma, 2nd ed. Philadelphia, W.B. Saunders, p. 1100, 1997.)*

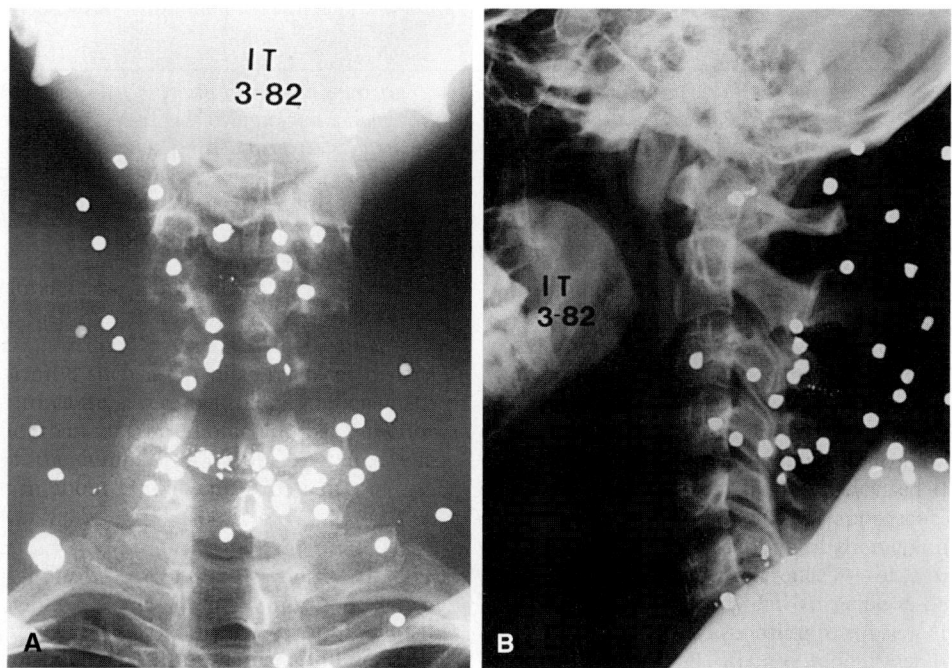

literature.[28] They show considerable variation, from relatively mild bone or ligament injuries to severe disruptions of the spinal column. Keith and Hall[28] noted that the spinal cord was often intact, although the patient had sustained a complete spinal cord injury. They assumed that this was due to contusion of the spinal cord. They also noted that with injuries to the posterior arch or pedicles, associated secondary fractures of the vertebral body were common. However, when the vertebral body was the primary site of gunshot injury, secondary injury to the posterior elements seldom occurred. They presumed that this was due to the vertebral body being composed primarily of cancellous bone, which is more easily deformed and hence transmits less energy to adjacent structures.

Klemperer and colleagues[32] investigated the pathology of indirect injuries to the spinal cord in an animal model. They produced gunshot injuries to the posterior spinous processes or interspinous ligaments in anesthetized animals. They found that whether spinal cord injury was achieved or not, and whether the spinal cord injury was complete or incomplete, showed a severe species variation. This most likely correlated with the size of the spinal canal relative to the size of the spinal cord. In subjects with extremely small canals, the incidence of spinal cord injury was extremely high. The pathologic sections of the spinal cord varied, as would be expected, but it was interesting that significant pathologic changes often were noted within the spinal cord even in some animals that had not sustained any paralysis.

Mirovsky and colleagues[45] performed a retrospective review of all patients with neurologic deficit following gunshot wounds that did not penetrate the spinal canal. They identified 26 cases with either complete or incomplete paraplegia that were managed from 1977 to 2003. They found three patients with complete paraplegia at the thoracic level who did not indicate any sign of canal compromise. At average follow-up of 4.1 years, none had any neurologic recovery. They did not comment on the size of the spinal canal; however, all injuries were at the thoracic level, where the ratio of spinal cord to canal size is the highest. Their results were similar with those of Stauffer and colleagues,[71] who reported on 185 patients with gunshot wounds of the spine. They had 106 patients with a complete lesion and 79 with an incomplete lesion. A total of 101 patients underwent laminectomy. They found that the spinal cord appeared normal in six patients with complete injury and in five patients with an incomplete injury. The most likely mechanism is that the kinetic energy of the passing bullet imparts a concussive injury to the spinal cord. In addition this energy may also disrupt or thrombose the vascular supply to the spinal cord.

PATIENT EVALUATION

The evaluation of patients with gunshot wounds of the spine should include the same detailed history, physical examination, and radiographic evaluation as would be performed for patients with other suspected spine injuries. Attention is first given to the ABCs of emergency treatment protocols.

The history should include a general description of the weapon (e.g., handgun, rifle, assault weapon). Very often this information is not available, but it can be helpful if known. The patient should also be questioned as to whether any paralysis or paresthesias occurred immediately following the injury. If the patient did indeed have an episode of transient paralysis, a more detailed neurologic follow-up is indicated.

The importance of the physical examination cannot be overemphasized. This should include examination of the entrance and exit wounds, and the tissue should be palpated to assess the presence of crepitance and the general turgor of the tissue. The presence of a very large exit wound and the presence of crepitance and increased tissue turgor are consistent with wounds that have a large permanent cavity and may very well have significant tissue necrosis.[14] The physical examination should also include a good, detailed neurologic examination. The presence of paralysis or any abnormal reflexes should be documented.

The radiographic evaluation of the patient is also extremely important. Attention should be paid to the fracture type and the degree of bone comminution. The radiograph should also be scrutinized to see if the bullet remains in the torso and to assess the extent of bullet fragmentation. Increased bone comminution and bullet fragmentation should alert the treating physician to a possible association with a significant permanent cavity. Such a case may be one of the few instances in which significant wound débridement is required.[14]

Computed tomography (CT) may help to further assess the extent of the spine injury and the extent of spinal canal encroachment by bone or bullet fragments. The stability of the spine can also be better assessed with the help of CT; this is addressed in the later discussion of spine stability. The general surgical team that is helping to assess the patient may recommend other studies to evaluate the extent of soft tissue injuries to structures adjacent to the spine.[3] These might include a barium swallow, arteriography, and intravenous pyelogram.

Klein and colleagues performed a retrospective analysis of 2450 patients who were treated for gunshot wounds at the Ryder Trauma Center in Miami from 1991 to 2001.[31] They found that 10 percent (244) had associated spine injuries, 13 percent of whom had significant spinal injuries but presented without any neurologic symptoms. They concluded that a complete radiographic spine evaluation is mandatory after gunshot wounds to the face, neck, or trunk even without neurologic deficit.

The use of magnetic resonance imaging (MRI) in the evaluation of wounds with retained metallic ballistic fragments remains controversial. In general, radiologists are reluctant to perform MRI for patients with retained metallic bullet fragments.[53,65,73] This reluctance is heightened for those patients with retained fragments near vital and susceptible anatomic structures such as the spinal cord. Finitsis and co-workers evaluated the spine in 19 patients with metallic bullet fragments using MRI.[16] Eighteen of the 19 patients had a previously acquired quadriplegia or paraplegia. The MRIs were obtained acutely in 6 patients with gunshot injuries, and in 13 patients who were from 1 month to several years from their injury. There were no complications with the imaging study. They noted that patients with fragments known to be strongly ferromagnetic, such as the ball-bearing or Prometheus type of air gun pellets,[49] were not included. MRI studies established diagnoses in 17 patients (5 acute/subacute and 12 chronic). In those two cases in which the MRI was deemed suboptimal, artifact precluded exclusion of a spinal lesion in the region of interest. Imaging artifacts in these two patients were the result of multiple small metallic fragments associated with a dominant (>1 cm) metallic fragment. In the six recently injured patients, two had a cord contusion and two had an epidural hematoma with cord compression that was subsequently treated surgically. In the 13 chronically injured patients, 4 studies yielded negative results for cyst, scarring, atrophy, or a compressive lesion. One patient had a bullet embedded in the cord with a cyst above and below it, and one patient was diagnosed with an epidural abscess that was subsequently treated surgically. One study was nondiagnostic because of extensive metallic artifact. The authors of this particular article support the use of MRI for patients with retained metallic ballistic fragments in the region of the spine if more information is needed to effectively treat the patient.[16] Readers of this chapter need to understand that this is an area of controversy and that there are at least potential risks with this diagnostic approach. A myelogram followed by immediate CT and a 4-hour delayed CT scan remains the traditional method to assess the spinal neural elements following a gunshot injury of the spine.

TREATMENT OF GUNSHOT WOUNDS OF THE SPINE

Wound Care

In some cases, performing local wound care is more appropriate in the emergency department, and in other cases it is more appropriate in the operating room. The operating room is more appropriate for treating large exit wounds and when physical and radiographic findings suggest the presence of large permanent cavities. Although this type of wound is uncommon in civilian practice, it is important to recognize that such cases exist.

Because of the proximity of the esophagus, the major blood vessels, and the larynx and trachea in wounds of the neck, general surgeons in the past were extremely aggressive with recommending operative exploration. The traditional recommendation had been to explore all penetrating neck wounds.[60] Now it is more often advocated that only those neck wounds with signs of serious injury be explored and those without specific warning signs of major injury be observed.[50,64] The same is true for penetrating injuries of the chest and abdomen.[3] The availability of emergency arteriography coupled with the use of intravascular hemostatic coils has also changed the indications for emergency exploratory surgery. Many cases previously requiring surgery to achieve hemostasis can now be managed with minimally invasive techniques (Fig. 32-9).

Wound cultures should always be taken from the bullet tract. If the wound has been contaminated by the passage of the bullet through the pharynx, esophagus, or colon, or if the wound has been contaminated following injury, it

is even more essential that appropriate cultures be taken. For routine uncontaminated cases, we would recommend 3 days of treatment with parenteral antibiotics, such as a second-generation cephalosporin, at maximal intravenous dosage. If the bullet first penetrated the pharynx,[61,62] the esophagus, or the colon,[58] or if the wound was otherwise contaminated, a different antibiotic regimen is recommended (see discussion in later section on Associated Injuries).

Steroids and Gunshot Wounds to the Spine

The second National Acute Spinal Cord Injury Study (NASCIS 2) was published in 1990. This study demonstrated statistically significant improvements in both motor and sensory function at 6 weeks and 6 months after acute blunt SCI in patients treated with high-dose methylprednisolone. This randomized, double-blind, placebo-controlled trial found no statistically significant increased risk in the complication rates among patients with SCI who received methylprednisolone. The exclusion criteria from NASCIS 2 included all GSW victims.[5] However, some have extrapolated from the results of the study to justify administering steroids to GSW victims. At the present time two retrospective studies are evaluating the efficacy of administration of steroids to SCI patients with GSWs, and neither study documents a benefit of their use. Heary and colleagues performed a retrospective review of 254 patients who were treated for GSWs to the spine.[23] Three subgroups were established: methylprednisolone (NASCIS 2 protocol), dexamethasone (initial dose, 10–100 mg), and no steroids. All patients that received steroids were initially treated at an outside hospital prior to transfer. No patients received steroids at the authors' institution. Of the patients transferred while receiving steroids, 95 percent were transferred within 48 hours of the gunshot injury. No statistically significant neurologic benefits were demonstrable from the use of steroids. The researchers measured neurologic recovery using the motor scales recommended by the American Spinal Injury Association (ASIA) and the Frankel grading system. Infectious complications were increased in both groups receiving steroids (not statistically significant). Gastrointestinal complications were significantly increased in the dexamethasone group, and pancreatitis was significantly increased in the methylprednisolone group. The mean duration of follow-up was 56.3 months. Levy and colleagues found similar results in their retrospective analysis of 236 patients.[40] They had 181 patients who did not receive steroids and 55 patients that were treated according to the NASCIS 2 protocol. The administration of methylprednisolone did not significantly improve functional outcomes in patients with GSW injuries to the spine or increase the number of complications experienced by patients during their hospitalizations. Based on these two studies we do not recommend treatment of these patients with steroids until the efficacy of such treatment is proven in a controlled study.

Assessment and Treatment of Spine Stability

The majority of civilian GSWs of the spine are stable. In assessing the stability in the cervical spine, it has been

FIGURE 32-9 *A, A lateral radiograph following a gunshot wound to the neck at the level of C3-C4. The patient's primary problem was significant bleeding. Angiography revealed an injury to the left vertebral artery. **B**, This lateral film was taken following insertion of a hemostatic coil into the left vertebral artery. This achieved complete hemostasis. **C**, This computed tomographic scan shows the location of the hemostatic coil within the left vertebral artery. (From Eismont, F.; Lattuga, S. Gunshot wounds of the spine. In: Browner, B.D.; Jupiter, J.B.; Levine, A.M.; et al., eds. Skeletal Trauma, 2nd ed. Philadelphia, W.B. Saunders, p. 1100, 1997.)*

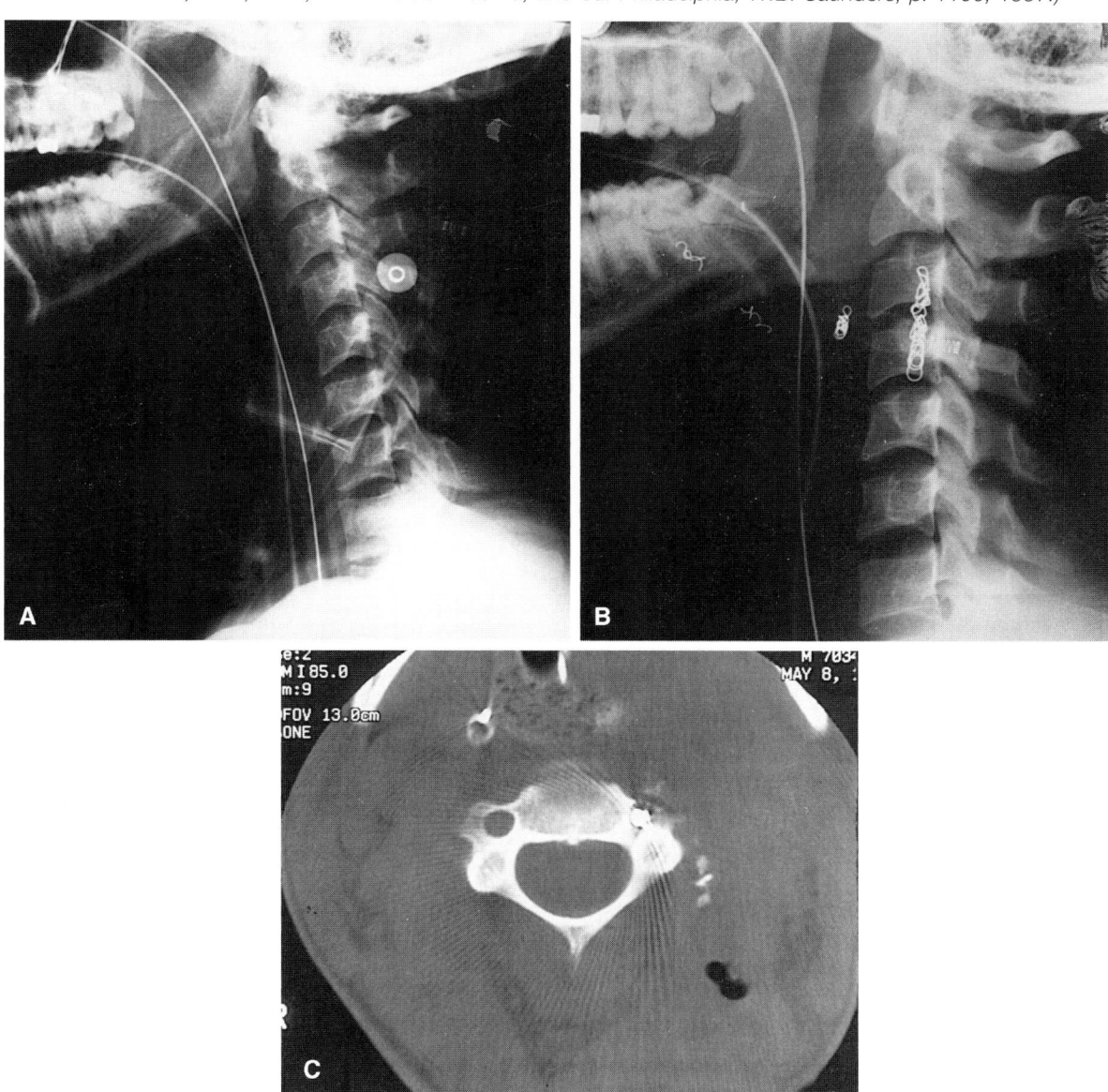

noted that 36 percent of the weight of the head is carried by the anterior vertebral bodies and disks, and 32 percent by each of the two posterolateral columns, which are composed of facet joints and lateral masses.[51]

If none of the three columns is compromised, then no immobilization is recommended. If one of the three columns is disrupted, then a rigid cervical collar is recommended. If two or three of the three columns are disrupted, then halo vest immobilization is recommended. In the thoracic and lumbar spine, the three-column concept of Denis can be applied, but the treating physician must understand that the mechanism of destruction is considerably different from that in the closed injuries for which this classification was designed.[11] If destruction is limited to one of the three columns, then no particular immobilization is needed. If two or three columns are compromised by the GSW, then use of a thoracolumbosacral orthosis (TLSO) is recommended whenever the patient is out of bed.

Unlike closed spinal cord injuries, it is only rarely necessary to operate on a GSW of the spine for purposes of establishing stability. The length of immobilization for these injuries of the cervical, thoracic, or lumbar spine is normally 6 to 8 weeks. At that time, flexion and extension plain film radiographs of the affected region are performed to establish whether the spine has adequately healed and is stable.

The most unstable injuries are seen in small children, in whom the size of the vertebrae is small relative to the size of the bullet. Other factors predisposing to a significant instability of the spine include injuries with severe bone comminution and bullet fragmentation and previous laminectomy.[71] Even in these cases, although the instability may be significant, surgical treatment is seldom indicated. The temporary use of skull-tong traction for severe instability of cervical spine injuries or Roto-Rest bed treatment for severe thoracic or lumbar injuries may be indicated for 2 to 3 weeks; this allows early healing before routine mobilization, using braces as previously described.

Associated Injuries

It is important to consider associated viscus injuries in patients with GSWs of the spine. If the bullet has first penetrated the pharynx,[61,62] esophagus, or colon,[58] then extra precautions should be taken to prevent spine infection. This is essential only when the bullet has first penetrated the viscus and then penetrated the spine, and it does not seem to be clinically important if the bullet first traversed the spine before perforating the viscus. It is surprising that the heat generated by the firing of the bullet does not autosterilize it.[80] The general surgical team normally performs emergency surgery to repair the viscus,[3] place adequate drains, and recommend broad-spectrum antibiotics to cover organisms normally found in the viscus. This is especially important for injuries of the pharynx, esophagus, and colon. It is less important for injuries of the stomach, duodenum, and small intestine, the contents of which are normally sterile; however, spine sepsis has also been rarely reported with GSWs to the other segments of the gastrointestinal tract.[21] In contrast to recommendations of 20 years ago, which promoted radical spine débridement,[59] the best results have been reported by Roffi and co-workers, who recommended minimal spine débridement and protection with 1 to 2 weeks of parenteral antibiotics.[58] The parenteral antibiotics should be broad-spectrum agents directed at the particular bacteria normally associated with injury of the viscus. If complications accompany the viscus repair, the length of time of antibiotic coverage may need to be extended. By following this treatment protocol, the incidence of spine infection has been dramatically decreased, and it is now in the range of 5 to 15 percent for severe injuries involving the pharynx, esophagus, or colon. It is important to remember that spine infections after a GSW can be insidious and that follow-up of at least 6 months is necessary before a patient can be considered free of spinal infection.[22,59]

Kumar and colleagues reported on 33 patients with GSWs to the spine and associated viscus injury, with an average follow-up of 29 months. In 13, the bullet passed through the colon or rectum prior to damaging the spine.[34] All patients had immediate exploratory laparotomy, but none had immediate laminectomy, débridement of the missile tract, or bullet removal. A colostomy was performed in 3 patients, and primary repair or resection and anastomosis was performed in 10 patients. The total duration of antibiotic treatment ranged from 2 to 43 days. Six patients received a single antibiotic (Cefotetan) and seven received multiple antibiotics. Antibiotic coverage

was extended depending on the complications encountered with the viscus repair or resection. Three patients developed peritonitis that required repeated wash-outs. There were no complications related to disk space infection, osteomyelitis, or retained bullet fragments.

Treatment of these transperitoneal colon injuries with a 2-day course of antibiotics plus irrigation of the missile tract at surgery has been recommended in the past.[29] However, considering both the findings of Roffi and colleagues and the small number of patients with colon injuries in this particular series, we would recommend the longer 1- to 2-week course of antibiotics.

Bullet in the Disk Space

Three factors must be considered in deciding whether surgery is indicated when the bullet is located in the disk space. The first consideration is whether lead poisoning will develop. Reports in the literature suggest that the lead is leached out of a bullet that is bathed in synovial fluid, and lead poisoning can subsequently occur.[20,72,79] One article in the literature has suggested that this may also be the case with a lead bullet located within the disk space.[9] At our institution we studied 12 patients that had bullet or bullet fragments within the intervertebral disk space.[63] One of the 12 patients did show evidence of plumbism. She presented 9 years after her injury with constipation and fatigue. Her serum lead level was 136 mg/dL. A normal blood lead level is 0; however, toxicity usually does not develop until the blood serum lead level exceeds 24 mg/dL (ref. 0–24.9 mg/dL). A peripheral blood smear stained with hematoxylin and eosin revealed basophilic stippling. The patient subsequently underwent a partial L4 and L5 laminectomy and diskectomy with excision of the bullet fragment. The patient's serum lead level normalized 6 months following bullet removal, and her complaints completely resolved 2 months postoperatively. A review of the literature does not indicate what percentage of patients with bullets in the disk space will develop lead poisoning in the future; hence, it is not possible to make a sound scientific decision about whether surgery should be recommended routinely. An alternative to routine surgical removal is to obtain a baseline serum lead level, and removal of the bullet is recommended if a rise to an abnormal serum lead level is later noted.

The second consideration includes the mechanical disruption of the motion segment by the presence of a bullet within the disk space. Medical experience for this problem is also anecdotal. This problem can also be followed on a clinical basis. If mechanical-type symptoms develop (e.g., worsening of local pain with upright posture and activity and decrease in local pain with recumbency), and if the symptoms were not present prior to the GSW, then consideration could be given to removal of the bullet combined with local fusion.

The third consideration regarding surgery is whether disk extrusion resulted from a GSW of the spine. If this has occurred, and if the disk extrusion is causing significant symptomatic neural compression, then surgery is indicated for removal of the disk fragments to achieve neural decompression. This occurrence is extremely uncommon, but it has been reported in the literature.[57]

Bullet in the Spinal Canal

Many articles have been written concerning removal of bullets from the spinal canal;[10,24,26,35,54,68,69,71,82] however, until recently, this problem had not been reviewed in a scientific fashion. For conclusions to be valid, the two groups must have equivalent pathology, with one group having bullets removed and the other group having bullets left in place. It is also important that this study be done on a prospective basis, recording adequate neurologic information as well as quantitative assessment of complaints of pain, for example. Such a review was performed by Waters and Adkins.[75] They reviewed cases of 90 patients, of whom 32 had bullet removals and 58 had bullets left in place. They were able to conclude that at the T12–L5 levels statistically significant neurologic motor improvement occurred with removal of the bullet from the spinal canal (Fig. 32-10). There was no difference, however, in sensation or in pain experienced by the patients. In thoracic spine injuries, from T1 to T11, no statistical difference was seen for either complete or incomplete injuries, whether or not the bullet was removed. Similarly, no difference was seen with bullet removal in the cervical spine; however, the authors suggest that the patient numbers were too small to be able to draw statistical conclusions about the cervical spine.

Adding our own subjective opinion to these data, we recommend that patients with cervical injuries undergo bullet removal, as this significantly decreases the degree of spinal cord compression.[7] We even recommend this in cervical complete injuries, not for cord function return, but rather for nerve root improvement at the adjacent level over a period of time. The rationale for doing this is the same as that for closed spinal cord injuries of the cervical spine accompanied by significant residual neural compression by bone or disk fragments, which can show local nerve root improvement following elective decompression.[1,4]

Everyone also agrees that surgery is indicated in patients with bullets in the spinal canal who are experiencing neurologic deterioration. We emphasize, however, that surgery should be performed only in patients in whom compression of the neural elements by bone, disk, bullet, or hematoma has been documented. Such deterioration is extremely uncommon but is occasionally seen (Fig. 32-11). We emphasize that surgery is indicated only with demonstrated compression, as it is also known that neurologic deterioration can occur on the basis of ascending spinal cord necrosis with no residual neural compression and that this particular pathology is not helped by surgery, and in fact, it may be worsened.

There have been a few reports of late neurologic sequelae after GSWs to the spine.[33,48,70,81] These particular reports describe an epidural chronic inflammatory mass as a result of the retained bullet fragment. Most of these cases were caused by a retained bullet in a disk space. Late onset of neurologic symptoms is extremely rare, and we do not recommend removal of retained foreign bodies near or in the spinal canal in order to prevent a possible neurologic deterioration at a later date.

Once the decision has been made to surgically remove the bullet from the spinal canal, it is essential that a scout radiograph be taken in the operating room before the incision is made. The reason for this is that the bullet can occasionally migrate within the spinal canal, depending on the position of the patient.[27,37,83] This is especially true for patients with large spinal canals and relatively small bullets.

Regarding the timing of surgery for removal of bullets from the spinal canal, we normally recommend that this surgery be performed at 7 to 10 days following the injury, because at this time such problems as cerebrospinal fluid (CSF) leakage and dural repair are simplified considerably (Fig. 32-12). This obviously does not apply in cases of significant neurologic deterioration, which, as stated previously, require immediate surgery.

Rate of Neurologic Recovery

We know from the established literature that most spinal cord injuries improve to some extent over time. Complete SCIs usually demonstrate root improvement at one or two levels over time. Incomplete SCIs have a chance for dramatic improvement over time. For incomplete injuries, this includes both improved spinal cord function as well as local root function. An early review of closed and open SCIs at the University of Miami in the early 1980s showed that patients with open SCIs (the majority of these were due to GSWs) still showed statistically significant neurologic improvement at 6 months follow-up, but the improvements started slightly later than in those with closed injuries. This was true for both incomplete and complete open SCIs.[19] This is illustrated in Figure 32-13.

COMPLICATIONS OF GUNSHOT WOUNDS OF THE SPINE

Cerebrospinal Fluid–Cutaneous Fistulas

CSF-cutaneous fistulas have been described after GSWs of the spine. These can sometimes be seen as a direct result of the GSW[76]; however, they are seen most commonly following acute surgical treatment with laminectomy (Fig. 32-14). Stauffer and co-workers[71] described their experience with 185 patients and noted that of those not having laminectomies, the incidence of CSF-cutaneous fistulas was 0 percent. In those treated with laminectomy, "spinal débridement," and bullet removal, the incidence was 6 percent.

Considering that most of the CSF-cutaneous fistulas are seen following acute surgical treatment, I would emphasize delaying the removal of the bullet for 7 to 10 days, as mentioned in the preceding section. When surgery is performed to remove the bullet, meticulous dural repair and meticulous closure of the paraspinous muscles and deep fascia and skin are necessary to minimize the chance of a postoperative CSF-cutaneous fistula.[12] At the time of repair of the dura, it should be checked with Valsalva's maneuvers to make certain that it is indeed water-tight. If a water-tight closure cannot be achieved, then a lumbar subarachnoid cutaneous drain (Fig. 32-15) should be placed to adequately decompress the dural sac to promote proper healing and to prevent such problems as CSF-cutaneous fistulas and subsequent meningitis.[30]

FIGURE 32-10   *A-C, This young man was shot through the flank, and the bullet lodged within the spinal canal at the L5-S1 level. He had normal motor function in his legs but some dysesthesia in the S1 nerve root distribution, and he had some urinary dysfunction with elevated postvoid residual volumes. He was taken to surgery 8 days after the injury was inflicted, and the bullet was easily removed. A small dural laceration was easily repaired. The patient had return of normal urologic function. (From Eismont, F.; Lattuga, S. Gunshot wounds of the spine. In: Browner, B.D.; Jupiter, J.B.; Levine, A.M.; et al., eds. Skeletal Trauma, 2nd ed. Philadelphia, W.B. Saunders, p. 1104, 1997.)*

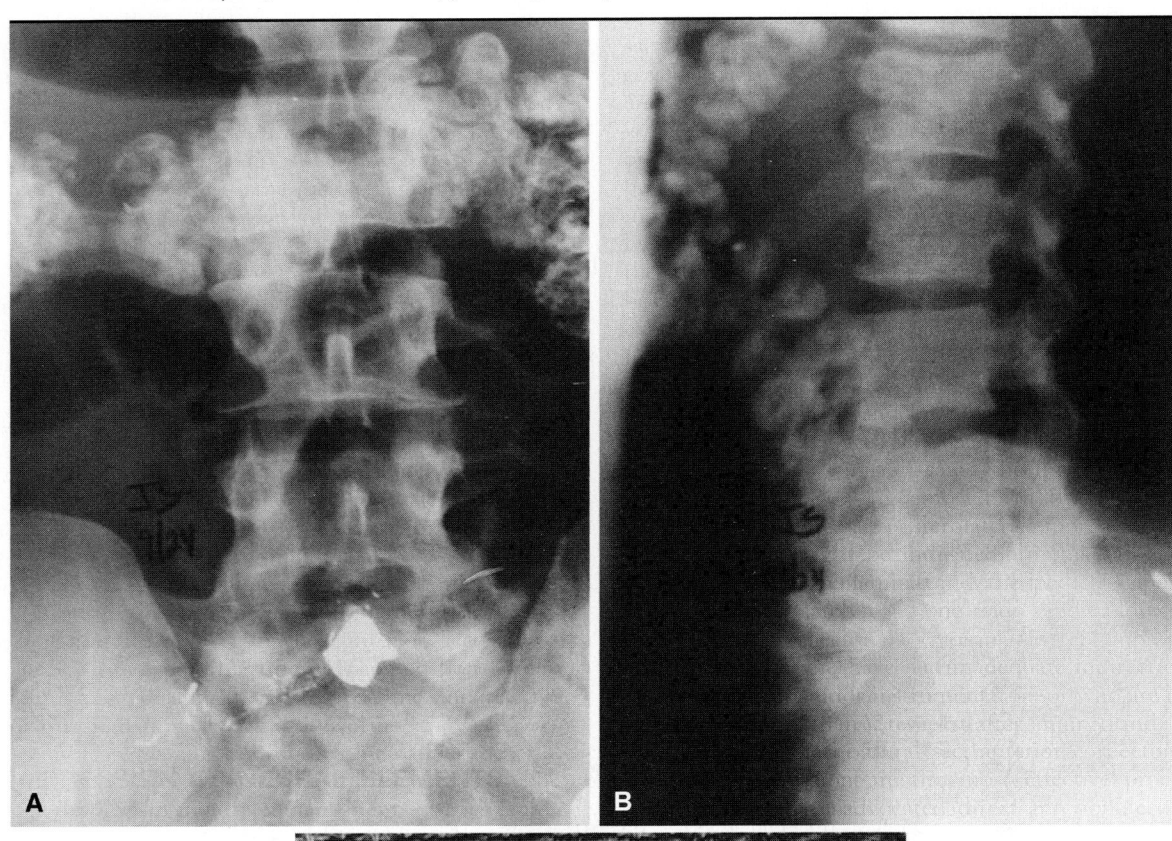

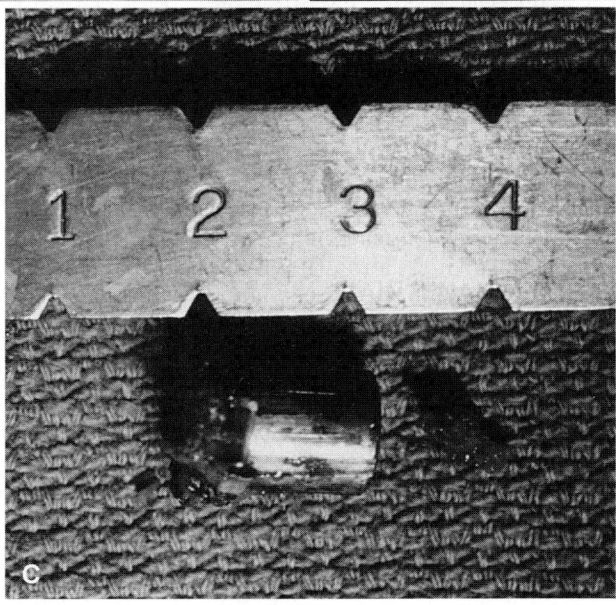

FIGURE 32-11 **A–D,** *This young boy was accidentally shot in the neck and had progressive quadriparesis. At 24 hours after injury he had lost all motor function in his legs. The plain films revealed that the bullet was filling the right side of the spinal canal. He was taken to surgery emergently and an anterior cervical procedure was performed. The trachea and esophagus were found to be intact. A corpectomy of C5 and C6 was performed to remove the bullet. An anterior cervical fusion was then performed using autologous iliac crest bone graft. The patient regained ambulation, and the only residual weakness involved the arms. (From Eismont, F.; Lattuga, S. Gunshot wounds of the spine. In: Browner, B.D.; Jupiter, J.B.; Levine, A.M.; et al., eds. Skeletal Trauma, 2nd ed. Philadelphia, W.B. Saunders, p. 1106, 1997.)*

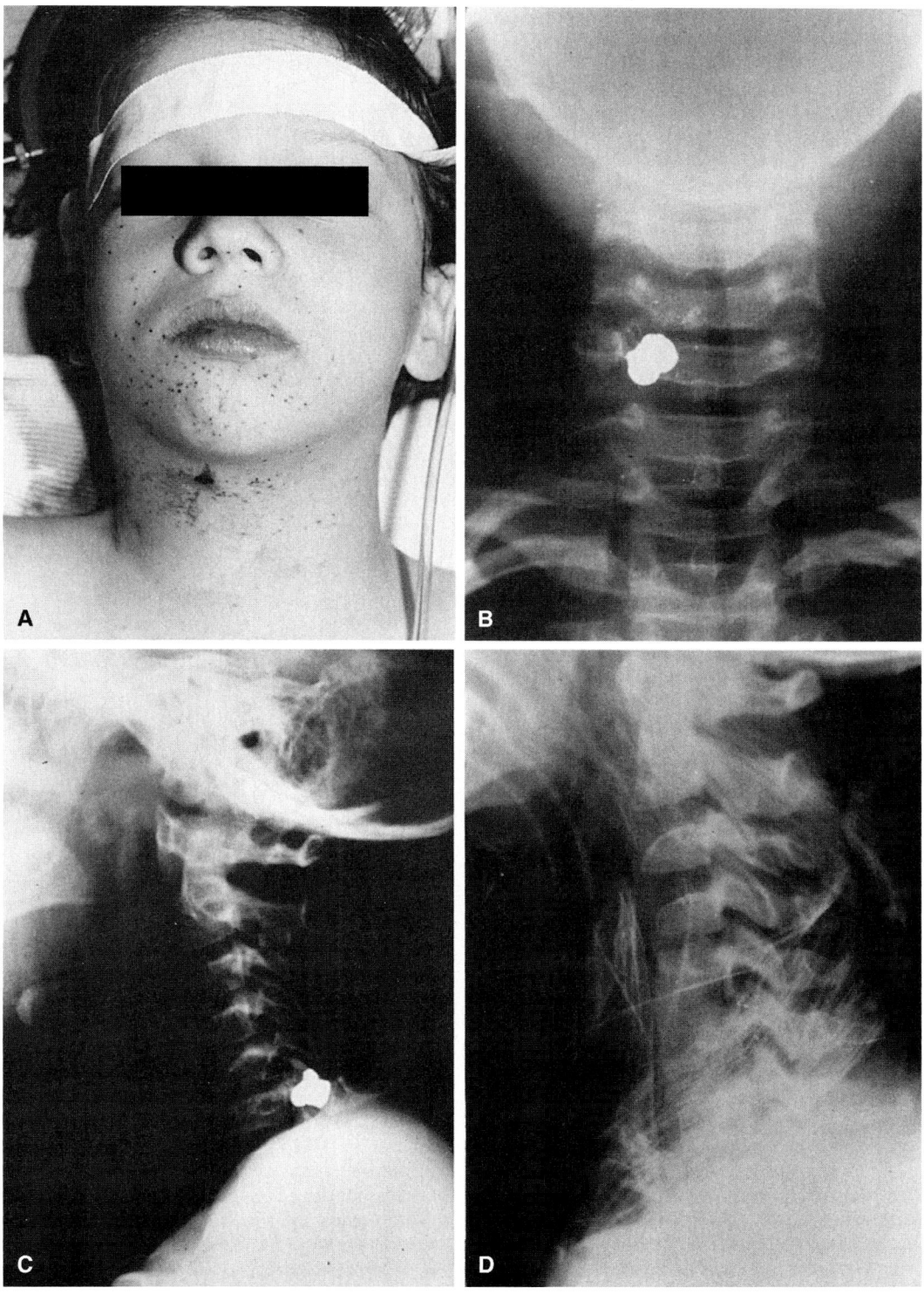

FIGURE 32-12 **A-C,** *This patient, who had been shot, presented to the emergency department with complete paraplegia, no bowel or bladder function, and no motor or sensory function below L1. His neurologic condition was unchanged for 1 week. He was taken to surgery for removal of the bullet, which was located within the dura. The goal of surgery was not to improve the function of the conus medullaris, but rather to maximize the chance for improvement of the L1-L4 nerve rootlets that traveled past the level of injury. (From Eismont, F.; Lattuga, S. Gunshot wounds of the spine. In: Browner, B.D.; Jupiter, J.B.; Levine, A.M.; et al., eds. Skeletal Trauma, 2nd ed. Philadelphia, W.B. Saunders, p. 1107, 1997.)*

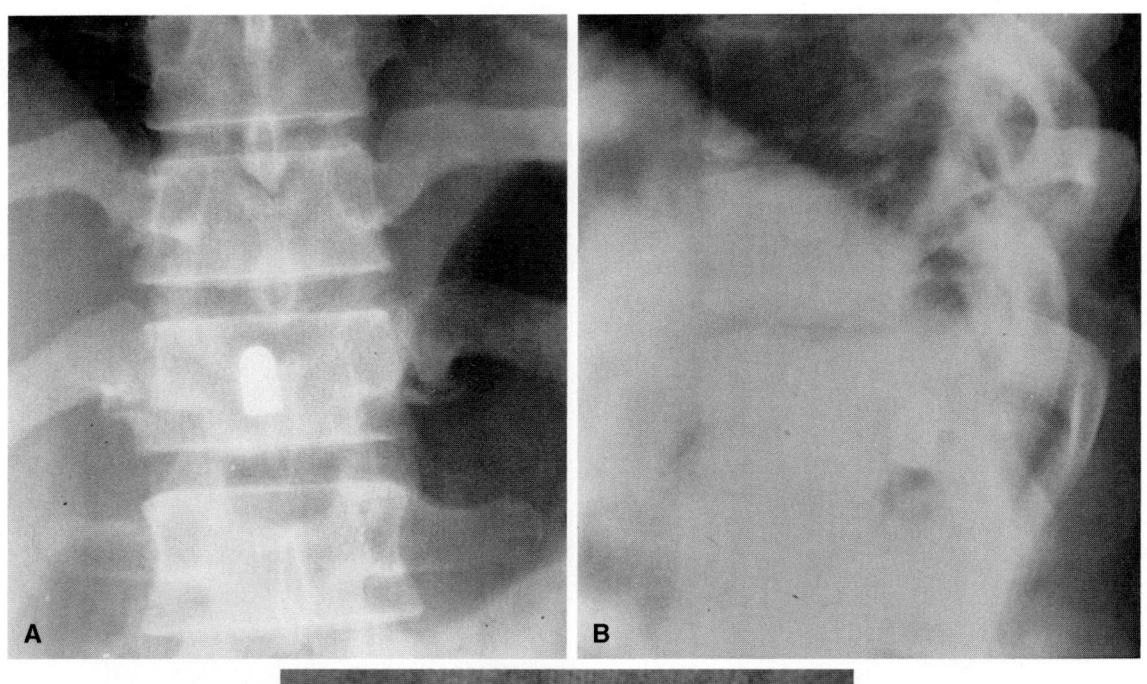

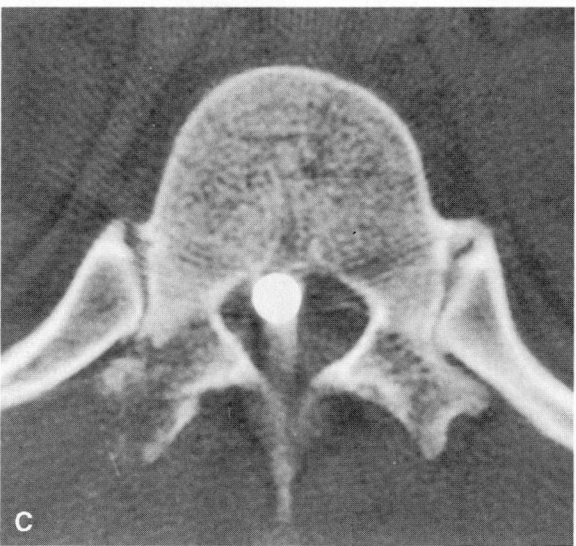

Spine Infections Following Gunshot Wounds

Spine infections occur infrequently following GSWs of the spine. Most follow injuries to the pharynx,[61,62] esophagus, or colon[58]; they very seldom occur after injury to any other organs, including the stomach or small bowel. Preceding sections have discussed methods of treatment to minimize this complication, including the routine use of prophylactic antibiotics for 72 hours after injury and for 7 to 14 days after injury of a contaminated viscus.[58,61,62] The choice of antibiotic was discussed earlier in the chapter.

The other common cause of infection following GSWs of the spine is iatrogenic infection following surgery. Stauffer and co-workers, in their review of patients treated with laminectomy for bullet removal, found that 4 percent of patients developed a postoperative wound infection,[71] which is treatable like any other postoperative infection of the spine.[17]

FIGURE 32-13 *This graph shows that the prognosis for recovery in penetrating injuries of the spine is worse than that for closed injuries. This is true for both complete and incomplete injuries. (From Green, B.A.; Eismont, F.J.; Klose, K.J.; et al. A Comparison of Open Versus Closed Spinal Cord Injuries During the First Year Post Injury. Presented at the Annual Meeting of the American Spinal Injury Association, New Orleans, 1981.)*

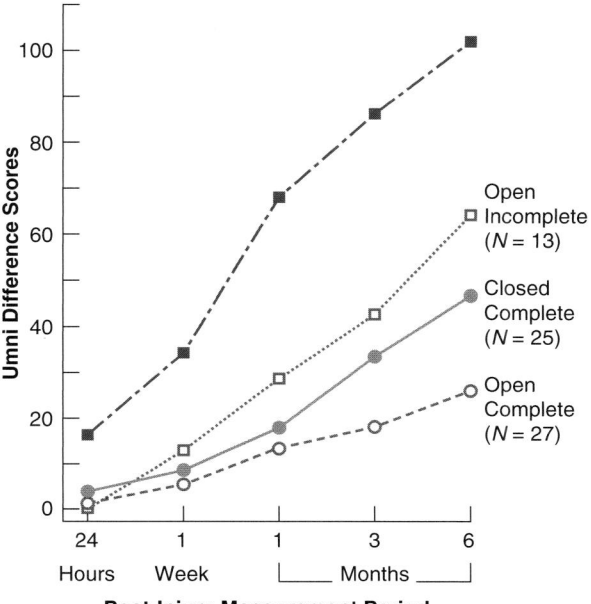

Open Incomplete (N = 13)
Closed Complete (N = 25)
Open Complete (N = 27)

FIGURE 32-14 *For legend see next page*

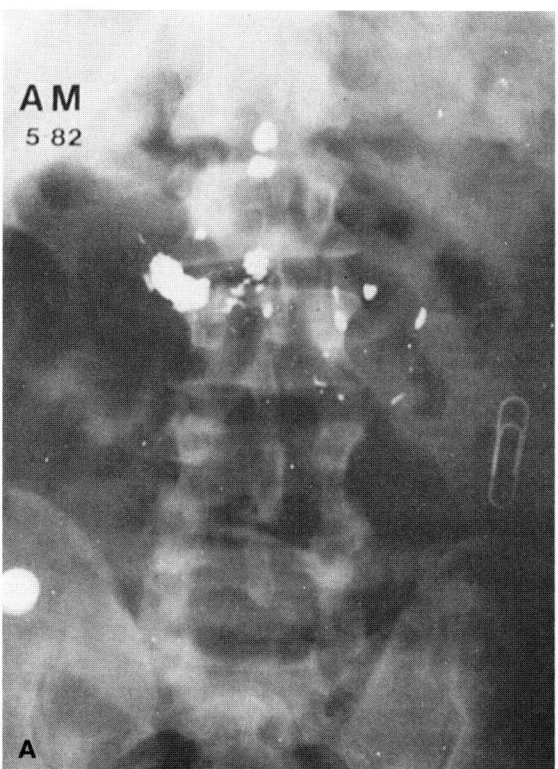

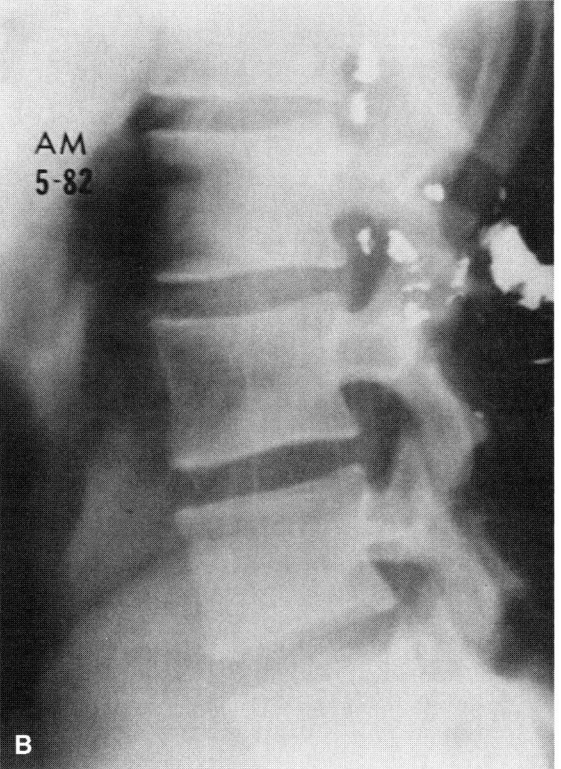

(Continued)

In patients with spine infections, significant fistula formation may be seen (Fig. 32-16). In patients with a contaminated viscus injury, a fistula may occur from the viscus to the spine. In these cases, it is not possible to effect resolution of the infection without adequate correction of the pharyngeal, esophageal, or bowel fistula. This may require such tactics as diversionary drainage and prolonged hyperalimentation. Occasionally, patients are seen with cutaneous fistulas leading to vertebral osteomyelitis–disk space infection, but it is much more common for this to occur in patients with a viscus fistula, as described earlier.

The reasons for surgical treatment of patients with spine infections following GSWs are the same as for patients with spine infection from other causes—progressive paralysis associated with the infection, progressive deformity, lack of a known organism, suspected foreign body associated with the infection, and failure of conservative treatment. In most cases, the spine infections are not noted until several weeks following the injury; at that time we normally recommend a CT-guided needle biopsy of the spine followed by a 6-week course with maximum-dose parenteral antibiotics. Open surgery would be reserved for the cases previously described.

FIGURE 32-14 | *(Continued) **A-C,** This patient was shot in the back and presented with complete paraplegia at the L1 level. He was taken to surgery emergently where a laminectomy was performed. Postoperatively the patient developed a cerebrospinal fluid (CSF)–cutaneous fistula through the site of the bullet wound. It is now appreciated that this type of surgery is ineffectual, because no major bullet fragment is present within the spinal canal. The chance of developing the CSF–cutaneous fistula was also heightened by performing the surgery immediately. Treatment now requires placement of a subarachnoid CSF shunt and revision surgery to treat the CSF–cutaneous fistula, the postoperative infection, and the secondary meningitis. (From Eismont, F.; Lattuga, S. Gunshot wounds of the spine. In: Browner, B.D.; Jupiter, J.B.; Levine, A.M.; et al., eds. Skeletal Trauma, 2nd ed. Philadelphia, W.B. Saunders, p. 1109, 1997.)*

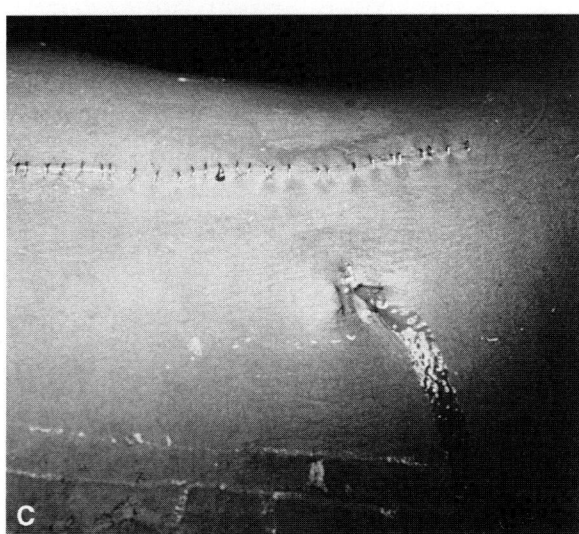

Pain Following Gunshot Wounds of the Spine with Associated Spinal Cord Injury

It is common for patients with SCIs secondary to GSWs of the spine to have problems with severe deafferent pain. Most commonly this is described as a searing, burning type of pain, which normally radiates into the paralyzed extremities. A local pain may also be present, which is described more commonly as an ache. These pains usually improve with the passage of time and the use of conservative measures, such as an aggressive course of nonsteroidal anti-inflammatory drugs in combination with amitriptyline (Elavil) or gabapentin (Neurontin).[36,56,78] Although amitriptyline has not, to our knowledge, been tested in patients with penetrating injuries of the spine, it has been proven to help with

FIGURE 32-15 | *This drawing shows the use of a CSF subarachnoid cutaneous shunt, which allows decompression of the dura and healing of the original CSF–cutaneous fistula. (From Kitchell, S.; Eismont, F.J.; Green, B.A. Closed subarachnoid drainage for management of cerebrospinal fluid leakage after an operation on the spine. J Bone Joint Surg [Am] 71:984–989, 1989.)*

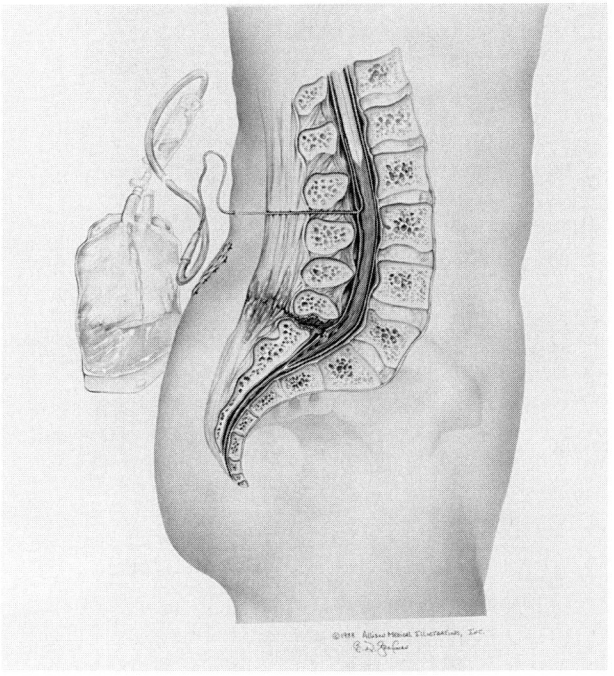

burning diabetic neuropathic pain[36] and with postherpetic neuralgia.[78] In our anecdotal experience, it seems helpful in patients with GSWs of the spine. If the amitriptyline is not successful, a course of gabapentin is normally utilized.

If the deafferent type of pain is still present and disabling, decompressive procedures are unlikely to significantly improve the symptoms (Fig. 32-17). The series by Waters and Adkins,[75] in which bullets were removed from the spinal canal of patients with gunshot spinal cord injury, has shown that although paralysis can be improved with bullet removal in the T12 to L5 region, no difference in pain is noted.[75] If surgery is contemplated for this type of deafferent pain, then use of a dorsal root entry zone (DREZ) procedure, using intraoperative computer assessment, can offer significant pain relief in some patients.[47] This is best utilized in patients without useful distal motor function, because of the risk of increasing distal neurologic deficit with this procedure.

In patients with persistent severe local pain and aching that seems out of proportion to what would normally be expected, evaluation should be undertaken to rule out underlying infection. This would include obtaining a sedimentation rate, C-reactive protein (CRP), and a CT scan. Interpretation of the CT scan under these

FIGURE 32-16 *A, B,* This patient sustained a gunshot wound with perforation of the colon, and the bullet traversed the L3 vertebral body. Chronic vertebral osteomyelitis developed, with a sinus draining through each flank. The sinogram reveals the significant vertebral destruction. Treatment for this problem requires assessment of the gastrointestinal tract to rule out any remaining bowel fistula. This should be followed by vigorous spine débridement and packing of the cavity with cancellous bone or viable soft tissue, followed by a protracted course of antibiotics. (From Eismont, F.; Lattuga, S. Gunshot wounds of the spine. In: Browner, B.D.; Jupiter, J. B.; Levine, A.M.; et al., eds. Skeletal Trauma, 2nd ed. Philadelphia, W.B. Saunders, p. 1111, 1997.)

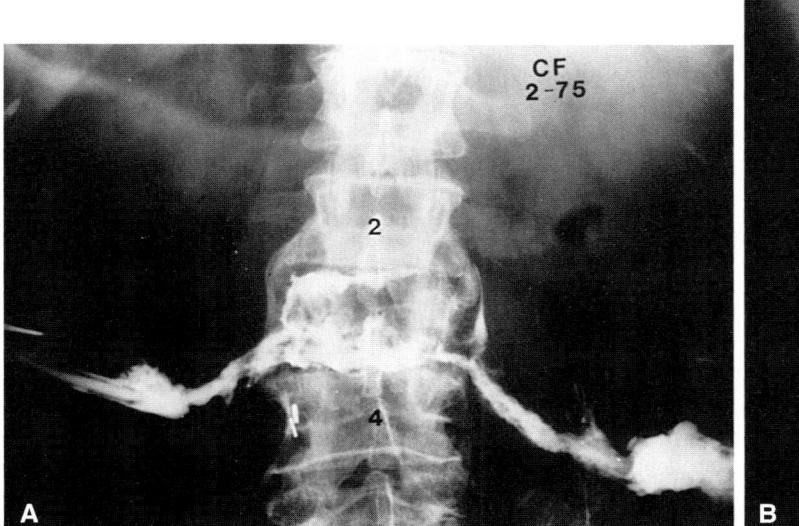
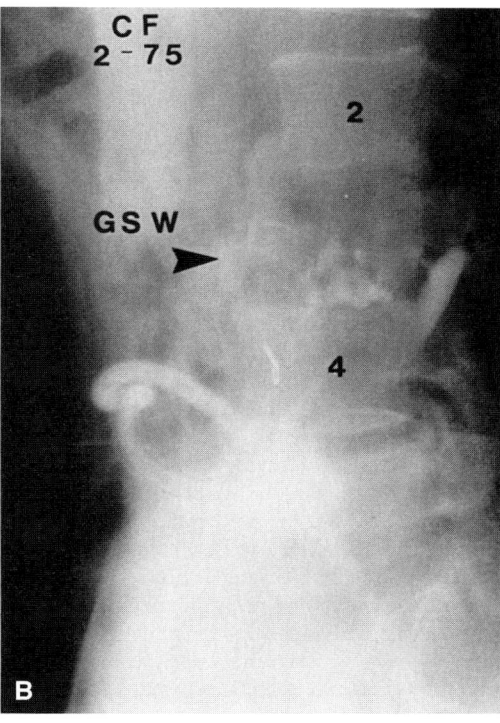

FIGURE 32-17 *A, B,* This patient had incomplete paraplegia following a gunshot wound to the spine. He had some function in almost every muscle group below the level of injury, but the main problem was severe pain radiating into the extremities. Passage of time and medical treatment with amitriptyline were unsuccessful. Following removal of the bullet, the patient had significant improvement of pain. Unfortunately, this type of positive response cannot be predicted with bullet removal. (From Eismont, F.; Lattuga, S. Gunshot wounds of the spine. In: Browner, B.D.; Jupiter, J.B.; Levine, A.M.; et al., eds. Skeletal Trauma, 2nd ed. Philadelphia, W.B. Saunders, p. 1108, 1997.)

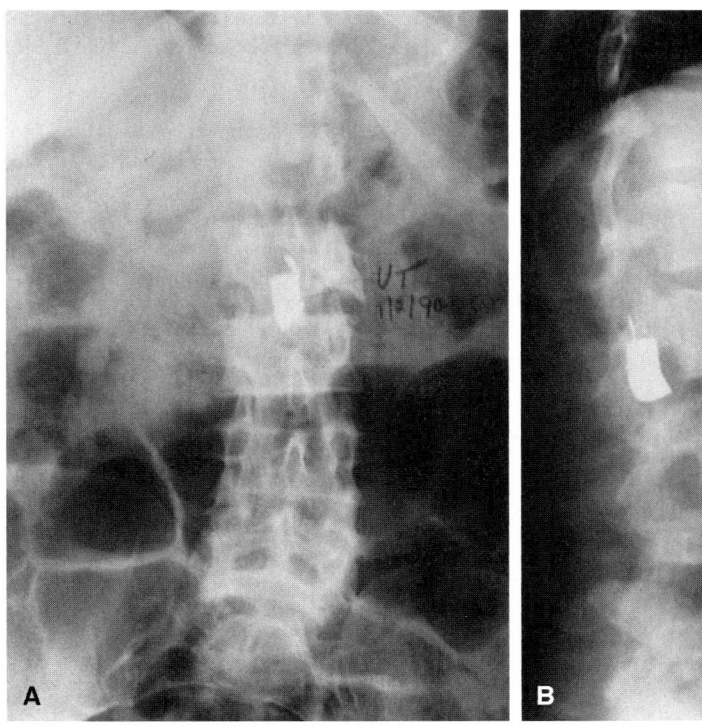
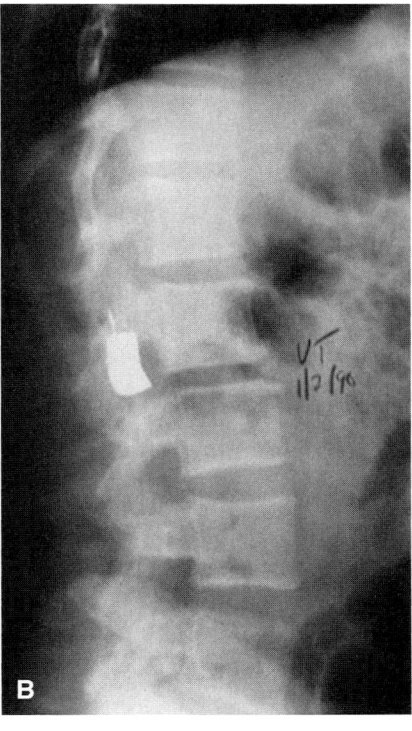

circumstances is always difficult, because the affected vertebra most commonly has sustained a fracture, and only signs of progressive bone destruction allow diagnosis of the infection.

Vascular Injuries

The vertebral arteries enter the transverse foramen at C6 as they travel cephalad within the cervical spine. At C2 they deviate posterolaterally and then continue their course on the posterior arch of C1 and up through the foramen magnum. A review of 110 patients with penetrating wounds to zone II revealed seven vertebral artery injuries (6%), none with neurologic deficits.[44] Unilateral occlusion of the vertebral artery secondary to a GSW has been reported in three separate series, totaling 58 cases.[18,43,55] Only one patient developed transient vertebrobasilar ischemia, and it was due to a vertebral arteriovenous fistula. Mohammed and colleagues presented 59 patients that had gunshot injuries to the neck.[46] Their objective was to prospectively determine the efficacy of physical exam alone versus angiography to diagnose a vascular injury. They found 23 patients who had vascular injury, including 13 patients with positive findings on physical examination (hematoma formation, current bleeding or history of bleeding, thrill, bruit, and pulse deficit) and 10 patients without clinical signs. A sensitivity of 57 percent, specificity of 53 percent, positive predictive value of 43 percent, and negative predictive value of 67 percent were calculated for physical examination alone in detecting vascular injury. They concluded that findings on physical examination are not good predictors of vascular injury in stable patients with GSWs to the neck, and that arteriography or ultrasonography is needed to identify vascular injuries. Le Roux presented another South African experience with 49 patients with gunshot injuries to the spine and found that 6 percent had vascular injury.[39] Reid and associates reviewed 43 cases of injury to the vertebral artery, most often as a result of gunshot or stab wounds associated with cervical spine fracture.[55] They did not have any patients develop neurologic sequelae attributable to vertebral–basilar ischemia. In their series, mortality related to a vertebral artery injury was only 4.7 percent, likely as a result of accurate diagnosis and prompt operative intervention.

Locked-in syndrome can result from injury or infarction of the ventral pons. This syndrome consists of a paralysis of voluntary movement, sparing only eyelid and vertical eye movement. Patients are quadriplegic and nonverbal, but alert and able to communicate through eye blinking.[52] This can occur with cervical GSW with bilateral occlusion of the vertebral arteries.

OTHER PENETRATING INJURIES OF THE SPINE

Impalement Injuries

Impalement injuries of the spine are uncommon. Trauma is usually massive, and gross wound contamination is more likely to be present than in other injuries to the spine.[25] Patients should be taken to surgery for spine débridement. Cultures for aerobes, anaerobes, and fungus should be carefully obtained. Unlike the relatively clean GSWs described earlier, these injuries require a minimum of 3 weeks of parenteral therapy with broad-spectrum antibiotics specific to the organisms found at the original débridement. It is not uncommon to find a combination of bacteria and fungi. With such injuries it is also extremely important to rule out significant presence of foreign bodies, such as pieces of clothing, which may have been driven into the spine at the time of the impalement injury (Fig. 32-18).

Patients with impalement injuries of the spine often have recurrent spine infections and spontaneous drainage from sinus tracts. Successful treatment usually requires sinography to define the course of the sinus, tomography or CT immediately after sinography to define the bone or disk pathologic characteristics, and surgery to débride the spinal source of infection as well as to excise the chronic sinus tract. The injection of methylene blue into the sinus tract helps to identify the tissue that requires excision (Fig. 32-19). Methylene blue should never be used if the possibility of a dural–cutaneous fistula exists; intrathecal injection of methylene blue is fatal.

Stabbing Injuries

Stabbing injuries of the spine are seen much less commonly than GSWs of the spine. In some countries, these are the most common type of penetrating injury of the spine. Radiographs should be taken immediately to make certain that no foreign bodies remain. Any remaining foreign bodies (Fig. 32-20) should be surgically removed. Unlike GSWs of the spine, which are normally sterile, foreign bodies are not sterile and can be the source of persistent late infections. Stab wounds are very often associated with Brown–Séquard-type paralysis; hence, they have the best prognosis for incomplete spinal injuries. The general prognosis for patients with stab injuries to the spine and incomplete paralysis is significantly better than that for patients with GSWs of the spine and a similar extent of paralysis.

FIGURE 32-18 *A, B, This patient was impaled on a reinforcing rod following a motorcycle accident. The rod was removed in the operating room with both anterior and posterior exposure of the spine provided. The spine was cultured and vigorously débrided at the time of initial emergency surgery. Despite 3 weeks' administration of broad-spectrum antibiotics, persistent vertebral osteomyelitis and pain developed and vertebral destruction continued (C). At 6 weeks after injury, the patient was returned to surgery for simultaneous anterior and posterior débridement, fusion, and stabilization D, E. Pieces of clothing were found within the vertebral body, and cultures at surgery revealed standard pyogenic organisms as well as a fungus infection. Radiographs taken 10 years after injury reveal complete resolution of the infection. Broken rods and a flat-back deformity are now appreciated, but the patient is asymptomatic and is able to participate in full wheelchair activities with no pain. (From Eismont, F.; Lattuga, S. Gunshot wounds of the spine. In: Browner, B.D.; Jupiter, J.B.; Levine, A.M.; et al., eds. Skeletal Trauma, 2nd ed. Philadelphia, W.B. Saunders, p. 1112, 1997.)*

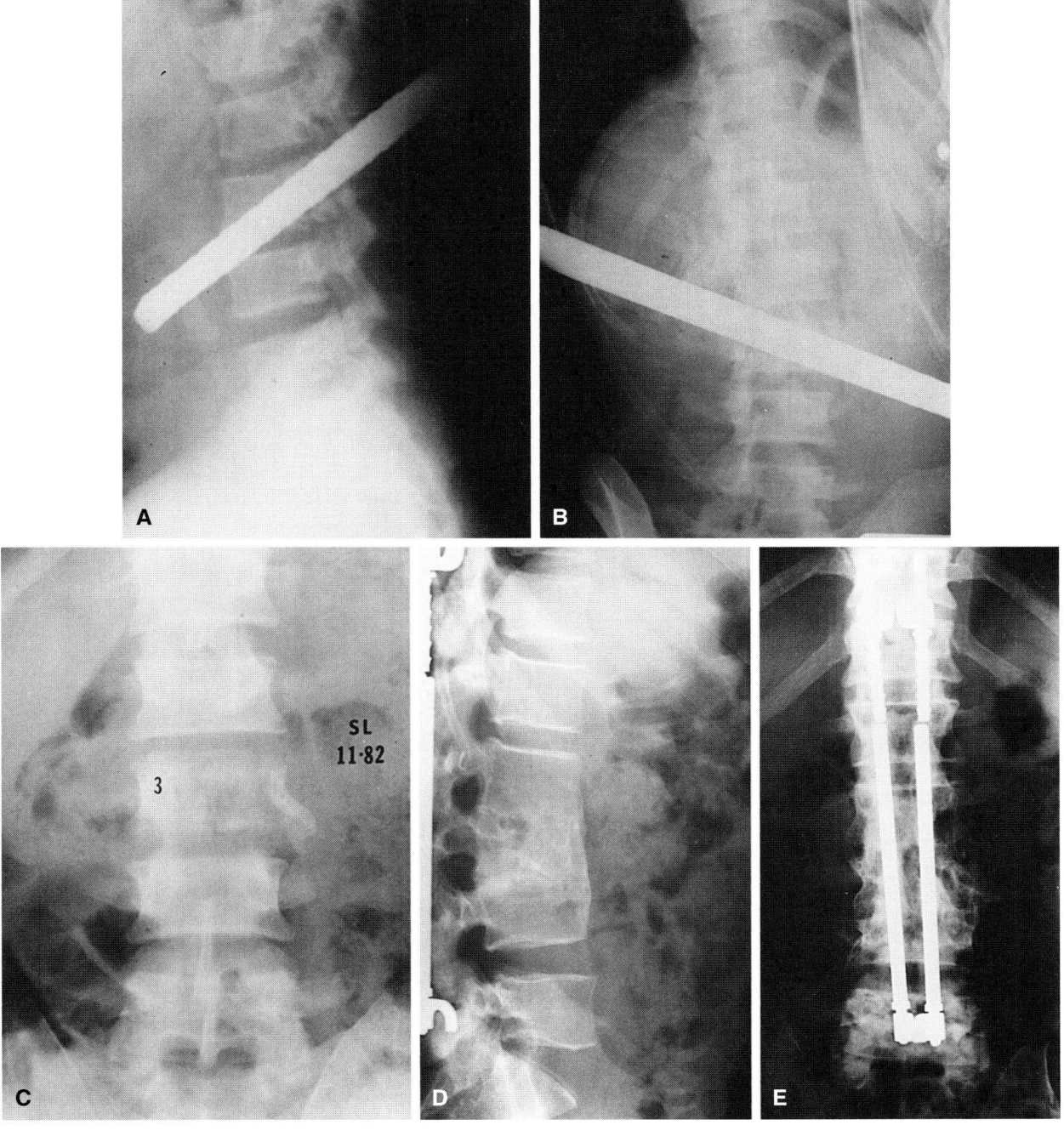

FIGURE 32-19 *This man fell at a construction site and landed on a reinforcing rod, which pierced the perineum and transverse colon and penetrated the sacral ala. He presented to us many months after injury with a persistent perineal fistula, after several courses of antibiotics and anterior abdominal operations failed. **A,** The anteroposterior (AP) tomogram of the sacrum shows the lytic tract in the ala caused by the penetrating rod and persistent infection (arrows). **B,** The AP view of the pelvis immediately after the sinogram shows that the fistulous tract ends in the right ala (arrows). **C,** The lateral sinogram also confirms the source of the infection in the sacral ala. This patient was successfully treated with a posterior lateral muscle splitting approach and wide débridement of the sacral ala followed by a 6-week course of antibiotics for all organisms cultured from the alar bone debris. (From Eismont, F.; Lattuga, S. Gunshot wounds of the spine. In: Browner, B.D.; Jupiter, J.B.; Levine, A.M.; et al., eds. Skeletal Trauma, 2nd ed. Philadelphia, W.B. Saunders, p. 1113, 1997.)*

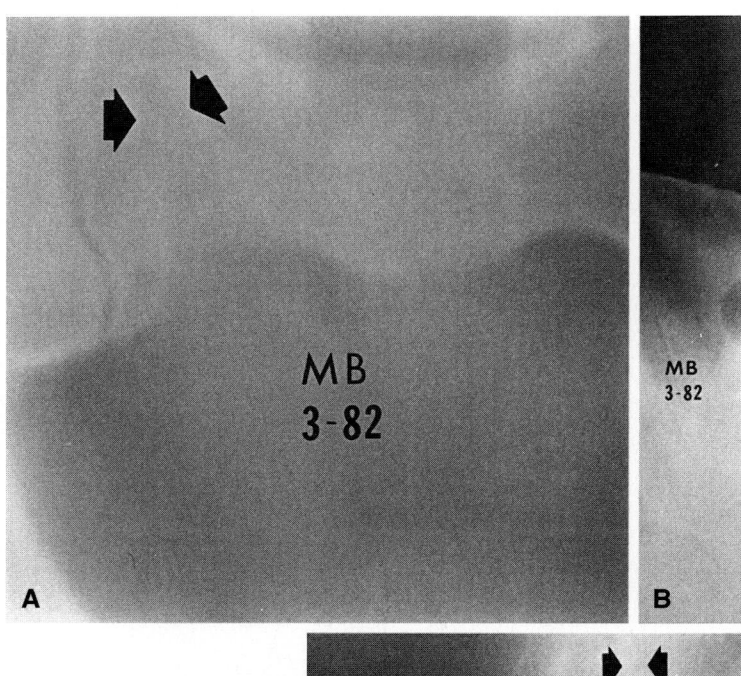

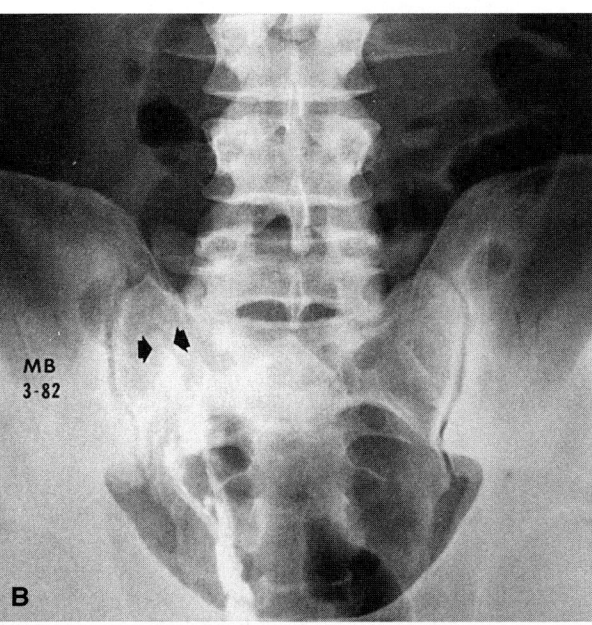

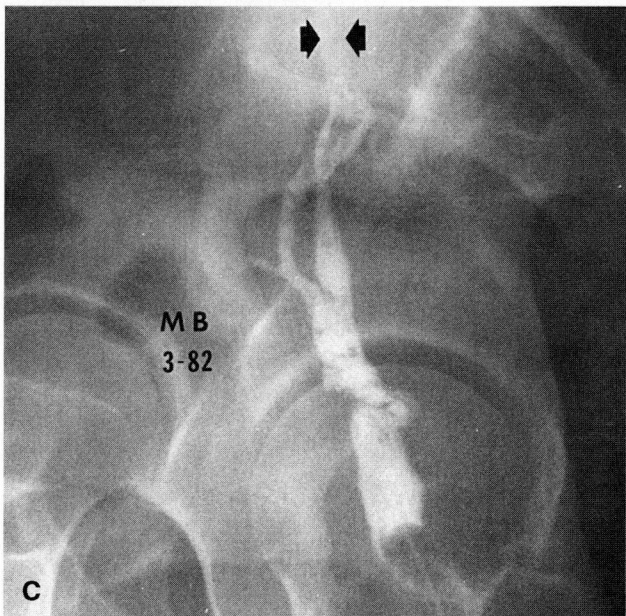

FIGURE 32-20 *This patient presented to the emergency department after being stabbed with a pair of scissors. After emergency treatment for a pneumothorax, anteroposterior (**A**) and lateral (**B**) chest films reveal a metallic foreign body adjacent to the thoracic spine. **C,** Computed tomography verifies the location of the foreign body. This patient was taken to surgery for removal of the foreign body to minimize the chance of development of a persistent infection. (From Eismont, F.; Lattuga, S. Gunshot wounds of the spine. In: Browner, B.D.; Jupiter, J.B.; Levine, A.M.; et al., eds. Skeletal Trauma, 2nd ed. Philadelphia, W.B. Saunders, p. 1114, 1997.)*

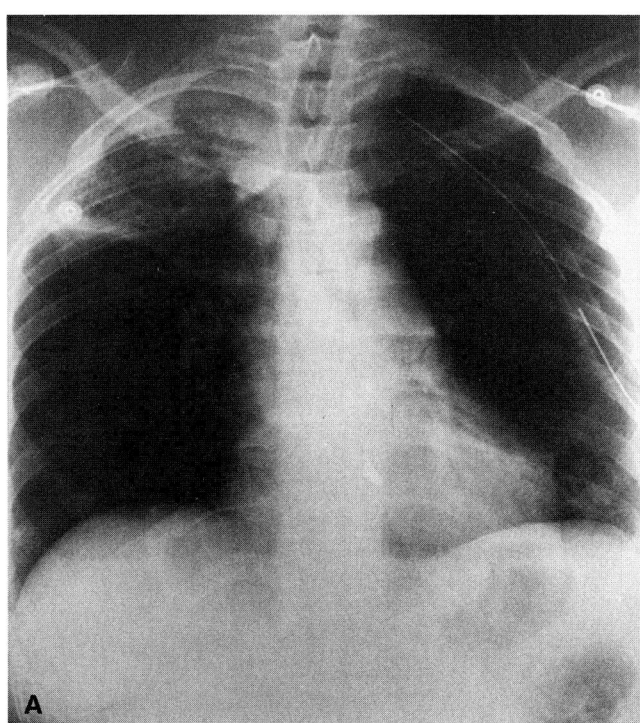
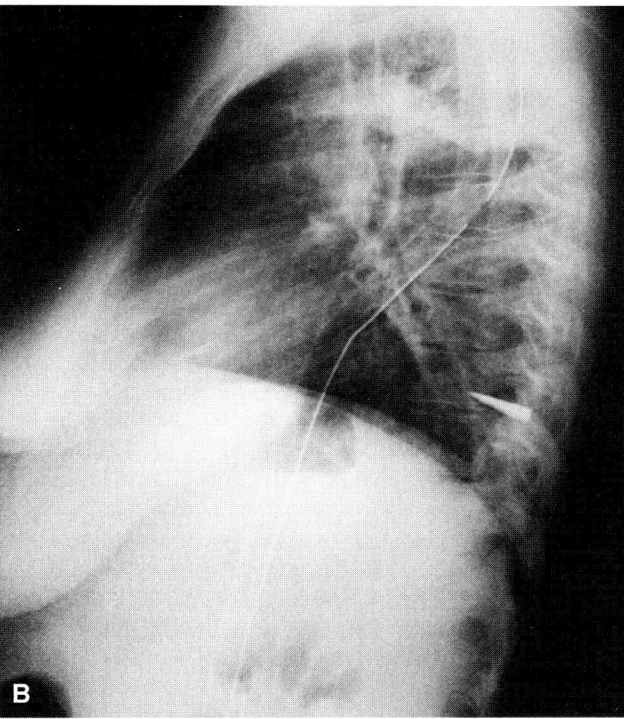
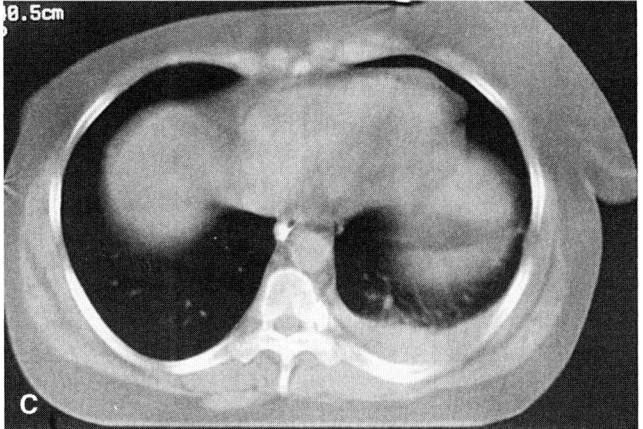

CONCLUSION

Unfortunately, the incidence of SCIs due to GSWs is rising. Because of this, it is necessary for all orthopaedic surgeons to be familiar with the evaluation and treatment of these injuries. The importance of a good history, physical examination, and radiographic evaluation is emphasized. The reader understands that most GSWs of the spine can be treated nonoperatively, but this does not apply to all cases. It is important not to miss the very rare injury that clinically resembles a typical war injury.

REFERENCES

1. Anderson, P.A.; Bohlman, H.H. Anterior decompression and arthrodesis of the cervical spine: Long-term motor improvement. Part II—Improvement in complete traumatic quadriplegia. J Bone Joint Surg [Am] 74:683–692, 1992.
2. Bahebeck, J.; Atangana, R.; Mboudou, E.; et al. Incidence, case-fatality rate and clinical pattern of firearm injuries in two cities where arm owning is forbidden. Injury 36:714–717, 2005.

3. Bishop, M.; Shoemaker, W.C.; Avakian, S.; et al. Evaluation of a comprehensive algorithm for blunt and penetrating thoracic and abdominal trauma. Am Surg 57:737–746, 1991.

4. Bohlman, H.H.; Anderson, P.A. Anterior decompression and arthrodesis of the cervical spine: Long-term motor improvement. Part I—Improvement in incomplete traumatic quadriparesis. J Bone Joint Surg [Am] 74:671–682, 1992.

5. Bracken, M.B.; Shoemaker, W.C.; Avakian, S.; et al. A randomized, controlled trial of methylprednisolone or naloxone in the treatment of acute spinal-cord injury. Results of the Second National Acute Spinal Cord Injury Study. N Engl J Med 322:1405–1411, 1990.

6. Breitenecker, R. Shotgun wound patterns. Am J Clin Pathol 52:250–269, 1969.

7. Cammisa, F.P.; Eismont, F.J.; Tolli, T. Penetrating injuries of the cervical spine. In Camins, M.B.; O'Leary, P., eds. Disorders of the Cervical Spine. Baltimore: Williams & Wilkins, pp. 317–322, 1992.

8. Coben, J.H.; Dearwater, S.R.; Forjuoh, S.N.; et al. A population-based study of fatal and nonfatal firearm-related injuries. Acad Emerg Med 33:126–127, 1997.

9. Cushid, J.G.; Kopeloff, L.M. Epileptogenic effects of metal powder implants in the motor cortex in monkeys. Int J Neuropsychiatry 3:24–28, 1968.

10. Cybulski, G.R.; Stone, J.L.; Kant, R. Outcome of laminectomy for civilian gunshot injuries of the terminal spinal cord and cauda equina: Review of 88 cases. Neurosurgery 24:392–397, 1989.

11. Denis, F. The three column spine and its significance in the classification of acute thoracolumbar spinal injuries. Spine 8:817–831, 1983.

12. Eismont, F.J.; Wiesel, S.W.; Rothman, R.H. Treatment of dural tears associated with spinal surgery. J Bone Joint Surg [Am] 63:1132–1136, 1981.

13. Fackler, M.L. Wound ballistics. A review of common misconceptions. JAMA 259:2730–2736, 1988.

14. Fackler, M.L.; Bellamy, R.F.; Malinowski, J.A. The wound profile: Illustration of the missile-tissue interaction. J Trauma 28(1 Suppl):S21–29, 1988.

15. Fackler, M.L.; Malinowski, J.A. The wound profile: a visual method for quantifying gunshot wound components. J Trauma 25:522–529, 1985.

16. Finitsis, S.N.; Falcone, S.; Green, B.A. MR of the spine in the presence of metallic bullet fragments: Is the benefit worth the risk? AJNR Am J Neuroradiol 20:354–356, 1999.

17. Gepstein, R.; Eismont, F.J. Postoperative spine infections. In Garfin, S.R., ed. Complications of Spine Surgery. Baltimore: Williams & Wilkins, pp. 302–322, 1989.

18. Golueke, P.; Sclafani, F.; Phillips, T.; et al. Vertebral artery injury—diagnosis and management. J Trauma 27:856–865, 1987.

19. Green, B.A.; Eismont, F.J.; Close, K.J.; et al. A comparison of open versus closed spinal cord injuries during the first year post injury. In Annual Meeting of the American Spinal Injury Association, New Orleans, 1981.

20. Grogan, D.P.; Bucholz, R.W. Acute lead intoxication from a bullet in an intervertebral disc space. A case report. J Bone Joint Surg [Am] 63:1180–1182, 1981.

21. Hales, D.D.; Duffy, K.; Dawson, E.G.; et al. Lumbar osteomyelitis and epidural and paraspinous abscesses. Case report of an unusual source of contamination from a gunshot wound to the abdomen. Spine 16:380–383, 1991.

22. Heary, R.F.; Vaccaro, A.R.; Mesa, J.J.; et al. Thoracolumbar infections in penetrating injuries to the spine. Orthop Clin North Am 27:69–81, 1996.

23. Heary, R.F.; Vaccaro, A.R.; Mesa, J.J.; et al. Steroids and gunshot wounds to the spine. Neurosurgery 41:576–583; discussion 583–584, 1997.

24. Heiden, J.S.; Weiss, M.H.; Rosenberg, A.W.; et al. Penetrating gunshot wounds of the cervical spine in civilians. Review of 38 cases. J Neurosurg 42:575–579, 1975.

25. Horowitz, M.D.; Dove, D.B.; Eismont, F.J.; et al. Impalement injuries. J Trauma 25:914–916, 1985.

26. Jacobson, S.A.; Bors, E. Spinal cord injury in Vietnamese combat. Paraplegia 7:263–281, 1970.

27. Karim, N.O.; Nabors, M.W.; Golocovsky, M.; et al. Spontaneous migration of a bullet in the spinal subarachnoid space causing delayed radicular symptoms. Neurosurgery 18:97–100, 1986.

28. Keith, A.; Hall, M.E. Specimens of gunshot injuries of the face and spine, contained in the army medical collection now on exhibition in the Museum of Royal College of Surgeons of England. Br J Surg 7:55–71, 1919.

29. Kihtir, T.; Ivatury, R.R.; Simon, R.; et al. Management of transperitoneal gunshot wounds of the spine. J Trauma 31:1579–1583, 1991.

30. Kitchel, S.H.; Eismont, F.J.; Green, B.A. Closed subarachnoid drainage for management of cerebrospinal fluid leakage after an operation on the spine. J Bone Joint Surg [Am] 71:984–987, 1989.

31. Klein, Y.; Cohn, S.M.; Soffer, D.; et al. Spine injuries are common among asymptomatic patients after gunshot wounds. J Trauma 58:833–836, 2005.

32. Klemperer, W.W.; Fulton, J.F.; Lamport, H.; et al. Indirect spinal cord injuries due to gunshot wounds of the spinal column in animal and man. Mil Surg 114:253–265, 1954.

33. Kuijlen, J.M.; Herpers, M.J.; Beuls, E.A. Neurogenic claudication, a delayed complication of a retained bullet. Spine 22:910–914, 1997.

34. Kumar, A.; Wood, G.W., 2nd; Whittle, A.P. Low-velocity gunshot injuries of the spine with abdominal viscus trauma. J Orthop Trauma 12:514–517, 1998.

35. Kupcha, P.C.; An, H.S.; Cotler, J.M. Gunshot wounds to the cervical spine. Spine 15:1058–1063, 1990.

36. Kvinesdal, B.; Molin, J.; Frøland, J.; et al. Imipramine treatment of painful diabetic neuropathy. JAMA 251:1727–1730, 1984.

37. Ledgerwood, A.M. The wandering bullet. Surg Clin North Am 57:97–109, 1977.

38. Leonard, M. The solution of lead by synovial fluid. Clin Orthop 64:255–261, 1969.

39. le Roux, J.C.; Dunn, R.N. Gunshot injuries of the spine—A review of 49 cases managed at the Groote Schuur Acute Spinal Cord Injury Unit. S Afr J Surg 43:165–168, 2005.

40. Levy, M.L.; Gans, W.; Wijesinghe, H.S.; et al. Use of methylprednisolone as an adjunct in the management of patients with penetrating spinal cord injury: Outcome analysis. Neurosurgery 39:1141–1148; discussion 1148–1149, 1996.

41. Magnuson, E. Seven deadly days. Time, July 17: 30–61, 1989.

42. May, M.; West, J.W.; Heeneman, H.; et al. Shotgun wounds to the head and neck. Arch Otolaryngol 98:373–376, 1973.

43. Meier, D.E.; Brink, B.E.; Fry, W.J. Vertebral artery trauma: Acute recognition and treatment. Arch Surg 116:236–239, 1981.

44. Menawat, S.S.; Dennis, J.W.; Laneve, L.M.; et al. Are arteriograms necessary in penetrating zone II neck injuries? J Vasc Surg 16:397–400; discussion 400–401, 1992.

45. Mirovsky, Y.; Shalmon, E.; Blankstein, A.; et al. Complete paraplegia following gunshot injury without direct trauma to the cord. Spine 30:2436–2438, 2005.

46. Mohammed, G.S.; Pillay, W.S.; Barker, P.; et al. The role of clinical examination in excluding vascular injury in haemodynamically stable patients with gunshot wounds to the neck. A prospective study of 59 patients. Eur J Vasc Endovasc Surg 28:425–430, 2004.

47. Nashold, B.S., Jr.; Ostdahl, R.H. Dorsal root entry zone lesions for pain relief. J Neurosurg 51:59–69, 1979.

48. Nino, H.E.; Leppick, I.E.; Lai, C.; et al. Progressive sensory loss one year after bullet injury of spinal cord. JAMA 240:1173–1174, 1978.

49. Oliver, C.; Kabala, J. Air gun pellet injuries: The safety of MR imaging. Clin Radiol 52:299–300, 1997.

50. Ordog, G.J.; Albin, D.; Wasserberger, J.; et al. 110 bullet wounds to the neck. J Trauma 25:238–246, 1985.

51. Pal, G.P.; Sherk, H.H. The vertical stability of the cervical spine. Spine 13:447–449, 1988.

52. Plum, F.; Posner, J.P.; Saper, C.B.; et al. Diagnosis of Stupor and Coma. New York, Oxford Univ. Press, 1966.

53. Pohost, G.M.; Blackwell, G.G.; Shellock, F.G. Safety of patients with medical devices during application of magnetic resonance methods. Ann N Y Acad Sci 649:302–312, 1992.

54. Pool, J.L. Gunshot wounds of the spine: Observations from an evacuation hospital. Surg Gynecol Obstet 81:617–622, 1945.

55. Reid, J.D.; Weigelt, J.A. Forty-three cases of vertebral artery trauma. J Trauma 28:1007–1012, 1988.

56. Richards, J.S. Pain secondary to gunshot wounds during the initial rehabilitation process in spinal cord injury patients. J Rehabil Res Dev (25 Suppl):75, 1989.

57. Robertson, D.P.; Simpson, R.K.; Narayan, R.K. Lumbar disc herniation from a gunshot wound to the spine. A report of two cases. Spine 16: 994–995, 1991.

58. Roffi, R.P.; Waters, R.L.; Adkins, R.H. Gunshot wounds to the spine associated with a perforated viscus. Spine 14:808–811, 1989.

59. Romanick, P.C.; Smith, T.K.; Kopaniky, D.R.; et al. Infection about the spine associated with low-velocity-missile injury to the abdomen. J Bone Joint Surg [Am] 67:1195–1201, 1985.

60. Saletta, J.D.; Lowe, R.J.; Lim, L.T.; et al. Penetrating trauma of the neck. J Trauma 6:579–587, 1976.

61. Schaefer, S.D.; Bucholz, R.W.; Jones, R.E.; et al. "How I do it"—Head and neck. Treatment of transpharyngeal missile wounds to the cervical spine. Laryngoscope 91:146–148, 1981.

62. Schaefer, S.D.; Bucholz, R.W.; Jones, R.E.; et al. The management of transpharyngeal gunshot wounds to the cervical spine. Surg Gynecol Obstet 152:27–29, 1981.

63. Scuderi, G.J.; Vaccaro, A.R.; Fitzhenry, L.N.; et al. Long-term clinical manifestations of retained bullet fragments within the intervertebral disk space. J Spinal Disord Tech 17:108–111, 2004.

64. Sheely, C.H., 2nd.; Mattox, K.L.; Ruel, G.J., Jr.; et al. Current concepts in the management of penetrating neck trauma. J Trauma 15:895–900, 1975.

65. Shellock, F.G.; Curtis, J.S. MR imaging and biomedical implants, materials, and devices: An updated review. Radiology 180:541–550, 1991.

66. Sherman, I. Brass foreign body in the brain stem. J Neurosurg 17:483–485, 1960.

67. Sights, W.B.; Bye, R.J. The fate of retained intracerebral shotgun pellets. J Neurosurg 33:646–653, 1970.

68. Simpson, R.K., Jr.; Venger, B.H.; Narayan, R.K. Treatment of acute penetrating injuries of the spine: A retrospective analysis. J Trauma 29:42–46, 1989.

69. Simpson, R.L.; Venager, B.H.; Narayan, R.K. Penetrating spinal cord injury in a civilian population: A retrospective analysis. Surg Forum 37:494–496, 1986.

70. Staniforth, P.; Watt, I. Extradural "plumboma." A rare cause of acquired spinal stenosis. Br J Radiol 55:772–774, 1982.

71. Stauffer, E.S.; Wood, R.W.; Kelly, E.G. Gunshot wounds of the spine: The effects of laminectomy. J Bone Joint Surg [Am] 61:389–392, 1979.

72. Switz, D.D.; Elmorshidy, M.E.; Deyerle, W.M. Bullets, joints, and lead intoxication. Arch Intern Med 136:939–941, 1976.

73. Teitelbaum, G.P.; Yee, C.A.; VanHorn, D.D.; et al. Metallic ballistic fragments: Imaging safety and artifacts. Radiology 175:855–859, 1990.

74. Tindel, N.L.; Marcillo, A.E.; Tay, B.K.; et al. The effect of surgically implanted bullet fragments on the spinal cord in a rabbit model. J Bone Joint Surg [Am] 83:884–890, 2001.

75. Waters, R.L.; Adkins, R.H. The effects of removal of bullet fragments retained in the spinal canal. A collaborative study by the National Spinal Cord Injury Model Systems. Spine 16:934–939, 1991.

76. Waters, R.L.; Sie, I.H. Spinal cord injuries from gunshot wounds to the spine. Clin Orthop Relat Res 408:120–125, 2003.

77. Waters, R.L.; Sie, I.H.; Adkins, R.H.; et al. Injury pattern effect on motor recovery after traumatic spinal cord injury. Arch Phys Med Rehabil 76:440–443, 1995.

78. Watson, C.P.; Evans, R.J.; Reed, K.; et al. Amitriptyline versus placebo in postherpetic neuralgia. Neurology 32:671–673, 1982.

79. Windler, E.C.; Smith, R.B.; Bryan, W.J.; et al. Lead intoxication and traumatic arthritis of the hip secondary to retained bullet fragment. J Bone Joint Surg [Am] 60:254–255, 1978.

80. Wolf, A.W.; Benson, D.R.; Shoji, H.; et al. Autosterilization in low-velocity bullets. J Trauma 18:63, 1978.

81. Wu, W.Q. Delayed effects from retained foreign bodies in the spine and spinal cord. Surg Neurol 25:214–218, 1986.

82. Yashon, D.; Jane, J.A.; White, R.J. Prognosis and management of spinal cord and cauda equina bullet injuries in sixty-five civilians. J Neurosurg 32:163–170, 1970.

83. Yip, L.; Sweeny, P.J.; McCarroll, K.A. Spontaneous migration of an intraspinal bullet following a gunshot wound. Am J Emerg Med 8:569–570, 1990.

84. Young, J.A.; Burns, P.E.; McCutchen, R. Spinal Cord Injury Statistics: Experience of the Regional Spinal Cord Injury Systems. Phoenix, Good Samaritan Medical Center, pp. 1–152, 1982.

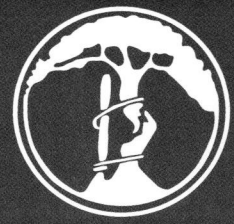

CHAPTER 33

Fractures in the Stiff and Osteoporotic Spine

Luke Madigan, M.D. and Jerome M. Cotler, M.D.

The structural integrity of the spinal column is due to a combination of both the bony elements and the supporting soft tissues. Diseases that adversely affect either of these two components lead to weakening of the spine. Pathologic processes that increase bone formation and produce heterotopic bone make the spine stiffer and more brittle and predispose it to fracture, even from relatively minor trauma. Disease states such as ankylosing spondylitis, diffuse idiopathic skeletal hyperostosis (DISH), osteoporosis, and other similar conditions can all lead to increased fracture risk and to characteristic fracture patterns. Complicating this patient population is the often chronic state of back and neck pain that can make the detection of new fractures more difficult. Standard imaging studies are often difficult to interpret secondary to the underlying disease process. It is important to recognize that these patients warrant special consideration and heightened awareness when they present with complaints of new or different pain, even in the face of relatively minor trauma. Due to their underlying disease process this patient population is at increased risk for neurologic deterioration and post-traumatic deformity, especially if diagnosis is delayed and external support for the patient is limited.

OSTEOPOROTIC SPINAL FRACTURES

Osteoporosis affects more than 200 million people worldwide.[30] In the United States it accounts for approximately 1.5 million fractures per year, of which 700,000 occur in the spine.[49] The lifetime risk of vertebral fracture secondary to osteoporosis is 16 percent for women and 5 percent for men, with a likely higher prevalence if asymptomatic fractures are taken into account.[34]

Osteoporosis is the progressive loss of bone mass in both the axial and appendicular skeleton. It is defined by the World Health Organization (WHO) as a bone mineral density T-score, as measured by decrease in dual energy x-ray absorptiometry (DEXA) scan, of greater than 2.5 standard deviations away from the mean for normals.[15] It is characterized radiographically by the deterioration of the microarchitecture, low bone mass, and increased susceptibility to fracture. Osteoporosis is divided into primary and secondary. Primary osteoporosis is further subdivided into

type I, or postmenopausal osteoporosis, and type II, age-related (or senile) osteoporosis. Type I osteoporosis is seen in postmenopausal or estrogen-deficient women, while type II affects both men and women after the age of 70 years. Secondary osteoporosis is caused by numerous medical conditions (including chronic renal disease, endocrinopathies, connective tissue disorders, gastrointestinal disorders, and hematopoetic disorders), medications (most commonly steroids), and nutritional deficiencies.[30]

The loss of trabecular bone in the vertebral bodies leads to a decrease in its compressive strength. This loss of strength leads to increased fracture risk with resultant kyphotic deformity of the spine. The upper thoracic spine is the most common site for an osteoporotic vertebral body fracture.[3] Patients usually present with spinal pain and point tenderness over the involved area. A history of trauma is not always present in these patients. Radicular symptoms or neurologic deterioration may occur days to weeks after the start of spinal pain and may herald continued collapse of the involved vertebral bodies with impingement of nerve roots or the spinal cord itself. Cord compression is decidedly uncommon and usually self-limited.[28]

Osteoporotic fractures are usually the result of compressive forces on the anterior half of the vertebral body. The ensuing loss of anterior vertebral height results in wedging the body and resultant kyphotic deformity. This deformity leads to increased stress being placed on the anterior aspects of adjacent vertebral bodies and increases the fracture risk at other vertebral levels.[44] Another fracture pattern that can be seen in the setting of osteoporosis is failure of both end plates with resulting shortening of the vertebral body and a distortion of the body's shape. Characterized by foreshortening of the apical spine, compression fractures usually caused by low-energy trauma or no apparent trauma at all rarely extend into the middle column and produce a burst fracture pattern.

Plain radiographic imaging of the spine is the mainstay in diagnosis of osteoporotic compression fractures. Concern for canal encroachment or any poorly visualized fractures warrants the use of computed tomography (CT) or magnetic resonance imaging (MRI). These latter technologies can better delineate the fracture pattern and assess any posterior cortical and spinal canal involvement.

1043

Evidence of nonacute spinal fractures includes sclerosis, rounding of the fracture edges, and cyst formation. If a determination of the age of the fracture is needed, a technetium-99 (^{99m}Tc)-labeled bone scan can be obtained; however, bone scans can remain positive for up to 18 months after a fracture[3] and are nonspecific for other than evidence of bony activity. A bone scan cannot differentiate among tumor, osteoporosis, and osteoarthritis. Technetium-99 bone scans have largely been supplanted by MRI of the affected area, since this study is more specific.[48] Any neurologic deficit mandates an MRI study of the spine. Also, if there is a question of pathologic or metastatic disease involvement, an MRI should be obtained, since it can better differentiate among tumor, infection, and fracture.

The traditional mainstay of treatment for osteoporotic compression fractures has been a short course of analgesia and immobilization. Prolonged bed rest should be avoided because it may further exacerbate preexisting osteopenia and can lead to pulmonary complications and deconditioning in the elderly. Older patients sometimes require admission to the hospital for control of their pain because it can be difficult to manage in an outpatient setting due to multiple comorbidities and a baseline decrease in cognition. Potent narcotics should be avoided in this elderly patient population due to these factors and also because of the increased risk of drug interactions. Once a patient is admitted he or she should be enrolled in an organized physical therapy program that focuses on mobilization. Treatment of the acute fracture as well as treatment of underlying medical conditions should be instituted when an osteoporotic fracture is recognized. The literature shows that as a medical community we undertreat osteopenia and osteoporosis.[30]

Though nonoperative care of these osteoporotic fractures is still the primary treatment approach, surgical intervention can be considered in certain cases. Indications for surgical intervention include progressive neurologic deficit, intractable pain refractory to conservative care, and progressive deformity, namely increased kyphosis. The osteoporotic spine makes surgical fixation difficult. Segmental instrumentation with fusion decreases the forces at any one level in the fusion but can lead to early transitional disease in adjacent levels due to the increased forces transmitted on them. Sublaminar wires can be used to maximize fixation area but can lead to cut-out through a weakened lamina.[22] Pedicle screw fixation should be done with the maximal screw diameter in order to attain the greatest purchase in the thinned pedicles. The use of bone cement for augmentation of pedicle screw constructs is controversial secondary to an unclear approval status for its use in the spine by the U.S. Food and Drug Administration (FDA). The highest pullout strength is obtained when pedicle screws are augmented by hooks at the same level.[20] Again, early transitional disease is a likely sequela as well as construct failure.

Treatment of vertebral compression fractures with injection of polymethylmethacrylate (PMMA) has gained more acceptance in recent years. In 2002, approximately 54,000 of these procedures were performed (38,000 vertebroplasties and 16,000 kyphoplasties).[39] Both vertebroplasties and kyphoplasties are minimally invasive procedures that involve placement of a large-bore needle into the vertebral body via a transpedicular or a lateral body approach. The main difference is that kyphoplasty involves the inflation of a balloon tamp inside the vertebral body prior to injection of the PMMA in an effort to reduce the fracture deformity to a more normal alignment. The technique of vertebroplasty was originally advocated to help in the setting of pathologic fractures, metastatic disease, multiple myeloma, or hemangiomas of the spine[14,44,45] (Fig. 33-1). Kyphoplasty is a relatively new technique, introduced in 1998, which sought to improve on vertebroplasty by effecting fracture reduction.[48] It is generally thought to create less cement extravasation than vertebroplasty due to the fact that the cement is placed into a preformed cavity.[48]

Both vertebroplasty and kyphoplasty have been shown to significantly decrease pain in the setting of a compression fracture.[29,44,45,48] Kyphoplasty has been shown to restore some of the vertebral height of the damaged body.[29,44,45,58] Lieberman and colleagues showed height restoration in 70 percent of the compression fractures in their series, with a mean restoration of 46.8 percent when treated with kyphoplasty.[29] Phillips and co-workers showed an improvement in kyphosis of 14° in reducible fractures in a series of 40 patients treated with kyphoplasty.[45] In a further study Phillips found that end plate elevation and height restoration were easier when compression fractures were treated within 1 month.[44] In a prospective nonrandomized comparison of the two techniques Grohs and colleagues found that kyphoplasty could decrease vertebral body kyphosis 6°, but vertebroplasty could not.[16] Both groups had a rapid decrease in pain after the procedures as measured by the Visual Analogue Scale, but the pain reduction was long-lasting (at 2-year follow-up) in only the kyphoplasty group. The Oswestry Disability Index (ODI) showed significant improvement in the kyphoplasty group at the 4-month and 1-year follow-up period but returned to baseline low back pain at the 2-year follow-up.

Complications in both procedures have been reported. It has been shown that cement extravasation occurs in 30 to 70 percent of patients undergoing vertebroplasty.[48] The vast majority of these incidents are of little consequence to the patient. In a review of the FDA database, Nussbaum and associates found 58 complications in 52 patients treated with either vertebroplasty or kyphoplasty.[39] During the collection period approximately 40,000 to 60,000 kyphoplasties, 130,000 to 160,000 transpedicular vertebroplasties, and 10,000 to 15,000 lateral vertebroplasties were performed. Complications were graded as either major (death, canal intrusion or cord compression, epidural hematoma, pulmonary embolism or anaphylaxis) or minor (equipment breakage or cement embolus with no clinical symptoms). Of the 52 patients, 33 had undergone kyphoplasty (21 major/12 minor complications) and 19 had undergone vertebroplasty (8 major/11 minor complications). In the vertebroplasty group four major complications arose in both the transpedicular and lateral approach groups. The kyphoplasty group had the greatest number of major complications, with 20 of the 21 patients having to undergo decompressive spinal surgery secondary to cord compression and 6 patients sustaining permanent neurologic injury.[39]

Eight deaths occurred in the cohort as a whole (seven in the vertebroplasty group and one in the kyphoplasty group). Of the four deaths in the lateral approach vertebroplasty

FIGURE 33-1 ** A, B,** *Sagittal and coronal computed tomography of a 77-year-old female who underwent vertebroplasty of a T12 fracture. The patient had retropulsion of posterior wall fragment (arrows) resulting in lower extremity paraplegia. (All images are reprinted with permission from Alexander R. Vaccaro, MD, Thomas Jefferson University Hospital, Philadelphia, PA.)*

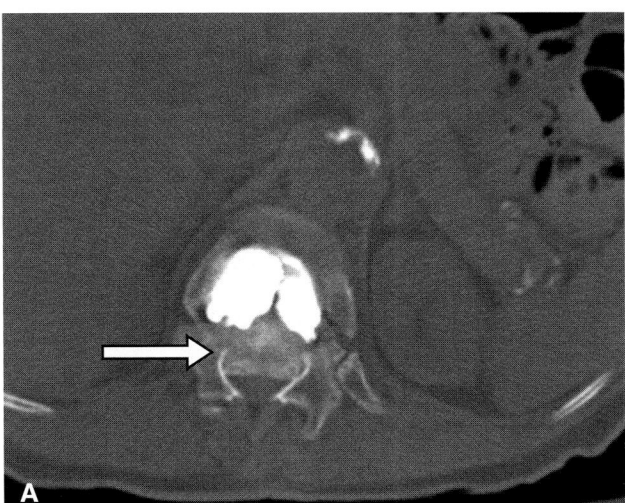

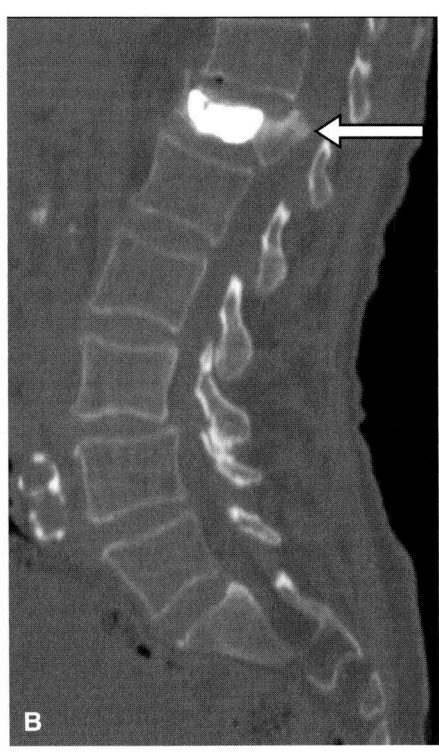

group one was due to an anaphylactic reaction to the bone cement, one to cement extravasation with resultant cord compression, and the other two deaths were after multilevel vertebroplasties (8 levels and 10 levels, respectively). The authors cited that this was far too many levels to do in one setting and that doing "more than eight levels simultaneously was not accepted medical practice." The three deaths that occurred in the transpedicular vertebroplasty were all related to anaphylaxis to the PMMA; the one death in the kyphoplasty patient was the result of a cardiac arrest during transfer from the operating room table.[39]

Another concern after undergoing either vertebroplasty or kyphoplasty is the risk of subsequent fracture. When the fractures are fixed with cement they become stiffer than the vertebral segments both cephalad and caudad. This in turn increases the forces that are seen by these adjacent vertebral bodies and their risk of fracture. Lindsay and co-workers showed that the chance of sustaining a vertebral compression fracture within the first year after having been diagnosed with one was 19.2 percent.[31] If a patient had two vertebral compression fractures, then the risk increased to 24 percent within the first year.[31]

This increased incidence is related to the patient's osteoporosis and can be decreased by use of bisphosphonates in this group. All patients with osteoporotic compression fractures should be appropriately screened for the severity of their osteoporosis. They should either be treated or referred for treatment to their internist or endocrinologist to prevent further fractures. Vertebroplasty has been shown in the literature to have a rate of subsequent fracture of 23 to 52 percent.[48]

Harrop and colleagues showed that rate of compression fracture postkyphoplasty was 22.6 percent per patient.[19] When they stratified the patients as having primary osteoporosis versus secondary steroid-induced osteoporosis, they found that the primary group had a rate of 11.25 percent versus 48.6 percent for the steroid-induced group.[19] They felt that kyphoplasty in patients with primary osteoporosis did not appear to increase their risk of facture and may have served to reduce their overall risk. In contrast, Fribourg and associates found a new fracture rate of 26 percent in their study of 38 patients who underwent kyphoplasty.[13] They felt that rate of fracture was higher after kyphoplasty than the natural history of vertebral compression fractures treated conservatively.

The role of both vertebroplasty and kyphoplasty is continuing to evolve in the treatment of vertebral compression fractures. The lack of any large or multicenter, double-blind, prospective studies comparing the two and the lack of long-term follow-up still mean that these procedures are unproven in the long run. The additional cost incurred with kyphoplasty (approximately 2.5 times that of vertebroplasty) as well as the additional time (patients more often require general anesthesia and sometimes a stay overnight), and additional radiation exposure to both patient and physician, have to be factored into the decision-making process.[39]

ANKYLOSING SPONDYLITIS

A seronegative spondyloarthropathy, ankylosing spondylitis (AS) is an inflammatory disease usually characterized by bilateral sacroiliitis that progresses in a cephalad direction. An enthesopathy of paravertebral joints of the spine generally develops after the initial involvement of the sacroiliac joints. This can lead to calcification of the joints and intervertebral disks and ultimately to fusion of the spine, or the so-called bamboo spine. The fusion of the spine can result in a fixed hyperkyphotic posture that compromises the patient's sagittal balance and makes ambulation as well as horizontal gaze difficult. Other extraspinal manifestations of the disease include hip and knee flexion contractures (which occur in compensation for the loss of sagittal balance as well as degenerative disease), cardiac conduction abnormalities, aortic valve insufficiency, pulmonary apical fibrosis, urethritis, and iridocyclitis.[27]

Ankylosing spondylitis typically affects young males in their thirties, with a male-to-female ratio of 3:1; it usually presents with insidious-onset low back pain and stiffness. It is worse in the morning or after long periods of rest. There is a strong family predilection with a 15 to 20 percent family history of the disease. AS has been linked to the HLA-B27 gene locus and is positive in 80 to 95 percent of patients, with carriers having an increased risk of 16 to 50 percent.[27] Patients who are HLA-B27-negative generally develop AS at an older age and lack the positive family history. Women who develop AS tend to do so at a later age, have less progressive symptoms, and frequent alternative sites of onset.[27]

A typical AS patient develops low back pain in the third to fourth decade. The classic feature is inflammation with bony destruction at the area of insertion of a tendon, or enthesopathy. This inflammation leads to new bone formation and leads to ankylosis of the joints. In the spine it results in calcification of the anterior longitudinal ligament, posterior longitudinal ligament, the ligamentum flavum, and interspinous ligaments. This calcification leads to squaring of the vertebral bodies and the creation of flowing syndesmophytes that bridge the disk spaces and link the vertebrae. Again, in its most severe form it results in the classic "bamboo spine" (Fig. 33-2).

Current medical management of AS continues to include nonsteroidal anti-inflammatory drugs (NSAIDs) as well as disease-modifying medications such as sulfasalizine, methotrexate, thalidomide, and antitumor necrosis factor-α agents.[27] The patient also needs to be educated about the natural history of the disease and counseled about correct posture, using only one pillow in bed, and the value of hyperextension stretching and physical exercise.

As ankylosis continues in AS patients their chest wall expansion decreases secondary to fusion of the rib articulations with the sternum and thoracic spine. This decrease in relative area can lead to restrictive lung disease. This restrictive process predisposes these patients to pulmonary problems whether they are treated operatively or nonoperatively.[7,23,54,55] Limited chest wall expansion during maximal inspiration is the most specific clinical diagnostic measure for AS.[3]

Though AS is a disease manifested by bone deposition in the soft tissues, patients afflicted with it have osteopenic or osteoporotic spines even in the very early stages of the disease.[37,47,52] It is hypothesized that the increased vascularity in conjunction with the underlying inflammatory nature of the disease is the precipitator of this decrease in vertebral bone density. Though ankylosis may extend

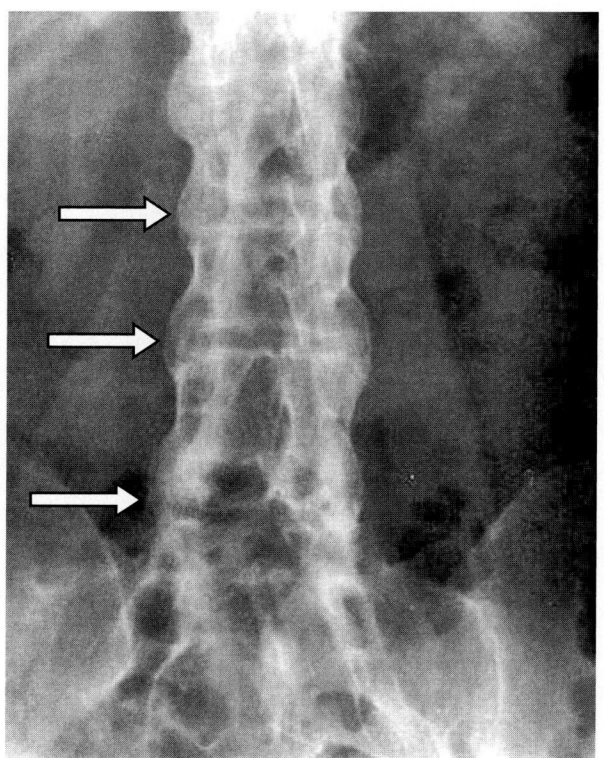

FIGURE 33-2 *Anteroposterior radiograph of a 62-year-old male with ankylosing spondylitis. The arrows point to the marginal syndesmophytes that are characteristic of this disease process. (All images are reprinted with permission from Alexander R. Vaccaro, MD, Thomas Jefferson University Hospital, Philadelphia, PA.)*

through the subaxial spine, the atlantoaxial and occipitocervical junctions are often spared or less severely affected. This junction with decreased ankylosis creates an area of increased force dispersion and along with inflammatory synovitis of these joints can lead to a relative hypermobility of these upper two cervical articulations. Traumatic atlantoaxial dislocation, odontoid fractures and occipitocervical dissociation are often seen in these patients.[18,24,25,32,36,42]

Patients who carry the diagnosis of AS are 3.5 times as likely to sustain a fracture of their spine.[7,12] The increased rigidity of their spinal column along with the decreased bone density makes traumatic spinal fractures more likely. The fused segments create long lever arms that lack the usual energy-dissipating ability of the intervertebral disks and ligaments. This ankylosis leads to a majority of the force being concentrated on a relatively narrow segment of the spinal column with bone that has decreased density and therefore a lessened resistance to failure. This results in relatively innocuous injuries, resulting from low-energy trauma or just from normal physiologic loads, creating severe fracture patterns all along the spinal column.

Traumatic spinal fractures in patients with AS are typically the result of hyperextension injuries most commonly manifesting themselves in the cervical spine[1] (Fig. 33-3). Fractures in the thoracic and lumbar spine also occur, and as

FIGURE 33-3 *A 67-year-old man with ankylosing spondylitis who fell, sustaining a hyperextension injury resulting in a fracture through the C6-C7 disk space.* **A,** *Anteroposterior cervical radiograph. The arrows show the obscure fracture line.* **B,** *Sagittal computed tomography demonstrating the fracture line (arrows) traversing the disk space of C6-C7.* **C,** *T1-weighted magnetic resonance image of the same patient showing widening of the intervertebral disk space (arrow).*

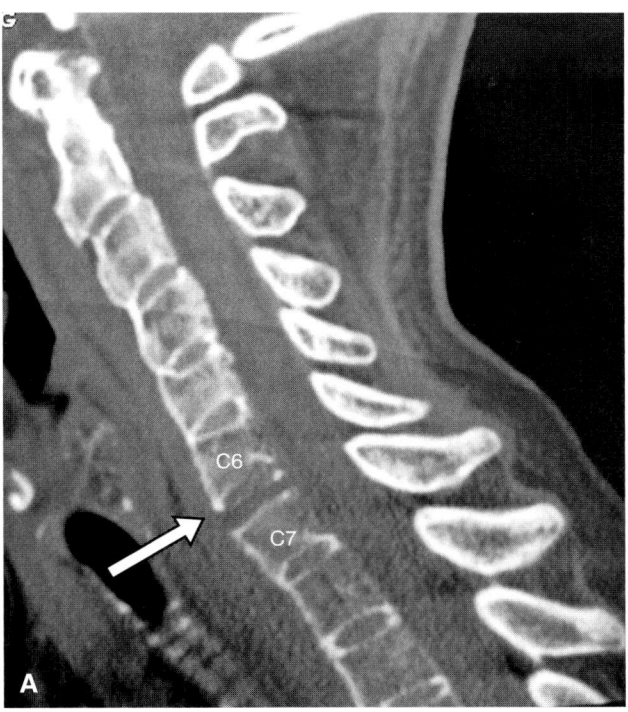

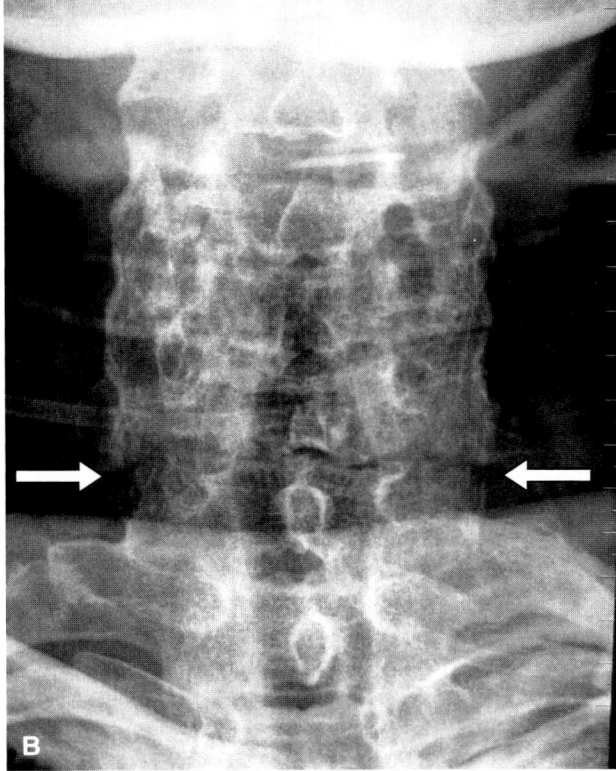

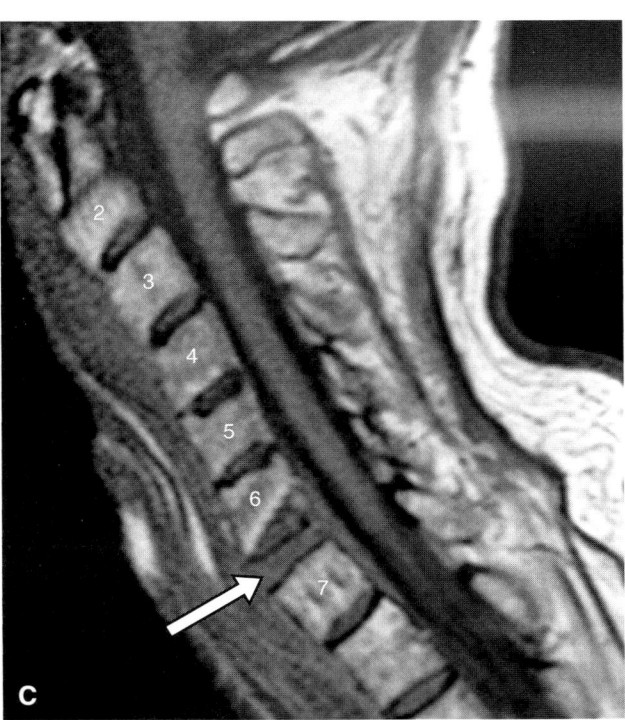

(Continued)

FIGURE 33-3   *(Continued)* **D, E,** *Postoperative radiographs after 360° fusion with anterior C7 corpectomy and graft stabilization with a bioabsorbable plate and posterior segmental fixation from C3 to T3. (All images are reprinted with permission from Alexander R. Vaccaro, MD, Thomas Jefferson University Hospital, Philadelphia, PA.)*

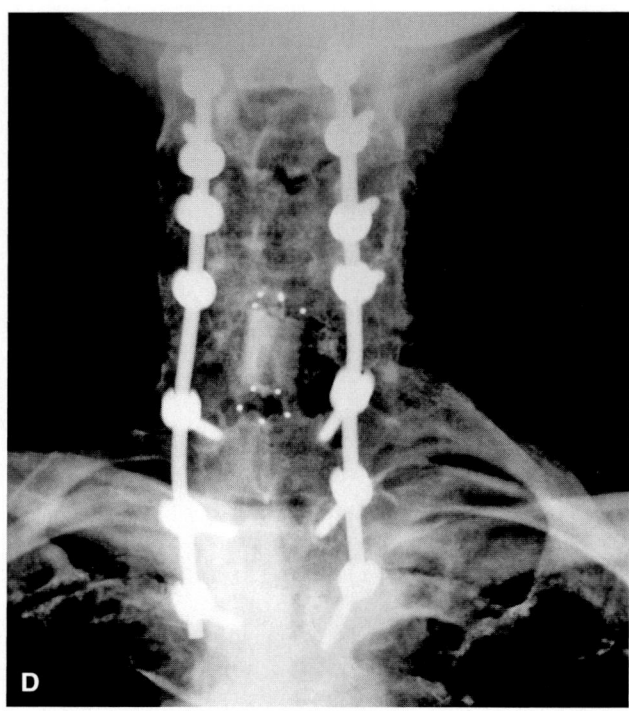

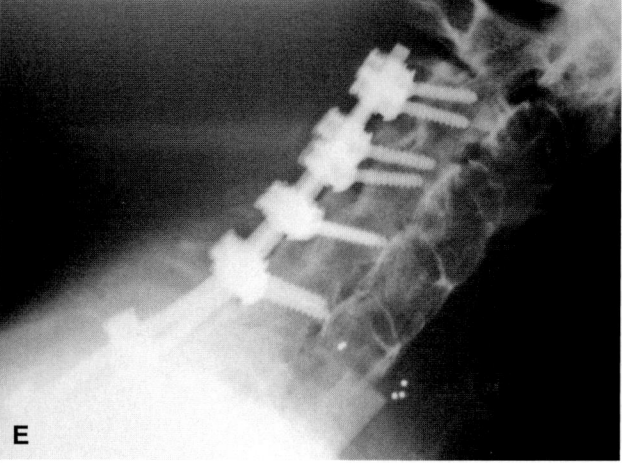

with all spine fractures other, *non-contiguous fractures* must also be sought.[7,12,41]

Neurologic deficit after spine fractures in patients with ankylosing spondylitis is common, up to 75 percent, and mortality following these injuries can be as high as 50 percent.[17,57] Ankylosing spondylitis has been found to be a significant predictor for mortality in cervical spine fractures.[40] Patients with AS are also predisposed to develop neurologic deficit in a delayed fashion.[53] Broom and Raycroft had five patients with AS who initially presented neurologically intact and subsequently developed a neurologic deficit, secondary to delay in diagnosis, development of epidural hematoma, or inability to adequately immobilize the fracture site.[4] These complications occurred at an average of 15 days after injury (range 2–35).[4]

Radiographic imaging of the spinal column in AS is difficult. Traumatic injuries can be obscured by the increased bony sclerosis and syndesmophytes that are present throughout the spine.[23] Vigilance needs to be increased when evaluating patients with AS for a spine fracture, because occult fractures can be present even if radiographs are interpreted as negative. Delay in diagnosis can have catastrophic neurologic sequelae and can lead to progressive spinal deformity.[4,10,11,46,57] Radiographic evaluation of these patients by CT, with sagittal and coronal reconstructions, after even minor trauma is mandatory if the patient has any subjective complaints of neck or back pain. Three-dimensional (3-D) CT has been shown to be more sensitive than standard CT.[56] The sensitivity of MRI has been found to be superior to conventional radiographs and 3-D CT with respect to delineating cord deformity, ligament damage

(especially posterior), soft-tissue disruptions, dural pathology, and epidural hematoma formation.[11,51,56]

The typical fracture pattern seen in patients with AS is a transdiscal fracture with posterior element involvement, with fractures into the vertebral body being less common.[26,51] The fusion of multiple segments of the spinal column results in the spine functioning like a long bone.[41] The forces transmitted through these long lever arms on the calcified discoligamentous complex, with its decreased ability to withstand even physiologic loads, result in this characteristic fracture pattern and prolonged healing potential.

Initial immobilization of these patients is important. Straightening of the neck or indiscriminant application of traction can result in worsening of the neurologic condition.[46] The neck should be immobilized in its preinjury position, which is usually hyperkyphotic. Displacement of fractures can ensue if a patient's neck is forced into extension, resulting in severe neurologic injury.[11,57] Manipulation of these fractures can lead to formation of epidural hematoma, to which these patients are predisposed, and worsening of any neurologic deficit. Use of orthoses in treating these patients must take into account their preexisting deformity, necessitating the use of a custom orthosis. Due to ankylosis around the articulations of the chest wall and its decreased excursion, it is important that pulmonary toilet be emphasized in these patients in order to decrease their susceptibility to pulmonary infections.

Nonoperative treatment of spinal column fractures in this patient population has been advocated by many authors.[17,23,50,57] Traction, collar, and halo–vest immobilization have all been used for AS patients with relatively nondisplaced fractures with or without neurologic compromise. Complications such as nonunion, pseudoarthrosis, and neurologic deterioration have all been seen when conservative care is the mainstay of treatment.[4,7,9,50,57] Most cervical spine fractures seen in patients with AS are three-column injuries, which are highly unstable and usually respond poorly with nonoperative care.

Operative management of spinal fractures may be the preferred treatment in patients with cervical spine injuries. The instability of some of these fracture types, as well as the inability of a patient with decreased pulmonary function to tolerate halo–vest immobilization, may make surgical stabilization optimal. Other factors such as worsening neurologic condition, increasing deformity, epidural hematoma, or widely displaced fractures may necessitate operative intervention.

Operative intervention in the setting of spinal fracture depends on the location of the fracture. The posterior approach is favored in thoracic spinal fractures due to the pre-existing decrease in pulmonary function that is present in these patients at baseline. Multiple points of fixation are often used so as to decrease the stress at any one level.[54] In the cervical spine a posterior-only approach can be used if patient deformity is so extreme (i.e., chin-on-chest deformity) that adequate anterior access cannot be attained. Anterior surgery can be done subsequent to posterior surgery if needed. If an anterior approach is to be used in the cervical spine it is often reinforced with a posterior fusion due to the tenuous nature of vertebral body fixation in the osteoporotic spine. Patient positioning during surgery should be done with extreme diligence so as to not exaggerate correction of a preexisting deformity. Neurologic monitoring is usually helpful in this situation.

Different construct types can be used in these patients. Calcification of the ligamentous structures of the spine can make passage of sublaminar wires or hooks difficult. Other forms of fixation such as transverse process hooks, spinous process wires, or pedicle screws should be considered. The two former types of fixation are not as strong as sublaminar hooks or wires, whereas the latter gives a more solid construct. As in an osteoporotic patient, a pedicle screw construct with supplemental sublaminar hooks would further increase the pullout strength.[20]

Patients with AS are predisposed to epidural hematoma formation after traumatic spinal column fractures. The reported rates of this complication have been as high as 20 percent.[23,55] It should be suspected whenever a patient suffers neurologic deterioration after an initial period of stability and mandates MRI of the affected fracture site and early decompression.

The syndrome of synovitis, acne pustulosis, and hyperostosis osteitis (SAPHO) can lead to spinal ankylosis similar to that seen in ankylosing spondylitis. The syndesmophytes again create a spinal column with long lever arms that predispose it to fractures from even minor trauma. Though similar to AS in spinal manifestations, there is no link to HLA-B27, and the ankylosis usually does not extend from the sacrum cephalad. Also, the extraspinal manifestations are not similar to AS and usually bear more resemblance to psoriatic arthritis. Cervical spinal column fracture with spinal cord injury (SCI) from a hyperextension mechanism has been reported with this syndrome.[6]

DIFFUSE IDIOPATHIC SKELETAL HYPEROSTOSIS

Diffuse idiopathic skeletal hyperostosis (DISH, Forestier disease, or ankylosing hyperostosis) is another disease that is manifested by spinal ankylosis. DISH commonly occurs in men in their fifth to sixth decade of life. It commonly results in a flowing fusion mass across the anterolateral aspect of the spinal column without the degenerative changes seen in AS. Radiographic criteria for diagnosis of DISH are having anterolateral intervertebral fusion across four segments with preservation of disk height without significant degenerative disease and without sacroiliac or apophyseal joint degeneration or fusion.[5] Though it can be seen throughout the spine, it is most commonly encountered on the right side of the thoracic spine.[5,35]

Similar to patients with AS, vertebral osteoporosis or osteopenia is seen in patients with DISH, though to a lesser degree.[35] Recent studies using DEXA studies have shown that in the peripheral skeleton the bone mineral density (BMD) is actually significantly higher than in age-matched controls.[8] This seemingly contradictory evidence stems from the fact that relative to AS, DISH has fewer if any extraskeletal manifestations and their severity is often less.[35]

Patients with DISH commonly complain of mild to moderate chronic back pain, with some aspect of spinal stiffness; the extreme spinal deformities seen in AS are not typically seen in DISH.[5,35] Skip lesions in the spine can also be seen in DISH. Medical comorbidities associated with DISH include diabetes mellitus, obesity, hypertension, and coronary artery disease.[35]

Though vertebral fusion masses may not be as widespread as in patients with AS, long-segment fusions can create areas of stiffness throughout the spine. These long lever arms can accentuate traumatic forces and make areas of the spine more susceptible to lower energy trauma.[2,21,24,35] Radiologic evaluation of patients with DISH is the same as that for patients with AS. Plain radiographs can be misinterpreted secondary to increased bone formation, so judicious use of CT and MRI is recommended to rule out occult fractures even in the setting of minor trauma.

Fractures in DISH historically have been described as traversing the vertebral body.[2,9,35,38,43] There are, however, many studies in which the majority of fractures occurred through the disk space.[5,21,24,33,43] Fractures are commonly seen at the end of a long fusion mass. These fractures are commonly caused by a hyperextension injury and result in a three-column spinal injury. Fractures in DISH are not as common as in AS, which is thought to be due to the occurrence of skip areas and the lack of ankylosis of the facet joint.[21] These skip area findings allow dissipation of forces through multiple sites in the spine, thus not concentrating traumatic forces at one distinct segment. As in AS, patients with DISH are at risk for neurologic complications[21,35,43] that can be as high as 87.5 percent.[43] Delay in diagnosis of a spinal fracture has also been seen in several studies,[21,43] whereas a mortality rate of 12.5 percent was also seen in one study.[43]

Management of fractures in patients with DISH is like that in patients with AS. Both nonoperative and operative management of these fractures can be utilized. Patients with nondisplaced thoracic or lumbar fractures can be treated with bed rest, followed by mobilization with an orthosis (thoracolumbosacral orthosis—TLSO). Nonoperative management has been shown to carry a high mortality rate, especially when there was a neurologic deficit.[35,38] Nonoperative management can also lead to neurologic deterioration and post-traumatic deformity.[5] Fractures involving all three columns and those with marked displacement or dislocation are more adequately treated with surgical intervention.[5,35,43] Segmental instrumentation and decompression with the avoidance of fracture site overdistraction are useful in these patients. The generally increased quality of bone lends itself to alternative forms of fixation.

CONCLUSION

Fracture fixation in the osteoporotic and stiff spine requires the surgeon to use the myriad of techniques at his or her disposal. New and emerging ways of treating vertebral compression fractures are being studied and becoming more widespread. In patients with AS or diffuse idiopathic skeletal hyperostosis the physician needs to be vigilant for fractures and not hesitate to order more advanced imaging studies if the circumstances warrant it (increased back pain, change in back pain, or pain after even minor trauma). These patients have a higher propensity for missed fractures or delay in diagnosis, which can lead to catastrophic outcomes.

REFERENCES

1. Amamilo, S.C. Fractures of the cervical spine in patients with ankylosing spondylitis. Orthop Rev 28:339–343, 1989.
2. Bernini, P.M.; Floman, Y.; Marvel, J.P.; et al. Multiple thoracic spine fractures complicating ankylosing hyperostosis of the spine. J Trauma 21:811–814, 1981.
3. Blam, O.G.; Cotler, J.M. Fractures of the stiff and osteoporotic spine. Skeletal Trauma, 3rd ed, Philadelphia, Saunders, 2002, pp. 1004–1011.
4. Broom, M.J.; Raycroft, J.F. Complications of fractures of the cervical spine in ankylosing spondylitis. Spine 13:763–766, 1998.
5. Burkus, J.K.; Denis, F. Hyperextension injuries of the thoracic spine in diffuse idiopathic skeletal hyperostosis. Report of four cases. J Bone Joint Surg [Am] 76:237–243, 1994.
6. Deltombe, T.; Nisolle, J.F.; Boutsen, Y.; et al. Cervical spinal cord injury in SAPHO syndrome. Spinal Cord 37:301–304, 1999.
7. Detwilder, K.N.; Loftus, C.M.; Godersky, J.C.; et al. Management of cervical spine injuries in patients with ankylosing spondylitis. J Neuorsurg 72:210–215, 1990.
8. Di Franco, M.; Maurceri M.T.; Sili-Scavalli, A.; et al. Study of peripheral bone mineral density in patients with diffuse skeletal hyperostosis. Clin Rheumatol 19:188–192, 2000.
9. Fardon, D.F. Odontoid fracture complicating ankylosing hyperostosis of the spine. Spine 3:108–112, 1978.
10. Farmer, J.; Vaccaro, A.R.; Albert, T.J.; et al. Neurologic deterioration after cervical spinal cord injury. J Spinal Disord 11:192–196, 1998.
11. Finkelstein, J.A.; Chapman, J.R.; Mirza, S. Occult vertebral fractures in ankylosing spondylitis. Spinal Cord 37:444–447, 1999.
12. Fox, M.W.; Onofrio, B.N. Neurological complications of ankylosing spondylitis. J Neurosurg 78:871–878, 1993.
13. Fribourg, D.; Tang, C.; Sra, P.; et al. Incidence of subsequent vertebral fracture after kyphoplasty. Spine 29:2270–2276, 2004.
14. Galibert, P.; Deramond, H.; Rosat, P.; et al. Preliminary note on the treatment of vertebral angioma by percutaneous acrylic vertebroplasty. J. Neurochirurgie 33:166–168, 1987.
15. Genant, H.K.; Cooper, C.; Poor, G.; et al. Interim report and recommendations of the World Health Organization task force for osteoporosis. Osteoporosis Int 10:259–264, 1999.
16. Groh, J.G.; Matzner, M.; Trieb, K.; et al. Minimal invasive stabilization of osteoporotic vertebral fractures. J Spinal Disord Tech 18:238–242, 2005.
17. Graham, B.; Peteghem, P.K. Fractures of the spine in ankylosing spondylitis: Diagnosis, treatment and complications. Spine 14:803–807, 1989.
18. Govender, S.; Charles, R.W. Fracture of the dens in ankylosing spondylitis. Injury 18:213–214, 1987.
19. Harrop, J.S.; Prpa, B.; Reinhardt, M.K.; et al. Primary and secondary osteoporosis' incidence of subsequent vertebral compression fractures after kyphoplasty. Spine 29:2120–2125, 2004.
20. Hasegawa, K.; Takahashi, H.E.; Uchiyama, S. An experimental study of a combination method using a pedicle screw and laminar hook for the osteoporotic spine. Spine 22:958–963, 1997.
21. Hendrix, R.W.; Melany, M.; Miller, F.; et al. Fracture of the spine in patients with ankylosis due to diffuse idiopathic skeletal hyperostosis: Clinical and imaging findings. AJR Am J Roentgenol 162:899–904, 1994.
22. Hu, S.S. Internal fixation in the osteoporotic spine. Spine 22:43S–48S, 1997.
23. Hunter, T.; Dubo, H. Spinal fractures complicating ankylosing spondylitis: A long-term follow-up study. Arthritis Rheum 26:751–759, 1983.
24. Israel, Z.; Mosheiff, R.; Gross, E.; et al. Hyperextension fracture–dislocation of the thoracic spine with paraplegia in a patient with diffuse idiopathic skeletal hyperostosis. J Spinal Disord 7:455–457, 1994.
25. Kaplan, S.L.; Tun, G.C.; Sarkarati, M. Odontoid fracture complicating ankylosing spondylitis: A case report and review of the literature. Spine 15:607–610, 1990.
26. Karasick, D.; Schweitzer, M.E.; Abidi, N.A.; et al. Fractures of the vertebra with spinal cord injuries in patients with ankylosing spondylitis. AJR Am J Roentgenol 165: 1205–1208, 1995.
27. Kubiak, E.N.; Moskovich, R.; Errico, T.J.; et al. Orthopaedic management of ankylosing spondylitis. J Am Acad Orthop Surg 13:267–278, 2005.

28. Lee, Y.L.; Yip, K.M. The osteoporotic spine. Clin Orthop 323:91–97, 1996.

29. Lieberman, I.H.; Dudeney, S.; Reinhardt, M.K.; et al. Initial outcome and efficacy of "kyphoplasty" in the treatment of painful osteoporotic vertebral compression fractures. Spine 26:1631–1638, 2001.

30. Lin, J.T.; Lane, J.M. Osteoporosis: A review. Clin Orthop 425:126–134, 2004.

31. Lindsey, R.; Silverman, S.L.; Cooper, C.; et al. Risk of new vertebral compression fracture in the year following a fracture. JAMA 285:319–323, 2001.

32. McCall, I.; El Masri, W.; Jaffrey D. Hangman's fracture in ankylosing spondylitis. Injury 16:483–484, 1985.

33. McKenzie, M.K.; Bartal, E.; Pay, N.T. A hyperextension injury of the thoracic spine in association with diffuse skeletal hyperostosis. Orthopedics 14:895–898, 1991.

34. Melton, L.J. III; Epidemiology of spinal osteoporosis. Spine 22:2S–11S, 1997.

35. Meyer, P.R., Jr. Diffuse idiopathic skeletal hyperostosis in the cervical spine. Clin Orthop 359:49–57, 1999.

36. Miller, F.H.; Rogers, L.F. Fractures of the dens complicating ankylosing spondylitis with atlantooccipital fusion. J Rheumatol 18:773–774, 1991.

37. Mitra, D.; Elvins, D.M.; Speden, D.J.; et al. The prevalence of vertebral compression fractures in mild ankylosing spondylitis and their relationship to bone mineral density. Rheumatology 39:85–89, 2000.

38. Mody, G.M.; Charles, R.W.; Ranchod, H.A.; et al. Cervical spine fracture in diffuse idiopathic skeletal hyperostosis. J Rheumatol 15:129–131, 1991.

39. Nussbaum, D.A.; Gailloud, P.; Murphy, K. A review of complications associated with vertebroplasty and kyphoplasty as reported to the food and drug administration medical device related web site. J Vasc Interven Radiol 15:1185–1192, 2004.

40. Olerud, C.; Andersson, S.; Svensson, B.; et al. Cervical spine fractures in the elderly. Acta Orthop Scand 70:509–513, 1999.

41. Osgood, C.P.; Abbasy, M.; Mathews, T. Multiple spine fractures in ankylosing spondylitis. Trauma 15:163–166, 1975.

42. Ozgocmen, S.; Ardicoglu, O. Odontoid fracture complicating ankylosing spondylitis. Spinal Cord 38:117–119, 2000.

43. Paley, D.; Schwartz, M.; Cooper, P.; et al. Fractures of the spine in diffuse idiopathic skeletal hyperostosis. Clin Orthop 267:22–32, 1991.

44. Philips, F.M. Minimally invasive treatments of osteoporotic vertebral compression fractures. Spine 28:S45–S53, 2003.

45. Philips, F.M.; McNally, T.; Wetzel, F.T.; et al. Early clinical and radiographic results of kyphoplasty for the treatment of osteopenic vertebral compression fractures. Eur Spine J 10:S7, 2001.

46. Podolosky, S.M.; Hoffman, J.R.; Pietrafesa, C.A. Neurologic complications following immobilization of cervical spine fracture in a patient with ankylosing spondylitis. Ann Emerg Med 12:578–580, 1983.

47. Ralston, S.H.; Urguhart, G.D.K.; Brzeski, M.; et al. Prevalence of vertebral compression fractures due to osteoporosis in ankylosing spondylitis. BMJ 300:563–565, 1990.

48. Rao, R.D.; Singrakhia, M.D. Painful osteoporotic vertebral fracture: Pathogenesis, evaluation, and roles of vertebroplasty and kyphoplasty in its management. J Bone J Surg [Am] 85:2010–2022, 2003.

49. Riggs, B.L.; Melton, L.J., III. The worldwide problem of osteoporosis: Insights afforded by epidemiology. Bone 17:505S–511S, 1995.

50. Rowed, D.W. Management of cervical spinal cord injury in ankylosing spondylitis. J Neurosurg 77:241–246, 1992.

51. Shih, T.T.; Chen, P.; Li, Y.; et al. Spinal fractures and pseudoarthrosis complicating ankylosing spondylitis: MRI manifestations and clinical significance. J Comput Assist Tomogr 25:164–170, 2001.

52. Spencer, D.G.; Park, W.M.; Dick, H.M.; et al. Radiologic manifestations in 200 patients with ankylosing spondylitis: Correlation with clinical features and HLA-B27. J Rheumatol 6:305–315, 1979.

53. Straiton, N. Fractures of the lower vertebral column in ankylosing spondylitis. Brit J Clin Prac 41:933–934, 1987.

54. Taggard, D.A.; Traynelis, V.C. Management of cervical spine fractures in ankylosing spondylitis with posterior fixation. Spine 25:2035–2039, 2000.

55. Tico, N.; Ramon, S.; Garcia-Ortun, F.; et al. Traumatic spinal cord injury complicating ankylosing spondylitis. Spinal Cord 36:349–352, 1998.

56. Wang, Y.; Teng, M.M.; Chang, C.; et al. Imaging manifestations of spinal fractures in ankylosing spondylitis. Am J Neuroradiol 26:2067–2076, 2005.

57. Weinstein, P.R.; Karpman, R.R.; Gall, E.P.; et al. Spinal cord injury, spinal fracture, and spinal stenosis in ankylosing spondylitis. J Neurosurg 57:609–616, 1982.

58. Wong, W.; Riley, M.A.; Garfin, S. Vertebroplasty/kyphoplasty. JWI 2:117–124, 2000.

CHAPTER 34

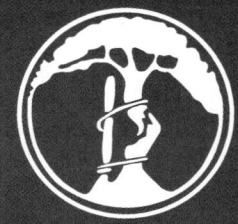

Complications in the Treatment of Spinal Trauma

**Robert K. Eastlack, M.D., Bradford L. Currier, M.D.,
Choll W. Kim, M.D., Ph.D., and Michael J. Yaszemski, M.D., Ph.D.**

Treatment of spinal trauma was described as early as the Hippocratic era. Hippocrates' famous extension bench, known as "scamnum" when popularized by Celsius, was used frequently for realignment of a fractured or deformed spine. In ancient and medieval times, forceful and brisk maneuvers accompanied by immobilization were the mainstay of spinal trauma treatment. A patient would often lie prone while attendants would pull on his ankles and axillae and a "physician" would sit or press on prominences such as a gibbus or palpable fracture deformity.

As recently as the late 1800s, Jean-Francis Calot and his contemporaries manipulated spinal deformities with their fists. In 1917, Hartmann (at the Accident Hospital for coal miners in Upper Silesia) treated a patient with a fracture-dislocation of the thoracolumbar junction by having two assistants suspend the patient by the armpits and pelvis while he performed reduction by forceful manipulation from below with his fists. Later, through the first four decades of the 20th century, methods of postural reduction by hyperextension were introduced. Davis, Rogers, and Bohlman were champions of such methods through the use of slings, frames, or similar devices.[63]

As one might imagine, such treatment led to unacceptably high rates of complications, including soft tissue breakdown, neurologic compromise, malunion, instability, and pulmonary compromise. Treatment of spinal trauma has changed significantly over the last two decades. However, despite better imaging, better understanding, better access to treatment, and the availability of internal fixation, challenging complications continue to exist today.

COMPLICATIONS OF NONOPERATIVE TREATMENT

Halo Vest Immobilization

Indications for use of the halo vest have evolved greatly since its description by Perry and Nickel in 1953. Initially described for postoperative immobilization of patients who had undergone cervical fusion for neck paralysis from poliomyelitis, Thompson and Freeman extended its use

to the treatment of fractures. Complications of halo vest immobilization can be divided into those related to application of the device and those related to its use. Traditionally, the use of plaster-molded vests carried a risk of cast syndrome, pressure sores, and respiratory problems in patients with limited respiratory reserves. Prefabricated padded plastic vests have helped decrease the incidence of these complications, but at the expense of decreased rigidity and increased cost. However, patient compliance has improved, and the incidence of pin loosening has decreased with these lightweight prefabricated vests.

The pins themselves pose problems as well. Pin site infection is not uncommon but may be minimized with daily pin site care, including twice-daily application of a dilute hydrogen peroxide solution (50% in water). The reported incidence of pin site infection ranges from 2 to 35 percent, although the rate seems to be substantially reduced by insertion of the pins at 8 in-lb of torque versus 6 in-lb in adults.[17,50,55,84] Oral antibiotics are usually effective, but if a pin is loose and infected, a new pin should be placed in a nearby hole in the halo ring. If the pins are incorrectly placed cephalad to the equator of the skull, halo slippage may occur (Fig. 34-1). The pins should be torqued to 8 in-lb in adults and 6 in-lb or less in children. In patients with osteoporosis or for those in whom the pins are inadvertently placed in the temporal areas, the skull can be perforated. Dural penetration has been reported and can lead to epidural abscess or cerebrospinal fluid (CSF) leakage.[78,104,120]

No orthosis can apply predictable and continuous traction to the cervical spine when the patient is not supine. When the patient is sitting or standing, a previously distracted cervical spine can become compressed by the force of gravity on the head and halo vest construct (Fig. 34-2). Such compression can lead to loss of reduction and possibly a new neurologic deficit. Likewise, rotational forces are poorly constrained by a halo vest orthosis. Treatment of a unilateral facet dislocation, for example, may lead to persistent root compression and failure of therapy. Whitehill and colleagues[144] described five cases of loss of reduction in patients with facet dislocations immobilized

FIGURE 34-1 *Failed halo pin sites. At follow-up, the halo pins of this gentleman had dislodged, and the vest and headpiece migrated proximally. His halo was removed and he was treated in a cervical collar for the remainder of treatment.*

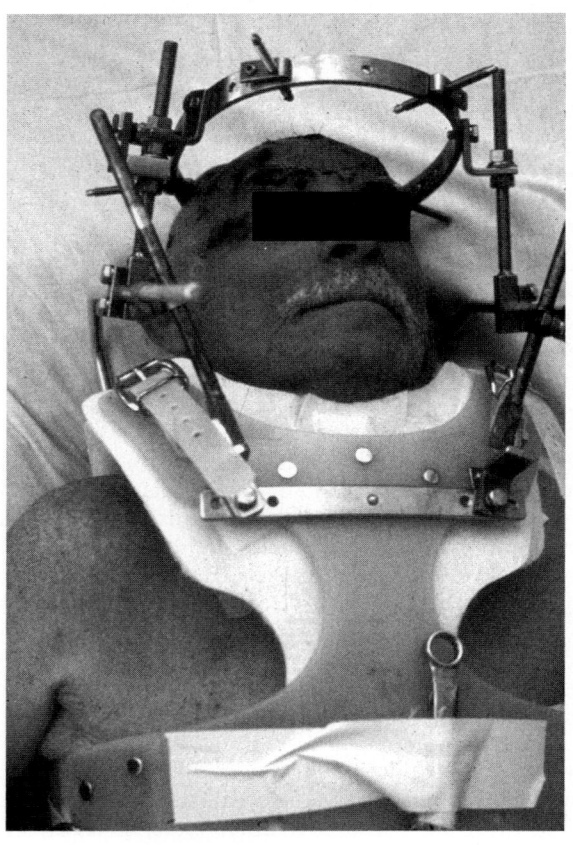

in a halo vest. Glaser and associates[55] and Bucholz and Cheung[20] documented loss of reduction in 10 percent of all patients and in 37 percent of patients with facet subluxation and dislocation.

Anderson and co-workers[5] evaluated upright and supine lateral radiographs after halo immobilization in 42 patients with 45 noncontiguous levels of cervical spine injury. At noninjured levels, an average of 3.9° of angular change was found between adjacent levels from the occiput to C6. The greatest motion occurred more proximally (8.0° between the occiput and C1). No significant translation was seen at the noninjured levels. At the injured level, sagittal-plane angulation averaged 7.0°, and the average translation was 1.7 mm. A significant amount of fracture site motion was defined as greater than 3° of sagittal angulation or more than 1 mm of translation and occurred in 78 percent of the 45 injured levels. Three patients experienced loss of reduction that required reapplication of traction after vest removal. Asymptomatic malunion developed in 11 patients. One may postulate that this motion contributes to such a high degree of nonunion in type II odontoid fractures treated in a halo vest.

Residual kyphosis of a post-traumatic cervical spine can lead to a multitude of complications (Fig. 34-3). Neural impairment can occur from compression of the spinal cord as it drapes over the apex of the deformity. Late neck pain may be seen as a result of the modified mechanics of the paraspinous musculature that occurs when the lever arm of the muscles is altered by the deformity. Additionally, facet degeneration of adjacent segments can ensue from hyperextension of adjacent vertebral levels in an attempt to compensate for the loss of cervical lordosis in a kyphotic cervical spine.[84]

Caution must be taken when using halo-vest immobilization in the elderly. A recent report on its use in patients older than age 65 demonstrated increases in

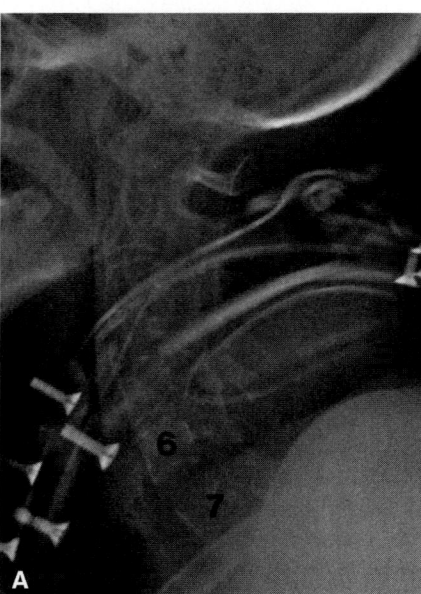

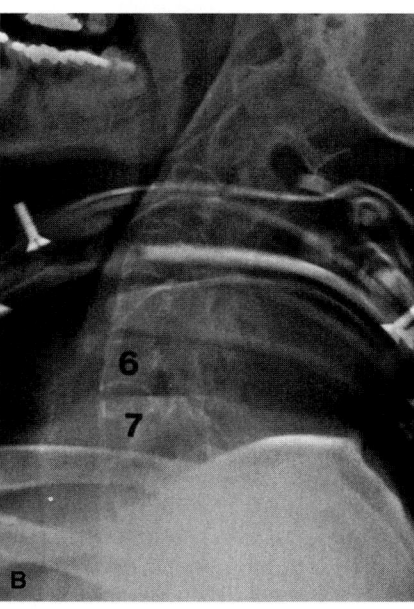

FIGURE 34-2 *Poor axial immobilization by halo. Immobilization in the axial plane is difficult with all external fixation systems, including the halo. In this patient with a fracture through a severely ankylosed cervical spine, the fracture is gapped open when supine (A) but compressed when upright (B).*

FIGURE 34-3 *Failed external immobilization for cervical facet fractures. This patient was evaluated 1.5 years after nonoperative treatment of an initially nondisplaced C6 lateral mass fracture. He complained of neck pain and paresthesia down the lateral aspect of his arm.* **A,** *Flexion radiographs showed subluxation and kyphosis.* **B,** *Treatment included anterior cervical diskectomy and fusion. Preoperative planning, however, included the possible need for circumferential fusion.*

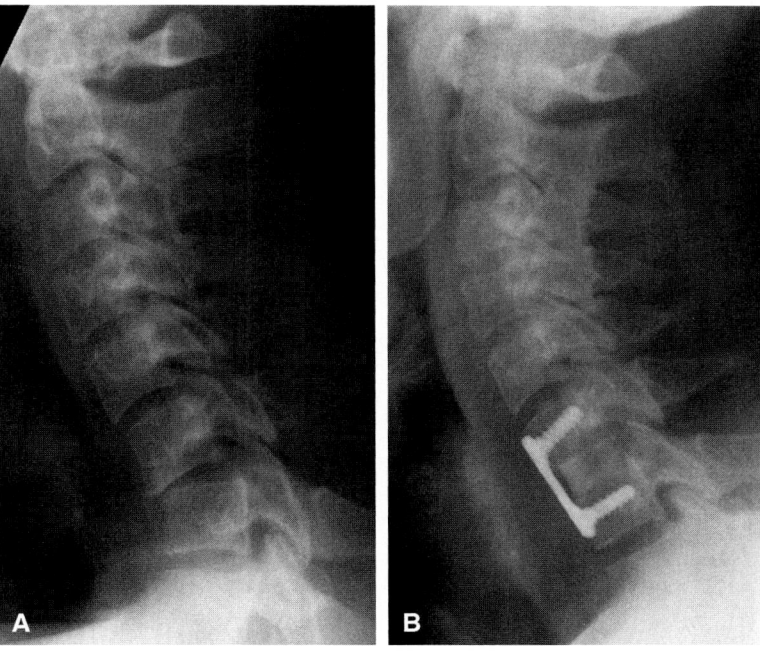

morbidity and mortality compared with treatment with a cervical orthosis.[134] In properly chosen patients, halo immobilization is an excellent treatment option that is associated with frequent but usually minor complications. However, nonunion and malunion can occur and should be considered markers of treatment failure. In patients with nonflexion-type injuries, the success rate of halo treatment approaches that of surgical fusion (87 vs. 95%).[118] However, in the group of patients with posterior ligamentous injury, the failure rate increases to as high as 46 percent.[22,118]

Braces or casts continue to play a substantial role in our treatment of thoracolumbar injuries. For stable burst fractures, such nonoperative management is generally successful, and the disadvantages of skin breakdown and progressive deformity can be mitigated by clinical and radiographic scrutiny following placement of the orthosis. Radiographs should be obtained early and often in the acute phase of treatment to ascertain any deleterious changes in spinal alignment. Mehta and associates demonstrated the value of taking these films in an upright or weight-bearing position, as collapse and worsened alignment resulted in a change of treatment in 25 percent of their patients.[95] In the literature, most authors report either rare or no neurologic deterioration in neurologically intact patients when employing nonoperative treatment.[99,125,141] However, Denis and colleagues reported a neurologic decline in 17 percent of their patients treated nonsurgically for burst fractures.[34] Most patients (>70%) in this particular study had fractures that involved three columns of injury.

Operative Versus Nonoperative Treatment

Comparisons of operative and nonoperative treatment in the treatment of spinal trauma are ubiquitous in the literature. For the purposes of this chapter, we limit our discussion to those in the more controversial areas.

Type II odontoid fractures in the elderly have been considered at higher risk for nonunion by a number of authors.[8,25,38] Because these patients do not tolerate halo-vest immobilization well and nonsurgical treatment may lead to higher nonunion rates, early surgical stabilization has been advocated.[82] However, some authors have demonstrated acceptable outcomes, including stable nonunions, using cervical orthosis immobilization alone.[60,64,98,107,121,134] Greene and associates suggest that the amount of initial displacement (>6 mm) or comminution plays a critical role in determining the benefit of surgical intervention.[60] Despite numerous studies on the subject, controversy remains on the most suitable treatment for the elderly patient with a type II odontoid fracture.

Wood and coauthors prospectively evaluated patients with stable (i.e., no radiographic evidence of posterior osseoligamentous complex involvement) thoracolumbar burst fractures undergoing operative or nonoperative treatment.[150] No differences in functional or radiographic outcome were demonstrated; however, the complication rates for operative intervention were considerably higher (67 vs. 9%). Importantly, the costs associated with operative intervention were nearly five times those incurred from nonoperative treatment.

Rechtine and colleagues[109] examined 235 patients with unstable thoracolumbar spine fractures who were given a choice of undergoing operative or nonoperative treatment. The groups were statistically similar in all respects. Although the length of stay in the hospital was 24 days greater in the nonoperative group, the incidence of complications (with the exception of wound infection) was similar for decubitus ulcers, pneumonia, deep vein thrombosis, pulmonary embolism, and death. Polytrauma was a risk factor for increased complications, and greater than 8 hours on a spine board almost universally led to sacral decubiti.[31]

Admittedly, many of the studies comparing operative and nonoperative management are retrospective in design, and most have some inherent selection bias. However, the combined experience demonstrated within these studies provides important guidance in the treatment of spinal trauma. Evolving techniques allow more advanced surgical options for many of these injuries, but we must temper our enthusiasm to implement them with the substantial morbidity and mortality associated with operative intervention. Additionally, economic considerations will undoubtedly play an ever-increasing role in our patient management. These issues are highlighted in the recent study by Wood and associates.[150]

COMPLICATIONS OF OPERATIVE TREATMENT

Patient Positioning

The potential for complications begins as early as or perhaps even before patient positioning on the operating table. Care must be taken to ensure that the airway is protected when the patient is transferred from a bed to the operating table, especially if the patient is also being turned from a supine to a prone position. In the prone position, the face must be padded evenly to avoid pressure ulceration. Prefabricated foam pads with holes for airway access are available and effective. Support devices with mirrored bases allow visual inspection of the facial structures throughout the operation. Direct pressure on the eye must be specifically avoided to prevent catastrophic retinal artery occlusion and loss of vision.[90,149] Direct pressure applied to the scalp has been associated with alopecia, which is usually reversible but is occasionally permanent. Slight rotation of the patient's head throughout the procedure, if not clinically contraindicated, helps prevent such complications. When the patient must remain prone for longer periods, we typically employ Mayfield tongs to minimize the effects of pressure on the face.

Meticulous padding of vulnerable areas, such as the elbows and knees, should help prevent neurapraxia or more serious nerve injuries to the ulnar and common peroneal nerves. The lateral femoral cutaneous nerves are easily injured by undue pressure at the proximal aspect of the thighs. The brachial plexus is at risk if the lateral decubitus or prone position is used. An axillary roll placed 5 to 10 cm distal to the axilla and avoidance of excessive abduction and forward flexion of the arm both help reduce the incidence of brachial plexopathy. In the prone position, shoulder abduction should be less than or equal to 90°, and upper extremity protraction (toward the floor) can be

taken to the lower limit of the arm board height, as long as the axillae remain free of impingement on the chest pad.

Venous return must be considered during patient positioning as well. The abdomen and chest should remain free of pressure to prevent vena cava obstruction. Low venous return can lead to loss of cardiac preload and subsequent hypotension. Obstruction of caval flow can produce increased venous pressure around the sinusoids of the spine and thereby cause unnecessary and often significant increases in blood loss. Venous obstruction has also been implicated in the rare but devastating complication of postoperative blindness.[74] The knee-chest position, in which the hips and knees are flexed, causes venous pooling in the lower extremities and has been associated with reports of lower extremity compartment syndrome requiring fasciotomy.[3]

VASCULAR AND SOFT TISSUE COMPLICATIONS

Cervical Spine

Injuries to the vascular and soft tissues of the neck may occur during surgery, but these injuries may result directly from the trauma, as well. In fact, several studies have demonstrated vertebral artery occlusion in approximately 20 percent of nonpenetrating cervical trauma.[54,133,137] Fortunately, most of these patients are not symptomatic, which is likely due to a usually generous intracranial and extracranial collateral circulation.

The common carotid artery and the contents of the carotid sheath are at risk during anterior exposure of the cervical spine. Blunt finger dissection and repeated, but gentle, palpation of the carotid artery to assess its location help decrease the likelihood of injury. Likewise, palpation of the nasogastric tube can identify the location of the esophagus. Mobilization of the longus colli muscles off the anterolateral vertebral bodies before placement of deep retractors also helps minimize vessel damage. Checking the temporal artery pulse of the patient during the procedure helps to assess whether excessive retraction is causing occlusion of the carotid artery. Carotid artery laceration, division, and thrombosis have been reported during anterior spinal fusion.[69] Some approaches to the cervical spine risk injury to either the internal or external jugular vein. Although in most circumstances these vessels can be ligated unilaterally with little clinical consequence, venous injury can lead to air embolism, which may cause pulmonary compromise, blindness, or death. Posterior placement of C1-C2 transarticular screws or C1 lateral mass screws can risk injury to the internal carotid artery as it passes just anterior to the lateral masses of C1.[30]

The vertebral artery is at risk from both anterior and posterior approaches to the cervical spine (Fig. 34-4), especially in C1-C2 transarticular arthrodesis, in which rates of arterial injury have ranged from 4 to 8 percent.[87,151] In a review of 1215 cases by Golfinos and colleagues,[58] these injuries occurred in 1 case from retraction of soft tissues, in 1 case during screw tapping, and in 2 cases from lateral decompression. Transarticular screws at C1-C2 should also be planned via preoperative computed tomography (CT). Although less devastating a complication, malposition of the screws has been a substantial problem. In a retrospective evaluation by Grob and co-workers, only 85 percent of

FIGURE 34-4 | *Vertebral artery injury. Instrumentation placed near the transverse foramen of C2, such as transarticular C1-C2 or C2 pars screws, may enter to the foramen and injure the vertebral artery. In this example, the left C2 pars screw (which is on the right side of the image) can be seen violating the left C2 transverse foramen in the CT axial (**A**) and sagittal reconstruction (**B**) images.*

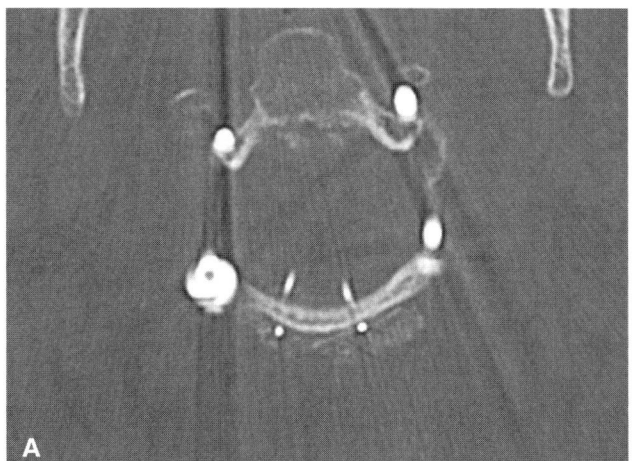
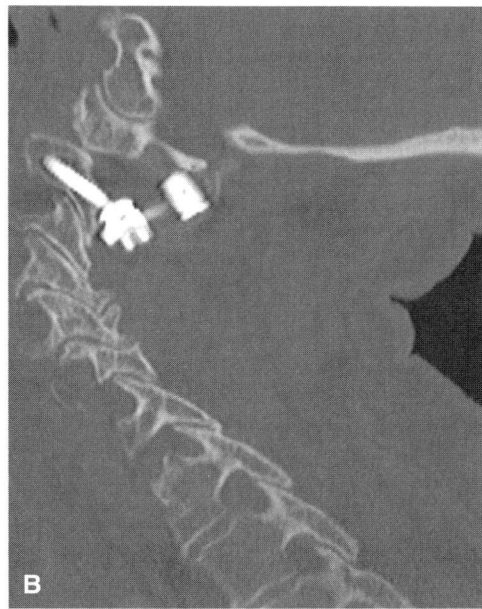

screws were ideally positioned, but the use of intraoperative advanced imaging techniques may eliminate many of these earlier problems.[62] The incidence of vertebral artery injury in anterior cervical surgery is approximately 0.3 to 0.5 percent and occurs most frequently with corpectomy.[21,125,127]

Most authors agree that the vertebral artery should not be repaired, but rather packed with thrombin-soaked absorbable gelatin sponges to achieve hemostasis through tamponade. When transarticular screw fixation is used, the contralateral side should not be instrumented if vertebral artery injury is suspected. In the rare case in which ligation is required for hemostasis, intraoperative angiography may be performed to assess the ability of the patient to tolerate such a procedure. However, in these cases, such studies are probably impractical, and, furthermore, some evidence indicates that sacrifice of one vertebral artery does not lead to permanent neurologic sequelae in most patients.[124] The ability of a patient to tolerate unilateral vertebral artery ablation is supported by a study of nine patients with traumatic occlusion of the vessel. In two of the nine, neurologic sequelae developed, but the findings were transient. However, Smith and associates[127] reported that in three of seven cases of vertebral artery ligation, symptomatic vertebrobasilar symptoms such as syncope, nystagmus, dizziness, and Wallenberg's syndrome developed. They supported repair of an injured vertebral artery whenever possible. As the use of lateral mass screw fixation expands, the number of vertebral artery injuries may increase. This complication from the placement of screws into the transverse foramen is best prevented by knowledge of the anatomy and intraoperative use of bony landmarks. Preoperative CT with angiography should be considered when planning for screw placement in C1 or C2 to assess the location of the C2 transverse foramen, vertebral arteries, and internal carotid arteries.

Complications from C1 lateral mass screws are largely related to neurovascular injury. The vertebral artery passes over the posterior arch near its junction with the lateral mass, this "pedicle analogue" can be quite thin (<4 mm in 20% and <3.5 mm in 8%) in many individuals.[24] Therefore the vertebral artery may be at considerable risk when inserting a screw through the posterior arch and into the lateral mass. Preoperative CT may be helpful in determining the dimensions available, but lateral mass screw insertion just below the arch alleviates much of the concern over vertebral artery injury. Anteriorly, the internal carotid arteries and hypoglossal nerves lie in close proximity to the ventral surface of C1 and can be injured by tools or screws that are too lengthy.

Occipital fixation has evolved over the past several decades to rely more heavily on screw and plate fixation. The bone in this area is thickest in the midline below the external occipital protuberance (EOP) and becomes substantially thinner lateral to the midline. Bicortical drilling in the thinner bone, found laterally or above 1 cm below the EOP, risks injury to the neurologic contents or penetration of the vascular sinuses.[116] Puncture of the inner dural wall of a sinus can lead to fatal subdural hematoma, and penetration of the outer dural wall can still cause substantial blood loss.

Esophageal perforation after anterior spinal trauma or surgery is uncommon but well recognized. Direct traumatic injury to the esophagus has been described with hyperextension injuries, in which traction on the esophagus occurs as well as entrapment between vertebral body fracture fragments during spontaneous reduction.[2,97,111,130] The largest series of esophageal perforations to date was reported by Gaudinez and coauthors.[51] Over a 25-year period, 44 patients with esophageal perforation were treated at that institution. Although most pharyngoesophageal perforations occur in the early postoperative period, delayed perforations in patients who had fully convalesced from the acute postoperative period have been reported.[75] The most frequently occurring symptoms are neck and throat pain, odynophagia, dysphagia, hoarseness, and aspiration. In the series by Gaudinez and colleagues,[51] cervical osteomyelitis or cervical abscess developed in half the patients. Clinical findings may include fever, cervical tenderness and induration, weight loss, tachycardia, crepitus from emphysema, and hematemesis. Though far less common, expectoration of necrotic bone has been reported as well. A high index of suspicion is required because diagnostic imaging often yields negative results. In addition, they showed that 22.7 percent of patients had false negative results from imaging studies. Endoscopy was 63.6 percent sensitive for definitive diagnosis in the 40 patients who underwent the procedure.[51]

Though not specifically addressed in the aforementioned series, a combination of direct visualization and a swallow study is regarded by most to have the highest diagnostic yield. Management of esophageal perforation varies. Conservative management includes observation, intravenous nutrition, a feeding tube or gastrostomy, appropriate antibiotic coverage, and aspiration precautions. These techniques may be effective for small, uncomplicated perforations. However, the literature suggests high morbidity and mortality with nonsurgical management of all but the smallest of perforations, especially with tears of the lower part of the esophagus. Consultation with a thoracic or esophageal surgical specialist is recommended in all cases. Prompt recognition of symptoms and pathology is paramount because a delay in diagnosis can lead to death. The esophagus should be examined carefully after any anterior cervical spinal operation, and any esophageal injury noted in the operative suite should be emergently repaired by an experienced surgeon. The repair can be augmented, when necessary, with a muscle flap, such as a proximally based medial pectoralis major rotational flap.

Thoracolumbar Spine

Anterior thoracolumbar surgery has a multitude of potential complications, including pneumothorax, hemothorax, and chylothorax. Respiratory functional restrictions following thoracotomy should be strongly considered when planning such an approach. Patients with lung contusions or other significant trauma-related pulmonary compromise should undergo thoracotomy beyond 2 weeks from the time of injury. Preoperative evaluation of the respiratory function can play an important role in timing decisions for surgery.

Massive hemothorax may occur from profuse vertebral body bleeding and can cause hemodynamic instability. It may require surgical tamponade of venous sinuses in the vertebral body with bone wax or ligation of bleeding segmental arteries.[105] Hemorrhage from a thoracic fracture causing persistent hemothorax has been reported in a patient with a complete neurologic injury induced by the fracture.[32] After more than 7 days of recurrent hemothorax, the patient underwent operative reduction and stabilization of the fracture, which led to the cessation of bleeding. This scenario defines an additional indication for early fixation of a high-energy thoracic vertebral fracture in patients with complete neurologic compromise.

The presence of a thoracic fracture should also alert the physician to the possibility of thoracic duct injury. The incidence of chylothorax in association with rib and thoracic fractures is increasing because of escalating numbers of vehicular accidents and nonpenetrating trauma. At least 13 patients with chylothorax secondary to thoracic fractures have been reported, and at least 2 of them died of the sequelae of the chylothorax itself, 1 from tension chylothorax.[152] Although most cases of traumatic chylothorax can be managed nonoperatively, the need for surgical intervention in the subset of patients with associated thoracic fractures is higher and approaches 50 percent.

Delayed appearance of a chylothorax results from the formation of a mediastinal chyloma, which then ruptures into a pleural cavity, usually 7 to 10 days after the injury. When a chylothorax is suspected, diagnostic thoracentesis and tube thoracostomy should be undertaken. Oral intake should be discontinued because even low-fat, clear liquids markedly increase chyle flow.[57] Historically, continuous chylous chest drainage despite 6 weeks of nonoperative therapy was an indication for surgical intervention. However, more recently, some authors have become more aggressive in preventing ongoing protein and lymphocyte losses and thereby minimizing the risk of infection. Some authors now recommend surgery if nonoperative management is unsuccessful after 2 weeks.[126] Most agree that a more aggressive approach is preferred in a patient with concomitant spinal fractures because of the high immunologic and nutritional cost of prolonged chest tube drainage.[126] Rare reports have mentioned iatrogenic chyle leaks after anterior thoracolumbar surgery, most of which indict surgical exposure as the cause, but some also suggest deformity correction as a potential cause.[100,101,108] Most, however, agree that microlymphatic disruption is inevitable, and it seems likely that clinically insignificant chyle leaks are undiagnosed and heal spontaneously.

Diaphragmatic rupture or herniation may occur after thoracolumbar exposure or after the crura of the diaphragm are taken down and repaired to improve exposure in the thoracolumbar region. The ureters and great vessels are at risk during retroperitoneal dissection, especially in the revision setting. Consideration should be given to preoperative ureteral stenting in revision procedures. Injury to the sympathetic plexus overlying the anterior aspect of the lower lumbar and upper sacral vertebrae may cause retrograde ejaculation.

Traditionally, much attention has been paid to the segmental blood supply of the thoracic cord. Specifically, the artery of Adamkiewicz is considered to be vital to cord perfusion. The transthoracic approach to the spine usually requires mobilization of the segmental vessels over a multitude of levels. Dwyer and Schafer,[39] however, have shown that ligation of multiple ipsilateral segmental arteries can be performed without neurologic compromise. DiChiro and colleagues[37] demonstrated in monkeys that even the arteria magna could be ligated without sequelae. However, if both this vessel and the anterior spinal artery were disrupted, paraplegia resulted. Much of the work and the case reports of neurologic compromise in the face of segmental artery disruption have been related to surgical treatment of deformity. The effect of deformity, especially if congenital, on the blood supply to the cord is unclear. In a polytrauma patient, cross-clamping of the aorta results in disruption of the segmental blood flow to the cord bilaterally, which may result in paralysis. Trauma to the cord and associated edema may make the spinal cord far more sensitive to the effects of mild ischemia.

The anterior approach to the lumbar spine for the operative treatment of spinal trauma is usually performed through the retroperitoneal or, less commonly, the transperitoneal approach. If the pathologic condition does not dictate approaching the spine on a particular side, most surgeons prefer the left side because the aorta is more forgiving and easier to mobilize than the vena cava. The left common iliac vein is the vessel most at risk during left-sided retroperitoneal and transperitoneal exposures. Regardless of the approach, instrumentation should be placed on the lateral side of the vertebral body and not in contact with the great vessels. Other potential injuries to adjacent structures during anterior approaches to the lumbar spine include visceral and ureteral lacerations. If these are recognized intraoperatively, they should be repaired at that time. Appropriate broad-spectrum antibiotic coverage is indicated in the setting of bowel injury, but there are no strict guidelines on duration of treatment.

Vascular complications during posterior lumbar spine surgery usually happen during diskectomy, most commonly at the L4-L5 level. Freeman[49] showed that the pituitary rongeur is the most frequent culprit. Mortality rates range from 15 to 65 percent, which underlines the concern for this particular iatrogenic injury, but the incidence is fortunately quite low (0.01–0.05%).[48,59,103,132] In the setting of trauma, one must be keenly aware of any disruption of the anterior longitudinal ligament. Incompetence of this ligament makes perforation of the great vessels more difficult to avoid. Unless acute hypotension occurs intraoperatively, these injures may initially go unnoticed. Late abdominal rigidity, abdominal pain, tachycardia, and anemia should alert the physician to the possibility of this complication, which may be avoided by limiting the depth of insertion of the pituitary rongeur during diskectomy. Vascular and neurologic injuries can also occur from placement of instrumentation. A pedicle screw placed too medially or inferiorly may violate the spinal cord, thecal sac, or exiting nerve root. During preparation of the vertebra for a pedicle screw, or during insertion of too lengthy a pedicle screw, life-threatening injury may occur to anterior structures, such as the great vessels (Fig. 34-5). This can result in immediate hemorrhage from the vessel, but the proud screw can also slowly erode through the vessel wall and result in a delayed hemorrhagic event. More unusual complications of pedicle screw fixation have been reported as well. Some surgeons insert markers or Kirschner wires into the pedicle holes to check position with a radiograph or image intensifier before screw placement. At least one case of fatal cardiac tamponade from myocardial violation with a Kirschner wire has been reported. Fluoroscopy was used to confirm the position of the wire, and no evidence of complications was noted during the procedure itself.[65]

The lateral extracavitary approach to the thoracolumbar spine deserves special mention. This approach, which is used to replace a two-incision front-back procedure, allows ventral decompression and dorsal fixation. However, the approach is technically demanding. Resnick and Benzel[113] reported a 55 percent incidence of morbidity in a series of 33 patients with acute fractures. The most common complication was hemothorax or effusion requiring tube thoracostomy, followed by pneumonia, which occurred in seven patients. Other authors have noted pseudohernias caused by sacrifice of the intercostal nerves. Although the morbidity associated with this procedure may be high, its risks should be weighed against the combined risk of a two-stage procedure.

Dural Tear

It is difficult, if not impossible, to know the true incidence of dural tears as a result of trauma. Certain injuries seem to have a predilection for causing dural tears, including lumbar burst fractures associated with lamina fractures. Aydinli and associates found that nearly 20 percent of patients with this particular injury were found to have dural tears, and a third of the subset with tears were neurologically intact.[11] In patients with high-energy injuries and complete paraplegia of the thoracic spine, actual severance of the cord and dural sac is possible. Likewise, a gunshot wound to the spine may cause disruption of the dura. Iatrogenic dural tears also occur, especially during attempted posterolateral decompression. CSF leaks may lead to positional headache, wound complications, meningitis, arachnoiditis, and pseudomeningocele.

The diagnosis of iatrogenic CSF leakage is fairly straightforward. Obvious egress of fluid from a visible tear in the dura is diagnostic. As the thecal sac decompresses because of a leak, the local extravascular pressure around the epidural veins decreases, leading to an increase in venous bleeding from the epidural space, which may be the first indication of a dural tear. Additionally, when the dural sac is decompressed, especially when reducing a kyphotic deformity, leakage may occur from a tear. Postoperatively, one must be alert for signs of clear drainage from the wound or the presence of a subcutaneous fluid collection. Severe headache exacerbated by an upright posture should alert the clinician to the possibility of a CSF leak. Large volumes of fluid may be seen inasmuch as the choroid plexus produces over 20 mL of CSF hourly. If it is unclear whether the fluid is CSF, testing for β_2-transferrin presence in drainage or fluid collections is diagnostic for CSF presence. A pseudomeningocele may develop if a dural tear occurs and is not repaired in watertight fashion.

Dural tears may be classified as dorsal, lateral, or ventral. Although the best treatment is prevention, most tears can be repaired primarily if they do occur. However, massive defects may be irreparable. The first step in repair is complete exposure of the dural rent. Magnification and adequate lighting are required. Dural elements must be returned to their intrathecal location and should not be incorporated into the repair inadvertently. The goal is a watertight repair that is free of tension. Usually, this objective can be accomplished with 6-0 polypropylene (Prolene) suture placed in a running locking stitch. The recommended location of the suture is 2 mm from the dural edge

FIGURE 34-5 *Pedicle screw malposition. Pedicle screws that are too long may penetrate the anterior cortex of the vertebral body and place the great vessels at risk, as seen on these computed tomographic scans (A-C). Alternatively, pedicle screws can be malpositioned outside the pedicle, as can be seen with this axial CT image of a medially placed screw within the spinal canal.*

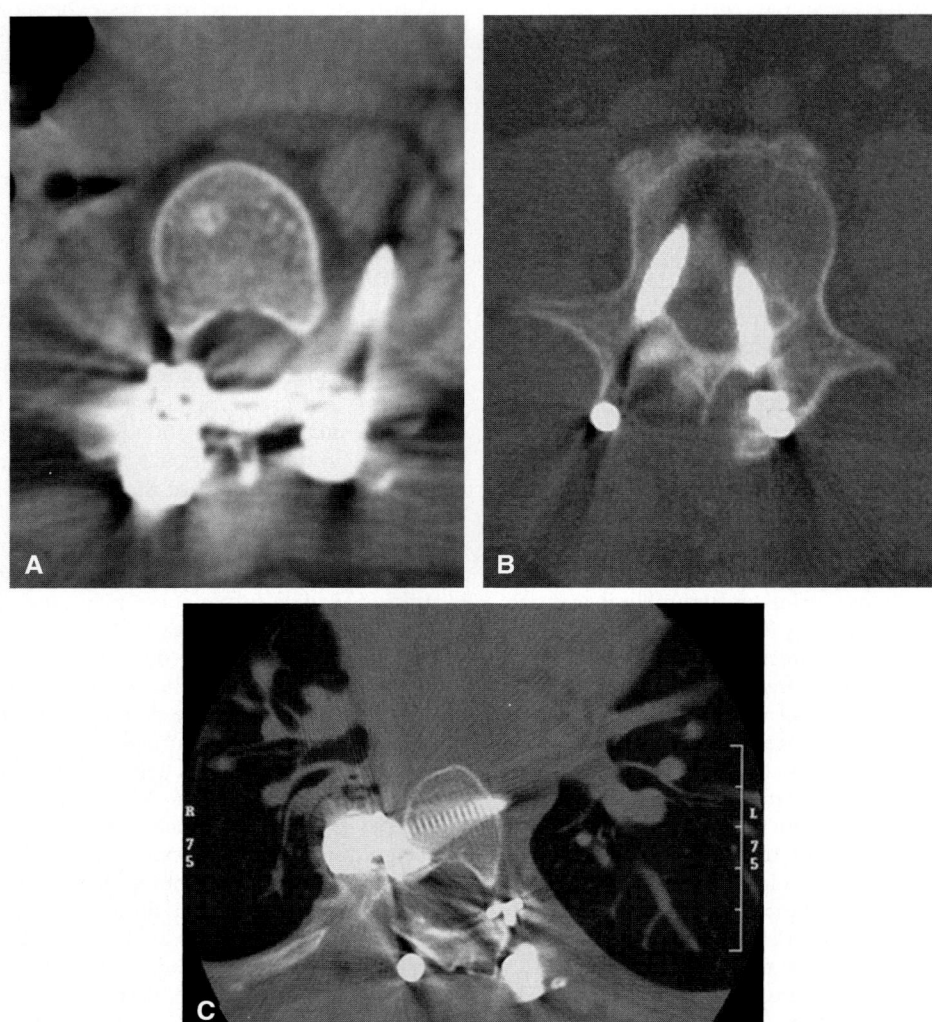

with 3 mm between sutures. A Valsalva maneuver may be simulated by the anesthesiologist after repair to assess for residual leak. If leakage occurs after repair, augmentation with additional suture, gelatin sponge, autogenous fat, or fibrin glue is required. More complex tears may require grafting with fascia lata or with commercially available dural patches. Meticulous watertight fascial closure is as important as the dural repair itself because the fascial barrier is relied on to prevent durocutaneous fistulas. Most surgeons avoid the use of intramuscular drains in the presence of a dural tear because negative pressure may encourage a persistent leak.

During a posterior approach, most posterior and lateral dural tears can be exposed directly. Below the level of the conus, an anterior tear may be approached through a posterior durotomy and gentle retraction of nerve roots to allow access to the anterior aspect of the dural tube. However, anterior tears during posterior exposure at cord levels may need to be treated indirectly.

Indirect repair is most commonly performed with fibrin glue, which is formed by mixing thrombin and cryoprecipitate that has been screened for human immunodeficiency and hepatitis virus. It forms a biologic glue with biomechanical "patchlike" properties, and it can seal tears that cannot be fully exposed for repair, or it can be used to augment tenuous repairs. Cooling the individual components before mixing may improve the biomechanical strength of the product.[146] In addition to repair, diversion of CSF through a subarachnoid drain for 4 to 5 days may allow the dura, fascia, and surgical incision to heal. Finally, maintaining the patient in a flat position on bed rest for several days has been advocated, especially with tenuous repairs; however, this practice is not universally supported and is probably unnecessary when the tear is well repaired.

Metabolic Changes

As a result of inactivity and changes in body composition, most patients with chronic spinal cord injury undergo important metabolic changes. Glucose intolerance occurs more frequently in these patients than in the general population. Baumann and Spungen[12,13] performed a 75-g oral glucose tolerance test on 100 veterans (50 with paraplegia and 50 with quadriplegia) and 50 able-bodied veteran controls. In the spinal cord-injured group, 22 percent of the subjects were diabetic by criteria established by the World Health Organization as compared with 6 percent in the control group. Normal oral glucose tolerance was noted in 82 percent of the controls, 50 percent of the paraplegics, and 38 percent of the quadriplegics. Insulin levels were lower in controls, thus indicating insulin resistance in the spinal cord-injured patients. This hyperinsulinemia may well play a role in the increased concentration of triglycerides and the decreased concentration of high-density lipoprotein cholesterol in spinal cord-injured patients. All these changes, coupled with inactivity, play a role in the high incidence of atherosclerosis seen in this group.

Spinal cord injury leads to unloading of the skeleton, and hypercalcemia and hypercalciuria quickly ensue. Restriction of dietary calcium does not treat the cause of the derangement, which is initially due to increased osteoclastic activity within the first 3 to 5 days and later involves a lifetime of decreased osteoblastic activity. Osteoporosis may lead to insufficiency or traumatic fractures, but these fractures may be markedly underdiagnosed and manifested as little more than swelling. Hypercalciuria may result in early nephrolithiasis and the recommendation that dietary calcium be forever avoided. However, such restriction often leads to deficiency and worsening of osteoporosis after the acute period of marked bone loss subsides, usually within 14 months.[115] Although their role still remains to be defined, bisphosphonates may be the best agent for management of this condition.[12,115]

Endogenous anabolic hormone levels have been demonstrated at depressed levels in a proportion of individuals with spinal cord injury, as well.[13] Such changes in serum testosterone, growth hormone, and insulin-like growth factor 1 (IGF-1) levels may worsen adverse metabolic changes, such as increased adiposity, lipid profile deterioration, and decreased exercise tolerance.

Some evidence supports the depression of endogenous anabolic hormones in spinal cord-injured patients. Decreased levels of serum testosterone, growth hormone, and IGF-1 may exacerbate the body composition changes seen in these patients. In addition, exercise tolerance and strength may be decreased. Thyroid dysfunction is seen as well. Depressed levels of triiodothyronine (T_3) and reverse T_3 have been demonstrated, and this effect may also contribute to fatigue and an increase in adiposity. However, some believe that it is due to associated illness and metabolic derangement, and as such, the use of replacement therapy for this type of "deficiency" in the presence of normal thyroid tissue is controversial.

Although the medical management of each of these metabolic derangements is beyond the scope of this chapter, the orthopaedic surgeon must be cognizant that such medical issues exist and must use an appropriate team to minimize the late sequelae of these abnormalities. Amelioration of these abnormalities promises to improve the longevity and quality of life of persons with spinal cord injury.

Postoperative Infection

Postoperative infections may result from inoculation during the index procedure or from hematogenous seeding. Infection after elective spinal surgery has been well studied, but surprisingly few papers in the literature specifically address infection after trauma-related spinal surgery. Blam and colleagues retrospectively evaluated 256 patients who underwent acute surgical intervention for spinal trauma and found an infection rate of approximately 9 percent.[15] This is consistent with the 10 percent rate demonstrated by Rechtine and co-workers, but it is distinctly higher than the well-documented 3 to 6 percent rate of infection commonly seen after elective spine surgery.[15,19,92,106,110] Risk factors include increased age, obesity, diabetes, smoking, immunosuppression, duration of preoperative hospitalization, spinal dysraphism, myelodysplasia, revision surgery, lengthy operative time, and the use of instrumentation, bone graft, or methyl methacrylate.[29,71,83,92,123,129,147]

The use of perioperative prophylaxis to prevent infection is widespread. Patients with instrumented fusions have a decreased infection rate with the use of prophylaxis compared with those undergoing surgery without prophylaxis. Commonly, the antibiotic is administered before the incision and for 24 hours postoperatively, although some surgeons prefer to administer antibiotics until suction drains or catheters are removed. The choice of antibiotic is guided by consideration of multiple factors, including host immunocompetence, the bacterial flora common in the region, the type of procedure, cost, and the side effects profile. Most commonly, a cephalosporin is used. Because of increasing concern regarding the development of bacterial resistance, drugs such as vancomycin should be discouraged for prophylaxis and reserved only for patients at increased risk of methicillin-resistant staphylococcal infections. Such patients include those with lymphopenia, recent or current hospitalization, postoperative wound drainage, and alcohol abuse.

Once the diagnosis of postoperative infection is made clinically, early surgical intervention is necessary because medical management is likely to fail. Débridement should proceed in a systematic fashion. Each layer is débrided and cultured before advancing deeper with the dissection. If gross deep drainage or purulence is encountered with subfascial aspiration, deep débridement is performed.

Although solidly fixed instrumentation is typically left in place in the early postoperative period, all other foreign bodies such as bone wax and hemostatic gelatin (Gelfoam) must be removed. Any hematoma should be thoroughly evacuated. Many authors retain bone grafts, especially if they are adherent. Others recommend removal of loose grafts and washing before replacement. If the graft is grossly purulent or necrotic, it should be discarded and another bone grafting procedure performed at a later débridement when the local infection is controlled. Hemostasis must be meticulous to prevent re-formation of a hematoma seeded with bacteria. Dead space must be obliterated, and the use of a rotation flap should be considered for dead space management. Primary wound closure over drains, often with retention sutures to prevent dehiscence, is favored when possible. Depending on the amount of devitalized tissue, routine serial débridement is often required. Simple wound infections may be packed open and allowed to close by secondary intention. More complex wound infections may require musculocutaneous flaps.

Postoperatively, antibiotic therapy is required for at least 10 to 14 days for straightforward soft tissue wound infections (without underlying hardware or bone involvement). Six weeks of parenteral antibiotic treatment is preferred in cases of bone involvement, deep infection, or retained foreign bodies (e.g., metal or graft). Continuation of oral antibiotics after the 6-week parenteral course may be required in cases of diminished nutritional reserves, and infectious disease consultation should be considered.

In all cases, nutritional assessment and repletion are of paramount importance. Up to 35 percent of hospitalized patients have evidence of protein-calorie malnutrition. Weight loss of more than 10 percent, a serum transferrin level less than 1.5 g/L, anergy, a serum albumin concentration less than 3 g/dL, or a total lymphocyte count less than 1200 should raise suspicion of malnutrition. Protein-calorie malnutrition causes decreased cardiac output and lower peripheral oxygen tension, as well as impaired pulmonary defenses, wound healing, and cell-mediated immune defenses. In addition to the treatment of malnutrition, its prevention must be considered in all hospitalized patients, especially those with increased metabolic demands because of fever, trauma, or surgery.

INSTRUMENTATION FAILURE

Cervical Spine

Treatment of cervical spine trauma with anterior diskectomy or corpectomy and fusion has historically been done with and without instrumentation. However, uninstrumented attempts at fusion led to higher rates of pseudarthrosis, disk space collapse, and postoperative kyphosis.[138] Anterior cervical instrumentation has evolved to the use of locking screw–plate technology, which has reduced the rate of failure seen with nonconstrained plates, but dislodgement of the graft or plate-screw failure still occurs with longer constructs.[86] Vaccaro and colleagues reported on a series of patients that underwent corpectomy, fibula strut-grafting, and anterior plate instrumentation, and found that 9 percent of two-level and 50 percent of three-level procedures had dislodgement of the graft or failure of the instrumentation.[136] For longer (>three levels) anterior corpectomy reconstructions, augmentation with posterior instrumentation should be strongly considered.[114,136]

Anterior odontoid screws have been advocated for the treatment of type II odontoid fractures that are reducible, noncomminuted, and commensurate with appropriate biomechanical considerations (i.e., fracture perpendicularity to the fixation). The primary complications of screw breakout and malposition occur in less than 5 percent of cases and may largely be related to osteopenic or comminuted bone[131] (Fig. 34-6). Andersson and co-workers recommend alternative treatment in the elderly and/or those with osteoporosis.[6]

Posterior cervical wiring has been done with less frequency since the emergence of cervical screw-rod and screw-plate technologies; however, wire techniques are still employed in various situations. Complications of interspinous and sublaminar wiring include wire breakage, wire pull-out, dural penetration, neurologic injury, and pseudarthrosis.

Lateral mass screws can be placed with a variety of different techniques. After using the An technique, Heller and associates retrospectively evaluated their patients for complications associated with a lateral mass screw-plate system. Iatrogenic foraminal stenosis and plate failure

---

FIGURE 34-6 *Anterior odontoid screw failure. Osteopenic bone increases the risk of cut-out with anterior odontoid screws, and in this case, a nonunion has resulted from such failure in the proximal fragment. The movement of the screw within the body of C2 and the base of the odontoid can be more easily appreciated on flexion* **(A)** *and extension* **(B)** *views.*

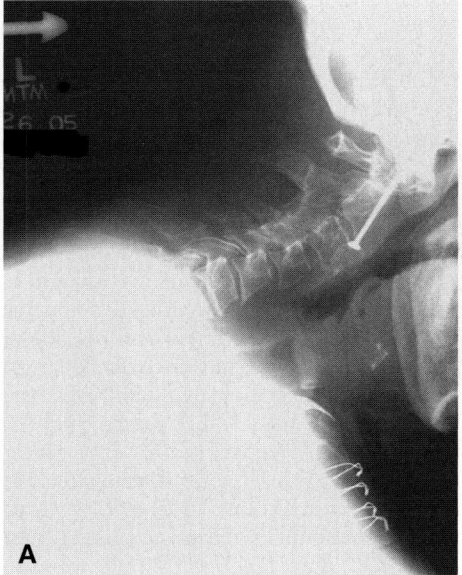
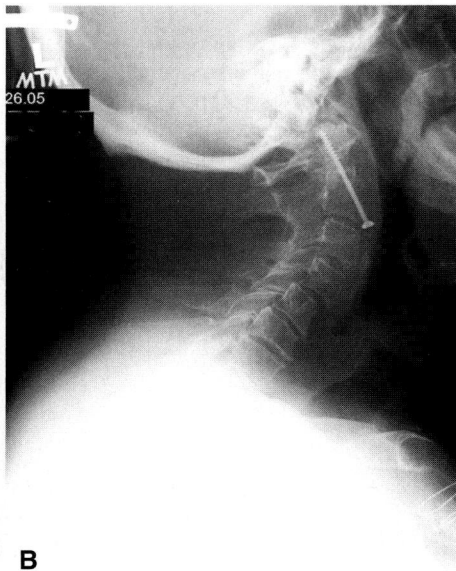

A

B

occurred in 2.6 percent and 1.3 percent of their patients, respectively.[66] Direct screw trauma caused nerve root injury in 0.6 percent of all screws that were placed, whereas facet violation occurred in only 0.2 percent. Vertebral artery injury was not reported in this series and remains rare, but it is a devastating complication of too little lateral angulation during screw placement (should be >10°). Lateral mass failure on placement of the screw remains a frustrating but not infrequent (6–7%) complication that may occur intraoperatively.[23] Lateral mass screws within the atlas are now an important tool for use in upper cervical stabilization. Pull-out strength for these screws tends to be similar to that of C2 pars interarticularis screws, and both are weaker than occiput screws (by approximately 40%).[70] Much like C1-C2 rod-screw constructs, transarticular C1-C2 screw constructs have very low rates of instrumentation failure, and their biomechanical strength is similar.[96]

Although cervical pedicle screws have demonstrated improvement in pull-out strength, placing them carries considerably higher risk than is found with lateral mass screws. Preoperative CT should be obtained and scrutinized prior to the use of cervical pedicle screws. The transverse foramen in C2 is often situated too medially for safe passage of a screw into the body, in which case a safer choice may be to employ a pars screw that stops short of the foramen. The medially located spinal cord and laterally positioned vertebral artery are at considerable risk with pedicle screw placement from C2 to C6, and great care must be taken to avoid these structures. Abumi and co-workers reported on 669 cervical pedicle screws and found that 45 (7%) violated the pedicle wall.[1] Nearly half of these breaches occurred medially. Because of the rare presence of the vertebral artery at the C7 level, pedicle screw use has been advocated with less trepidation at the cervicothoracic junction.[3]

Craniocervical fixation has evolved over the years from wiring and onlay-grafting techniques to plate-screw configurations. Most of these techniques have seemingly been successful in achieving arthrodesis without hardware failure, but early techniques were often supplemented by lengthy use of external immobilization.[4] Improvements in implant fixation and rigidity have allowed a reduction on the reliance on external immobilization, and implant failure has not been commonly seen.[122]

Thoracolumbar

Loss of stabilization may result from error in surgical technique, improper preoperative planning, or poor implant selection. Systems using rods and hooks may fail from hook pull-out, hook-rod disengagement, or rod fracture. Hook pull-out may be due to improper placement or osseous fracture. Lamina fracture may be associated with aggressive laminotomy, osteoporotic bone, or overdistraction (Fig. 34-7). Hook dislodgment is the most commonly reported complication of posterior Harrington rod instrumentation after spinal trauma.[14,28,43,46,52] Edwards and colleagues[42] noted four factors that account for hook dislodgment: rigidity of fixation, the anatomic level, hook design, and rod clearance. The rate of hook dislodgment depends on the spinal level, with the rate varying from 5 percent at L4 to 20 percent at S1.[52,140] In older, semirigid Harrington models, rod clearance greater than 1 cm was needed to prevent rod-hook disengagement during

flexion and rotation. The advent of segmental multihook fixation has decreased the incidence of hook failure. However, care must be taken to fully tighten the hooks on the rod to prevent motion at this interface.

Pedicle screw fixation has dramatically expanded the surgical armamentarium for treating spinal trauma. Though largely avoidable, the potential complications associated with pedicle screw use can be significant. A short screw or a screw placed laterally has suboptimal fixation, whereas a medially placed screw may violate the canal and cause a dural tear or neurologic injury. A screw that is excessively long may violate the anterior aspect of the vertebral body and can cause potentially life-threatening perforation of the great vessels. Pedicle screws can fracture the pedicle on insertion and can potentially loosen, break, or pull out. Although a larger diameter screw has greater biomechanical pull-out strength, judgment is needed to avoid pedicle blowout.[148,155] If the screw is larger than the inner pedicle diameter or greater than 80 percent of the total pedicle diameter, perforation of the pedicle wall is quite likely. The medial wall of the pedicle, particularly in the thoracic spine, is two to three times thicker than the lateral wall. This typically leads to fracture blowout through the lateral wall of the pedicle. In a large series of 4790 pedicle screws in 875 patients, Lonstein and co-workers[85] showed that in experienced hands, the rate of complications is quite low. In their series, reoperation was necessary for 11 screws (0.2%) because of nerve root irritation, and 25 (0.5%) screws were fractured at follow-up. Preoperative CT with careful planning and intraoperative fluoroscopy can help in avoiding more significant errors in pedicle screw placement.

For many years, some surgeons have used translaminar or facet screws to facilitate fusion.[77,88] Although violation of the canal or nerve root is possible, the reported rate of complications is low. The screws should be placed only after decortication and cancellous packing of the facets have been performed to maximize fusion rates and avoid screw notching.

Postoperative Deformity

Fixation failure, loss of reduction, and subsequent deformity are some of the more frequent complications seen after spinal trauma. Additionally, the application of spinal instrumentation has been the direct cause of spinal deformity, such as with flat back syndrome. Flat back syndrome is a condition associated with loss of normal lumbar lordosis. It is frequently the result of distraction instrumentation within the posterior spine that ends caudal to L3 (Fig. 34-8). Although solid arthrodesis may be achieved, the flat back deformity can be problematic.[35,80] Sagittal plane deformity and imbalance may occur, and muscular strain and chronic pain are often reported as patients attempt to maintain their lordosis and balance. Additionally, compensatory hyperlordosis above and below the fusion often causes degenerative spondylosis and stenosis. Avoidance of overdistraction and the use of appropriately contoured segmental fixation help prevent this complication. Flattening the lumbar lordosis facilitates decompression procedures by increasing the interlaminar distance, but if fusion is performed, normal lumbar lordosis

FIGURE 34-7   *Hook failure. This patient has significant osteoporosis contributing to fractures of the lamina at the site of the proximal (T10) hooks as shown on a lateral radiograph **(A)** and computed tomographic scan **(B)**. Treatment included proximal extension of the fusion with pedicle screw instrumentation **(C)**.*

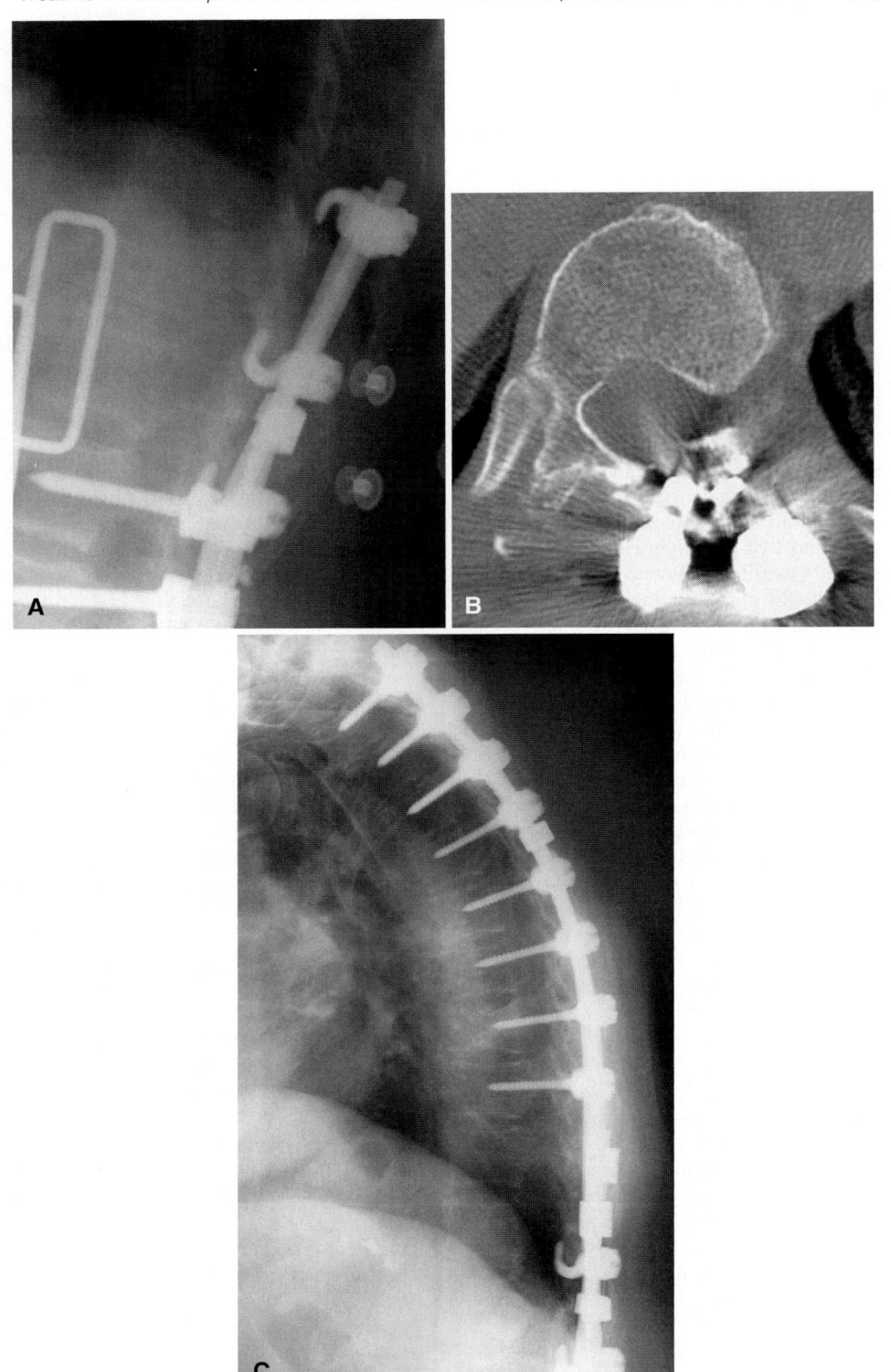

FIGURE 34-8 *Post-traumatic flat back deformity. This patient sustained an L3 burst fracture 11 years previously. Progressive bilateral lower extremity weakness, right leg pain, and early fatigue prompted the current medical evaluation. **A,** Standing radiographs show significant sagittal imbalance and loss of lumbar lordosis. **B,** Treatment included anterior discectomy and interbody fusion, followed by removal of previous instrumentation, pedicle subtraction osteotomy, and instrumented fusion.*

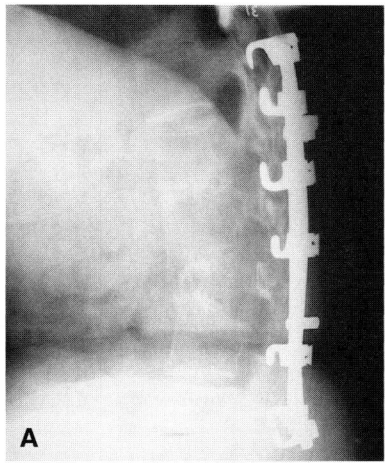
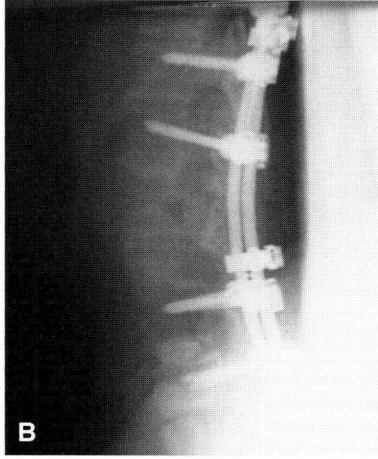

must be reestablished prior to final fixation. Lumbar lordosis is increased by hip extension and decreased by hip flexion, as occurs when patients are placed in the knee-chest position or positioned on a four-post frame. Although hyperlordosis is much less common, it can lead to complications as well. Iatrogenic foraminal stenosis and nerve root impingement can be caused by excessive lordosis.[128]

The best treatment of iatrogenic deformity is avoidance, but if diagnosed early, it can be treated by realignment. Delay in diagnosis or treatment ultimately results in the need for more extensive realignment procedures, such as pedicle subtraction or Smith-Peterson osteotomies. Many patients with iatrogenic deformity present a diagnostic dilemma, as the source of chronic back pain can be from a variety of other sources.

Late Deformity

Late and progressive deformity and chronic pain as a result of spinal trauma can lead to significant disability. Although these sequelae can occur despite proper management, each injury pattern and each patient must be considered individually to minimize complications. Patient age, lifestyle, and preexisting deformity may all play a role, but the initial stability of the injury and early management are probably paramount in predicting future decompensation and deformity.[89]

The most common postoperative deformity after trauma-related cervical decompression is kyphosis. At the time of initial treatment, careful consideration of disrupted osseoligamentous structures anteriorly or posteriorly should dictate the appropriate reconstruction and stabilization technique. Although pain relief after the index operation can be considerable, failure to address loss of structural integrity can lead to progressive deformity, increasing neck pain, or recurrent neurologic symptoms.

The thoracolumbar junction is the most common site for acute fractures and the development of late post-traumatic deformity. The abrupt change between the more mobile lumbar spine and the more rigid thoracic spine with its stabilizing ribs and sternum places the thoracolumbar junction at high risk for decompensation. However, no area of the spine is immune to deformity, and decompensation is not limited to the sagittal plane; a complex three-dimensional deformity may be located anywhere from the occiput to the sacrum.

The most important aspect of managing spinal deformity is prevention, and to avert the development of such deformity, the initial injury must be well understood. Osseous destruction is only part of the equation; ligamentous injury and disk disruption must be evaluated as well. Andreychik and associates[7] attributed an increase in postoperative kyphosis without an increase in vertebral body compression to structural failure of adjacent disk spaces resulting from the initial injury. Because fractures extending into the disk space may not be appreciated on routine supine radiographs, physiologic loading may be required to fully assess stability.

Missed posterior ligamentous injury can cause subsequent progressive deformity, as well. Burst fractures, for example, typically settle less than $10°$ before the kyphotic deformity is check-reined by the posterior ligamentous structures. However, if these structures are disrupted, severe deformity can ensue.

Most clinicians agree that the goal of treatment is to restore normal alignment in an unstable spine for a period sufficient to allow healing through either spontaneous bony healing or surgical arthrodesis. Bed rest, casting, and bracing have all proven effective in the treatment of specific injury patterns and patient subgroups. If the injury, the patient's compliance, and the potential for healing permit the use of nonoperative management, close follow-up is critical. Clinical evaluation and serial standing radiographs should be carried out early and frequently to detect the progression of instability or deformity.

The deleterious effects of laminectomy alone for neural decompression in the presence of spinal trauma are well documented (Fig. 34-9). Complete spondyloptosis and severe deformity have been reported.[145] Malcolm and coworkers[89] reported on 48 patients with post-traumatic

FIGURE 34-9 | *Postlaminectomy cervical kyphosis.* **A,** *This patient sustained posterior element fractures of the lower cervical spine and had an incomplete spinal cord injury. Advanced imaging studies showed canal compromise from the posterior element fractures. He was treated with laminectomy of C5 and C6 and halo immobilization.* **B, C,** *Serial radiographs showed gradual loss of reduction, with the development of kyphosis. The patient was eventually treated with corpectomy and fusion.*

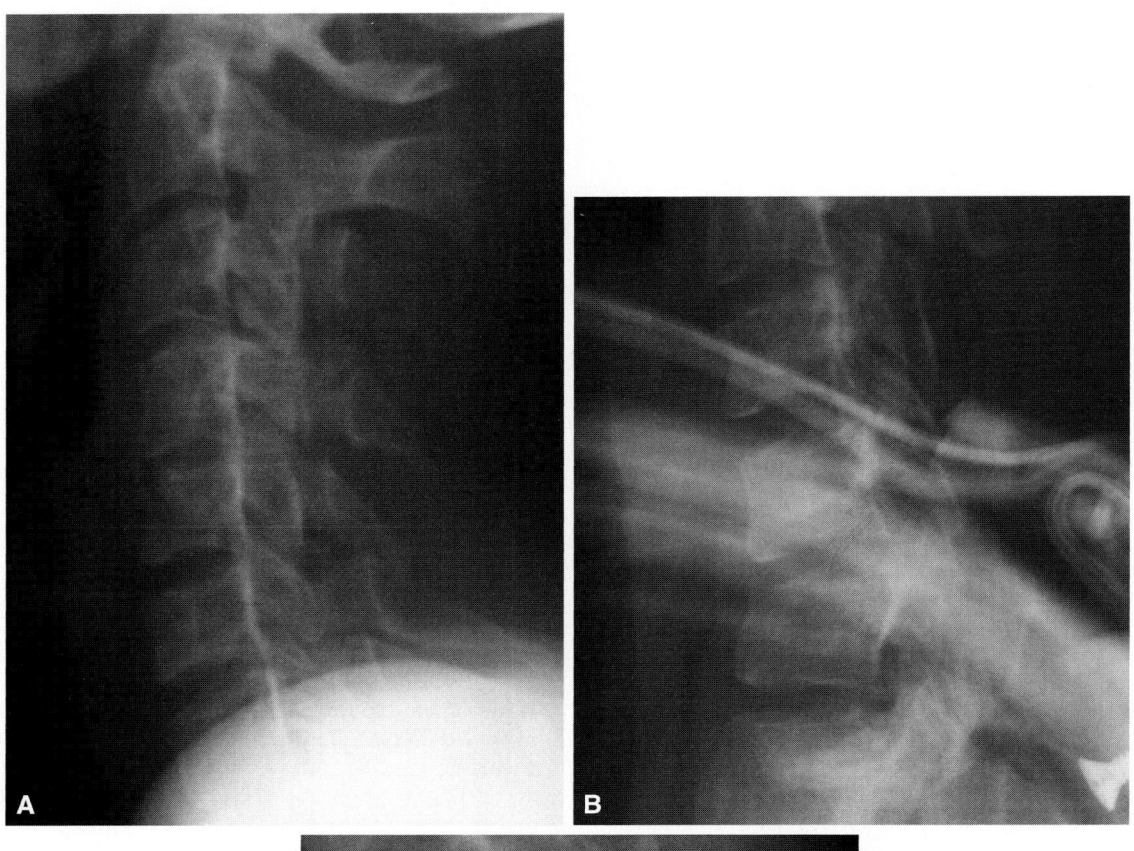

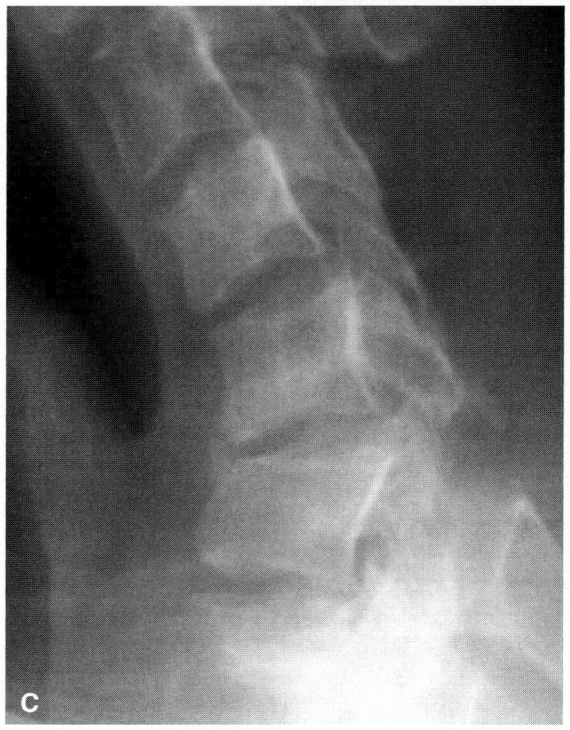

kyphosis. Half of these patients had an isolated laminectomy at the time of injury, and detrimental effects were seen at all levels of the spine. In the thoracic spine, the kyphotic deformity was 15° greater in the group that underwent decompression with laminectomy. At the thoracolumbar junction and lumbar spine, the kyphotic deformities were 13° and 11° more severe, respectively.

Technical errors can precipitate deformity even in the face of posterior instrumentation. A fusion that is too short and does not span the zone of injury is more likely to lead to a junctional deformity, especially if the arthrodesis ends at the cervicothoracic or thoracolumbar junction or at the apex of the thoracic kyphosis (Fig. 34-10). Additionally, a short fusion that spans the defect but is placed posterior to destroyed anterior elements is more likely to fail unless the anterior column is restored (Fig. 34-11). Parker and others have developed and validated a classification scheme to help determine when an anterior strut graft is required to supplement a short posterior construct for thoracolumbar fractures.[105]

CLINICAL FEATURES OF LATE DEFORMITY

Symptoms attributable to deformity may be insidious in onset and may follow a painless period of indeterminate length. As many as 70 to 90 percent of patients experience some chronic pain at the region of the fracture regardless of the type of treatment or the degree of deformity.[33,73,102,153] As many as 20 percent may be permanently disabled, and 40 percent report functional limitations. Debilitating pain is often the initial symptom and is the most common cause

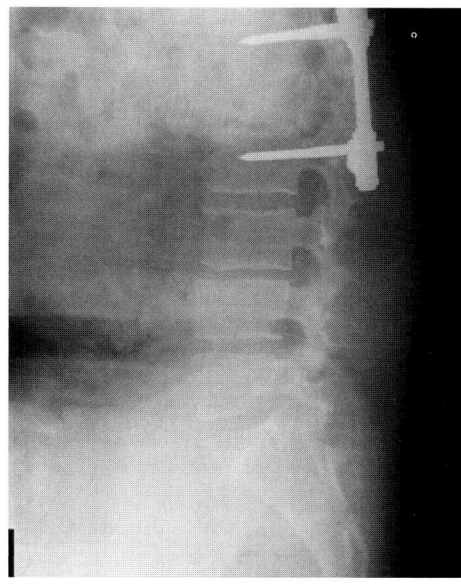

FIGURE 34-11 *Failure of the anterior column. This patient underwent short-segment fixation of an L1 burst fracture with substantial vertebral body comminution. The short-segment fixation has begun to fail by progressive collapse of L1 and pull-out of the L2 screws, leading to worsening focal kyphosis at the injured segment.*

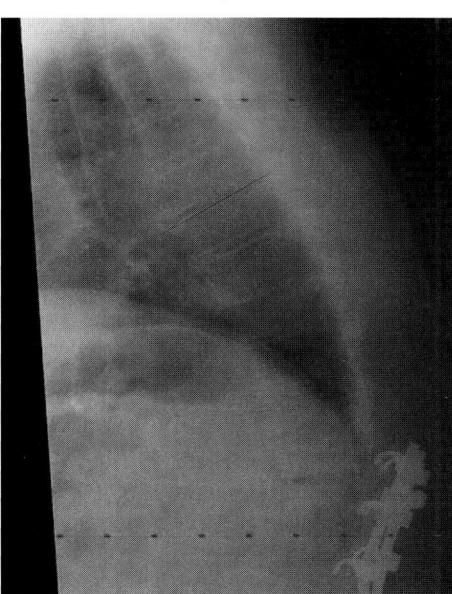

FIGURE 34-10 *Junctional kyphosis. This patient underwent an L1-L5 posterior instrumented fusion, and a decade later developed progressive kyphosis at the level above the fusion (T12-L1). She required a pedicle subtraction osteotomy and extensive revision posterior spinal arthrodesis to the upper thoracic spine.*

of reconstructive surgery for post-traumatic deformity. Though challenging, the clinician must try to isolate the cause of the patient's symptoms. Instability or nonunion is more amenable to surgical intervention than is mechanical back pain. "Mechanical back pain" in this setting is an activity-related pain that may be muscular, diskogenic, or arthritic in nature. Alternatively, it may be due to stress fractures of adjacent vertebrae secondary to excessive loads caused by the deformity.

No consensus has been reached on the specific severity of kyphosis that leads to pain and symptoms. Farcy and co-workers[44] showed that at the thoracolumbar junction, a threshold of 25° is tolerated before symptoms are likely to occur. The lumbar spine tolerated only 15° of deformity. However, Andreychik and co-workers[7] did not find any correlation between symptoms and the degree of deformity in their series of 55 burst fractures of the lumbar spine. Most authors, however, agree that more sedentary patients tolerate a greater degree of deformity than do active laborers or athletes, which is not surprising when one considers the muscular work involved in maintaining posture in the presence of deformity.

In a paraplegic patient, poor sitting balance because of progression of deformity may be of more concern than pain. Altered sitting balance can lead to soft tissue complications at the gibbus and in the buttock region. It can also impair the ability to power a wheelchair with the upper part of the body and arms. Additionally, subtle deformity may rapidly overcome the ability of weakened paraspinal muscles in patients with higher neurologic compromise.

Finally, some patients may be seen primarily with a progressive neurologic deficit. Malcolm and coauthors reported that approximately 27 percent of patients had a progressive neurologic deficit.[89] The neurologic deficit appears to be a function of the degree of deformity and the amount of canal compromise due to retropulsed bone. Fidler[45] showed that typically bone fragments in the canal are resorbed over time, but that severe angular deformity and abnormal transmission of stress may alter this remodeling process. Additionally, hypertrophic remodeling from segmental instability and perhaps the development of a post-traumatic syrinx can worsen the stenosis at a given level. The deformity of the spine may be quite complex and must be appreciated in three dimensions. Full-length, standing (or sitting) radiographs should be obtained. It is often helpful to obtain the full-length radiograph with the patient's knees extended to correct for any sagittal imbalance compensation occurring in the lower extremity joints. In addition, bending films can be used to assess flexibility. If pseudarthrosis is suspected, flexion and extension views may assist in the diagnosis of segmental instability. If the levels adjacent to the deformity are not flexible enough to compensate for kyphosis, a crouched gait may develop and lead to flexion contractures of the hips. These flexion deformities of the lower extremities should be addressed before correction of the spinal deformity.

CLASSIFICATION OF LATE DEFORMITY

In 1993, Denis and Burkus proposed that post-traumatic deformity fell into three categories, each of which included three subtypes.[35] This classification helps in planning the surgical approach and instrumentation, but it does not distinguish deformities on the basis of their relative magnitudes (Table 34-1).

SURGICAL MANAGEMENT OF LATE DEFORMITY

Surgical indications for correction of deformity include incapacitating pain, progressive deformity, new or progressive neurologic deficit, or failure of a significant neurologic deficit to improve in the face of residual deformity and neural compression. Because the risks of extensive surgical interventions are significant, one should not consider cosmetic deformity by itself to be a relative indication for surgical intervention.

CERVICAL SPINE   When post-traumatic kyphosis of the cervical spine requires correction, preoperative halo or cranial traction may be helpful in correcting at least a portion of the malalignment. This can be accomplished over the course of several days before the operative intervention. Realignment of the kyphotic deformity involves a relative lengthening of the anterior column or shortening of the posterior column. Rigid deformities may require a release of the posterior structures, usually via facet osteotomy, before correction can be expected with anterior column resection (diskectomy or corpectomy) and reconstruction. Should decompression be necessary, it can be performed initially, and the cervical spine can then be placed into more lordotic alignment prior to final fixation.

In the cervical spine, Vaccaro and colleagues[136] showed that long anterior reconstructions with static plates have an unacceptably high failure rate. In a retrospective, multicenter study examining the use of an anterior cervical locking plate and strut graft for a three-level corpectomy, the failure rate was 50 percent when a posterior construct was not used, as opposed to a 9 percent rate of graft or plate dislodgment when a two-level corpectomy was fused in a similar fashion. A higher incidence of graft failure was seen with increased age, failure to lock the screws into the plate, and the use of a peg-in-hole bone graft construct. The type of postoperative immobilization and violation of end plates with screws had no statistically significant effect on failure rates. However, no comparison was made between traumatic and nontraumatic causes, and therefore it is unclear whether subclinical posterior ligamentous injury may increase the risk of failure.

McAfee and Bohlman[93] reviewed the results of 15 patients with multiple-level cervical corpectomies and an anterior-posterior cervical fusion with instrumentation. No patient in their series experienced dislodgment of either the instrumentation or graft material. It seems logical that a posterior tension band construct would help decrease the bending moment experienced by the anterior plate and strut graft, but further study into such biomechanics is still needed before recommendations regarding the best construct can be made.

THORACOLUMBAR SPINE   For Denis and Burkus type IA thoracolumbar deformities of less than 15° that meet the criteria for surgical intervention, posterior spinal fusion is indicated. If the overall sagittal balance of the spine is acceptable and the patient's symptoms are located at the apex of the deformity, a short fusion with instrumentation will probably suffice, especially if pseudarthrosis or limited segmental instability is the source of the pain. As the magnitude of the deformity increases, an anterior procedure preceding the posterior fusion becomes necessary in assisting correction of the deformity. However, Edwards and Rhyne[41] demonstrated that late correction of up to 30° of kyphosis is feasible through a posterior approach in the absence of an anterior bony bridge. These authors apply three-point loading through posterior constructs to cause

	Table 34-1		
	Classification of Late Deformity		
Type	**Level**	**Neurologic Deficit**	**Distant Kyphotic Deformity**
IA	Cephalad to T11	No	No
IB	Cephalad to T11	No	Yes
IC	Cephalad to T11	Yes	Yes
IIA	T12-L1	No	No
IIB	T12-L1	No	Yes
IIC	T12-L1	Yes	Yes
IIIA	L2-L4	No	No
IIIB	L2-L4	No	Yes
IIIC	L2-L4	Yes	Yes

Source: Denis, F.; Burkus, J.K. Classification and treatment of posttraumatic kyphosis in the thoracic and lumbar spine. Semin Spine Surg 5:187–198, 1993.

viscoelastic relaxation of the anterior scar and ligaments. An osseous bridge anteriorly would require a limited anterior release before correction posteriorly. In the thoracic spine, assuming that infection has been eliminated from the differential diagnosis, a posterior compression construct is usually adequate to repair a pseudarthrosis. In the presence of neurologic compromise (type IC), it may be possible to decompress the neural elements by correcting the deformity from a posterior approach if the deformity and compression are mild. This approach requires a longer construct with multiple attachment sites. However, compression from larger deformities or retropulsed bone in the canal mandates anterior decompression before a posterior approach.

Regardless of the approach, the goal is restoration of 40° or less of kyphosis from T2 through T12, which may necessitate the use of a longer posterior construct in patients with type IB deformities. If correction of kyphosis cannot be fully achieved through combined anterior and posterior approaches, wedge-type osteotomies, such as an eggshell or pedicle subtraction osteotomy, may be performed (typically in the lumbar spine below the level of the conus medullaris). Ending a fusion at a level of disk disease or instability should be avoided during the selection of fusion levels.

The thoracolumbar junction deserves special attention. Small deformities (e.g., less than 20°) with no neurologic deficit (type IIA) can be treated with a short posterior construct that preserves lumbar motion segments. In type IIB deformities with associated hyperkyphosis of the thoracic spine, the construct must be extended and may require either a limited anterior release for a flexible deformity or a more extensive release if the upper thoracic deformity is fixed. Type IIC deformities with neurologic deficit and canal compromise of more than 25 percent require anterior decompression. Occasionally, short-segment decompression with a strut graft and anterior instrumentation may obviate the need for a posterior construct, but any residual posterior instability or the absence of a stable anterior reconstruction would mandate a staged procedure. The use of an anterior strut, however, may allow one to preserve lower lumbar motion segments when considering the required fixation points for a posterior approach alone.

McBride and Bradford[94] reported on their series of six patients with a mean thoracolumbar junctional kyphosis of 38° and a range of 20° to 83°. Five of the six had a neurologic deficit, and all had canal encroachment of 25 to 57 percent. All patients were treated by transthoracic vertebrectomy and an allograft strut augmented with a vascularized pedicle tenth rib graft. The mean correction was 26°, or 68 percent. All neurologically incomplete patients improved, and although one patient required revision for graft displacement, no pseudarthroses were reported. The authors note that such treatment requires a competent posterior osteoligamentous complex or the addition of either solid anterior instrumentation or a staged posterior construct.

In the lumbar spine, true kyphosis is rarely seen. Rather, kyphosis typically refers to the loss of lordosis, also called flat back deformity, or hypolordosis. This condition can be particularly symptomatic for patients, and surgical correction often requires osteotomy of the spine. The first report of osteotomy of the spine for kyphosis was made by Smith-Petersen and colleagues.[128] Distraction and deformity of neural and vascular structures and subsequent complications led to investigation of alternative corrective procedures.

The method preferred today is an eggshell osteotomy, also called a pedicle subtraction osteotomy. This technique shortens rather than lengthens the vertebral column.[81,135,139] This osteotomy involves transpedicular fixation above and below the level to be osteotomized, usually at the apex of the deformity, and correction of the deformity through removal of cancellous bone from the vertebral body. Asymmetrical decancellation can correct both coronal and sagittal deformities. Up to 50° of sagittal correction and 40° of coronal correction can be achieved. The osteotomy is started only after instrumentation is completed because the blood loss from the procedure can be severe and may necessitate expeditious closure of the bony osteotomy site. The osteotomy is closed by extension bending at the decancellation site, which is accomplished by extending the table. Reduction can be facilitated by positioning the patient on a hinged frame so that the table can be extended to help close the osteotomy (Fig. 34-12). Adjacent nerve roots above and below the osteotomy then

---

FIGURE 34-12 *Pedicle subtraction osteotomy is facilitated by the use of a hinged four-post frame **(A)**, which allows gentle and gradual reduction of the osteotomy site **(B)**. The inset shows the extent of bone resection for a pedicle subtraction osteotomy, which produces approximately 30° to 35° of correction.*

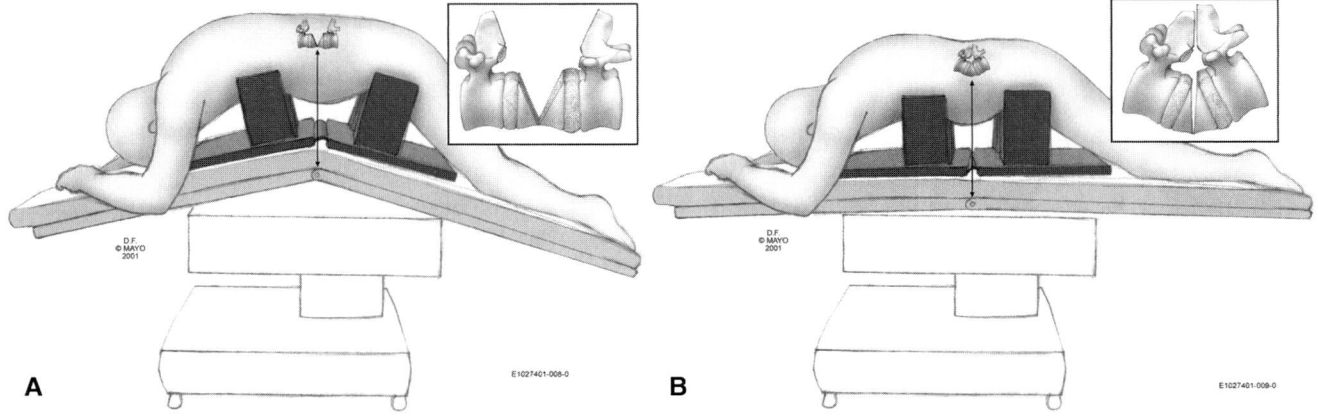

A   **B**

share a common foramen created by removal of the pedicle. Meticulous care must be used to avoid entrapment of nerve roots or dura. This procedure should be effective for most type III deformities.[112]

Adjacent-Segment Disease

Adjacent-segment disease should be a concern for all surgeons who perform spinal fusions. Many reports have highlighted the accelerated degeneration that occurs above and below the level of a rigid fusion.[72,79] Study of this phenomenon in the cervical spine has demonstrated uncertainty about the true role fusion plays in the development of adjacent-segment disease. Most series indicate an annual incidence of 3 percent per year following cervical fusion, but there are still doubts as to whether this indeed represents an increased rate over the natural history of cervical spondylosis.[68]

In the thoracolumbar spine, adjacent segment disease has been more readily linked to fusion procedures.[53] Additionally, it seems that instrumented fusions are more prone to adjacent-segment disease than are fusions without instrumentation. In their series, Ghiselli and co-workers found that 37 percent of the patients in their cohort would require adjacent-segment disease-related surgery within 10 years of the index fusion, and that "floating lumbar fusions" (not including the sacrum or the thoracic spine) were most likely to result in development of adjacent disease. The cause of this phenomenon in the thoracolumbar spine is still somewhat unclear, but it may be due to direct impingement of instrumentation on the facet joints. Some believe that denervation of the surrounding tissues, especially the facet capsule, if injured, leads to neuropathic destruction of the facet. One can minimize this degeneration by protection of the facet capsule in joints outside the region of the fusion, and by not terminating a fusion in a region of stenosis, spondylolisthesis, posterior column deficiency, or an abnormal disk. This type of preoperative planning, however, is less feasible in the setting of trauma than in the setting of elective fusion for degenerative disease. Extending a fusion to a "normal" level may decrease the incidence of one complication in exchange for a further decrease in mobility of the spine.

Several studies have reported stress fractures of the pelvis in patients with long lumbosacral fusions.[61,150] This phenomenon is most likely to occur in older osteoporotic women. The fracture typically occurs on the side from which bone graft is harvested and is probably due to a stress riser created in the ilium at graft acquisition (Fig. 34-13). Symptoms of stress fractures are usually seen in the first few months after surgery, and protected weight bearing is generally adequate for resolution of the symptoms.

Pseudarthrosis

Pseudarthrosis is a complication of both instrumented and noninstrumented fusions and refers to failure of arthrodesis after an attempt at bony fusion. Rates of pseudarthrosis after posterior spinal fusion vary widely in the literature, from as low as 0 percent to as high as 30 percent.[10,142] The major sequela of pseudarthrosis is pain, but the diagnosis of pseudarthrosis can be challenging in a patient with pain after fusion. Instrumentation often obscures radiographic evaluation, and back pain may be a mechanical phenomenon in

FIGURE 34-13 *Pelvic fracture during iliac crest bone graft harvesting. In the setting of osteoporosis, aggressive bone graft harvesting may lead to fracture of the ilium.* **A,** *This 72-year-old woman with rheumatoid arthritis underwent bone graft harvest from the iliac crest. Pain developed in her hip area. Radiographs revealed a fracture at the bone graft site with subsequent pubic rami insufficiency fractures and pelvic instability.*

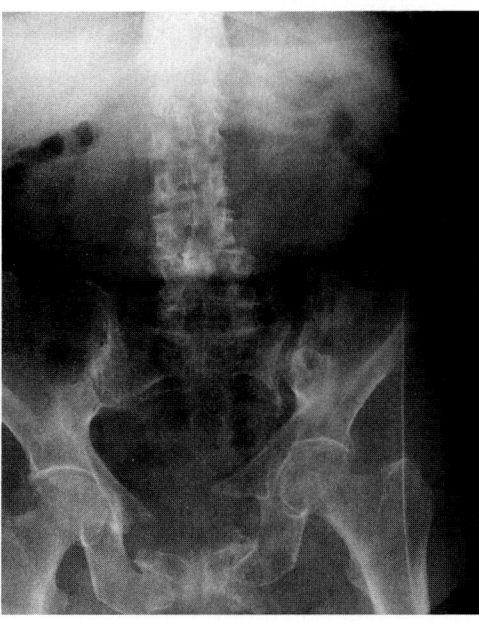

a patient with a solid fusion. Implant failure is a strong indicator of fusion failure, and radiolucency about the fixation (e.g., pedicle screws) can support this diagnosis as well. Most orthopaedic surgeons agree that a change of more than $5°$ at a single functional spinal unit on flexion-extension radiographs is worrisome for pseudarthrosis.

In the cervical spine, pseudarthrosis may occur following treatment of odontoid fractures with an anterior screw. Fountas and colleagues demonstrated a nonunion rate of 13 percent in patients treated for type II and rostral type III odontoid fractures using this technique.[47] Risk of nonunion when using the anterior odontoid screw is more common with osteoporosis, fracture comminution, and unfavorable fracture alignment (nonperpendicular to screw trajectory). Salvage is most reliably performed through posterior C1-C2 arthrodesis. Nonunions with anterior cervical arthrodesis range in incidence rates from 4 to 50 percent in various studies, with higher rates seen in multilevel procedures.[9,27,36,91,117,143]

The rate of pseudarthrosis increases with the number of levels being fused.[26,76] Additionally, advanced age, malnutrition, obesity, and the use of nonsteroidal anti-inflammatory medications have been associated with decreased rates of fusion. Brown and associates[18] showed that tobacco smoking decreases rates of fusion. In a comparison of patients undergoing lumbar laminectomy and fusion, pseudarthrosis developed in 40 percent of smokers, whereas nonunion developed in only 8 percent of nonsmokers.

Recently, Glassman and colleagues showed that if patients stop smoking for at least 6 months after lumbar fusion surgery, the rate of nonunion is comparable to that of non-smokers.[56] For smokers who did not stop smoking, the nonunion rate was 26.5 percent, whereas nonsmokers had a nonunion rate of 14.2 percent. Similarly, Rogozinski and co-workers[119] looked at fusion rates in nonsmokers, preoperative smokers, and postoperative smokers. Although the fusion rate in the postoperative smoker group was less than 60 percent, the study indicated that nonsmokers and preoperative smokers had nearly the same rate of fusion. The negative effect of tobacco smoking on spinal arthrodesis has also been shown in the cervical spine.[67] In the setting of trauma, it is impossible to ask patients to stop smoking before surgery, but cessation of smoking after arthrodesis seems to confer a benefit. Autograft in some studies has also been shown to be superior to allograft as fusion material.[5] However, although autograft is generally incorporated more quickly, the rate of successful fusion is no different with the use of allograft in single-level anterior fusions in the cervical spine.[154]

The incidence of pseudarthrosis in the setting of trauma seems to be lower than that in the setting of degenerative disease or deformity. In 1979, Bohlman[16] reported on a large series of cervical spine fractures treated operatively without a single pseudarthrosis. Flesch and associates[46] reported only 1 nonunion in 40 patients with thoracolumbar spine fractures treated with Harrington instrumentation and fusion. Edwards and Levine[40] reported a 2 percent pseudarthrosis rate in 200 injuries of the thoracolumbar spine; the rate was almost four times higher at the lumbosacral junction. They noted that many of these pseudarthroses were due to technical error. However, Kim and co-workers also demonstrated a higher pseudarthrosis rate when attempting arthrodesis to the sacrum versus L5, or a more cephalad level.[76] Fusion rates can be enhanced with meticulous decortication of the transverse processes while trying to avoid fracture of these processes. Copious application of autograft and placement of graft beneath the posterior implants are recommended. Many spine surgeons favor the use of a gouge for decortication because of the potential for thermal necrosis that may occur during bur decortication.

SUMMARY

The complications of spinal trauma are numerous and challenging. They may occur as a direct result of the injury, because of a lack of appreciation of the injury and subsequent improper treatment, or as a result of the inherent risk of the treatment itself. Successful treatment of these complications relies on prompt recognition. Complications that occur as a result of spinal trauma are often related to immobilization. Prolonged bed rest leads to deconditioning, poor pulmonary function, and decubitus ulcers. Vigilance must be paid to these mundane, but clinically important issues, and proper understanding of the injury pattern provides another avenue by which to avoid complications. Spinal stability must be scrutinized with an eye toward potential deformity. Whether external or internal immobilization is used, all fractures should be monitored closely so that loss of reduction can be discovered early and treated expeditiously. Inadequate fixation

techniques, neglecting to support the anterior column, and failing to restore normal alignment are the causes of most iatrogenic deformities. Meticulous attention to detail during all phases of treatment, combined with attentive medical care, will prevent most of the complications associated with spinal trauma.

REFERENCES

1. Abumi, K.; Shono, Y.; Ito, M.; et al. Complications of pedicle screw fixation in reconstructive surgery of the cervical spine. Spine 25:962–969, 2000.
2. Agha, F.P.; Raji, M.R. Oesophageal perforation with fracture dislocation of cervical spine due to hyperextension injury. Br J Radiol 55:369–372, 1982.
3. Albert, T.J.; Klein, G.R.; Joffe, D.; et al. Use of cervicothoracic junction pedicle screws for reconstruction of complex cervical spine pathology. Spine 23:1596–1599, 1998.
4. An, H.S.; Coppes, M.A. Posterior cervical fixation for fracture and degenerative disc disease. Clin Orthop Relat Res 335:101–111, 1997.
5. Anderson, P.A.; Budorick, T.E.; Easton, K.B.; et al. Failure of halo vest to prevent in vivo motion in patients with injured cervical spines. Spine 16 (Suppl):501–505, 1991.
6. Andersson, S.; Rodrigues, M.; Olerud, C. Odontoid fractures: High complication rate associated with anterior screw fixation in the elderly. Eur Spine J 9:56–59, 2000.
7. Andreychik, D.A.; Alander, D.H.; Senica, K.M.; et al. Burst fractures of the second through fifth lumbar vertebrae. Clinical and radiographic results. J Bone Joint Surg 78A:1156–1166, 1996.
8. Apuzzo, M.L.; Heiden, J.S.; Weiss, M.H.; et al. Acute fractures of the odontoid process. An analysis of 45 cases. J Neurosurg 48:85–91, 1978.
9. Aronson, N.; Filtzer, D.L.; Bagan, M. Anterior cervical fusion by the Smith-Robinson approach. J Neurosurg 29:396–404, 1968.
10. Axelsson, P.; Johnsson, R.; Stromqvist, B.; et al. Posterolateral lumbar fusion. Outcome of 71 consecutive operations after 4 (2–7) years. Acta Orthop Scand 65:309–314, 1994.
11. Aydinli, U.; Karaeminogullari, O.; Tiskaya, K.; et al. Dural tears in lumbar burst fractures with greenstick lamina fractures. Spine 26:E410–415, 2001.
12. Bauman, W.A.; Spungen, A.M. Disorders of carbohydrate and lipid metabolism in veterans with paraplegia or quadriplegia: A model of premature aging. Metabolism 43:749–756, 1994.
13. Bauman, W.A.; Spungen, A.M. Metabolic changes in persons after spinal cord injury. Phys Med Rehabil Clin N Am 11:109–140, 2000.
14. Benzel, E.C.; Kesterson, L.; Marchand, E.P. Texas Scottish Rite Hospital rod instrumentation for thoracic and lumbar spine trauma. J Neurosurg 75:382–387, 1991.
15. Blam, O.G.; Vaccaro, A.R.; Vanichkachorn, J.S.; et al. Risk factors for surgical site infection in the patient with spinal injury. Spine 28:1475–1480, 2003.

16. Bohlman, H.H. Acute fractures and dislocations of the cervical spine. An analysis of three hundred hospitalized patients and review of the literature. J Bone Joint Surg 61A:1191–1142, 1979.

17. Botte, M.J.; Byrne, T.P.; Garfin, S.R. Application of the halo device for immobilization of the cervical spine utilizing an increased torque pressure. J Bone Joint Surg Am 69:750–752, 1987.

18. Brown, C.W.; Orme, T.J.; Richardson, H.D. The rate of pseudarthrosis (surgical nonunion) in patients who are smokers and patients who are nonsmokers: A comparison study. Spine 11:942–943, 1986.

19. Brown, E.M.; Pople, I.K.; de Louvois, J.; et al. Spine update: Prevention of postoperative infection in patients undergoing spinal surgery. Spine 29:938–945, 2004.

20. Bucholz, R.D. Halo vest versus spinal fusion for cervical injury: Evidence from an outcome study. J Neurosurg 70:884–892, 1989.

21. Burke, J.P.; Gerszten, P.C.; Welch, W.C. Iatrogenic vertebral artery injury during anterior cervical spine surgery. Spine J 5:508–514; discussion 514, 2005.

22. Chan, R.C.; Schweigel, J.F.; Thompson, G.B. Halothoracic brace immobilization in 188 patients with acute cervical spine injuries. J Neurosurg 58:508–515, 1983.

23. Choueka, J.; Spivak, J.M.; Kummer, F.J.; et al. Flexion failure of posterior cervical lateral mass screws. Influence of insertion technique and position. Spine 21:462–468, 1996.

24. Christensen, D.; Lynch, J.; Currier, B.; et al. C1 anatomy and dimension relative to lateral mass screw placement. 28th Annual Meeting of the Cervical Spine Research Society. Charleston, South Carolina, 2000.

25. Clark, C.R.; White, A.A., 3rd. Fractures of the dens. A multicenter study. J Bone Joint Surg Am 67:1340–1348, 1985.

26. Cleveland, M.; Bosworth, D.; Thompson, F. Pseudarthrosis in the lumbosacral spine. J Bone Joint Surg 30A:302–312, 1948.

27. Connolly, E.S.; Seymour, R.J.; Adams, J.E. Clinical evaluation of anterior cervical fusion for degenerative cervical disc disease. J Neurosurg 23:431–437, 1965.

28. Cotler, J.M.; Vernace, J.V.; Michalski, J.A. The use of Harrington rods in thoracolumbar fractures. Orthop Clin North Am 17:87–103, 1986.

29. Currier, B.L. Spinal infections. In An, H.S., ed. Principles and Techniques of Spine Surgery. Baltimore, Williams & Wilkins, 1998, pp. 567–603.

30. Currier, B.L.; Todd, L.T.; Maus, T.P.; et al. Anatomic relationship of the internal carotid artery to the C1 vertebra: A case report of cervical reconstruction for chordoma and pilot study to assess the risk of screw fixation of the atlas. Spine 28:E461–467, 2003.

31. Curry, K.; Casady, L. The relationship between extended periods of immobility and decubitus ulcer formation in the acutely spinal cord-injured individual. J Neurosci Nurs 24:185–189, 1992.

32. Dalvie, S.S.; Burwell, M.; Noordeen, M.H. Haemothorax and thoracic spinal fracture. A case for early stabilization. Injury 31:269–270, 2000.

33. Denis, F. The three column spine and its significance in the classification of acute thoracolumbar spinal injuries. Spine 8:817–831, 1983.

34. Denis, F.; Armstrong, G.W.; Searls, K.; et al. Acute thoracolumbar burst fractures in the absence of neurologic deficit. A comparison between operative and nonoperative treatment. Clin Orthop Relat Res 189:142–149, 1984.

35. Denis, F.; Burkus, J.K. Classification and treatment of posttraumatic kyphosis in the thoracic and lumbar spine. Semin Spine Surg 5:187–198, 1993.

36. DePalma, A.F.; Rothman, R.H.; Lewinnek, G.E.; et al. Anterior interbody fusion for severe cervical disc degeneration. Surg Gynecol Obstet 134:755–758, 1972.

37. DiChiro, G.; Fried, L.C.; Doppman, J. Experimental spinal cord angiography. Br J Radiol 43:19–30, 1970.

38. Dunn, M.E.; Seljeskog, E.L. Experience in the management of odontoid process injuries: An analysis of 128 cases. Neurosurgery 18:306–310, 1986.

39. Dwyer, A.F.; Schafer, M.F. Anterior approach to scoliosis. Results of treatment in fifty-one cases. J Bone Joint Surg 56B:218–224, 1974.

40. Edwards, C.; Levine, A. Complications associated with posterior instrumentation in the treatment of thoracic and lumbar injuries. In Garfin, S.R., ed. Complications of Spine Surgery. Baltimore, Williams & Wilkins, 1989.

41. Edwards, C.; Rhyne, A.L. Late treatments of posttraumatic kyphosis. Semin Spine Surg 2:63–69, 1990.

42. Edwards, C.; York, J.E.; Levine, A.; et al. Determinants of spinal dislodgement. Orthop Trans 10–8, 1986.

43. Edwards, C.C.; Levine, A.M. Early rod-sleeve stabilization of the injured thoracic and lumbar spine. Orthop Clin North Am 17:121–145, 1986.

44. Farcy, J.P.; Weidenbaum, M.; Glassman, S.D. Sagittal index in management of thoracolumbar burst fractures. Spine 15:958–965, 1990.

45. Fidler, M.W. Remodelling of the spinal canal after burst fracture. A prospective study of two cases. J Bone Joint Surg 70B:730–732, 1988.

46. Flesch, J.R.; Leider, L.L.; Erickson, D.L.; et al. Harrington instrumentation and spine fusion for unstable fractures and fracture-dislocations of the thoracic and lumbar spine. J Bone Joint Surg 59A:143–153, 1977.

47. Fountas, K.N.; Machinis, T.G.; Kapsalaki, E.Z.; et al. Surgical treatment of acute type II and rostral type III odontoid fractures managed by anterior screw fixation. South Med J 98:896–901, 2005.

48. Franzini, M.; Altana, P.; Annessi, V.; et al. Iatrogenic vascular injuries following lumbar disc surgery. Case report and review of the literature. J Cardiovasc Surg (Torino) 28:727–730, 1987.

49. Freeman, D. Major vascular complications of lumbar disk surgery. West J Surg Gynecol Obstet 69:175–177, 1961.

50. Garfin, S.R.; Botte, M.J.; Waters, R.L.; et al. Complications in the use of the halo fixation device. J Bone Joint Surg Am 68:320–325, 1986.

51. Gaudinez, R.F.; English, G.M.; Gebhard, J.S.; et al. Esophageal perforations after anterior cervical surgery. J Spinal Disord 13:77–84, 2000.

52. Gertzbein, S.D.; Macmichael, D.; Tile, M. Harrington instrumentation as a method of fixation in fractures of the spine. J Bone Joint Surg 64B:526–529, 1982.

53. Ghiselli, G.; Wang, J.C.; Bhatia, N.N.; et al. Adjacent segment degeneration in the lumbar spine. J Bone Joint Surg Am 86-A:1497–1503, 2004.

54. Giacobetti, F.B.; Vaccaro, A.R.; Bos-Giacobetti, M.A.; et al. Vertebral artery occlusion associated with cervical spine trauma. A prospective analysis. Spine 22:188–192, 1997.

55. Glaser, J.A.; Whitehill, R.; Stamp, W.G.; et al. Complications associated with the halo-vest. A review of 245 cases. J Neurosurg 65:762–769, 1986.

56. Glassman, S.D.; Anagnost, S.C.; Parker, A.; et al. The effect of cigarette smoking and smoking cessation on spinal fusion. Spine 25:2608–2615, 2000.

57. Goins, W.R.; Rodriguez, A. Traumatic chylothorax. In Turney, S.; Rodriguez, A.; Cowley, R., eds. Management of Cardiothoracic Trauma. Baltimore, Williams & Wilkins, 1990, pp. 383–386.

58. Golfinos, J.G.; Dickman, C.A.; Zabramski, J.M.; et al. Repair of vertebral artery injury during anterior cervical decompression. Spine 19:2552–2556, 1994.

59. Goodkin, R.; Laska, L.L. Vascular and visceral injuries associated with lumbar disc surgery: Medicolegal implications. Surg Neurol 49:358–370; discussion 370–352, 1998.

60. Greene, K.A.; Dickman, C.A.; Marciano, F.F.; et al. Acute axis fractures. Analysis of management and outcome in 340 consecutive cases. Spine 22:1843–1852, 1997.

61. Grimm, J.; Jackson, R. Stress fracture of the pelvis: A complication following instrumented lumbar fusion. Paper presented at the 27th Annual Meeting of the Scoliosis Research Society, Kansas City, Missouri, 1992.

62. Grob, D.; Jeanneret, B.; Aebi, M.; et al. Atlanto-axial fusion with transarticular screw fixation. J Bone Joint Surg Br 73:972–976, 1991.

63. Guttmann, L. Spinal deformities in traumatic paraplegics and tetraplegics following surgical procedures. Paraplegia 7:38–58, 1969.

64. Hanigan, W.C.; Powell, F.C.; Elwood, P.W.; et al. Odontoid fractures in elderly patients. J Neurosurg 78:32–35, 1993.

65. Heini, P.; Scholl, E.; Wyler, D.; et al. Fatal cardiac tamponade associated with posterior spinal instrumentation. A case report. Spine 23:2226–2230, 1998.

66. Heller, J.G.; Silcox, D.H., 3rd; Sutterlin, C.E., 3rd. Complications of posterior cervical plating, Spine 20:2442–2448, 1995.

67. Hilibrand, A.S.; Fye, M.A.; Emery, S.E.; et al. Impact of smoking on the outcome of anterior cervical arthrodesis with interbody or strut-grafting. J Bone Joint Surg 83A:668–673, 2001.

68. Hilibrand, A.S.; Robbins M. Adjacent segment degeneration and adjacent segment disease: The consequences of spinal fusion? Spine J 4 Suppl:190S–194S, 2004.

69. Hohf, R.P. Arterial injuries occurring during orthopaedic operations. Clin Orthop 28:21–37, 1963.

70. Hong, X.; Dong, Y.; Yunbing, C.; et al. Posterior screw placement on the lateral mass of atlas: An anatomic study. Spine 29:500–503, 2004.

71. Horwitz, N.H.; Curtin, J.A. Prophylactic antibiotics and wound infections following laminectomy for lumber disc herniation. J Neurosurg 43:727–731, 1975.

72. Hsu, K.; Zucherman, J. The long term effect of lumbar spinal fusion: Deterioration of adjacent motion segments. In Yonenobu K.O.; Takemitsu, Y., eds. Lumbar Fusion and Stabilization. Berlin, Springer-Verlag, 1993, pp. 54–64.

73. Jodoin, A.; Dupuis, P.; Fraser, M.; et al. Unstable fractures of the thoracolumbar spine: A 10-year experience at Sacre-Coeur Hospital. J Trauma 25:197–202, 1985.

74. Kamming, D.; Clarke, S. Postoperative visual loss following prone spinal surgery. Br J Anaesth 95:257–260, 2005.

75. Kelly, M.F.; Spiegel, J.; Rizzo, K.A.; et al. Delayed pharyngoesophageal perforation: A complication of anterior spine surgery. Ann Otol Rhinol Laryngol 100:201–205, 1991.

76. Kim, Y.J.; Bridwell, K.H.; Lenke, L.G.; et al. Pseudarthrosis in adult spinal deformity following multisegmental instrumentation and arthrodesis. J Bone Joint Surg Am 88:721–728, 2006.

77. King, D. Internal fixation for lumbosacral fusions. J Bone Joint Surg 30A:560–565, 1948.

78. Kostuik, J.P. Indications for the use of the halo immobilization. Clin Orthop 154:46–50, 1981.

79. Krag, M. Biomechanics of transpedicle spinal fixation. In Weinstein J.W., S., ed. The Lumbar Spine. Philadelphia, W.B. Saunders, 1990.

80. Lagrone, M.O.; Bradford, D.S.; Moe, J.H.; et al. Treatment of symptomatic flatback after spinal fusion. J Bone Joint Surg 70A:569–580, 1988.

81. Lehmer, S.M.; Keppler, L.; Biscup, R.S.; et al. Posterior transvertebral osteotomy for adult thoracolumbar kyphosis. Spine 19:2060–2067, 1994.

82. Lennarson, P.J.; Mostafavi, H.; Traynelis, V.C.; et al. Management of type II dens fractures: A case-control study. Spine 25:1234–1237, 2000.

83. Levi, A.D.; Dickman, C.A.; Sonntag, V.K. Management of postoperative infections after spinal instrumentation. J Neurosurg 86:975–980, 1997.

84. Levine, A.M.; Edwards, C.C. Complications in the treatment of acute spinal injury. Orthop Clin North Am 17:183–203, 1986.

85. Lonstein, J.E.; Denis, F.; Perra, J.H.; et al. Complications associated with pedicle screws. J Bone Joint Surg 81A:1519–1528, 1999.

86. Lowery, G.L.; McDonough, R.F. The significance of hardware failure in anterior cervical plate fixation. Patients with 2- to 7-year follow-up. Spine 23:181–186; discussion 186–187, 1998.

87. Madawi, A.A.; Casey, A.T.; Solanki, G.A.; et al. Radiological and anatomical evaluation of the atlantoaxial transarticular screw fixation technique. J Neurosurg 86:961–968, 1997.

88. Magerl, F. Stabilization of the lower thoracic and lumbar spine with external skeletal fixation. Clin Orthop 189:125–141, 1984.

89. Malcolm, B.W.; Bradford, D.S.; Winter, R.B.; et al. Post-traumatic kyphosis. A review of forty-eight surgically treated patients. J Bone Joint Surg 63A:891–899, 1981.

90. Manfredini, M.; Ferrante, R.; Gildone, A.; et al. Unilateral blindness as a complication of intraoperative positioning for cervical spinal surgery. J Spinal Disord 13:271–272, 2000.

91. Martins, A.N. Anterior cervical discectomy with and without interbody bone graft. J Neurosurg 44:290–295, 1976.

92. Massie, J.B.; Heller, J.G.; Abitbol, J.J.; et al. Postoperative posterior spinal wound infections, Clin Orthop Relat Res 284:99–108, 1992.

93. McAfee, P.C.; Bohlman, H.H. One-stage anterior cervical decompression and posterior stabilization with circumferential arthrodesis. A study of twenty-four patients who had a traumatic or a neoplastic lesion. J Bone Joint Surg 71A:78–88, 1989.

94. McBride, G.G.; Bradford, D.S. Vertebral body replacement with femoral neck allograft and vascularized rib strut graft. A technique for treating post-traumatic kyphosis with neurologic deficit. Spine 8:406–415, 1983.

95. Mehta, J.S.; Reed, M.R.; McVie, J.L.; et al. Weight-bearing radiographs in thoracolumbar fractures: Do they influence management? Spine 29:564–567, 2004.

96. Melcher, R.P.; Puttlitz, C.M.; Kleinstueck, F.S.; et al. Biomechanical testing of posterior atlantoaxial fixation techniques. Spine 27:2435–2440, 2002.

97. Morrison, A. Hyperextension injury of the cervical spine with rupture of the oesophagus. J Bone Joint Surg Br 42-B:356–357, 1960.

98. Muller, E.J.; Schwinnen, I.; Fischer, K.; et al. Non-rigid immobilisation of odontoid fractures. Eur Spine J 12:522–525, 2003.

99. Mumford, J.; Weinstein, J.N.; Spratt, K.F.; et al. Thoracolumbar burst fractures. The clinical efficacy and outcome of nonoperative management. Spine 18:955–970, 1993.

100. Nagai, H.; Shimizu, K.; Shikata, J.; et al. Chylous leakage after circumferential thoracolumbar fusion for correction of kyphosis resulting from fracture. Report of three cases. Spine 22:2766–2769, 1997.

101. Nakai, S.; Zielke, K. Chylothorax—A rare complication after anterior and posterior spinal correction. Report on six cases. Spine 11:830–833, 1986.

102. Nicoll, E. Fractures of the dorso-lumbar spine. J Bone Joint Surg 31A:376–394, 1949.

103. Papadoulas, S.; Konstantinou, D.; Kourea, H.P.; et al. Vascular injury complicating lumbar disc surgery. A systematic review. Eur J Vasc Endovasc Surg 24:189–195, 2002.

104. Papagelopoulos, P.J.; Currier, B.L.; Stone, J.; et al. Biomechanical evaluation of occipital fixation. J Spinal Disord 13:336–344, 2000.

105. Parker, J.W.; Lane, J.R.; Karaikovic, E.E.; et al. Successful short-segment instrumentation and fusion for thoracolumbar spine fractures: A consecutive 4½-year series. Spine 25:1157–1170, 2000.

106. Picada, R.; Winter, R.B.; Lonstein, J.E.; et al. Postoperative deep wound infection in adults after posterior lumbosacral spine fusion with instrumentation: Incidence and management. J Spinal Disord 13:42–45, 2000.

107. Polin, R.S.; Szabo, T.; Bogaev, C.A.; et al. Nonoperative management of types II and III odontoid fractures: The Philadelphia collar versus the halo vest. Neurosurgery 38:450–456; discussion 456–457, 1996.

108. Rames, R.D.; Schoenecker, P.L.; Bridwell, K.H. Chylothorax after posterior spinal instrumentation and fusion. Clin Orthop Relat Res 261:229–232, 1990.

109. Rechtine, G.R., 2nd; Cahill, D.; Chrin, A.M. Treatment of thoracolumbar trauma: Comparison of complications of operative versus nonoperative treatment. J Spinal Disord 12:406–409, 1999.

110. Rechtine, G.R.; Bono, P.L.; Cahill, D.; et al. Postoperative wound infection after instrumentation of thoracic and lumbar fractures. J Orthop Trauma 15:566–569, 2001.

111. Reddin, A.; Mirvis, S.E.; Diaconis, J.N. Rupture of the cervical esophagus and trachea associated with cervical spine fracture. J Trauma 27:564–566, 1987.

112. Reeg, S.; Boachie-Adjei, O. Management of late deformity after spine trauma. In Capen, D.; Haye, W., eds. Comprehensive Management of Spine Trauma. St. Louis, C.V. Mosby, 1998.

113. Resnick, D.K.; Benzel, E.C. Lateral extracavitary approach for thoracic and thoracolumbar spine trauma: Operative complications. Neurosurgery 43:796–802, 1998.

114. Riew, K.D.; Sethi, N.S.; Devney, J.; et al. Complications of buttress plate stabilization of cervical corpectomy. Spine 24:2404–2410, 1999.

115. Roberts, D.; Lee, W.; Cuneo, R.C.; et al. Longitudinal study of bone turnover after acute spinal cord injury. J Clin Endocrinol Metab 83:415–422, 1998.

116. Roberts, D.A.; Doherty, B.J.; Heggeness, M.H. Quantitative anatomy of the occiput and the biomechanics of occipital screw fixation. Spine 23:1100–1107; discussion 1107–1108, 1998.

117. Robinson, R.A. Anterior and posterior cervical spine fusions. Clin Orthop Relat Res 35:34–62, 1964.

118. Rockswold, G.L.; Bergman, T.A.; Ford, S.E. Halo immobilization and surgical fusion: Relative indications and effectiveness in the treatment of 140 cervical spine injuries. J Trauma 30:893–898, 1990.

119. Rogozinski, C.; Rogozinksi, A.; Weiss, H. Effect of cigarette smoking on instrumented lumbosacral fusion. Paper presented at the Annual Meeting of the American Academy of Orthopaedic Surgeons. Orlando, Florida, 1996.

120. Rosenblum, D.; Ehrlich, V. Brain abscess and psychosis as a complication of a halo orthosis. Arch Phys Med Rehabil 76:865–867, 1995.

121. Ryan, M.D.; Taylor, T.K. Odontoid fractures in the elderly. J Spinal Disord 6:397–401, 1993.

122. Sasso, R.C.; Jeanneret, B.; Fischer, K.; et al. Occipitocervical fusion with posterior plate and screw instrumentation. A long-term follow-up study. Spine 19:2364–2368, 1994.

123. Schulitz, K.P.; Assheuer, J. Discitis after procedures on the intervertebral disc. Spine 19:1172–1177, 1994.

124. Sen, C.; Eisenberg, M.; Casden, A.M.; et al. Management of the vertebral artery in excision of extradural tumors of the cervical spine. Neurosurgery 36:106–115, 1995.

125. Shen, F.H.; Samartzis, D.; Khanna, N.; et al. Comparison of clinical and radiographic outcome in instrumented anterior cervical discectomy and fusion with or without direct uncovertebral joint decompression. Spine J 4:629–635, 2004.

126. Silen, M.L.; Weber, T.R. Management of thoracic duct injury associated with fracture-dislocation of the spine following blunt trauma. J Trauma 39:1185–1187, 1995.

127. Smith, M.D.; Emery, S.E.; Dudley, A.; et al. Vertebral artery injury during anterior decompression of the cervical spine. A retrospective review of ten patients. J Bone Joint Surg Br 75:410–415, 1993.

128. Smith-Petersen, M.N.; Larson, C.B.; Aufranc, O.E. Osteotomy of the spine for correction of flexion deformity in rheumatoid arthritis. Clin Orthop Relat Res 66:6–9, 1969.

129. Stambough, J.L.; Beringer, D. Postoperative wound infections complicating adult spine surgery. J Spinal Disord 5:277–285, 1992.

130. Stringer, W.L.; Kelly, D.L., Jr.; Johnston, F.R.; et al. Hyperextension injury of the cervical spine with esophageal perforation. Case report. J Neurosurg 53:541–543, 1980.

131. Subach, B.R.; Morone, M.A.; Haid, R.W., Jr.; et al. Management of acute odontoid fractures with single-screw anterior fixation. Neurosurgery 45:812–819; discussion 819–820, 1999.

132. Szolar, D.H.; Preidler, K.W.; Steiner, H.; et al. Vascular complications in lumbar disk surgery: Report of four cases. Neuroradiology 38:521–525, 1996.

133. Taneichi, H.; Suda, K.; Kajino, T.; et al. Traumatically induced vertebral artery occlusion associated with cervical spine injuries: Prospective study using magnetic resonance angiography. Spine 30:1955–1962, 2005.

134. Tashjian, R.Z.; Majercik, S.; Biffl, W.L.; et al. Halo-vest immobilization increases early morbidity and mortality in elderly odontoid fractures. J Trauma 60:199–203, 2006.

135. Thiranont, N.; Netrawichien, P. Transpedicular decancellation closed wedge vertebral osteotomy for treatment of fixed flexion deformity of spine in ankylosing spondylitis. Spine 18:2517–2522, 1993.

136. Vaccaro, A.R.; Falatyn, S.P.; Scuderi, G.J.; et al. Early failure of long segment anterior cervical plate fixation. J Spinal Disord 11:410–415, 1998.

137. Vaccaro, A.R.; Klein, G.R.; Flanders, A.E.; et al. Long-term evaluation of vertebral artery injuries following cervical spine trauma using magnetic resonance angiography. Spine 23:789–794; discussion 795, 1998.

138. Wang, J.C.; McDonough, P.W.; Endow, K.K.; et al. Increased fusion rates with cervical plating for two-level anterior cervical discectomy and fusion. Spine 25:41–45, 2000.

139. Weatherley, C.; Jaffray, D.; Terry, A. Vascular complications associated with osteotomy in ankylosing spondylitis: A report of two cases. Spine 13:43–46, 1988.

140. Weber, S.C.; Benson, D. A comparison of segmental fixation and Harrington instrumentation in the management of unstable thoracolumbar spine fractures. Orthop Trans 9:36, 1985.

141. Weinstein, J.N.; Collalto, P.; Lehmann, T.R. Thoracolumbar "burst" fractures treated conservatively: A long-term follow-up. Spine 13:33–38, 1988.

142. West, J.L., 3rd; Ogilvie, J.W.; Bradford, D.S. Complications of the variable screw plate pedicle screw fixation. Spine 16:576–579, 1991.

143. White, A.A., 3rd; Southwick, W.O.; Deponte, R. J.; et al. Relief of pain by anterior cervical-spine fusion for spondylosis. A report of sixty-five patients. J Bone Joint Surg Am 55:525–534, 1973.

144. Whitehill, R.; Richman, J.A.; Glaser, J.A. Failure of immobilization of the cervical spine by the halo vest. A report of five cases. J Bone Joint Surg 68A:326–332, 1986.

145. Whitesides, T.E., Jr. Traumatic kyphosis of the thoracolumbar spine. Clin Orthop Relat Res 128:78–92, 1977.

146. Wiegand, D.A.; Hartel, M.I.; Quander, T.; et al. Assessment of cryoprecipitate-thrombin solution for dural repair. Head Neck 16:569–573, 1994.

147. Wimmer, C.; Gluch, H.; Franzreb, M.; et al. Predisposing factors for infection in spine surgery: A survey of 850 spinal procedures. J Spinal Disord 11:124–128, 1998.

148. Wittenberg, R.H.; Lee, K.S.; Shea, M.; et al. Effect of screw diameter, insertion technique, and bone cement augmentation of pedicular screw fixation strength. Clin Orthop Relat Res 296:278–287, 1993.

149. Wolfe, S.W.; Lospinuso, M.F.; Burke, S.W. Unilateral blindness as a complication of patient positioning for spinal surgery. A case report. Spine 17:600–605, 1992.

150. Wood, K.B.; Geissele, A.E.; Ogilvie, J.W. Pelvic fractures after long lumbosacral spine fusions. Spine 21:1357–1362, 1996.

151. Wright, N.M.; Lauryssen, C. Vertebral artery injury in C1-2 transarticular screw fixation: Results of a survey of the AANS/CNS section on disorders of the spine and peripheral nerves. American Association of Neurological Surgeons/Congress of Neurological Surgeons. J Neurosurg 88:634–640, 1998.

152. Wright, P.; Gardner, A. Traumatic chylothorax: A case after dislocation of the thoracic spine. J Bone Joint Surg 34B:64, 1952.

153. Young, M.H. Long-term consequences of stable fractures of the thoracic and lumbar vertebral bodies. J Bone Joint Surg 55B:295–300, 1973.

154. Zdeblick, T.A.; Ducker, T.B. The use of freeze-dried allograft bone for anterior cervical fusions. Spine 16:726–729, 1991.

155. Zindrick, M.R.; Wiltse, L.L.; Widell, E.H.; et al. A biomechanical study of intrapeduncular screw fixation in the lumbosacral spine. Clin Orthop Relat Res 203:99–112, 1986.

Pelvis

Section Editor: Alan M. Levine, M.D.

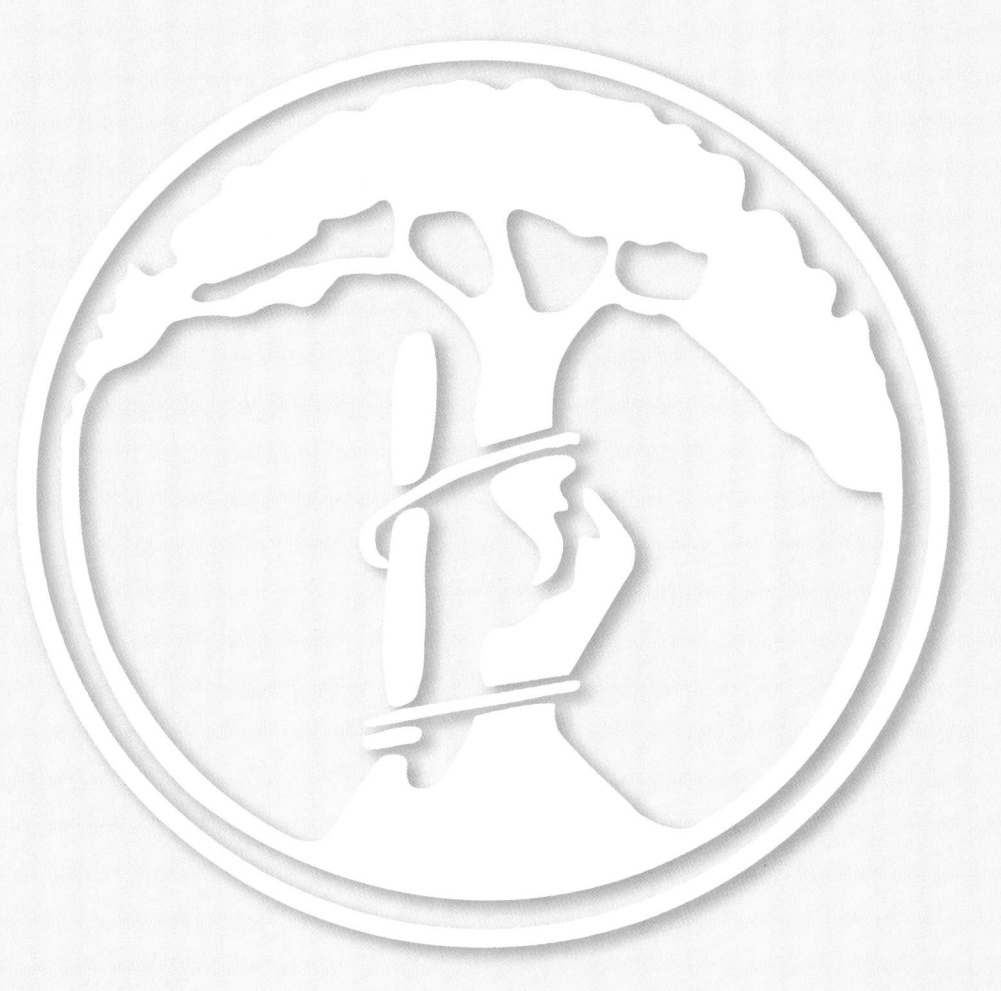

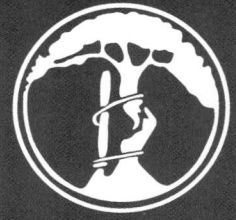

CHAPTER 35

Fractures of the Sacrum

Alan M. Levine, M.D.

Treatment of injuries to the sacrum requires consideration of a number of additional factors beyond those relevant to injuries of the thoracic and lumbar spine. These factors are related to the anatomic complexity of the sacrum, the mobility of the lumbosacral junction, and the difficulty inherent in fixation to the sacrum. Additionally, relatively large forces are necessary to achieve and maintain reduction of either transverse upper and midsacral fractures or vertical fractures involving the sacral ala and sacroiliac joints. Finally, sacral fractures encompass a wide variety of entities that range in severity from a simple buckle fracture of the sacral ala to a severely comminuted fracture associated with major injury to the pelvis. The spectrum is also broad when the causes of the injury are considered along with the epidemiology of the affected individuals. These fractures may be the result of high-energy trauma such as from motor vehicle and motorcycle accidents or suicide attempts involving younger individuals or result from low-energy insufficiency fractures or falls involving elderly persons.

Throughout the 1970s and 1980s, the lack of satisfactory techniques for reduction and stabilization of injuries in the sacrum frequently resulted in less than optimal treatment results and led some authors to espouse nonoperative techniques as a better alternative.[17,28,29] Occasional reports, however, suggested that an operative approach yielded better anatomic results and perhaps even better functional outcomes.[51,76] Even with the more widely accepted use of pedicle screw fixation in the lumbar spine and various methods of sacral fixation used in North America, some early, poorly conceptualized operative approaches to fractures in this region also led to early failure.[3,4,45,88] These results caused some surgeons to accept chronic pain and the failure to return to preinjury occupation as the norm in this very young group of patients.

The lumbosacral junction in particular must resist a number of large forces, but it must also permit a significant amount of motion. It has therefore been difficult to obtain anatomic reduction and reconstruction of the lumbar spine and sacrum until the most recent advances in instrumentation. This difficulty has led many authors to suggest either limited procedures and goals or "benign neglect" as the methods of treatment of sacral injuries. In addition, in the sacrum, failure to recognize the nature of the injuries and their severity has resulted in a lack of organized treatment schemes. The normal kyphotic sagittal configuration

of the sacrum and the many overlying structures have made imaging difficult, even with the use of standard two-dimensional computed tomography (CT). Fixation to the bone of the sacrum has been even more problematic. These numerous features and problems distinguish fractures of the sacrum from the more abundant and common fractures at the thoracolumbar junction.

More accurate diagnostic imaging studies, as well as advances in instrumentation techniques, now allow us to treat sacral injuries with the greater degree of accuracy and competence typical of approaches for the more proximal spinal injuries. Recently, however, more controversy has arisen concerning the optimal treatment method for both transverse and vertical sacral fractures. Some have advocated attempts at decompression and anatomic reduction while others have advocated bypassing the injured sacrum and regaining stability by fixing the lower lumbar spine to the ilium.[60,82,83] To this end, however, we must have a clear understanding of the anatomic and functional differences that distinguish the sacrum from the remainder of the more proximal areas of the spine.

Treatment goals for spine trauma in general are (1) anatomic reduction of the injury, (2) rigid fixation of the fracture, and, when necessary, (3) decompression of the neural elements. For treatment of the sacral spine, we must add the considerations of (4) maintenance of sagittal alignment, and (5) prevention of frequent complications (e.g., loss of sacral fixation, failure to attain decompression and reduction, and pseudarthrosis). As the characteristics of the sacrum are reviewed, it will become evident that techniques that were discussed in previous sections of the book for the treatment of cervical, thoracic, thoracolumbar, and lumbar spine injuries are not applicable to the treatment of sacral injuries.

ETIOLOGY AND EPIDEMIOLOGY

Sacral fractures can be subdivided into several major categories based on cause. The most common cause of sacral fractures is high-energy trauma resulting in major pelvic disruption, which has a high incidence of associated sacral fractures. Pohlemann and associates[69] found that 28 percent of patients with pelvic ring injuries had sacral fractures (377 sacral fractures/1350 pelvic fractures), and Denis and colleagues reported a 30 percent incidence (236 sacral/776 pelvic).[21] Most of these fractures are vertical in orientation and may be either unilateral or bilateral; in addition, they may occasionally have a transverse component. Isolated sacral fractures are much more uncommon and represent approximately 5 to 10 percent of all traumatic injuries that occur as a result of high-energy accidents. Most of the isolated fractures are transverse and result from direct trauma such as occurs because of a fall from a height.[86] Occasionally these transverse fractures may be due to direct trauma, but when that occurs the injury is usually more distal (S3). The final type of sacral fracture is an insufficiency fracture, which occurs either spontaneously or after a trivial episode of trauma.[81] Most patients in whom insufficiency fractures of the sacrum develop have predisposing factors such as osteopenia, chronic steroid use, or pelvic irradiation.[58,81] The actual incidence of this type of fracture is unknown because recognition and diagnosis have not been frequently emphasized. Although more than 500 cases have been reported in the literature,[27,43] the incidence is considerably higher because insufficiency fractures are an unrecognized cause of back pain in elderly female patients.[19,36]

ANATOMIC FEATURES

The sacrum forms both the terminal portion of the spine and the central portion of the pelvis. Its five fused vertebrae give rise to an overall kyphotic sagittal alignment that influences the alignment of the mobile spine above it. The normal kyphosis of the thoracic spine falls within a range of 15 to 49°,[98] whereas normal lumbar lordosis is generally thought to be less than 60°. These values are in part determined by the slope of the sacral base, which averages approximately 45° from the horizontal. This angle is critical in determining the amount of shear force[87] to which the lumbosacral junction is subjected. Anatomic differences in the structure of the lumbar vertebrae and sacrum influence therapeutic decisions and make attachment of fixation devices necessarily different from that for proximal levels in the thoracic and lumbar spine.

The sacroiliac joint, which joins the sacrum to the rest of the pelvis, includes the lateral portions of S1, S2, and part of S3, with the more caudal portions of the sacrum remaining free. The stability of the sacroiliac joint is maintained by strong ligamentous attachments such as the anterior and posterior sacroiliac ligaments, the sacrotuberous ligaments, and the sacrotransverse ligaments. The strength of this ligamentous complex helps determine the location of fractures of the sacrum, with transverse fractures commonly occurring at the midportion of S3 at the end of the sacroiliac attachment. Similarly, vertical fractures occur through the ala rather than through the joint as a result of the strength of the sacroiliac joint in resisting disruption.

With caudal descent in the lumbar spine, the overall dimensions of the canal enlarge, whereas the area occupied by the neural elements decreases. The cord in the thoracic region measures approximately 86.5 mm² and is housed within a canal that is generally 17.2 × 16.8 mm². Thus, in the thoracic region, the cord occupies about 50 percent of the canal area. In the thoracolumbar region, the conus broadens, as does the canal. The spinal cord usually terminates at approximately L1. In the lumbar region, the canal is typically large (23.4 × 17.4 mm²).[24,72] Here, the roots of the cauda equina are the only contents. In the sacrum, however, the diameter of the canal again begins to narrow and flatten. In addition, with the normal, slightly kyphotic angle at the midpoint of the sacrum (S2-S3), the roots are tethered in a relatively fixed location. This tethering of the roots allows less flexibility in placing any fixation devices within the canal in the sacrum. The sacral roots are responsible for urinary continence, micturition, fecal continence, defecation, and sexual function. After emanating from the conus medullaris, the sacral roots traverse the canal of the lumbar spine in a relatively posterior location and exit through the ventral and dorsal foramina. Fractures through the sacral ala can also result in an L5 root injury as demonstrated by Denis and colleagues.[21] This root exits the foramen and traverses over the top of the sacral ala such that displacement of the alar fracture can cause injury to the root. Denis and co-workers also evaluated the frequency of injury to individual sacral roots and found that root injury at the ventral foramen was less likely at S3 and S4 than at S1 and S2 because of a significant difference in the root-to-foramen ratio in the two areas. Because innervation of bowel and bladder function is by bilateral sacral roots, injury to one side does not disrupt sphincter function, whereas bilateral injury does.[37]

With the increasing emphasis on innovative methods of fixation for injuries in the low lumbar spine and sacrum, an understanding of the pertinent anatomic dimensions takes on new significance. Previously, with hook fixation or sublaminar wiring to the posterior elements, the only important consideration was the posterior topographic anatomy. However, the dimensions, position, and orientation of the pedicles, as well as the shape of the vertebral body, are likewise critical. The initial anatomic description of pedicle morphology with respect to pedicle screw fixation was presented by Saillant[79] in 1976 and confirmed by two later studies from North America.[46,100] The critical features are the sagittal and transverse width of the pedicles, pedicle length, pedicle angle, and chord length (depth to the anterior cortex along a fixed orientation). Understanding the three-dimensional anatomy of the various sacral levels, as well as the position of the neurovascular structures applied to the anterior surface of the sacrum, is critical to the conceptualization of adequate and safe fixation to the sacrum.

The anatomic constraints of the sacrum are quite severe, with its overall sagittal contour being gradually kyphotic at about 25° with the apex at S3. The sacral laminae are extremely thin and might be absent in some areas. At their maximal thickness, the sacral alae are between 40 and 45 mm. The area of maximal bone thickness is in the vestigial pedicle of each sacral segment, and this area rapidly decreases in size with progression to the distal segments. At S3 or S4, the maximal thickness may only be 20 mm. The anatomic structures that may be encountered at the level of the S1 body are the internal iliac vein, the lumbosacral plexus, and the sacroiliac joint. A safe zone about 2 cm wide and bordered by the sacral promontory medially and the iliac vein laterally is present and invariably entered with orientation of a screw along the S1 pedicle.[56] Screws can be directed only medially at the

S1 level because the critical neurovascular structures will then lie lateral to the sacral promontory. Screws placed laterally at either 30 or 45° are aimed at a smaller lateral safe zone. The more lateral orientation provides for a longer screw length of 44 mm.[56] The S1 level is the only segment that will allow simultaneous screw placement in the lateral and medial directions. Screw placement should be bicortical for maximal purchase. At the S2 level, the only vulnerable structure is the sigmoid colon on the left side. Penetration through the cortex by more than 1 cm is usually necessary to produce an injury. At the S2 level, the thickness of the sacral bone has decreased significantly compared with that at the S1 level, and thus, the holding power of the bone in an axis parallel to placement of S1 would be significantly less. To compensate for these deficiencies, orientation of fixation devices proximally and laterally will significantly increase the length of screw purchase and therefore pull-out strength. Variations in the amount of cancellous and cortical bone mass in different regions of the sacrum significantly affect fixation possibilities and the risks associated with fixation. Because of increased bone mass, sacrum fixation is more secure in the ala or vertebral bodies than in the very thin posterior laminar structures.

Anatomic considerations are different for vertical sacral alar fractures that require fixation. Iliosacral fixation is dependent on visualizing the anterior border of the ala on the inlet view, which can be difficult. As a result of the concavity of the ala, it is easy to misdirect screws anterior to the ala and jeopardize neurovascular structures. The starting point for percutaneous iliosacral screws is based on landmarks on the lateral aspect of the ilium. Preoperative planning based on CT allows accurate assessment of the anatomic relationships. The use of image intensification for screw guidance requires accurate identification of the anterior and superior aspects of the sacrum to avoid exiting the ala anteriorly and then reentering it more medially. As a result of the contour of the body, passage of screws is safer at S1 than at S2, and use of S2 should be reserved only for patients with severe comminution of the S1 ala. It has been shown, however, that these relationships and the margin for error can dramatically change with the accuracy of the fracture reduction. For zone 2 fractures the cross-sectional contact area decreased by 30, 56, 81, and 90 percent with 5, 10, 25, and 20 mm of displacement, respectively.[73] Thus not only is the anatomy critical, but also the distortion of the anatomy by the fracture must be clearly taken into account.

The iliac wing as a fixation site for lumbopelvic stabilizations in the pelvis is the other anatomic configuration important in the treatment of sacral fractures. Several studies[7,84] have evaluated the optimal path as well as the maximum screw diameter and length using both cadavers and three-dimensional CT reconstructions. The distance between the posterior superior iliac crest and the anterior inferior iliac spine is approximately 140 mm in males and 130 mm in females and allows an 8-mm screw in males and a 6- to 7-mm screw in females. The cortical thickness averages about 5 mm in males and 4.7 mm in females. Other paths do not provide as optimal a trajectory. These screws can be placed using a fluoroscopic lateral and obturator oblique-outlet view.

SACRAL INJURY PATTERNS
Facet Fractures and Dislocations

Facet injuries to the lumbar spine occur infrequently. Levine and colleagues noted that bilateral facet dislocations below L1-L2 represent only 10 percent of the total cases,[50] and those at the lumbosacral junction are even less common. The important feature of this type of flexion-distraction injury is that it is mainly a soft tissue injury that results in complete disruption of the posterior ligamentous complex, as well as the intravertebral disk. The bony architecture of the facets may remain intact in many cases, but they are totally juxtaposed and dislocated. The minor compression of the anterior portion of the inferior body is merely a result of the severe ligamentous injury and does not contribute to the overall instability of the injury. The posterior walls of the vertebral bodies remain intact, and canal compromise results from translation of one intact vertebral ring in relation to the adjacent ring. This injury must be differentiated from a facet fracture, which is a different injury mechanically and consists of comminution of the facets and sometimes also the laminae, pars interarticularis, and vertebral body.

The severe translation observed with facet dislocations may lead to partial or complete cauda equina syndrome. This severe translation is a result of posterior ligamentous disruption combined with severe disk disruption. Denis[20] suggested that complete posterior disruption is insufficient to account for the degree of flexion instability seen in this injury. Only incompetence of the posterior longitudinal ligament, annulus fibrosus, and disk could produce such a degree of translational instability. The anterior longitudinal ligament is often stripped from the anterior portion of the inferior body but remains intact. A number of authors[41,52,54,96] suggest that this might be a flexion-distraction injury with the axis of rotation posterior to the anterior longitudinal ligament.

Radiographs of facet fractures and dislocations at the lumbosacral junction are usually diagnostic. They demonstrate an intact posterior wall at L5 with significant translation, lesser degrees of anterior compression, and loss of disk height (Fig. 35-1). Anteroposterior (AP) radiographs of the lumbar spine often reveal dislocation of the facets. CT confirms the pathology and demonstrates an empty facet sign,[63] as well as the severity of canal compromise on sagittal reconstructions.[32]

Although unilateral facet dislocations and fracture-dislocations are rare in the thoracic or lumbar spine, unilateral facet injuries have been reported to occur to a disproportionate degree at the lumbosacral junction.[14,16,18,22,40,47,59,80,101] For unilateral facet dislocations to occur, a combination of flexion-rotation and distraction is required. Facet fracture-dislocations can occur when the extent of distraction is not sufficient to allow the inferior facet to clear the superior facet. An element of shear is present in both unilateral and bilateral facet fracture-dislocations. It is of note that in the more recent literature, a number of case reports have documented the combination of a unilateral lumbosacral facet dislocation and an associated sacral fracture.[16,23,38,93] Recognition of these unusual high-energy injuries is predominantly due to improved imaging of the sacrum. The combination of a facet dislocation and a sacral fracture,

FIGURE 35-1   *Unilateral facet dislocations in the lumbar spine are exceedingly rare and have a rotational abnormality that is often diagnostic.* **A,** *On a lateral radiograph, rotational malalignment is indicated by the step-off between the posterior walls of L5 and S1 (dotted lines).* **B,** *Anteroposterior radiograph demonstrating asymmetry of the disk space, as well as a suggestion of widening of the facet at L5 and S1 (arrow).* **C,** *Computed tomography demonstrating a dislocated facet with the inferior articular process of L5 lying anterior to the superior articular process of S1 (arrow). (From Kramer, K.M.; Levine, A.M. Unilateral facet dislocation of the lumbosacral junction. A case report and review of the literature. J Bone Joint Surg [Am] 71:1258–1261, 1989.)*

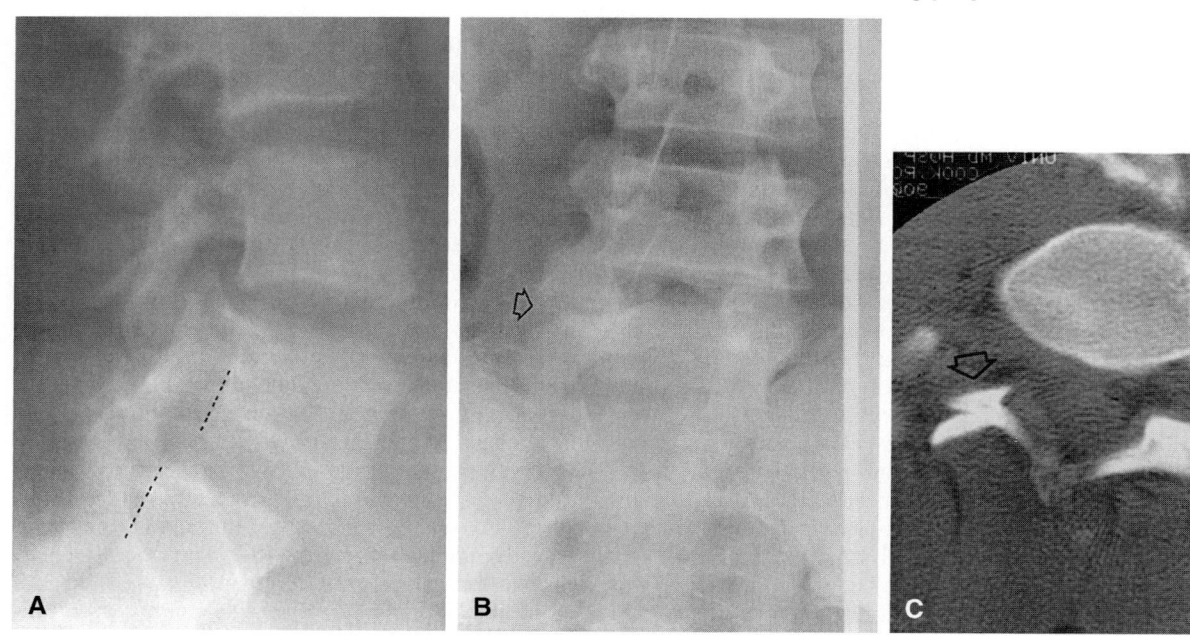

especially if comminuted, can complicate fixation at the lumbosacral junction. The implications for postreduction stability are significantly different for a true facet dislocation (intact facets) and a fracture-dislocation. Unilateral dislocations or fracture-dislocations differ from bilateral dislocations in that on the AP view, a significant rotatory component can be seen in the former. In addition, in unilateral dislocations and fracture-dislocations, avulsion of the transverse processes may be seen. Lumbosacral facet insufficiency can occur in combination with vertical fractures of the sacrum as the fracture extends into the base of the superior articular process of the sacrum, thus effectively creating a total incompetent lumbosacral junction. When it occurs bilaterally in association with severe comminution of the upper sacrum, lumbopelvic stabilization may be necessary to restore stability between the spine and pelvis.[6,60,82,92]

Sacral Fractures

Until recently, fractures of the sacrum were combined with fractures of the pelvis,[31] although they were first mentioned by Malgaine in 1847. Bonnin[8] was one of the first to attempt to characterize these injuries. He identified six different types of sacral fracture from a review of 44 pelvic injuries, 45 percent of which were also associated with sacral fractures. He also provided a discussion of the mechanisms of injury, as well as the occurrence of neurologic deficit. Although a number of reports have been published,[11,13,25,26,30,55,71,97] less than 5 percent of all sacral fractures occur as isolated injuries. As mentioned previously, in addition to the association with pelvic fractures, the combination of lumbosacral dislocation with facet

injury and sacral fracture is a relatively common pattern.[16,38,93] Similarly, a more recent study[93] identified 17 patients with concomitant noncontiguous thoracolumbar and sacral fractures. The implications are significant in that five of the sacral fractures were missed initially, thus resulting in the possibility of continued or additional injury to the distal roots. Two reports[21,85] attempted to classify sacral fractures by manageable criteria so that they could be correlated with the fracture pattern, neurologic deficit, and treatment options. Sacral fractures can be caused by direct trauma to the sacrum, but most result from indirect forces acting on the pelvis or lumbar spine.

Sacral fractures are usually classified according to the direction of the fracture line; thus, fractures can be vertical, transverse, or oblique (Fig. 35-2). Most sacral injuries, however, are vertical. After reviewing the literature and their own series, these fractures were classified in a useful fashion by Schmidek and colleagues[85] into indirect and direct patterns. Indirect patterns of vertical fractures include (1) lateral mass fracture, (2) juxta-articular fracture, (3) cleaving fracture, and (4) avulsion fracture (Fig. 35-3). In addition, they included high transverse as the final type of indirect mechanism and considered gunshot wounds and low transverse fractures to be direct mechanisms of injury. Sabiston and Wing suggested a simpler three-part classification[78] (Fig. 35-4).

Denis and colleagues[21] classified 236 sacral fractures into zones based on both clinical and 35 anatomic cadaveric studies of the sacrum. The three zones that they thought had clinical significance were zone 1, which was the sacral ala up to the lateral border of the neural foramen;

FIGURE 35-2 *Fractures of the sacrum can be classified in a number of different ways. One of the most common is that of the direction of the fracture line within the sacrum. Therefore, fractures can be vertical **(A)**, oblique **(B)**, or transverse **(C)**. These fractures can occur at any level in the sacrum. Vertical fractures may occur in the alae or through the foramina. Similarly, oblique fractures may occur at any location. Transverse fractures are less common and are found more frequently at the apex of the sacral kyphosis between S2 and S3, but they may also occur as a high transverse fracture at S1 or S2.*

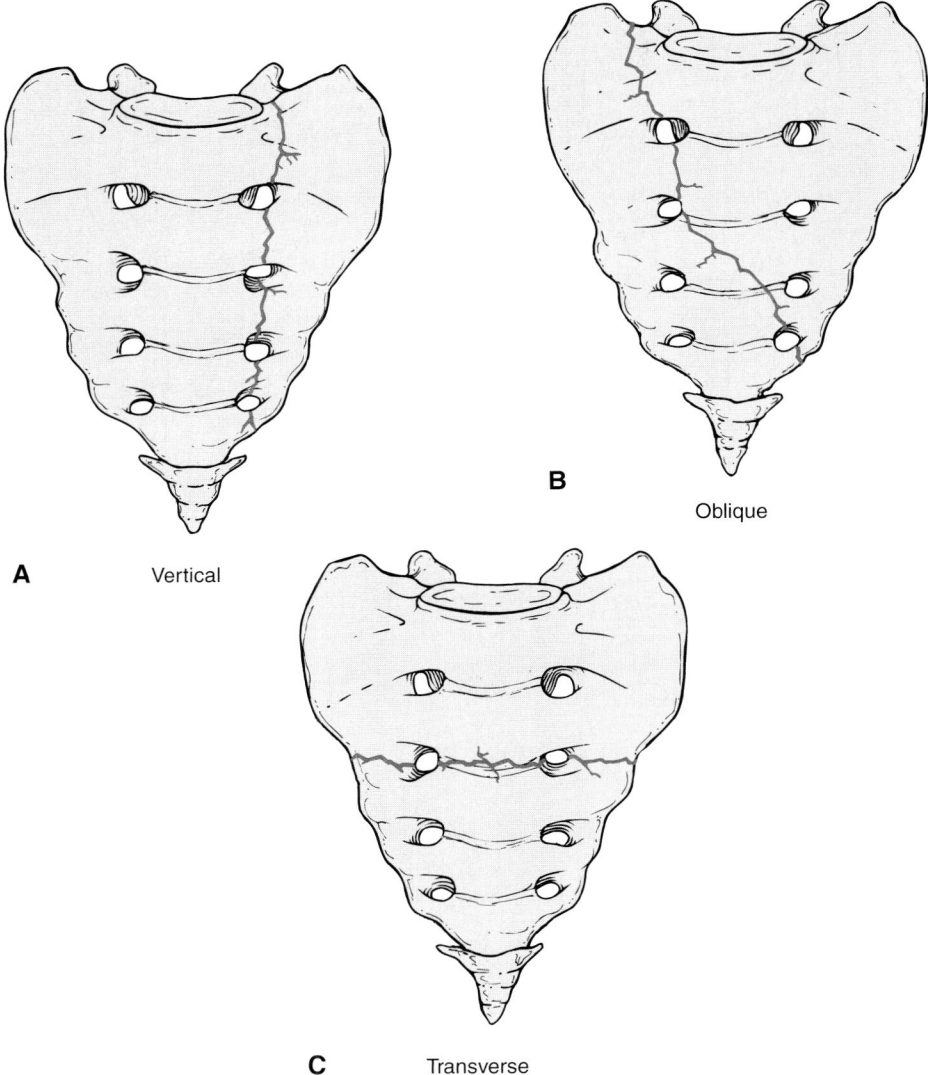

A   Vertical

B

Oblique

C   Transverse

zone 2, which was the neural foramen; and zone 3, which included the central portion of the sacrum and the canal (Fig. 35-5). In this series, 118 patients had fractures in zone 1, 5.9 percent of whom had neurologic deficits. These injuries were frequently fractures caused by lateral compression of the pelvis, vertical shear fractures, or sacrotuberous avulsions.[21] The next group was zone 2, or foraminal fractures. These fractures involved one or more foramina, and the fracture line exited through the sacral canal without involvement of the central neural canal. This type of fracture was found in 81 of 236 patients, and 28.4 percent of these patients had some neurologic findings. Zone 2 injuries often resulted from vertical shear fractures. The final group of patients had zone 3, or central sacral canal, involvement. These injuries were seen less frequently, in only

21 of 236 patients, but had a high rate of neurologic deficit (56.7%). This group included some patients who had a transverse component of the fracture.

Oblique fractures most often combine some element of a transverse fracture with that of a vertical fracture. In addition, an oblique fracture is the type that may involve both the sacrum and the lumbosacral junction. Thus, an oblique component ends proximally in a fracture at the base of the S1 facet or goes directly through the facet joint. As a result, the level and complexity of the instability are increased. Isler[42] proposed a classification of injuries that extend into the lumbosacral junction (Fig. 35-6). Type A are lateral to the L5-S1 facet and do not alter lumbosacral stability. Type B destroys the articulation, and type C extends into the canal, and both of these types are unstable and highly complex.

FIGURE 35-3 *Schmidek and colleagues classified vertical fractures into four fracture patterns, including lateral mass fractures **(A)**, juxta-articular fractures **(B)**, cleaving fractures **(C)**, and avulsion fractures **(D)**. (Redrawn from Schmidek, H.H.; Smith, D.A.; Kristiansen, T.K. Sacral fractures. Neurosurgery 15:735–746, 1984.)*

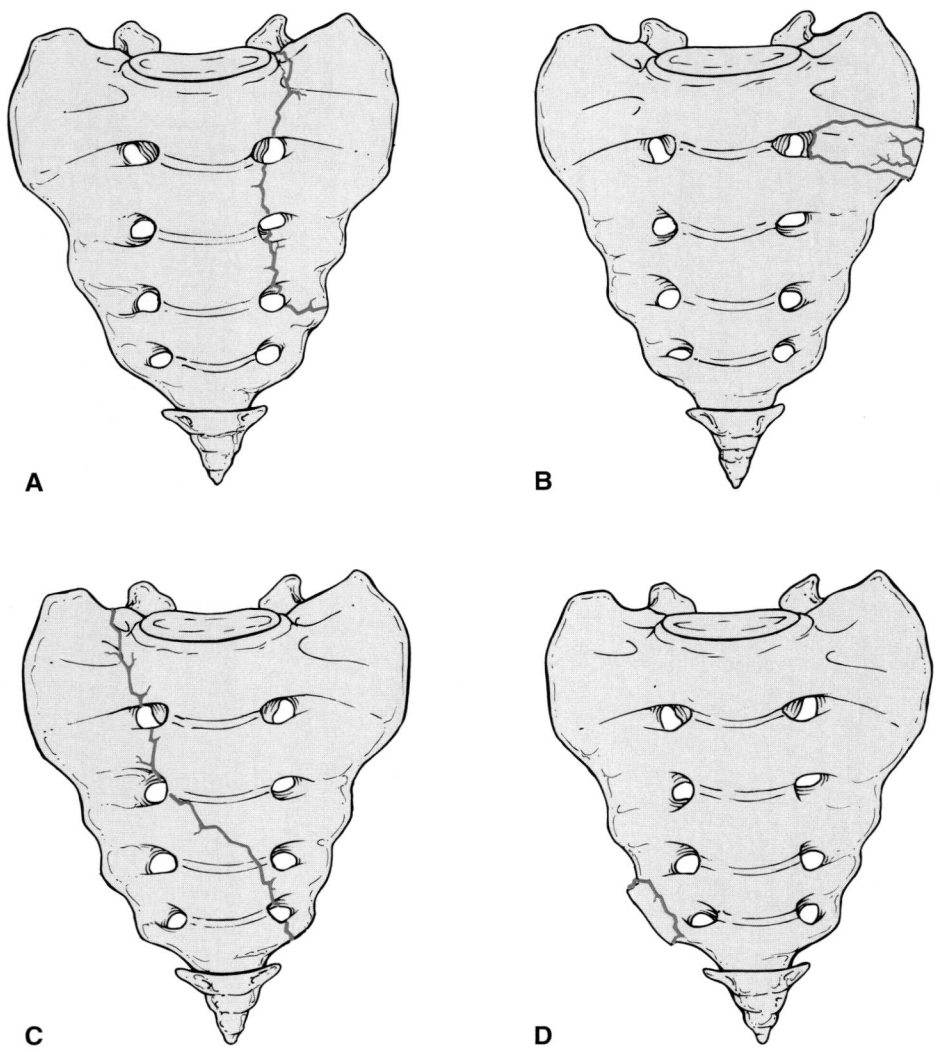

A

B

C

D

Transverse fractures of the sacrum occur less frequently than vertical fractures[8,28,76] and account for approximately 4.5 to 10 percent of each series. They most commonly result from high-energy injuries, such as falling from a height onto the lower extremities. As characterized by Roy-Camille and co-workers[76] from their own series of 13 patients and extensive cadaveric studies, these fractures are generally high transverse fractures (S1 or S2) with anterior bending (kyphosis) between the superior and the inferior fragments and verticalization of the distal fragment. They are frequently associated with bilateral alar fractures and fractures of the L5 transverse process. Displacement and tilting of the fragments can be related to the relative flexion or extension of the hips at the moment of impact. Direct blows to the sacrum can result in low transverse fractures (S3 or S4) by levering on the distal segments below the point of fixation by the sacroiliac joints. Three distinct types of fractures were identified. Type I was a flexion injury without significant deformity, type II was a flexion injury with

posterior displacement of the cephalad fragment, and type III was caused by extension with anterior displacement of the cephalad fragment. Depending on displacement, these transverse fractures can be associated with rectal perforation or cerebrospinal fluid leakage. They are frequently associated with neurologic deficits, including bowel and bladder dysfunction and perineal numbness. No motor weakness is usually detected. These fractures are, therefore, the most easily missed and have the gravest implications for significant neurologic deficit. Generally found in the S2-S3 region, they may be responsible for complete loss of bowel and bladder function. The diagnosis is usually very difficult to make based only on plain radiographs and may also be missed on CT because the fracture is parallel to the axial cuts and thus may not be well visualized even with two-dimensional reconstruction. Interestingly, the most predictable method of visualization for this particular type of sacral fracture seems to be magnetic resonance imaging (MRI) (Fig. 35-7).

FIGURE 35-4 *Sabiston and Wing's classification of sacral fractures had three main types. Type A included vertical fractures, type B consisted of transverse fractures below the level of the sacroiliac joint, and type C fractures were transverse at the level of the sacroiliac joint with vertical components. (Redrawn from Sabiston, C.P.; Wing, P.C. Sacral fractures: Classification and neurologic implications. J Trauma 26:1113–1115, 1986.)*

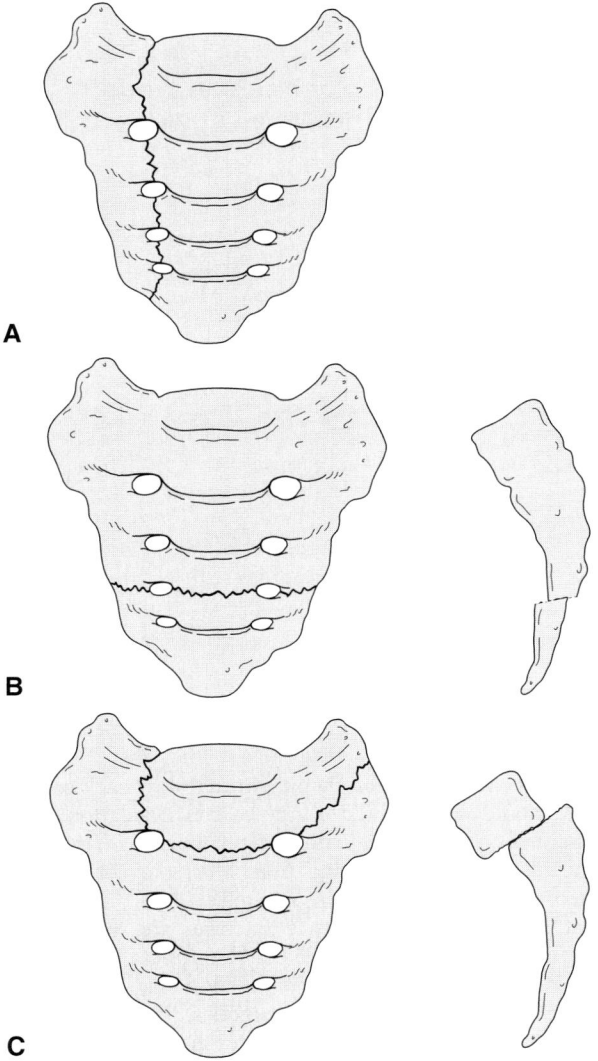

A

B

C

Most recently an attempt has been made to standardize the various measurements so as to characterize sacral fractures.[48] Kuklo and associates reviewed 67 papers in the English literature that dealt with measurements related to sacral fractures. They concluded that the critical measurements were (1) AP displacement, (2) vertical translation, (3) AP translation, (4) sagittal angulation, (5) sacral kyphosis, (6) horizontal displacement, and (7) anal occlusion. Optimal radiographic studies and measurement methods were suggested. These methods have not been validated for reproducibility nor have they been shown to

be in anyway prognostic or helpful in selecting appropriate therapy for an individual patient. However, the study does point out the huge variability in reporting and the effort needed to standardize diagnostic methods.

Recognition plus description of the patterns observed in sacral insufficiency fractures is a relatively recent occurrence that is in large part due to the use of MRI. Because the fractures are visualized infrequently on plain radiographs, the observer must often depend on areas of edema and compaction observed on MRI to find all the fracture lines. MRI allows a number of different patterns to be seen, including a single vertical line parallel to the sacroiliac joint,[15,35] but the most commonly described pattern is the "H" or "Honda" sign.[9,66] Peh and coauthors[66]

FIGURE 35-5 *Denis and associates classified 236 fractures of the sacrum into zones. Zone 1 was the region of the ala, and fractures in this area occurred in 118 patients, 5.9% of whom had neurologic deficits. Zone 2 was the foraminal region, where the fracture line involved one or more foramina and exited without involvement of the central neural canal. This group comprised 81 patients, 28.4% of whom had neurologic findings. The final group of patients had zone 3 injuries, or central canal involvement. This pattern was seen in only 21 patients, but they had an extremely high rate of neurologic deficit (56.7%). (Redrawn from Denis, F.; Davis, S.; Comfort, T. Sacral fractures: An important problem. Retrospective analysis of 236 cases. Clin Orthop Relat Res 227:67–81, 1988.)*

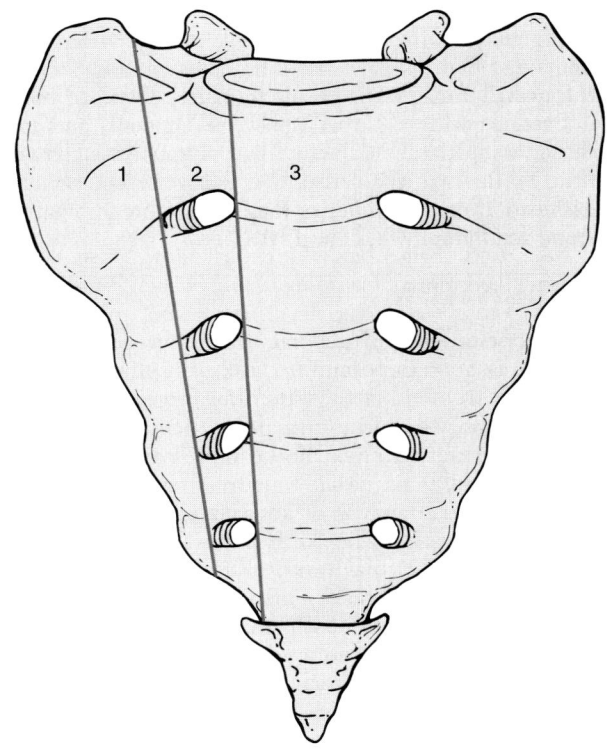

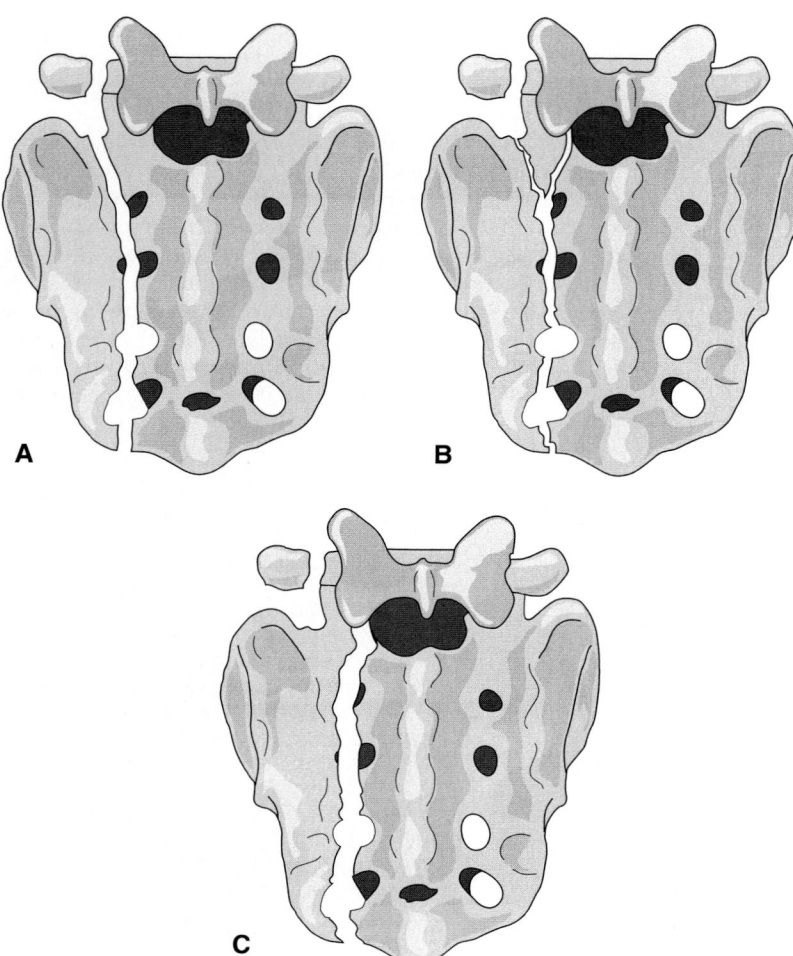

FIGURE 35-6 *Classification of injuries involving the lumbosacral junction as proposed by Isler.[42] **A,** The fracture line goes lateral to the L5-S1 facet and does not destabilize it. The L5-S1 facet is destabilized when the fracture line either goes on both sides **(B)** or just medial to it **(C).***

A

B

C

described a series of 21 patients with insufficiency fractures of the sacrum, 9 of whom had the "H" configuration. Four patients had high bilateral sacral fractures without the bar, and four had unilateral sacral ala fractures. Two had bilateral fractures with a partial transverse element, and one each had a unilateral ala fracture with a transverse component. The final patient had only a transverse component. Classification of these injuries may require a combination of bone scintigraphy, CT, and MRI.

EVALUATION

After resuscitation and general evaluation of a trauma victim, it is very important to ascertain the details of the accident from either the patient or the rescue personnel. High-energy decelerating injuries such as falls from a height or ejection from a motor vehicle or motorcycle have the potential for either a pelvic ring fracture combined with a sacral injury or an isolated sacral fracture. Physical examination should include palpation of the entire spinal column, pelvis, and sacrum, as well as visual inspection for ecchymosis or bruising. As part of the routine physical examination, the perineum and especially the anus should be assessed for normal sensation and tone. In patients with significant trauma to the urethra or the rectum, rectal perforation may be present. Rectal perforation may also occur in association with a transverse

fracture of the sacrum without any other injury to the pelvis, depending on the direction of displacement of the sacral fracture.

Assessment of an elderly patient with low back or sacral pain should also include a very careful evaluation of the sacral region. A clinical history of previous irradiation, significant osteopenia resulting from a drug effect, or senile osteoporosis should also be elicited.[19,36,58,94] Neurologic complications of insufficiency fractures are rare,[43] but a careful history of bowel and bladder function should be obtained. Such a history may be confusing, especially if the patient has been taking narcotics for the pain and now has constipation secondary to the pain medication obscuring changes in bowel function. In view of the low yield of plain radiographs in these patients, a technetium-labeled bone scan should be performed early in the course of reviewing the patient's symptoms.

Neurologic Deficit

Sacral injuries may be associated with neurologic deficit, depending on the type of injury and the direction of the fracture line. Patients with vertical fractures involving the sacral roots on just one side can have normal bowel and bladder function and only subtle sensory deficits, unless the S1 root is involved. Transverse fractures of the sacrum with translation, however, are accompanied by neurologic

FIGURE 35-7 *This young man had a tree fall directly on his sacrum, causing the fracture at the level of S3-S4 as noted in the lateral radiograph (A) and sagittal computed tomographic reconstruction (B). The sacral fracture did not heal and caused severe pain. It is of note that his follow-up postinjury MRI (C) showed a meningocele dissecting subcutaneously (arrows). Although he had bowel and bladder sensation and function it was not completely normal and his preoperative sphincter electromyogram suggested dysfunction consistent with distal root transection. Intraoperatively he had a meningocele (D) but no further active dural leak. The S3 roots were intact but distal to that were completely transected. The distal portion of the sacrum was completely resected as the fragment was too small to fix. He achieved complete pain relief and was able to go back to work with retention of relatively normal bowel and bladder function.*

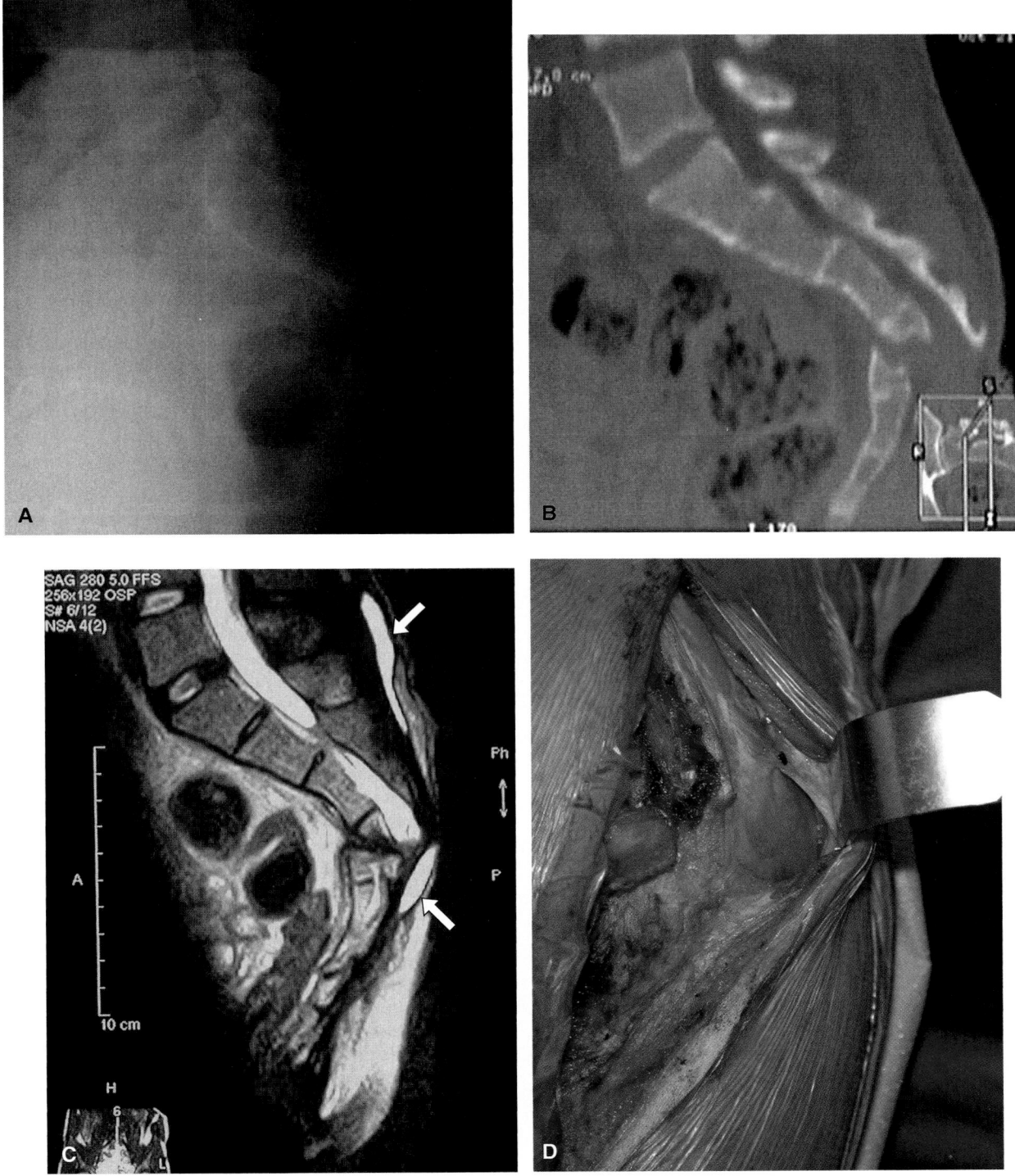

deficit in almost all patients. In fact it has been shown that up to 35 percent of all patients with transverse fracture have root transections, and many have several dural lacerations. Depending on the series 15 to 40 percent of all patients with high-energy sacral fracture will have significant neurologic deficit.[99] Zone 1 vertical alar fractures are associated with neurologic deficit in 5.9 percent of patients, and the deficit usually involves only the sciatic nerve or the L5 root and is generally minor. Zone 2 sacral fractures are associated with neurologic deficit in approximately 28.4 percent of patients, a small proportion of whom have bowel and bladder involvement. The remainder have sciatica associated with L5, S1, or S2. The L5 root can be associated with a displaced vertical shear fracture and fracture of the transverse process of L5, a combination that has been termed the *traumatic far-out syndrome*.[21] This injury is most frequently associated with footdrop. Zone 3 fractures involve the central sacral canal and are associated with neurologic deficit in at least 50 percent of patients. Most of these patients have bowel, bladder, and sexual dysfunction. The remainder of patients with injury at this level have L5 or S1 findings. With neurologic injury from S2 to S5, impairment of bowel and bladder function can occur, but patients might not have functional incontinence with preservation of at least one of the two S2 and S3 roots. Bilateral root disruption invariably leads to severe deficits.

Cystometry performed in conjunction with sphincter electromyography can be useful in correlating findings from clinical examination. With all sacral fractures, however, a complete investigation should be carried out because it is often difficult to ascertain whether the root involvement is a result of the pelvic fracture or the associated sacral fracture.

Neurologic complications of insufficiency fractures are exceedingly rare. In the few reported cases, the onset of neurologic deficit was delayed in relation to the onset of fracture symptoms.[43,64] Urinary retention, as well as numbing and tingling of the feet, has been reported. The mechanism of onset of neurologic symptoms associated with this entity is unclear in that the onset is not always associated with displacement. Surgery is not generally required because resolution of the neurologic symptoms seems to occur spontaneously with resolution of the back symptoms. However, MRI is recommended for patients who do have a deficit; surgery for decompression is reserved for those with severe compression and displacement; and nonoperative treatment is given to the majority.[43]

Radiologic Evaluation

Radiographic diagnosis of sacral injuries is usually quite difficult. Every patient who sustains high-energy trauma should have an AP radiograph of the pelvis in accordance with the advanced trauma life support (ATLS) guidelines. Plain AP and even lateral radiographs of either the pelvis or sacrum are often not helpful in visualizing fractures of the sacrum. Detail is often overlaid by soft tissue shadows and bowel gas, and in addition, the lumbar lordosis and kyphotic sagittal contour of the sacrum make the fracture lines oblique to the plane of the radiograph (Fig. 35-8). The Ferguson view is the best view of the upper portion of the sacrum and can

demonstrate foraminal involvement. Lateral radiographs can help diagnose transverse fractures of the sacrum. Denis and co-workers reported that up to 50 percent of patients in their series who were neurologically intact had a delay in diagnosis of the sacral fracture. Such delay still occasionally occurs even in patients with neurologic deficit. Plain radiographs show only 30 percent of sacral fractures in most series. L5 transverse process fractures can be seen in up to one half of all patients with pelvic and sacral fractures. Even with careful retrospective study, only another 35 percent of these injuries can be detected. A sacral fracture should be suspected in every patient with a pelvic fracture and neurologic deficit. Thus, clinical suspicion coupled with the mechanism of injury should trigger the use of ancillary studies for both acute traumatic injury and insufficiency fractures. In all patients in whom a sacral fracture is suspected, however, a lateral view of the sacrum as well as an inlet view (35 to 40° of caudal tilt of the radiographic tube) and an outlet view (45° of cranial tilt of the tube) should be obtained. Thin-cut CT with coronal and sagittal reconstructions has become the standard for evaluation of both pelvic and sacral fractures[21,44,48,94] (Fig. 35-9). It provides better visualization of especially difficult fractures lateral to the sacral ala.[57] Transverse sacral fractures are difficult to delineate because they are parallel to the coronal plane of the primary CT scan and require sagittal and coronal reconstructions for demonstration. The role of the various measurements that can be made directly from the CT scan is unclear, but standardization should be a goal in describing these fractures.[48] In addition, MRI can be helpful in delineating both the areas of neural compression in the sacrum and displacement of the fracture fragments. Whereas myelography was used previously to evaluate patients with neurologic deficit, MRI is now the study of choice for acute sacral injuries with deficit. MRI not only assesses the area of compression but also gives clear images of the displacement because the information is gathered primarily in both the axial and sagittal planes without reformatting (see Fig. 35-8).

Evaluation of an elderly patient with a suspected insufficiency fracture of the sacrum is more complicated. In this instance, the use of plain radiographs is generally unrewarding but such radiographs should not be overlooked because they are helpful in ruling out other lumbosacral pathology. A technetium-99 bone scan is the initial study and can be of help in these patients (Fig. 35-10). It will generally show activity in one of the patterns previously described, soon after the onset of symptoms.[34,36,58,66] Standard imaging for a bone scan is an anterior and posterior projection, with the posterior view being more effective in demonstrating activity in these fractures. However, activity in the sacrum can sometimes be obscured by residual activity in the bladder, so an outlet view can be helpful in those circumstances. Although a bone scan is highly sensitive, it is not specific, and accurate confirmation of the fracture along with delineation of the pattern is more optimally achieved with CT. Proper alignment of the gantry and thin cuts (2 mm) allowing for reconstruction are critical to obtaining the maximal amount of data from the study. Routine CT of the pelvis does not permit diagnostic resolution of this problem. Vertical fractures are viewed as a combination of the fracture line and sclerosis. The transverse component, when it exists, is best seen on a reconstruction. Additionally, other helpful changes are evident on CT besides the fracture lines and sclerosis in older

FIGURE 35-8 *A 19-year-old woman was involved in a motor vehicle accident and sustained a transverse sacral fracture. The fracture was not visualized well on either the initial lateral (**A**) or the initial anteroposterior (AP) (**B**) radiograph and was thus not recognized at first. The lateral plain film shows only a slight break in the round sagittal contour (arrow). On the AP view only the vertical component of the fracture is visible. Although the patient had loss of both bowel and bladder function, this also was not initially appreciated. When the neural deficit was recognized, a computed tomographic scan was obtained. **C,** The axial view shows only the vertical component of the fracture, not the transverse. **D,** Midsagittal reconstruction does not demonstrate clearly the configuration of the fracture.*

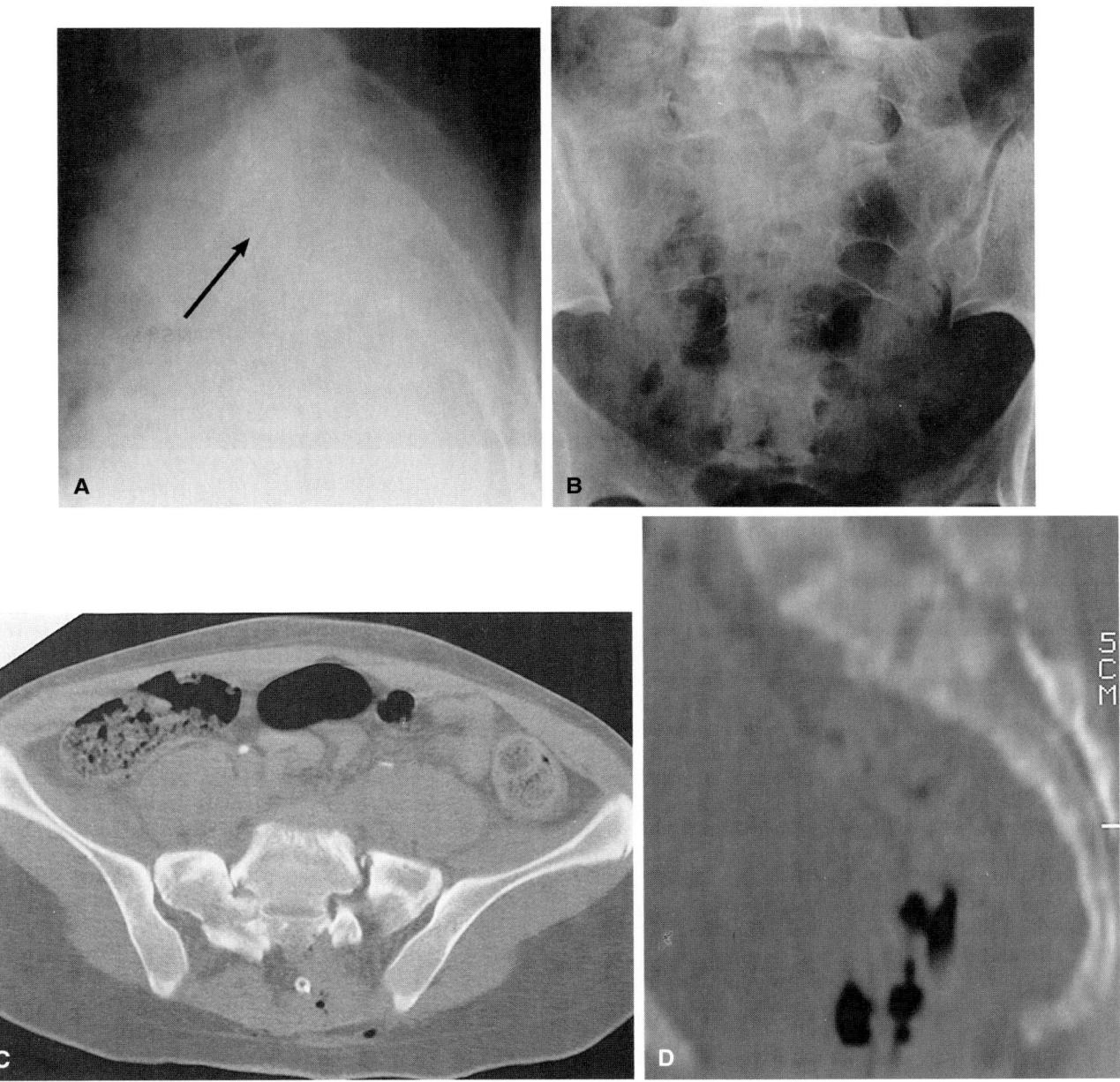

(Continued)

fractures. A vacuum phenomenon can sometimes be appreciated both within the sacroiliac joint and within the fracture site (intraosseous).[67,87] MRI can be used either as a screening tool in a symptomatic patient or to define the fracture. It is often helpful in a patient with previous irradiation to help rule out recurrence. MRI can both visualize and define the fracture with a single study. The fracture lines are defined as bands of decreased signal intensity on T1-weighted images, whereas on T2-weighted and short tau inversion recovery (STIR) images, the lines can be seen as areas of edema around the ala or body of the sacrum. Some authors believe that MRI is sensitive but nonspecific and suggest confirmation with CT, but recently it has been shown that the finding of fluid within the fracture seems to be helpful in confirming the diagnosis.[64]

FIGURE 35-8 *(Continued)* **E,** *The magnetic resonance image, however, showed an angulated fracture in the S2 region. The fracture was in kyphosis with the superior fragment displaced posterior to the inferior fragment. The patient underwent operative reduction and decompression with plate fixation as shown on lateral **(F)** and AP **(G)** views. The double-screw fixation in S1 stabilized the proximal fragment, with the cephalad screw directed medially and the next screw directed laterally. The patient regained bowel and partial bladder function and return of perineal sensation.*

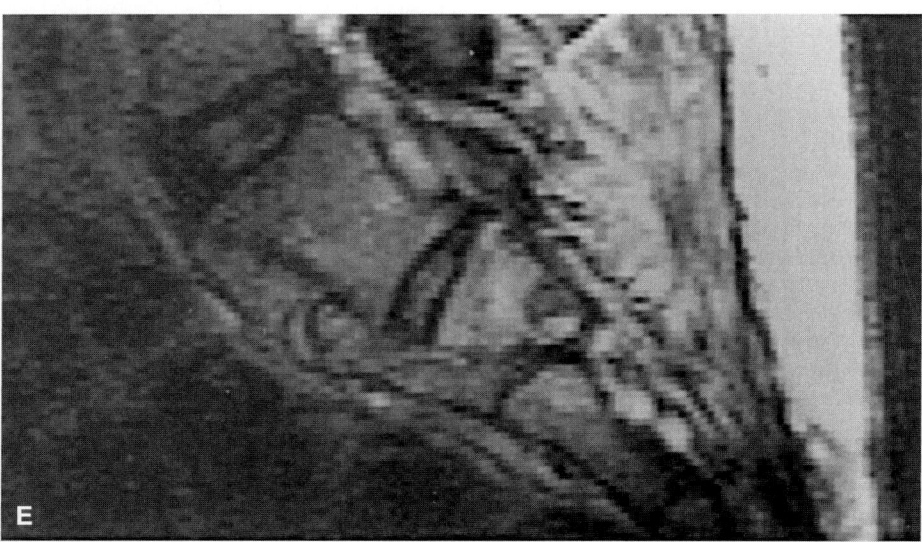

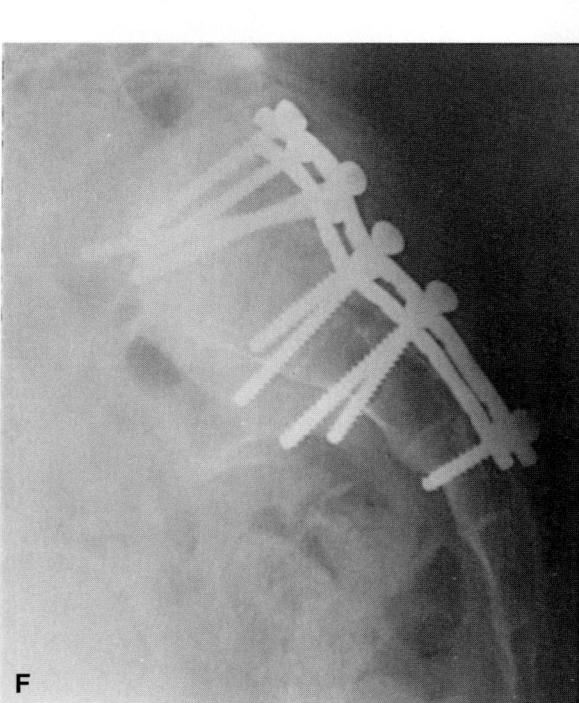

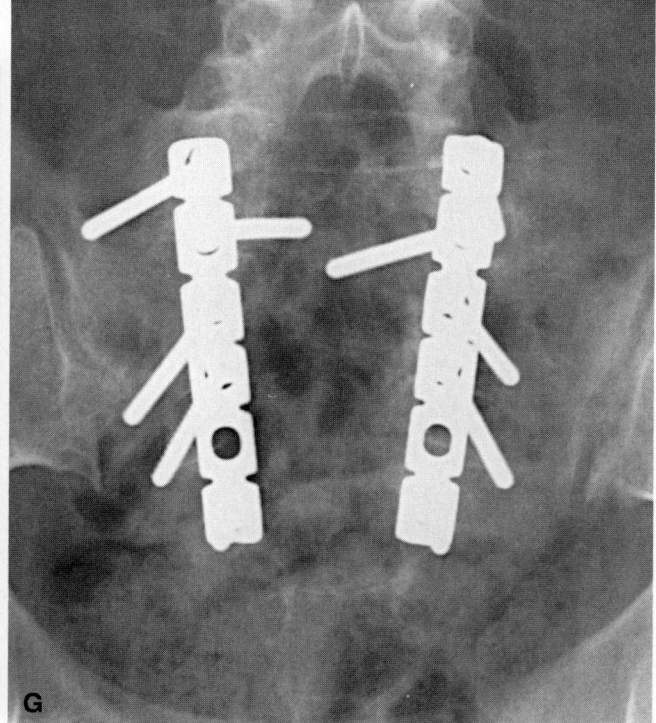

MANAGEMENT

Indications

Various systems have been devised in an attempt to classify spinal injuries according to both mechanism and degree of instability. In addition, a number of definitions have been proposed—for example, stable versus unstable. A generic definition of spinal stability includes fracture patterns that are not likely to change position with physiologic loads and will therefore not cause additional neurologic deficit or increasing deformity. Although many systems that are applicable to lumbar spine injuries have been proposed, no pragmatic system has been devised that clearly groups the injuries so that treatment approaches can be differentiated.

FIGURE 35-9 *A 24-year-old woman sustained pelvic trauma in a motor vehicle accident. **A,** An anteroposterior radiograph of her pelvis demonstrates a fracture of her right pubis and ischium with an indistinct fracture through the sacrum. **B,** Computed tomography clearly shows the fracture line (arrows) traversing the neural foramina; thus, it is classified as a zone 2 fracture. This patient had radicular deficits in the S2 and S3 distributions.*

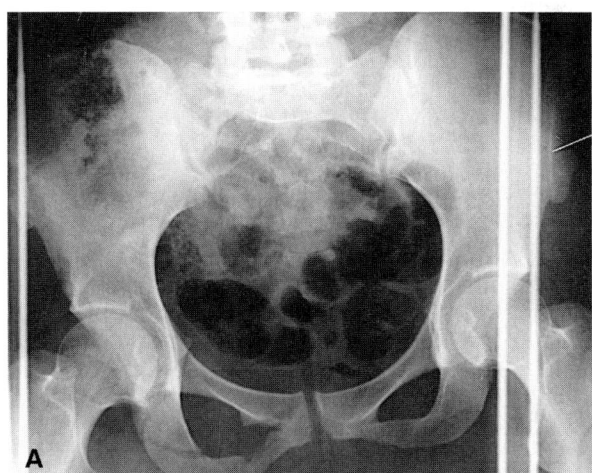
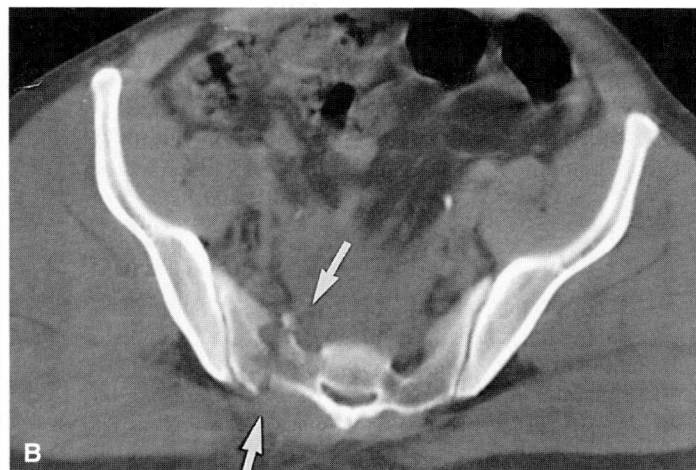

In general terms, surgical indications for sacral injuries are the following: (1) the presence of detectable motion at the fracture site that cannot be controlled by nonoperative methods (instability), (2) neurologic deficit, or (3) severe disruption of axial or sagittal spinal alignment. With a large canal-to-neural-element ratio, significant translation or angulation must take place to cause a neural injury.

Because vertical sacral fractures usually occur in combination with other pelvic ring fractures, some options for treatment of instability are discussed later with the remainder of pelvic fractures. The occurrence of lumbosacral dissociation, however, especially in the presence of Isler B and C fractures,[42] can require stabilization of this gross instability pattern either alone or in combination with anterior pelvic fixation.[6,39,60,82,83] This also can restore the patient to early weight-bearing by rigid fixation of the spine to the pelvis, which in the polytrauma victim can be more beneficial than prolonged bed rest. The rate of complications needs to be balanced again the overall patient benefit.[6] Transverse fractures of the sacrum are generally of two types. A greenstick type, which increases sacral kyphosis without translational deformity, is generally stable (Fig. 35-11). Proximal transverse fractures of the sacrum with neurologic deficit are often accompanied by gross translational instability for which no nonoperative solution is available. Additionally if distal fractures go on to nonunion, the degree of pain and stability can be significant (see Fig. 35-7). Although direct fixation is rarely possible at the level of L3 and distally, excision of the distal portion of the sacrum can give marked pain relief.

The second criterion that constitutes an indication for treatment is neurologic deficit. Considerable controversy has arisen concerning the benefits of operative treatment of spinal injury with respect to neurologic recovery for cord level injuries. No level I evidence suggests that operative management of neurologic deficit related to sacral injuries is more effective than nonoperative management, but several small series have evaluated the benefit of

decompression of the roots on return of function. In the small group of patients with high transverse sacral fractures, kyphosis, and neurologic deficit, reduction of deformity, laminectomy, and decompression of the involved roots are indicated and often provide return of neural function,[28,76] although one very small series (four patients) suggests that an unspecified group can regain some function with nonoperative treatment.[68] Gibbons and colleagues,[33] in a series of 23 patients with neurologic deficits from sacral fractures, showed that 88 percent regained some function with operative treatment, whereas only 20 percent regained any function with nonoperative treatment.

In a nonrandomized comparison of 13 patients those with surgical decompression had statistically improved motor function and overall outcome but similar results in return of bowel and bladder, relief of radicular pain, and return of sensation.[99] A second series of 19 patients with sacral fracture-dislocations and spinopelvic dissociation underwent both decompression and lumbopelvic reconstruction. Of the 15 with complete cauda equina syndrome 7 regained full bowel and bladder function, and this was much more likely to happen if there was no sacral root discontinuity (6/7patients).[82] Other neurologic injuries that accompany fractures of the sacrum are less likely to respond to direct operative intervention. A significant portion of these injuries are root avulsions, and the remainder are neuropraxias, which frequently respond to nonoperative treatment.

The next indication for treatment is severe sagittal- or coronal-plane deformity. Most fractures of the sacrum result in kyphotic deformities and may be accompanied by translational and rotational abnormalities. Because maintenance of normal sagittal alignment is critical for the normal weight-bearing axis of the body and therefore for optimal function of the paraspinous musculature, restoration to normal is a criterion for treatment of many fractures in the spine but to date has not been applied to the sacrum. However, this statement has not been fully

FIGURE 35-10 | *This 87-year-old man was working in his garden and began to have severe low back pain without a history of trauma. **A,** A plain anteroposterior (AP) radiograph of his pelvis was unremarkable, but the intensity of his pain continued to escalate. A bone scan showed increased activity in the S1 joints on the AP view **(B)** and a "Honda" sign on the posteroanterior view **(C)**. Axial computed tomography images **(D, E)** showed the fracture line (**D,** arrow), with coronal reconstruction **(E)** most effectively demonstrating the fracture pattern. Magnetic resonance imaging also helped to define the problem.*

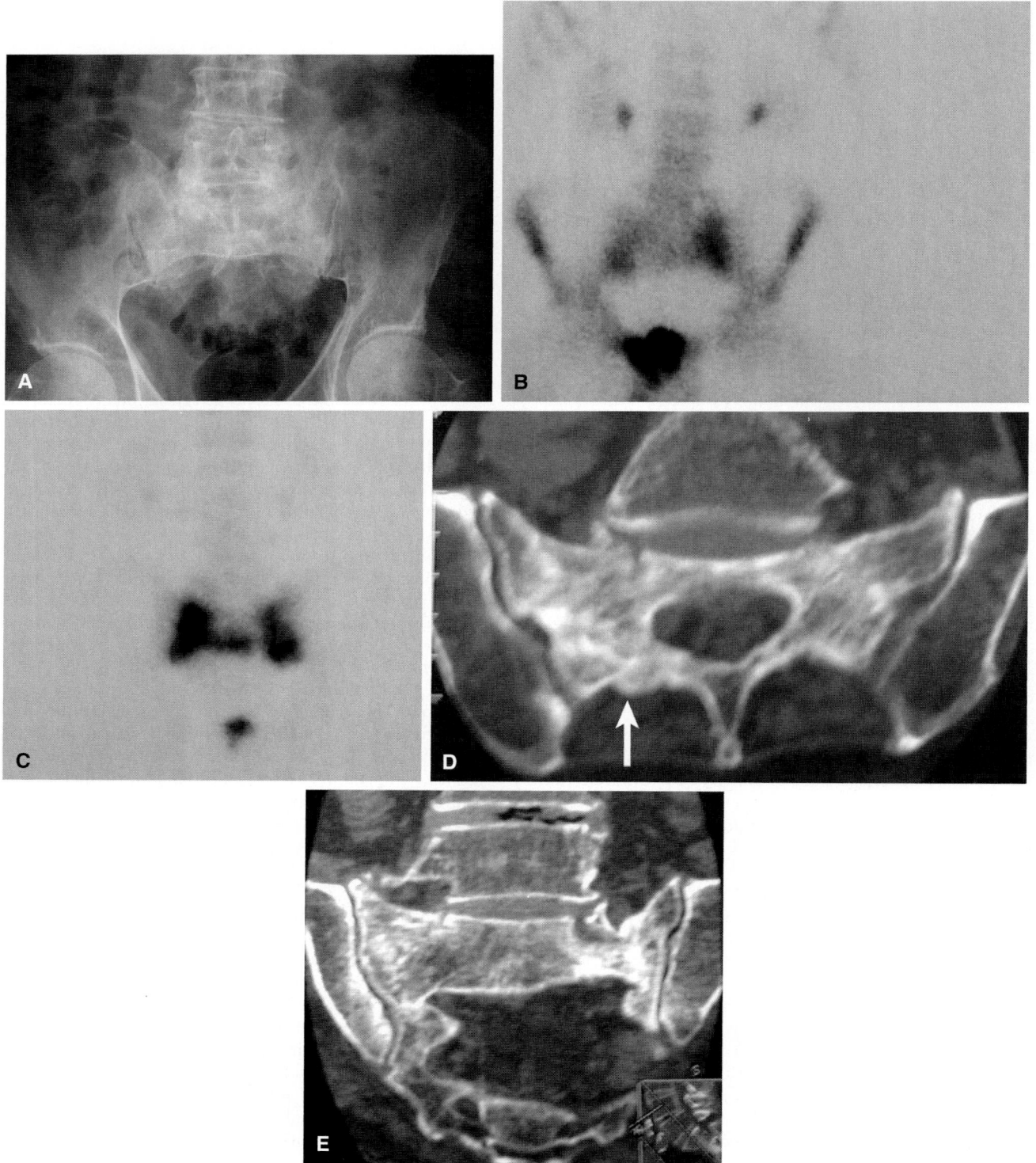

FIGURE 35-11 *This patient fell from a height and landed on his buttocks. **A,** A lateral radiograph shows an increase in kyphosis and comminution of the anterior cortex (arrow). **B,** On an anteroposterior view, the fracture line was seen to occur at the level of the termination of the sacroiliac joint and its attachment to the sacrum (arrows). **C,** A computed tomographic scan shows minimal comminution with fracturing of only the anterior cortex (arrow).*

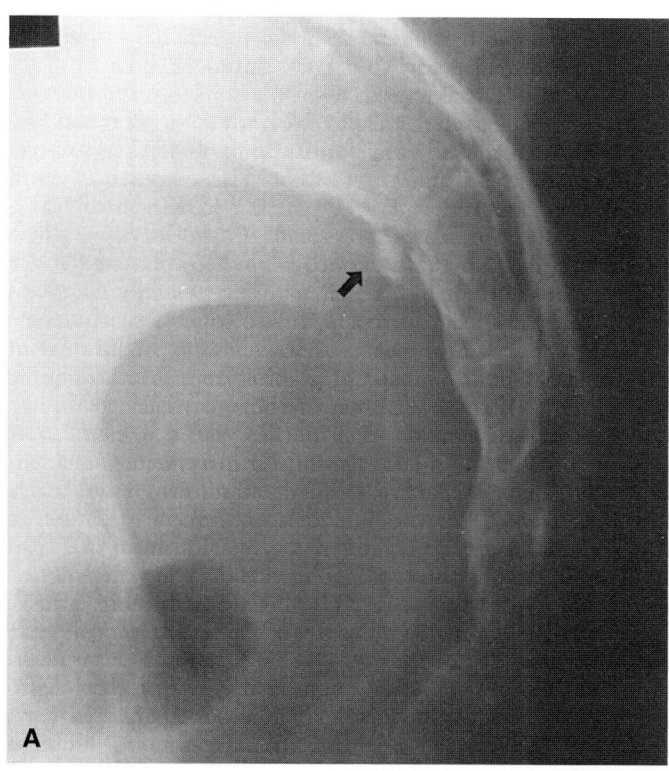

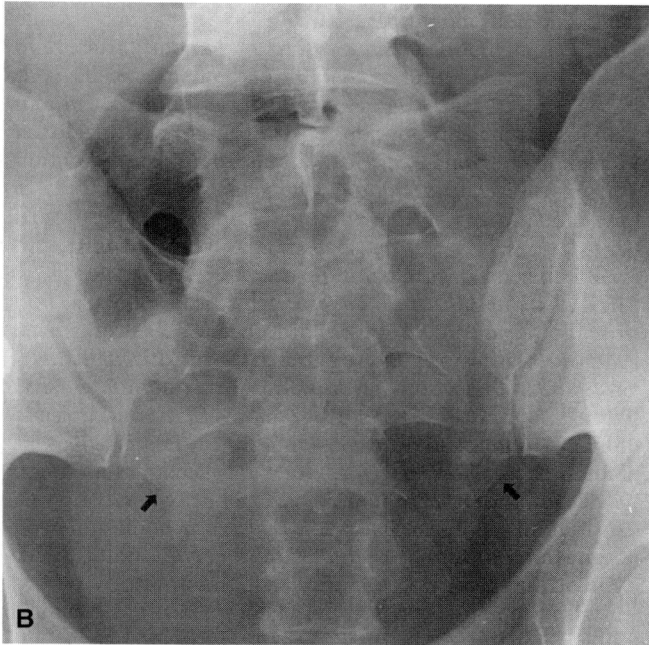

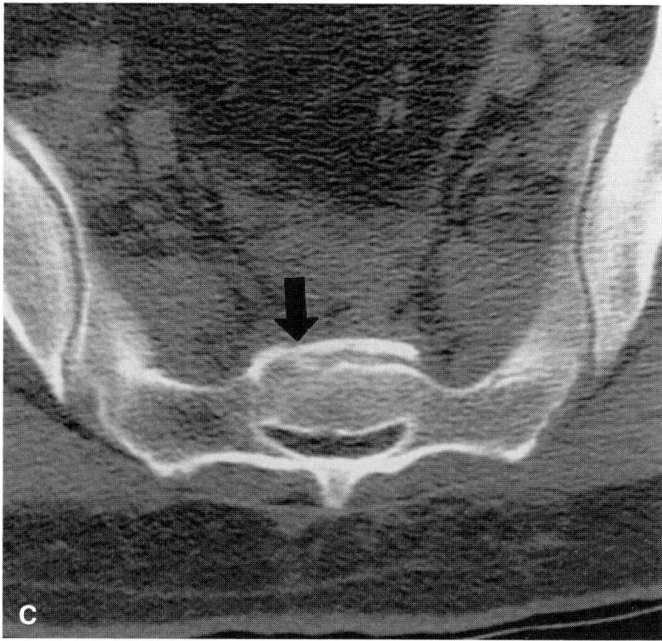

verified because most of these injuries occur in relatively young individuals and the follow-up in most operative and nonoperative series is still relatively short. In the absence of neurologic deficit, clinically stable fractures that do not have significant associated kyphosis can be optimally treated nonoperatively.

Thus, in summary, fractures and dislocations involving the lumbosacral junction that result in neurologic deficit, instability, or deformity need to have operative treatment. This group includes oblique sacral fractures that destroy the stability of the lumbosacral articulation on either side. Reestablishment of pelvic stability when the sacral fracture is combined with a more significant pelvic injury is a critical goal of treatment and can be accomplished either operatively or nonoperatively. Finally, transverse sacral fractures that are either traumatic or insufficiency in type and cause marked root compression and deficit, especially with severe fracture site angulation or translation, also require surgical intervention. The paramount consideration for operative versus nonoperative treatment of traumatic sacral injuries is the presence or absence and the type of neurologic deficit. Patients with vertical fractures and some patients with oblique fractures who have an isolated root deficit are treated on the basis of the instability of the injury and not the deficit. Transverse fractures and some oblique fractures with loss of bowel and bladder function are treated with an attempt to recover these functions. Although nonoperative treatment can be considered in the latter circumstance,[68] other studies have suggested that decompression either indirectly by realignment or directly by removing the compression fragment yields better results.

Treatment Options

A number of treatment measures can be used for the management of sacral fractures and generally involve either nonoperative or operative treatment. Nonoperative treatment generally consists of bed rest or postural reduction (or both) in combination with external orthotic immobilization. Nonoperative treatment has some role in the treatment of low-energy sacral fractures (insufficiency fractures) but little role in high-energy injuries. Although external fixation may have a significant role in the acute and definitive treatment of pelvic fractures, the role in sacral fractures and lumbosacral instability is distinctly limited or almost nonexistent. Appropriate operative intervention can involve various procedures, including (1) resection of the distal sacrum, (2) decompression of the neural elements from a posterior or posterolateral approach, (3) direct reduction and stabilization of the sacral fracture, and finally (4) reduction and stabilization of lumbosacral instability with lumbopelvic fixation. Additionally combinations of these may be used together or even with anterior stabilization of the pelvis.

NONOPERATIVE TREATMENT

Patients with intact neurologic function and minimally displaced or angulated fractures (zone 1 or 2 in combination with a stable pelvic fracture) may require only a short period of bed rest followed by early mobilization with or without an orthosis (see Fig. 35-9). Weight-bearing is progressively increased, depending on the fracture pattern and displacement. Occasionally, an external fixator is necessary for the anterior portion of the ring, whereas the interdigitation of the fragments may provide sufficient stability posteriorly.

Fractures of the sacrum occurring through S3 and distally do not create intrinsic weight-bearing instability, although depending on the severity of the injury, the distal fragment may have relatively little attachment to the proximal fragment (see Fig. 35-7). Initial operative management is infrequently indicated even in the presence of neurologic deficit. Since there is innervation redundancy for bowel and bladder function and since severe injuries

at this level often result in root transection, early exploration-decompression is of little benefit. Initial treatment should therefore consist of mobilization with protection of the area in sitting to observe whether there is return of function and relief of pain. Operative treatment should be considered only in the setting of persistent nonunion with pain after 6 months and completion of sphincter electromyographic (EMG) evaluation.

Most insufficiency fractures of the sacrum can be treated nonoperatively, even those accompanied by neurologic deficit (see Fig. 35-10). The necessity of using bed rest as the initial portion of the treatment has, however, been a matter of debate. In fact, the use of bed rest initially does not preclude the subsequent development of a neurologic deficit.[43] Many reports, however, have advocated the use of bed rest[34,43,61,65,66,95] despite the many complications associated with a period of bed rest in the elderly, including increased osteopenia; deep venous thrombosis; decreased muscle strength; and cardiac, gastrointestinal, and genitourinary complications.[5] Currently, however, no evidence is available in the literature to advocate one methodology over another. No published series has suggested that patients treated with bed rest have an unacceptable rate of complications; in addition, however, no evidence has indicated that the time to healing and relief of symptoms is shorter when an initial period of bed rest is used before progressive ambulation is initiated. Most studies demonstrate a prolonged period of symptoms lasting at least 3 months and often as long as 9 months before complete relief of symptoms and return to full function.[19,34,36,66] Those with a previous history of irradiation may require an even longer period before resolution of symptoms, in some cases up to and exceeding 1 year.[58] Few reported patients had adverse outcomes; however, the duration of disability and symptoms was prolonged. Even those with neurologic symptoms who were treated nonoperatively had reasonable functional outcomes.[43]

The role of operative treatment in sacral insufficiency fractures has not been thoroughly explored. However, several recent small case series[10,12,70] have evaluated the role of percutaneous sacroplasty in the treatment of sacral insufficiency fractures. None of the series looked at indications, but the obvious clinical situation would be the elderly patient who continues to have severe incapacitating pain that restricts mobility after 3 months of nonoperative treatment. In all of the series the patients had the sacroplasty done under CT guidance with at least one needle placed in the fracture on each side with about 4 mL of methylmethacrylate injected on each side. There was no occurrence of neural impingement and only one instance of a small amount of soft tissue extrusion. Most patients had at least some moderate improvement of pain, and several had complete relief of pain. This technique requires further investigation but might be considered in the patient with severely limited mobility secondary to pain after 3 months of nonoperative treatment.

For vertically unstable fractures in zone 1, the displacement should be initially reduced with the use of skeletal traction, followed by anterior or posterior fixation (or a combination of both). Fixation can be achieved with the use of anterior plating of the symphysis and posterior techniques such as posterior iliosacral plating, sacral bars, and tension band plates across the ilium. The use of iliosacral screws placed percutaneously has allowed stable fixation with less extensive surgery.[62,74,75,90,91] The method for that technique is well described in Chapter 36 and will not be repeated here. Satisfactory outcomes depend on achieving reduction of the sacral fracture before initiating the procedure and on obtaining adequate visualization of the sacrum with image intensification to ascertain that the screws remain within the sacrum.[74,75]

For patients with either isolated transverse or oblique fractures with or without involvement of the L5-S1 articulation, either bilateral plating[49,76] or other techniques[89] can be considered. These measures should not be considered for minimally displaced fractures.

Surgical Techniques for Specific Types of Injuries

RESECTION

Little has been written about resection as an alternative for treatment of sacral fractures except in coccygeal fractures where the results are quite equivocal because of the mixed indications for its use. Although its utility is distinctly limited, it does have a role in relieving pain in patients with distal sacral fractures that have failed nonoperative treatment and have gone on to nonunion or to painful malunion. Before proceeding with resection it is critical to understand the status of the distal roots. Severe displacement of the distal fragment (see Fig. 35-7) suggests that the roots are severed and discontinuous. Evidence of a meningocele on MRI and abnormality on voiding cystometrogram and sphincter EMG reinforce this clinical conclusion. However, the surgeon must be prepared either to completely resect the distal fragment or to take it out in pieces while preserving the continuity of any remaining roots.

FIXATION TECHNIQUES

Beginning with the work of Louis[53] and Roy-Camille and associates,[77] systems of spinal plates fixed with pedicle screws have been used for fractures. Their use is most appropriate for fixation of both the lumbosacral junction and the sacrum. Especially for the sacrum, they not only provide a mode of fixation for sequential screws but, by proper bending of the plating, can also control displacement and angulation. The strength of these plates lies in the fact that they can achieve rigid fixation of the spine with limited length of instrumentation. Roy-Camille plates for the lumbar spine allow two pedicle screws to be placed at each level, which is especially important at S1. For localized fixation only at the lumbosacral junction, the use of a screw-rod construct is optimal. Screws are placed into the pedicle of L5, and after reduction of the dislocation or fracture-dislocation, the rods can be attached to screws directed either medially in S1 or laterally into the ala. Their utility is somewhat diminished if fixation needs to be carried to S2 to stabilize an oblique fracture line because the construct has a higher profile and somewhat less versatility than plate fixation on the sacrum proper. With severe comminution an iliolumbar construct may be considered as described in the following section.

LUMBOSACRAL FACET INJURIES AND DISLOCATIONS

The patient should be placed in the prone position with the table flexed at the level of the hips to allow easy reduction of the dislocation. After the dislocation is reduced, the table is extended to lock the reduction before beginning stabilization. A posterior incision is made from the midportion of the spinous process of L4 down to the level of S2. Care is taken during dissection to avoid disruption of the L4-L5 interspinous ligament or the facet capsules of the same level. Careful dissection of the L5-S1 facets is performed to ascertain whether any fracture lines have occurred through the articular processes or through the base of the S1 articular process and obliquely into the sacrum. If no fracture lines are present, reduction can be accomplished by applying distraction through towel clips placed on the spinous processes of L5 and S1 to disengage them (see Fig. 35-1). If reduction cannot be readily accomplished, additional flex is added to the table. Once the articular processes are disengaged, those of L5 are pulled posteriorly and inferiorly to lock them into the appropriate position. Usually, they do not completely engage until the table is switched from flexion to slight extension. It is inadvisable to resect the tips of the articular processes to perform the reduction maneuver because such resection compromises the stability of the final reduction. If it is difficult to achieve complete reduction or hold it because the spinous processes tend to spread apart, an interspinous wire can be placed temporarily to maintain the reduction until the final instrumentation is placed. Care should be taken to not attempt to compress the interspace with either the wire or the final construct because of the potential for compression of the disk, which can result in nerve root impingement. After reduction is achieved, the posterior aspect of the disk should be palpated to ensure that disk herniation and root impingement have not occurred. If such is the case, diskectomy should be performed at this point after the initial reduction.

After the interspace is checked, pedicle screws should then be placed in routine fashion in L5 and S1. Medial placement of the screws at S1 is somewhat easier with this injury, and the final position of the hardware should be in only slight compression, just enough to maintain the reduction. Fusion is done with iliac crest graft. In patients with fractures through the tips of the articular processes, the fragments should be removed before attempting to achieve the reduction. The final reduction may not be as rotationally stable and may require wire fixation before placing the final construct. If a fracture line goes through the base of an articular process and then obliquely into the sacrum, the articular processes of that side may not have even been juxtaposed by the translation achieved by displacement. Therefore, reduction may be accomplished on the affected side simply by translating the fractured fragment posteriorly. This technique does not allow for stable reduction before the application of instrumentation. In this instance, a plate construct should be used as described later, with one screw in L5 and two in S1 and the plate extended as far distally as necessary to fully stabilize the oblique nature of the fragment.

SACRAL FRACTURES

Several methods of surgical treatment of sacral injuries have been shown to provide significant benefit to the patient. Prior to that, surgical treatment was restricted to sacral laminectomies and decompression. Only rarely was an indication for reduction of any sacral deformities noted because no adequate methods of sacral stabilization existed. However, more recently it has been appreciated that transverse fractures with severe kyphosis might be improved by manipulation and stabilization to prevent skin compromise in thin individuals and afford decompression to compromised sacral roots. Vigorous manipulation of the fragments can carry the risk of rectal perforation and should be considered with great caution.

Patients with transverse fractures of the sacrum and neurologic deficit undeniably benefit from surgical decompression and stabilization.[2,76,89] Compression of the sacral roots may be due to combined causes. Most transverse fractures angulate into increased kyphosis and may indeed translate (Fig. 35-12). Thus, the sacral roots may be tented over the exaggerated kyphosis. Sacral laminectomy alone certainly fails to decompress the roots because the kyphosis still remains. In addition, if decompression is achieved by removing or tamping the apex of the kyphosis down without stabilization, the impingement can recur with additional translation (see Fig. 35-12). Thus, in that instance, reduction of the distal fragment to the proximal fragment is accomplished, followed by plate stabilization, and subsequent removal of any unreduced fragments. If the fracture is more impacted and comminuted and not as angulated, compression of the roots is generally due to retropulsion of fragments into the canal. In that instance, reduction is not necessary because the impacted fragments should not be disturbed. Stabilization in situ should be performed and decompression then accomplished.

The technique for reduction and stabilization of an angulated transverse fracture of the sacrum is reasonably straightforward (Fig. 35-13). Most transverse fractures occur between S1 and S3. A radiolucent operating table is necessary for screw placement. For a transverse fracture

---

FIGURE 35-12 *This patient, a 30-year-old man, fell from a height of 35 ft, landed on both feet, and fell backward onto his buttocks; he sustained multiple injuries to both feet and an oblique sacral fracture with a complete neural injury at the S2 level. **A,** An anteroposterior radiograph did not clearly demonstrate the oblique nature of the fracture line (dashed line) with extension into the L5-S1 articulation on one side. **B,** A lateral view shows the increase in kyphosis apparent at the fracture site (arrow). **C,** An axial computed tomographic scan clearly shows the oblique nature of the fracture line as it courses through the floor of the canal into the neural foramen and the ventral surface of the sacrum. **D,** The nature of the displacement is better seen on magnetic resonance imaging, with the proximal fragment displaced anteriorly and the distal fragment posteriorly. The fracture traversed the base of the S1 facet on the right and therefore required plating to the L5 pedicle **(E, F)** to achieve reduction and stabilization.*

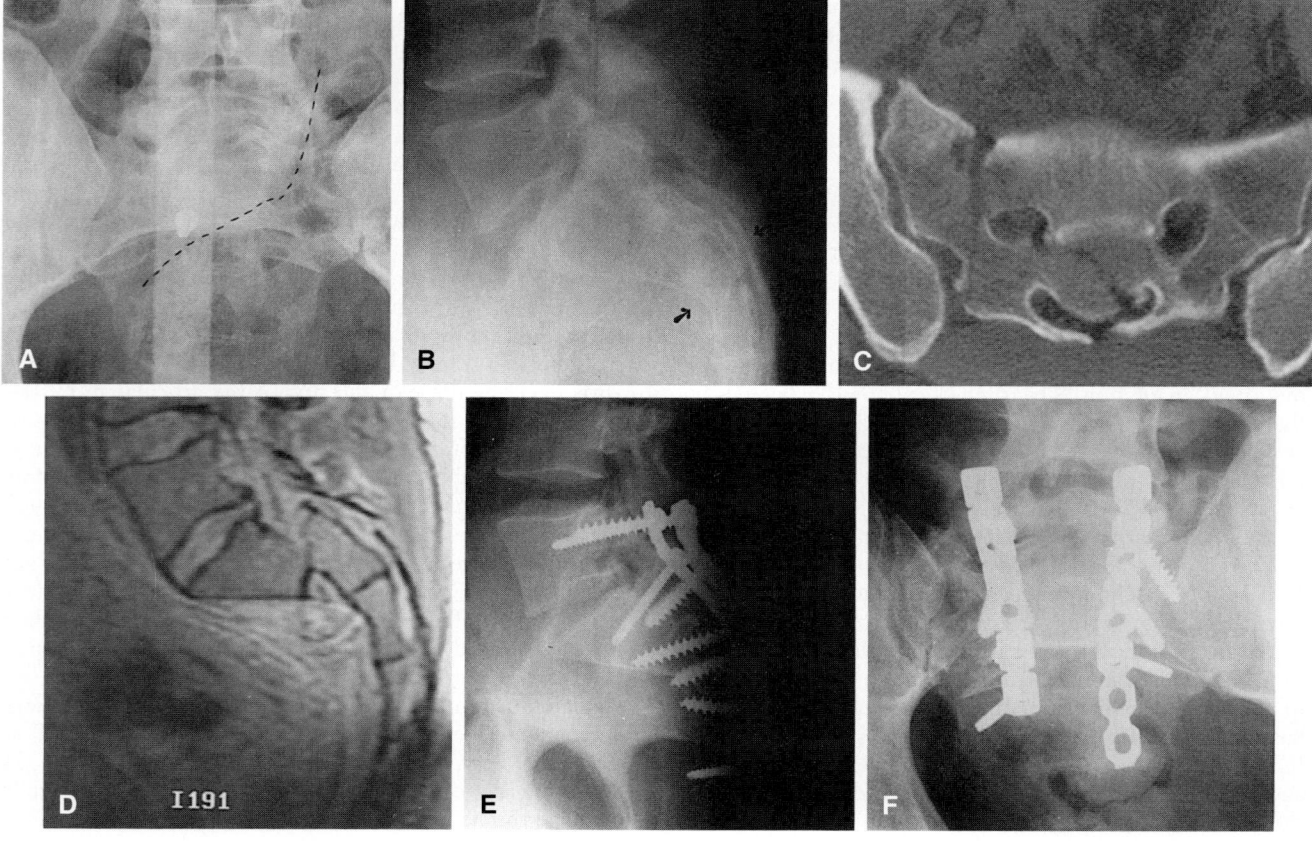

FIGURE 35-13 *Technique of reduction and plate fixation of transverse sacral fractures. A transverse fracture line in the sacrum usually occurs at the region of the second or third dorsal foramen. **A,** A lateral view of the model demonstrates kyphosis of the fracture, as well as translational deformity. Most transverse sacral fractures occur in the most kyphotic area of the sacrum, S2-S3. After an appropriate workup to delineate the direction of the fracture and the area of maximal sacral root compression, the patient is placed in the prone position with the hips flexed 45°. The incision runs from the inferior tip of the L4 spinous process to the region of S4. Although the sacrum is approached through a midline incision and the posterior aspect is stripped subperiosteally, exposure is often insufficient. Detaching the inferior-most attachment of the paraspinal musculature from the sacrum at S3-S4 can broaden the exposure. **B,** The first step in reduction is to expose the complete fracture line and then perform a laminectomy approximately 2.5 cm in length and centered on the fracture line to clearly visualize the neural elements. It should be carried far enough laterally to extend out into the dorsal foramen. **C,** After the nerve roots are clearly delineated, the fracture line is opened on both sides of the sacrum, first with a small curette and then with a small Cobb elevator inserted gently in each side to pry apart the impacted fracture. By using the elevators to gently lever the fracture, the kyphosis and translation can be at least partially reduced **(D)**. If the proximal fragment is posteriorly displaced*

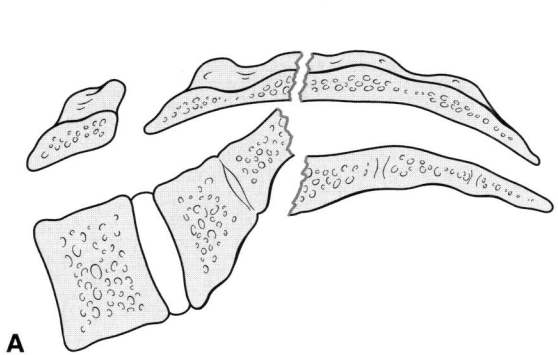

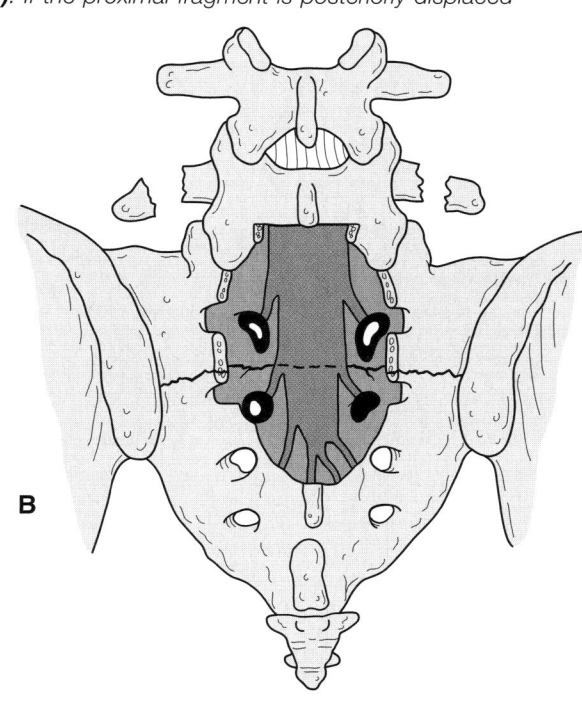

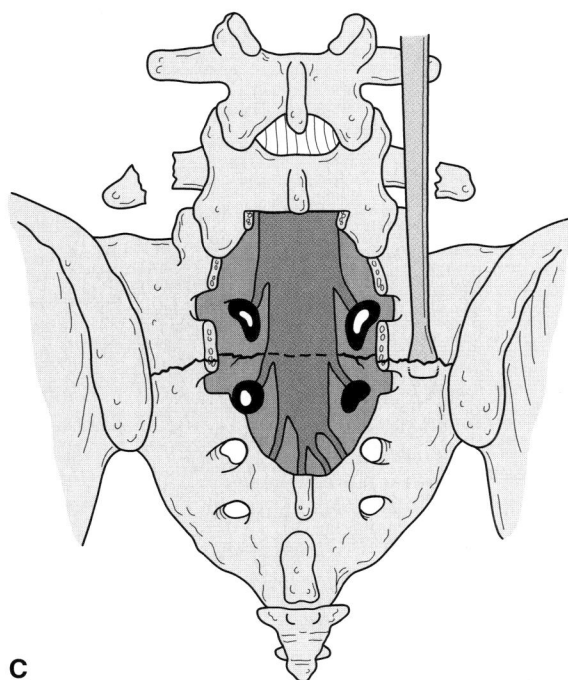

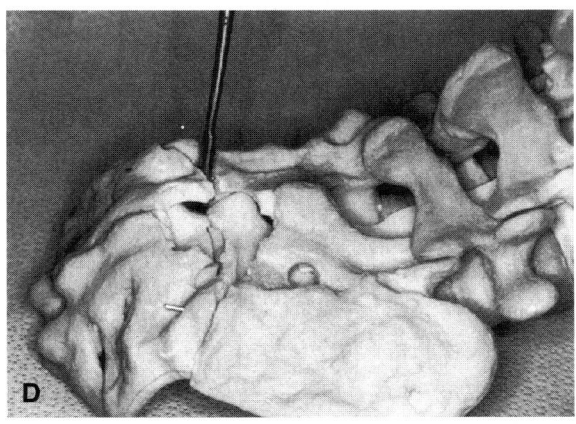

(Continued)

FIGURE 35-13 *(Continued) **E,** the instrument should be placed under the ventral surface of the distal fragment. Separation of the fracture fragments and at least partial reduction are critical before plate fixation is begun. A 3.5- or 4.5-mm pelvic reconstruction plate is selected on the basis of hole spacing and the size of the sacrum. If anatomic positioning is achieved manually, the plate is contoured to directly match the contour of the posterior aspect of the sacrum; if the position is less than anatomic, the plate is slightly undercontoured. If the fracture is more oblique and shortened, a temporary screw can be placed in both the proximal and distal fragments and a distraction tool applied to achieve length while the final plate is being positioned. **F,** With the exception of the S1 segment, plate placement and screw starting points lie on a line along the dorsal foramen with the screw directed laterally into the residual pedicle. Two screws are placed at S1, the more proximal screw directed laterally from the dimple at the base of the S1 facet. **G,** A bicortical hole is drilled and tapped, and then the screw inserted. **H,** The second screw in S1 is inserted and directed medially into the body. The screw hole is likewise tapped and the screw inserted either to the full depth of the body or bicortically.*

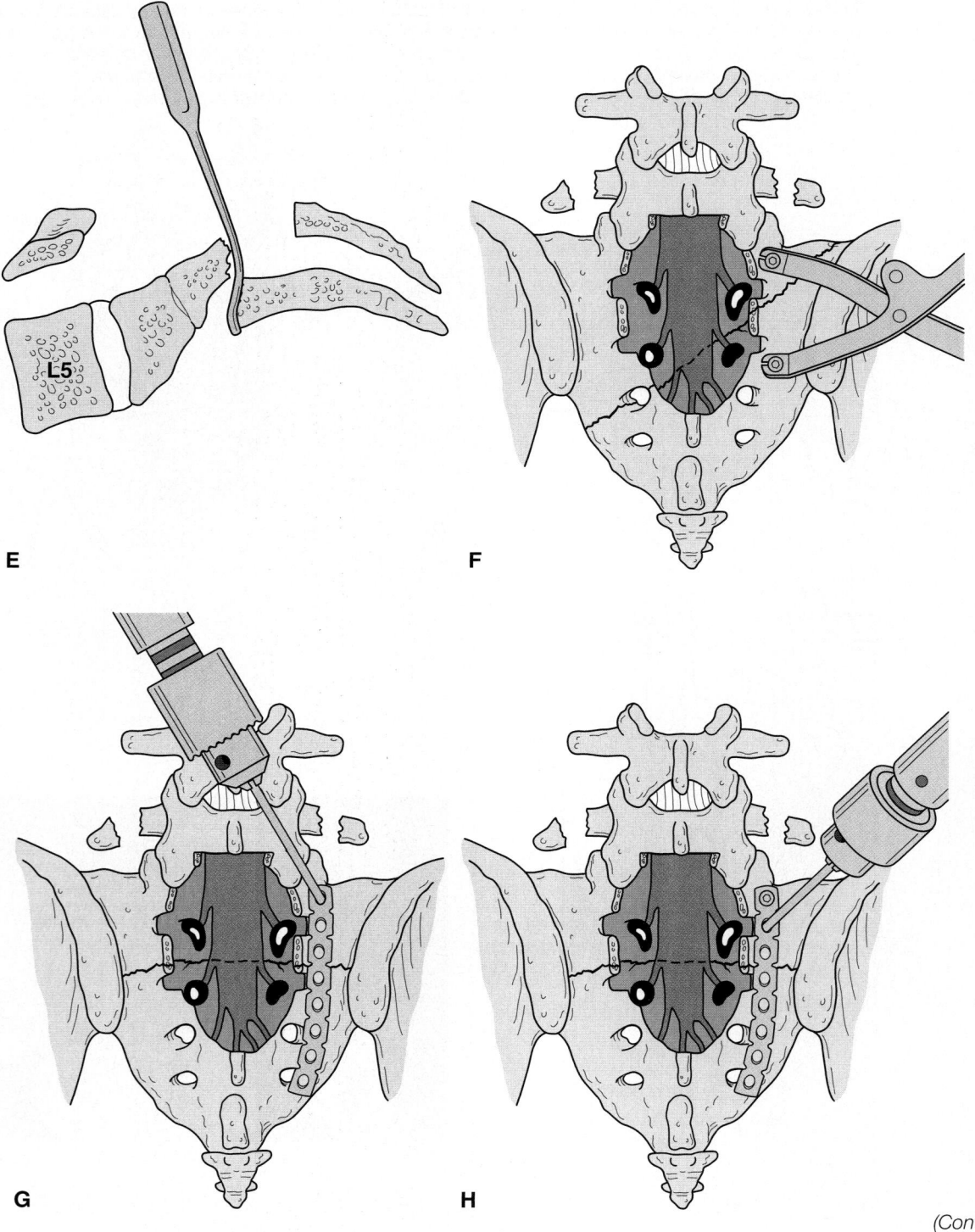

E

F

G

H

(Continued)

FIGURE 35-13 *(Continued)* ***I,*** *The starting site for the most distal screw is selected. A minimum of two and preferably three points of fixation need to be present distal to the fracture line. These screws are angled obliquely parallel to the sacroiliac joint for maximal length and fixation. An attempt should be made to place pairs of adjacent screws so that they converge in the caudocephalad direction for maximal pull-out strength. The distal-most screws rarely exceed 20 mm, whereas the more proximal screws average between 35 and 45 mm. The screw is tightened into position but is not used to achieve fracture reduction. If the reduction is not complete and the plate is completely in contact with the posterior aspect of the sacrum, further manual reduction is done before final tightening of all screws. Screws are then placed in every hole that does not fall directly over a dorsal foramen* ***(J).*** *The contralateral side is plated in a similar fashion.*

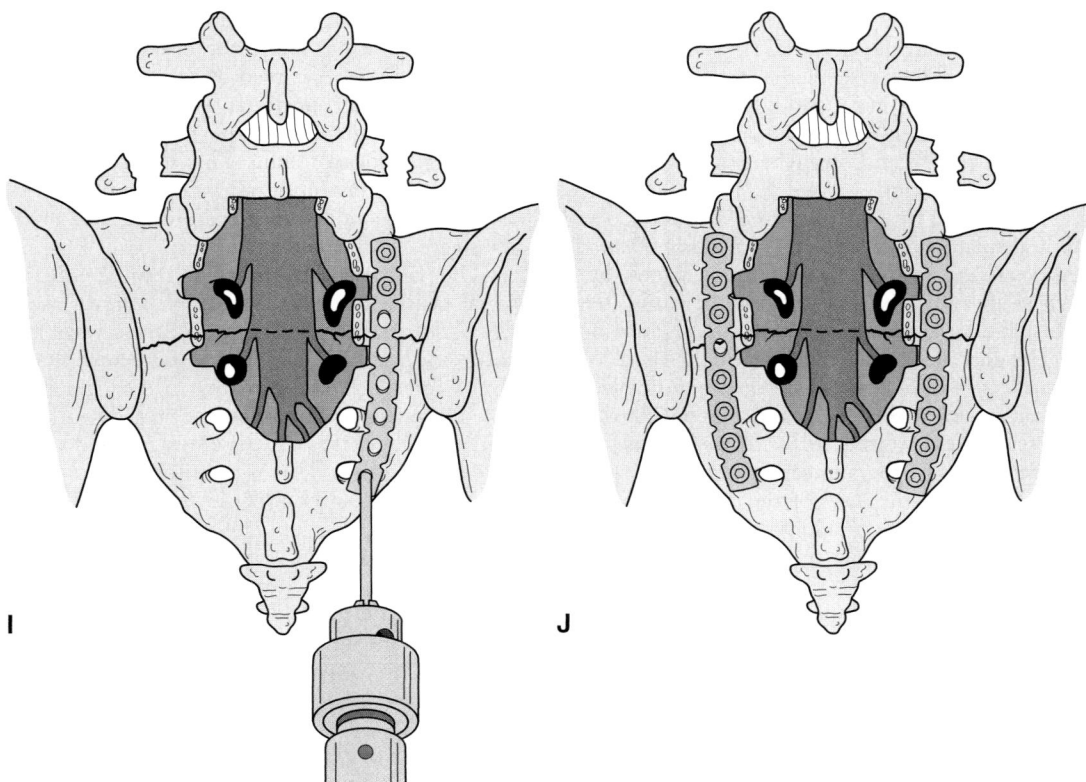

or even one with an oblique component, the patient is placed on the operating table in the prone position with the hips and knees slightly flexed. A longitudinal incision is used for exposure from the L5 spinous process (sparing the L5-S1 facet capsule) to the S4 level if there is no involvement of the L5-S1 facet on either side. If the fracture is more oblique, exposure to the L4 level is necessary to include the L5 pedicle in the instrumentation. Removing the distal attachment of the paraspinous musculature subperiosteally from the posterior aspect of the sacrum at its terminal position at S3 to S4 can facilitate exposure of the posterior aspect of the sacrum.

A sacral laminectomy is performed from S1 to S4 to expose the sacral roots (see Fig. 35-13), with dissection continued laterally to fully delineate the transverse fracture. The laminectomy is initiated at the proximal end of the sacrum, where the canal is larger, and directed distally until the fracture line is encountered. The decompression is extended laterally to identify the takeoff of the ventral roots and the bone of the vestigial pedicles. Although complete decompression is not necessary at this point,

the fracture line may be entered with a curette laterally and the sacral canal partially undercut to remove the bone at the apical point of the kyphosis and prevent impingement of the roots after reduction (see Fig. 35-13). The fracture is disimpacted by opening the fracture line with Cobb elevators gently placed on both sides of the fracture or by using a distraction device temporarily placed proximal and distal to the fracture to distract it. If the proximal fragment lies posteriorly, the Cobb elevator can be gently placed within the fracture lines laterally anterior to the ventral surface of the distal fragment to lever it posteriorly and correct the kyphosis. If the fracture is easily reduced by levering it with the Cobb elevators, the spine is prepared for fixation. In cases in which the fracture line passes through the canal at an oblique angle (20–40°), the sacrum may become foreshortened by sliding obliquely. Length can be regained by using a pelvic reduction clamp placed on two unicortical screws.

If the fracture does not involve the L5-S1 articulation, screw placement is begun in the area of the pedicles at each level from S1 to S4. The most proximal screw at the medial border of the S1 facet is directed 30° medially into the body of S1. The next screw just proximal to the first dorsal foramen is directed laterally at about 40° into the sacral ala. This technique allows two screws to be placed in S1, and a screw is then placed in each subsequent pedicle running parallel to the sacroiliac joint. At a point midway between each dorsal foramen and in a line just medial to the level of the foramen, a 2-mm drill bit is angled laterally between 30 and 45°, and a hole is drilled through both cortices. Each hole is depth-gauged and tapped for the use of a cancellous screw. A malleable titanium or stainless steel plate (pelvic reconstruction plate) of correct length (about 40 mm in S1 and decreasing sequentially to 20 mm at S4) is then selected and its holes spaced to accommodate the predrilled holes when the sacral fracture is in the reduced position.

The fracture is reduced by gentle leverage with the Cobb elevators, and both plates are placed simultaneously. *Do **not** use the plates to achieve fracture reduction!* All screws are placed on both sides and tightened down sequentially (see Fig. 35-13). In patients with comminution, screws may be placed in the sacroiliac joint and posterior of the ilium or extended up to the L5 pedicle for more proximal involvement or for involvement of the L5-S1 articulation. At this point, if compression of the ventral surface of the roots is still occurring after reduction of the angular deformity, excavation lateral to the canal at the level of the fracture should be performed. Such excavation allows the bone to be removed with a pituitary rongeur from under the canal. The bone should not be tamped down but, instead, removed to ascertain that the decompression is complete. Bone grafting of the fracture is not necessary in the body of the sacrum; however, if the construct is extended to L5, routine posterolateral graft application is indicated. The paraspinous musculature is then reapproximated over a drain. The patient is immobilized in a lumbosacral orthosis with the leg included for 3 months. Recovery of bowel and bladder function may be slow and take up to 12 to 18 months.

If the fractures of the sacrum are vertical through the neuroforamina or involve the lumbosacral articular, alternative methods need to be utilized to regain stability. Clearly sacral plating is insufficient and additionally fixation into the severely comminuted sacrum is compromised. In that instance fixation from the lumbar spine directly into the ilium bypasses the comminuted sacrum and stores stability between the spine and the pelvis but does not control the fragments of the sacrum. Direct decompression can accompany the iliolumbar stabilization but must achieve root decompression by bone removal that does not require reduction of deformity or stabilization of fragments to maintain the reduction.[82]

Surgical technique for this procedure requires a midline incision from the inferior tip of the L3 spinous process to the region of S4. If decompression is to be done a midline approach is utilized, but if only stabilization is necessary then a modified posterior approach can be used. As the midline incision is made down to the level of the spinous process and fascia over the sacrum, flaps are elevated just above the fascia out to the iliac crests from S1 to S3. The paraspinous muscles are not detached distally where

they insert into the sacrum between S3 and S4. Dissection of L4 and L5 is done in a standard fashion to allow insertion of pedicle screws at L4 and L5 without disruption of the L3-L4 facet joint capsule. Over the sacrum three vertical incisions are made: one in the midline from L5 to S3 and one over each iliac crest. Subperiosteal dissection is done under each muscle mass from S1 to S3, and the iliac crest on each side is stripped on both its inner and outer surfaces to the level of the sacrum. At S3 the posterior aspect of the ilium is at the level of the posterior aspect of the sacrum, but at S1 the ilium is stripped to a depth of about 1.5 cm. A curved osteotome is then used to make a cut flush to the posterior aspect of the sacrum from S3 to S1 removing the entire posterior iliac crest on each side as a single block of bone. This has two purposes: the first is to harvest sufficient graft for the lumbopelvic fusion and the second is to decrease the prominence of the posterior hardware.

The L4 and L5 pedicle screws are inserted in the usual fashion with variable-angle screws used in at least L5 if not in both levels. Two iliac screws are placed on each side starting with the distal screw. Its entry site is approximately 1 cm proximal to the cut end surface of the ilium (approximately the region of the posterior superior iliac crest [PSIS]) aiming at the anterior inferior iliac crest (AIIS). This is monitored on fluoroscopy using obturator inlet and outlet views as well as a lateral view of the ilium and iliac oblique views. A smooth K-wire can be used to establish the correct tract in the absence of a specially manufactured pedicle finder or probe of 140 mm in length. The path should be confirmed on fluoroscopy on both sides, and a minimum depth of 80 mm is necessary for purchase with a maximum depth of as much 140 mm in males and 130 mm in females. After the placement of markers for the first screw on each side, the second is placed parallel and proximal in the cut surface of the ilium by 1.5 cm. Generally the two proximal screws should be at least 10 to 20 mm shorter than the distal screw. All four screws are then inserted without use of a tap to a depth that buries the screw to the level of the rod slot into the iliac cancellous bone to minimize hardware prominence.

Assembly of the rod-screw construct can be done in one of two ways. If the system does not have connectors, then the rod needs to be contoured to attach to the L4 and L5 screw heads, bending both over the prominence of the sacrum and flaring laterally to allow attachment to the iliac screws (Fig. 35-14C). The construct is more easily assembled if the rod does not have to be flared laterally to attach to the screws but can be attached with lateral connectors between the rod and the iliac screw heads (see Fig. 35-13D). All of the hardware is placed under the elevated paraspinous musculature, thereby decreasing prominence and soft tissue wound problems. The amount of contouring can be decreased when using direct fixation to the iliac screws by placing the pedicle screws in L4 and L5 in a lateral-to-medial direction and using variable-angle screws. Wound closure is achieved over a drain by closing all three of the vertical fascial incisions followed by a standard skin closure.

FIGURE 35-14 | *This patient with a comminuted fracture through S1-S2 with lumbosacral dissociation (A) underwent iliolumbar stabilization (B, C).*

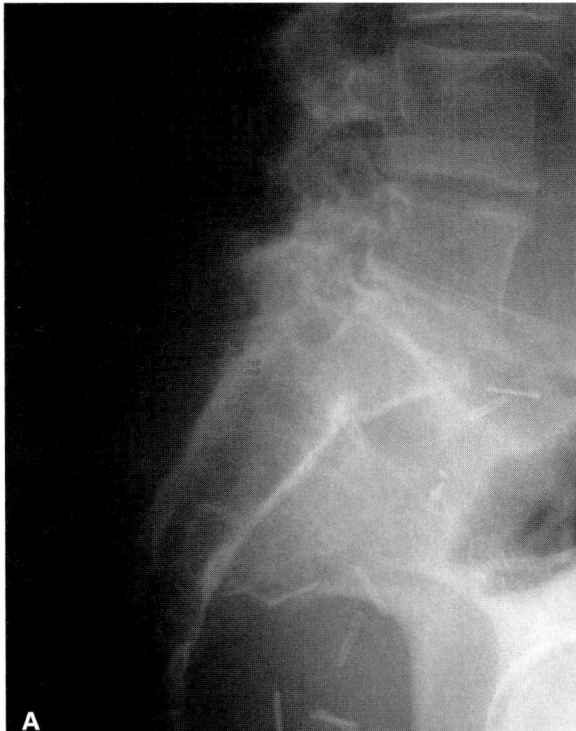

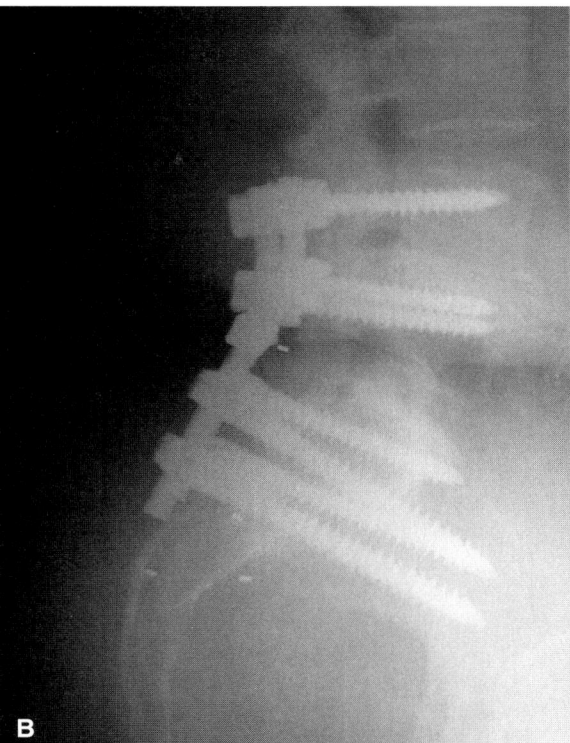

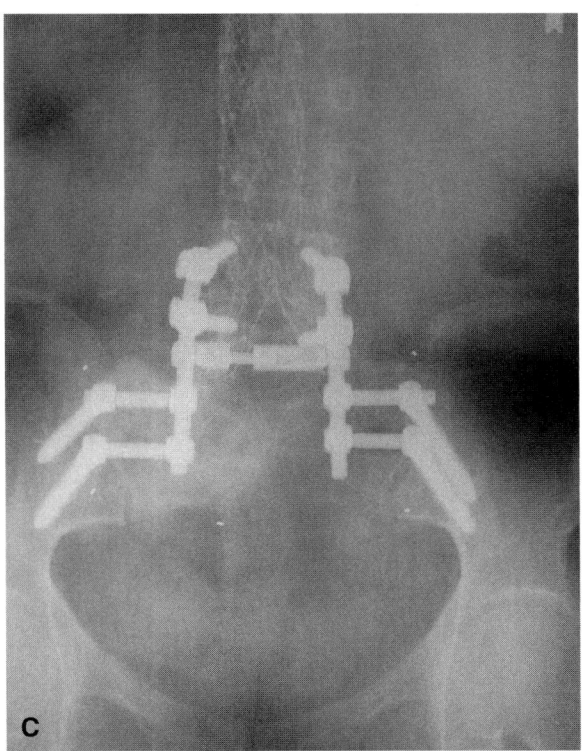

(Continued)

FIGURE 35-14 *(Continued)* **D,** *Iliac screw fixation is done through three fascial incisions—one midline and two over the iliac crests. Subperitoneal dissection of each iliac crest is done, the crest is resected flush with the back of the sacrum of S2/3, the paraspinous muscle is left attached distally but elevated between the midline incision and the iliac crest incision.* **E,** *The lumbar can be attached directly to the iliac screws using variable axis heads and a medial trajectory or* **(F)** *by continuing the rod.* **G,** *A rod can also be used with connectors or the iliac screws.*

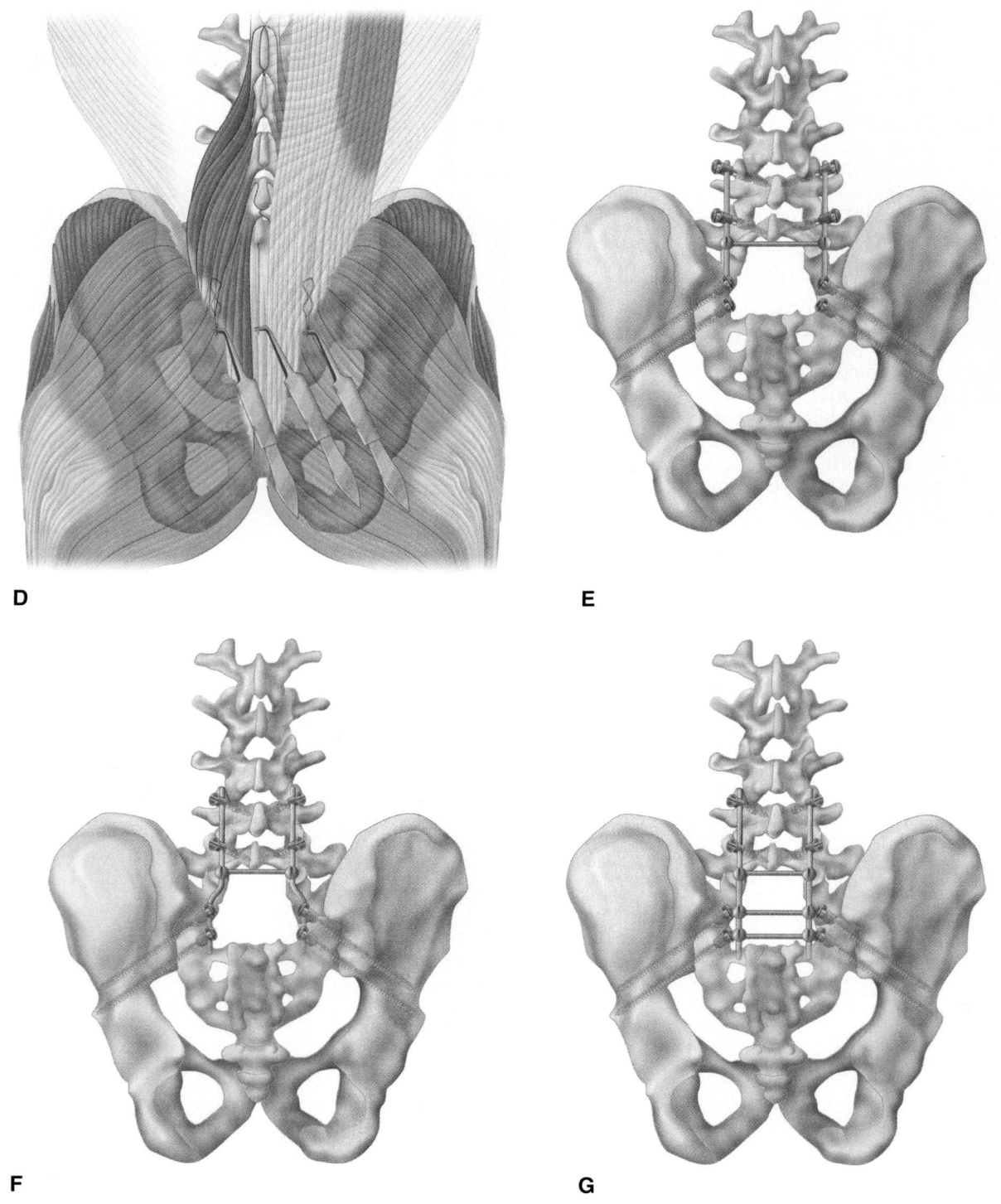

D

E

F

G

COMPLICATIONS

Few complications specific to these injuries are encountered. However, failure of recognition is the most common problem in both insufficiency fractures and traumatic injuries. In an elderly patient with an insidious onset of back pain and disability, the use of a bone scan or MRI will usually lead to the diagnosis. In a patient with acute trauma, careful evaluation of sphincter function is critical along with MRI if the neurologic assessment is not consistent in a patient with a history conducive to such an injury. Only one series[6] has specially evaluated the rate of complications in iliolumbar stabilization for spinopelvic instability. They found a 16 percent infection rate, 11 percent wound complication, 31 percent hardware failure, and 42 percent of patients requiring an unplanned return to the operating room. Neurologic complications were very infrequent, with the exception of incomplete return of function secondary to traumatic root avulsion.

SUMMARY

Recognition of the importance of sacral fractures both in patients with pelvic injuries and in patients with isolated traumatic fractures or insufficiency fractures is a relatively late occurrence. With increased awareness has come improved recognition of the natural history and the development of improved treatment methodologies.

REFERENCES

1. Akbarnia, B.A.; Crandall, D.G.; Burkus, K.; et al. Use of long rods and a short arthrodesis for burst fractures of the thoracolumbar spine. A long-term follow-up study. J Bone Joint Surg [Am]76:1629–1635, 1994.
2. Albert, T.J.; Levine, M.J.; An, H.S.; et al. Concomitant noncontiguous thoracolumbar and sacral fractures. Spine 18:1285–1291, 1993.
3. An, H.S.; Simpson, J.M.; Ebraheim, N.A.; et al. Low lumbar burst fractures: Comparison between conservative and surgical treatments. Orthopedics 15:367–373, 1992.
4. An, H.S.; Vaccaro, A.; Cotler, J.M.; et al. Low lumbar burst fractures. Comparison among body cast, Harrington rod, Luque rod, and Steffee plate. Spine 16:S440–S444, 1991.
5. Babayev, M.; Lachmann, E.; Nagler, W. The controversy surrounding sacral insufficiency fractures: To ambulate or not to ambulate? Am J Phys Med Rehabil 79:404–409, 2000.
6. Bellabarba, C.; Schildhauer, T.A.; Vaccaro, A.R.; et al. Complications associated with surgical stabilization of high-grade sacral fracture dislocations with spino-pelvic instability. Spine 31:S80–S88, 2006.
7. Berry, J.L.; Stahurski, T.; Asher, M.A. Morphometry of the supra sciatic notch intrailiac implant anchor passage. Spine 26:E143–E148, 2001.
8. Bonnin, J.G. Sacral fractures and injuries to the cauda equina. J Bone Joint Surg [Br] 27:113–127, 1945.
9. Brahme, S.K.; Cervilla, V.; Vint, V.; et al. Magnetic resonance appearance of sacral insufficiency fractures. Skeletal Radiol 19:489–493, 1990.
10. Brook, A.L.; Mirsky, D.M.; Bello, J.A. Computerized tomography guided sacroplasty: A practical treatment for sacral insufficiency fracture: Case report. Spine 30:E450–E454, 2005.
11. Bucknill, T.M.; Blackburne, J.S. Fracture–dislocations of the sacrum. Report of three cases. J Bone Joint Surg [Br] 58:467–470, 1976.
12. Butler, C.L.; Given, C.A.; Michel, S.J.; et al. Percutaneous sacroplasty for the treatment of sacral insufficiency fractures. AJR Am J Roentgenol 184:1956–1959, 2005.
13. Byrnes, D.P.; Russo, G.L.; Ducker, T.B.; et al. Sacrum fractures and neurological damage. Report of two cases. J Neurosurg 47:459–462, 1977.
14. Carl, A.; Blair, B. Unilateral lumbosacral facet fracture–dislocation. Spine 16:218–221, 1991.
15. Chen, C.K.; Liang, H.L.; Lai, P.H.; et al. Imaging diagnosis of insufficiency fracture of the sacrum. Zhonghua Yi Xue Za Zhi (Taipei) 62:591–597, 1999.
16. Connolly, P.J.; Esses, S.I.; Heggeness, M.H.; et al. Unilateral facet dislocation of the lumbosacral junction. Spine 17:1244–1248, 1992.
17. Court-Brown, C.M.; Gertzbein, S.D. The management of burst fractures of the fifth lumbar vertebra. Spine 12:308–312, 1987.
18. Das, D.S.; McCreath, S.W. Lumbosacral fracture-dislocations. A report of four cases. J Bone Joint Surg [Br] 63:58–60, 1981.
19. Dasgupta, B.; Shah, N.; Brown, H.; et al. Sacral insufficiency fractures: An unsuspected cause of low back pain. Br J Rheumatol 37:789–793, 1998.
20. Denis, F. The three column spine and its significance in the classification of acute thoracolumbar spinal injuries. Spine 8:817–831, 1983.
21. Denis, F.; Davis, S.; Comfort, T. Sacral fractures: An important problem. Retrospective analysis of 236 cases. Clin Orthop Relat Res 227:67–81, 1988.
22. Dewey, P.; Browne, P.S. Fracture–dislocation of the lumbo-sacral spine with cauda equina lesion. Report of two cases. J Bone Joint Surg [Br] 50:635–638, 1968.
23. Ebraheim, N.A.; Savolaine, E.R.; Shapiro, P.; et al. Unilateral lumbosacral facet joint dislocation associated with vertical shear sacral fracture. J Orthop Trauma 5:498–503, 1991.
24. Elliot, H.C. Cross sectional diameters and areas of human spinal cord. Anat Rec 93:287–293, 1945.
25. Fardon, D.F. Displaced fracture of the lumbosacral spine with delayed cauda equina deficit: Report of a case and review of literature. Clin Orthop Relat Res 120:155–158, 1976.
26. Fardon, D.F. Displaced transverse fracture of the sacrum with nerve root injury: Report of a case with successful operative management. J Trauma 19:119–122, 1979.
27. Finiels, H.; Finiels, P.J.; Jacquot, J.M.; et al. [Fractures of the sacrum caused by bone insufficiency. Meta-analysis of 508 cases]. Presse Med 26:1568–1573, 1997.

28. Fountain, S.S.; Hamilton, R.D.; Jameson, R.M. Transverse fractures of the sacrum. A report of six cases. J Bone Joint Surg [Am] 59:486–489, 1977.

29. Fredrickson, B.E.; Yuan, H.A.; Miller, H. Burst fractures of the fifth lumbar vertebra. A report of four cases. J Bone Joint Surg [Am] 64:1088–1094, 1982.

30. Fredrickson, B.E.; Yuan, H.A.; Miller, H.E. Treatment of painful long-standing displaced fracture-dislocations of the sacrum. A case report. Clin Orthop Relat Res 166:93–95, 1982.

31. Furey, W.W. Fractures of the pelvis with special reference to associated fractures of the sacrum. Am J Roentgenol Radium Ther 47:89–96, 1942.

32. Gellad, F.E.; Levine, A.M.; Joslyn, J.N.; et al. Pure thoracolumbar facet dislocation: Clinical features and CT appearance. Radiology 161:505–508, 1986.

33. Gibbons, K.J.; Soloniuk, D.S.; Razack, N. Neurological injury and patterns of sacral fractures. J Neurosurg 72:889–893, 1990.

34. Gotis-Graham, I.; McGuigan, L.; Diamond, T.; et al. Sacral insufficiency fractures in the elderly. J Bone Joint Surg [Br] 76:882–886, 1994.

35. Grangier, C.; Garcia, J.; Howarth, N.R.; et al. Role of MRI in the diagnosis of insufficiency fractures of the sacrum and acetabular roof. Skeletal Radiol 26:517–524, 1997.

36. Grasland, A.; Pouchot, J.; Mathieu, A.; et al. Sacral insufficiency fractures: An easily overlooked cause of back pain in elderly women. Arch Intern Med 156:668–674, 1996.

37. Gunterberg, B. Effects of major resection of the sacrum. Clinical studies on urogenital and anorectal function and a biomechanical study on pelvic strength. Acta Orthop Scand Suppl 162:1–38, 1976.

38. Hanley, E.N., Jr.; Knox, B.D.; Ramasastry, S.; et al. Traumatic lumbopelvic spondyloptosis. A case report. J Bone Joint Surg [Am] 75:1695–1698, 1993.

39. Harma, A.; Inan, M. Surgical management of transforaminal sacral fractures. Int Orthop 29:333–337, 2005.

40. Herron, L.D.; Williams, R.C. Fracture–dislocation of the lumbosacral spine. Report of a case and review of the literature. Clin Orthop Relat Res 186:205–211, 1984.

41. Holdsworth, F.W.; Hardy, A. Early treatment of paraplegia from fractures of the thoraco-lumbar spine. J Bone Joint Surg [Br] 35:540–550, 1953.

42. Isler, B. Lumbosacral lesions associated with pelvic ring injuries. J Orthop Trauma 4:1–6, 1990.

43. Jacquot, J.M.; Finiels, H.; Fardjad, S.; et al. Neurological complications in insufficiency fractures of the sacrum. Three case-reports. Rev Rheum Engl Ed 66:109–114, 1999.

44. Kaehr, D.M.; Anderson, P.A.; Mayo, K.; et al. Classification of sacral features based on CT imaging. J Orthop Trauma 3:163, 1989.

45. Knight, R.Q.; Stornelli, D.P.; Chan, D.P.; et al. Comparison of operative versus nonoperative treatment of lumbar burst fractures. Clin Orthop Relat Res 293:112–121, 1993.

46. Krag, M.H.; Weaver, D.L.; Beynnon, B.D.; et al. Morphometry of the thoracic and lumbar spine related to transpedicular screw placement for surgical spinal fixation. Spine 13:27–32, 1988.

47. Kramer, K.M.; Levine, A.M. Unilateral facet dislocation of the lumbosacral junction. A case report and review of the literature. J Bone Joint Surg [Am] 71:1258–1261, 1989.

48. Kuklo, T.R.; Potter, B.K.; Ludwig, S.C.; et al. Radiographic measurement techniques for sacral fractures consensus statement of the Spine Trauma Study Group. Spine 31:1047–1055, 2006.

49. Levine, A.M. Fixation of fractures of the sacrum. Operative Techn Orthop 7:221–231, 1997.

50. Levine, A.M.; Bosse, M.; Edwards, C.C. Bilateral facet dislocations in the thoracolumbar spine. Spine 13:630–640, 1988.

51. Levine, A.M.; Edwards, C.C. Low lumbar burst fractures. Reduction and stabilization using the modular spine fixation system. Orthopedics 11:1427–1432, 1988.

52. Lewis, J.; McKibbin, B. The treatment of unstable fracture–dislocations of the thoraco-lumbar spine accompanied by paraplegia. J Bone Joint Surg [Br] 56:603–612, 1974.

53. Louis, R. Fusion of the lumbar and sacral spine by internal fixation with screw plates. Clin Orthop Relat Res 203:18–33, 1986.

54. McAfee, P.C.; Yuan, H.A.; Fredrickson, B.E.; et al. The value of computed tomography in thoracolumbar fractures. An analysis of one hundred consecutive cases and a new classification. J Bone Joint Surg [Am] 65:461–473, 1983.

55. Meyer, T.L.; Wiltberger, B. Displaced sacral fractures. Am J Orthop 4:187, 1962.

56. Mirkovic, S.; Abitbol, J.J.; Steinman, J.; et al. Anatomic consideration for sacral screw placement. Spine 16:S289–S294, 1991.

57. Montana, M.A.; Richardson, M.L.; Kilcoyne, R.F.; et al. CT of sacral injury. Radiology 161:499–503, 1986.

58. Moreno, A.; Clemente, J.; Crespo, C.; et al. Pelvic insufficiency fractures in patients with pelvic irradiation. Int J Radiat Oncol Biol Phys 44:61–66, 1999.

59. Morris, B.D. Unilateral dislocation of a lumbosacral facet. A case report. J Bone Joint Surg [Am] 63:164–165, 1981.

60. Mouhsine, E.; Wettstein, M.; Schizas, C.; et al. Modified triangular posterior osteosynthesis of unstable sacrum fracture. Eur Spine J 15:857–863, 2006.

61. Newhouse, K.E.; el-Khoury, G.Y.; Buckwalter, J.A. Occult sacral fractures in osteopenic patients. J Bone Joint Surg [Am] 74:1472–1477, 1992.

62. Nork, S.E.; Jones, C.B.; Harding, S.P.; et al. Percutaneous stabilization of U-shaped sacral fractures using

iliosacral screws: Technique and early results. J Orthop Trauma 15:238–246, 2001.

63. O'Callaghan, J.P.; Ullrich, C.G.; Yuan, H.A.; et al. CT of facet distraction in flexion injuries of the thoracolumbar spine: The "naked" facet. AJR Am J Roentgenol 134:563–568, 1980.

64. Peh, W.C. Intrafracture fluid: A new diagnostic sign of insufficiency fractures of the sacrum and ilium. Br J Radiol 73:895–898, 2000.

65. Peh, W.C.; Khong, P.L.; Ho, W.Y. Insufficiency fractures of the sacrum and os pubis. Br J Hosp Med 54:15–19, 1995.

66. Peh, W.C.; Khong, P.L.; Ho, W.Y.; et al. Sacral insufficiency fractures. Spectrum of radiological features. Clin Imaging 19:92–101, 1995.

67. Peh, W.C.; Ooi, G.C. Vacuum phenomena in the sacroiliac joints and in association with sacral insufficiency fractures. Incidence and significance. Spine 22:2005–2008, 1997.

68. Phelan, S.T.; Jones, D.A.; Bishay, M. Conservative management of transverse fractures of the sacrum with neurological features. A report of four cases. J Bone Joint Surg [Br] 73:969–971, 1991.

69. Pohlemann, T.; Gansslen, A.; Tscherne, H. [The problem of the sacrum fracture. Clinical analysis of 377 cases]. Orthopade 21:400–412, 1992.

70. Pommersheim, W.; Huang-Hellinger, F.; Baker, M.; et al. Sacroplasty: A treatment for sacral insufficiency fractures. AJNR Am J Neuroradiol 24:1003–1007, 2003.

71. Purser, D.W. Displaced fracture of the sacrum. Report of a case. J Bone Joint Surg [Br] 51:346–347, 1969.

72. Rauschning, W. In Post, J.D. (ed). Computed Tomography of the Spine. Baltimore, Williams & Wilkins, pp. 20–67, 1984.

73. Reilly, M.C.; Bono, C.M.; Litkouhi, B.; et al. The effect of sacral fracture malreduction on the safe placement of iliosacral screws. J Orthop Trauma 17:88–94, 2003.

74. Routt, M.L., Jr.; Simonian, P.T. Closed reduction and percutaneous skeletal fixation of sacral fractures. Clin Orthop Relat Res 329:121–128, 1996.

75. Routt, M.L., Jr.; Simonian, P.T.; Agnew, S.G.; et al. Radiographic recognition of the sacral alar slope for optimal placement of iliosacral screws: A cadaveric and clinical study. J Orthop Trauma 10:171–177, 1996.

76. Roy-Camille, R.; Saillant, G.; Gagna, G.; et al. Transverse fracture of the upper sacrum. Suicidal jumper's fracture. Spine 10:838–845, 1985.

77. Roy-Camille, R.; Saillant, G.; Mazel, C. Plating of thoracic, thoracolumbar, and lumbar injuries with pedicle screw plates. Orthop Clin North Am 17:147–159, 1986.

78. Sabiston, C.P.; Wing, P.C. Sacral fractures: Classification and neurologic implications. J Trauma 26:1113–1115, 1986.

79. Saillant, G. Etude anatomique des pedicules vertebraux, application chirurgicales. Chir Orthop Traumatiol 62:582–586, 1995.

80. Samberg, L.C. Fracture–dislocation of the lumbosacral spine. A case report. J Bone Joint Surg [Am] 57:1007–1008, 1975.

81. Saraux, A.; Valls, I.; Guedes, C.; et al. Insufficiency fractures of the sacrum in elderly subjects. Rev Rhum Engl Ed 62:582–586, 1995.

82. Schildhauer, T.A.; Bellabarba, C.; Nork, S.E.; et al. Decompression and lumbopelvic fixation for sacral fracture–dislocations with spino-pelvic dissociation. J Orthop Trauma 20:447–457, 2006.

83. Schildhauer, T.A.; Josten, C.; Muhr, G. Triangular osteosynthesis of vertically unstable sacrum fractures: A new concept allowing early weight-bearing. J Orthop Trauma 20:S44–S51, 2006.

84. Schildhauer, T.A.; McCulloch, P.; Chapman, J.R.; et al. Anatomic and radiographic considerations for placement of transiliac screws in lumbopelvic fixations. J Spinal Disord Tech 15:199–205, 2002.

85. Schmidek, H.H.; Smith, D.A.; Kristiansen, T.K. Sacral fractures. Neurosurgery 15:735–746, 1984.

86. Singh, H.; Rao, V.S.; Mangla, R.; et al. Traumatic transverse fracture of sacrum with cauda equina injury—A case report and review of literature. J Postgrad Med 44:14–15, 1998.

87. Stabler, A.; Steiner, W.; Kohz, P.; et al. Time-dependent changes of insufficiency fractures of the sacrum: Intraosseous vacuum phenomenon as an early sign. Eur Radiol 6:655–657, 1996.

88. Stephens, G.C.; Devito, D.P.; McNamara, M.J. Segmental fixation of lumbar burst fractures with Cotrel-Dubousset instrumentation. J Spinal Disord 5:344–348, 1992.

89. Strange-Vognsen, H.H.; Kiaer, T.; Tondevold, E. The Cotrel-Dubousset instrumentation for unstable sacral fractures. Report of 3 patients. Acta Orthop Scand 65:219–220, 1994.

90. Taguchi, T.; Kawai, S.; Kaneko, K.; et al. Operative management of displaced fractures of the sacrum. J Orthop Sci 4:347–352, 1999.

91. Templeman, D.; Goulet, J.; Duwelius, P.J.; et al. Internal fixation of displaced fractures of the sacrum. Clin Orthop Relat Res 329:180–185, 1996.

92. Vaccaro, A.R.; Kim, D.H.; Brodke, D.S.; et al. Diagnosis and management of sacral spine fractures. Instr Course Lect 53:375–385, 2004.

93. Van Savage, J.G.; Dahners, L.E.; Renner, J.B.; et al. Fracture–dislocation of the lumbosacral spine: Case report and review of the literature. J Trauma 33:779–784, 1992.

94. Verhaegen, M.J.; Sauter, A.J. Insufficiency fractures, an often unrecognized diagnosis. Arch Orthop Trauma Surg 119:115–116, 1999.

95. Weber, M.; Hasler, P.; Gerber, H. Insufficiency fractures of the sacrum. Twenty cases and review of the literature. Spine 18:2507–2512, 1993.

96. Whitesides, T.E., Jr. Traumatic kyphosis of the thoracolumbar spine. Clin Orthop Relat Res 128:78–92, 1977.

97. Wiesel, S.W.; Zeide, M.S.; Terry, R.L. Longitudinal fractures of the sacrum: Case report. J Trauma 19:70–71, 1979.

98. Winter, R.B. Congenital Deformities of the Spine. New York, Thieme-Stratton, 1983.

99. Zelle, B.A.; Gruen, G.S.; Hunt, T.; et al. Sacral fractures with neurological injury: Is early decompression beneficial? Int Orthop 28:244–251, 2004.

100. Zindrick, M.R.; Wiltse, L.L.; Doornik, A.; et al. Analysis of the morphometric characteristics of the thoracic and lumbar pedicles. Spine 12:160–166, 1987.

101. Zoltan, J.D.; Gilula, L.A.; Murphy, W.A. Unilateral facet dislocation between the fifth lumbar and first sacral vertebrae. Case report. J Bone Joint Surg [Am] 61:767–769, 1979.

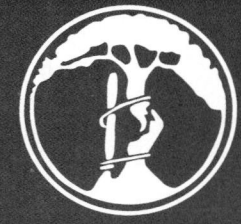

CHAPTER 36

Pelvic Ring Disruptions

Michael D. Stover, M.D., Keith A. Mayo, M.D., and James F. Kellam, M.D., F.R.C.S.(C.)

The pelvis is the key link between the axial skeleton and the major weight-bearing locomotive structures, the lower extremities. The forces resulting from activities such as sitting and ambulating are transferred through its bony structure to the spine. Major structures of the vascular, neurologic, genitourinary, and gastrointestinal systems pass through or across its ring. Because of the energy necessary to disrupt the pelvis, it has important consequences for injury to other organ systems. The potential for death or significant disability is high. Orthopaedic surgeons treating any multiply injured patient must understand and be prepared to deal with the consequences of major pelvic disruption.*

Following treatment of the pelvic injury, residual deformity or associated injuries can create significant problems in functional recovery.[44,60] Pain is a common complaint after major pelvic disruptions. Holdsworth[49] reported that 15 of 27 patients with sacroiliac (SI) joint dislocations were unable to return to work. He concluded that displacement of the SI joint was a significant cause of this disability. Peltier[87] emphasized the posterior weight-bearing capacity of the SI area and its importance in mortality and morbidity in multiply injured patients. Raf,[94] Dunn and Morris,[26] and Huittinen and Slatis[50] all confirmed that displacement through the weight-bearing arch of the pelvis, particularly the SI joint, can lead to long-term problems of pain and inability to regain function and resume the previous lifestyle.

A review by Tile[120] showed a significant difference between fractures that were classified as stable and those that were classified as unstable. The unstable group had a significant increase over the stable group in the incidence of pain in the posterior SI region. Malunion causing leg length inequalities was significantly higher in the unstable group. Persistent instability including nonunion of the pelvis was a problem, particularly in injuries that involved the SI joint. Patients in the series who had open anatomic reduction and stabilization of the pelvic ring appeared to do better. The subdivision of pelvic fractures into two groups—stable and unstable—seems to be validated by most studies.[11,20,28] Stable fractures more commonly do well and are less likely to cause disability, whereas patients with unstable fractures have more significant problems, such as a higher mortality rate[9,21,30,66] and a higher rate of dysfunction secondary to pain, malunion, and occasionally, nonunion.[43,45]

Therefore, to optimize outcomes following pelvic injuries, a multidisciplinary approach to treatment is necessary. The role of the orthopaedist should be based on an understanding of the anatomy and biomechanics of the pelvis, with particular attention regarding stability. Identification of the anatomic injury, recognition of specific patterns and their associated injuries, can guide emergent treatment as well as definitive reconstruction. The ultimate goal is to restore the displaced pelvic ring to an anatomic position while minimizing complications.

ANATOMY

The pelvis is a ring structure made up of three bones: the sacrum and two innominate bones. The three bones and three joints composing the pelvic ring have no inherent stability without vital ligamentous structures.[106] The innominate bone is formed from the fusion of three ossification centers: the ilium, the ischium, and the pubis (Fig. 36-1). These three centers coalesce at the triradiate cartilage of the acetabulum and, when fused, form the complete innominate bone. The innominate bones meet the sacrum posteriorly at the two SI joints. Anteriorly, they meet one another at the pubic symphysis. The SI joint is made up of two parts. The caudal portion consists of the articular surface of the joint; the upper, more dorsal portion, between the posterior tuberosity of the ilium and the sacrum, contains the fibrous or ligamentous parts of the joint (interosseous ligaments) (Fig. 36-2). The anterior portion of this synovial joint is covered with articular cartilage on the sacral side and fibrocartilage on the iliac side (Fig. 36-3). The joint itself has a small ridge on the sacral side that provides minimal stability. The symphysis pubis consists of two opposed surfaces of hyaline cartilage. These surfaces are covered with fibrocartilage and surrounded by a thick band of fibrous tissue.

The strongest and most important ligamentous structures are in the posterior aspect of the pelvis. These ligaments connect the sacrum to the innominate bones. The stability provided by the posterior ligaments must withstand the forces of weight-bearing transmitted across the

---

*See references 7, 21, 30, 35, 39, 60, 68, 71, 73, 76, 85, 86, 89, 90, 92, 104, 105.

FIGURE 36-1 | *The bony architecture of the pelvis consists of the sacrum and the two innominate bones. Without their ligamentous attachments, these bones provide no inherent stability.*

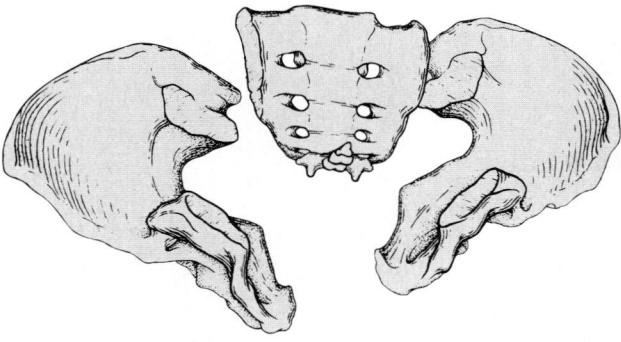

SI joints from the lower extremities to the spine. The posterior SI ligaments are divided into two components: short and long (see Fig. 36-2). The short posterior ligaments are oblique and run from the posterior ridge of the sacrum to the posterior superior and posterior inferior spines of the ilium. The long posterior ligaments are longitudinal fibers that run from the lateral aspect of the sacrum to the posterior superior iliac spines (PSIS) and merge with the sacrotuberous ligament. The long ligaments lie posterior and superficial to the short ligaments.

The anterior SI ligaments run from the ilium to the sacrum. This structure provides some stability, but less than that provided by the posterior ligaments (Fig. 36-2). The symphysis is reinforced inferiorly by muscle insertions

and the arcuate ligament. The thickest portion of this fibrous joint is usually superior and anterior.

In addition to the interosseous ligaments that span these joints, connecting ligaments join various portions of the pelvic ring. The sacrotuberous ligament is a strong band running from the posterolateral aspect of the sacrum and the dorsal aspect of the posterior iliac spine to the ischial tuberosity. Its medial border thickens to form a falciform tendon, which blends with the obturator membrane at the ischial tuberosity. It also merges into the posterior origin of the gluteus maximus. This ligament, in association with its ipsilateral posterior SI ligaments, is especially important in maintaining vertical stability of the pelvis.

The sacrospinous ligament is triangular. It runs from the lateral margins of the sacrum and coccyx and the sacrotuberous ligament to insert on the ischial spine. It divides the posterior column of the pelvis into the greater and lesser sciatic notches. The sacrospinous ligament may be important in maintaining rotational control of the pelvis if the posterior SI ligaments are intact (see Fig. 36-2).

Several ligaments run from the spine to the pelvis. The iliolumbar ligaments secure the pelvis to the lumbar spine. They originate from the L4 and L5 transverse processes and insert on the posterior iliac crest. The lumbosacral ligaments run from the transverse process of L5 to the ala of the sacrum. They form a strong ridge anteriorly and abut the L5 root.

If its ligamentous structures are intact, the pelvis is a stable ring. The posterior SI ligaments form a posterior tension band for the pelvis. The transversely placed ligaments, including the short posterior SI and the anterior SI along with the iliolumbar and sacrospinous ligaments,

FIGURE 36-2 | *Ligamentous complexes of the pelvis. **A,** Posteriorly, the major ligaments noted in the region of the sacroiliac joint are the posterior sacroiliac ligaments, both long and short. The long blend with the sacrospinous and the sacrotuberous ligaments. **B,** In cross section, the orientation of the very thick posterior interosseous sacroiliac ligaments is noted.*

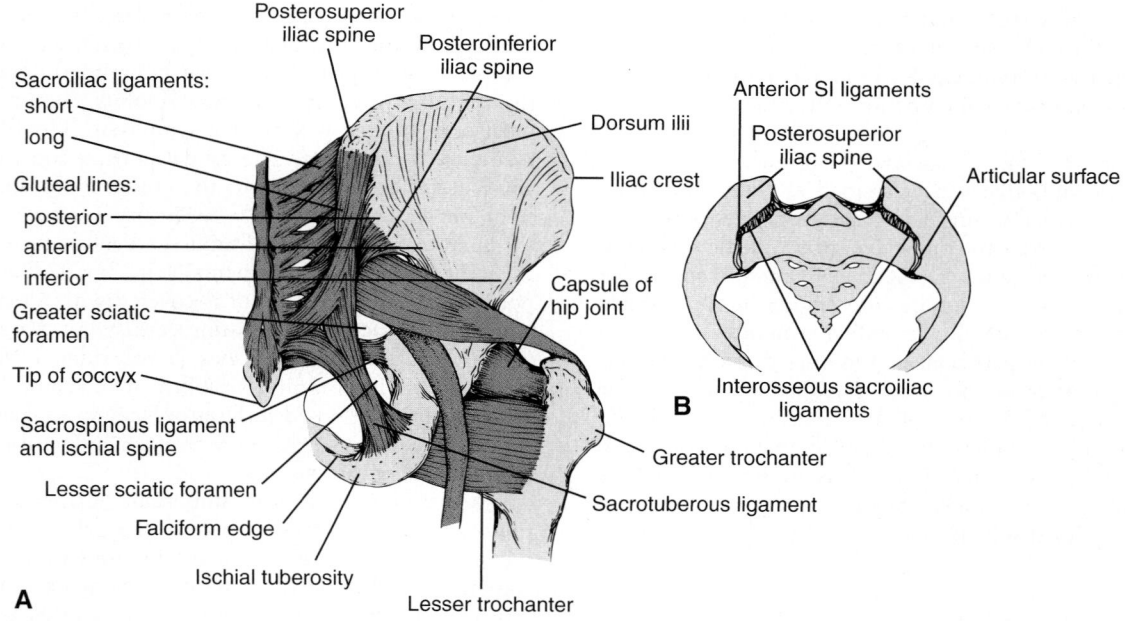

*The sacroiliac joint. **A,** Iliac side of the sacroiliac joint, as well as the remainder of the innominate bone and the important bony landmarks. **B,** Sacral side. The two portions of the sacroiliac joint can best be appreciated on these views. The articular surface of the sacroiliac joint on the sacrum has a ridge and is covered by articular cartilage. The posterior portion is filled with ligamentous structures.*

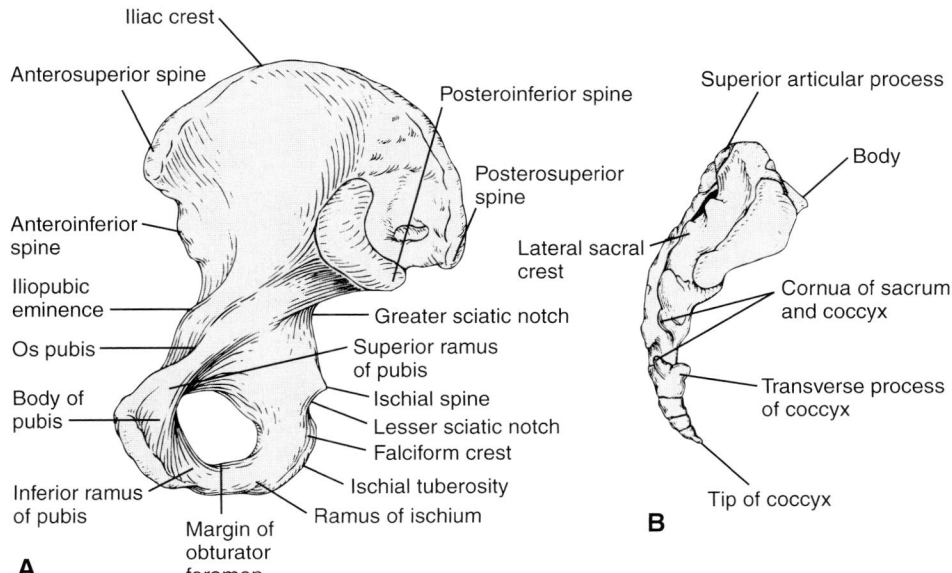

resist rotational forces. The vertically placed ligaments, including the long posterior SI, sacrotuberous, and lateral lumbosacral ligaments, may resist vertical shear or vertical migration.

The intact pelvis defines two major anatomic areas. The false pelvis and the true pelvis are divided by the pelvic brim, which runs from the sacral promontory along the junction between the ilium and the ischium onto the pubic ramus. No major muscular structures cross the pelvic brim. Above the brim, the false pelvis (greater pelvis) is contained by the sacral ala and the iliac wings. The false pelvis is lined laterally by the iliopsoas muscle. It forms part of the abdominal cavity. The true pelvis (lesser pelvis) lies below the brim, and its lateral wall consists of portions of the pubis, ischium, and a small triangular portion of the ilium. The obturator foramen, which is covered by muscles and membrane, also defines the boundary of the true pelvis. The foramen opens superiorly and laterally for passage of the obturator nerve and vessels. The obturator internus takes its origin from the membrane and curves out through the lesser sciatic notch to attach to the proximal end of the femur. The obturator internus tendon is an important structure because it serves as a guide to access the posterior column (Fig. 36-4). The piriformis originates from the lateral aspect of the sacrum and is key to understanding the sciatic nerve. Commonly, the sciatic nerve leaves the pelvis anterior to the piriformis and enters the greater sciatic notch (Fig. 36-5). Occasionally, the peroneal division leaves through or posterior to the piriformis. The floor of the true pelvis consists of the coccyx, the coccygeal and levator ani muscles, and the urethra, rectum, and vagina, which pass through them.

The lumbosacral coccygeal plexus is made up of the anterior rami of T12 through S4. The most pertinent for pelvic anatomy and injury include the L4 to S1 roots.

The lumbar roots L4 and L5 enter the true pelvis from the false pelvis, whereas the sacral roots are part of the true pelvis. The L4 root merges with L5 to form the lumbosacral trunk at the sacral promontory (12 mm from the SI joint). The L5 root is 2 cm away from the SI joint as it exits the intervertebral foramen.[3] The sacral roots pass through the sacral foramen and join the plexus. Numerous branches extend to the major muscles within the pelvis. The superior gluteal and inferior gluteal nerves leave ventral to the piriformis and exit the pelvis through the greater sciatic notch.

Major blood vessels lie on the inner wall of the pelvis. The median sacral artery is situated on the anterior aspect of the midline of the sacrum. The superior rectal artery is a major branch lying midline and posterior. The common iliac divides and gives off the internal iliac, which runs past the pelvic brim into the true pelvis. A branch of the internal iliac, the superior gluteal artery, crosses over the anterior and caudal portion of the SI joint to exit the greater sciatic notch. As it sweeps around the notch, it lies directly on bone. The external iliac artery runs cranial to the pelvic brim (pubic ramus), exiting the pelvis posterior to the inguinal ligament were it becomes the common femoral artery. These arteries and associated veins can all be injured and represent a potential source for significant hemorrhage during pelvic disruption (Fig. 36-6).

The major components of the genitourinary system contained with in the pelvis are the ureters, bladder, and urethra. The bladder is situated cranial to the pelvic floor (i.e., coccygeal and levator ani muscles). These muscles arise in continuity from the ischial spines, obturator membrane, and pubis and insert into the coccyx and anal coccygeal raphe. They form a muscular diaphragm with a gap anteriorly through which pass the urethra, vagina, rectum,

FIGURE 36-4 *Internal aspect of the pelvis. **A,** The inner aspect of the pelvis consists of the true pelvis, which is below the pelvic brim, and the false pelvis above it. The sacrotuberous and sacrospinous ligaments are attached to their appropriate structures and form the basis of the pelvic floor. **B,** The major structures in the inner aspect of the pelvis are the lumbosacral plexus, which originates from the L5 and the sacral roots and leaves the pelvis through the greater sciatic notch as the sciatic nerve, and the superior gluteal artery. The obturator internus originates from the obturator membrane and loops out through the lesser sciatic notch. Note that no muscles cross the pelvic brim.*

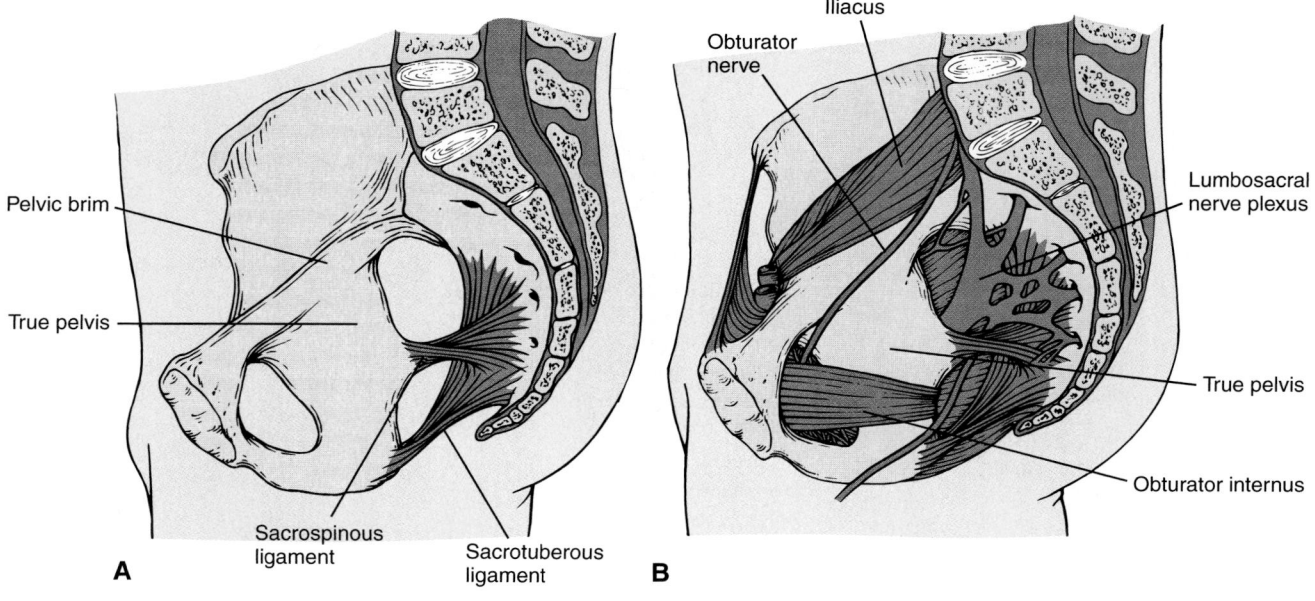

FIGURE 36-5 *The outer aspect of the pelvis shows how the piriformis originates from the inner aspect of the pelvis and attaches to the greater trochanter. Cranial to this structure, the superior gluteal artery and vein lie very close to bone in the sciatic notch. This proximity to bone makes these vessels vulnerable to injury in pelvic disruptions. Below the piriformis, the sciatic nerve usually disappears and runs extremely close to the ischium.*

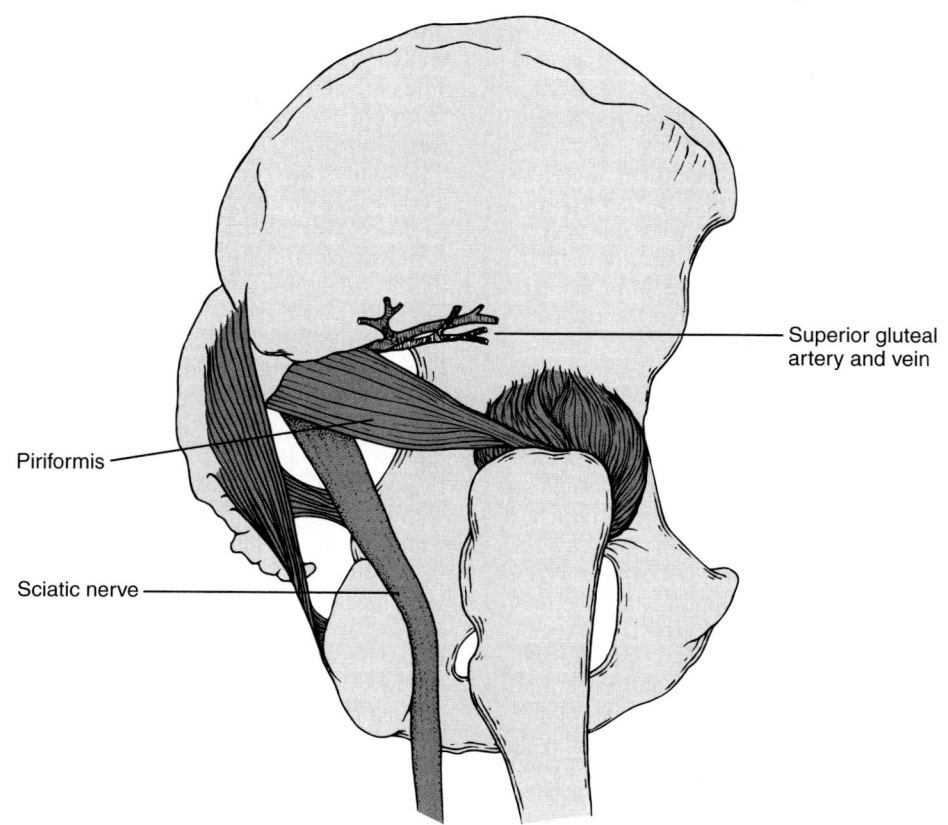

FIGURE 36-6 *Internal aspect of the pelvis showing the great vessels and the lumbosacral plexus, as well as the pelvic floor, bladder, and rectum.*

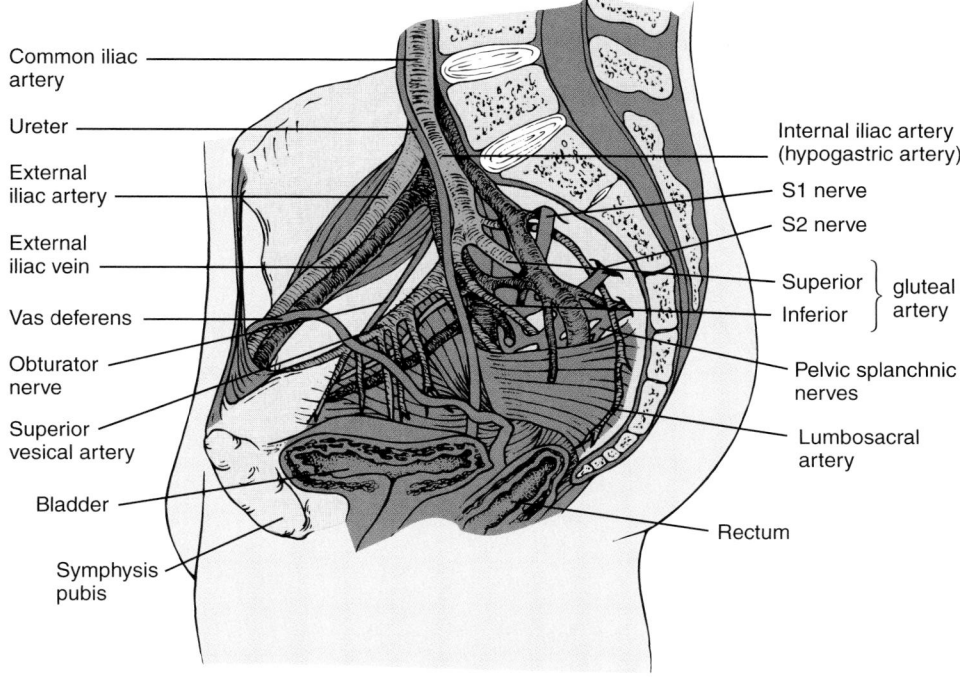

Common iliac artery
Ureter
External iliac artery
External iliac vein
Vas deferens
Obturator nerve
Superior vesical artery
Bladder
Symphysis pubis
Internal iliac artery (hypogastric artery)
S1 nerve
S2 nerve
Superior
Inferior } gluteal artery
Pelvic splanchnic nerves
Lumbosacral artery
Rectum

and their supporting ligaments. The fascia of the pelvic floor is loose and mobile. In males, the prostate lies between the bladder and pelvic floor and is invested by a dense fascial membrane. The urethra passes through the prostate and before it exits below the pelvic floor. The junction between the prostate and the pelvic floor is strong, as is the membranous urethra. The weak link in this area is the urethra below the pelvic diaphragm in its bulbous portion. Colapinto has shown that when the bladder is pulled forcefully, the urethra ruptures in its bulbous portion, which is the most common site of urethral rupture below the pelvic floor.[15] Occasionally, the membranous portion of the urethra ruptures at the upper surface of the pelvic floor. In females, the urethral injury is near the bladder neck. Urinary continence depends on the external (striated muscle) sphincter at the membranous urethra (midurethra in females) and the bladder neck (smooth muscle) in both males and females. Structures also passing through the urogenital diaphragm are the pudendal arteries and veins, the pudendal nerve (S2-S4), and the autonomic nerves of the pelvis (S2-S4). These are all responsible for normal sexual function.

PELVIC STABILITY

A stable pelvic injury can be defined as one that can withstand normal physiologic forces without abnormal deformation. In the upright position, the weight of the body pushes the sacrum down between the iliac wings and causes approximately 5° dorsoventral rotation.[79] The innominate bones move posteriorly and a flexion rotation occurs as the posterior ring moves caudally and the pubic rami swing cranially.[60] Tile and Hearn[121] also

demonstrated using a physiologic mechanical testing system that with sitting or standing, the symphysis is in tension and the posterior complex is compressed. In single stance, the symphysis is compressed and the posterior complex is distracted. For these actions to occur, the pelvic ring must maintain its integrity through its ligamentous and bony components.[113]

Sequential sectioning of the pelvic ligaments can help define the relative contribution of individual components to the spectrum of pelvic stability.[113] If only the symphysis is sectioned, mechanical testing of the pelvis reveals a symphyseal diastasis no greater than 2.5 cm (Fig. 36-7A). Further opening is inhibited by the sacrospinous and anterior SI ligaments. If the symphysis, pelvic floor ligaments and anterior SI ligaments are sectioned, more than 2.5 cm of external rotation (diastasis) is noted (Fig. 36-7B). Abutment of the posterior iliac spines against the sacrum stops the pelvis from any further rotation. These investigators noted that cranial or posterior displacement did not occur because the posterior longitudinal ligaments and sacrotuberous ligaments remained intact. In this situation, the pelvis is only rotationally unstable and can therefore be restored to its anatomic integrity by reduction and stabilization of the anterior ring, using the intact posterior osseous ligamentous hinge.

With sectioning all of the symphysis, sacrospinous, sacrotuberous, and posterior SI ligaments, the pelvis becomes globally unstable and is free to translate or rotate in any direction (see Fig. 36-7C). Keep in mind that some bone injuries produce instability equivalent to that caused by disruption of the posterior ligaments. Fractures through the iliac wing, fracture dislocations of the SI joint, or some complete fractures of the sacrum bypass the

FIGURE 36-7   *A, Division of the symphysis pubis allows the pelvis to open to approximately 2.5 cm with no damage to any posterior ligamentous structures. B, Division of the anterior sacroiliac and sacrospinous ligaments, either by direct division of their fibers (right) or by avulsion of the tip of the ischial spine (left), allows the pelvis to rotate externally until the posterior superior iliac spines abut the sacrum. Note, however, that the posterior ligamentous structures (e.g., the posterior sacroiliac and iliolumbar ligaments) remain intact. Therefore, no displacement in the vertical plane is possible. C, Division of the posterior band ligaments, that is, the posterior sacroiliac, as well as the iliolumbar, causes complete instability of the hemipelvis. Note that global displacement is now possible.*

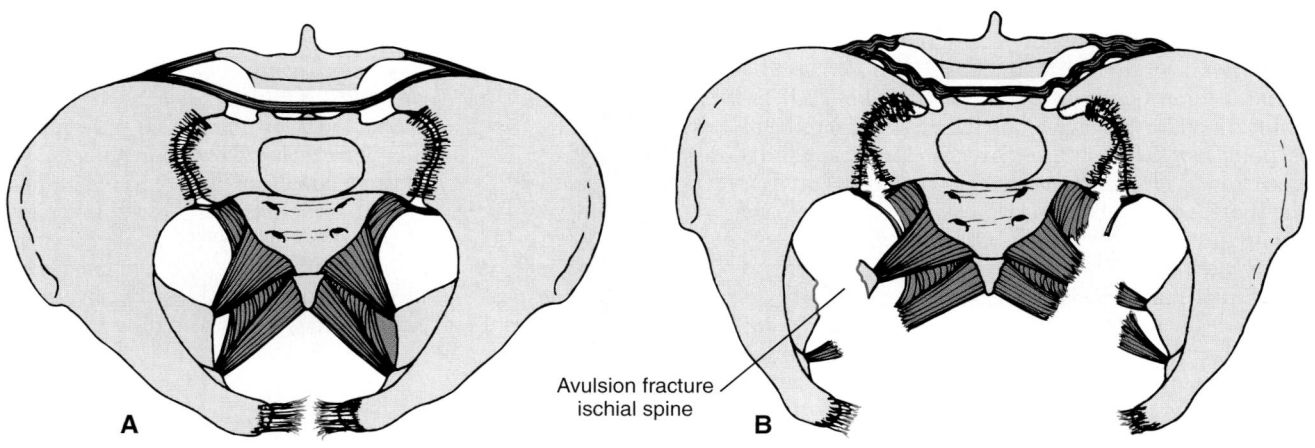

Avulsion fracture
ischial spine

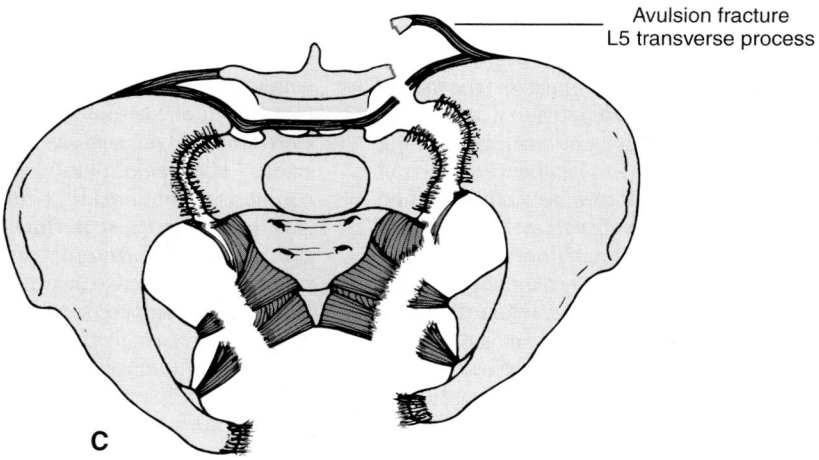

Avulsion fracture
L5 transverse process

ligamentous structures and, hence, may represent globally unstable posterior injuries. Avulsion fractures of the ischial spine, ischial tuberosity, or lateral sacrum can indicate injuries equivalent to ligamentous disruption of the pelvic floor. Holographic analysis of pelvic stability following more selective ligament sectioning has shown that removal of the sacrotuberous or sacrospinous ligaments, or both, has no effect on patterns of pelvic deformation. However, if the SI interosseous ligaments are excised, the sacrum becomes wedged deeply into the pelvis on erect loading.[119] If the symphysis remains intact while only the posterior ligaments are sectioned, little posterior instability occurs because the posterior bony complex is compressed.[11]

Radiographic Anatomy of the Pelvis

The pelvis is a complex three-dimensional structure that is most commonly represented with two-dimensional images. A single anteroposterior (AP) radiograph of the pelvis can convey a significant amount of information regarding pelvic stability and associated injuries, and in the majority of cases, can be sufficient to initiate treatment in emergency situations. Therefore it is important to be familiar with normal AP imaging and some of the most common variants.

TECHNIQUES

An AP radiograph of the pelvis should be centered just cranial (1–2 cm) to the pubic symphysis. The umbilicus serves as a reliable midline landmark with the beam generated approximately 40 cm from the film. The radiographic field should be cleared of all foreign materials and debris.

Evaluation can begin from either posterior or anterior and work around the pelvic ring. A systematic way of reviewing the radiograph should be undertaken each time so that injuries are not missed, especially in the circumstance of other obvious injuries that may distract the surgeon. The pelvis in its entirety can vary in size and shape, depending on the individual and gender, but it is most commonly a symmetrical structure and differences from side to side must therefore be investigated and explained. For instance, the iliac wings, acetabulum, and obturator rings should be of a similar shape, size, and orientation. The acetabuli should be equidistant from the midline.

EVALUATION

We usually begin our evaluation posterior and midline with the lower lumbar spine and the lumbosacral junction. The spinous processes should be midline and the pedicles symmetrically placed on either side. The transverse processes of the lower lumbar segments are perpendicular to the beam, and therefore easily visible. Without complete lumbar films, it may be difficult to distinguish L5 from S1. The lumbar spine has a typical lordosis, and the angle between it and the sacrum and can vary between 30 and 60° (sacral inclination, sacrovertebral angle), making the

sacrum appear differently between individuals on an AP pelvis. There are typically five lumbar and sacral segments. Normally, L5 and S1 bodies are completely segmented but may be incomplete with one side or both unsegmented (Fig. 36-8). This lumbosacral dysmorphism can be present in up to 21 percent of individuals.[117,122] The sacral foramina are then evaluated for cortical disruptions. The width of sacral ala of S1 is compared with the contralateral side. This is followed by evaluation of the SI joints, looking for asymmetries or widening. The evaluation of the posterior pelvis continues by following the iliac crest from the posterior spine to the anterior superior iliac spine (ASIS), anterior inferior iliac spine (AIIS), and the roof of the acetabulum. The ilium itself should be examined for fracture lines, width, and deformity. Completing the posterior pelvic evaluation, the brim or iliopectineal line is followed posteriorly and should project medially past the SI joint to the cranial cortical margin of the S2 foramen. This is described as the arcuate line and may help in identifying cranial displacement of the hemipelvis or cortical irregularities of the second sacral foramen (see Fig. 36-8). The six acetabular lines of Judet should be

FIGURE 36-8 *Anteroposterior and cranial (inlet) views of the pelvis. **A,** Note the sacral dysmorphism with incomplete segmentation of the transverse process of L5. Continuation of the pelvic brim extends onto the roof of the S2 foramen. **B,** Complex injuries of the pelvic ring and acetabulum may detract from evaluation of sacral dysmorphism appreciated on the inlet view.*

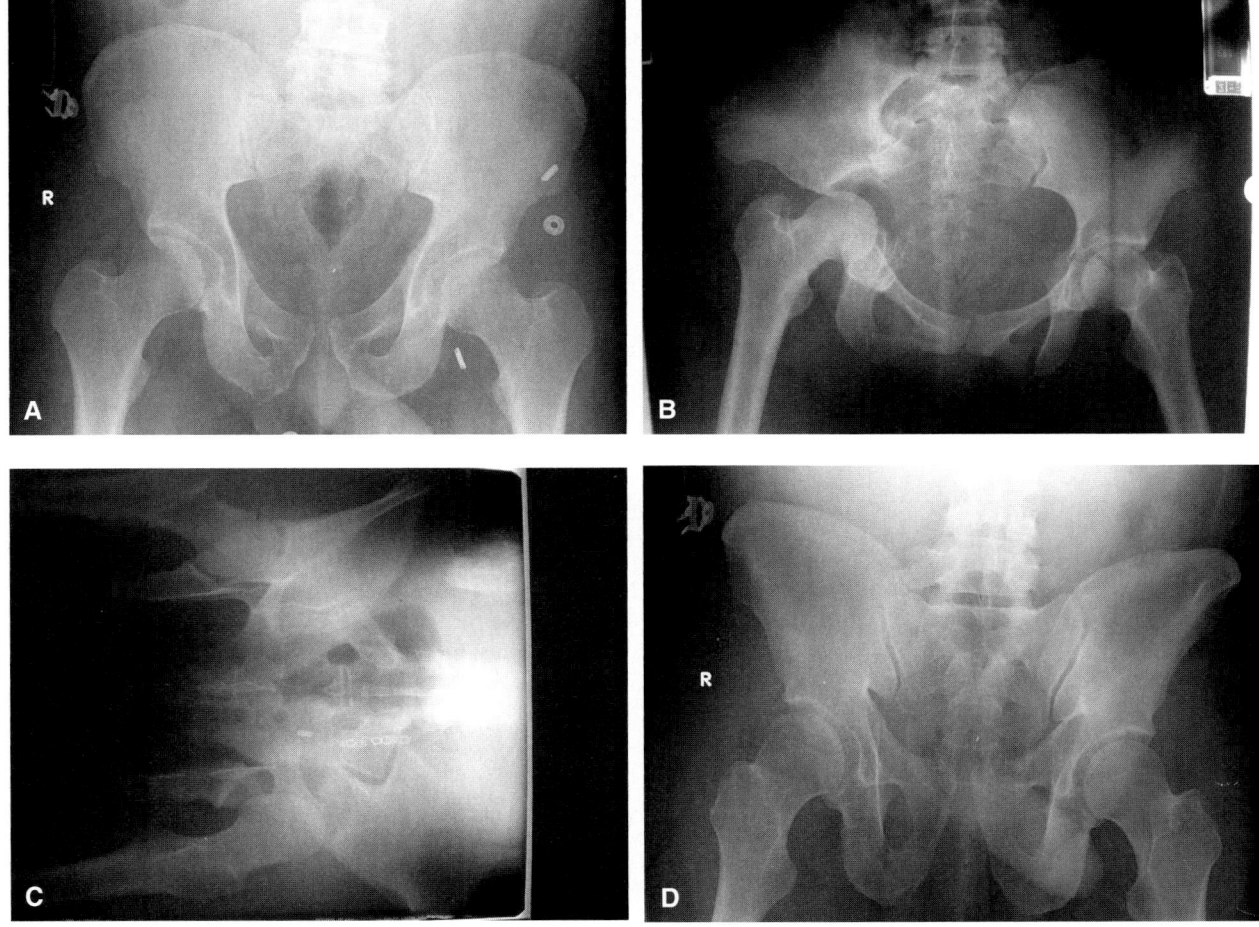

evaluated next to determine if fractures of the acetabulum are present (see Chapter 37 for more detail). The pubic and ischial rami, the pubic body, along with the shape and size of the obturator ring define injury or post-traumatic deformity of the anterior ring. Finally the symphysis pubis is scrutinized for abnormal width, overlap, or discrepancies in height of either pubic body relative to the other.

Depending on the injury and force application, deformation or displacement of the pelvis occurs through zones of injury, whether fractures of the bony pelvis or ligamentous disruptions. Theoretically, displacement could occur in any direction, and the resultant deformity be defined anatomically in planes of translation (cranial–caudad,

anterior–posterior, medial–lateral) and rotation (commonly thought of in terms of flexion–extension, abduction–adduction, and internal–external). Following full cataloging of anatomic injuries, residual displacement or deformity should be critically analyzed. A vertical line down the middle of the lumbar spinous processes to the tip of the coccyx is drawn to start the process. Perpendiculars are then added to determine the relative cranial–caudal translation of the ischium, acetabular roof, and inferior SI joint facet compared with the intact hemipelvis (Fig. 36-9). Relative displacements of anterior-to-posterior structures from the midline or perpendiculars can also define medial lateral plane translation and help evaluate

FIGURE 36-9 **A–C** *depict common methods for evaluation and descriptions for hemipelvic displacement.*

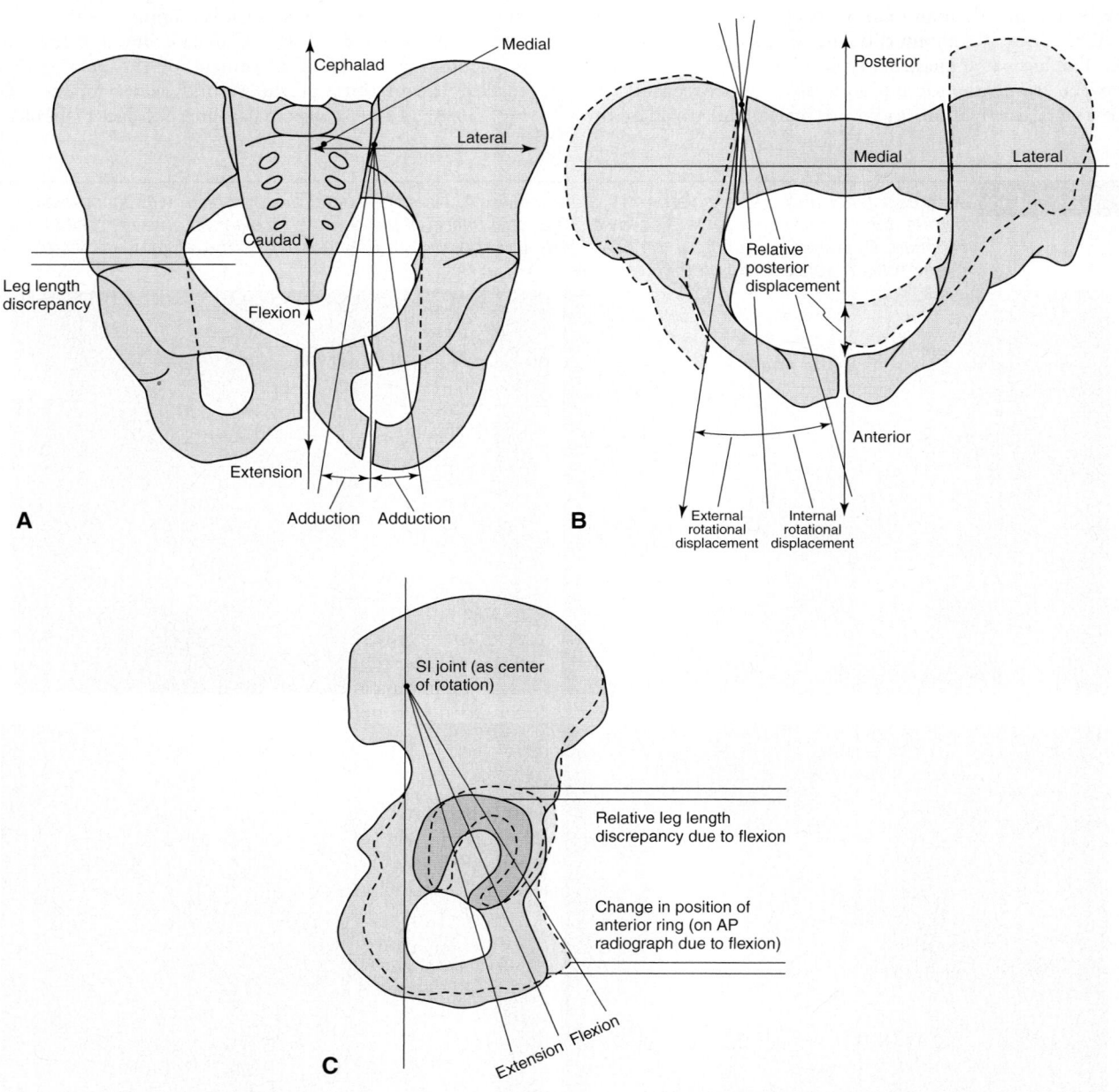

for rotational deformities. In rotationally unstable injuries, the center of rotation is typically near the posterior ring injury. Therefore by convention, in globally unstable injuries, rotational deformities are described in this fashion as well. Other than specific measurements, the overall appearance of the hemipelvis also provides clues to rotational deformity. A wider iliac wing and a smaller obturator foramen are typical for external rotation deformity. Cranial displacement of the acetabular roof with a larger obturator foramen and less cranial displacement of the posterior iliac crest may be associated with flexion–rotation of the hemipelvis rather than complete posterior ring instability.

Evaluation of the AP pelvis for determination of anatomic zones of injury and deformity recognition is important throughout the treatment of a patient with a pelvic fracture. From initial resuscitation, determination of stability, and, finally, reconstruction, an understanding of deformity helps guide treatment. Final reduction and restoration of stability in the reconstructive phase depends on it.

PATHOMECHANICS AND MECHANISMS OF PELVIC DISRUPTION

Pelvic disruptions are commonly felt to occur secondary to four types of force application. The first two, AP compressions and lateral compression, are applied directly to the pelvic ring, whereas abduction–external rotation and shear may be transmitted indirectly to the pelvic ring. Each force application can result in characteristic deformities of the pelvic ring.

Anteroposterior Force Pattern

The AP force pattern typically causes external rotation of the hemipelvis. As a result of a posteriorly directed force, the pelvis is usually disrupted at the pubic symphysis and springs open, injuring the pelvic floor and anterior SI ligaments, hinging on the intact posterior ligaments. This force more commonly results in only rotational instability because the posterior ligamentous complex remains intact (see Fig. 36-7B).

Lateral Compression Force Pattern

The most common force pattern of pelvic fractures is lateral compression. Depending on the point of application and the magnitude of this force, different lateral compression injuries are seen. If force is applied to the posterior aspect of the pelvis it is typically parallel to the trabeculae of the sacrum, creating compression or impaction of the cancellous bone of the sacrum. It causes minimal soft tissue disruption because the posterior ligamentous structures relax as the hemipelvis is driven inward. Because the force of injury is essentially parallel to the ligament fibers and trabeculae of the bone, it produces a very stable fracture configuration.

In the second type of lateral compression, the force is directed over the anterior half of the iliac wing. This force tends to rotate the hemipelvis inward, with the pivot point being the anterior SI joint or anterior ala. Consequently, the anterior portion of the sacrum is crushed,

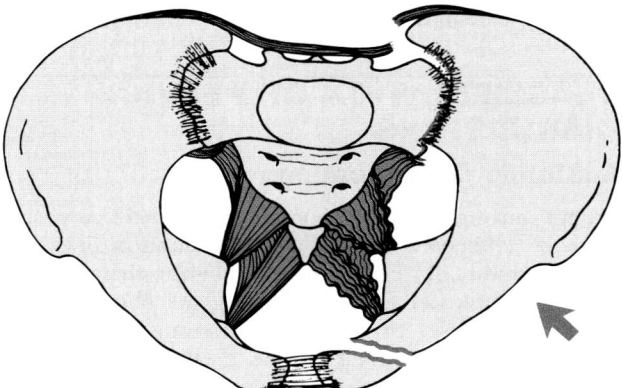

FIGURE 36-10 *Lateral compression—unstable. In this mechanism, the force (arrow) is directed over the anterior aspect of the hemipelvis. The hemipelvis pivots around the anterior portion of the sacroiliac joint, thus compressing the sacrum or fracturing through the ilium (or both). Posteriorly, the posterior interosseous hinge is now disrupted and the pelvis is unstable in internal rotation. It may exhibit some degree of vertical instability. Vertical instability is limited by the intact sacrotuberous ligaments.*

and disruption of the posterior SI ligament complex may follow.[21,124] This injury becomes more unstable as disruption of the posterior osseous or ligamentous structures become more severe. However, the sacrospinous and sacrotuberous ligaments remain intact along with the pelvic floor, thereby limiting translational instability (Fig. 36-10). This force can continue to push the hemipelvis across to the opposite side, producing a lateral compression injury on the side of force application and an external rotation injury on the contralateral side.[124] The resulting anterior pelvic lesions may be any combination of ramus fractures or fracture–dislocations through the symphysis. The fractures of the pubic rami are typically horizontal in orientation. Finally, a force applied over the greater trochanteric region also produces a lateral compression injury, usually associated with an acetabular fracture.

External Rotation–Abduction Force Patterns

The third force, common in motorcycle accidents, is an external rotation–abduction force. This force is usually applied indirectly through the femoral shafts and hips. The leg is caught and externally rotated and abducted, a mechanism that tends to tear the hemipelvis from the sacrum.

Shear Force Pattern

Shear fractures are the result of high-energy forces usually applied perpendicular to the bony trabeculae; these forces quite commonly lead to unstable fractures or dislocations or both. The exact fracture pattern depends on both the amount of force applied and the bone strength in relation to the ligamentous structures. In general, if bone strength is less than ligamentous strength, the bone fails first. In the setting of shear force, this failure commonly results in sacral fractures and vertically oriented rami fractures, as opposed to the horizontal pattern seen in lateral compression. Conversely, if the bone strength is relatively greater, ligamentous injuries usually occur and manifest with pubic symphysis and SI joint disruptions.[40]

In conclusion, the mechanism of injury can be obtained from history and may be inferred from fracture pattern, but not always.[64a] The fracture pattern, displacement, deformity, and clinical exam provide clues to pelvic stability. Subsequent diagnostic tests and classifications are aimed at categorization of the stability to enable logical treatment decisions.

CLASSIFICATION OF PELVIC DISRUPTIONS

Anatomic Classifications

Several anatomic classifications have been proposed. Bucholz[12] proposed a pathologic classification based on autopsy studies. Five sites of injury were characterized: (1) anterior vertical fractures dividing the obturator ring or adjacent bodies of the pubis, (2) transiliac fractures extending from the crest of the greater sciatic notch, (3) trans-sacral fractures either outside or inside the foramina, (4) pure separation of the symphysis, and (5) pure disruption of the SI joint.

Letournel and Judet[64] suggested a more comprehensive classification based on the site of injury (Fig. 36-11). These include injuries to the posterior ring (i.e., sacral fractures, SI joint fracture–dislocations, SI joint dislocations, and iliac wing fractures), acetabulum, and anterior ring (rami fractures, pubic body fractures, and symphyseal disruptions). Regardless of which classification scheme a surgeon subsequently uses, identification of specific anatomic injuries from complete evaluation of the radiographs as outlined by Letournel is necessary. This classification still serves as the most descriptive system and is commonly used in conjunction with current classification schemes to define a specific patient's injury.

Mechanism-of-Injury Classification (Young and Burgess)

A classification by Young and Burgess[134] based on the mechanisms of injury previously discussed alerts the surgeon to potential associated injuries and resuscitation requirements that may be associated with pelvic fractures. The classification has three major components (Fig. 36-12).

The first component in the Young and Burgess classification is a lateral compression injury.[134] A lateral compression type I injury results from a posteriorly applied force that causes sacral impaction. It is stable. Patients with these injuries usually have minimal problems with resuscitation. A lateral compression type II injury follows a more anteriorly directed force with resultant disruption of the posterior osseous–ligamentous structures but maintenance the pelvic floor. The result is rotational instability. It may be associated with an anterior sacral crush injury. Lateral compression type II injuries are often associated with head injuries and intra-abdominal trauma. A lateral compression type III injury results from a laterally directed force that has continued to cross the pelvis to produce an external rotation injury to the contralateral hemipelvis. This is usually the result of an isolated direct impact (crush) to the pelvis. A common example is being run over by a car. The injury is usually isolated to the pelvis and has a minimum of significant associated injuries.

The second is an AP compression injury,[134] which is divided into three types. Type I is characterized by less than 2.5 cm of anterior ring diastasis and consists of vertical fractures of the pubic rami or disruption of the symphysis. Because no posterior injury of significance occurs, problems with resuscitation are minimal. An AP compression type II injury has greater than 2.5 cm of anterior ring diastasis with opening of the SI joints, resulting in rotational instability. An AP compression type III injury is a complete disruption anteriorly and posteriorly. Type II and type III have significant resuscitation requirements. The type III fracture is globally unstable with significant associated injuries.

The final component is a vertically unstable or shear injury and a combined mechanism injury leading to unstable fracture patterns with significant retroperitoneal hemorrhage and major associated injuries.[21,134]

Arbeitsgemeinschaft für Osteosynthesefragen System– Orthopaedic Trauma Association Comprehensive Pelvic Classification (Modified After Tile)

This classification combines both the mechanism of injury and the degree of pelvic stability and can be used as an aid in determining the prognosis and treatment options.[43,112]

FIGURE 36-11 *The Letournel and Judet classification of pelvic fractures is anatomic. A, Iliac wing fractures; B, ilium fractures with extension to the sacroiliac joint; C, trans-sacral fractures; D, unilateral sacral fractures; E, sacroiliac joint fracture–dislocation; F, acetabular fractures; G, pubic ramus fractures; H, ischial fractures; I, pubic symphysis separation. Combinations of all of these injuries can occur.*

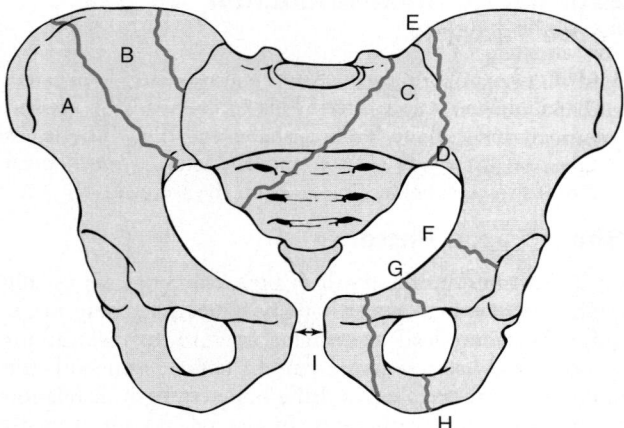

FIGURE 36-12 *Young and Burgess classification.* **A,** *Lateral compression force. Type I: A posteriorly directed force causing a sacral crushing injury and horizontal pubic ramus fractures ipsilaterally. This injury is stable. Type II: A more anteriorly directed force causing horizontal pubic ramus fractures with an anterior sacral crushing injury and either disruption of the posterior sacroiliac joints or fractures through the iliac wing. This injury is ipsilateral. Type III: An anteriorly directed force that is continued and leads to a type I or type II ipsilateral fracture with an external rotation component to the contralateral side; the sacroiliac joint is opened posteriorly, and the sacrotuberous and spinous ligaments are disrupted.* **B,** *Anteroposterior (AP) compression fractures. Type I: An AP-directed force opening the pelvis but with the posterior ligamentous structures intact. This injury is stable. Type II: Continuation of a type I fracture with disruption of the sacrospinous and potentially the sacrotuberous ligaments and an anterior sacroiliac joint opening. This fracture is rotationally unstable. Type III: A completely unstable or a vertical instability pattern with complete disruption of all ligamentous supporting structures.* **C,** *A vertically directed force or forces at right angles to the supporting structures of the pelvis leading to vertical fractures in the rami and disruption of all the ligamentous structures. This injury is equivalent to an AP type III or a completely unstable and rotationally unstable fracture. (Redrawn from Young, J.W.R.; Burgess, A.R. Radiologic Management of Pelvic Ring Fractures. Baltimore, Munich, Urban & Schwarzenberg, 1987.)*

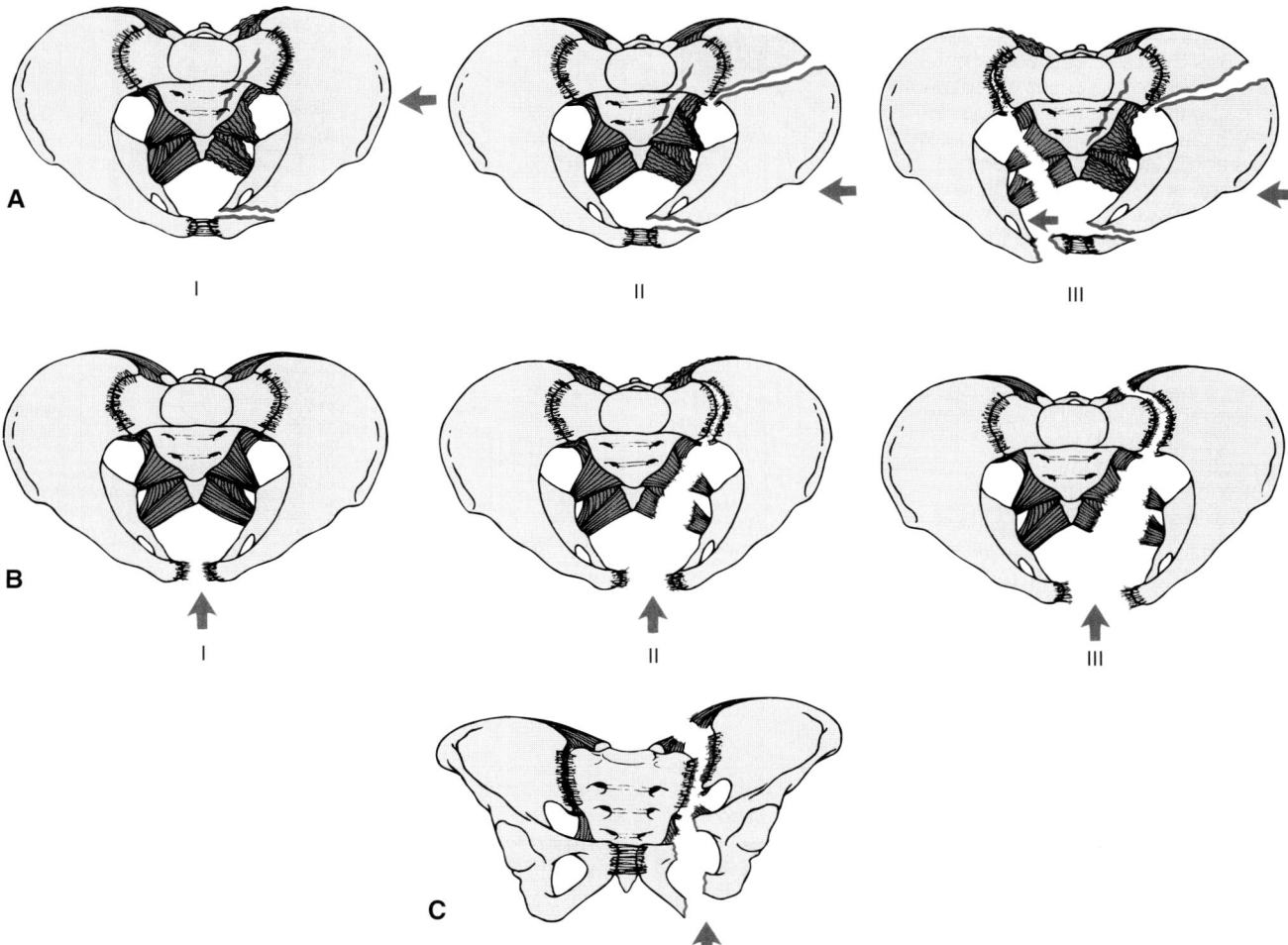

A   I   II   III

B   I   II   III

C

Determination of pelvic stability with regard to rotational or global displacement, the history and mechanism of injury, and assessment of soft tissue injuries facilitates a complete classification.

Type A injuries preserve the bony and ligamentous integrity of the posterior complex of the pelvis and the pelvic floor and therefore never cause pelvic ring instability (Fig. 36-13). Surgical reduction and fixation may still be indicated in some. A type A1 injury consists of avulsion of the pelvic apophyses by a sudden muscular pull; these injuries usually require only symptomatic care. Type A2 injuries represent isolated iliac wing fractures. Because they have not violated the posterior osseous ligamentous hinge, they remain completely stable. This group includes a spectrum of injuries resulting from direct blows. The undisplaced low-energy injuries are usually seen in osteoporotic bone, and the high-energy direct blows in younger individuals can result in open fractures (Fig. 36-14). A type A3 injury is a fracture of the sacrum and coccyx that does not involve the posterior supporting elements (below S2). As shown by Denis and colleagues[24] and Kaehr and co-workers,[51] appropriate neurologic assessment of these sacral fractures

FIGURE 36-13 | *Modified Tile AO Müller classification. Type A: Stable posterior arch with intact pelvic ring injuries. Group 1 represents avulsion fractures of the iliac spine (A1.1), iliac crest (A1.2), and ischial tuberosity (A1.3). Group 2 represents fractures of the innominate bone or injuries from direct blows: iliac wing (A2.1), unilateral anterior arch (A2.2), and bifocal anterior arch (A2.3). Group 3 represents transverse fractures of the sacrum caudal to S2: Sacrococcygeal dislocation (A3.1), sacrum undisplaced (A3.2), and sacrum displaced (A3.3). (Redrawn from Müller, E., ed. Comprehensive Classification of Pelvis and Acetabulum Fractures. Bern, Switzerland, Maurice E. Müller Foundation, 1995.)*

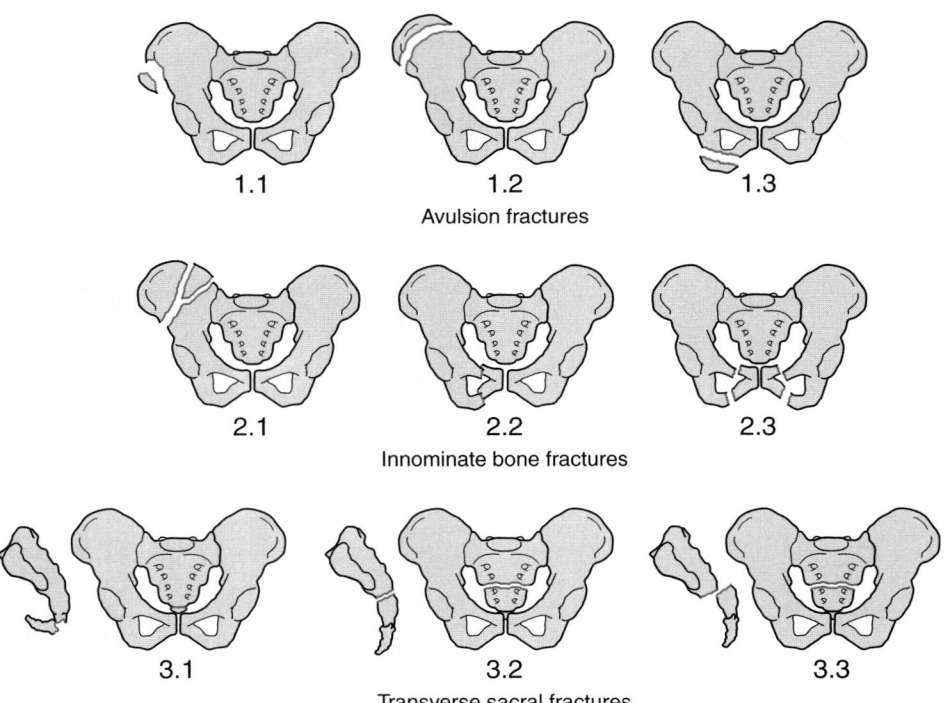

is necessary to determine whether decompression may be required. If the sacral fracture extends into the S1 and S2 vertebrae and is associated with an anterior injury, it is more appropriately classified as a pelvic ring disruption.

Type B fractures are incomplete disruptions of the posterior arch that allow rotation of the hemipelvis (Fig. 36-15A). A B1 injury is a unilateral external rotation (open-book B1.1) or tension failure fracture through the sacrum (B1.2). A variable degree of rotational instability may be present with these injuries and may require further clinical or radiographic analysis to determine the degree (Fig. 36-15B–D).

FIGURE 36-14 | *Type A injuries. Avulsion fracture of the ischial spine occurring in a skeletally immature athlete. A high-energy direct blow to the iliac wing resulting in an open fracture of the iliac wing.*

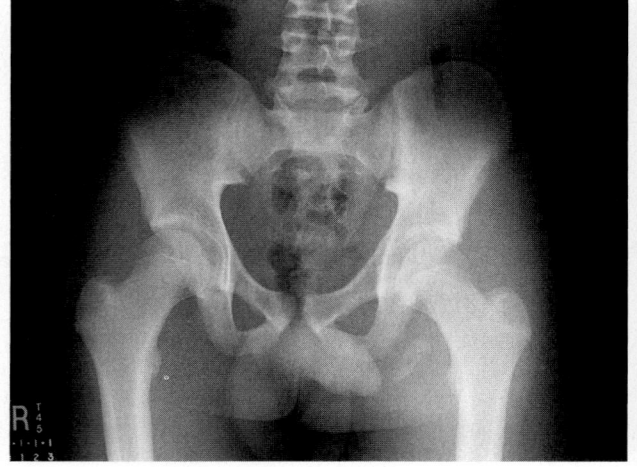 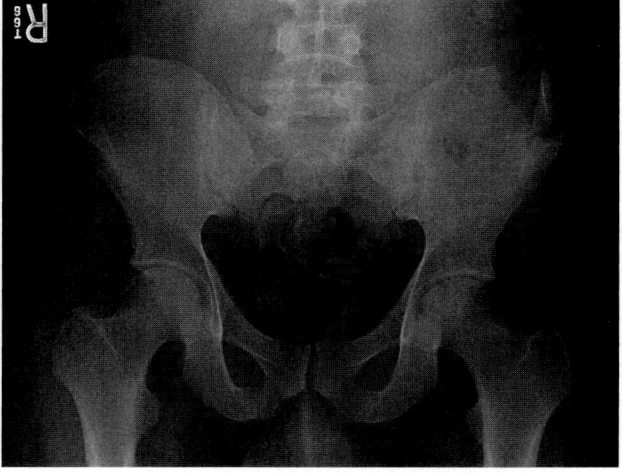

FIGURE 36-15 | *A, Examples of B type injuries, all with anterior symphyseal disruptions. Anterior injuries can also include unilateral or bilateral rami fractures. **B,** B1.1 with injury to the anterior sacroiliac (SI) joint. Note air density within the joint, which may indicate rotational injury through the joint. Physical exam may confirm the instability. **C,** B1.1 injury with obvious instability. Computed tomography confirms unilateral injury through the SI joint with concomitant tensile sacral fracture.*

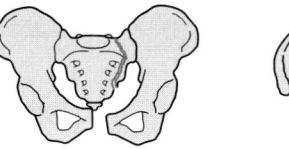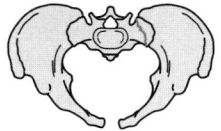

1.1
Through anterior SI joint

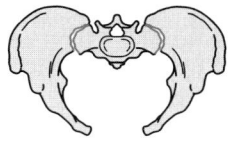

1.2
Sacral fracture

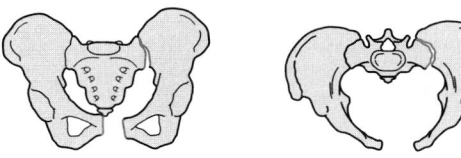

A   **B3.1**

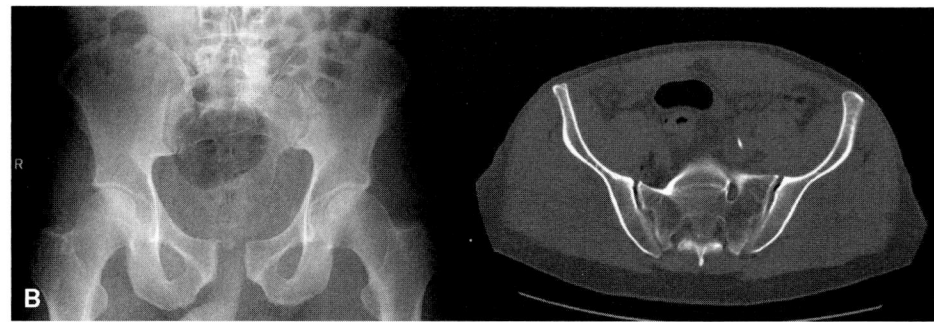

B

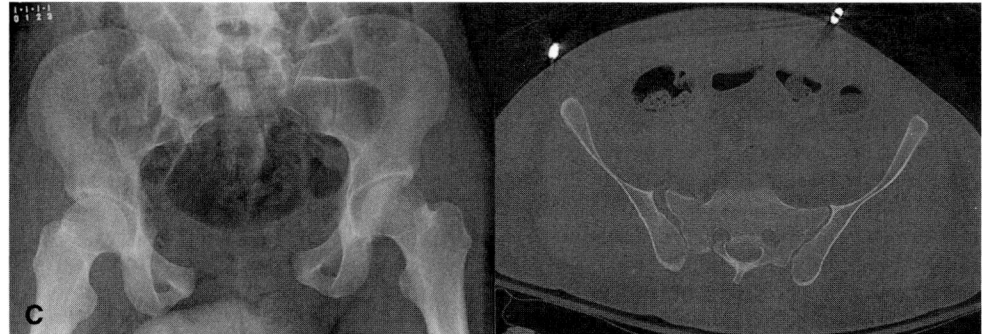

C

(Continued)

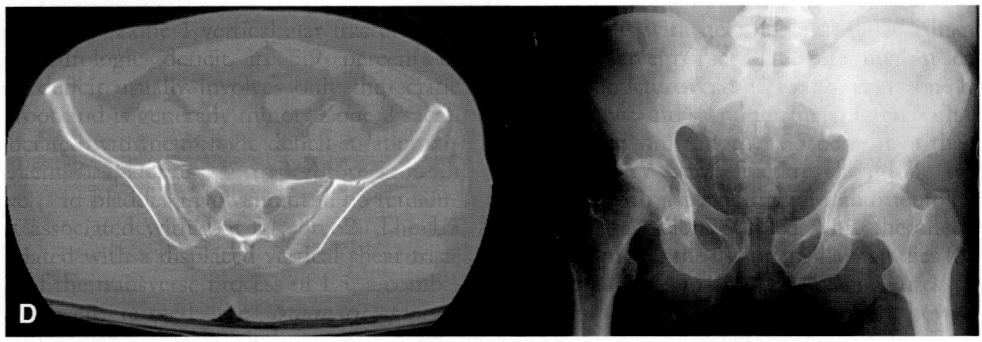

Type B2 injuries are produced by lateral compression or internal rotation and are also only rotationally unstable (Fig. 36-16). A type B2.1 injury is caused by a force directed over the posterior iliac wing. This results in a sacral impaction injury and most commonly with horizontally oriented rami fractures (Fig. 36-17A). As noted earlier, this does not result in injury to the posterior pelvic or pelvic floor ligaments. A B2.2 injury is produced by a lateral compression force and involves a partial fracture–subluxation of the SI joint, associated with anterior ring fractures or fracture dislocations of the pubic symphysis. The typical posterior fracture pattern extends from the iliac wing into the SI joint, with ligamentous disruption of the caudal SI joint. A portion of the cranial iliac wing and SI joint remain attached to the sacrum. These rotationally unstable injuries are the equivalent of the Young and Burgess lateral compression type II injuries. Because the force of injury is applied in an oblique fashion across the pelvis, the involved portion of the pelvis is flexed, adducted, and internally rotated, positioning the femoral head cranially; these can be associated with a leg length discrepancy (see Fig. 36-17B).

Less common anterior arch injuries associated with B2 injuries can be a locked symphysis or a tilt fracture. A locked symphysis injury disrupts the symphysis rather than fracturing the rami as it drives one side of the symphysis behind the other (Fig. 36-18A). A tilt fracture is an unusual anterior variant associated with a lateral compression mechanism in which the superior pubic ramus is fractured at the pubic root near the acetabulum and through the ischial ramus; continued medial displacement of the hemipelvis causes dislocation of the symphysis or fracture of the pubic body, allowing the fragment to tilt caudally and anteriorly into the perineum. This injury is seen more commonly in females than males. The major problem with this fracture is its position within the perineum, where the fragment can protrude into the vagina with resulting dyspareunia (Fig. 36-18B).

Type B3 injury is a bilateral posterior ring injury with neither side vertically unstable and each side possibly having a different mechanism of injury. A type B3.1 injury

FIGURE 36-16 *Modified Tile AO Müller classification. Type B: Incomplete disruptions (internal rotation). Internally directed or lateral compression forces cause anterior sacral compression injuries (B2.1), partial fracture–subluxations of the sacroiliac joint (B2.2), and incomplete posterior iliac wing fractures (B2.3). (Redrawn from Müller, E., ed. Comprehensive Classification of Pelvis and Acetabulum Fractures. Bern, Switzerland, Maurice E. Müller Foundation, 1995.)*

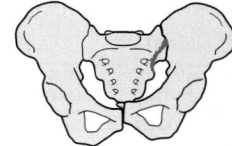 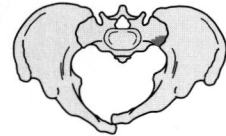

2.1

Anterior sacral compression injury

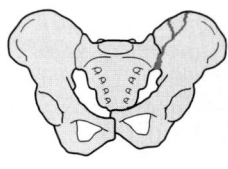 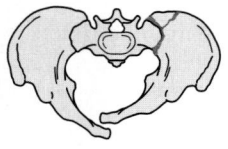

2.2

Partial fracture subluxation of sacroiliac joint

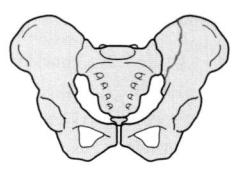 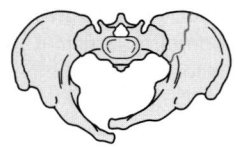

2.3

Incomplete posterior iliac fracture

FIGURE 36-17 *Clinical example of lateral compression-type injuries. **A,** B2.1 Anterior sacral compression fracture associated with contralateral segmental parasymphyseal fracture. **B,** Crescent fracture. Note the fracture entering the caudal portion of the sacroiliac joint with dislocation.*

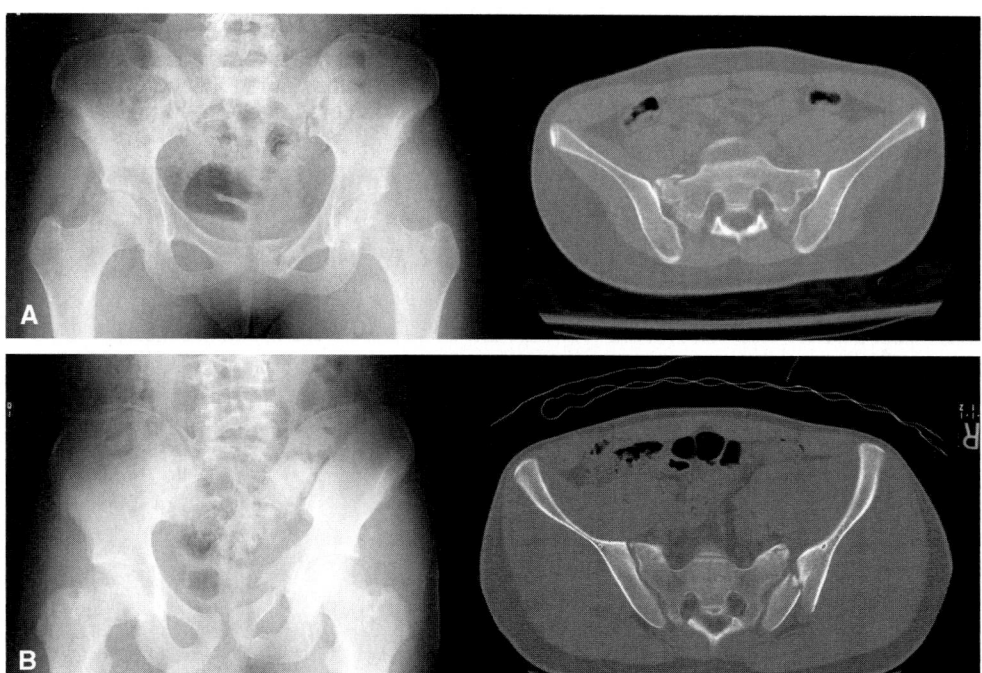

is a bilateral external rotation injury with greater than 2.5 cm of symphyseal displacement (Fig. 36-19A). Type B3.2 and 3.3 injuries are secondary to lateral compression causing external rotation of the contralateral hemipelvis (Fig. 36-19B) or on both sides of the pelvis sustaining a lateral compression mechanism, respectively. By definition, both sides of the injury are unstable only in rotation. In B3.2 and 3.3 injuries, the pelvic floor remains competent and the posterior ligaments are intact, resulting in only rotational instability. If global instability is present, the injury is classified as a type C injury.

A type C injury is globally unstable due to the complete disruption of the bone or ligaments that stabilize the hemipelvis to the axial skeleton (Fig. 36-20). Further subdivision is based on the nature of the posterior lesion. C1.1 is an iliac fracture, C1.2 is an SI dislocation or fracture–dislocation, and C1.3 is a fracture through the sacrum (Fig. 36-21). C2 injuries are bilateral disruptions in which one hemipelvis is rotationally unstable (B types) and the other side is globally unstable (C types). C3 injuries represent bilateral, globally unstable hemipelvi (Fig. 36-22).

FIGURE 36-18 *A, A locked symphysis with one pubic body displaced behind the other. B, A tilt fracture occurs when the superior pubic body has dislocated from the symphysis and rotates into the perineum around a fracture of the ipsilateral public root.*

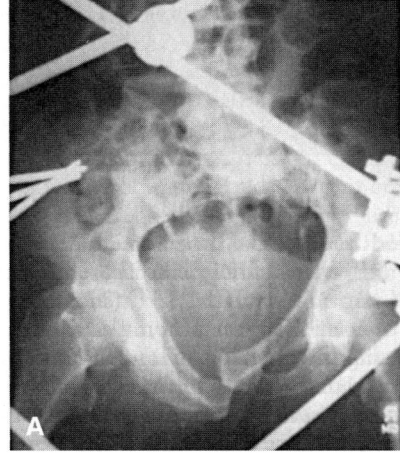 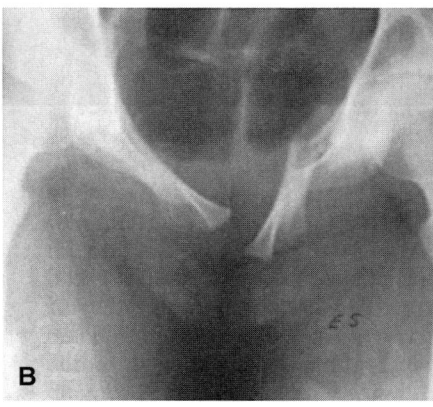

FIGURE 36-19 *Clinical examples of B3 injuries.* **A,** *B3.1 Bilateral rotational injuries occurring through both sacroiliac (SI) joints.* **B,** *B3.2 A windswept deformity with internal rotation of the left hemipelvis through the SI joint and partial disruption of the anterior right SI joint and external rotation of the hemipelvis.*

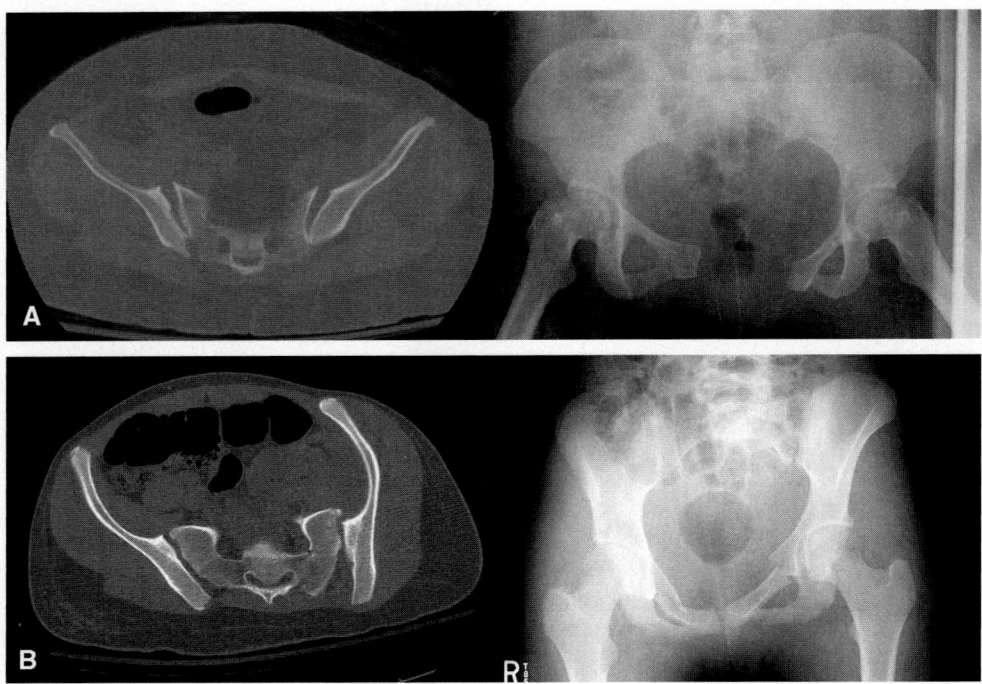

ASSESSMENT OF PELVIC DISRUPTION

Acute Management

First responders can play a pivotal role in the early management of unstable pelvic ring injuries. Advanced trauma life support (ATLS) protocols determine general evaluation and primary interventions. High-energy mechanism and field exam may suggest pelvic injury. Lower limb deformity without obvious associated fracture or dislocation and pelvic motion on stress may be present. However, the lower extremity findings may only consist of subtle rotational asymmetry. The utility of manual examination is experience-based, can be complicated by field logistics, and carries with it at least the theoretical risk of clot disruption. For these reasons, a reasonable approach in the setting of high-energy trauma is routine use of some type of pelvic stabilization device.[31] A concern with application of a pelvic circumferential compression device (PCCD) has been potential accentuation of lateral compression injury deformity resulting in soft tissue injury (bladder, urethra, and vagina). Bottlang and colleagues demonstrated that this is not likely to occur.[8] It appears safe to apply a PCCD to all patients with high-energy mechanisms, especially if an unstable pelvic ring injury is suspected. Vermeulen and Hoffmeyer reported on the application of a PCCD in the field to 19 patients who were thought by the paramedics to have an unstable pelvic injury.[127] Application time was 30 seconds and much faster than with a pneumatic garment. Radiographic evaluation in the emergency room showed that two patients had no injury until the PCCD was removed, when repeat films showed symphyseal widening and sacral fracture.

Emergency and trauma unit assessment of the patient must include evaluation of the immediate life-threatening problems associated with pelvic fractures (Fig. 36-23). A pelvic ring injury is considered a signpost leading to other concomitant life-threatening injuries,[20,21,30,66] including major head, chest, abdominal, and retroperitoneal vascular injuries.[9,30,35,66,78] A history of the injury may also provide insight into the energy absorbed. Low-energy pelvic injury is produced by a fall from a low height (<1 m), such as occurs with tripping. This injury type is often seen in elderly, osteoporotic patients. High-energy injuries are usually caused by vehicular or industrial trauma or by falls from greater heights (>1 m).

Low-energy pelvic ring injuries may be isolated, but high-energy injuries are often associated with important anatomically local and remote pathology. Significant pelvic hemorrhage may occur in up to 75 percent of patients,[66] urogenital injuries in 12 percent, and lumbosacral plexus injuries in about 8 percent.[14,66,80] The likelihood of aortic rupture is eight times greater in high-energy pelvic ring trauma than in blunt trauma injury overall.[74,78] The mortality rate in the high-energy group is about 15 to 25 percent.[21,66] Sixty percent to 80 percent of patients with a high-energy pelvic fracture have other associated musculoskeletal injuries.[66] This complex setting mandates a planned method of simultaneous assessment and treatment. Management is optimized by an interdisciplinary team that includes a general or trauma/critical care surgeon, an emergency department physician when appropriate, an anesthesiologist, and an orthopaedic surgeon.

FIGURE 36-20 *Modified Tile AO Müller classification. Type C: Complete disruptions. Complete disruptions can be unilateral or bilateral. Unilateral disruptions occur through the iliac wing (C1.1), through the sacroiliac joint (C1.2), and through the sacrum (C1.3). Bilateral injuries are combinations of incomplete, complete, and totally complete injuries and are not shown in this figure. (Redrawn from Müller, E., ed. Comprehensive Classification of Pelvis and Acetabulum Fractures. Bern, Switzerland, Maurice E. Müller Foundation, 1995.)*

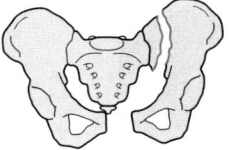 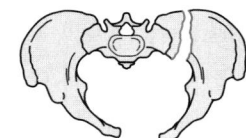

1.1
Through iliac wing

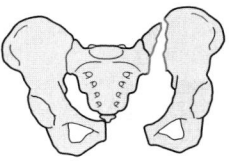 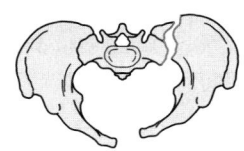

1.2
Through sacroiliac joint

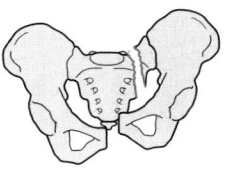 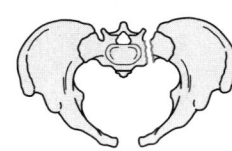

1.3
Through sacrum

Standardized resuscitation priorities provide the core of the ATLS protocols, which are discussed in greater detail in Chapter 6. It is important that the orthopaedic surgeon be involved in the primary resuscitation and care of these patients to provide input to the group on the severity and stability of the pelvic fracture. This can greatly assist in decision making. Second, it is important that the pelvis be thoroughly assessed acutely so that any evidence of instability can be documented and appropriate treatment planned and instituted early on rather than later.

Bladder catherization per ATLS guidelines is indicated in the hypotensive patient to help monitor resuscitation. This should be preceded in a male by exam for evidence of blood at the urethral meatus, evaluation for scrotal hematomas, and rectal assessment for a high riding prostate. In females, a vaginal examination as well as inspection of the urethral meatus is performed. If any evidence of pelvic instability is noted in addition to any of the preceding findings, urinary catheterization should not be undertaken before urethrography unless it is truly needed for the monitoring of the patient's resuscitation. Serum lactate or base deficit to assess adequacy of resuscitation may provide an additional window before bladder catherization is required. The risk of completing an incomplete urethral tear exists in these settings with significant late sequalae. Lowe and associates reported that 57 percent of men with urethral injury secondary to a pelvic fracture had none of the classic signs.[65]

Physical signs of pelvic instability include deformity of a lower extremity without a long bone fracture. This usually presents as shortening or malrotation (or both) on the side of the unstable hemipelvis. Flank or buttock contusions and swelling may herald significant hemorrhage. Visual inspection of the posterior part of the pelvis is done when the patient is logrolled for examination of the spine. Palpation of the posterior aspect of the pelvis may reveal a closed degloving injury, large hematoma, or more rarely a palpable displacement through a posterior ring injury site (ilium, SI joint, or sacrum). Similarly, palpation of the symphysis may lead to recognition of a gap. A single manual pelvic stress exam by an experienced surgeon may be useful if questions of pelvic stability persist after the secondary survey. This exam should not be undertaken, however, if a circumferential sheet or PCCD has been applied and the patient remains hemodynamically unstable. Additional signs of potential instability include an open pelvic fracture, scrotal hematomas, and lower extremity neurologic deficits potentially attributable to lumbosacral plexus injury. As an adjunct to the secondary survey, an AP radiograph of the pelvis is mandatory in all patients who have a depressed level of consciousness, who fail to respond to fluids when no intra-abdominal or thoracic source of bleeding is noted, or who complain of pain or tenderness on examination of the pelvis.[53]

Once the patient is assessed and resuscitation is underway, the surgical team must be prepared to act efficiently if ongoing pelvic bleeding is observed or suspected.[30,35,66,71,116] The usual cause of ongoing pelvic bleeding is disruption of the posterior pelvic (presacral) venous plexus. Much less commonly, bleeding from a large vessel such as the common, external, or internal iliac may occur. Injury to large vessels usually is associated with rapid, massive bleeding and loss of distal pulses. The severity of the hemorrhage determines the appropriate management path. The five areas of potential hemorrhage are external, thoracic, intraperitoneal, retroperitoneal, and extremity fractures. A standardized protocol involving the orthopaedic surgeon and trauma surgeon is necessary to distinguish an intraperitoneal from a retroperitoneal source of hemorrhage. In an acutely injured patient, abdominal examination is unreliable. Therefore, rapid determination of the presence of intra-abdominal blood by ultrasonography, computed tomography (CT), or supraumbilical diagnostic peritoneal lavage is mandatory.[73] Infraumbilical minilaparotomy is fraught with problems because the pelvic hematoma may track up through the anterior fascial planes and contaminate the specimen.

The major aim of the orthopaedic surgeon in controlling pelvic bleeding is stabilization of the unstable

FIGURE 36-21 *Examples of C1 injuries. **A,** Posterior injury occurring through the sacroiliac joint. **B,** Sacrum. **C,** Ilium.*

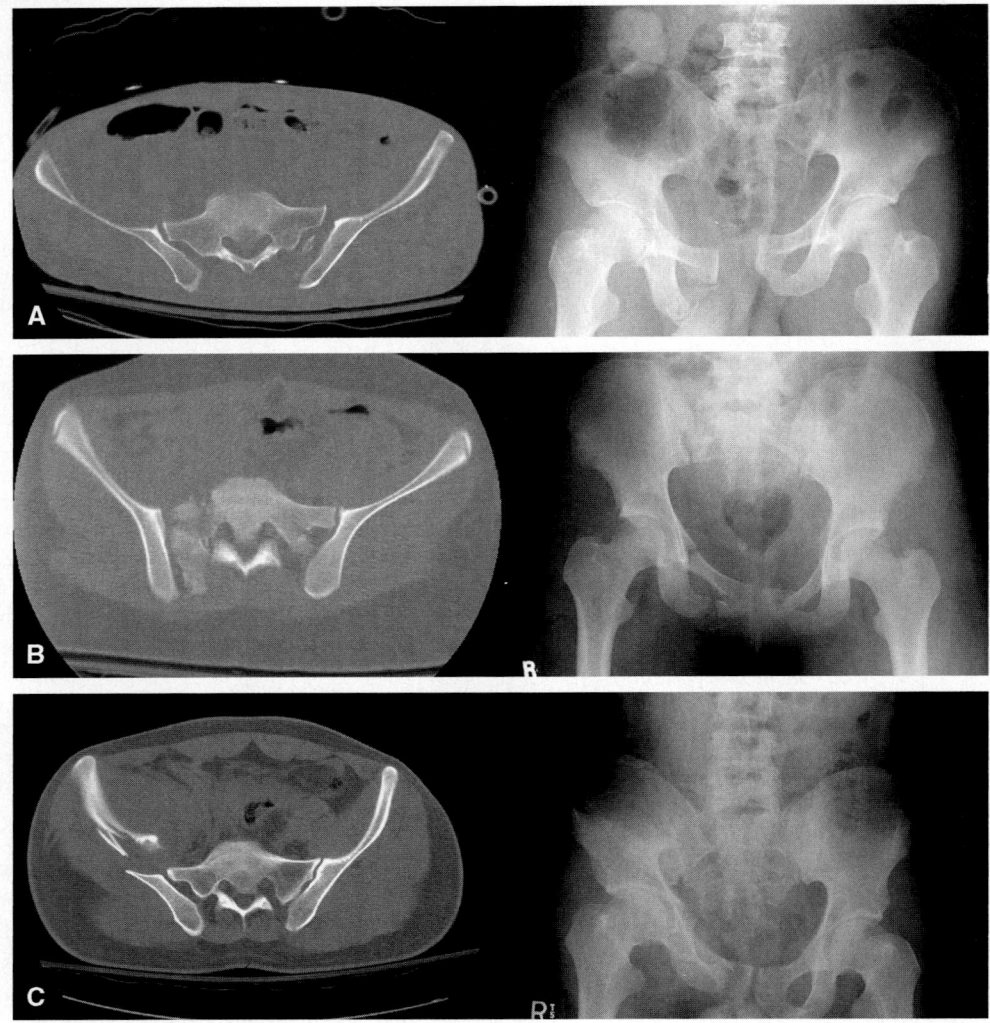

pelvic injury.[19,35,49,66,71,73] Stabilization of the pelvic injury can maintain or decrease retroperitoneal volume and thereby facilitate tamponade of the bleeding vessels. The timing of placement of operative acute pelvic stabilization devices should be a decision made in consultation with the general or trauma/critical care surgeon in charge of the resuscitation.[72] Before placement of the these devices, the pelvic AP radiograph should be assessed. This radiograph reveals several clues regarding the exact nature of the injury and the potential for ongoing bleeding. A lateral compression injury usually has a horizontal (coronal) fracture through the rami with evidence of an anterior sacral impaction injury. The sacral injury is best appreciated by following the arcuate line between the sacral promontory and the iliopectineal line. A line drawn vertically through the midline of the sacrum can also reveal a significant rotational deformity of the hemipelvis. This deformity usually is characterized by medial rotation, but also may include a component of flexion as evidenced by an ischial height asymmetry.[124] An AP injury is usually recognized by the presence of vertical fractures through the rami that tend to be separated but not vertically displaced. Posterior displacement of the hemipelvis can be inferred with the use of the second sacral arcuate line.[124] Vertical instability with or without translation can be recognized by displacement greater than 1 cm through the posterior SI joint, fracture diastasis through the sacrum, or by an avulsion fracture of the sacrum.

The key clinical correlates of injury type are the association of lateral compression and vertical shear injuries with major intra-abdominal and head injuries.[134] Also, unstable AP compression injuries and completely unstable injuries have a far greater incidence of retroperitoneal hemorrhage than intra-abdominal bleeding. Given these correlations it is reasonable to expect that most lateral compression injuries do not usually benefit from emergency stabilization techniques. Unstable AP and vertical shear injuries, however, remain an important focus in the acute setting and can be managed by a variety of techniques. In cases where prehospital administration of a PCCD has not been undertaken, this is a logical first step and has been shown to safe and effective.[8] An inexpensive alternative in the trauma bay is a circumferential compressive linen sheet.[58]

FIGURE 36-22 *Bilateral injuries.* **A,** *C2. Complete of the left sacroiliac (SI) joint and subtle rotational displacement of the right SI joint, confirmed on computed tomography.* **B,** *Left trans-sacral fracture and obvious complete dislocation of the right SI joint, both injuries are globally unstable posteriorly.*

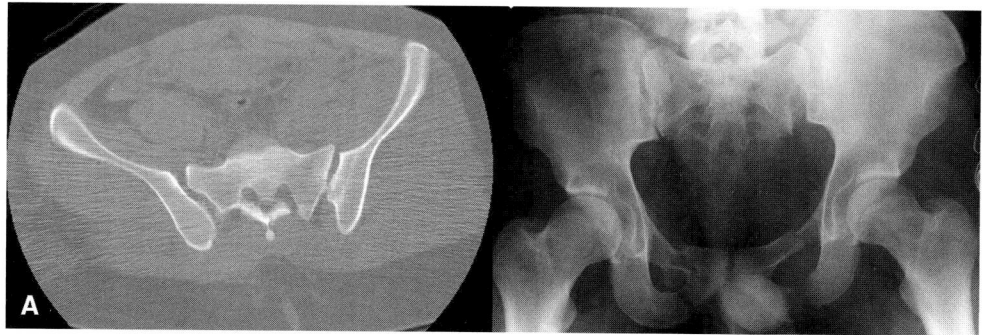

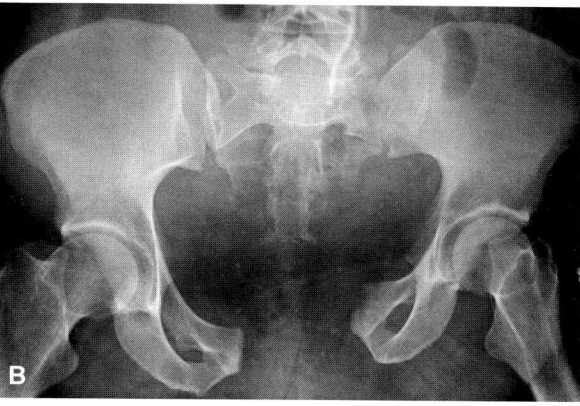

The sheet can be configured to encompass the thighs as well, assisting in reduction of the pelvis. This is particularly true if there is some remaining posterior ligamentous continuity and the intact lower extremities have been manually internally rotated prior to application. Any circumferential construct risks pressure-induced skin breakdown when applied for long periods, and routine surveillance therefore is a requisite component of use. Vacuum body splints provide another effective alternative for emergency pelvic stabilization and have been employed in the field in many locales. They can be applied to the patient's flanks to maintain access to the abdomen and groin. They are also useful as a splint for lower extremity injuries and spine.

Skeletal traction can be a useful adjunct for these techniques. A small-diameter Kirschner wire (K-wire) and traction bow without elaborate slings or supports is all that is needed. Ten to 15 kg of traction through a distal femoral pin can reduce translational displacement significantly, particularly in the acute setting. Combining this with circumferential compression provides a noninvasive strategy for emergent stabilization that optimizes the chance for tamponade.

The oldest form of emergency pelvic stabilization is the pneumatic antishock garment (PASG).[35] This inflatable garment is placed over the lower extremities and around the abdomen and inflated until blood pressure is stabilized. The garment works by increasing peripheral vascular resistance and by providing an autotransfusion from the lower extremities to the body core. However, in this situation of pelvic trauma, the abdominal component of the trousers can act as a pneumatic splint to potentially decrease pelvic

volume and minimize continued motion of the pelvic ring injury. This decrease in motion prevents any further disruption of the pelvic veins or the clots that have formed. At present, PASGs are largely of historical interest due to simpler alternatives and concerns regarding lower extremity compartment syndromes due to prolonged inflation times.[35,65]

In selected cases a more efficient method of emergency pelvic stabilization is the application of specialized pelvic clamps.[12,36] These clamps can be applied in the emergency department, operating theater, or ICU. The pelvic C-clamp[36] is designed for use in C type injuries in the hemodynamically unstable patient with significant displacements through disrupted SI joint(s) or sacral fracture. It addresses the site of instability by a direct compressive force applied to the ilium lateral to the SI joints. It is important that placement follows closed reduction maneuvers and is usually preceded or accompanied by a circumferential sheet or PCCD at the thighs. If a sheet is already in place, a window can be made for clamp placement. As an alternative, a pelvic clamp is applied to either the posterior ring or the anterior pelvis in the cancellous bone above the acetabulum.[7,9]

For the past several decades, the default option for stabilization of the pelvis in the hemodynamically unstable patient has been the application of an anterior external fixation frame.[50,88,90] Whenever feasible, the frame should be used in conjunction with traction through the ipsilateral femur to control cranial and posterior displacement. Application of the frame requires operative intervention, and it

FIGURE 36-23 *Algorithm for resuscitation after pelvic disruption.* Abbreviations: *Fx, fracture; RPH, retroperitoneal hematoma; R/O, rule out.*

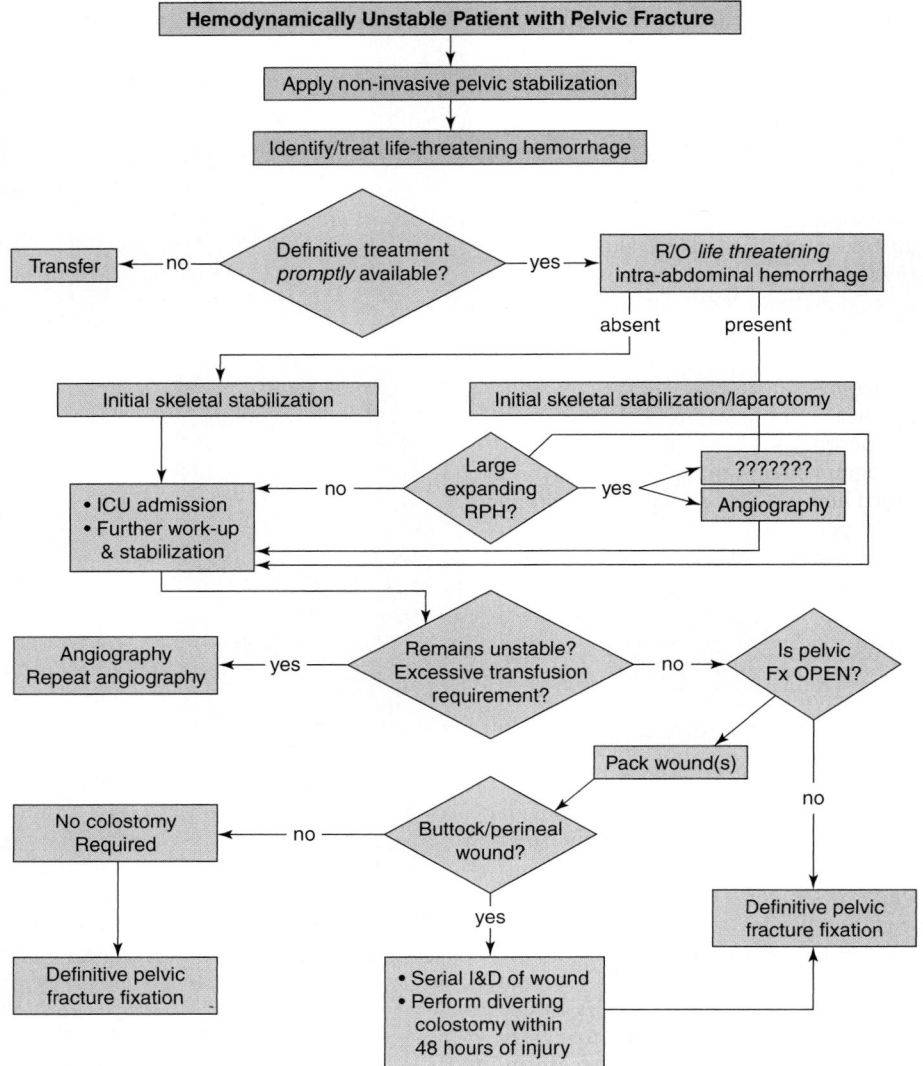

must be applied expeditiously. A hemodynamically stable patient does not require temporary stabilization unless it is thought that motion of the pelvic fracture may lead to recurrence of the hemorrhage. Earlier and more effective use of circumferential compression techniques may well lead to fewer indications for acute pelvic external fixation.

Decision making can be guided by the patient's response to resuscitation.[41] A patient with injuries that fail to respond to appropriate fluid resuscitation and who does not have intra-abdominal and thoracic hemorrhage is likely bleeding from a named retroperitoneal arterial source. This type of patient may benefit from angiography to localize the bleeding source and determine whether embolization can be used to stop the bleeding. Temporary balloon occlusion of large-caliber arteries may be lifesaving until definitive control can be achieved by surgery. Some type of pelvic stabilization should be undertaken before angiography.

Many institutions routinely use CT for abdominal and pelvic evaluation of the trauma patient. If the patient is stabilized and able to undergo CT, it should be contrast-enhanced. A patient with contrast extravasation on CT has a 40:1 likelihood of significant arterial bleeding requiring embolization.[110] Therefore, even in facilities where ultrasound is the primary modality for identification for intra-abdominal bleeding, early contrast-enhanced CT may be useful in the patient who is a transient responder or has a pelvic ring injury pattern at higher risk for arterial blood loss.

Diagnostic and therapeutic angiography in patients with pelvic hemorrhage is difficult even in experienced hands. Selective embolization is most effective in controlling bleeding from small-diameter vessels (i.e., ≤3 mm). Angiography may assist in localizing large-vessel bleeding, but only if time and hemodynamic stability permit.[101] Compromising delays in resuscitation and treatment can occur if the angiography response time is slow or the angiographer is inexperienced. The radiology department must have the necessary equipment available to administer lifesaving procedures in the event of cardiopulmonary collapse when performing embolization in these high-risk patients.[52] Under optimum circumstances, in one study arteriographic embolization was 100 percent effective in stopping bleeding and saving lives if done within 3 hours of injury.[1]

A positive test for intra-abdominal blood in a patient who fails to respond to standard resuscitation protocols mandates an exploratory laparotomy as part of a coordinated treatment plan. This plan should provide for pelvic stability during the abdominal procedure. Since sheet wraps and PCCDs encroach on the surgical field, they should be moved distally to the proximal thighs and replaced by external fixation, pelvic clamp or occasionally percutaneous image-guided posterior ring fixation. During laparotomy, if the retroperitoneal hematoma is expanding, packing of the presacral area and retro pubic space is carried out. Transperitoneal digital or visual assessment and improvement of the posterior ring reduction has been reported.[84] This may improve the efficacy of pelvic packing. If the patient remains hypotensive despite emergent pelvic stabilization, control of abdominal bleeding, and retroperitoneal packing, then angiography should be performed immediately. Any clotted vessel seen during angiography should be treated by embolization to prevent delayed hemorrhage if the clot is dislodged or reabsorbed. In open pelvic fractures that are hemorrhaging through an open wound, packing of the area plus a circumferential compressive dressing are needed to assist in controlling bleeding.

The use of extraperitoneal pelvic packing has become popular especially in Europe and recently in North America. This technique requires external bony pelvic fixation followed by packing of the pelvic retroperitoneal space via an extraperitoneal route. The rationale for the technique is that the majority of severe bleeding is venous from the pelvic plexus and cancellous bone surfaces. By applying a direct tamponade with the packs this bleeding is effectively controlled. It is performed through a midline incision from the pubic symphysis superiorly. The peritoneum is left intact, and the space between the peritoneum and bony pelvis is bluntly opened bilaterally. Three sponges are packed below the pelvic brim on each side directed back toward the SI joint. The incision is then closed. Packing is removed at 24 to 48 hours depending on the patient's stability. If after the packing hypotension persists, then angiography is performed. The proponents of this technique believe that it is a more efficient use of resources and time than angiography first and then surgery. No evidence supports either approach as better. It is up the hospital trauma and orthopedic surgeons to decide what protocol best fits their resources.[20,61]

After the patient has been stabilized, further assessment of the other intraperitoneal pelvic structures must be carried out. If any indication of an unstable fracture is noted, urethrography should be performed in male patients.[14,71] This technique is accomplished by inserting a small catheter into the urethral meatus, inflating the balloon, and injecting approximately 25 to 30 mL of a radiopaque dye to outline the urethra. If no leak is evident, a catheter is inserted. It is best to do the radiograph of the pelvis in an oblique plane (e.g., as in a Judet view of the full pelvis) to put the urethra into full relief. However, in most situations, this view is difficult to obtain, and a standard AP radiograph is satisfactory. After urethrography, a cystogram should be obtained by filling the bladder with 400 mL of dye and taking a radiograph.

After evacuation of the dye, a postvoid view is taken to determine any occult extraperitoneal bladder rupture. If these investigations do not reveal a cause of the hematuria, an intravenous pyelogram should be obtained. In female patients, urethrography is rarely helpful and usually omitted. A thorough physical examination, including a vaginal examination, is performed before the catheter is placed, and even then a vaginal injury may be missed in up to 50 percent of cases.[83]

An open pelvic fracture further complicates assessment and diagnosis.[83,88,89] The wound must be adequately evaluated. Wounds occurring in the anterior aspect of the pelvis or over the flank are relatively clean and can be treated like most open fractures. However, wounds that occur in the buttock and groin regions and any wound in the perineal region require exact assessment. Because of the risk of fecal contamination, any wounds that involve the rectum or the perineal or buttock regions must be débrided and an external fixation device applied. Performance of a colostomy to divert the fecal stream should be given serious consideration for this group of open pelvic fractures. Other fractures that do not involve these areas but are clean can be débrided, and then appropriate fixation can be instituted.

Occasionally, in a hemodynamically stable patient, external fixators are applied in the acute phase to facilitate care.[112,113] The frame adequately stabilizes the pelvic disruption to allow patient mobility and nursing care.[90]

Definitive Management

After stabilization of an acutely injured patient, assessment of multiple factors will help to determine definitive management. This evaluation is necessary to decide the appropriate management based on the balance between our ability to decrease the chance of late pain, malunion, and nonunion following pelvic injuries and the need to avoid complications of the injury or subsequent treatment.[44,46,73,84,91,104,112] This assessment begins with a clinical determination of pelvic stability, precise definition of the skeletal injuries on the pelvis radiographs, followed by classification of the injury. Despite suspicion of instability based on mechanism, exam, or radiographs, definitive treatment may be determined or modified based on patient factors such as associated injuries, status of the soft tissue in and around the zone of injury, or comorbidities.

HISTORY

Accident site information, patient history, and radiographic data can all be used to help in determining the mechanism of injury. Direct application of force or crushing injuries to the pelvis can cause serious soft tissue disruption, which can lead to degloving lesions and possibly soft tissue or wound complications. Indirectly applied force usually spares the soft tissue. Knowledge of the patient's age, occupation, and expectations is necessary if the surgeon and the patient are to have a common treatment goal.

PHYSICAL EXAMINATION

Once neurologic, cardiovascular, and respiratory issues have stabilized, a secondary complete orthopaedic survey should be completed. Specifically regarding the pelvis, the surgeon should take into account prior abdominal or visceral interventions. Is the abdominal wound closed or still open above the fascia? Have osteomies been performed and what are their locations? Has a suprapubic catheter been placed around the perineal area, and for what injury? Is an indwelling Foley catheter in place for resuscitation or an associated lower genitourinary injury? Evaluation of open pelvic wounds for location, contamination, and residuals of prior intervention should be noted. Is there a scrotal or labial hematoma indicative of disruption of the pelvic floor? Any leg length discrepancies should be measured and any internal and external rotational abnormalities evaluated. Areas of abrasions or ecchymosis may be associated with soft tissue degloving injuries. After inspection, palpation of the areas of injury should be carried out to determine soft tissue disruption, bony gaps, and hematomas. A full neuromuscular and vascular examination of the lower extremities should be repeated.

Rotational instability can be assessed by pushing on the anterior superior iliac wings both internally and externally to determine whether the pelvis opens and closes. Palpation of the posterior pelvic ring is sensitive to determining the presence of a posterior pelvic ring injury. This assessment is best done when the patient is initially examined; however, if the stability of the pelvis is at all in doubt, examination under anesthesia is mandatory.[49] Confirmation can be obtained with radiographs or image intensification with the patient anesthetized.

Radiographic Assessment

Before definitive treatment decisions are made, a complete radiographic assessment of the pelvis should be done. As mentioned, a trauma AP pelvis film can help initiate treatment in the vast majority of cases. Additional images need not be obtained in the acute phase following injury as this may introduce an unnecessary delay in treatment. Complete evaluation of the pelvis requires AP, inlet, and outlet views. CT of the pelvis is also felt to be mandatory in high-energy injuries or in patients in whom a posterior injury is suspected and the posterior ring is poorly visualized on the standard three

radiographs. The surgeon should develop a systematic approach to evaluating these radiographs much like that for the AP pelvic film. Technological advances, such as the 64-slice CT scanners, have made possible the rapid acquisition of volumetric data that can be manipulated into high-resolution two- and three-dimensional images. To date, no studies have been published to determine if these are able to substitute for plain radiography. Also inherent with these new techniques is exposure to high doses of radiation. Each surgeon should currently weigh the risks and benefits of this new technology as it will likely prove helpful for some select complex injuries and truly aid in evaluation and reconstruction.

It is important to remember that the pelvis, in the supine position, lies 45 to 60° oblique to the long axis of the skeleton. Consequently, an AP radiograph is essentially an oblique radiograph of the pelvis. To appropriately determine displacement, it is mandatory to evaluate two radiographs taken at right angles, which has led to development of the inlet and outlet views by Pennal and Sutherland.[28,88]

ANTEROPOSTERIOR RADIOGRAPH

The AP radiograph (Fig. 36-24) is very useful in providing an overview of the pelvic injury. A repeat AP pelvic film should be obtained following stabilization of the patient if the initial radiograph is of poor quality. Full evaluation should proceed as described. Subsequent radiographs should confirm injuries documented on the AP radiograph, better define their location, and help in determining hemipelvic displacement in translation and rotation.

INLET RADIOGRAPH

The inlet view (Fig. 36-25) is taken with the patient in the supine position. The tube is directed from the head toward the feet at 60°.[82] It is therefore perpendicular to the pelvic brim, and the radiographic view is a true inlet picture of the pelvis. On this view the pelvic brim, the pubic rami, the SI joints, and the ala and body of the sacrum can be

FIGURE 36-24 *A,* For the anteroposterior (AP) projection, the beam is directed perpendicular to the midpelvis and the radiologic plate. *B,* Radiographic appearance of the pelvis in the AP plane.

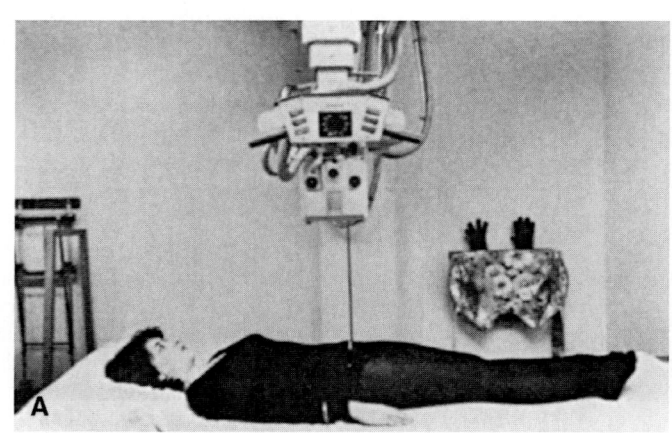

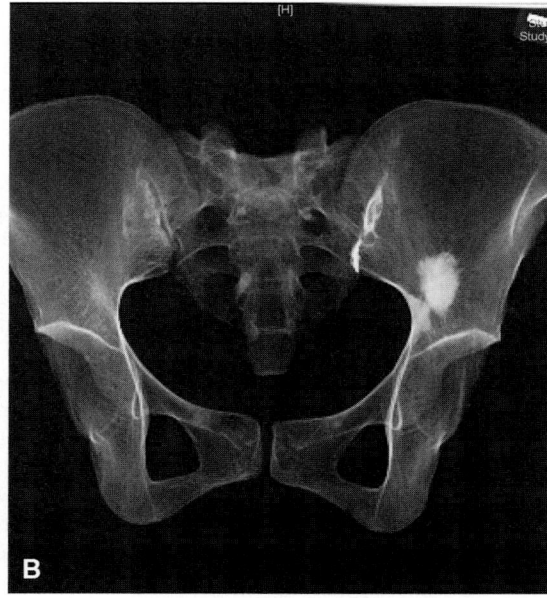

FIGURE 36-25   **A,** For the inlet projection, the beam is directed from the head to the midpelvis at an angle of 60° to the plate. **B,** Radiographic appearance in the inlet projection.

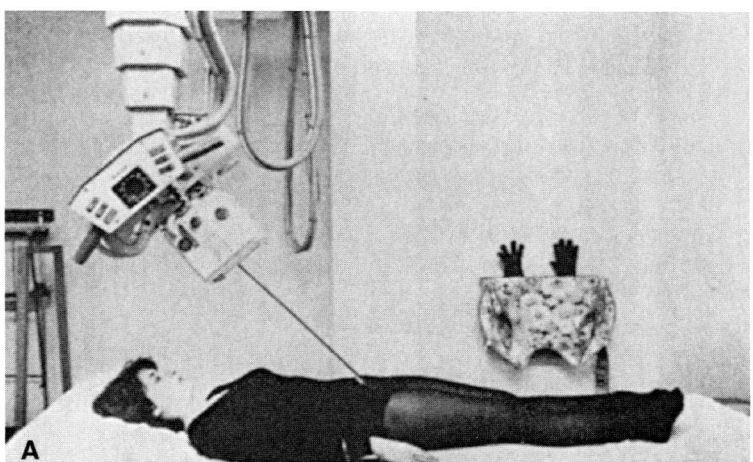

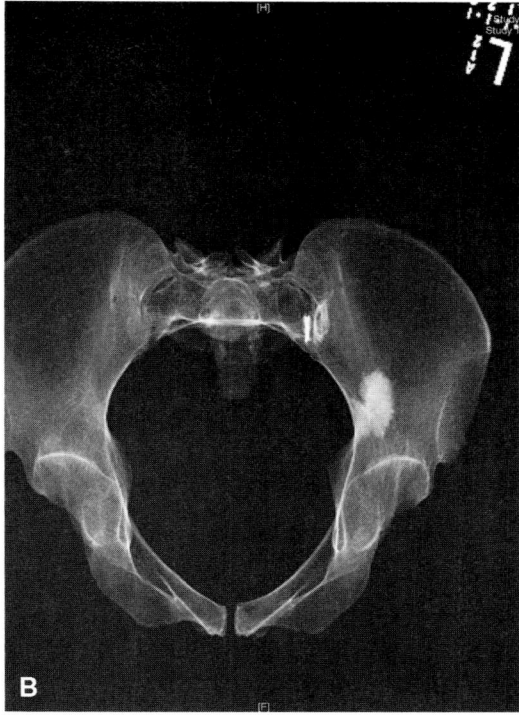

seen, as well as the posterior iliac spine. This view is useful for determining displacement of the SI joint, iliac wing, or fractures through the sacrum. Inspection of the sacral ala, particularly along the arcuate line, demonstrates sacral impaction, which is best seen in this projection. This is visualized as a buckling through this line or a shortening of the sacrum on one side compared with the other. Ischial spine avulsions can also be seen on this view. The axial plane component of rotation (internal or external) may be best appreciated with this view. The oblique or horizontal morphology of rami fractures may also be more apparent with this projection.

OUTLET RADIOGRAPH

The outlet view (Fig. 36-26) is taken with the tube directed 45° to the long axis of the patient, but at the foot of the

FIGURE 36-26   **A,** For the outlet projection, the beam is directed from the foot to the symphysis at an angle of 40° to the plate. **B,** Radiographic appearance in the outlet projection.

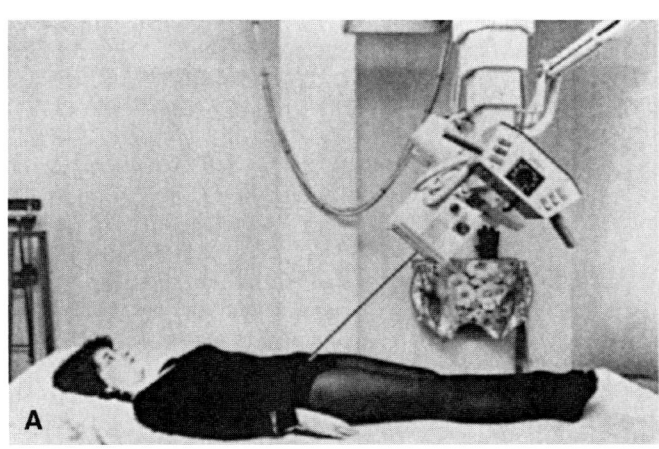

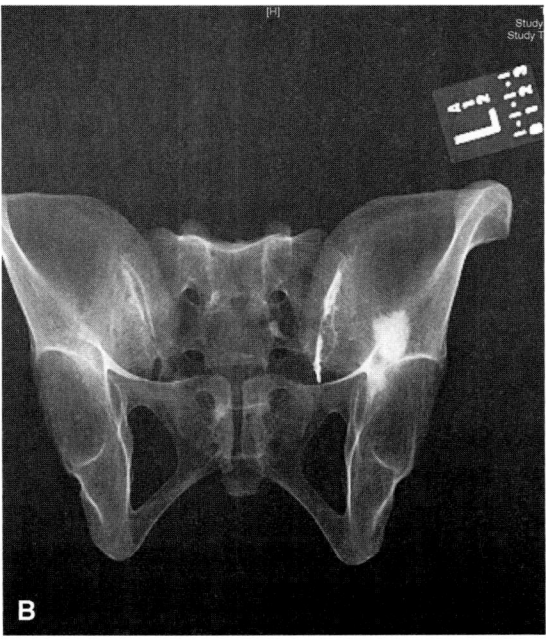

patient.[82] The tube is directed toward the head. This radiograph is very useful for determining displacement of the hemipelvis, noted at the ischium, acetabulum, or caudal SI joints. An excellent view of the first two or three sacral segments and foramina are profiled in this view. Complete visualization of the bony boundaries of the obturator foramen are outlined, and the vertical orientation of rami fractures are profiled. The coronal and sagittal plane components of rotation (abduction–adduction, flexion–extension, respectively) are also seen and better understood with evaluation of this projection.

Computed Tomography

The use of CT has revolutionized assessment of the posterior osseous ligamentous structures of the pelvis. It is mandatory for determining the exact nature of a posterior injury (Fig. 36-27A). It reveals whether an injury through the sacrum is a crushing injury or a shearing injury with a large gap. Sacroiliac joint displacement is valuable in determining the stability of this posterior injury. Anterior opening of the joint with a closed posterior portion represents a rotationally unstable injury with intact posterior ligaments (type B). If the joint is open throughout its course, the posterior ligaments are disrupted and the injury is globally unstable (type C). CT is also helpful in defining acetabular injuries. Many pubic ramus fractures that occur near the base of the anterior column enter the acetabulum, and the CT allows for appropriate assessment of these injuries. Close scrutiny of the upper sacral vertebral bodies and lumbosacral junction must be done to assess the anatomic abnormalities in preparation for posterior stabilization and treatment of L5-S1 facet joint injuries. Advances in technology have shown that two- and three-dimensional reconstructions of CT scans may provide a more useful evaluation of fracture morphology and of the overall displacement of a pelvic fracture than plain film radiography (see Fig. 36-27B).

FIGURE 36-27   *High-quality 64-slice computed tomographic (CT) scans obtained for a complex injury.* **A,** *Anteroposterior pelvis.* **B,** *Axial CT cuts revealing complex sacral fracture–dislocation.* **C,** *Two-dimensional reconstructions reveal an associated fracture of L5.*

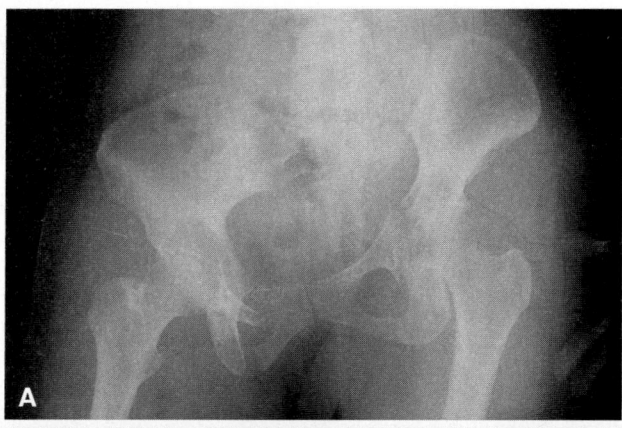

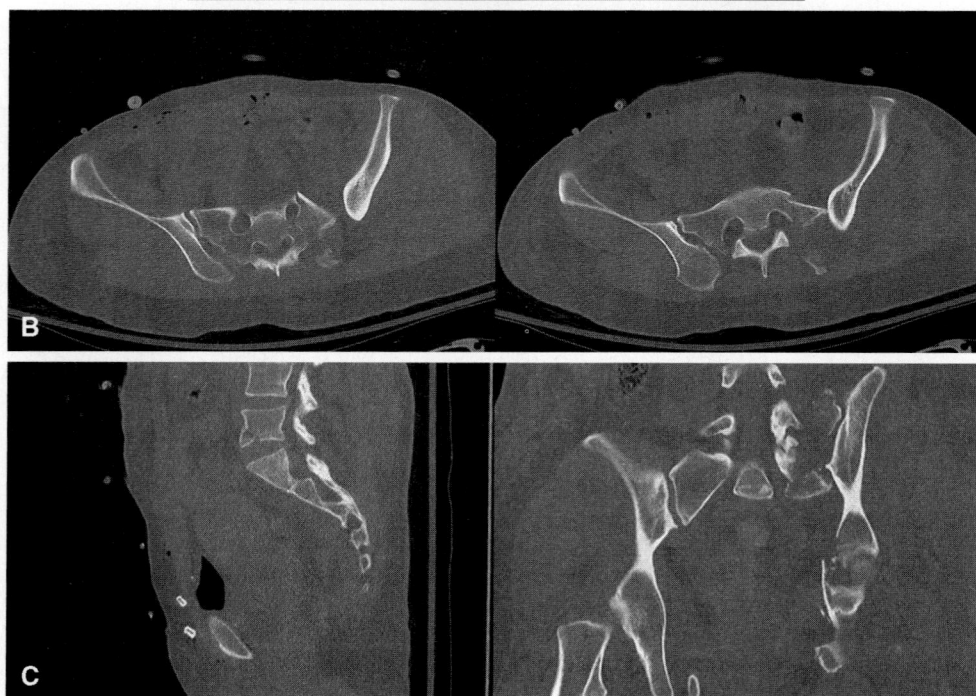

FIGURE 36-27 *(Continued)* **D,** *Three-dimensional surface-rendered images help define injury and deformity.*

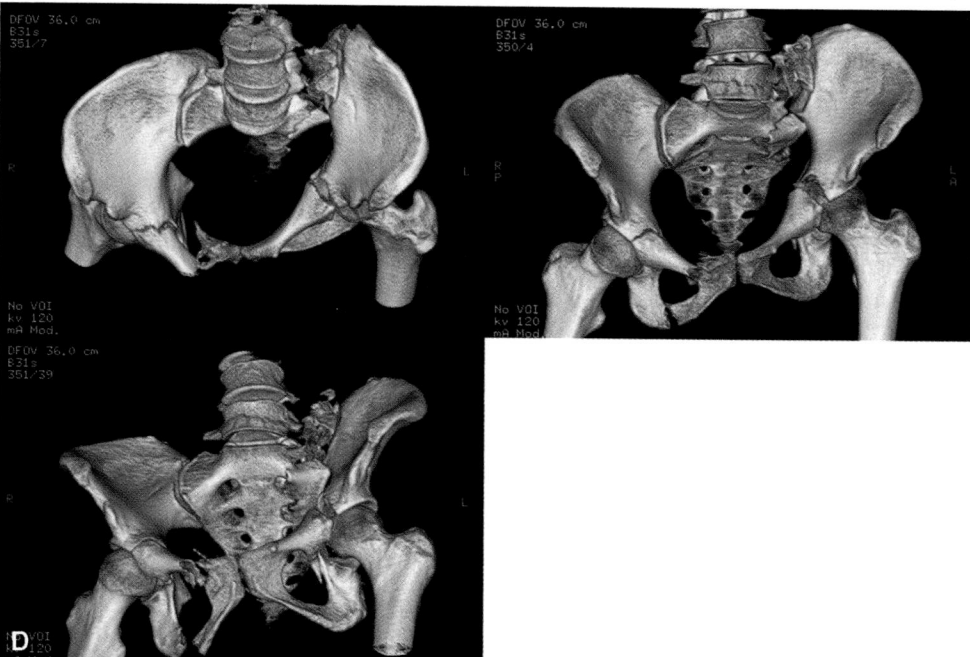

Examination Under Anesthesia

If after all these investigations the true instability pattern of the pelvis is unclear, the physician should not hesitate to examine the patient under anesthesia within the first 5 to 7 days after injury because the results may dictate major changes in treatment.

DECISION MAKING

After a full assessment of the pelvic injury is complete, a decision can be made regarding appropriate treatment[17] (Fig. 36-28). As with any skeletal injury, two key factors will drive treatment decisions: instability and displacement. The benefit of the comprehensive classification system is that it can be used, along with experience of the surgeon, to determine the natural history of pelvic ring injuries until union. The first component to be considered is instability. The vast majority of dislocations are by definition unstable and require reduction and stabilization. Fractures of the posterior ring may be stable if minimally displaced, but will be mobile and may heal in an unacceptable position if initially displaced. Nonsurgical treatment of pelvic ring injuries demand close early clinical and radiographic follow-up to identify instability or subsequent displacement.

B-type fractures that are stable include AP compression injuries with less than 2.5 cm of displacement (type B1.1) and lateral compression injuries with sacral impaction (type B2.1). It is unlikely that these injuries will displace further, but plain imaging is only a static evaluation of the dynamic injury process. If patients are difficult to mobilize, if there is significant internal rotation of the ring with associated injuries to the genitourinary system, or an air density is detected in the SI joint along with possible anterior SI ligament injury, evaluation under anesthesia may be warranted.

Displacement of the symphysis disruption[106,113] of more than 2.5 cm is an indication for operative stabilization.

Fractures and dislocations through the SI joint have a high incidence of sequelae such as long-term pain, discomfort, and nonunion.[43,44,46,49,55,93,102,105] To avoid these problems, operative stabilization of the pelvis is indicated to ensure reduction and stability. Extra-articular SI joint fractures occurring through the iliac wing (C1.1) or sacrum are globally unstable and have the potential for further displacement. If initial displacement is acceptable, these may be closely monitored with radiographs as the patient is mobilized. If initial displacement is deemed unacceptable, closed reduction, application of an external fixator to control the rotatory abnormality, and possible traction may be able to correct deformity but may limit patient mobility[50,51] (Table 36-1). Unless medically contraindicated, these displaced fractures of the posterior ring should be treated operatively if the patient understands the risks and benefits of reduction and stabilization. Indications for surgical stabilization may be expanded if it is felt the patient would benefit from early mobilization due to associated injuries. It may be argued that this helps to diminish pain, instability, or subsequent displacement during early rehabilitation, but has not been substantiated in the literature.

Significant displacement is defined as:

- Leg length discrepancy of greater than 1 cm.
- Significant internal rotation abnormality with no external rotation of the lower extremity past neutral. Similarly, the lack of internal rotation in an external rotation-type fracture is significant.

Obviously, a tilt fracture leads to a significant deformity, particularly in females, who may be subject to dyspareunia because of a displaced fragment near the vagina. If a stable fracture is significantly displaced, intervention may be required.

Treatment of associated injuries, particularly injuries to the acetabulum or long bones of the lower extremity, must

FIGURE 36-28 *Algorithm for management of pelvic fractures. Abbreviations: C.R.I.F., closed reduction internal fixation; CT, computed tomography; E.U.A., examination under anesthesia; Ex fix, external fixation; O.R.I.F., open reduction and internal fixation; PCCD, pelvic circumferential compression device; SI, sacroiliac.*

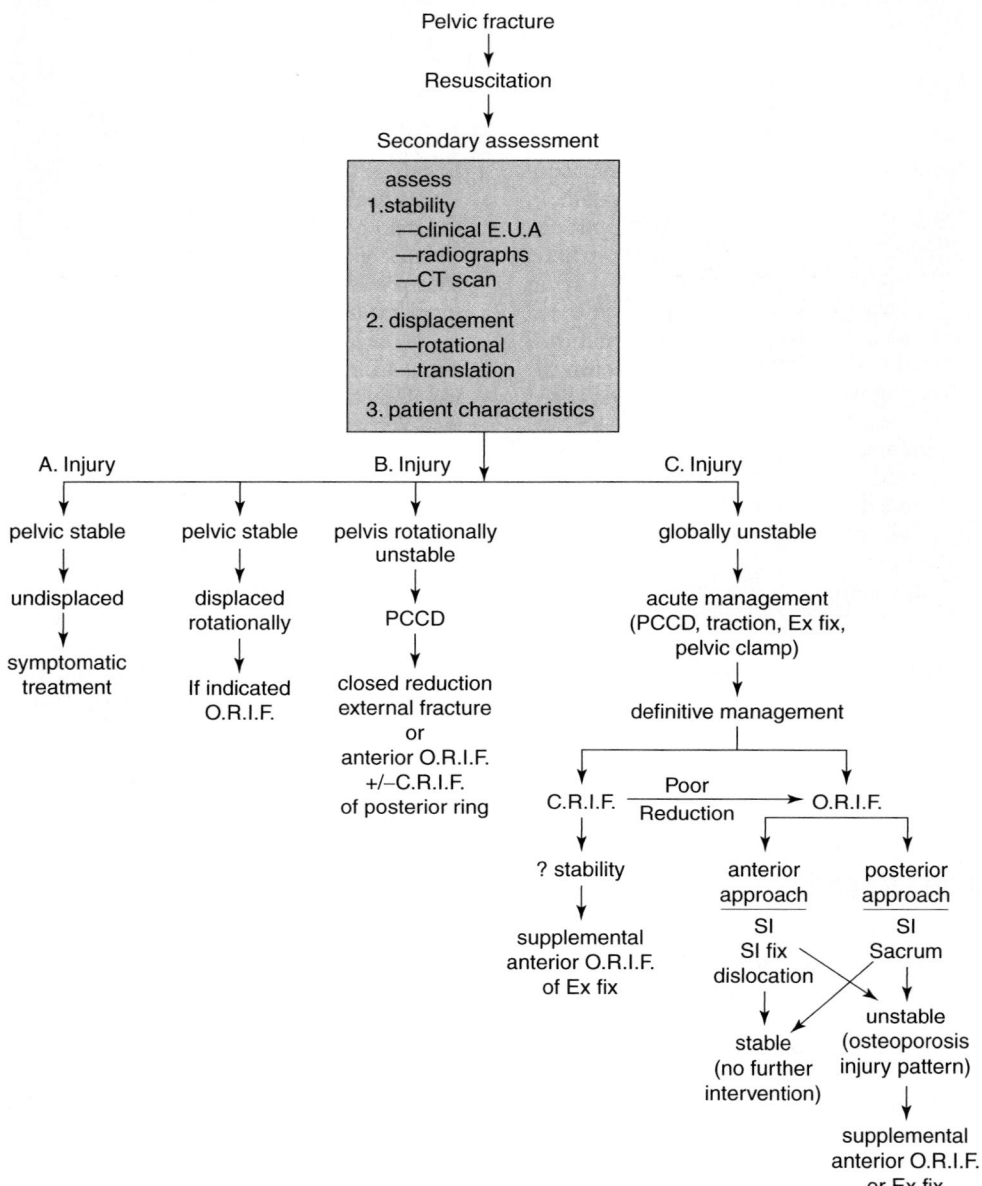

Table 36-1
Indications for External Fixation
Resuscitation
Rotationally unstable fractures
Open-book fracture
Bucket-handle fracture
Adjunct to traction in unstable fractures (type C)

also be considered when planning operative procedures. A femoral shaft fracture associated with a major pelvic disruption treated by traction may lead to significant knee stiffness. This combination of a pelvic fracture and an ipsilateral femur fracture leads to a higher mortality rate than either

injury does alone. The presence of multiple lower limb long bone fractures associated with a pelvic fracture is usually an indication for surgery to maximize functional rehabilitation.

REDUCTION AND FIXATION TECHNIQUES

Biomechanics of Pelvic Fixation

Logical decisions regarding the stabilization of pelvic disruptions require knowledge of the mechanical stability of different internal and external techniques. A mechanical study showed that in bilateral unstable posterior injuries, the anterior external fixator frame does not afford enough stabilization to allow weight-bearing.[121] Mears and

Rubash[74] attempted to improve the mechanical stability of external fixation by using pelvic transfixation pins, but this technique led to insertional difficulties and problems with nursing care. By adding another cluster of pins to the anterior inferior spine region, Mears and Rubash achieved increased stability.[74] McBroom and Tile[68] suspended a pelvis from the sacrum, which allowed full triplanar motion and showed that all existing external frames would stabilize the pelvic ring sufficiently to allow mobilization of the patient if the posterior osseous ligamentous hinge remained intact. With disruption of this posterior hinge, unstable pelvic disruptions could not be stabilized with any of the existing external frames. The best external frame design was a rectangular construct mounted on two to three 5-mm pins spaced 1 cm apart and inserted into the iliac crest.

Using a similar model, McBroom and Tile showed that internal fixation could significantly increase the force resisted by the pelvic ring when compared with external fixation.[68] In stable injuries, failure was ultimately caused by screw pull-out; therefore, in stable open-book fractures, anterior fixation allowed early mobilization. However, in an unstable injury with a disrupted posterior hinge, anterior symphysis plates did not stabilize the pelvic ring. A moderate increase in stability could be achieved by anterior symphysis plating and a trapezoidal external frame. However, the only direct method of stabilizing this unstable pelvic ring injury was by posterior and anterior fixation. The strongest available fixation was achieved by two plates at right angles across the symphysis along with posterior screw fixation or transiliac bar fixation. From mechanical studies, it is recommended that for iliac wing fractures, open reduction and stable internal fixation with interfragmental compression and neutralization plates be performed. For unilateral SI dislocation, direct fixation across the joint with cancellous screws or anterior SI fixation with plates failed at similar loads.[109] Tile and Hearn showed that iliosacral lag screws have the best pull-out strength if they have a 32-mm thread length and are positioned in the sacral body.[121] Posterior iliosacral screws that have purchase in the sacral body (S1) provide a suitable technique, but insertion may be complicated by neurologic or vascular injury. Pohlemann and colleagues[90] achieved sacral fixation with 3.5-mm plates. They tested osteosynthesis with the plate versus sacral rods and an internal spinal fixator. The results showed that plates failed at 74 percent of body weight and sacral rods failed at 85 percent of body weight. Albert and co-workers[2] described the use of a 4.5-mm reconstruction plate fixed to the posterior tubercles and iliac wings. Mechanical testing showed that this construct failed at an average of 1000 N. Although these results are the best reported, they were done in plastic bone.[50] If the anterior injury is easily amenable to surgery, plate fixation of the symphysis is the best treatment. If it is not amenable to surgery and the anterior injury remains displaced and unstable, external fixation to control the anterior injury may be helpful. In bilateral posterior unstable disruptions, fixation of the displaced portion of the pelvis to the sacral body is necessary and can be accomplished only through posterior screw fixation.

The results of all mechanical studies are routinely reported in newtons. A newton is equal to 0.22 lb of force. Failure of posterior SI joint plating at 387 N is equal to failure at 85.14 lb of force, which is much less than the body weight of an average adult. Caution must be exercised in the postoperative period to not overstress the internal fixation construct by weight-bearing or an upright position.

ANTERIOR APPROACHES TO THE PELVIS: EXPOSURE AND REDUCTION

SYMPHYSEAL REDUCTION AND STABILIZATION

Disruption of the pubic symphysis is most often related to an AP or external (lateral) rotation injury to the pelvis. Consequently, the principle of reduction is to close the pelvic ring by internal (medial) rotation. This can be accomplished by a variety of closed techniques. Application of a PCCD or sheet in the field or before treatment in the trauma bay often provides a reasonable initial reduction and should be adjusted or removed carefully, especially in the hemodynamically unstable patient. When a satisfactory reduction exists, a PCCD may be translated to the proximal thigh, often without loss of compression, to allow access for C-clamp or external fixator placement when needed. Alternatively, "windows" can be placed in a sheet for the same purpose. A local prep and drape is adequate and appropriate in this setting. An additional important closed reduction aid is manual internal rotation of the intact lower extremities by an assistant. The hip capsule provides an effective fulcrum for this maneuver in most cases.

C-type injuries with symphysis disruption and significant initial posterior and cranial displacement usually require application of distal traction to the involved hemipelvis through the lower extremity as well. Although manual traction may suffice in some cases with an anesthetized patient, 10 to 15 kg of force applied through a distal femoral traction pin with the hip flexed 30 to 45° is generally far more effective.

Other closed reduction methods include medially directed manual compression at the iliac crests and the use of external fixator pins placed in the iliac crest or supra-acetabular region that can be used as "joysticks" for manipulation of the displaced hemipelvis.

APPLICATION OF EXTERNAL FIXATION TO THE PELVIS

As noninvasive early pelvic stabilization techniques become universal, it is likely that the need for external fixator placement in the acute phase will wane. Nonetheless, orthopaedic trauma surgeons should remain comfortable with and competent in efficient application of an external frame.[123] During the resuscitation phase, this device may have to be applied quickly, in as little as 20 to 30 minutes (Fig. 36-29).

It is important to use 5-mm pins (Schanz screws) with the threads buried in the thick anterior portion of the iliac crest or supra-acetabular area. Traditional guidelines have called for the placement of two to three iliac crest pins per side. One reliable pin in each inominate bone is sufficient for primary external fixation in the acute setting, which is done to reduce and stabilize an AP compression injury, reestablishing normal pelvic volume and allowing for potential tamponade. The addition of multiple pins may increase the likelihood that one is secure, but provides little in the way of incremental stability. A standard rectangular, triangular or circular frame is all that is needed in most situations. Supra-acetabular pin placement offers

FIGURE 36-29 | *Application of external fixation to the pelvis.* **A,** *Landmarks are the iliac crest and the anterior superior iliac spine.* **B,** *The iliac wing is palpated to determine its orientation. It may also be determined by the use of an open technique or by spinal needles to outline both the inner and the outer aspects of the pelvis.* **C,** *Appropriate orientation of the iliac wing; note the pin orientation on an angle to the body.*

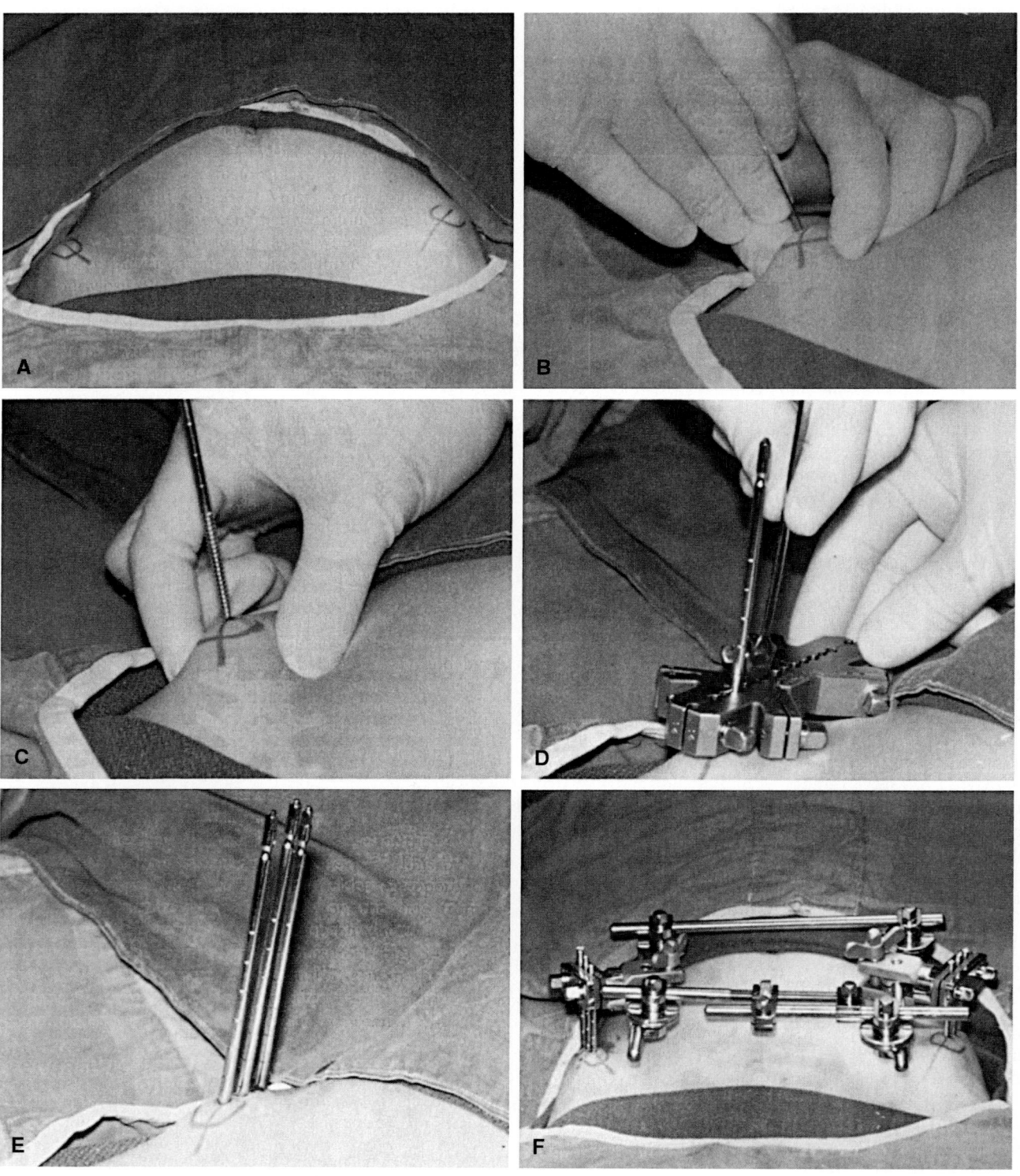

some advantages with regard to soft tissue clearance and conversion to definitive open surgery where appropriate;[31,55] however, it does require fluoroscopic control in most cases.

Application of the external fixation frame requires consideration of the deformity and subsequent reduction techniques outlined earlier. Once a preliminary reduction is achieved, small incisions for the pins can be made that will not be subjected to significant shear after the frame is assembled. Percutaneous technique preserves the best soft tissue environment for subsequent anterior surgical approaches. Since most frames are still used during acute and early phase management, removal can be considered in 2 to 5 days. Use of a bulky, soft tissue immobilizing dressing and pin clamp will minimize the effect of residual skin tension over this short interval. If a percutaneous method is to be used, some surgeons feel it is advantageous to use transverse incisions angled across the iliac crest at 90° and directed toward the umbilicus. If a later iliac crest incision is planned, standard stab wounds parallel to the crest are preferred to minimize compromise of the incision by these wounds. If multiple iliac crest pins are utilized, the most anterior pin is positioned 2 cm dorsal to the anterior superior iliac spine to avoid the lateral femoral cutaneous nerve. Regardless of whether a percutaneous closed or an open method is used, it is imperative to understand the anatomy of the inominate bone. The normal orientation of the iliac wing is 45° oblique to the sagittal and coronal body axes. Additionally, the iliac crest has a lateral overhang and the iliac fossa present a concave internal surface. A model pelvis in the operating room can help the surgeon determine the exact pin orientation. A small-diameter smooth K-wire can be placed along the medial aspect of the iliac crest to act as a directional finder for the drill and the pin. Image intensification oriented in the plane of the crest helps guide pin placement. When placing the pins, it is important to start the pin just medial to the midline of the iliac crest. After the starting point is identified, a drill bit is directed in the appropriate orientation as determined by the guide. A drill hole that just perforates the iliac crest is made. The size of the drill hole is determined by the system in use. Normally, for 5-mm pins, a 3.2- to 3.5-mm drill bit is required. Once the pin has been seated in the predrilled hole, it is gently turned by hand and allowed to seek its way between the inner and outer cortical tables of the inominate bone at an orientation approximately perpendicular to the crest (Fig. 36-30).

The complete threads of the pin should be buried within the iliac bone. Once the pins have been placed into both hemipelves, they can be used cautiously as a handle to assist in reduction of the hemipelvis. If the patient's condition permits, pin placement should be checked before the patient leaves the operating room. The outlet view reveals whether the pin is out of the crest. The obturator oblique view is tangential to the crest and shows whether the pins are between the two tables. A combination of both views provides excellent visualization of the iliac crest to guide insertion (Fig. 36-31).

| **FIGURE 36-30** | *Improper pin position. It can be seen from the pelvic radiograph that the pins have gone through the iliac wing and out the lateral aspect (arrow). Note that the orientation of these pins is far too perpendicular and, therefore, the direction of the iliac wing has been forgotten. These pins are inadequate for long-term use and would have to be replaced.* |

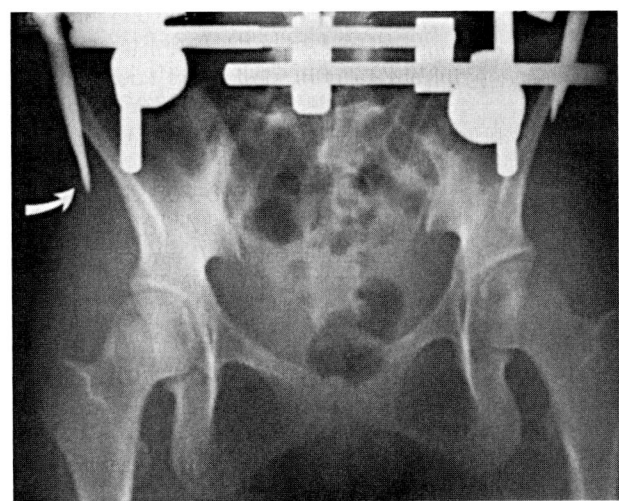

FIGURE 36-31 *Clinical (A) and radiographic (B) images of pelvic external fixator constructed with 5.5-mm Schanz screws placed just cranial and lateral to the hip joint. These are connected by a curved carbon fiber rod, which is under tension as evidenced by the Schanz screw deflection. The bulky dressing minimizes soft tissue shear against the pins.*

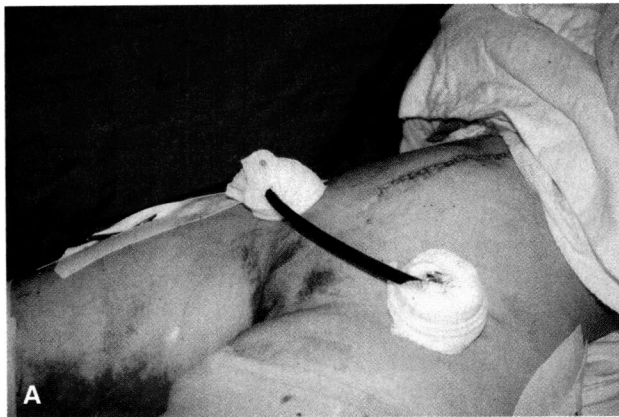

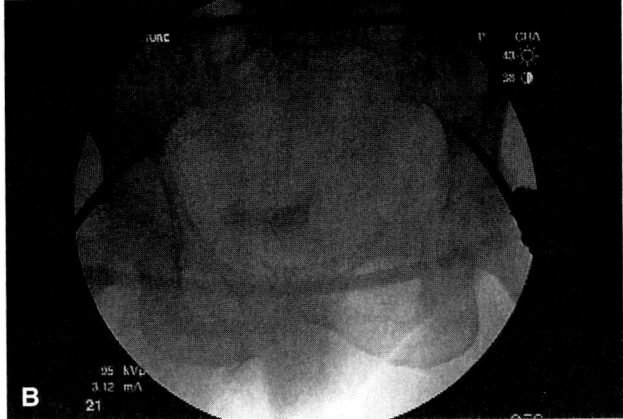

Use of supra-acetabular pins requires fluoroscopic control. A pilot smooth K-wire is inserted approximately 5 cm distal and 2 to 3 cm lateral to the ASIS. This ideally should localize a starting point approximately 2 cm proximal to the hip joint and slightly lateral to the AIIS. This position is verified using combined obturator outlet and iliac inlet views, and the K-wire is seated with a mallet. Once the starting point is established, a small longitudinal incision is made and a drill/pin sleeve is passed over the guide wire. A drill bit is then passed to create an aperture directed posteriorly toward the greater sciatic notch. The exact trajectory is determined by the anticipated needs for hip flexion and abdominal clearance. The pin is then inserted by hand through the retained sleeve. The frame is then assembled.

After pin placement and verification, the frame can be constructed. A simple frame with adequate thigh and abdominal clearance is the goal and can be achieved with a variety of different constructs (see Fig. 36-32,A,B). Once the frame has been applied, final fluoroscopically controlled adjustments in the reduction are carried out and the frame is tightened.

OPEN REDUCTION AND INTERNAL FIXATION OF THE SYMPHYSIS: TECHNIQUE
A Foley catheter is inserted for bladder decompression.[49,54] The approach to the symphysis can be made through a midline or Pfannenstiel incision. The Pfannenstiel incision is usually centered approximately 2 cm cranial to the symphysis and extends a total distance of 10 to15 cm, depending on body habitus. Irrespective of the skin incision, the deep exposure is the same. After the skin and subcutaneous tissues have been incised, the fascia over the rectus abdominis muscles and the external oblique muscle are identified. The Pfannenstiel approach requires carefully dissected proximal and distal subcutaneous flaps. The spermatic cord in men and round ligament in women (with the adjacent ilioinguinal nerve) should be protected. In many cases of symphyseal disruption, the rectus abdominis is partially or completely avulsed from one or both pubic bodies. In these cases, the deep exposure can be carried out relatively easily. The inferior 8 to 10 cm of the linea alba is split down to the symphysis. More proximal dissection of the linea alba may lead into the peritoneal cavity. The insertion of the recti onto the pubic bodies should be preserved when present (Fig. 36-33).

Dissection of the anterior aspect of the pubis is rarely needed and in males usually sacrifices the suspensory ligaments of the penis. Posteriorly, the space of Retzius is opened, and the Foley bulb is palpated for bladder location, but no additional dissection in this area is warranted. By remaining on the pubic bodies, the exposure can be extended laterally to expose the superior pubic rami to the iliopectineal eminence. This is facilitated by placement of a Hohman retractor posterior to the rectus through the fascia of the pectineus muscle over the anterior aspect of the superior ramus. Beware that the standard midline laparotomy incision does not extend the incision distally enough to expose the symphysis. An orthopaedic surgeon must be present if the trauma surgeon is making the incision so that the appropriate length is achieved.

Once the exposure has been completed, a variety of reduction techniques can be employed. The simplest and least invasive method utilizes a pointed reduction (Weber) clamp that can be applied through the soft tissues to the anterior pubic bodies just caudal and lateral to the pubic tubercle (Fig. 36-33). The clamp can be placed obliquely to address small step-offs at the symphysis. It is usually unnecessary to place clamps through the obturator externus and membrane into the medial margin of the obturator foramen. A more powerful and invasive alternative is the Juengbluth clamp placed on the anterior pubic bodies with anterior-to-posterior screw positions, usually accompanied by a nut on at least one side.

Once a satisfactory reduction is achieved, an appropriate plate is contoured and applied to the superior aspect of the pubic bodies. Plate choice depends on the type of associated posterior ring injury as well as the presence and security of posterior fixation. If the posterior osseous ligament hinge is intact (a stable AP compression injury), the use of a single plate placed on the superior aspect of the pubic bodies and crossing the symphysis is adequate.[49,54,107,108] If the posterior osseous ligamentous hinge is disrupted and will not be stabilized internally, the use of a second plate (four holes or more) placed on the anterior pubic bodies may provide a small incremental increase in stability. However, if posterior stabilization will be carried out, single-plate fixation is satisfactory. A two-hole or greater, 3.5- or 4.5-mm plate is used to provide suitable stability. A wide assortment of plates are available, including specifically designed symphyseal plates, some which offer a locking screw plate interface for use in osteoporotic individuals. The symphysis cycles in tension and compression, depending on the patient's position. For this reason, both the surgeon and patient need to be aware that all symphyseal fixation constructs ultimately loosen or fail or both. Clinically and radiographically, these failures are often subtle, but they can be more dramatic as well, particularly when mobilization limitations are exceeded. Ultimately, determination of plate size should be based on the plate that best fits the pubic bodies.[54]

Once the plate is positioned, palpation of the posterior aspect of the pubic body determines the orientation of the drill so that the screw can be placed through the full length of the pubic body. Usually, a 50- to 60-mm screw can be placed into the body of the pubis (Fig. 36-34). More lateral screws are shorter, but they may be directed to engage the primary pubic body screw to provide additional fixation in porotic bone. In the unusual setting where a second plate is deemed useful, it can be contoured along the anterior aspect of the pubic bodies and the screws placed in an anterior-to-posterior direction between the superiorly placed plate screws. These screws must not be left long to avoid erosion into the bladder. After fixation has been achieved, the incisions are closed over drains while making sure that the rectus abdominis is well apposed to its insertion. This is best achieved with complete muscle. The use of suture anchors may be beneficial when a portion of the rectus insertion has been avulsed. The external oblique aponeurosis must be repaired, and if the external ring has been entered, care must be taken to repair it anatomically so that an inguinal hernia does not develop.

FIGURE 36-32 **A,** *Midline transverse incision positioned just cranial to the symphysis and centered on the midline.* **B,** *Cutaneous flaps are raised in the midline cranially and caudally to better define and incise the linea alba.* **C,** *Retractors are placed over the anterosuperior pubic ramus to maintain rectus attachments to the anterior pelvic ring. A malleable retractor is placed posterior to the anterior pelvic ring to protect the bladder and retract the abdominal contents.* **D,** *Typical positioning of pointed reduction forceps to achieve reduction of the anterior ring. More substantial reduction tools may be necessary on the setting of complete (C type) posterior injuries to effect reduction.* **E,** *In the setting of poor bone material, typical cranially positioned plates may be supplemented with an anterior plate or posterior fixation (or both) to improve the mechanical stability of a rotational injury after reduction.*

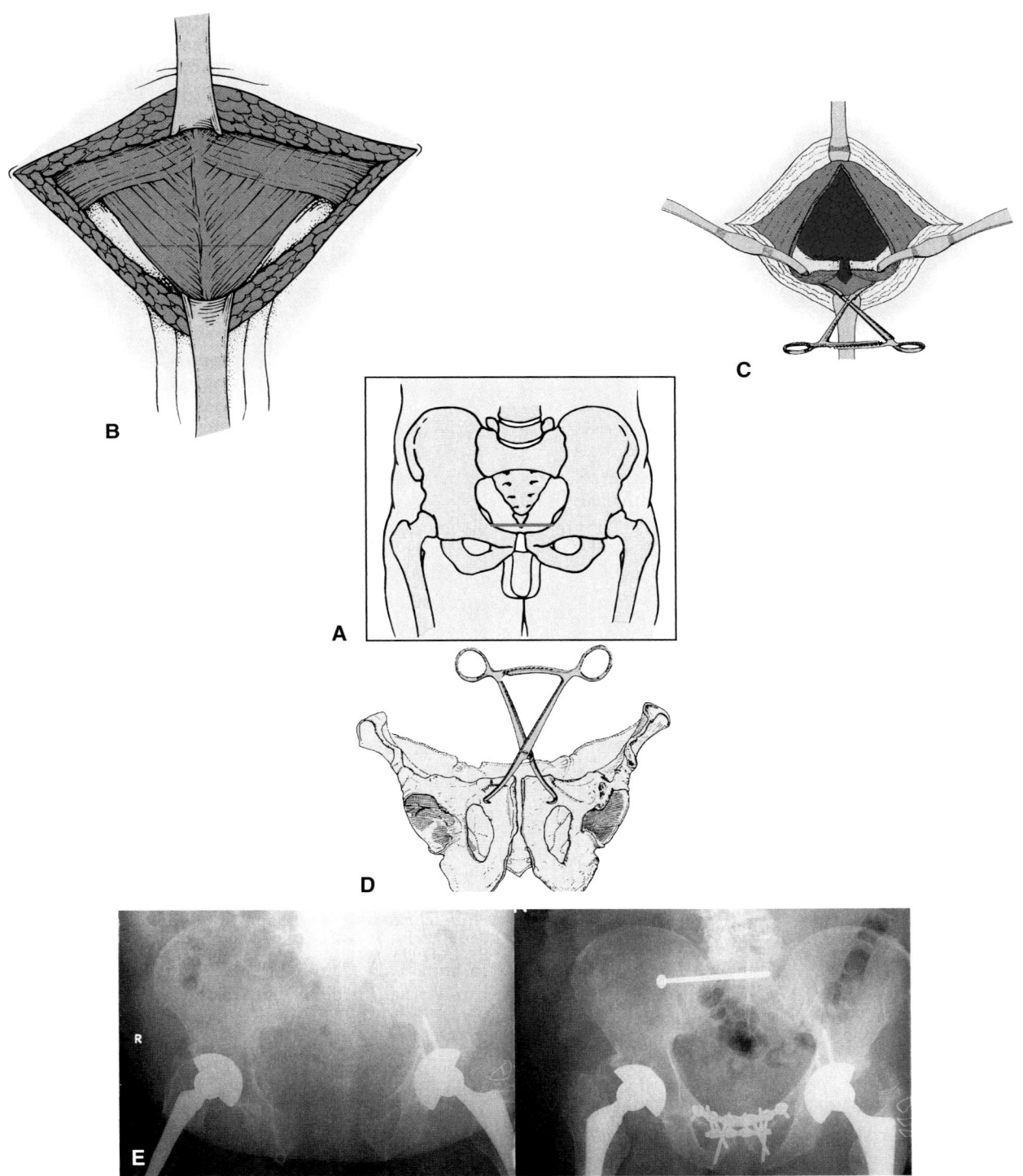

FIGURE 36-33 Series of radiographs demonstrating typical stabilization of open-book (B1.3) injury. **A,** Injury films depicting pubic symphysis dislocation and rotational injury to the sacroiliac (SI) joint. **B,** Despite obvious anterior diastasis, note the subtle opening of the left SI joint on computed tomography. **C,** Postreduction and healing. Four-to-six-hole small-fragment plates are typically sufficient anterior symphyseal fixation in rotationally unstable injuries.

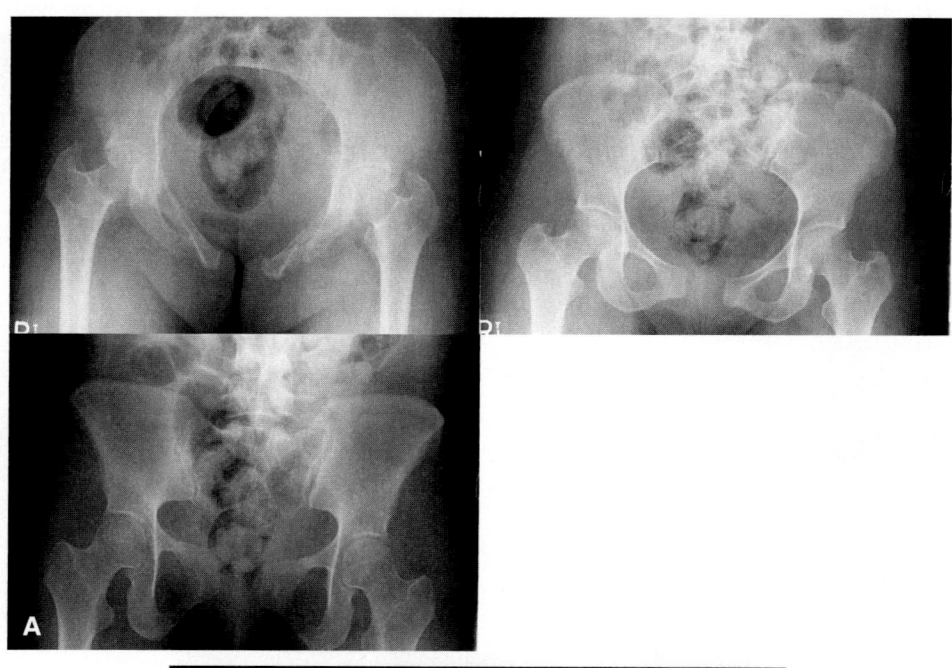

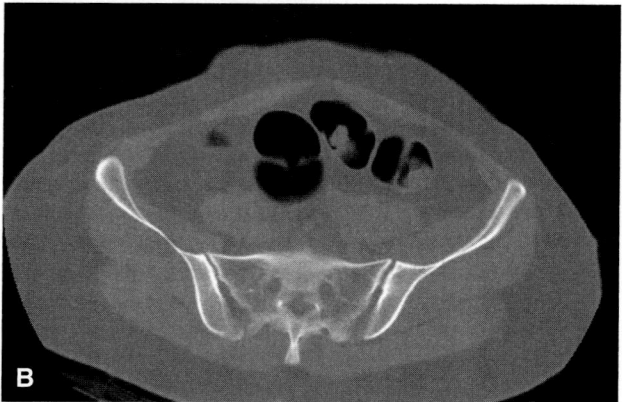

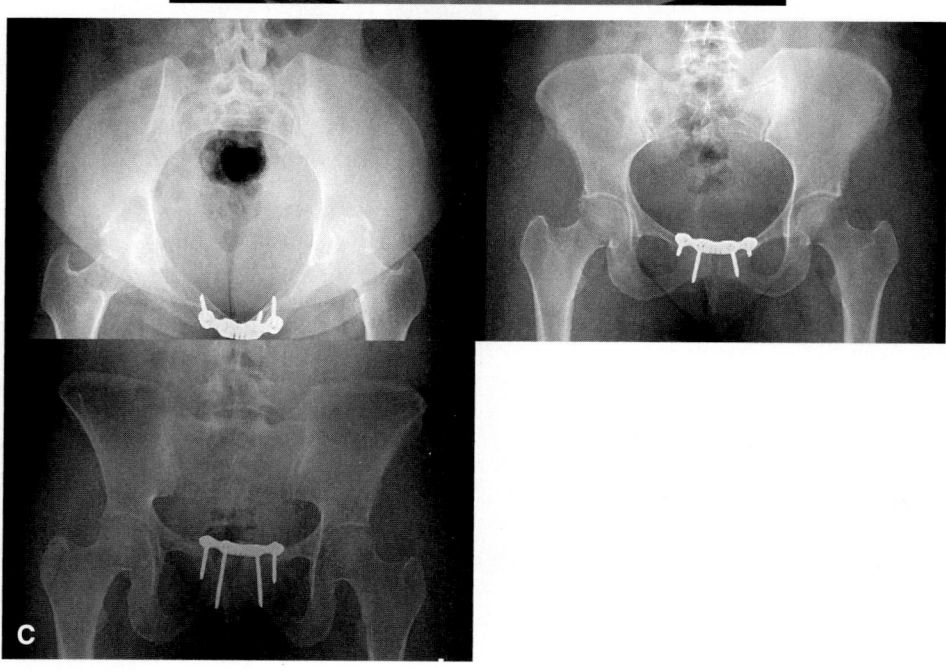

FIGURE 36-34 | *A,* A tilt-type injury. *B,* Computed tomography reveals complete sacral injury with impaction on the left side. *C,* Anterior ring fixation includes a retrograde pubic screw. This intermedullary screw can be used in an attempt to block internal rotation deformation of the pelvis.

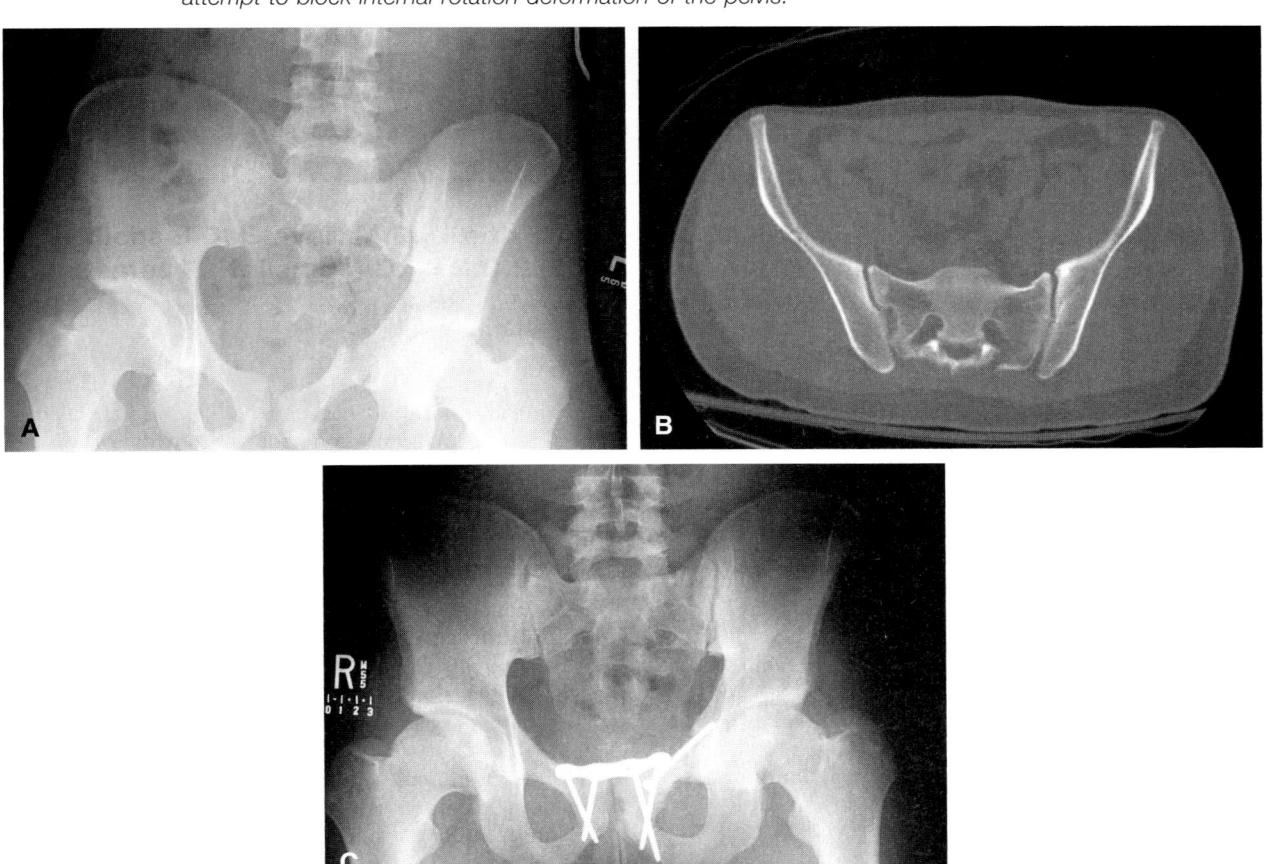

If a pubic ramus fracture requires exposure, it can be done by extending the surgical exposure along the pubic ramus. The reduction can be accomplished, and stabilization of the symphysis will usually control displacement of the pubic ramus. If the displacement is within the first 4 cm lateral to the body of the pubis, the plate may be extended out onto this area to achieve plate fixation. If an extensile approach is required for reduction and stabilization of a pubic ramus fracture, particularly at the root of the acetabulum, it is accomplished with an ilioinguinal anterior approach, as described by Letournel.[64,121] This approach allows adequate exposure of the whole anterior aspect of the pelvis and appropriate plate fixation with a well-contoured 3.5-mm reconstruction plate (Figs. 36-36 and 36-37).

An alternative anterior exposure is the modified Stoppa approach to the inner aspect of the pelvis.[16,45] With the patient in the supine position and the involved extremity draped free, a transverse incision is made 2 cm above the symphysis similar to the Pfannenstiel incision. The recti are split along the linea alba and sharply elevated from the pubic body and rami. The rectus and neurovascular structures are retracted laterally and anteriorly. With the surgeon standing on the opposite side of the table from the fracture, the vascular anastomoses between the inferior

epigastrics or external iliacs and the obturator vessels are ligated. Full access is achieved by dividing the iliopectineal fascia posteriorly and the obturator internus fascia inferiorly. Before elevation of the posterior iliacus, it may be necessary to cauterize the iliolumbar artery branch(es) that perforate the internal iliac fossa just lateral to the anterior aspect of the SI joint capsule. This exposure will allow access to the quadrilateral surface and entire pelvic brim posteriorly as far as the SI joint. Flexion of the ipsilateral leg facilitates the exposure by decreasing the tension on the psoas and iliac vessels. The obturator nerve and vessel must be protected throughout this approach. An identical exposure can be incorporated into a traditional ilioinguinal approach by expanding the dissection from the medial window. This is most useful when the anterior ring injury is accompanied by a displaced acetabular fracture.

The standard fixation is plate osteosynthesis. Screws inserted at or lateral to the iliopectineal eminence will be in the hip joint. Retrograde intramedullary screw fixation of ramus fractures has been reported by Letournel[64] and recently popularized by Routt.[105] The role of the retrograde pubic screw has been poorly defined, but may provide adjunctive stability especially in rotationally unstable injuries (Fig. 36-35).

FIGURE 35-35 *Anteroposterior pelvis radiograph **(A)** and computed tomographic image **(B)** showing pelvic ring injury consisting of wide symphyseal diastasis and left-sided zone 2 sacral fracture in 67-year-old female. **C,** Closed reduction techniques, and **D,** Open reduction of symphysis using a pointed reduction forceps (Weber clamp). **E,** Final reduction and fixation construct consisting of two iliosacral screws and six-hole pubic symphysis plate.*

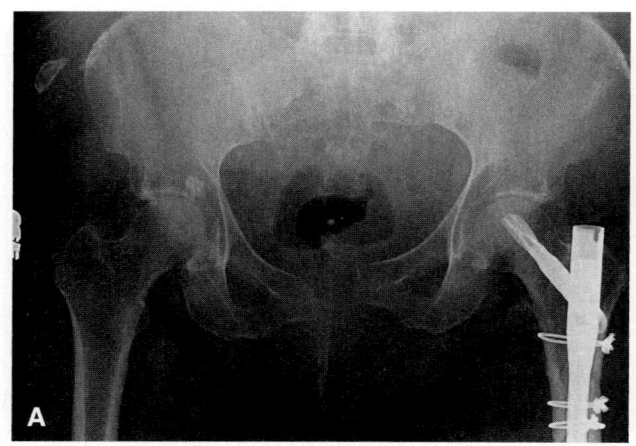

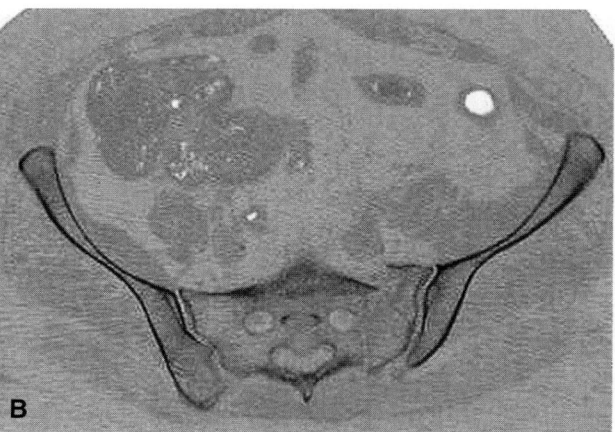

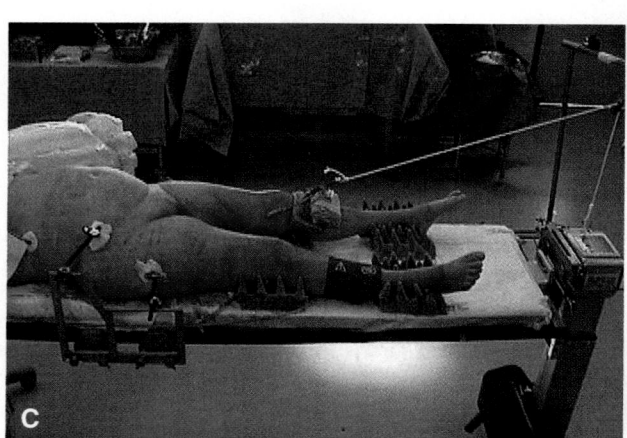

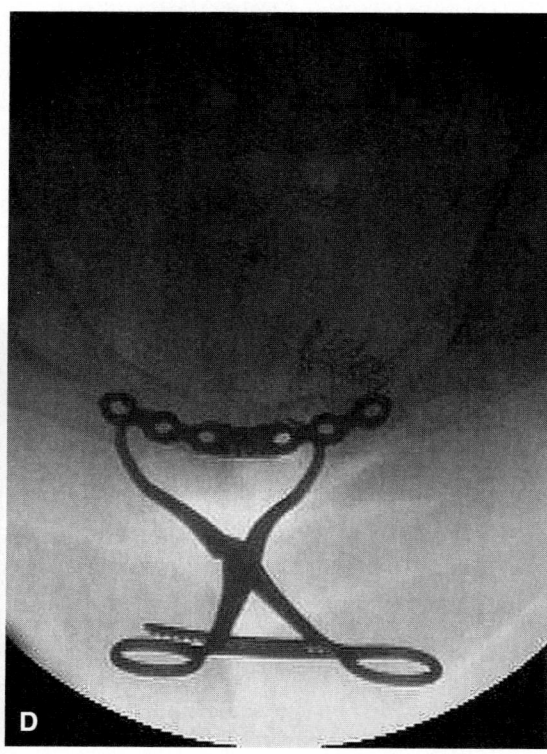

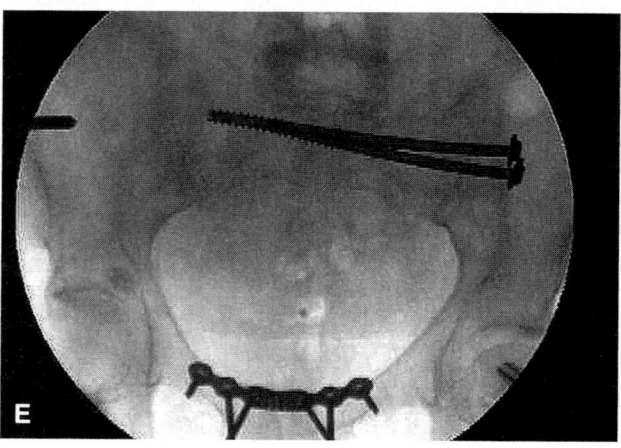

FIGURE 36-36 *Anterior approach to the sacroiliac joint.* **A,** *Anterior approach to the sacroiliac (SI) joint is positioned along the iliac crest and should extend past the anterosuperior iliac spine for 2 to 3 cm.* **B,** *The deep layer is extended medially through the inguinal ligament similar to the ilioinguinal approach. This improves mobilization of the iliopsoas and visualization of the SI joint from anterior.*

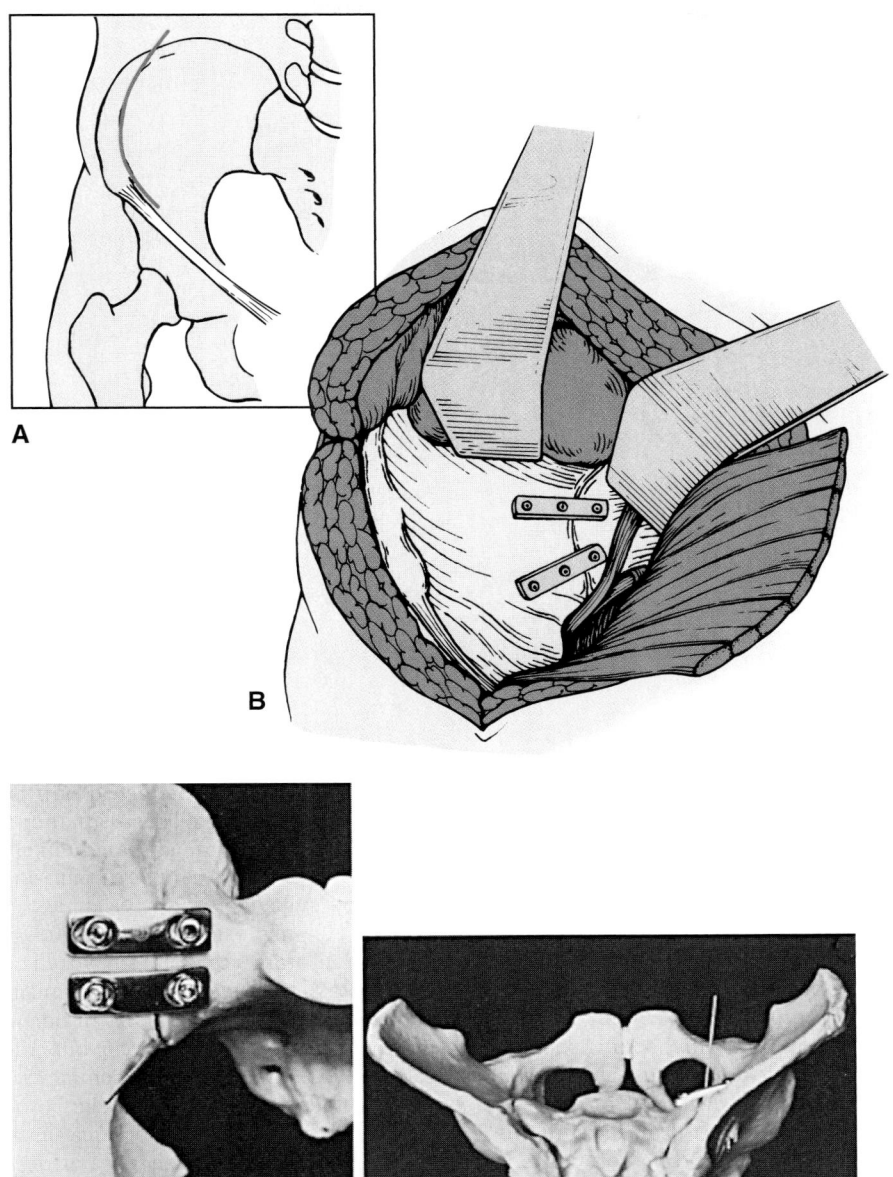

APPROACH TO POSTERIOR PELVIC RING INJURIES

Iliac fractures, dislocations, or fracture–dislocations through the SI joint can be reduced and stabilized either anteriorly or posteriorly.[49,61,64,99,109] Advantages of the anterior approach include better visualization of the cranial and anterior SI joint, which can then be reduced under direct visualization.[109] It may be easier to denude the articular cartilage of the SI joint to facilitate the insertion of a bone graft for potential fusion of this joint.[49,109] Anterior

approach to the SI joint may also be advantageous for rotationally unstable SI joint injuries with open or complex anterior ring injuries (Fig. 36-38). The disadvantage of this approach is the close relationship of the L4, L5, and lumbosacral trunk to the SI joint. The L4 nerve root runs between the L5 root and the SI joint and merges with the L5 root to form the lumbosacral trunk an average of 11.49 mm from the joint line at the level of the sacral promontory. It is at risk for a traction palsy if adequate exposure is not obtained and excessive retraction is necessary.[3,47] Reduction of the caudal portion of the SI joint

*Reduction technique for sacroiliac dislocation—anterior approach. **A**, Use of a pointed reduction clamp to apply traction and control rotation. **B**, A Schanz screw in the iliac crest to apply traction, produce translation, and control rotation. **C**, A pointed reduction clamp may be used to maintain reduction through a previously drilled hole in the sacrum and the iliac wing, or a large asymmetric pointed clamp may be placed onto the anterior aspect of the sacrum, just medial to the sacroiliac joint, and then passed over the posterior aspect of the iliac crest (not shown). **D**, Preinsertion of two screws on either side of the sacral iliac joint. The reduction may be performed with a Farabeuf clamp. **E, F**, Pelvic reduction clamp. **G**, Reduction may also be achieved indirectly by using a plate attached to the sacrum with one screw and, subsequently, using a second screw to pull the pelvis up and in. The flat plate is inserted into the sacrum and fixed. A gap is left under the sacroiliac joint but will be reduced when the iliac screw (arrow) is tightened. (From Tile, M., ed. Fractures of the Pelvis and Acetabulum, 2nd ed. Baltimore, Williams & Wilkins, 1995.)*

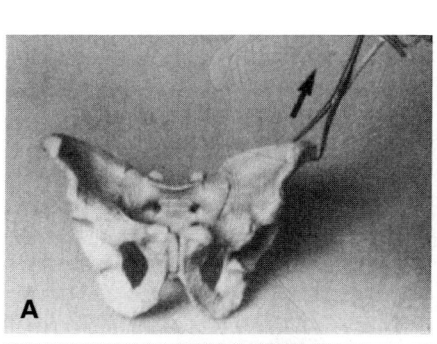
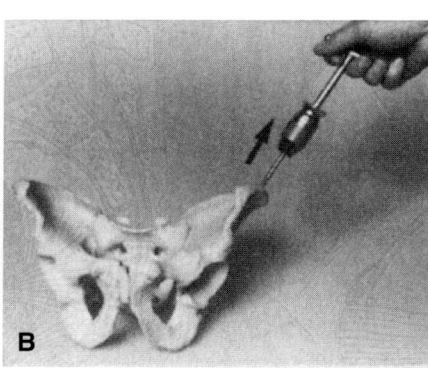
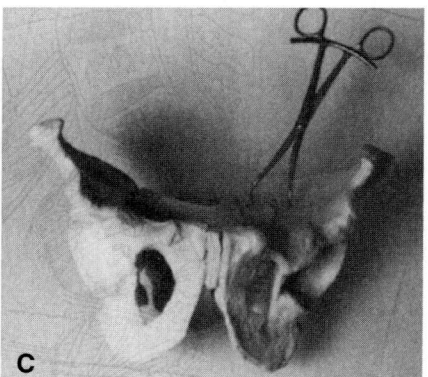
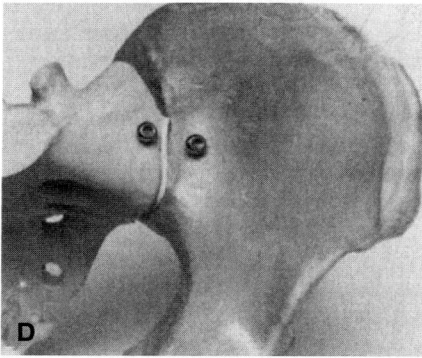
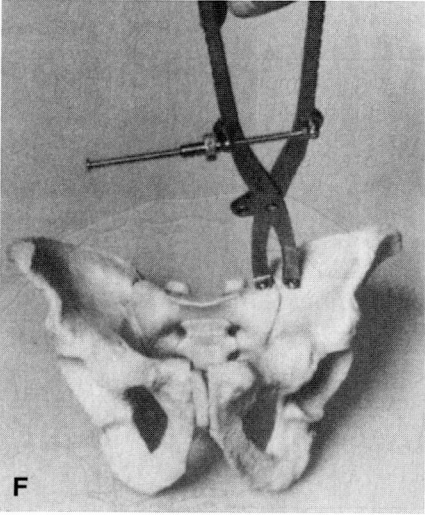
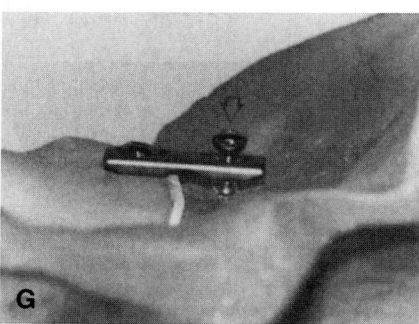
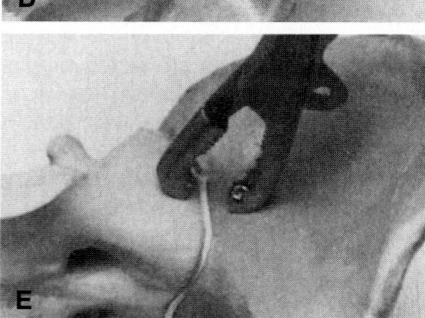

*Rotational injury with complex anterior ring fractures is an indication for an anterior approach to the sacroiliac (SI) joint. **A**, Rotational injury to the left SI joint with multifragmentary bilateral rami fractures. **B**, Stabilization of the SI joint using an anterior approach.*

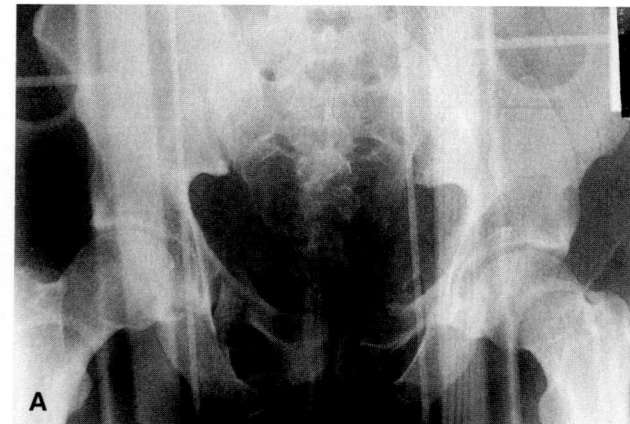
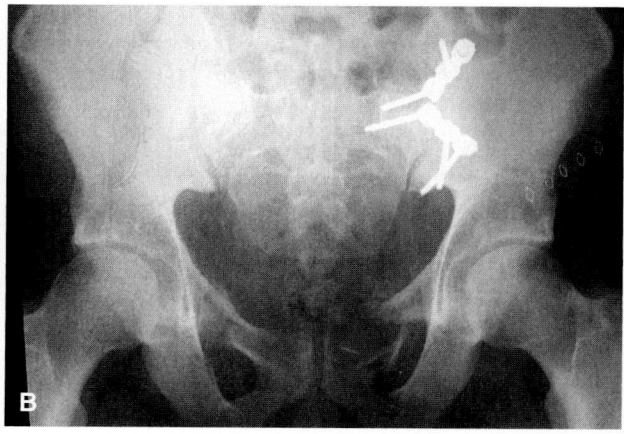

may also be difficult from the anterior approach when the SI joint is globally unstable. Careful CT evaluation of the SI articulation is also imperative prior to SI joint reduction from an anterior approach. In a lateral compression mechanism, the anterior SI joint may be impacted and reduction and fixation made difficult or impossible from an anterior approach.

The advantages of the posterior approach are its simplicity in exposing the iliac wing and SI joint and its ability to completely visualize and directly reduce all injuries to the posterior pelvic ring including either sacral or SI dislocations and fracture–dislocations.[64] The major disadvantage of this approach is that the patient must be turned prone, which may be difficult in a multiply injured patient. Damage to the anterior vascular structures in front of the sacrum or to the cauda equina by inadvertent perforation with the screws must also be avoided. Posterior soft tissue crush injuries or significant skin loss may also cause problems.[49]

Both techniques carry a risk for significant complications, of which the surgeon must be well aware, but neither approach has been definitely proven better. As long as appropriate precautions are taken, both approaches provide adequate reduction and stabilization of fractures or fracture–dislocations of the SI joint.

The decision regarding which approach to use is determined by the characteristics of the soft tissue injury and the fracture. The anterior approach is indicated for SI joint dislocations and fracture–dislocations involving the ilium, for iliac wing fractures, and when either of these injuries occurs in conjunction with an associated anterior pelvic ring injury that requires fixation. The anterior approach is not indicated for sacral fractures or when the risk of infection from an external fixator pin, colostomy, suprapubic catheter, or overhanging abdominal pannus is high. The posterior approach can be used for all posterior pelvic injuries, including sacral fractures, fracture–dislocations involving the SI joint, and fractures of either the ilium or sacrum and the iliac wing. Contraindications to a posterior approach are crush or degloving injuries to the posterior skin or wounds that communicate with the perineum and ischiorectal area.

For all internal fixations of the pelvis, the use of an image intensifier and a radiolucent operating table is mandatory. The C-arm is necessary to confirm reduction and screw placement. Familiarity with the three pelvic radiographic views is necessary. Patient size, bowel gas, and radiographic dye may hinder the ability to obtain quality radiographs and force a change in treatment or radiographic technique.

ANTERIOR APPROACH TO THE SACROILIAC JOINT: EXPOSURE AND REDUCTION

The patient is placed in the supine position on a radiolucent table. A small radiolucent roll may be placed just lateral to the midline on the involved side to elevate the involved hemipelvis for easier manipulation[109] (see Fig. 36-36). The involved leg is draped free so that it is available to assist in the reduction. This approach can also be performed with the patient in the lateral decubitus position. The incision starts approximately 6 cm behind the highest point of the iliac crest and is best carried anteriorly 3 to 5 cm past the anterior superior iliac spine. Posteriorly, the muscles of the lateral abdominal wall are split in the

direction of their fibers to expose the posterior half of the iliac crest. The iliac fascia and the insertions of the external muscles of the abdomen onto the iliac crest are sharply elevated from the iliac crest, and the iliacus muscle is then elevated subperiosteally from the internal iliac wing. The external oblique is then incised medial to the ASIS for 3 to 5 cm and reflected caudally. The inguinal ligament is incised for this distance over the iliopsoas muscle similar to developing the lateral window of the ilioinguinal. This provides for improved exposure and visualization of the anterior SI joint (Fig. 36-39). The lateral femoral cutaneous nerve is located just medial to the anterior superior spine and must be protected in this approach. At this point, with flexion and internal rotation of the hip to relax the psoas and iliacus, careful dissection along the iliac wing will bring the SI joint into view. Because the iliac wing usually displaces posteriorly, the sacrum is generally found anterior to the iliac wing. Care should be taken to avoid going through the iliacus onto the sacrum and damaging the L5 root. By following the displaced iliac wing, the articular cartilage of the SI joint can be identified, and by moving both superiorly and posteriorly, the sacral ala can be identified. Subperiosteal dissection is then carried along the ala. Care should be taken to gently retract the soft tissues medially, including the L4 and L5 roots. The L5 root normally lays 2 to 3 cm medial to the S1 joint in a small groove and then goes over the anterior aspect of the sacrum to drop into the pelvis. After the superior aspect of the sacral ala has been identified, dissection continues along the anterior aspect of the ala and the pelvic brim down inside the true pelvis to identify the notch. The surgeon must take care that the dissection remains subperiosteal and avoid injury to the superior gluteal artery. If bleeding does occur, packing of the area can usually control it. After the dislocation or fracture–dislocation has been identified, the SI joint may be denuded of cartilage on its sacral side and the subchondral plate roughened if fusion of the joint is desired. A small bone graft can be taken from the anterior iliac crest. The fracture or dislocation is then reduced.

Reduction is best accomplished by placing bone-holding forceps on the iliac wing through the interval between the ASIS and AIIS to grasp the hemipelvis and pull it forward. The use of 5-mm Schanz pins in the iliac crest is helpful in obtaining the correct rotational position of the hemipelvis. By pulling the pelvis forward with the bone-holding clamp and rotating it with the Schanz pins, reduction is obtained at the level of the SI joint (see Fig. 36-38). By using an asymmetrical pelvic reduction clamp, the SI joint can be reduced and stabilized provisionally. One arm of the clamp is placed on the posterior aspect of the iliac crest and the other on the anterior aspect of the sacral ala. The direction of force is such that the joint is pushed anteriorly and closed down posteriorly. With a fracture through the iliac wing, this maneuver helps reduce the dislocation. Reduction may also be accomplished by placing one screw into the sacral ala and one into the iliac wing and then applying the pelvic reduction clamps. Provisional stabilization is achieved by placing a 3.2-mm Steinmann pin percutaneously through the iliac wing into the ala. Before reduction, this pin may be inserted through the ilium into the iliac side of the SI joint so that its position

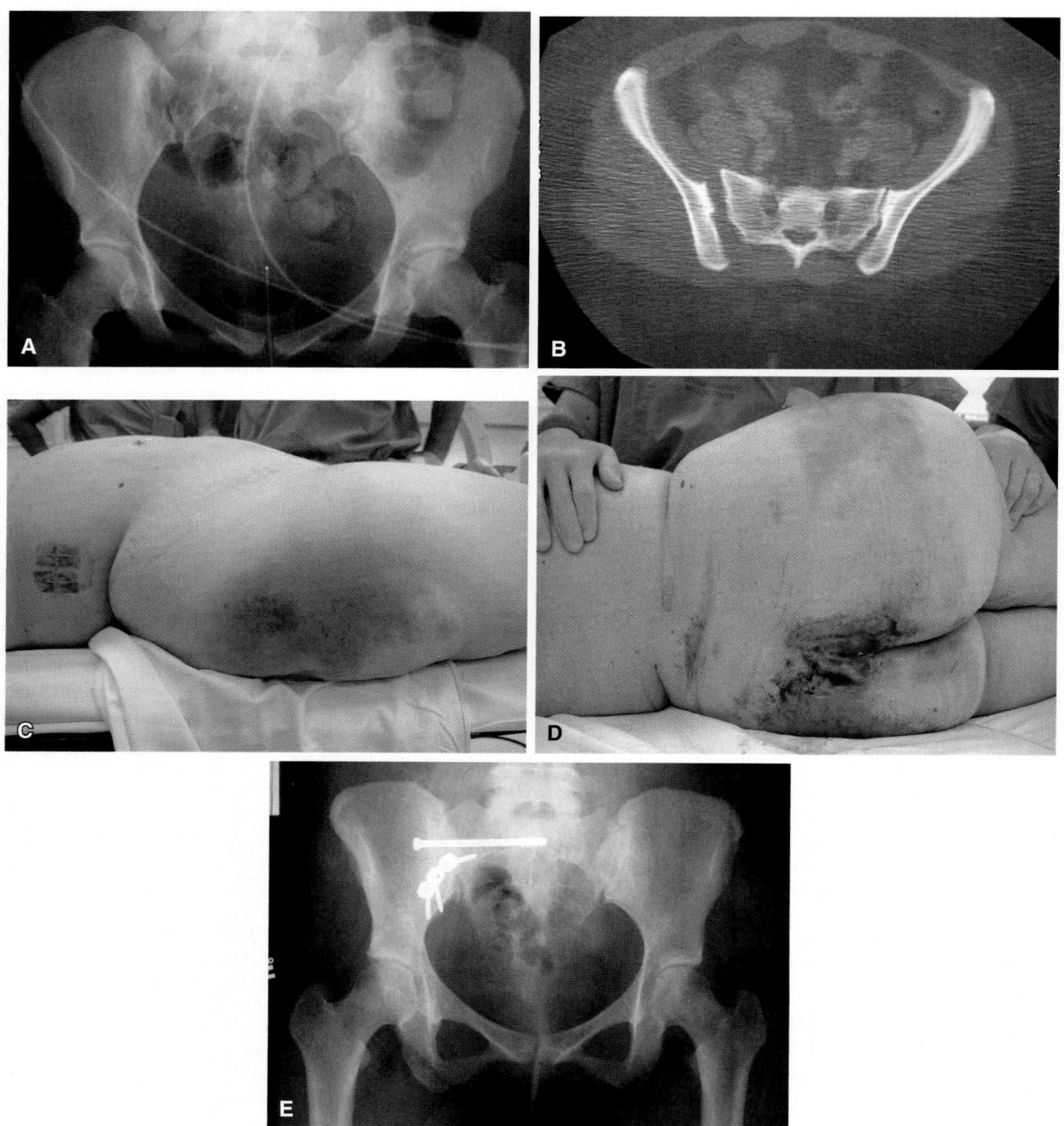

FIGURE 36-39 | *Poor soft tissues are an indication for an anterior approach to the sacroiliac (SI) joint. A moderately obese individual pinned between two objects. **A,** Anteroposterior view of the pelvis with right SI joint side location, left minimally displaced transverse acetabulum fracture. **B,** Computed tomography confirms posterior injury. **C,** Right flank ecchymosis and clinical exam were consistent with degloving injury. **D,** Posterior abrasions in the area where the bar struck the patient and posterior soft tissues. **E,** Fixation after anterior approach achieved with plate and percutaneous SI screw to secure caudal joint.*

is confirmed under direct vision. A staple across the SI joint may also be used as a temporary stabilization device.[57]

A 3.5- or 4.5-mm three- or four-hole reconstruction plate is then contoured. One screw is placed into the sacral ala and directed parallel to the SI joint. The direction of the screw can be determined by placing a 1.6-mm K-wire in the joint at the time of reduction. These screws are usually 30 to 40 mm long. The plate is attached to the iliac wing by fully threaded cancellous screws, which usually traverse the length of the posterior tubercle (see Fig. 36-38). The pelvic reduction clamp can then be removed and replaced by a second plate. Specialized plates have been developed for SI joint stabilization, but they do not allow incorporation of iliac wing fracture fixation.[109] At times, a small ridge may overgrow the SI joint on either the iliac or the sacral side. This ridge may make reduction and plate fixation difficult and can be removed. A final way of stabilizing the joint once reduction is achieved is by insertion of a percutaneous cancellous screw into the sacral body and neutralization with a three- or four-hole 3.5- or 4.5-mm anterior SI plate (Fig. 36-40). After image intensification or plain radiographs confirm reduction, the wound is closed in the appropriate fashion. Similar reduction and fixation techniques are utilized to reduce and stabilize the caudal portion of the SI joint component of a fracture–dislocation. This should proceed first as the joint should take precedence. Direct reduction and interfragmentary fixation of the fractures of the iliac wing followed by neutralization plating complete the fixation construct (Fig. 36-41).

POSTERIOR APPROACH TO THE PELVIS: EXPOSURE AND REDUCTION

Of the posterior approaches to pelvic ring injuries, the paramedian approach as described by Letournel is the most utilitarian and can be used for SI joint fracture–dislocations, SI joint dislocations, and sacral fractures and has extensive utility in delayed reconstruction or repair of malunions and nonunions of the pelvic ring.[64,100] Careful

preoperative evaluation of the posterior soft tissue envelope helps to avoid such soft tissue complications as infection or skin breakdown.

The patient is traditionally placed in a prone position on a radiolucent table with the hip extended to neutral and the knees flexed to protect the sciatic nerve. Adequate fluoroscopic images are obtained prior to the prep and drape. The gluteal cleft is isolated from the operative field, and the skin is antiseptically prepared. The use of commercially available radiolucent tables and devices that facilitate stabilization of a stable hemipelvis to the table allows for longitudinal traction to be applied to the unstable hemipelvis without the potential of deformity introduced by the use of a perineal post (Fig. 36-42). Once the field is draped, an adhesive occlusive drape (3M Ioband) is used to isolate the area of the incision. A longitudinal incision is made 2 cm lateral to the PSIS (see Fig. 36-42A). This incision may be curved slightly in its cephalad extent if more anterior exposure of the iliac crest is needed. Cutaneous flaps are then raised off of fascia of the gluteus maximus to the midline. The abductors are released from their origin on the posterior iliac crest to the PSIS; (see Fig. 36-42B). The origin of the gluteus maximus is released from the PSIS and the

---

FIGURE 36-40 *A,* Sacroiliac (SI) fracture–dislocation with anterior extension. *B,* Note the sacral impaction on computed tomography.

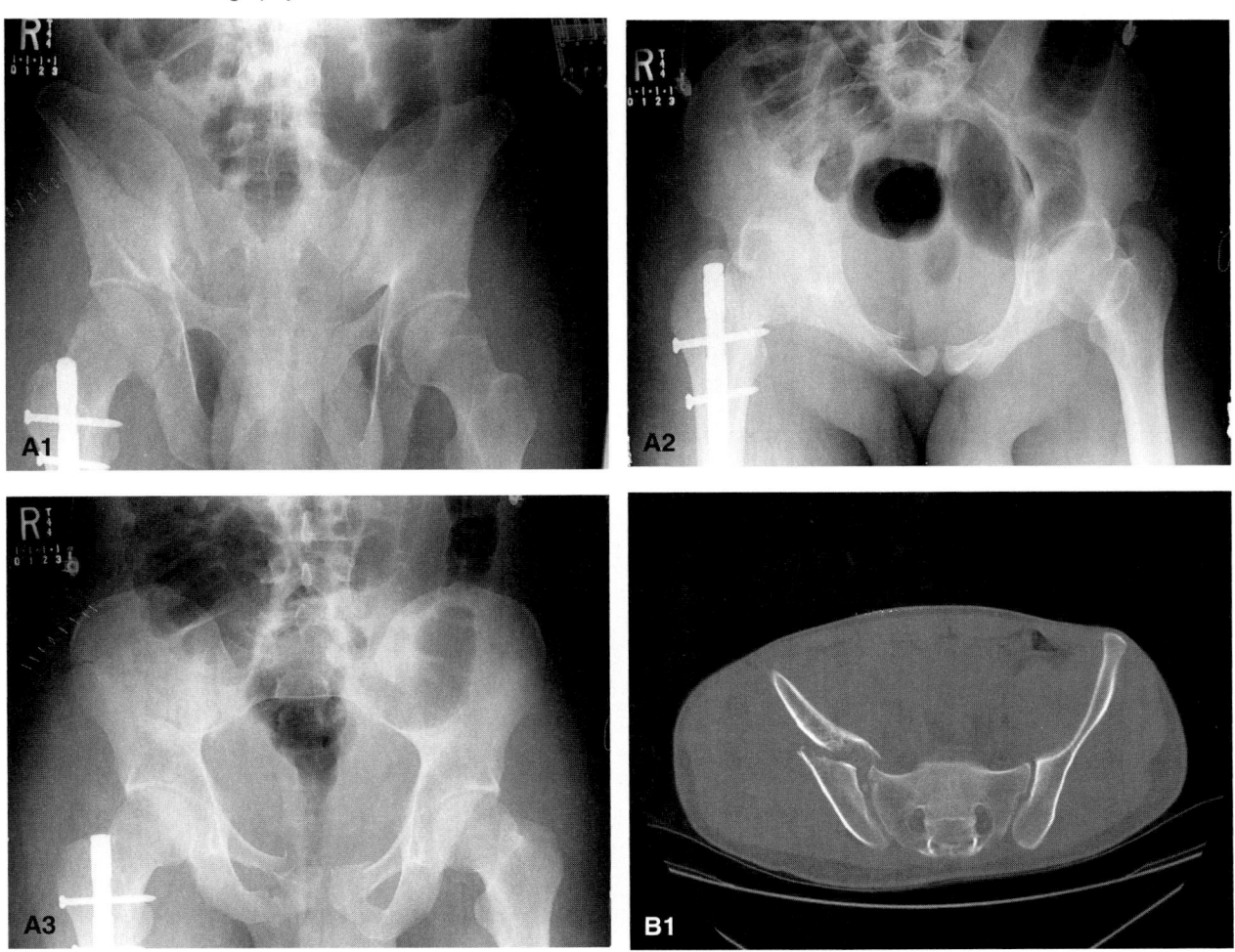

FIGURE 36-40 *(Continued)* ***C,*** *SI reduction neutralized with a fully threaded cancellous screw due to impaction of the sacrum. Screw and plate fixation of multifragmentary iliac component.*

FIGURE 36-41 *Positioning prone with pelvic stabilizer attached to contralateral intact pelvis. This allows traction to be directly applied to the injured hemipelvis. This can easily be incorporated into the surgical field.*

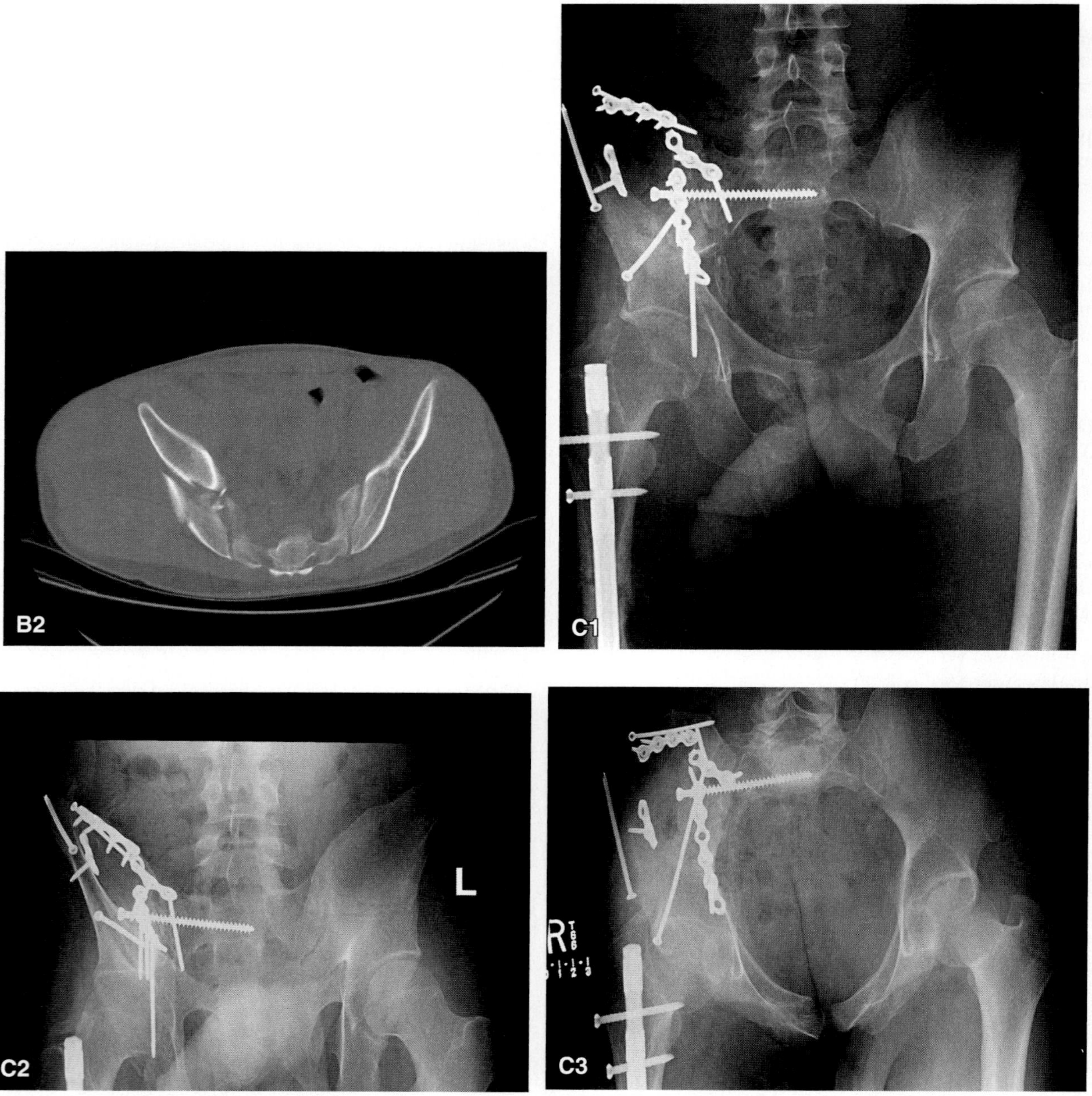

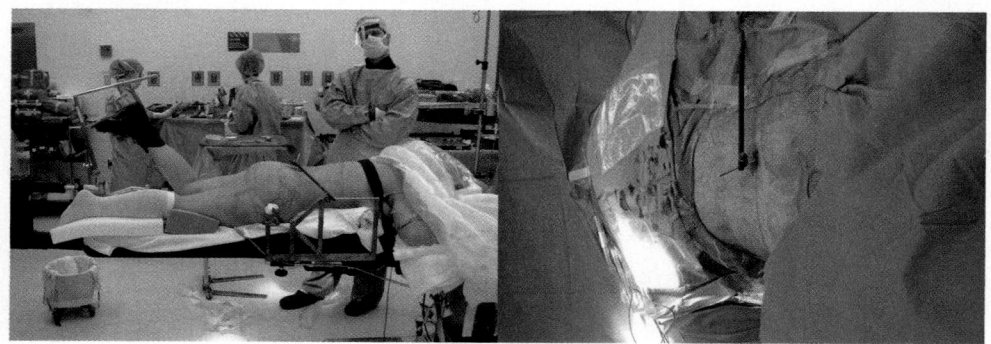

FIGURE 36-42 *Posterior approach to the pelvic ring. **A,** Incision lateral to the posteroinferior iliac spine. **B,** Elevation of the gluteus from the posterior crest and midline. **C,** Cranial and caudal extent to gluteus maximus past the posterior iliac crest. **D,** Deep exposure after elevation of the glutei from the ilium and erector spinae from the sacrum, allowing access to all injuries of the posterior pelvic ring.*[67a]

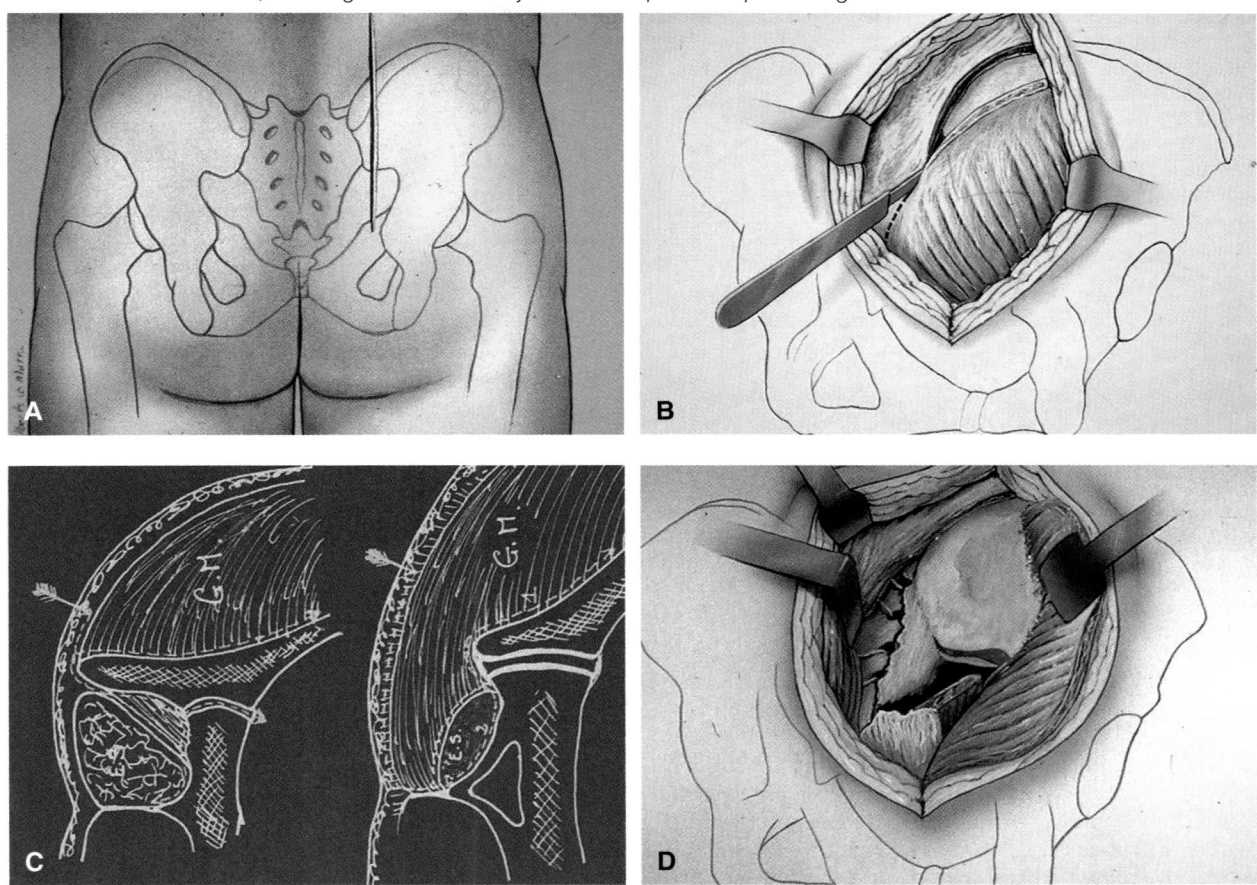

dorsal fascia of the multifidis. Care should be taken during the dissection to preserve this origin to facilitate later repair of the glutei. The glutei are then elevated as a flap based on the superior and interim gluteal artery and nerve from the external surface of the ilium. If not already disrupted by the injury, access to the SI joint and sacrum can be accomplished by elevation of the erector spinae from the dorsal sacrum (Fig. 36-42D). Entrance into the true pelvis through the greater sciatic notch is initially gained by release of the sacrotuberous and sacrospinous ligament attachments to the lateral sacrum. Care should be taken when dissecting along the lateral and ventral notch to protect the superior gluteal neurovascular pedicle.

SACROILIAC JOINT

Use of a lamina spreader allows the joint or fracture to be distracted and débrided. On completion of débridement of the joint or fracture, reduction is accomplished with the use of pointed reduction clamps, a femoral distractor, and pelvic reduction forceps. Reduction of the SI joint can be confirmed by palpation anteriorly and direct visualization of the caudal portion of the joint. Palpation along the superior border of the sacral ala and the iliac crest

can also be carried out. Confirmation of a satisfactory reduction by radiographs or image intensification is recommended The cranial reduction of the SI joint dislocation can be performed with the use of a clamp from the sacrum to the posterior spine. Rotational reduction of the SI can be achieved with a Schanz pin in the posterior spine and held with an angled clamp placed through the greater notch After the SI dislocation has been reduced, iliosacral screw fixation is performed. As an open procedure, the guide wire or drill starts on the outer aspects of the iliac crest 1.5 cm anterior to a line from the posterior superior to the posterior inferior spine (crista glutea) and 2.5 cm above the greater sciatic notch.[75] The use of a specific point on the iliac wing demands that the SI joint be anatomically reduced and there is minimal sacral dysmorphism (Fig. 36-43). This position should be used merely as a guide to identifying an appropriate starting point. Before advancing into the sacrum, position of the drill or wire should be confirmed radiographically. AP and inlet views determine the AP position of the screw, the outlet view is used to determine the superoinferior position of the screw, and guide wire or drill bit placement is confirmed to be aimed into the sacral body (Fig. 36-44). The authors recommend using an oscillating drill, slowly advancing the

FIGURE 36-43 *Starting position for posterior screw fixation of pelvic disruptions.* ***A,*** *The proper starting position is approximately 15 mm from the elevated attachment of the gluteus maximus muscles on a line drawn from the top of the greater sciatic notch on the iliac crest.* ***B,*** *Another similar location, found by starting approximately 2.5 cm (2 to 3 fingerbreadths) lateral to the posterior superior iliac spine and 2 fingerbreadths cranial to the greater sciatic notch. Both these starting positions require anatomic reduction of the disruption.*

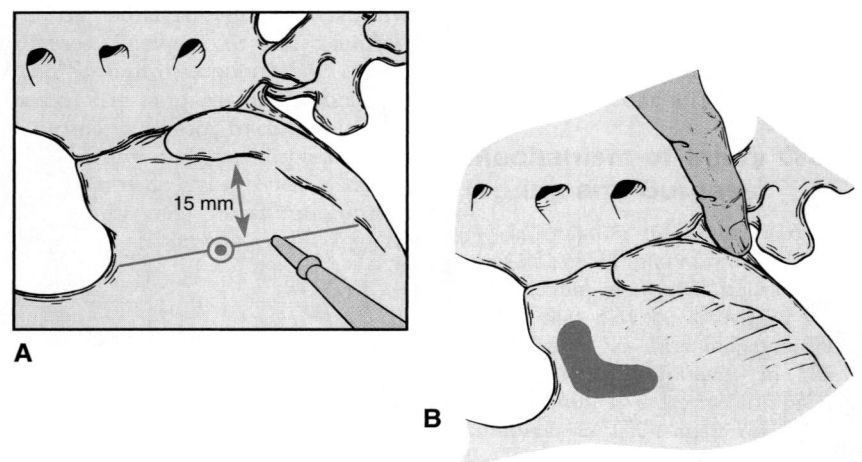

FIGURE 36-44 *To make sure that the screw fixation into the sacrum or sacral ala is placed safely, the use of image intensification is mandatory. On a radiolucent table, an image intensifier is brought in so that anteroposterior 40° caudal and 40° cephalad views can be obtained. The screws can then be directed under direct radiographic control into the sacral ala and body superior to the S1 foramen and thereby avoid the cauda.*

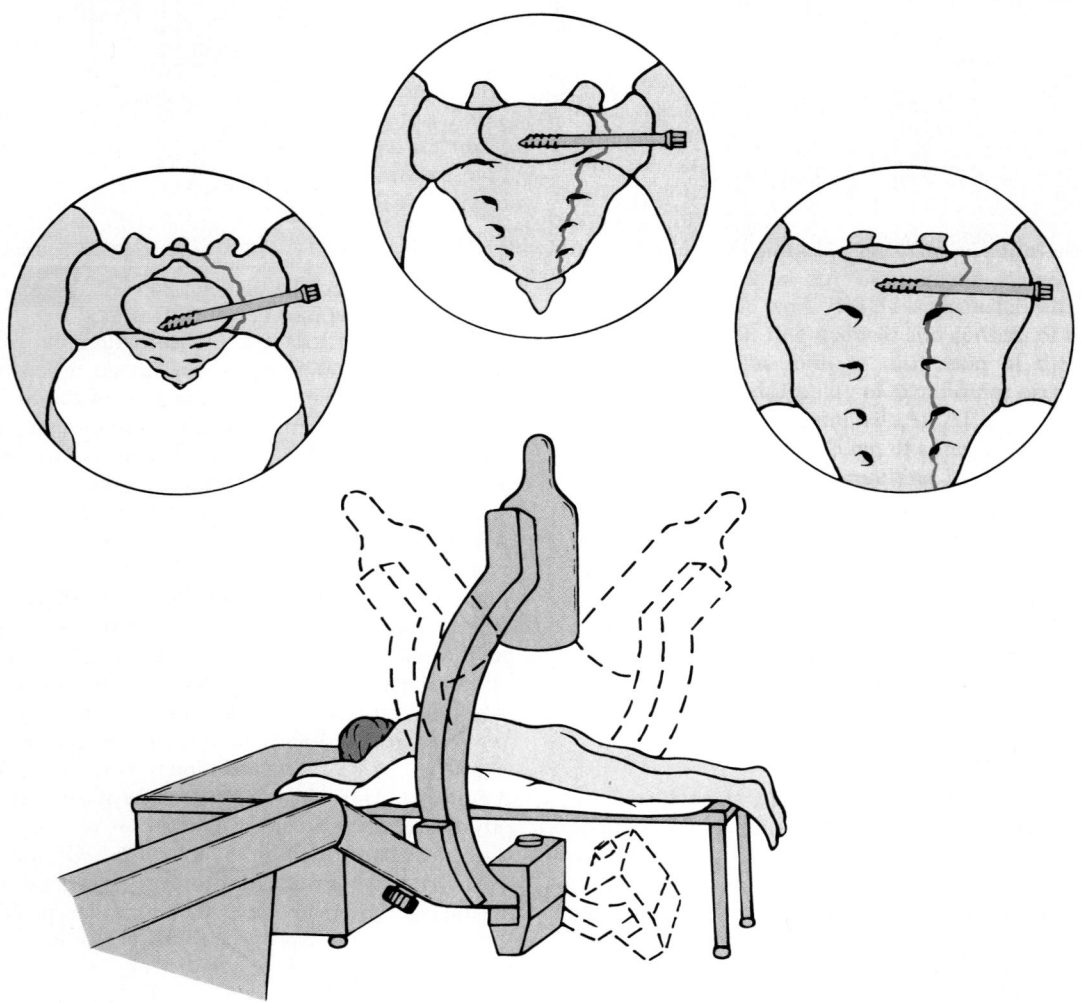

tip using a pistoning motion. This helps to ensure that the drill bit remains in bone. Three cortical barriers should be crossed (i.e., the outer iliac wing, the iliac side of the SI joint, and the sacral subchondral bone). If a fourth cortical barrier is encountered, the drill bit is about to leave the sacrum, with potential danger either to the cauda equina or to the anteriorly placed neurologic and vascular structures. If the position of the drill or guide wire is not correct, it is withdrawn completely and redirected. A small two- or three-hole plate can be applied to the outer aspect of the iliac wing, or a washer can be used to prevent penetration of the screws into the iliac bone. In SI dislocations, cancellous screws with a 16- or 32-mm thread length and a 6.5- or 7.3-mm diameter are normally used (see Fig. 36-43). However, the surgeon should make sure that the threads cross into the sacral body in order to obtain purchase in the best available bone. Mechanically, a screw with a 16-mm thread length may be more beneficial than a screw with a 32-mm thread length because the junction of the screw shaft and threads is further from the potentially mobile dislocation or fracture site. The 32-mm thread has been shown to provide more stability in cadaver models. Although screw position can be evaluated by direct visualization posteriorly and by palpation of the ala superiorly and anteriorly, it is mandatory that C-arm fluoroscopy be used to confirm its safe position.

SACRAL FRACTURES

Fractures through the sacrum are probably the most difficult to reduce and stabilize.[47,112] Open reduction and internal fixation can be performed via a paramedian, or midline approach may be utilized, depending on the type of fracture or planned fixation. With an open technique, the fracture can be opened with a laminar spreader and the sacral roots visualized and decompressed if necessary. A femoral distractor applied to both posterior tubercles can be helpful in controlling and maintaining the reduction.[63] Reduction is usually accomplished by traction to reduce vertical displacement and by direct manipulation with reduction clamps or Schanz pins to correct anterior, posterior, and rotational displacement. Fine adjustments are made with the pointed reduction forceps and maintained in place for provisional fixation.[63,83] Three basic methods of stabilization can be used. The first is the posterior iliosacral screw fixation method described previously. The screw fixation must enter the sacral body. If a lag screw technique is selected, direct visualization of the fracture for transforaminal fractures allows safe compression. The threads must not cross the fracture if compression is to be effective. If nerve root impingement is a possibility, a fully threaded position screw may be used to maintain the reduction, but adjunctive fixation may be necessary in the absence of compression. In the setting of fractures involving the central body of S1 or in revision situations, a screw placed through the sacrum to the contralateral ilium can be utilized. Safe placement of the screw into this corridor can be difficult (Fig. 36-45).[6a]

The second method of fixation is the use of plate fixation. This may supplement screw fixation in comminuted sacral fractures. Through similar incisions on both sides,

one being smaller on the stable hemipelvis, the gluteus maximus can be elevated from its origin. A tunnel is then made under the erector spinae muscle just above the level of the SI joint and through the spinous of S3. A 3.5- or 4.5-mm reconstruction plate can be slid across the posterior aspect of the sacrum and subsequently continued on to both iliac wings (Fig. 36-46). Screws placed through the plate and between the tables of the ilium provide initial fixation and compression posteriorly. One to two further screws into each ilium complete the fixation (Figs. 36-47 and 36-48).

Pohlemann and colleagues described alternative midline approaches for reduction and fixation of sacral fractures with small-fragment plates.[90] The operative approach is through a single dorsal incision with the patient in the prone position. The important landmarks for the skin incision are the L4 and L5 spinous processes, the posterior iliac crests, and the upper gluteal cleft. Unilateral sacral fractures are approached through an incision midway between the sacral spines and the posterior iliac crest on the involved side. For bilateral sacral ala exposure, an incision slightly lateral to the sacral spines is used. Deep exposure of unilateral fractures is achieved by incising the lumbodorsal fascia close to the sacral spines and elevating the muscle from the sacrum. If a more extensile approach is needed, the erector spinae can be elevated completely by detaching its distal and lateral attachments to the sacrum and posterior iliac crest. For bilateral exposure, the unilateral approach can be performed on both sides. Reduction is accomplished as described previously. Screws placed laterally into the ala and medially into the sacral bone between the posterior foramina attach the posterior sacral plates as close to the SI joint as allowed by the attachments of the iliosacral ligaments (Fig. 36-49). The lateral alar screws are safely placed if their orientation is parallel to the plane of the SI joint, as identified by a K-wire placed into the joint posteriorly. Plunging with the drill bit is dangerous because of the anteriorly placed internal iliac vessels and lumbosacral trunk. The S1 alar screw must not exit the superior surface of the ala. Palpation of this surface is possible between the L5 transverse process and the sacrum. The medial screw at S1 is placed directly inferior to the distal border of the L5-S1 facet. Enough room is available to insert two 3.5-mm screws. The screw is oriented in the sagittal plane and parallel to the cranial sacral lamina for lateral fractures. For transforaminal fractures, the screw is angulated 20° laterally in the horizontal plane and parallel to the cranial sacral lamina in the sagittal and frontal planes. It is aimed at the sacral promontory, so it has an average length of 50 to 80 mm. For S2-S4 medial screws, the entry point is along an imaginary vertical line through the foramina and in the midpoint between them. The direction of placement is perpendicular to the posterior sacral lamina. A more medial direction would be dangerous because the screw would enter the central canal. The implants used are standard small-fragment plates that are cut to fit. Each fracture line must be crossed by at least two plates, preferably at S1, S3, or S4. For transalar fractures, H-plates are used at the S1 and lower levels. If the fragmentation extends too far laterally for secure screw placement, the plate must extend onto the ilium. If a medial screw cannot be inserted, a dynamic compression

FIGURE 36-45 *This man had a disruption of his left sacroiliac joint fixed by posterior screw fixation. **A,** This patient was struck from behind by a truck and suffered a displaced fracture through the sacroiliac joint and pubic rami anteriorly. **B,** Inlet view confirming posterior displacement at the sacroiliac joint on the left side. **C,** Anteroposterior view demonstrating posterior screw fixation of the pelvis. Note how the screws have been placed across and into the body of the sacrum. Such placement is necessary for sacral fractures, but it also gains good purchase in sacroiliac joint dislocations. The screws are above the first sacral foramen. **D,** Good screw placement is noted on the inlet view, which shows that reduction has been achieved and adequate fixation has occurred with screws in the ala and body of the sacrum. **E,** Outlet view again confirming proper position of the screws.*

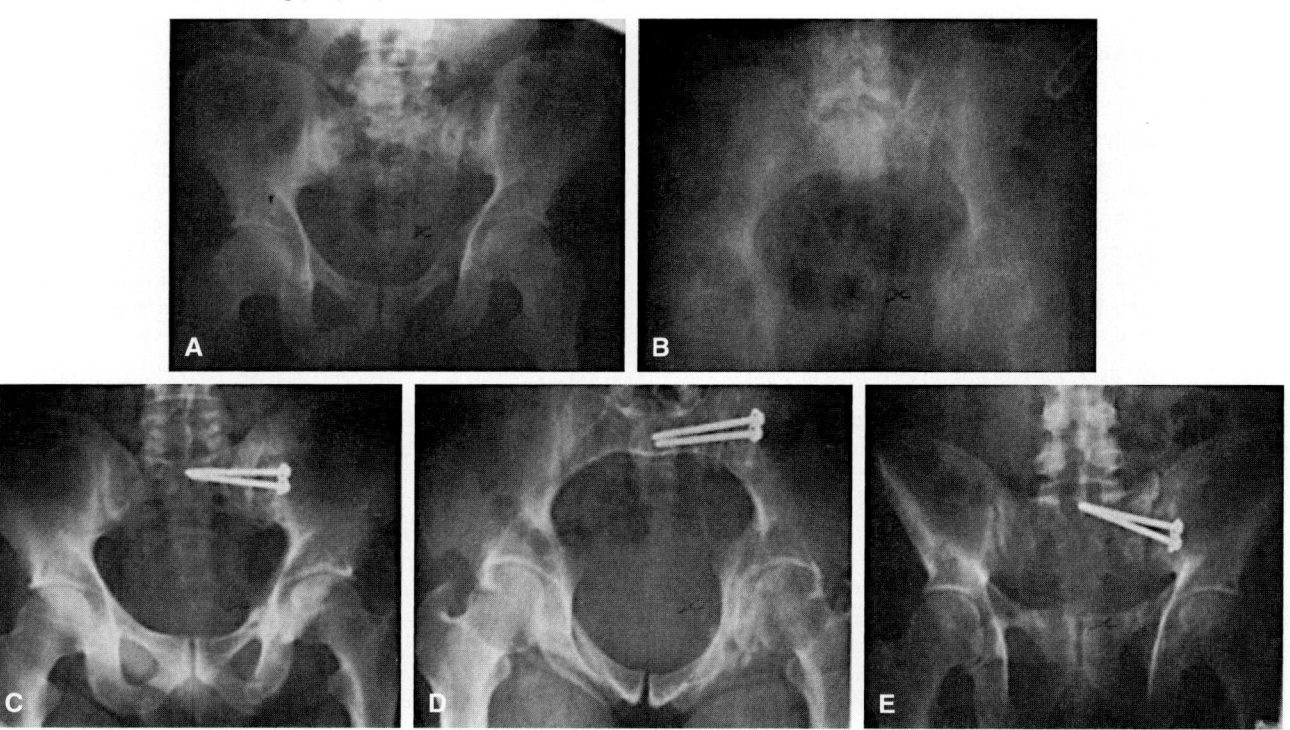

plate must cross the midline to the opposite ala. Transforaminal fractures are stabilized in a similar manner. Two dynamic compression plates parallel to each other at S1 and S3 stabilize bilateral (zone 3) fractures. These plates cross the midline and are fixed to the alar region. Supplemental thinner plates such as H-plates or one third tubular plates may be added, depending on the fracture pattern. After posterior fixation, anterior pelvic stabilization is necessary to supplement this tension band-type fixation. Such stabilization may be accomplished by symphyseal plating or anterior external fixation based on the anterior injury.

Historically, transiliac bars have also been used for posterior pelvic ring fixation. This technique does not provide for direct interfragmentary fixation and is positioned eccentrically from posterior ring injuries. Its use as a sole method of posterior ring fixation has been replaced by the previously discussed methods, but can still can be considered for supplemental fixation of the posterior ring, much like the posterior tension band plate. Techniques for open or percutaneous placement of cannulated screws through both iliac wings has been described but care must be taken to avoid penetration of the caudal sacral canal.

SACROILIAC JOINT FRACTURE DISLOCATIONS AND FRACTURES OF THE ILIAC WING

Fixation is achieved by interfragmental compression and the application of neutralization plates. Commonly, surgical treatment of SI joint fracture–dislocations is from the posterior approach, as the entirety of the fracture line can be visualized on the lateral aspect of the ilium. Following reduction, initial interfragmentary fixation is obtained in the bone between the tables of the ilium. Next, plates are applied along the outer aspect of the bone to neutralize internal rotation forces. Normally, the application of a plate should be just under the crest and along the sciatic buttress where the bone is more dense. Thick bone is also present posteriorly, where the tubercle is available for plate fixation (Fig. 36-50).

A similar approach using the lateral position can provide more anterior iliac access for reduction and fixation of SI joint fracture–dislocations or iliac fractures. By placing the patient in the lateral decubitus position and carrying the incision along the iliac crest to the posterior tubercle and then distal as described previously, the surgeon can mobilize the gluteal mass from the outer aspect of the pelvic ring. Then, by detaching the abdominal musculature and iliacus from their attachments to the inner aspect of the iliac crest, the SI joint

FIGURE 36-46 *Transiliac screw.* **A,** *Trans-sacral fracture with pubic symphysis dislocation.* **B,** *Medial extension with minor fragmentation of a sacral fracture.* **C,** *Intraoperative confirmation of positioning of the transiliac screw.* **D,** *Postoperative film following open reduction and internal fixation of the anterior pelvic ring with closed reduction and percutaneous pinning fixation of the sacral fracture.* **E,** *Follow-up after 6 months with moderate loss of position of the sacral fracture at union.*

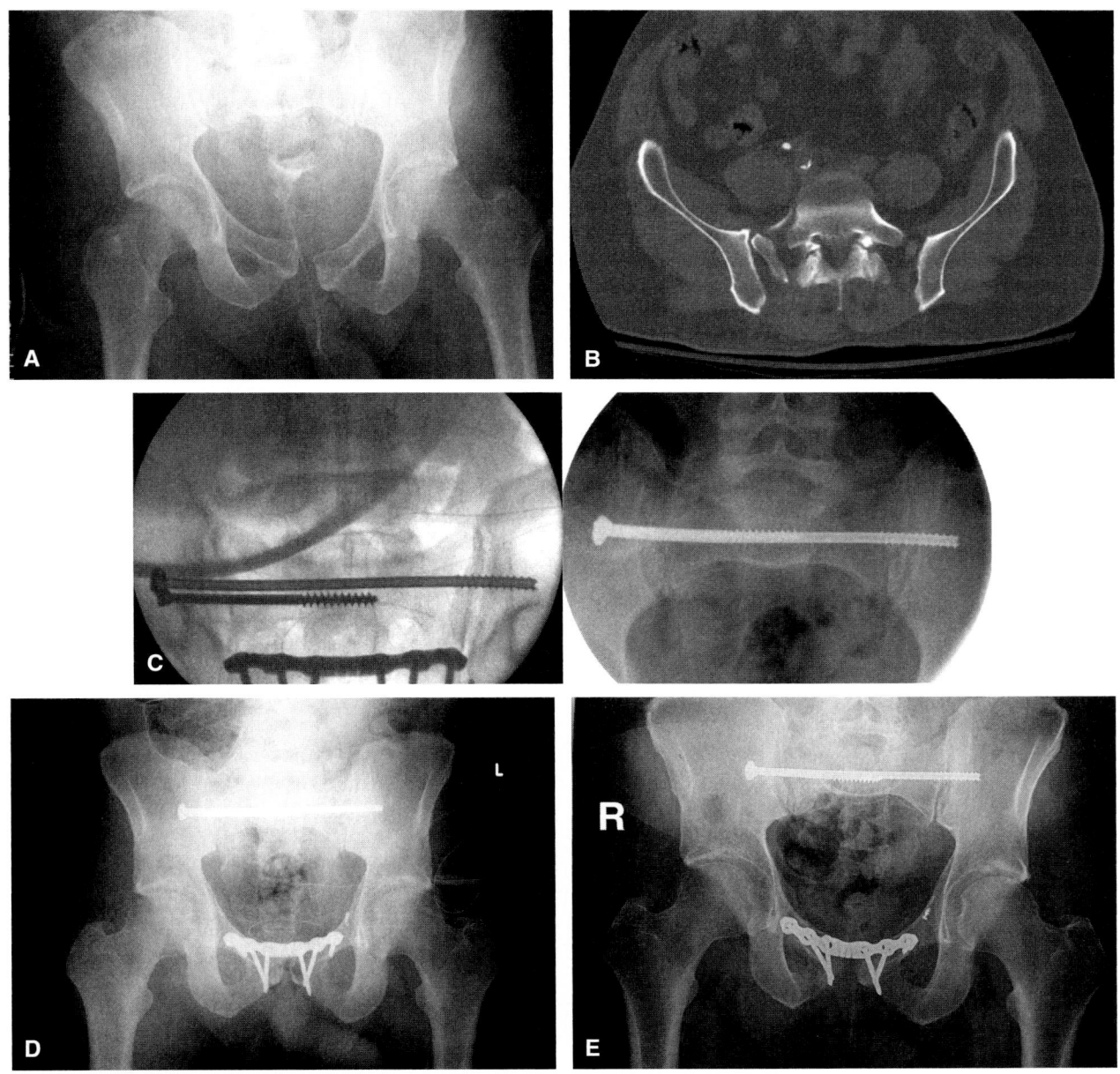

and sacral ala may be visualized. Care must be taken not to devascularize the iliac wing if both sides of the bone are elevated; in addition detachment of the abductor mass has been associated with a higher incidence of heterotopic ossifications (Fig. 36-51).

PERCUTANEOUS ILIOSACRAL SCREW FIXATION UNDER FLUOROSCOPIC CONTROL

The potential for severe soft tissue complications accompanying an open posterior pelvic ring exposure has led to the development of closed reduction and a percutaneous stabilization technique.[25,64,94,99,111] This technique is suitable for stabilization of some SI joint dislocations and sacral fractures. To use this method, the fracture must be reduced and the surgeon must understand the radiographic anatomy of the sacrum, posterior iliac wing, and related soft tissues.

Accurate ilosacral screw placement is critical to achieving maximal stability and avoiding complications. The screw must start on the outer aspect of the iliac wing, cross the SI joint, follow the S1 pedicle mass into the body of S1, and remain completely in bone. Safe placement

FIGURE 36-47 *Line drawing of posterior pelvic plate position and screw placement.*

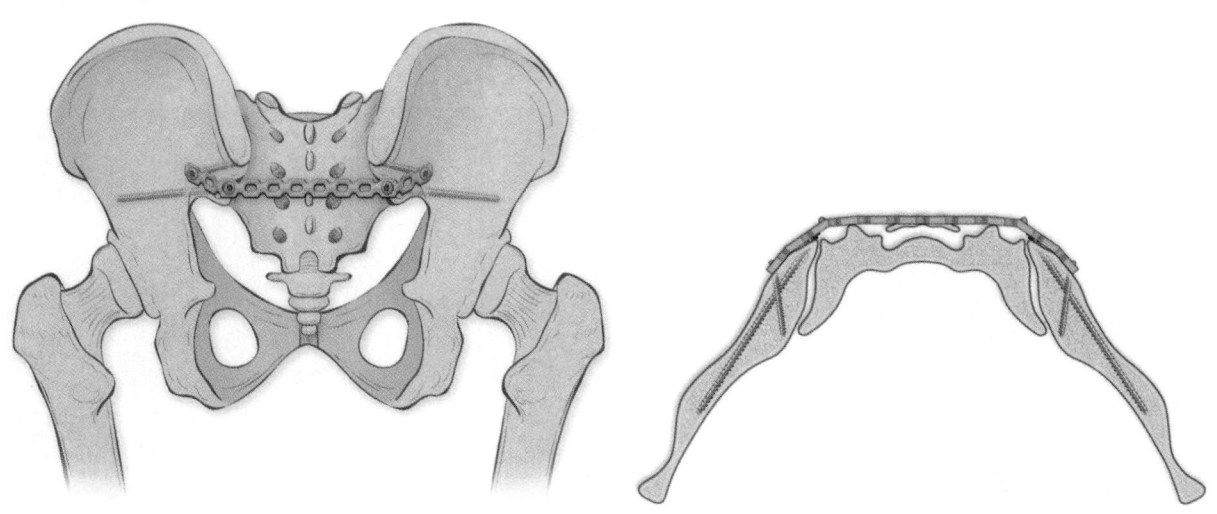

FIGURE 36-48 *Complex posterior ring injury including comminuted midline sacral fracture and contralateral sacroiliac (SI) joint rotational injury.* **A,** *Anteroposterior view of the pelvis.* **B,** *Cranial computed tomography (CT) depicts midline extension, caudal CT defines contralateral rotational injury.* **C,** *Postoperative film demonstrates long iliosacral screw for initial compression followed by tension band plate for stability. Left SI joint was approached initially from the anterior to control rotation and limit deformity to this hemipelvis after posterior TB plate. Note that anterior ring fixation or external fixation is unnecessary in the setting of stable posterior ring fixation.*

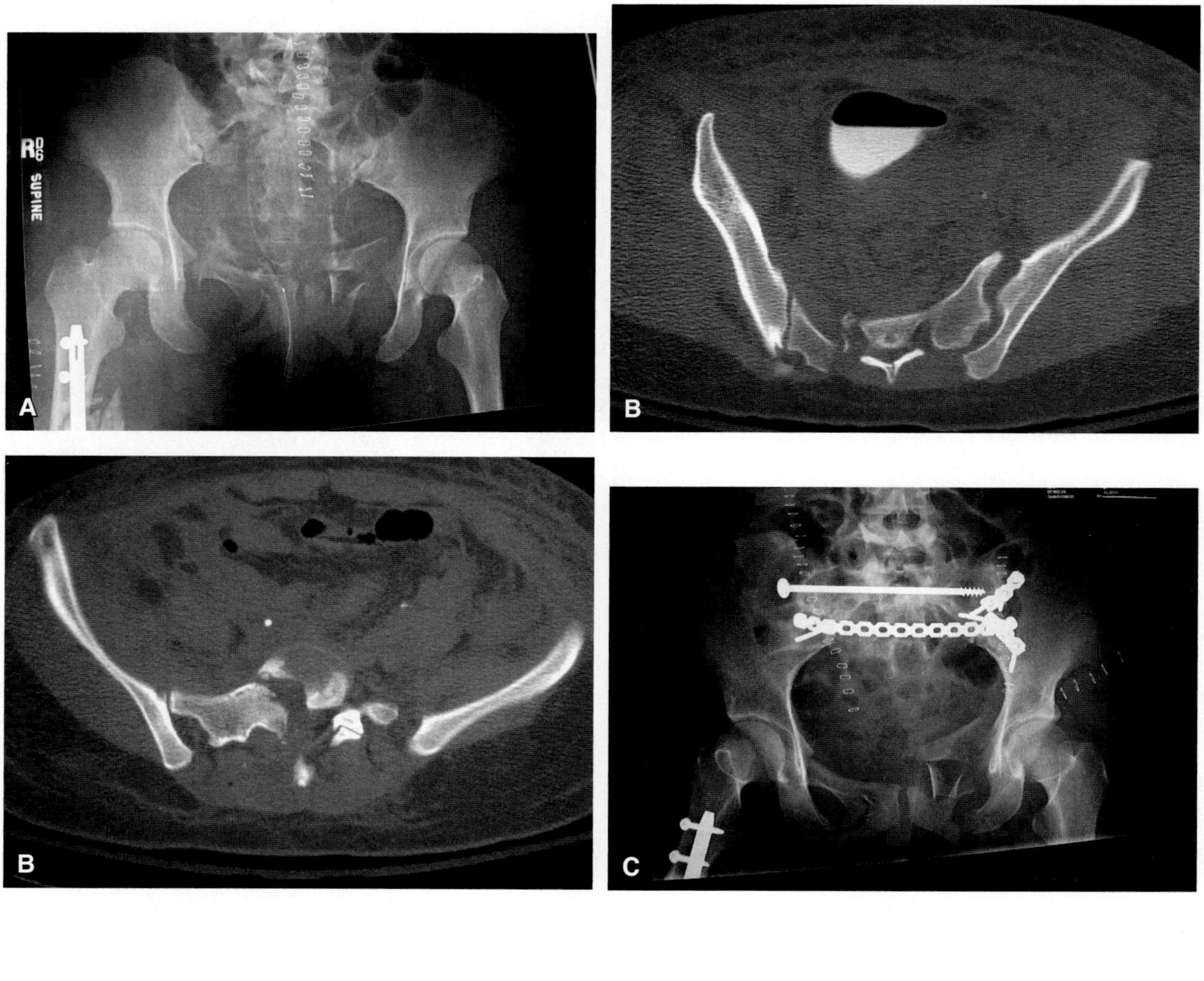

Anatomy of the upper part of the sacrum (S1-S2). **A,** This diagram represents the course of the L5 root (arrow) going over the gutter of the sacral ala and descending in front of the sacroiliac joint and the course of the S1 root in a medial-to-lateral direction. One can see where the safe position is for screw placement. **B,** This diagram shows the area that must be taken into account for placement of a percutaneous screw from outside the iliac wing into the body of the sacrum. **C,** From above the promontory the concavity of the ala can again be appreciated, as can the location of the posterior sacral wall. **D,** This cross section through the sacrum demonstrates the promontory of S1 and the concavity of the sacral ala. Safe placement of screws is marked by the white area. (**B–D,** From Tile, M., ed. Fractures of the Acetabulum and Pelvis, 2nd ed. Baltimore, Williams & Wilkins, 1995. **A,** From Chip, M.; Chip, L., Jr.; Simonian P.T.; et al. Radiographic recognition of the sacral alar slope for optimal placement of iliosacral screws: A cadaveric and clinical study. J Orthop Trauma 10:171–177, 1996.)

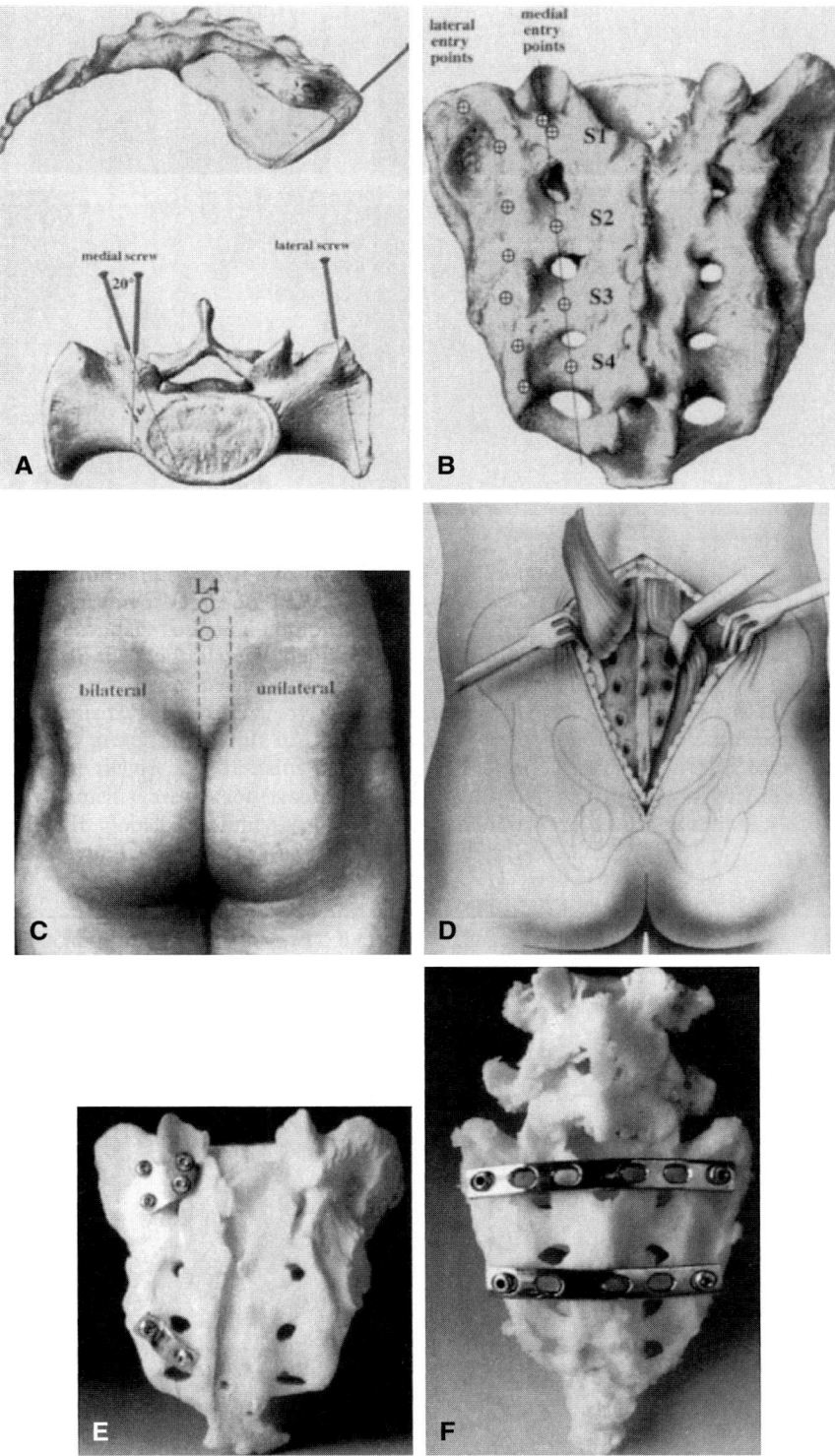

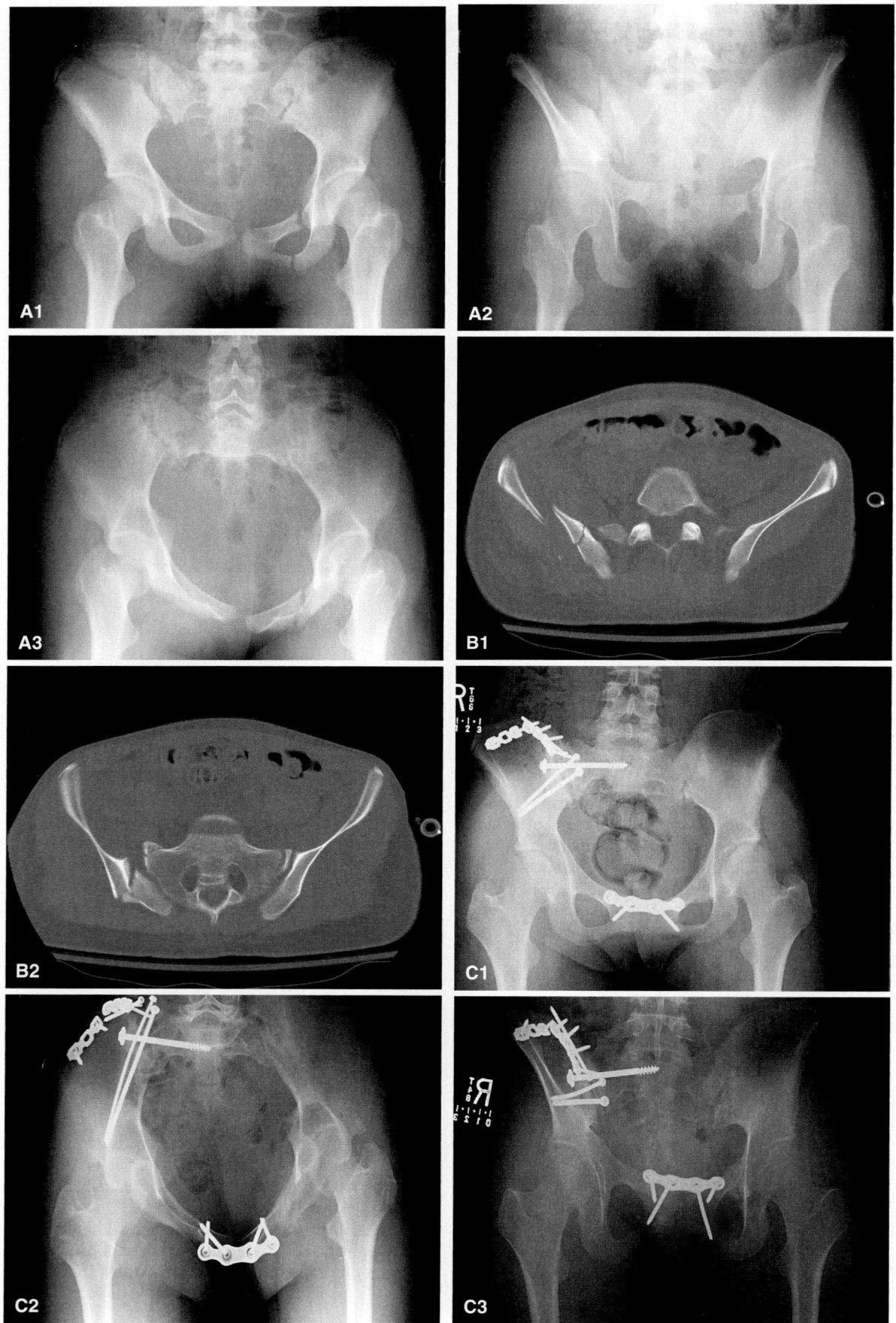

FIGURE 36-50 *Fracture–dislocation approached and stabilized posteriorly. Note that the interfragmentary screws were placed between the inner and outer tables of the ilium. Due to a small intact cranial fragment of the intact ilium, fixation was augmented with iliosacral screws.*

A1

A2

A3

B1

B2

C1

C2

C3

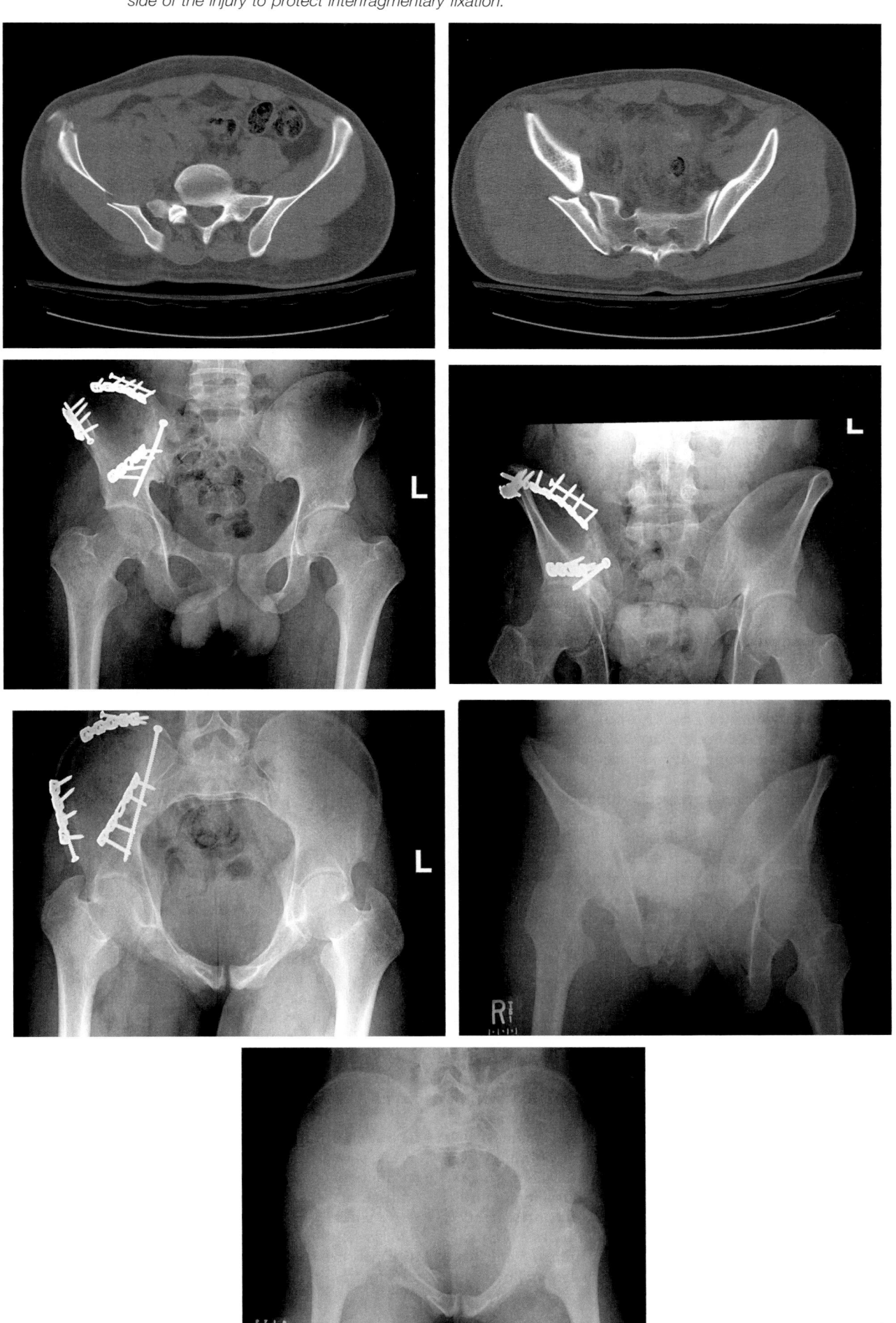

FIGURE 36-51 Iliac fracture with anterior extension stabilized through a lateral approach. Plates were placed on the tension side of the injury to protect interfragmentary fixation.

demands thorough understanding of sacral radiographic anatomy because this technique is performed completely percutaneously, with no options to guide or confirm screw placement by palpation or visualization. The S1 pedicle is bordered inferiorly by the S1 root canal and foramen. The pedicle is approximately 28 mm (width) by 28 mm (height) in cross section. The superior surface slopes downward in a posterior-to-anterior direction at an angle of 45°, with a gutter for the L5 root located 2 cm medial to the SI joint.[77] The internal iliac artery lies anterior to the ala and gives off its largest branch, the superior gluteal artery, anterior to the SI joint.[96] These three structures are at risk of injury if the drill bit, guide wire, or screw penetrates through the ala. The body of the sacrum joins both alae through the pedicles and is surrounded by the cauda equina posteriorly, the pelvic viscera anteriorly, the L5-S1

intervertebral disk superiorly, and the fused S1-S2 disk space inferiorly. The S1 body has an anteriorly protruding bony prominence, the sacral promontory, that is anterior to the sacral ala (Fig. 36-52). Screws aimed toward the promontory will not traverse the bony sacral pedicular canal and may cause injury to the neurovascular structures that lie anterior to the pedicle/ala (Fig. 36-53). More than half of the S1 root canal is filled by the S1 nerve root. It runs inferiorly and laterally to the anterior S1 foramen. Because of this inferior, sloping course, the posterior half of the body of S1 is not available for screw placement because the screw could traverse the S1 root canal. Only the middle portion of the S1 body is therefore left for screw placement near the upper S1 end-plate. For safe placement of the screws, only the sacral landmarks should be used; the iliac landmarks are important to confirm reduction. The sacral landmarks are

FIGURE 36-52 *Anatomy of the upper part of the sacrum (S1-S2). **A,** This cross section through the sacrum demonstrates the promontory of S1 and the concavity of the sacral ala. Safe placement of screws is marked by the white area. **B,** From above the promontory the concavity of the ala can again be appreciated, as can the location of the posterior sacral wall. **C,** This diagram represents the course of the L5 root (arrows) going over the gutter of the sacral ala and descending in front of the sacroiliac joint and the course of the S1 root in a medial-to-lateral direction. One can see where the safe position is for screw placement. **D,** This diagram shows the area that must be taken into account for placement of a percutaneous screw from outside the iliac wing into the body of the sacrum. (**A, B, D,** From Tile, M., ed. Fractures of the Acetabulum and Pelvis, 2nd ed. Baltimore, Williams & Wilkins, 1995. **C,** From Chip, M.; Chip, L., Jr.; Simonian P.T.; et al. Radiographic recognition of the sacral alar slope for optimal placement of iliosacral screws: A cadaveric and clinical study. J Orthop Trauma 10:171–177, 1996.)*

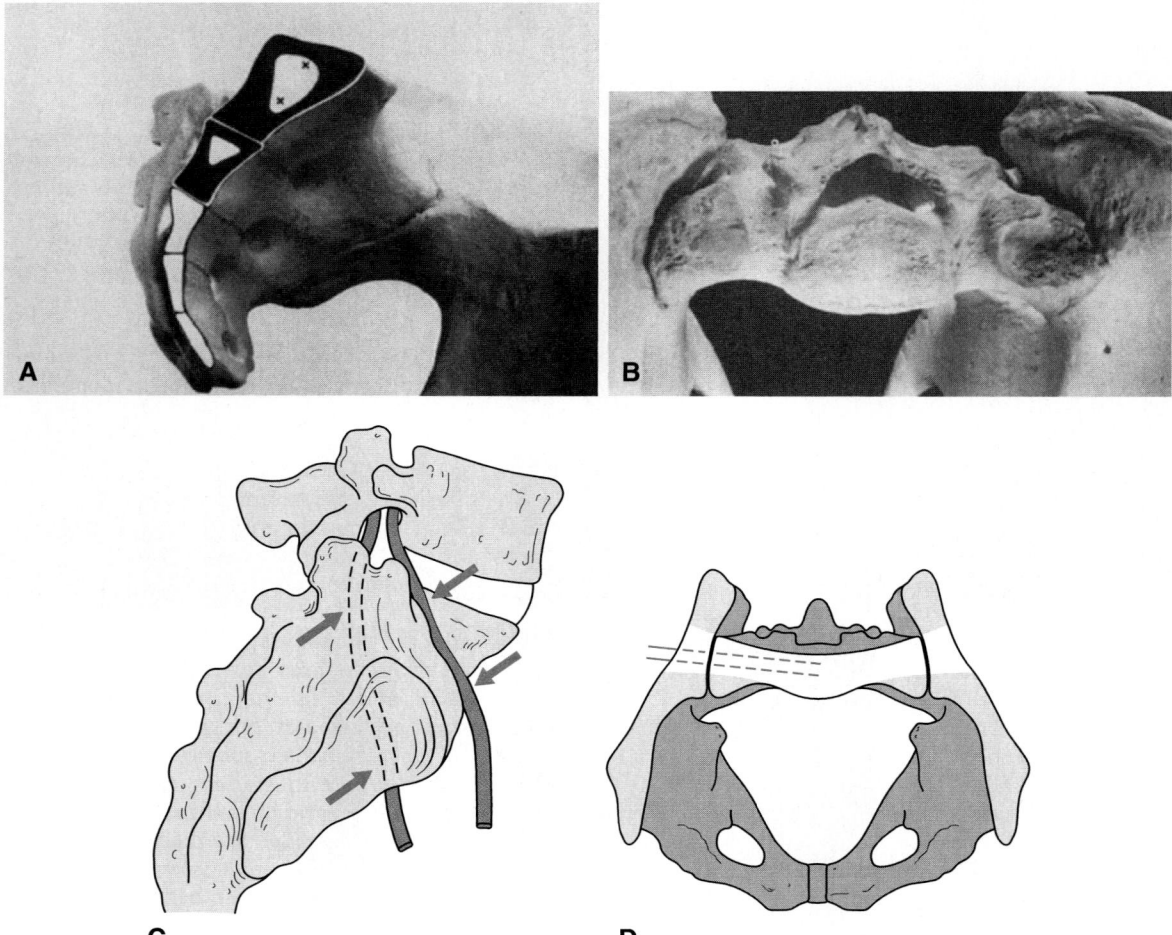

FIGURE 36-53 *Penetration of the ala with screw placement. Inlet (**A**) and outlet (**B**) views of the pelvis show that the screw appears to be intraosseous. **C,** A postoperative computed tomographic scan shows that the anterior cephalad screw is extraosseous. The patient's left L5 nerve root was injured. **D, E,** A plastic model shows how this injury can occur. (**A–C,** From Chip, M.; Chip, L., Jr.; Simonian P.T.; et al. Radiographic recognition of the sacral alar slope for optimal placement of iliosacral screws: A cadaveric and clinical study. J Orthop Trauma 10:171–177, 1996. **D, E,** From Tile, M., ed. Fractures of the Acetabulum and Pelvis, 2nd ed. Baltimore, Williams & Wilkins, 1995.)*

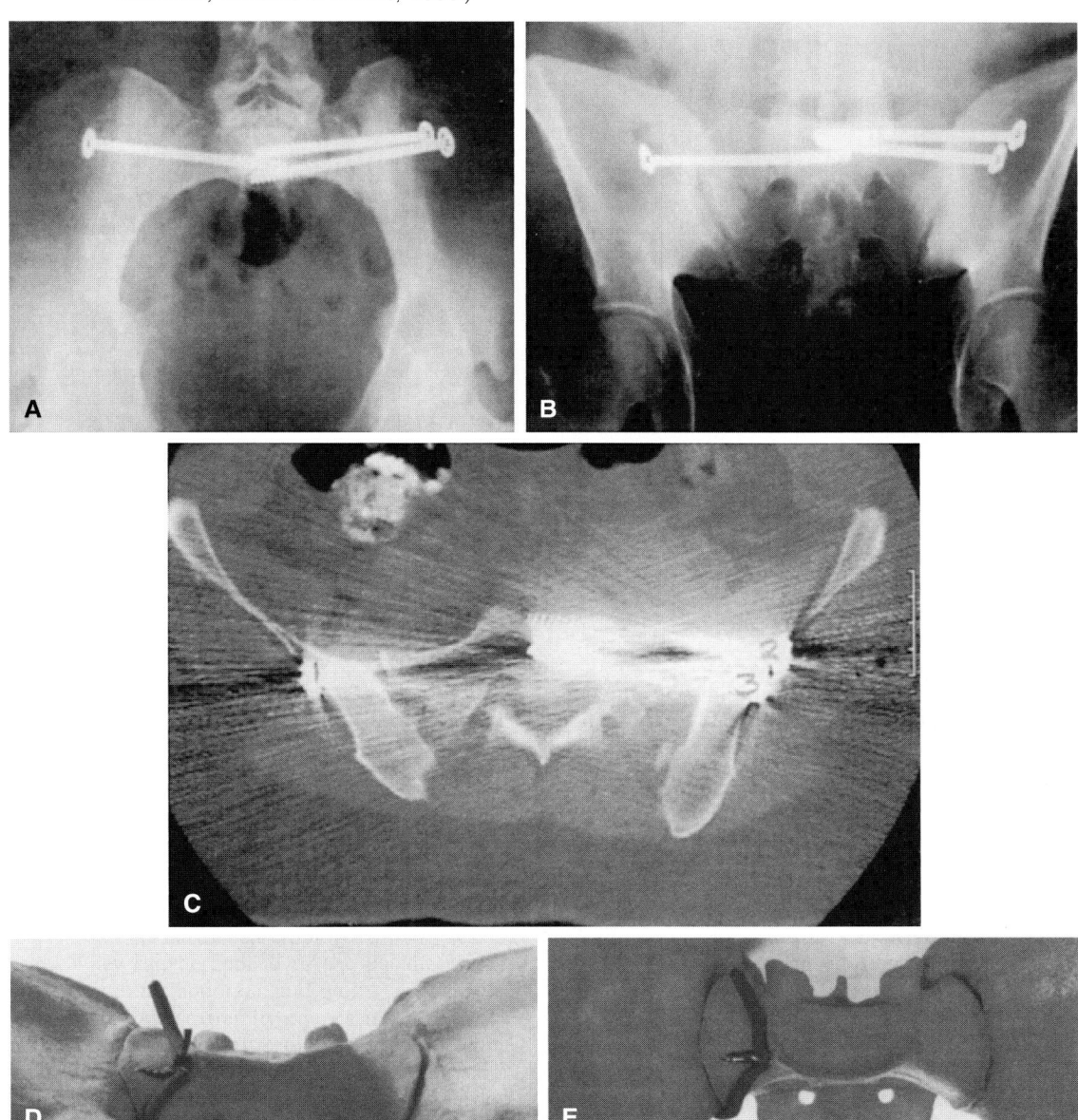

identified by using four fluoroscopic views of the pelvis: the AP, the inlet and outlet (tangential), and the lateral sacral views[93,94,96,111] (Fig. 36-54).

INDICATIONS Compelling clinical indications for closed reduction/percutaneous fixation management are severe open or closed pelvic ring soft tissue injury, abdominal compartment syndromes with an open abdomen, or colostomy associated with visceral injury or bowel diversion for posterior open pelvic fracture wounds. Anatomically, the lesions that can be addressed are SI dislocations, SI fracture–dislocations in which iliosacral screws will restore adequate stability, and extra foraminal (Denis zone I) sacral fractures. The use of these techniques in Denis zone II sacral fractures carries the risk of neural injury associated with small residual malreductions or impingement by foraminal debris. In some settings, this risk may be warranted. Here the technique can be considered a postresuscitation phase emergency

FIGURE 36-54 *Important radiographic landmarks for the insertion of percutaneous iliosacral screws. **A,** Cross section of the pelvis showing the sacral promontory and important aspects as visualized on a lateral sacral radiograph. The sacral promontory and the alar slope should be recognized in these views. **B,** Inlet view of the pelvis showing both the bony pelvis and the radiographic appearance of the anterior cortex of S1 and S2 superimposed. **C,** Inlet view of the bony pelvis and radiographic image showing that increasing the angle on the C-arm allows the anterior cortex of S2 to be visualized, but the posterior cortex of the sacral spinal canal is now seen. **D,** Outlet pelvic view and radiographic image showing the pubic tubercles just below the S1 foramen. (From Tile, M., ed. Fractures of the Acetabulum and Pelvis, 2nd ed. Baltimore, Williams & Wilkins, 1995.)*

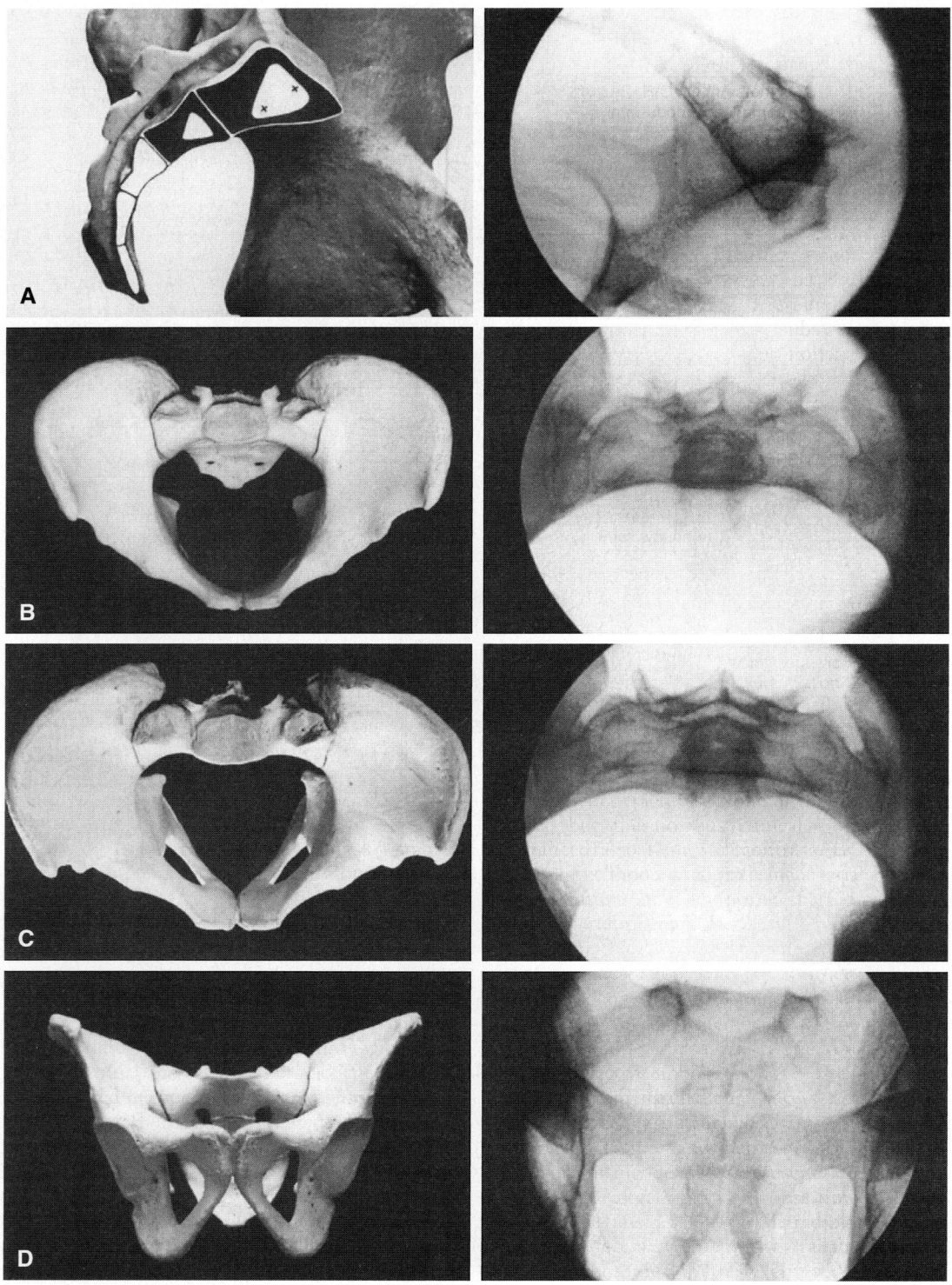

stabilization modality analogous to a pelvic clamp. Subsequent open revision may be needed for definitive management.

Early postinjury use of traction to minimize cranial/posterior displacements of the involved hemipelvis extends the length of time during which closed reduction techniques may be employed. Interim external fixation or pelvic clamps may also be useful. Nonetheless, once the patient is stable enough to tolerate a general anesthetic, earlier intervention is always preferred. Delays beyond 5 to 7 days limit the utility of these techniques.

LIMITATIONS Successful use of closed reduction/percutaneous fixation techniques for the posterior pelvic ring is predicated on good intraoperative imaging and the achievement of a satisfactory reduction. Osteoporosis also limits the stability of iliosacral screw fixation. This may warrant a modified mobilization plan or supplemental anterior ring internal or external fixation that would not be necessary in persons with normal bone density. Additionally, bilateral displaced injuries are generally not amenable to closed techniques, although it may be possible to carry out an open reduction on one side to restore a basis for closed reduction of the remaining hemipelvis injury. Lastly, presence of sacral dysmorphism[95,96] (transitional vertebra), which occurs in approximately 20 percent of people, may complicate assessment of reduction and safe screw placement. Careful preoperative planning based on plain radiographs and axial CT with appropriate sagittal, coronal, and three-dimensional reconstructions is required to assess whether a safe corridor for screw placement exits in these cases.

TECHNIQUE Closed reduction and percutaneous fixation is usually performed with the patient in the supine position because of the ease of reduction and to enable simultaneous anterior ring fixation when appropriate. Prone positioning is necessary if open reduction of the sacrum is anticipated. It may also be the surgeon's preference. For the supine position, the patient is placed on a soft radiolucent support beneath the lumbosacral spine to elevate the buttocks off the table and ensure access to the lateral aspect of the flank and buttock so that the starting point for the screw is not compromised. An entirely radiolucent table is preferred. The fluoroscopy unit is brought in on the side opposite the surgeon, and satisfactory inlet, outlet, and AP pelvis imaging as well as lateral sacral views centered at S1 are verified to be of satisfactory quality. To obtain the inlet view, the C-arm is tilted so that the anterior cortex of S1 overlaps that of S2. If such visualization is not done, the concavity of the sacrum will not be appreciated and the screw may exit anteriorly. However, the posterior cortex of S1 is best seen if the anterior cortex of S1 is over the coccyx. This projection is needed to ensure that the screw does not exit posteriorly. The outlet view is obtained by rotating the C-arm approximately 90° so that the pubic tubercles lie just inferior to the S1 foramen and the symphysis overlies the midline of the sacrum.[64] The floor positions for the fluoroscopy base and appropriate inlet and outlet angles are marked by the radiology technician for easy reproduction.

After complete radiographic visualization has been obtained, fracture reduction can be undertaken after induction of muscle-relaxing anesthesia. Closed reduction is usually possible within 2 to 5 days of the injury. Closed reduction requires knowledge of the displacement of the fracture. A completely unstable hemipelvis is displaced cranially and posteriorly and is externally rotated. However, depending on the mechanism of injury, the displacements may differ, so preoperative review of the radiographic studies provides the basis for intraoperative reduction maneuvers. The patient is prepared from the costal margins to the knees on both sides and down to the table on the involved side. The involved leg is prepared and draped free to allow manipulation. The first displacement to be corrected is the axial malposition, which is accomplished by longitudinal skeletal traction through a traction pin inserted in the distal end of the femur. Traction counter force may not be needed in the large patient or with early intervention. However, if greater force (more than 10–15 kg) is required because of delay or the patient is small, stabilization of the uninvolved hemipelvis may be needed. This can be done indirectly with a foot plate and soft thigh strap on the contralateral side as well as chest bolster on the side of the intervention. The most effective way to stabilize the intact pelvis to facilitate closed reduction is to secure the ilium and proximal femur to the table with a modified external fixation frame utilizing iliac as well as proximal femoral Schanz screws (see Fig. 36-37). If the fracture is posteriorly displaced, the traction is directed anteriorly by flexing the hip. Rotational displacement is corrected by placing one or two Schanz screws into the involved iliac crest or supra-acetabular area and using them to manipulate the hemipelvis into place. The external fixator or universal distractor can be used to reduce this component as well. These reduction maneuvers may require one or two assistants. Open reduction of a concomitant symphyseal disruption may also lead to at least a partial indirect reduction of the posterior ring (see Fig. 36-35). Once the reduction is achieved, it is confirmed by C-arm visualization with the three views of the hemipelvis. Provisional fixation follows with a prepositioned K-wire inserted into the ala or S1 body.

The superficial skin location for screw insertion is approximately 2 cm posterior to the intersection of a line from the femoral shaft and a line dropped from the ASIS. However, these coordinates may be distorted by soft tissue trauma or the femoral position change related to traction. The guide wire or drill bit is placed through a punctate wound down to the posterolateral aspect of the ilium. The inlet and outlet views show that this device is aimed into the S1 body and perpendicular to the SI joint. At this point, the C-arm is used to visualize the lateral part of the sacrum. The position of the drill bit or guide wire is confirmed to be in the middle of the S1 body. It is important to make sure that the screw is placed so that it is below the cortical projection of the sacral ala, which is seen only on the lateral view.[94,96,111] If the position is correct, the incision can be enlarged to between 1 and 1.5 cm, and the drill bit or guide wire is advanced toward the body of S1. It is useful to halt insertion of the pin when the tip reaches the superior aspect of the lateral border of the first sacral foramen on the outlet view. A true lateral view of the sacrum is obtained again to confirm that the tip of the pin is in the alar safe zone (pedicle). The progress of the drilling is watched on the three pelvic views (Fig. 36-55). The drill bit or guide wire perforates three cortical barriers (outer part of the ilium, inner iliac side of the SI joint, and sacral side of the SI joint). If a fourth cortical barrier is encountered, insertion is stopped and the drill bit or guide wire is realigned because it is potentially about to leave the safe channel and injure a major structure. Usually, misdirected drill bits or guide wires must be completely removed and restarted to create a new tract. However, occasionally it may be possible to reinsert through the same starting point with the guide wire or drill in reverse and gentle medial pressure. Once the position of the drill bit or guide wire is confirmed, the screw is inserted. A lag screw is used to fix a SI dislocation or zone I sacral fracture so that any residual gap can be closed. In transforaminal or body fractures of the sacrum, a fully threaded position screw can be used to maintain the reduction without fracture compression. However, he stability of a position screw construct is clearly reduced. Screw head position is confirmed by over-rotating the anteroposteriorly positioned C-arm 20 to 30° toward the involved side. This view shows the outer cortex of the ilium so that the position of the screw head is confirmed to abut the cortex. This relationship can also be seen on the inlet view centered on the screw head. Longer screw, placement past midline, is more difficult because of superimposition of the opposite-side alar cortical slope. Care must be taken if the screw is inserted past the midline to avoid the risk of perforation of the anterior sacral surface (see Fig. 36-55).

POSTOPERATIVE PLAN

The postoperative plan for these patients is ideally one of early mobilization. However, such mobilization must be tempered by the ability to achieve stable fixation of the fracture and the quality of bone. If bone quality is good and stable fixation is achieved in a rotationally unstable injury, the patient can be mobilized within 3 to 5 days on crutches, with full weight-bearing on the uninvolved side. Partial weight-bearing can be allowed between 3 and 6 weeks, with progression to full weight-bearing at 8 to 10 weeks and off all aids by 3 months if gait is normalized.

For globally unstable injuries, however, a more cautious approach may be needed. Early bed to reclining chair transfers are important, especially in the multiply injured patient. Stable posterior and anterior fixation can allow limited ambulation with a maximum of 20 kg weight-bearing on the involved side. Progression of weight-bearing should be avoided until fracture healing is observed in bony injuries, and it may be necessary to avoid full weight-bearing for 3 to 4 months. If the fixation is unstable because of injury pattern or bone density, the use of postoperative traction to protect the fixation for 4 to 6 weeks should be considered. Traction takes some of the force off the fixation, thereby decreasing the possibility of fixation failure. However, this technique is useful only for an isolated pelvic fracture, which is uncommon. The use of external fixation as a supplement to internal fixation may allow the patient to be in the upright position in bed or in a chair.

Radiographic follow-up is usually done in the early postoperative phase before hospital discharge, at 6 weeks, and at 3 months. At 3 months, the healing is usually satisfactory to allow full weight-bearing, and no further radiographs are necessary until 6 months to 1 year. After this interval, radiographs are necessary only if indicated by patient complaints.

Generally, removal of pelvic internal fixation is not done. The only fixation that usually causes local irritation problems is that placed just below or on the iliac crest or on the symphysis. Such fixation may require removal if it causes symptoms. Women of reproductive age may elect to have symphyseal fixation removed to avoid potential problems with labor, although the risk of retaining these implants has not been well established. Lastly, consideration should be given to iliosacral screw removal if significant posterior pelvic ring pain persists, particularly in the younger patient with obvious radiographic evidence of loosening.

GENITOURINARY INJURIES

Management of genitourinary injuries requires a team approach. The urologist and orthopaedic surgeon need to have a protocol to handle these injuries effectively. Extraperitoneal bladder ruptures are usually managed nonoperatively unless the pelvic ring injury requires operative intervention. In this case, open bladder repair is recommended to prevent infection of the fixation or persistent fistula formation. This repair is usually performed as early as the patient is stable and is combined with pelvic fracture osteosynthesis.

Treatment of urethral rupture is more controversial. Three options exist: immediate exploration and realignment over a catheter, primary urethroplasty, and suprapubic cystostomy drainage with delayed urethroplasty. Timing is dictated by the magnitude of the injury and complicating injuries to adjacent structures. The most important factor appears to be related to avoiding further surgical damage to the pelvic floor to keep the incidence of stricture and impotence low. Recent indirect open realignment procedures have been effective in early care with limited complications.[56,97]

In women, urinary complaints were more frequent in patients with residual pelvic displacement (≥ 5 mm), as was dyspareunia. Other than a higher incidence of cesarean section in displaced pelvic fractures (≥ 5 mm), no difference in occurrences of miscarriage or infertility were noted.[18]

OPEN PELVIC FRACTURES

An open pelvic fracture is defined as any fracture of the pelvic ring in which the fracture site is or has the potential for bacterial contamination as a consequence of the injury. This concept includes a fracture site open to the external environment, as well as a fracture site communicating with a vaginal or rectal laceration. For this injury to occur, a massive amount of energy must be transferred to the

FIGURE 36-55 *Technique for insertion of percutaneous iliosacral screws. **A,** The prone position on a radiolucent table. Similarly, screw insertion may be accomplished with the patient in a supine position with access by the C-arm for all three views. **B,** Alignment of the guide wire or drill for placing a screw into the sacrum. Note that the alignment is behind the S2 cortex in the central portion of the body to avoid the pedicles and the promontory and is below the alar slope line. **C,** Inlet view with S1 and S2 superimposed to show the position of the guide pins in place and avoid penetration of the ala and the posterior cortex of the sacrum. The outlet view confirms the appropriate position in the S1 body to avoid the S1 foramen. **D,** Final placement of screws in the safe zone of the sacrum. (From Tile, M., ed. Fractures of the Acetabulum and Pelvis, 2nd ed. Baltimore, Williams & Wilkins, 1995.)*

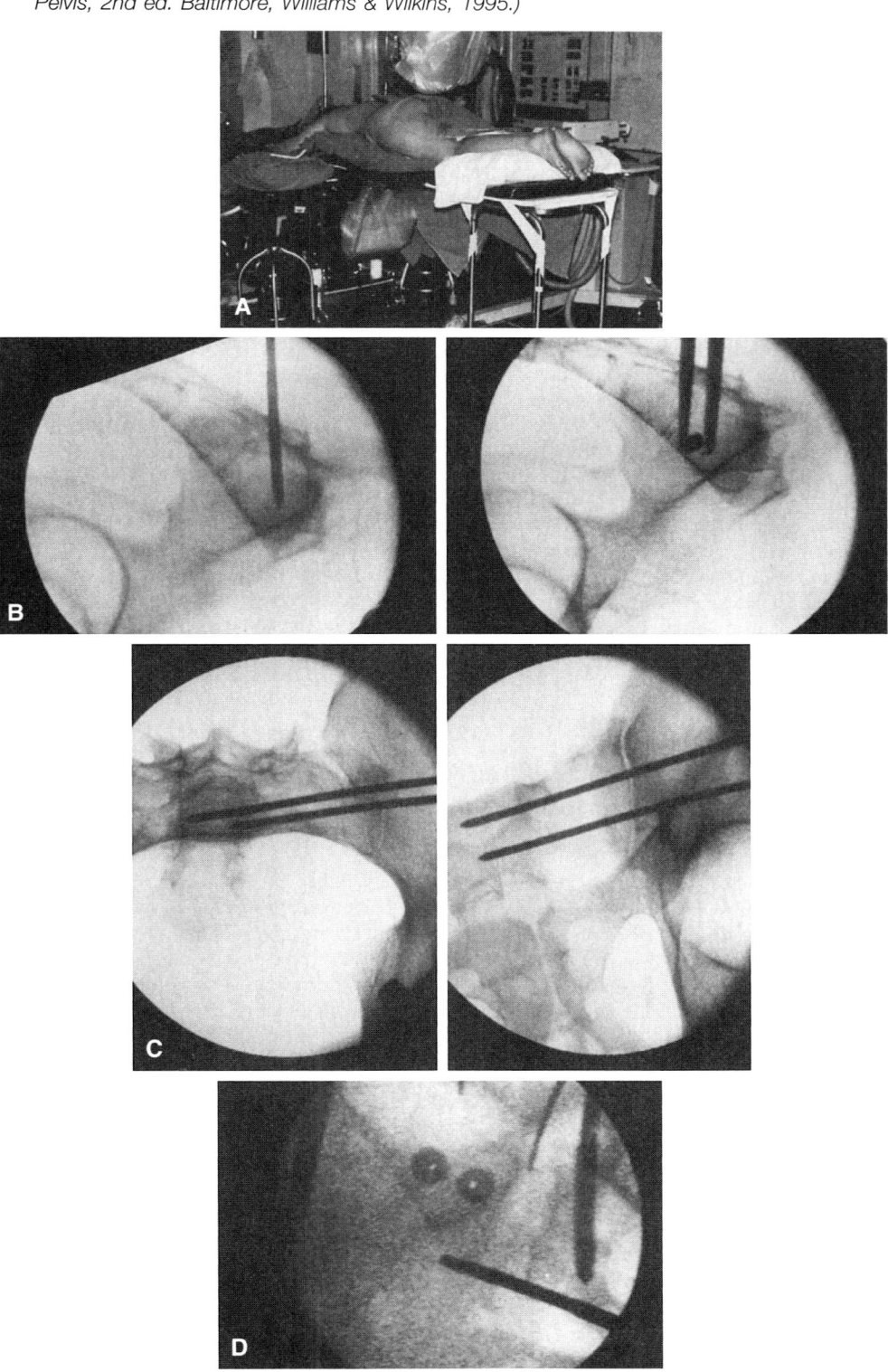

pelvis. This type of injury pattern leads to significant bony disruption and, more importantly, to severe soft tissue damage and resultant susceptibility to infection and late disabiity.[8] Raffe and Christensen[95] described 26 patients with open pelvic fractures. Disruption of the genitourinary system occurred in 12 and disruption of the gastrointestinal system in 7. Perry[89] and Richardson and associates[96] have emphasized the potential for major vessel disruption and resultant fatal hemorrhage as one of the most important early complications of this injury.

Assessment

Assessment of a patient with an open pelvic fracture must be meticulous. The best method of determining the extent of soft tissue damage is to describe the exact injury. Anteriorly or laterally directed wounds in the flank usually occur through muscle and do not involve rectal or genitourinary contamination. Wounds that occur in the perineum with extension into the rectum posteriorly and wounds that extend into the rectal or genitourinary region are contaminated by a rectal tear or have the potential for contamination at a later date.[27] Faringer and colleagues[35] attempted to delineate the location of the wound by dividing the pelvic region and upper part of the thighs into three distinct zones. Zone 1 is the perineum and extends from the lower anterior abdominal wall posteriorly over the sacrum. Zone 2 is the medial aspect of the thigh from the anterior midline to the posterior midline. Zone 3 is the flank and posterolateral region of the buttock.

A urethrogram and a cystogram reveal the genitourinary involvement. Rectal and vaginal examinations are mandatory in all patients with pelvic fractures. The presence of blood on either examination is an indication for visual inspection of that orifice to rule out an open injury.[76] Evaluation of neurologic status must also be undertaken immediately to determine which structures are not functioning.[122] Finally, contamination of the wound from both external and internal (intestinal) sources must be determined. After evaluation of the soft tissue injuries, appropriate radiographic evaluation of the pelvic fracture must be undertaken.

Management

Treatment of these patients must be well coordinated and meticulous because they can die early of hemorrhage. Rapid resuscitation with universal-donor blood and prompt noninvasive pelvic immobilization, such as with PASG trousers, in association with packing of the open wound, will help control major vessel bleeding.[1,19] These injuries may rarely represent internal traumatic hemipelvectomies and, in fact, conversion to an actual hemipelvectomy may be lifesaving in some patients. Once hemodynamic stabilization has occurred, appropriate débridement of the wounds is necessary. This procedure may involve consultation with general surgeons, urologists, and gynecologists so that the wounds can be explored adequately. If any wound enters the perineum (zone 1), especially if it has rectal involvement, a diverting colostomy should be performed.[32] This intervention should probably be a loop colostomy placed in the area of the transverse colon so that it is well out of the way of any surgical access

to the pelvis. Distal colonic washout should be undertaken so that the colon, from the colostomy site through to the rectum, is immediately cleansed. Broad-spectrum antibiotics with adequate coverage for bowel contamination should be started immediately and used prophylactically for 24 to 48 hours.

One very serious injury that occurs to the soft tissues is shearing and avulsion of the skin and subcutaneous tissue from the underlying muscle. In a sense, the skin has become devascularized by the loss of its blood supply from the underlying muscle. In these situations, a decision must be made regarding the extent of débridement required. These avulsions can be massive, and determination of their extent is usually guided by an evaluation of the skin and subcutaneous bleeding. All tissue that is dead and thought to be potentially nonviable must be removed. If débridement is inadequate and a large quantity of devitalized soft tissue remains, sepsis may result and compromise the patient's outcome. If the exact amount and extent of devitalized tissue are not initially evident, repetitive débridement is mandatory.

In fractures with significant contamination involving the perineum or rectum and in situations in which it is impossible to obtain a clean surgical wound, external fixation should be used. Such fixation provides a relatively stable pelvic ring so that the patient can be mobilized and repeat débridement can be performed. After the soft tissues have demonstrated viability and healing is progressing, definitive stabilization can then be carried out.

If the wound does not involve the perineum and is not significantly contaminated and if a clean surgical wound can be achieved, the use of primary internal fixation to stabilize the fracture is possible. Often, the open wound may allow reasonable access to these areas. This technique can also be supplemented by external fixation. The use of minimal lag screw fixation along with external fixation may be the best method for obtaining stability with this injury.

If the urethra or bladder is involved and the abdomen has been opened, stabilization of the anterior injury can be done by internal fixation if the fracture pattern is amenable.

In females with an open fracture into the vagina, débridement of the open fracture, usually through the vagina, is all that is required. If the vaginal laceration is clean, it can be closed primarily. Any potentially contaminated vaginal wound should be left open to heal secondarily. In these settings, anterior stabilization of the pelvis in the acute phase is best accomplished by external fixation.

Follow-Up Care

After the patient is hemodynamically stable and the pelvis has been stabilized, definitive fracture care can be undertaken. Further soft tissue treatment can be carried out, such as repair of the genitourinary system, and the colostomy can be closed at 6 to 12 weeks, after the soft tissue and rectal injuries have healed.

With aggressive care of patients with pelvic fractures, the nominal mortality rate of up to 50 percent can be reduced to 20 percent, This is equivalent to the mortality associated with a closed but completely unstable pelvic ring injury (type C).[8] Richardson and associates[96] showed that with very aggressive surgical intervention, early colostomy, and extensive débridement, the treatment results of open pelvic fracture could be markedly improved.

COMPLICATIONS

Because of the systemic nature of the injury and the wide spectrum of methods of treatment required, complications of pelvic fractures are often frequent and severe. The polytrauma setting and the systemic nature of the injury make the patient susceptible to the development of adult respiratory distress syndrome, thromboembolic disease, pneumonia, and multiple organ failure.

Early Complications

INFECTION

Postoperative infection can occur after either external or internal fixation. Infection with the use of external fixation devices usually occurs around the pin tracts. Pin tract infection can generally be managed adequately by appropriate release of the skin about the pins and changing dressings as required to maintain drainage from the pin tracts. Antibiotic coverage may be appropriate if drainage is excessive or cellulitis develops and is unresponsive to pin tract release and local dressing changes. Cultures in these open wounds are generally colonized with multiple organisms, and therefore broad-spectrum suppressive therapy is needed. Pin tract loosening may occur with persistent local sepsis. The clamps around the pins must be released and the pins checked for stability within the bone. If a pin is loose, it is inadvisable to reinsert it because of the localized infection. Consequently, the fixator may have to be removed, or alternative placement of the pins may be necessary. If the fixator has been placed in the standard iliac crest position, it is usually safe to place these new pins between the anterior superior and anterior inferior iliac spines. Most pin tract infections resolve with removal of the pins and débridement of the pin tract itself.

Postoperative infections after internal fixation usually occur secondary to significant soft tissue integrity or healing problems. These complications are common after a posterior approach in which an incision has been made through devitalized and nonviable skin and muscle. Very careful evaluation of the soft tissue injury must be undertaken. Even if this problem occurs anteriorly, the approach must be altered to operate and stabilize through viable soft tissue.[49]

If a postoperative infection does develop around the fixation, the same treatment principles apply as for acute postoperative infections after internal fixation. Incision and drainage plus débridement must begin early. The wound should be left open and the fixation evaluated for stability. If it is solidly fixed to bone, it can be left in place. If it is loose and not maintaining stability, it must be removed and supplemented or changed to an alternative. Pelvic osteomyelitis is a rare but disastrous complication. Repetitive débridement is the only treatment method.

Vacuum dressings are a useful adjunct to wound management and usually accelerate the secondary healing or establishment of a wound that can be covered by a local flap. In rare cases it may be necessary to excise major portions of the iliac crest to control the osteomyelitis.

LOSS OF FIXATION

Loss of fixation often occurs when the expected degree of healing cannot be achieved during the early phase of pelvic fixation. Honest assessment of the stability of the fixation must be made at the end of any surgical intervention. The use of external fixation or traction to supplement internal fixation must always be considered. If the adequacy of the fixation is uncertain, it is better to maintain the patient on bedrest with external fixation or traction and to delay mobilization until bony union or ligamentous healing has occurred. Early mobilization with loss of reduction and fixation may compromise the end result. Routt and co-workers[100] reported the complications associated with the percutaneous technique of insertion of an iliosacral lag screw. They evaluated 244 screws in 159 patients. Malreduction was noted in 19 of 159 patients. An inability to adequately image the posterior of the pelvis occurred in 18 patients because of obesity or residual intestinal contrast. Five screws were malpositioned because of failure to understand the value of the lateral sacral view. Fixation failure occurred in 7 patients.

NEUROLOGIC INJURY

Permanent nerve damage is a common disability after pelvic disruption, with an incidence of about 10 to 15 percent overall.[122] In unstable, double vertical-type fractures, the incidence rises to 46 percent. Huittinen and Slatis,[50] in their series of 85 patients, reported that a significant number had L5 or S1 root involvement. These appeared to be traction injuries, but anatomic studies suggested that root avulsions may actually occur. Recent interest has led to the development of a classification of sacral fractures[22] that may lead to a better understanding of the injury patterns and the injury site. Fractures through or medial to the foramina are associated with a high incidence of neurologic injury, as are transverse fractures of the sacrum with a kyphotic deformity. Reduction and stabilization of these pelvic injuries may improve recovery. Decompression of any sacral transverse fracture with a kyphotic deformity or any burst fracture of the sacrum that appears to compromise the root posteriorly may be of some value (see Chapter 35). However, the long-term results are disheartening.

Causalgia resulting from injuries to the L5 or S1 root (or both) or to the sciatic nerve can be particularly difficult to manage, both acutely and on a long-term basis, because of an inability to control pain. The use of specific medications has not been a great help. However, it appears that early intervention with a lumbar sympathetic block to break the pain cycle may be of some value. Consultation with pain management physicians should be carried out to determine an approach to alleviate some of the long-term disability. Lumbar sympathetic blocks may also help control chronic causalgia pain. If these blocks are effective, phenol or surgical obliteration of the sympathetic plexus may help.

Iatrogenic nerve injury secondary to operative treatment may occur. Attempts to modify its incidence by nerve-monitoring techniques have not reliably decreased its incidence.[42] The use of electromyographic monitoring techniques might be beneficial.[70,120]

Neurologic damage should be managed with an appropriate splint or brace, and surgical intervention should be carried out if indicated. Repair or decompression of the sciatic nerve has not to date been done with great success. Repair of the femoral nerve, which has a shorter travel route than the sciatic nerve, may be indicated if the nerve has been lacerated.

THROMBOEMBOLISM

Thromboembolic complications may occur more commonly in patients with a major pelvic disruption, especially those with associated lower extremity fractures.[10,13,29,37] Screening has not been successful in determining the at-risk group because most clots are located in the internal pelvic venous plexus, which is not amenable to standard screening methods. At the present time, it is suggested that some method of prophylaxis based on the patient's overall clinical situation be considered. Many different protocols are used, but none has proved more effective than another or even better than no prophylaxis in the prevention of fatal pulmonary emboli.[6,33,34,117]

Late Complications

PAIN

Pain can develop from malunion, nonunion, or osteoarthritis of the SI joint. Some patients, despite having had anatomic reduction and adequate fracture union (or a fused SI joint), continue to complain of discomfort and pain. The pain is usually localized to the area of the SI joint. Evaluation of the lower lumbar spine must be carried out, initially and late, to ensure that no occult fractures are present in this area or involvement of facet joints (30%). Other causes of this pain include significant soft tissue injury, particularly to the muscles and neurologic structures.

MALUNION

Malunion of the pelvic ring can be a source of chronic pain and dysfunction. Most problems stem from pelvic obliquity with accompanying sitting imbalance, compensatory scoliosis, relative leg length inequality and secondary gait abnormalities. Deformities occurring through or adjacent to the SI joint appear to be the most disabling. Patients usually experience pain in the low back or SI joint or both. Additionally, pain may localize over the ischial tuberosities, which are at an unequal level and, therefore, subjected to excessive pressure. Occasionally, severely displaced lateral compression fractures (type B2) can result in an internal rotational deformity that can encroach on the vaginal vault, bladder, or anterior soft tissue of the pelvis. Careful evaluation of the patient's functional and physical disability is mandatory. Chronic pain sequelae are common and may require a multidisciplinary approach. Complex deformity correction often requires a multiple-stage approach with significant surgical risk. Pain

relief and deformity correction are usually incomplete, but in carefully selected patients the improvements warrant the risks. Symptomatic malunion of the SI joint with modest deformity is a more straightforward problem that is usually treated by SI fusion.

NONUNION

Nonunion is an uncommon but well-recognized complication of globally unstable pelvic disruptions. Pelvic pain and instability are the most common initial symptoms. Lateral compression injuries may lead to anterior ramus nonunion, which is usually relatively asymptomatic. Complete evaluation of the patient's symptoms and bony pelvic abnormalities is mandatory. The principles of surgical treatment are stable pelvic ring fixation and bone grafting of the nonunion. Most cases require stable fixation both anteriorly and posteriorly, accompanied by osteotomy or takedown of the nonunion to allow correction of any significant malposition.[26]

RESULTS

Although the techniques of reduction and internal fixation of a disrupted pelvis are being refined, little proof has been presented that these techniques provide the patient any better result than closed reduction and stabilization by traction or external fixation. Riemer and colleagues[97] showed that the functional outcome in unstable pelvic disruptions treated by closed reduction and external fixation, as measured by the SF36, is no different from the result achieved with a stable pelvic ring fracture. This result was again demonstrated by Nepola and co-workers, who showed that functional outcomes using validated scores did not differ when related to residual vertical displacement.[81] Scheid and co-workers,[111] in a review of unstable pelvic ring injuries treated by internal fixation, found that 52 percent of patients experienced pain and a change in lifestyle. This percentage was similar to that reported by Kellam and associates[54] for a similar group of patients from the same institution with the same surgeons. These results were correlated with the location of the fracture, with sacral fractures and pure SI dislocation having the worst results. Dujardin and colleagues reviewed two consecutive cohorts of patients with unstable pelvic ring injuries by using anatomic measures and the validated pelvic outcome score of Majeed.[25] One group was treated by external fixation and the other by internal fixation based on protocol. The overall functional result depended on the location of the posterior lesion and the ability to reduce it anatomically. Pure SI joint dislocations fared poorly if anatomic reduction was not achieved. Fractures of the iliac wing or associated fracture–dislocations of the wing and SI joint did very well because they were easily reduced and stabilized. Sacral fractures did poorly despite good reduction because functional outcome was related to the associated nerve injury. Cole and associates[17] and Tornetta and Matta[124] have also shown that although anatomic reduction plus stable internal fixation is possible in completely unstable pelvic ring injuries and leads to excellent anatomic results, the final functional outcome is usually determined by the associated soft tissue injury or other nonorthopaedic traumatic injuries. In the rotationally unstable group, the results of internal fixation are much better, with up to 96 percent of patients having no pain on strenuous exercise.[114] There is probably little disagreement that patients with unreduced SI joint injuries do not do well unless the injuries are reduced and stabilized, but it cannot be guaranteed that this result is as consistent as the results of operative treatment of SI joint fracture–dislocation or iliac wing fractures. Until a randomized prospective trial is conducted to determine which method of treatment of a sacral fracture, fracture–dislocation of the SI joint, and fracture of the iliac wing (crescent) is most effective, surgeons must treat the patient's injury with prompt recognition of any problems, reduction of the displacement, and stabilization. If such treatment is not possible, referral to appropriate care is mandatory.

SUMMARY

Treatment of pelvic ring injuries requires an in-depth understanding of the anatomy of the pelvis and the mechanisms of injury. With this understanding and precise clinical and radiographic evaluation of the injury, appropriate management can be chosen. Analysis of pelvic stability and deformity provide the foundation for decision making. Surgical approaches to the anterior and posterior pelvic ring require a subspecialty training foundation and careful assessment of the injury to enveloping soft tissues. Surgical intervention based on these tenets is usually the best method of achieving a satisfactory outcome for a patient with an unstable or badly deformed pelvic ring injury. The complications of management of these injuries are formidable, but they can be mitigated by appropriate evaluation, planning, and surgical technique.

REFERENCES

1. Agolini, S.F.; Shah, K.; Gaffe J.; et al. Arterial immobilization is a rapid and effective technique for controlling pelvic fracture hemorrhage. J Orthop Trauma 43:395–399, 1997.
2. Albert, M.J.; Miller, M.E.; MacNaughton, M.; et al. Posterior pelvic fixation using a transiliac 4.5 mm reconstruction plate: A clinical and biomechanical study. J Orthop Trauma 7:226–232, 1993.
3. Altoona, D.; Tekdemir, I.; Ates, Y.; et al. Anatomy of the anterior sacroiliac joint with reference to lumbosacral nerves. Clin Orthop Rel Res 376:236–241, 2000.
4. American College of Surgeons. Advanced Trauma Life Support Manual. Chicago, American College of Surgeons, 1989.
5. Anglen, J.O.; DiPasquale, T. The reliability of detecting screw penetration of the acetabulum by intraoperative auscultation. J Orthop Trauma 8:404–408, 1994.
6. Asprinio, D.E.; Helfet, D.L.; Tile, M. Complications. In Tile, M., ed. Fractures of the Pelvis and Acetabulum. Baltimore, Williams & Wilkins, pp. 243–245, 1984.

6a. Beaule, P.E.; Antoniades, J.; Matta, J.M. Trans-sacral fixation for failed posterior fixation of the pelvic ring. Arch Orthop Trauma Surg 126(1):49–52, 2006.
7. Bone, L.B.; McNamara, K.; Shine, B.; et al. Mortality in multiple trauma patients with fractures. J Trauma 37:262–264, 1994.
8. Bottlang, M.; Krieg, J.C.; Mohr, M.; et al. Emergent management of pelvic ring fractures with the use of circumferential compression. J Bone Joint Surg [Am] 84(Suppl)2:43–47, 2002.
9. Brennerman, F.D.; Katyal, D.; Boulanger, B.R.; et al. Long-term outcomes in open pelvic fractures. J Trauma 42:773–777, 1997.
10. Brown, J.J.; Greene, F.L.; McMillin, R.D. Vascular injuries associated with pelvic fractures. Am Surg 50:150–154, 1984.
11. Browner, B.D., ed. Internal fixation of pelvic ring disruptions. Techn Orthop, Vol. 9, 1994.
12. Bucholz, R.W. The pathological anatomy of the Malgaigne fracture dislocation of the pelvis. J Bone Joint Surg [Am] 63:400–404, 1981.
13. Buckle, R.; Browner, B.D.; Morandi, M. A new external fixation device for emergent reduction and stabilization of displaced pelvic fractures associated with massive hemorrhage. J Orthop Trauma 7:177–178, 1993.
14. Buerger, P.M.; Peoples, J.B.; Lemmon, G.W.; et al. Risk of pulmonary emboli in patients with pelvic fractures. Am Surg 59:505–508, 1993.
15. Colapinto, V. Trauma to the pelvis: Urethral injury. Clin Orthop 151:46–55, 1980.
16. Cole, J.D.; Bolhofner, B.R. Acetabular fracture fixation via a modified Stoppa limited intrapelvic approach. Clin Orthop 305:112–123, 1994.
17. Cole, J.D.; Blum, D.A.; Ansel, L.J. Outcome after fixation of unstable posterior ring injuries. Clin Orthop Rel Res 329:160–179, 1996.
18. Connolly, J.F. Closed treatment of pelvic and lower extremity fractures. Clin Orthop Rel Res 240:115–128, 1989.
19. Copeland, C.E.; Bosse, M.J.; McCarthy, M.L.; et al. Effect of trauma and pelvic fracture on female genitourinary, sexual and reproductive function. J Trauma 11:23–81, 1997.
20. Cothren, C.C.; Osborn, P.M.; Moore, E.E.; et al. Preperitoneal pelvic packing for hemodynamically unstable pelvic fractures: A paradigm shift. J Trauma 62:4 834–842, 2007.
21. Cotler, H.B.; LaMont, J.G.; Hansen, S.T. Immediate spica cast for pelvic fractures. J Orthop Trauma 2:222–228, 1988.
22. Cryer, H.M.; Miller, F.B.; Evers, M.; et al. Pelvic fracture classification: Correlation with hemorrhage. J Orthop Trauma 28:973–980, 1988.
23. Delal, S.; Burgess, A.; Young, J.; et al. Pelvic fracture: Classification by force vector in relationship to associated injuries. Paper presented at an Orthopaedic

Trauma Association Meeting, Dallas, October 27–28, 1988.

24. Denis, F.; Davis, S.; Comfort, T. Sacral fractures: An important problem. Clin Orthop Rel Res 227:67–81, 1988.

25. Dujardin, F.H.; Hossenbaccus, M.; Duparc, F.; et al. Long-term functional prognosis of posterior injuries in high-energy pelvic disruptions. J Trauma 12:345–350, discussion 150–151, 1998.

26. Dunn, A.W.; Morris, H.D. Fractures and dislocations of the pelvis. J Bone Joint Surg [Am] 50:1639–1648, 1968.

27. Duwelius, P.J.; Van Allen, M.; Bray, T.J.; et al. Computed tomography guided fixation of unstable posteriorpelvic ring disruptions. J Orthop Trauma 6:420–426, 1992.

28. Ebraheim, N.A.; Biyani, A.; Wong, F. Nonunion of pelvic fractures. J Trauma 44:102–204, 1998.

29. Ebraheim, N.A.; Savolainen, E.R.; Rusin, J.R.; et al. Occult rectal perforation in a major pelvic fracture. J Orthop Trauma 2:340–343, 1988.

30. Edeiken-Monroe, B.S.; Browner, B.D.; Jackson, H. The role of standard roentgenograms in the evaluation of instability of pelvic ring disruption. Clin Orthop Rel Res 240:63–76, 1989.

31. Egbers, H.J.; Draijer, F.; Havemann, D.; et al. Stabilizing the pelvic ring with the external fixator. Biomechanical studies and clinical experiences. Orthopäde 21:6 363–372, 1992.

32. Ellison, M.; Timberlake, G.A.; Kerstein, M.D. Impotence following pelvic fracture. J Orthop Trauma 28:695–696, 1988.

33. Evers, M.B.; Cryer, H.M.; Miller, F.B. Pelvic fracture hemorrhage. Arch Surg 124:422–424, 1989.

34. Falcone, R.E., Thomas, B.W. "Bean bag" pelvic stabilization. Ann Emerg Med 28:458, 1996.

35. Faringer, P.D.; Mullins, R.J.; Feliciano, P.D.; et al. Selective fecal diversion in complex open pelvic fractures from blunt trauma. Arch Surg 129:958–964, 1994.

36. Fisher, C.G.; Blachut, P.A.; Salvian, A.J.; et al. Effectiveness of pneumatic leg compression devices for the prevention of thromboembolic disease in orthopaedic trauma patients: A prospective, randomized study of compression alone versus no prophylaxis. J Orthop Trauma 9:1–7, 1995.

37. Fishmann, A.J.; Greeno, R.A.; Brooks, L.R.; et al. Prevention of deep vein thrombosis and pulmonary embolism in acetabular and pelvic fracture surgery. Clin Orthopä 305:133–137, 1994.

38. Flint, L.M.; Brown, A.; Richardson, J.D. Definitive control of bleeding from severe pelvic fractures. Ann Surg 189:709–716, 1979.

39. Ganz, R.; Krushell, R.J.; Jakob, R.P.; et al. The antishock pelvic clamp. Clin Orthop 267:71–78, 1991.

40. Geertz, W.H.; Code, K.I.; Jay, R.M.; et al. A prospective study of venous thromboembolism after major trauma. N Engl J Med 331:1601–1606, 1994.

41. Ghanayem, A.J.; Wilbur, J.H.; Leiberman, J.M.; et al. The effect of laparotomy and external fixator stabilization on pelvic volume in an unstable pelvic ring injury. J Trauma 38:396–401, 1995.

42. Gilliland, M.D.; Ward, R.E.; Barton, R.M.; et al. Factors affecting mortality in pelvic fractures. J Orthop Trauma 22:691–693, 1982.

43. Gokcen, E.C.; Burgess, A.R.; Siegel, J.H.; et al. Pelvic fracture mechanism of injury in vehicular trauma patients. J Trauma 36:789–796, 1994.

44. Gruen, G.S.; Leit, M.E.; Gruen, R.J.; et al. The acute management of hemodynamically unstable multiple trauma patients with pelvic ring fractures. J Trauma 36:706–713, 1994.

45. Helfet, D.L.; Koval, K.J.; Hissa, E.A.; et al. Intraoperative somatosensory evoked potential monitoring during acute pelvic fracture surgery. J Orthop Trauma 9:28–34, 1995.

46. Helfet, D.L. Pelvic ring, the three "types." In Müller, M.E., ed. Comprehensive Classification of Pelvis and Acetabulum Fractures. Bern, Switzerland, Maurice E. Müller Foundation, 1995, p. 61.

47. Henderson, R.C. The long-term results of nonoperatively treated major pelvic disruptions. J Orthop Trauma 3:41–47, 1988.

48. Hirvensalo, E.; Lindahl, J.; Bostman, O. A new approach to the internal fixation of unstable pelvic fractures. Clin Orthop Rel Res 297:28–32, 1993.

49. Holdsworth, F.W. Dislocation and fracture dislocation of the pelvis. J Bone Joint Surg [Br] 30:461–466, 1948.

50. Huittinen, V.M.; Slatis, P. Fractures of the pelvis, trauma mechanism, types of injury and principles of treatment. Acta Chir Scand 138:563–569, 1972.

51. Kaehr, D.; Anderson, P.; Mayo, K.; et al. Classification of sacral fractures based on CT imaging. Paper presented at an Orthopaedic Trauma Association Meeting, Dallas, October 27–28, 1988.

52. Kellam, J.F.; McMurtry, R.Y.; Tile, M. The unstable pelvic fracture. Orthop Clin North Am 18:25–41, 1987.

53. Kellam, J.F. The role of external fixation in pelvic disruptions. Clin Orthop Rel Res 241:66–82, 1989.

54. Kellam, J.F.; Boyer, M.; Dean, R.; et al. Results of external fixation of the pelvis. Paper presented at the 12th International Congress on Hoffman External Fixation, Garmisch Partenkirchen Murnau, Bavaria, West Germany, October 9–10, 1986.

55. Kim, W.Y.; Hearn, T.C.; Seleem, O.; et al. Effect of pin location on stability of pelvic external fixation. Clin Orthop Rel Res 361:237–244, 1999.

56. Kiting, J.F.; Wearier, J.; Blackout, P.; et al. Early fixation of the vertically unstable pelvis: The role of iliosacral screw fixation in the management of the vertically unstable pelvis. J Trauma 13:107–113, 1999.

57. Koury, H.I.; Peschiera, J.L.; Welling, R.E. Selective use of pelvic roentgenograms in blunt trauma patients. J Trauma 34:236–237, 1993.

58. Krieg, J.C.; Mohr, M.; Ellis, T.J.; et al. Emergent stabilization of the pelvic ring injuries by controlled circumferential compression: A clinical trial. J Trauma 59:3, 659–664, 2005.

59. Lange, R.H.; Hansen, S. Pelvic ring disruptions with symphysis pubis diastasis. Indications, techniques and application of anterior internal fixation. Clin Orthop Rel Res 201:130–137, 1985.

60. Latenser, B.A.; Gentilello, L.M.; Tarver, A.A.; et al. Improved outcome with early fixation of skeletally unstable pelvic fractures. J Trauma 31:28–31, 1991.

61. Legothetopulos, K. Eine absolute sichere blutillungsmethode bei vaginalen und abdominalengynakologischen operationen. Zentrailbl Gynäkol. 50:3202, 1926.

62. Lee, J.; Abrahamson, B.S.; Harrington, T.G.; et al. Urologic complications of diastasis of the pubic symphysis: A trauma case report and review of world literature. J Trauma 48:133–136, 2000.

63. Leighton, R.K.; Waddell, J.P. Techniques for reduction and posterior fixation through the anterior approach. Clin Orthop Rel Res 329:115–120, 1996.

64. Letournel, E. Acetabular fractures: Classification and management. Clin Orthop Rel Res 151:81–106, 1980.

64a. Linnau, K.F.; Blackmore, C.C.; Kaufman, R.; et al. Do initial radiographs agree with crash site mechanism of injury in pelvic ring disruptions? A pilot study. J Orthop Trauma 21(6):375–380, 2007.

65. Lowe, M.A.; Mason, J.T.; Luna, G.K.; et al. Risk factors for urethral injuries in men with traumatic pelvic fractures. J Urol 140:506–507, 1988.

66. MacKenzie, E.J.; Cushing, B.M.; Jurkovich, G.J.; et al. Physical impairment and functional outcomes six months after severe lower extremity fractures. J Trauma 34:528–539, 1993.

67. Matta, J.M.; Saucedo, T. Internal fixation of pelvic ring fractures. Clin Orthop Rel Res 242:83–97, 1989.

67a. Matta, J.M.; Yerasimides, J.G. Table-skeletal fixation as an adjunct to pelvic ring reduction. J Orthop Trauma 21(9):647–656, 2007.

68. McBroom, R.; Tile, M. Disruptions of the pelvic ring. Presented at the Canadian Orthopaedic Research Society Convention. Kingston, Ontario, Canada. June, 1982.

69. McCoy, G.F.; Johnstone, R.A.; Kenwright, K. Biomechanical aspects of pelvic and hip injuries in road traffic accidents. J Orthop Trauma 3:118–123, 1989.

70. McLaren, A. Internal fixation in fractures of the pelvis and acetabulum. In Tile, M., ed. Fractures of the Pelvis and Acetabulum, 2nd ed. Baltimore, Williams & Wilkins, 1995, pp. 183–189.

71. McLellan, B.A.; Phillips, J.P.; Hunter, G.A.; et al. Bilateral lower extremity amputations after prolonged application of the PASG. A case report. J Surg 30:55–56, 1987.

72. McMurtry, R.Y.; Walton, D.; Dickinson, D.; et al. Pelvic disruption in the polytraumatized patient. A management protocol. Clin Orthop Rel Res 151:22–30, 1980.

73. Mears, D.C.; Capito, C.P.; Deleeuw, H. Posterior pelvic disruptions managed by the use of the double cobra plate. Instr Course Lect 37:143–150, 1988.

74. Mears, D.C.; Rubash, H.E. Pelvic and Acetabular Fractures. Thorofare, NJ, Slack, 1986.

75. Miranda, M.A.; Riemer, B.L.; Butterfield, S.L.; et al. Pelvic ring injuries: A long-term functional outcome study. Clin Orthop Rel Res 329:152–159, 1996.

76. Moed, B.R.; Hartman, M.J.; Ahmad, B.K.; et al. Evaluation of intraoperative nerve monitoring during insertion of an iliosacral implant in an animal model. J Bone Joint Surg [Am] 81:1529–1537, 1999.

77. Moreno, C.; Moore, E.E.; Rosenberger, A.; et al. Hemorrhage associated with major pelvic fracture: A multispecialty challenge. J Trauma 26:987–994, 1986.

78. Murr, P.C.; Moore, E.E.; Lipscomb, R.; et al. Abdominal trauma associated with pelvic fracture. J Trauma 20:919–923, 1980.

79. Nallathambi, M.N.; Ferreiro, J.; Ivatury, R.R.; et al. The use of peritoneal lavage and urological studies in major fractures of the pelvis—A reassessment. Br J Accident Surg 18:379–383, 1987.

80. Nelson, D.W.; Duwelius, P.J. CT-guided fixation of sacral fractures and sacroiliac joint disruptions. Radiology 180:527–532, 1991.

81. Nepola, J.V.; Trenhaile, S.W.; Miranda, M.A.; et al. Vertical shear injuries: Is there a relationship between residual displacement and functional outcome? J Trauma 46:1024–1030, 1999.

82. Niemi, T.A.; Norton, L.W. Vaginal injuries in patients with pelvic fractures. J Trauma 25:547–551, 1985.

83. Noojin, F.K.; Malkani, A.L.; Haikal, L.; et al. Cross-sectional geometry of the sacral ala for safe insertion of iliosacral lag screws: A computed tomography model. J Trauma 14:31–35, 2000.

84. Ochsner, M.G.; Hoffman, A.P.; DiPasquale, D.; et al. Associated aortic rupture pelvic fracture: An alert for orthopedic and general surgeons. J Trauma 33:429–434, 1992.

85. Oonishi, H.; Isha, H.; Hasegawa, T. Mechanical analysis of the human pelvis and its application to the artificial hip joint by means of the three-dimensional finite element method. J Biomech 16:427–444, 1983.

86. Pattimore, D.; Thomas, P.; Dave, S.H. Torso injury patterns and mechanisms in car crashes: An additional diagnostic tool. Injury 23:123–126, 1992.

87. Peltier, L.F. Complications associated with fractures of the pelvis. J Bone Joint Surg [Am] 47:1060–1069, 1965.

88. Pennal, G.F.; Sutherland, G.O. Fractures of the Pelvis. Motion picture. Chicago, American Academy of Orthopaedic Surgeons Film Library, 1961.

89. Perry, J.F. Pelvic open fractures. Clin Orthop Rel Res 151:41–45, 1980.

90. Pohlemann, T.; Bosch, U.; Gansslen, A.; et al. The Hannover experience in management of pelvic fractures. Clin Orthop 305:69–80, 1994.

91. Pohlemann, T.; Gänsslen, A.; Bosch, U.; et al. The technique of packing for control of hemorrhage in complex pelvic fractures. Tech Orthop 9:267–270, 1995.

92. Poole, G.V.; Ward, E.F. Causes of mortality in patients with pelvic fractures. Orthopedics 17:691–696, 1994.

93. Poole, G.V.; Ward, E.F.; Muakkassa, F.F.; et al. Pelvic fracture from major blunt trauma. Ann Surg 213:532–539, 1991.

94. Raf, L. Double vertical fractures of the pelvis. Acta Chir Scand 131:298–305, 1966.

95. Raffe, J.; Christensen, M. Compound fractures of the pelvis. Am J Surg 132:282–286, 1976.

96. Richardson, J.D.; Harty, J.; Amin, M. Open pelvic fractures. J Trauma 22:533–538, 1982.

97. Riemer, B.L.; Butterfield, S.L.; Diamond, D.L.; et al. Acute mortality associated with injuries to the pelvic ring: The role of early patient mobilization and external fixation. J Trauma 35:671–677, 1993.

98. Robinson, D.; Hendel, D.; Halperin, N. An overlapping pubic dislocation treated by closed reduction: Case report and review of the literature. J Trauma 29:883–885, 1989.

99. Rothenberg, D.A.; Fischer, R.P.; Strate, R.G. The mortality associated with pelvic fractures. Surgery 84:356–361, 1978.

100. Routt, M.L.C.; Kregor, P.J.; Mayo, K. Early results of percutaneous iliosacral screws placed with the patient in the supine position. J Orthop Trauma 9:207–214, 1995.

101. Routt, M.L.C.; Meier, M.C.; Kregor, P.J. Percutaneous iliosacral screws with the patient supine technique. Op Techn Orthop 3:35–45, 1993.

102. Routt, M.L.; Nork, S.E.; Mills, W.J. Percutaneous fixation of pelvic ring disruptions. Clin Orthop Rel Res 375:15–29, 2000.

103. Routt, M.L.C.; Simonian, P.T.; Agnew, S.G.; et al. Radiographic recognition of the sacral alar slope for optimal placement of iliosacral screws: A cadaveric and clinical study. J Orthop Trauma 10:171–177, 1996.

104. Routt, M.L.; Simonian, P.T.; Defalco, A.J.; et al. Internal fixation in pelvic fractures and primary repairs of associated genitourinary disruptions: A team approach. J Trauma 40:784–790, 1996.

105. Routt, M.L.C.; Simonian, P.T.; Grujic, L. The retrograde medullary superior pubic ramus screw for the treatment of anterior pelvic ring disruptions: A new technique. J Orthop Trauma 9:35–44, 1995.

106. Routt, M.L.C.; Simonian, P.T.; Inaba, J. Iliosacral screw fixation of the disrupted sacroiliac joint. Techn Orthop 9:300–314, 1994.

107. Ruedi, T.; von Hochstetter, A.H.C.; Schlumpf, R. Surgical Approaches for Internal Fixation. Berlin, Springer-Verlag, 1984, pp. 77–83.

108. Saibel, E.A.; Maggisano, R.; Witchell, S.S. Angiography in the diagnosis and treatment of trauma. J Can Assoc Radiogr 34:218–227, 1983.

109. Sachatzker, J.; Tile, M. Rationale of Operative Fracture Care. New York, Springer-Verlag, 1987, p. 165.

110. Scheid, D.K. Internal fixation. In Tile, M., ed. Fractures of the Pelvis and Acetabulum, 2nd ed. Baltimore, Williams & Wilkins, p. 197, 1995.

111. Scheid, D.K.; Kellam, J.F.; Tile, M. Open reduction and internal fixation of pelvic ring fractures. J Orthop Trauma 5:226, 1991.

112. Semba, R.T.; Yasukawa, K.; Gustilo, R.B. Critical analysis of results of 53 Malgaigne fractures of the pelvis. J Trauma 23:535–537, 1983.

113. Simonian, P.T.; Routt, M.L.C.; Harrington, R.M.; et al. Biomechanical simulation of the anteroposterior compression injury of the pelvis. Clin Orthop Rel Res 309:245–256, 1994.

114. Simonian, P.T.; Routt, M.L.C.; Harrington, R.M.; et al. Box plate fixation of the symphysis pubis: Biomechanical evaluation of a new technique. J Orthop Trauma 8:483–489, 1994.

115. Simonian, P.T.; Routt, M.L.C.; Harrington, R.M.; et al. Internal fixation of the unstable anterior pelvic ring: A biomechanical comparison of standard plating techniques and the retrograde medullary superior pubic ramus screw. J Orthop Trauma 8:476–482, 1994.

116. Simpson, L.A.; Waddell, J.P.; Leighton, R.K.; et al. Anterior approach and stabilization of the disrupted sacroiliac joint. J Trauma 27:1332–1339, 1987.

117. Southworth JD.; Bersack SR. Anomalies of the lumbosacral vertebrae in five hundred fifty individuals without symptoms referable to low back pain. AJR Am J Roentgenol 1950;64:624–634.

118. Stephen, D.J.; Kreder, H.J.; Day, A.C.; et al. Early detection of arterial bleeding in acute pelvic trauma. J Trauma 47:638–642, 1999.

119. Tile, M. Internal fixation. In Tile, M., ed. Fractures of the Pelvis and Acetabulum, 2nd ed. Baltimore, Williams & Wilkins, pp. 189–193, 1995.

120. Tile, M. Pelvic ring fractures. Should they be fixed? J Bone Joint Surg [Br] 70:1–12, 1988.

121. Tile, M.; Hearn, T. Biomechanics. In Tile, M., ed. Fractures of the Pelvis and Acetabulum, 2nd ed. Baltimore, Williams & Wilkins, 1995, pp. 22–36.

122. Tini, P.G.; Wieser, C.; Zinn, W.M. The transitional vertebra of the lumbosacral spine: Its radiological classification, incidence, prevalence, and clinical significance. Rheumatol Rehabil 16:180–185, 1977.

123. Tornetta, P.; Dickson, K.; Matta, J.M. Outcome of rotationally unstable pelvic ring injuries treated operatively. Clin Orthop Rel Res 329:147–151, 1996.

124. Tornetta, P.; Matta, J.M. Outcome of operatively treated unstable posterior pelvic ring disruptions. Clin Orthop Rel Res 329:186–193, 1996.

125. Trunkey, D.D.; Chapman, M.W.; Lim, R.C. Management of pelvic fractures and blunt traumatic injury. J Trauma 14:912–923, 1974.

126. Velmahos, G.C.; Kern, J.; Chan, L.S.; et al. Prevention of venous thromboembolism after injury: An evidence-based report—Part I: Analysis of risk factors and evaluation of the role of vena caval filters. J Trauma 49:132–139, 2000.

127. Vermeulen, B.P.; Hoffmeyer, P. Prehospitalization stabilization of pelvic disruption: A new strap belt to provide hemodynamic stabilization. Swiss Surg 5:43–46, 1999.

128. Vrahas, M.; Gordon, R.G.; Mears, D.C.; et al. Intraoperative somatosensory evoked potential monitoring of pelvic and acetabular fractures. J Orthop Trauma 6:50–58, 1992.

129. Vukicevic, S.; Marusic, A.; Stavljenic, A.; et al. Holographic analysis of the human pelvis. Spine 16:209–214, 1991.

130. Webb, L.X.; de Araujo, W.; Donofrio, P.; et al. Electromyography monitoring for percutaneous placement of iliosacral screw. J Trauma 14:245–254, 2000.

131. Weber, T.G.; Mast, J.W. The extended ilioinguinal approach for specific both column fractures. Clin Orthop Rel Res 305:106–111, 1994.

132. Weis, E.B. Subtle neurological injuries in pelvic fractures. J Trauma 24:983–985, 1984.

133. Wild, J.J.; Hanson, G.W.; Tullos, H.S. Unstable fractures of the pelvis treated by external fixation. J Bone Joint Surg [Am] 64:1010–1020, 1982.

134. Young, J.W.R.; Burgess, A.R. Radiological Management of Pelvic Ring Fractures. Baltimore, Urban & Schwarzenberg, 1987, pp. 22, 27, 41, 55.

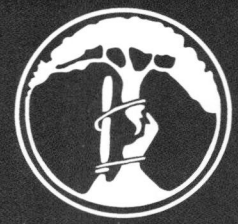

CHAPTER 37

Surgical Treatment of Acetabular Fractures

···

Milton Lee (Chip) Routt, Jr., M.D.

Acetabular fractures are uncommon and complex injuries that usually result from high-energy traumatic events. The rarity of these fractures makes it difficult for most physicians to become familiar with them. These injuries challenge even the most experienced physicians because of their deep and complex anatomy and associated primary organ system injuries. Over the past three decades, a great deal of information has been gathered regarding these injuries and their treatments.

EPIDEMIOLOGY

Acetabular fractures occur when the lower extremity, specifically the proximal femur, is excessively loaded. The resultant acetabular fracture pattern details are determined by the hip position at impact, the local bone quality, and the force of the applied load. As the load is further transmitted, the acetabular fracture displaces, and the femoral head may dislocate from the hip joint in line with the applied force. Two different age groups of patients typically sustain acetabular fractures.[107] Young adults with active and perhaps reckless lifestyles tend to be involved in high-energy traumatic accidents resulting in acetabular injuries. More senior but not necessarily less active patients sustain acetabular injuries from lower energy events such as falling from a standing height. The injury most likely results from insufficient bone quality. Certainly acetabular fractures can occur at any age, even in children, but these two populations account for the majority of such injuries.

The mechanisms of injury are usually automobile and motorcycle accidents, pedestrians struck by motor vehicles, falls from significant heights, and crush injuries. Legislation directed at seatbelt wear and enforcement has been shown to decrease the incidence and severity of acetabular injuries.[1] Conversely, some studies have suggested that mandatory helmet laws have improved patient survivability after motor cycle accidents and therefore increased the number and complexity of acetabular trauma.[43]

OSTEOLOGY

Normal pelvic osteology is quite confusing, and displaced acetabular fractures further complicate understanding. The acetabulum is a hemisphere-shaped recess located between the ilium, ischium, and pubis. It develops from the triradiate cartilage and matures into a variety of appearances. Some acetabuli are shallow and termed "dysplastic," and others are deeper. On radiographs, the dysplastic acetabuli are situated peripherally relative to the ilium, whereas deeper ones appear medially located. All of these anatomic factors are important when treating acetabular injuries.

Other than the region of the fossa acetabuli, the concave acetabular surface is covered with hyaline cartilage and surrounded on its periphery by the labrum. The peripheral labrum is attached to both the acetabular rim and the joint capsule. The fossa acetabuli is filled with fat and anchors the ligamentum teres along with its blood vessels. The fossa acetabuli's cortical backing is the quadrilateral surface. The transverse acetabular ligament borders the caudal aspect of the acetabulum.

The articular regions of the acetabulum include the anterior wall, dome, and posterior wall. The anterior wall's chondral surface is small relative to the other two areas. The cortical surface of the anterior wall area is almost completely composed of the iliopectineal eminence. The iliopsoas tendon passes lateral to the iliopectineal eminence (IPE) and just above the anterior wall region. The iliopsoas tendon travels along the iliopsoas gutter, where a bursa is located. Medially, the dense cortical pelvic brim borders the anterior wall, and anteriorly the cortical surface of the pectineal sulcus neighbors the anterior wall area. The acetabular dome is the superior articular area located directly beneath the anterior inferior iliac spine. The posterior wall region is the largest surface area of the three articular zones and comprises the remainder of the acetabular articular surface. All three articular zones are backed by a topographically complex corticocancellous bony anatomy. The surrounding bony "hills and valleys" represent the acetabular fault lines that allow fracture propagation (Fig. 37-1).

The acetabular two-column concept was introduced by Letournel. Using his conceptual model, the articular acetabulum is located between and as a part of two surrounding bony limbs representing an inverted Y shape. The anterior limb, or supporting column, includes the symphysis pubis, superior pubic ramus, anterior acetabular wall,

A, *The pelvic model reveals the complicated cortical bone surface anatomy surrounding the acetabulum. Specific fracture lines occur along these bony ridges and within the recesses.* **B,** *The different areas of pelvic osteology are specifically named to facilitate communication and improved understanding of acetabular injuries and their locations.*

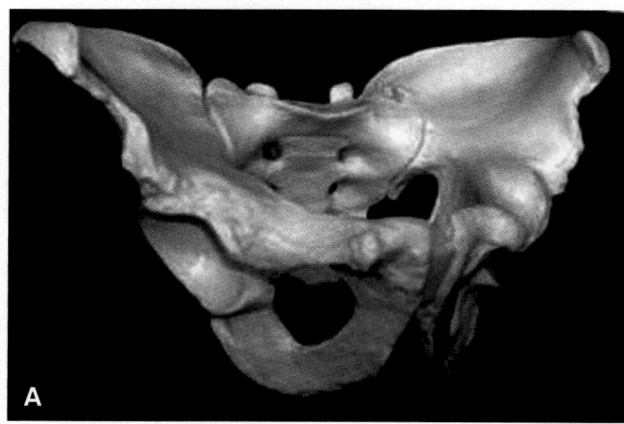

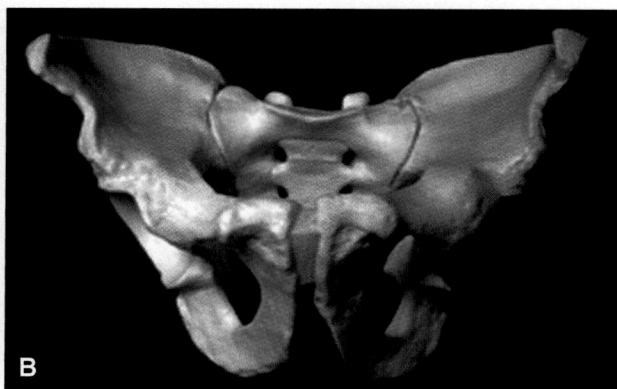

the anterior halves of the dome and fossa acetabuli, the anterior half of the quadrilateral surface, and anterior ilium including both anterior iliac spines and crest. The posterior limb, or supporting column, includes the entire posterior wall, the posterior portions of the dome and fossa acetabuli, the caudal portion of the greater sciatic notch, the ischial spine, the entire lesser sciatic notch, and the posterior half of the quadrilateral surface (Fig. 37-2).

The two-column model was intended to simplify the acetabular osseous architecture so that clinicians could better understand the injury patterns. But for some it became confusing especially when the fracture patterns and classification scheme were defined using most of the same osteologic terminology. In the two-column acetabular

model, the anterior column area includes the anterior wall, and the posterior column area includes the entire posterior wall. This confuses some clinicians since the walls are components of the supporting columns but separate from them as individual fracture patterns. For example, an elementary posterior column acetabular fracture pattern divides the posterior wall, extends through the greater sciatic notch, progresses through the quadrilateral surface, exits the caudal aspect of the fossa acetabuli, and exits the inferior ramus. The osteologic, two-column model and fracture pattern terminologies use shared words, yet are truly distinct from one another. To resolve the confusion, the anatomic acetabular areas, two-column model components, and the individual fracture patterns must be

A, *Letournel's two-column concept is demonstrated schematically by this illustration depicting the acetabulum between two supporting "columns" of an inverted Y shape.* **B,** *The anatomic correlation of the inverted Y model demonstrates the anterior column consisting of iliac and pubic components, and the posterior column consists of ischial components. The quadrilateral surface and fossa acetabuli are divided. The acetabulum is situated between the two limbs of the inverted Y-shaped support. The anterior and posterior wall regions are portions of their respective supporting columns.*

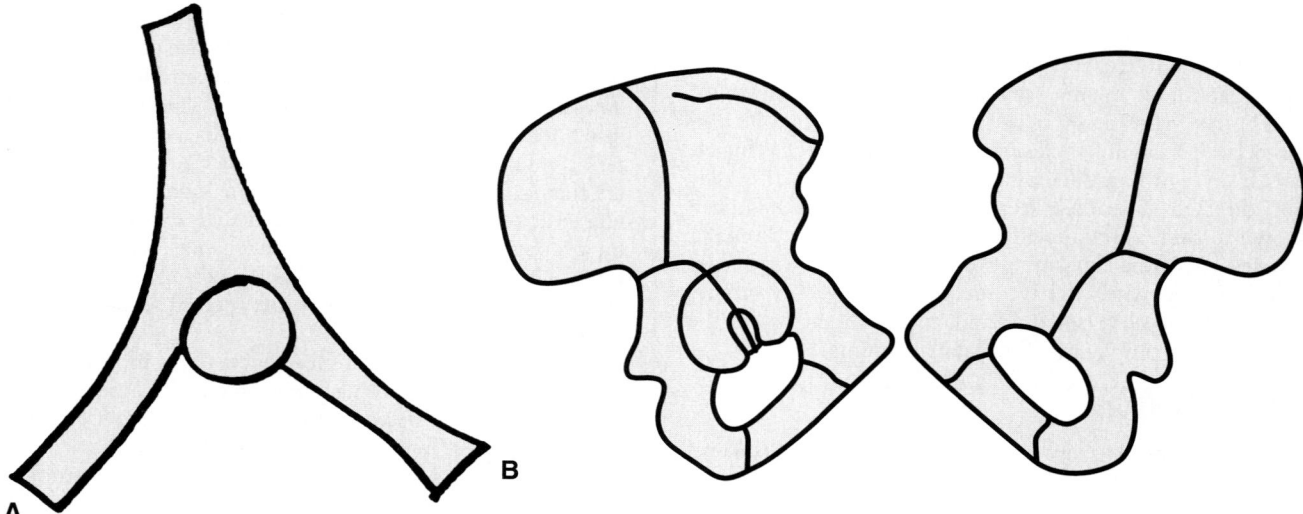

FIGURE 37-3 *This model shows that the anterior wall area is a portion of the anterior column, and the posterior wall area is a portion of the posterior column.*

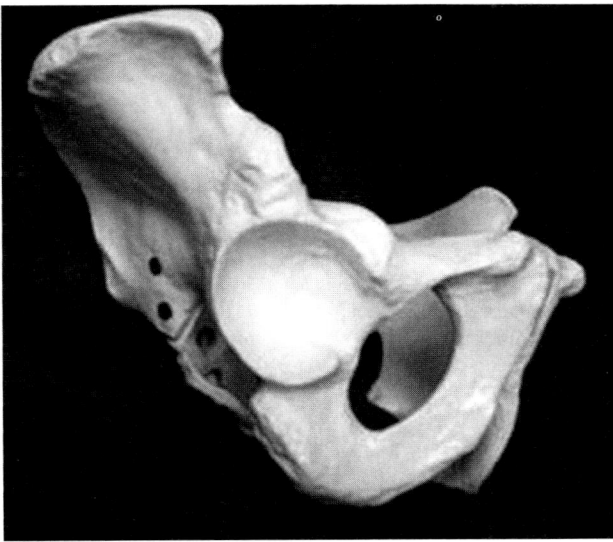

considered while respecting and consolidating all of this information (Fig. 37-3).

RADIOLOGY

Pelvic radiology is even more complex than pelvic osteology, but is the essential key to understanding acetabular fractures. Acetabular fracture diagnosis and classification schemes are based on the radiographic findings and Letournel's two-column acetabular concept. The screening anteroposterior (AP) plain pelvic radiograph is usually the first imaging study that alerts the treating physician to an acetabular injury. For this reason, certain radiographic osseous landmarks were introduced by Letournel and still serve as the foundation of acetabular imaging. Many clinicians evaluate the uninjured side initially to review the relevant landmarks and then compare them and their asymmetry with the injured side.

The normal radiographic markers represent bony cortical edges revealed by tangential x-ray beams. These cortical lines include the peripheral edges of both the anterior and posterior walls; the dense line representing the pelvic brim and superior pubic ramus edge; the dense line representing the pelvic brim and quadrilateral surface; the dome region's subchondral arc; and the acetabular "teardrop" representing the fossa acetabuli, obturator sulcus, and a portion of the quadrilateral surface. These six radiographic markers help clinicians to better understand and mark the two walls, the two supporting columns, the weight-bearing dome, and the caudal joint (Fig. 37-4).

Clinicians should learn normal acetabular radiology first and while holding and handling a pelvic model. The osseous model helps correlate osteology and radiology. Three-dimensional radiographic modeling may also facilitate pelvic and acetabular radiographic correlations and learning. Normal radiology should be mastered first, then the clinician moves on to displaced fracture imaging.

Normally, the anterior wall is medially located relative to the more peripheral posterior wall on the AP pelvic film. The anterior wall has an undulating edge anatomy attributed to the iliopsoas gutter, iliopectineal eminence, and pectineal cortical sulcus. Imaging of the anterior wall area reveals it to appear more radiodense than the posterior wall because of the superimposed (stacked) osseous anatomy. The posterior wall edge anatomy is convex and located peripherally relative to the anterior wall.

The anterior acetabular supporting column is represented on the AP pelvic film by the iliopectineal (iliopubic) line. This radiodense line is formed from tangential imaging of the pelvic brim cortical bone as it extends from the sacroiliac (SI) area to the pubis. The superior and posterior cortical edge of the superior pubic ramus in continuity with the pelvic brim cortical bone form the iliopectineal line. The iliopectineal line representing the supporting acetabular anterior column is only imaged on the AP plain pelvic radiograph.

The posterior acetabular supporting column is represented on the AP pelvic film by the ilioischial line. This radiodense line is formed from the tangential imaging of the pelvic brim, quadrilateral surface, and medial ischial cortical bone. As with the iliopectineal line, the ilioischial line is only seen on the AP plain pelvic radiograph.

Normally, the acetabular dome's subchondral arc is seen cranial to and congruent with the femoral head. It represents the weight-bearing area of the articular acetabulum and is vital to assessing hip joint congruity.

The acetabular "teardrop" is probably the most difficult radiographic landmark of the six to understand, but its value is relevant, especially when assessing the accuracy of surgical repair. The medial cortical portion of the teardrop is formed by the obturator neurovascular sulcus and a portion of the quadrilateral surface. The lateral cortical boundary represents the cortical surface of the fossa acetabuli.

These six AP pelvic radiographic acetabular markers represent acetabular supporting columns, walls, and the dome area. On the injured side, depending on the specific fracture details, the walls, columns, and the dome arc may be divided by fracture lines, impacted, or displaced along with certain fracture fragments.[109]

Once an acetabular fracture is identified, further radiographic assessments are indicated after any dislocations have been reduced. Biplanar imaging is obtained by placing the radiographic cassette beneath the patient's pelvis as for an AP image but then logrolling the patient approximately 45° onto the uninjured side for the film, and then rolling similarly onto the injured side using the same imaging technique. Rolling the patient onto the injured acetabular side usually causes pain and should be performed last. These two biplanar images identify the columns and walls more specifically and are named according to the injured side. When the injured side is rolled up, the obturator foramen is relatively perpendicular to the x-ray beam so the image is termed an "obturator oblique." The obturator oblique image demonstrates the anterior column and the posterior wall. Similarly when the injured side is rolled down, the iliac fossa is essentially

FIGURE 37-4 *A, This plain pelvic anteroposterior (AP) radiograph demonstrates the six important acetabular lines. The dome arc, the anterior wall, the posterior wall, the iliopectineal (or iliopubic) line, ilioischial line, and teardrop are noted. The dome line represents a subchondral region of the weight-bearing area. The anterior wall is medially located and undulating relative to the more peripheral and convex posterior wall. The anterior wall appears denser than the posterior wall because of the bony stacking of the two walls and femoral head. The peripheral posterior wall only radiographically stacks the femoral head and posterior wall. The iliopectineal (or iliopubic) line is a condensation of cortical bone shadows from the greater sciatic notch and pelvic brim ("ilio-") and superior pubic ramus ("pectineal or pubic"). This line represents the supporting anterior column. The ilioischial line shares the "ilio-" component with the previous line, but then diverges, representing the quadrilateral surface cortical bone imaged tangentially for its "ischial" component. The ilioischial line represents the posterior acetabular column. The teardrop is the last landmark and indicates the fossa acetabuli, quadrilateral surface, and obturator sulcus. B, Image alteration of this AP pelvic radiograph accentuates the ilioischial lines and teardrops bilaterally. C, This AP plain pelvic film demonstrates the radiographic appearance of a displaced posterior wall acetabular fracture. Five landmark lines are intact, but the peripheral posterior wall line is lost due to the displaced fracture. Also, a radiolucency is noted in the area where the posterior wall should be, and the displaced peripheral posterior wall fracture–displacement is seen.*

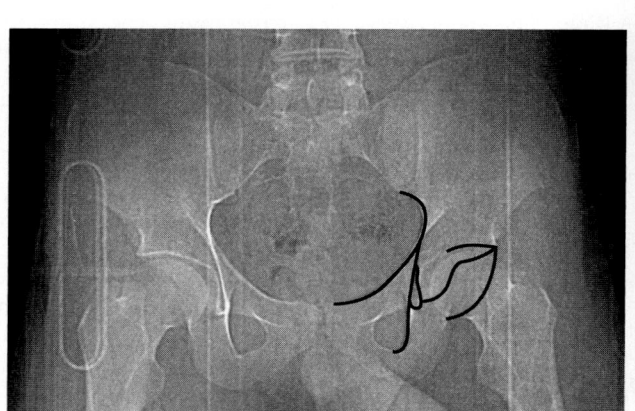
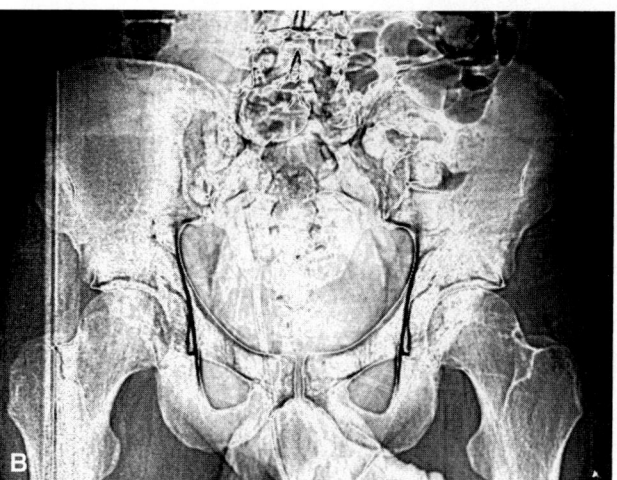
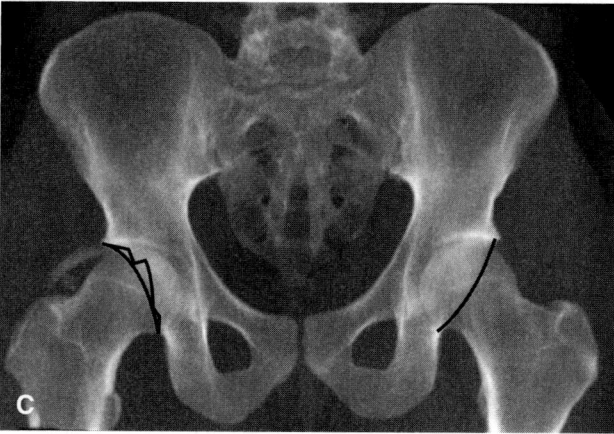

perpendicular to the x-ray beam, and the image is named an "iliac oblique" view. The iliac oblique film reveals the anterior wall and the posterior column (Fig. 37-5).

Rolling the patient for the oblique images not only causes pain but often reveals fracture instability sites that may not have been apparent on the AP plain pelvic film. The oblique acetabular images should not be obtained with the hip dislocated. The displaced fracture fragments and femoral head will obstruct important anatomic landmarks. Routine reduction maneuvers should be performed prior to the oblique films.

Other plain pelvic radiographs, such as inlet and outlet images, are indicated for those patients with pelvic ring injuries coupled with acetabular fractures. Such combination injuries are unusual but the additional imaging is recommended to completely identify the injury zones.

Pelvic computed tomography (CT) imaging further delineates acetabular injuries. Two-dimensional (2-D) pelvic CT scans are usually obtained in 5-mm axial slices from the iliac crest to the acetabular dome. From the dome region through the caudal articular areas, 3-mm images are recommended, and then 5-mm axial slices through the

FIGURE 37-5 **A,** *This patient has a significantly displaced left-sided acetabular fracture. On this oblique image, the patient's right side was rolled up and the injured left side down while the oblique radiograph was obtained. Since the x-ray beam is essentially perpendicular to the iliac fossa on the injured side, this is the iliac oblique image. This imaging can be a very painful for the patient, so patients are often less rotated as a result. Alert patients complain as body weight is applied onto the injured side.* **B,** *Now the injured left side has been rolled up and the normal right side is down. On the injured left side, the obturator foramen is essentially perpendicular to the x-ray beam, making this an obturator oblique image.*

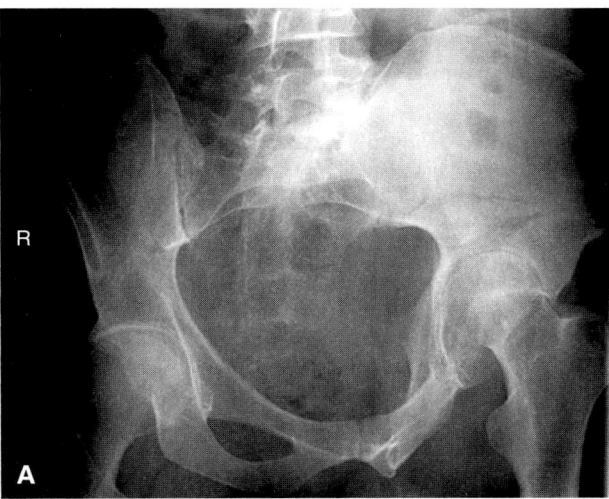
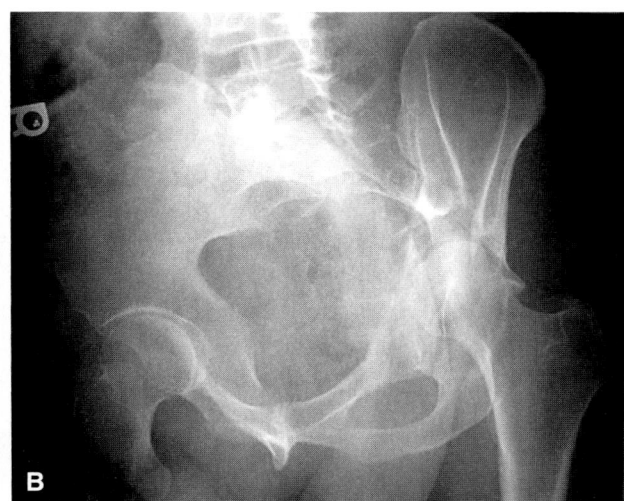

ischium. Two-dimensional pelvic CT provides information regarding bone quality, body habitus, surrounding soft tissue injury, occult posterior pelvic injury, and other acetabular details.[21,96] Related local osseous findings may include acetabular or femoral head impaction injuries, intra-articular debris, and subtle incongruity, among other findings. Numerous studies have demonstrated the need for CT when evaluating acetabular fractures.[97,115–117,119,151]

Recent computer imaging software allows the operator to produce "plain films" from the data acquired during pelvic CT. These pelvic images can then be rotated and manipulated on the monitor to provide the necessary oblique images.[149] The treating physicians must remember that such computer-generated and rotated oblique films are not obtained by rolling the patient as the routine oblique films are performed. Because of this, occult fracture instability will not be identified as it is with the traditional oblique films (Fig. 37-6).

Three-dimensional (3-D) pelvic CT techniques have been refined, thus improving the model quality and decreasing the radiographic exposure needed. The 3-D acetabular images provide the treating physician with a more realistic understanding of the overall acetabular pattern. The displacements and fracture line specifics are revealed on a radiographic model.[40] Such modeling should facilitate understanding and treatment planning. Many surgeons prefer the 3-D images for obvious reasons but be aware that certain 3-D imaging software packages may smooth some fracture lines. The 2-D pelvic CT remains the radiographic standard for acetabular fracture imaging and planning (Fig. 37-7).

Other radiographic studies have been advocated to better understand acetabular fractures. Dynamic acetabular imaging using angiographic fluoroscopic equipment was shown to improve understanding of certain complex fracture patterns. However, these methods were advocated prior to current CT imaging techniques.[158]

Pelvic angiography is indicated in hemodynamically unstable patients with acetabular fractures who have not responded to routine resuscitation techniques and evaluations. The angiograher should access the pelvic arterial tree using the contralateral side from the acetabular injury since fracture displacements may alter the groin vascular anatomy. Similarly, contrast agent leakage or hematoma in the ipsilateral groin area often cause significant dermatitis. These conditions in turn can adversely affect acetabular fracture treatment. Strategic embolizations can be lifesaving but also influence treatment decisions such as surgical exposure choice. The embolization procedure and its details should be documented in the permanent medical record. The treating surgeon should also remember that angiographic images are often of the highest quality and should be reviewed when possible.

The angiography suite is often an ideal location for closed manipulative reduction of acetabular fracture–dislocations. Typically the patients are sedated, and the reductions can be performed under real-time imaging if desired. Using the angiographic imaging equipment, the biplanar oblique plain radiographs can be obtained without moving the patient since the radiographic beam rotates around the patient.

Magnetic resonance imaging (MRI) has thus far had limited indications in patients with acetabular fractures due to acute trauma. Insufficiency fractures of the peripheral pubic ramus and related acetabular stress fractures have been identified using MRI.

FIGURE 37-6 *A–C,* These anteroposterior (AP) and biplanar oblique acetabular images were generated from routine pelvic computed tomography (CT) data. Such computer-generated images do not reflect fracture instability due to patient positioning as routine oblique acetabular plain radiographs do because the acquired axial CT imaging information is manipulated to create these images. The AP image identifies the extensive injuries to both the pelvic ring and left acetabulum. The iliac oblique view shows the posterior column and anterior wall areas of injury. The obturator oblique identifies the posterior wall and anterior column areas of involvement.

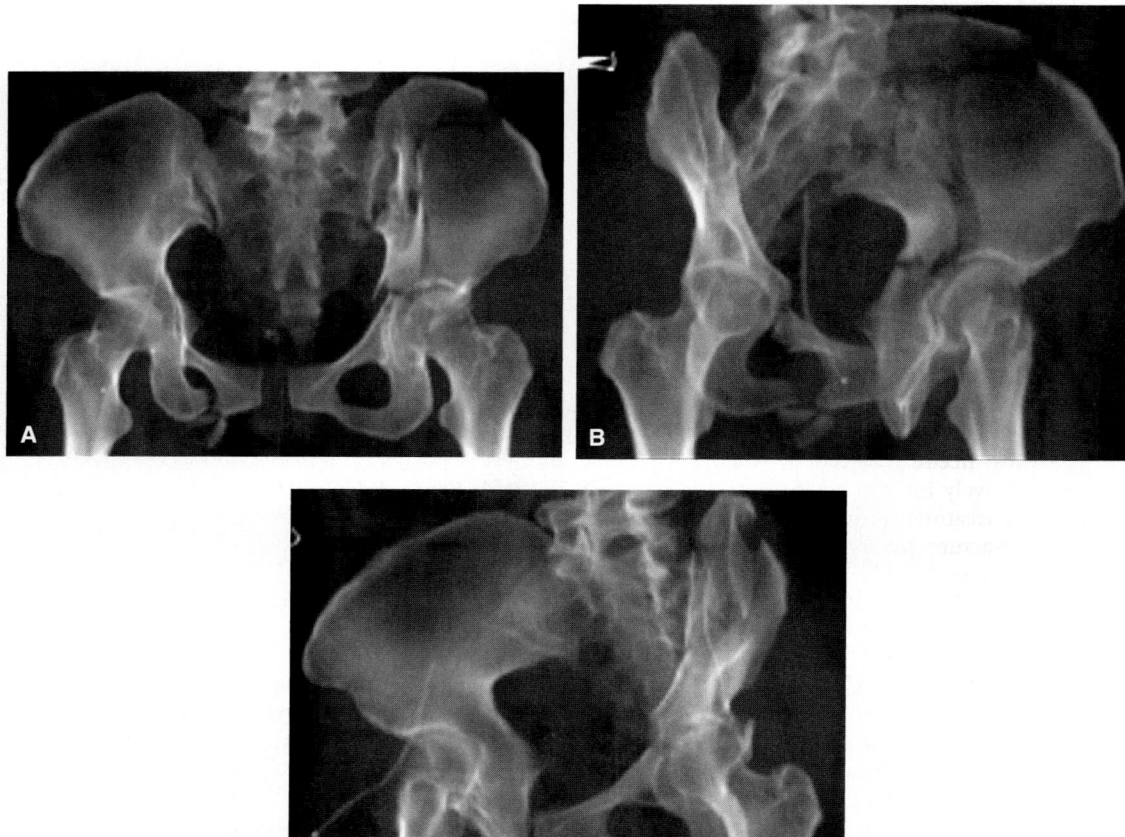

FIGURE 37-7 *A,* This pelvic anteroposterior film generated from the computed tomography data reveals the medial acetabular dome impaction and the quadrilateral surface fracture–displacement due to femoral intrusion. *B,* The three-dimensional imaging of the same patient perhaps better defines the quadrilateral surface fracture location and displacement. Unfortunately, the dome impaction is not seen using 3-D modeling, which highlights the need for all imaging methods to be studied carefully in order to assess the injury completely.

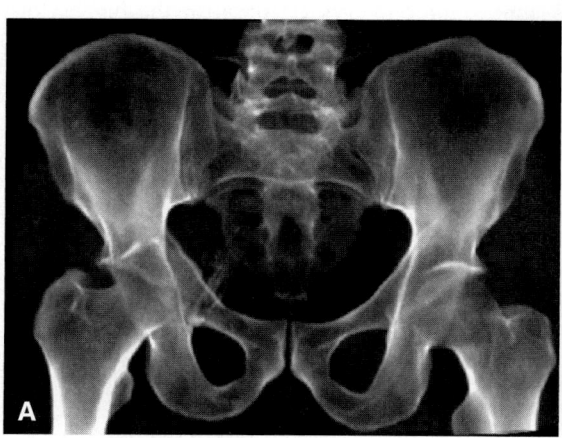
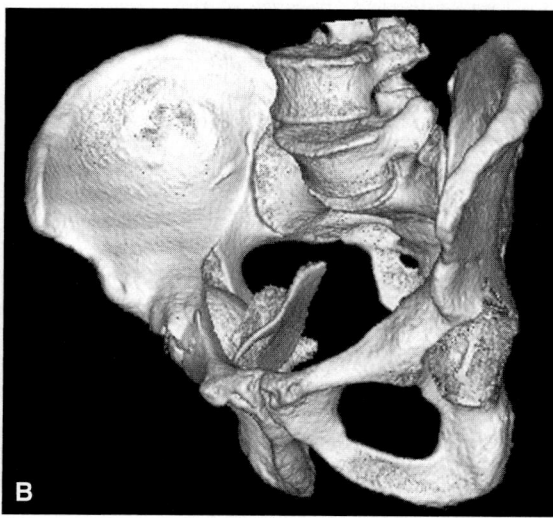

CLASSIFICATION

Acetabular fracture classification is confusing because the same terms used to describe the anatomic walls and supporting columns are used again to define certain fracture patterns. The treating physician must comprehend that anatomic areas and fracture patterns are related and similar, but are not the same. An anatomic area is an anatomic area, and the named fracture pattern involves that anatomic area.

Classifications are assigned based on radiographic criteria.[68–70,109,160] The AP pelvic film provides certain clues that are then refined on the oblique images and CT scans. When the iliopectineal line is disrupted or displaced but the ilioischial line is not, the fracture is likely an anterior column fracture pattern. The pelvic oblique views and CT images reveal the fracture details needed to define the classification pattern. When only the ilioischial line is disrupted or displaced on the AP film, then a posterior column pattern is presumed and further investigated.

Letournel's acetabular classification scheme was devised to help surgeons select an appropriate surgical exposure for those fractures needing operative management.[109] The scheme is relatively inclusive and easy to remember, but does not direct treatment nor is it prognostic.[15]

Ten common fracture patterns divided between two groups of five each were described. The "elementary" fractures included five different patterns, with the common theme being simplicity of the singular fracture plane. The elementary fractures include posterior wall, posterior column, anterior wall, anterior column, and transverse patterns. The transverse pattern is the only one of the five elementary patterns to not involve a single wall or single column. Instead, the transverse pattern fracture extends though the anterior wall and column areas as well as the pelvic brim, and the posterior wall and posterior column areas. The transverse pattern is a single fracture surface, however, and for the reason of fracture "purity," it was placed in the elementary group.

The five "associated" fractures were more complicated fractures, combining some of the elementary patterns.[58] The associated patterns often have numerous fracture planes and details that make them distinct, but also more difficult to understand and sort. These five associated patterns are termed posterior column with associated posterior wall, transverse with associated posterior wall, anterior column with associated posterior hemitransverse, T-type, and associated both column. Simply from their individual names, it is clear that the five associated acetabular fracture patterns complicate the complexity level of the injury and therefore the evaluation and management (Fig. 37-8).

Posterior Wall

The most common fracture pattern occurs in the posterior wall.[14,109] These injuries tend to occur when the flexed hip loads the posterior wall and a portion of the posterior wall is displaced away from its base.[2] These injuries are often seen after automobile accidents when the seated motorist rapidly decelerates and the flexed knee contacts the dashboard causing the flexed hip to load the posterior acetabular wall to failure. Because of this mechanism, knee-related

injuries such as patellar fractures, traumatic arthrotomy, and posterior cruciate ligament injuries may be related. In drivers contacting the steering mechanism with or without airbag protection, thoracic aortic injuries must be ruled out.

Like all acetabular fractures, posterior wall patterns have a variety of appearances, depending on the limb's position at load, the local bone quality, and the normal anatomy of the acetabulum.[18,172,207] Most surgeons would like to believe that "a posterior wall is a posterior wall and they are simple," but nothing is further from the truth. Posterior wall acetabular injuries range from superior dome area wall displacements, to more common posterior wall displacements, to more caudal wall displacements, to "barn door" comminuted wall injuries, among other configurations. In some patients, the posterior wall fragment fractures incompletely, and the femoral head crushes several chondrocancellous articular fragments into the intact posterior column cancellous bone, thereby producing an "intra-articular" posterior wall variant fracture–dislocation. Experienced clinicians recognize the variety of posterior wall injuries due to impact loading as well as those seen with the more complex associated acetabular fracture patterns in which the posterior wall fracture fragment is caused by capsular avulsion.

Posterior wall fractures can be comminuted or associated with osteochondral impaction injuries along the fracture margin of the stable posterior column fragment, or they can involve both.[30] Marginal impaction is not the only local chondro-osseus problem related to these fractures. Displaced posterior wall fractures imply that the patient experienced an associated dislocation. For this reason, the femoral head should be evaluated for resultant impaction or cleavage injuries and the hip joint inspected for debris.[100] Common sites for debris include the fossa acetabuli, between the femoral head and acetabular dome, and between the anterior femoral head and capsule. Debris can be fragments of cartilage, cancellous bone, cortical bone, or any combination of the three. Capsular and labral tissues may also be mislocated within the hip joint.

Routine posterior wall fractures are best identified on the obturator oblique image, especially when displaced. Usually, the displaced wall fragment yields in tension caudally along with the local capsule and labral tissues while the superoanterior labrum and capsule remain intact. The superior cortical aspect of the fracture is often comminuted since it yields in compression as the wall displaces. The displaced fragment damages the superior gemellus muscle and the lower portions of the gluteus minimus muscle as well. With dramatic injuries, the piriformis muscle belly is transected by the wall's sharp cortical edge. Not surprisingly, the sciatic nerve may be damaged by direct injury from the displaced wall fragment, the extruded femoral head at the time of dislocation, or by other direct or indirect factors. The piriformis anatomy is variable and its relationship with the sciatic nerve bundles may be responsible for nerve injury also (Figs. 37-9 and 37-10).

Posterior Column

Posterior column fractures occur infrequently but are relatively predictable in their appearance. As an elementary

FIGURE 37-8 | *This illustration demonstrates the five elementary **(A)** and five associated acetabular **(B)** fracture patterns.*

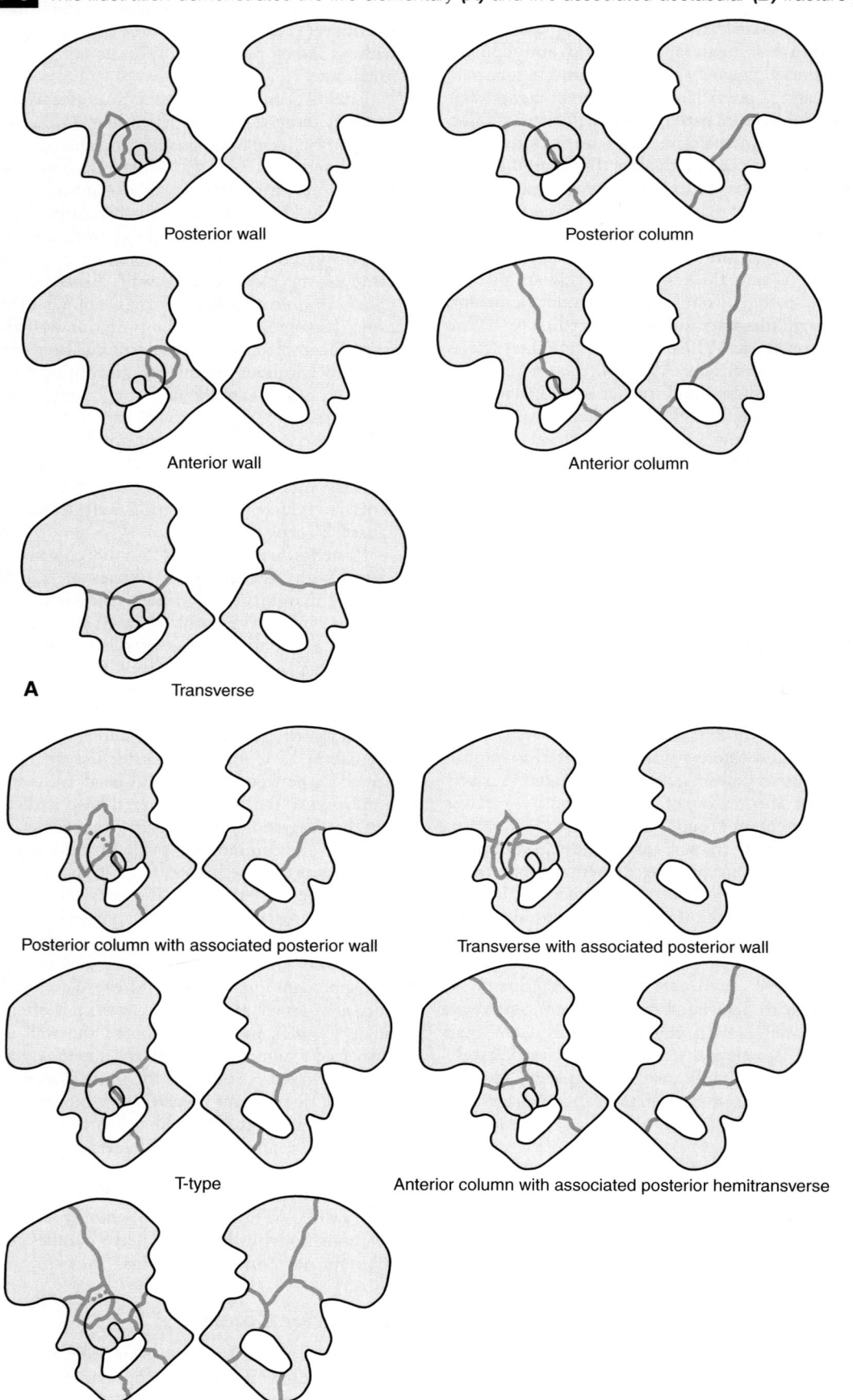

Posterior wall

Posterior column

Anterior wall

Anterior column

A Transverse

Posterior column with associated posterior wall

Transverse with associated posterior wall

T-type

Anterior column with associated posterior hemitransverse

B Associated both column

FIGURE 37-9 **A,** *The obturator oblique plain pelvic image demonstrates a displaced posterior wall fracture–dislocation. This film was obtained after a screening anteroposterior film had diagnosed the fracture–dislocation, but before orthopedic consultation. Manipulative reduction of the fracture–dislocation is recommended once diagnosed, and prior to complete radiographic evaluation.* **B,** *The corresponding acetabular computed tomography image reveals marginal impaction of chondrocancellous fragments into the intact posterior column area. As the femoral head dislocates, these chondrocancellous impaction fractures occur along the fracture edge. Less frequently, the articular surface of the displaced posterior wall may have impaction or comminution.*

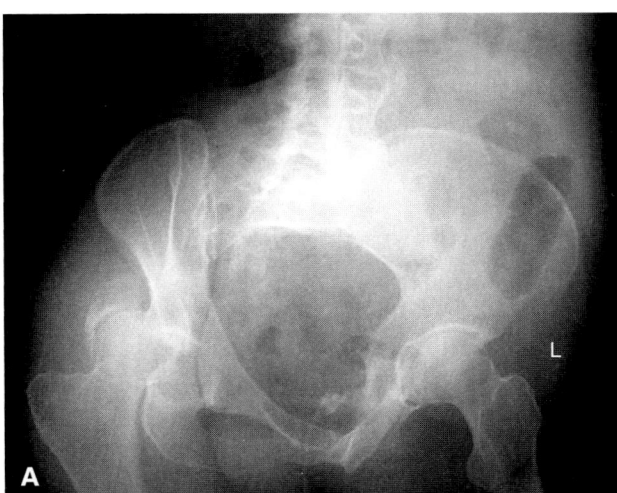

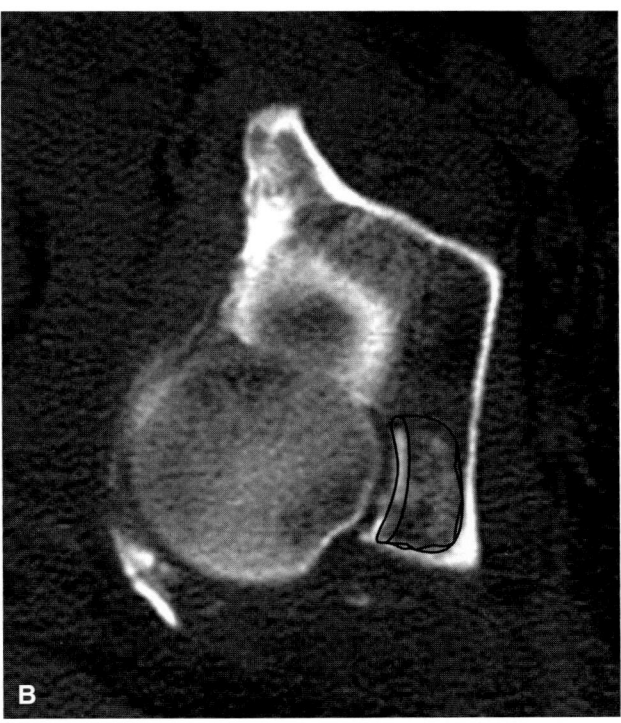

FIGURE 37-10 *This patient has a left-sided displaced posterior wall acetabular fracture with a common displacement pattern.*

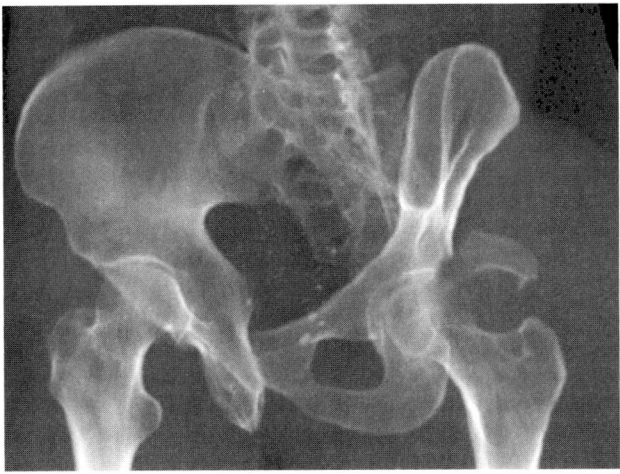

pattern, the fracture plane is singular, descending from the greater sciatic notch, with the lateral cortical disruption splitting the posterior column and wall areas while the medial cortical line divides the quadrilateral surface. The fracture plane progresses through the dome area, exits the caudal posterior wall and fossa acetabuli, and terminates through the ischium–inferior ramus junction. It is not unusual for dome chondrocancellous pyramidal-shaped fragments to be displaced and associated with this pattern. Similarly, torn labral tissues may be mislocated between the femoral head and weight-bearing dome with this fracture pattern. The displaced posterior column fracture fragment may injure the superior gluteal neurovascular bundle, especially when the fracture line is located high in the greater sciatic notch. This is important to remember both before and during surgery since arterial injury may cause ongoing bleeding and require embolization. At surgery, the superior gluteal neurovascular bundle should be visually identified to ensure that it is not displaced between the fracture fragments. If it is displaced, it should be carefully retracted as the fracture is reduced and clamped. Commonly, displaced posterior column fractures obstruct venous flow of the superior gluteal vein, causing its tributaries locally to engorge and dilate throughout the gluteal muscle bellies. These enlarged veins are fragile and often require ligation individually to control bleeding if they tear. It is important to spare the superior gluteal nerve during these ligations. The surgeon must resist the urge to simply apply a large vascular clip that could inadvertently damage the artery, vein, and nerve.

The sciatic nerve can also be injured by displaced posterior column acetabular fractures. These are usually traction injuries noted at patient presentation. Some may be related to direct contusion or stretch, and some may be related to piriformis muscle anatomic abnormalities that divide and tether the nerve, making it less able to displace along with the fracture fragment. Sciatic nerve injury can also result from the closed reduction. This occurs because the sciatic nerve course parallels certain displaced posterior column fracture planes and can become trapped within it as the displaced fracture–dislocation is reduced. This happens rarely but must be remembered and not missed or justified as an injury-related occurrence. For this reason, the pre- and postreduction nerve assessments are carefully detailed and documented. If the sciatic nerve exam changes after closed reduction of any acetabular fracture, then urgent exploration, neuroplasty, and fracture fixation are recommended.

Posterior column acetabular fractures are best seen on the iliac oblique and anteroposterior plain pelvic radiographs. The pelvic CT scan reveals detailed displacement information, identifies comminution, dome fragmentation, and loose bodies within the joint, and also shows impaction injuries that may occur along the fracture line (Fig. 37-11).

Anterior Wall

Anterior wall acetabular fractures are the least common of all types. The unnatural limb position needed to load the anterior wall coupled with the tiny surface area of the anterior wall make this pattern the most unlikely. Simply because of their anatomy, these fractures are quite small and associated with anterior dislocations. The iliac vasculature and femoral nerve can be injured in association with anterior wall fracture–dislocations.

The area of the anterior wall is often involved in pelvic ring fractures when the fracture lines of the peripheral superior pubic ramus extend into the anterior wall. This pelvic ring injury, however, should not be misclassified as an anterior acetabular wall fracture.

FIGURE 37-11 *A–C, The anteroposterior (AP) and oblique plain pelvic radiographs identify the posterior column acetabular fracture. On the AP film, the ilioischial line is disrupted. The oblique films further delineate the fracture. A dome chondrocancellous fracture fragment was displaced into the primary fracture surface. The superior gluteal neurovascular bundle was not located between the fracture surfaces.*

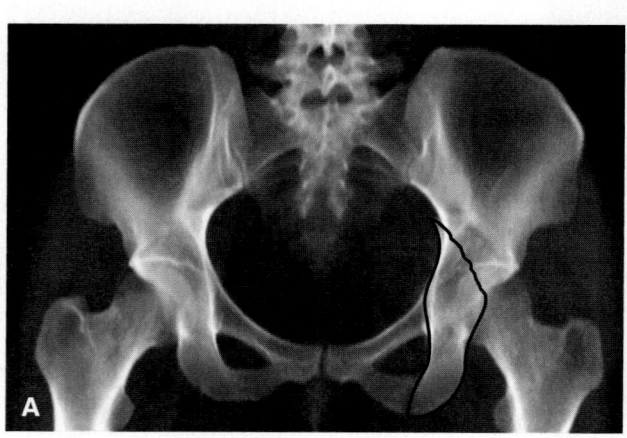
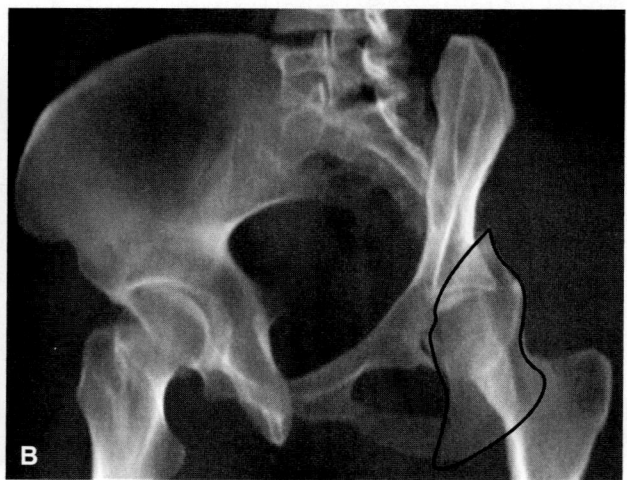
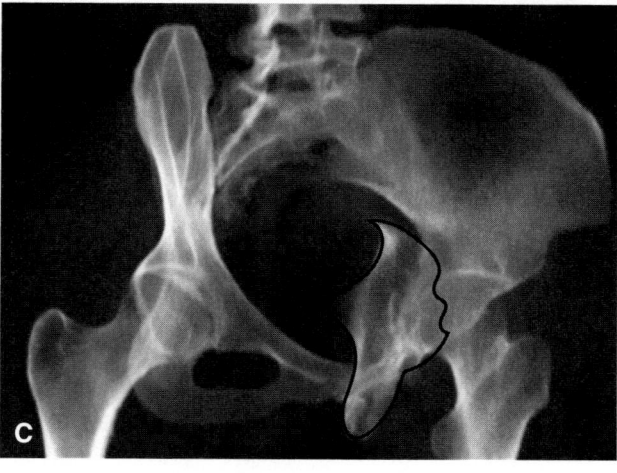

Anterior wall acetabular fractures may involve a small portion of the iliopectineal line on the AP film. The obturator oblique image may show subluxation of the femoral head, whereas the iliac oblique demonstrates the anterior wall fragment displacement.

Anterior Column

Anterior column acetabular fractures disrupt the iliopectineal line on the AP film and have a variety of appearances depending on their peripheral exit points. As an elementary pattern, the fracture plane is singular. These fractures were subclassified according to their iliac exit site. "High" anterior column fractures include those in which the iliac crest is the peripheral exit point. "Intermediate" patterns have their exit points in the region of the anterior superior iliac crest, and "low" patterns exit adjacent to the anterior inferior iliac spine. "Very low" patterns only involve the region medial to the iliopectineal eminence. The fracture displacement depends on the subclassification type. The high types have the tensor and sartorius muscle forces to cause displacement. Because of this displacement, the lateral femoral cutaneous nerve may be injured in association with this particular fracture type. The other patterns have variable deformities depending on the fracture specifics. Displaced intermediate and low types risk associated femoral and obturator neurovascular injuries.

The iliac oblique image usually best demonstrates displaced anterior column acetabular fractures. These fractures are often missed on the screening AP film. The iliac oblique film reveals the peripheral exit points well, especially for the high patterns. The radiolucent fracture gap along the pelvic brim is also apparent. The femoral head typically remains congruent with the displaced anterior column fracture fragment, which usually indicates a disrupted ligamentum teres (Fig. 37-12).

Transverse

Transverse acetabular fractures often confuse clinicians because of their inclusion in the elementary fracture group despite involving the two supporting columns. Transverse fracture patterns occur in a variety of orientations and obliquities but remain a singular fracture surface. Because of their singular fracture plane "purity," transverse fractures were included in the elementary group.

A common transverse fracture pattern begins at the anterior wall anatomic area, extends through the iliopsoas gutter and anterior wall articular surface, progresses across the pelvic brim and anterior column, through the quadrilateral surface dividing the upper and lower halves of the fossa acetabuli, and exits the posterior column and posterior wall's edge. The labrum is also injured, especially in displaced transverse patterns. The torn labrum or portions of it can intrude into the joint, causing further incongruity between the femoral head and intact dome region.[112,170]

Transverse fractures are the only elementary pattern to extend through both wall areas and both acetabular supporting column zones. The terminology can be confusing because the fracture involves "both of the acetabular columns" but is not an "associated both-column" pattern. As previously stated, fracture patterns and anatomic areas share terminology but should not be confused with each other nor the terms used synonymously.

The transverse pattern splits the acetabulum into two halves. The upper or cephalad half is almost always the stable portion of the fracture, whereas the caudal segment is mobile and displaced. The caudal fragment mobility is due to the fracture plane and the fact that the symphysis pubis ligaments function as a hinge for it (Fig. 37-13).[154,201,209]

The acetabular dome is involved to some extent by the transverse fracture plane. Letournel subclassified transverse fractures depending on their dome involvement. Transtectal transverse fractures involve the weight-bearing dome, whereas juxtatectal transverse fractures preserve the dome and exit at the junction of the dome and fossa acetabuli. Infratectal transverse patterns divide the fossa acetabuli. Typically, more intact dome before fracture involvement correlates with improved hip stability, congruity, and outcome. In cadaveric mechanical evaluations, step malreductions of transverse acetabular fractures in the superior

FIGURE 37-12 *A, This plain pelvic image shows a displaced anterior column acetabular fracture. The femoral head is displaced from the intact acetabulum and remains congruent with the anterior column fragment. B, These computed tomography axial images further define the fracture details in the dome region.*

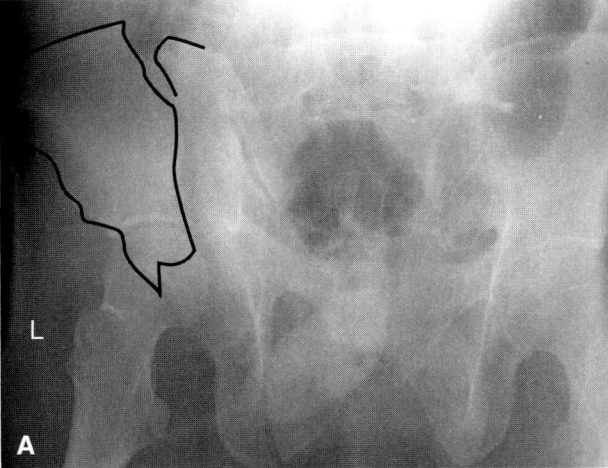

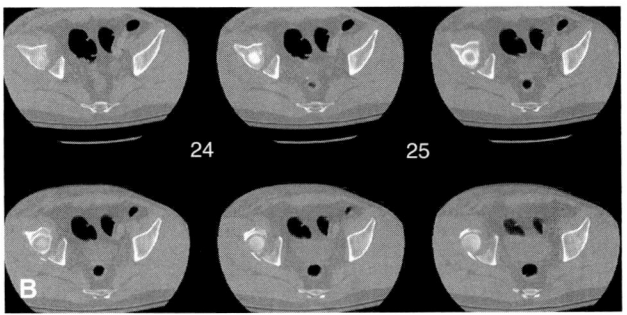

FIGURE 37-13 *In transverse acetabular fracture patterns, the ilioischial and iliopectineal lines are disrupted on the anteroposterior pelvic film. The remaining amount of dome determines stability after closed reduction. The caudal fragment of most transverse acetabular fractures is the unstable portion hinging on the symphyseal ligaments. In this example, the femoral head remains in congruity with the displaced caudal segment. The related symphyseal injury for this patient is also noted. Impaction injuries of the superolateral femoral head as well as along the transverse acetabular fracture surface are noted with such fracture lines and displacement patterns.*

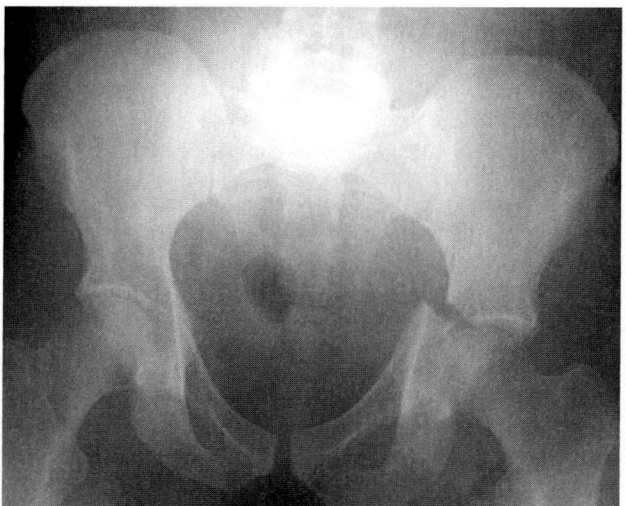

articular surface resulted in abnormally high contact forces that in clinical practice should predispose to the development of post-traumatic arthritis.[64,118]

Certain transverse acetabular fractures are associated with intrapelvic displacement of the femoral head along with the caudal fracture fragment. As the fracture displacement occurs, the femoral head can sustain a superolateral impaction fracture and/or the intact upper portion of the acetabular fracture line can be crushed.

In these fractures, the femoral head may remain beneath the weight-bearing dome or follow the caudal segment's displacement depending on several factors. For transtectal patterns, there may be insufficient intact dome for the femoral head to remain stable. Muscular spasm causes displacement of the femoral head through the fracture. As the intact dome coverage expands with juxtatectal and infratectal transverse patterns, femoral head stability improves.

Rarely, a transverse acetabular fracture occurs in association with an ipsilateral posterior pelvic ring injury. In these situations, both the upper and lower portions of the transverse fracture are unstable. The upper fracture fragment of such a transverse acetabular fracture pattern

is displaced and unstable because the ipsilateral SI joint is disrupted or an unstable ipsilateral sacral fracture is present. In this unusual scenario, the transverse acetabular fracture behaves as an associated both-column acetabular pattern since there is no articular component in continuity with the intact hemipelvis.

Transverse Fractures with Associated Posterior Wall Involvement

Transverse acetabular fractures with associated posterior wall involvement are common patterns combining the elementary transverse fracture plane with a posterior wall component. The AP film demonstrates both iliopectineal and ilioschial line disruptions, along with the loss of the posterior wall convex edge due to its displacement. Often the displaced wall is noted superimposed on the dome area on this film. If the film is examined carefully, the transverse fracture plane's displacement through the anterior wall area is seen as a lucent gap. On the AP film, the femoral head has several location options with these injuries. The simplest occurs when the femoral head is noted to be congruent with the dome. Another displacement pattern occurs when the femoral head follows the posterior wall displacement. Another pattern occurs when the femoral head follows the transverse caudal segment and is displaced medially. The oblique images are obtained after closed reduction of the femoral head beneath the dome. The iliac oblique image shows the posterior column exit point of the transverse fracture line. The obturator oblique image demonstrates the anterior column exit point of the transverse fracture as well as the displaced posterior wall fracture fragment and the defect left due to its displacement. It is not unusual in unstable patterns for the femoral head to redislocate as the patient is turned for each image and the body weight or limb weight is applied onto the injury. After closed reduction, an AP film in traction may reveal a previously missed superolateral femoral head impaction fracture.

The pelvic CT scan reveals the transverse fracture orientation and specific exit sites as well as any loose bodies within the joint or marginal impaction associated injuries. Posterior wall comminution is not always obvious on the plain images and is best seen on the CT scan. The CT scan may also confirm femoral head impaction lesions (Fig. 37-14).

Posterior Column Fracture with Associated Posterior Wall Involvement

In these uncommon injuries the ilioischial line is disrupted and the posterior wall defect and displacement are seen on the AP film. The iliac oblique image shows the posterior column component's exit through the greater sciatic notch, whereas the obturator oblique view identifies the displaced posterior wall fracture fragment. The pelvic CT scan should be examined not only for the specific fracture-related details but also for the local soft tissues. An injury to the superior gluteal artery or vein may cause deep buttock asymmetry on the scan due to local bleeding. The details cited earlier regarding both posterior column and posterior wall fracture elementary patterns are also relevant here.

FIGURE 37-14 *This unfortunate patient sustained an unusual hip injury consisting of both a comminuted proximal femur fracture as well as a displaced transverse fracture with an associated posterior wall acetabular component. The obturator oblique image shows the transverse acetabular fracture dividing the acetabulum into two fragments, as well as the displaced posterior wall component.*

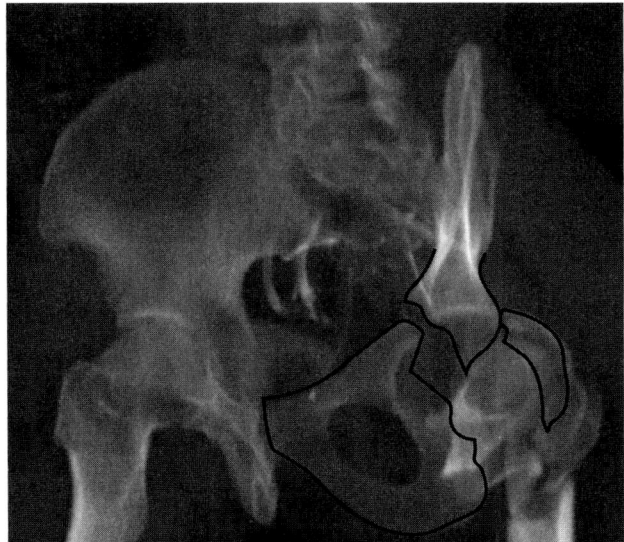

Anterior Column with Fracture with Associated Posterior Hemitransverse Injury

Acetabular fracture patterns that involve the anterior column as well as associated posterior hemitransverse injuries combine any variety of anterior column fracture with an additional fracture line that splits the posterior column, usually through the greater sciatic notch. Both the iliopectineal and ilioischial lines are disrupted on the plain AP film. The iliac oblique pelvic film reveals the anterior column fracture component's exits both along the iliac crest and through the anterior wall area, as well as the posterior hemitransverse fracture component's exit point, usually through the greater sciatic notch. These injuries can be unstable although each fracture component and the oblique x-ray films demonstrate the instability and displacement sites. Just like for anterior column elementary patterns, the anterior column component of the fracture is variable. The posterior hemitransverse component predictably divides the greater sciatic notch.

T-Type

The T-type acetabular fracture is simply a transverse fracture plane but with the unstable caudal segment split into two individual unstable segments. When viewed laterally, this acetabular fracture patterns is shaped like the letter T. For example, the anterior column portion of the fracture line begins at the anterior wall area and extends along the iliopsoas gutter across the pelvic brim and descends the

quadrilateral surface. The posterior column portion of the fracture line begins at the greater sciatic notch and descends to split the posterior wall area and meets the anterior column fracture line at the quadrilateral surface. The fracture line that divides the quadrilateral surface is a common fracture line. It is the vertical fracture line that descends from the transverse component to make this a T-type fracture pattern.

The low anterior column component is unstable due to the symphyseal hinge. The posterior column component is tethered by the sacrospinous and sacrotuberous ligaments. These injuries often have central displacement of the femoral head between the fracture fragments, or the femoral head can remain attached to the posterior column fragment if the ligamentum teres is intact.

On the AP film, both iliopectineal and ilioischial lines are disrupted, and the femoral head may be dislocated away from the intact dome. The ischial fracture may be minimally displaced and not always obvious. The iliac oblique image reveals the posterior column exits at the greater sciatic notch and ischial ramus. The obturator oblique identifies the anterior column exit site and displacements. CT details the each component location (Fig. 37-15).

Associated Both-Column Fracture

The associated both-column acetabular fracture pattern is thought by many surgeons to be the most difficult of all 10 acetabular fracture types. In these injuries, the articular dome and all other articular fracture fragments are without connection to the intact hemipelvis. In all nine other

FIGURE 37-15 *This patient has a displaced and very unstable T-type fracture pattern. The ilioischial and iliopectineal lines are disrupted, and the caudal segment is further divided into two separate fragments. Based on this image, the posterior column component and the proximal femur are displaced more than the anterior column fragment. There is a crush injury at the medial aspect of the dome. Because of the fracture location and deforming muscular forces, the manipulative reduction could not be maintained. She underwent urgent open reduction and stable internal fixation.*

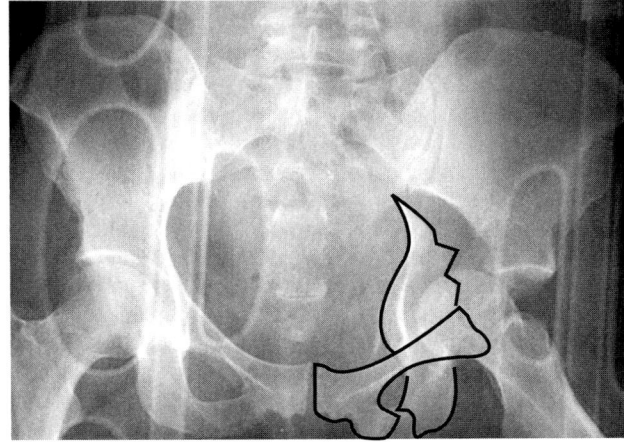

FIGURE 37-16   *A, The obturator oblique image demonstrates a "spur sign" or the caudal extent of the stable ilium, which when seen identifies an associated both-column acetabular fracture. The spur becomes visible when the acetabular articular fracture fragments displace medially away from it. In some associated both-column patterns, the articular fragments are minimally displaced from the intact ilium and a spur sign is not obvious. B, The displaced posterior wall fracture is also best seen on the obturator oblique but represents the displaced wall, not the intact ilium of an associated both-column fracture pattern. The displaced posterior wall fragment should not be confused with a spur sign.*

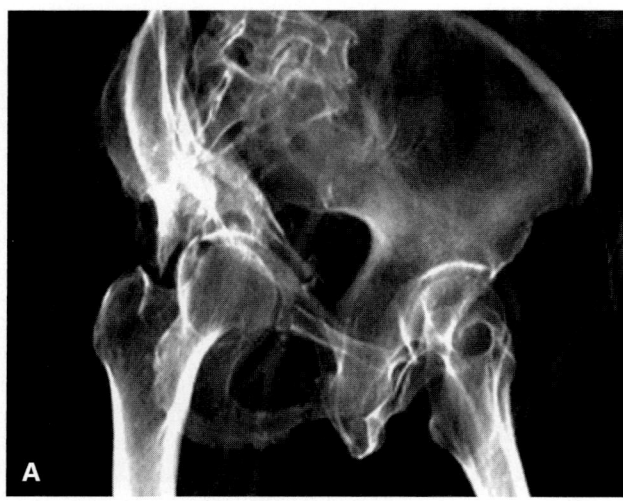
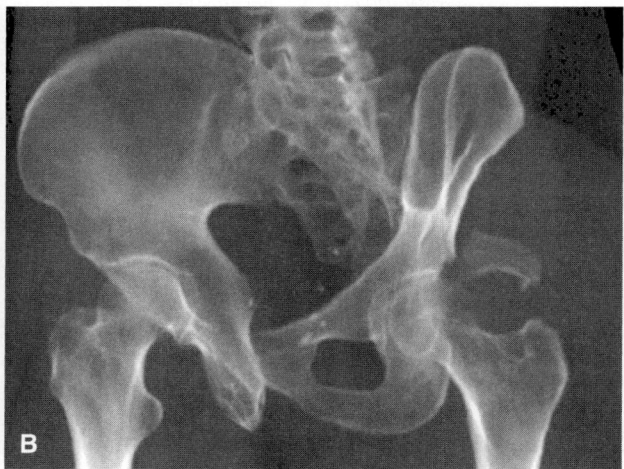

patterns, at least some portion of the articular acetabulum remains attached to the intact hemipelvis. Because of this traumatic fracture–separation of the articular fragments from the stable ilium, some use the term "floating acetabulum" for these patterns. Because this term is misleading and not descriptive, most surgeons do not use it.

Associated both-column acetabular fractures have several consistent fracture fragments. The intact iliac piece is the stable component. Its caudal extent represents the "spur sign," so named because it resembles a cockspur on the obturator oblique image, as the unstable articular fragments displace from it medially. Such medial articular fragment displacements cause the intact ilium's caudal extent (the "spur") to appear prominent as it remains in its normal site. When seen on the obturator oblique film, this spur sign is indicative of an associated both-column acetabular fracture. Inexperienced surgeons may confuse a displaced posterior wall acetabular fracture with the spur sign of an associated both-column fracture since both are seen on the obturator oblique image (Fig. 37-16).

When articular fragment displacement is minimal yet there is still no articular connection to the intact iliac segment, no spur sign is obvious, but an associated both-column acetabular fracture pattern is the correct diagnosis. In some patients, the intact iliac caudal extent is obvious even on the AP and iliac oblique films, so it is possible to see the spur on these other images. It is easy for the clinician to see that which he or she knows to look for.

Besides the intact iliac component, associated both-column fractures have several other consistent components. The upper anterior column fracture fragment usually contains the majority of the dome and may be incomplete at its iliac crest exit point. If so, the anterior column fragment may be displaced and relatively stable because of the deformed yet incomplete fracture along the crest. The lower anterior column fracture fragment

typically includes the articular anterior wall and pubic ramus limbs. The posterior column component typically exits the greater sciatic notch and ischial areas. It is not unusual for the pelvic brim to have some degree of cortical comminution. In some patterns as detailed in the earlier section on posterior wall fracture, the posterior wall fracture component is an avulsion injury due to medial displacement of the proximal femur (Fig. 37-17).

Variant Patterns

Certain acetabular fractures do not fit Letournel's classification system. These variant patterns exist and must be recognized after routine patterns have been ruled out. Unusual position of the lower extremity at injury, poor bone quality, or extreme loading conditions are responsible causes for

FIGURE 37-17   *This associated both-column fracture is further complicated by its pelvic brim/greater sciatic notch fragment displacement.*

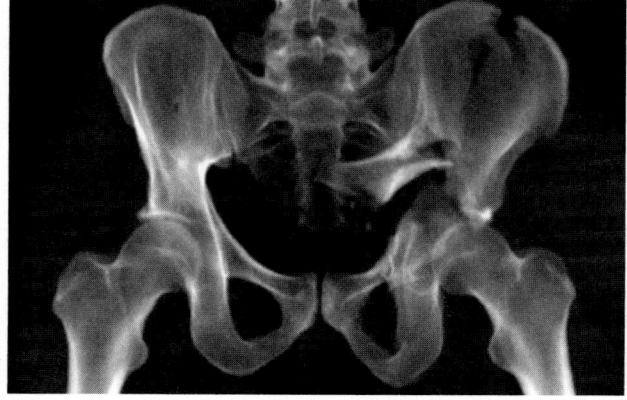

FIGURE 37-18 | *This patient has a combination injury consisting of an unstable pelvic ring disruption and a left-sided variant pattern acetabular fracture.*

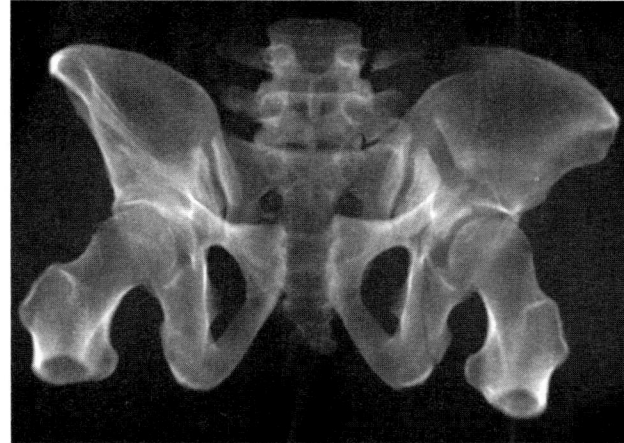

FIGURE 37-19 | *A, B, This anteroposterior film demonstrates a low anterior column fracture–dislocation of the left acetabulum. The iliopectineal line is disrupted, but the majority of the displaced fracture fragment comprises the anterior wall. This pattern is often confused with an anterior wall fracture. Further inspection of the plain film reveals a complete sacroiliac (SI) dislocation that renders the entire hemipelvis unstable. The SI injury is confirmed by the pelvic computed tomography. Because the sacrum is the "stable" hemipelvis, this acetabular fracture is a "behavioral" associated both-column variant pattern.*

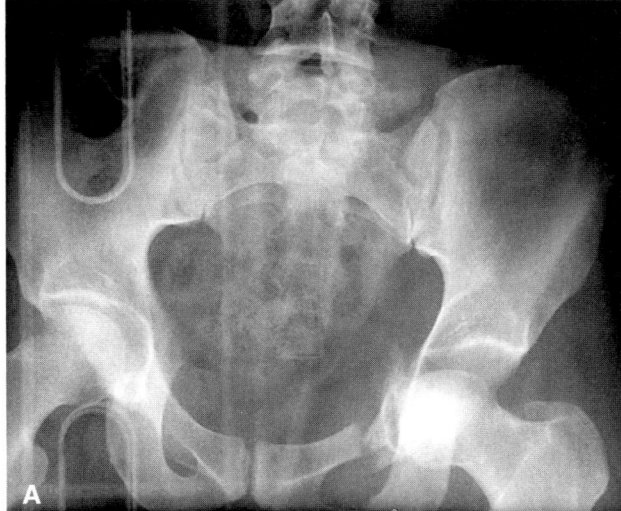

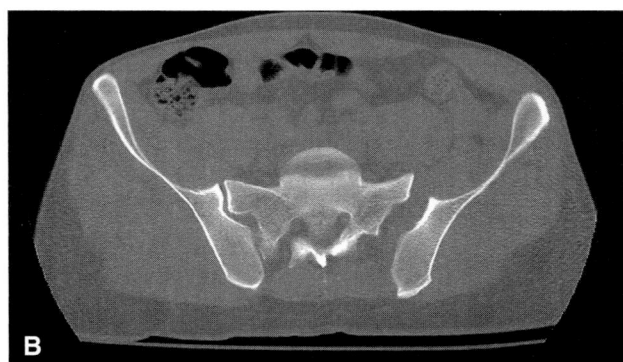

these injuries. Variant patterns are assessed and managed routinely. Their fracture specifics may necessitate more extensile exposure or special fixation tools. Dramatic impaction injuries for example may demand allograft bone or other suitable material to fill the defects. Acetabular fractures in association with unstable pelvic ring injuries are included as variant patterns as well (Figs. 37-18 and 37-19).

DECISION MAKING

The management goal for acetabular fractures is a painless and functional hip joint without complications.[22,79,95,189,200] Selecting the best treatment option is a complex clinical decision based on numerous factors related to the patient, the physician, the facility, and others.

The following questions arise when determining treatment:

1. Is the patient medically stable? If not, how can he or she be made stable?
2. Could the patient withstand any planned operation, much less an extensive one?
3. Could the patient withstand traction management or prolonged bedrest?
4. Are there patient-related medical, physical, psychosocial, or other issues that adversely affect either operative or nonoperative management? For example, is noncompliant behavior anticipated despite the treatment choice?
5. Is the fracture stable or unstable?
6. Is the fracture displaced or not? If displaced, where specifically are the displacement sites and to what extent?
7. If displaced, is there sufficient relative (secondary) congruity of the fracture fragments with the femoral head?
8. Is there ample bone to allow routine reduction and stable fixation techniques, or are special considerations indicated?
9. Will the fracture pattern specifics allow for accurate reduction, or will fracture-related issues, such as extensive dome comminution or crush injury, prevent reduction or stable fixation?

10. Will associated femoral head superolateral or other zone impaction fractures adversely affect the result apart from the acetabular repair?
11. Does the surgeon, a colleague, or regional referral center have sufficient experience and expertise in treating similar acetabular fractures?
12. Does the medical facility have sufficient ancillary support (e.g., intraoperative imaging technicians) and the necessary equipment?

Even though clinicians would rather have some absolute radiographic measurement to guide their acetabular management decision, the individual patient's overall medical condition is the primary determinant. First and foremost, the patient must be able to endure the chosen treatment.[139,153,210] Although many clinicians begin with the specific fracture pattern when choosing a treatment plan, the overall patient condition guides treatment considerations. Once that issue is resolved, the surgeon should focus on the fracture pattern and associated local soft tissue injuries. Fracture stability is related to several factors—the primary one is how much weight-bearing dome or intact acetabulum remains for the femoral head to articulate with. Biomechanical studies have shown that acetabular fracture stability decreases with higher applied loads across fracture surfaces and with a less intact dome. Because of this dome coverage issue, roof arc measurements are recommended to quantify in three radiographic views and on CT scanning the amount of intact dome.

Roof arc angles are measured on the AP and two oblique films. A line is first drawn on the film to set the horizontal standard and correct for patient positioning error on the x-ray cassette. For elementary patterns, the ischial tuberosities on each side are reliable as long as the injured side remains uninvolved by the fracture–displacement. In associated patterns, some other intact osseous landmark is used to set the horizontal standard. Next, a perpendicular vertical line is drawn from the horizontal standard line through the center of the hip joint, which, depending on its displacement, may or may not be the center of the femoral head. The next line is drawn from the center of the hip joint/ femoral head to the acetabular fracture's articular edge on that particular view. The roof arc angle is measured between the vertical line and the articular edge line. As the roof arc angle expands, so does the acetabular dome coverage and in turn so does the hip joint congruity and perhaps stability. Mechanical and clinical studies have offered a variety of roof arc angle limits for improved results (Fig. 37-20).

FIGURE 37-20 | *A–C, The measurements of acetabular fracture roof arc angles are shown on these three pelvic films. A, On the anteroposterior (AP) pelvic film, the right ischial tuberosity is involved by the fracture, so the horizontal standard line must be estimated. The femoral head is slightly subluxated on the AP view, so the center hip joint determination accounts for this. A vertical perpendicular line is drawn from the horizontal standard line through the hip joint center. Next and from the hip center, a line is drawn to the acetabular fracture edge. The angle between the perpendicular vertical and fracture edge lines is the roof arc angle. B, C, The process is repeated for the obturator and iliac oblique images.*

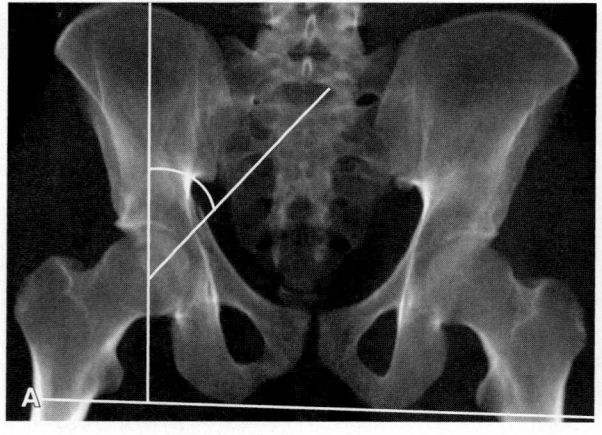
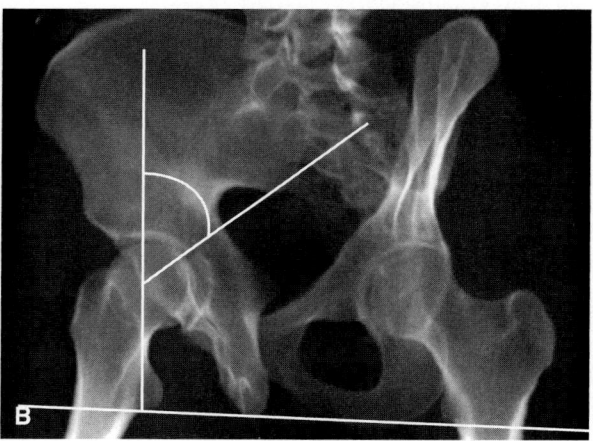
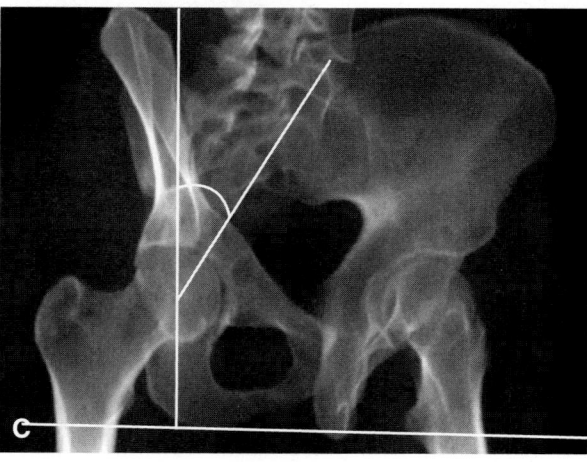

The physician measuring the roof arc angles must remember that the center of the hip joint is not always the femoral head itself since the head may be displaced from the anatomic hip joint center. If this occurs, then the hip is incongruent and the fracture is displaced sufficiently that roof arc measurements are in fact likely unwarranted.

Closed treatment of acetabular fractures should be based on hip congruity and fracture instability. Stability is determined from the history reflecting the energy of the traumatic event and from the radiographs. Final determination may require an examination of the fracture under anesthesia and fluoroscopy. The fluoroscopic examination under anesthesia should be performed using the anteroposterior as well as both oblique views. The C-arm must be positioned correctly in order to view possible instability sites without obstructing the necessary limb movements. For posterior wall acetabular assessment, the C-arm is positioned on the ipsilateral side to injury so the obturator oblique image is obtained and the unit does not obstruct hip flexion, adduction, and internal rotation. For fractures involving the posterior column, the C-arm unit is positioned on the opposite side to allow the iliac oblique view without obstructing limb movements. The AP view has limited use other than for medial instability assessment since the fluoroscope obstructs most limb movements other than central loading.

If the fracture is congruent and stable, protected weight-bearing and serial radiographic follow up to ensure no further displacement is recommended.[202,203] If the hip is congruent yet unstable without traction, then skeletal traction is used to maintain the reduction while the fracture heals. The traction pin is best inserted during this same anesthetic examination, using the C-arm to perfectly position the pin. A threaded pin of sufficient diameter is recommended when several weeks of traction is anticipated. The distal femoral traction pin is inserted to avoid the knee joint and local vascular structures.

If traction is selected, the patient is committed to a prolonged 6- to 8-week period of bed confinement. If traction is chosen, it is also important to know if the fracture reduction is maintained while the patient is upright in bed. A portable AP pelvic film with the patient awake and in traction confirms this fact and ensures that the hip is not overdistracted by excessive weight. An upright chest allows the patient to avoid problems associated with recumbency.

Operative repair of acetabular fractures is difficult, can be extensive, and is associated with numerous problems including operative bleeding. Because of this fact, the patient's cardiopulmonary and medical condition should be capable of withstanding surgery.

Some patients may refuse to receive blood or blood products based on their religious beliefs and therefore may not be candidates for open fracture reconstructive techniques. Blood salvage systems during surgery diminish this potential problem if the patient will allow such system to be used.[49,59]

If there are no patient-related issues, then the fracture pattern is evaluated for displacement and instability. Treating physicians must remember that displacement and stability are not necessarily linked. Certain displaced fractures may demonstrate relative stability, especially when the peripheral portions of the fractures are incomplete. Conversely, nondisplaced or minimally displaced fractures are not necessarily stable. For example, certain transverse acetabular fractures may have essentially no displacement on the AP radiograph, but the oblique films reveal their displacements and instability. In these situations, the patient's body weight along with gravity cause fracture displacement. Examination of the hip under anesthesia and fluoroscopy can also identify dramatic fracture instability in minimally displaced injuries (Figs. 37-21 and 37-22).

FIGURE 37-21 *A, B, This acetabular fracture's instability is revealed by the oblique images.*

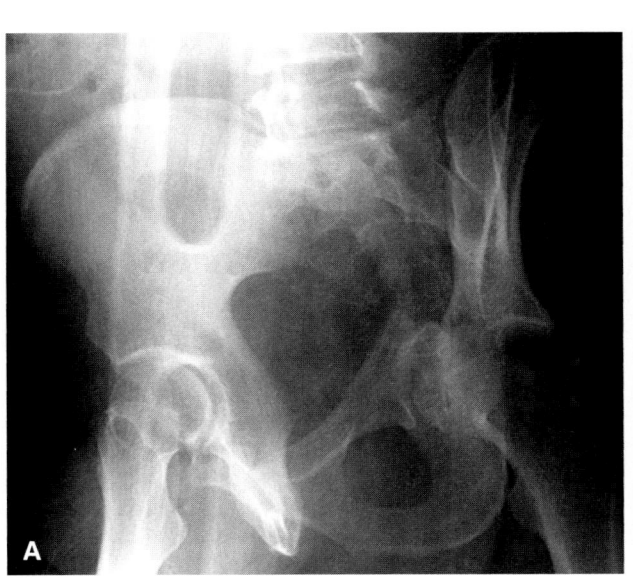
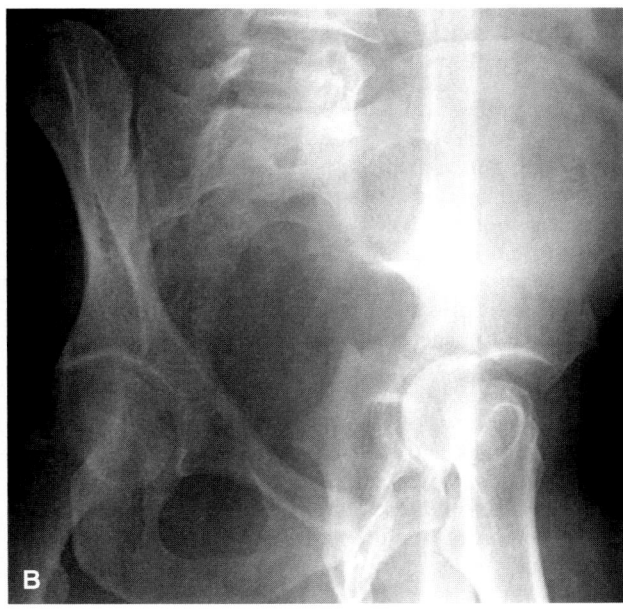

FIGURE 37-22 *A, B, This patient had a small, peripheral posterior wall acetabular fracture and an unstable pelvic ring injury. During the same anesthetic session as the pelvic ring stabilization, the acetabular fracture was examined under fluoroscopy and noted to be unstable, with 30° of passive hip flexion. The extra-articular medullary ramus screw is located posterior to the hip joint on this view.*

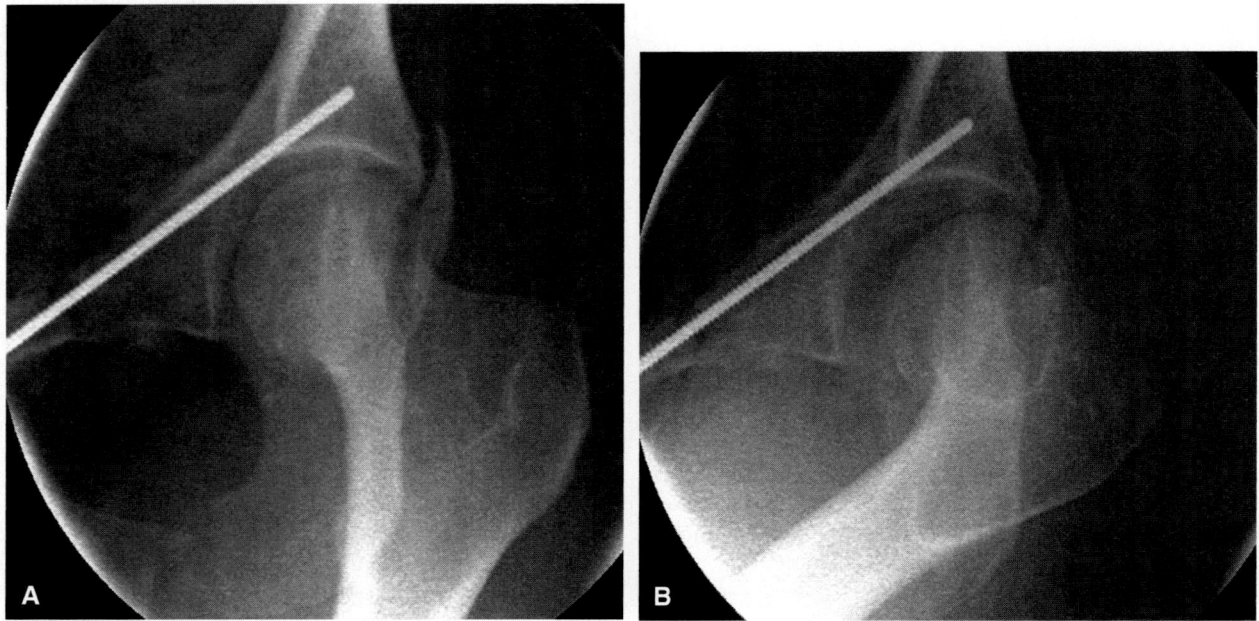

For stable fractures, some clinicians measure roof arc angles on the pelvic plain films and the subchondral arcs on the pelvic CT to determine congruity between the femoral head and acetabular dome region. As the intact dome area expands, thereby improving femoral head coverage, the roof arc angle increases and better results are anticipated.

Bone quality issues are important factors to consider prior to surgery.[7] Usually this problem is seen most in elderly patients and those with other bone diseases such as osteogenesis imperfecta.[44,77,129,188,204] The cortical surfaces may not be sufficient to hold a reduction clamp and support fixation plates. Children and adolescent patients with acetabular fractures warrant special considerations also.[72,73,92,117,159]

Special equipment has value when treating such "bone-deficient" fractures operatively. Bone graft substitutes, improved fixation constructs, and newer implant technology may all be needed to manage these injuries.

Articular chondrocancellous crush injuries along the primary fracture lines are difficult to reduce accurately. Small focal impaction fractures are elevated, reduced to the femoral head after the primary fracture lines are reduced and stabilized, and the defects supported with bone graft. Extensive impaction fractures including more zones of injury and more comminution are more difficult to accurately reduce and support, and therefore correlate directly with post-traumatic arthritic changes (Fig. 37-23).

Operative management restores articular congruity and provides stable fixation.[53] These factors should improve the clinical result by decreasing the incidence of post-traumatic arthritis and allowing early patient and joint mobility. Operative management is advocated for patients with displaced and unstable acetabular fractures who are appropriate surgical candidates.

Operative Timing

Operative treatment of an acetabular fracture occurs when the patient is medically stable, when the surgeon understands the fracture and its treatment details, and

FIGURE 37-23 *Patients with both medial acetabular dome and superolateral femoral head impaction injuries warrant special consideration during planning and treatment.*

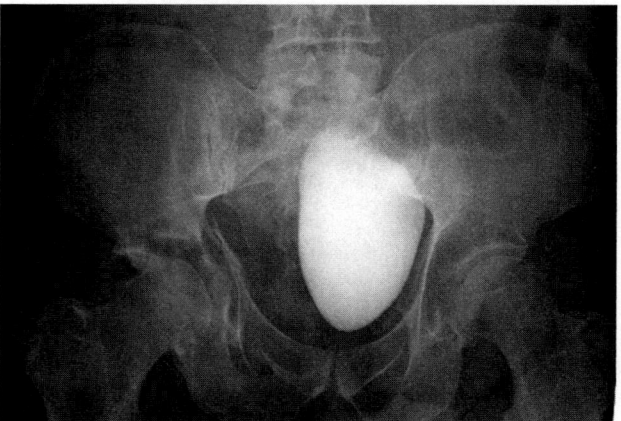

when the appropriate operative team is available. Usually this interval is between 2 and 5 days after injury.[29,161] Some surgeons believe that earlier operative intervention allows the fracture surfaces and local tissues to bleed more than if surgery occurs several days after injury. Although this assumption seems intuitive, it has not been proven. The surgeon must also remember that fracture surface cancellous bone bleeding halts when the fracture surfaces are reduced and stabilized. Knowing this, the surgeon performs the surgical exposure, prepares the fracture fragments for clamp and implant applications, and does so without disturbing the fracture surface clots. Removing the fracture surface clots immediately before reducing the fracture decreases operative blood loss. A blood salvage suction system is also advocated to recycle surgically related blood loss. Recent investigations suggest that blood salvage systems may not be worth the additional expense.

Urgent operative management is recommended for those unusual patients with open fractures, irreducible fracture–dislocations, nerve changes after closed reduction, and buttock or iliac compartmental syndrome. Open acetabular fractures occur rarely and can be staged as an initial irrigation and débridement procedure. The reduction and fixation is performed either during the initial anesthetic or as a subsequent procedure. Certain fractures are at risk for sciatic nerve changes after manipulative reduction. These include any pattern involving displacement through the posterior column or wall areas, especially when the fracture plane parallels the nerve course. Compartmental syndrome can occur at the buttock and iliac areas. Buttock compartmental syndrome has been linked to superior gluteal vascular injury due to displaced acetabular fractures involving the greater sciatic notch. The physical exam demonstrates buttock asymmetry and dramatic swelling. These findings are more difficult in obese patients, but the pelvic CT scan demonstrates the buttock asymmetrical swelling and soft tissue density. Prior to operative compartment release, angiographic evaluation and embolization of the potentially injured artery should be considered. Patients with iliac compartmental syndrome due to acetabular fracture usually have minimal fracture displacement but significant bleeding into the iliopsoas muscle or internal iliac fossa. They present with femoral nerve dysfunction but otherwise their physical exam may be unremarkable. Pelvic CT demonstrates the asymmetrical swelling and soft tissue density. Prior to surgical release, a routine screening coagulation panel is obtained and any abnormalities corrected.

Delayed patient referrals delay operative management and should be avoided. Early referral of a patient with an acetabular fracture to an experienced surgeon allows routine management to proceed. In some specialty centers dedicated to acetabular fracture care, aggressive early management of even complex acetabular fractures is standard and uncomplicated. Fracture reduction and fixation is easier when performed routinely and soon after injury. Early intervention avoids more extensile exposures. Dealing with fracture clots and mobile fragments several days after injury is much simpler than débriding fracture callus from relatively immobile fragments several weeks after injury. It is also quite common for the patient's overall clinical status to improve after early operative management.

Initial Management

The initial management of acetabular fractures follows routine evaluation and resuscitation guidelines similar to those with pelvic ring injuries. The patient's airway is secured, oxygenation confirmed, and vital signs assessed. Volume resuscitation begins with intravenous fluids while laboratory evaluations proceed. Just as for pelvic ring injuries, laboratory testing for patients with acetabular fractures should include routine serology along with serial hematocrits and a hemorrhage panel. A toxicology screen may aid both initial and subsequent treatments.

As mentioned previously, pelvic angiography is indicated when the resuscitation is thorough and adequate, yet unexplained bleeding is noted. Certain acetabular fracture patterns, such as those involving the greater sciatic notch (superior gluteal) and pubic ramus (iliac) areas, have been associated with vascular injuries. Similarly, acetabular injuries can occur in association with pelvic ring injuries. Targeted angiographic embolization halts pelvic arterial bleeding.

For less dramatic injuries, initial management assumes that the diagnosis is recognized by the evaluating physician. The injury history may include a description of hip subluxation and spontaneous reduction, or described dislocation that was reduced by an initial responder. Most commonly, missed or delayed acetabular fracture diagnosis occurs for peripheral or minimally displaced posterior wall fracture patterns. These are missed because the displaced fracture fragments are superimposed on the normal anatomy and additional oblique films are not obtained. The hip joint articular symmetry is lost on a plain AP film when the femoral head is no longer located beneath the dome. This particular finding is an indication for further imaging including a pelvic CT scan.

Once the diagnosis is confirmed, the femoral head should be located beneath the acetabular dome. This may require manipulative reduction. Adequate patient sedation and fluoroscopy facilitate the manipulative reduction and allow the physician to easily assess congruity and stability. Once reduced, skeletal traction can be used to maintain the reduction, offset local muscular spasm, and provide comfort, as well as alerting the medical personnel of the injury. An AP plain pelvic radiograph in traction ensures reduction and that the weight amount is appropriate. Overdistraction of the hip joint is not recommended.

SURGICAL EXPOSURES

The selection of a surgical exposure is a very important factor in the operative management of acetabular fractures. The exposure must allow the surgeon to sufficiently clean and reduce the fracture surfaces, as well as maintaining the reduction initially with clamps and then applying definitive and stable fixation. The operative table, surgical exposure, and patient positioning are chosen so that intraoperative fluoroscopic imaging is possible.

KOCHER–LANGENBECK The Kocher–Langenbeck exposure is recommended for posterior wall, posterior column, transverse, transverse-posterior wall, and some T-type fractures. It provides direct surgical access to the posterior column and wall regions, and with dissection through the greater sciatic notch, digital and clamp access to the quadrilateral surface. The exposure should be performed with the patient positioned prone, but the lateral position can also be used. A standard radiolucent operating table is recommended, although some surgeons prefer a traction table. In the past, traction tables have been associated with significant complications (Fig. 37-24).[66]

The injured extremity and both buttock areas are included in the sterile prepared area. The lower portion of the exposure parallels the upper lateral femoral shaft to the level of the greater trochanter where it curves so that the upper incisional component is directed toward the posterior iliac spine. The skin and fat are divided, and the fascia lata incision is made anterior to the gluteus maximus muscle's femoral insertion. The fascia lata incision is continued superiorly and posteriorly to include the gluteus maximus fascia. The gluteus maximus muscle bundles are bluntly split, preserving crossing neurovascular bundles. The trochanteric bursa is divided, and the gluteus medius is retracted anteriorly and superiorly. The piriformis muscle is isolated, tenotomized at its insertion, and tagged with a suture. The sciatic nerve is then exposed and its anterior relationship to the piriformis muscle is detailed. The piriformis muscle commonly has ancillary muscle bellies that penetrate through the sciatic nerve bundles yet share a common insertion tendon with the normal dorsal piriformis muscle. These ancillary muscle bellies should be excised to avoid inadvertent sciatic nerve injury when the piriformis is retracted. The sciatic nerve should be freed from any local tethering tissues. Hip extension and knee flexion relax the sciatic nerve within the field during the procedure. Next the obturator internus muscle tendon is identified and tenotomized at its insertion. The adjacent superior and inferior gemellus muscle bellies should be excised from the tendon after they have been elevated with subperiosteal dissection from the ischial area adjacent to the lesser sciatic notch. The quadratus femoris muscle is not disturbed throughout this exposure in order to preserve the femoral head's blood supply.

The caudal portion of the gluteus minimus is then either retracted from its superior acetabular origin or more preferably excised to the level of its caudal neurovascular bundle. The dissection continues if necessary through the greater sciatic notch. The periosteum along the edge of the greater sciatic notch is quite dense, and excision of this tissue is recommended. The dissection proceeds superiorly within the notch to the level of the superior gluteal neurovascular bundle, and inferiorly to the ischial spine. With the nerve relaxed and carefully retracted medially, subperiosteal dissection through the greater sciatic notch of the obturator muscle belly away from the quadrilateral surface is safely accomplished.

After reduction and fixation, multiplanar fluoroscopic imaging ensures the reduction quality and implant safety. The residual necrotic tissues are excised, the wound is irrigated, the tenotomies are repaired and closure proceeds in layers (Fig. 37-25).

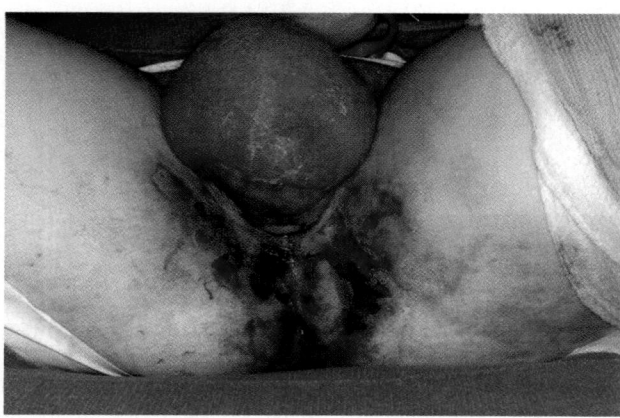

FIGURE 37-24 *This male patient underwent acetabular repair while positioned on a traction table. Sustained traction caused significant necrosis of his perineum and scrotum. Traction tables are rarely needed for patients undergoing acetabular surgery.*

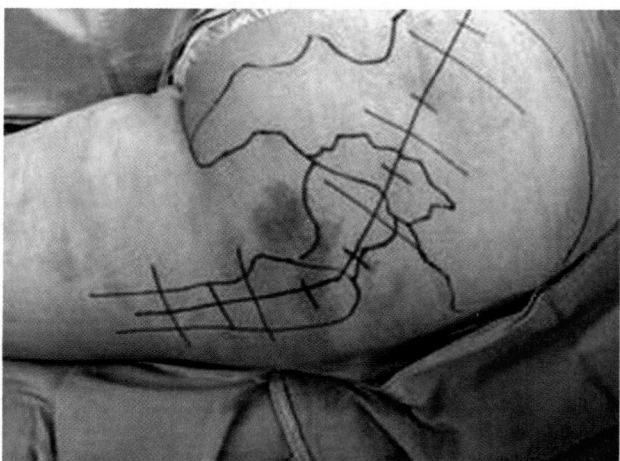

FIGURE 37-25 *The Kocher–Langenbeck planned skin incision along with bony landmarks are marked on this patient.*

ILIOINGUINAL The ilioinguinal exposure is an interesting exposure that can be divided into three main access intervals, or "windows"—lateral (iliac), middle (vascular), and medial (Stoppa).[78,111] Anatomic terms are preferred since numbering these surgical intervals is confusing and not advocated. Via these surgical intervals, the ilioinguinal exposure provides direct access to the anterior SI joint, the internal iliac fossa and iliac crest, the superior pubic ramus and symphysis pubis areas, and the quadrilateral surface. The ilioinguinal exposure is therefore indicated for anterior column and anterior wall fractures, anterior column with associated posterior hemitransverse patterns, certain T-type fractures, transverse fractures, and associated both-column acetabular fractures. If necessary, associated SI injuries are addressed using this exposure also.

The ilioinguinal exposure should be performed with the patient positioned supine, preferably on a radiolucent operating table. The patient's pelvis should be elevated on a soft lumbosacral support such as a folded blanket. The perineal area should be shaved and cleansed completely. The entire abdomen, bilateral flanks, and ipsilateral injured lower extremity are included in the sterile field. The draping isolates the perineum but allows access to the pubis, inguinal area, and flank areas, as well as the entire ipsilateral lower extremity. Hip flexion during the operation relaxes the iliopsoas muscle as well as the iliacfemoral vessels.

Traction tables are not recommended due to their expense, inventory, size, need for specially trained unscrubbed assistants to manipulate the table, imaging obstruction, and the potential for traction-related skin and nerve problems.[66]

It is important for the surgeon to identify both in the history and on physical examination if the patient has had previous inguinal operations such as hernia repair, appendectomy, caesarian section delivery, or open bladder procedures, among others. If so, prior infections are ruled out. Hernia repairs, especially those with mesh reinforcement, complicate the ilioinguinal exposure. Similarly, the preoperative exam and pelvic CT scan should be evaluated for inguinal hernia (Fig. 37-26).

Prior to skin incision, the surgeon determines which surgical intervals or windows are needed to expose, clean, reduce, and stabilize the fracture. If all three windows are to be used, the skin incision begins at the ipsilateral iliac crest, parallels the inguinal ligament, and ends just above the symphysis pubis. Osseous landmarks are difficult to determine in obese patients and those with significant displacements of the iliac crest fracture fragments. The contralateral normal-sided osseous landmarks may be used for symmetry, or the fluoroscope can be used if needed. Some surgeons consider the ilioinguinal skin incision in three individual segments: a Pfannenstiel portion, an iliac portion, and a connecting inguinal portion (Fig. 37-27A).

The skin and subcutaneous fat are incised and the spermatic cord or round ligament is identified and protected. Some surgeons prefer to place rubber drains around these structures in an attempt to protect them during the operation. Inadvertent or sustained retraction using the rubber drains can injure the spermatic cord (Fig. 37-27B–F).

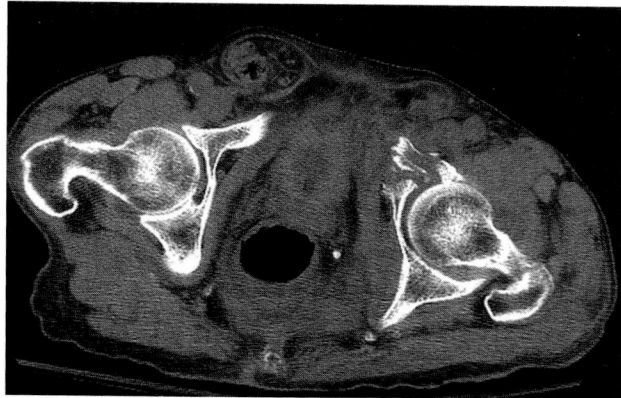

FIGURE 37-26 *This computed tomography image demonstrates a notable inguinal hernia. The hernia repair was performed using the ilioinguinal exposure at the time of acetabular fracture operative reduction and fixation.*

To open the lateral or iliac window, the abdominal oblique muscular insertions onto the iliac crest are incised, leaving a small stump for subsequent repair. The external oblique insertion can be incised posteriorly around the iliac crest, or its fascia split midway along the iliac crest and the posterior portion of the muscle left intact. The internal oblique and transverses abdominus insertions along the iliac crest are next divided from the anterior superior iliac crest to the posterior aspect of the crest. The iliacus muscle is elevated subperiosteally and retracted medially. Hip flexion eases this dissection by relaxing the iliopsoas muscle dramatically. This deep dissection can be delayed until the remainder of the exposure is performed if excessive bleeding from the iliac fracture components is anticipated.

The medial window is simply a Pfannenstiel surgical exposure that can be extended to a Stoppa exposure when needed. The midline rectus abdominus muscular raphe is divided superiorly from the pubis approximately 6 cm, and the local hematoma is removed from the space of Retzius. The ipsilateral rectus abdominus muscle is retracted anteriorly and laterally. The bladder is retracted posteriorly with a malleable retractor. The surgeon should stand on the uninjured side and use headlamp illumination for the deep pelvic dissection. Visualization of the posterior surface of the injured side superior pubic ramus will identify any communicating conduits between the obturator and inferior epigastric or iliac vascular systems.[199] These arteries and veins are ligated or cauterized depending on their diameter. The deep dissection should proceed after the inguinal dissection is complete so the medial window is packed with a sponge.

The inguinal dissection is the portion of the procedure that intimidates most surgeons, but should not. It simply connects the other two portions of the exposure, liberates the iliac vascular structures as they cross the anterior pelvis, further mobilizes the iliopsoas muscle, and allows direct visualization of the superior pubic ramus and a portion of the quadrilateral surface. The inguinal interval provides another window for clamp and implant application also.

FIGURE 37-27   ***A,*** *The perineum is cleansed thoroughly and isolated with barrier draping, and the ilioinguinal skin is marked on this patient's skin.* ***B,*** *The skin and subcutaneous fat are incised, the abdominal obliques have been tenotomized from the iliac crest, and the anterior abdominal fascia is incised from the anterior superior iliac spine medially to the external inguinal ring. The external inguinal ring remains intact in this example but can also be opened when needed. The caudal flap of the anterior abdominal fascia is retracted carefully, revealing the ilioinguinal nerve and inguinal ligament.* ***C,*** *The inguinal ligament is then divided, extending from the anterior superior iliac spine to the iliopectineal fascia. The lateral femoral cutaneous nerve penetrates the inguinal ligament just medial to the anterosuperior iliac spine in most patients. The inguinal ligament sharp division can proceed to the pubic tubercle if necessary.* ***D,*** *In this photograph, the inguinal ligament has been divided and blunt dissection on each side of the iliopectineal fascia allows retractor placement. The iliopectineal fascia separates the iliopsoas muscle and femoral nerve laterally from the iliac blood vessels medially. This patient has a small vein which pierces the iliopectineal fascia and should be ligated prior to dividing the iliopectineal fascia. The fascia is incised to the iliopectineal eminence and then elevated from the pelvic brim.*

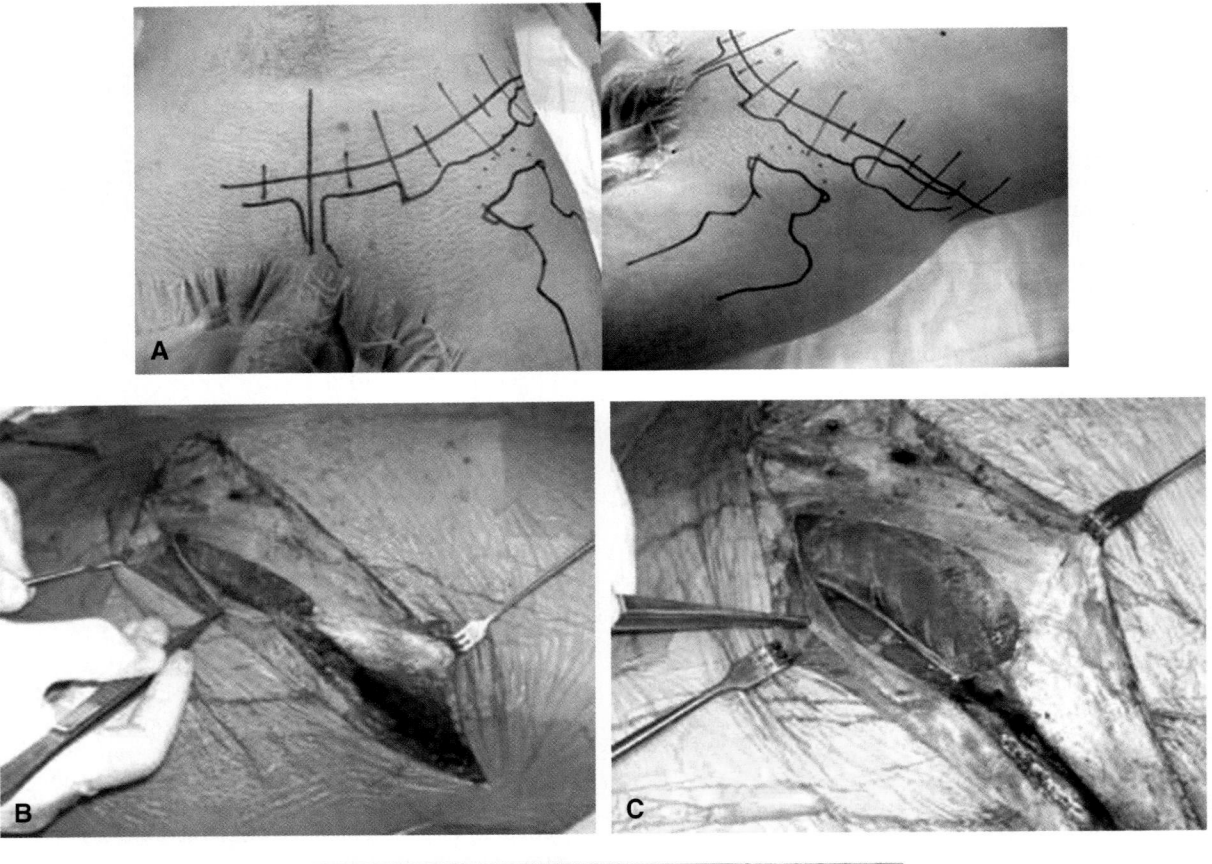

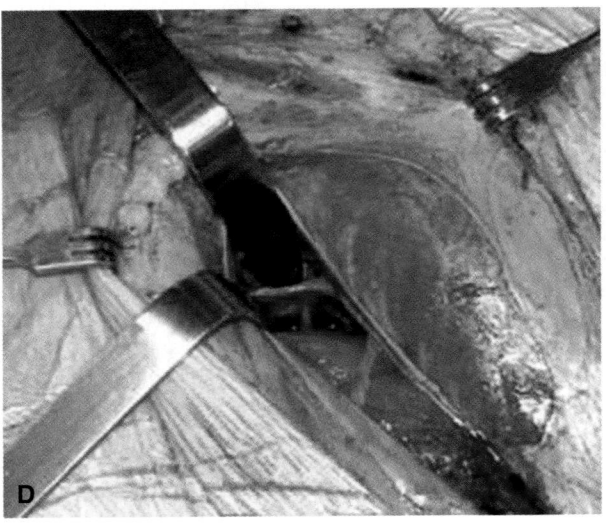

(Continued)

FIGURE 37-27 *(Continued)* **E,** *The lateral iliac interval is opened by elevating the iliacus muscle and then retracting the iliopsoas muscle unit medially. The malleable retractors are positioned medial to the pelvic brim and expose the internal iliac fossa. In this photograph, the fracture has been repaired with plates and screws.* **F,** *The Stoppa interval is opened by incising the rectus abdominus midline fascia, retracting the bladder, and incompletely elevating the ipsilateral rectus abdominus tendon insertion from the anterior parasymphyseal bone. The surgeon should stand on the uninjured side when developing this interval. Retraction of the bladder posteriorly and the injured side rectus abdominus muscle anteriorly reveals the pubic ramus. The periosteum is elevated after examining for and ligating any communicating vessels along the posterior aspect of the pubic ramus. The periosteal elevation proceeds to include the quadrilateral surface so that all three surgical intervals are in continuity. The obturator neurovascular bundle is visualized using the Stoppa interval. The iliac vessels are easily relaxed by hip flexion and are then retracted anteriorly. In this example, the deep pelvic view is what the surgeon sees when standing on the uninjured side. An intrapelvic plate has been applied using this Stoppa interval.*

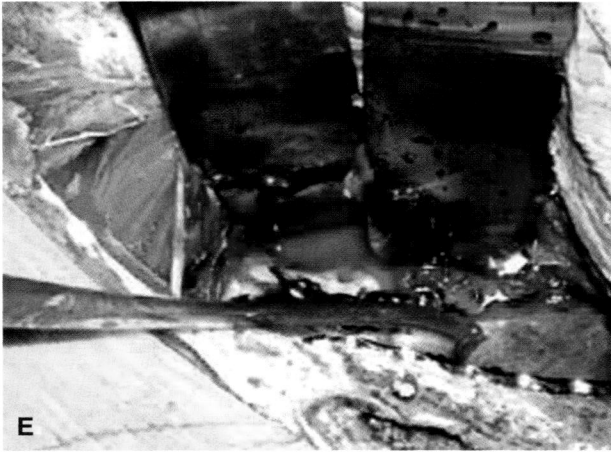
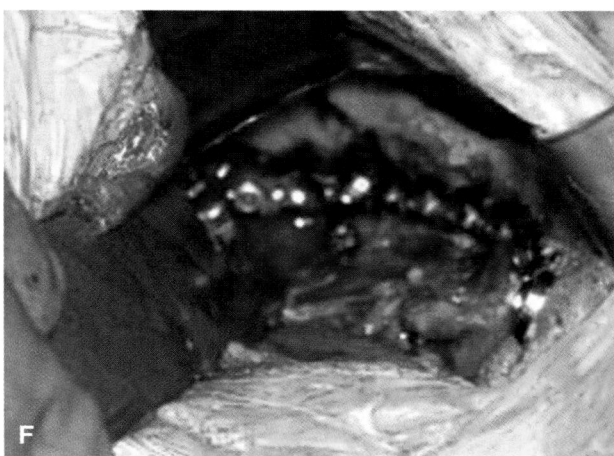

The inguinal portion of the dissection begins simply by inspecting and assessing the anterior abdominal fascia's local condition. Often due to fracture–displacement and associated local trauma, this anterior abdominal fascia is contused and ecchymotic. It may even be frayed and its fascial bundles traumatically separated. The anterior abdominal fascia should be incised 1 cm cranial to and paralleling the underlying yet palpable inguinal ligament. This fascial incision can include or use bands of traumatic separation when necessary. This fascial incision extends from and connects with the prior abdominal oblique incision adjacent to the anterior superior iliac spine (ASIS), and then proceeds medially and caudally toward the pubis. This fascial incision extends to and can even include the external inguinal ring (EIR) if the surgeon chooses. Some surgeons note the diameter of the EIR before opening it sharply in order to facilitate its accurate repair at closure. Other surgeons realize that opening the EIR is unnecessary to complete a safe and effective inguinal window dissection. Whether the EIR is opened or spared is unimportant. What is important is to repair it accurately if you choose to open it. The abdominal fascial incision paralleling and just above the inguinal ligament should now expose the ilioinguinal nerve seen penetrating anteriorly through the deep tissues and traveling parallel to the inguinal ligament toward the spermatic cord or round ligament. The nerve should be identified and protected, especially during closure of the abdominal fascial layer.

The inguinal ligament becomes visible when the caudal flap of the abdominal fascia is retracted inferiorly. The inguinal ligament is almost always intact. The inguinal ligament is then divided. Some surgeons prefer to split it from its pubic insertion to the ASIS origin. Others divide it only from the level of the iliopectineal fascia to the ASIS. Regardless of the chosen technique, the inguinal ligament is divided at least to the iliopectineal fascia.

The lateral femoral cutaneous nerve (LFCN) penetrates through the inguinal ligament usually only millimeters medial to the ASIS. The LFCN has an accompanying vascular system. It is wise to seek the nerve carefully as the inguinal ligament surgical division proceeds near the ASIS. Not every patient has an LFCN several millimeters medial to the ASIS, but most do. Some have branches of the LFCN located more medially just superficial to the femoral nerve and iliac vascular system.[47] The surgeon should protect the LFCN when possible. The LFCN can be excised to avoid injury if significant stretch injury is anticipated due to retraction.

Once the inguinal ligament is surgically divided, the iliopectineal fascia (IPF) is next isolated. The IPF is a confusing oblique "curtain" of dense tissue that separates the false from the true pelvis. Lateral to this fascial curtain is the iliopsoas muscle and the femoral nerve, while the iliac vessels and pelvic contents are medial to it. The IPF is attached to the inguinal ligament, and anchored to pelvic brim by blending with the local periosteum there. It is isolated easily either by digital or blunt instrument dissection medially and laterally. During this dissection, the surgeon inspects for penetrating vessels from the iliac system into the iliopsoas muscle. These small-diameter yet high-flow conduits should be isolated and ligated as necessary. Once the iliac vessels are carefully retracted medially and the iliopsoas muscle–femoral nerve unit is retracted laterally, the IPF is divided from inguinal ligament to pelvic brim and then divided from or elevated along with the pelvic brim periosteum. It is unnecessary to expose the iliac artery and vein directly. They simply should be mobilized as a unit to allow safe retraction for deep visualization of the acetabular anatomy. In some patients, the traumatic injury disrupts the iliac vessels surrounding soft tissues and consequently the vessels are obvious within the wound.

Once the IPF is divided and elevated and the iliac vessels mobilized, the deep dissection of the medial window resumes. Standing again on the uninjured side, the surgeon detaches the rectus abdominus tendon incompletely from its anterior parasymphyseal insertion until sufficient visualization is achieved. It is not necessary to completely tenotomize the rectus abdominus insertion since incomplete release always provides excellent deep exposure and facilitates the repair. With the rectus insertion retracted, the periosteum of the superior pubic ramus is elevated along with a portion of the pectineus muscle fascial origin. The iliac vessels are retracted along with the rectus tendon. Ipsilateral hip flexion eases and improves the retraction and hence the deep exposure. The superior pubic ramus periosteal elevation proceeds laterally until it meets the previous site of the IPF elevation at the IPE via the middle surgical interval.

Progressing more deeply, the obturator neurovascular bundle is identified and retracted medially. This bundle is often displaced medially by the quadrilateral surface fracture fragment's displacement. Rarely the obturator neurovascular bundle is found within the fracture site and despite its contused and distorted appearance should be carefully removed from the fracture and protected thereafter. The quadrilateral surface is next exposed by elevating the obturator internus muscle subperiosteally.

At this point in the operation, the three windows have been connected. The surgeon can stand on the uninjured side using the Stoppa interval; retract the bladder posteromedially along with the obturator neurovascular bundle; retract the rectus abdominus muscle and iliac vessels anterolaterally; and directly visualize the upper half of the quadrilateral surface, the pelvic brim, the superior pubic ramus, the anterior wall, and symphysis pubis. By standing on the injured side using the inguinal interval, the surgeon can retract the iliac vessels medially; retract the iliopsoas and femoral nerve laterally; and directly visualize the anterior wall, midportion of the pubic ramus, the iliopsoas gutter, a portion of the internal iliac fossa, and the upper aspect of the quadrilateral surface. And standing on the injured side using the iliac window, the surgeon can retract the iliacus muscle medially and visualize the entire iliac crest, internal iliac fossa, pelvic brim, SI joint, iliopsoas gutter, and AIIS.

Several details are relevant. The surgeon should sequence the deep interval dissections according to anticipated fracture bleeding so that the deep area of most anticipated fracture bleeding is exposed last. Similarly, fracture surface clots should be removed as the last phase of site preparation. Once these clots are removed, the fracture surface bleeding is often impressive and can only be halted by fracture reduction. It is important to remember that fracture fragment displacements can alter the palpable anatomy of the iliac crest and pubis. Because of this fact, the skin incision should be located where these palpable landmarks should be rather than where they may be when displaced. Similar to scarring from prior local operations, displaced fracture fragments distort the soft tissue anatomy and thereby complicate the dissection. Identifying the appropriate anatomy is vital for a successful procedure. Mobilizing the iliac vessels is an important step in the ilioinguinal exposure and frightens many surgeons. The critical step is to isolate the iliopectineal fascia and then make sure to divide it and then elevate it from the pelvic brim and IPE. If the IPF is left even incompletely attached, then mobilization and retraction of the iliac vessels is compromised. Hip flexion during the dissection relaxes the local anatomy and eases retraction. The surgeon should also remember that the iliac vessels may have small branches that penetrate through the IPF before they enter or exit the iliopsoas muscle. Palpation along the IPF before blunt dissection reveals these penetrating small-diameter yet high-flow conduits. They should be controlled with ligation and then divided.

Avoid plunging retractors anterior and deep to the bladder. Such maneuvers are unnecessary and can disrupt the local anterior bladder venous plexus, causing bleeding.

The communicating vessels between the obturator system and iliac or inferior epigastric system, the so-called corona mortis, also causes much surgical concern. These branches are quite common unless fracture comminution or displacement has destroyed them. The surgeon should simply look for them during the initial blunt dissection along the superior pubic ramus. Once seen, vessels of sufficient diameter should be isolated and controlled with ligation or clipping. Similarly, the obturator vascular bundle may be injured by fracture comminution at its sulcus beneath the lateral aspect of the superior pubic ramus. Fracture-related bleeding in this zone responds to local packing. Rarely, the iliac vein can be injured by sharp superior pubic ramus fracture fragments. This becomes apparent during the Stoppa wound interval dissection and is controlled by manual pressure. The surgeon must take care to apply enough pressure to stop the iliac venous bleeding yet not apply too much pressure causing arterial flow disruption and arterial thrombus formation. Once the iliac vein is repaired (preferably by a vascular surgeon), the ipsilateral peripheral pulses should be monitored throughout the remainder of the operation.

EXTENDED ILIOFEMORAL   This surgical exposure has been advocated for delayed acetabular reconstruction and for those patterns that demand direct visualization of the articular surface during the repair.[4,61,88,120] Since the mobilized flap is based on the superior gluteal vascular supply, some angiographic studies advocate a preoperative assessment of these vessels to ensure their patency.[25,89,198] Clinical studies have not supported such preoperative angiography, citing few problems related to flap necrosis.[129,169]

For this extensile acetabular approach, the patient is positioned laterally, and the entire lower extremity and flank are prepared in the sterile field after the perineum is cleaned and isolated. The surgical incision parallels the iliac crest from posterior to anterior, curving at the ASIS and following the palpable interval between the sartorius and tensor muscles. The lateral ilium is elevated subperiosteally, and the gluteus medius, gluteus minimus, piriformis, and obturator internus muscles are tenotomized at their insertions. The hip abductor muscle mass is retracted carefully to protect the superior gluteal neurovascular bundle and sciatic nerve. A hip joint capsulotomy is performed along its periphery at the labral edge, and the proximal femur is retracted to expose the articular fracture fragments. The proximal femur is retracted using a greater trochanteric bone hook or a sturdy pin inserted at the level of the lesser trochanter. The fracture reductions begin at the articular surfaces and expand toward the iliac crest from central to peripheral. The fragments are cleaned, manipulated, clamped, and secured with lag screws and supporting plates applied to the lateral ilium and posterior column.

The closure is performed with the hip abducted to relax tension on the proximal femoral tendon insertion repairs and abductor origin repair along the crest. Prolonged operative times are related to flap swelling, which complicates closure. Some form of ectopic bone prophylaxis is advocated for this extensile exposure.

COMBINED ANTERIOR AND POSTERIOR EXPOSURES

Combined and simultaneous anterior and posterior surgical exposures during the same anesthetic administration were designed to improve reduction quality of associated fracture patterns by improving fracture visualization.[173,179] With two surgeons working simultaneously, operative times were diminished. Unfortunately, the Stoppa surgical interval of the ilioinguinal exposure cannot be developed in the mobile or floppy lateral position. Similarly, the Kocher–Langenbeck exposure cannot be developed to its full extent due to the positioning.

In some patients with associated or variant fracture patterns, sequential use of an ilioinguinal exposure with the patient positioned supine followed by a Kocher–Langenbeck exposure with the patient positioned prone has merit.[142] For example, in a patient with an associated both-column acetabular fracture that has a large posterior wall component and an ipsilateral anterior SI joint disruption, the SI joint and primary column fractures are reduced and stabilized initially. Then the patient is turned prone either during the same anesthesia or subsequently for a prone Kocher–Langenbeck exposure to reduce and stabilize the posterior wall fracture (Fig. 37-28).

If this sequential exposure tactic is selected, the surgeon should not obstruct the subsequent reduction with initial procedure implants. All acetabular repairs should be carefully planned preoperatively, but sequential exposures demand the best planning since poorly located screws applied during the initial procedure can obstruct the subsequent reductions and fixations.

OTHER EXPOSURES

Several other exposures have been described for acetabular surgery.* The modified extended iliofemoral exposure employs an iliac crest osteotomy to improve visualization and therefore reduction–fixation while maintaining some

---

FIGURE 37-28 *This patient had sequential ilioinguinal (supine) and then Kocher–Langenbeck (prone) exposures during the same anesthetic session to treat his displaced associated both-column acetabular fracture. There was a large posterior wall component of the fracture. The posterior column screws were inserted using the initial ilioinguinal exposure and positioned carefully so as to not obstruct the subsequent posterior wall reduction from the posterior exposure. Because of the associated risk of ectopic bone with two exposures, oral indomethacin was used for 6 weeks after surgery.*

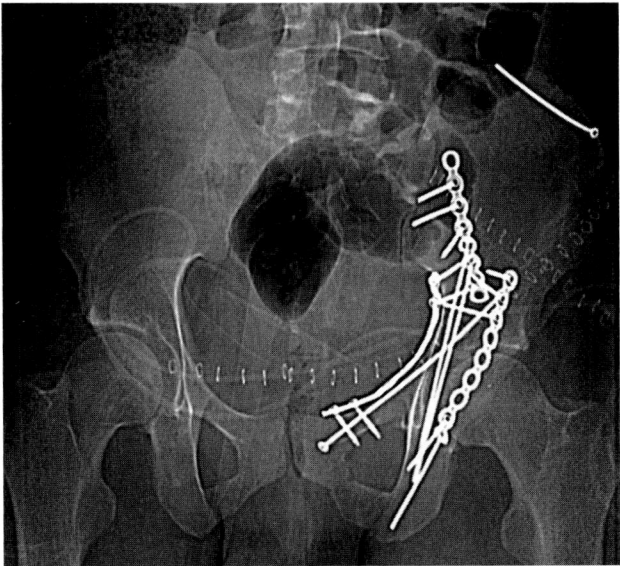

local soft tissue attachments. Using this approach, both the inner and outer iliac areas are exposed.[170,196]

The "trochanteric flip" exposure has been advocated recently as a less extensive dissection that allows surgical dislocation of the femoral head from the acetabulum in order to improve direct articular visualization. The greater trochanteric osteotomy avoids tenotomies. This procedure is usually done with the patient positioned laterally and like many "new" techniques has become recently popular as surgeons explore indications and related complications that remain undefined.[182–184]

MANIPULATIVE REDUCTION/PERCUTANEOUS FIXATION

Some acetabular fractures may be amenable to percutaneous treatment.[42,143,157,171] For these fractures, screws are inserted through small wounds across the fracture surfaces using aiming devices and intraoperative fluoroscopy, or other imaging-guidance systems.[11,28,80] This technique seems best suited for minimally displaced fractures that are unstable.[82,99] It may also have a role for those medically unstable patients who cannot undergo more extensive operations or those with unsuitable soft tissues that prevent open procedures. Accurate fracture reduction without subluxation is required prior to percutaneous fixation. The treating physician must remember that fracture reduction quality is more important than screw

---

*See references 4, 8, 16, 27, 57, 71, 83, 85, 93, 98, 130, 182, 196, 211, 212.

insertion techniques. Malreductions should not be accepted only in order to use percutaneous fixation techniques.[191,192] Surgeon experience, improved manipulative devices, and refined intraoperative imaging have allowed this technique to progress. Critical assessments of this technique and its indications are ongoing.

Exposure, Reduction, and Fixation by Fracture Pattern

POSTERIOR WALL

Routine posterior wall fractures are reduced and stabilized using Kocher–Langenbeck exposures.[5,109,156] The displaced wall fragment may stretch the sciatic nerve, may be impaled on the undersurface of the gluteus minimus muscle, or extruded between the muscle intervals. Often the piriformis, obturator internus, and gemellus muscles are anteriorly located relative to the displaced posterior wall fragment. The necrotic gluteus minimus muscle should be excised, preserving the related neurovascular bundles.[166] The wall fragment edge and cancellous surface are cleansed of debris and hematoma, and then the fracture site is likewise prepared. The wall fragment often has a caudal labral remnant that can be excised. The hip is distracted to remove loose bodies and chondral debris using either a bone hook on the greater trochanter or a hip distractor. Once the femoral head is located beneath the dome, chondrocancellous impaction injuries are then elevated using the reduced femoral head and dome as templates, and these fragments are supported with bone grafting into their related defects as needed (Fig. 37-29).[30,151]

Before reducing the wall fragment, the surgeon should mark the articular limits of the joint in order to avoid inadvertent drilling into the joint during implant application. Once the wall is reduced, the upper and lower joint limits are not visible as they are when the wall is displaced. The wall fragment is reduced using the cortical edges to refine the reduction and protecting the sciatic nerve from the sharp fracture edge. The fracture is clamped or impacted and then held with extra-articular thin wires remote from planned plate application sites. Lag screws can be used individually or through the plate.[24] Unfortunately the quadrilateral surface is not the sturdiest of bones, so these lag screws often have questionable fixation power. A slightly undercontoured pelvic reconstruction plate is applied in a balanced location along the cortical surface of the wall fragment and secured above and below the joint with screws of appropriate length after predrilling and accurate depth assessment. A balanced plate is located between the labral edge and the cortical fracture line. Usually a seven- or eight-hole standard 3.5-mm pelvic reconstruction plate is sufficient for most routine posterior wall fractures.[60,81] Undercontouring the plate produces compressive fixation as the screws above and below the fracture are tightened. Plate compression demands a balanced implant since an unbalanced plate applied in compression causes fracture displacement. The two caudal plate screws are inserted into the ischium, and the superior screws are located just above the dome. The surgeon should remember that the wall fixation fails due to caudal tension, so the lower screws must be securely fixated in the bone. Similarly, if the plate is located too medially or not firmly

---

FIGURE 37-29 *A, B, The chondrocancellous impaction fragments are seen by these computed tomography images both before and after reduction and fixation. Cancellous allograft was used to fill the defect and support the elevated fragment.*

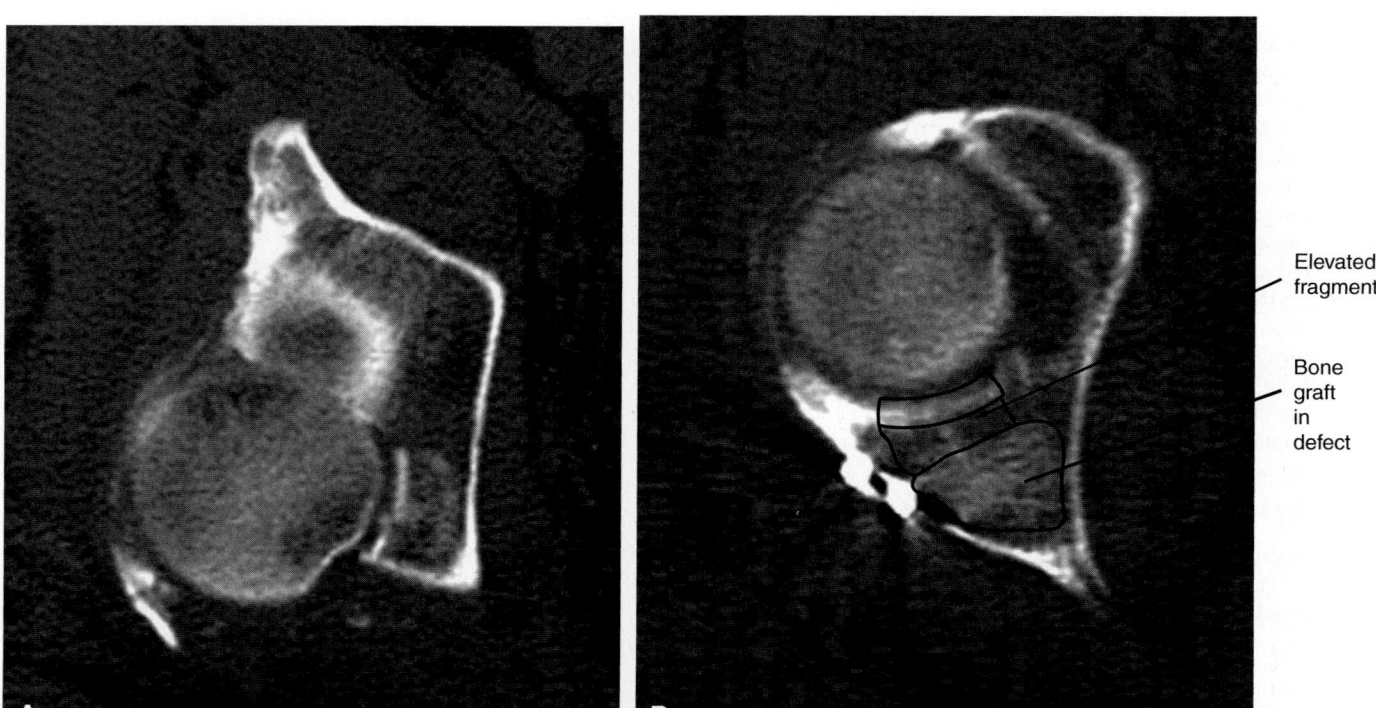

Elevated fragment

Bone graft in defect

applied, the wall fragment will displace from beneath the plate.[169] The fixation construct is stressed by moving the hip through a full range of motion while directly observing the fracture line. Any residual instability is addressed immediately. Identified intraoperative instability risks fixation failure if not corrected.[104,138,150] Biplanar fluoroscopic images ensure the reduction quality and implant safety prior to wound closure (Figs. 37-30 through 37-33).

POSTERIOR COLUMN

Posterior column acetabular fractures are reduced and stabilized using a Kocher–Langenbeck exposure with the patient positioned either supine or prone. The sciatic and superior gluteal nerves are protected during the exposure and fracture reduction. The surgeon should first distract the primary fracture and anatomically reduce any chodrocancellous dome fracture fragments. The posterior column fracture is then reduced and clamped through the greater sciatic notch according to the preoperative plan and based on the radiographic imaging. Some surgeons use a reduction clamp anchored to the unstable fracture fragment and intact pelvis using cortical screws. If applied properly, the clamp manipulates the unstable fragment and secures the reduction as the definitive implants are applied. It is important to locate the clamp remote from anticipated surgical implant sites and with extra-articular screws that are not inadvertently placed into the fracture plane or hip joint. The clamp should not cause tension on the sciatic nerve.

Lag screw fixation for a reduced posterior column fracture is usually directed from the area of the greater sciatic notch anteriorly. This screw insertion requires medial retraction of the sciatic nerve. A malleable pelvic reconstruction plate is recommended to supplement the posterior column fracture fixation, but remember that the screws into the caudal segment are important for stability (Fig. 37-34).

ANTERIOR WALL

Anterior wall acetabular fractures are exposed, cleaned, reduced, and stabilized using an ilioinguinal exposure. The middle (vascular) surgical interval reveals the fracture beneath the iliac vessels and iliopsoas tendon. The reduction is held with clamps or thin wires while the supporting plate fixation is applied. The surgeon should take care drilling and inserting screws using the middle surgical interval since the iliac vessels are medially located, the femoral nerve is laterally located, and the obturator neurovascular bundle is medial and deep to the joint. The surgeon should not plunge with the drill or depth gauge when aiming toward the obturator neurovascular bundle. A drill sleeve of sufficient length to protect the local soft tissues is recommended during drilling within this interval. The anterior wall has a limited cortical surface that makes fixation challenging. Fortunately, these are rare injuries.

ANTERIOR COLUMN

The ilioinguinal exposure is used for anterior column acetabular fractures. A manipulation pin in the iliac crest allows the surgeon to externally rotate the displaced fracture

FIGURE 37-30 *This peripheral posterior wall fracture fragment was initially reduced and then stabilized using a reconstruction plate applied directly to the fracture in a balanced and secure manner. Unfortunately, rotation of the hip in the operating room under direct visualization after the initial fixation caused fragment displacement, indicating insufficient fixation by the reconstruction plate alone. The fragment was too small and peripheral for interfragmentary screw fixation. A spring–hook plate was fashioned from a three-hole one-third tubular plate by first flattening the implant and then cutting away a portion of the peripheral hole. The resulting plate tips were bent to form a hook on the end of the plate. Then the plate was overcontoured so that when the central screw was inserted, the plate would flatten, causing the hooks to secure the peripheral wall fragment. The hooks are located on the posterior wall fragment's edge rather than on the labrum. The reconstruction plate was then reapplied dorsally to finalize the construct.*

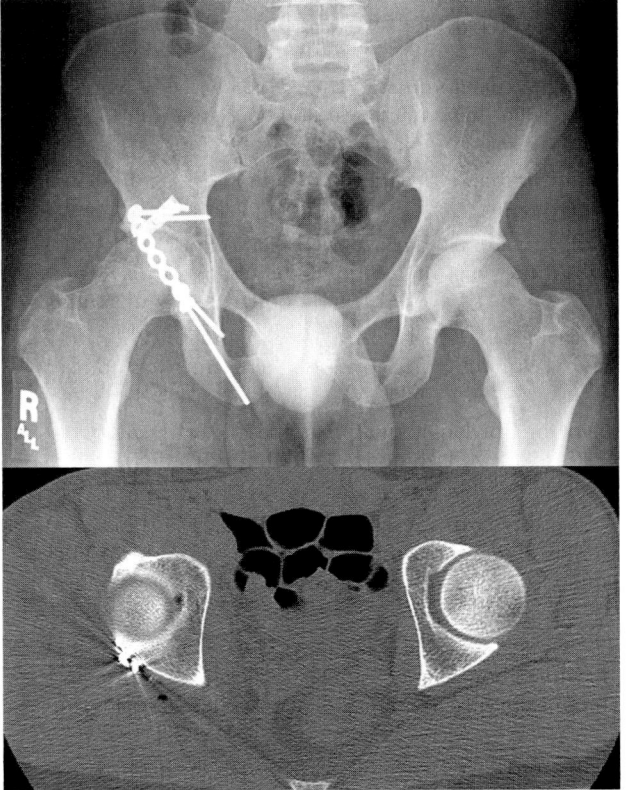

fragment in order to better clean the fracture surfaces. The pin can also be used to internally rotate and manipulate the fragment for reduction. Lag screws are applied along the pelvic brim into the superior ramus, posterior column, greater sciatic notch, posterior ilium, or iliac crest depending on the specific fracture details. A plate is used when

FIGURE 37-31 *Customized spring–hook implants for peripheral wall fixation are easy to fashion from one-third tubular plates. First flatten the implant and then overcontour it. This causes compression as the central screw is inserted and tightened. The hooks should contact the bone rather than the capsule or labrum in order to avoid inadvertent hook contact with the femoral head.*

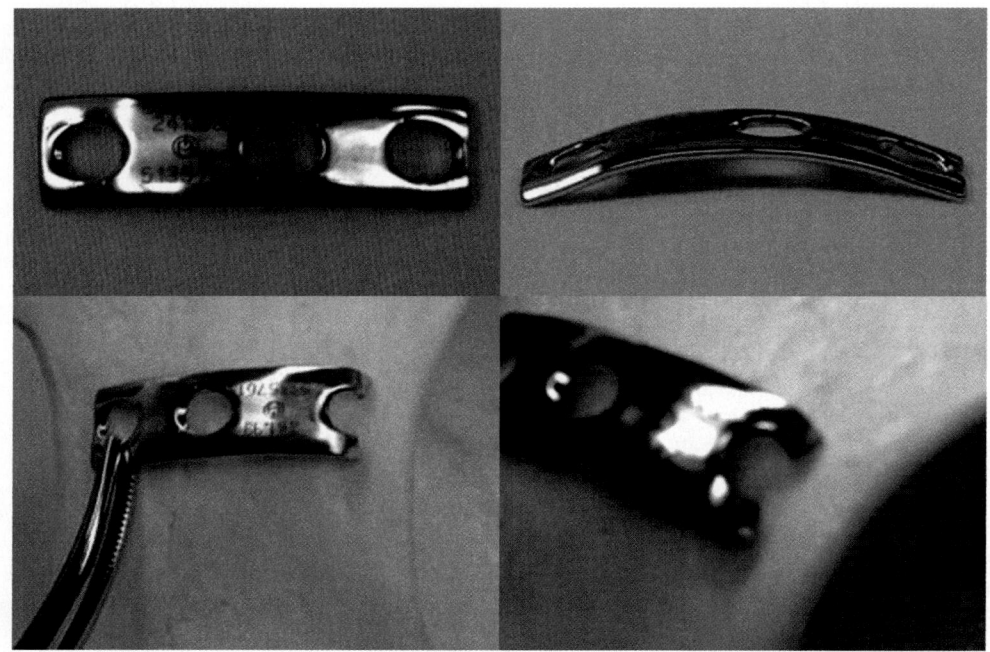

necessary to support the lag screws, serve as a washer for the screws, and offset the deforming forces caused by the tensor muscle and hip abductors (Fig. 37-35).[101,102]

TRANSVERSE

Transverse acetabular fractures are difficult to group because of their variety. Patient factors such as obesity and fracture details such as impaction injuries dictate which exposure is selected.[148,175]

Many transverse acetabular fractures can be accurately reduced and stabilized using a Kocher–Langenbeck exposure with the patient positioned prone. The prone position eliminates the weight of the ipsilateral limb causing unwanted displacement of the fracture and also facilitates dissection through the greater sciatic notch along the quadrilateral surface for fracture cleaning and clamp application. The prone position demands the hip to be in neutral position. As the knee is flexed to relax the sciatic nerve, the rectus femoris muscle becomes taut and in certain fracture patterns causes the transverse fracture to further displace, despite adequate pharmacologic muscle relaxation and traction. The surgeon must be alert to this potential problem and know that it is best remedied with slight knee extension until the femoral head easily reduces beneath the weight-bearing dome. The knee is supported in that position while the sciatic nerve is carefully retracted to allow the transverse fracture to be reduced and clamped. Once clamped satisfactorily, the knee can be flexed again to relax the nerve without effect on the reduction (Fig. 37-36).

After reduction and clamping, the transverse fracture is supported with lag screws from the supra-acetabular area into the superior pubic ramus.[34,183] These screws are inserted either through the wound or more commonly percutaneously using fluoroscopic biplanar guidance. The transverse fracture is supported using a plate, the surgeon remembering that the caudal screws hold the unstable fracture along with the lag screw into the ramus (Fig. 37-37).

For some transverse patterns in certain patients, an ilioinguinal exposure is selected. The fracture is cleaned, reduced, clamped, and stabilized using lag screws, and a plate is applied along the anterior column. An intrapelvic plate is selected when medial displacement of the caudal fracture fragment is significant. The intrapelvic plate is anchored to the intact bone through the Stoppa surgical interval just above the greater sciatic notch and to the unstable segment along the posterior superior aspect of the superior pubic ramus (Fig. 37-38).[41]

TRANSVERSE FRACTURE WITH ASSOCIATED POSTERIOR WALL INVOLVEMENT

The transverse fracture with associated posterior wall acetabular involvement is usually reduced and stabilized using a Kocher–Langenbeck surgical exposure with the patient positioned prone. This has the advantages noted earlier and also allows access to the wall fracture. In these patients, the debris within the joint is removed initially. Usually the wall can be retracted superolaterally and the unstable caudal portion of the transverse fracture displaced medially to remove intra-articular loose bodies. Then the

FIGURE 37-32 *A,* This patient had a comminuted posterior wall fracture with intra-articular debris noted on the injury computed tomography scan within the fossa acetabuli. At surgery, manual distraction of the hip failed to allow sufficient joint visualization for removal of the fragments within the fossa. A joint distractor was applied, and the debris was thought to be completely removed. The retrieved fragments corresponded to the preoperative fragment length measurements. Then the comminuted posterior wall fragments were reassembled and secured with extra-articular Kirschner wires, but the fracture fragments did not reduce appropriately and there were missing cortical fragments. Fluoroscopic imaging revealed an incongruous femoral head–dome relationship and residual debris within the joint. *B, C,* The wires were removed, the distractor was reapplied, the residual debris was identified and removed, and the reduction and fixation then proceeded routinely.

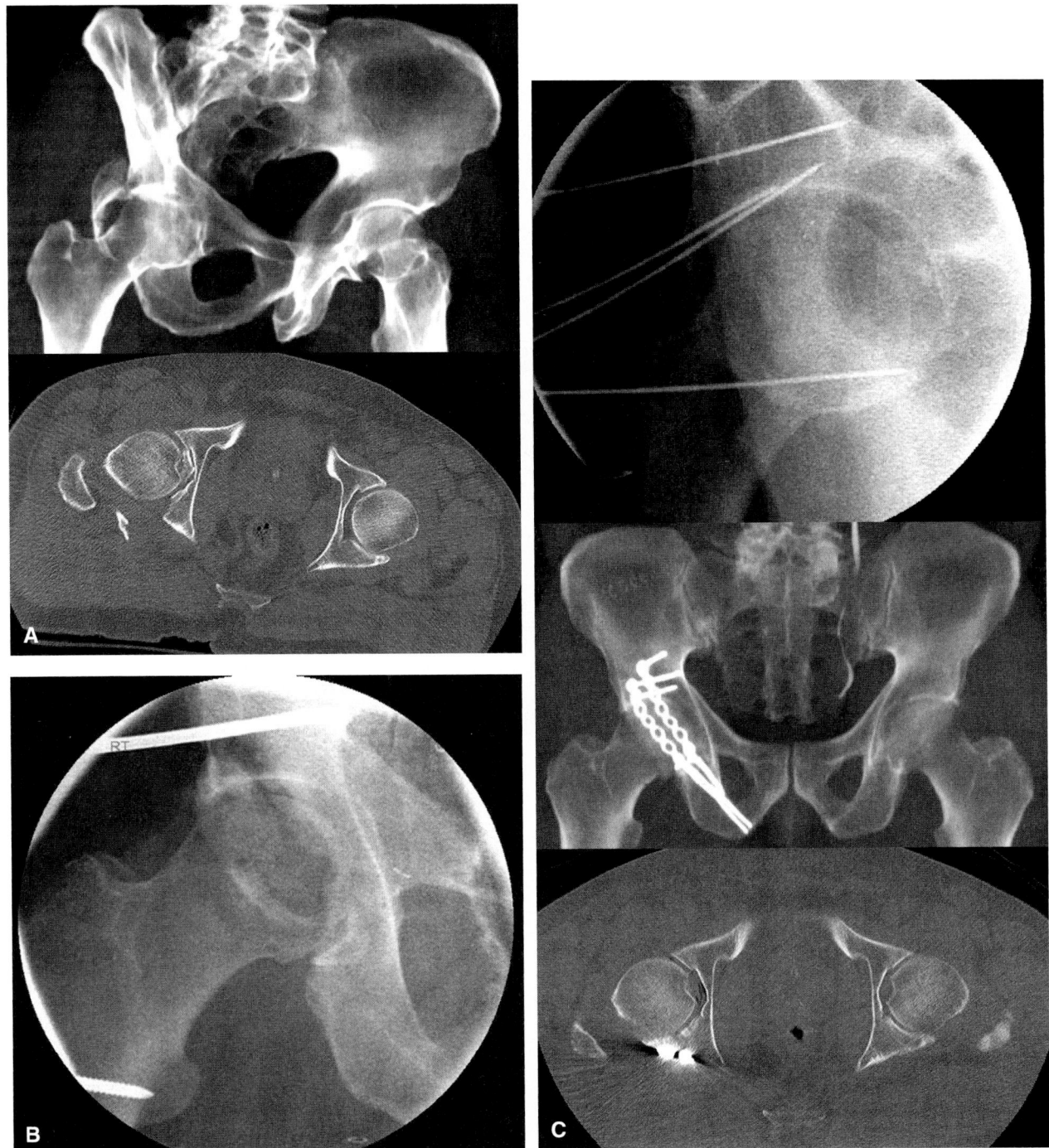

FIGURE 37-33   *A, This patient's posterior wall fracture was accurately reduced, but the surgeon mistakenly applied the plates too medially and did not perform an intraoperative hip stability assessment after fixation. B, The patient returned to the clinic complaining of hip pain and deformity. This obturator oblique film demonstrates that the fixation implants remained intact as the fracture fragment redisplaced and the hip dislocated once again. C, He was referred for operative repair consisting of plate removal, reduction, and fixation with a balanced peripheral plate and supplementary lag screw through the plate.*

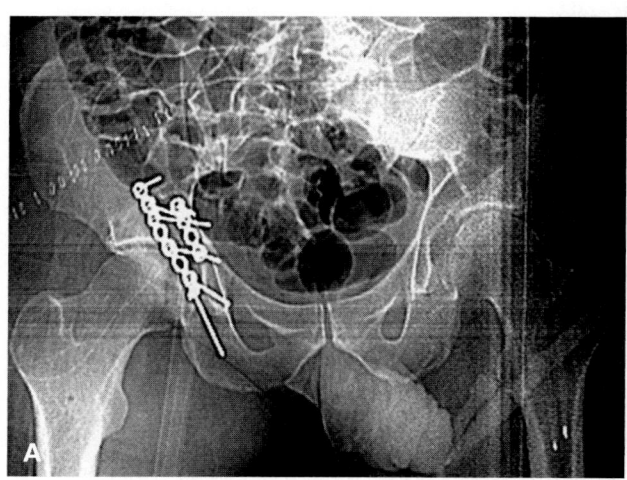
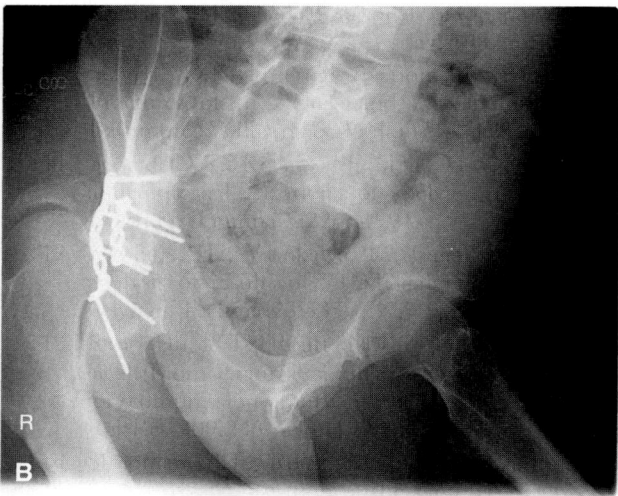

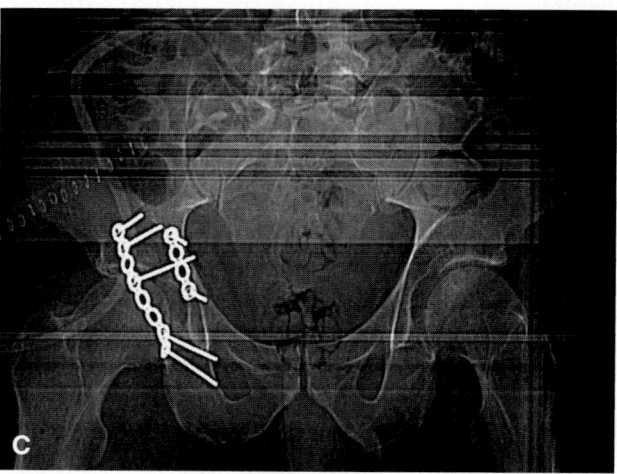

transverse fracture plane is cleansed, reduced, and clamped. Since the posterior wall fracture fragment is displaced, the transverse fracture is more difficult to accurately reduce because of the displaced wall defect. Similarly, a clamp using two independent screws to manipulate and hold the reduction is much more complicated to apply than simply clamping through the greater sciatic notch.

Just as with transverse patterns, knee flexion in these patients may also cause a tight rectus femoris muscle to displace the primary transverse fracture line. The same remedy works for this pattern and the transverse is reduced, clamped, and stabilized through its anterior column using a lag screw into the superior pubic ramus from the supra-acetabular surface. With a displaced posterior wall associated fracture, the femoral head can now be distracted to visually assess the transverse plane reduction.

This is not possible for elementary transverse patterns without a wall fracture. Once the reduction is stabilized and approved, the wall fragment is cleansed, any impaction segments are elevated, reduced, and supported with bone graft, and then the wall is reduced and held with thin wires or clamped.

If the wall fragment does not reduce perfectly, it is obstructed, usually by a malreduction of the transverse fracture, or too much graft material has been packed into the defects in supporting the impaction fragments. Once corrected and the reduction achieved, the wall and posterior column component of the transverse fracture line are stabilized using a contoured malleable pelvic reconstruction plate. Lag screws can be applied through the plate or remote from it to further support the wall fracture as indicated (Fig. 37-39).

FIGURE 37-34   **A,** *A displaced posterior column acetabular fracture is shown on this iliac oblique image.* **B,** *The injury computed tomography (CT) axial image reveals a large chondrocancellous dome fragment trapped between the primary fracture surfaces. A Kocher–Langenbeck exposure allowed distraction of the primary fracture initially, reduction of the dome fragment, and then reduction and fixation of the posterior column fracture.* **C,** *The postoperative CT image demonstrates the reduction and fixation.*

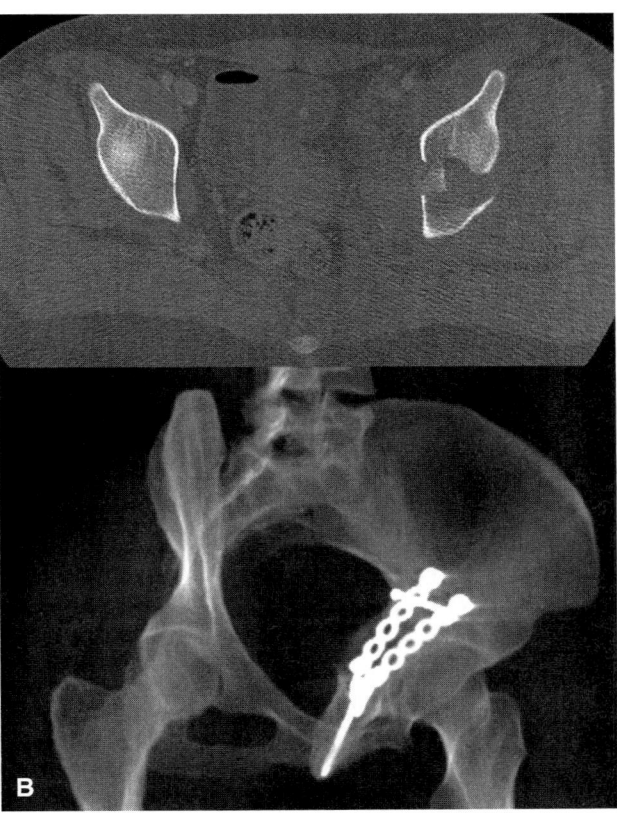

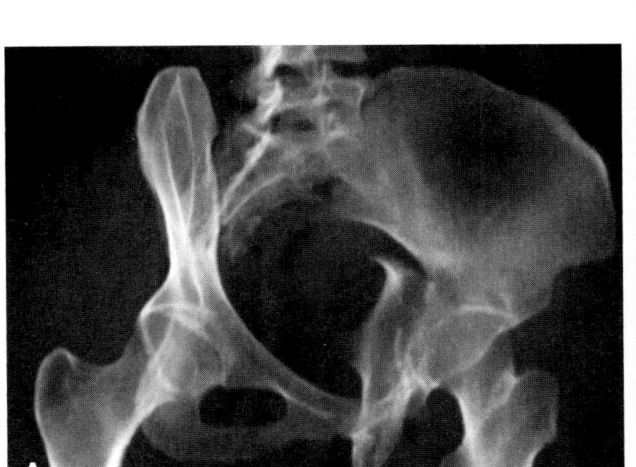

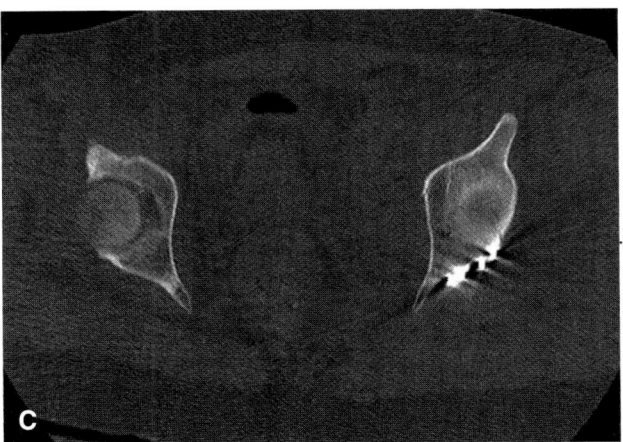

POSTERIOR COLUMN FRACTURE WITH ASSOCIATED POSTERIOR WALL INVOLVEMENT

Posterior column fractures with associated posterior wall involvement are treated using a Kocher–Langenbeck exposure with the patient positioned prone. The same details as noted earlier for the elementary posterior column pattern and elementary posterior wall pattern apply. Similar to the transverse fracture with associated posterior wall involvement, the posterior column reduction is complicated by the displaced wall defect at the time of posterior column reduction. Palpation through the greater sciatic notch along the quadrilateral surface cortical fracture line and intraoperative fluoroscopic imaging are used to guarantee the reduction accuracy. The posterior column reduction is initially clamped, and then the wall fragment is reduced and clamped or held with thin wires. The fracture is stabilized with one or two supporting plates. Lag screws are applied as needed.[216]

FIGURE 37-35 | *A, The iliac oblique image demonstrates the displaced anterior column acetabular fracture as well as significant vascular calcifications. B, The ilioinguinal exposure was planned but because of the patient's overall medical condition and fracture-related bleeding intraoperatively, only the lateral iliac interval was developed. This limited the fracture exposure and cleaning and, ultimately, the reduction accuracy. The postoperative iliac oblique view reveals the reduction to be imperfect.*

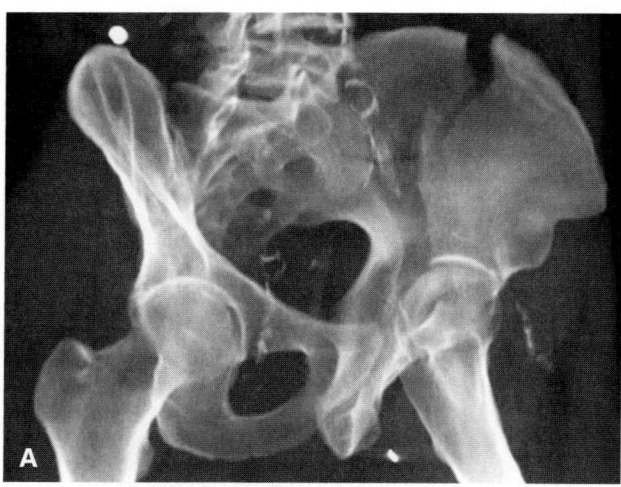 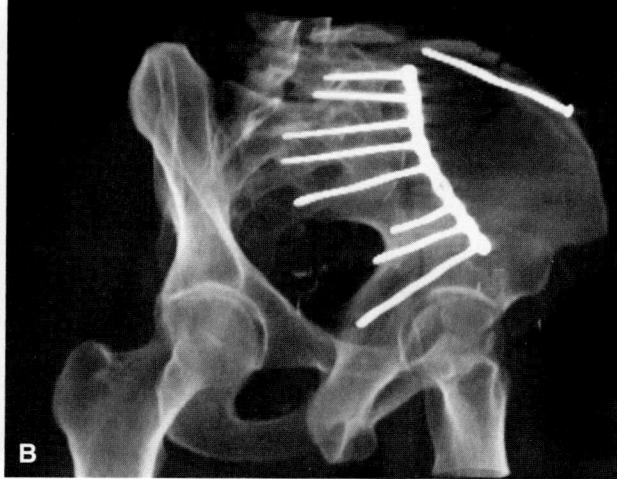

ANTERIOR COLUMN FRACTURE WITH ASSOCIATED POSTERIOR HEMITRANSVERSE INVOLVEMENT

These fractures have a variety of appearances but can usually be reduced and fixed using an ilioinguinal exposure.

The anterior column component is reduced and stabilized initially with lag screws and appropriate plates, but the surgeon is careful not to inadvertently place screws that obstruct the posterior hemitransverse fracture line. The posterior hemitransverse fracture is reduced using the middle and Stoppa surgical intervals, clamped, and then

FIGURE 37-36 | *Various clamp applications are possible for transverse acetabular fractures. Using a Kocher–Langenbeck exposure with the patient positioned prone, the clamp can be positioned through the greater sciatic notch onto the quadrilateral surface, avoiding the sciatic and obturator nerves. A different reduction clamp that is applied dorsally using two independent screws is also shown. All clamps should be positioned to secure the reduction but not obstruct implant applications.*

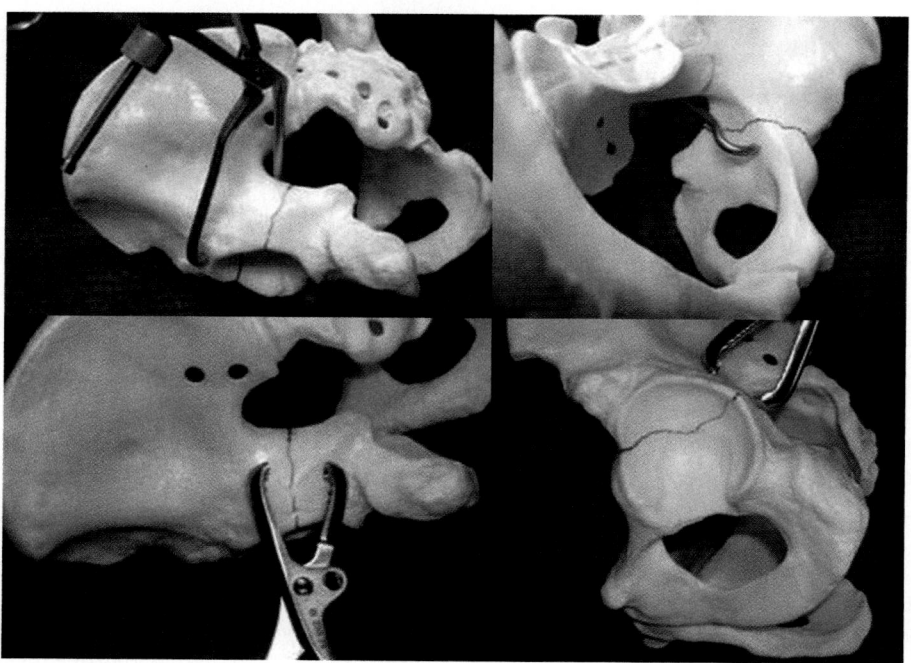

FIGURE 37-37 *A–C, This displaced transverse acetabular fracture–dislocation was initially treated with manipulative reduction and skeletal traction. Once the patient was medically cleared, open reduction was performed using a Kocher–Langenbeck exposure, and the fracture was clamped through the greater sciatic notch. The fluoroscopic inlet and obturator–outlet views were used to insert the medullary ramus screw through a separate stab incision, thereby securing the anterior column component of the transverse fracture initially. The plate further supports the fixation construct.*

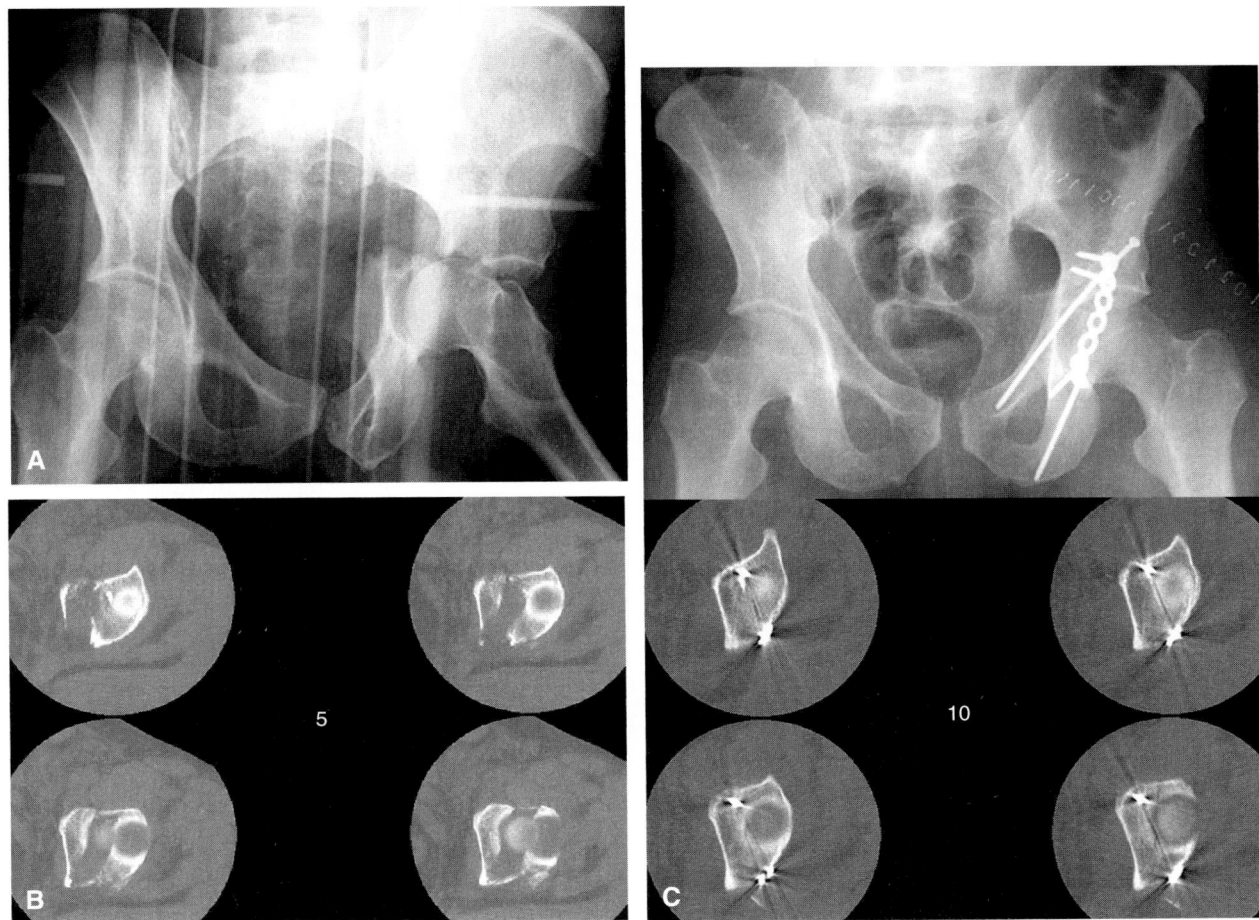

secured with screws inserted from the internal iliac fossa along the pelvic brim into the ischium. Biplanar fluoroscopy is recommended to guide insertion of these screws into the ischium and remote from the hip joint.

T-TYPE

These fractures have many variables. When the anterior column fracture articular component is low and minimally displaced, a Kocher–Langenbeck exposure is selected to address the posterior column displaced fracture component.

When both fracture components are displaced and involve significant portions of the joint, an ilioinguinal exposure is used to reduce and stabilize them. Fixation implants are tailored to the fracture specifics.

In some patients, an initial supine ilioinguinal exposure addresses the anterior column component, and a subsequent prone Kocher–Langenbeck exposure is used for the posterior column component.[187] Some surgeons advocate simultaneous anterior and posterior surgical

exposures, but the floppy lateral positioning limits the extent of each exposure and gravity deforms the fracture.

ASSOCIATED BOTH-COLUMN FRACTURE

Associated both-column acetabular fractures have numerous variables and details that determine the proper exposure or exposures necessary to achieve accurate reduction and stable fixation. For those fracture patterns in which the posterior column component is located in the upper portion of the greater sciatic notch, an ilioinguinal exposure is indicated. Typically, the anterior column fracture components are first reduced to the intact ilium. The dome articular anterior column fracture fragment may be incomplete at its iliac crest exit site and require local osteotomy to complete the fracture. This allows the fragment to be sufficiently mobilized for cleaning and reduction. Incomplete fractures cannot be accurately reduced without completing the fracture. When stabilizing the fracture components, the surgeon must be careful to locate

FIGURE 37-38 *Clamp application for a transverse acetabular fracture using an ilioinguinal exposure is shown. The clamp is applied to the quadrilateral surface through the middle surgical interval and lateral to the anterior inferior iliac spine. Anterior column medullary ramus screw(s) can be inserted using fluoroscopic imaging or under direct visualization.*
Interfragmentary screws from the internal iliac fossa into the ischium can also be used. It is difficult to apply plate fixation while the clamp is holding the reduction.

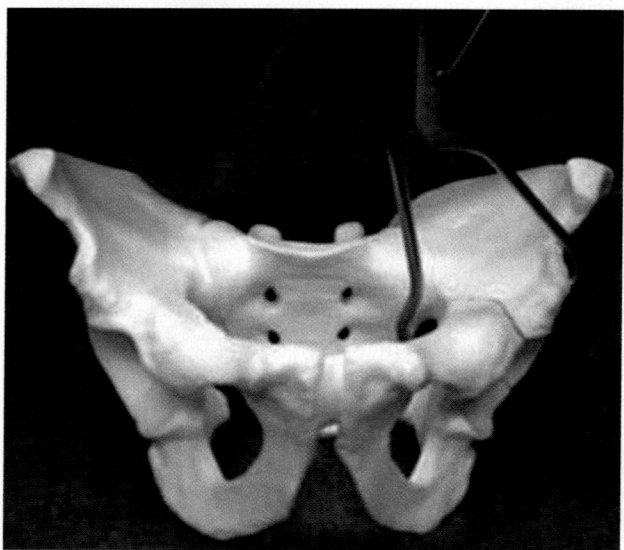

the fixation screws so they do not obstruct the subsequent columnar fragment reduction.

The posterior column fracture surface is best seen either through the ilioinguinal's middle surgical interval or in some instances the Stoppa interval. Using the Stoppa interval, the posterior column fracture component can be manipulated using a spiked pusher while a clamp is applied to maintain the reduction. Once the intruded posterior column fragment is reduced, the Stoppa interval provides access to the intact ilium adjacent to and above the greater sciatic notch. This area of intact ilium is the site where an intrapelvic plate is securely attached when indicated.

The posterior column fracture fragment is routinely reduced to the intact ilium and anterior column fracture together. Fixation is achieved using screws directed from the internal iliac fossa adjacent to the pelvic brim into the ischium. These screws anchor at both the intact ilium and anterior column fracture component, depending on the fracture details. Intraoperative fluoroscopy is used to ensure that these screws are located remote from the joint yet deep into the posterior column fracture fragment. Plate fixation supports the reductions. Short-length plates support the interfragmentary screws and are easily contoured. Longer plates can span several fracture zones but are more difficult to accurately contour (Fig. 37-40).

For certain associated both-column acetabular fracture patterns with low posterior column fracture planes or posterior wall components, other surgical exposures are selected. Sequential supine ilioinguinal followed by a subsequent prone Kocher–Langenbeck exposure may be indicated for such fractures.

The extended iliofemoral approach is selected for those patients with variant fracture patterns or delayed presentation.

TECHNICAL NOTE: OPERATIVE MANAGEMENT OF A TRANSVERSE FRACTURE WITH ASSOCIATED POSTERIOR WALL ACETABULAR COMPONENT USING A KOCHER–LANGENBECK EXPOSURE AND THE PATIENT POSITIONED PRONE

Once the exposure is completed, the fracture surfaces are cleansed of organizing hematoma and debris. With the patient relaxed, the hip joint can be distracted, using either a bone hook placed at the greater trochanter or a distractor device applied through bone pins. If a distraction device is selected, one bone pin should be located above the joint yet adjacent to the greater sciatic notch remote from anticipated future fixation implants. The other pin is inserted into the femur at or just above the level of the lesser trochanter. The distraction device should be positioned so as not to obstruct wound access yet providing the needed joint visualization. The distraction should be applied carefully and without tension on the sciatic nerve. Ipsilateral knee flexion during the distraction process usually relaxes the nerve sufficiently. The amount and duration of distraction should be limited to that needed to remove loose bodies, clean the fracture surfaces, or assess the reduction. Distraction should never be sustained longer than several minutes, unless reliable nerve monitoring is being used.

The dominant fracture surfaces are reduced after the joint debris is removed. The femoral head should be located beneath the stable weight-bearing dome fragment. The fracture fragments are maneuvered using a variety of techniques. A pointed dental pick or other similar device is useful for manipulating the fragments without disrupting their soft tissues excessively. Clamps or extra-articular wires temporarily stabilize the fracture until definitive lag screws or a contoured plate is applied. Impaction fractures are elevated and reduced using the femoral head articular surface as a mold. Elevation of marginal impaction fragments leaves a residual cancellous defect that is then filled with bone graft material to support the elevated osteochondral piece. Small volumes of cancellous autograft are available at the greater trochanter within the surgical exposure. The interval between the hip abductor muscular insertion and vastus lateralis muscular origin is exposed and an elliptical corticotomy is predrilled and fashioned with a narrow osteotome. The corticotomy is sized according to the anticipated amount of graft material needed to pack the defect. The cancellous trochanteric donor bone graft is then packed into the acetabular juxta-articular defect, preventing collapse of the elevated articular fragment.

Once the primary fracture lines are reduced and the impaction fragments elevated and supported, the posterior

FIGURE 37-39 | **A, B,** This patient has a transverse fracture with an associated posterior wall acetabular component with chondrocancellous impaction fractures along the fracture margin. The transverse fracture component is more displaced through the posterior than the anterior column. **C, D,** The Kocher–Langenbeck exposure was used with the patient positioned prone to reduce and stabilize the fracture. The debris was removed from the joint, the head was located beneath the dome, and the transverse fracture was reduced and stabilized with a medullary ramus screw. The impaction segments were then elevated to fit the femoral head and supported with greater trochanteric donor cancellous autograft. Then the wall fragment was reduced and the entire construct supported with plate fixation.

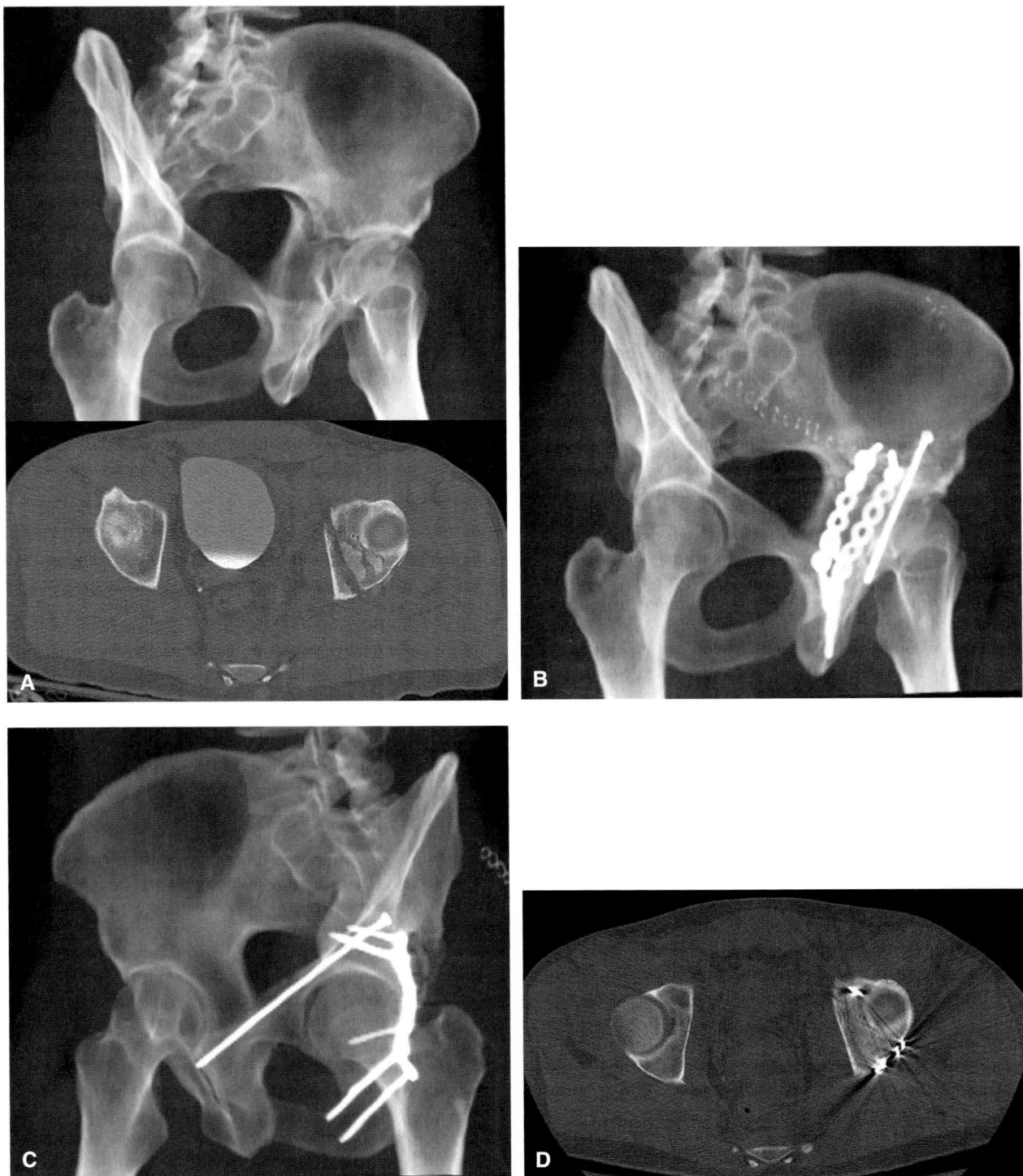

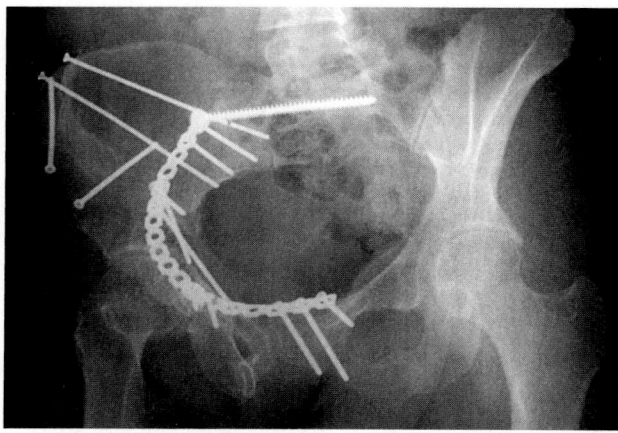

FIGURE 37-40 *This image was obtained 9 years after surgery for an associated both-column fracture. A long plate was used to secure the reduction. These implants are difficult to contour and apply.*

wall fracture component is reduced and secured with wires. The temporary fixation wires should be located to maintain the reduction without interfering with subsequent definitive fixation. Wires are not used as definitive implants for acetabular fractures. Reports describe migration of acetabular wires primarily to the thorax.[103,127]

Malleable plates have the benefit of being easily contoured to fit the complex acetabular topography while maintaining stability when applied properly. For posterior wall fractures, the malleable plate must contact the cortical surface of the wall uniformly and be located in a balanced manner. Balancing the plate indicates that the implant is located equidistant between the labral edge and the cortical fracture line of the wall. The plate should be slightly undercontoured to provide compression as it is anchored above and below the fracture using extra-articular screws. The caudal plate fixation screws are directed deep into the ischium since they must resist tension failure, while the supra-acetabular fixation screws are positioned just above the wall fracture line.

TECHNICAL NOTE: APPLICATION OF AN INTRAPELVIC PLATE TO SUPPORT THE QUADRILATERAL SURFACE FRACTURE COMPONENT

Intrapelvic plating is a demanding and detailed yet beneficial procedure.[41,162,164] The intrapelvic plate is applied using the Stoppa interval of an ilioinguinal exposure and after the quadrilateral surface fracture component has been reduced and clamped. The technique requires that the iliac bone anterior to the SI joint and cranial to the greater sciatic notch be stable since this is the attachment site for the implant. The implant extends from this stable iliac area to the symphyseal region. A 9- or 10-hole 3.5-mm pelvic reconstruction plate is chosen for most adult patients and is slightly overcontoured to provide a buttressing effect once applied. The implant can be contoured to a model pelvis preoperatively and

sterilized during the procedure. The screws which attach the plate to the stable iliac bone are inserted obliquely simply due to the local soft tissue anatomy. For this reason, these two or three most proximal plate holes should be obliquely sculptured with a 3.5-mm drill to allow the eventual oblique screw insertions to occur without them impinging on the plate and therefore being misdirected by the plate. The initial drill hole for the first screw is drilled in the perfect location for plate application before the implant is placed. This drill hole depth is measured, and several millimeters of additional length are added to accommodate the plate thickness. The plate is then placed and the predrilled screw is inserted. As the initial oblique screw is tightened, the plate may rotate as the screw impinges on it; therefore, the plate should be held by a sturdy clamp to prevent this potentially dangerous plate movement. The plate flexion can be adjusted to fit the pelvic brim medially before the initial oblique screw is finally tightened into the stable iliac component. Once the plate is adjusted it is clamped to the parasymphyseal area. The implant's overcontouring produces compression along its contact with the quadrilateral surface, if well contoured and applied. Next the parasymphyseal screws are inserted after predrilling and accurate depth assessment. Another iliac area screw can be inserted at this point, and lag screw fixation is also used when needed through the plate (Fig. 37-41).

AFTERCARE

Rehabilitation after acetabular fracture depends on the injury details, patient condition, and the selected treatment.[23,35,46] A licensed physical therapist helps guide the prescribed rehabilitation program that is designed to not only restore hip range of motion and strength but also improve coordination and overall fitness. For the initial 6 weeks after injury, protected weight-bearing using assistive devices such as crutches or a walker is indicated. Isometric exercises are used to maintain muscle strength. Passive range-of-motion exercises or devices usually provide patient comfort and may improve acetabular cartilage healing.[33,124] Progressive partial weight-bearing and light resistance exercises are instituted 6 weeks after injury with the goal of independent ambulation 3 months after injury. After 3 months, most patients discontinue using ambulation assistance devices and increase their strengthening and conditioning programs accordingly.[48] Some patients, such as those with contralateral lower extremity injuries, are not able to ambulate because of their associated injuries. Rehabilitation programs are tailored to meet each patient's individual needs.

COMPLICATIONS

Complications related to acetabular fractures and their treatments are certainly not uncommon.[54,56,67] Surgeon-related complications include patient selection errors, decision errors, and technical mistakes among others.[13,37,50,52,81,86,91,163,195] Patient-related complications often stem from associated medical comorbidities, other primary system injuries, noncompliance, and obesity.[65,155,206,215] Certain problems have multifactorial etiologies.[12,17,36,38,75,94,105,106,110,140,176,177]

FIGURE 37-41 | ***A,*** *This male adult patient fell from a ladder and was unable to ambulate because of right hip pain. The AP pelvic film and axial 2D CT scan demonstrated the fracture and displacement patterns.* ***B,*** *The Stoppa surgical interval was used to reduce and then stabilize the fracture. Working through the fracture, the dome impaction was reduced, and then the quadrilateral surface was reduced. An intrapelvic plate supported the reduction.*

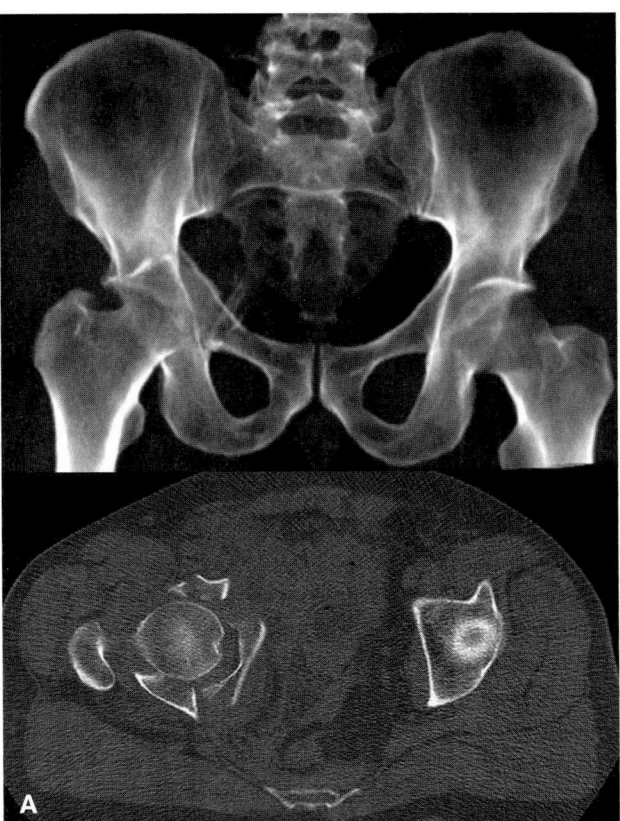
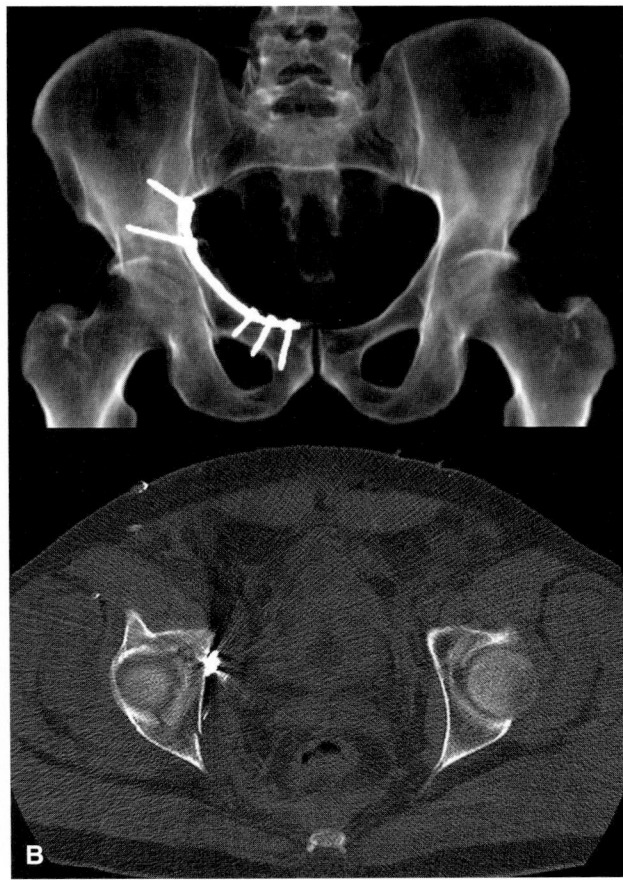

Malreduction

In numerous clinical series, inaccurate acetabular fracture reduction correlates with poorer clinical results.* Mechanical cadaveric studies have substantiated these clinical findings in that even 2 mm or more of articular dome stepoff caused significant articular peak pressure differences.

Acetabular malreduction happens due to poor treatment selection, inexperience, insufficient exposure, poor fracture surface cleaning, misaligned clamp or implant application, delayed surgery, comminution, insufficient fixation, and other factors. Regardless of its reason, acetabular malreduction is directly related to hip degeneration. Other than situations of significant impaction and comminution, malreduction should be avoidable. Simple solutions include developing a sufficient exposure, mobilizing and cleaning each fracture surface, and being patient with the reduction maneuvers and sequence. Inaccurate initial reductions are not acceptable, and the surgeon must take the time to correct such errors during the initial procedure. Intraoperative fluoroscopy confirms obvious malreductions but also identifies more subtle misalignments.

*See references 19, 39, 51, 74, 84, 113, 114, 121–123, 138, 145, 174, 205, 213, 214.

Nerve Injury

Several nerves surround the acetabulum and can be injured due to the acetabular fracture fragments' displacement or operative management. Anteriorly, the femoral, lateral femoral cutaneous, and ilioinguinal nerves are most at risk. The femoral nerve courses along with the iliopsoas muscle through the false pelvis and travels beneath the inguinal ligament as it enters the thigh bordered medially by the iliopectineal fascia. Certain acetabular fracture patterns involve the peripheral pubic ramus area and can injure the femoral nerve due to their anterior displacements.[67] The femoral nerve can also be damaged during ilioinguinal surgical exposures, usually due to sustained or vigorous retraction and clamp application using the middle interval between the iliac vessels and femoral nerve. One study of femoral nerve injury demonstrated that good functional motor–sensory recovery could be expected.[62]

The lateral femoral cutaneous nerve pierces the inguinal ligament usually several millimeters medial to the anterior superior iliac spine. In some patients, the nerve is situated more medially. One anatomic study documented this variant location in 25 percent of the cadaveric specimens. This cutaneous nerve can be injured during ilioinguinal exposures. Routine retraction of the iliopsoas muscle medially may cause excessive stretching of the nerve. Some surgeons recommend segmental excision of the nerve prior to stretch injury to avoid resultant meralgia paresthetica; others preserve the lateral femoral cutaneous nerve.

During the inguinal dissection of the ilioinguinal exposure, the ilioinguinal nerve is exposed as the deep fascia is incised. This nerve is at most risk during this portion of the exposure and then again at closure of the same fascia. The nerve is often adherent to the undersurface of the anterior abdominal fascia and should be freed from it prior to closure. This process avoids inadvertent suturing of the nerve during the fascial closure.

The obturator nerve travels deep within the pelvis located only a few millimeters medial to the quadrilateral surface. Displaced fractures through this zone injure the obturator nerve. It is difficult to examine the obturator nerve motor function in patients with acetabular fractures because hip adduction is painful, but the sensory evaluation of the medial thigh should be performed and noted, especially preoperatively. During ilioinguinal exposures using the Stoppa interval, retraction of the obturator neurovascular bundle may be necessary to visualize, clean, and reduce the posterior column fracture lines and remove debris from the medial aspect of the fracture and hip. Excessive or sustained retraction can similarly injure the obturator nerve and should be avoided. Although it seems far-fetched, the nerve can likewise be injured from deep intrapelvic reduction clamp application through the greater sciatic notch via a posterior exposure. Some transverse and many transverse with associated posterior wall fracture patterns are treated operatively using a posterior exposure. The transverse fracture plane reduction is maintained using a clamp with one limb positioned through the greater sciatic notch onto the quadrilateral surface. The other clamp limb is located at the supra-acetabular area. The clamp application onto the quadrilateral surface risks obturator nerve injury. The other clamp limb must be situated to avoid stretching the sciatic nerve.

The sciatic nerve is most at risk during posterior surgical exposures. The nerve may be traumatically injured by posterior fracture–dislocations from stretch or direct contusion. The sciatic nerve is rarely lacerated by sharp fracture fragment edges. Sciatic nerve injuries have also been noted immediately after manipulative reduction of posterior wall fracture–dislocations due to entrapment of the nerve between the posterior wall fragment and its posterior column fracture plane. Progressive sciatic nerve injuries are known to occur in association with vertical fractures through the posterior column region. For these reasons, the function of the sciatic nerve is detailed prior to manipulative reduction maneuvers and should be monitored along with the patient's vital signs during each nursing shift. The sciatic nerve can also be injured during posterior acetabular repairs. Even in situations of the most dramatic displacements, the sciatic nerve can reliably be found on the dorsal surface of the quadratus femoris muscle and then traced and liberated progressing proximally to the greater sciatic notch. The piriformis muscle is commonly dorsal to the sciatic nerve, but variant muscle bundles of the piriformis are common. For this reason, the nerve and its relationship with the piriformis are fully exposed. Any muscle bundles located anterior to the nerve or those piercing the nerve are excised. In comminuted posterior fractures, small bone and chondral fragments may be impaled within the nerve or its epineurium. These fragments are identified and removed before manipulating or retracting the nerve. The sciatic nerve is relaxed during the operation by positioning the hip in extension and the knee in flexion. In some patients, the rectus femoris muscle is tight such that knee flexion will produce unwanted hip flexion. This can frustrate reduction since the hip flexion force is transferred to the acetabular fracture, allowing the femoral head to displace the fracture fragments. In such situations, the knee is extended and the reduction proceeds, taking care to avoid sciatic nerve stretch. Special retractors have been designed to protect the sciatic nerve during posterior acetabular exposures. The retractor is positioned in the lesser sciatic notch and oriented to be parallel to the sciatic nerve course. The surgeon monitors the retractor position at all times since tilting of the retractor compresses the nerve. The nerve is visualized and protected during the exposure, fracture surface cleaning, reduction, clamp application, and implant placement. A concise preoperative plan outlining the operative details of reduction sequence and implant location diminish the amount of time that the sciatic nerve retraction is needed, further decreasing the risk of injury. Finally, the implants are positioned and located to avoid nerve injury. Screw-and-plate application, especially along the caudal aspect of the posterior column adjacent to the lesser sciatic notch and hamstring origin, should be done under direct visualization to avoid inadvertent sciatic nerve injury.

Intraoperative nerve monitoring has had mixed results in acetabular fracture surgery.[10,63,76,208] Most studies have focused on the sciatic nerve injury during surgery. Spontaneous electromyography (EMG) has been shown to be superior to somatosensory evoked potential monitoring in detecting intraoperative sciatic nerve compromise in acute acetabular surgery. Spontaneous EMG allows more rapid detection and therefore more rapid response to the offending maneuver that should prevent permanent nerve problems. One study demonstrated that routine visualization and protection of the sciatic nerve during surgery obviated the need for intraoperative electrodiagnostic modalities.[132]

The superior gluteal nerve is often forgotten in the grand scheme of acetabular surgery. Most surgeons tenotomize the piriformis muscle once they have ensured its normal dorsal relationship with the sciatic nerve, but they neglect to protect the superior gluteal nerve, especially from stretch injury. The superior gluteal nerve can be injured in a variety of ways. The simplest is due to fracture displacements in the upper aspect of the greater sciatic notch. Not infrequently, the superior gluteal neurovascular bundle is found in continuity but displaced into the fracture surface that has divided the greater sciatic notch. The surgeon can manipulate the unstable fracture fragment and protect the bundle as the fracture surfaces are reduced and clamped. The superior gluteal nerve can also be damaged by excessive or sustained retraction of the gluteus medius and gluteus minimus muscles anterosuperiorly within the surgical wound. Excessive anterior or superior dissection beyond the supra-acetabular region causes stretch injury of the nerve. Surgical exposure alternatives are used when anterosuperior acetabular access is necessary. As long as it does not adversely affect the fracture reduction, hip abduction during the surgical exposure and retraction is helpful to relax the superior gluteal nerve.

Deep Venous Thrombosis

Patients with acetabular fractures are at risk for deep venous thrombosis (DVT). Clinical exam seeking this diagnosis is performed at least daily. Special investigations such as venography, MRI venography, and duplex exams have been advocated. Each method has its associated problems.[20,141,190,197]

The DVT risk is diminished with anticoagulant medications or with mechanical methods such as sequential pneumatic compression.[6] Low-molecular-weight heparin (LMWH) when begun without delay is an effective method of thromboprophylaxis, especially in high-risk patients with acetabular fractures.[194] Some surgeons note increased wound problems in patients treated with LMWH after acetabular fracture surgery.

However, some patients have contraindications to systemic anticoagulation and cannot use sequential limb compression devices because of limb injuries or other reasons. Vena caval filters do not prevent nor treat DVT but do decrease the risk of pulmonary embolus. Recent advances include easier insertion techniques and the development of temporary and removable vena caval filters. Removable filters protect the patients during their most vulnerable clinical phase and are then removed once the risk has normalized. The filters do require the risk of a second procedure for removal.[3,108]

Infection

Fortunately, wound infections after acetabular operations are rare. The infection may be superficial or deep. Deep infections involving the joint are devastating when septic necrosis of the femoral head occurs. Hip irritability is a clinical sign of deep infection involving the joint. Expeditious and thorough surgical wound débridement allows accurate cultures to be obtained. The wound is débrided of necrotic tissues and irrigated appropriately. In most circumstances, the wound is closed over drains and specific antibiotic therapy is directed at the offending organism. The patient's overall medical condition is optimized. Some surgeons recommend halting physical therapy, including range-of-motion exercises, until the wound is sealed and secure. Prior to operative débridement, pelvic radiographs are obtained to rule out fixation failure related to the infection. If recurrent wound infection ensues after surgical débridement and appropriate antibiotics, the surgeon should repeat the wound cultures to assess the potential for superinfection. Open wound management is used for those rare patients with recurrent infections despite adequate débridement and specific antibiotic therapy. Surgical implants may be colonized but should not be considered for removal until the fracture has healed (Figs. 37-42 and 37-43).

Ectopic Bone Formation

Regional ectopic bone formation after acetabular fracture surgery varies in its severity and location.[45,55,87,90,137,166] Craniocerebral trauma and combined simultaneous surgical exposures are two known risk factors. Ectopic bone occurs commonly after posterior and extensile exposures, but rarely after ilioinguinal exposures alone. More severe forms of ectopic bone limit hip movement and therefore impair function. In some patients, ectopic bone forms

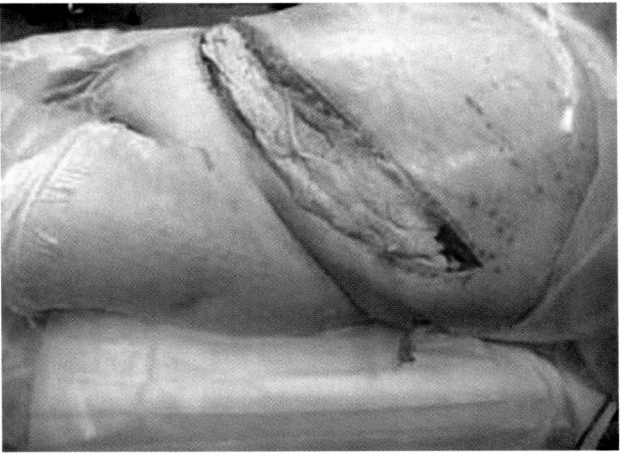

FIGURE 37-42 *This patient developed an acute and deep wound infection after his ilioinguinal exposure for acetabular fracture repair. Initial irrigation and débridement and specific antibiotics failed to control the infection. Open wound management was then used, followed by delayed primary closure.*

around the sciatic nerve and may cause the nerve to be irritable or have altered function.

Clinical studies substantiate the use of oral indomethacin as ectopic bone prophylaxis after acetabular fracture surgery.[125,128,134,136] Similarly, targeted low-dose irradiation decreases the incidence and severity of ectopic bone formation after acetabular surgery.[9,26,32,135] Some patients are unable to take or tolerate oral indomethacin such that rectal administration is considered when appropriate. Irradiation is more costly and time-consuming, and some clinicians are concerned about its short-term effect on wound healing and long-term oncogenic potential.[31]

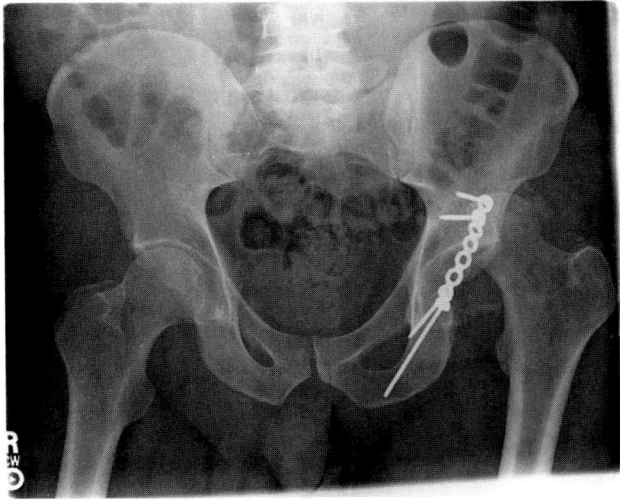

FIGURE 37-43 *This patient had a septic hip dislocation postoperatively. The posterior wall fracture fixation remained intact while the femoral head extruded through the traumatic capsular injury.*

FIGURE 37-44 | *These patients developed excessive ectopic bone after their acetabular fractures. Early excision of the hip region ectopic bone is recommended if the new bone is preventing functional hip movement or is injuring the sciatic nerve.*

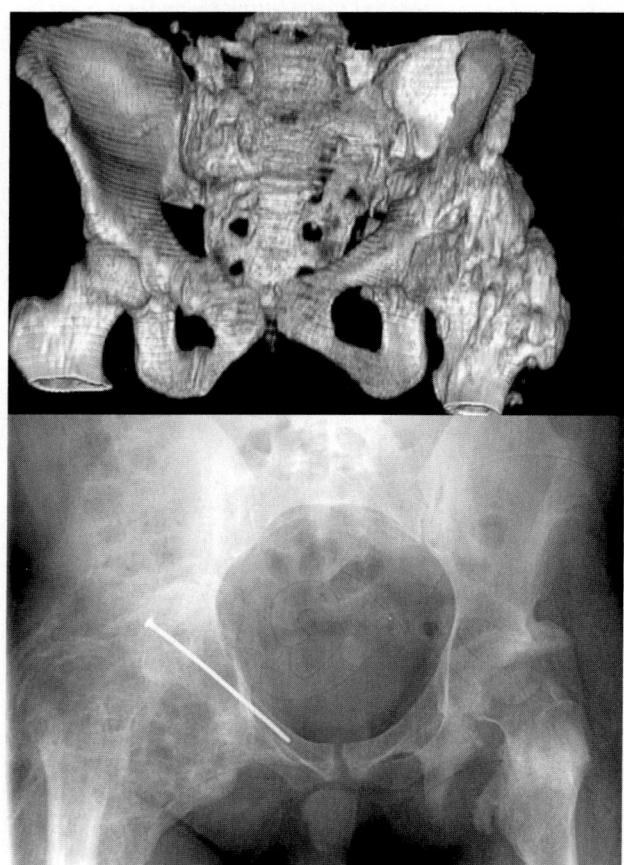

Early surgical excision of ectopic bone is recommended when functional hip range of motion is limited. Since acetabular and femoral head articular cartilage viability is dependant on joint movement, early surgical excision of offending ectopic bone is necessary. Special studies such as bone scans and blood tests to assess ectopic bone maturity prior to excision are not indicated in these patients. Similarly, when the nerve function is adversely affected by ectopic bone, the offending bone is excised and a neuroplasty performed to liberate the nerve and regain function (Fig. 37-44).

Aseptic Necrosis of the Femoral Head

Aseptic femoral head necrosis is an unusual but significant problem after acetabular fracture, especially in young patients. The unique femoral head blood supply is theoretically injured by the traumatic event, causing the necrosis. Hip dislocations and acetabular fracture–dislocations may damage the medial femoral circumflex or lateral epiphyseal vasculature and cause such necrosis.[217] Injury to these blood vessels can also occur during surgery. The quadratus femoris muscle contains the medial femoral circumflex vessels and must be protected and preserved during surgical exposures. During surgery, manipulative devices such as bone hooks along the femoral neck and greater trochanteric regions may also damage these vessels. Patients should be counseled regarding the potential development of aseptic necrosis and its clinical symptoms in order to improve early detection. MRI evaluations are compromised somewhat by the local acetabular fixation devices.

Arthritis

Post-traumatic arthritis causes hip stiffness, pain, and a poor clinical result.[165] Most studies agree that improved fracture reduction decreases the incidence and severity of post-traumatic arthritis.[109,131,133] Chondral injury, especially of the acetabular dome, is directly related to arthritic changes (Fig. 37-45).

Fixation Error

Fixation errors usually follow insufficient exposure and reduction.[146,147,178,180,181] The mechanical features of each fixation construct should be planned preoperatively and then critically assessed prior to wound closure. It is often helpful to draw each fracture fragment and its related fixation construct on a sterile towel to ensure that each fracture fragment has achieved sufficient stability before closing the wound. The hip should be stressed under direct visualization to guarantee stability (Fig. 37-46).

FIGURE 37-45 | *This patient developed symptomatic hip arthritis less than 1 year after his acetabular fracture repair.*

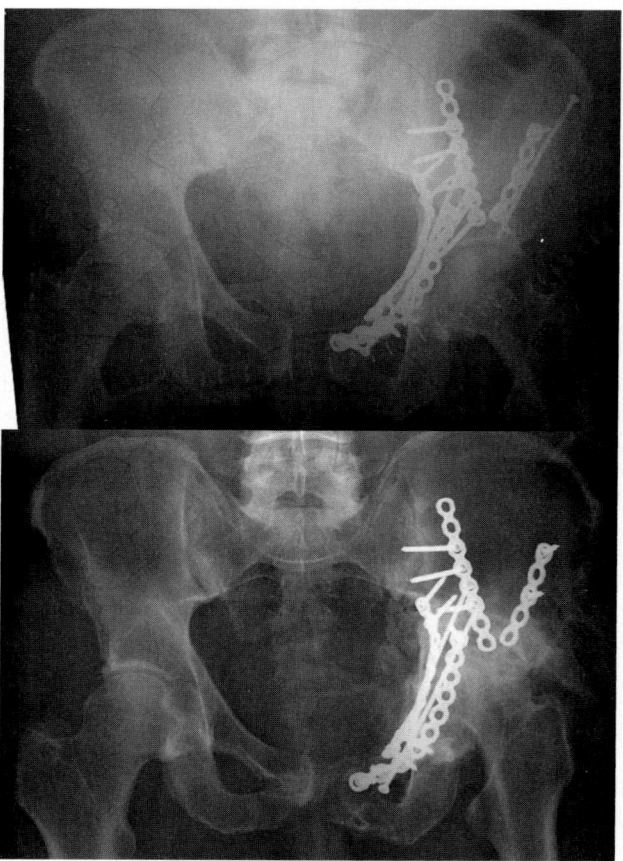

FIGURE 37-46 *A, B, This patient presented with hip pain several months after attempted repair of his transverse fracture with an associated posterior wall acetabular component. The anteroposterior radiograph identifies fixation failure, redislocation, and fracture displacement. The film highlights several important facts. The fracture may or may not have been well reduced. The implant was not well positioned on the wall component to maintain fixation. The fixation of the caudal unstable transverse fragment was similarly insufficient. Perhaps longer screws into the ischium or another plate would have added to the construct. Perhaps fixation of the anterior column component of the transverse fracture using a medullary screw would have been helpful. The reconstruction procedure required an initial anterior exposure to remove the fracture callus, followed by a posterior exposure for sciatic neuroplasty, and reduction of the head, wall, and transverse components. A sciatic nerve injury resulted from the reconstructive procedure.*

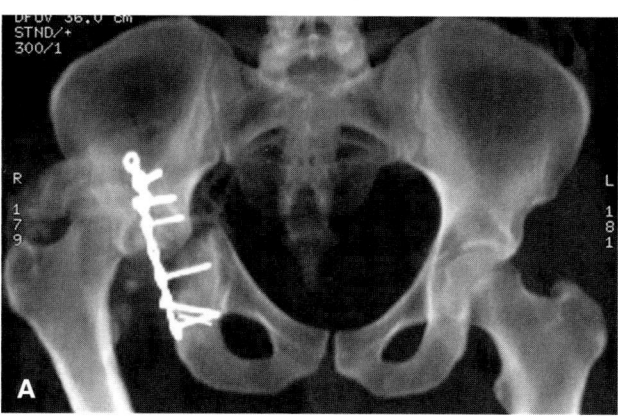

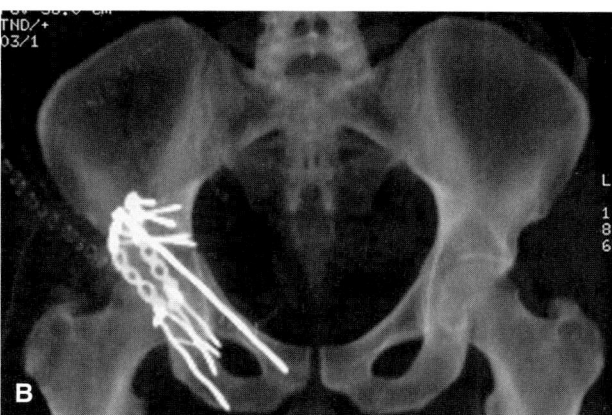

SUMMARY

Acetabular fractures occur rarely and are quite variable. The anatomy and radiology are complex but critical to understanding the injuries and their classification. Early management follows routine resuscitation protocols, and fracture–dislocations should be reduced expediently. Operative reduction and stable fixation is advocated for displaced and unstable fractures. An appropriate surgical exposure facilitates an accurate fracture reduction, which is vital for improved outcomes. Stable fixation is mandatory to allow early rehabilitation of the joint and patient. A variety of complications are well known and should be avoided when possible. The treatment of acetabular fractures is challenging for orthopedic surgeons in many ways, but experience and modern technologies should continue to advance this clinical area.

REFERENCES

1. al-Qahtani, S.; O'Connor, G. Acetabular fractures before and after the introduction of seatbelt legislation. Can J Surg 39:317–320, 1996.
2. Alexander, R.D.; Grimm, L.; Vrahas, M.S. The effect of knee immobilization on degree of hip flexion: A clinical correlation with posterior wall acetabular fractures. Am J Orthop 26:345–347, 1997.
3. Allen, T.L.; Carter, J.L.; Morris, B.J.; et al. Retrievable vena cava filters in trauma patients for high-risk prophylaxis and prevention of pulmonary embolism. Am J Surg 189:656–661, 2005.
4. Alonso, J.E.; Davila, R.; Bradley, E. Extended iliofemoral versus triradiate approaches in management of associated acetabular fractures. Clin Orthop Relat Res 305:81–87, 1994.
5. Alonso, J.E.; Volgas, D.A.; Giordano, V.; et al. A review of the treatment of hip dislocations associated with acetabular fractures. Clin Orthop Relat Res 377:32–43, 2000.
6. Anglen, J.O.; Bagby, C.; George, R. A randomized comparison of sequential-gradient calf compression with intermittent plantar compression for prevention of venous thrombosis in orthopedic trauma patients: Preliminary results. Am J Orthop 27:53–58, 1998.
7. Anglen, J.O.; Burd, T.A.; Hendricks, K.J.; et al. The "Gull Sign": A harbinger of failure for internal fixation of geriatric acetabular fractures. J Orthop Trauma 17:625–634, 2003.
8. Anglen, J.O.; Hughes, M. Trochanteric osteotomy for incarcerated hip dislocation due to interposed posterior wall fragments. Orthopedics 27:213–216, 2004.
9. Anglen, J.O.; Moore, K.D. Prevention of heterotopic bone formation after acetabular fracture fixation by single-dose radiation therapy: A preliminary report. J Orthop Trauma 10:258–263, 1996.

10. Arrington, E.D.; Hochschild, D.P.; Steinagle, T.J.; et al. Monitoring of somatosensory and motor evoked potentials during open reduction and internal fixation of pelvis and acetabular fractures. Orthopedics 23:1081–1083, 2000.

11. Attias, N.; Lindsey, R.W.; Starr, A.J.; et al. The use of a virtual three-dimensional model to evaluate the intraosseous space available for percutaneous screw fixation of acetabular fractures. J Bone Joint Surg [Br] 87:1520–1523, 2005.

12. Bacarese-Hamilton, I.A.; Bhamra, M. Small bowel entrapment following acetabular fracture. Injury 22:242–244, 1991.

13. Bartlett, C.S.; DiFelice, G.S.; Buly, R.L.; et al. Cardiac arrest as a result of intraabdominal extravasation of fluid during arthroscopic removal of a loose body from the hip joint of a patient with an acetabular fracture. J Orthop Trauma 12:294–299, 1998.

14. Baumgaertner, M.R. Fractures of the posterior wall of the acetabulum. J Am Acad Orthop Surg 7:54–65, 1999.

15. Beaule, P.E.; Dorey, F.J.; Matta, J.M. Letournel classification for acetabular fractures. Assessment of interobserver and intraobserver reliability. J Bone Joint Surg [Am] 85:1704–1709, 2003.

16. Beaule, P.E.; Griffin, D.B.; Matta, J.M. The Levine anterior approach for total hip replacement as the treatment for an acute acetabular fracture. J Orthop Trauma 18:623–629, 2004.

17. Berg, E.E. Charcot arthropathy after acetabular fracture. J Bone Joint Surg [Br] 79:742–745, 1997.

18. Berton, C.; Bachour, F.; Migaud, H.; et al. [A new type of acetabular fracture: "True" posterosuperior fracture, a case report]. Rev Chir Orthop Reparatrice Appar Mot 93:93–97, 2007.

19. Bhandari, M.; Matta, J.; Ferguson, T.; et al. Predictors of clinical and radiological outcome in patients with fractures of the acetabulum and concomitant posterior dislocation of the hip. J Bone Joint Surg [Br] 88:1618–1624, 2006.

20. Borer, D.S.; Starr, A.J.; Reinert, C.M.; et al. The effect of screening for deep vein thrombosis on the prevalence of pulmonary embolism in patients with fractures of the pelvis or acetabulum: A review of 973 patients. J Orthop Trauma 19:92–95, 2005.

21. Borrelli, J., Jr.; Goldfarb, C.; Catalano, L.; et al. Assessment of articular fragment displacement in acetabular fractures: A comparison of computerized tomography and plain radiographs. J Orthop Trauma 16:449–456; discussion 456–457, 2002.

22. Borrelli, J., Jr.; Goldfarb, C.; Ricci, W.; et al. Functional outcome after isolated acetabular fractures. J Orthop Trauma 16:73–81, 2002.

23. Borrelli, J., Jr.; Ricci, W.M.; Anglen, J.O.; et al. Muscle strength recovery and its effects on outcome after open reduction and internal fixation of acetabular fractures. J Orthop Trauma 20:388–395, 2006.

24. Bosse, M.J. Posterior acetabular wall fractures: A technique for screw placement. J Orthop Trauma 5: 167–172, 1991.

25. Bosse, M.J.; Poka, A.; Reinert, C.M.; et al. Preoperative angiographic assessment of the superior gluteal artery in acetabular fractures requiring extensile surgical exposures. J Orthop Trauma 2:303–307, 1988.

26. Bosse, M.J.; Poka, A.; Reinert, C.M.; et al. Heterotopic ossification as a complication of acetabular fracture. Prophylaxis with low-dose irradiation. J Bone Joint Surg [Am] 70:1231–1237, 1988.

27. Bray, T.J.; Esser, M.; Fulkerson, L. Osteotomy of the trochanter in open reduction and internal fixation of acetabular fractures. J Bone Joint Surg [Am] 69: 711–717, 1987.

28. Brown, G.A.; Willis, M.C.; Firoozbakhsh, K.; et al. Computed tomography image-guided surgery in complex acetabular fractures. Clin Orthop Relat Res 370:219–226, 2000.

29. Brueton, R.N. A review of 40 acetabular fractures: The importance of early surgery. Injury 24:171–174, 1993.

30. Brumback, R.J.; Holt, E.S.; McBride, M.S.; et al. Acetabular depression fracture accompanying posterior fracture dislocation of the hip. J Orthop Trauma 4:42–48, 1990.

31. Burd, T.A.; Hughes, M.S.; Anglen, J.O. Heterotopic ossification prophylaxis with indomethacin increases the risk of long-bone nonunion. J Bone Joint Surg [Br] 85:700–705, 2003.

32. Burd, T.A.; Lowry, K.J.; Anglen, J.O. Indomethacin compared with localized irradiation for the prevention of heterotopic ossification following surgical treatment of acetabular fractures. J Bone Joint Surg [Am] 83:1783–1788, 2001.

33. Caterini, R.; Farsetti, P.; Potenza, V.; et al. Immediate passive mobilization of the hip after internal fixation of acetabular fractures. Chir Organi Mov 85:243–249, 2000.

34. Chang, J.K.; Gill, S.S.; Zura, R.D.; et al. Comparative strength of three methods of fixation of transverse acetabular fractures. Clin Orthop Relat Res 392:433–441, 2001.

35. Chelly, J.E.; Casati, A.; Al-Samsam, T.; et al. Continuous lumbar plexus block for acute postoperative pain management after open reduction and internal fixation of acetabular fractures. J Orthop Trauma 17:362–367, 2003.

36. Chen, A.L.; Wolinsky, P.R.; Tejwani, N.C. Hypogastric artery disruption associated with acetabular fracture. A report of two cases. J Bone Joint Surg [Am] 85:333–338, 2003.

37. Chen, C.M.; Chiu, F.Y.; Lo, W.H.; et al. Cerclage wiring in displaced both-column fractures of the acetabulum. Injury 32:391–394, 2001.

38. Cheng, S.L.; Rosati, C.; Waddell, J.P. Fatal hemorrhage caused by vascular injury associated with an acetabular fracture. J Trauma 38:208–209, 1995.

39. Chiu, F.Y.; Chen, C.M.; Lo, W.H. Surgical treatment of displaced acetabular fractures—72 cases followed for 10 (6–14) years. Injury 31:181–185, 2003.

40. Cimerman, M.; Kristan, A. Preoperative planning in pelvic and acetabular surgery: The value of advanced computerised planning modules. Injury 38:442–449, 2007.

41. Cole, J.D.; Bolhofner, B.R. Acetabular fracture fixation via a modified Stoppa limited intrapelvic approach. Description of operative technique and preliminary treatment results. Clin Orthop Relat Res 305:112–123, 1994.

42. Crowl, A.C.; Kahler, D.M. Closed reduction and percutaneous fixation of anterior column acetabular fractures. Comput Aided Surg 7:169–178, 2002.

43. Dakin, G.J.; Eberhardt, A.W.; Alonso, J.E.; et al. Acetabular fracture patterns: Associations with motor vehicle crash information. J Trauma 47:1063–1071, 1999.

44. Darmanis, S.; Bircher, M. Fractures of the acetabulum in osteogenesis imperfecta. J Bone Joint Surg [Br] 88:670–672, 2006.

45. Daum, W.J.; Scarborough, M.T.; Gordon, W., Jr.; et al. Heterotopic ossification and other perioperative complications of acetabular fractures. J Orthop Trauma 6:427–432, 1992.

46. Davoli, O.; Bilotta, T.W.; Villani, S.; et al. The opportunity of rehabilitation treatment in acetabular fractures treated by osteosynthesis. Chir Organi Mov 83:237–247, 1998.

47. de Ridder, V.A.; de Lange, S.; Popta, J.V. Anatomical variations of the lateral femoral cutaneous nerve and the consequences for surgery. J Orthop Trauma 13:207–211, 1999.

48. Dickinson, W.H.; Duwelius, P.J.; Colville, M.R. Muscle strength testing following surgery for acetabular fractures. J Orthop Trauma 7:39–46, 1993.

49. DiPasquale, T.; Greiwe, R.M.; Simmons, P.; et al. Temporary partial intra-iliac balloon occlusion for the treatment of acetabulum fracture in a Jehovah's Witness: A case report. J Orthop Trauma 19: 415–419, 2005.

50. Ebraheim, N.A.; Savolaine, E.R.; Hoeflinger, M.J.; et al. Radiological diagnosis of screw penetration of the hip joint in acetabular fracture reconstruction. J Orthop Trauma 3:196–201, 1989.

51. Epstein, H.C. Posterior fracture–dislocations of the hip; long-term follow-up. J Bone Joint Surg [Am] 56:1103–1127, 1974.

52. Fassler, P.R.; Swiontkowski, M.F.; Kilroy, A.W.; et al. Injury of the sciatic nerve associated with acetabular fracture. J Bone Joint Surg [Am] 75:1157–1166, 1993.

53. Fica, G.; Cordova, M.; Guzman, L.; et al. Open reduction and internal fixation of acetabular fractures. Int Orthop 22:348–351, 1998.

54. Frank, J.L.; Reimer, B.L.; Raves, J.J. Traumatic iliofemoral arterial injury: An association with high anterior acetabular fractures. J Vasc Surg 10:198–201, 1989.

55. Ghalambor, N.; Matta, J.M.; Bernstein, L. Heterotopic ossification following operative treatment of acetabular fracture. An analysis of risk factors. Clin Orthop Relat Res 305:96–105, 1994.

56. Giannoudis, P.V.; Da Costa, A.A.; Raman, R.; et al. Double-crush syndrome after acetabular fractures. A sign of poor prognosis. J Bone Joint Surg [Br] 87:401–407, 2005.

57. Gorczyca, J.T.; Powell, J.N.; Tile, M. Lateral extension of the ilioinguinal incision in the operative treatment of acetabulum fractures. Injury 26:207–212, 1995.

58. Goulet, J.A.; Bray, T.J. Complex acetabular fractures. Clin Orthop Relat Res 240:9–20, 1989.

59. Goulet, J.A.; Bray, T.J.; Timmerman, L.A.; et al. Intraoperative autologous transfusion in orthopaedic patients. J Bone Joint Surg [Am] 71:3–8, 1989.

60. Goulet, J.A.; Rouleau, J.P.; Mason, D.J.; et al. Comminuted fractures of the posterior wall of the acetabulum. A biomechanical evaluation of fixation methods. J Bone Joint Surg [Am] 76:1457–1463, 1994.

61. Griffin, D.B.; Beaule, P.E.; Matta, J.M. Safety and efficacy of the extended iliofemoral approach in the treatment of complex fractures of the acetabulum. J Bone Joint Surg [Br] 87:1391–1396, 2005.

62. Gruson, K.I.; Moed, B.R. Injury of the femoral nerve associated with acetabular fracture. J Bone Joint Surg [Am] 85:428–431, 2003.

63. Haidukewych, G.J.; Scaduto, J.; Herscovici, D., Jr.; et al. Iatrogenic nerve injury in acetabular fracture surgery: A comparison of monitored and unmonitored procedures. J Orthop Trauma 16:297–301, 2002.

64. Hak, D.J.; Hamel, A.J.; Bay, B.K.; et al. Consequences of transverse acetabular fracture malreduction on load transmission across the hip joint. J Orthop Trauma 12:90–100, 1998.

65. Hak, D.J.; Olson, S.A.; Matta, J.M. Diagnosis and management of closed internal degloving injuries associated with pelvic and acetabular fractures: The Morel-Lavallee lesion. J Trauma 42:1046–1051, 1997.

66. Hammit, M.D.; Cole, P.A.; Kregor, P.J. Massive perineal wound slough after treatment of complex pelvic and acetabular fractures using a traction table. J Orthop Trauma 16:601–605, 2002.

67. Hardy, S.L. Femoral nerve palsy associated with an associated posterior wall transverse acetabular fracture. J Orthop Trauma 11:40–42, 1997.

68. Harris, J.H., Jr.; Coupe, K.J.; Lee, J.S.; et al. Acetabular fractures revisited: Part 2, a new CT-based classification. AJR Am J Roentgenol 182:1367–1375, 2004.

69. Harris, J.H.; Coupe, K.J.; Lee, J.S.; et al. Acetabular fractures revisited: A new CT-based classification. Semin Musculoskelet Radiol 9:150–160, 2005.

70. Harris, J.H., Jr.; Lee, J.S.; Coupe, K.J.; et al. Acetabular fractures revisited: Part 1, redefinition of the Letournel anterior column. AJR Am J Roentgenol 182:1363–1366, 2004.

71. Heck, B.E.; Ebraheim, N.A.; Foetisch, C. Direct complications of trochanteric osteotomy in open reduction and internal fixation of acetabular fractures. Am J Orthop 26:124–128, 1997.

72. Heeg, M.; de Ridder, V.A.; Tornetta, P., 3rd; et al. Acetabular fractures in children and adolescents. Clin Orthop Relat Res 376:80–86, 2000.

73. Heeg, M.; Klasen, H.J.; Visser, J.D. Acetabular fractures in children and adolescents. J Bone Joint Surg [Br] 71:418–421, 1989.

74. Heeg, M.; Klasen, H.J.; Visser, J.D. Operative treatment for acetabular fractures. J Bone Joint Surg [Br] 72:383–386, 1990.

75. Heeg, M.; Zimmerman, K.W.; Klasen, H.J. Entrapment of the ureter following indirect reduction of an acetabular fracture. A case report. J Bone Joint Surg [Am] 76:913–915, 1994.

76. Helfet, D.L.; Anand, N.; Malkani, A.L.; et al. Intraoperative monitoring of motor pathways during operative fixation of acute acetabular fractures. J Orthop Trauma 11:2–6, 1997.

77. Helfet, D.L.; Borrelli, J., Jr.; DiPasquale, T.; et al. Stabilization of acetabular fractures in elderly patients. J Bone Joint Surg [Am] 74:753–765, 1992.

78. Helfet, D.L.; Schmeling, G.J. Management of complex acetabular fractures through single non-extensile exposures. Clin Orthop Relat Res 305:58–68, 1994.

79. Hesp, W.L.; Goris, R.J. Conservative treatment of fractures of the acetabulum. Results after longtime follow-up. Acta Chir Belg 88:27–32, 1988.

80. Huegli, R.W.; Staedele, H.; Messmer, P.; et al. Displaced anterior column acetabular fracture: Closed reduction and percutaneous CT-navigated fixation. Acta Radiol 45:618–621, 2004.

81. Im, G.I.; Shin, Y.W.; Song, Y.J. Fractures to the posterior wall of the acetabulum managed with screws alone. J Trauma 58:300–303, 2005.

82. Jacob, A.L.; Suhm, N.; Kaim, A.; et al. Coronal acetabular fractures: The anterior approach in computed tomography-navigated minimally invasive percutaneous fixation. Cardiovasc Intervent Radiol 23:327–331, 2000.

83. Jakob, M.; Droeser, R.; Zobrist, R.; et al. A less invasive anterior intrapelvic approach for the treatment of acetabular fractures and pelvic ring injuries. J Trauma 60:1364–1370, 2006.

84. Jimenez, M.L.; Tile, M.; Schenk, R.S. Total hip replacement after acetabular fracture. Orthop Clin North Am 28:435–446, 1997.

85. Jimenez, M.L.; Vrahas, M.S. Surgical approaches to the acetabulum. Orthop Clin North Am 28:419–434, 1997.

86. Johnson, E.E.; Eckardt, J.J.; Letournel, E. Extrinsic femoral artery occlusion following internal fixation of an acetabular fracture. A case report. Clin Orthop Relat Res 217:209–213, 1987.

87. Johnson, E.E.; Kay, R.M.; Dorey, F.J. Heterotopic ossification prophylaxis following operative treatment of acetabular fracture. Clin Orthop Relat Res 305:88–95, 1994.

88. Johnson, E.E.; Matta, J.M.; Mast, J.W.; et al. Delayed reconstruction of acetabular fractures 21–120 days following injury. Clin Orthop Relat Res 305:20–30, 1994.

89. Juliano, P.J.; Bosse, M.J.; Edwards, K.J. The superior gluteal artery in complex acetabular procedures. A cadaveric angiographic study. J Bone Joint Surg [Am] 76:244–248, 1994.

90. Kaempffe, F.A.; Bone, L.B.; Border, J.R. Open reduction and internal fixation of acetabular fractures: Heterotopic ossification and other complications of treatment. J Orthop Trauma 5:439–445, 1991.

91. Kang, C.S.; Min, B.W. Cable fixation in displaced fractures of the acetabulum: 21 patients followed for 2–8 years. Acta Orthop Scand 73:619–624, 2002.

92. Karunakar, M.A.; Goulet, J.A.; Mueller, K.L.; et al. Operative treatment of unstable pediatric pelvis and acetabular fractures. J Pediatr Orthop 25:34–38, 2005.

93. Karunakar, M.A.; Le, T.T.; Bosse, M.J. The modified ilioinguinal approach. J Orthop Trauma 18:379–383, 2004.

94. Karunakar, M.A.; Shah, S.N.; Jerabek, S. Body mass index as a predictor of complications after operative treatment of acetabular fractures. J Bone Joint Surg [Am] 87:1498–1502, 2005.

95. Kebaish, A.S.; Roy, A.; Rennie, W. Displaced acetabular fractures: long-term follow-up. J Trauma 31:1539–1542, 1991.

96. Keith, J.E., Jr.; Brashear, H.R., Jr.; Guilford, W.B. Stability of posterior fracture–dislocations of the hip. Quantitative assessment using computed tomography. J Bone Joint Surg [Am] 70:711–714, 1988.

97. Kellam, J.F.; Messer, A. Evaluation of the role of coronal and sagittal axial CT scan reconstructions for the imaging of acetabular fractures. Clin Orthop Relat Res 305:152–159, 1994.

98. Kloen, P.; Siebenrock, K.A.; Ganz, R. Modification of the ilioinguinal approach. J Orthop Trauma 16:586–593, 2002.

99. Konig, B.; Schaser, K.; Schaffler, A.; et al. [Percutaneous reduction and stabilization of a dislocated acetabular fracture: Case report.]. Unfallchirurg 109:328–331, 2006.

100. Konrath, G.A.; Hamel, A.J.; Guerin, J.; et al. Biomechanical evaluation of impaction fractures of the femoral head. J Orthop Trauma 13:407–413, 1999.

101. Konrath, G.A.; Hamel, A.J.; Sharkey, N.A.; et al. Biomechanical evaluation of a low anterior wall fracture: Correlation with the CT subchondral arc. J Orthop Trauma 12:152–158, 1998.

102. Konrath, G.A.; Hamel, A.J.; Sharkey, N.A.; et al. Biomechanical consequences of anterior column fracture of the acetabulum. J Orthop Trauma 12:547–552, 1998.

103. Kottmeier, S.; Born, C.T.; Saul, H. Laparoscopic retrieval of a migrating intrapelvic pin: Case report and review of the literature. J Trauma 35:952–955, 1993.

104. Kreder, H.J.; Rozen, N.; Borkhoff, C.M.; et al. Determinants of functional outcome after simple and complex acetabular fractures involving the posterior wall. J Bone Joint Surg [Br] 88:776–782, 2006.

105. Kregor, P.J.; Templeman, D. Associated injuries complicating the management of acetabular fractures: Review and case studies. Orthop Clin North Am 33:73–95, viii, 2002.

106. Kuhlman, J.E.; Fishman, E.K.; Ney, D.R.; et al. Nonunion of acetabular fractures: Evaluation with interactive multiplanar CT. J Orthop Trauma 3:33–40, 1989.

107. Laird, A.; Keating, J.F. Acetabular fractures: A 16-year prospective epidemiological study. J Bone Joint Surg [Br] 87:969–973, 2005.

108. Lam, R.C.; Bush, R.L.; Lin, P.H.; et al. Early technical and clinical results with retrievable inferior vena caval filters. Vascular 12:233–237, 2004.

109. Letournel, E. Acetabulum fractures: Classification and management. Clin Orthop Relat Res 151:81–106, 1980.

110. Letournel, E. Diagnosis and treatment of nonunions and malunions of acetabular fractures. Orthop Clin North Am 21:769–788, 1990.

111. Letournel, E. The treatment of acetabular fractures through the ilioinguinal approach. Clin Orthop Relat Res 292:62–76, 1993.

112. Leunig, M.; Sledge, J.B.; Gill, T.J.; et al. Traumatic labral avulsion from the stable rim: A constant pathology in displaced transverse acetabular fractures. Arch Orthop Trauma Surg 123:392–395, 2003.

113. Levine, R.G.; Renard, R.; Behrens, F.F.; et al. Biomechanical consequences of secondary congruence after both-column acetabular fracture. J Orthop Trauma 16:87–91, 2002.

114. Liebergall, M.; Mosheiff, R.; Low, J.; et al. Acetabular fractures. Clinical outcome of surgical treatment. Clin Orthop Relat Res 366:205–216, 1999.

115. Mack, L.A.; Harley, J.D.; Winquist, R.A. CT of acetabular fractures: Analysis of fracture patterns. AJR Am J Roentgenol 138:407–412, 1982.

116. Magid, D.; Fishman, E.K.; Brooker, A.F., Jr.; et al. Multiplanar computed tomography of acetabular fractures. J Comput Assist Tomogr 10:778–783, 1986.

117. Magid, D.; Fishman, E.K.; Ney, D.R.; et al. Acetabular and pelvic fractures in the pediatric patient: Value of two- and three-dimensional imaging. J Pediatr Orthop 12:621–625, 1992.

118. Malkani, A.L.; Voor, M.J.; Rennirt, G.; et al. Increased peak contact stress after incongruent reduction of transverse acetabular fractures: A cadaveric model. J Trauma 51:704–709, 2001.

119. Martinez, C.R.; Di Pasquale, T.G.; Helfet, D.L.; et al. Evaluation of acetabular fractures with two- and three-dimensional CT. Radiographics 12:227–242, 1992.

120. Matta, J.M. Fractures of the acetabulum: Accuracy of reduction and clinical results in patients managed operatively within three weeks after the injury. J Bone Joint Surg [Am] 78:1632–1645, 1996.

121. Matta, J.M. Operative treatment of acetabular fractures through the ilioinguinal approach: A 10-year perspective. J Orthop Trauma 20(1 Suppl):S20–S29, 2006.

122. Matta, J.M.; Anderson, L.M.; Epstein, H.C.; et al. Fractures of the acetabulum. A retrospective analysis. Clin Orthop Relat Res 205:230–240, 1986.

123. Matta, J.M.; Merritt, P.O. Displaced acetabular fractures. Clin Orthop Relat Res 230:83–97, 1988.

124. Matta, J.M.; Olson, S.A. Factors related to hip muscle weakness following fixation of acetabular fractures. Orthopedics 23:231–235, 2000.

125. Matta, J.M.; Siebenrock, K.A. Does indomethacin reduce heterotopic bone formation after operations for acetabular fractures? A prospective randomised study. J Bone Joint Surg [Br] 79:959–963, 1997.

126. Mayo, K.A.; Letournel, E.; Matta, J.M.; et al. Surgical revision of malreduced acetabular fractures. Clin Orthop Relat Res 305:47–52, 1994.

127. McCardel, B.R.; Dahners, L.E.; Renner, J.B. Kirschner wire migration from the pelvis to the heart and a new method of fixation of articular fracture fragments, acetabular reconstruction. J Orthop Trauma 3:257–259, 1989.

128. McLaren, A.C. Prophylaxis with indomethacin for heterotopic bone. After open reduction of fractures of the acetabulum. J Bone Joint Surg [Am] 72:245–247, 1990.

129. Mears, D.C. Surgical treatment of acetabular fractures in elderly patients with osteoporotic bone. J Am Acad Orthop Surg 7:128–141, 1999.

130. Mears, D.C.; Velyvis, J.H. Acute total hip arthroplasty for selected displaced acetabular fractures: Two to twelve-year results. J Bone Joint Surg [Am] 84:1–9, 2002.

131. Mears, D.C.; Velyvis, J.H.; Chang, C.P. Displaced acetabular fractures managed operatively: Indicators of outcome. Clin Orthop Relat Res 407:173–186, 2003.

132. Middlebrooks, E.S.; Sims, S.H.; Kellam, J.F.; et al. Incidence of sciatic nerve injury in operatively treated acetabular fractures without somatosensory evoked potential monitoring. J Orthop Trauma 11:327–329, 1997.

133. Moed, B.R.; Carr, S.E.; Gruson, K.I.; et al. Computed tomographic assessment of fractures of the posterior wall of the acetabulum after operative treatment. J Bone Joint Surg [Am] 85:512–522, 2003.

134. Moed, B.R.; Karges, D.E. Prophylactic indomethacin for the prevention of heterotopic ossification after

acetabular fracture surgery in high-risk patients. J Orthop Trauma 8:34–39, 1994.

135. Moed, B.R.; Letournel, E. Low-dose irradiation and indomethacin prevent heterotopic ossification after acetabular fracture surgery. J Bone Joint Surg [Br] 76:895–900, 1994.

136. Moed, B.R.; Maxey, J.W. The effect of indomethacin on heterotopic ossification following acetabular fracture surgery. J Orthop Trauma 7:33–38, 1993.

137. Moed, B.R.; Smith, S.T. Three-view radiographic assessment of heterotopic ossification after acetabular fracture surgery. J Orthop Trauma 10:93–98, 1996.

138. Moed, B.R.; Willson Carr, S.E.; Watson, J.T. Results of operative treatment of fractures of the posterior wall of the acetabulum. J Bone Joint Surg [Am] 84:752–758, 2002.

139. Moed, B.R.; Yu, P.H.; Gruson, K.I. Functional outcomes of acetabular fractures. J Bone Joint Surg [Am] 85:1879–1883, 2003.

140. Mohanty, K.; Taha, W.; Powell, J.N. Non-union of acetabular fractures. Injury 35:787–790, 2004.

141. Montgomery, K.D.; Potter, H.G.; Helfet, D.L. The detection and management of proximal deep venous thrombosis in patients with acute acetabular fractures: A follow-up report. J Orthop Trauma 11:330–336, 1997.

142. Moroni, A.; Caja, V.L.; Sabato, C.; et al. Surgical treatment of both-column fractures by staged combined ilioinguinal and Kocher–Langenbeck approaches. Injury 26:219–224, 1995.

143. Mouhsine, E.; Garofalo, R.; Borens, O.; et al. Percutaneous retrograde screwing for stabilisation of acetabular fractures. Injury 36:1330–1336, 2005.

144. Mullis, B.H.; Dahners, L.E. Hip arthroscopy to remove loose bodies after traumatic dislocation. J Orthop Trauma 20:22–26, 2006.

145. Murphy, D.; Kaliszer, M.; Rice, J.; et al. Outcome after acetabular fracture. Prognostic factors and their inter-relationships. Injury 34:512–517, 2003.

146. Norris, B.L.; Hahn, D.H.; Bosse, M.J.; et al. Intraoperative fluoroscopy to evaluate fracture reduction and hardware placement during acetabular surgery. J Orthop Trauma 13:414–417, 1999.

147. O'Shea, K.; Quinlan, J.F.; Waheed, K.; et al. The usefulness of computed tomography following open reduction and internal fixation of acetabular fractures. J Orthop Surg (Hong Kong) 14:127–132, 2006.

148. Oh, C.W.; Kim, P.T.; Park, B.C.; et al. Results after operative treatment of transverse acetabular fractures. J Orthop Sci 11:478–484, 2006.

149. Ohashi, K.; El-Khoury, G.Y.; Abu-Zahra, K.W.; et al. Interobserver agreement for Letournel acetabular fracture classification with multidetector CT: Are standard Judet radiographs necessary? Radiology 241:386–391, 2006.

150. Olson, S.A.; Bay, B.K.; Chapman, M.W.; et al. Biomechanical consequences of fracture and repair of the posterior wall of the acetabulum. J Bone Joint Surg [Am] 77:1184–1192, 1995.

151. Olson, S.A.; Bay, B.K.; Pollak, A.N.; et al. The effect of variable size posterior wall acetabular fractures on contact characteristics of the hip joint. J Orthop Trauma 10:395–402, 1996.

152. Olson, S.A.; Matta, J.M. The computerized tomography subchondral arc: A new method of assessing acetabular articular continuity after fracture (a preliminary report). J Orthop Trauma 7:402–413, 1993.

153. Oransky, M.; Sanguinetti, C. Surgical treatment of displaced acetabular fractures: Results of 50 consecutive cases. J Orthop Trauma 7:28–32, 1993.

154. Ovre, S.; Madsen, J.E.; Roise, O. Transitional transverse acetabular fractures: Differences between fractures with a large posterio-superior fragment and the inverse T-fracture—A report of 10 unusual cases. Acta Orthop 76:803–808, 2005.

155. Pals, S.D.; Brown, C.W.; Friermood, T.G. Open reduction and internal fixation of an acetabular fracture during pregnancy. J Orthop Trauma 6:379–381, 1992.

156. Pantazopoulos, T.; Nicolopoulos, C.S.; Babis, G.C.; et al. Surgical treatment of acetabular posterior wall fractures. Injury 24:319–323, 1993.

157. Parker, P.J.; Copeland, C. Percutaneous fluoroscopic screw fixation of acetabular fractures. Injury 28:597–600, 1997.

158. Patel, N.H.; Hunter, J.; Weber, T.G.; et al. Rotational imaging of complex acetabular fractures. J Orthop Trauma 12:59–63, 1998.

159. Peterson, H.A.; Robertson, R.C. Premature partial closure of the triradiate cartilage treated with excision of a physical osseous bar. Case report with a fourteen-year follow-up. J Bone Joint Surg [Am] 79:767–770, 1997.

160. Petrisor, B.A.; Bhandari, M.; Orr, R.D.; et al. Improving reliability in the classification of fractures of the acetabulum. Arch Orthop Trauma Surg 123:228–233, 2003.

161. Plaisier, B.R.; Meldon, S.W.; Super, D.M.; et al. Improved outcome after early fixation of acetabular fractures. Injury 31:81–84, 2000.

162. Ponsen, K.J.; Joosse, P.; Schigt, A.; et al. Internal fracture fixation using the Stoppa approach in pelvic ring and acetabular fractures: Technical aspects and operative results. J Trauma 61:662–667, 2006.

163. Probe, R.; Reeve, R.; Lindsey, R.W. Femoral artery thrombosis after open reduction of an acetabular fracture. Clin Orthop Relat Res 283:258–260, 1992.

164. Qureshi, A.A.; Archdeacon, M.T.; Jenkins, M.A.; et al. Infrapectineal plating for acetabular fractures: A technical adjunct to internal fixation. J Orthop Trauma 18:175–178, 2004.

165. Ragnarsson, B.; Mjoberg, B. Arthrosis after surgically treated acetabular fractures. A retrospective study of 60 cases. Acta Orthop Scand 63:511–514, 1992.

166. Rath, E.M.; Russell, G.V., Jr.; Washington, W.J.; et al. Gluteus minimus necrotic muscle debridement diminishes heterotopic ossification after acetabular fracture fixation. Injury 33:751–756, 2002.

167. Reilly, M.C.; Olson, S.A.; Tornetta, P., 3rd; et al. Superior gluteal artery in the extended iliofemoral approach. J Orthop Trauma 14:259–263, 2000.

168. Reinert, C.M.; Bosse, M.J.; Poka, A.; et al. A modified extensile exposure for the treatment of complex or malunited acetabular fractures. J Bone Joint Surg [Am] 70:329–337, 1988.

169. Richter, H.; Hutson, J.J.; Zych, G. The use of spring plates in the internal fixation of acetabular fractures. J Orthop Trauma 18:179–181, 2004.

170. Roffi, R.P.; Matta, J.M. Unrecognized posterior dislocation of the hip associated with transverse and T-type fractures of the acetabulum. J Orthop Trauma 7:23–27, 1993.

171. Rommens, P.M. Is there a role for percutaneous pelvic and acetabular reconstruction? Injury 38: 463–477, 2007.

172. Rommens, P.M.; Gimenez, M.V.; Hessmann, M. Posterior wall fractures of the acetabulum: Characteristics, management, prognosis. Acta Chir Belg 101:287–293, 2001.

173. Routt, M.L., Jr.; Swiontkowski, M.F. Operative treatment of complex acetabular fractures. Combined anterior and posterior exposures during the same procedure. J Bone Joint Surg [Am] 72:897–904, 1990.

174. Ruesch, P.D.; Holdener, H.; Ciaramitaro, M.; et al. A prospective study of surgically treated acetabular fractures. Clin Orthop Relat Res 305:38–46, 1994.

175. Ruggieri, F.; Zinghi, G.F.; Montanari, G.; et al. Transverse fractures of the acetabulum. Ital J Orthop Traumatol 12:25–40, 1986.

176. Ruotolo, C.; Savarese, E.; Khan, A.; et al. Acetabular fractures with associated vascular injury: A report of two cases. J Trauma 51:382–386, 2001.

177. Russell, G.V., Jr.; Nork, S.E.; Chip Routt, M.L., Jr. Perioperative complications associated with operative treatment of acetabular fractures. J Trauma 51: 1098–1103, 2001.

178. Sawaguchi, T.; Brown, T.D.; Rubash, H.E.; et al. Stability of acetabular fractures after internal fixation. A cadaveric study. Acta Orthop Scand 55:601–605, 1984.

179. Schmidt, C.C.; Gruen, G.S. Non-extensile surgical approaches for two-column acetabular fractures. J Bone Joint Surg [Br] 75:556–561, 1993.

180. Schopfer, A.; DiAngelo, D.; Hearn, T.; et al. Biomechanical comparison of methods of fixation of isolated osteotomies of the posterior acetabular column. Int Orthop 18:96–101, 1994.

181. Schopfer, A.; Willett, K.; Powell, J; et al. Cerclage wiring in internal fixation of acetabular fractures. J Orthop Trauma 7:236–241, 1993.

182. Senegas, J.; Liorzou, G.; Yates, M. Complex acetabular fractures: A transtrochanteric lateral surgical approach. Clin Orthop Relat Res 151:107–114, 1980.

183. Shazar, N.; Brumback, R.J.; Novak, V.P.; et al. Biomechanical evaluation of transverse acetabular fracture fixation. Clin Orthop Relat Res 352: 215–222, 1998.

184. Siebenrock, K.A.; Gautier, E.; Woo, A.K.; et al. Surgical dislocation of the femoral head for joint debridement and accurate reduction of fractures of the acetabulum. J Orthop Trauma 16:543–552, 2002.

185. Siebenrock, K.A.; Gautier, E.; Ziran, B.H.; et al. Trochanteric flip osteotomy for cranial extension and muscle protection in acetabular fracture fixation using a Kocher–Langenbeck approach. J Orthop Trauma 12:387–391, 1998.

186. Siebenrock, K.A.; Gautier, E.; Ziran, B.H.; et al. Trochanteric flip osteotomy for cranial extension and muscle protection in acetabular fracture fixation using a Kocher–Langenbeck approach. J Orthop Trauma 20(1 Suppl):S52–S56, 2006.

187. Simonian, P.T.; Routt, M.L., Jr.; Harrington, R.M.; et al. The acetabular T-type fracture. A biomechanical evaluation of internal fixation. Clin Orthop Relat Res 314:234–240, 1995.

188. Spencer, R.F. Acetabular fractures in older patients. J Bone Joint Surg [Br] 71:774–776, 1989.

189. Stannard, J.P.; Alonso, J.E. Controversies in acetabular fractures. Clin Orthop Relat Res 353:74–80, 1998.

190. Stannard, J.P.; Singhania, A.K.; Lopez-Ben, R.R.; et al. Deep-vein thrombosis in high-energy skeletal trauma despite thromboprophylaxis. J Bone Joint Surg [Br] 87:965–968, 2005.

191. Starr, A.J.; Jones, A.L.; Reinert, C.M.; et al. Preliminary results and complications following limited open reduction and percutaneous screw fixation of displaced fractures of the acetabulum. Injury 32 (Suppl 1):SA45–50, 2001.

192. Starr, A.J.; Reinert, C.M.; Jones, A.L. Percutaneous fixation of the columns of the acetabulum: A new technique. J Orthop Trauma 12:51–58, 1998.

193. Starr, A.J.; Watson, J.T.; Reinert, C.M.; et al. Complications following the "T extensile" approach: A modified extensile approach for acetabular fracture surgery-report of forty-three patients. J Orthop Trauma 16:535–542, 2002.

194. Steele, N.; Dodenhoff, R.M.; Ward, A.J.; et al. Thromboprophylaxis in pelvic and acetabular trauma surgery. The role of early treatment with low-molecular-weight heparin. J Bone Joint Surg [Br] 87:209–212, 2005.

195. Stockle, U.; Hoffmann, R.; Nittinger, M.; et al. Screw fixation of acetabular fractures. Int Orthop 24:143–147, 2000.

196. Stockle, U.; Hoffmann, R.; Sudkamp, N.P.; et al. Treatment of complex acetabular fractures through a modified extended iliofemoral approach. J Orthop Trauma 16:220–230, 2002.

197. Stover, M.D.; Morgan, S.J.; Bosse, M.J.; et al. Prospective comparison of contrast-enhanced computed tomography versus magnetic resonance venography

in the detection of occult deep pelvic vein thrombosis in patients with pelvic and acetabular fractures. J Orthop Trauma 16:613–621, 2002.

198. Tabor, O.B., Jr.; Bosse, M.J.; Greene, K.G.; et al. Effects of surgical approaches for acetabular fractures with associated gluteal vascular injury. J Orthop Trauma 12:78–84, 1998.

199. Teague, D.C.; Graney, D.O.; Routt, M.L., Jr. Retropubic vascular hazards of the ilioinguinal exposure: A cadaveric and clinical study. J Orthop Trauma 10:156–159, 1996.

200. Templeman, D.C.; Olson, S.; Moed, B.R.; et al. Surgical treatment of acetabular fractures. Instr Course Lect 48:481–496, 1999.

201. Thomas, K.A.; Vrahas, M.S.; Noble, J.W., Jr.; et al. Evaluation of hip stability after simulated transverse acetabular fractures. Clin Orthop Relat Res 340:244–256, 1997.

202. Tornetta, P., 3rd. Non-operative management of acetabular fractures. The use of dynamic stress views. J Bone Joint Surg [Br] 81:67–70, 1999.

203. Tornetta, P., 3rd. Displaced acetabular fractures: Indications for operative and nonoperative management. J Am Acad Orthop Surg 9:18–28, 2001.

204. Tornkvist, H.; Schatzker, J. Acetabular fractures in the elderly: An easily missed diagnosis. J Orthop Trauma 7:233–235, 1993.

205. Triantaphillopoulos, P.G.; Panagiotopoulos, E.C.; Mousafiris, C.; et al. Long-term results in surgically treated acetabular fractures through the posterior approaches. J Trauma 62:378–382, 2007.

206. Tseng, S.; Tornetta, P., 3rd. Percutaneous management of Morel-Lavallee lesions. J Bone Joint Surg [Am] 88:92–96, 2006.

207. Vailas, J.C.; Hurwitz, S.; Wiesel, S.W. Posterior acetabular fracture–dislocations: Fragment size, joint capsule, and stability. J Trauma 29:1494–1496, 1989.

208. Vrahas, M.; Gordon, R.G.; Mears, D.C.; et al. Intraoperative somatosensory evoked potential monitoring of pelvic and acetabular fractures. J Orthop Trauma 6:50–58, 1992.

209. Vrahas, M.S.; Widding, K.K.; Thomas, K.A. The effects of simulated transverse, anterior column, and posterior column fractures of the acetabulum on the stability of the hip joint. J Bone Joint Surg [Am] 81:966–974, 1999.

210. Webb, L.X.; Bosse, M.J.; Mayo, K.A.; et al. Results in patients with craniocerebral trauma and an operatively managed acetabular fracture. J Orthop Trauma 4:376–382, 1990.

211. Weber, T.G.; Mast, J.W. The extended ilioinguinal approach for specific both column fractures. Clin Orthop Relat Res 305:106–111, 1994.

212. Wey, J.; DiPasquale, D.; Levitt, L.; et al. Operative treatment of acetabular fractures through the extensile Henry approach. J Trauma 46:255–260, 1999.

213. Wright, R.; Barrett, K.; Christie, M.J.; et al. Acetabular fractures: Long-term follow-up of open reduction and internal fixation. J Orthop Trauma 8: 397–403, 1994.

214. Ylinen, P.; Santavirta, S.; Slatis, P. Outcome of acetabular fractures: A 7-year follow-up. J Trauma 29:19–24, 1989.

215. Yosipovitch, Z.; Goldberg, I.; Ventura, E.; et al. Open reduction of acetabular fracture in pregnancy. A case report. Clin Orthop Relat Res 282:229–232, 1992.

216. Yu, J.K.; Chiu, F.Y.; Feng, C.K.; et al. Surgical treatment of displaced fractures of posterior column and posterior wall of the acetabulum. Injury 35:766–770, 2004.

217. Yue, J.J.; Sontich, J.K.; Miron, S.D.; et al. Blood flow changes to the femoral head after acetabular fracture or dislocation in the acute injury and perioperative periods. J Orthop Trauma 15:170–176, 2001.

Index

Note: Page numbers followed by *f* refer to figures; page numbers followed by *t* refer to tables; and *b* refer to boxes.

Metacarpal fracture (*Continued*)
  treatment of, 1227–1228, 1227*t*,
      1242–1274
    anesthesia in, 1226–1227, 1226*f*
    splintage in, 1227, 1228*f*
  unstable, 1228, 1228*t*
Metacarpophalangeal joint, 1221, 1223*f*
  dislocation of, 1317–1320, 1317*f*, 1319*f*
  thumb, 1222
Metal(s), 83. *See also* Metal implant
  atomic structure of, 83, 84*f*
  brittle, 85
  bullet, 1022–1023, 1023*f*, 1024*f*
  casting of, 84
  cold-forging of, 84
  cold-working of, 84, 84*f*
  corrosion of, 84–85
  ductility of, 85
  elasticity of, 85
  endurance limit of, 85
  fatigue of, 85–86, 87*f*
  fatigue strength of, 85
  forging of, 84
  hardness of, 85
  mechanics of, 85–86, 86*f*, 87*f*, 88*f*
  modulus of elasticity of, 85, 86*f*
  passivation of, 84
  plastic deformation of, 85
  processing of, 84
  shot-peening of, 84
  stiffness of, 85
  stress-strain curve for, 85, 86*f*
  toughness of, 85, 86*f*
  types of, 86–89
  ultimate stress of, 85, 86*f*
  wrought, 84
  yield point of, 85, 86*f*
Metal detectors, implant on, 91
Metal implant, 83–92
  bacterial adherence to, 91, 92*f*
  biocompatibility of, comparative studies
      of, 91
  cobalt-chromium alloy, 88*t*, 89
    biocompatibility of, 91
    comparative studies of, 89–91
  comparative studies of, 89–91, 90*f*
  failure of
    fatigue curve of, 87*f*
    high-stress, low-cycle, 85, 87*f*
    low-stress, high-cycle, 85, 87*f*
    tear zone of, 85
  imaging of, comparative studies of, 91
  infection with, 91, 92*f*
  on metal detectors, 91
  radiation therapy interaction with, 91
  stainless steel, 87–89, 88*f*, 88*t*
    biocompatibility of, 91
    comparative studies of, 89–91, 90*f*
    radiation therapy interaction with,
        91
  titanium, 88*t*, 89
    biocompatibility of, 91
    comparative studies of, 89–91, 90*f*
    radiation therapy interaction with, 91
  titanium alloy, 88*t*, 89
Metastatic disease, 453. *See also at specific*
    bones
  bone scan in, 462–463

Metastatic disease (*Continued*)
  computed tomography in, 463, 464*f*,
      466*f*
  diagnosis of, 460–464
  fracture with. *See* Pathologic fracture(s),
      metastasis-related
  incidence of, 453–454
  magnetic resonance imaging in,
      463–464, 467*f*
  mechanisms of, 455–459
  new bone formation with, 459–460
  pain in, 460
  positron emission tomography in,
      462–463, 463*f*
  prognosis for, 454–455
  radiography in, 460–462, 461*f*, 462*f*,
      463, 465*f*
  treatment of, 460, 464–501
    bisphosphonates in, 453, 464–465
    chemotherapy in, 465
    hormonal agents in, 465
    nonoperative, 464–465, 465–467
    radiation therapy in, 465–467
    zoledronate in, 464–465
Metatarsal(s), 2703
  first
    plantar-flexed, 2749, 2751*f*
    reconstructive surgery on, 2758,
        2758*f*
  fracture of. *See* Metatarsal fracture
  lesser, osteotomy of, 2758, 2759*f*
Metatarsal fracture, 2703–2713
  anatomy of, 2703
  classification of, 2704
  complications of, 2708
  epidemiology of, 2703
  evaluation of, 2704, 2704*f*, 2705*f*
  fifth metatarsal, 2709–2713
    anatomy of, 2709
    avulsion, 2710
    classification of, 2709–2710, 2710*f*
    mechanism of, 2709
    metadiaphyseal (Jones), 2710–2712,
        2711*f*
      outcomes of, 2712
    proximal diaphyseal (stress),
        2712–2713
    shaft, 2713
  first metatarsal, 2706–2707, 2706*f*
  gunshot-related, 449*f*, 450
  incidence of, 2703
  malunion of, 2758–2759, 2758*f*, 2759*f*
  mechanism of, 2704
  nonunion of, 2758–2759, 2758*f*, 2759*f*
  second, third, fourth metatarsals, 2707,
      2707*f*, 2708*f*
  tarsometatarsal fracture and, 2694,
      2697*f*
  treatment of, 2704–2709. *See also at*
      Metatarsal fracture, fifth metatarsal
    indications for, 2704
    nonoperative, 2704–2706
    operative, 2706–2707
      care after, 2707
      first metatarsal, 2706–2707, 2706*f*
      outcomes of, 2708–2709
      second, third, fourth metatarsals,
          2707, 2707*f*, 2708*f*

Metatarsophalangeal joint injury,
    2713–2718
  first joint, 2713–2716
    anatomy of, 2713–2714
    dislocation, 2715–2716, 2716*f*, 2718*f*
    evaluation of, 2714
    mechanism of, 2714
    sprain, 2714–2715
    treatment of, 2714–2715
    turf toe, 2714–2715
  lesser joints, 2716–2718
    anatomy of, 2716–2717
    treatment of, 2718
Methadone
  equivalent doses of, 255*t*
  intravenous dose of, 256
  in opioid withdrawal, 279
  in pain, 257
  preprocedure use of, 255–256
Methyl methacrylate spacer, in metacarpal
    fracture, 1320, 1320*f*
Methylprednisolone, in spinal cord injury,
    742–743, 743*t*
Metronidazole, 260*t*, 262*t*, 263*t*, 539*t*
Mexiletine, in neuropathic pain, 258*t*
Miami J collar, 799–800, 799*f*, 800*f*, 801*f*
Microcapillary infusion technique, for
    compartment pressure, 349–351
Midcarpal instability, 1392–1393, 1393*f*
  secondary (adaptive), 1393–1394, 1394*f*
Midcarpal shift test, 1377
Midfoot. *See also* Tarsometatarsal joint
  amputation at, 2875–2876, 2876*f*
  sprain of, 2687
Minimally invasive percutaneous plate
    osteosynthesis (MIPPO), 170–172,
    172*t*, 173*t*, 2093–2094, 2094*f*,
    2105–2108, 2107*f*
Minocycline, 260*t*, 261, 263*t*
Missed injury, 575–576, 575*f*
Mitral regurgitation, hip fracture treatment
    and, 1822
MODEMS (Musculoskeletal Outcomes
    Date Collection and Management
    System) questionnaires, 722, 722*t*
Monocytes, in multiple organ failure, 557
Monteggia fracture, 1481–1486, 1484*f*,
    1486*f*
  classification of, 1482, 1483*f*
  complications of, 1485
  malunion of, 1486
  misdiagnosis of, 1484
  nonunion of, 1486, 1486*f*
  reverse. *See* Galeazzi fracture
  treatment of, 1484, 1485, 1485*f*
Morphine, 255*t*, 256
  adverse effects of, 256
  equivalent doses of, 255*t*
  patient-controlled, 254*t*
  preoperative, 255*t*
Morphine 6-glucuronide, 256
Morrey/Mayo Clinical Performance Index
    for the Elbow, 719*t*
Motor Index Score, in spinal cord injury,
    734–735, 736*f*
Motor nerve conduction studies, in
    peripheral nerve injury, 566–568
Moxifloxacin, 260*t*, 263*t*

Neurapraxia, 563, 565, 565*t*
  electromyography in, 566, 567*t*
  nerve conduction study in, 567*t*
Neurologic examination
  in fat embolism syndrome, 546
  in pelvic ring disruption, 1128
  in tibial plateau fracture, 2212–2213
  in tibial shaft fracture, 2335
  in trauma patient, 187
Neurologic injury. *See also* Brain injury;
    Peripheral nerve injury; Spinal cord
    injury
  in knee dislocation, 2177
  in lumbar spine fracture, 990–992, 993,
      998, 1013, 1013*f*
  in occipitoatlantal dislocation, 818
  in odontoid fracture, 829–830
  in pelvic ring disruption, 1163–1164
  in sacral fracture, 1080, 1084,
      1086–1088, 1091
  in thoracolumbar injury, 967–970
Neuroma, amputation-related, 2879
Neurotmesis, 563–564, 565*t*
  electromyography in, 566, 567*t*
  nerve conduction study in, 567*t*
Neurovascularly intact injury, 566,
    568–569
Nicotine, nonunion and, 617
Nicotine replacement therapy, 275
Nifedipine, in complex regional pain
    syndrome type I, 572, 572*t*
Nightstick fracture, 1460, 1462*f*
Nonsteroidal anti-inflammatory drugs
    (NSAIDs)
  bone healing and, 254
  in complex regional pain syndrome
      type I, 571
  contraindications to, 254
  glomerular filtration rate and, 1823
  nonunion and, 617–618, 619
  in pain management, 253–254
Nonunion, 615–708. *See also at specific
    fractures*
  age and, 618, 659, 661*f*
  albumin deficiency and, 618
  alcohol use/abuse and, 618
  anatomic location of, 639–641
  ankle fracture, 2530–2531, 2577–2578
  atrophic, 624, 634*t*, 636, 636*f*, 638*f*
    bone graft for, 673
    treatment of, 635*t*, 636, 638*f*
  blood supply and, 616
  bone-to-bone contact and, 616, 625*f*
  calcaneal fracture, 2663
  with Charcot neuropathy, 653, 657*f*
  cigarette smoking and, 617, 619
  clavicular fracture, 655*f*, 1771*f*,
      1773–1777, 1773*f*, 1774*f*, 1775*f*
  cuboid fracture, 2757–2758
  definition of, 615
  depression with, 631
  diaphyseal, 621, 641, 643*f*
    angular deformity with, 625, 626*f*
    treatment of, 641, 643*f*
  distal femoral fracture, 2122, 2123*f*,
      2289–2291
  distal humeral fracture, 1573, 1574*f*,
      1575*f*, 1576*f*

Nonunion (*Continued*)
  distal radial fracture, 654*f*, 1443
  epiphyseal, 621, 640, 641*f*
    angular deformity with, 625
    treatment of, 640, 641*f*
  etiology of, 616–618, 619*t*
  evaluation of, 618–632, 634*t*, 696–697
    angiography in, 628
    bone scan in, 627–628, 633*f*, 634*t*
    cineradiography in, 622*f*, 628
    computed tomography in, 627,
        631*f*, 632*f*
    consultations for, 629–632
    deformity in, 620, 623*f*, 624–627,
        626*f*, 627*f*, 628*t*, 629*f*
      angular, 625, 626*f*, 627*f*, 629*f*
      length-type, 625
      rotational, 625, 627
      translational, 627, 629*f*
    Doppler ultrasonography in, 628
    fluoroscopy in, 628
    laboratory studies in, 628–629, 634*t*
    magnetic resonance imaging in, 628
    neurovascular examination in, 619,
        621*f*, 622*f*, 631
    patient history in, 619, 620*f*
    physical examination in, 619–621,
        621*f*, 622*f*
    previous implants in, 624
    radiography in, 621–627, 623*f*, 624*f*,
        626*f*, 627*f*, 629*f*, 630*f*, 634*t*
    sinography in, 628
    surface characteristics in, 624, 625*f*
    ultrasonography in, 628, 634*f*
    worksheet for, 620*f*
  femoral neck fracture, 1852, 1892–1894
  femoral shaft fracture, 693*f*, 2067–2070,
      2068*f*
  greater tuberosity fracture, 1746, 1746*f*
  humeral shaft fracture, 656*f*, 657*f*,
      1617–1620, 1618*f*
  hypertrophic, 622–624, 634*t*, 635–636,
      636*f*, 637*f*, 638*f*
    elephant foot type of, 622–624,
        636*f*
    horse hoof type of, 622–624, 636*f*
    painless, 653, 655*f*
    stiff, 657, 693*f*
    treatment of, 635–636, 635*t*, 637*f*,
        638*f*
    vascular characteristics of, 622–624,
        624*f*
  in impairment assessment, 713
  infected, 616–617, 619, 634*t*, 636–639,
      636*f*
    allograft for, 671*f*, 676, 679*f*
    antibiotic in, 631
    bone graft for, 673
    draining, 637–638, 639*f*
    evaluation of, 629
    exchange nailing for, 682, 683*f*
    external fixation for, 690
    nondraining, 638–639, 639*f*
    quiescent, 639, 639*f*
    treatment of, 635*t*, 636–639, 639*f*,
        682, 683*f*
  lax, 657, 660*f*
  lumbar spine fracture, 1013

Nonunion (*Continued*)
  mechanical instability and, 616, 617*f*
  metacarpal fracture, 1322, 1329–1330
  metaphyseal, 621, 640, 642*f*
    angular deformity with, 625
    bone marrow injection for, 640
    external fixation for, 640, 642*f*
    intramedullary nail fixation for, 640,
        642*f*
    plate-and-screw stabilization for, 640,
        642*f*
  metatarsal fracture, 2758–2759, 2758*f*,
      2759*f*
  mobility of, 657
  Monteggia fracture, 1486, 1486*f*
  navicular fracture, 2681, 2756–2757,
      2757*f*
  nonviable, 622, 624, 633*f*
  NSAIDs and, 617–618, 619
  oligotrophic, 622–624, 634*t*, 636, 636*f*,
      638*f*, 657, 660*f*, 688*f*
    bone graft for, 671
    treatment of, 635*t*, 636, 638*f*
  pain in, 631
  painless, 653–655, 655*f*, 656*f*, 657*f*
  patellar fracture, 666*f*, 2310–2312, 2310*f*
  pelvic fracture, 1164
  phalangeal fracture, 1322, 1329–1330,
      1330*f*
  predisposing factors for, 616
  proximal femoral fracture, 1948–1949,
      1950*f*, 2024–2030, 2028*f*, 2029*f*
  proximal humeral fracture, 1746–1747,
      1746*f*, 1747*f*, 1748*f*, 1749*f*,
      1751–1752
  proximal tibial fracture, 627*f*, 2296–2299
  radial shaft fracture, 1490–1494, 1493*f*,
      1495*f*
  radiolucent lines in, 621–622
  scaphoid fracture, 1351–1360
  segmental bone defects with, 641–649,
      643*f*, 644*f*, 649*f*, 649*t*, 651*t*
    acute compression treatment for,
        642–646, 644*f*, 645*f*, 646*f*
    bone graft for, 694
    circumferential (complete), 642, 643*f*,
        644–646, 644*f*, 645*f*, 646*f*, 651*t*
    exchange nailing for, 681
    external fixation for, 316–317, 316*f*,
        317*f*, 318*f*, 646–649, 647*f*, 648*f*,
        690, 694
    gradual compression treatment for,
        646–649, 647*f*, 648*f*
    partial (incomplete), 642, 643*f*, 647,
        649*f*
    splinter (sliver) bone transport for,
        647, 649*f*
    static treatment for, 642
  stiff, 651, 657
  subtrochanteric femoral fracture,
      2024–2030, 2028*f*, 2029*f*
  vs. synovial pseudarthrosis, 627–628
  talar neck fracture, 2606–2607,
      2754–2755
  tibial pilon fracture, 2502–2503, 2507
  tibial plateau fracture, 2279
  tibial shaft fracture, 682*f*, 2418–2422,
      2419*f*

Osteomyelitis (*Continued*)
  computed tomography in, 595–597
  culture in, 593, 599, 600
  definition of, 589
  diabetes mellitus and, 590
  diagnosis of, 593–597, 593*f*, 594*f*, 595*f*, 596*f*
  diffuse, 592, 592*f*
  epidemiology of, 589–590
  etiologic classification of, 592
  hematogenous, 589, 590
  host factors in, 590, 592
  in impairment assessment, 713
  indium-labeled leukocyte imaging in, 595, 596*f*
  laboratory tests in, 594
  localized, 592, 592*f*
  magnetic resonance imaging in, 595–597, 596*f*
  medullary, 592, 592*f*
  pathogenesis of, 590–591
  patient history in, 593
  physical examination in, 593, 593*f*, 594*f*
  post-traumatic (exogenous), 589–590
  radiography in, 593–594
  radionuclide imaging in, 594–595, 595*f*, 596*f*
  risk factors for, 590
  sulfur colloid marrow scan in, 595, 596*f*
  superficial, 592, 592*f*
  terminology for, 589
  treatment of, 597–609
    amputation in, 597–598, 598*f*
    antibiotic beads in, 600–601, 601*f*
    antibiotics in, 608–609
    bone stabilization in, 600, 600*f*
    cancellous bone graft in, 601
    complementary modalities in, 609
    cultures in, 600
    dead space in, 600–601
    débridement in, 599, 599*f*
    decision for, 597
    electrical stimulation in, 609
    external fixation in, 600, 600*f*, 602
    fracture type and, 597
    hyperbaric oxygen in, 609
    limb reconstruction in, 602–608
      acute shortening and relengthening for, 602–605, 603*f*, 604*f*, 605*f*, 606*f*
      bone transport for, 605–608, 607*f*, 608*f*
      case studies of, 602–608
    limb salvage in, 598–609
    muscle transfer in, 601–602, 601*f*
    overview of, 597
    soft tissue coverage in, 601–602, 601*f*
    vascularized flap in, 426–427
Osteonecrosis. *See* Avascular necrosis
Osteopenia, 516, 516*t*.
    See also Osteoporosis
  ankle fracture and, 2564
  bone augmentation in, 137
  fracture fixation in, 135–137
  intertrochanteric fracture and, 1913
  lumbar spine fracture with, 985
  nonunion treatment in, 656, 658*f*, 659*f*

Osteopenia (*Continued*)
  Singh index of, 1850, 1851*f*, 1858
  subtrochanteric femoral fracture and, 2021
Osteophytes, spinal, 779–780
Osteoporosis. *See also* Osteopenia
  bisphosphonates in, 1828
  bone formation markers in, 515
  calcitonin in, 1828
  calcium supplementation in, 1828
  classification of, 1043
  computed tomography in, 515, 1043–1044
  DC plate and, 108–110, 110*f*
  definition of, 515, 1043
  DEXA scan in, 514*t*, 515, 516
  diagnosis of, 515–516, 516*t*, 1827
  epidemiology of, 513, 1043
  estrogen replacement therapy in, 1828
  fracture in, 58–59, 59*f*
    financial aspects of, 513
    healing of, 514–515
    hip, 58–59, 59*f*, 514, 519
    mechanism of, 514, 514*t*
    risk for, 514
    treatment of, 518–520
    vertebral, 519–520, 789, 1043–1045
      imaging of, 1043–1044
      lumbar, 1001
      mechanism of, 1043
      nonoperative treatment of, 1044, 1045
      operative treatment of, 1044–1045, 1045*f*
      symptoms of, 1043
  humeral shaft fracture nonunion and, 1619
  magnetic resonance imaging in, 1043–1044
  parathyroid hormone in, 42
  prevention of, 516–518
  proximal femoral fracture treatment and, 1827–1828
  proximal femur, 1850–1852
  raloxifene in, 1828
  risk factors for, 1827
  teriparatide in, 1828
  trabecular bone changes in, 514
  treatment of, 516–518
  type I, 514
  type II, 514
  ultrasonography in, 515
  vitamin D in, 1828
Osteosynthesis, 14
Osteotomy
  in ankle arthrosis, 2763, 2763*f*
  calcaneal, 2769–2771, 2771*f*
  clavicular, 1776*f*, 1777
  distal femoral. *See* Femoral fracture (distal), malunion of, osteotomy for
  in distal radial fracture malunion, 1442–1443, 1443*f*, 1444*f*, 1445*f*, 1446*f*, 1447*f*, 1448*f*
  fibular, 2608–2610, 2763
  greater tuberosity, 1744, 1744*f*
  in intertrochanteric hip fracture, 1925, 1926*f*

Osteotomy (*Continued*)
  in lower extremity deformity. *See* Lower extremity deformity, osteotomy for
  metatarsal, 2758, 2759*f*
  in nonunion treatment, 669–670
  phalangeal, 1323–1330, 1325*f*, 1326*f*
  in subtalar arthrosis, 2769–2771, 2771*f*
  tibial. *See* Tibial fracture (proximal), malunion of, osteotomy for
  tibial tubercle, 2092
  ulnar, 1392
Outcomes research, 717–726
  clinical vs. patient-oriented, 717–718
  end results in, 717
  goals of, 717
  guidelines for, 723–724
  instruments for, 718–723, 719*t*
    development of, 718
    disease-specific, 719*t*, 722
    generic, 719–722, 719*t*
    joint-specific, 719*t*, 722–723
    pain, 719
    patient-specific, 723
    region-specific, 722, 722*t*
    web sites for, 722*t*
  nonvalidated scales in, 718
  reliability in, 718
  small area analysis in, 717
Oxacillin, 260*t*, 263*t*
Oxcarbazepine, in neuropathic pain, 258*t*
Oxycodone, 255*t*, 256
  preoperative, 255*t*
Oxygen
  cerebral, in head injury, 212
  hyperbaric, in osteomyelitis, 609
Oxygen therapy, 185
  in blast lung, 231
  in disaster-related evacuation, 230
  in fat embolism syndrome prevention, 548–549
  perioperative, 533–534

P

Padget-Schroetter syndrome, 551
Paget, Sir James, 7
Pain, 253–258
  in ankylosing spondylitis, 1046
  assessment of, 253
  in calcaneal fracture, 2652, 2662
  in compartment syndrome, 343–344, 344*f*
  complex regional. *See* Complex regional pain syndrome
  etomidate-related, 182
  in external fixation, 313–314
  in femoral neck fracture, 1852
  after gunshot injury, 1034–1036, 1035*f*
  in metastatic disease, 460–462
  in navicular fracture, 2681
  neuropathic, 257–258, 258*t*
  in nonunion, 631
  patient expectation for, 253
  in pelvic ring disruption, 1164
  post-amputation, 2874, 2874*f*, 2879
  in posterior process talar fracture, 2586–2587
  scales for, 253, 719
  somatic, 253

Pelvis. *See also* Sacrum
  anatomy of, 1107–1111, 1108*f*, 1109*f*,
    1110*f*, 1111*f*
  external fixation for, 1134–1139, 1135*f*,
    1136*f*, 1137*f*, 1138*f*
  false, 1109
  fracture of. *See* Pelvic fracture; Pelvic
    ring disruption
  gunshot injury of, 432*f*, 443–445, 443*f*,
    444*f*
    intestinal contamination with,
      443–445
    intra-articular effects of, 443
  hemorrhage in, 187
  injury to. *See* Pelvic fracture; Pelvic ring
    disruption
  metastatic disease of, 463, 464*f*,
    483–484, 484–487, 486*f*, 487*f*
  radiography of, 1109*f*, 1112–1115,
    1113*f*, 1128–1129
    anteroposterior view for, 1109*f*,
      1112–1113, 1113–1114, 1113*f*,
      1114–1115, 1128, 1129*f*
    inlet view for, 1128–1129, 1129*f*
    outlet view for, 1129, 1130*f*
    stability of, 1109*f*, 1111–1115, 1112*f*,
      1113*f*
    true, 1109, 1110*f*
Penicillins, 260*t*, 262*t*, 263*t*
Percutaneous intra-arterial digital
    subtraction arteriography, 327
Percutaneous transluminal coronary
    angioplasty, hip fracture treatment
    and, 1821
Perforating peroneal artery, 2589, 2589*f*
Pericardiocentesis, 187, 187*f*
Perilunate dislocation, 1346, 1380–1383,
    1381*f*, 1382*f*
  diagnosis of, 1381
  trans-scaphoid, 1380–1381, 1383–1384,
    1383*f*, 1384*f*
  transtriquetral, 1384
  treatment of, 1381–1383
    closed reduction in, 1382, 1382*f*
    open reduction and internal fixation
      in, 1382, 1383
    percutaneous pinning in, 1382–1383
Perilunate instability, 1380–1383
  progressive, 1375, 1376*f*
Peripheral nerve, cross-section of, 565*f*
Peripheral nerve injury, 563–569. *See also at*
    specific nerves and fractures
  causalgia with, 568
  classification of, 563–565, 565*t*
  degrees of, 565
  in distal radial fracture, 1439
  electromyography in, 566, 567*t*
  evaluation of, 566–568, 566*t*, 567*t*
  external fixation and, 293–306
  historical perspective on, 563
  in impairment assessment, 714
  incidence of, 565–566
  mixed, 565
  nerve conduction studies in, 566–568,
    567*t*
  nonunion with, 658–659, 660*t*
  partial, 565
  prognosis for, 568

Peripheral nerve injury (*Continued*)
  projectile-related, 568
  somatosensory-evoked potentials in, 568
Periprosthetic fracture
  acetabular, 2844, 2844*f*, 2845*f*
  distal femur, 2850–2853
    classification of, 2851
    incidence of, 2850–2851
    intraoperative, 2851
    revision total knee arthroplasty for, 2853
    risk factors for, 2851
    treatment of, 2119–2120, 2851–2853,
      2852*f*, 2853*f*
  femoral shaft, 2063–2064, 2065*f*
  greater trochanter, 2846, 2847*f*
  proximal femur, 2844–2845
    classification of, 2845–2846, 2846*f*
    falls and, 2845
    implant loosening and, 2845
    intraoperative, 2846
    prevalence of, 2844–2845
    risk factors for, 2845
    treatment of, 2846–2849
    type A, 2846, 2846*f*, 2847*f*
    type B1, 2846*f*, 2847–2848, 2848*f*
    type B2, 2848, 2849*f*
    type B3, 2848–2849, 2850*f*
    type C, 2849
  proximal tibia, 2853–2856
    classification of, 2854–2855, 2854*f*
    risk factors for, 2854
    treatment of, 2855–2856
    type I, 2855
    type II, 2855
    type III, 2855–2856
Peritoneal lavage, 190
Perkins, George, 10
Peroneal artery injury, 324*t*
Peroneal nerve injury, 2177
Peroneus brevis tendon, 2518–2519, 2518*f*
  dislocation of, 2575
    in calcaneal fracture, 2664–2665
  evaluation of, 2525, 2752*f*, 2753, 2753*f*
  impingement of, in calcaneal fracture,
    2663–2664, 2664*f*
  injury to, 2732
Peroneus longus tendon, 2518–2519, 2518*f*
  dislocation of, 2575
    in calcaneal fracture, 2664–2665
  evaluation of, 2525, 2752*f*, 2753, 2753*f*
  injury to, 2732
    in cuboid fracture, 2700–2702
Personal protective equipment, 250
  in disaster management, 229–230
Petaling, in nonunion treatment, 674, 675*f*
Petechiae, in fat embolism syndrome, 546,
    546*t*
Phalangeal fracture (fingers), 1227–1228,
    1227*t*, 1274–1311
  complications of, 1322–1330
  condylar, 1284–1294
    anatomy of, 1284–1287, 1288*f*
    bicondylar, 1290–1294, 1292*f*
      open reduction and internal fixation
        for, 1291–1294, 1294*f*, 1295*f*,
        1296*f*
      tension band wire fixation for,
        1290–1291, 1293*f*

Phalangeal fracture (fingers), condylar
    (*Continued*)
    unicondylar, 1287–1290, 1292*f*
      closed reduction for, 1288, 1289*f*
      nondisplaced, 1288, 1289*f*
      open reduction and internal fixation
        for, 1288, 1290, 1290*f*, 1291*f*,
        1292*f*
  contracture after, 1323
  deformity after, 1323–1330
  delayed union of, 1322
  distal, 1301–1311
    anatomy of, 1301–1302, 1304*f*
    avulsion, 1308–1311, 1309*f*, 1310*f*
    base (physeal), 1306–1308, 1306*f*,
      1307*f*, 1308*f*
      in children, 1307, 1308, 1308*f*,
        1309*f*
    classification of, 1304, 1305*f*, 1305*t*
    comminuted, 1305*f*
    mechanism of, 1302–1311
    shaft, 1306
    treatment of, 1304–1308
    tuft, 1304–1305, 1305*f*
  epidemiology of, 1221, 1222*t*
  evaluation of, 1223–1225, 1225*f*
  incidence of, 1274–1275, 1275*t*
  infection of, 1322
  malunion of, 1322, 1322*f*, 1323–1330,
    1325*f*, 1328*f*
    in children, 1329
    osteotomy in, 1323–1330, 1325*f*,
      1326*f*
  middle, 1280–1284
    base, 1295–1300
      classification of, 1295, 1297*f*
      coban wraps for, 1295, 1296*f*
      comminuted, 1296–1297, 1297–
        1298
      dorsal, 1299–1300, 1300*f*
      dynamic traction for, 1296, 1298*f*
      dynamic traction splint for,
        1296–1297
      force couple splint for, 1297, 1298*f*
      impaction, 1300, 1301*f*
      lateral plateau, 1300, 1302*f*, 1303*f*
      stability of, 1295, 1297*f*
      volar plate arthroplasty for,
        1297–1298, 1299*f*
    diaphyseal, 1280–1283, 1280*f*, 1280*t*,
      1286*f*
    outcome of, 1300
  neck, 1284, 1287*f*
    in children, 1329
  nonunion of, 1322, 1329–1330, 1330*f*
  open, 1320
    antibiotic spacer in, 1320, 1320*f*
  osteoarthritis after, 1322–1323
  proximal, 1275–1279, 1280–1284
    diaphyseal, 1280–1283, 1280*f*
      closed, aligned, stable, 1280, 1280*t*
      closed, malaligned, comminuted,
        unstable, 1280*t*, 1281–1282,
        1283*f*
      closed, malaligned, stable,
        1280–1281, 1280*t*
      closed, malaligned, unstable, 1280*t*,
        1281, 1281*f*, 1282*f*

Phalangeal fracture (fingers), proximal
(*Continued*)
    open reduction and internal fixation
        for, 1285*f*, 1286*f*, 1287*f*
    extra-articular base, 1275, 1275*f*
    intra-articular base, 1276–1279
        avulsion, 1276–1277, 1276*f*, 1277*f*,
            1278*f*
        comminuted, 1276
        compression, 1276*f*, 1277, 1278*f*,
            1279*f*
        vertical shear, 1276, 1276*f*, 1278,
            1279*f*
    stable, 1227–1228, 1228*t*
    treatment of, 1227–1228, 1227*t*
        complications of, 1322–1330
        compression screws for, 1239–1240,
            1239*f*, 1240*f*, 1240*t*, 1241*f*
        external fixation for, 1240–1242,
            1242*t*, 1243*f*, 1244*f*
        functional casting for, 1229–1231,
            1229*f*, 1230*f*, 1231*t*
        intraosseous wires for, 1233–1236,
            1236*f*, 1236*t*, 1237*f*, 1237*t*,
            1238*f*, 1238*t*
        Kirschner wires for, 1231–1233,
            1232*f*, 1233*f*, 1234*f*, 1235*f*,
            1235*t*
        plate fixation for, 1240, 1242*t*
        splintage in, 1227, 1228*f*
        tension band wiring for, 1237–1238,
            1238*f*, 1239*t*
    unstable, 1228, 1228*t*
Phalangeal fracture (toes)
    first, 2718–2719, 2719*f*
    lesser, 2720, 2721*f*
Phalanges (fingers). *See also* Phalangeal
        fracture (fingers)
    alignment of, 1223–1224
    anatomy of, 1222–1223, 1222*f*, 1224*f*
    complex injury to, 1321–1322
    length of, 1222
    mallet injury of, 1311–1314
        bony, 1312–1314, 1313*f*, 1313*t*, 1314*f*
        tendinous, 1311–1312, 1311*f*
Phantom limb sensation, 2879
Pharynx, gunshot injury to, 1028
Phenoxybenzamine, in complex regional
        pain syndrome type I, 572, 572*t*
Philadelphia collar, 799–800, 800*f*, 801*f*
Phlegmasia cerulea dolens, 554
Phosgene intoxication, 226*t*
Physical impairment. *See* Impairment
Physical status classification, 526–527, 528*t*
Physical therapy
    in complex regional pain syndrome
        type I, 572
    after femoral neck fracture, 1890
    in nonunion, 631
    after proximal humeral fracture,
        1699–1704, 1700*f*, 1701*f*, 1702*f*,
        1703*f*
Piggyback method, of hip reduction,
        1799–1800, 1800*f*
Piperacillin/tazobactam, 260*t*, 263*t*
Piriformis, 1109, 1110*f*, 1915
    sciatic nerve relationship to, 1783–1784,
        1784*f*

Pisiform fracture, 1366
Plafond impaction, with supination-
        adduction ankle fracture, 2531, 2532*f*,
        2533*f*
Plague, 225*t*
Plantar nerves, 2525
Plantar reflex, 739
Plasmacytoma, bone metastasis in, 502*f*
Plaster of Paris, 39
    historical perspective on, 5–7, 6*f*, 7–8
Plate(s), 68–71, 384–385. *See also at specific*
        fractures
    angled, 111–112
        95-degree, 112, 114*f*
        130-degree, 111–112
    anti-glide, 106–107, 108*f*
    biomechanics of, 68–69, 69*f*, 70*f*
    blade, 114*f*
    bone interaction with, 68
    bridge, 103–104, 106*f*
        indirect reduction and, 133–135, 136*f*
    buttress, 102–103, 104*f*
    compression, 103, 106*f*
    DC, 108–110, 109*f*, 110*f*
        buttress mode of, 108
        compressive mode of, 108, 109*f*
        double loading of, 108, 109*f*
        incline opposition with, 110
        neutral mode of, 108
        osteoporosis with, 108–110, 110*f*
        shortcomings of, 108–110, 110*f*
        uneven stiffness with, 110, 110*f*
    design of, 68, 68*f*
    empty holes in, 94–95
    failure of, 115
        empty holes and, 94–95, 96*f*
    fracture healing study of, 69–71, 70*f*, 75
    historical perspective on, 13–17, 13*f*, 14*f*,
        15*f*, 16*f*, 17*f*
    LCDC, 110, 111*f*
    neutralization, 102, 103*f*
    one-third tubular, 110, 112*f*
    porosis under, 71
    quarter-tubular, 110, 112*f*
    reconstruction, 110–111, 113*f*
    rigidity of, 68
    Schuli device for, 110, 112*f*
    screws for. *See* Screw(s)
    semi-tubular, 110, 112*f*
    sliding screw system with, 112–115,
        115*f*, 116*f*
    spring, 102–103, 104*f*
    static compression with, 124–125, 130*f*,
        131*f*
    tension band principles and, 104–106
    wave, 104, 106*f*
    working length of, 68, 69*f*
Plâtre coulé, 5–6, 6–7, 6*f*
Pneumatic antishock garment, in pelvic
        ring disruption, 1125
Pneumonia, postoperative, 1822
Pneumothorax
    clavicular fracture and, 1768
    open, 186
    tension, 185, 186*f*
Point contact fixator, 144, 144*f*
Pointe métallique, 17–18
Poirier, space of, 1369

Polyaxial locking head screw, 146–148,
        147*f*
Polymethyl methacrylate (PMMA)
    for antibiotic carrier, 374–376, 375*f*,
        376*f*
    in intertrochanteric hip fracture, 1938
    for osteopenic bone, 137, 656, 659*f*
Polytetrafluoroethylene (PTFE) graft
    in arterial repair, 330
    in venous repair, 332–333
Polytrauma. *See* Multiple-trauma patient
Popliteal artery injury, 324*t*, 560
    iatrogenic, 325*t*
    knee dislocation and, 326, 326*f*,
        2176–2177, 2176*f*
    tibial shaft fracture and, 2328–2329,
        2328*f*
    treatment of, 331*f*, 333*f*, 334, 334*f*
Popliteal fibular ligament injury, 2222,
        2222*f*
Popliteus tendon injury, 2222, 2223*f*
Positron emission tomography, in
        metastatic disease, 462–463, 463*f*
Post-thrombotic syndrome, 264–265
Posterior cord syndrome, 735*f*, 736–737,
        736*t*
Posterior cruciate ligament, 2203, 2204*f*
    evaluation of, 2171–2172, 2171*f*
    injury to, 2176, 2176*t*, 2180–2181,
        2180*f. See also* Knee dislocation
        tibial plateau fracture and, 2220–2222
    treatment of, 2184
    reconstruction of, 2184–2188, 2186*f*,
        2187*f*
    rehabilitation after, 2188–2189
Posterior inferior tibiofibular ligament,
        2517–2518, 2517*f*
    disruption of, 2573–2574
        pronation-abduction injury and,
            2534–2536, 2537*f*
        supination–external rotation injury
            and, 2533, 2535*f*
    repair of, 2548, 2552*f*
Posterior interosseous nerve injury, in
        forearm fracture, 1487
Posterior ligamentous complex, disruption
        of, with lumbar spine fracture, 984,
        985*f*, 999, 1000*f*
Posterior longitudinal ligament, 865*f*, 866,
        920
Posterior talofibular ligament, 2515, 2518*f*
Posterior tibial tendon, 2519, 2519*f*
    evaluation of, 2525, 2753
    rupture of, 2530, 2575, 2752*f*
Posterior vertebral body angle, in
        thoracolumbar compression fracture,
        946
Postphlebitic syndrome, 554
Potassium, serum, succinylcholine effects
        on, 183
Pott, Percival, 11
Powers ratio, in occipitoatlantal dislocation,
        817–818, 818*f*
Prednisone, in complex regional pain
        syndrome type I, 572*t*
Preexisting conditions, in impairment
        assessment, 714
Pregabalin, in neuropathic pain, 258*t*

Spinal cord injury (*Continued*)
blast-type, 227
Brown-Séquard syndrome in, 735*f*, 736*t*, 737
cell death in, 732, 733*f*
central cord syndrome in, 735*f*, 736, 736*t*
in children, 748
classification of, 733–737, 735*f*, 735*t*, 736*f*
complete, 733, 734
deep venous thrombosis with, 553
in elderly patient, 748–749
etiology of, 729, 730*f*
Frankel classification of, 734–735, 735*t*, 737
glucose intolerance in, 1060–1061
gunshot. *See* Gunshot injury, spinal
hypercalcemia in, 1061
hypercalciuria in, 1061
hypotension with, 737, 738
imaging of, 782–789. *See also* Cervical spine injury, imaging of
impalement, 1036, 1037*f*, 1038*f*
incidence of, 729–730
incomplete, 733, 735–737, 735*f*, 736*t*
sacral sparing in, 733–734, 734*f*
ischemia in, 732
low-molecular weight heparin prophylaxis in, 553
magnetic resonance imaging in, 743–744, 776–778, 778*f*, 780
management of, 737–748
accident scene, 737
airway in, 737, 738
algorithm for, 744, 745*f*
anal wink in, 739
assessment for, 738–740, 739*f*, 740*f*, 741*f*, 742*f*
bulbocavernosus reflex in, 739
computed tomography in, 740
cremasteric reflex in, 739
extremity examination in, 738, 739*f*, 740*f*
Gardner-Wells tongs for, 744, 746*f*, 747*f*
halo ring for, 744–748, 748*f*
imaging for, 740–742
magnetic resonance imaging in, 740–741, 741–742
pharmacologic, 742–743, 743*t*
physical interventions for, 743–748
plantar reflex in, 739
positioning for, 737, 738, 741–742, 744, 1056
radiography in, 739–740
resuscitation for, 737–738
sensory examination in, 738, 741*f*
specialized centers for, 729–730
stretch reflexes in, 738–739, 742*f*
transport for, 737, 741–742
metabolic changes in, 1060–1061
Motor Index Score in, 734–735, 736*f*
in multiple-trauma patients, 738, 749
pathophysiology of, 730–732, 732*f*, 733*f*
penetrating trauma and, 737
posterior cord syndrome in, 735*f*, 736–737, 736*t*

Spinal cord injury (*Continued*)
prevention of, 729
regeneration after, 733
sacral sparing in, 733–734, 734*f*
secondary, 732, 732*f*
shock with, 734, 737, 738
stabbing, 1036–1038, 1039*f*
tibial shaft fracture and, 2327
Spinal deformity
postoperative, 1063–1065, 1065–1070, 1065*f*, 1066*f*
cervical, 1054, 1055*f*, 1065–1067, 1066*f*, 1068
classification of, 1068, 1068*t*
clinical features of, 1067–1068
late, 1065–1070, 1066*f*, 1067*f*
classification of, 1068, 1068*t*
clinical features of, 1067–1068
treatment of, 1068–1070, 1069*f*
thoracolumbar, 1067, 1067*f*, 1068–1070, 1069*f*
sacral fracture and, 1091–1093
Spinal injury, 727–752. *See also* Spinal cord injury *and specific spinal injuries*
epidemiology of, 729–730, 730*f*
etiology of, 729, 730*f*
gunshot. *See* Gunshot injury, spinal
imaging of, 753–792
computed tomography for, 766–772. *See also at* Computed tomography (CT)
magnetic resonance imaging for, 772–782. *See also* Magnetic resonance imaging (MRI), spinal
radiography for, 753–766
cervical, 753–763. *See also* Cervical spine, radiography of
lumbar, 764–765, 766*f*
sacral, 766
thoracic, 764, 765*f*, 766*f*
impalement, 1036, 1037*f*, 1038*f*
management of, 737–748
at accident scene, 737
algorithm for, 745*f*
assessment in, 738–740, 739*f*, 740*f*, 741*f*, 742*f*
in children, 748
in elderly patient, 748–749
in multiple-trauma patient, 749
orthoses in. *See* Spinal orthoses
resuscitation in, 737–738
prevention of, 729
stabbing, 1036–1038, 1039*f*
Spinal nerve roots, 1109
injury to, 736*t*, 737
in cervical spine, 768, 770*f*
in lumbar spine fracture, 990–992
in sacral fracture, 1080, 1086–1088, 1087*f*
Spinal orthoses, 793–812. *See also* Brace/bracing
cervical, 798, 798*f*, 799–800, 799*f*
biomechanics in, 793
cervicothoracic
high, 799–800, 799*f*, 800*f*, 801*f*
low, 801–803, 801*f*, 802*f*
complications of, 794
design of, 794

Spinal orthoses (*Continued*)
historical perspectives on, 793
indications for, 793
lumbar, 803–810, 803*f*, 804*f*, 806*f*, 807*f*, 809*f*
biomechanics in, 793
in fracture, 996
patient factors in, 793–794
nerve compression with, 794
thoracic, 801–803, 801*f*, 802*f*, 803–810, 804*f*, 808*f*
biomechanics in, 793
patient factors in, 793–794
Spinal shock, 734
Spine. *See also* Cervical spine; Lumbar spine; Sacrum; Thoracic spine; Thoracolumbar spine
ankylosing spondylitis of. *See* Ankylosing spondylitis
bamboo, 1046, 1046*f*
computed tomography of, 766–772
in pathologic conditions, 787–789
fracture of. *See at* Cervical spine; Lumbar spine; Thoracic spine; Thoracolumbar spine injury
gunshot injury to. *See* Gunshot injury, spinal
infection of
after gunshot injury, 1032–1033, 1035*f*
after impalement injury, 1036, 1038*f*
injury to. *See* Spinal cord injury; Spinal injury *and specific spinal injuries*
magnetic resonance imaging of, 772–782. *See also* Magnetic resonance imaging (MRI), spinal
metastatic disease of, 459*f*, 460, 487–501, 493*f*, 497*f*.
See also Pathologic fracture, metastasis-related
asymptomatic, 490–493, 497*f*
classification of, 490–493, 497*f*
clinical manifestations of, 460
diagnosis of, 463–464, 465*f*, 466*f*, 467*f*, 468*f*
neurologic deficit with, 495–496, 498*t*
surgical treatment of, 496–497
symptomatic, 493–495, 497*f*
osteophytes of, 779–780
radiography of, 753–766.
See also Cervical spine, radiography of; Lumbar spine, radiography of; Thoracic spine, radiography of
radionuclide imaging of, 781–782
stenosis of, 779–780
three-column model of, 927, 933*f*
Spinolaminar line, 758*f*
Spinous process split, in lumbar burst fracture, 986, 990–992, 990*f*
Spiral vein graft, 332–333
Spleen
embolization of, 191
injury to, 191
Splint/splinting
abduction, in humeral shaft fracture, 1598*t*, 1599
coaptation, in humeral shaft fracture, 1598*t*, 1599

Tibial fracture (distal), soft tissue injury
  with (*Continued*)
    flaps for, 418–419, 420*f*, 421*f*, 422*f*,
      423*f*
Tibial fracture (proximal). *See also* Tibial
    plateau fracture
  femoral shaft fracture and, 2060–2063,
    2063*f*
  gunshot-related, 449
  less invasive stabilization system (LISS)
    in, 157*f*, 158, 160*f*, 160*t*
  malunion of, 2299–2309
    conservative treatment of, 2299–2301
    diagnosis of, 2299
    osteotomy for, 2301–2309
      closing-wedge, 2301*f*, 2302–2303,
        2302*f*, 2303*f*
      combined intra- and extraarticular,
        2304–2305, 2305*f*, 2306*f*
      fibular head osteotomy with,
        2305–2307, 2307*f*
      indications for, 2301
      monocondylar, 2305–2307, 2307*f*
      opening-wedge, 2303–2304, 2304*f*,
        2305*f*, 2307, 2308*f*
      results of, 2309
      valgus deformity and, 2303–2304,
        2303*f*
  nonunion of, 627*f*, 2296–2299
    diagnosis of, 2296
    external fixation for, 690*f*
    intramedullary nail fixation for, 669,
      673*f*
    treatment of, 647*f*, 2296–2299, 2300*f*
  periprosthetic, 2853–2856
    classification of, 2854–2855, 2854*f*
    risk factors for, 2854
    treatment of, 2855–2856
    type I, 2855
    type II, 2855
    type III, 2855–2856
  soft tissue injury with, 388*f*, 389*f*
    flaps for, 416–417, 418*f*
  vascular injury with, 378*f*
Tibial nerve, 2519, 2519*f*
  injury to, 2530
    in calcaneal fracture, 2663
Tibial pilon fracture, 2453–2514
  arthrosis after, 2503, 2504*f*, 2505*f*,
    2506*f*, 2508–2509, 2749
  axial compression in, 2453
  classification of
    AO-OTA, 2455–2456, 2456*f*, 2457*f*,
      2458*f*
    Lauge-Hansen, 2454
    Mast et al., 2454–2455
    Ruëdi and Allgöwer, 2454, 2455*f*
  computed tomography of, 2454, 2454*f*,
    2456, 2458*f*, 2463*f*, 2466*f*, 2476*f*,
    2480*f*, 2487*f*, 2494*f*, 2506*f*
  definition of, 2453
  evaluation of, 2462
  fibula fracture with, 2453–2454
  foot position and, 2453, 2454*f*, 2458*f*,
    2485*f*, 2487*f*, 2491*f*
  fracture blisters with, 2475, 2485*f*
  historical perspective on, 2458–2462
  infection after, 2461, 2502, 2503–2508

Tibial pilon fracture (*Continued*)
  initial treatment of, 2462
  lipodermatosclerosis after, 2508
  malunion of, 2502–2503
  mechanism of, 2453–2454, 2454*f*
  nonoperative treatment of, 2464, 2465
  nonunion, 2507
  nonunion of, 2502–2503
  operative treatment of, 2464–2465,
    2465–2467
    ambulation after, 2500
    amputation in, 2501, 2501*f*
    anterolateral incision for, 2474, 2476*f*
    anteromedial incision for, 2467–2474,
      2474*f*
    approach in, 2467–2474
    arthrodesis in, 2500, 2501, 2503,
      2505*f*, 2506*f*, 2507–2508
    care after, 2500
    closure for, 2499
    complications of, 2459–2460,
      2501–2508
      arthrotic, 2503
      early, 2501–2502
      infectious, 2502, 2503–2508,
        2506*f*
      late, 2502–2508
      malunion, 2502–2503
      nonunion, 2502–2503, 2507
      soft tissue, 2501, 2502
      thrombotic, 2502
    deep venous thrombosis after, 2502
    external fixation in, 2493–2499,
      2493*f*, 2494*f*
      complications of, 2502
      joint-spanning frames for,
        2494–2497
      outcomes of, 2459–2460
      tensioned-wire, 2465, 2471*f*,
        2472*f*, 2494*f*, 2498–2499,
        2498*f*
    incision for, 2467–2474, 2474*f*,
      2475*f*, 2476*f*
    mini-arthrotomy for, 2463*f*, 2466*f*,
      2472*f*, 2474, 2474*f*, 2476*f*,
      2491*f*
    modified lateral approach to, 2474
    in open fracture, 2499–2500
    open reduction and internal fixation
      in, 2458–2462, 2483–2499,
      2486*f*, 2487*f*, 2491*f*, 2492*f*
      AO distractor in, 2484–2486,
        2487*f*, 2491*f*
      complications of, 2459–2460
      en peigne technique in, 2492–2493,
        2492*f*
      fibular fixation in, 2484, 2486*f*,
        2494*f*
      hybrid plating in, 2492
      length restoration in (step 1),
        2484–2486, 2486*f*, 2494*f*
      metaphyseal defect bone grafting in
        (step 3), 2490–2492
      metaphyseal shell reconstruction in
        (step 2), 2486–2490, 2486*f*
      metaphysis-diaphysis reattachment
        in (step 4), 2486*f*, 2492–2499
      outcomes of, 2458–2462

Tibial pilon fracture, operative treatment of
  (*Continued*)
    plate fixation in, 2457*f*, 2458*f*,
      2468*f*, 2469*f*, 2476*f*, 2480*f*,
      2485*f*, 2486*f*, 2487*f*, 2491*f*,
      2492–2493, 2492*f*
    soft tissue injury and, 2492–2493,
      2492*f*
    spanning external fixation in, 2476*f*,
      2484, 2485*f*, 2491*f*, 2493*f*
  outcomes of, 2508, 2508*t*
  percutaneous, 2467, 2477
  plates for, 2461–2462, 2462*f*, 2463*f*,
    2465, 2466*f*, 2468*f*, 2469*f*, 2476*f*,
    2487*f*, 2491*f*
  posterolateral incision for, 2474
  posteromedial-anterior approach to,
    2474, 2480*f*, 2485*f*
  radiography after, 2500
  soft tissue injury and, 2467, 2475–2477,
    2492–2493, 2499, 2501, 2502
  staging of, 2466*f*, 2467, 2469*f*, 2476*f*,
    2477–2479, 2479–2483, 2480*f*,
    2485*f*, 2487*f*
    outcomes of, 2460–2461
  supramalleolar nonunion and, 2503
  tibialis anterior tendon in, 2474
  timing of, 2474–2475, 2484*f*
  type B, 2465
  type B3, 2480*f*, 2485*f*
  type C1, 2465
  type C2, 2465, 2466*f*, 2468*f*, 2469*f*,
    2471*f*, 2476*f*, 2491*f*
  type C3, 2465, 2467, 2487*f*, 2494*f*,
    2505*f*, 2506*f*
  osteomyelitis after, 2503–2508
  plaster immobilization in, 2465
  prognosis for, 2508–2509
  radiography of, 2454
  shearing component in, 2453
  soft tissue injury with, 2475–2477
  traction in, 2465
  type A, 2455–2456, 2456*f*
  type B, 2455–2456, 2456*f*
    treatment of, 2465
  type B2, 2455–2456, 2456*f*, 2457*f*
  type B3, 2455–2456, 2456*f*, 2458*f*,
    2480*f*, 2485*f*
    treatment of, 2480*f*, 2485*f*
  type C, 2455–2456, 2456*f*
  type C1, 2455–2456, 2456*f*
    with diaphyseal extension, 2465
    treatment of, 2463*f*, 2465
    without diaphyseal extension, 2465
  type C2, 2455–2456, 2456*f*
    with diaphyseal extension, 2465,
      2469*f*, 2471*f*
    treatment of, 2465, 2466*f*, 2468*f*,
      2469*f*, 2471*f*, 2476*f*, 2491*f*
    without diaphyseal extension, 2465,
      2468*f*, 2491*f*
  type C3, 2455–2456, 2456*f*
    with diaphyseal extension, 2465,
      2472*f*
    treatment of, 2465, 2467, 2487*f*,
      2494*f*, 2505*f*, 2506*f*
    without diaphyseal extension, 2465,
      2487*f*

INDEX **153**

Tibial shaft fracture, treatment of (*Continued*)
   lag screws in, 2393
   limb shortening after, 2428
   limited motion after, 2430–2431
   low-intensity pulsed ultrasound therapy in, 45
   malunion after, 2422–2428, 2426*f*, 2427*f*, 2429*f*
   in multiple-trauma patient, 2340–2341
   nerve injury and, 2429–2430
   nonoperative, 2353–2356
     alignment loss after, 2356
     bracing for, 2354–2356, 2355*f*, 2357*f*
   nonunion after, 2418–2422, 2419*f*
     intramedullary nailing for, 2419–2422, 2419*f*, 2420*f*, 2421*f*
     plate fixation for, 2422, 2423*f*
     tension band plating for, 2422, 2424*f*
     wave or bridge plating for, 2321*f*, 2422, 2424*f*
   in open fracture, 2346–2350, 2347*f*
   outcome scales for, 2404–2406, 2406*t*
   plate fixation in, 2382–2395, 2383*f*
     angular stable plate for, 2390, 2391*f*, 2392*f*
     approaches to, 2383–2389, 2384*f*
     bone grafting with, 2393, 2394*f*
     hardware removal after, 2395
     implant type for, 2389
     minimally invasive approaches to, 2384–2389, 2387*f*, 2388*f*
     plate length for, 2390–2393
     reduction for, 2389, 2389*f*, 2390*f*
     rehabilitation after, 2393–2395
     results of, 2395
     screw density for, 2390–2393
     wound management for, 2393
   pressure sores with, 2428–2429
   provisional immobilization in, 2350–2351
     cast for, 2339–2340, 2351–2353, 2352*f*, 2353*f*
     external fixator for, 2351
     splint for, 2350–2351, 2353
   reflex sympathetic dystrophy after, 2430
   refracture after, 2428
   results of, 2402–2406, 2403*t*, 2404*f*, 2405*f*
   revascularization in, 2344
   rotational deformity after, 2428, 2429*f*
   ultrasound in, 2399, 2401*f*
   vascular problems and, 2430
   weight-bearing for, 662, 663*f*
   wound slough and, 2407–2408
  vascular injury with, 2329, 2339, 2342–2344, 2343*f*, 2430
  wound slough with, 2407–2408
Tibial tubercle
  avulsion of, 2138, 2162, 2162*f*
  fracture of, 2241, 2242*f*

Tibial tubercle, fracture of (*Continued*)
  tibial plateau fracture and, 2218, 2219*f*
Tibial tubercle osteotomy, 2092
Tibiofibular bone bridge, in transtibial amputation, 2868–2871, 2871*f*
Tibiofibular diastasis, 2574, 2574*f*
Tibiofibular joint
  distal, 2323
  proximal, 2323
    injury to, 2433–2434, 2434*f*
Tibiofibular syndesmosis. *See also* Anterior inferior tibiofibular ligament; Posterior inferior tibiofibular ligament
  anatomy of, 2517–2518, 2517*f*, 2523, 2523*f*
  instability of, 2523, 2524*t*, 2530, 2576–2577, 2577*f*
    evaluation of, 2526
  synostosis of, 2577
  transfixation of, 2548–2550, 2550–2554, 2555*f*, 2556*f*, 2557*f*, 2558*f*
Tibioperoneal trunk injury, 324*f*, 324*t*
Tibiotalar arthrodesis, 2500, 2501, 2503, 2505*f*, 2506*f*, 2507–2508
Ticarcillin/clavulanate, 260*t*, 263*t*
Tigecycline, 260*t*, 261–264, 263*t*
Tilt fracture, 1120, 1121*f*, 1135, 1140*f*
Tinel sign, in shoulder gunshot injury, 434
Tip-apex distance, in intertrochanteric fracture fixation, 1946–1947, 1947–1948, 1947*f*, 1948*f*
Tizanidine, in neuropathic pain, 258*t*
Tobramycin, 260*t*, 263*t*
  calcium sulfate pellet coating with, 539–540
Toe(s). *See also* Metatarsal(s); Phalangeal fracture (toes)
  ray resection in, 2875, 2875*f*
Toenail injury, 2721
Tolerance, substance, 270*t*
Tongs, Gardner-Wells, 744, 746*f*, 747*f*, 794–795, 794*f*, 795*f*
Tornado, injury from, 369
Toronto Extremity Salvage Score, 722
Toronto Salvage Score, 719*t*
Trachea, trauma to, 189
Traction, 384
  in acetabular fracture, 1187
  cervical spine, 794–798. *See also* Cervical spine, traction for
  in distal femoral fracture, 2078, 2087–2088, 2088*f*
  in femoral head fracture, 1839–1840, 1840–1841, 1842, 1843*f*
  in femoral shaft fracture, 208, 208*f*, 2044–2047, 2045*f*, 2046*f*
  halo ring. *See* Halo ring traction
  historical perspective on, 8–10, 9*f*, 10*f*
  in humeral shaft fracture, 1598*t*, 1599
  in intertrochanteric hip fracture, 1921
  in lower cervical facet dislocation, 898, 899–900, 900–901, 900*f*, 901*f*
  in open forearm fracture, 1477, 1477*f*
  in pelvic ring disruption, 1125
  in phalangeal fracture, 1296–1297, 1298*f*
  in proximal humeral fracture, 1653
  in radial shaft fracture, 1477, 1477*f*

Traction (*Continued*)
  in subtrochanteric femoral fracture, 1987–1988
  in tibial pilon fracture, 2465
  in tibial plateau fracture, 2227–2228
  in ulnar shaft fracture, 1477, 1477*f*
Tramadol, 255*t*, 256–257
Transarticular approach and retrograde plate osteosynthesis (TARPO) with lateral parapatellar arthrotomy, 2092–2093, 2093*f*, 2108
Transcutaneous electrical stimulation, in complex regional pain syndrome type I, 573
Transforming growth factor-β, in bone healing, 34, 42
Transportation
  in disaster management, 230–231
  in trauma patient, 206
Transposition flap, 405, 405*f*
Transverse atlantal ligament, 814–815, 814*f*
  rupture of, 823–826
Trapezium fracture, 1366, 1369*f*, 1370*f*
Trapezoid fracture, 1367, 1371*f*
Trauma. *See* Fracture(s); Injury; Mangled extremity; Multiple-trauma patient; Spinal cord injury
Trauma Care Systems and Development Act, 178
Trauma system, 178
  level of, 178, 179*t*
Trauma team, 178, 198, 198*f*
Traumatic far-out syndrome, with sacral fracture, 1086–1088
Triage, 227–229
  accuracy of, 228–229
  categories for, 228
  miscategorization in, 228–229, 229*f*
Tricalcium phosphate, in bone repair, 38
Triclosan
  for surgical antisepsis, 528–529, 531*t*
  suture coating with, 540
Tricyclic antidepressants, in neuropathic pain, 258*t*
Trimethoprim-sulfamethoxazole, 260*t*, 262*t*, 263*t*
Triquetrolunate ballottement test, 1377
Triquetrum fracture, 1366, 1367*f*, 1368*f*
  chisel-type, 1366, 1367*f*
Trochanteric fracture. *See* Femoral fracture (proximal), intertrochanteric
d-Tubocurarine, in airway establishment, 184
Tularemia, 225*t*
Tumor necrosis factor, 204*t*
  glucose hemostasis and, 531
Turf toe, 2714–2715
Tympanic membrane, rupture of, 225, 231–232

U

UCLA Shoulder Rating Scale, 719*t*, 723
Ulna. *See also* Radius
  fracture of. *See* Ulnar fracture
  gunshot injury of, 438–439, 439–440, 439*f*
  surgical anatomy of, 1459, 1460*f*